AF556949

EQUINE REPRODUCTION

ANGUS O. McKINNON, BVSc, MSc
Diplomate ACT and ABVP
Goulburn Valley Equine Hospital
Shepparton, Victoria;
Senior Research Fellow
Center for Early Human Development
Monash University
Clayton, Victoria
Australia

JAMES L. VOSS, DVM, MS
Dean, College of Veterinary Medicine and Biomedical Sciences
Colorado State University
Fort Collins, Colorado
USA

EQUINE REPRODUCTION

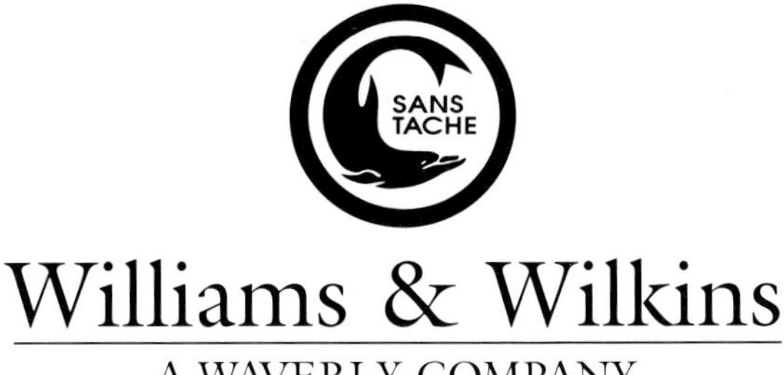

Williams & Wilkins
A WAVERLY COMPANY

BALTIMORE • PHILADELPHIA • LONDON • PARIS • BANGKOK
BUENOS AIRES • HONG KONG • MUNICH • SYDNEY • TOKYO • WROCLAW

Williams & Wilkins
Rose Tree Corporate Center, Building II
1400 North Providence Road, Suite 5025
Media, PA 19063-2043 USA

Executive Editor: Carroll C. Cann
Developmental Editor: Tanya Lazar
Editor: Dorothy DiRienzi
Production Manager: Samuel A. Rondinelli

Library of Congress Cataloging-in-Publication Data
Equine reproduction / [edited by] Angus O. McKinnon, James L. Voss
p. cm.
Includes index.
ISBN 0-8121-1427-2
1. Horses--Reproduction. 2. Horses--Breeding. I. McKinnon, A. O. II. Voss, J.L. (James L.)
SF768.2.H67E68 1992
636.1'08982--dc20
91-29283
CIP

PRINTED IN THE UNITED STATES OF AMERICA

Print number: 5 4

ISBN 0-8121-1427-2

This Book Is Dedicated To The Horse

PREFACE

This text was generated by our desire to create a useful addition to the available literature on all aspects of equine reproduction. Our idea was that practicing equine veterinarians needed a text devoted exclusively to equine reproduction, which while showing due respect to historical perspectives, should collate current information in a clear, concise, and easily accessible form. In addition, a perceived disproportionate interest in reproductive physiology of the mare should be addressed by inclusion of sections on the stallion and neonate.

The practice of veterinary medicine is progressing rapidly toward species specialization; within this, discipline specialization now occurs. However, the nature of our service necessitates talented general practitioners, and for the foreseeable future, they will remain the backbone of the profession. At the same time, education of the client has improved through greater access to information, and many clients have become more demanding and critical of veterinary services. This has placed many of us in unenviable situations. How do we remain cognizant of all the latest and pertinent research findings? Publication of most current research, at best, is scattered widely through many research and veterinary educational journals. Researchers without a veterinary educational background have contributed greatly to recent discoveries and have published reports, albeit unwittingly, in journals beyond our usual access. How many practicing veterinarians routinely scrutinize journals such as *Biology of Reproduction, Animal Science,* or even *Reproduction and Fertility,* apart from special supplements? Similarly, how many basic and applied equine researchers read the *Proceedings of the American Association of Equine Practitioners* or articles in popular equine magazines and have a real understanding of the relative importance of problems of the equine industry?

A need seemed to exist to combine recent information within the discipline of equine reproduction into a format useful for practicing equine veterinarians. Veterinarians in mixed practice, veterinary students, basic and applied scientists, and graduate students may benefit from the breadth and specificity of the information presented here in 118 well referenced chapters.

The text is divided into three main sections: the mare, the stallion, and the neonate. Each is equally important to veterinarians involved in equine reproductive practice. Too often, interest in the mare wanes once her pregnancy is diagnosed. Monitoring of pregnancy and neonatal care are areas of prime importance, because presumably the aim of any breeding program is to produce viable offspring. In addition, education regarding stallion reproductive physiology and management is alarmingly sparse, and the stallion is often neglected despite being half the fertility equation. The discussions of the mare and stallion are divided into the following topics: anatomy, physiology, and endocrinology; breeding management; diseases of the reproductive tract; and reproductive surgery. Additional topics in the section on the mare are pregnancy, parturition, and the puerperal period. Discussion of the neonate is divided into neonatal care and diseases according to body systems.

Ninety-five authors and co-authors have contributed to this work. The number of North American authors reflects our affiliations; however, readers should note chapters by numerous internationally recognized educators from both Northern and Southern Hemispheres.

Editing the contributions has been an enriching experience for both of us. The satisfaction from learning something new in each chapter has been incalculable. We are pleased to note that all proceeds that would normally be due contributors of this text will be allocated by common agreement to equine reproductive research.

Sheppartown, Victoria, Australia Angus O. McKinnon
Fort Collins, Colorado, USA James L. Voss

ACKNOWLEDGMENTS

The editors acknowledge and extend a special thanks to the individuals at Colorado State University and in Australia who contributed so much to the successful completion of this textbook: Ann Blackstone, who designed the line drawings appearing on the front cover and at the beginning of each chapter; Brian Evans, medical illustrator, who drew many of the illustrations for authors at Colorado State University; Janice Brown, Helen Mawhiney and Sandra Swets, who assisted by typing manuscripts and correspondence to authors (a special thanks to Janice Brown who assumed a major role in communicating with co-authors); JoEllen Linderer, who assisted in typing and mailing of manuscripts and page proofs to the publisher. Also, a special thanks goes to Michelle Goulding, who communicated all of the correspondence from Australia to those in the United States.

CONTRIBUTORS

Wilbur A. Aanes, DVM, MS
Professor Emeritus
Department of Clinical Sciences
Colorado State University
Fort Collins, CO 80523

Helen M. Acland, BVSc
Associate Professor of Pathology
Laboratory of Large Animal Pathology
School of Veterinary Medicine
University of Pennsylvania
New Bolton Center
Kennett Square, PA 19348

Ragan Adams, MA, DVM
Research Associate
Department of Clinical Sciences
Colorado State University
Fort Collins, CO 80523

Susan L. Alexander, MS, PhD
Research Scientist
Equine Research Unit
Lincoln University
Canterbury
New Zealand

W.R. (Twink) Allen, BVSc, PhD, DESM, MRCVS
Director, Thoroughbred Breeders' Association
Equine Fertility Unit
Mertoun Paddocks, Woodditton Road
Newmarket, Suffolk CB8 9BH
United Kingdom

Rupert P. Amann, PhD
Animal Reproduction and Biotechnology Laboratory
Colorado State University
Fort Collins, CO 80523

D.F. Antczak, VMD, PhD
Director, Cornell Equine Genetics Center
James A. Baker Institute for Animal Health
New York State College of Veterinary Medicine
Cornell University
Ithaca, NY 14853

A.C. Asbury, DVM
Professor, Department of Large Animal Clinical Sciences
University of Florida
Gainesville, FL 32610

Ernest Bailey, PhD
Professor
M.H. Gluck Equine Research Center
Department of Veterinary Science
University of Kentucky
Lexington, KY 40546-0099

Barry A. Ball, DVM, PhD, Diplomate ACT
Assistant Professor of Theriogenology
New York State College of Veterinary Medicine
Cornell University
Ithaca, NY 14853

T.L. Blanchard, DVM, MS, Diplomate ACT
Professor of Theriogenology
Department of Large Animal Medicine and Surgery
Texas Veterinary Medical Center
Texas A&M University
College Station, TX 77843-4475

William T.K. Bosu, DVM, MSc, PhD
Professor and Chairman
Department of Medical Sciences
School of Veterinary Medicine
University of Wisconsin
Madison, WI 53706

Ann Trommershausen Bowling, PhD
Adjunct Professor
Department of Reproduction and Serology Laboratory
School of Veterinary Medicine
University of California-Davis
Davis, CA 95616

Steven P. Brinsko, DVM, MS, Diplomate ACT
New York State College of Veterinary Medicine
Cornell University
Ithaca, NY 14853

Frank Bristol, BVSc, MSc, Diplomate ACT
Professor
Department of Herd Medicine and Theriogenology
University of Saskatchewan
Saskatoon, Saskatchewan S7N 0W0
Canada

Derek Brook, BVMS, MSc, FRCVS, Diplomate ABVP
President, Veterinary Dynamics
San Luis Obispo, CA 93401

T. Douglas Byars, DVM, Diplomate ACVIM
Hagyard-Davidson-McGee, PSc
848 V Nandino Boulevard
Lexington, KY 40511

Claire E. Card, DVM, MVSc, PhD, Diplomate ACT
Assistant Professor
Department of Herd Medicine and Theriogenology
University of Saskatchewan
Saskatoon, Saskatchewan S7N 0W0
Canada

Elaine M. Carnevale, DVM, MS
Research Assistant
Department of Veterinary Science
University of Wisconsin
Madison, WI 53706

Brian D. Cleaver
Horse Research Center
University of Florida
Gainesville, FL 32611

Gail T. Colbern, DVM, MS, Diplomate ACT
Medical Research Institute
2330 Clay Street
San Francisco, CA 94115

M.J. Cooper, BVM&S, PhD, MRCVS
Cooper and Partners, Veterinary Surgeons
55 Balance Street
Uttoxeter, Staffs ST14 8JQ
United Kingdom

E. Gus Cothran, PhD
Director
Equine Blood Typing Research Laboratory
Department of Veterinary Science
University of Kentucky
Lexington, KY 40546

Marcelo A. Couto, DVM, PhD
Department of Reproduction
School of Veterinary Medicine
University of California-Davis
Davis, CA 95616

J.E. Cox, BSc, B Vet Med, PhD, FRCVS
Senior Lecturer
Division of Equine Studies
Department of Veterinary Clinical Science
University of Liverpool Veterinary Field Station
Leahurst Neston, South Wirral L64 7TE
United Kingdom

Peter F. Daels, DVM, PhD
Assistant Professor, Theriogenology
Department of Clinical Sciences
New York State College of Veterinary Medicine
Cornell University
Ithaca, NY 14853

Steven D. Davis
Horse Research Center
University of Florida
Gainesville, FL 32611

Stanley M. Dennis, BVSc, PhD, FRCVS, FRC Path, Diplomate ACT
Professor, Department of Pathology
Kansas State University
Manhattan, KS 66506

Paul J. DeVries, DVM
Vierhouten Equine Clinic
Vosbergerweg 40
8181 JJ Heerde
The Netherlands

Thomas J. Divers, DVM, Diplomate ACVIM
Associate Professor of Medicine
New York State College of Veterinary Medicine
Cornell University
Ithaca, NY 14853

Paul A. Doig, DVM, MSc
Director, Veterinary Medical Affairs
Boehringer Ingelheim (Canada) Ltd
Burlington, Ontario L7L 5H4
Canada

Jack Easley, DVM, MS, Diplomate ABVP (Equine Specialty)
Equine Veterinary Practice
Shelbyville, KY 40065

Peter F. Flood, BVSc, MSc, PhD, MRCVS
Professor and Head
Department of Veterinary Anatomy
University of Saskatchewan
Saskatoon S7N 0W0
Canada

James K. Graham, PhD
Animal Reproduction and Biotechnology Laboratory
Colorado State University
Fort Collins, CO 80523

Kathryn A. Graves
Assistant Research Professor
Equine Blood Typing Research Laboratory
Department of Veterinary Science
University of Kentucky
Lexington, KY 40546-0099

A.L. Hallowell, DVM
Private Practioner
Auburn, WA 98002

Robert B. Hillman, AB, DVM, MS, Diplomate ACT
Senior Clinician
Department of Clinical Sciences
New York State College of Veterinary Medicine
Cornell University
Ithaca, NY 14853

H.F. Hintz, PhD
Professor of Animal Nutrition
New York State College of Veterinary Medicine
Cornell University
Ithaca, NY 14853

John P. Hughes, DVM
Professor
Department of Reproduction
School of Veterinary Medicine
University of California-Davis
Davis, CA 95616

John H. Hyland, BVSc, PhD, FACVSc
Department of Veterinary Science
University of Melbourne
Werribee
Victoria 3030
Australia

Clifford H.G. Irvine, FACVSc, DSc, DSc(Hon), DVSc
Professor Emeritus
Director, Equine Research Unit
Lincoln University
Canterbury
New Zealand

Robert A. Kainer, DVM, MS
Professor Emeritus
Department of Anatomy and Neurobiology
Colorado State University
Fort Collins, CO 80523

Jay F. Kirkpatrick, PhD
Senior Staff Scientist
Deaconess Research Institute
Billings, MT 59102

Julia H. Kydd, MSc, PhD
Animal Health Trust Equine Virology Unit
Lanwades Hall
Kennett
Newmarket, Suffolk CB8 7PN
United Kingdom

Michelle M. LeBlanc, DVM, Diplomate ACT
Associate Professor
Department of Large Animal Clinical Sciences
University of Florida
Gainesville, FL 32610

Horst W. Leipold, Dr med vet, MS, PhD
Distinguished Professor of Veterinary Medical Genetics
Department of Pathology
Kansas State University
Manhattan, KS 66506

Robert M. Löfstedt, BVSc, MS, Diplomate ACT
Associate Professor of Health Management
Atlantic Veterinary College
Prince Edward Island
Canada C1A 4P3

Cheryl Lopate, MS, DVM
Bluff Country Veterinary Service
Houston, MN 55943

Sara K. Lyle, DVM, MS
Private Practitioner
Largo, FL 34640

Mark D. Markel, DVM, PhD, Diplomate ACVS
Assistant Professor of Surgery
School of Veterinary Medicine
University of Wisconsin, Madison
Madison, WI 53706

Jill J. McClure, DVM, MS, Diplomate ACVIM and ABVP
Professor of Equine Medicine
Department of Veterinary Clinical Sciences
Louisiana State University
Baton Rouge, LA 70803

Patrick M. McCue, DVM
Department of Reproduction
School of Veterinary Medicine
University of California-Davis
Davis, CA 95616

Sue M. McDonnell, PhD
Research Assistant Professor
Section of Reproductive Studies
Head, Reproductive Behavior Program
School of Veterinary Medicine
University of Pennsylvania
New Bolton Center
Kennett Square, PA 19348

Angus O. McKinnon, BVSc, MSc, Diplomate ABVP (Equine), Diplomate ACT
Goulburn Valley Equine Hospital
Shepparton, Victoria, 3630;
Senior Research Fellow
Center for Early Human Development
Monash University
Clayton, Victoria 3168
Australia

Eduardo Brum Medici, DVM Med Vet
Barao Do Truinfo 1557
Bage-RS-Brazil
CEP 96,400

Henry Q Murphy
Manager, Donerail Farm
Lexington, KY 40577

Ray Nachreiner, DVM, PhD
College of Veterinary Medicine
Michigan State University
East Lansing, MI 48823

Terry M. Nett, PhD
Animal Reproduction and Biotechnology Laboratory
Colorado State University
Fort Collins, CO 80523

Gordon D. Niswender, PhD
University Distinguished Professor
Animal Reproduction and Biotechnology Laboratory
Colorado State University
Fort Collins, CO 80523

Eric Palmer, PhD
Ingenieur Agronome
Director of Research Unit on Equine Reproduction
INRA
Nouzilly, France

B.W. Pickett, PhD
Animal Reproduction and Biotechnology Laboratory
Colorado State University
Fort Collins, CO 80523

R.A. Pierson, MS, PhD
Associate Professor
Reproductive Biology Research Unit
Department of Obstetrics and Gynecology
University of Saskatchewan
Royal University Hospital
Saskatoon, Saskatchewan S7N 0X0
Canada

Virginia B. Reef, DVM, Diplomate ACVIM (Internal Medicine)
Associate Professor of Medicine in the Widener Hospital
Director of Large Animal Cardiology and Diagnostic Ultrasonography
School of Veterinary Medicine
University of Pennsylvania
New Bolton Center
Kennett Square, PA 19348

Sidney W. Ricketts, BSc, BVSc, DESM, FRCVS
Rossdale and Partners MsRCVS
Beaufort Cottage Stables
High Street
New Market, Suffolk CB8 8JS
England

Steven M. Roberts, DVM, MS, Diplomate ACVO
Associate Professor
Department of Clinical Sciences
Colorado State University
Fort Collins, CO 80523

Jeffrey L. Rubin, DVM, MS
Department of Clinical Studies
School of Veterinary Medicine
University of Pennsylvania
New Bolton Center
Kennett Square, PA 19348

Harold C. Schott, II, DVM, PhD
Instructor in Equine Medicine
Department of Veterinary Clinical Medicine and Surgery
Washington State University
Pullman, WA 99164

Jim Schumacher, DVM, MS, Diplomate ACVS
Department of Large Animal Medicine and Surgery
Texas Veterinary Medical Center
Texas A&M University
College Station, TX 77845-4475

Krista L. Seltzer, DVM
Large Animal Hospital
New York State College of Veterinary Medicine
Cornell University
Ithaca, NY 14853

Patricia L. Sertich, MS, VMD, Diplomate ACT
Marion Dilley and David George Jones Scholar
Section of Reproductive Studies
School of Veterinary Medicine
University of Pennsylvania
New Bolton Center
Kennett Square, PA 19348

Dan C. Sharp, PhD
Professor of Physiology
Horse Research Center
University of Florida
Gainesville, FL 32611

Robert K. Shideler, DVM, Diplomate ACT
Professor, Department of Clinical Sciences
Colorado State University
Fort Collins, CO 80523

Craig A. Smith, DVM, PhD, Diplomate ACT
Assistant Professor and Theriogenology Section Head
Department of Medical Sciences
School of Veterinary Medicine
University of Wisconsin
Madison, WI 53706

Michael S. Spensley, DVM
Manager, Clinical Development
Department of Pharmaceutical Development
Solvay Animal Health
Mendota Heights, MN 55120

F.P. Sprinkle, MS, DVM
Private Practitioner
LaGrange, KY 40031

Edward L. Squires, PhD
Professor
Animal Reproduction and Biotechnology Laboratory
Colorado State University
Fort Collins, CO 80523

Ted S. Stashak, DVM, MS, Diplomate ACVS
Department of Clinical Sciences
Colorado State University
Fort Collins, CO 80523

Francesca Stewart, PhD
Thoroughbred Breeders' Association
Equine Fertility Unit
AFRC Institute of Animal Physiology and Genetics Research
Babraham, Cambridge CB2 4AT
United Kingdom

Tex S. Taylor, DVM, MS
Professor
Department of Large Animal Medicine and Surgery
Texas Veterinary Medical Center
Texas A&M University
College Station, TX 77843

Walter R. Threlfall, DVM, PhD, Diplomate ACT
Department of Veterinary Clinical Sciences
The Ohio State University
Columbus, OH 43210

Josie L. Traub-Dargatz, DVM, MS, Diplomate ACVIM
Associate Professor
Department of Clinical Sciences
Colorado State University
Fort Collins, CO 80523

Gayle W. Trotter, DVM, MS, Diplomate ACVS
Associate Professor
Department of Clinical Sciences
Colorado State University
Fort Collins, CO 80523

John W. Turner, Jr., PhD
Associate Professor
Department of Physiology
Medical College of Ohio
Toledo, OH 43699

N.W. Umphenour, DVM
Resident Veterinarian
Gainesway Farm
Lexington, KY 40577

Wendy E. Vaala, VMD, Diplomate ACVIM (Internal Medicine)
Assistant Professor of Medicine in the Widener Hospital
School of Veterinary Medicine
University of Pennsylvania, New Bolton Center
Kennett Square, PA 19448

Steven D. VanCamp, DVM, Diplomate ACT
Associate Professor of Theriogenology
Department of Food Animal and Equine Medicine
North Carolina State University
Raleigh, NC 27606

Prof. Dr. M. Vandeplassche, DVM
Beekstraat 4
Ghent 9910, Belgium

Dickson D. Varner, DVM, MS, Diplomate ACT
Texas Veterinary Medical Center
Texas A&M University
College Station, TX 77843-4475

James R. Vasey, BVSc, Diploma Veterinary Surgery, FASVSc (Equine Surgery)
Goulburn Valley Equine Hospital
Shepparton, Victoria
Australia

J.T. Vaughan, DVM, MS, Diplomate ACVS
Dean, College of Veterinary Medicine
Auburn University
Auburn, AL 36849

James L. Voss, DVM, MS
Dean, College of Veterinary Medicine and Biomedical Sciences
Colorado State University
Fort Collins, CO 80523

Rudolf O. Waelchli, DVM, MSc, Privatdozent
Department of Reproduction
Veterinary College
University of Zurich
Winterthurerstrasse 260
Zurich 8057
Switzerland

Barbara Brewer Welsch, MA, DVM, Diplomate ACVIM and ACVECC
Associate Professor
Large Animal Medicine and Neurology
University of Florida
Gainesville, FL 32611

G.L. Woods, DVM, PhD
Department of Veterinary Science
University of Idaho
Moscow, ID 83843

Annalisa Young, BVetMed, MS, CertESM, MRCVS
Rossdale and Partners MsRCVS
Beaufort Cottage Stables
High Street
Newmarket, Suffolk CB8 8JS
England

CONTENTS

PART I. THE MARE

SECTION A. ANATOMY

SECTION B. PHYSIOLOGY/ENDOCRINOLOGY

HORMONES

PART II. THE STALLION

SECTION A. ANATOMY, PHYSIOLOGY, AND ENDOCRINOLOGY

SECTION B. BREEDING MANAGEMENT

PART III. THE NEONATE

SECTION A. CARE OF THE MARE AND FOAL IN THE NEONATAL PERIOD

SECTION B. DISEASES OF FOALS DURING THE NEONATAL PERIOD

PART I

THE MARE

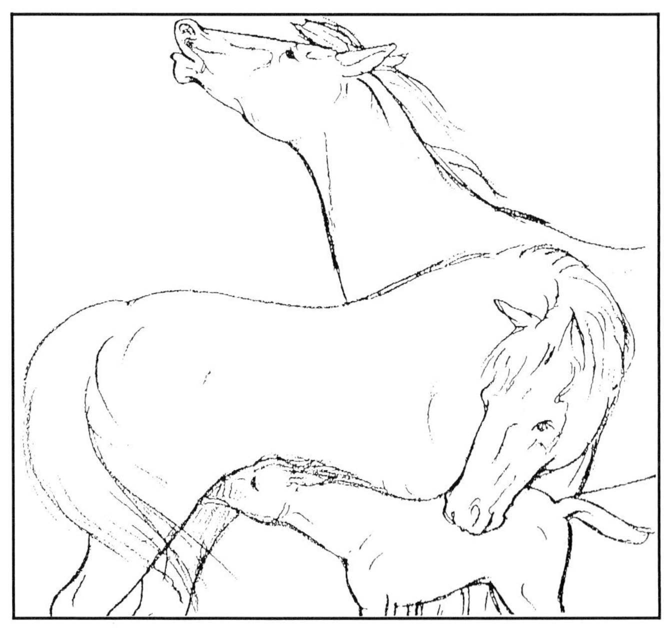

SECTION A

ANATOMY

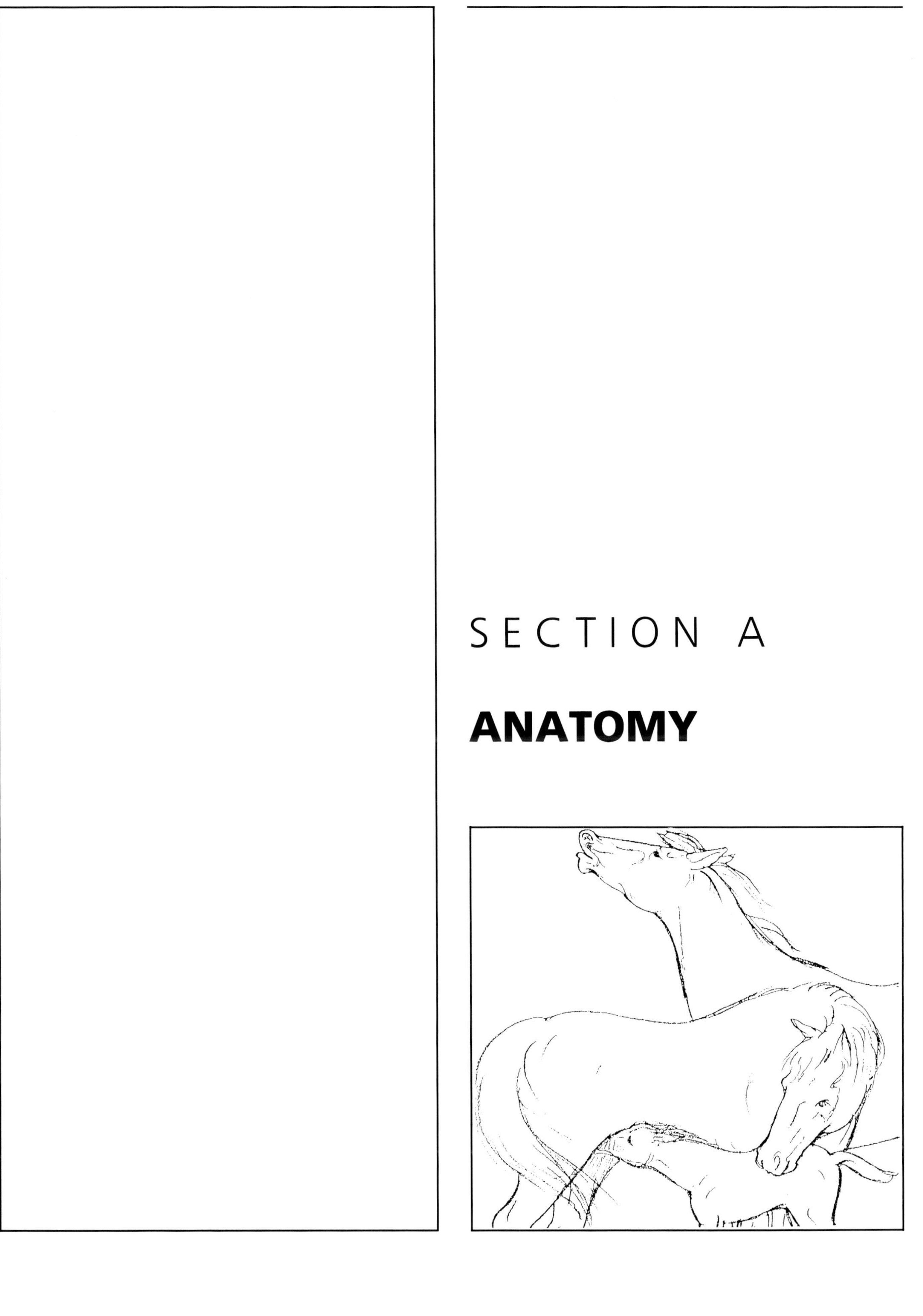

CHAPTER 1

REPRODUCTIVE ORGANS OF THE MARE

R.A. Kainer

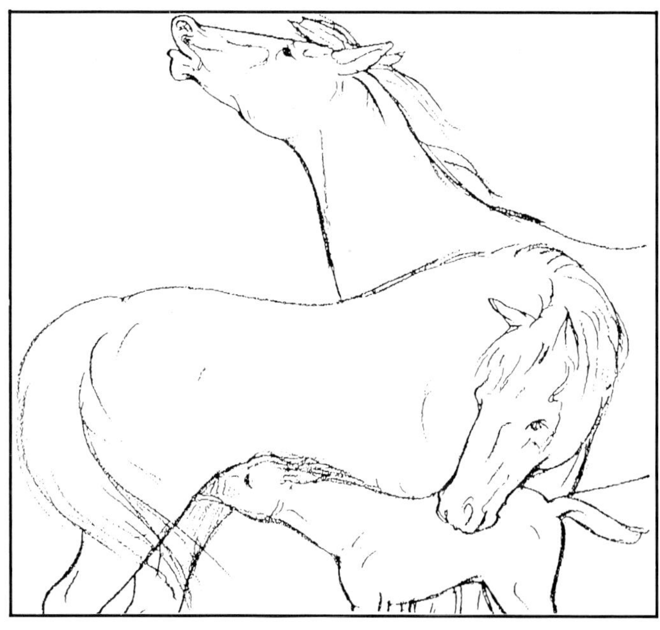

NEUROENDOCRINE CONTRIBUTORS

Neural and endocrine functions of three regions of the diencephalon—pineal gland, hypothalami, and pituitary gland—contribute to the development and cyclic physiology of the reproductive system of the mare. Interactions with other parts of the nervous system and with hormones produced by organs of the reproductive tract influence sexual behavior, pregnancy, parturition, and lactation.

PINEAL GLAND

Unlike its human counterpart, which is shaped somewhat like a pinecone (hence, pineal), the equine pineal gland is a dark brownish red, ovoid projection from the epithalamus occupying a median position between the rostral colliculi and thalami. Its short stalk contains the pineal recess of the third ventricle, and a suprapineal recess covers the gland dorsally (Fig. 1-1).[1]

Septa extending into the pineal gland from a capsule of pia mater separate masses of epithelial cells derived from ependyma. Melatonin secreted by these cells is considered to exert an antigonadotropic effect in the control of reproductive photoperiodicity via action on the hypothalamo-pituitary-gonadal axis.[2] Light inhibits the organ's activity, thus stimulating reproduction. In a report on pony mares, pineal activity was highest during late fall and winter and lowest during spring, summer, and early fall, and the percentage of ovulatory mares was inversely related to pineal hydroxyindole-*O*-methyltransferase activity.[3]

Blood supply to the pineal gland is from branches of the deep cerebral arteries that terminate in the formation of a rete pinealis. Venous blood drains into the ventral longitudinal sinuses.[4] Nerve fibers in the stroma of the gland are probably of sympathetic origin. It is believed that impulses from the retina travel via the rostral accessory optic tract to the hypothalamic tegmental tract, then to the thoracic spinal cord, and up to the cranial cervical ganglion.[4] Nerve fibers from the latter follow arteries to end on pineal epithelial cells.[4]

HYPOTHALAMI

Contralateral hypothalami face each other across the third ventricle. They join basally to form the tuber cinereum, and caudal to this region, the fused mammillary bodies (Fig. 1-1). The tuber cinereum is continuous with the infundibulum of the hypophysis.

Nuclei of nerve cell bodies occur in each hypothalamus. Supraoptic, paraventricular, preoptic, and rostral hypothalamic nuclei contain cell bodies of neurosecretory cells. Large, magnocellular neurosecretory cells in supraoptic nuclei (dorsal to the optic chiasm) are the source of vasopressin (antidiuretic hormone), whereas magnocellular cells in the paraventricular nuclei (in lat-

Illustrated by T.O. McCracken and B.R. Evans.

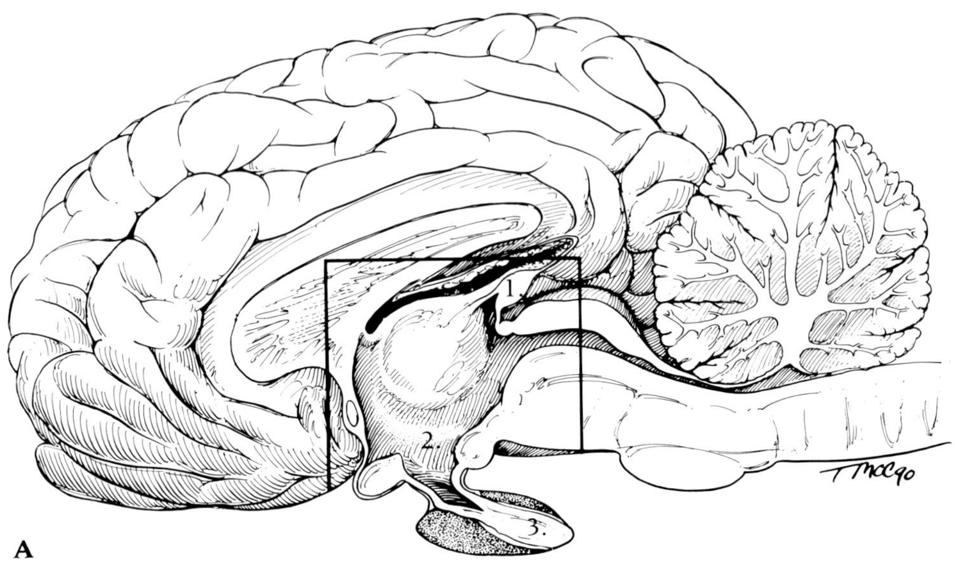

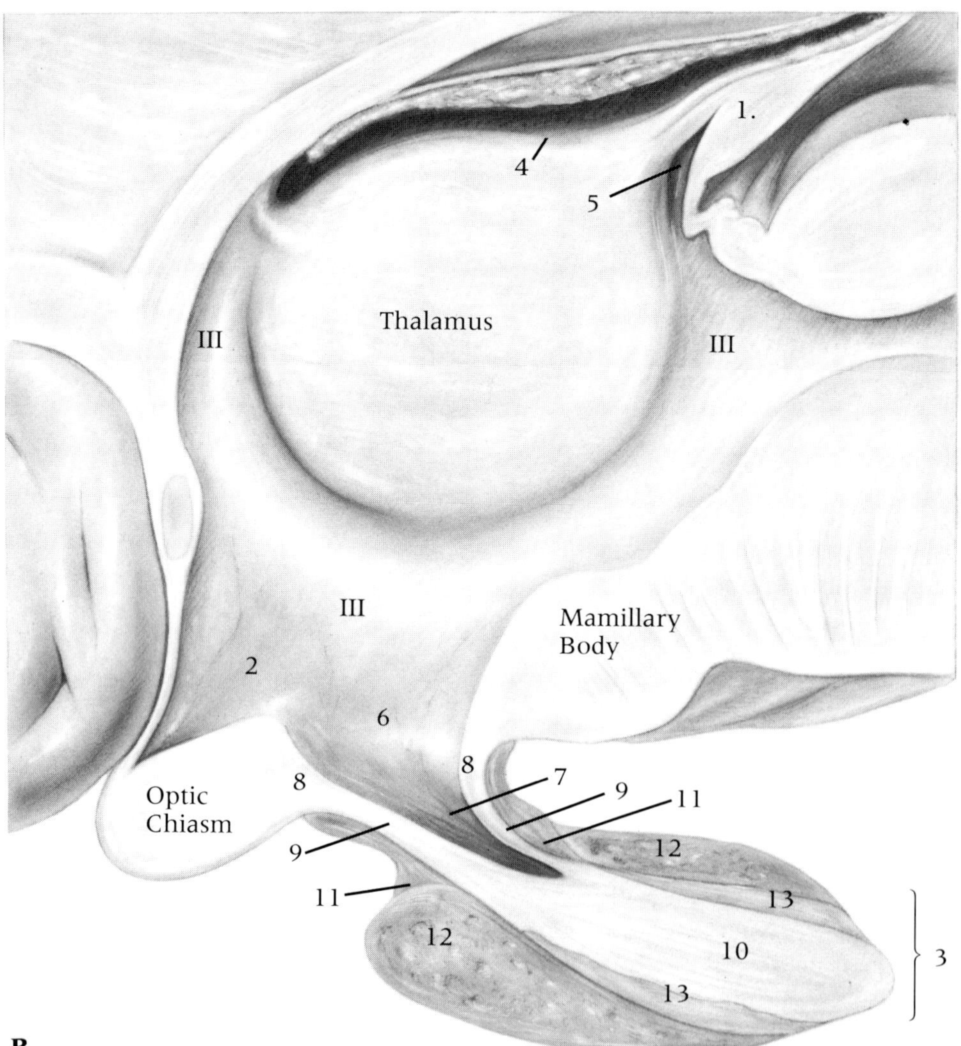

FIG. 1–1. *A,* Neuroendocrine contributors of the diencephalon to the reproductive system. *B,* Enlargement of a median section through the diencephalon. 1, Pineal gland; 2, hypothalamus; 3, hypophysis cerebri; III, third ventricle; 4, suprapineal recess of III; 5, pineal recess of III; 6, tuber cinereum; 7, infundibular recess of III; 8, median eminence; 9, infundibular stalk; 10, neural lobe; (8, 9, 10 = neurohypophysis); 11, pars tuberalis; 12, pars distalis; 13, pars intermedia; (11, 12, 13 = adenohypophysis).

eral walls of the third ventricle) produce both vasopressin and oxytocin. Processes of magnocellular secretory cells project to the neurohypophysis, terminating in its neural lobe. Smaller, parvicellular neurosecretory cell bodies in preoptic nuclei (rostral to the optic chiasm) produce gonadotropin-releasing hormone; parvicellular neurosecretory cell bodies in rostral hypothalamic nuclei (caudal to preoptic nuclei) produce thyrotropin-releasing hormone.[5] These and other releasing hormones are carried by processes of parvicellular neurosecretory cells to the median eminence region of the hypophysial infundibulum, where they end in association with dorsal and ventral capillary plexuses.[6]

Hypothalamic blood supply is derived from rostrodorsal hypophysial (infundibular) arteries and branches from caudal communicating and internal carotid arteries.[7] Venous blood drains into cavernous and intercavernous sinuses.

Central nervous system connections to the hypothalami include input from the limbic system, cerebral cortex, thalami, and reticular-activating system. The hypothalami have autonomic connection with the spinal cord and direct input from the accessory optic tract.

HYPOPHYSIS (PITUITARY GLAND)

Most of the hypophysis lies within the hypophysial fossa of the turkish saddle (sella turcica) of the basisphenoid bone. In the horse, the long axis of this dorsoventrally flattened, oval mass is almost horizontal to the hypothalamic base (Fig. 1-1). The hypophysis is held in place by the sellar diaphragm of dura mater. A foramen in the diaphragm admits passage of the hypophysial stalk.

Two major parts comprise the hypophysis—the neurohypophysis, derived from the developing diencephalon, and the adenohypophysis, derived from a pouch of oral ectoderm. The infundibulum of the neurohypophysis descends from the hypothalamic tuber cinereum. An outpocketing of the third ventricle, the infundibular recess, extends into the proximal part of the infundibular stalk. The well-vascularized median eminence region of the infundibulum is continued distad by the infundibular stalk, which terminates in an expanded neural lobe (human "posterior pituitary").

The bulk of the adenohypophysis, the pars distalis (human "anterior pituitary"), and the contiguous pars intermedia enclose nearly all of the neural lobe with only a small area of the caudal surface of the latter exposed. The pars tuberalis of the adenohypophysis ascends to enclose the infundibular stalk and the median eminence. Together the infundibular stalk and the tuberal part comprise the hypophysial stalk.

Axons and telodendria of parvicellular neurosecretory cells, vessels of the primary capillary plexus, and origins of hypophysial portal veins are present in the median eminence and in the proximal part of the infundibular stalk. Axons of magnocellular neurosecretory cells pass through the median eminence and infundibular stalk on their way to terminate in the neural lobe. Supportive neuroglial cells are present in the neurohypophysis. The tuberal part of the adenohypophysis consists of follicles or cords of weakly basophilic cells and numerous hypophysial portal veins. Clumps of basophilic cells in the pars intermedia are the source of melanocyte-stimulating hormone.

The pars distalis consists of clumps and cords of granular acidophils and basophils and agranular chromophobes. On proper stimulation, specific cell types secrete somatotropin, prolactin, adrenocorticotropic hormone, follicle-stimulating hormone, luteinizing hormone, thyrotropin, and lipoproteins. Sinusoidal capillaries and smaller efferent capillaries are present among the groups of cells.

Vascular Relationships

The internal carotid arteries give origin to rostroventral infundibular (hypophysial) arteries, which supply the ventral region of the primary capillary plexus in the median eminence (Fig. 1-2). The caudal communicating branches detach rostrodorsal infundibular arteries, which supply the dorsal region of the plexus. Superficial and deep, looped capillaries are linked together in the median eminence and extend caudad as far as the end of the infundibular recess. Ventral and dorsal groups of hypophysial portal vessels, descending from the primary capillary plexus through the tuberal part, constitute the sole blood supply to the distal part of the adenohypophysis. There the portal vessels terminate in a sinusoidal capillary network (Fig. 1-3). It has been suggested, but not substantiated, that ventral and dorsal groups of portal vessels are functionally related to specific zones of the median eminence and to certain regions of the distal part of the adenohypophysis.[6]

Right and left caudal infundibular arteries arise from the caudal intercarotid artery (or from internal carotid arteries) within the intercavernous sinus. They pierce the wall of the sinus and run in the dural sheath, sending branches to the dura mater and capsule of the hypophysis, and terminate in capillaries of the neural lobe and distal infundibular stalk.[6]

Venous drainage is mainly from the caudal aspect of the hypophysis to the right and left cavernous sinuses. From each sinus, two courses exist: (1) a caudoventral course to the ventral petrosal sinus and thence to the foramen lacerum and (2) a rostrolateral course to emissary veins in the orbital fissure—the ophthalmic vein and deep facial vein.[8] Continuity with the deep facial vein provides a route for catheterization to obtain samples of blood coming from the hypophysis. A catheter may be passed into the facial vein, then through the deep facial vein into the cavernous sinus.

Hypothalamo-Hypophysial Connections

In the median eminence, neurohemal organs—junctions between telodendria at the ends of processes of parvicellular neurosecretory cells descending from nuclei in the hypothalamus and capillaries of the primary

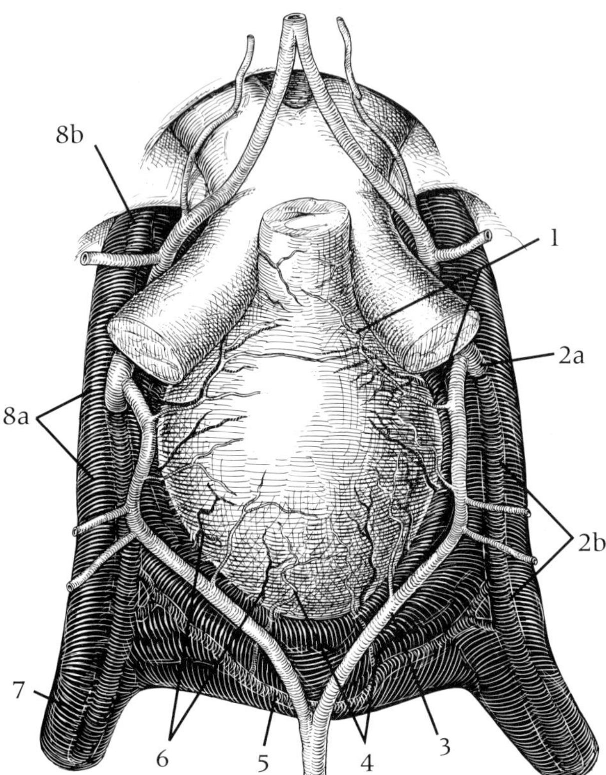

FIG. 1–2. Blood supply to and venous drainage from the hypophysis. Dorsal view of hypophysis and optic chiasm. 1, Rostroventral hypophysial arteries; 2a, internal carotid artery emerging from cavernous sinus; 2b, internal carotid artery within cavernous sinus; 3, caudal communicating branch; 4, caudal hypophysial arteries; 5, intercarotid artery within intercavernous sinus; 6, hypophysial veins; 7, ventral petrosal sinus; 8a, cavernous sinus; 8b, cavernous sinus exiting through orbital fissure. (Adapted in part from Vitums, A.: Observations on the equine hypophysial portal system. Anat. Histol. Embryol., *4*:149–161, 1975.)

plexus—are the sites of transfer of releasing and inhibitory hormones to the blood. Hypophysial portal veins coursing distad from the primary capillary plexus carry blood through the tuberal part to the distal part of the adenohypophysis where the veins terminate by branching into the sinusoidal (secondary) capillary plexus (Fig. 1-3). Releasing and inhibitory hormones leave the capillaries and contact target cells in the distal part of the adenohypophysis. Hormones produced by the target cells enter efferent capillaries that carry blood to veins draining to the cavernous sinuses.

Axons of magnocellular neurosecretory cells descend from hypothalamic nuclei through the median eminence and infundibular stalk to the neural lobe of the neurohypophysis (Fig. 1-3). Secretory granules (Herring bodies), consisting of prohormones, enzymes, and carrier molecules (neurophysins), migrate distad through the axons to neurohemal organs where hormones (oxytocin and antidiuretic hormone) are transferred through capillary walls into the blood.[5] Veins drain to the cavernous sinuses.

REPRODUCTIVE TRACT OF THE MARE

GENERAL RELATIONSHIPS

The mare's reproductive tract—ovaries, uterine tubes, uterus, vagina, and vulva—extends from the approximate position of the ovaries, ventrally to the fourth or fifth lumbar vertebra and caudally through the pelvic cavity to the vulva (Figs. 1-4 and 1-5). Contralateral ovaries, uterine tubes, and uterine horns lie on either side of the descending colon and its mesocolon; the uterine body and cervix are ventral to the terminal part of the descending colon and the rectum. The bladder is located ventrally to the uterine body and cervix with the urethra coursing caudad ventral to the vagina and emptying into the vestibule at the urethral orifice. The vagina is related bilaterally to the sacrotuberous ligaments, dorsally to the rectum, and ventrally to the urethra. The vestibule of the vagina, according to the *Nomina Anatomica Veterinaria (NAV)*,[9] is related dorsally to the anus and extends caudoventrad over the ischiatic arch to the vulva. The vestibule and vulva are related dorsally to the muscles and fascia of the perineal body. Laterally the vestibule and vulva are covered by the perineal fascia in apposition with the semimembranosus muscles.[10]

Variations in distension and the movement of the intestines and the bladder as well as pregnancy influence the positions of the internal genitalia. In the nonpregnant mare, ovaries, uterine tubes, and uterine horns may be in contact with the dorsal abdominal wall or may be located among intestinal coils. Distension of the bladder or descending colon can displace the uterine body to one side. It has been suggested that intestinal temperature and motility may affect the function of the reproductive organs in contact with the intestines.[11]

When the intestinal mass is removed, the internal genitalia droop into the emptied abdominal cavity, stretching the broad ligament on each side (Fig. 1-5). Broad ligaments are connecting double peritoneal sheets extending along lateral sublumbar and lateral pelvic walls from the third or fourth lumbar vertebra to the level of the fourth sacral vertebra. They become continuous with the serous tunics enclosing the ovaries, uterine tubes, and uterus. The portion of the broad ligament suspending the ovary, the mesovarium, detaches the mesosalpinx from its lateral surface. The mesosalpinx suspends the uterine tube (oviduct or salpinx). Most of the broad ligament is mesometrium, the connecting peritoneum extending to and continuous with the perimetrium, the serous tunic enclosing the uterus. In their abnormally suspended position, uterine horns are slung in a V-shaped configuration with the mesometrial attachment dorsally. Each stretched broad ligament provides for visualization of the contained ovarian vessels near its cranial edge, uterine vessels in its middle, and the round ligament of the uterus, on its lateral aspect. The round ligament of the uterus, the homologue of the gubernaculum testis, extends from its rounded, blunt end to the internal inguinal ring. Also contained between the two layers of the broad ligament

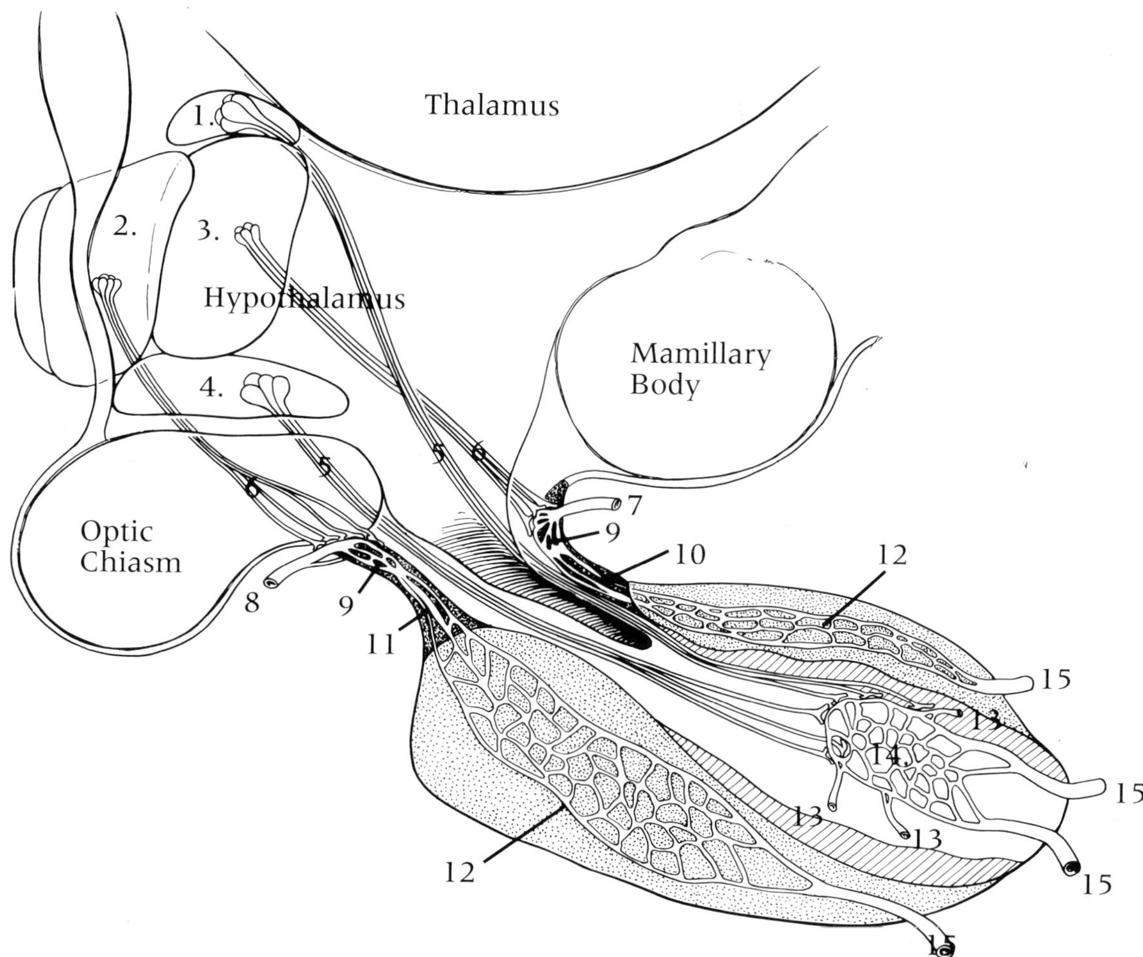

FIG. 1–3. Hypothalamo-hypophysial relationships. 1, Paraventricular nucleus; 2, preoptic nucleus; 3, rostral hypothalamic nucleus; 4, supraoptic nucleus; 5, processes of magnocellular neurosecretory cells; 6, processes of parvicellular neurosecretory cells; 7, branch of rostrodorsal hypophysial (infundibular) artery; 8, branch of rostroventral hypophysial (infundibular) artery; 9, primary capillary plexus within median eminence; 10, dorsal group of hypophysial portal vessels; 11, ventral group of hypophysial portal vessels; 12, sinusoidal capillary network within pars distalis; 13, branches of caudal hypophysial arteries; 14, capillaries of neural lobe; 15, hypophysial veins. (Adapted in part from Vitums, A.: Observations on the equine hypophysial portal system. Anat. Histol. Embryol., *4*:49–161, 1975; and Krieger, D.T.: The hypothalamus and neuroendocrinology. *In* Neuroendocrinology. Edited by D.T. Krieger and J.C. Hughes. Sunderland, Sinauer Associates, 1980, pp. 3–12.)

are lymphatic vessels, loose collagenous and adipose tissues, and sheets of smooth muscle continuous with the outer muscular layer of the uterine tube and uterus. During pregnancy, thickening of the broad ligaments restraining the descending gravid uterus is a result of enlargement of blood and lymphatic vessels and an increase in the smooth muscle mass.

Cystic remnants of mesonephric tubules and ducts (epoöphoron and paraoöphoron) occur commonly in the mesovarium and mesosalpinx. They tend to regress with age.[12] The long broad ligaments of the mare permit exteriorization of the ovaries, uterine tubes, and uterine horns through a midventral celiotomy.[11] An ovary may be exteriorized through an incision in the paralumbar fossa.[13]

Caudal to where the broad ligaments become continuous with the lateral ligaments of the bladder, two dorsoventrally flattened peritoneal pouches project into the pelvic cavity. Peritoneum reflects from the rectum onto the vagina, forming the rectogenital pouch, and from the bladder onto the vagina, forming the vesicogenital pouch that extends farther caudad. The extent of the vagina covered varies inversely with distension of the rectum and bladder.[14] When the latter are nearly empty, enough peritoneum (8 to 10 cm) covers the vagina so that the rectogenital pouch can be entered surgically through the dorsolateral wall of the vaginal fornix in the procedure of ovariectomy via colpotomy.[15] Farther caudally, a rectovaginal septum separates the rectum and vagina.

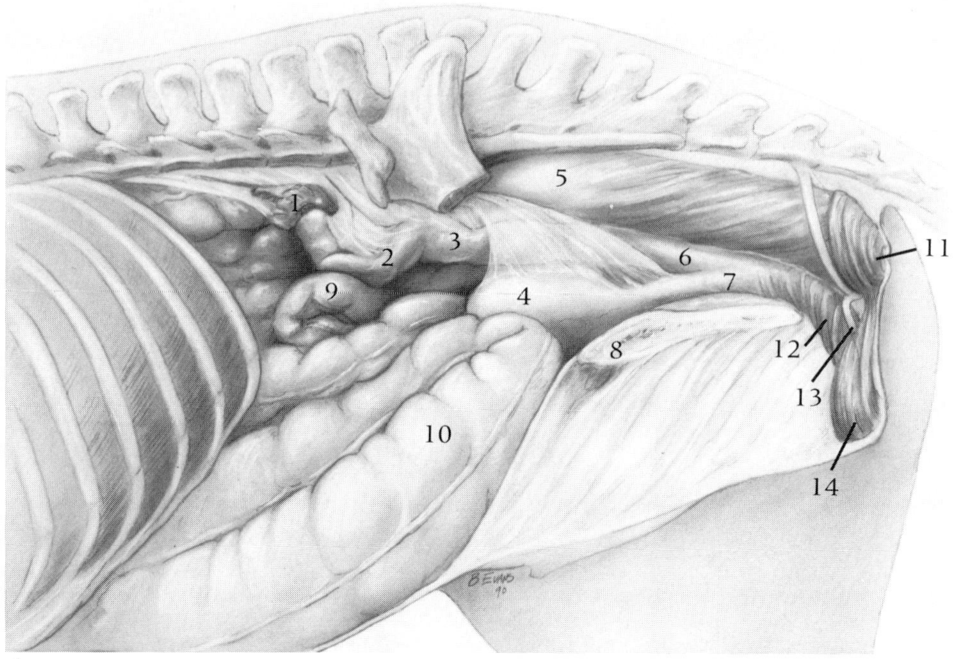

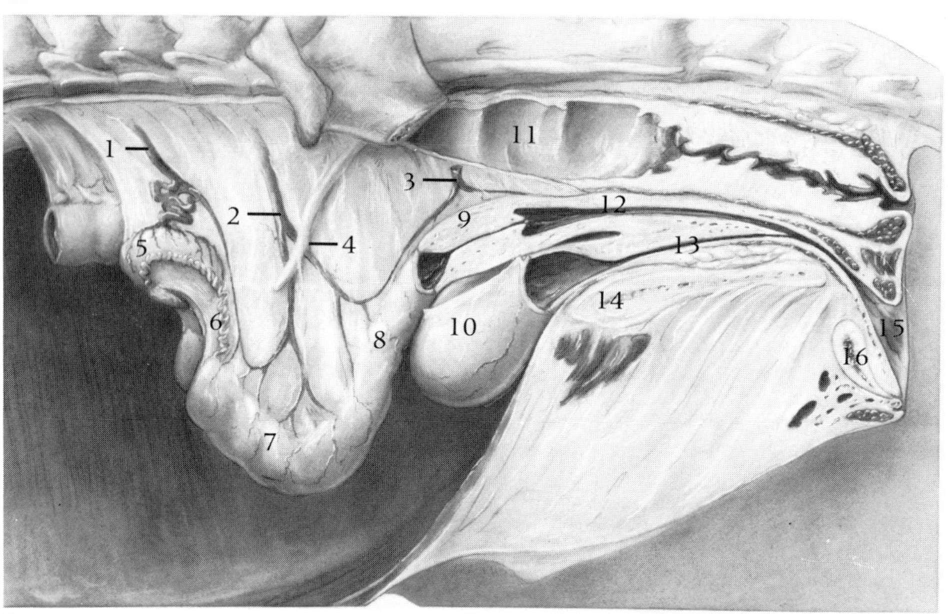

FIG. 1–4. *A,* Left lateral view of mare's reproductive tract with intestines in situ. Left laterocaudal abdominal and lateral pelvic walls removed. 1, Left ovary; 2, left uterine horn; 3, uterine body; 4, bladder; 5, ampulla of rectum; 6, vagina; 7, urethra; 8, pelvic brim; 9, descending colon; 10, left ventral colon; 11, external anal sphincter muscle; 12, vestibular constrictor muscle; 13, clitoral retractor muscle; 14, vulvar constrictor muscle. *B,* Left lateral view of mare's reproductive tract with intestinal mass removed. Rectum, uterine cervix, bladder, urethra, vaginal vestibule, and clitoris in median section. 1, Ovarian artery; 2, uterine artery; 3, vaginal artery; 4, round ligament of uterus; 5, left ovary; 6, left uterine tube; 7, left uterine horn; 8, uterine body; 9, uterine cervix; 10, bladder; 11, ampulla of rectum; 12, vagina proper; 13, urethra; 14, pelvic brim; 15, vaginal vestibule; 16, corpus cavernosum clitoridis.

OVARIES

As described above, the position of the ovaries is variable largely because of the extensive mesovarium that permits the ovary a wide range of passive movement. An ovary may lie on top of the intestinal mass in contact with the dorsal abdominal wall or it may be situated among the intestinal coils roughly on a plane through the fourth or fifth lumbar vertebra. The left ovary is caudal to the right, but it is closer to the ipsilateral kidney. The distance from the ovaries to tips of the uterine horns also varies. During pregnancy, the ovaries

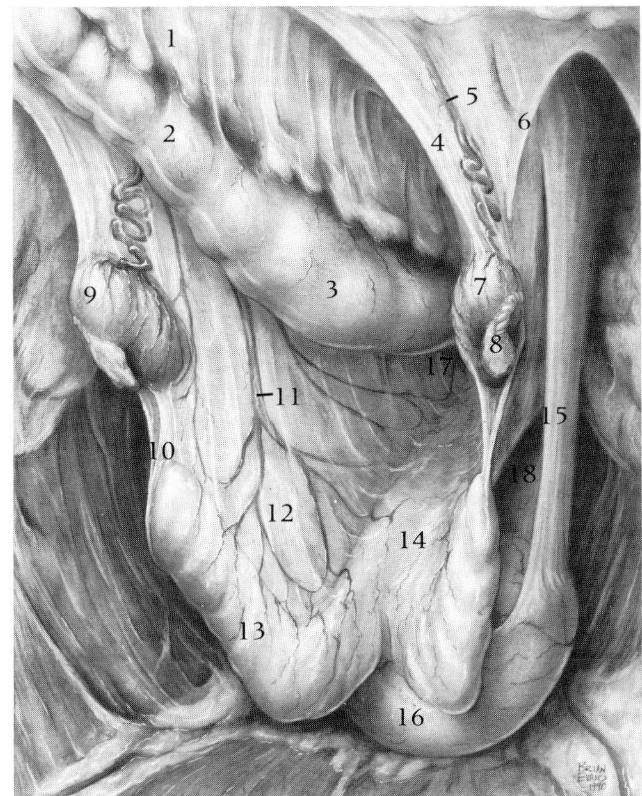

FIG. 1–5. Frontolateral view of a mare's reproductive tract with intestinal mass removed. 1, Mesocolon; 2, descending colon; 3, ampulla of rectum; 4, mesovarium; 5, ovarian artery; 6, round ligament of uterus; 7, left ovary; 8, left uterine tube; 9, right ovary; 10, proper ligament of ovary; 11, uterine artery; 12, mesometrium; 13, right uterine horn; 14, uterine body; 15, left lateral ligament of bladder; 16, bladder; 17, rectogenital pouch; 18, vesicogenital pouch.

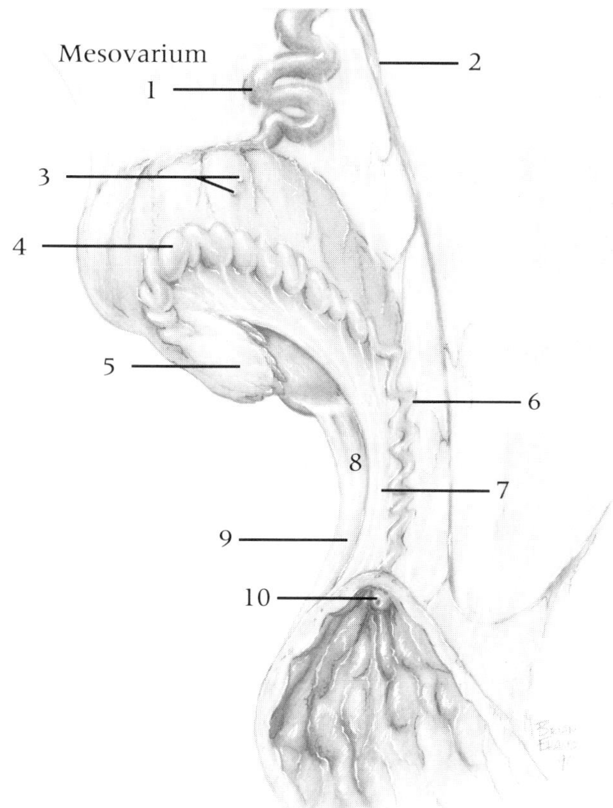

FIG. 1–6. Left ovary, uterine tube, ovarian bursa, and opened tip of left uterine horn. 1, Ovarian branch of left ovarian artery; 2, uterine branch of left ovarian artery; 3, adrenocortical nodules; 4, ampulla of left uterine tube; 5, infundibulum of uterine tube covering ovulation fossa; 6, isthmus of uterine tube; 7, mesosalpinx; 8, ovarian bursa; 9, left proper ligament of ovary; 10, uterine ostium of uterine tube (slightly exaggerated).

are pulled cranioventrad as well as mediad, an important position to recall when palpating per rectum.

The large ovaries (averaging 7 to 8 cm along the long axis) of the mare are reniform with a convex dorsal border attached to the mesovarium and a sharply concave ventral free border indented by an ovulation fossa (*NAV*—ovarian fossa). Medial and lateral surfaces are covered by visceral peritoneum continuous with the mesovarium and contain prominent parallel branches from the ovarian vessels. Yellow, grapelike clusters of adrenocortical nodules (1 to 2 mm in diameter) may be present in loose connective tissue on the surface of the ovary.[16] A variable amount of adipose tissue also occurs in the loosely adherent serosa.

From the caudal pole of the ovary, the proper ligament of the ovary—a band of smooth muscle within the broad ligament—extends to the tip of the uterine horn. The cranial pole of the ovary is attached, in part, to the uterine tube's infundibulum, which overlays the ovulation fossa (Fig. 1-6). Polygonal cells of the superficial epithelium ("germinal epithelium") lining the ovulation fossa impart a darker color than the contiguous mesothelial cells covering the rest of the organ.[1,14]

The histologic structure of the equine ovary is unique among domestic mammals in that it has a peripheral collagenous connective tissue vascular zone around a central parenchymatous zone, containing developing and atretic ovarian follicles, corpora lutea, and corpora albicantia. The parenchymatous zone surfaces at the ovulation fossa, and during folliculogenesis, maturing follicles move toward the fossa, enlarging to a diameter of 4.5 to 6 cm. Mature ovarian follicles become less turgid immediately before ovulation. A corpus hemorrhagicum commonly forms following ovulation. The developing reddish corpus luteum does not bulge from the ovary, but it may project slightly into the ovulation fossa. Later, the corpus luteum becomes yellow. The primary corpus luteum of pregnancy is supplemented by secondary corpora lutea that begin to form around day 40 of gestation, developing from follicles that continue to grow rapidly during the first couple of months of gestation. Luteinization takes place in follicles that have ovulated and in anovulatory follicles.[11] Secondary corpora lutea are spherical, irregular, or gourdlike with a tract leading to the ovulation fossa. Many corpora lutea have a central cavity.[17] Corpora lutea continue to function until the sixth month of gestation, and then regression occurs.

The mare's large ovaries are eclipsed in size by the developing fetal ovaries at midgestation. Fetal ovaries later regress, and by the time of parturition, they are one-tenth their greatest fetal size.[1] Their shape at birth is oval, with superficial ("germinal") epithelium covering the entire free surface. Observed as early as 5 months of age,[18] indentation of the free border to form the ovulation fossa continues until puberty when the growth of the organ is accelerated. The ovary is larger in young mares, and it tends to become more fibrous in older mares.

UTERINE TUBES (OVIDUCTS OR SALPINGES)

Each uterine tube consists of an expansive infundibulum covering the ovary's ovulation fossa, a highly tortuous ampulla about 6 mm in diameter, and a less tortuous isthmus half the diameter of the ampulla (Fig. 1-6). The isthmus terminates at a small uterine ostium on a papilla within the end of the uterine horn. Based on measurements made with the loops effaced and free of the suspending mesosalpinx, equine uterine tubes are from 20 to 30 cm long with the ampulla comprising about half the length.[1,14]

Irregular fimbriae are present along the margin of the funnel-shaped infundibulum. Some are attached to the cranial pole of the ovary, allowing the rest of the infundibulum to spread over the ventral aspect and cover the ovulation fossa. At the edges of the fimbriae, their serosal covering is contiguous to the mucous membrane. The latter is highly folded, especially in the ampulla where secondary and tertiary ridges branch from longitudinal folds. The lining of simple columnar epithelium is intermittently ciliated. Ciliogenesis and ciliary motion (toward the uterus) reflect stages of the sexual cycle. A thin, well-vascularized lamina propria supports the epithelium. Inner, circularly disposed smooth muscle fibers are covered by outer, longitudinally arranged fibers that continue into the mesosalpinx.

The abdominal ostium in the center of the infundibulum is about 6 mm in diameter; the uterine ostium of the tube, 2 to 3 mm in diameter.[14] The inner circular muscle increases to form a sphincter at the tubouterine junction. Unfertilized ova are retained for a considerable duration in the uterine tubes (up to several months), parthogenetic cleavage occurring in some of them.[19]

The ovarian bursa of the mare is a peritoneal pouch extending from the ovulation fossa caudad to the cranial aspect of the uterine horn. Laterally it is bounded by the uterine tube and mesosalpinx. A fold of broad ligament containing the proper ligament of the ovary forms the medial wall of the ovarian bursa.

UTERUS

Two uterine horns, diverging sharply from a small intercornual ligament, are located entirely within the abdominal cavity, lying on or intermingling with intestinal coils. The body of the uterus becomes continuous caudally with the uterine cervix in the cranial part of the pelvic cavity. Length of the uterine horns ranges from 20 to 25 cm. They are asymmetrical in parous mares. The diameter of the horns increases from their blunt tips to their junction with the body. The body averages 18 to 20 cm in length; the cervix, 5 to 7 cm.[14] Mesometrium attaches to the dorsal borders of the horns and follows to the lateral aspects of the body and cervix. In situ before manipulation, the walls of the horns and body of the uterus are flaccid and intestine-like. Handling causes the uterus to contract rapidly, the decrease in length and increase in diameter imparting the sausage shape of the horns observed after removal of the uterus from the abdominal cavity.[11]

Internally, the uterine ostium of a uterine tube opens on a small papilla in the endometrium in the tip of each horn. The sphincter of circular muscle at the tubouterine junction serves as a valve, preventing reflux of uterine contents through the uterine ostium. A short median septum is present where the uterine horns join the body. The lumen of the uterus is practically obliterated by its flaccid walls and 12 to 15 large longitudinal folds of reddish brown endometrium with collagenous connective tissue cores. Only capillary spaces occur between the endometrial folds.[20]

The epithelial layer of the endometrium of the uterine body and horns is simple columnar epithelium (pseudostratified during estrus) with cuboidal to tall cells, depending on stage of the estrous cycle. Fewer than half of the cells are ciliated. Branched tubular glands extend from the surface through a compact layer of connective tissue cells and reticular fibers into a fibrous and vascularized spongy layer of lamina propria.[20] The myometrium of the uterine wall consists of an inner circular layer of smooth muscle, a middle vascular layer, and an outer longitudinal layer of smooth muscle. The latter two layers are coextensive with the vasculature and musculature of the mesometrium. Enclosing visceral peritoneum, the perimetrium, is continuous with the two peritoneal sheets of the mesometrium (Fig. 1-7).

The constricted, thick-walled cervix is traversed by the cervical canal, which extends from the internal uterine orifice and opens into the body to the external uterine orifice in the protruding vaginal portion of the cervix (Fig. 1-8). The wall contains an increased amount of collgenous connective tissue and a sphincter of smooth muscle derived from the inner layer of myometrium. Longitudinal mucosal folds in the cervical canal are continuous with those in the endometrium of the body and tend to bulge caudad at the external uterine orifice. A fold may continue onto the vaginal floor as a frenulum.[11] The endometrium of the cervical canal is grossly paler. Tubular glands do not project from the epithelial layer, which consists of both ciliated and mucigenous cells.

CYCLIC UTERINE ANATOMY

Uterine Anatomy during Estrus

During estrus, the uterine wall thickens, muscular tone increases, vascularity becomes greater, and proliferated endometrial glands are active. Vaginoscopic examina-

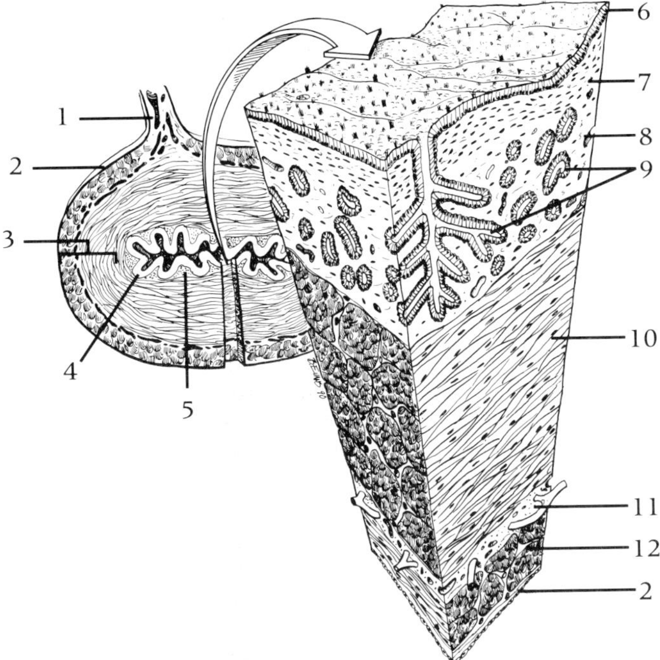

FIG. 1–7. Cross section of uterine horn. 1, Mesometrium; 2, perimetrium; 3, myometrium; 4, endometrium; 5, collagenous connective tissue core; 6, surface epithelium; 7, compact layer of lamina propria; 8, spongy layer of lamina propria; 9, endometrial glands; 10, internal (circular) layer of myometrium; 11, middle (vascular) layer of myometrium; 12, external (longitudinal) layer of myometrium.

tions of the vaginal portion of the cervix reveal functional anatomic variations that correlate with ovarian activity and behavioral changes during the estrous cycle.[21] In proestrus, the cervix and its folds begin to enlarge and the mucous membrane becomes unevenly congested. During estrus, the cervix is completely relaxed and droops ventrad; the folds protrude farther from the enlarging external uterine orifice, which will eventually admit three or four fingers (Fig. 1-9A). Mucosal congestion is even and deep, and cervical secretions are abundant.[21] Manipulation of the cervix tends to restore some of its turgidity.

Uterine Anatomy during Diestrus

In diestrus, the thickness of the uterine wall decreases and muscular tone and endometrial glandular activity subside. The cervical canal constricts as the cervix becomes firmer and protrudes caudad (Fig. 1-9B). It is occluded by a plug of mucus. Mucosal folds protrude less and are no longer congested.[16]

Uterine Anatomy during Pregnancy

During pregnancy, the developing embryo, and then fetus, causes enlargement of the horn, then the body, and finally, the contralateral horn. The mesometrium, enlarging in response to distension of vessels and increased muscular mass, exerts tension on the enlarging

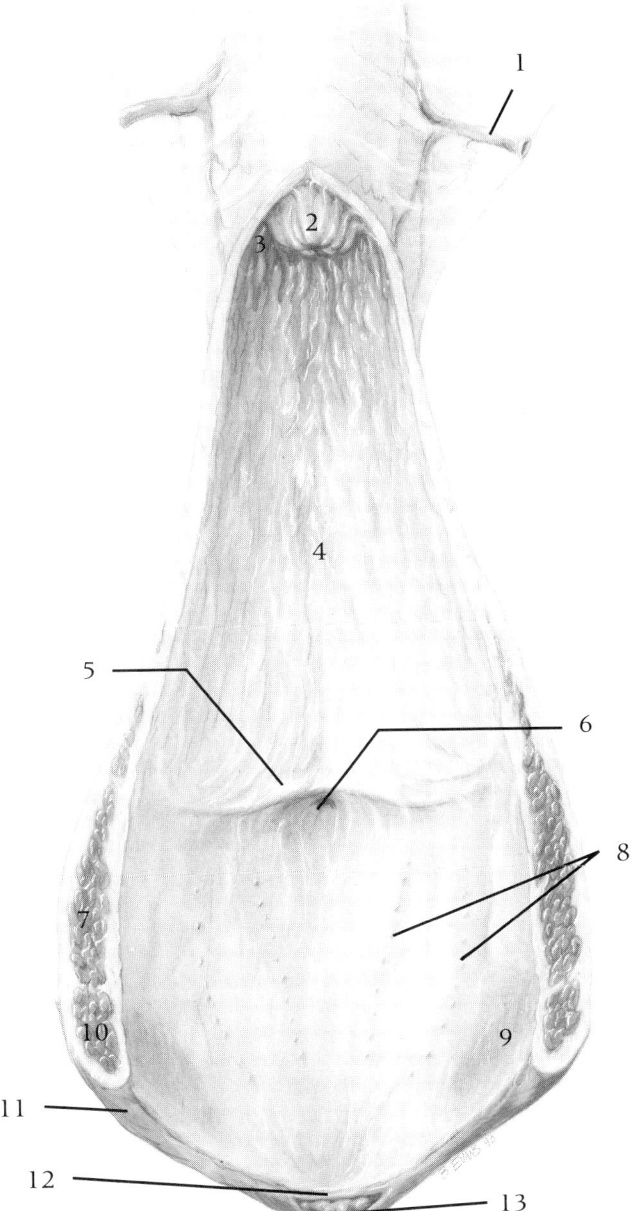

FIG. 1–8. Dorsal view of opened vagina and vulva. 1, Vaginal artery; 2, vaginal portion of cervix; 3, vaginal fornix; 4, ventral vaginal wall; 5, transverse fold; 6, urethral orifice; 7, vestibular constrictor muscle; 8, orifices of vestibular glands; 9, locus of submucosal vestibular bulb; 10, vulvar constrictor muscle; 11, vulvar labium; 12, transverse frenular fold (clitoral prepuce); 13, clitoral glans.

horns, causing them to flex somewhat. As the uterus descends to the abdominal floor, the myometrium becomes thinner, except in the then-firm cervix, which is pulled craniad out of the pelvic cavity. The cervical canal is filled with a thick mucous plug, and the external uterine orifice is contracted to a slit. The arrangement of collagenous, elastic, and smooth muscle fibers in the wall permit extreme dilation of the cervix, accommodating passage of the foal during parturition. It has been

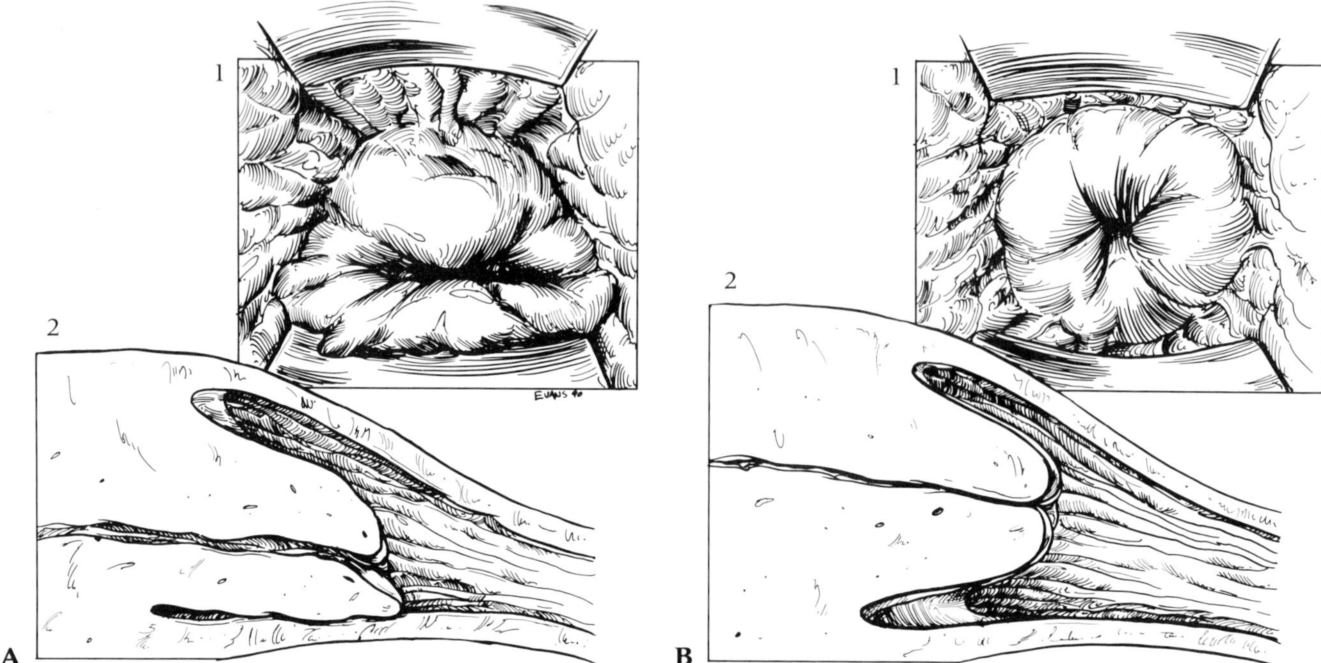

FIG. 1–9. Vaginal portion of uterine cervix. *A*, during estrus and *B*, during diestrus. 1, Vaginoscopic view; 2, median section.

suggested that collagenase is involved in the process of labor.[22]

The endometrium becomes thicker and more vascular during the formation of the yolk-sac placenta and then the diffuse, microcotyledonous, epitheliochorial placenta of the mare is formed. A ring of endometrial cups develops, starting about day 37 of gestation. Slow regression begins around day 70 and is complete by 130 days.[23] Endometrial cups are formed by hypertrophy of endometrial glands and the subsequent invasion of the endometrium by chorionic epithelial cells.[24] These cells develop into cup cells, which produce pregnant mare serum gonadotropin (equine chorionic gonadotropin).

VAGINA

The vaginal fornix is an anular recess formed by the junction of the cranial vaginal walls with the caudally projecting vaginal portion of the cervix. The vagina, including its vestibule *(NAV)*, extends caudad from the fornix to the labia of the vulva (Fig. 1-8). Some authors include the vestibule as part of the vulva in keeping with the designation of the shallow human vestibule and the embryonic origin of these parts of the reproductive tract. The thin-walled vagina proper (averaging about 20 cm in length) ends caudally at the transverse fold above the external urethral orifice. This fold is a remnant of the hymen, which partitioned the vestibule from the vagina proper. It may extend for a variable distance up the lateral walls, and occasionally a persistent hymen is present.[11]

Stratified squamous epithelium covers the well-vascularized lamina propria of the longitudinally folded vaginal mucous membrane. An abrupt junction exists with the simple columnar epithelium on the protruding cervical folds at the external uterine orifice. During estrus, an increased amount of mucus on the pale mucosal surface comes from the cervical canal. The equine vagina proper is aglandular. Cornification of the superficial layer of the epithelium is minimal during estrus and cannot be used as a cytological criterion for determining different stages of the estrous cycle.

Longitudinal folds of the vaginal mucous membrane are effaced when the organ is distended. Exposure to air tends to darken the mucous membrane. The fibroelastic tissue and smooth muscle in the wall permit distension of the vagina to the limits of the pelvic wall during passage of the foal. At other times, compression from feces in the rectal ampulla causes dorsoventral collapse of the vaginal wall, reducing the lumen to a horizontal slit. The vagina is enclosed by a loose collagenous connective tissue adventitia, containing numerous sympathetic ganglia, a venous plexus, and adipose tissue. As noted earlier, the extent of the cranial part of the vagina covered by peritoneum is related inversely to the fullness of the rectum and bladder.

VESTIBULE

The vestibule (whether vaginal or vulvar) has a short, straight dorsal wall and a longer (10 to 12 cm), sloping ventral wall extending to the labia of the vulva just beyond the ischiatic arch. From the ventral commissure of the labia inward, this configuration gives the vestibular vault a ventrodorsal slope (Fig. 1-4B).

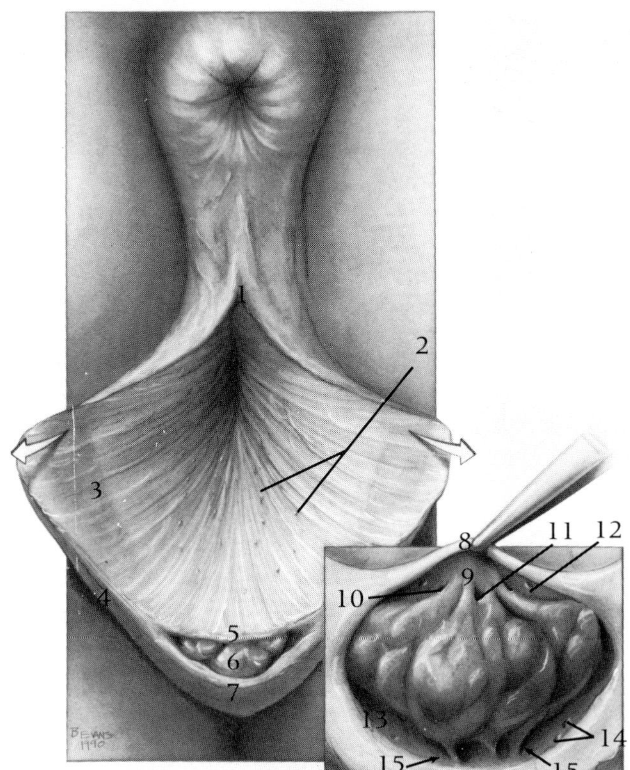

FIG. 1–10. View of vulva and vestibule through parted vulvar labia. 1, Dorsal commissure; 2, orifices of vestibular glands; 3, location of vestibular bulb (beneath darker mucous membrane); 4, vulvar labium; 5, transverse frenular fold (clitoral prepuce); 6, clitoral glans; 7, ventral commissure. Inset: clitoral glans. 8, Transverse frenular fold retracted; 9, frenulum; 10, openings of lateral sinuses; 11, opening of median sinus; 12, locations of frenular sinuses; 13, clitoral fossa; 14, labial recesses; 15, locations of ventral sinuses. (Locations of sinuses adapted in part from McAllister, R.A., and Sack, W.O.: Identification of anatomic features of the equine clitoris as potential growth sites for Taylorella equigenitalis. J. Am. Vet. Med. Assoc., *196*:1965–1966, 1990.)

Parting the vulvar labia reveals a pink to brownish red, folded mucous membrane of the vestibule (Fig. 1-10). Stratified squamous epithelium continues as the epithelial lamina of the mucous membrane. A layer of encircling smooth muscle fibers lies deep to the proper lamina. The latter contains elastic fibers and lymph nodules.[25] A ventral row and a lateral row of openings of branched tubular, mucous vestibular glands extend along each side. A darker region of mucous membrane on each lateral wall just cranial to the vulvar labium lays over a vestibular bulb, a mass of erectile tissue approximately 7 by 3 cm (Figs. 1-8 and 1-10). The vestibular bulb is related laterally to the constrictor muscle of the vestibule.

The constrictor muscle of the vestibule arises from the levator fascia and the lateral edges of the perineal septum, which covers the roof of the vestibule.[10] Some of the muscle's fibers attach to the retractor muscle of the clitoris (suspensory ligament of the anus). Here the clitoral retractor is a band of smooth muscle descending from a decussation ventral to the subanal loop of the muscle and extending dorsocaudal to the vestibular constrictor toward the vulvar labium.[10] The sides and ventral aspect of the vestibule are covered by the vestibular constrictor muscle that blends caudally with the vulvar constrictor muscle (Fig. 1-4A).

VULVA

Projecting caudad over the ischiatic arch, the vulva consists of two labia and the clitoris. The labia are in apposition at the vulvar cleft, uniting at the sharp angle of the dorsal commissure and at the rounded ventral commissure. At the mucocutaneous junction, the aglandular mucous membrane meets the smooth, highly glandular, usually pigmented skin covering the labia. The mucocutaneous junction continues onto the transverse frenular fold (clitoral prepuce[9]). The vulvar constrictor muscle and, on each side, the smooth muscle of the clitoral retractor are contained within the labia. Dorsally, the vulvar constrictor muscle is continuous with the caudal part of the external anal sphincter muscle; ventrally, it sweeps under the clitoris. On its way toward the clitoris, each band of the clitoral retractor muscle is covered by superficial fascia and a few fibers of the vulvar constrictor muscle.[10] Contractions of the vulvar constrictor function with the vestibular constrictor during copulation. The former muscle also causes eversion of the clitoris ("winking") following urination or during the flow of fluids during estrus.[11] The arrangement of the tissues within the labia permit their wide expansion during delivery of the foal.

The wrinkled, creased skin of the large clitoral glans is observed when the labia are parted at the ventral commissure (Fig. 1-10). The clitoral glans presents a central part separated partially by grooves from two lateral parts. A clitoral fossa surrounds the sides and vental aspect of the glans, and the transverse frenular fold of integument covers the glans dorsally. A median frenulum extends from the clitoral glans to the transverse frenular fold.

A constant median clitoral sinus (about 1 cm deep) and two shallow (2 to 3 mm deep) lateral sinuses present in 75% of clitorides are located in creases in clitoral skin immediately ventral to the transverse frenular fold (Fig. 1-10). In 30% of clitorides examined, the orifice of the median sinus could be seen without displacing the transverse frenular fold.[26] Frenular recesses at the junction of the transverse frenular fold with the medial labial walls and the glans and ventral recesses in the deepest part of the clitoral fossa are 7 to 8 mm deep. Shallower labial recesses, 2 mm deep, may be observed in the medial labial walls. All of these invaginations contain a variable amount of smegma (from sebaceous glands in clitoral skin). The significance of this detailed anatomy is that although smegma may be sponged from frenular, ventral, and labial recesses it is retained in the median and lateral sinuses. But the lateral sinuses are considered too shallow to support the growth of anaero-

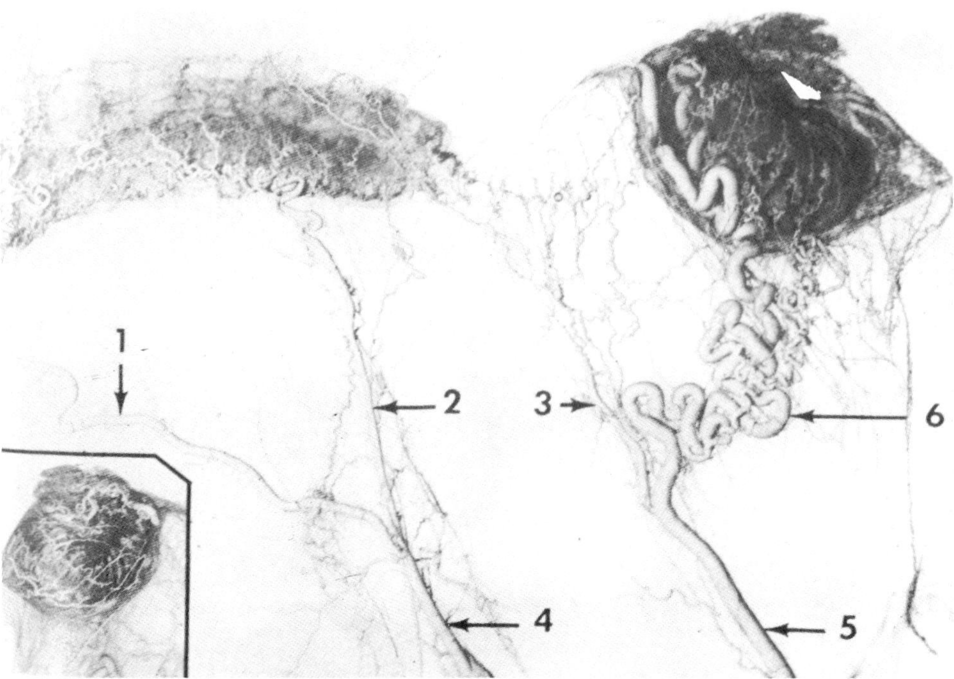

FIG. 1–11. Dorsal view of latex casts of arteries to uterine horn and ovary in the mare. Insert: ventral view of ovary. 1, Caudal branch of uterine artery; 2, cranial branch of uterine artery; 3, uterine branch of ovarian artery; 4, uterine artery; 5, ovarian artery; 6, ovarian branch of ovarian artery. (From Ginther, O.J., Garcia, M.C., Squires, E.L., and Steffenhagen, W.P.: Anatomy of the vasculature of the uterus and ovaries in the mare. Am. J. Vet. Res., *33*:1561–1568, 1972.)

bic bacteria, in particular Taylorella equigenitalis.[26]

The body of the mare's large clitoris contains an erectile tissue mass, the corpus cavernosum clitoridis. Two crura extend caudad to attach on the ischiatic arch.

VASCULAR AND NEURAL RELATIONSHIPS OF THE REPRODUCTIVE TRACT

Arterial Supply and Venous Drainage

The ovary is supplied by the tortuous ovarian branch of the ovarian artery coursing ventrolaterad from the abdominal aorta. A smaller uterine branch of this artery anastomoses with the cranial branch of the main blood supply to the uterus, the uterine artery, descending from the external iliac artery. These vessels supply blood to the uterine tube and cranial part of the uterine horn. The caudal branch of the uterine artery anastomoses with the uterine branch of the vaginal artery (from the internal pudendal artery), providing the blood supply to the caudal part of the uterine horn and the uterine body (Figs. 1-11 and 1-12).

Blood from the ovary drains through several smaller veins that converge to form the ovarian branch of the ovarian vein. While satellite veins accompany the arteries, the main venous drainage of the uterus is via the ovarian vein. Interconnecting veins from the ovary and cranial part of the uterus form an extensive utero-ovarian plexus, but the close intertwining of the ovarian vein and artery observed in other species (e.g., the ewe) does not exist in the mare.[27]

The main blood supply to the caudal part of the reproductive tract is from the internal pudendal artery.[28] A small branch from the umbilical artery courses craniad along the ureter into the broad ligament. The first part of the uterine branch of the vaginal artery (which may also arise from the umbilical or cranial gluteal artery) supplies the vagina, and its vestibular branch supplies the rest of the vagina and courses ventrad around the vestibule. The next branch, the ventral perineal artery, gives a dorsal labial branch to the vulva (Fig. 1-13) and occasionally sends one to the vestibular bulb. The termination of the internal pudendal artery is the artery of the vestibular bulb. It courses to the ventral surface of the vulva, providing small branches to the vestibular bulb. A second blood supply to this region, the obturator artery, terminates by entering the root of the clitoris, dividing into deep and dorsal arteries of the clitoris.

Satellite veins carry blood from the caudal part of the reproductive tract. Veins from the clitoris communicate with the vestibular bulb.

Lymphatic Drainage

Lymph flows from the ovaries, uterine tubes, and uterus to lumbar aortic lymph nodes.[29] Lymphatic vessels from the uterus, vagina, and vulva are afferent to medial iliac lymph nodes. A uterine lymph node occurs occasionally in the broad ligament.

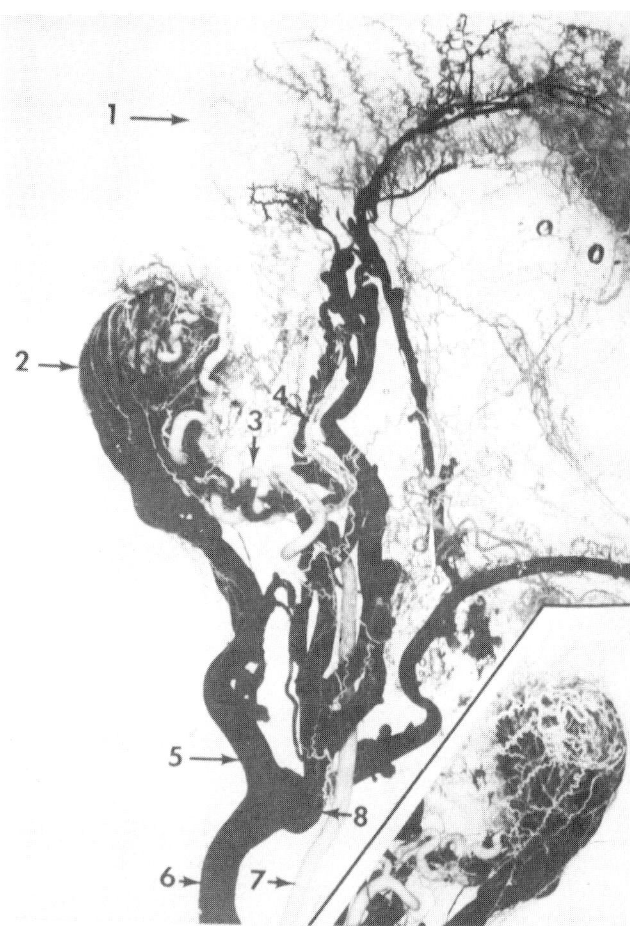

FIG. 1–12. Dorsal view of intervascular relationships of the vessels to the ovary and uterine horn. Latex casts of main arteries (gray) and veins (black). Venous branches to uterine horn incompletely injected. Insert: Ventral view of blood supply to ovary. 1, Uterine horn; 2, ovary; 3, ovarian branch of ovarian artery; 4, uterine branch of ovarian artery; 5, ovarian branch of ovarian vein; 6, ovarian vein; 7, ovarian artery; 8, uterine branch of ovarian vein. (From Ginther, O.J., Garcia, M.C., Squires, E.L., and Steffenhagen, W.P.: Anatomy of the vasculature of the uterus and ovaries in the mare. Am. J. Vet. Res., *33*:1561–1568, 1972.)

Innervation

Renal, aortic, uterine, and pelvic plexuses supply sympathetic fibers to the ovaries, uterine tubes, uterus, and vagina.[14] Pudendal and caudal rectal nerves (derived from the third and fourth sacral nerves) innervate the muscles of the vestibule and vulva and the vulvar skin. They both contribute to the formation of superficial perineal nerves, which emerge ventrolateral to the anus and supply the labia (Fig. 1-13).[10]

THE MARE'S UDDER

The small, inconspicuous udder of the virgin mare lies caudal to two prominent folds of abdominal skin extending to the bases of two small, laterally flattened teats. In some mares each fold of skin continues caudad

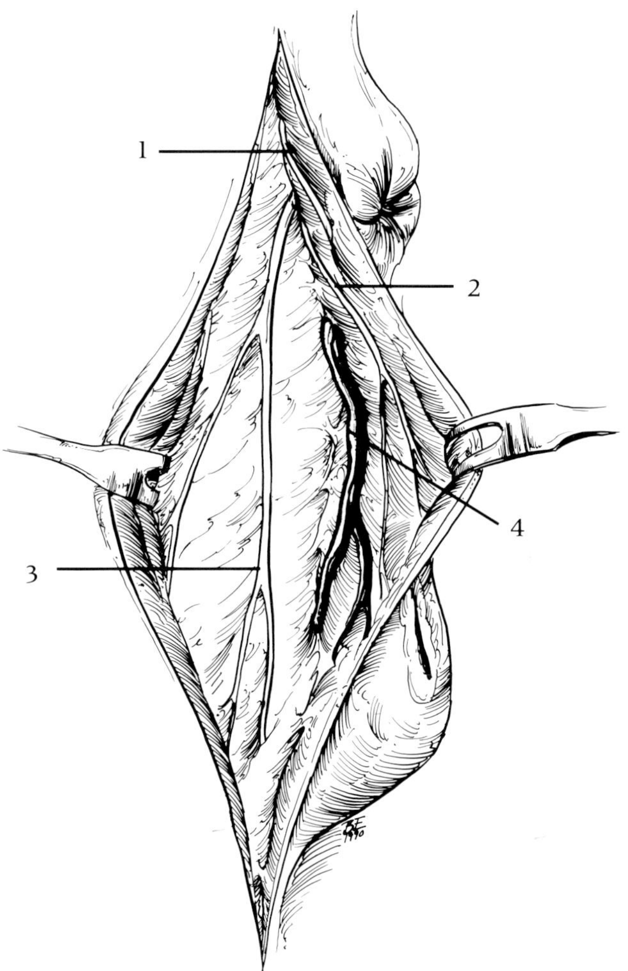

FIG. 1–13. Nerve and blood supply to vulvar labium. 1, 2, and 3, Superficial perineal nerves; 4, ventral perineal artery and vein. Size of nerves and vessels slightly exaggerated. (Adapted in part from Habel, R.: The perineum of the mare. Cornell Vet., *43*:249–278, 1953.)

lateral to the teat (Fig. 1-14). The longitudinal intermammary groove dividing the right and left halves of the organ contains wrinkled skin covered with a layer of dark colored sebum that can be peeled away. In very young fillies, a few hairs protrude from the orifices at the tips of the teats, but they soon regress.

As the ducts, secretory alveoli and their enclosing myoepithelial cells, and supportive tissues develop during gestation, the udder enlarges, effacing cutaneous folds. The teats of the roughly flattened hemispherical halves (mammae) of the udder elongate and become conical. Two (sometimes three) ostia (orifices)—one caudal to the other—open into a depression at the apex of the teat. Each orifice leads to a separate papillary duct (streak canal). Continuing from each papillary duct, a separate papillary part (teat cistern) leads into the glandular part (gland cistern) of the lactiferous sinus. Thus there are two (or three) closely associated lactiferous duct systems in the glandular complex of each half of the mare's udder with the cranial system being the largest (Fig. 1-14).

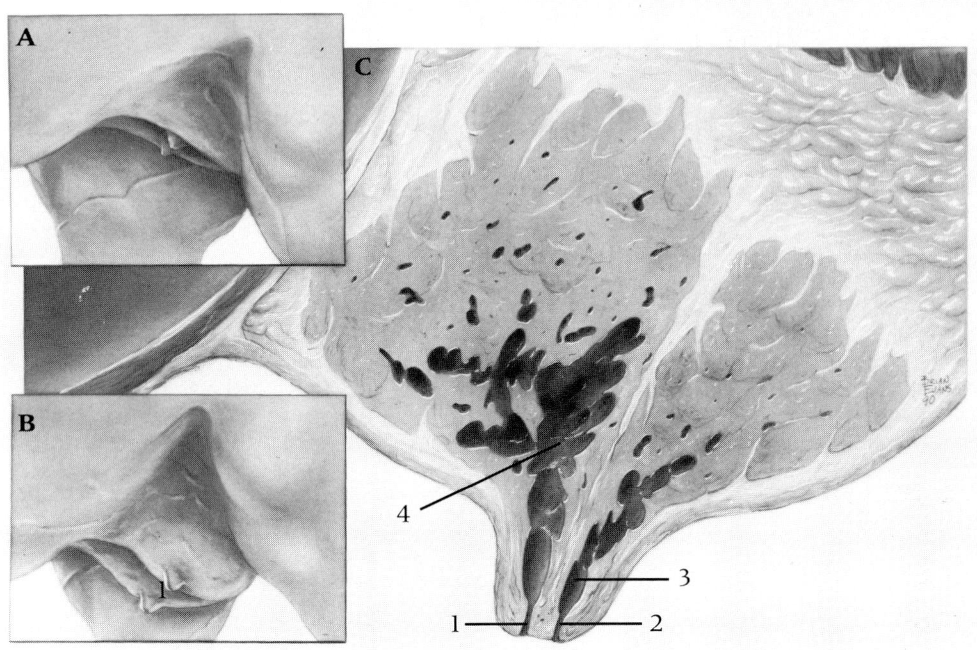

FIG. 1–14. Gross anatomy of the equine udder. *A*, Udder of a virgin mare. *B*, Lactating udder. 1, Intermammary groove. *C*, Sagittal section of a lactating udder. 1, Cranial papillary duct (streak canal); 2, caudal papillary duct; 3, papillary part of caudal lactiferous sinus (teat cistern); 4, glandular part of cranial lactiferous sinus (gland cistern).

At its junction with the teat cistern, the stratified squamous epithelium of the folded lining the papillary duct gradually changes to the bistratified columnar epithelium, which lines most of the lactiferous duct system. Smaller ducts leading from the alveoli are formed by simple columnar epithelium. Smooth muscle, fibroelastic tissue, and blood vessels comprise the bulk of the teat wall. The apex of the teat lacks an organized sphincter.[30]

Support for each half of the udder is provided by a fibrous lateral suspensory ligament and a more elastic medial ligament. The medial suspensory ligament is separated from the contralateral ligament by loose collagenous connective tissue.[14] Supporting trabeculae projecting inward from the ligaments enclose ill-defined lobes and branch into finer lobular connective tissue surrounding the ducts and alveoli.

The sparsely haired skin of the udder, including the teats, is slightly thicker than the average for equine skin.[31] Numerous sebaceous glands and apocrine tubular sweat glands are present, increasing toward the apices of the teats. Sebum in the intermammary groove protects the halves of the udder against friction during locomotion.[30] Concentrations of sebaceous glands occur peripheral to each papillary duct ostium. "Waxing" at the tips of the teats is a phenomenon presaging impending parturition. It is caused essentially by increased secretion of sebum plus small amounts of cellular debris and colostrum.

Each external pudendal artery descends through an inguinal canal and enters the caudal part of the udder, branching into cranial and caudal mammary arteries. An interconnecting venous plexus on either side of the base of the udder drains principally to contralateral external pudendal veins. Blood also drains from the plexus craniad in the caudal superficial epigastric vein, which connects with a superficial vein of the thoracic wall (especially during the first lactation[1]). The plexus also connects caudally with the obturator vein or with branches of the internal pudendal vein.[30]

Lymph from the udder flows through lymphatic vessels afferent to a conglomerate of superficial inguinal (mammary) lymph nodes at the base of the udder. Afferents may come from the subcutis to accessory mammary lymph nodes that drain to main mammary nodes.[29]

Genitofemoral nerves coursing through the inguinal canals provide the main innervation to the udder. The skin of the udder is supplied by nerves of the flank and a descending branch from the pudendal nerve.[1]

An average-size lactating mare produces around 10 L of milk daily.[30] The milk fat content of equine milk is quite low (1.6%); the lactose content is high (6.1%).[32]

REFERENCES

1. Dyce, K.M., Sack, W.O., and Wensing, C.J.G.: Textbook of Veterinary Anatomy. Philadelphia, W.B. Saunders, 1987.
2. Reiter, R.J.: Pineal control of reproduction. Eleventh International Congress of Anatomy: Advances in the Morphology of Cells and Tissues. Edited by E.A. Vidrio and M.A. Galina. New York, Alan R. Liss, 1981, pp. 349–355.
3. Wesson, J.A., Orr, E.L., Quay, W.B., and Ginther, O.J.: Seasonal relationship between pineal hydroxindole-*O*-methyl-transferase (HIOMT) activity and reproductive activity in the pony. Gen. Comp. Endocrinol., *38*:46–52, 1979.
4. Venzke, W.G.: Endocrinology. *In* Sisson and Grossman's The Anatomy of the Domestic Animals. Vol. 1. 5th ed. Edited by R. Getty. Philadelphia, W.B. Saunders, 1975, pp. 550–551.
5. Krieger, D.T.: The hypothalamus and neuroendocrinology. *In* Neuroendocrinology. Edited by D.T. Krieger and J.C. Hughes. Sunderland, Sinauer Associates, 1980, pp. 3–12.
6. Vitums, A.: Observations on the equine hypophysial portal system. Anat. Histol. Embryol., *4*:149–161, 1975.
7. Nanda, B.S.: Blood supply to the brain. *In* Sisson and Grossman's The Anatomy of the Domestic Animals. Vol. 1. 5th ed. Edited by R. Getty. Philadelphia, W.B. Saunders, 1975, p. 579.
8. Vitums, A.: Development of the venous drainage of the equine hypophysis cerebri. Anat. Histol. Embryol., 7:120–128, 1978.
9. Nomina Anatomica Veterinaria. 3rd ed. Ithaca, World Association of Veterinary Anatomists, 1983.
10. Habel, R.: The perineum of the mare. Cornell Vet., *43*:249–278, 1953.
11. Ginther, O.J.: Reproductive Biology of the Mare: Basic and Applied Aspects. Ann Arbor, McNaughton, Gunn, 1979.
12. Warszawsky, L.F., Parker, W.G., First, N.L., and Ginther, O.J.: Gross changes of the internal genitalia during the estrous cycle in the mare. Am. J. Vet. Res., *33*:19–26, 1972.
13. Witherspoon, D.M.: The site of ovulation in the mare. J. Reprod. Fertil. Suppl., *23*:329–330, 1975.
14. Sisson, S.: Female genital organs. *In* Sisson and Grossman's The Anatomy of the Domestic Animals. Vol. 1. 5th ed. Edited by R. Getty. Philadelphia, W.B. Saunders, 1975, pp. 542–549.
15. Scott, E.A., and Kunze, D.J.: Ovariectomy in the mare: Presurgical, surgical and postsurgical considerations. J. Equine Med. Surg., *1*:5–12, 1977.
16. Ono, H., Satoh, H., Miyake, M., and Fujimoto, Y.: On the development of "ovarian adrenocortical cell nodule" in the horse. Exp. Reprod. Equine Health Lab., *6*:59–90, 1969.
17. Squires, E.L., Douglas, R.H., Steffenhagen, W.P., and Ginther, O.J.: Ovarian changes during the estrous cycle and pregnancy in mares. J. Anim. Sci., *38*:330–338, 1974.
18. Prickett, M.E.: Pathology of the equine ovary. Proc. Am. Assoc. Equine Pract., pp. 145–154, 1966.
19. Van Niekerk, C.H., and Gerneke, W.H.: Persistence and parthogenetic cleavage of tubal ova in the mare. Onderstepoort J. Vet. Res., *33*:195–232, 1966.
20. Kenney, R.M.: Cyclic and pathologic changes in the mare endometrium as detected by biopsy, with a note on early embryonic death. J. Am. Vet. Med. Assoc., *172*:241–262, 1978.
21. Lieux, P.: Relationship between the appearance of the cervix and the heat cycle in the mare. Vet. Med. Small Anim. Clin., *65*:859–866, 1970.
22. Hafez, E.S.E.: Reproduction in Farm Animals. 3rd ed. Philadelphia, Lea & Febiger, 1974, p. 51.
23. Clegg, M.T., Boda, J.M., and Cole, H.H.: The endometrial cups and allantochorionic pouches in the mare with emphasis on the source of equine gonadotropin. Endocrinology, *54*:448–463, 1954.
24. Allen, W.R., Hamilton, E.W., and Moor, R.M.: Origin of equine endometrial cups. II. Invasion of the endometrium by trophoblast. Anat. Rec., *177*:485–502, 1973.
25. Krölling, O., and Grau, H.: Lehrbuch der Histologie und vergleichenden mikroskopischen Anatomie der Haustiere. Berlin, Paul Parey, 1960.
26. McAllister, R.A., and Sack, W.O.: Identification of anatomic features of the equine clitoris as potential growth sites for Taylorella equigenitalis. J. Am. Vet. Med. Assoc., *196*:1965–1966, 1990.
27. Ginther, O.J., Garcia, M.C., Squires, E.L., and Steffenhagen, W.P.: Anatomy of the vasculature of the uterus and ovaries in the mare. Am. J. Vet. Res., *33*:1561–1568, 1972.
28. Goshal, N.G.: Equine heart and arteries. *In* Sisson and Grossman's The Anatomy of the Domestic Animals. Vol. 1. 5th ed. Edited by R. Getty. Philadelphia, W.B. Saunders, 1975, pp. 605–607.
29. Saar, L.I., and Getty, R.: Equine lymphatic system. *In* Sisson and Grossman's The Anatomy of the Domestic Animals. Vol. 1. 5th ed. Edited by R. Getty. Philadelphia, W.B. Saunders, 1975, pp. 625–627.
30. Schummer, A., Wilkens, H., Vollmerhaus, B., and Habermehl, K.-H.: *In* R. Nickel, A. Schummer and E. Seiferle's Anatomy of the Domestic Animals. Vol. 3. The Circulatory System, the Skin, and the Cutaneous Organs of the Domestic Mammals. New York, Paul Parey, 1981, pp. 538–540.
31. Talukdar, A.H., Calhoun, M.L., and Stinson, A.W.: Microscopic anatomy of the skin of the horse. Am. J. Vet. Res., *33*:2365–2390, 1972.
32. Jacobson, N.L., and McGilliard, A.D.: The mammary gland and lactation. *In* Dukes' Physiology of Domestic Animals. 10th ed. Edited by M.J. Swenson. Ithaca, Comstock Publishing Associates, 1984, p. 871.

CHAPTER 2

EXTERNAL PERINEAL CONFORMATION

J. Easley

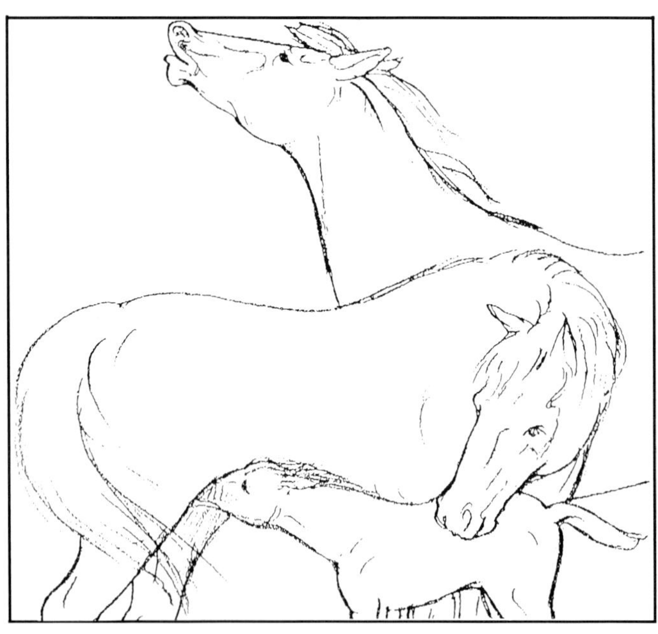

The external genitalia of the mare have received much attention because of their importance to overall genital health. As early as 1937, Caslick described abnormal perineal conformation that could lead to pneumovagina, cervicitis, endometritis, and subfertility in mares.[1] Since then, efforts have been made to assess normal form and function of the mare's vulvar and perineal structures and to determine more accurately their role in comprehensive reproductive health. The following discussion is intended to call the practitioner's attention to conformational and anatomic design of the external genitalia of the mare and describe various deviations commonly seen.

PERINEAL FORM AND FUNCTION

The external genitalia of the mare are composed of the perineum and vulva. The perineum has been defined as a body wall encompassing the outlet of the pelvis and surrounding the urogenital passage and anal canal. At the embryonic stage of development, the cloacal membrane and the urorectal septum form the primitive perineum (which later becomes the perineal body), subdividing the anal membrane dorsally from the urogenital membrane ventrally. The perineum is bounded dorsally by the base of the tail and coccygeal muscles, laterally, by the sacrosciatic ligaments, and semimembranous muscles, and ventrally by the ischial arch and udder.

Motor control of the muscles in this region is supplied by the deep perineal nerves. Fibers of the caudal rectal and pudendal nerves, arising from the spinal cord in sacral segments three through five, produce branches to the rectal and anal sphincters and superficial perineal areas.[2,3] Sensation to the ventral and lateral region of the area is furnished by the caudal cutaneous femoral nerve emanating from the spinal cord at segments S1 and S2. This nerve distribution pattern accounts for variable effects of anesthetic agents, dosages, and needle placement seen with epidural anesthesia in the mare.

The equine vulva consists of the clitoris and the labia. The labia contain the mucocutaneous vulvar lips and the constrictor muscles, which form an acute angle above (known as the dorsal commissure) and a rounded junction below (the ventral commissure). The opening of the vulvar cleft between the dorsal and ventral commissures is usually 12 to 15 cm long. Physiological changes in total vulvar length are under hormonal influence. Progesterone causes an increase in vulvar muscle tone and a shortening of vulvar length. Under the influence of estrogen the vulva relaxes and lengthens. The vulvar length is greatest during estrus or close to parturition and decreases during pregnancy. The vulvar constrictor muscle is tightly apposed on its deep surface to the constrictor vestibuli and the retractor clitoridis muscles (see Chapter 1). These muscles function as a unit to invert the clitoris when the mare is exhibiting signs of estrus and "winks" (Fig. 2-1).

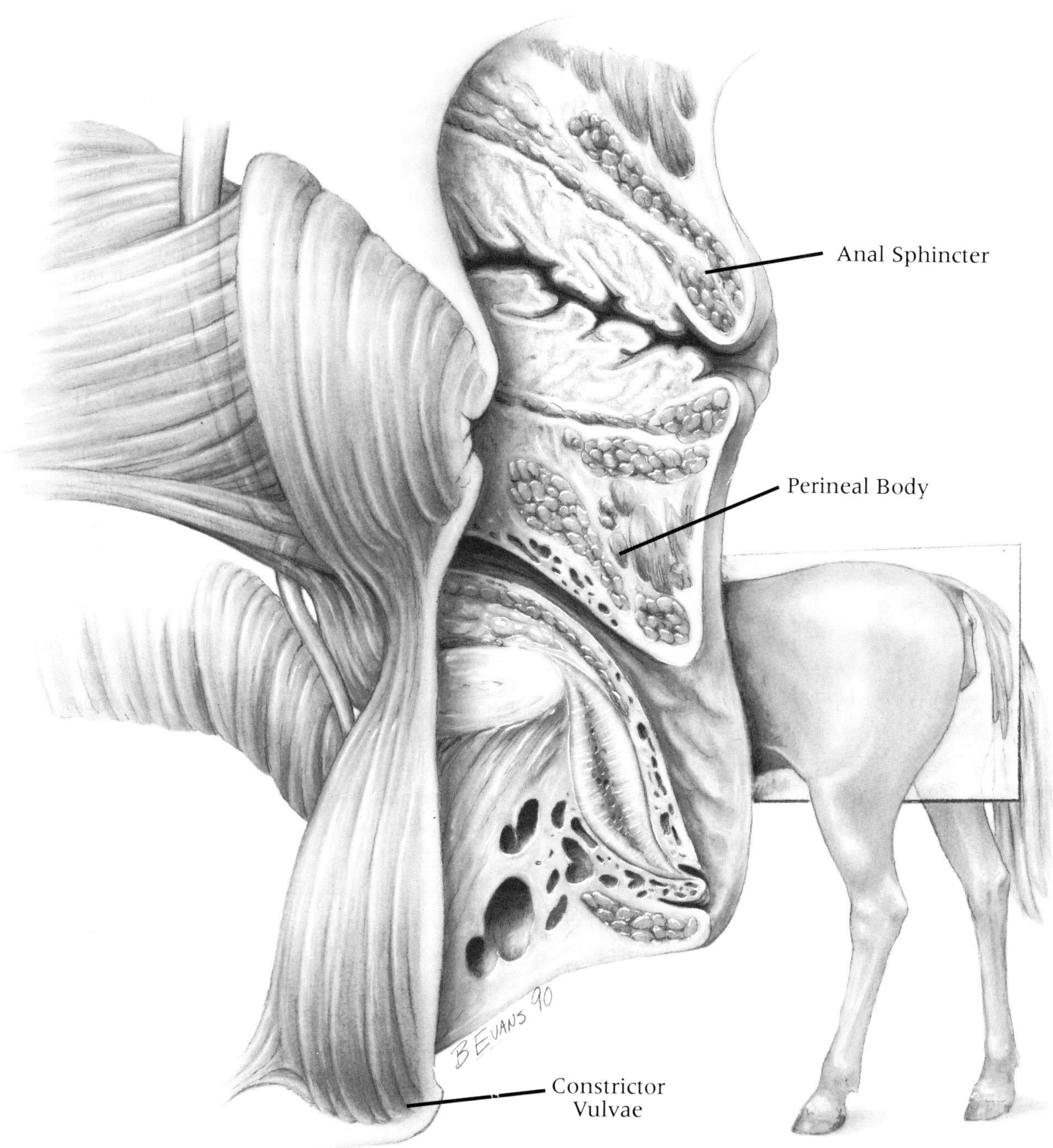

FIG. 2–1. Caudolateral and median cross section of the mare's perineum. (Courtesy of G.W. Trotter and B.R. Evans, Colorado State University.)

OPTIMAL PERINEAL CONFORMATION

The right and left vulvar lips should meet evenly and appear full and firm, functioning as a seal and forming the first protective barrier between external environment and the uterus. The other anatomical barriers present in the mare's reproductive tract are the transverse fold and the cervix.[4]

The vulva extends over the ischial arch of the pelvis. For maximal reproductive function, the dorsal commissure of the vulva should be no more than 4 cm above the pelvic floor (meaning that approximately two-thirds of the vulvar cleft should lie below the pelvic floor).[4] The vulvar lips should be in a vertical position with a cranial-to-caudal slope of no more than 10 degrees from vertical (Fig. 2-2).

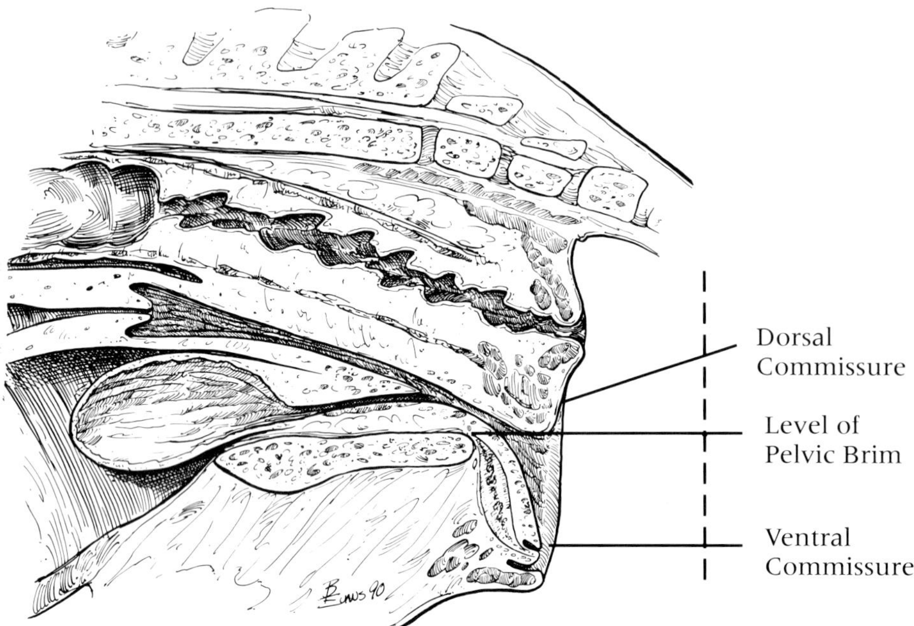

FIG. 2–2. Cross section of normal (Type I) mare perineum. The vulvar lips are in a vertical position with less than 10° of declination, or slope. The effective vulvar length is less than 4 cm, with less than one-third of the vulvar cleft above the pelvic brim. The Caslick Index is less than 50. (Courtesy of G.W. Trotter and B.R. Evans, Colorado State University.)

PERINEAL CONFORMATIONAL VARIATIONS

Certain variations in conformation of the vulvoperineal area can predispose to reproductive failure, most notably a distance of more than 4 cm between the dorsal commissure of the vulva and the pelvic floor, and/or an angle of more than 10 degrees in the declination of the vulvar lips.

A proper vulvar seal to prevent pneumovagina (wind sucking) in mares is important for maximum reproductive efficiency. Pascoe developed a formula to forecast a mare's predisposition to reproductive difficulties related to conformation.[5] Using a computation that multiplied the effective length, in centimeters, of the mare's vulva (distance between the dorsal commissure and pelvic floor) by the angle of declination of the vulva in degrees, he obtained a number termed the Caslick Index.[5] Mares with a Caslick Index of more than 150 (Fig. 2-3) experienced more numerous and severe reproductive problems, principally pneumovagina and urovagina, compared with those with an index of less than 50.

In studies of vulvar length and angle of declination on more than 9000 mares, Pascoe confirmed that vulvar conformation had an effect on pregnancy rates in those mares.[5] He recognized three distinct vulvoperineal conformational types, based on the anatomic positions of the anus, tail setting, and brim of the pelvis. The types are as follows:

Type I mares (Fig. 2-2) have less than 2 to 3 cm of the vulva dorsal to the pelvic brim, and rarely require a Caslick operation (see Chapter 48), even when aged.

Type II mares exhibit an effective length between the dorsal commissure and the pelvic floor of 6 to 7 cm and a Caslick Index of more than 50. It is often possible to predict which mares will develop this conformation by their third year. With age, the effective length and the angle of declination of the vulva increases because of the general relaxation of organs and muscles in the pelvic region, resulting in an index higher than 150.

Type III mares (Fig. 2-3) measure 5 to 9 cm between the dorsal commissure and the pelvic floor, and often require a Caslick operation at an early age. As time goes on, the vulval conformation becomes more and more horizontal, with the brim of the pelvis located in the lowest region of the measurement. Those mares experience serious reproductive problems; sometimes the Caslick operation is ineffective because when sutured to a point lower than the pelvic brim so little of the vulva remains open that natural breeding is impossible and urine retention seems unavoidable.[5]

Variations in perineal conformation have many causes, and it is undoubtedly inherent in some mares. A flat croup, elevated tail set, underdeveloped vulvar lips, and sunken anus all contribute to faulty perineal conformation. Poor physical condition intensifies the problem and can precipitate abnormal structure even in mares with normal conformation; as the muscles deteriorate, the anus sinks farther forward and the vulva shifts from its vertical position to a more horizontal orientation. As mares age, the effective length of the vulva is increased.[4–7]

Because structure that is not conducive to reproduction by its very nature inhibits its own perpetuation, it appears that the use of the Caslick operation may per-

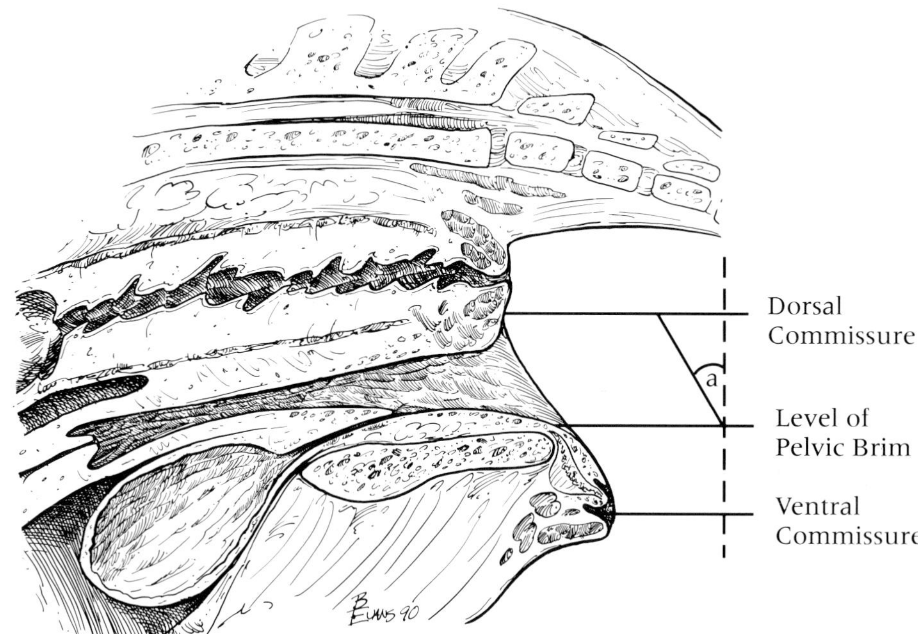

FIG. 2–3. Cross section of mare perineum with Type III conformation. The vulvar lips are sloped dorsal to the pelvic brim, making the angle of declination of the vulva (a) greater than 30°. The effective vulvar length is greater than 5 cm from the level of the pelvic brim to the dorsal commissure. The Caslick Index is more than 150. (Courtesy of G.W. Trotter and B.R. Evans, Colorado State University.)

petuate conformational faults by enabling mares to become pregnant that otherwise would be unable to conceive. In the United States, where a Caslick operation (see Chapter 48) has been widely used, it has become a virtual necessity in Thoroughbreds. However, in breeds and countries where the surgery has not been widely used, there appear to be relatively few cases that require the surgical procedure.

Another common cause of abnormal perineal conformation is trauma, particularly from foaling. In multiparous mares, repeated stretching and occasional tearing of the reproductive tract alters muscular control of the vulva, vestibule, and vagina. When the barrier of the vulvar labia is compromised, pneumovagina can result.[4,5]

External trauma to the vulvar labia can also cause a breach in the vulva barrier, as can inversion of one labium relative to the other, a condition generally found in overweight mares. In older mares, splanchnoptosis can precipitate perineal abnormalities, as the organs of the pelvic and abdominal cavities relax and sink. The vulvar constrictor and constrictor vestibuli muscles then stretch to accommodate the shifted organs, and the anus moves craniad, pulling the vulvar labia into a more horizontal position (Figs. 2-2 and 2-3).[4]

Changes in size and shape of the clitoris are observed in normal mares when the clitoris becomes edematous and slightly everted under the influence of estrogens. Anabolic steroid therapy has also been reported as a cause of clitoral enlargement and protrusion.[8] The degree of clitoral development was dose and drug dependent. Intersexed foals have been reported to exhibit an enlarged clitoris with or without partially sealed vulvar lips and/or a prominent perineal raphe (Fig. 2-4).[9] An abnormal structure resembling a penis can been seen with hermaphroditism or pseudohermaphroditism. These animals are sterile, but their appearance can be improved by surgically removing the abnormal appendage. The clitoris and the clitoral sinuses may be absent due to surgical removal in mares that have been imported into the United States from nations endemic for contagious equine metritis.

CONSEQUENCES OF VARIATIONS IN PERINEAL CONFORMATION

Abnormal perineal structure such as described above results in the compromise of the vulvar seal, the first protective barrier in the reproductive tract. This precipitates the onset of pneumovagina, or the aspiration of air and fecal material into the vestibule.[4–6]

Pneumovagina can lead to urovagina (urine pooling). If the urethral orifice is pulled craniad to the ischium, urine cannot be completely voided through the caudal vagina and vulvar lips. A "splash back" of urine occurs, and a pool is formed in the anterior portion of the vaginal canal.

Both pneumovagina and urovagina can lead to cervicitis, vaginitis, or endometritis. The chronic irritation from urine, air, or fecal material alters the pH of vaginal

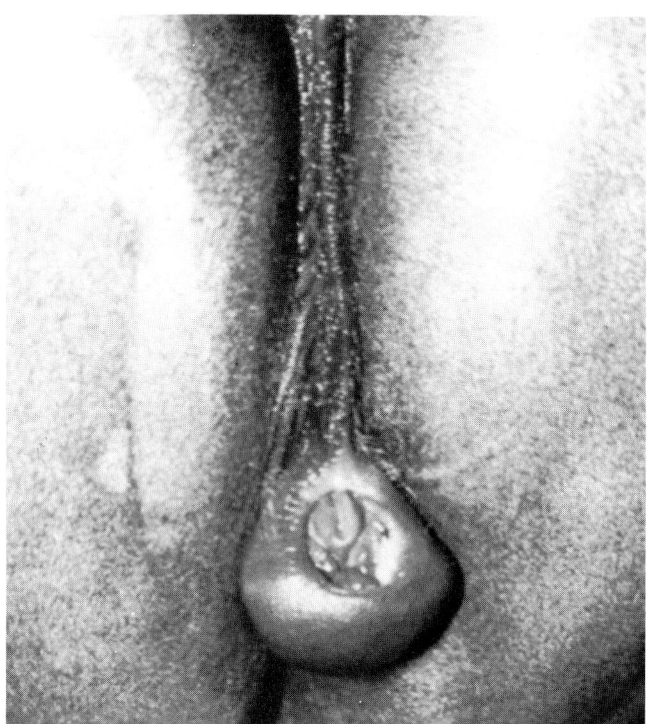

FIG. 2–4. Perineum of an intersex foal. The dorsal labia are underdeveloped. The clitoris is enlarged and protruding beyond the margins of the ventral vulvar labia.

tissues and affects sperm viability, which decreases the mare's ability to conceive.

Pneumovagina also leads to constant or intermittent bacterial contamination of the caudal reproductive tract, which is a leading predisposing factor to bacterial vaginitis, cervicitis, and endometritis. See Chapters 48 and 49 for correction of these problems.

Vaginal contamination can cause early embryonic death and subsequent infertility. During the late stages of gestation, mares with poor perineal conformation are susceptible to aspiration of air leading to placentitis. This can cause fetal septicemia and lead to abortion or neonatal sepsis.

CONCLUSION

The anatomic makeup and proper function of the mare's perineum are important for reproductive soundness. Proper neuromuscular and hormonal control of these structures are crucial for all stages of reproduction from copulation, fertilization, and conception through pregnancy maintenance and parturition. It is important that mares be evaluated for proper perineal conformation. An effort should be made to select breeding stock with conformational characteristics that promote reproductive health.

REFERENCES

1. Caslick, E.A.: The vulva and the vulvo-vaginal orifice and its relationship to genital health of the Thoroughbred mare. Cornell Vet., *27*:178–187, 1937.
2. Rooney, J.R., Sack, W.O., and Habel, R.E.: Guide to the Dissection of the Horse. Ithaca, W.O. Sack, 1967, pp. 63–70.
3. Schumacher, J., Bratton, G.R., and Williams, J.W.: Pudendal and caudal rectal nerve blocks in the horse—An anesthetic procedure for reproductive surgery. Theriogenology, *24*:457–464, 1985.
4. Trotter, G.W., and McKinnon, A.O.: Surgery for abnormal vulvar and perineal conformation in the mare. Vet. Clin. North Am. Equine Pract., *4*:389–405, 1988.
5. Pascoe, R.R.: Observations of the length and angle of declination of the vulva and its relation to fertility in the mare. J. Reprod. Fertil. Suppl., *27*:299–305, 1979.
6. Ansari, M.M.: The Caslick operation in mares. Compend. Contin. Educ. Pract. Vet., *5*:S107–S111, 1983.
7. Pouret, E.J.M.: Surgical techniques for correction of pneumo- and urovagina. Equine Vet. J., *14*:249–250, 1982.
8. Maher, J.M., Squires, E.L., Voss, J.L., and Shideler, R.K.: Effect of anabolic steroids on reproductive function of young mares. J. Am. Vet. Med. Assoc., *183*:519–524, 1983.
9. Power, M.M., and Leadon, D.P.: Diploid-Triploid Chimaerism (64,XX/96,XXY) in an intersex foal. Equine Vet. J., *22*(B):211–214, 1990.

SECTION B

PHYSIOLOGY/ ENDOCRINOLOGY

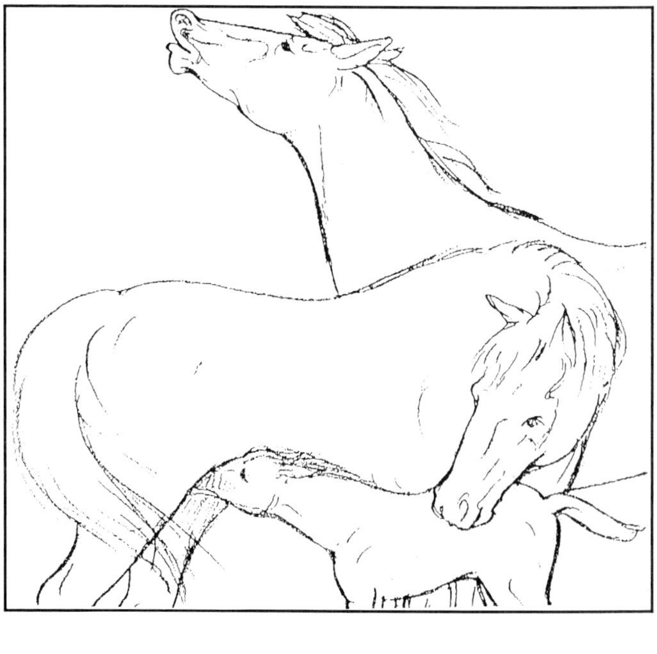

CHAPTER 3

MECHANISMS OF HORMONE ACTION

G.D. Niswender

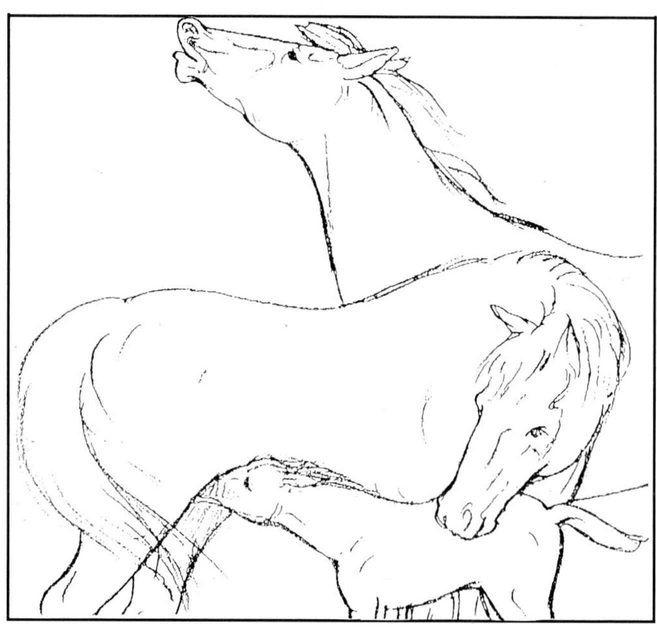

DEFINITION OF HORMONE ACTIONS

Until recent times hormones were defined as chemical substances secreted by specialized ductless glands, carried by the bloodstream to specific target cells where they altered the function of these cells. This defines the classic endocrine effect of hormones, i.e., they are carried to target organs via the bloodstream. With the advent of more sophisticated procedures, however, it has recently become apparent that hormones are also used for cell-to-cell communication within an organ. When hormones are secreted by one cell and influence the activities of neighboring cells it is called a paracrine effect. An example is the reduced secretion of glucagon and insulin by α and β cells of the pancreas as a result of increased somatostatin release by Δ cells. Finally, there are also cases when a hormone is secreted by a cell that influences the activities of that same cell, called an autocrine effect. An example of this is the secretion of somatostatin by the parafollicular cells of the thyroid, which then decreases calcitonin secretion from these same cells. Thus the scope of actions of hormones has been considerably broadened as a result of these new discoveries.

PEPTIDE AND PROTEIN HORMONES

There are more peptide hormones, containing from three to many amino acids, than any other class of hormones. For example, thyrotropin-releasing hormone (TRH) is composed of a sequence of 3 amino acids, gonadotropin-releasing hormone (GnRH) has 10 amino acids, and adrenocorticotropin (ACTH) consists of 39 amino acids. There are other peptide hormones too numerous to mention, including additional hypothalamic-releasing hormones, various growth factors such as epidermal growth factor and insulinlike growth factor, and several gut hormones. Insulin (51 amino acids) and glucagon (29 amino acids) are other examples of peptide hormones. Protein hormones are big peptides composed of many amino acids. Two important examples of protein hormones are growth hormone and prolactin, which are composed of approximately 200 amino acids.

GLYCOPROTEIN HORMONES

Protein hormones may contain carbohydrate moieties attached to the protein backbone. These glycoprotein hormones—include luteinizing hormone (LH), follicle-stimulating hormone (FSH), equine chorionic gonadotropin (eCG), previously named pregnant mare serum gonadotropin (PMSG), and human chorionic gonadotropin (hCG)—which are important as endogenous or exogenous regulators of equine reproduction. The remaining glycoprotein hormone is thyroid-stimulating hormone (TSH).

The glycoprotein hormones are composed of two subunits, an α-subunit that contains 89 amino acids and a β-subunit that contains from 112 to 142 amino acids. The α-subunits for all hormones within a species have identical amino acid compositions. For example, the α-subunits of equine LH, FSH, TSH, and eCG are identical as are the α-subunits of human LH, FSH, TSH and CG. The β-subunit of the glycoproteins have different amino acid compositions except for the β-subunits of equine LH and eCG, which are identical. Thus LH and eCG are identical hormones produced by different tissues in the mare (see Chapter 9). It is the β-subunit that confers hormonal specificity on the intact hormone and the subunits themselves have little, if any, biological activity.

STEROID HORMONES

Essentially all steroid hormones are derived from a common precursor, cholesterol (Fig. 3-1). Substituents at the 3, 11, 17, 18, 20, and 21 carbons determine the biological nature of the steroid hormone. Examples of each major class of steroid hormones are also depicted in Fig. 3-1. The mineralocorticoids, glucocorticoids, and progestins all have 21 carbons. Oxygenated substituents at the carbon atom at the 11 position are required for corticosteroid activity and further changes at the 18 and 21 carbon atoms ultimately define the type of biological activity of the steroid hormone. The androgens have 19 carbon atoms, whereas the estrogens are composed of 18 carbon atoms. The phenolic A ring (Fig. 3-1) is required for estrogenic activity.

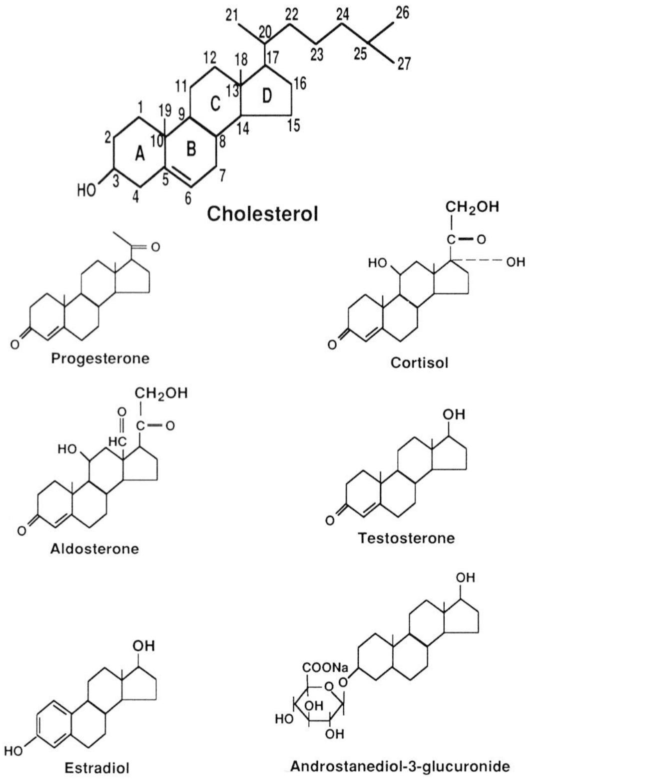

Cholesterol
Progesterone
Cortisol
Aldosterone
Testosterone
Estradiol
Androstanediol-3-glucuronide

FIG. 3–1. Chemical structure of cholesterol with lettering of the four-ring structures and numbering for each carbon atom. The chemical structure for the major steroid hormone in each class, including progesterone (progestins), cortisol (glucocorticoids), aldosterone (mineralocorticoids), and testosterone (androgens); estradiol-17β (estrogens) is also depicted. An example of a reduced steroid (androstanediol) conjugated to glucuronic acid via the 3 carbon atom for excretion is also presented.

PROSTAGLANDINS

Prostaglandins are also lipid hormonal molecules that are synthesized from arachidonic acid. The two most important prostaglandin (PG) molecules for regulating the reproductive processes are $PGF_2\alpha$, which is produced by the uterus and plays a role in luteal regression at the end of the reproductive cycle in most animals, and PGE_2.[1] PGE_2 has a positive effect on progesterone secretion by the corpus luteum and prevents many of the negative effects of $PGF_2\alpha$.

SYNTHESIS AND SECRETION OF HORMONES

PROTEINACEOUS HORMONES

Protein hormones are synthesized just as other proteins are synthesized. The peptide chain is synthesized on the ribosomes of the rough endoplasmic reticulum as a prohormone. As for other proteins made for secretion, initially the "leader sequence"—usually an 18 to 21 amino acid lipophilic peptide—is synthesized, which allows penetration of the endoplasmic reticular membrane. The rest of the peptide chain then passes through the membrane as it is synthesized. The hormone is enzymatically cleaved from the prohormone and transported to the Golgi apparatus where it is packaged into membrane-bound secretory granules. In the case of glycoproteins, carbohydrate is added either in the endoplasmic reticulum or the Golgi apparatus, depending on the particular carbohydrate to be added. Proteinaceous hormones are stored as granules near the cell membrane until the appropriate stimulus is received for secretion. Granules are released from the cell by the process of exocytosis. Extracellular hormone then enters the bloodstream and is carried to the appropriate target tissues.

Synthesis of hormones that are modified amino acids is much less complex and in all cases involves a series of sequential enzymatic alterations of the amino acid. In the case of thyroid hormones these reactions occur in thyroid follicle cells, and the resultant hormones are part of the thyroglobulin molecule. In the case of the catecholamines, epinephrine and norepinephrine, these reactions occur in several tissues, particularly the adrenal medulla. Melatonin is synthesized from tryptophan primarily in the pineal gland.

STEROID HORMONES

For steroid hormone synthesis by the adrenal glands or the gonads, cholesterol in the form of lipoprotein is taken into the appropriate cell type by receptor-mediated endocytosis. Cholesterol is then cleaved from the lipoprotein by enzymes within the lysosome and the free cholesterol is esterified for storage as lipid droplets or converted to the appropriate steroid (i.e., adrenal or gonadal) by a series of enzymatic steps in the mitochondrion and smooth endoplasmic reticulum. Because steroids are soluble in the lipid cellular membrane, they are thought simply to diffuse out of the cell. Thus there is very little, if any, storage of steroid hormones in the cells where they are synthesized. Changes in the rates of secretion of steroid hormones reflect changes in the rates of synthesis.

The pathway for prostaglandin synthesis is depicted in Figure 3-2. The enzymes required for these conversions are present in many tissues in the body, and it is the relative proportion of each enzyme that determines the levels of the ultimate secretory product. For example, the nonpregnant uterus secretes primarily $PGF_2\alpha$ during the time of luteolysis, whereas the pregnant uterus and/or embryo secretes PGE_2.

CONTROL OF HORMONE SECRETION

The primary function of hormones is to regulate body functions and maintain homeostasis. A complex series of physiologic mechanisms have evolved to control secretion of hormones. There are two feedback systems (negative and positive) that are of particular importance for the reproductive system. For example, GnRH secreted by the hypothalamus stimulates secretion of LH and FSH from the anterior pituitary. In males, LH stimulates testosterone secretion from the testes, and in females LH stimulates estradiol secretion from the follicle and/or progesterone from the corpus luteum. The control for this system is provided by a long-loop negative feedback system. The sex steroid (i.e., testosterone, estradiol, or progesterone) feeds back at the level of the hypothalamus and pituitary, and when "normal" blood levels of sex steroid are reached the secretion of GnRH and LH is inhibited. This completes the negative feedback loop and ensures homeostatic regulation of the gonads. Obviously both the hypothalamus and anterior pituitary must monitor serum levels of sex steroids if this system is to work. These tissues are target organs for these steroids and, therefore, have specific sex steroid hormone receptors that initiate the appropriate response to the differing levels of the gonadal steroids. Control of the thyroid gland and the adrenal cortex by the hypothalamus and anterior pituitary also occurs via a long-loop negative feedback system. Some evidence for a short-loop negative feedback system also exists for these endocrine systems (i.e., gonads, thyroid, and adrenal cortex). In this case, hormone from the anterior pituitary gland is proposed to feed back directly on the hypothalamus and reduce secretion of the appropriate hypothalamic-releasing hormone.

This is also one case of a positive endocrine feedback loop. In females that are cycling normally, LH enhances estradiol production from the preovulatory follicle. This enhanced estradiol secretion stimulates GnRH secretion from the hypothalamus and increases the number of receptors for GnRH on the gonadotrophs in the anterior pituitary. In this case, the result of the increased estradiol is a major surge of LH, which causes ovulation. Physical reorganization of the ruptured follicle and luteinization of the steroid-secreting cells prevent further secretion of estradiol. This is the only case of a purely endocrine positive feedback system.

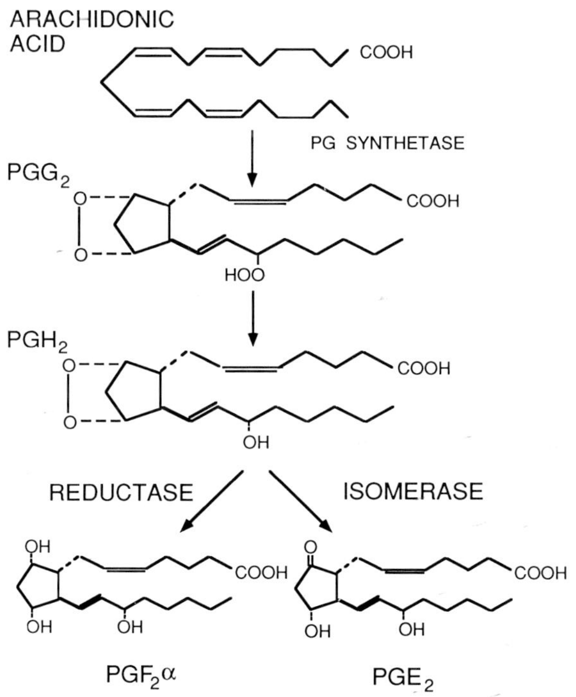

FIG. 3-2. Synthetic pathway for the biosynthesis of prostaglandins $PGF_2\alpha$ and PGE_2. Arachidonic acid is converted to PGG_2 by the enzyme prostaglandin synthetase. PGG_2 is converted to PGH_2 which is further modified by prostaglandins reductase to $PGF_2\alpha$ or by prostaglandins isomerase to PGE_2. These reactions occur in numerous tissues in the body, particularly the reproductive tract.

MECHANISMS OF HORMONE ACTION

RECEPTORS

Hormones influence the activity of target cells by binding to specific receptor molecules. Receptors are protein or glycoprotein molecules and many have a multiple subunit structure.[2] In some cases the receptor also has inherent enzymatic activity.[2] The cellular location of the receptor depends, in general, on the chemical nature of the hormone that it binds. Proteinaceous hormones (with thyroxine and tri-iodothyronine as exceptions), which are not soluble in the limiting membranes of target cells, must act from outside the cell. Therefore, receptors for these hormones are located within the plasma membrane, and binding of hormone results in modification of the activity of second messenger systems within the cell. These second messenger systems will be discussed in more detail in the next section and are ultimately responsible for modifying hormonally regulated cellular activities.

There are a number of factors that influence the quantity of receptors for hormones on target cells, including other hormones (heterologous regulation), and in most cases, the hormone itself (homologous regulation). For example, follicle-stimulating hormone and estradiol have been shown to increase the number of receptors for LH in follicular granulosa cells.[3] Luteinizing hormone causes down regulation of LH receptors[4] by receptor-mediated endocytosis and recently has been shown to reduce the quantity of messenger RNA encoding for the receptor[5] and thus synthesis of new receptors. Receptor-mediated endocytosis appears to be the primary mechanism for the relatively rapid decrease in receptors following exposure to large quantities of hormone (i.e., down regulation). In ovine luteal cells, life of the receptor on the membrane appears to be a single binding of hormone.[6] The hormone receptor complex is then internalized, the hormone degraded, and the receptor likely recycled. Interestingly, when hCG binds to the LH receptor, the receptor is immobilized, apparently because of some interaction between the hormone, a transmembrane protein, and the cytoskeleton.[7] This immobilization of the hCG-LH receptor complex results in a dramatically prolonged biological response.[8] Although studies have not been performed, it seems likely that equine chorionic gonadotropin will have similar biological properties. The prolonged down regulation of receptors after exposure to high doses of LH or hCG is a result of reduced expression of the gene encoding for the LH receptor in target cells.[5] Precise regulation of receptor numbers appears to be physiologically important. For example, in the corpus luteum it is well known that LH stimulates secretion of progesterone, yet circulating concentrations of LH are lowest when progesterone concentrations are highest. As the corpus luteum develops there is a dramatic increase in the numbers of receptors for luteinizing hormone.[9,10] The result is a high degree of correlation among number of receptors for LH, number of receptors occupied by LH, and serum concentrations of progesterone. Thus responsiveness of the target organ (i.e., number of receptors) to a hormone may be more important than circulating concentrations of the hormone. Interestingly, in a response that appears to be unique to the mare, affinity of the luteal receptor for LH also increases as progesterone secretion increases during the estrous cycle.[10]

In the case of steroids and thyroid hormones, receptors appear to be intracellular. These hormones enter the cell and bind to specific receptors, which alter gene transcription and translation in the nucleus.[2] Exceptions to this general statement exist: progesterone has been shown to stimulate cyclic adenosine monophosphate (cAMP) production in frog oocytes and estrogens have been shown to exert actions at the level of the cell membrane in nervous tissues.[11] Thus, in general, hormones that cannot diffuse through the plasma membrane act from outside the cell via second messenger systems whereas those that can enter the cell act at the genomic level.

INTRACELLULAR SECOND MESSENGER SYSTEMS

Various mechanisms are used by target cells to respond to hormone binding to a plasma membrane-bound receptor. This is a relatively new area of investigation and understanding of second messenger systems and how they interact to control cellular responses is rapidly expanding. In general, hormone binding to receptor either activates an intracellular enzyme or causes an influx of calcium. A receptor is specific for a single hormone, but a cell may have receptors for a number of different hormones. For example, granulosa cells in the preovulatory follicle are known to have receptors for insulin, thyroxine, LH, FSH, prolactin, estradiol, and prostaglandin. Most of the hormones act via different intracellular second messenger systems and the cells' activity is ultimately regulated by complex interactions of all of these systems.

The molecular structures of receptors for LH and FSH have recently been elucidated.[12,13] These receptors have large extracellular domains (approximately 350 amino acids) and seven transmembrane elements attached to an intracellular segment, which activates an inner-membrane guanosine triphosphate (GTP) binding or G-protein. The general feature of seven transmembrane domains is characteristic of a number of receptors, including those for epinephrine and rhodopsin, which activate G-proteins.[12] Binding of hormone to the extracellular domain of the receptor results in an interaction of the intracellular domain with G-protein, resulting in GTP binding and activation of this protein. There are activated G-proteins (G_s) that stimulate the activity of adenylate cyclase, G-proteins (G_i) that inhibit adenylate cyclase, and others that regulate the activity of ion channels.[14] Adenylate cyclase catalyzes the conversion of adenosine triphosphate to cyclic adenosine monophosphate.

Adenylate Cyclase/cAMP/Protein Kinase A System

The most widely studied and thoroughly characterized (Fig. 3-3) messenger system is the adenylate cyclase/cAMP/protein kinase A system.[15,16] A stimulatory hormone binding to its receptor activates a stimulatory G-protein via GTP binding. The active G-protein stimulates adenylate cyclase, and the elevated intracellular levels of cAMP result in activation of protein kinase A. There are at least two types of protein kinase A, both of which are activated by cAMP binding to the cAMP-binding subunit, causing release of the active catalytic subunit. The catalytic subunit phosphorylates proteins through serine or threonine residues which modifies activity of the protein. There are at least four intracellular sites of action of protein kinase A. First, the activity of many key regulatory enzymes (two examples are phosphorylase,[17] involved in energy regulation, and cholesterol esterase,[18] involved in steroid biosynthesis) is regulated by the state of phosphorylation. Phosphorylation enhances activity of most enzymes, but decreases activity of others.

Second, ribosomal proteins are also phosphorylated

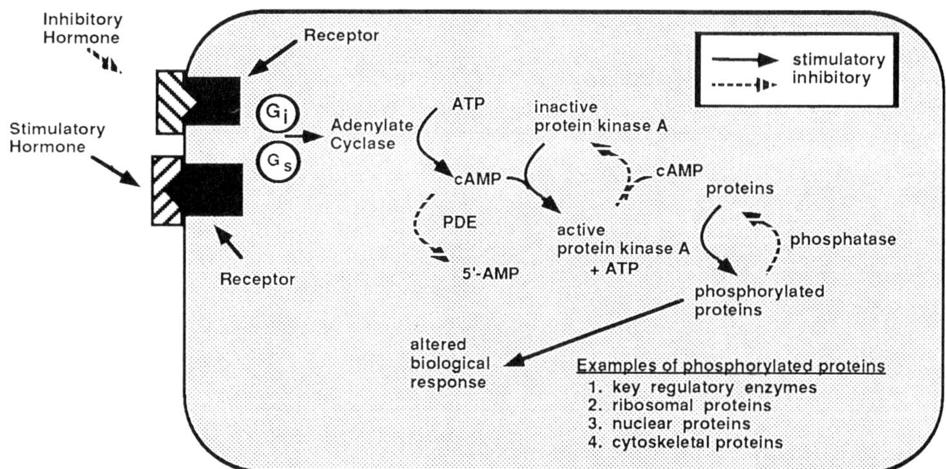

FIG. 3–3. A diagram of the protein kinase A second messenger system. Stimulation of this system is initiated by hormone binding to its receptor, activation of the stimulatory G-protein (G_s) via GTP binding results in activation of adenylate cyclase with increased conversion of ATP to cAMP. The cAMP activates protein kinase A, which phosphorylates protein substrates leading to an altered biological response. Examples of phosphorylated proteins are listed in the figure and discussed in the text. The hatched arrows depict the pathway for inhibition of this system. Binding of some hormones inhibits adenylate cyclase activity via an inhibitory G_i-protein. In addition, phosphodiesterase converts cAMP to 5′-AMP, which is inactive. Dissociation of cAMP from protein kinase A inactivates this enzyme, and protein phosphatases inactivate (dephosphorylate) the activated, phosphorylated proteins.

by protein kinase A, leading to enhanced protein synthesis. For a variety of proteins, including many of the regulatory enzymes, the rate of synthesis is enhanced after phosphorylation of ribosomal proteins. A third major action of protein kinase A is phosphorylation of nuclear proteins, resulting in enhanced RNA production and ultimately protein synthesis. Interestingly, cAMP can also bind to a response element on certain genes and modify transcription and translation and thus RNA production directly.[19] Finally, cytoskeletal proteins can be phosphorylated, resulting in modification of cell shape and functions of microtubules and microfilaments.[20] All of these actions result in alteration of the biological response of the target cell.

Several mechanisms play a role in inactivating the intracellular mechanisms stimulated by hormones via the protein kinase A system (Fig. 3-3). Hormones that inhibit adenylate cyclase activity and cAMP production via an inhibitory G_i protein have already been mentioned. The G-protein has also slow GTPase activity and thus inactivates itself over time. In addition, phosphodiesterase converts cAMP to 5′-AMP, an inactive metabolite. Cyclic AMP can also dissociate from the binding subunit of protein kinase A, allowing recombination with the catalytic subunit, which results in inactivation of protein kinase A. Finally, specific protein phosphatases can dephosphorylate proteins, altering their active state. All mechanisms are important for limiting or reversing effects of hormonal stimulation of the protein kinase A system.

A specific example of a hormone that acts through the protein kinase A system is the effect of LH on progesterone secretion by the corpus luteum (Fig. 3-4). In this case, LH binding to its receptor enhances activity of adenylate cyclase, resulting in increased intracellular levels of cAMP and activation of protein kinase A.[6] The protein kinase A phosphorylates cholesterol esterase[18] and thus increases cholesterol availability for steroidogenesis. In addition, a component of the cholesterol side-chain cleavage complex (the P450 component) is also phosphorylated, and the rate of side-chain cleavage is enhanced.[21] This appears to be the rate-limiting step in progesterone biosynthesis. Some evidence suggests that cholesterol transport to the mitochondria is influenced by microfilaments and that protein kinase A affects this process.[22] Thus several steps in the progesterone biosynthetic pathway appear to be stimulated by LH binding and enhanced protein kinase A activity.

Protein Kinase C

Binding of a number of hormones to their receptors results in activation of calcium-independent phospholipase C (Fig. 3-5). This enzyme catalyzes the breakdown of phosphatidylinositol 4,5-bisphosphate (PIP_2) to diacylglycerol and de-*myo*-inositol 1,4,5-triphosphate (IP_3). Diacylglycerol enhances the affinity of protein kinase C for calcium. The IP_3 releases calcium from intracellular stores, and calcium binding to protein kinase C results in activation of this enzyme. Active protein kinase C phosphorylates proteins at serine and threonine residues and influences intracellular activity of target cells via mechanisms similar to those for protein kinase A. However, actions of the protein kinase C second messenger system are often antagonistic to the protein kinase A system. For example, in luteal cells, $PGF_2\alpha$ ac-

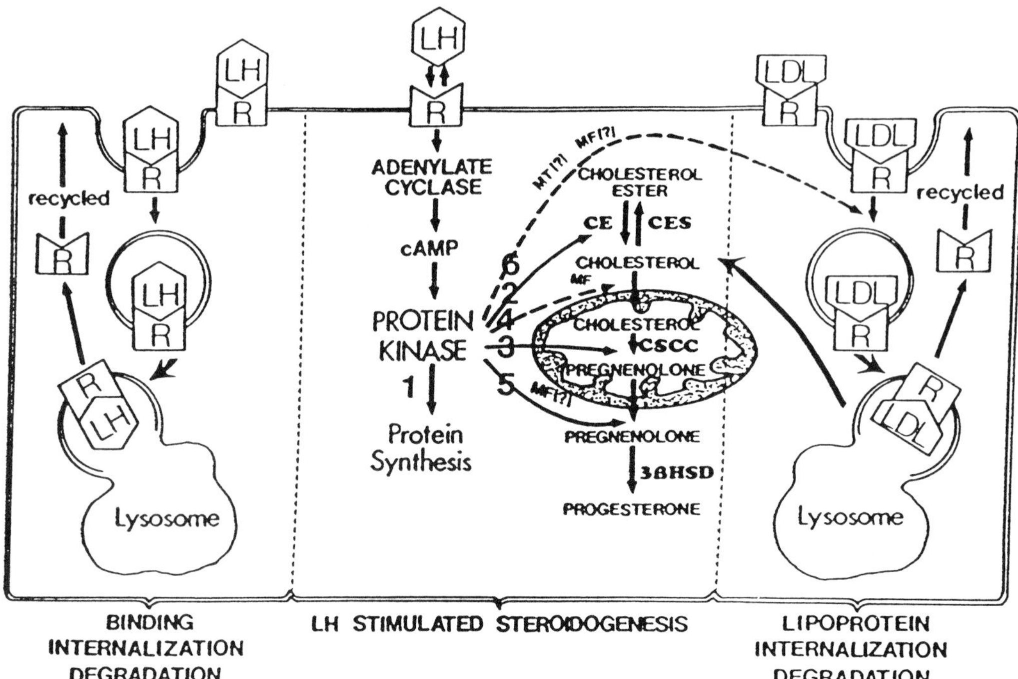

FIG. 3–4. Schematic representation of the intracellular events involved in LH-stimulated steroidogenesis. LH binds to its receptor (R) in the cell membrane and activates adenylate cyclase, resulting in increased intracellular levels of cAMP and activation of protein kinase A. The active protein kinase (1) stimulates protein synthesis, (2) phosphorylates cholesterol esterase (CE), (3) activates cholesterol side-chain cleavage complex (CSCC), (4) stimulates transport of cholesterol into the mitochondrion, (5) may stimulate transport of pregnenolone out of the mitochondrion, and/or (6) may stimulate the uptake of low-density lipoprotein (LDL), thus increasing cholesterol for substrate. In some species high-density lipoprotein is the preferred moiety for cholesterol uptake. Luteinizing hormone and its receptor are internalized, and the LH is degraded in lysosomes. The receptors for LH and LDL are probably recycled to the plasma membrane.

tivates protein kinase C, which inhibits protein kinase A–stimulated secretion of progesterone after stimulation by luteinizing hormone.[23]

Protein Kinase G and Tyrosine Kinase

Two additional protein kinase systems modulate hormonal actions. The guanylate cyclase/cGMP/protein kinase G second messenger system acts similarly to the protein kinase A system and often provides antagonistic actions to the protein kinase A system. In this case, hormone binding stimulates activity of guanylate cyclase and enhances cGMP production and protein kinase G activation. Another system is the tyrosine kinase system in which the hormone receptor itself has kinase activity and phosphorylates proteins through tyrosine residues. To date, no significant examples of reproductive hormone activation of the protein kinase G or tyrosine kinase systems exist. However, the receptor for insulin and many of the growth factor receptors are tyrosine kinases,[2] and activity of these hormones in reproductive tissues is mediated via this second messenger system. The tyrosine kinase second messenger system is a rather recent discovery and is assuming greater importance daily.

Calcium

Intracellular levels of the divalent cation calcium can also serve as a second messenger system for hormones. Hormone binding to receptor may cause calcium influx through ligand-gated calcium channels. For example, prostaglandin $F_2\alpha$ treatment of luteal cells not only activates protein kinase C but also causes a sustained elevation of intracellular levels of calcium, presumably through a $PGF_2\alpha$-gated calcium channel.[24] The increased levels of intracellular calcium can then have a number of effects. The intracellular calcium binding protein calmodulin can be activated by binding of up to four molecules of calcium.[2] Active calmodulin can influence activity of some enzymes directly, and a calmodulin-dependent protein kinase can cause protein phosphorylation with actions similar to those described for other protein kinases.

Evidence suggests that prolonged elevation of intracellular levels of calcium can also be cytotoxic. High intracellular calcium initiates events within the nucleus that eventually lead to programmed cell death.[25] This process appears to be important for the normal demise of the corpus luteum.[26]

In summary, Figure 3-6 depicts some of the complex interactions of the protein kinase A, protein kinase C,

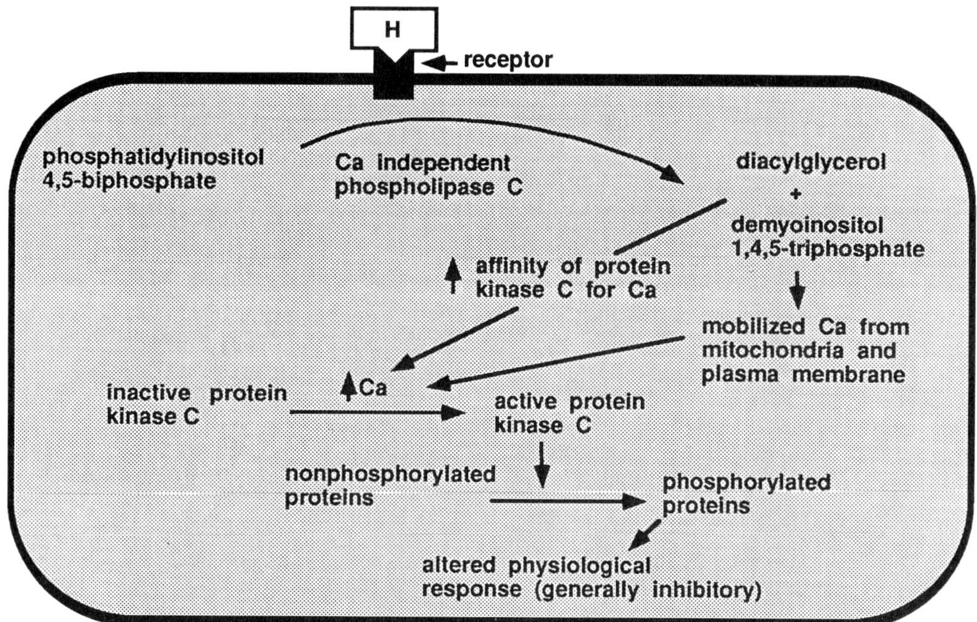

FIG. 3–5. Mechanisms for activation of the protein kinase C second messenger system. Hormone binding to receptor activates phospholipase C, which converts phosphatidylinositol 4,5-biphosphate (PIP_2) to diacylglycerol and de-*myo*-inositol 1,4,5-triphosphate (IP_3). The diacylglycerol binds to a specific site on protein kinase C and increases its affinity for calcium. The IP_3 mobilizes calcium from intracellular stores, and calcium binding to protein kinase C activates its catalytic actions. The active protein kinase C phosphorylates proteins leading to an altered physiologic response.

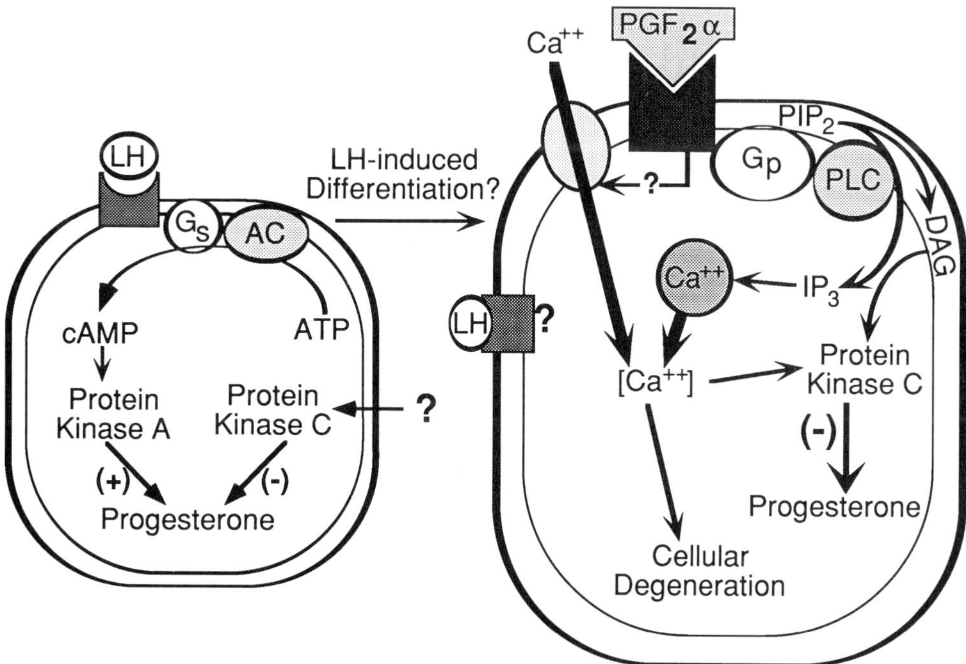

FIG. 3–6. Regulation of progesterone secretion from the two steroidogenic luteal cell types. In small luteal cells (left) binding of LH activates the protein kinase A system and stimulates synthesis of progesterone (see Fig. 3-2). Activation of protein kinase C is inhibitory to progesterone synthesis, although it is not clear what hormone activates this system in small cells. Binding of LH to small cells may also cause them to differentiate into large cells. In large luteal cells (right) binding of LH does not appear to activate any second messenger system. Binding of $PGF_{2}\alpha$ results in activation of the protein kinase C system and inhibition of progesterone secretion and also causes calcium influx and eventual cellular degeneration. This model is based on data obtained with ovine luteal cells.

and calcium second messenger systems in regulating progesterone secretion from ovine luteal cells. This is a single, simplified example of the complex interactions of these second messenger systems in regulating functions of target cells.

Steroid Hormones

For the last two to three decades, the generally accepted mode of action for steroid and thyroid hormones has been that they diffuse through the plasma membranes of all cells in the body and that target cells have cytosolic receptors for these hormones.[27] In the case of steroids, binding of the hormone to these intracellular receptors resulted in retention of the steroid, and the hormone receptor complex under went "activation" and was transported to the nucleus where it bound to chromatin and stimulated transcription and translation, resulting in synthesis of steroid hormone–dependent protein[2] (Fig. 3-7). We now know that the steroid receptor complex occurred only in the nucleus and that this complex binds to specific areas of chromatin, called response elements, and regulates transcription of specific genes. For example, the estradiol-estrogen receptor binds to a control region on the genes encoding for the two subunits of LH and suppresses their activity[28] (Fig. 3-8). As can be seen in Figure 3-7, a complex interaction of the protein kinase A, protein kinase C, and estradiol receptor systems regulates the function of the gonadotroph.

In some instances, steroid hormones directly influence activity of second messenger systems controlled by proteinaceous hormones. For example, estradiol has been shown to enhance the quantities of protein kinase C present in target cells,[29] presumably via enhancement of transcription and translation of one of the genes encoding for this protein.

Prostaglandins

The intracellular mechanism of action of the prostaglandins has only recently been determined. In luteal cells, $PGF_2\alpha$ treatment activates the protein kinase C second messenger system[23] and also results in dramatic increases in intracellular calcium concentrations.[24] The mechanism of action of PGE_2 has not been elucidated.

HORMONE METABOLISM

The routes for metabolism and excretion of hormones in horses have not been studied in great detail; however, it seems likely that these processes are similar to those in most other species. For proteinaceous hormones there are two important mechanisms involved in hormone metabolism. First, in most cases a relatively small percentage of the hormone secreted into the bloodstream is ultimately bound to receptors on target cells. Depending on the hormone and its affinity for its receptor, either it is internalized into the target cell by receptor-mediated endocytosis[6] and degraded, or it eventually dissociates from the receptor and returns to the circulatory system. Once the hormone receptor complex has been internalized, it is transported to lipo-

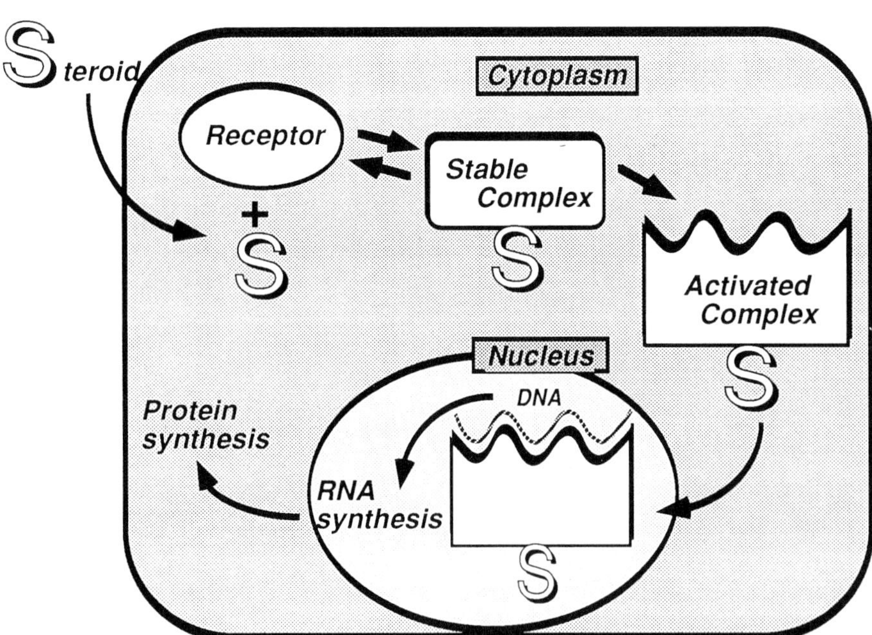

FIG. 3–7. Classic model depicting the mechanisms of action of steroid hormones. The steroid diffuses into the cell and binds to a cytoplasmic receptor, which becomes "activated," migrates to the nucleus, interacts with DNA, and results in enhanced RNA and protein synthesis. The increased protein synthesis results in the eventual biologic response to the hormone. The mechanisms whereby steroid hormones enter cells and the presence of cytoplasmic receptors is currently controversial.

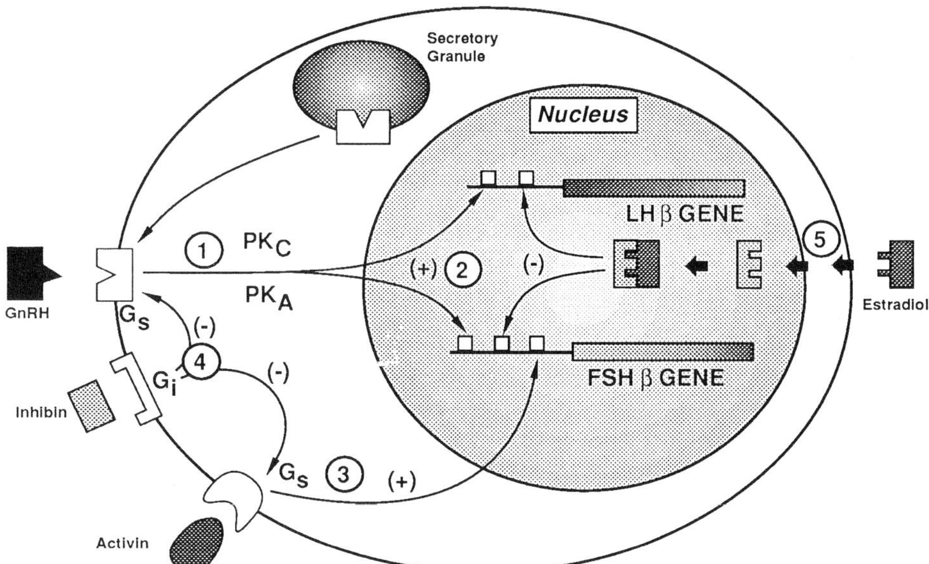

FIG. 3–8. Hypothetical model for regulation of expression of the genes encoding for the β-subunits of LH and FSH. GnRH binds to its receptor and activates (1) the protein kinase C (PK_C) or protein kinase A (PK_A) second messenger system. Evidence suggests that GnRH activates both of these pathways, depending on the species and experimental protocol. PK_A and/or PK_C may interact with specific-response elements to regulate gene transcription (2). Activin also activates a stimulatory G-protein and PK_A leading to alteration in gene transcription of the gene for the β-subunit of FSH (3). Inhibin likely activates an inhibitory G-protein, which negatively influences the actions of GnRH and activin (4). The receptor for GnRH is probably recycled to the plasma membrane via gonadotropin-containing secretory granules. Finally , (5) estradiol exerts a negative effect via interaction of the estradiol-estradiol receptor complex with the estradiol response element on the genes.

somes where the hormone dissociates and is degraded. The receptor is, at least in part, recycled to the plasma membrane. For example, considerably less than 1% of the cardiac output is distributed to the ovary. Thus if every molecule of LH and FSH that reached the ovary was bound, internalized, and degraded, blood levels of gonadotropins would not be significantly affected.

Peptide, protein, and glycoprotein hormones present in the bloodstream are inactivated and degraded by elements in the blood, liver, and kidney and excreted. The chemical nature of the hormone has a dramatic effect on the rate of loss from the circulation. For example, the time required to lose one-half ($t_{1/2}$) of an injected dose of GnRH (10 amino acids) from the blood of ewes is 3.7 min.[30] In general, the larger the peptide and/or protein, the longer the half-life in blood. The presence and chemical composition of the carbohydrate moieties present in glycoproteins also influences the time required for clearance from the bloodstream. For example, LH contains less carbohydrate than FSH and the $t_{1/2}$ in blood for LH is ± 30 min whereas the $t_{1/2}$ for FSH is at least 2 h. The $t_{1/2}$ for clearance of hCG, which contains substantially more carbohydrate than LH or FSH is 2 to 5 days, depending on the species studied. Differences in the rates of clearance of the proteinaceous hormones obviously have important implications for therapeutic use of these compounds.

Steroid hormones are all degraded and excreted via a similar mechanism. In general, the oxygenated substituents are reduced. These reduced forms are filtered efficiently by the kidney but are also efficiently reabsorbed. Therefore, in the liver, and in some cases the kidney, the reduced steroids are conjugated, primarily via the 3-hydroxy position, to a sulfate or glucuronide derivative that is not reabsorbed by the kidney. Thus the excreted form of steroids are generally sulfated or glucuronidated derivatives.

Most tissues in the body appear to metabolize prostaglandins to some extent. For example, more than 90% of $PGF_2\alpha$ in the blood is metabolized to 13,14-dihydro-15-keto $PGF_2\alpha$ on a single pass through the lungs. Thus the lung is the major site of metabolism, although other tissues such as the uterus also play a significant role.

REFERENCES

1. Knickerbocker, J.J., Wiltbank, M.C., and Niswender, G.D.: Mechanisms of luteolysis in domestic animals. Domest. Anim. Endocrinol., 6:91–107, 1988.
2. Bolander, F.F.: Molecular Endocrinology. San Diego, Academic Press, 1989.
3. Richards, J.S., et al.: Ovarian follicular development in the rat: Hormone receptor regulation by estradiol, follicle

stimulating hormone and luteinizing hormone. Endocrinology, *99*:1562–1570, 1976.

4. Suter, D.E., et al.: Alterations in the number of ovine luteal receptors for LH and progesterone secretion induced by homologous hormone. Biol. Reprod., *22*:205–210, 1980.
5. LaPolt, P.S., et al.: Ligand-induced down-regulation of testis LH receptors: Differential inhibition of alternatively processed LH receptor messages. Biol. Reprod., *42*(Suppl. 1):84 (#131), 1990.
6. Niswender, G.D., et al.: Regulation of luteal function in domestic ruminants: New concepts. Recent Prog. Horm. Res., *41*:101–142, 1985.
7. Roess, D.A., Niswender, G.D., and Barisas, B.G.: Cytoskeletal modulation of the lateral mobility of hCG-occupied LH receptors in ovine luteal cells. Endocrinology, *122*:261–269, 1988.
8. Bourdage, R.J., Fitz, T.A., and Niswender, G.D.: Differential steroidogenic response of ovine luteal cells to ovine luteinizing hormone and human chorionic gonadotropin. Proc. Soc. Exp. Biol. Med., *175*:483–486, 1984.
9. Diekman, M.A., O'Callaghan, P., Nett, T.M., and Niswender, G.D.: Validation of methods and quantification of luteal receptors for LH throughout the estrous cycle and early pregnancy in ewes. Biol. Reprod., *19*:999–1009, 1978.
10. Roser, J.F., and Evans, J.W.: Luteal luteinizing hormone receptors during the postovulatory period in the mare. Biol. Reprod., *29*:499–510, 1983.
11. Duval, D., Durant, S., and Homo-Delarche, F.: Non-genomic effects of steroids. Interactions of steroid molecules with membrane structures and functions. Biochim. Biophys. Acta, *737*:409–442, 1983.
12. Segaloff, D.L., et al.: The structure of the lutropin/choriogenotropin receptor as determined by biochemical approaches and by cDNA cloning. *In* Glycoprotein Hormones. Edited by W.W. Chin and I. Boime. Norwell, Serono Symposia, 1990, pp. 377–384.
13. Sprengel, R., et al.: The testicular receptor for follicle-stimulating hormone: Structure and functional expression of cloned DNA. Mol. Endocrinol., *4*:525–530, 1990.
14. Brown, A.M., and Birnbaumer, L.: Direct G protein gating of ion channels. Am. J. Physiol., *245*:H401–H410, 1988.
15. Marsh, J.: The role of cAMP in gonadal function. Adv. Cyclic Nucleotide Res., *6*:137–199, 1975.
16. Birnbaumer, L., et al.: Regulation of hormone receptors and adenylyl cyclases by guanine nucleotide binding N proteins. Recent Prog. Horm. Res., *41*:41–99, 1985.
17. Gilman, A.G.: G proteins and dual control of adenylate cyclase. Cell, *36*:577–579, 1984.
18. Caffrey, J.L., et al.: The activity of ovine luteal cholesterol esterase during several experimental conditions. Biol. Reprod., *21*:601–680, 1979.
19. Kennedy, G., Andersen, G., Hamernik, D.L., and Nett, T.M.: Transcriptional interaction of the URE, CRE, and a downstream regulatory element in the gene encoding the α-subunit of human glycoprotein hormone. *In* Glycoprotein Hormones. Edited by W.W. Chin and I. Boime. Norwell, Serono Symposia, 1990, pp. 259–268.
20. Gospodarowicz, D., and Gospodarowicz, F.: The morphological transformation and inhibition of growth of bovine luteal cells in tissue culture induced by luteinizing hormone and dibutyryl cyclic AMP. Endocrinology, *96*:458–467, 1975.
21. Caron, M.G., Goldstein, S., Savard, K., and Marsh, J.: Protein kinase stimulation of a reconstituted cholesterol side chain cleavage enzyme system in the bovine corpus luteum. J. Biol. Chem. *250*:5137–5149, 1975.
22. Hall, P.F.: Trophic stimulation of steroidogenesis: In search of the elusive trigger. Recent. Prog. Horm. Res. *41*:1–39, 1985.
23. Wiltbank, M.C., Diskin, M.G., Flores, J.A., and Niswender, G.D.: Regulation of the corpus luteum by protein kinase C. II. Inhibition of lipoprotein-stimulated steroidogenesis by prostaglandin $F_2\alpha$. Biol. Reprod., *42*:239–245, 1990.
24. Wiltbank, M.C., et al.: Hormonal regulation of free intracellular calcium concentrations in small and large ovine luteal cells. Biol. Reprod., *41*:771–778, 1989.
25. Kerr, J.F.R., Wyllie, A.H., and Currie, A.R.: Apoptosis: A basic biological phenomenon with wide-ranging implications in tissue kinetics. Br. J. Cancer, *26*:239–244, 1972.
26. Sawyer, H.R., Niswender, K.D., Braden, T.D., and Niswender, G.D.: Nuclear changes in ovine luteal cells in response to $PGF_2\alpha$. Domest. Anim. Endocrinol., *7*:229–238, 1990.
27. Jensen, E.V., and Jacobson, H.I.: Fate of steroid estrogens in target tissues. *In* Biological Activities of Steroids in Relationship to Cancer. Edited by G. Pincus and E.P. Vollmer. New York, Academic Press, 1960, pp. 161–178.
28. Shupnik, M.A., et al.: Estrogen regulation of the rat LHβ gene. *In* Glycoprotein Hormones. Edited by W.W. Chin and I. Boime. Norwell, Serono Symposia, 1990, pp. 251–258.
29. Drouva, S.E., et al.: Estradiol modulates proteinkinase C activity in the rat pituitary in vivo and in vitro. Endocrinology, *126*:536–544, 1990.
30. Nett, T.M., et al.: A radioimmunoassay for gonadotropin-releasing hormone (GnRH) in serum. J. Clin. Endocrinol. Metab., *36*:880–885, 1973.

CHAPTER 4

GnRH

C.H.G. Irvine
S.L. Alexander

A great deal of research has been done on hypothalamic-pituitary-gonadal relationships since Geoffrey Harris first postulated that pituitary hormone secretion was regulated by releasing hormones transported from the hypothalamus. Nevertheless this concept has held up more strongly for the reproductive axis than for any other. Clinical applications of this knowledge continue to expand; unfortunately the empirical use of gonadotropin-releasing hormone (GnRH) in many forms of infertility of nonhypothalamic origin continues to expand as well. The objective of this review is to present updated information on the physiology of GnRH so that it may be more logically used in equine reproductive management.

CHEMISTRY

The brain exerts control of the reproductive axis through release of the decapeptide GnRH from the hypothalamus. When first extracted and sequenced by Schally and co-workers[1] it was called luteinizing hormone-releasing hormone (LH-RH) because it induced marked release of luteinizing hormone in all species. Subsequently it was found to induce follicle-stimulating hormone (FSH) release in many species.[2] The evidence for a separate FSH-RH is not convincing, and it is generally agreed that there is only one releasing hormone for the gonadal axis in all mammals, hence the term GnRH.

Molecular techniques have shown that GnRH is synthesized as part of a larger molecule (Fig. 4-1). Before secretion, GnRH is split off from the remainder of the molecule, a 56 amino acid peptide called gonadotropin-releasing hormone associated peptide (GAP), which is secreted concurrently with the decapeptide.[3] Fragments of GAP and GAP itself also can stimulate gonadotropin secretion from pituitary cells in culture, but are less potent than GnRH.[3] The physiologic role of GAP is unclear.

ANALOGUES

Modifications of the GnRH molecule have been made, and many of the analogues have clinically useful agonist or antagonist properties. In general, substitution of glycine at the 6 position with D-alanine, tryptophan, or serine confers more structural and metabolic stability to the molecule so that its action is prolonged.[4,5] Removal of the 10-terminal glycine with amidation of the 9-proline also increases agonist activity.[5] Some agonists are up to 100 times more potent than native GnRH, although the relative potencies in the rat—which is the usual test animal—may be quite different in the horse. However, after administration for several days, agonists may become antagonists by induction of refractoriness. This is caused by (1) receptor loss (down regulation), (2) uncoupling of remaining receptors from their intracellular response mechanism, and (3) inhibition of hormone synthesis.[6] Refractoriness may also be induced by prolonged exposure to high levels of the native hor-

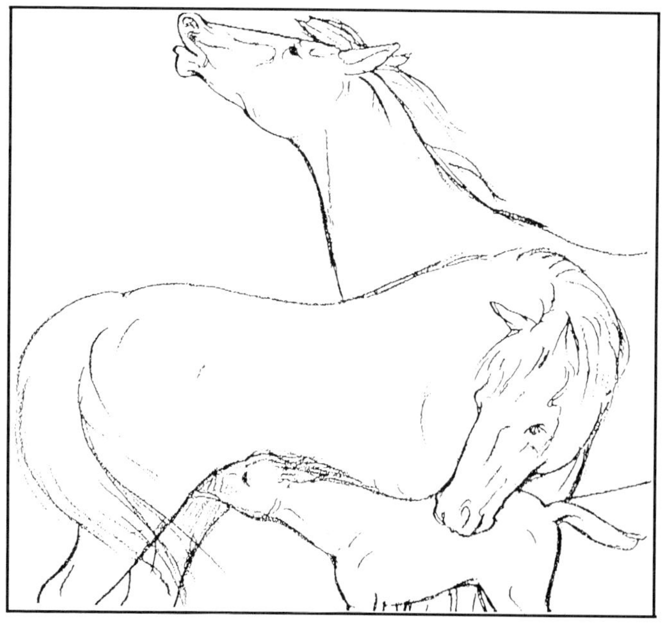

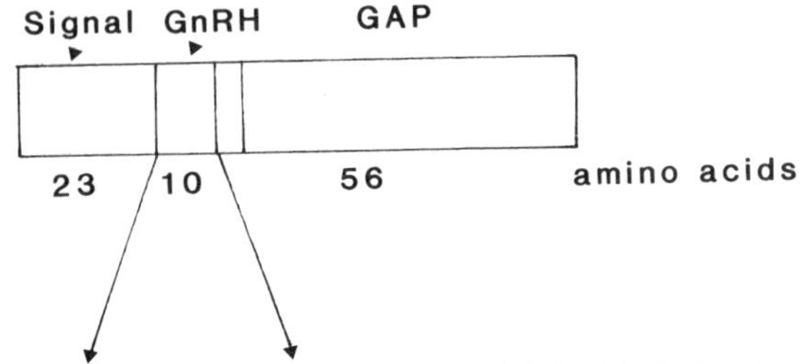

FIG. 4–1. The large precursor molecule (pre-pro GnRH) which is cleaved to yield gonadotropin-releasing hormone (GnRH) and gonadotropin-releasing hormone associated peptide (GAP). The number of amino acids in each segment of the molecule is shown beneath the diagram. The amino acid sequence of GnRH is shown at the bottom of the figure. In the finished product, the first amino acid, glutamine, is converted to pyroglutamic acid and the terminal amino acid, glycine, is amidated.

mone.[7] The horse seems to be relatively resistant to refractoriness (see below). Substitutions near the N-terminal, particularly of histidine in position 2, produce antagonist analogues, which bind to the GnRH receptor without activating gonadotrophin secretion.[5] At appropriate doses these analogues can compete with natural GnRH for its receptors and, therefore, suppress its effect. An attempt is being made to formalize the nomenclature of releasing hormones as "-relins," e.g., GnRH is gonadorelin, its tertiary butyl serine substitution at the 6 position is buserelin, and so on. Some U.S. journals prefer the name LH-RH and some British journals insist on luliberin. In this review GnRH is used.

SITES OF SYNTHESIS, SECRETION, AND ACTION

In some species, GnRH synthesis is restricted to a network of neurons located in discrete areas of the hypothalamus, e.g., arcuate nucleus in the monkey,[7] but in the horse GnRH is relatively evenly distributed throughout the hypothalamus.[8] The GnRH axons that leave the hypothalamus pass mainly to the external capillary plexus of the median eminence, where they store their secretory product in terminal granules. When the neuron is depolarized, GnRH is discharged and enters fenestrated capillaries for transport via portal vessels to the pituitary where it binds to receptors on the gonadotrope. Some axons that travel to the median eminence have branches that terminate in higher centers of the brain and presumably release GnRH simultaneously in both areas.[9] Axons from approximately 20 to 30% of the GnRH cells in the hypothalamus travel only to higher centers.[10] Receptors for GnRH are found in the hippocampus in proximity to these GnRH axon terminals.[9] Evidence suggests that exogenous GnRH administration stimulates areas in the brain responsible for sexual behavior in gonadectomized rams[11] and rats.[12] In the gelding given subeffective doses of testosterone, injection of GnRH causes a significant increase in several aspects of sexual behavior.[13] Studies have shown that endogenously induced GnRH release also stimulates sexual behavior and thus coordinates the endocrine and behavioral sexual responses as well as contributing to the cascade of events that terminates in orgasm.[9,12]

Although the major function of GnRH is to stimulate gonadotropin secretion, it also stimulates production of its own receptor.[6] Gonadotropin-releasing hormone is synthesized in other tissues (e.g., in the gonads of rodents, but not other species, and in the placenta of many species), but has no defined physiological role in these organs. Exogenous GnRH does not influence equine chorionic gonadotropin (eCG) secretion in the mare.[14]

REGULATION OF SECRETION

MODE OF SECRETION

Experimental Models

The mode of GnRH secretion has proved difficult to study because after GnRH is released from nerve endings at the median eminence, it travels in fine portal venules within the cranial cavity to the pituitary gland. The picomolar concentrations in portal blood are diluted to subfemtomolar concentrations in peripheral blood.[15] Because peripheral concentrations of GnRH are immeasurably low, information about GnRH requires sampling of portal blood from almost inaccessible vessels. Surgical techniques for this have been developed in the rat,[16], monkey,[17] and sheep.[18] They require removal of part of the skull, exposure and incision of the portal vessels, and collection by suction of the blood that leaks from them. Sampling time rarely exceeds 6 to 12 h and is done under deep anesthesia in all but sheep. Although the data obtained have been criticized on methodologic[19] and physiologic[15] grounds, most information available on GnRH secretion has come from this model. Levine and Ramirez[20] have used a push-pull perfusion system on the medial basal hypothalamus, a method that has been adapted to the horse by Sharp and Grubaugh.[21] Irvine and Alexander have developed in the horse a method for collecting blood that perfuses the pituitary and exits via veins that may be cannulated by a relatively atraumatic procedure.[15] This method has some advantages, in particular the collection of blood containing many simultaneously secreted hypothalamic and pituitary hormones, which permits study of interactions.[15]

Experimental Results

The earliest information on the *mode* of secretion of GnRH came from the elegant, although indirect, experiments of Knobil's group on female monkeys.[7] He concluded that GnRH secretion is "obligatorily intermittent," with episodes of secretion being essentially separated by periods of nonsecretion. Continuous secretion exposes GnRH receptors to continuous stimulation, which results in refractoriness which may be the result of receptor down regulation and other factors (see above). In the horse, however, continual infusion of GnRH for 24 h induces a steady increase in LH,[22] and osmotic minipumps that deliver GnRH constantly for 28 days also maintain LH secretion.[23] Similarly, implants that release a GnRH agonist continuously over 28 days induce prolonged gonadotropin secretion without refractoriness,[24] even at relatively large doses. [25] Recently Montovan et al.[26] showed that daily administration of up to 50 mg/day of a potent GnRH agonist has no suppressive effect on LH levels, sexual behavior, or semen characteristics in stallions; in mares, luteal levels of LH are maintained, and although follicular development is suppressed, this requires up to 30 days of treatment. These experiments show that, in horses, gonadotropin secretion is much less readily suppressed by persistence of high GnRH levels. They also show that the pituitary can respond to a continuous GnRH signal, but the studies do not show that the hypothalamus generates such a signal.

In the stallion having no sexual stimulation[27] and in the anestrous mare,[15] GnRH secretion is pulsatile in pituitary venous blood with long periods when GnRH is undetectable (Fig. 4-2). However, in estrous mares, GnRH secretion is continuous with superimposed pulses increasing from every 2 h to twice hourly during estrus[28] (see Chapter 5). Likewise, in stallions during the breeding season GnRH secretion is continuous with superimposed pulses up to twice hourly[29] (Fig. 4-3). Using push-pull perfusion of the medial basal hypothalamus of the mare, Sharp and Grubaugh[21] found that GnRH secretion is irregularly episodic with intervening periods of no secretion in anestrous, transitional, and diestrous mares, but is continuous during estrus. They also found a marked increase in GnRH secretion with passage into the breeding season but no change in frequency of peaks. Thus in the horse both continuous and discontinuous modes of GnRH secretion occur.

TIMING OF SECRETION

In the horse, timing of the GnRH signals that induce FSH and LH release is important, because it determines whether or not any hormone is released and the relative amounts released of each hormone.[25,29] If the GnRH signal is insufficient to release more than one gonadotropin pulse per day, the mare remains anestrous.

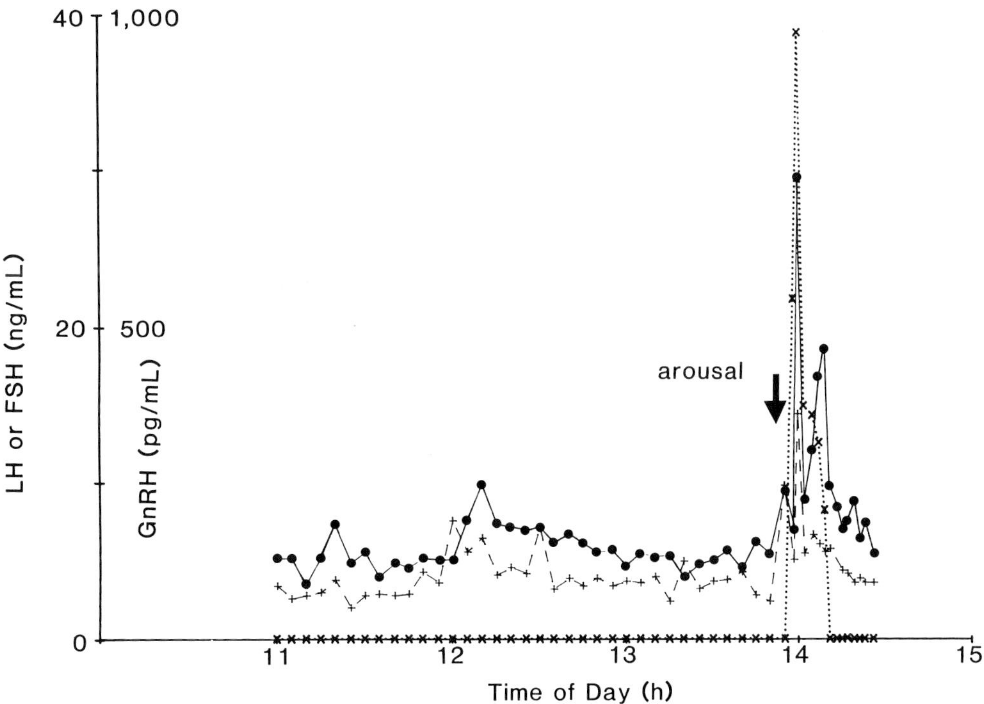

FIG. 4–2. Concentrations of GnRH (x···x), LH (●——●) and FSH (+——+) in pituitary venous blood collected every 5 min from a stallion at the end of the breeding season. The stallion was presented with an estrous mare at the time marked by the arrow and was allowed to tease the mare across a 1.2 meter gate until the end of the sampling period. The stallion was sexually aroused by this procedure, as shown by penile erection, flehmen, and vocalizations. Before arousal, concentrations of GnRH, LH, and FSH were similar in pituitary venous and jugular blood, indicating that no secretion was occurring. Arousal, however, stimulated secretion of all three hormones. (Adapted from Irvine, C.H.G. and Alexander, S.L.: Effect of sexual arousal on gonadotropin-releasing hormone, luteinizing hormone and follicle-stimulating hormone secretion in the stallion. J. Reprod. Fertil. Suppl., *44*:135–143, 1991.

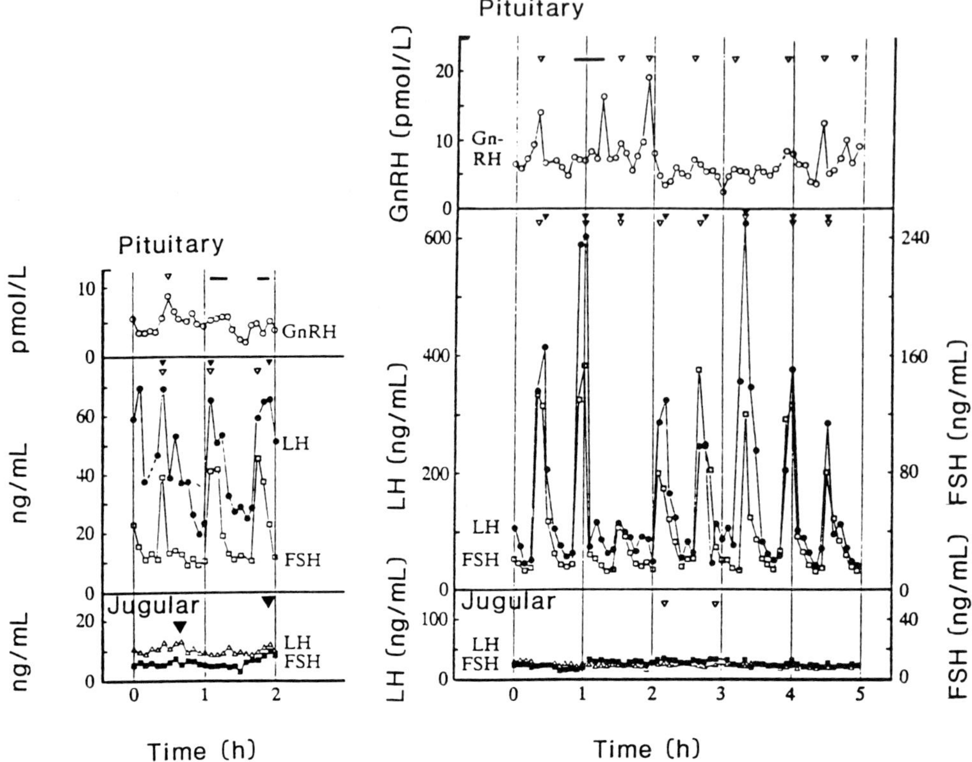

FIG. 4–3. Concentrations of GnRH (○) in pituitary venous blood, testosterone (T; ■) in jugular blood, and LH (●) and FSH (△) in pituitary venous blood and concurrent jugular blood samples collected at frequent intervals from two stallions (*a* and *b*) in the breeding season. These stallions had regular contact with estrous mares. Pulses of GnRH and LH are marked by solid arrowheads and FSH pulses by open arrowheads. Solid horizontal bars indicate prolonged secretory episodes. The open bar along the horizontal axis of each upper panel shows the detection limit of the GnRH radioimmunoassay (RIA) in which each set of samples was assayed. (From Irvine, C.H.G. and Alexander, S.L.: Secretion rates and short-term patterns of gonadotrophin-releasing hormone, FSH and LH in the normal stallion in the breeding season. J. Endocrinol., *117*:197–206, 1988.)

If the signal induces two to four gonadotropin pulses per day, FSH release predominates and induces follicular development. If GnRH signals are of sufficient frequency or size to induce gonadotropin pulses at intervals of 2 h or less, LH release predominates and induces ovulation. Thus changes in the intensity of the GnRH signal play an important role in the annual and ovulatory cycles of the mare.[28,30,31] However, ovarian hormones have an important modulating influence on the pituitary response to GnRH stimulation.

Most dogma on GnRH pulse frequency is derived from LH pulse frequency, which is believed to reflect GnRH pulses.[18] This appears to be true at circhoral (approximately hourly) pulse frequencies found in the periovulatory mare[28] and breeding season stallion[29] (Fig. 4-3), as it does in other species. However, it may not be true at slower gonadotropin pulse frequencies observed in diestrous and anestrous mares. Preliminary experiments have shown GnRH pulse frequency remains relatively rapid in such mares, with many GnRH pulses unaccompanied by gonadotropin pulses.[31] Similarly, in the luteal-phase ewe fewer than 30% of the GnRH pulses induce LH pulses.[32] Although it appears that in the luteal-phase mare, and to a lesser extent in the ewe, most GnRH pulses are ineffective in inducing gonadotropin secretion, frequent GnRH pulses may serve to maintain gonadotropin synthesis.[33]

AMPLITUDE OF SECRETION

The concentration of GnRH in blood perfusing the pituitary is important information for rational replacement or other treatment. Apart from very brief spikes the concentration of GnRH in the pituitary venous blood of the horse during gonadotropin pulses is up to 15 pg/mL but it is likely that the concentration at the gonadotrope is about twice that because pars distalis blood is subsequently diluted with blood from the partes nervosa and intermedia before sampling. Exogenous doses of 3 μg GnRH that, after distribution in the extracellular space, induce plasma concentrations of approximately 24 pg/mL also induce pulses of gonadotropin secretion that simulate endogenously driven pulses.[34]

REGULATION BY INTRAHYPOTHALAMIC INFLUENCES

Knobil postulated that there is a zeitgeber (time giver) in the arcuate nucleus of the hypothalamus of the monkey that discharges regularly in the absence of any external influence.[7] Hypothalamic cells in vitro release GnRH spontaneously in pulses; for example, GnRH is released at 48 ± 7-min intervals in hypothalami from diestrous rats.[35] Data from sheep,[32] rat,[20] and horse[28,29] indicate that the GnRH discharges that induce gonadotropin pulses rarely occur at intervals of less than 30 min. This suggests that if a zeitgeber does exist, it may contain a network of cells with a drifting membrane potential with a period of approximately 30 min, somewhat analogous to the sinoatrial node. Although the GnRH-containing neurons are separated by other cells they connect with each other as a network and depolarize simultaneously. Knobil showed that in multiunit recording from an array of arcuate nucleus cells in the ovariectomized mobile monkey, bursts of electrical activity lasting about 14 min occur hourly and are correlated with LH secretion.[36] In the intact monkey, however, bursts last for only 2 min. The frequency of bursts is inversely correlated with estradiol and is very low during the periovulatory period when LH is highest.

In the rat and pig, knife cuts placed in various parts of the hypothalamus have demonstrated that inputs from the anterior basal hypothalamus, but not the posterior basal hypothalamus, are essential for surges of GnRH release, although tonic release is not suppressed. This has led to the hypothesis that in the female, ovulatory gonadotropin surges are driven from a center anatomically and physiologically distinct from that inducing tonic release. Other interpretations of the disconnection experiments are possible. Furthermore, species differences occur so the mechanism that operates in the mare is uncertain.

NEUROTRANSMITTER CONTROL OF GnRH SECRETION

Such a vast and conflicting literature can be found on this subject that it is difficult to present a coherent scheme. Considerable species differences occur but an unfortunate lack of data exists for the horse. Most evidence suggests that main stimulatory inputs are from local nonadrenergic neurons and major inhibitory inputs are dopaminergic. Administration of many neurotransmitters and blockers has shown that cholinergic, serotonergic, and GABA-ergic pathways may also be important. Recent findings on the mode of action of progesterone illustrate some of the interactions involved. In the horse, like most species, the basic circhoral LH pulse frequency is slowed by progesterone (see Chapter 5). At luteolysis, the LH pulse frequency, which has been restrained to two to four per day by progesterone, increases in the horse, at least in part, as a result of an increase in GnRH pulse frequency.[31] In several species, progesterone increases local production of an opioid neuromodulator, possibly β-endorphin, which slows down GnRH pulse frequency. This probably happens in the horse because administration of the opioid antagonist naloxone increases GnRH and LH pulse frequency.[21] One of the many local inhibitory actions of opioids is to suppress release of norepinephrine in the vicinity of GnRH-secreting neurons. This removes a stimulus to GnRH secretion. Thus a simplified scheme of the action of progesterone on pulse frequency involves (in sequence) opioid, norepinephrine, GnRH, and luteinizing hormone. Although the major effect of opioids is on suppression of GnRH secretion at the hypothalamus, some evidence indicates that opioids may also act at the pituitary by reducing responsiveness to gonadotropin-releasing hormone.[37] This might account for the discrepancy between GnRH and LH pulse frequency during the luteal phase.[31]

REGULATION BY EXTRAHYPOTHALAMIC HORMONAL INFLUENCES

Apart from the neural connections that affect GnRH secretion, evidence shows (see previous section) that circulating hormones impinge on these circuits as part of the hormonal feedback control. Receptors for estradiol and progesterone have been found in the hypothalamus. Although there is agreement that progesterone is inhibitory to pulse frequency and consequently stimulatory to pulse amplitude, the role of estradiol is complex and controversial.[38] A short-loop feedback of LH on GnRH secretion has been postulated[39] but also discounted, at least in the monkey.[40] Furthermore, no LH receptors, which are essential for an action of LH, could be found in the ovine hypothalamus.[41] Many of the inhibitory influences on GnRH secretion (e.g., corticotropin-releasing factor and progesterone) are generally believed to act via the opioid-mediated suppression of GnRH secretion described above. In all species studied thus far, the inhibitory influence of inhibin on FSH release is exerted solely at the pituitary.

REGULATION BY ENVIRONMENTAL INFLUENCES

Many of the environmental factors that influence gonadotropin secretion are presumed to act via GnRH secretion. The best documented environmental signal is increased melatonin secretion during darkness, which conveys information on photoperiod to the endocrine system (see Chapter 11). These melatonin patterns allow seasonally breeding animals like the horse to link their breeding season to a particular time of year. In stallions and mares, secretion of both gonadotropins increases as the breeding season approaches.[30,42] However, melatonin does not appear to act directly via GnRH because there are no melatonin receptors in the hypothalamus, although they are in high concentration in the pars tuberalis, which forms a "collar" around the pituitary stalk.[43] Because short portal vessels carry blood from the pars tuberalis to the pars distalis, where most of the gonadotropes are located, a melatonin-influenced pathway exists by which photoperiodic signals could regulate the breeding season independently from gonadotropin-releasing hormone.

Olfactory, tactile, auditory, visual, and psychogenic signals have been shown to advance the onset of the breeding season in seasonal animals or to increase LH or testosterone in other species.[44,45] These signals probably act by increasing GnRH secretion; however, because of the difficulty in measuring basal GnRH secretion in the unperturbed, uninvaded subject, this has been demonstrated experimentally in only a single situation. In the stallion, brief sexual arousal has recently been shown to induce marked increases in the concentration of GnRH in pituitary venous blood[27] (Fig. 4-2). It is unknown whether the stimulating signal in this case is olfactory, tactile, auditory, or visual. The episode of GnRH secretion induced by arousal is accompanied by an increase in gonadotropin concentrations in pituitary venous blood but not in jugular blood.[27] It seems highly likely that more prolonged contact between the stallion and mare, or copulation itself, would induce a more prolonged increase in GnRH and gonadotropin secretion so that jugular LH and FSH levels would rise. One study demonstrated that jugular LH in mares and stallions is higher after copulation.[46] These observations could have relevance to mare and stallion management. Luteinizing hormone stimulates ovulation as well as testosterone secretion, and release of spermatozoa from the seminiferous tubules. Therefore, lowered LH concentrations as a result of inadequate exposure of stallions to sexually arousing situations could affect both libido and fertility.

RATE OF GnRH SYNTHESIS, SECRETION, AND DEGRADATION

Concentrations of GnRH in the median eminence are much greater than in any other area (total median eminence GnRH content equals 4 to 6 ng). The total amount in the remainder of the hypothalamus of the mare is 4 to 6 ng.[47] Because the ovulatory surge concentration in pituitary venous blood is approximately 10 pg/mL when blood flow is 30 mL/min, GnRH secretion rates are of the order of .3 ng/min.[28] Therefore, turnover is rapid, and synthesis and secretion are probably tightly coupled. Because jugular blood flow in the horse is approximately 6 L/min a 200-fold dilution of pituitary effluent occurs immediately in jugular blood and a further 5-fold dilution in the first passage through the heart. This is further rapidly diluted 6-fold by passage into the extravascular, extracellular fluid. Although equilibrium conditions are probably never attained, the highest concentration in peripheral blood probably never exceeds 2 fg/mL (2 fmol/L), which is immeasurably low with current methodology. Thus kinetic studies with physiologic concentrations are difficult to perform, although information about the disposal of an exogenous GnRH dose may be useful. Many enzymes are capable of GnRH degradation. In neural tissue, the major site of cleavage of GnRH is between the fifth and sixth amino acids.[48] Removal of the pyroglutamic acid in position 1 or splitting at position 9 by a postproline-cleaving enzyme also occurs. Degradation is faster in horse plasma at 37° C than in most other species.[49] The N- and C-terminals of GnRH (but not of most of its analogues) are brought into close proximity by hydrogen bonding, through which the molecule may bind to a hydrophobic site on albumin, thus delaying its loss from plasma. It seems likely that the final half-life of GnRH in the horse is no less than 30 min. Therefore, large exogenous doses can exert a prolonged effect. The known degradation products or derivatives of GnRH have no biologic action, unlike those of some other oligopeptides, e.g., arginine vasopressin.[50]

REFERENCES

1. Matsuo, H., et al.: Structure of the proposed porcine luteinizing hormone- and follicle-stimulating hormone-releasing hormone. Biochem. Biophys. Res. Commun., *43*:1334–1339, 1971.
2. Schally, A.V.: Aspects of hypothalamic regulation of the pituitary gland. Science, *202*:18–26, 1978.
3. Mason, A.J., Nikolics, K., Stewart, T.A., and Seeburg, P.H.: The mammalian GnRH gene: A central role in mammalian reproduction. *In* Neuroendocrine Control of the Hypothalamo-pituitary System. Edited by H. Imura. Tokyo, Karger, 1988, pp. 3–11.
4. Monahan, M.W., Amoss, M.S., Anderson, H.A., and Vale, W.: Synthetic analogs of the hypothalamic luteinizing hormone-releasing factor with increased agonist or antagonist properties. Biochemistry, *12*:4616–4620, 1973.
5. Sandow, J., et al.: Structure-activity relationships in the LH-RH molecule. *In* Control of Ovulation. Edited by D.B. Crighton, N.B. Haynes, N.B. Foxcroft, G.R. and G.E. Lamming. London, Butterworth, 1978, pp. 49–70.
6. Clayton, R.N.: Gonadotrophin-releasing hormone: Its actions and receptors. J. Endocrinol., *120*:11–19, 1989.
7. Knobil, E.: The neuroendocrine control of the menstrual cycle. Rec. Progr. Horm. Res., *36*:53–88, 1980.
8. Strauss, S.S., Chen, C.L., Kalra, S.P., and Sharp, D.C.: Localization of gonadotropin-releasing hormone (GnRH) in the hypothalamus of ovariectomized pony mares by season. J. Reprod. Fertil. Suppl., *27*:123–129, 1979.
9. Leblanc, P., et al.: Characterization and distribution of receptors for gonadotropin-releasing hormone in the rat hippocampus. Neuroendocrinology, *48*:482–488, 1988.
10. Merchenthaler, I., et al.: Combined retrograde tracing and immunocytochemical identification of luteinizing hormone-releasing hormone- and somatostatin-containing neurons projecting to the median eminence of the rat. Endocrinology, *125*:2812–2821, 1989.
11. Schanbacher, B.D., and Lunstra, D.D.: Acute and chronic effects of gonadotropin releasing hormone on reproductive characteristics of rams during the nonbreeding season. J. Anim. Sci., *44*:650–655, 1977.
12. Moss, R.L.: Actions of hypothalamic hormones on the brain. Ann. Rev. Physiol., *41*:617–631, 1979.

13. Pozor, M.A., McDonnell, S.M., Kenney, R.M., and Tischner, M.: GnRH facilitates copulatory behavior in geldings treated with testosterone. J. Reprod. Fertil. Suppl., 4:666–667, 1991.
14. Thompson, D.L., Reville, S.I., and Derrick, D.J.: Short-term mode of secretion of equine chorionic gonadotropin and the effect of GnRH. Theriogenology, *18*:583–591, 1982.
15. Irvine, C.H.G., and Alexander, S.L.: A novel technique for measuring hypothalamic and pituitary hormone secretion rates from collection of pituitary venous effluent in the normal horse. J. Endocrinol., *113*:183–192, 1987.
16. Porter, J.C., and Smith, K.R.: Collection of hypophysial stalk blood in rats. Endocrinology, *81*:1182–1185, 1967.
17. Carmel, P.W., Antunes, J.L., and Ferin, M.: Collection of blood from pituitary stalk and portal veins in monkeys and from the pituitary sinusoidal system of monkeys and man. J. Neurosurg., *50*:75–80, 1979.
18. Clarke, I.J., and Cummins, J.T.: The temporal relationship between gonadotropin-releasing hormone and luteinizing hormone secretion in ovariectomized ewes. Endocrinology, *111*:1737–1739, 1982.
19. Gibbs, D.M.: Collection of pituitary portal blood: A methodological analysis. Neuroendocrinology, *38*:97–101, 1984.
20. Levine, J.E., and Ramirez, V.D.: Luteinizing hormone-releasing hormone release during the rat estrous cycle and after ovariectomy as estimated with push-pull cannulae. Endocrinology, *111*:1439–1448, 1982.
21. Sharp, D.C., and Grubaugh, W.R.: Use of push-pull perfusion techniques in studies of gonadotrophin-releasing hormone secretion in mares. J. Reprod. Fertil. Suppl., *35*:289–296, 1987.
22. Garcia, M.C., and Ginther, O.J.: Plasma luteinizing hormone concentration in mares treated with gonadotropin-releasing hormone and estradiol. Am. J. Vet. Res., *36*:1581–1584, 1975.
23. Hyland, J.H., et al.: Infusion of gonadotrophin releasing hormone (GnRH) induces ovulation and fertile oestrus in mares during seasonal anoestrus. J. Reprod. Fertil., Suppl., *36*:211–220, 1987.
24. Allen, W.R., et al.: Induction of ovulation in anoestrous mares with a slow-release implant of a GnRH analogue (ICI 118 630). J. Reprod. Fertil. Suppl., *36*:469–478, 1987.
25. Turner, J.E., and Irvine, C.H.G.: The effect of various gonadotrophin-releasing hormone regimens on gonadotrophins, follicular growth and ovulation in deeply anoestrous mares. J. Reprod. Fertil. Suppl., *44*:213–225, 1992.
26. Montovan, S.M., et al.: The effect of a potent GnRH agonist on gonadal and sexual activity in the horse. Theriogenology, *33*:1305–1321, 1990.
27. Irvine, C.H.G., and Alexander, S.L.: Effect of sexual arousal on gonadotrophin-releasing hormone, luteinizing hormone and follicle-stimulating hormone secretion in the stallion. J. Reprod. Fertil. Suppl., *44*:135–143, 1991.
28. Alexander, S.L., and Irvine, C.H.G.: Secretion rates and short-term patterns of GnRH, FSH and LH throughout the periovulatory period in the mare. J. Endocrinol., *114*:351–362, 1987.
29. Irvine, C.H.G., and Alexander, S.L.: Secretion rates and short-term patterns of gonadotrophin-releasing hormone, FSH and LH in the normal stallion in the breeding season. J. Endocrinol., *117*:197–206, 1988.
30. Alexander, S.L., and Irvine, C.H.G.: Control of onset of breeding season in the mare and its artificial regulation by progesterone treatment. J. Reprod. Fertil. Suppl., *44*:307–319, 1991.
31. Irvine, C.H.G., and Alexander, S.L.: Neuroendocrine control of reproduction in the mare. Proc. Endocrine Soc. Aust., *S7*:1–4, 1989.
32. Clarke, I.J., Thomas, G.B., Yao, B., and Cummins, J.T.: GnRH secretion throughout the ovine estrous cycle. Neuroendocrinology, *46*:82–88, 1987.
33. Clarke, I.J., and Cummins, J.T.: The significance of small pulses of GnRH. J. Endocrinol., *113*:413–418, 1987.
34. Alexander, S.L., and Irvine, C.H.G.: Effect of graded doses of gonadotrophin-releasing hormone on serum LH concentrations in mares in various reproductive states: comparison with endogenously generated LH pulses. J. Endocrinol., *110*:19–26, 1986.
35. Dluzen, D.E., and Ramirez, V.D.: Transient changes in the in vitro activity of the luteinizing hormone releasing hormone pulse generator after ovariectomy in rats. Endocrinology, *118*:1110–1113, 1986.
36. Knobil, E.: The electrophysiology of the GnRH pulse generator in the rhesus monkey. J. Steroid Biochem., *33*:669–671, 1989.
37. Blank, M.S., Fabbri, A., Catt, K.J., and Dufau, M.L.: Inhibition of luteinizing hormone release by morphine and endogenous opiates in cultured pituitary cells. Endocrinology, *118:*2097–2101, 1986.
38. Kalra, S.P., and Kalra, P.S.: Do testosterone and estradiol-17 enforce stimulation or stimulation of luteinizing hormone-releasing hormone secretion. Biol. Reprod., *41*:557–570, 1989.
39. Naylor, A.M., Porter, D.W.F., and Lincoln D.W.: Inhibitory effect of central LHRH on LH secretion in the ovariectomized ewe. Neuroendocrinology, *49*:531–536, 1989.
40. Kesner, J.S., Kaufman, J.-M., Wilson, R.C., and Knobil, E.: On the short-loop feedback regulation of the hypothalamic luteinizing hormone releasing hormone "pulse generator" in the rhesus monkey. Neuroendocrinology, *42*:109–116, 1986.
41. Lengoc, C.M., and Irvine, C.H.G.: Inability to detect LH/hCG receptors in sheep hypothalamus [abstr.]. Proc. Endocrine Soc. Aust., *27*(Suppl.):53, 1984.
42. Harris, J.M., Irvine, C.H.G., and Evans, M.J.: Seasonal changes in serum levels of FSH, LH and testosterone and in semen parameters in stallions. Theriogenology, *19*:311–322, 1983.
43. Morgan, P.J. et al.: Melatonin receptors on ovine pars tuberalis: Characterization and autoradiographical localization. J. Neuroendocrinol. *1*:1–4, 1989.
44. Karsch, F.J., and Wayne, N.L.: Interplay of endogenous rhythms and environmental cues in organizing the seasonal reproductive cycle of the ewe. Proceedings of the Eleventh International Congress on Animal Reproduction and Artificial Insemination. Vol. 5. 1988, pp. 221–227.
45. Lincoln, G.A., Libre, E.A., and Merriam, G.R.: Long term reproductive cycles in rams after pinealectomy or superior cervical ganglionectomy. J. Reprod. Fertil., *85*:687–704, 1989.
46. Irvine, C.H.G., Alexander, S.L., and Hughes, J.P.: Effect of copulation on plasma LH and sex steroid hormone levels in horses. Proceedings of the Tenth International Congress on Animal Reproduction and Artificial Insemination. Vol. 2. 1984, pp. 1–4.
47. Hart, P.J., Squires, E.L., Imel, K.J., and Nett, T.M.: Seasonal variation in hypothalamic content of gonadotropin releasing hormone (GnRH), pituitary receptors for GnRH, and pituitary content of luteinizing hormone and follicle

stimulating hormone in the mare. Biol. Reprod., *30*:1055–1062, 1984.

48. Krause, J.E., Advis, J.P., and McKelvey, J.F.: Characterization of the site of cleavage of luteinizing hormone-releasing hormone under conditions of measurement in which LHRH degradation undergoes physiologically related change. Biochem. Biophys. Res. Commun., *108*:1475–1481, 1982.

49. Nett, T.M., and Adams, T.E.: Further studies on the radioimmunoassay of gonadotrophin-releasing hormone: Effect of radioiodination, antiserum and unextracted serum on levels of immunoreactivity in serum. Endocrinology, *101*:1135–1144, 1977.

50. DeWied, D.: Vasopressin related peptides in behavior. *In* Frontier in Neuroendocrinology. Edited by W.F. Ganong and L. Martini. London, Oxford, pp. 97–140, 1969.

CHAPTER 5

FSH AND LH

S.L. Alexander
C.H.G. Irvine

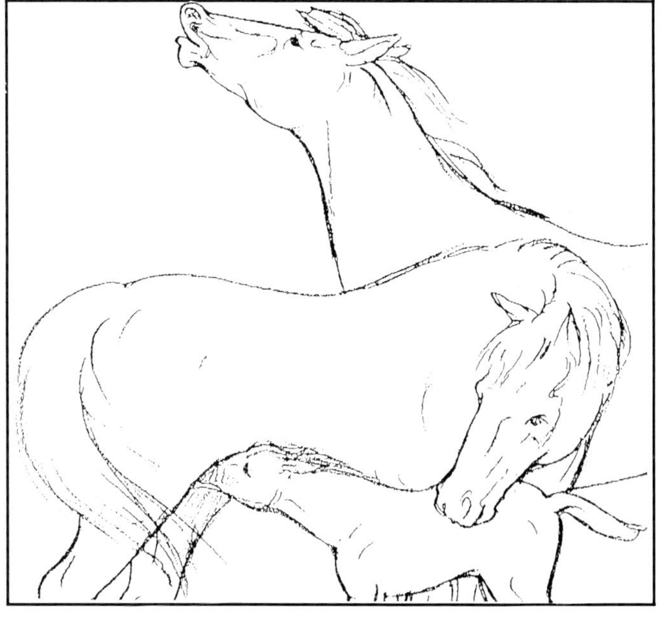

The gonadotropins, follicle-stimulating hormone (FSH), and luteinizing hormone (LH), are considered together in this chapter, because they are structurally similar, are regulated similarly, and work in concert to achieve fertility in both the male and female. These hormones are products of the pars distalis and pars tuberalis of the pituitary.

CHEMISTRY

The gonadotropins, FSH, and LH as well as thyroid-stimulating hormone (TSH) and equine chorionic gonadotropin (eCG) are glycoprotein hormones consisting of two dissimilar subunits, called α and β. The α-subunit is species specific and is essentially identical in all four hormones. By contrast, the β-subunit seems to confer on each hormone its specific biologic function.[1] The subunits are products of separate genes, which in the mouse and human are located on different chromosomes. Consequently, the subunits are synthesized separately within the cell but spontaneously associate to form the entire molecule. The rate-limiting step in production of the gonadotropins seems to be synthesis of the β-subunit. The α-subunit is made in excess and can be secreted, particularly when secretion rate is rapid.[2] However, dissociated subunits have little or no biologic activity.

Equine gonadotropins have been isolated, purified, and sequenced. Early work has shown that the two hormones have approximately the same molecular weight (i.e., 34,000).[3] Both hormones are glycoproteins, each containing about 25% carbohydrate by weight.[4] The terminal sugar on a large number of the carbohydrate side chains of both hormones is sialic acid. Sialic acid, which has a strongly negative charge, affects binding of the hormones to receptors and thus influences both biologic activity and circulatory half-life. Equine LH appears to be unique among mammalian luteinizing hormones in several respects. First, it contains more carbohydrate and is more heavily sialylated than any other species of LH studied. Second, the β-subunit of equine LH is longer than that of other LHs, being extended at the C-terminal by 28 amino acids. This C-terminal extension carries all but one of the carbohydrate side chains attached to the β-subunit and therefore contributes markedly to the overall acidity of the molecule. Studies have shown that the protein structure of the LH β-subunit[5] is identical to that of equine chorionic gonadotropin.[6] As might be expected from this observation, the horse has a single gene coding for this common β-subunit.[7] By contrast, other species that make chorionic gonadotropins, like the human, have evolved separate genes for the β-subunit of their luteotrophic pregnancy hormone. Third, equine LH (like eCG) has been found to have FSH activity in other species,[8] although not in the horse. This anomaly is undoubtedly related to the unique features of equine LH, discussed above, that make the hormone more similar to the FSH of other species than to the luteinizing hormone.

POLYMORPHISM AND SIALIC ACID

Each equine gonadotropin exists in the pituitary as a family of molecular forms that can be separated on the basis of charge[3] (Fig. 5-1). This heterogeneity stems largely from varying degrees of sialylation of carbohydrate side chains.[9–11] When present, sialic acid masks penultimate galactose residues and prevents the hormones from binding to galactose receptors in the liver, thus delaying their degradation. For this reason, equine LH, which contains more sialic acid than LHs of other species, also has a longer circulatory half-life (5 h compared with 25 min for ovine LH, which is not sialylated). The half-life of eCG, the circulating form of which contains even more sialic acid than circulating equine LH, is 6 days.[12] Sialic acid also influences binding of hormones to target tissue receptors. Accordingly, the variously charged isoforms of equine FSH and LH found in the pituitary have been shown to differ in relative receptor binding and in vitro biologic potencies.[9–11] In general, these studies found potency to increase with acidity; however, these results should be interpreted cautiously for two reasons. First, receptor binding and biologic activity were measured in rodent tissues; the isoforms of equine LH may interact differently with equid and nonequid receptors. Second, the absolute amount of hormone present was measured by radioimmunoassay with the assumption that the antibody would have equal affinity for all isoforms. However, this may not be true, because sialic acid can also influence antigenicity of glycoproteins.

This complex question of gonadotropin polymorphism might be of purely academic interest if the various forms of hormone were found only in the pituitary and merely represented various stages in the synthetic process, with just one isoform being secreted. However, in other species circulating gonadotropins have also been found to be polymorphic, with the distribution of isoforms varying with steroid milieu or after gonadotropin-releasing hormone (GnRH) stimulation. Likewise, in the horse, the forms of both circulating LH (Fig. 5-2)[13] and FSH[14] vary during the ovulatory cycle. These observations suggest the gonadotropic signal can vary in both quantity and quality and that the polymorphism of LH and FSH has physiologic relevance. Most importantly, in humans, some cases of infertility have been associated with the presence of abnormal forms of circulating gonadotropins. Therefore, it is important to understand the source and regulation of gonadotropin polymorphism. In the horse, investigation of this question is just beginning. Recent work has shown that the form of LH secreted by mares at estrus is much more alkaline than the bulk of the hormone found in the pituitary (Fig. 5-3).[15] The selection of this form occurs at the instant of secretion as shown by characterization of hormonal isoforms in pituitary venous effluent. The reason that this particular form is chosen for secretion is not known. Because of its alkalinity it is likely to contain less sialic acid and, therefore, have a shorter circulatory half-life than other LH isoforms. Possibly a short-acting LH signal is desired for final follicular maturation. As will be discussed later, both gonadotropins have several physiologic roles, and it may be that the various isoforms subserve these different functions.

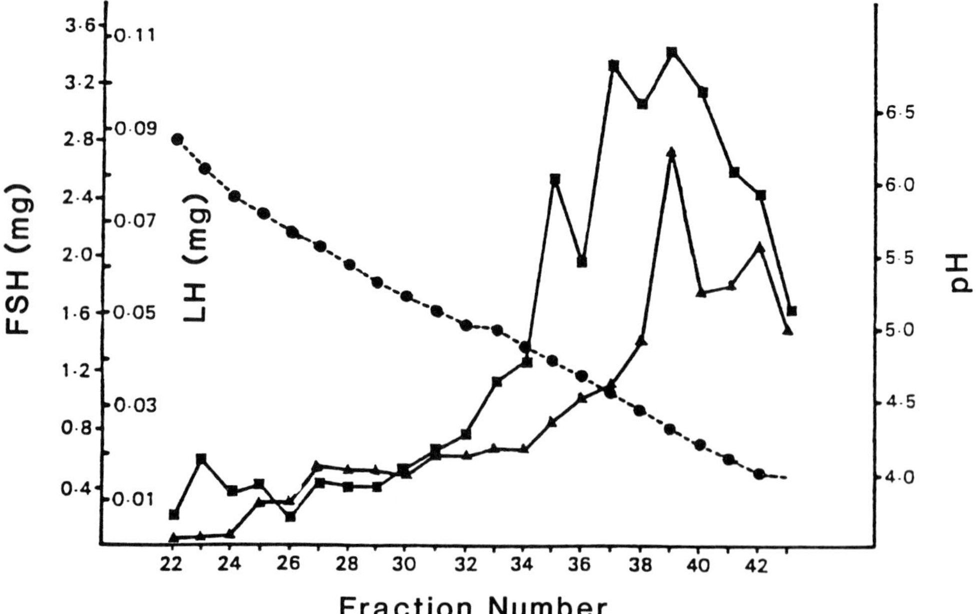

FIG. 5–1. Fractionation of an extract of horse pituitaries using isoelectric focusing, which separates molecules on the basis of their isoelectric point. Molecules that focus at a low pH value are negatively charged at physiologic pH. The charge heterogeneity shown by both gonadotropins is a result of presence of variable amounts of sialic acid on carbohydrate side chains. ● indicates pH, ■ indicates LH as measured by in vitro assay, and ▲ indicates FSH as measured by radioreceptor assay. (Adapted from Irvine, C.H.G.: Kinetics of gonadotrophins in the mare. J. Reprod. Fertil. Suppl., *27*:131–141, 1979.)

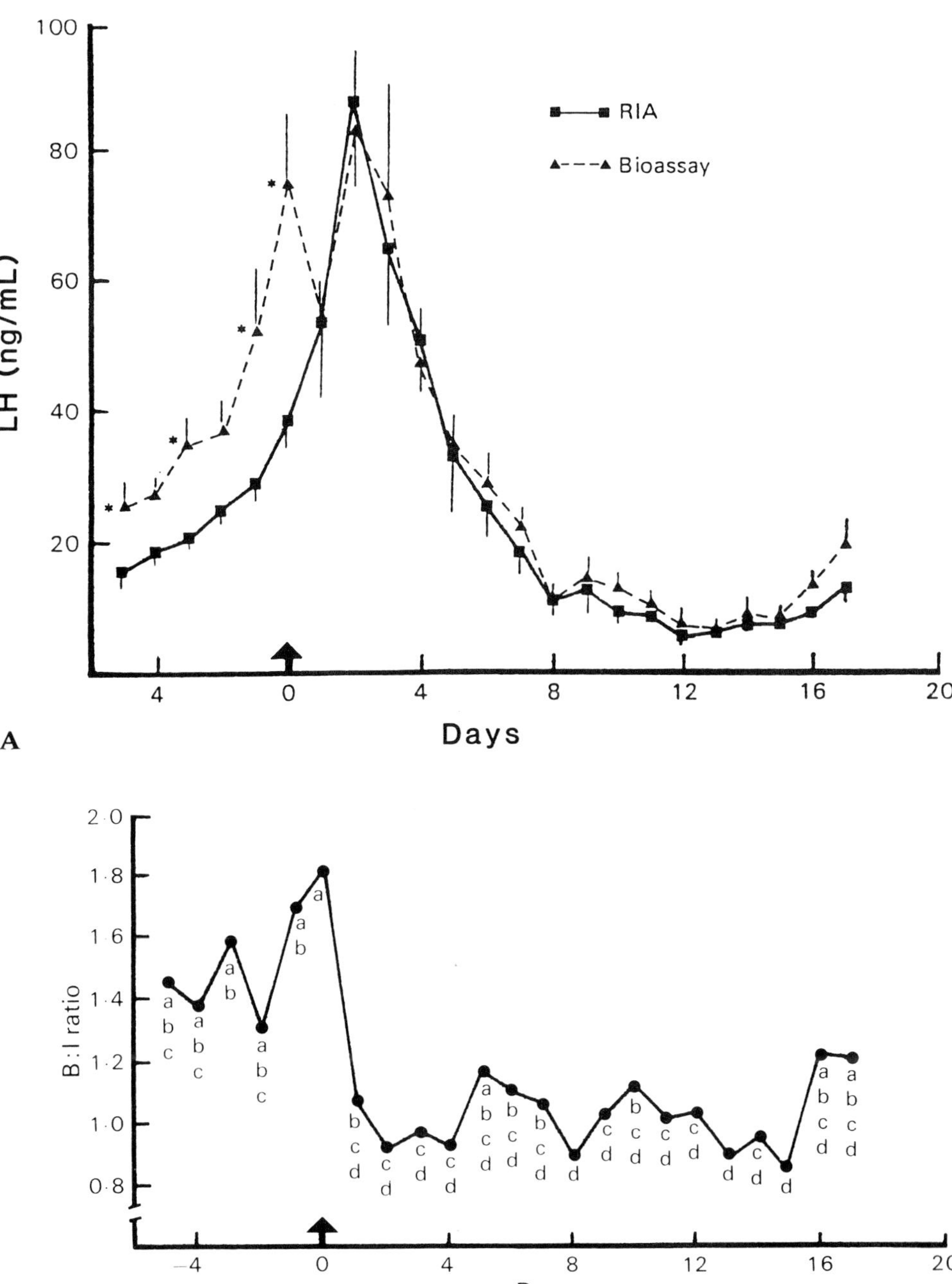

FIG. 5–2. *A,* Mean (± s.e.m.) concentrations of LH measured by radioimmunoassay and in vitro bioassay in jugular blood samples collected daily throughout the ovulatory cycle from eight mares. Day O is day of ovulation. Values with a * are significantly different from corresponding immunoassay values ($p < .05$). *B,* Geometric mean ratios of biologic to immunologic (B:I) LH activity in serum of eight mares throughout the ovulatory cycle. Values without a common subscript are significantly different ($p < .01$). Because the different isoforms of LH differ in relative potency in radioimmunoassay and in vitro bioassay, the changes in the B:I ratio throughout the ovulatory cycle provide indirect evidence that the forms of LH in circulation have also changed. (From Alexander, S.L., and Irvine, C.H.G.: Radioimmunoassay and in vitro bioassay of serum LH throughout the equine oestrous cycle. J. Reprod. Fertil., Suppl., *32*:253–260, 1982.)

PATTERNS THROUGHOUT THE OVULATORY CYCLE OF THE MARE

In the early 1970s radioimmunoassays were developed to measure equine LH[16] and FSH[17] and profiles of these hormones were measured in jugular blood samples collected daily throughout the ovulatory cycle. For LH, concentrations are low during the midluteal phase, but rise in a prolonged ovulatory surge beginning a few days before the onset of estrus, peaking usually on the day after ovulation and returning gradually over several days to midluteal phase values. Thus the ovulatory

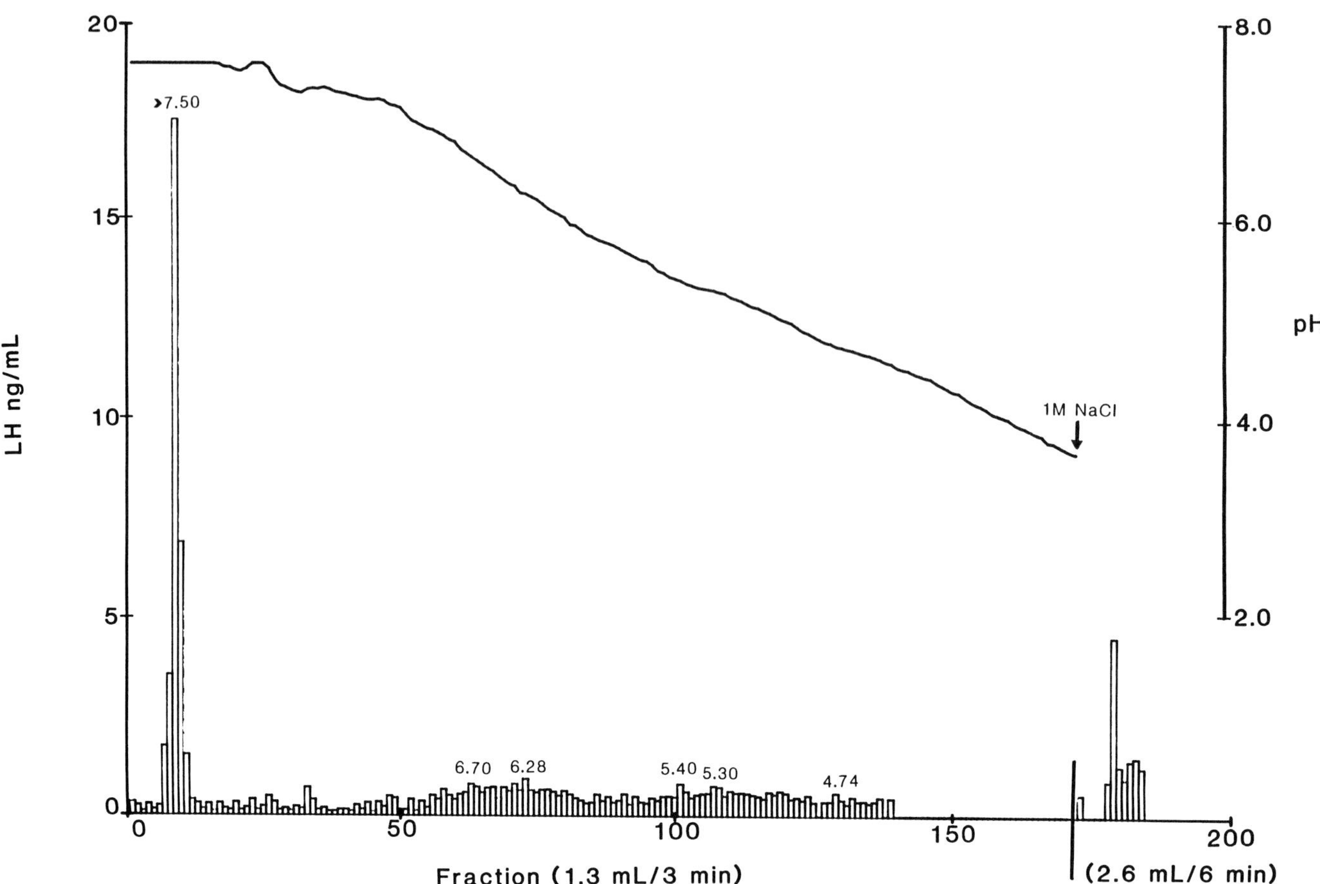

FIG. 5–3. Fractionation of pituitary venous plasma using chromatofocusing, a technique similar to isoelectric focusing, which separates molecules on the basis of their isoelectric point. The pituitary venous blood focused was collected from an estrous mare. Over 80% of the LH in the sample had just been secreted as assessed by the concentration gradient between pituitary venous and jugular blood. Notice that in contrast to pituitary extract (Fig. 5-1) the majority of LH in pituitary venous plasma focuses above a pH value of 6. (Adapted from Shand, N., Alexander, S.L., and Irvine, C.H.G.: Comparison of the microheterogenicity of horse LH and FSH in the pituitary with that secreted into pituitary venous blood at oestrus. J. Reprod. Fertil. Suppl., *44*:1–11, 1991.)

surge can last well over a week, which is uniquely long compared with other studied mammals. Unlike LH, FSH shows a biphasic profile during the cycle, with surges at 10- to 12-day intervals. One surge occurs at or just after ovulation and the second during mid- to late luteal phase, approximately 10 days before the next ovulation. In early estrus, FSH concentrations reach their lowest value in the cycle. As can be seen, the gonadotropins can be secreted differentially, as in early estrus (FSH falling and LH rising) and the midluteal phase (FSH rising and LH low). The regulation of this differential secretion will be discussed below.

MODE OF SECRETION

Early workers assumed that the gonadotropins were secreted continuously so that daily blood samples would be adequate to define the pituitary signal to the gonads. However, studies in other species have shown that LH appears in peripheral blood in distinct pulses, the frequency of which is slow in the luteal phase and rapid in the follicular phase. These pulses are thought to reflect the mode of GnRH secretion (see Chapter 4). Subsequently, in the mare, frequent blood sampling has revealed distinct LH and FSH pulses during the luteal phase[18] (Fig. 5-4), seasonal acyclicity, and the transitional period into the breeding season.[19,20] During these times, pulse frequency is slow (approximately one to five pulses per day). More than 90% of FSH and LH pulses occur coincidentally. From sampling jugular blood, it has not been possible to demonstrate convincingly pulsatile gonadotropin secretion during the ovulatory surge.[21] Even when jugular blood is collected at 5-min intervals, pulses cannot be unequivocally identified, although low-amplitude fluctuations (approximately 30% peak increase) have been described as occurring every 45 to 60 min (Fig. 5-5).[18] However, measurement of FSH and LH in pituitary venous blood shows beyond doubt that secretion is pulsatile during

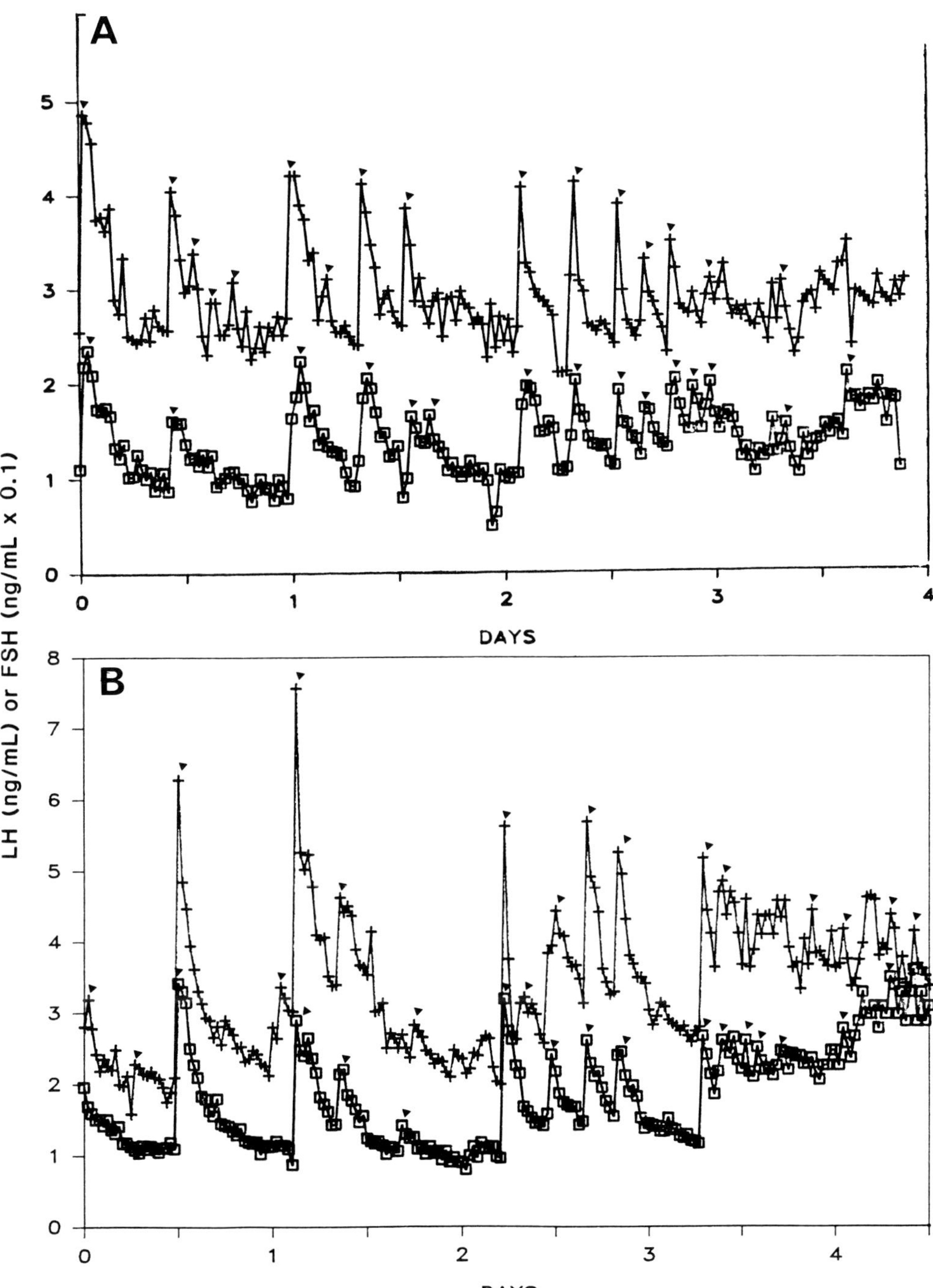

FIG. 5–4. Concentrations of LH (□) and FSH (+) in jugular blood samples collected from two mares every 30 min for approximately 4 days beginning 14 to 15 days after ovulation. During this period, the mare Dolly *(B)* lysed her corpus luteum, causing progesterone levels to fall so that she was in estrus at the end of the experiment. By contrast, in the mare Big Red *(A)*, progesterone levels showed only a transient decline, and she did not return to estrus. Pulses of LH and FSH are marked with arrowheads.

the ovulatory surge, with gonadotropin pulses occurring synchronously at a frequency that increases from every 2 h to twice per hour just before ovulation (Fig. 5-6).[22] The most likely reason that pulses cannot be detected in peripheral blood is that the long circulatory half-life of the gonadotropins maintains a large peripheral pool when secretion rate is rapid, which serves to dampen individual pulses. Collection of pituitary venous blood has also been useful in demonstrating pulsatile LH and FSH secretion in sexually active stallions in the breeding season.[23] An interesting aspect of these highly stimulated states in both the mare and the stal-

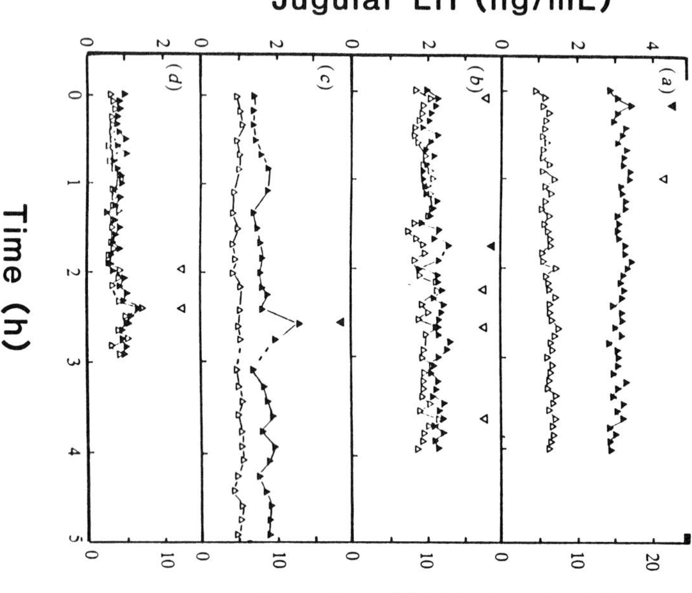

FIG. 5–5. Concentrations of LH (▲) and FSH (△) in jugular blood samples collected from four mares (*a–d*) every 5 to 10 min for 3 to 5 h early in estrus. Pulses of LH and FSH are marked with arrowheads; however, few gonadotropin pulses could be identified. (From Alexander, S.L., and Irvine, C.H.G.: Secretion rates and short-term patterns of gonadotrophin-releasing hormone, FSH and LH throughout the periovulatory period in the mare. J. Endocrinol., *114*:351–362, 1987.)

lion is that gonadotropin secretion appears to continue between pulses. Thus pulses are superimposed on a background of tonic secretion.

CONTROL OF SECRETION

In the horse, secretion of both LH and FSH is stimulated by GnRH, a decapeptide produced by the hypothalamus, and has been shown by administering GnRH to horses.[24,25] Furthermore, active immunization of mares against GnRH results in significant decreases in the gonadotropins.[26] GnRH can be measured in pituitary venous blood, and pulses of GnRH do occur coincidentally with gonadotropin pulses in periovulatory mares and sexually active stallions.

Gonadotropin-releasing hormone binds to specific receptors in the membrane of the gonadotrope, which may secrete both gonadotropins. Cells containing both LH and FSH have been identified in rat pituitaries; however, cells containing either FSH or LH are also observed. The number of cell types responsible for synthesizing FSH and LH in the horse is unknown. The availability of free receptors can be a limiting factor in response, although additional receptors can be induced by estradiol and by low concentrations of GnRH itself. By contrast, exposure to continuous or high concentrations of GnRH is deleterious because this down regulates or uses up receptors. The postreceptor-transduction mechanism also seems to be disrupted by such treatment, and eventually gonadotropin secretion is inhibited by the very signal that originally stimulated the response.[27] This phenomenon of down regulation may have evolved to protect the cell from exhaustion in the event of repetitive stimulation.[27] The phenomenon should be remembered when developing GnRH administration regimens. However, the horse may be more resistant to GnRH receptor down regulation than other species, because ovulation has been induced by GnRH treatments at dose rates that would be contraceptive in humans.[28]

Synthesis of the gonadotropins is also stimulated by gonadotropin-releasing hormone. Within seconds of receptor binding, calcium is mobilized within the gonadotrope, possibly by influx of extracellular calcium,[29] and this ion appears to be the initial intracellular carrier of the GnRH signal. Receptor binding also leads to changes in phospholipid metabolism within the cell, with accumulation of diacylglycerol, which activates the phosphorylating enzyme protein kinase C. Contrary to earlier theories, cyclic adenosine monophosphate (cAMP) is not directly involved in transducing the GnRH signal within the cell.[27] Other work suggests that the message conveyed by these two intracellular pathways may differ, with the initial rise in intracellular calcium signaling gonadotropin secretion, which is immediate, and the protein kinase C path signaling synthesis, which is delayed.[29]

DIFFERENTIAL FSH AND LH SECRETION

Secretion of GnRH is pulsatile (see Chapter 4), and modulation of pulse frequency can signal to the pituitary to release preferentially FSH or LH, independently from any feedback from the gonads. In ovariectomized monkeys and sheep, in which the hypothalamic input to the pituitary has been destroyed, replacement of GnRH pulses at a high frequency (e.g., hourly) and results in a greater rise in LH than in FSH concentrations.[30,31] Conversely, a slow frequency of stimulation (e.g., one GnRH pulse every 3 to 4 h) favors FSH secretion.[30,31] In the mare, similar results have been obtained with GnRH treatments during seasonal acyclicity, when LH and FSH pulse frequency are profoundly suppressed and the ovaries can be very small and inactive. Under these conditions, GnRH pulses given every 45 min cause predominantly LH secretion, whereas GnRH pulses given every 6 h increase FSH secretion.[28] Measurement of GnRH and the gonadotropins in pituitary venous blood from stallions shows that when the interval between gonadotropin pulses falls below 30 min, there is a significant reduction in amplitude of the second FSH, but not the second LH, pulse.[23] The intracellular basis for this difference between FSH and LH responses to GnRH stimulation is unknown. In sheep, however, a greater proportion of pituitary content of FSH than of LH is released per day, and the release of FSH may be more closely related to the rate of synthesis

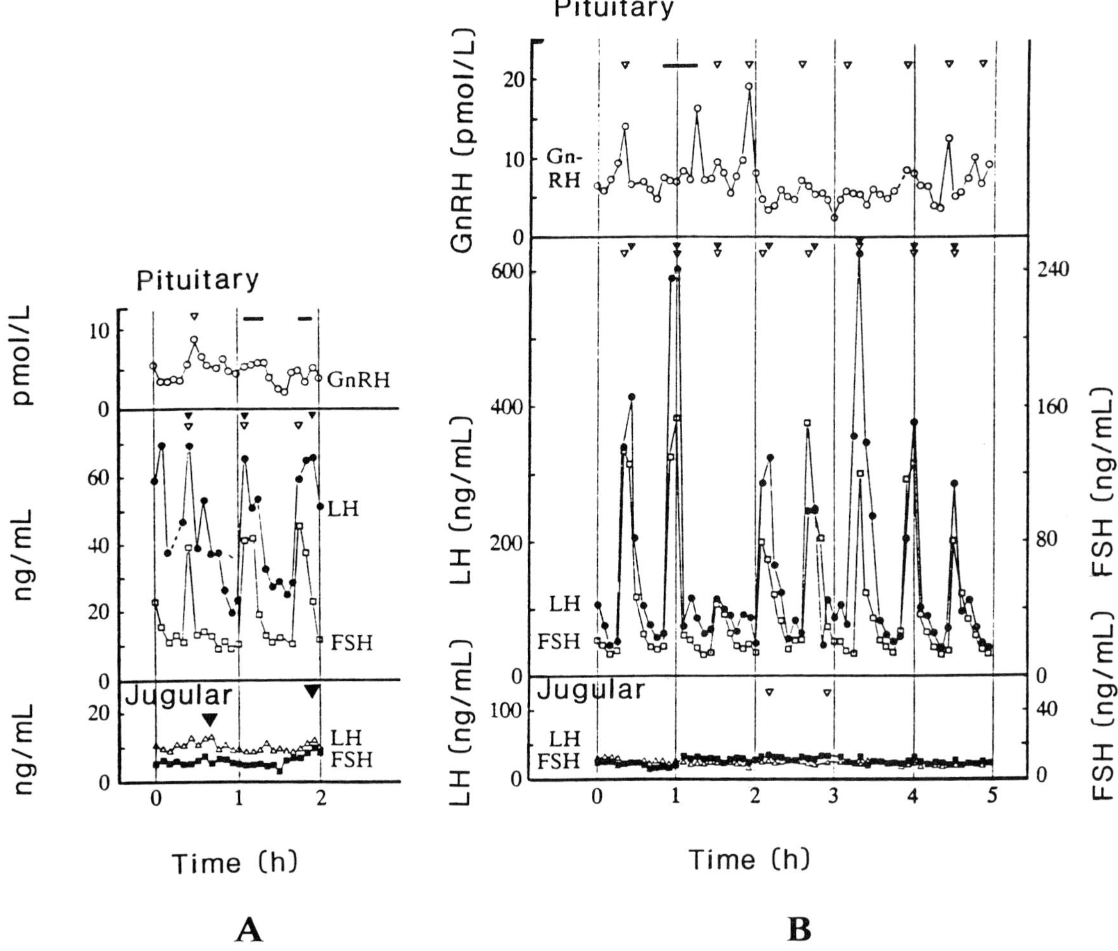

FIG. 5–6. Concentrations of GnRH, LH, and FSH in pituitary venous blood, and of LH and FSH in concurrent jugular blood samples collected every 5 min for 2 to 5 h from a mare on: A, the day before ovulation and B, the day of ovulation. Pulses of GnRH and FSH are marked by open arrowheads and LH by solid arrowheads. Horizontal bars indicate prolonged secretory episodes. (From Alexander, S.L., and Irvine, C.H.G.: Secretion rates and short-term patterns of gonadotrophin-releasing hormone, FSH and LH throughout the periovulatory period in the mare. J. Endocrinol., *114*:351–362, 1987.)

than that of luteinizing hormone.[32,33] If this is the case, it might be easier to exhaust the releasable pool of FSH than that of LH by repeated GnRH stimulation.[32] Thus in the mare, periods of differential FSH and LH secretion during the normal ovulatory cycle may be explained, at least in part, by changes in frequency of stimulation. During estrus, GnRH pulse rate increases to a maximum frequency of two per hour as measured in pituitary venous blood.[22] At that time, LH rises and FSH is suppressed. Conversely, in the midluteal phase, gonadotropin pulses occur approximately twice daily. Preliminary measurements of GnRH in pituitary venous blood show that pulse rate is lower at that time than during the periovulatory surge; however, the decline in GnRH frequency is not as great as that in gonadotropin frequency, and a large percentage of GnRH pulses are not effective in stimulating gonadotropin release.[34] Similarly, in the portal blood of sheep, ineffective, or "silent," GnRH pulses occur.[35] It is thought that these silent pulses may be important in inducing gonadotropin synthesis or GnRH receptors. In any case, in the luteal-phase mare, GnRH pulse frequency is reduced, and at that time, FSH is elevated whereas LH remains low.

GONADAL HORMONE FEEDBACK

Changes in GnRH pulse frequency are not the only means by which LH and FSH may be differentially regulated. Gonads produce both steroid and protein hormones; the most widely studied of these in the mare are the steroids estradiol (E_2) and progesterone and the protein hormone inhibin. These hormones act at either the hypothalamus or pituitary to influence gonadotropin secretion.

Progesterone is produced by the corpus luteum. Concentrations of the hormone rise after ovulation, and high levels are maintained until approximately 3 days before estrus, when the corpus luteum is lysed. In the sheep, progesterone acts at the hypothalamus[36] to slow GnRH pulse frequency and does not affect responsiveness of the pituitary to GnRH stimulation. In ovariectomized mares, progesterone administration suppresses LH levels, as assessed by daily blood samples, in the breeding season but not in the nonbreeding season.[37] The reason for this seasonal difference in response may be that LH levels in ovariectomized mares are high in the breeding season because LH pulse frequency is rapid (approximately 13 pulses per day).[38] Suppression of pulse frequency by progesterone at that time would result in a readily measured drop in mean LH levels.

By contrast, LH levels in the ovariectomized mare in the nonbreeding season are low because pulse frequency is slow (approximately 1 pulse per day).[38] The effect of any additional suppression of pulse frequency by progesterone on mean LH levels, which are already profoundly lowered, might be difficult to detect. Like LH, FSH levels in ovariectomized mares in the nonbreeding season are not altered by progesterone treatment. However, in the breeding season, FSH levels in ovariectomized mares are raised, although not to the point of statistical significance, by progesterone.[37] Likewise, FSH levels in mares in shallow acyclicity can be elevated by treatment with the synthetic progestagen allyl trenbolone.[39,40] These effects are probably mediated through a drop in GnRH pulse frequency, which increases the FSH to LH concentration ratio, as discussed above.

Estradiol is produced by the maturing ovarian follicle. In the mare concentrations are exceedingly low (2 to 15 pg/mL), and thus strain the measuring ability of even the best assays. As best as can be determined, estradiol begins to increase 6 to 8 days before ovulation (i.e., approximately at the start of estrus) rising progressively to peak about 2 days before ovulation. Low luteal-phase values are regained within a day or two after ovulation.[41] In other species, the effect of E_2 on LH and FSH secretion is complex and depends on the concentration attained and the duration of exposure. High E_2 concentrations initially inhibit LH, but then trigger an ovulatory LH surge. Most work suggests that the inhibitory effect of E_2 is exerted at the gonadotrope, because the amount of LH secreted per pulse is reduced but pulse rate is not altered during the negative-feedback phase. Correspondingly, LH responses to exogenous GnRH are also initially decreased by E_2 administration. The pulse frequency of GnRH in portal blood of sheep is not initially suppressed by E_2 treatment;[35,42] however, long-term treatment may eventually do so.[36] In many species, ovariectomy results in chronically elevated LH levels, which can be normalized by E_2 replacement. Paradoxically, in the rat these events do not seem to involve the anticipated changes in GnRH secretion. Ovariectomy is accompanied by a fall in net GnRH secretion rate, and E_2 therapy, although restoring LH to intact values, does not affect GnRH secretion patterns.[43] By contrast, there is no doubt that E_2 acts at the hypothalamus to trigger an ovulatory surge, because this effect can be blocked by disconnecting the hypothalamus from the pituitary,[44] and an increase in GnRH concentrations can be measured in portal blood accompanying the E_2-induced LH surge in anestrous ewes.[42] Low concentrations of E_2 seem to increase both LH and FSH secretion, possibly by inducing GnRH receptors or gonadotropin synthesis. Estradiol can also affect the heterogeneity of luteinizing hormone. The exact nature of this effect is controversial and it may vary with sex and species. In general, E_2 seems to favor synthesis and secretion of more alkaline LH isoforms.

In the mare, unlike other species, E_2 administration does not lead to an ovulatory LH surge nor does it cause marked LH suppression. Long-term treatment of ovariectomized mares with E_2 raises LH levels for the duration of treatment in both the breeding and nonbreeding seasons.[37] There is some evidence that E_2 in concert with GnRH can influence the form of circulating LH in the mare. Treatment of seasonally acyclic mares with E_2 followed by hourly pulses of GnRH results in a sustained increase in the relative in vitro biologic activity of plasma-luteinizing hormone.[45] Treatment with either hormone alone does not alter LH bioactivity in seasonally acyclic mares.[45] The combined E_2-GnRH treatment was designed to mimic hormonal events during the periovulatory period when the relative bioactivity of plasma LH increases.[13] Results suggest that the interaction between E_2 and GnRH may produce this normal increase in bioactivity.

Effects of E_2 on FSH have not been investigated as thoroughly as has LH in other species, possibly because satisfactory assays for FSH have been more difficult to develop, particularly in sheep. It is generally agreed that administration of E_2 suppresses FSH in women, monkeys, and sheep.[32] Similarly, immunization of sheep against E_2 raises FSH and increases follicular development. This is used as a technique for superovulation in this species. In the ovariectomized mare, contradictory FSH results have been obtained with E_2 treatment. Some workers have found no effect of E_2 on FSH either in the breeding or nonbreeding season,[37] whereas others have found FSH suppression as observed in other species.[46]

Inhibin is a large (molecular weight 32,000) glycosylated protein consisting of two subunits linked by disulfide bridges. It is synthesized by the granulosa cells of developing follicles and is secreted into follicular fluid, but can also be measured in peripheral blood. Inhibin specifically inhibits FSH synthesis and basal secretion and blocks the response of both gonadotropins to GnRH stimulation. The production of inhibin is stimulated by FSH, thereby forming a tight feedback circuit. Inhibin was initially believed to be the principal inhibitor of FSH secretion. If this were the case, plasma inhibin and FSH concentrations might be expected to be inversely correlated. However, some evidence from sheep shows that during the follicular phase FSH and inhibin fall in parallel, while E_2 rises.[47] Furthermore, in both sheep and women, inhibin increases at the time of the preovulatory FSH surge.[32] These results are not surprising when it is considered that inhibin secretion depends on FSH stimulation. However, this relationship makes it likely that inhibin acts together with some other factor, probably E_2, to suppress FSH during the follicular phase.

Inhibin has not been purified from equine follicular fluid, so its structure is unknown. However, equine follicular fluid contains a proteinaceous substance that when administered to mares depresses FSH.[48] Furthermore, equine follicular fluid is very potent in a specific radioimmunoassay for ovine inhibin.[34] Inhibin-like activity can also be measured in mare jugular plasma. In the midluteal phase, pulses of FSH are followed by pulses of inhibin, suggesting that FSH stimulates inhibin production as in other species. During the periovulatory period, inhibin and FSH concentrations are positively correlated,[34] as observed in sheep. On the day following ovulation, there is a dramatic rise in plasma inhibin levels that is possibly the result of expulsion of inhibin-rich follicular fluid into the peritoneal cavity at ovulation, with the subsequent absorption of inhibin. These results suggest that in the mare, as in the sheep and women, inhibin may not be the sole inhibitor of FSH, but may act synergistically with estradiol.

FUNCTIONS OF FSH AND LH

The gonadotropins exert their effects by binding to specific ovarian receptors, which leads to activation of the membrane-bound enzyme adenylyl cyclase and thence to increased production of the intracellular messenger cAMP (see Chapter 3). It is possible that the gonadotropins may also be translocated into target cells where LH is able to stimulate the enzyme glucose-6-phosphate dehydrogenase, which provides NADPH for steroid hydroxylation and other biosynthetic purposes.[49] Luteinizing hormone also may activate RNA polymerases.[49]

Cyclic ovarian function depends totally on the gonadotropins, because removal of the pituitary results in loss of fertility with arrest of the ovaries in a juvenile state. Growth of preovulatory follicles, ovulation, and the establishment of a corpus luteum can only be restored by replacing both gonadotropins.

Receptors for FSH are found mainly on the granulosa cells in ovarian follicles. Small, preantral follicles have only FSH receptors, and they respond to FSH stimulation by producing progesterone, which under most circumstances is rapidly metabolized to androstenedione.[50] Under the influence of FSH, granulosa cells proliferate rapidly. In preantral follicles, receptors for LH are confined to the thecal cells and other types of ovarian interstitial cell. However, after antrum formation, LH receptors also appear on granulosa cells. Both antrum formation and the induction of LH receptors require the presence of FSH and estradiol.[51] As the follicle matures, thecal and granulosa cells cooperate to secrete estradiol. In response to LH, thecal cells produce androgens that are aromatized to estrogens by the granulosa cells. Activity of aromatase, the aromatizing enzyme, is induced by FSH, as is secretion of inhibin, as discussed earlier. Follicle-stimulating hormone is also involved in increasing follicular vascularity. Improved circulation helps serve the follicle's rising metabolic demands and allows steroidal products (e.g., estradiol) to escape into the bloodstream. Surprisingly, FSH has a role in ovulation through inducing granulosa cells to secrete tissue plasminogen activator into follicular fluid. This enzyme converts plasminogen, which is found in follicular fluid and is presumably derived from plasma, into plasmin, which is a protease. Exposure of follicular wall strips to plasmin weakens their tensile strength, and this may be a mechanism involved in follicular wall rupture at ovulation.

In the mare, follicles can develop up to 1 cm in diameter without pituitary hormones. However, further development to 2.5 to 3 cm in diameter depends on follicle-stimulating hormone. The presumptive ovulatory follicle can be identified in mare ovaries by several markers, including an increased number of LH receptors in the granulosa cell layer and high follicular fluid estradiol concentrations.[52] Ovulatory follicles are also more vascular and, by estrus, are the largest follicle present in the ovaries.[52] Most of these characteristics are FSH dependent. Accordingly, seasonally acyclic mares can be induced to develop preovulatory follicles by twice daily administration of a crude pituitary extract containing equine FSH and LH, but not by an LH-like substance alone (human chorionic gonadotropin).[53] Furthermore, if FSH is administered to mares in the late-luteal phase–early estrus, at the time when FSH levels decline in the normal cycle, induction of multiple preovulatory follicles ensues.[54] However, these follicles do not ovulate. It may be that LH is needed for this to occur or that crowding at the ovulation fossa blocks ovulation from occurring. These observations on raising FSH concentrations suggest that the FSH nadir early in estrus is important in selecting a single follicle for ovulation. Data on follicular development in the mare[17] have been interpreted as showing that the rise in FSH occurring around the time of ovulation accelerates development of a group of small, preantral follicles. One of these is subsequently "primed" by the late-luteal phase FSH surge to provide the next ovulatory follicle, while the remaining follicles in the cohort become atretic. Apparently these follicles can be rescued by prolonging the late-luteal phase FSH surge.

Final follicular maturation and ovulation are thought to require luteinizing hormone. Steroidogenesis is stimulated by LH by enhancing the conversion of cholesterol esters to pregnenolone. In other species, it has been shown that just before ovulation, LH induces the granulosa cells to switch from making estradiol as the final product to progesterone. In the periovulatory follicle, progesterone becomes the predominant steroid in follicular fluid. This switch in steroidogenesis is important for ovulation, which is blocked by administration of the steroid hormone synthesis inhibitor cyanoketone. In the mare, however, this switch has not been demonstrated. The major steroid in equine follicular fluid from the presumptive ovulatory follicle is estradiol.[52] The exact mechanism by which LH acts to cause ovulation is unknown. It can stimulate prostaglandin production by granulosa cells, and in the rat, administration of the prostaglandin synthethase inhibitor indomethacin can block ovulation. Luteinizing hormone can also stimulate histamine release from cells in the ovarian stroma, and this may contribute to increased capillary permeability in the thecal layer and hyperemia observed before ovulation. Luteinizing hormone is also essential for formation and maintenance of the corpus luteum. However, normal function of the corpus luteum also depends on adequate follicular maturation before ovulation, which relies in turn on appropriate priming by follicle-stimulating hormone.

In the mare, the role of LH in final follicular maturation and ovulation is supported by the following observation: The rate of development of the preovulatory follicle accelerates 3 to 6 days before ovulation when plasma FSH is falling, while LH is rising. At this time, administration of an antiserum against a crude gonadotropin preparation inhibits both follicular development and ovulation.[55] Conversely, treatment with an LH-like substance (human chorionic gonadotropin) shortens time to ovulation, possibly by increasing follicular maturation rate. Finally, when the periovulatory LH rise is suppressed by progesterone administration, follicles develop to approximately 3 cm in diameter but have a low frequency of ovulation.[56] On the other hand, the importance of an LH surge in inducing ovulation has been questioned by recent research in which the LH surge was blocked by desensitizing the pituitary to GnRH stimulation by administering massive doses of a potent GnRH analogue.[57] Two of four treated mares ovulated despite the absence of any LH rise.[57] Furthermore, ovulation can occur in the luteal phase when LH concentrations are relatively low.[58] These intriguing observations warrant further study. In neither situation is LH suppressed to immeasurably low levels, and it is possible that although LH is necessary for ovulation, in some mares, a marked surge of the hormone is not required. Alternatively, in the mare, LH may not have as precise a relationship to ovulation as is observed in other species.[57] The role of LH in corpus luteum establishment and maintenance in the mare is supported by the tight coupling of LH and progesterone pulses early in the luteal phase. However, other workers have not confirmed this observation.[59] On the other hand, antibodies to a crude gonadotropin preparation when given to mares at various times during the luteal phase reduce the weight of the corpus luteum, which macroscopically appears to be regressing.[60]

Because LH and, to a lesser extent, FSH have a range of actions, and, as discussed earlier, also circulate in several different forms, it is tempting to speculate that each form subserves a different function. However, this hypothesis requires further investigation.

REFERENCES

1. Pierce, J.C., and Parsons, T.F.: Glycoprotein hormones: Structure and function. Annu. Rev. Biochem., *50*:465–495, 1981.
2. Hagan, C., McNatty, K.P., and McNeilly, A.S.: Immunoreactive and subunits of luteinizing hormone in human peripheral blood and follicular fluid throughout the menstrual cycle, and their effect on the secretion rate of progesterone by human granulosa cells in culture. J. Endocrinol., *69*:33–46, 1976.
3. Braselton, W.E., and McShan, W.H., Jr.: Purification and properties of follicle-stimulating and luteinizing hormones from horse pituitary glands. Arch. Biochem. Biophys., *139*:45–58, 1970.
4. Landefeld, T.D., and McShan, W.H., Jr.: Equine luteinizing hormone and its subunits. Isolation and physicochemical properties. Biochemistry, *13*:1389–1393, 1974.
5. Bousfield, G.R., Liu, W.-K., Sugino, H., and Ward, D.N.: Structural studies on equine glycoprotein hormones; Amino acid sequence of equine lutropin β subunit. J. Biol. Chem., *262*:8610–8617, 1987.
6. Sugino, H., Bousfield, G.R., Moore, W.T., and Ward, D.N.: Structural studies on equine glycoprotein hormones: Amino acid sequence of equine chorionic gonadotropin β subunit. J. Biol. Chem., *262*:8603–8609, 1987.
7. Stewart, F., and Maher, J.K.: Analysis of horse and donkey gonadotrophin genes using Southern blotting and DNA hybridization techniques. J. Reprod. Fertil. Suppl., *44*:19–26, 1991.
8. Licht, P., et al.: Biological and binding activities of equine pituitary gonadotrophins and pregnant mare serum gonadotrophin. J. Endocrinol., *83*:311–322, 1979.
9. Irvine, C.H.G.: Kinetics of gonadotrophins in the mare. J. Reprod. Fertil. Suppl., *27*:131–141, 1979.
10. Matteri, R.L., and Papkoff, H.: Characterization of equine luteinizing hormone by chromatofocusing. Biol. Reprod., *36*:262–269, 1987.
11. Matteri, R.L. and Papkoff, H.: Microheterogeneity of equine follicle-stimulating hormone. Biol. Reprod., *38*:324–331, 1988.
12. Catchpole, H.R., Cole, H.H., and Pearson, R.B.: Studies on the rate of disappearance and fate of mare gonadotropic hormone following intravenous injection. Am. J. Physiol., *112*:21–26, 1935.
13. Alexander, S.L., and Irvine, C.H.G.: Radioimmunoassay and in-vitro bioassay of serum LH throughout the equine oestrous cycle. J. Reprod. Fertil. Suppl., *32*:253–260, 1982.
14. Alexander, S.L., Irvine, C.H.G., and Turner, J.E.: Comparison by three different radioimmunoassay systems of the polymorphism of plasma FSH in mares in various reproductive states. J. Reprod. Fertil. Suppl., *35*:9–18, 1987.
15. Shand, N., Alexander, S.L., and Irvine, C.H.G.: Comparison of the microheterogenicity of horse LH and FSH in the pituitary with that secreted into pituitary venous blood at oestrus. J. Reprod. Fertil. Suppl., *44*:1–11, 1991.
16. Whitmore, H.L., Wentworth, B.C., and Ginther, O.J.: Circulating concentrations of luteinizing hormone during oestrous cycles of mares as determined by radioimmunoassay. Am. J. Vet. Res., *34*:631–636, 1973.
17. Evans, M.J., and Irvine, C.H.G.: Serum concentrations of FSH, LH and progesterone during the oestrous cycle and early pregnancy in the mare. J. Reprod. Fertil. Suppl., *23*:193–200, 1975.
18. Alexander, S.L., and Irvine, C.H.G.: Effect of graded doses of gonadotrophin-releasing hormone on serum LH concentrations in mares in various reproductive states: Comparison with endogenously generated pulses. J. Endocrinol., *110*:19–26, 1986.
19. Fitzgerald, B.P., et al.: Changes in LH pulse frequency and

amplitude in intact mares during the transition into the breeding season. J. Reprod. Fertil., *79*:485–493, 1987.

20. Alexander, S.L., and Irvine, C.H.G.: Control of onset of breeding season in the mare and its artificial regulation by progesterone treatment. J. Reprod. Fertil. Suppl., *44*:307–319, 1991.

21. Fitzgerald, B.P., I'Anson, H., Legan, S.J., and Loy, R.G.: Changes in patterns of luteinizing hormone secretion before and after the first ovulation in the postpartum mare. Biol. Reprod., *33*:316–323, 1985.

22. Alexander, S.L., and Irvine, C.H.G.: Secretion rates and short-term patterns of gonadotrophin-releasing hormone, FSH and LH throughout the periovulatory period in the mare. J. Endocrinol., *114*:351–362, 1987.

23. Irvine, C.H.G., and Alexander, S.L.: Secretion rates and short-term patterns of gonadotrophin-releasing hormone, FSH and LH in the normal stallion in the breeding season. J. Endocrinol., *117*:197–206, 1988.

24. Evans, M.J., and Irvine, C.H.G.: Measurement of equine FSH and LH: Response of anestrous mares to gonadotropin-releasing hormone. Biol. Reprod., *15*:477–484, 1976.

25. Evans, M.J., and Irvine, C.H.G.: Induction of follicular development, maturation and ovulation by gonadotropin releasing hormone administration to acyclic mares. Biol. Reprod., *16*:452–462, 1977.

26. Garza, F., Jr., et al.: Active immunization of intact mares against gonadotropin-releasing hormone: differential effects on secretion of luteinizing hormone and follicle-stimulating hormone. Biol. Reprod., *35*:347–352, 1986.

27. Clayton, R.N.: Gonadotrophin-releasing hormone: Its actions and receptors. J. Endocrinol., *120*:11–19, 1989.

28. Turner, J.E., and Irvine, C.H.G.: The effect of various gonadotrophin-releasing hormone regimens on gonadotrophins, follicular growth and ovulation in deeply anoestrous mares. J. Reprod. Fertil. Suppl., *44*:213–225, 1991.

29. Conn, P.M., McArdle, C.A., Andrews, W.V., and Huckle, W.R.: The molecular basis of gonadotropin-releasing hormone (GnRH) action in the pituitary gonadotrope. Biol. Reprod., *36*:17–35, 1987.

30. Pohl, C.R., et al.: Hypophysiotropic signal frequency and the functioning of the pituitary-ovarian system in the rhesus monkey. Endocrinology, *112*:2076–2080, 1983.

31. Clarke, I.J., et al.: Effects on plasma luteinizing hormone and follicle-stimulating hormone of varying the frequency and amplitude of gonadotropin-releasing hormone pulses in ovariectomized ewes with hypothalamo-pituitary disconnection. Neuroendocrinology, *39*:214–221, 1984.

32. McNeilly, A.S.: The control of FSH secretion. Acta Endocrinol. (Copenh), *119*(Suppl. 288):31–40, 1988.

33. Chappel, S.C., Ulloa-Aguirre, A., and Coutifaris, C.: Biosynthesis and secretion of follicle-stimulating hormone. Endocr. Rev., *4*:179–212, 1983.

34. Irvine, C.H.G., and Alexander, S.L.: Neuroendocrine control of reproduction in the mare. Proc. Endocrine Soc. Aust., *S7*:1–4, 1989.

35. Clarke, I.J., and Cummins, J.T.: Increased gonadotropin-releasing hormone pulse frequency associated with estrogen-induced luteinizing hormone surges in ovariectomized ewes. Endocrinology, *116*:2376–2383, 1985.

36. Karsch, F.J., Cummins, J.T., Thomas, G.B., and Clarke, I.J.: Steroid feedback inhibition of pulsatile secretion of gonadotropin-releasing hormone in the ewe. Biol. Reprod., *36*:1207–1218, 1987.

37. Garcia, M.C., Freedman, L.J., and Ginther, O.J.: Interaction of seasonal ovarian factors in the regulation of LH and FSH secretion in the mare. J. Reprod. Fertil. Suppl., *27*:103–111, 1979.

38. Fitzgerald, B.P., I'Anson, H., Loy, R.G., and Legan, S.J.: Evidence that changes in LH pulse frequency may regulate the seasonal modulation of LH secretion in ovariectomized mares. J. Reprod. Fertil., *69*:685–692, 1983.

39. Turner, D.D., Garcia, M.C., Webel, S.K., and Ginther, O.J.: Influence of follicular size on the response of mares to allyl trenbolone given before the onset of the ovulatory season. Theriogenology, *16*:73–84, 1981.

40. Squires, E.L., et al.: Relationship of altrenogest to ovarian activity, hormone concentrations and fertility of mares. J. Anim. Sci., *56*:901–910, 1983.

41. Noden, P.A., Oxender, W.D., and Hafs, H.D.: The cycle of oestrus, ovulation and plasma levels of hormones in the mare. J. Reprod. Fertil. Suppl., *23*:189–192, 1975.

42. Clarke, I.J.: Gonadotrophin-releasing hormone secretion (GnRH) in anoestrous ewes and the induction of GnRH surges by oestrogen. J. Endocrinol., *117*:355–360, 1988.

43. Kalra, S.P., and Kalra, P.S.: Do testosterone and estradiol-17 enforce inhibition or stimulation of luteinizing hormone-releasing hormone secretion? Biol. Reprod., *41*:557–570, 1989.

44. Clarke, I.J., and Cummins, J.T.: Direct pituitary effects of estrogen and progesterone on gonadotropin secretion in the ovariectomized ewe. Neuroendocrinology, *39*:267–274, 1984.

45. Alexander, S.L., and Irvine, C.H.G.: Alteration of relative bio-immunopotency of serum LH by GnRH and estradiol treatment in the mare. Proceedings of the Tenth International Congress of Animal Reproduction and Artificial Insemination. Vol. 2. 1984, pp. 1–4.

46. Garza, F. Jr., Thompson, D.L. Jr., St. George, R.L., and French, D.D.: Androgen and estradiol effects on gonadotropin secretion and response to GnRH in ovariectomized pony mares. J. Anim. Sci., *62*:1654–1659, 1980.

47. Tsonis, C.G., McNeilly, A.S., and Baird, D.T.: Inhibin secretion by the sheep ovary during the luteal and follicular phases of the oestrous cycle and following stimulation with FSH. J. Endocrinol., *117*:283–291, 1988.

48. Miller, K.F., Wesson, J.A., and Ginther, O.J.: Changes in concentrations of circulating gonadotropins following administration of equine follicular fluid to ovariectomized mares. Biol. Reprod., *21*:867–872, 1979.

49. McKerns, K.W.: Regulation of gene expression in the nucleus by gonadotropins. *In* Structure and Function of the Gonadotropins. Edited by K.W. McKerns. New York, Plenum, 1978, pp. 315–338.

50. Roy, S.K., and Greenwald, G.S.: In vitro steroidogenesis by primary to antral follicles in the hamster during the periovulatory period: Effects of follicle-stimulating hormone, luteinizing hormone, and prolactin. Biol. Reprod., *37*:39–46, 1987.

51. Ross, G.T., and Vande Wiele, R.L.: The ovaries. *In* Textbook of Endocrinology. 5th ed. Edited by R.H. Williams. Philadelphia, W.B. Saunders, 1974, pp. 368–419.

52. Fay, J.E., and Douglas, R.H.: Changes in thecal and granulosa cell LH and FSH receptor content associated with follicular fluid and peripheral plasma gonadotrophin and steroid hormone concentrations in preovulatory follicles of mares. J. Reprod. Fertil. Suppl., *35*:169–181, 1987.

53. Lapin, D.R., and Ginther, O.J.: Induction of ovulation and multiple ovulations in seasonally anovulatory and ovulatory mares with an equine pituitary extract. J. Anim. Sci., *44*:834–842, 1977.

54. Irvine, C.H.G.: Endocrinology of the estrous cycle of the mare: Application to embryo transfer. Theriogenology *15*:85–104, 1981.

55. Pineda, M.H., and Ginther, O.J.: Inhibition of estrus and ovulation in mares treated with an antiserum against an equine pituitary fraction. Am. J. Vet. Res., *33*:1775–1780, 1972.

56. Evans, M.J., Loy, R.G., Taylor, T.B., and Barrows, S.P.: Effects of exogenous steroids on serum FSH and LH and on follicular development in cyclic mares. J. Reprod. Fertil. Suppl., *32*:205–212, 1982.

57. Montovan, S.M., et al.: The effect of a potent GnRH agonist on gonadal and sexual activity in the horse. Theriogenology, *33*:1305–1321, 1990.

58. Geschwind, I.I., et al.: Plasma LH levels in the mare during the oestrous cycle. J. Reprod. Fertil. Suppl., *23*:207–212, 1975.

59. Evans, J.W.: Biorhythms in plasma progesterone concentrations and absence of correlation to LH biorhythms during different stages of the equine oestrous cycle. J. Reprod. Fertil. Suppl., *44*:684–685, 1991.

60. Pineda, M.H., Ginther, O.J., and McShan, W.H.: Regression of the corpus luteum in mares treated with an antiserum against an equine pituitary fraction. Am. J. Vet. Res., *33*:1767–1773, 1972.

CHAPTER 6

PROGESTERONE

E.L. Squires

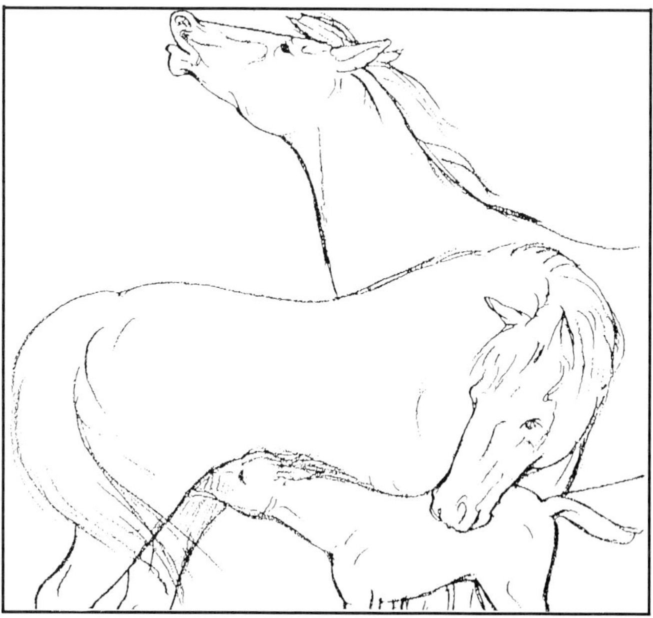

Progesterone is one of the key hormones controlling reproductive function in the mare. Its use by the horse breeder and veterinarian will be discussed in more detail in subsequent chapters. Secretion of progesterone from the corpus luteum (CL) is required for normal pregnancy in all domestic species. Control of CL function has been the focus of investigations for several years. If pregnancy does not occur following estrus and mating, progesterone secretion from the CL must be terminated to allow the reproductive cycle to be repeated. Artificially providing the mare with progesterone has numerous practical applications for the equine practitioner (Chapter 33).

CHEMISTRY

In general, steroid hormones such as progesterone are derived from a common precursor molecule, cholesterol. The chemical term steroid refers to a variety of lipid compounds, all possessing the basic four-carbon ring. All steroid hormones are synthesized from cholesterol, a 27-carbon steroid (see Fig. 7-2). Cholesterol is synthesized from acetate in the liver and is released into the blood as lipid droplets, or cholesterol can be obtained by de novo synthesis in the smooth endoplasmic reticulum of steroid-secreting cells.[1] The first series of steps in the biosynthesis of steroid hormones involves side-chain hydrolysis to yield a 21-carbon intermediate, pregnenolone. Many steroidogenic tissues produce more than one class of steroid. It is often difficult to distinguish whether the steroid is present as a precursor or whether the given steroid is secreted into the blood as a hormone. Administration of a certain steroid to an animal might lead to conversion to other steroids. For example, progesterone may be converted to corticosteroids, androgens, or estrogens. Once transported into the mitochondria, cholesterol is converted to pregnenolone by side-chain cleavage enzyme. Pregnenolone is then converted to progesterone (see Fig. 7-2) by the enzyme 3β-hydroxy-Δ^5-steroid dehydrogenase (3β-HSD).

Within the equine ovary are two primary structures: follicles and corpora lutea. The equine follicle is composed of both granulosa and thecal cells. Apparently, both cell types are essential for normal steroidogenesis. It is proposed that only granulosa cells contain 3β-HSD and conversion of pregnenolone to progesterone occurs in granulosa cells. Progesterone then passes to the thecal cells where it is converted to estradiol.[2,3] Concentrations of estradiol and androgens rise in follicular fluid prior to ovulation, and at the time of atresia, concentrations of androgens and estrogens in follicular fluid decrease.[3–5] The presumptive ovulatory follicle was shown to contain more thecal-luteinizing hormone receptors than nonovulatory follicles, and concentrations of luteinizing hormone (LH) were highest in presumptive ovulatory follicles in mares on day 4 of estrus.[5] The preovulatory surge of gonadotropins induces a change in follicular compartments, resulting in release of an ovum and transformation of the follicle into a corpus luteum. Progesterone in follicular fluid has been suggested as having a role in follicular rupture at ovulation.[6] After ovulation, granulosa cells become luteinized and conversion of progesterone to 17α-hydroxyprogesterone is retarded and progesterone accumulates with some conversion to 20α-dihydroxyprogesterone. The ketone group at carbon 3 and the double bond between carbons 4 and 5 are believed to be necessary for biologic activity of progesterone.

MORPHOLOGY OF CORPUS LUTEUM

The tissues of the growing, secreting, and regressing CL of 35 cycling and early pregnant mares were studied by light microscopy.[7] Results showed the regression of thecal cells within 24 h after ovulation. Two types of luteal cell were found in the CL: a large light-staining cell and a small dark-staining cell. In a more recent study, CL were collected from mares during early (day 4 to 5), mid- (day 8 to 9), and late (day 12 to 13) diestrus.[8] Dispersed cell suspensions were obtained by enzymic digestion of tissue. Isolated cells consisted mainly of three cell types: (1) large luteal (LL) cells, (2) small luteal (SL) cells, and (3) endothelial cells. The proportion of LL cells decreased between mid and late diestrus, and the proportion of SL cells significantly increased as age of CL advanced. Luteal tissue from cow,[9] sheep, and goats[10] has been shown to consist of at least two morphologically and biochemically distinct cell types that can be separated according to difference in size and their ability to secrete progesterone. The majority of receptors for LH have been reported to be on the SL cells. Apparently in sheep, the granulosa cells give rise to LL cells and theca cells, to SL cells,[9] but SL cells may also give rise to some LL cells. On a per cell basis, LL cells produce more progesterone than do SL cells, but SL cells are stimulated more by luteinizing hormone. In addition, only LL cells contain secretory granules. Oxytocin is synthesized and secreted from these granules in LL cells. Relaxin has also been found in LL cells of cattle CL, but apparently similar studies have not been conducted in horses. Watson and Sertich demonstrated the production of prostaglandin (PG) F, PGE_2, and 6-keto-$PGF_1α$, by luteal cells incubated for 24 h.[8] The role of these compounds in controlling production of progesterone has not been elucidated for the mare. They suggested that perhaps the change in ratio of PGF: PGE_2 throughout the cycle may be of significance in luteolysis (see Chapter 18).

CONTROL OF PROGESTERONE SECRETION

Progesterone is a primary secretory product of the corpus luteum. Other products that may interfere with measurement of progesterone in a radioimmunoassay are 17α-hydroxyprogesterone and 20α-hydroxyprogesterone. Luteinizing hormone is a major pituitary luteotropin in most domestic species. Following LH stimulation, theca interna synthesize androgens, which subsequently diffuse through the basement membrane. Within granulosa cells, androgens are converted to estradiol-17β by aromatase enzyme. The aromatase enzyme is under the control of follicle-stimulating hormone (FSH). Furthermore, FSH is associated with granulosa cell proliferation, antrum formation, maintenance of granulosa cell viability, and synthesis of gonadotropin receptors.[11] Unique to the mare, LH remains quite high for several days after ovulation. It is thought that elevated concentrations of LH after ovulation may be important for the development of the corpus luteum.[12] When antibodies to LH were administered to mares, CL weight for antiserum-treated mares was less than that of controls.[13] This indicates that endogenous pituitary factors which were inhibited by the antiserum, presumably LH, were necessary for development of the corpus luteum. However, during the time of high concentrations of progesterone, LH levels are depressed. In contrast, progesterone has little, if any, effect on FSH secretion.[14] This may explain why considerable follicular activity occurs in mares exposed to elevated progesterone levels for extended periods, such as during pregnancy. Although addition of LH in vitro stimulates progesterone secretion from bovine luteal slices,[15] the addition of ovine LH to slices of corpora lutea from seven mares did not result in a significant increase in progesterone.[16] These authors suggested that the equine CL was more refractory to exogenous stimulation than the bovine corpus luteum.

In one review,[17] five new concepts concerning control of the CL function in the cow were reported: (1) Prostacyclin (PGI_2) plays a luteotrophic role in the bovine CL; (2) Luteal cells arise from two sources (SL cells are of thecal origin and LL cells, in early diestrus, are of granulosa cell origin, but by day 10 of the cycle, nearly half of the LL cells are of thecal origin; (3) Oxytocin of luteal cell origin plays a role in CL development and regression. Oxytocin may, in fact, interfere with the luteotrophic role of prostacyclins. Oxytocin released from the corpus luteum reaches the uterus where it causes a release of $PGF_2α$, which in turn causes luteal regression. Conversely, administration of a luteolytic dose of $PGF_2α$ to a cow at day 12 of the cycle causes immediate release of oxytocin from the corpus luteum into the bloodstream; (4) Second-messenger system for control of progesterone synthesis in the CL of the cow may include protein kinase C activation in calcium mobilization; (5) Progesterone synthesis in the small theca-derived cell is primarily controlled by cyclic adenosine monophosphate *(cAMP)* dependent mechanisms, and elevated intracellular calcium inhibits progesterone synthesis in these cells. Factors that drastically elevate intracellular calcium serve to turn off the progesterone synthesis in these cells. Although control of CL function has been investigated extensively in the cow and sheep, limited studies have been conducted in the mare. A recent review on control of CL function provided convincing evidence that prostaglandin secretion from the uterine endometrium is involved in luteolysis.[18] However, the exact trigger for prostaglandin secretion is not clear. The early conceptus is responsible for suppression of prostaglandin release, such that progesterone secretion can continue and pregnancy is maintained. Further studies are needed to determine the role of prostaglan-

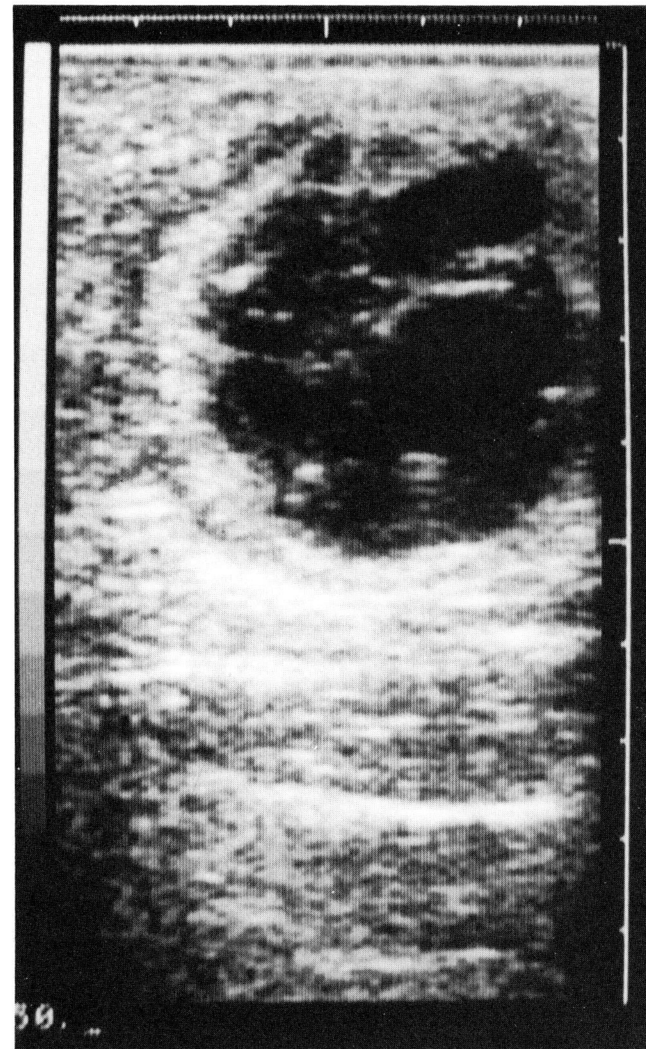

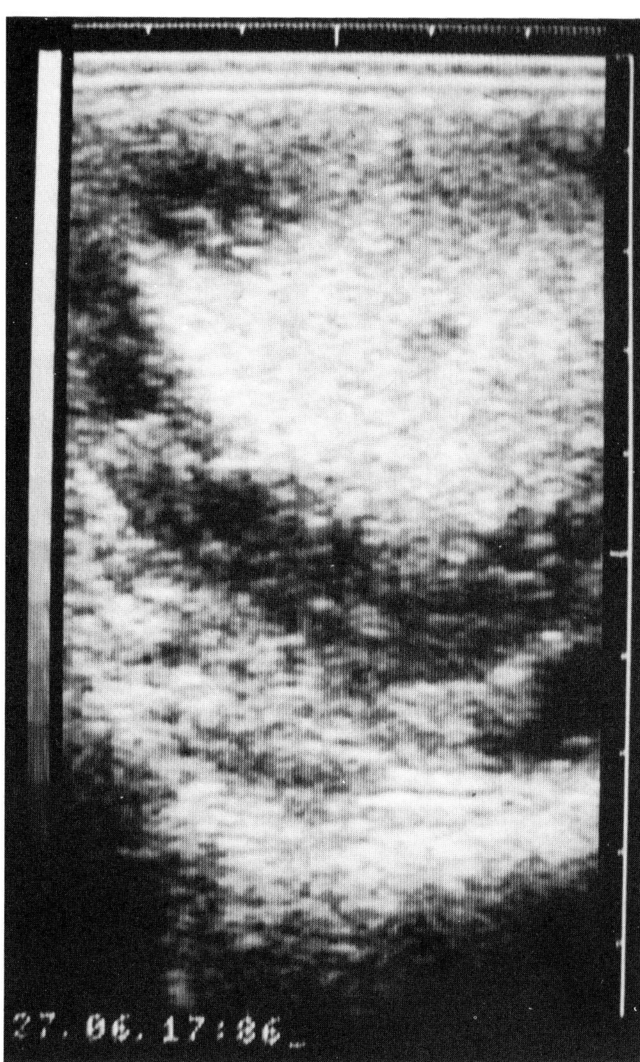

FIG. 6–1. Ultrasonographic image of centrally nonechogenic corpus luteum *(A)* and uniformly echogenic corpus luteum *(B)*

dins, prostacyclin, oxytocin, relaxin, estradiol, and other compounds in the luteotropic and luteolytic process of the mare. Another study reported PGE_2 tended to be the predominant prostaglandin released by the early CL, rather than a metabolized prostacyclin.[8] However, administration of PGE to cyclic mares did not prolong the lifespan of the corpus luteum.[18] Both calcium ionophore and cAMP stimulate prostaglandin synthesis by luteal cells of other species,[17] but neither were stimulatory when added to horse luteal cells.[8]

ULTRASONOGRAPHIC EVALUATION OF THE EQUINE CORPUS LUTEUM

Recent development of ultrasonographic technology has permitted accurate, visual observation of the development, maintenance, and regression of the CL in mares.[19,20] Although it was once thought that the ruptured follicle initially filled with blood and became a corpus hemoragicum, it is now known that only 50% of CLs contain fluid or clots.[19] In a subsequent experiment, CLs were classified into those centrally nonechogenic fluid-filled luteal glands (Fig. 6-1A) and uniformly echogenic luteal glands (Fig. 6-1B).[20] No significant difference in progesterone concentration was found between these types of CL in the first 5 days of luteal development. Thus fluid-filled CL did not differ from nonfluid-filled CL in regard to production of progesterone. Although concentrations of progesterone in jugular blood were not correlated to the size of the CL, as assessed by ultrasonography, evaluation of the corpus luteum of recipient mares prior to embryo transfer has been suggested.[21]

SECRETION OF PROGESTERONE

During estrus, concentrations of progesterone are generally below the detectable concentration for radioimmunoassay.[22] Secretion of progesterone from the CL of the mare occurs earlier than in other domestic farm an-

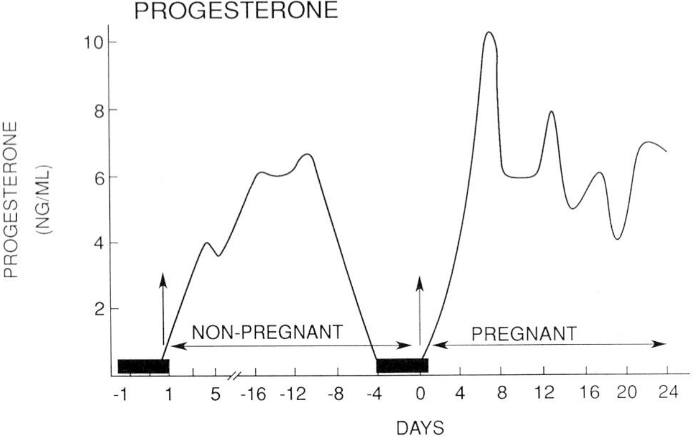

FIG. 6–2. Concentrations of progesterone in jugular blood throughout the mare's estrous cycle. Solid bars represent estrus. Vertical arrow represents ovulation.

imals. This results in systemic levels above 1 ng/mL by 2 to 3 days after ovulation (Fig. 6-2). Concentrations of progesterone continue to rise and peak on approximately day 6. In the nonpregnant mare, the CL continues to produce progesterone until approximately 14 to 15 days after ovulation.[12,23–25] Secretion of $PGF_2\alpha$ from the uterus is responsible for the regression of the corpus luteum.[26] Concentrations of progesterone were not different for mares with one or two corpora lutea. However, when two ovulations occurred, progestin concentrations did not increase until 24 h after the second ovulation.[2] In cattle, progesterone is secreted in pulses and progesterone pulses occur most frequently with LH pulses.[11] The mode of secretion of progesterone in the mare apparently has not been investigated extensively. Although the possibility of diurnal variation in concentration of progesterone was suggested, supporting data were not evident.[2] Recently, a study was conducted to describe the pattern of progesterone secretion during the different stages of the equine estrous cycle and to determine the correlation of progesterone concentrations to LH concentrations.[27] Blood samples from mares in early (day 3), mid- (day 7), and late (day 15) diestrus were obtained at 3-min intervals for 2 h and at 15-min intervals for an additional 6 h. Ultradian rhythms were detected in the 3- and 15-min samples in all mares except those that had experienced luteolysis prior to day 15 postovulation. The mean number of secretory episodes was 3.6 and 3.5 for the 8-h period, respectively. The mean interpeak interval and the mean peak duration were less for the day-7 group when compared with the day-3 and day-15 groups. The day-15 group had larger maximum heights and mean peak heights than the other two groups. Thus the pattern of progesterone secretion changes during different stages of diestrus. The observed secretory episodes explained the day-to-day variation in concentrations previously reported by many laboratories for daily blood samples. Shideler reported that one daily blood sample was not adequate to assess progesterone deficiency in pregnant mares and that at least two samples taken frequently were needed to assess mean concentrations of progesterone.[28] The biologic half-life of exogenous progesterone when injected intravenously into an ovariectomized mare was reported to be 2.5 and 20 min, respectively, for the first two components of the decay curve.[29] The conclusion was that blood plasma of mares lacked specific binding proteins for progesterone. Thus progesterone injected into mares or endogenous progesterone disappears quite rapidly from the circulation.

ROLE OF PROGESTERONE

GONADOTROPIN SECRETION

The role of gonadal steroids in the regulation of gonadotrophin secretion has been extensively studied in cattle, sheep, and laboratory animals. It has been the subject of several reviews.[30–32] The two steroid hormones estrogen and progesterone are major components of negative- and positive-feedback systems that control the release of several pituitary hormones, including prolactin, FSH, and luteinizing hormone. Evidence from one study indicated that the gonadotropins are released in a pulsatile mode in most domestic species, including the horse.[33] Direct evidence for a pulsatile pattern of gonadotropin-releasing hormone (GnRH) released into the pituitary cavernous sinus was obtained. In sheep, studies have demonstrated that each pulse of LH from the pituitary is coincident with a pulse of GnRH from the hypothalamus. However, episodes of GnRH secretion may exist that are not accompanied by LH pulses.[30] A more detailed discussion of GnRH-induced LH release is presented in Chapter 5. The intent of this review is to emphasize the role of progesterone in controlling LH and FSH secretion. Administration of progesterone can have both inductive and suppressive effects on gonadotropin secretion, and as for estradiol, the nature of these effects is time and dose dependent. Although the stimulatory action of acute increases in progesterone may contribute to the LH surge in some species, such as humans,[34] the most common effect of progesterone on the LH-pulse–generating system is a negative-feedback action. During the luteal phase of the menstrual cycle, plasma progesterone and estrogen concentrations are elevated and pulse frequency is slow. In contrast, LH pulse frequency increases during the early follicular phase when plasma estrogen and progesterone are lower.[34] The inverse relationship between LH pulse frequency and circulating levels of progesterone has also been demonstrated in the cow[35] and sheep.[30] The frequency of LH pulses in the ewe is highest shortly after ovulation when progesterone secretion is low. Frequency decreases during early luteal to midluteal phases as progesterone increases and is minimal at the time of the midluteal phase when progesterone secretion is maximal. Finally, the pace of LH pulse increases markedly at the time of luteal regression when progesterone falls. Karsch suggested that progesterone acts on the brain to reduce LH pulse frequency by increasing the interval between episodes of GnRH release.[30] Studies on the feedback mechanisms for gonadotropin secretion in the horse are somewhat limited. Because estradiol peaks proceed the LH peak by about 2 days, this steroid has been implicated as being responsible for preovulatory LH secretion.[36] A working hypothesis was presented for the regulation of LH secretion in the mare. Two components were proposed to be involved, the primary central nervous system, or the pituitary, component—which was independent of ovarian influence—and the estradiol component.[37] Ovariectomy during diestrus in summer was followed by an increase in plasma concentrations of LH, which indicated the ovarian influences were predominantly inhibitory to LH at that time. These results were in contrast to more recent results in which long-term ovariectomized mares were used to determine the effect of progesterone on FSH and LH concentrations.[38] Treatment of mares with progesterone had no effect on daily LH secretion but increased daily FSH secretion. Differences in the two studies may have been the result of the duration of time from ovariectomy to treatment. Others have reported an inverse relationship between plasma progesterone and LH concentrations in mares.[25] Another study[39] was designed to investigate the role of ovarian steroids in the control of gonadotropin secretion of cycling mares. Mares were either administered 150 mg progesterone, 150 mg progesterone and 10 mg estradiol-17β, 10 mg estradiol-17β, or cottonseed oil vehicle from day 1 to day 28 after ovulation. Blood samples were collected daily. Administration of exogenous progesterone prevented the preovulatory rise in LH at the expected time. These authors suggested a negative feedback of progesterone at the level of hypothalamus to suppress gonadotropin-releasing hormone. This was similar to the suppressive effect of progesterone given to ovariectomized mares during the breeding season.[37] Mares administered both progesterone and estradiol had lower concentrations of LH, but concentrations of FSH were similar to those that received progesterone only. More recently, a study was done to determine the effect of progesterone administration and withdrawal on secretion of FSH and LH during the transitional season.[40] Jugular blood was collected through indwelling canula from 12 deeply anestrous mares every 30 min for 12 h. This regime was repeated every 2 weeks until ovulation occurred. At the beginning of spring, six of these mares were randomly chosen to receive 150 mg progesterone daily for 12 days. Intensive blood sampling of all 12 mares was done immediately, before the first progesterone treatment, after 1 week of treatment and 1 week after progesterone withdrawal. Distinct pulses in plasma concentrations of LH and FSH were detected in all 12 mares. Mean LH pulse frequency increased progressively during spring to summer and was associated with a steady rise in ovarian activity. In contrast, mean pulse frequency of FSH increased, but not significantly during spring. When pulse frequency before progesterone treatment had been rapid (greater than three pulses per 12 h) and mean concentrations of LH were elevated (greater than 1 ng/mL), progesterone reduced both parameters, therefore decreasing the variability between mares. Further studies are needed to define more clearly the role of progesterone in controlling the pulsatile release of LH and FSH, particularly during the transitional period. In addition, studies are needed in which frequent samples are collected to determine if progesterone secretion is pulsatile and if the secretion pattern of progesterone changes throughout the cycle.

UTERINE SECRETIONS

Secretions from the uterus, termed uterine milk, are apparently important in nurturing the early conceptus. The ability of the endometrium to provide adequate amounts of appropriate secretions depends to a large extent on progesterone. The total protein content of uterine secretion throughout the estrous cycle of mares has been studied, and results indicated that total protein content decreases abruptly as progesterone declines.[41] In contrast, with luteal maintenance and continued progesterone production, protein content of uterine secretions remain elevated.[41] The sheep uterus, under progesterone influence, also secretes two major glycoproteins called uterine milk proteins (UTMP).[42] In a subsequent study with mares, eight ovariectomized pony mares were used to test the effect of various doses of progesterone (0, 50, 150, and 450 mg per day in oil, I.M., for 10 days) on total protein and uteroferrin in uterine secretions.[43] Progesterone increased uteroferrin but there was no difference among doses of progesterone. Progesterone treatment decreased LH and tended to increase total protein. Eighteen additional ovariectomized mares were given vehicle, 10 mg estradiol, 150 mg progesterone, or progesterone plus estradiol daily for 28 days. Both progesterone and progesterone plus estradiol increased total protein, uteroferrin, and uterine secretions compared to vehicle or estradiol alone.

Several studies have demonstrated that ovariectomized mares administered progesterone can become pregnant and remain pregnant after embryo transfer.[44] However, if intact mares were exposed to endogenous progesterone or ovariectomized mares to exogenous progesterone for longer than approximately 9 days prior to embryo transfer, pregnancy rates were dramatically decreased. This indicated that changes in the uterine environment occur after several days of progesterone treatment, which may adversely affect embryo survival. Zavy et al. reported that uterine protein profiles in ovariectomized mares administered progesterone for 21 days were similar to those found in intact mares in early diestrus or early pregnancy.[45] In a subsequent study, the effects of different durations of progesterone treatment on total protein content, acid phosphatase, and activity and pattern of uterine protein secretion were determined in an attempt to relate differences in uterine environment of the recipient mare to survival of transferred embryos.[46] Ovariectomized mares were assigned to one of two groups: (1) synchronous mares given progesterone from 2 days after ovulation of a potential donor mare or (2) asynchronous mares administered progesterone from 5 to 7 days before the predicted time of ovulation of a potential donor mare. Four procedures were performed using both synchronous and asynchronous mares: (1) no transfer; (2) sham transfer at day 7; (3) embryo transfer at day 7; resulting in a pregnancy on day 14; and (4) embryo transfer on day 7, resulting in no pregnancy at day 14. Uterine fluid was collected from the recipient mares, either at day 7 or 7 days after embryo or sham transfer (day 14). This schedule resulted in uterine fluid being recovered after mares had been treated with progesterone for 5, 12 to 15, and 19 to 21 days. Total concentration of protein in uterine fluid tended to increase with duration of progesterone treatment and acid phosphatase, and protein content of uterine flush, was significantly affected by duration of treatment, being tenfold higher after 19 to 21 days of treatment than after 5 days of treatment. Similarly, in sheep, uterine milk proteins were at low levels after 6 days of progesterone treatment and increased as duration of progesterone treatment continued.[42]

UTERINE TONE

Circulating concentrations of ovarian steroids have been shown to have a prominent influence on uterine resistance to infection. During the time of progesterone domination, the uterus is highly susceptible to establishment of infection of invading organisms. Whereas under the influence of estrogen, pathogens are usually rapidly eliminated. A study, designed to determine the effect of ovarian steroids on antibody production,[47] found that progesterone treatment reduced titers of specific IgG and IgA in uterine secretions of mares administered progesterone daily for 14 days compared to those administered estradiol or vehicle only. Therefore, administration of progesterone to a mare susceptible to uterine infection is contraindicated, and penetration of a mare's cervix during the time of high progesterone concentration may result in induction of uterine infection, even in normal mares.

Clinicians are quite aware of the effects of progesterone on uterine tone. In fact, exogenous progesterone has been used to improve uterine tone in mares with poor tone during early pregnancy. Berg and Ginther injected progesterone into ovariectomized and ovarian-intact mares and determined uterine tone.[48] Administration of progesterone produced uterine thickness or tone characteristic of diestrus; uterine tone was not as great as that occurring during pregnancy. In a further experiment during the anovulatory season, pony mares were treated with estradiol and progesterone. Results indicated the extensive uterine tone in early pregnancy, and sometimes in pseudopregnancy, is not solely attributed to production of progesterone, because addition of a small amount of estradiol increased thickness and tone to a point comparable to that occurring in pregnant and pseudopregnant mares. This was in contrast to a study in which uterine tone was similar in ovariectomized pregnant embryo transfer recipients that had received either progesterone or progesterone plus estradiol.[44]

The concentration of progesterone has also been shown to effect mobility, fixation, orientation, and survival of the equine embryonic vesicle.[49] Embryonic vesicles in mares that had luteal progesterone removed by ovariectomy or by treatment with prostaglandin, moved to a different uterine segment less frequently than in mares with luteal or exogenous progesterone. In a subsequent study, progesterone administration resulted in elevated uterine contractile activity scores, but not until after 14 days of treatment.[50] The authors concluded that progesterone plays a role in the mobility of the conceptus, but other factors are also involved in the extensive mobility that occurs on days 11 to 14.

REFERENCES

1. Norris, D.O.: The chemistry of steroid hormones. *In* Vertebrate Endocrinology. 2nd ed. Edited by D. Norris. Philadelphia, Lea & Febiger, 1985, pp. 202–215.
2. Ginther, O.J.: Reproductive Biology of the Mare: Basic and Applied Aspects. Ann Arbor, McNaughton, Gunn, 1979.
3. Meinecke, B., Gips, H., and Meinecke-Tillmann, S.: Progestogen, androgen and oestrogen levels in plasma and ovarian follicular fluid during oestrous cycle of the mare. Anim. Reprod. Sci., *12*:255–265, 1987.
4. Kenney, R.M., Condon, W., Ganjam, V.K., and Channing, C.: Morphological and biochemical correlates of equine ovarian follicles as a function of their state of viability or atresia. J. Reprod. Fertil. Suppl., *27*:103–171, 1979.
5. Fay, J.E., and Douglas, R.H.: Changes in thecal and granulosa cell LH and FSH receptor content associated with follicular fluid and peripheral plasma gonadotropin and steroid hormone concentrations in preovulatory follicles of mares. J. Reprod. Fertil. Suppl., *35*:169–181, 1987.
6. Tsafrui, A., Abisogun, A.O., and Reigh, R.: Steroids and follicular rupture at ovulation. J. Steroid Biochem., *27*:359–363, 1987.
7. Van Niekerk, C.H., Morgenthal, J.C., and Gerneke, W.H.: Relationship between the morphology of and progesterone production by the corpus luteum of the mare. J. Reprod. Fertil. Suppl., *23*:171–175, 1975.
8. Watson, E.D., and Sertich, P.L.: Secretion of prostaglandins and progesterone by cells from corpora lutea of mares. J. Reprod. Fertil., *88*:223–229, 1990.
9. O'Shea, J.D.: Heterogeneous cell types in the corpus luteum of sheep, goats and cattle. J. Reprod. Fertil. Suppl., *34*:71–85, 1987.
10. Schwall, R.H., Sawyer, H.R., and Niswender, G.D.: Differential regulation by LH and prostaglandins of steroidogenesis in small and large luteal cells of the ewe. J. Reprod. Fertil., *76*:821–829, 1986.
11. Smith, M.F.: Recent advances in corpus luteum physiology. J. Dairy, Sci., *69*:911–926, 1986.
12. Noden, P.A., Oxender, W.D., and Hafs, H.D.:The cycle of oestrus, ovulation and plasma levels of hormones in the mare. J. Reprod. Fertil. Suppl., *23*:189–192, 1975.
13. Pineda, M.H., Ginther, O.J., and McShan, W.H.: Regres-

sion of corpus luteum in mares treated with an antiserum against an equine pituitary fraction. Am. J. Vet. Res., *33*:1767–1773, 1972.

14. Garcia, M.C., and Ginther, O.J.: LH control by estradiol and progesterone in mares. J. Anim. Sci., *43*:285, 1976.

15. Mason, N.R., Marsh, J.M., and Savard, K.: An action of gonadotropin in vitro. J. Biol. Chem., *237*:271–278, 1962.

16. Condon, W.A., Ganjam, V.K., and Kenney, R.M.: Cataecholamines and equine luteal progestagens. J. Reprod. Fertil. Suppl., *27*:199–203, 1979.

17. Hansel, W., and David, J.P.: New concepts of the control of corpus luteum function. J. Reprod. Fertil., *78*:755–768, 1986.

18. Sharp, D.C., McDowell, K.J., Werthenauer, J., and Thatcher, W.W.: The continuum of events leading to maternal recognition of pregnancy in mares. J. Reprod. Fertil. Suppl., *37*:101–107, 1989.

19. Pierson, R.A., and Ginther, O.J.: Ultrasonic evaluation of the corpus luteum of the mare. Theriogenology, *23*:795–806, 1985.

20. Townson, D.H., Pierson, R.A., and Ginther, O.J.: Characterization of plasma progesterone concentrations for two distinct luteal morphologies in mares. Theriogenology, *32*:197–204, 1989.

21. McKinnon, A.O., Squires, E.L., and Voss, J.L.: Ultrasonic evaluation of the mare's reproductive tract: Part I. Compend. Contin. Educ. Pract. Vet., *9*:336–345, 1987.

22. Plotka, E.D., et al.: Periovulatory changes in peripheral plasma progesterone and estrogen concentrations in the mare. Am. J. Vet. Res., *36*:1359–1362, 1975.

23. Allen, W.E., and Hadley, J.C.: Blood progesterone concentrations in pregnant and nonpregnant mares. Equine Vet. J., *6*:87–93, 1974.

24. Evans, M.J., and Irvine, C.H.G.: Serum concentrations of FSH, LH and progesterone during the estrous cycle and early pregnancy in the mare. J. Reprod. Fertil. Suppl., *23*:193–200, 1975.

25. Nett, T.M., Pickett, B.W., Seidel, G.E., Jr., and Voss, J.L.: Levels of luteinizing hormone and progesterone during the estrous cycle and early pregnancy in mares. Biol. Reprod., *14*:412–415, 1976.

26. Douglas, R.H., and Ginther, O.J.: Concentrations of prostaglandins F in uterine venous plasma of anesthetized mares during the estrous cycle and early pregnancy. Prostaglandins, *11*:251–260, 1976.

27. Evans, J.W.: Biorhythms in plasma progesterone concentrations and absence of any correlation to LH biorhythms during different stages of the equine oestrous cycle. J. Reprod. Fertil. Suppl., *44*:684–685, 1991.

28. Shideler, R.K., et al.: Progestogen therapy of ovariectomized pregnant mares. J. Reprod. Fertil. Suppl., *32*:459–464, 1982.

29. Ganjam, V.K., Kenney, R.M., and Flickinger, G.: Effect of exogenous progesterone on its endogenous levels: Biological half-life of progesterone and lack of progesterone-binding in mares. J. Reprod. Fertil. Suppl., *23*:183–188, 1975.

30. Karsch, F.S.: Central action of ovarian steroids in the feedback regulation of pulsatile secretion of luteinizing hormone. Annu. Rev. Physiol., *49*:365–382, 1987.

31. Mahesh, V.B., and Muldoon, T.G.: Integration of the effects of estradiol and progesterone in the modulation of gonadotropin secretion. J. Steroid Biochem., *27*:665–675, 1987.

32. Fink, G.: Oestrogen and progesterone interactions in the control of gonadotropin and prolactin secretion. J. Steroid Biochem., *30*:169–178, 1988.

33. Alexander, S.L., and Irvine, C.H.G.: Effect of graded doses of gonadotropin-releasing hormone on serum LH concentrations in mares in various reproductive states: Comparison with endogenously generated pulses. J. Endocrinol., *110*:19–26, 1986.

34. Nippoldt, T.B., et al.: The roles of estradiol and progesterone in decreasing luteinizing hormone pulse frequency in the luteal phase of the menstrual cycle. J. Clin. Endocrinol. Metab. *69*:67–76, 1989.

35. Rahe, C.H., et al.: Pattern of plasma luteinizing hormone in the cyclic cow: Dependence upon the period of the cycle. Endocrinology, *107*:498–503, 1980.

36. Pattison, M.L., Chen, C.L., Kelley, S.T., and Brandt, G.W.: Luteinizing hormones and estradiol in peripheral blood of mares during the estrous cycle. Biol. Reprod., *11*:245–250, 1974.

37. Garcia, M.C., Freedman, L.S., and Ginther, O.J.: Interaction of seasonal and ovarian factors in the regulation of LH and FSH secretion in the mare. J. Reprod. Fertil. Suppl., *27*:103–111, 1979.

38. McNeill-Wiest, D.R., Thompson, D.L., and Wiest, J.J.: Gonadotropin secretion in ovariectomized pony mares treated with dexamethasone or progesterone and subsequently with dihydrotesterone. Domest. Anim. Endocrinol., *5*:149–154, 1988.

39. Evans, M.J., Loy, R.G., Taylor, T.B., and Barrows, S.P.: Effect of exogenous steroids on serum FSH and LH and on follicular development in cyclic mares. J. Reprod. Fertil. Suppl., *32*:205–212, 1982.

40. Alexander, S.L., and Irvine, C.H.G.: Control of onset of breeding season in the mare and its artificial regulation by progesterone treatment. J. Reprod. Fertil. Suppl., *44*:307–319, 1991.

41. Zavy, M.T., et al.: An investigation of the uterine luminal environment of non-pregnant and pregnant pony mares. J. Reprod. Fertil. Suppl., *27*:403–411, 1979.

42. Ing, N.H., et al.: Progesterone induction of uterine milk proteins: Major secretory proteins of sheep endometrium. Biol., Reprod., *41*:643–654, 1989.

43. McDowell, K.J., Sharp, D.C., and Grubaugh, W.: Comparison of progesterone and progesterone + oestrogen on total and specific uterine proteins in pony mares. J. Reprod. Fertil. Suppl., *35*:335–342, 1987.

44. McKinnon, A.O., Squires, E.L., Carnevale, E.M., and Hermenet, M.J.: Ovariectomized steroid-treated mares as embryo transfer recipients and as a model to study the role of progestins in pregnancy maintenance. Theriogenology, *29*:1055–1063, 1988.

45. Zavy, M.T., et al.: Identification of stage-specific and hormonally induced polypeptides in the uterine protein secretions of the mare during the oestrous cycle and pregnancy. J. Reprod. Fertil., *64*:199–207, 1982.

46. Hinrichs, K., Kenney, R.M., and Sharp, D.C.: Differences in protein content of uterine fluid related to duration of progesterone treatment in ovariectomized mares used as embryo recipients. Equine Vet J. Suppl., *8*:49–55, 1989.

47. Watson, E.D.: The influence of estrogen and progesterone on antibody synthesis by the endometrium of the mare. Proceedings of the 5th International Conference of Equine Infectious Disease. Edited by D.G. Powell, Lexington, University Press of Kentucky, 1988, pp. 181–185.

48. Berg, S.L., and Ginther, O.J.: Effect of estrogens on uterine tone and life span of the corpus luteum in mares. J. Anim. Sci., *47*:203–208, 1978.

49. Kastelic, J.P., Adams, G.P., and Ginther, O.J.: Role of progesterone in mobility, fixation, orientation and survival of the equine embryonic vesicle. Theriogenology, *27*:655–663, 1987.

50. Cross, D.T., and Ginther, O.J.:The effect of estrogen, progesterone and prostaglandin $F_2\alpha$ on uterine contractions in seasonally anovulatory mares. Domest. Anim. Endocrinol., *44*:271–278, 1987.

CHAPTER 7

ESTROGENS

T. M. Nett

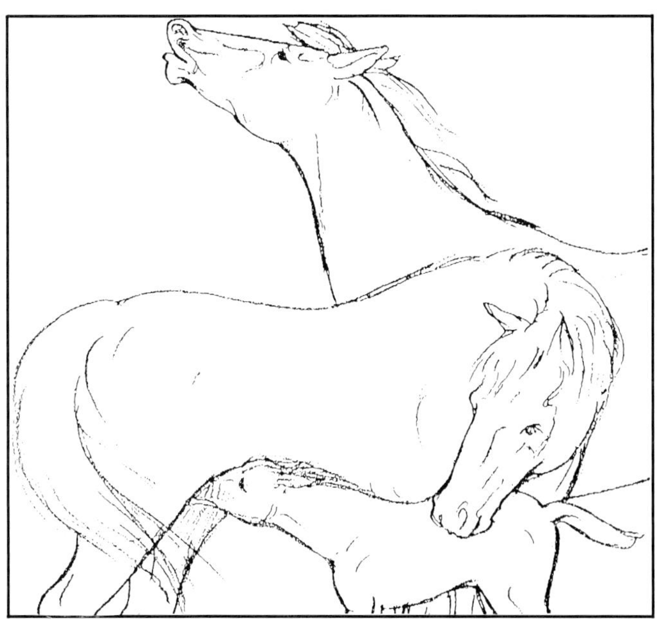

Structures of unconjugated estrogens found in the blood of horses are depicted in Figure 7-1. In nonpregnant mares, the predominant estrogen present in follicular fluid and in the circulation is estradiol.[1] A small amount of estrone is present in follicular fluid and the peripheral circulation, but the concentration of estrone in the circulation does not appear to vary with stage of the estrous cycle.[2] Therefore, it would appear that estradiol is the primary estrogen responsible for estrogenic effects noted in mares during the estrous cycle.

During pregnancy, the fetal-placental unit becomes the major source of estrogens in the mare. In addition to estradiol and estrone, B ring unsaturated estrogens—equilin, equilenin, 17β-dihydroequilin, 17α-dihydroequilin, 17β-dihydroequilenin, and 17α-dihydroequilenin—appear in the circulation during gestation and increase in amount as pregnancy progresses. These B ring unsaturated estrogens do not appear to be formed via the classic steroid biosynthetic pathway.

The stallion testis produces and secretes estrone and estradiol. The concentration of estrone in the peripheral circulation exceeds that of estradiol.[3] Circulating concentrations of estradiol vary with season in the stallion, but those of estrone do not. Therefore, as in the mare, it would seem that estradiol is responsible for the biologic effects attributed to estrogens in the stallion.

BIOSYNTHESIS OF ESTROGENS

Two alternate pathways have been proposed for biosynthesis of steroid hormones in the follicle of the mare.[4] These pathways are generally referred to as the Δ^4 or Δ^5 pathways and are depicted in Figure 7-2. Based on an analysis of steroids present in follicular fluid of mares, it is believed that the Δ^4 pathway is the major route of estrogen biosynthesis.[5,6]

The cell types responsible for the various steps in estrogen biosynthesis in the equine follicle have not been definitively determined. Both theca cells and granulosa cells in tissue culture have the ability to synthesize estrogens. Granulosa cells have a much higher concentration of the enzyme 3β-hydroxy-Δ^5-steroid dehydrogenase than theca cells. This enzyme is responsible for the conversion of pregnenolone to progesterone.[7] Furthermore, granulosa cells produce much more progesterone than do theca cells when cultured under identical conditions; however, similar quantities of estradiol were produced by each cell type.[8] When theca cells and granulosa cells were cultured together, the amount of estradiol produced was much greater than when either cell type was cultured alone.[9] Therefore, for the efficient production of estradiol the presence of both cell types may be required. Based on this information, a two-cell hypothesis for synthesis of estradiol by the equine follicle has been proposed in which progesterone is produced by the granulosa cells and then transferred across the basement membrane to theca cells where it is converted to estradiol.[5]

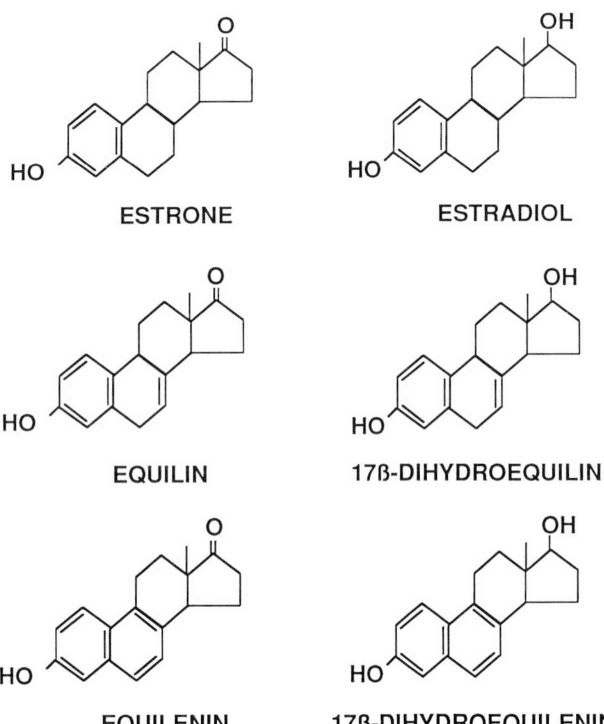

FIG. 7–1. Structures of biologically active estrogens detected in the blood of equids. Estrone and estradiol are produced by the follicle and testis. The placenta produces each of the estrogens depicted.

During pregnancy, the equine placenta is a major source of estrogens. In addition to estradiol and estrone, which appear to be synthesized via the classic steroid pathway depicted in Figure 7-2, there is another yet-to-be-defined pathway via which the B ring unsaturated estrogens (Fig. 7-1) are synthesized. These unique estrogens are produced from acetate but do not use androstenedione, cholesterol, or squalene as intermediates.[10,11]

Nyman et al. demonstrated that the stallion testis is capable of synthesizing estrogens.[12] Biosynthesis of estrogens can apparently occur via either the Δ^4 or Δ^5 pathways in the stallion testis,[13] although the majority of steroid biosynthesis appears to occur via the Δ^4 pathway. Both Leydig cells and Sertoli cells have been reported to synthesize estrogens in males. However, to date the cell type responsible for production of estrogens in the stallion testis has not been determined.

BIOLOGICAL FUNCTIONS OF ESTROGENS

As noted above, estradiol appears to be responsible for estrogenic activity observed in both mares and stallions. In mares, estradiol is responsible for estrous behavior. Injections of estradiol into ovariectomized mares induces estrous behavior within a matter of hours.[14] Likewise, administration of estradiol to mares during seasonal anestrus induces estrous behavior, presumably by binding to estrogen receptors in the brain and inducing behavioral changes. Estradiol also is responsible for inducing an increase in secretion of LH that occurs during estrus and causes rupture of the follicle. This appears to occur via two separate actions of estradiol. First, an increase in secretion of GnRH from the hypothalamus during estrus occurs[15] and, second, the number of receptors for GnRH increases in the anterior pituitary gland,[16] which sensitizes the anterior pituitary to gonadotropin-releasing hormone. Together these effects lead to the increase in LH observed during estrus that is responsible for ovulation.

Systematic studies of the effects of estradiol on the tubular genitalia of the mare have not been reported. Based on changes in uterine tone that occur during the estrous cycle of the mare,[17] estradiol does not seem to produce an increase in fluid accumulation in the uterus characteristically noted in other species. Estradiol does appear to induce a relaxation of the cervix and to increase the diameter of the cervical canal during estrus.[18] Likewise, there is increased secretion of oviductal fluid[19] and increased production of fluid with high lubricating properties by the cervix and vagina during estrus,[18] presumably induced by the high concentrations of estradiol present at that time.

The functions of estrogens, during pregnancy in the mare are unclear. Nishikawa suggested that estrogens during midpregnancy may be luteotropic in mares and suggested that the high concentrations of estrogens noted at that time may be responsible for prolonging the function of the secondary corpora lutea.[20] This concept was tested by administering the synthetic estrogen diethylstilbestrol (DES) to mares from days 84 to 142 of gestation. Such treatment increased excretion of prenanediol in the urine of mares and mares so treated had a lower percentage of spontaneous abortions.[20] In contrast, in a more recent study, Nett and Pickett did not observe any alteration in serum concentrations of progesterone in mares treated with DES compared to control mares.[21] Therefore, the validity of this hypothesis is questionable.

In stallions, the biologic functions of estradiol are largely unknown. Administration of estradiol to geldings was able to restore libido but did not influence weight of accessory sex organs nor was it able to restore the ability of geldings to ejaculate.[22] Therefore, it appears that estradiol is involved in stimulating sexual behavior at central neural centers, but it does not appear to affect the genital tract of the stallion directly.

REFERENCES

1. Younglai, E.V.: Steroid content of the equine ovary during the reproductive cycle. J. Endocrinol., *50*:589–597, 1971.
2. Noden, P.A., Oxender, W.D., and Hafs, H.D.: The cycle of oestrus, ovulation and plasma levels of hormones in the mare. J. Reprod. Fertil. Suppl., *23*:189–192, 1975.
3. Thompson, D.L., Jr., Pickett, B.W., and Nett, T.M.: Effect of season and artificial photoperiod on levels of estradiol-17β and estrone in blood serum of stallions. J. Anim. Sci., *47*:184–187, 1978.

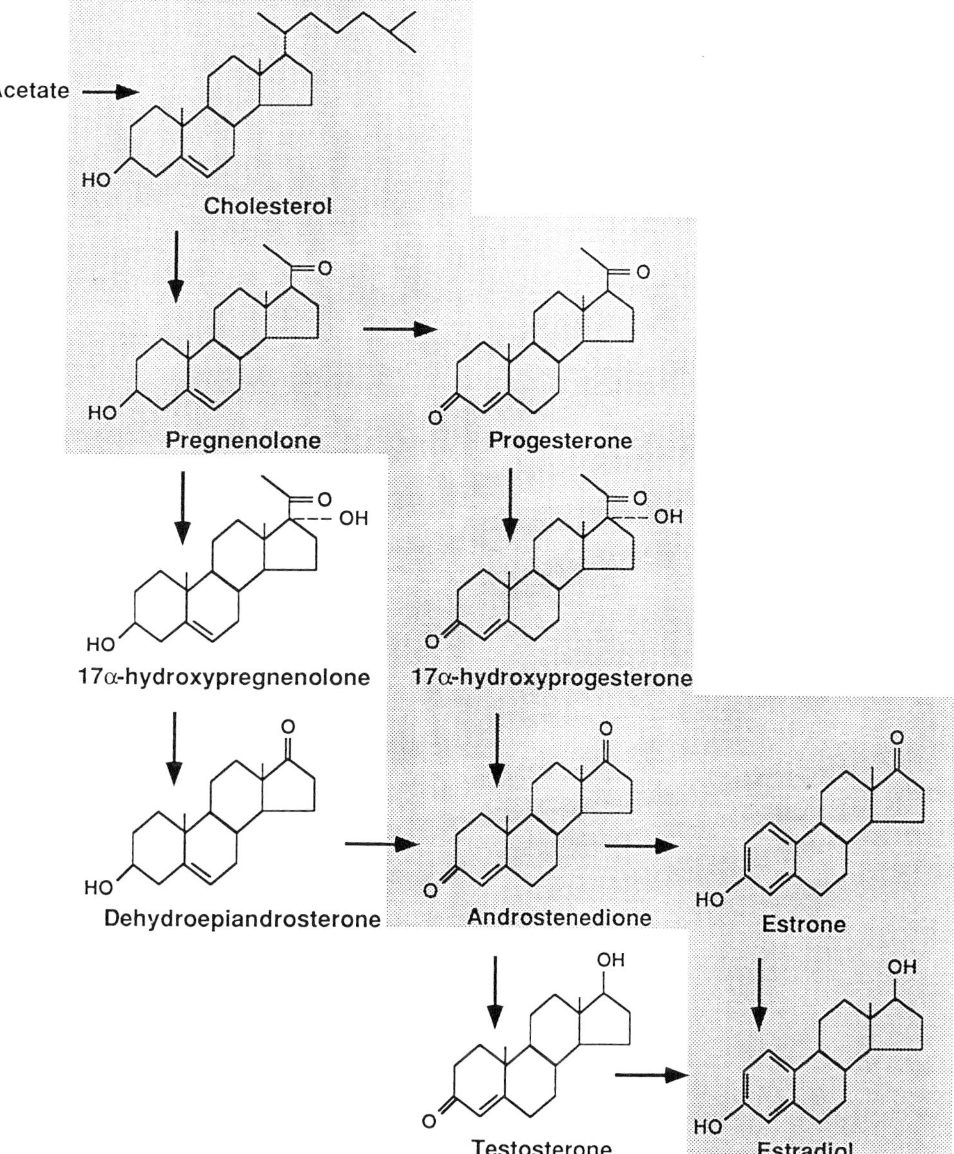

FIG. 7–2. Pathways for the biosynthesis of estrogens in equids. Both the Δ^4 and Δ^5 pathways are depicted and may be used for synthesis of estrogens. The preferred pathway for biosynthesis of estrogens in the testis and in the follicle is the Δ^4 pathway (shaded).

4. Short, R.V.: Δ^5 3β-Hydroxy steroids in the follicular fluid of the mare. J. Endocrinol., *23*:277–283, 1961.
5. Short, R.V.: Steroids in the follicular fluid and corpus luteum of the mare. A "two-cell type" theory of ovarian steroid synthesis. J. Endocrinol., *24*:59–63, 1962.
6. Younglai, E.V., and Short, R.V.: Pathways of steroid biosynthesis in the intact Graafian follicle of mares in oestrus. J. Endocrinol., *47*:321–331, 1970.
7. Hay, M.F., Allen, W.R., and Lewis, I.M.: The distribution of Δ^5-3β-hydroxysteroid dehydrogenase in the Graafian follicle of the mare. J. Reprod. Fertil. Suppl., *23*:323–327, 1975.
8. Channing, C.P., and Grieves, S.A.: Studies on tissue culture of equine ovarian cell types: Steroidogenesis. J. Endocrinol., *43*:391–402, 1969.
9. Mahajan, D.K., and Samuels, L.T.: The steroidogenic ability of various cell types of the equine ovary. Steroids, *24*:713–730, 1974.
10. Bhavnani, B.R., Short, R.V., and Solomon, S.: Formation of estrogens by the pregnant mare. II. Metabolism of ^{14}C-acetate and ^{3}H-cholesterol injected into the fetal circulation. Endocrinology, *85*:1172–1179, 1971.
11. Bhavnani, B.R., and Short, R.V.: Formation of steroids by the pregnant mare. III. Metabolism of ^{14}C-squalene and ^{3}H-dehydroisoandrosterone injected into the fetal circulation. Endocrinology, *92*:657–666, 1973.
12. Nyman, M.A., Geiger, J., and Goldzieher, J.W.: Biosynthesis of estrogen by the perfused stallion testis. J. Biol. Chem., *234*:16–21, 1959.
13. Ganjam, V.K.: Episodic nature of the Δ^4-ene and Δ^5-ene steroidogenic pathways and their relationship to the adreno-gonadal axis in stallions. J. Reprod. Fertil. Suppl., *27*:67–71, 1979.
14. Ginther, O.J.: Reproductive Biology of the Mare: Basic and Applied Aspects. Ann Arbor, McNaughton and Gunn, 1979, pp. 72–75.

15. Irvine, C.H.G., and Alexander, S.L.: A novel technique for measuring hypothalamic and pituitary hormone secretion rates from collection of pituitary venous effluent in the normal horse. J. Endocrinol., *113*:183–192, 1987.
16. Silvia, P.J., Squires, E.L., and Nett, T.M.: Changes in the hypothalamic-hypophyseal axis of mares associated with seasonal reproductive recrudescence. Biol. Reprod., *35*:897–905, 1986.
17. Van Niekerk , C.H.: Early clinical diagnosis of pregnancy in mares. J. S. Afr. Vet. Med. Assn., *36*:51–58, 1965.
18. Andrews, F.N., and McKenzie, F.F.: Estrus, ovulation and related phenomena in the mare. Univ. Missouri Agri. Exp. Sta. Res. Bull., *329*:1–117, 1941.
19. Engle, C.C., Witherspoon, D.M., and Foley, C.W.: Technique for continuous collection of equine oviduct secretions. Am. J. Vet. Res., *31*:1889–1896, 1970.
20. Nishikawa, Y.: Studies on Reproduction in Horses. Tokyo, Japan Racing Assoc., 1959.
21. Nett, T.M., and Pickett, B.W.: Effect of diethylstilboestrol on the relationship between LH, PMSG, and progesterone during pregnancy in the mare. J. Reprod. Fertil. Suppl., *27*:465–470, 1979.
22. Thompson, D.L., Jr., et al.: Sexual behavior, seminal pH and accessory sex gland weights in geldings administered testosterone and(or) estradiol-17β. J. Anim. Sci., *51*:1358–1366, 1980.

CHAPTER 8

PROSTAGLANDINS

W.R. Allen
M.J. Cooper

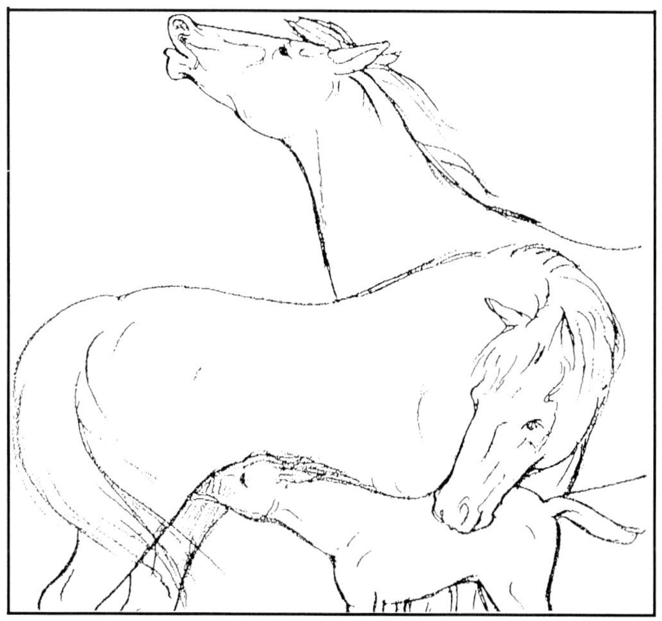

The first indication that prostaglandin $F_2\alpha$ ($PGF_2\alpha$) might be the elusive luteolytic substance that controls the lifespan of the corpus luteum (CL), and hence the length of the estrous cycle, in laboratory and domestic farm animal species is attributed to Pharriss and Wyngarden.[1] They reported that both the size and the progesterone content of CL in pseudopregnant rats diminished rapidly following a single intramuscular injection of $PGF_2\alpha$. A considerable array of carefully planned and well-executed experiments had been performed on the ewe and other species earlier in the 1960s, all of which had shown that the uterus controls luteal lifespan in the cycling animal through release of a soluble lytic factor toward the end of the diestrous interval. Moor and Rowson demonstrated that bilateral hysterectomy in the cycling ewe prolonged CL function significantly.[2] Hemihysterectomy did likewise, but only when the half of the uterus ipsilateral to the ovary containing the CL was removed.[3,4] Similar unilateral effects of the uterus on luteal lifespan and secretory activity were demonstrated using partial hysterectomy in the pig[5,6] and in the guinea pig.[7]

These early hysterectomy studies were followed by a parallel set of experiments involving the transfer of one or more embryos in sheep and pigs to surgically isolated portions of the uterus that were either ipsilateral or contralateral to the ovary bearing the CL.[8–11] Together, these elegant preparations demonstrated convincingly that a viable conceptus must be present in the uterus to prevent cyclical luteolysis by no later than day 12 after ovulation in the sheep and day 14 in the pig, that the embryo must be ipsilateral to the CL if placed in a surgically isolated uterine horn in both species, and that in the intact uterus in the pig a minimum of four conceptuses evenly spaced throughout the uterine horns are necessary to inhibit the lytic action of the uterus and ensure luteal maintenance for the continuation of pregnancy. An important experiment carried out during the same period demonstrated that infusion of frozen-thawed homogenates of day-14, but not day-25, sheep embryonic membranes daily from day 10 of diestrus into the uterine lumen of the cycling ewe for 4 to 6 days suppressed the lytic effect of the uterus and allowed prolongation of CL function to day 25 and beyond.[12]

Thus by 1969 the stage was set for Pharriss and Wyngarden's discovery.[1] A wealth of good experimental evidence had then proved that the release of a uterine luteolytic hormone directly to the ipsilateral ovary was the mechanism controlling the duration of the estrous cycle in the nonpregnant animal. Furthermore, the release of another soluble factor from the developing conceptus, termed the maternal recognition of pregnancy signal by Short,[13] was the key that prevented release of uterine luteolysin and so permitted the CL to remain functional and maintain the progestational requirements of pregnancy. Upon publication of the paper by Pharriss and Wyngarden[1] a flurry of research activity took place throughout the world to confirm that $PGF_2\alpha$

was similarly luteolytic when administered to other animal species. This proved to be the case in the cow,[14] the mare,[15] the ewe,[16] and the sow,[17] and very quickly, pharmaceutical companies turned their attention to synthesis of molecules structurally related to $PGF_2\alpha$ to produce analogues in which the balance of luteolytic- and smooth-muscle–stimulating properties were different from the naturally occurring prostaglandin. It was generally believed then, and remains basically true today, that the ability of these substances to induce contraction of various types of smooth muscle is associated with their toxicity in many species. As early as 1972, ICI Pharmaceuticals Division had synthesized two such analogues, cloprostenol and fluprostenol, both of which exhibited greatly enhanced luteolytic properties when compared with the naturally occurring hormone.[18] The former proved to be the drug of choice for synchronizing estrus in cattle,[19] whereas the latter proved efficacious for inducing luteolysis in mares.[20] It is of some historic interest that, because of the high incidence of spontaneously prolonged luteal function in nonpregnant mares and the need for a simple and efficacious method in treating the condition, fluprostenol was the first synthetic prostaglandin to be marketed commercially for therapeutic purposes (Equimate; ICI Pharmaceuticals, Cheshire, UK).

SYNTHESIS AND METABOLISM OF $PGF_2\alpha$ IN THE MARE

Prostaglandin $F_2\alpha$ is just one of a large family of 20-carbon fatty acids derived from arachidonic acid. The latter is released in free form as a result of the hydrolysis of membrane phospholipids by the enzyme phospholipase A. It is then converted to prostaglandins and related compounds via the cyclo-oxygenase pathway, using a microsomal enzyme complex known collectively as prostaglandin synthetase.[21] Prostaglandin $F_2\alpha$, and its close relative prostaglandin E_2 (PGE_2) are the two prostaglandins most closely associated with reproduction in mammals and both may be released by various cell types within the reproductive tract in response to a variety of endocrine, neural, and physical stimuli.[22]

Endogenous prostaglandins are metabolized very rapidly in the body, both at the site of production and also in the lungs, liver, and kidneys.[23] In the mare, PGF_2 is metabolized first to 15-keto-$PGF_2\alpha$, then to 13, 14-dihydro-15-keto-$PGF_2\alpha$ and, finally, to a range of 11-ketotetranor-PGF compounds.[24] Although the 13,14-dihydro-15-keto metabolite (PGFM) has a biological half-life of only 5 min in the peripheral circulation, it is considerably more stable in plasma or serum when separated from the red blood cells. For this reason there has been widespread acceptance over the years that measurement of PGFM concentrations in peripheral blood gives an accurate reflection of the amount and rate of release of $PGF_2\alpha$ from tissues.[25–29]

$PGF_2\alpha$ IN THE CYCLING MARE

Although little, if anything, is known about the possible role of PGE_2 in equine reproduction, firm evidence exists that $PGF_2\alpha$ is the uterine luteolytic hormone which controls luteal lifespan and function and hence the duration of the estrous cycle in the nonpregnant mare. Following the original demonstrations of the potent luteolytic properties of exogenous $PGF_2\alpha$[15] and PGF analogues[30] in the mare,[31] Douglas and Ginther were the first to demonstrate a rise in uterine release of endogenous PGF_2 in the mare associated with luteolysis during the estrous cycle.[31] By measuring $PGF_2\alpha$ concentrations in individual samples of uterine vein blood recovered from cycling and pregnant mares under general anaesthesia, they found that concentrations were significantly higher on day 14 after ovulation in pregnant than in cycling mares and the concentrations were higher at this stage than at days 10 and 18 in the nonpregnant animals (Fig. 8-1).

Neely et al.[32] and Stabenfeldt et al.[27] further examined $PGF_2\alpha$ release in cycling mares by measuring PGFM concentrations in peripheral plasma. The study by Neely et al.[32] involved the recovery of jugular vein samples every 3 to 6 h continuously over a 4-month period from seven cycling mares, and it established three important parameters. First, as in the ewe and other farm species,[16] $PGF_2\alpha$ is released from the endometrium in pulsatile bursts of short duration. These releases occur over days 14 to 17 after ovulation during a typical cycle in the mare and the first pulse of $PGF_2\alpha$ precedes the first measurable decline in plasma progesterone concentrations by 3 to 4 h (Fig. 8-1). Progesterone concentrations take only 24 to 48 h to fall to baseline values (i.e., < 1 ng/mL) but substantial, and still pulsatile, releases of $PGF_2\alpha$ may continue for 1 to 2 days after luteolysis is complete. Second, in nonpregnant mares that spontaneously maintain the CL beyond its normal lifespan (prolonged diestrus), the pulsatile releases of $PGF_2\alpha$ are depressed or completely absent around days 14 to 16. This condition of prolonged diestrus occurs more frequently in mares than in other domestic livestock species,[33] and it does not appear to be associated with any particular abnormality or pathologic change in the uterus (Fig. 8-2). The persisting luteal tissue is sensitive to the luteolytic action of exogenous $PGF_2\alpha$ or its analogues.[20]

The third, and not altogether unexpected finding in the study by Neely et al.[32] was the release of $PGF_2\alpha$ by the endometrium in response to filling the uterus with a large volume of saline. Prior to the advent of injectable preparations of $PGF_2\alpha$ and PG analogues in the early 1970s, nonpregnant mares that stopped cycling during the breeding season had been treated by intrauterine saline irrigation in an attempt to induce estrus and renewed follicular growth. This therapy appeared to work well in some mares but not in others,[34,35] and when it was realized by the increased use of progesterone assays that noncyclicity during the spring and summer months was almost always a result of the affected mare having passed spontaneously into prolonged diestrus,[36] it was

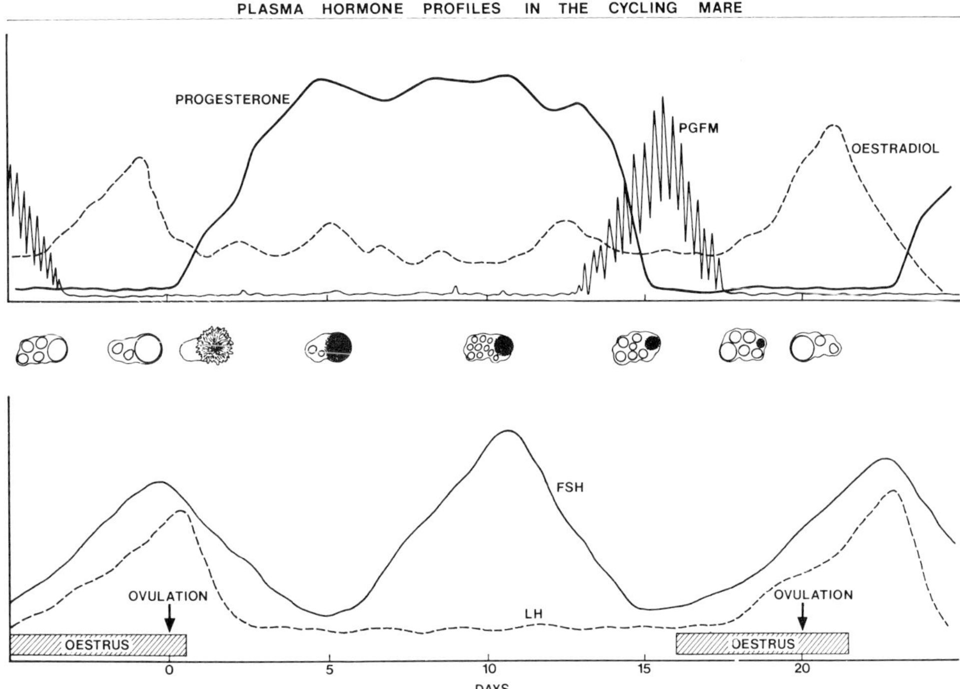

FIG. 8–1. Diagrammatic summary of the peripheral plasma profiles of FSH, LH, progesterone, estradiol, and 13,14-dihydro-15-keto-$PGF_2\alpha$ (PGFM) measured in the mare during an estrous cycle.

assumed, quite reasonably, that intrauterine irrigation stimulated release of endometrial $PGF_2\alpha$ which, in turn, induced lysis of the persisting luteal tissue. This was confirmed when Neely et al. demonstrated a rapid rise in plasma PGFM concentrations within minutes of infusing saline into the uteri of diestrous mares.[32] However, Pascoe subsequently examined the whole question of intrauterine saline infusion in more detail, and he made two important discoveries.[37] First, he noted that the rapid release of $PGF_2\alpha$ immediately after saline treatment only occurred if the saline being infused was slightly acidic and, therefore, caused mild irritation of the endometrium; infusion of physiologic saline with a neutral pH gave only a very muted PGFM response or none at all. Second, an infusion of neutral pH saline was sometimes followed by a second and more prolonged release of $PGF_2\alpha$, beginning 48 to 72 h after infusion. However, this secondary rise in PGFM concentrations only occurred when using saline that contained no antibiotics so that a low-grade bacterial endometritis commenced shortly after treatment.

Thus it has become clear that untoward release of $PGF_2\alpha$ from the mare's uterus, in large enough quantities and over a long enough period to induce premature luteolysis, can be stimulated by chemical and/or bacterial inflammation of the endometrium. Various mechanical stimuli, such as dilation of the cervix and the manipulative and pressure effects associated with nonsurgical embryo recovery using physiologic media containing antibiotics, may stimulate a rapid but brief rise in plasma PGFM concentrations,[28,38] but this is only rarely of sufficient magnitude and duration to cause luteolysis unless followed by bacterial endometritis.[37,39,40] Similarly, manual compression of the uterus per rectum when attempting to rupture one of twin conceptuses between days 18 and 30 of gestation stimulates a rapid but brief rise in plasma PGFM concentrations in some mares that is not accompanied by any immediate change in peripheral plasma progesterone profile[41] and which, judging by the high rate of success of the manipulation in mares carrying bicornuate twins,[41,42] is not followed by luteolysis at a later stage. Surgical hysterotomy performed between days 40 and 65 of gestation via a ventral midline abdominal incision under general anesthesia stimulates a large and steep rise in plasma PGFM concentrations when the uterus is incised with the scalpel. However, this release of $PGF_2\alpha$ is also relatively short lived (i.e., < 4 h) and would, therefore, be unlikely to induce luteolysis.[43]

$PGF_2\alpha$ IN THE PREGNANT MARE

Three unusual features of early pregnancy in the mare seem to set it apart from other large domestic species in terms of the mechanism involved in maternal recognition of pregnancy and maintenance of luteal function beyond the duration of cyclical diestrus (Fig. 8-3). First, as indicated originally by hysterectomy and hemihysterectomy experiments carried out in mares by Ginther and First,[44] and confirmed subsequently by perfusion of postmortem mare reproductive tracts with colored latex,[45] the mare does not possess the characteristic intertwining of the uterine vein and ovarian artery in the

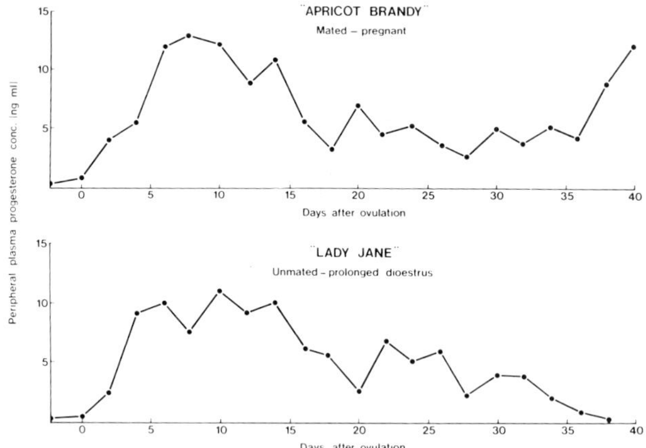

FIG. 8–2. The common occurrence of spontaneous prolongation of luteal function in the mare. Peripheral plasma progesterone concentrations measured in two Welsh Pony mares during the first 40 days after ovulation (day 0). "Apricot Brandy" was mated and conceived whereas "Lady Jane" was not mated but passed simultaneously into prolonged diestrus. Note the similarity of the two profiles between days 5 and 30.

ovarian pedicule that enables direct countercurrent perfusion of endometrial $PGF_2\alpha$ into the ovarian artery as occurs in the ewe and other species.[16] Thus endometrial $PGF_2\alpha$ released during days 14 to 17 in the cycling mare can only reach the ovary by passing through the cardiovascular system in which it is subject to rapid metabolism in the lungs and other organs.[46] This lack of a local utero-ovarian transport system in the mare is perhaps the underlying reason for the increased sensitivity, on a dose per body weight basis compared with other species, of the equine CL to the luteolytic effects of exogenous $PGF_2\alpha$ and PGF analogues.[20,36]

A second fascinating, and apparently unique, feature of the pregnant mare is the maintenance, until relatively late in gestation, of the spherical form of the conceptus[47] and its great mobility within the uterine lumen.[48] In the sheep, cow, and most dramatically, in the pig, the trophectoderm of the blastocyst undergoes tremendous growth and elongation between days 10 to 14 after ovulation (Fig. 8-4). In the pig, for example, the spherical blastocyst that measures approximately 5 to 10 mm in diameter at day 10, transforms within the space of the next 3 days into an elongated, thread-like structure of more than 1 m in length.[49] This elongation phase in the ruminants and suids means that, at the critical time for transmission of the fetal signal to prevent release of endometrial $PGF_2\alpha$, trophoblast tissue is in close contact with a large area of the endometrial surface. This, in turn, enables direct passage of the fetal message from the organ of supply, the trophoblast, to the target organ, the maternal endometrium (Fig. 8-4).

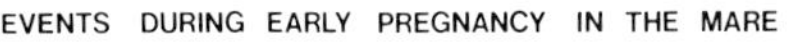

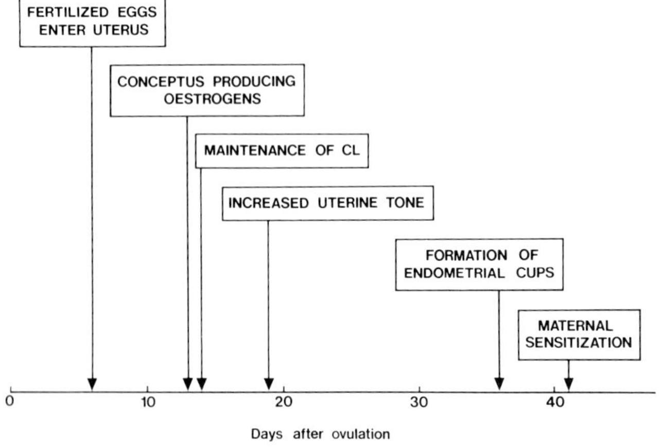

FIG. 8–3. Summary of some of the significant events associated with the maternal recognition of pregnancy in the mare.

The horse conceptus similarly sends its antiluteolytic maternal recognition of pregnancy signal to the endometrium between days 14 and 16 after ovulation.[50,51] However, because of the lack of any ipsilateral utero-ovarian local transport mechanism, the conceptus, if tempted to elongate like the other species, would face the seemingly impossible task of expanding sufficiently over the space of only 2 or 3 days to have trophoblast cells in contact with virtually the entire endometrial surface of the whole uterus. It seems to have solved this problem by remaining spherical, staying completely unattached to the endometrium[52,53] and moving continually throughout the uterus. By comparing the known side of ovulation with the eventual side of implantation in Thoroughbred mares it had been realized for many years that transuterine migration of the conceptus occurred in approximately 50% of equine pregnancies.[54–56] However, the full extent and the back-and-forth movement of the conceptus throughout the uterus before, during, and after the crucial period for release of the maternal recognition of pregnancy signal was not fully appreciated until Ginther carried out an exhaustive series of experiments that involved long, unbroken periods of transrectal ultrasonography of the uteri of mares between days 10 and 25 of gestation.[48,57–59] These prolonged examinations revealed that the equine conceptus remains "on the move" from the time it emerges from the uterotubal papilla at day 5 or 6[39] until it becomes "fixed" in the eventual site of implantation at the base of one uterine horn around day 17 or 18[58] by the dramatic increase in myometrial tone that commences at day 16 or 17.[60]

The third unique feature of the young equine conceptus that may play a role in the maternal recognition of pregnancy is the development of the so-called equine blastocyst capsule. This constitutes a thin, translucent, amorphous, acellular layer that closely invests the external surface of the trophoblast cells and completely envelops the conceptus (Fig. 8-5).[61,62] It appears to be composed of heavily glycosylated proteins, is remarkably resistant to solubilization and enzyme degradation,[63] and persists intact until at least day 25 of gestation.[64] Although its exact function is not known, many have speculated that it plays some role in the maternal recognition of pregnancy, perhaps acting simply as a physical shield to protect the conceptus from the pressure of the myometrial contractions which move it so rapidly around the uterus. Or it may possibly function as some sort of filter of

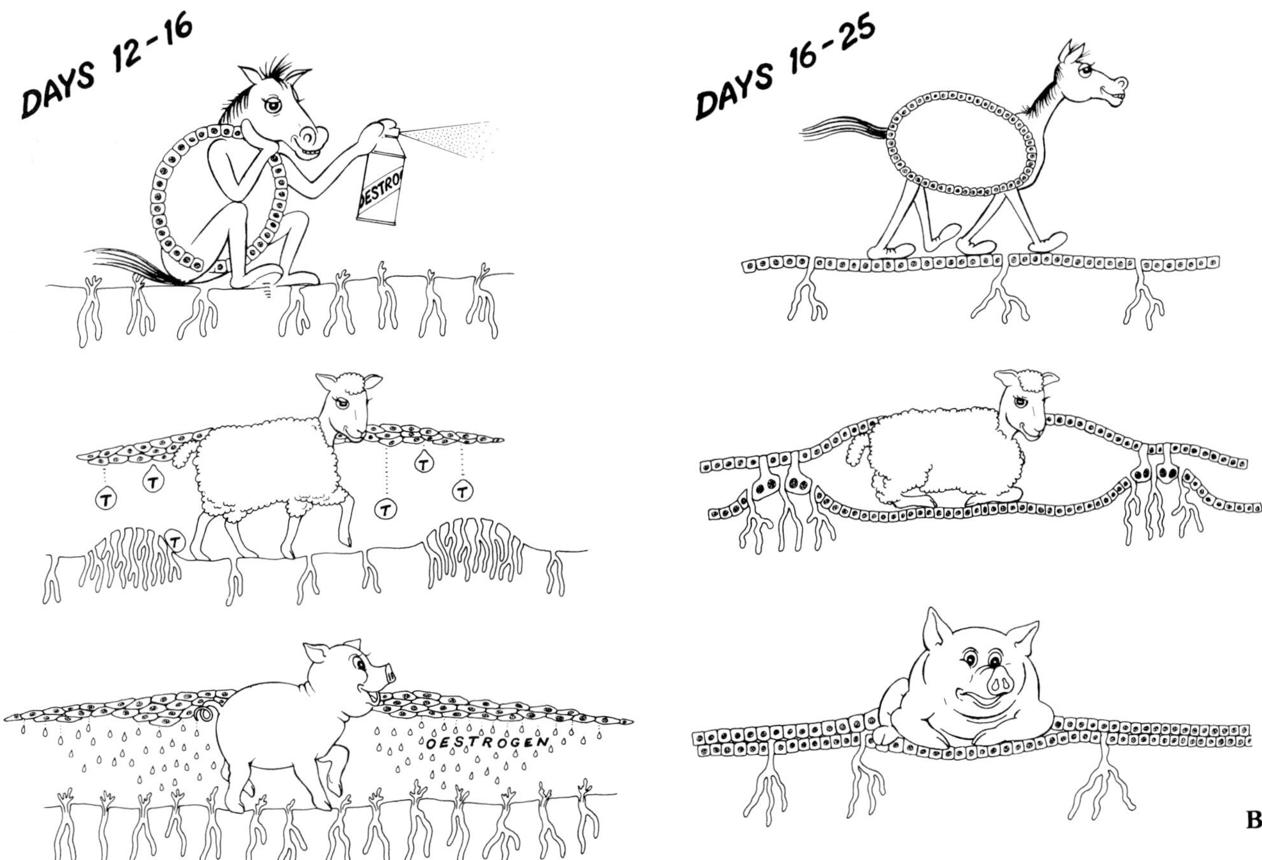

FIG. 8–4. Cartoons depicting the striking morphologic and development differences among horse, sheep, and pig conceptuses during *(A)* the period associated with maternal recognition of pregnancy at days 12 to 16 after ovulation and *(B)* the period associated with implantation at days 16 to 25 in the sheep and pig.

the chemical signal from the conceptus before this reaches the endometrium.

Whatever role the blastocyst capsule may play, some difference of opinion exists about mechanisms involved in its initial development. In a study involving the bisection of morulae for the production of monozygotic (identical) twins, Skidmore et al.[65] observed that when the resulting demiembryos were cultured in vitro for 48 to 96 h, they developed into expanding blastocysts that were devoid of a capsule. This occurred regardless of whether a capsule had already existed when the morulae were bisected originally. On the other hand, when intact morulae were cultured for the same periods of time they developed into hatched blastocysts surrounded by apparently normal capsules. Skidmore and colleagues[65] argued that the difference indicated an obligatory role for the zona pellucida in "molding" capsule precursor proteins and organs to the spherical form of the embryo before cross-linking and a general "setting" or solidification process gave rise to the capsule per se. However, in a similar study involving the culture of morulae in vitro, McKinnon and colleagues[66] noted that if the capsule was not already visible microscopically between the zona pellucida and the clump of blastomeres when the morula was placed in culture, it failed to develop during the subsequent culture period. Furthermore, they transferred a pair of demiembryos from a bisected morula to recipient mares and subsequently flushed the uteri of the recipients 8 days later (day 14 after ovulation). An ongoing conceptus was recovered from both mares, and in each case, it was surrounded by an apparently normal capsule. Since neither demiembryo was invested in a zona pellucida at the time of transfer, this finding indicated that the zona is not, after all, necessary to mold the capsule constituents to the shape of the embryo. Furthermore, the lack of capsule development or precapsular morulae cultured in vitro, and the development of new capsules on the demiembryos growing in vivo, suggests the possibility that endometrial proteins or other uterine factors play an important part in capsule development. Betteridge[64] eloquently discussed the possible mechanisms involved in the development of the equine blastocyst capsule and compared the situation to the formation of the neozona on the inside and the gloiolemma on the outside of the microprotein coat laid down on the surface of the rabbit embryo during its passage through the oviduct as proposed by Denker.[67] The results of further current studies on the subject by Betteridge and colleagues should prove of great interest.

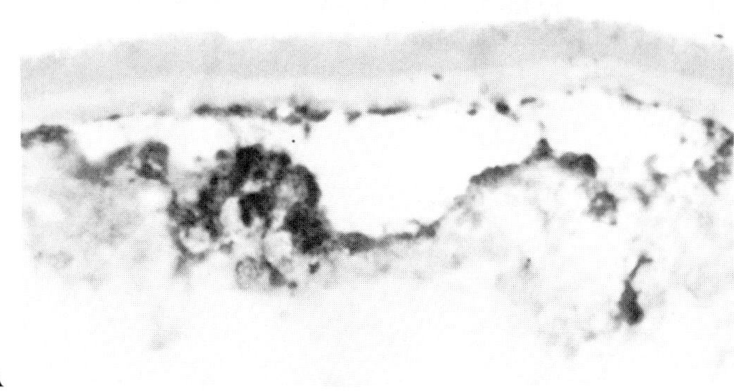

A

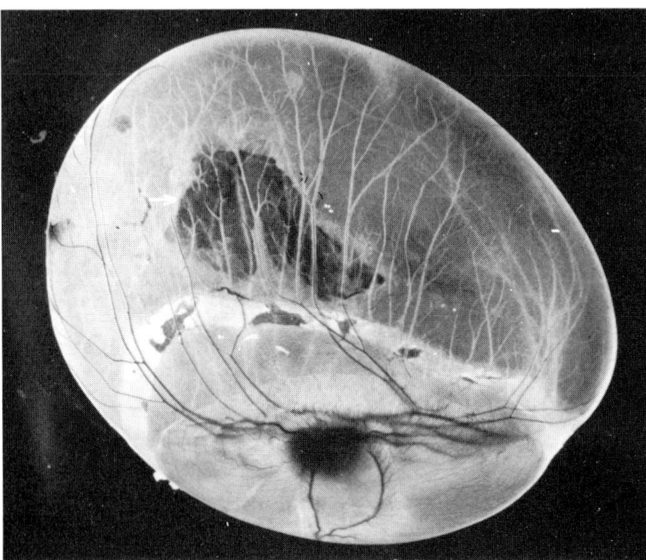

B

FIG. 8–5. The equine blastocyst capsule. *A*, Section of a day-12 horse conceptus stained with a monoclonal antibody (102.1) specific for equine trophoblast. The bilaminar capsule is seen closely investing the trophectoderm (× 280). (Reproduced with permission from Dr. J.G. Oriol.) *B*, Intact horse conceptus at day 35 after ovulation. The blotchy, whitish, hazy appearance of the allantochorion (arrow) is caused by the persisting remnants of the disintegrating blastocyst capsule.

Thus it appears that the horse embryo has played some neat evolutionary tricks to ensure the maintenance of luteal function in its mother and, hence, its own survival in a progesterone-dominated uterus. In the absence of evidence to the contrary it seems reasonable to suppose that during its wanderings within the uterine lumen the conceptus continually releases its chemical signal onto the endometrium to restrain the latter from liberating its stores of $PGF_2\alpha$ to bring about luteolysis. Presumably, the conceptus must achieve direct, or very near, contact with a high proportion of the total endometrial surface to achieve this objective and, indeed, McDowell et al. demonstrated that surgical compartmentalization of the mare's uterus to restrict conceptus mobility between days 12 and 20 results in luteolysis unless the conceptus is left with the uterine body, one complete horn, and the majority of the other horn in which to wander about, regardless of which side the CL is situated.[51] It remains a matter of speculation as to which, if any, of these unusual features of luteal maintenance in equids may have imposed evolutionary pressure on the others to develop. Did the absence in the mare of the local utero-ovarian vascular connection that forms such a vital part of the maternal recognition of pregnancy mechanism in ruminants and other large species drive the conceptus to remain spherical, produce a protective capsule, and stay mobile to deliver its antiluteolytic signal to those parts of the uterus which its trophoblast would otherwise be unable to reach? Or did a mobile conceptus, able to cast its message efficiently into all corners of the uterine domain, obviate the need for a local utero-ovarian pathway to develop?

The chemical nature of the fetal luteostatic signal in the pregnant mare remains unknown, although there is now ample evidence that it functions primarily in an antiluteolytic, rather than a luteotrophic, manner. The concentration of receptors for $PGF_2\alpha$ in luteal tissue in pregnant mares between days 12 and 18 after ovulation is equal to, or even higher than, the concentration in the CL at the same stage of the cycle,[68] and the pulsatile releases of PGFM measured in the peripheral circulation between days 14 and 17 in the nonpregnant mare[32] are muted or completely absent in the pregnant mare at this stage.[69] Furthermore, concentrations of $PGF_2\alpha$ measured in the uterine lumenal fluids of mares are appreciably lower at day 14 of gestation than at the same stage of the cycle,[70,71] whereas the production of $PGF_2\alpha$ in vitro by explants of endometrial tissue is equivalent with endometrium recovered from pregnant and nonpregnant mares at days 14 and 16, but is depressed when either nonpregnant or pregnant endometrium explants are coincubated with conceptus tissues.[70]

In ruminants such as the sheep and cow, it is now firmly established that the antiluteolytic factor released by the conceptus is an acidic polypeptide of approximately 19,000 molecular weight which is termed, respectively, ovine and bovine trophoblast protein (OTP and BTP)[72] (Fig. 8-4A). This protein shows a remarkable degree of homology with the antiviral factor interferon-α[73,74] and it appears to function in the uterus both by directly suppressing the release of $PGF_2\alpha$ from the endometrium[75] and by preventing the induction of receptors in the endometrium to limit the $PGF_2\alpha$-stimulating properties of oxytocin released from the corpus luteum.[76]

In the pig, on the other hand, the experiments of Bazer and Thatcher[77] and others provided a convincing argument that the large quantities of estrogens secreted by the porcine trophoblast[78] are the antiluteolytic factor in this species and that they function by redirecting the $PGF_2\alpha$, which is normally secreted by the lumenal and glandular epithelium in an endocrine manner into the uterine venous drainage, into an exocrine type of secretion that enters the uterine lumen[77] (Fig. 8-4A). Supportive evidence for such a concept comes from finding a tenfold or more increase in the concentrations of $PGF_2\alpha$ in intralumenal fluids on days 14 to 18 of pregnancy compared with the same stage of the estrous cycle[77] and an absence of any trophoblastin-like proteins with antiluteolytic properties in porcine trophoblast tissues.[79] Furthermore, a single injection of estradiol benzoate given to cycling gilts between days 10 and 12 of diestrus will significantly prolong luteal lifespan.[80]

Like the porcine conceptus, and in contrast to the embryos of a wide range of small and large domestic and wild animal species examined to date,[78] the still-spherical equine conceptus begins to secrete large quantities of estrogens from as early as day 12 after ovulation.[81,82] Furthermore, attempts to identify a trophoblastin-like molecule with interferon-like properties,[83] or mRNA for equine interferons,[84] in days 13 to 20 horse conceptus tissues have met with no success. It is, therefore, tempting to speculate that the horse conceptus, like the pig, prevents release of endometrial $PGF_2\alpha$ and, hence, achieves luteostasis by means of its early and excessive production of estrogens (Fig. 8-4A). However, three pieces of evidence seem to argue against such a possibility. First, intralumenal uterine fluid concentrations of $PGF_2\alpha$ are lower, rather than higher, around day 14 in pregnant as compared with nonpregnant mares.[71] Second, single or multiple injections of estradiol given to cycling mares from day 10 of diestrus do not prolong luteal lifespan as in the pig.[85] Third, coincubation of endometrial explants with conceptus tissues restrained in dialysis tubing of varying molecular pore sizes indicated that the conceptus product which is able to suppress $PGF_2\alpha$ release by the endometrium has a molecular weight between 1,000 and 12,000.[86] This is appreciably above the molecular weight of estrogen or any other steroid hormone.

In attempting to summarize the situation concerning the maternal recognition of pregnancy and luteostasis in the pregnant mare, one can speculate with a parable. The spherical, encapsulated, estrogen-secreting day-14 conceptus motors its way around the uterus liberating unknown quantities of an endometrial $PGF_2\alpha$-suppressing low-molecular-weight molecule, rather in the manner of a man distributing fertilizer by hand onto a lawn in springtime. A sizable release of $PGF_2\alpha$ from the endometrium is necessary toward the end of diestrus to survive the metabolic wastage caused by its passage to the ovaries via the peripheral rather than a local circulatory route. Similarly, a good dose of fertilizer is needed to make up for that which will be washed into the drains by the rain before it has gained access to the roots of the grass plants. But, rather like the heavy thunderstorm that can so easily ablate the gardener's best intentions with the fertilizer, the $PGF_2\alpha$ release-and-response mechanism in the mare is so finely tuned that it requires only a minor disturbance for insufficient $PGF_2\alpha$ to reach the ovary to bring about complete luteolysis. Hence, the syndrome of spontaneous prolonged diestrus occurs commonly in nonpregnant cycling mares. But, tit for tat, the mechanism for inducing luteostasis during pregnancy is equally hair-triggered and is easily switched on. Thus the equine conceptus gets away, under normal circumstances, with its seemingly nomadic and indifferent lifestyle and the vague distributing about the uterine environment of its maternal recognition of pregnancy hormone. Perhaps it is the specificity of this signal, not its quantity or method of delivery, that is the key.

PROSTAGLANDIN SECRETION IN LATER PREGNANCY

Once luteostasis of the primary corpus luteum has been achieved around day 16 after ovulation in the pregnant mare, $PGF_2\alpha$ seems to largely disappear from the mare's blood and from the mind's eye for the next 10 months. There are, however, two aspects involving $PGF_2\alpha$ release in the intervening period that deserve brief mention. Endotoxemia, resulting from the sudden release into the circulation of lipopolysaccharide endotoxin from the cell wall of gram-negative bacteria, can cause abortion in rodents,[87] pigs,[88] and mares[22,89] through the luteolytic action of a pronounced release of $PGF_2\alpha$ stimulated by the endotoxin. In the mare, Daels et al. demonstrated that a single bolus injection of endotoxin causes a rapid and biphasic rise in plasma PGFM concentrations of 4- to 6-h duration that is followed by luteolysis with abortion occurring 2 to 3 days later in pregnant mares up to, but not beyond, day 55 of gestation.[22] This endotoxin-induced surge of $PGF_2\alpha$ release can be prevented by simultaneous administration of the prostaglandin synthetase inhibitor flunixin meglumine, provided this is given either before, or within only a few minutes after, the injection of endotoxin.[90]

The other interesting and, as yet unexplained, observation concerning untoward release of $PGF_2\alpha$ during early pregnancy in the mare is the abortion that frequently follows one or more injections of 3000 IU human Chorionic Gonadotrophin (hCG) given between days 20 and 30 after ovulation[91] and which can be prevented by the simultaneous administration of exogenous progesterone.[92] Urwin re-examined this question by measuring progesterone concentrations in serial jugular vein blood samples recovered at four hourly intervals from day-20 to day-30 pregnant mares before and after hCG treatment.[93] She observed a precipitous drop in concentrations that commenced within 4 h after the hCG injection and, hence, was reminiscent of the steep decline in plasma progesterone values that occurs in diestrous mares after an injection of exogenous prostaglandin $F_2\alpha$ analogue.[36] Unfortunately, she did not measure plasma PGFM concentrations in the hCG-treated mares but, in view of the clear evidence of luteolysis coupled with earlier observation that abortion can be prevented by exogenous progesterone,[90] the likelihood is great that the event is stimulated by an untoward release of $PGF_2\alpha$ from the endometrium. Why such a thing should occur in response to a single injection of an otherwise innocuous gonadotropin preparation that is used routinely to hasten ovulation in estrous mares[94] remains a mystery.

Prostaglandin $F_2\alpha$ returns to prominence in the pregnant mare during the final stages of gestation. Concentrations of PGFM in peripheral plasma increase slowly

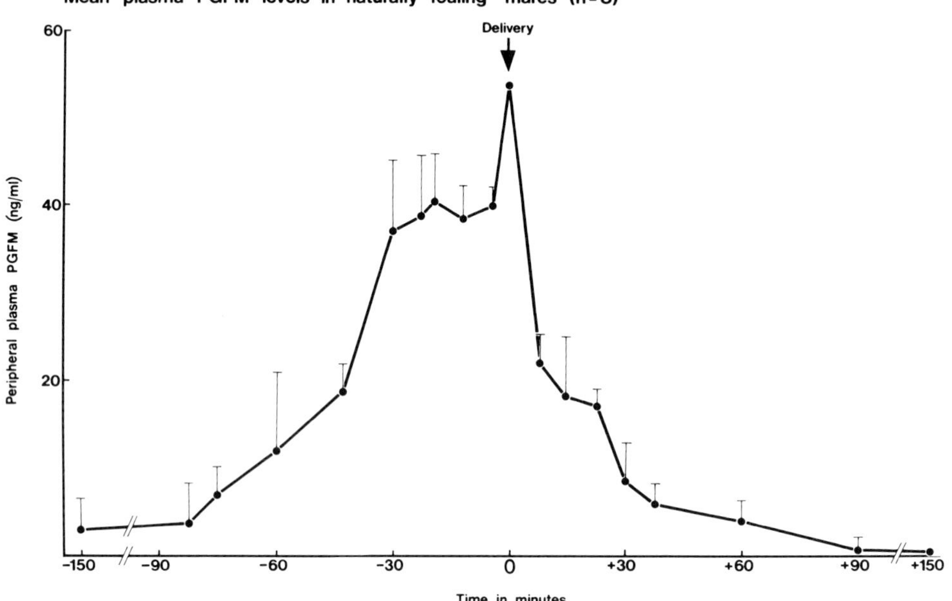

FIG. 8–6. Mean plasma 13,14-dihydro,15-keto-PGF$_{2\alpha}$ (PGFM) concentrations measured in eight pony mares during spontaneous foaling. Note the coincidence of the peak with passage of the foal through the birth canal. (From Pashen, R.L.: Studies on the endocrinology of pregnancy in the mare. Ph.D. thesis, University of Cambridge, Cambridge, 1980.)

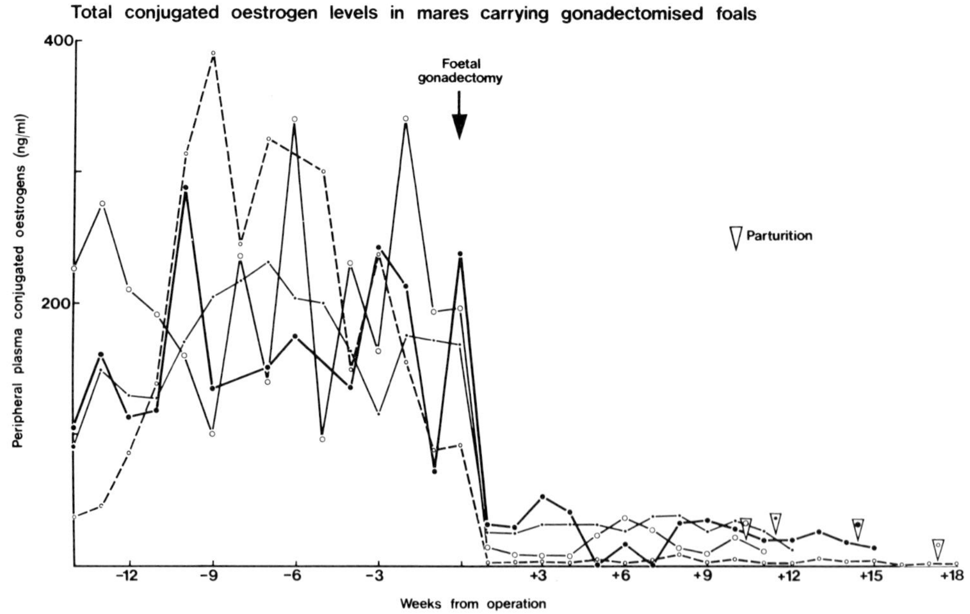

FIG. 8–7. Total conjugated estrogen concentrations measured in the peripheral plasma of four pony mares before and after bilateral gonadectomy of their fetuses between days 197 and 353 of gestation. (From Pashen, R.L.: Studies on the endocrinology of pregnancy in the mare. Ph.D. thesis, University of Cambridge, Cambridge, 1980.)

and steadily during the last month before foaling with an explosive rise that commences with the onset of first-stage labor and reaches a sharp and well-defined peak of around 40 to 60 ng/mL coincidentally with maximum expulsive effort during second-stage labor (Fig. 8-6). The concentrations then fall steeply again and have usually reached baseline values of < 1 ng/mL by as soon as 1 to 2 h after the end of third-stage labor and expulsion of the placenta.[26,29,95] Similar, and equally steep, rises in plasma PGFM concentrations accompany parturition induced in mares at term by either a low dose (5 to 10 IU) of oxytocin[96] or a single intramuscular injection of either of the $PGF_2\alpha$ analogues fluprostenol and cloprostenol.[97,98] If the mare is fully at term when the treatment is given, the foal is born within 45 to 90 min and the PGFM peak in maternal plasma coincides closely with second-stage labor as in spontaneous parturition. If fetal readiness for birth has not yet been fully achieved, however, the interval between treatment and foaling increases and a less well defined peak of PGFM in maternal blood may occur prior to the onset of second-stage labor.[97]

The available evidence indicates that a steady buildup in the capacity of the uterus to synthesize, store, and release $PGF_2\alpha$ occurs in parallel with maturation of the fetus and/or placenta leading to foaling. The stimulus for this fairly rapid increase in $PGF_2\alpha$ synthesizing capacity and the trigger for the explosive release of prostaglandin at foaling are not well understood, although estrogens produced by the fetoplacental unit may play at least a priming role in the process. Bilateral fetal gonadectomy carried out in four mares between days 197 and 253 of gestation resulted in an immediate fall to baseline values of the high concentrations of phenolic and B ring unsaturated estrogens present in the blood and urine of mares during the second half of pregnancy[26] (Fig. 8-7). Although parturition commenced spontaneously between days 294 and 323 in all four mares carrying gonadectomized fetuses, the pattern of uterine contractions was weak and abnormal such that three of the foals required manual traction to complete their passage through the birth canal. Serial blood samples were obtained from two of the mares during parturition and these showed no evidence of the typical surge in PGFM concentrations that accompanies normal foaling (Fig. 8-8).

These unexpected findings indicated a strong influence of estrogens on the synthesis and/or release of prostaglandins in the pregnant equine uterus. Estrogens are considered essential in the normal process of prostaglandin synthesis in many species. In the sheep and goat, for example, temporal relationships have been demonstrated among the prepartum estrogen surge, the increase in uterine $PGF_2\alpha$ synthesis, the decrease in the oxytocic threshold of the myometrium, and the increase in spontaneous activity of the uterus.[99,100] At first glance the horse would seem not to comply to this general pattern because the mare shows a steady fall in plasma and urinary estrogen concentrations during the last two months of gestation[101] and does not exhibit any secondary rise associated with parturition that is so characteristic of ruminants and other large domestic

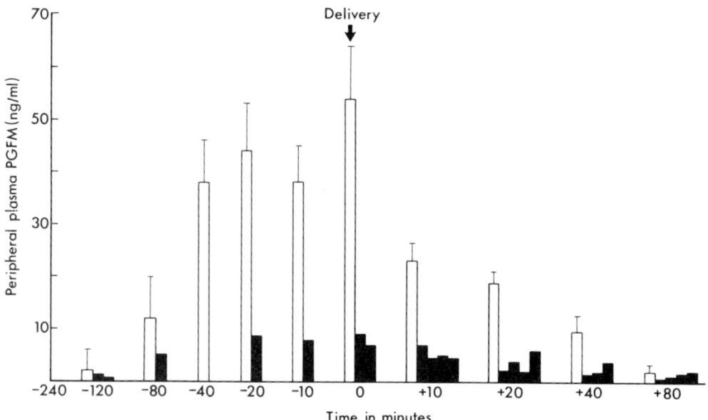

FIG. 8–8. Comparison of the mean plasma 13,14-dihydro-15-keto-$PGF_2\alpha$ (PGFM) concentrations measured in eight pony mares carrying intact fetuses around the time of foaling (open bars) with the levels in two mares carrying bilaterally gonadectomized fetuses that commenced parturition spontaneously (solid bars). (From Pashen, R.L.: Studies on the endocrinology of pregnancy in the mare. Ph.D. thesis, University of Cambridge, Cambridge, 1980.)

species.[102] On the other hand, a completely different mechanism for the regulation of prostaglandin synthesis could exist in the mare which relies fundamentally on the maintenance of a definite threshold concentration of estrogens for preparing and priming the tissues involved in other endocrine and/or enzyme changes that are, in turn, responsible for $PGF_2\alpha$ production during labor. The estrogens could act either directly on the major sites of prostaglandin synthesis or indirectly via the control of prostaglandin and/or oxytocin receptor numbers. Any reduction in the number of oxytocin binding sites that occurred as a result of decreased estrogen secretion would certainly reduce oxytocin-induced release of $PGF_2\alpha$.[97,103] This would then result in severe disruption of the changes during labor that depend on normal $PGF_2\alpha$ production, including myometrial contractions and cervical dilation.

REFERENCES

1. Pharriss, B.B., and Wyngarden, L.J.: The effect of prostaglandin $F_2\alpha$ on the progestagen content of ovaries from pseudopregnant rats. Proc. Soc. Exp. Biol. Med., *130*:92–94, 1969.
2. Moor, R.M., and Rowson, L.E.A.: Influence of the embryo and uterus on luteal function in the sheep. Nature, *201*:522–523, 1964.
3. Rowson, L.E.A., and Moor, R.M.: Effect of partial hysterectomy on the length of the dioestrous interval in sheep. Proceedings of the First International Congress on Animal Reproduction and Artificial Insemination. 1964, pp. 6–13.
4. Moor, R.M., and Rowson, L.E.A.: Local uterine mechanisms affecting luteal function in the sheep. J. Reprod. Fertil., *11*:307–310, 1966.
5. Du Mesnil du Buisson, F.: Regression unilaterale des corpes jaunes apres hysterectomie partielle chez la truie.

Ann. Biol. Anim. Biochim. Biophys., *1*:106–109, 1961.

6. Anderson, L.L., Rathmacher, R.P., and Melampy, R.M.: The uterus and unilateral regression of corpora lutea in the pig. Am. J. Physiol., *210*:611–616, 1966.
7. Heap, R.B., Perry, J.S., and Rowlands, I.W.: Corpus luteum function in the guinea pig; arterial and luteal progesterone levels, and the effect of hysterectomy and hypophysectomy. J. Reprod. Fertil., *13*:537–554, 1967.
8. Du Mesnil du Buisson, F., and Rombauts, P.: Reduction experimentale du nombre de foetus an cours de la gestation de la trui et mantien des corps jaunes. Ann. Biol. Anim. Biochim. Biophys., *3*:445–449, 1963.
9. Moor, R.M., and Rowson, L.E.A.: The corpus luteum of the sheep: Relationships between morphology and function during the oestrous cycle. Acta Endocrinol. (Copenh.), *51*:245–263, 1966.
10. Anderson, L.L.: Pituitary-ovarian relationships in pigs. J. Reprod. Fertil. Suppl., *1*:21–28, 1966.
11. Dhindsa, D.S., and Dzuik, P.J.: Effect of position of embryos on pregnancy in pigs. J. Anim. Sci., *25*:1266–1271, 1966.
12. Rowson, L.E.A., and Moor, R.M.: The influence of embryonic tissue homogenate infused into the uterus, on the life-span of the corpus luteum in the sheep. J. Reprod. Fertil., *13*:511–516, 1967.
13. Short, R.V.: Implantation and the maternal recognition of pregnancy. *In* Ciba Foundation Symposium on Foetal Autonomy. Edited by G.E.W. Wolstenholme and M. O'Connor. London, J. & A. Churchill, 1969, pp. 2–26.
14. Rowson, L.E.A., Tervitt, R., and Brand, A.: Synchronization of oestrus in cattle by means of prostaglandin. Proceedings of the Seventh International Congress on Animal Reproduction and Artificial Insemination. Vol. 2. 1972, pp. 865–869.
15. Douglas, R.H., and Ginther, O.J.: Effect of prostaglandin $F_2\alpha$ on length of diestrus in mares. Prostaglandins, *2*:265–268, 1972.
16. McCracken, J.A., et al.: Prostaglandin $F_2\alpha$ identified as a luteolytic hormone in sheep. Nature (New Biol.), *238*:129–134, 1972.
17. Guthrie, H.D., and Polge, E.J.C.: Luteal function and oestrus in gilts treated with a synthetic analogue of prostaglandin $F_2\alpha$ (ICI-79,939) at various times during the oestrous cycle. J. Reprod. Fertil., *48*:423–425, 1976.
18. Binder, B.: 16-Aryloxyprostaglandins; A new class of potent luteolytic agent. Prostaglandins, *6*:98–90, 1974.
19. Cooper, M.J.: Control of oestrous cycles of heifers with a synthetic prostaglandin analogue. Vet. Rec., *95*:200–203, 1974.
20. Allen, W.R., et al.: Further studies on the use of synthetic prostaglandin analogues for inducing luteolysis in mares. Equine Vet. J., *6*:31–35, 1974.
21. Samuelsson, B.: Prostaglandins, thromboxanes and leucotrienes: Formation and biological roles. Harvey Lect., *75*:1–40, 1981.
22. Daels, P.F. et al.: Effect of Salmonella typhimurium endotoxin on $PGF_2\alpha$ release and fetal death in the mare. J. Reprod. Fertil. Suppl., *35*:485–492, 1987.
23. Angåard, E., Larsson, C., and Samuelsson, B.: The distribution of 15-hydroxyprostaglandin dehydrogenase and prostaglandin[13] reductase in tissues of the swine. Acta Physiol. Scand., *81*:391–404, 1971.
24. Goff, S.A., Basu, S., and Kindahl, H.: Measurements of 11-ketotethanon PGF metabolites: An approach for monitoring prostaglandin-$F_2\alpha$ release in the mare. Theriogenology, *21*:887–896, 1984.
25. Kindahl, H., Edqvist, L.E., Bane, A., and Granstrøm, E.: Blood levels of progesterone and 15-keto 13,14-dihydroprostaglandin $F_2\alpha$ during the normal oestrous cycle and early pregnancy in heifers. Acta Endocrinol. (Copenh.), *82*:134–149, 1976.
26. Pashen, R.L., and Allen, W.R.: The role of the fetal gonads and placenta in steroid production, maintenance of pregnancy and parturition in the mare. J. Reprod. Fertil. Suppl., *27*:499–509, 1979.
27. Stabenfeldt, G.H. et al.: Control of luteolysis in the mare. Acta Vet. Scand. Suppl., *77*:159–170, 1981.
28. Betteridge, K.J., Renard, A., and Goff, A.K.: Uterine prostaglandin release relative to embryo collection, transfer procedure and maintenance of the corpus luteum. Equine Vet. J. Suppl., *3*:25–33, 1985.
29. Haluska, G.J., and Currie, W.B.: Variation in plasma concentrations of oestradiol-17β and their relationship to those of progesterone, 13,14-dihydro 15-keto prostaglandin $F_2\alpha$ and oxytocin across pregnancy and at parturition in pony mares. J. Reprod. Fertil., *84*:635–646, 1988.
30. Allen, W.R., and Rowson, L.E.A.: Control of the mare's oestrous cycle by prostaglandins. J. Reprod. Fertil., *33*:539–543, 1973.
31. Douglas, R.H., and Ginther, O.J.: Concentrations of prostaglandin F in uterine venous plasma of anaesthetised mares during estrous cycle and early pregnancy. Prostaglandins, *11*:251–260, 1976.
32. Neely, D.P., et al.: Prostaglandin release patterns in the mare: Physiological, patho-physiological and therapeutic responses. J. Reprod. Fertil. Suppl., *27*:181–189, 1979.
33. Stabenfeldt, G.H., Hughes, J.P., Evans, J.W., and Geschwind, I.I.: Unique aspects of the reproductive cycle of the mare. J. Reprod. Fertil. Suppl., *23*:155–160, 1975.
34. Arthur, G.H.: Influence of intrauterine saline infusion upon the oestrous cycle of the mare. J. Reprod. Fertil. Suppl., *23*:231–234, 1975.
35. Neely, D.P., Hughes, G.H., Stabenfeldt, G.H., and Evans, J.W.: The influence of intrauterine saline infusion on luteal function and cyclical activity in the mare. J. Reprod. Fertil. Suppl., *23*:235–239, 1975.
36. Allen, W.R., and Cooper, M.J.: The use of synthetic analogues of prostaglandins for inducing luteolysis in mares. Ann. Biol. Anim. Biochim. Biophys., *15*:461–469, 1975.
37. Pascoe, D.R.: Single embryonic reduction in the mare with twin conceptuses: Studies of hormone profiles and drug therapies using a physiological model, and manual and surgical reduction technique in vivo. Ph.D. thesis, University of California, Davis, 1986.
38. Sirois, J., Betteridge, K.J., and Goff, A.K.: $PGF_2\alpha$ release, progesterone secretion and conceptus growth associated with successful and unsuccessful transcervical embryo transfer and reinsertion in the mare. J. Reprod. Fertil. Suppl., *35*:419–427, 1986.
39. Allen, W.R.: Embryo transfer in the horse. *In* Mammalian Egg Transfer. Edited by C.E. Adams, Boca Raton, CRC Press, 1982, pp. 135–154.
40. Bowen, M.J., Salsbury, J.M., Bowen, J.M., and Kraemer, D.C.: Non-surgical auto transfer in the mare. Equine Vet. J. Suppl., *3*:100–102, 1985.
41. Pascoe, D.R. et al.: Management of twin conceptuses by manual embryonic reduction: Comparison of two techniques and three hormone treatments. Am. J. Vet. Res., *48*:1594–1599, 1987.
42. Allen, W.R. et al.: Modern veterinary management of twin pregnancy in Thoroughbred mares. Thoroughbred Breeder, pp. 96–98, Nov. 1989.
43. Pascoe, D.R., and Stover, S.M.: Surgical removal of one

conceptus from 15 mares with twin conceptuses. J. Vet. Surg., *18*:141–145, 1989.

44. Ginther, O.J., and First, N.L.: Maintenance of the corpus luteum in hysterectomised mares. Am. J. Vet. Res., *32*:77–89, 1971.

45. Ginther, O.J., Garcia, M.C., Squires, E.L., and Steffenhagen, W.P.: Anatomy of vasculature of uterus and ovaries in the mare. Am. J. Vet. Res., *33*:1561–1568, 1972.

46. Samuelsson, B.: Structures, biosynthesis and metabolism of prostaglandins. *In* Lipid Metabolism. Edited by S.J. Wakil, New York, Academic Press, 1970, pp. 107–153.

47. Van Niekerk, C.J. and Allen, W.R.: Early embryonic development in the horse. J. Reprod. Fertil. Suppl., *23*:495–498, 1975.

48. Ginther, O.J.: Dynamic physical interactions between the equine embryo and uterus. Equine Vet. J. Suppl., *3*:41–47, 1985.

49. Perry, J.S., Heap, R.G., and Amoroso, E.C.: Steroid hormone production by pig blastocysts. Nature, *245*:45–47, 1973.

50. Hershman, L., and Douglas, R.H.: The critical period for the maternal recognition of pregnancy in mares. J. Reprod. Fertil. Suppl., *27*:395–401, 1979.

51. McDowell, K.J. et al.: Restricted conceptus mobility results in failure of maternal recognition of pregnancy in mares. Biol. Reprod., *39*:340–348, 1988.

52. Ewart, J.C.: Studies on the development of the horse. I. The development during the third week. Trans. R. Soc. Edinb., *51*:287–329, 1915.

53. Amoroso, E.C.: Placentation. *In* Marshall's Physiology of Reproduction. Vol. 2. 3rd ed. Edited by A.S. Parkes. London, Longmans Green, 1952, pp. 127–297.

54. Bain, A.M.: The ovaries of the mare during early pregnancy. Vet. Rec., *80*:229–231, 1957.

55. Butterfield, R.M., and Mathews, R.G.: Ovulation and the movement of the conceptus in the first 35 days of pregnancy in Thoroughbred mares. J. Reprod. Fertil. Suppl., *27*:447–452, 1979.

56. Pascoe, R.R.: Transuterine migration of the fetus in the mare between Day 42 and parturition. J. Reprod. Fertil. Suppl., *32*:441–446, 1982.

57. Ginther, O.J.: Mobility of the equine conceptus. Theriogenology, *19*:603–611, 1983.

58. Ginther, O.J.: Fixation and orientation of the early equine conceptus. Theriogenology, *19*:613–623, 1983.

59. Ginther, O.J.: Intrauterine movement of the early conceptus in barren and post partum mares. Theriogenology, *21*:633–644, 1984.

60. Van Niekerk, C.H.: The early diagnosis of pregnancy, the development of the foetal membranes and nidation in the mare. J. S. Afr. Vet. Med. Assoc., *36*:453–488, 1965.

61. Betteridge, K.J. et al.: Development of horse embryos up to twenty-two days after ovulation: Observations on fresh specimens. J. Anat., *135*:191–209, 1982.

62. Bousquet, D., Guillomot, M., and Betteridge, K.J.: Equine zona pellucida and capsule: Some physicochemical and antigenic properties. Gamete Res., *16*:121–132, 1987.

63. Oriol, J.G., Beresford, B., Sharom, F., and Betteridge, K.J.: Biochemical composition of the equine capsule: a preliminary report. J. Reprod. Fertil. Suppl., *44*:639–641, 1991.

64. Betteridge, K.J.: The structure and function of the equine capsule in relation to embryo manipulation and transfer. Equine Vet. J. Suppl., *8*:92–100, 1989.

65. Skidmore, J., Boyle, M.S., Cran, D., and Allen, W.R.: Micromanipulation of equine embryos to produce monozygotic twins. Equine Vet. J. Suppl., *8*:126–128, 1989.

66. McKinnon, A.O. et al.: Bisection of equine embryos. Equine Vet. J. Suppl., *8*:129–133, 1989.

67. Denker, H.W.: Basic aspects of ovoimplantation. Obstet. Gynecol. Ann. *12*:15–42, 1983.

68. Vernon, M.W. et al.: Specific $PGF_2\alpha$ binding by the corpus luteum of the pregnant and non-pregnant mare. J. Reprod. Fertil. Suppl., *27*:421–429, 1979.

69. Kindahl, H., Knudsen, D., Madeh, A., and Edqvist, L.E.: Progesterone, Prostaglandin $F_2\alpha$, PMSG and oestrone sulphate during early pregnancy in the mare. J. Reprod. Fertil. Suppl., *32*:353–359, 1982.

70. Berglund, L.A., Sharp, D.C., Vernon, M.W., and Thatcher, W.W.: Effect of pregnancy and collection techniques on prostaglandin-F in the uterine lumen of pony mares. J. Reprod. Fertil. Suppl., *32*:335–341, 1982.

71. Zavy, M.T. et al.: Effect of exogenous gonadal steroids and pregnancy on uterine luminal prostaglandin F in mares. Prostaglandins, *27*:311–320, 1984.

72. Bazer, F.W., Vallet, J.L., Gross, T.S., and Thatcher, W.W.: Comparative aspects of maternal recognition of pregnancy between sheep and pigs. J. Reprod. Fertil. Suppl., *37*:85–89, 1989.

73. Imchawa, K. et al.: Interferon-like sequence of ovine trophoblast protein secreted by embryonic trophectoderm. Nature, *330*:377–379, 1987.

74. Stewart, H.J. et al.: Sheep anti-luteolytic interferon cDNA sequence and analysis of mRNA levels. J. Mol. Endocrinol., *2*:65–70, 1989.

75. Bazer, F.W. et al.: The role of ovine conceptus secretory proteins in the establishment of pregnancy. *In* Cell and Molecular Biology of the Uterus. Edited by W.W. Leavitt. New York, Plenum Press, 1987, pp. 221–231.

76. Flint, A.P.F., and Sheldrick, E.L.: Continuous infusion of oxytocin prevents induction of uterine oxytocin receptor and blocks luteal regression in cyclic ewes. J. Reprod. Fertil., *75*:623–631, 1985.

77. Bazer, F.W., and Thatcher, W.W.: Theory of maternal recognition of pregnancy in swine based on estrogen controlled endocrine versus exocrine secretion of prostaglandin $F_2\alpha$ by the uterine endometrium. Prostaglandins, *14*:347–401, 1977.

78. Gadsby, J.E., Heap, R.B., and Burton, R.D.: Oestrogen production by blastocyst and early embryonic tissue of various species. J. Reprod. Fertil., *60*:409–417, 1980.

79. La Bonnardiere, C., et al.: Production of two species of interferon by large white and Meishan pig conceptuses during the pre-attachment period. J. Reprod. Fertil., *91*:469–478, 1991.

80. Caldwell, B.V., et al.: The relationship between day of formation and functional life span of induced corpora lutea in the pig. J. Reprod. Fertil., *18*:107–113, 1969.

81. Flood, P.F., Betteridge, K.J., and Irvine, D.S.: Oestrogens and androgens in blastocoelic fluid and cultures of cells from equine conceptuses of 10–22 days gestation. J. Reprod. Fertil. Suppl., *27*:412–420, 1979.

82. Heap, R.B., Hamon, M., and Allen, W.R.: Studies on oestrogen synthesis by the preimplantation equine conceptus. J. Reprod. Fertil. Suppl., *32*:343–352, 1982.

83. Sharp, D.C., et al.: Is an interferon-like protein involved in the maternal recognition of pregnancy in mares? Equine Vet. J. Suppl., *8*:6–9, 1989.

84. Baker, C.B., Adams, M.H., and McDowell, K.J.: Lack of expression of alpha or omega interferons by the base conceptus. J. Reprod. Fertil. Suppl., *44*:439–443, 1991.

85. Woodley, S.L., Burns, P.J., Douglas, R.H., and Oxender, W.D.: Prolonged interovulatory interval after oestradiol treatment in mares. J. Reprod. Fertil. Suppl., *27*:205–209, 1979.

86. Weithenhauer, J., et al.: Characterization of the equine conceptus prostaglandin-inhibitory product. Biol. Reprod. Suppl., *1*:329, 1989.

87. Skarnes, R.C., and Harper, M.J.K.: Relationship between endotoxin-induced abortion and the synthesis of prostaglandin F. Prostaglandins, *1*:191–203, 1972.

88. Cort, N., and Kindahl, H.: The effect of a bacterial endotoxin or cloprostenol on the clinical status and hormonal levels in 80–100 day pregnant gilts. Acta Vet. Scand., *27*:145–148, 1986.

89. Kindahl, H., et al.: Experimental models of endotoxaemia related to abortion in the mare. J. Reprod. Fertil. Suppl., *44*:509–516, 1991.

90. Daels, P.F., Stabenfeldt, G.H., Kindahl, H., and Hughes, J.P.: Prostaglandin release and luteolysis associated with physiological and pathological conditions of the reproductive cycle of the mare: A review. Equine Vet. J. Suppl., *8*:29–34, 1989.

91. Allen, W.E.: Pregnancy failure induced by human Chorionic Gonadotrophin in pony mares. Vet. Rec., *96*:88–90, 1975.

92. Allen, W.E.: The pregnancy protecting effect of progesterone against human chorionic gonadotrophin challenge in mares. Ir. Vet. J., *30*:23–27, 1976.

93. Urwin, V.E.: Gonadotrophic control of ovarian function in pregnant mares. Ph.D. thesis, University of Cambridge, Cambridge, UK 1985.

94. Michel, T.H., Rossdale, P.D., and Cash R.S.G.: Efficacy of human Chorionic Gonadotrophin and Gonadotrophin-releasing Hormone for hastening ovulation in Thoroughbred mares. Equine Vet. J., *18*:438–442, 1986.

95. Stewart, D.R., Kindahl, H., Stabenfeldt, G.H., and Hughes, J.P.: Concentrations of 15-keto, 13,14 dihydro prostaglandin $F_2\alpha$ in the mare during spontaneous and oxytocin-induced foaling. Equine Vet. J., *16*:270–274, 1984.

96. Pashen, R.L.: Low doses of oxytocin can induce foaling at term. Equine Vet. J., *12*:85–87, 1980.

97. Pashen, R.L.: Studies on the endocrinology of pregnancy in the mare. Ph.D. thesis, University of Cambridge, 1980.

98. Leadon, D.P., Rossdale, P.D., Jeffcott, L.B., and Allen, W.R.: A comparison of agents for inducing parturition in mares in the pre-viable and premature periods of gestation. J. Reprod. Fertil. Suppl., *32*:597–602, 1982.

99. Thorburn, G.D. et al.: Parturition in the goat and sheep: Changes in corticosteroids, progesterone, estrogens and prostaglandin F. J. Reprod. Fertil. Suppl., *16*:61–84, 1972.

100. Flint, A.P.F. et al.: Control of utero-ovarian venous prostaglandin F during labour in sheep—Acute effects of vaginal and cervical stimulation. J. Endocrinol., *63*:67–87, 1974.

101. Raeside, J.I., and Kptrap, R.M.: Patterns of urinary oestrogen excretion in individual pregnant mares. J. Reprod. Fertil. Suppl., *23*:469–475, 1975.

102. Bedford, C.A. et al.: The role of oestrogens and progesterone in the onset of parturition in various species. J. Reprod. Fertil. Suppl., *16*:1–23, 1972.

103. Barnes, R.J. et al.: Foetal and maternal plasma concentrations in 13,14-dihydro-15-oxo-prostaglandin F in the mare during late pregnancy and at parturition. J. Endocrinol., *78*:201–215, 1978.

CHAPTER 9

EQUINE CHORIONIC GONADOTROPIN

W.R. Allen
F. Stewart

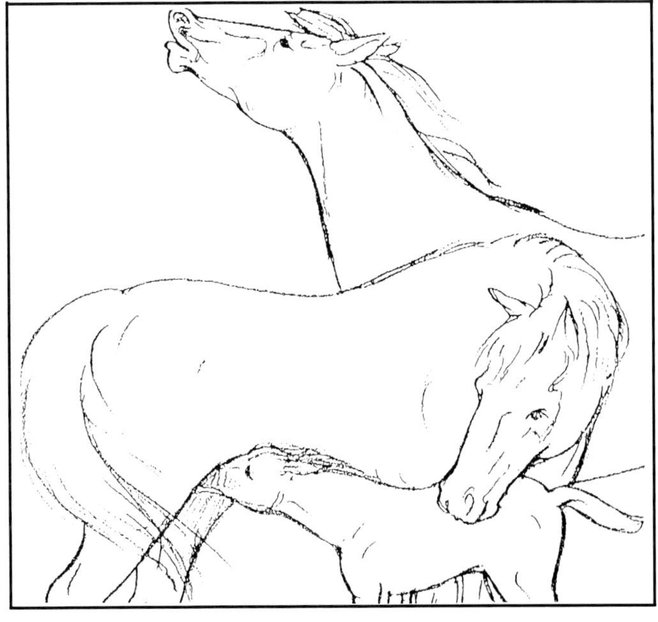

It is not difficult to imagine the air of excitement that would have pervaded the Department of Animal Science of the University of California at Davis in 1930 when two of its young scientists, the late Professors Harold Cole and George Hart, first discovered the existence of equine Chorionic Gonadotropin (eCG).[1] Until recently, their discovery was known as Pregnant Mare Serum Gonadotropin (PMSG). Three years before the discovery, German obstetricians Aschheim and Zondek had dropped a bombshell into the then-embryonic field of reproductive endocrinology with the publication of their paper showing that the urine and blood serum of women in the first trimester of pregnancy contained large quantities of a gonadotropic hormone.[2] This discovery of what later came to be termed human Chorionic Gonadotropin (hCG) stimulated a flurry of activity in many other laboratories around the world. Endocrinologists hurriedly injected samples of urine and blood serum from all sorts of pregnant and nonpregnant animal species—including laboratory rodents, cows, ewes, sows, bitches, and cats—into immature mice and rats, but all with a disappointingly negative result. The animal science group at Davis was in the thick of this worldwide search for other sources of pregnancy-associated gonadotropic activity, and they too suffered the disappointment of negative findings, including a lack of response in rats injected with samples of urine from mares in early pregnancy (H.H. Cole, personal communication). But when, at last, the group determined if any activity might be present in the serum of pregnant mares, they hit the jackpot. And even more exciting, whereas by this time it had become apparent from further studies that the gonadotropic activity in human pregnancy urine was restricted to the Luteinizing Hormone (LH) component of the two fractions being extracted from pituitary glands,[3,4] the activity in pregnant mare serum was more like that of the second gonadotropic fraction present in pituitary tissue and subsequently termed Follicle-Stimulating Hormone (FSH).[5] Thus injection of as little as 0.1 mL of crude serum from a pregnant mare at day 60 of gestation into an immature rat stimulated not only a wave of follicular growth in the ovaries and the accompanying uterine enlargement and vaginal cytologic changes induced by estrogen secreted by the maturing follicles, it also stimulated ovulation of the follicles and the development of mature corpora lutea. Clearly then, pregnant mare's serum contained high concentrations of what appeared, on the face of it, to be a mixture of both FSH and LH, which were then known to be secreted in a rhythmic manner by the pituitary gland in nonpregnant animals. It was indeed a momentous discovery, because it provided for the first time a readily available, easily extractable source of potent gonadotropic hormone which, in turn, enabled a wide variety of experiments to be undertaken in subsequent years on the biologic properties of eCG in particular and gonadotropic hormones in general.

In their classic paper announcing the discovery of eCG, Cole and Hart demonstrated, with remarkable accuracy, the general pattern of secretion of the hormone during pregnancy.[1] Using 18- to 23-day-old prepubertal rats as the test animals, they injected serum recovered from 14 mares between mating and 222 days of gestation and compared the increase in utero-ovarian weight 4 days after injection with controls injected with up to 4 mL of nonpregnant mare serum. In this way they showed that gonadotropic activity first appears in peripheral serum between 37 and 41 days after ovulation and levels rise steeply to reach a peak between days 60 and 80. Thereafter, concentrations begin to fall again steadily until activity disappears completely from the serum between days 120 and 160. Many other similar studies undertaken since then to monitor eCG secretion patterns in pregnant mares and other equids, using a wide variety of in vivo biologic,[6–10] hemagglutination-inhibition,[11–13] radioimmunologic,[14,15] and in vitro radioreceptor[16,17] assay methods have all confirmed the essential shape of the secretion curve and the variability between individual animals in terms of the peak concentration of eCG measurable in blood (Fig. 9-1).

Cole and his colleagues in Davis remained active and pre-eminent in the general field of eCG during the following 30 years. They modified, refined, and increased the accuracy, sensitivity, and speed of their in vivo bioassay method to measure concentrations of eCG in serum and partially purified extracts of hormone,[18–20] investigated thoroughly the essential physicochemical[21–23] and biologic[24,25] properties of hormone; examined the relationships between the secretion of eCG and other morphologic and endocrinologic events in the pregnant mare;[26–28] and studied, and eventually discovered, the source of eCG in the pregnant mare.[29–31] They also determined the half-life of the hormone in horse blood[32,33] and confirmed the finding of the team led by the late Professor Wadslaw Bielanski[34] of the profound influence of fetal genotype on the rate of eCG production in early pregnancy.[35] Thus Cole's group carried out most of the basic investigative work on this intriguing, and still puzzling, hormone. Subsequent studies have merely used modern technology to apply layers of icing and the odd candle to their rich and well-baked cake.

This chapter is dedicated to the memory of Professor Harold H. Cole and his band of dedicated coworkers who made such valuable use of their good fortune to have lived and worked in the golden age of endocrinologic discovery. It is also intended to give a personalized review of the present knowledge of this most perplexing of gonadotropic hormones—what it consists of; where it comes from; and what it does biologically, both inside and outside the pregnant mare.

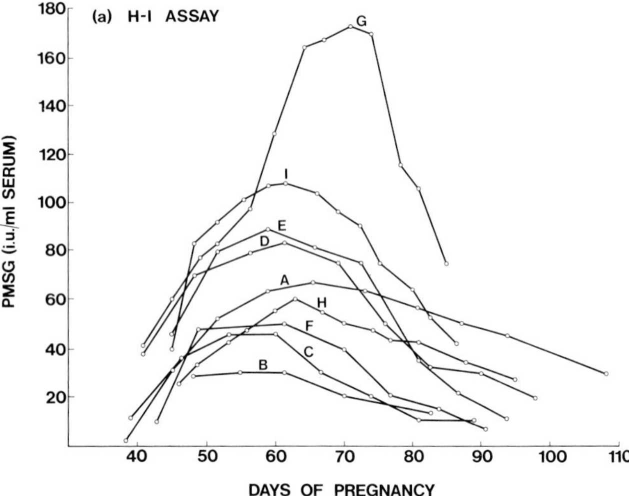

FIG. 9–1. Concentrations of eCG (PMSG) measured by hemagglutination-inhibition (H-I) assay in the serum of nine pony mares between 40 and 110 days of gestation. Note the individual variation between mares in the peak concentrations (31 to 173 IU/mL) reached between days 54 and 73.

PHYSICOCHEMICAL PROPERTIES OF eCG

Equine Chorionic Gonadotropin is a high molecular weight (≈ 70,000) acidic glycoprotein with an abnormally high carbohydrate content (≈ 45%) consisting mainly of sialic acid, galactose, and glucosamine.[24,36–42] It has a low isoelectric point of only 2.4 and is remarkably resistant to acid hydrolysis.[37,43] It is extracted most easily from horse serum by initial precipitation with metaphosphoric acid or acetone, followed by further precipitation "cuts" with graded concentrations of alcohol.[36,44] This level of initial extraction and purification yields a product with a potency of 2,000 to 3,000 IU/mg protein, which is suitable for administration to laboratory and farm animal species as a gonadotropin to induce follicular development and ovulation. Further purification using column chromatography yields a final extract of highly purified hormone that exhibits a specific gonadotrophic potency of 13,500 to 15,000 IU/mg protein.[41,45] The recognized International Standard for eCG is a partially purified extract from horse serum, which is maintained at the National Centre for Medical Research, Mill Hill, London. It was prepared and assayed in the early 1960s by 16 different laboratories using a variety of in vivo bioassay methods, and the product was assigned a potency of 1,600 IU per vial containing 1.6 mg protein.[46] Clearly, this standard must be replaced by a more highly purified and better characterized product.

Like the pituitary and chorionic gonadotrophins and Thyroid-Stimulating Hormone (TSH) in all the mammalian species, eCG is a heterodimeric glycoprotein that consists of an α- and a β-subunit joined noncovalently.[47] The α-subunits are identical within each species, whereas the β-subunits differ, indicating that the specificity of action must reside in the β-subunit. This has been confirmed experimentally by interchanging the α-subunits between some of the hormones, including between different species, without altering their specificity of action. In all species so far examined, including the horse,[48] the α-subunit has been shown to be encoded by a single gene. The amino acid sequence of the α-subunit is highly homologous across the species and the horse sequence shows a 68 to 79% homology with the other available mammalian α-subunits sequences. However, it shows several unique substitutions, including transposition between tyrosine and histidine at positions 87 and 93,[49] which may be related to some of the unusual properties of the equine gonadotropins.[48] In general, each β-subunit is also encoded by a single gene, which together form a family of closely related genes that have clearly arisen through gene duplication.

It was discovered some time ago that both horse and human CG β-subunits are longer at the C-terminal by about 30 residues than all of the pituitary β-subunits. This implied a possible evolutionary linkage between primate and equine CG, but it has now been established that these hormones evolved independently. The primate CG β-subunit gene(s) have apparently arisen via duplication of the LH β gene, followed by a mutation leading to the C-terminal extension and further gene duplication,[50,51] probably before divergence of baboons and humans.[52] This has given rise to a single pituitary LH β gene and a family of six or seven placental CG β genes, some of which are pseudogenes and are not expressed, but all of which show the C-terminal extension.[50] The first indication that the story in equids was different came with the discovery that the horse LH β-subunit also has a C-terminal extension,[53] and 2 years later, Bousfield and colleagues showed that the horse LH β-subunit is, in fact, identical in amino acid sequence to the horse CG β-subunit.[54,55] This provided an explanation for the previous somewhat surprising observation that horse LH exhibits the same intrinsic FSH-like activity as eCG when administered to nonequine species.[56,57] Hence, equids, instead of having evolved separate genes for the purpose, simply express their pituitary gene in the placenta. Gene mapping has recently confirmed this by demonstrating that horse and donkey DNA have only a single copy of the β-subunit gene.[58] The reason for the β-subunit C-terminal extension in primates and equids remains a mystery but it seems likely to be related in some way to expression and/or secretion of the hormone in placental tissues. Or it may simply serve to increase the biologic half-life of the hormones. It is interesting that the gene mutations giving rise to the C-terminal extension (a single-base deletion in primates and a 10-base deletion in equids) occurred in the same area of the gene in each case.[59,60]

As mentioned, eCG contains a much higher carbohydrate content than any of the other known mammalian pituitary and chorionic gonadotropins, including hCG.[36,40,41,61] Recent studies have shown that approximately 20% of the α-subunit and more than 50% of the β-subunit of eCG comprises carbohydrate moieties, each having a mixture of N- and O-linked carbohydrate chains.[61–63] In addition to having a higher total amount of carbohydrate, a much higher proportion of this carbohydrate in eCG is in the form of sialic acid, compared with the gonadotropins of other species.[40]

BIOLOGIC PROPERTIES OF eCG

Perhaps the most unusual and interesting feature of the eCG molecule is its unique ability to express both FSH-like and LH-like biologic activities when administered to other mammalian species.[1,24] This property is in contrast to hCG and the CGs of other primate species, which can induce only LH-like responses.[64] Human Menopausal Gonadotropin (hMG) likewise expresses dual FSH-like and LH-like activities in vivo but this arises from a mixture of pituitary FSH and LH, which are secreted in large quantities when the pituitary gland escapes in older age from the negative feedback effects of ovarian steroids.[65]

The first indication that donkey CG also exhibits FSH-like activity in nonequine species came with the development of the very useful radioreceptor assay technique. Employing rat testicular FSH and LH receptors and a variety of radioactively labeled gonadotropins, donkey CG was shown to possess significant, but considerably less, FSH-receptor binding activity than horse CG.[17] For example, the FSH to LH ratio of horse CG is approximately 1.0 compared with 0.1 for donkey CG, and the horse × donkey hybrid conceptuses (mules and hinnies) produce an FSH to LH ratio midway between the two parental extremes (around 0.5).

A number of studies have confirmed that donkey CG expresses much less FSH-like activity than horse CG[57,66] and that zebra CG is more like donkey CG than horse CG. Donkey LH has also been shown to be chemically and biologically similar to donkey CG,[67] which is not surprising because they are almost certainly, as in the horse, encoded by the same genes.[58] Donkey CG has a C-terminal extension similar in length to horse CG[60] but, due to a frame shift in the DNA sequence, shows only 21% amino acid sequence homology.

The structural basis for the dual biologic and therefore dual receptor binding, activities of eCG (and LH) remains unclear. It presumably lies within the β-subunit which, apart from the C-terminal extension, is understandably LH-like, showing approximately 70% homology with other species' LH β sequences, including human CG. Its ability to bind to FSH as well as LH receptors in nonequine species is, therefore, probably the result of minor amino acid differences within the β-subunit. Although the carbohydrate moeties of the gonadotropin molecules contribute to biologic half-life, and possibly receptor binding affinity and/or signal transduction, evidence does not exist to support their involvement in receptor binding specificity.

The FSH-like properties of eCG have resulted in the wide-scale use of partially purified extracts of the hormone as the cheapest and most readily available form of exogenous gonadotropin to stimulate follicular growth and ovulation in laboratory animals and in the larger domestic and farm animal species. It can be used at lower doses as an adjunct to progestagen withdrawal or other forms of estrous synchronization to induce normal rates of ovulation in adult or prepubertal animals. Alternatively, when administered in higher doses, its FSH-like component stimulates the development of multiple follicles, which are then ovulated by the LH-like component to give the superovulation that is required in embryo recovery and transfer programs.[68,69] In this latter use, however, the exceptionally long half-life of the eCG molecule can be disadvantageous in that a single injection of hormone can stimulate two or more asynchronous waves of follicular growth in the animal's ovaries. Furthermore, the LH-like component of the eCG may ovulate a partly mature follicle existing in the ovaries of the recipient at the time of the eCG injection, and the progesterone secreted by the resulting CL can interfere with ovulation of the subsequent wave of follicles stimulated by the FSH-like component of the eCG.[70] Because of these difficulties, most modern embryo transfer programs in cattle prefer to treat donor animals during days 10 to 14 of diestrus with repeated injections over a 4-day period of lower doses of purified pituitary FSH with a luteolytic dose of prostaglandin $F_2\alpha$ given 48 h after starting the gonadotropin therapy.[71,72]

SOURCE OF eCG IN THE MARE

Cole's group discovered the source of eCG in the pregnant mare—the unique and still puzzling placental outgrowths now known universally as endometrial cups;[30] but this important finding was not made without some problems along the way.

Two of Cole's graduate students, Catchpole and Lyons, were assigned the task of locating the source and demonstrating the method of secretion of eCG,and they set out to do so in the light of papers published at that time by Zondek,[73] Phillip,[3] Collip,[4] and others, which had demonstrated convincingly that hCG in pregnant women is produced by the fetal component of the placenta. Catchpole and Lyons carried out an exhaustive study over 2 years that involved driving many hundreds of miles between widely scattered horse abattoirs in California on the off-chance of being able to recover uteri from pregnant mares.[29] They carried out painstaking dissections of these hard-won specimens and made crude saline extracts of known weights of fetal, placental, and endometrial tissues taken from various parts of the uterus (H.R. Catchpole, personal communication). They submitted the extracts to their rat utero-ovarian weight bioassay to measure gonadotropic activity and, not surprisingly when viewed in hindsight, they found higher concentrations of hormone at 40 to 80 days of gestation in the endometrium of the gravid uterine horn in direct contact with the developing fetal membranes than in the empty nongravid horn. Furthermore, because they did not specifically identify and assay the endometrial cups within the selected samples of endometrium, they tended to find higher levels of gonadotropic activity in extracts of the allantochorion than in those of the endometrium. They concluded, quite naturally, that like hCG in human pregnancy, eCG was probably secreted by the trophoblast cells of the developing placenta and was taken up by, and accumulated selectively in, the underlying endometrium.[29]

The subject rested at that point for the following 9 years until once again, Cole came to the fore with his "rediscovery" of the endometrial cups. Some 40 years previously the German anatomist W. Schauder had mentioned the existence of a series of saucer-shaped endometrial protruberances in the gravid uterine horn of mares during the first half of pregnancy.[74] These structures, which appeared to Schauder to have no physical or other significant function in terms of placentation and the maintenance of pregnancy, each had a distinct depression or crater-like appearance in the middle of which was found a honey-colored, sticky material. He gave them the name endometrial cups.

Cole and Goss looked afresh at Schauder's endometrial cups, and to their surprise, they found the cup tissue itself, and even more so the associated exocrine secretion, contained concentrations of eCG that were orders of magnitude higher than those in the adjacent normal endometrium or in any parts of the fetal placenta.[30] They concluded, quite rightly, that the endometrial cups were the fount of eCG and that the hormone entered the maternal bloodstream via a complex of large lymph sinuses which existed in the endometrial stroma beneath each cup.[30] Thus it now seemed that eCG, unlike hCG in primates, was actually maternal in origin.

Two further elucidative errors were to be made before the real source of eCG was to come to light. In its next substantial paper on the subject, the Davis group gave a detailed morphologic description of the development and regression of the endometrial cups, from the time of their first appearance on the endometrium at day 40 of gestation to their degeneration and sloughing from the endometrial surface at days 130 to 150.[31] The researchers noted each mature cup at days 60 to 70 was composed of a mass of large epithelioid-type cells that were similar in appearance to the large glycogen-filled decidual cells of rodent and human placentas.[75] Occasional blood vessels and distended endometrial glands were interspersed throughout the tight knot of decidual-like cells. Because the endometrial cups appeared to have no direct physical connection to the overlying epitheliochorial placenta, Clegg et al.[31] concluded that the decidual-like cells were maternal in origin, having differentiated from endometrial stromal cells in a manner similar to the development of the decidual reaction in pregnant or pseudopregnant rodent uteri in response to pregnancy or an appropriate mechanical stimulus.[76] Furthermore, they stained sections of endometrial cups with periodic acid-Schiff (PAS) solution, which was considered to be specific for glycoprotein molecules.[77] Whereas the decidual-like cells stained only faintly, the epithelial cells lining the dilated endometrial glands within the cup and the exocrine secretion within the glands and accumulated on the surface of the cup stained intensely. Because this endometrial cup secretion was extremely potent in eCG activity, and because eCG was known to be a large glycoprotein molecule with an unusually high carbohydrate content,[24,36] the Davis group concluded that eCG was secreted by the epithelium of the dilated glands within the cup.[31]

These errors were compounded during the next 15 years, first by Amoroso when discussing immunologic aspects of the endometrial cups at various stages of gestation[78] and again by Allen when describing the relationship between the annulate chorionic girdle region of the fetal membranes and the development of the endometrial cups at day 36 of gestation.[79] In this latter study it was wrongly concluded, on the basis of histo-

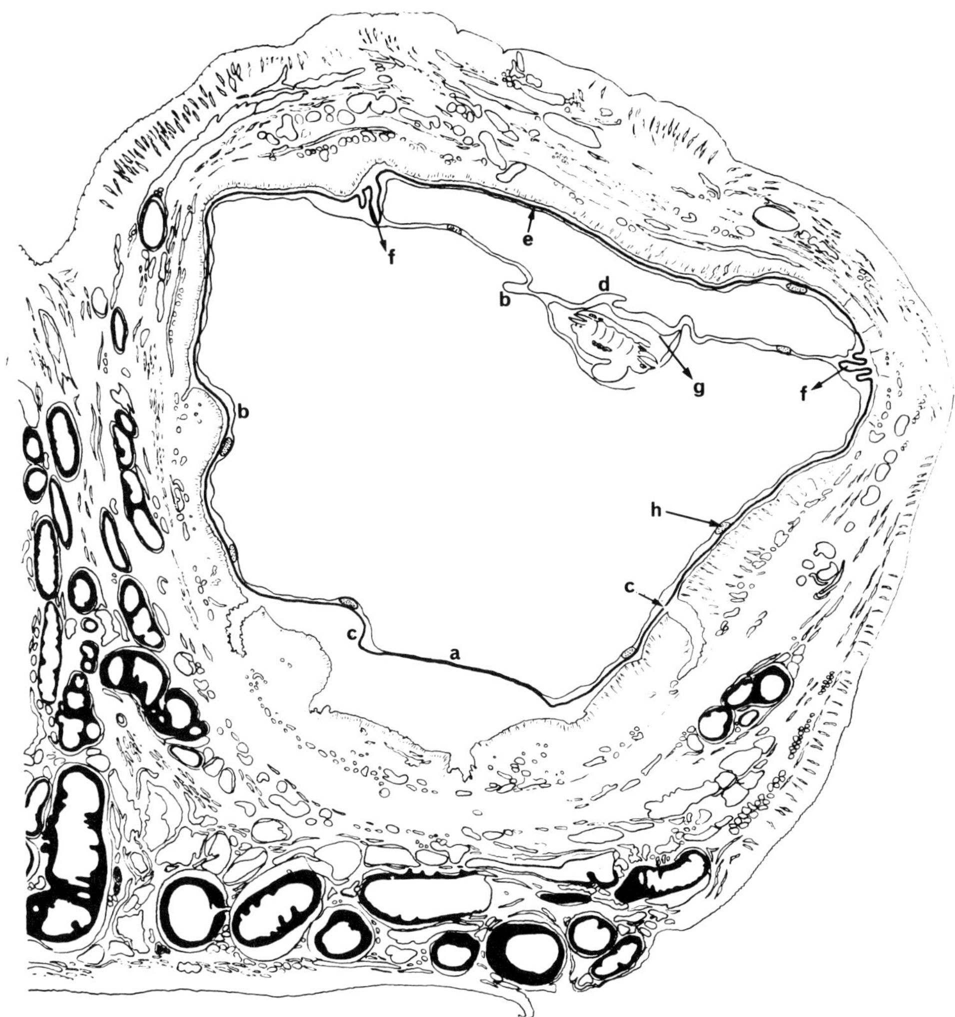

FIG. 9–2. Diagrammatic facsimile of a transverse histologic section through the conceptus in the perfuse-fixed gravid uterine horn of a mare on day 25 after ovulation. a, nonvascularized bilaminar omphalopleure at the abembryonic pole; b, yolk sac membrane; c, chorionic membrane; d, allantoic membrane; e, fused allantochorion at embryonic pole; f, commencing development of the chorionic girdle at the abutment of the allantoic and yolk sac membranes; g, amniotic membrane; h, embryonic blood vessel of the mesoderm.

logic evidence gleaned from perfuse-fixed pregnant horse uteri (Fig. 9-2), that the chorionic girdle secreted a humoral fetal "factor," which passed down the glands in the adjacent area of endometrium and induced undifferentiated stromal cells within the glands to undergo a decidualization response and so transform into endometrial cup cells.

Two years later the true picture at last began to emerge. Chorionic girdle tissue was dissected from horse conceptuses recovered intact at days 34 to 36 of gestation by surgical hysterotomy. The tissue was minced finely with scissors and when cultured in vitro as simple explants produced stable colonies of large, epithelioid binucleated cells that secreted high concentrations of eCG into the culture medium for >180 days. The cultured girdle cells showed all the morphologic characteristics of endometrial cups in vivo, and they transformed similarly when transplanted to extrauterine sites such as the testis.[80] Subsequently, a light microscopic and ultrastructure study of the placental interface in mares between days 34 and 40 of gestation demonstrated migration of the specialized chorionic girdle cells into the endometrium at days 36 to 38, followed by their rapid transformation into the large eCG-secreting decidual-like cells of the endometrial cup.[81] Thus the original conclusions of Catchpole and Lyons[29] were vindicated. Fetal trophoblast cells indeed secrete eCG but only those specialized ones of the chorionic girdle when they migrate into the endometrium at days 36 to 38 to form the endometrial cups.

DEVELOPMENT AND INVASION OF THE CHORIONIC GIRDLE

The development of the progenitor tissue of the equine endometrial cups, the chorionic girdle, is a strange and little understood phenomenon. The girdle was first described by Ewart as constituting a "complex whitish band, nearly a quarter of an inch in width, placed nearly equatorially on the embryonic sac which is concerned in fixing the embryo to the uterine surface and which may be a means of absorbing additional nourishment."[82] The girdle was not really mentioned again in the literature until remarked on by van Niekerk[83] and was then described in more detail by van Niekerk and Allen[84] following the discovery of its role in endometrial cup formation. It has received much more attention since then, especially from Antczak and colleagues in their search for the source of paternally derived Major Histocompatibility Complex (MHC) and other foreign fetal antigens that stimulate maternal humoral and cell-mediated antibody responses during pregnancy.[85,86]

The girdle comprises a narrow and discrete thickening of the trophoblast that develops around the circumference of the spherical conceptus at the point where the enlarging allantoic and regressing yolk sac membranes abut each other (Figs. 9-3 and 9-4). It first appears histologically at around day 25 after ovulation as a series of shallow ridges in the single-cell layer of trophoblast (Fig. 9-2). During the next 10 days, the trophoblast cells toward the top of these folds multiply rapidly so that the ridges and intervening folds grow and deepen to form elongated flap-like projections (Fig. 9-5A). These become flattened on the apical surface by the pressure of the opposing endometrium, thereby making in cross-section a thickened, stratified type of trophoblast some 8 to 10 cells deep that contains gland-like structures created by the surface epithelium of adjacent folds. These simple glands secrete a mucoid material that helps to bind lumenal surface of the girdle to the endometrium (Fig. 9-5B).

The invasion of endometrium by the chorionic girdle to form the endometrial cups is summarized diagrammatically in Figure 9-6. Between days 36 and 38 the hyperplastic trophoblast cells on the surface of the girdle begin to vigorously invade and destroy endometrium epithelium. They do this by extending blunt pseudopodia-like processes which force their way between, and sometimes straight through, the epithelial cells on the lumenal surface, which they occasionally phagocytose during the destructive process. When the girdle cells reach the basement membrane of the epithelium, they continue to migrate down the openings of endometrial glands, dislodging the glandular epithelium as they go (Fig. 9-7A). After a brief delay they then breach the basement membrane by the same method of pseudopodium extrusion and they pass off into the endometrial stroma, both vertically downward from the lumenal surface and laterad from the lumena of the glands. Within as little as 24 to 48 h after entering the stroma, the girdle cells cease their migration, round up, enlarge greatly so that they become tightly packed together, and transform into mature eCG-secreting endometrial cups cells.[81]

The entire chorionic girdle becomes detached from the underlying chorion at the time of migration into the endometrium.[81] The integrity of the fetal membranes is maintained by a single layer of apparently undifferenti-

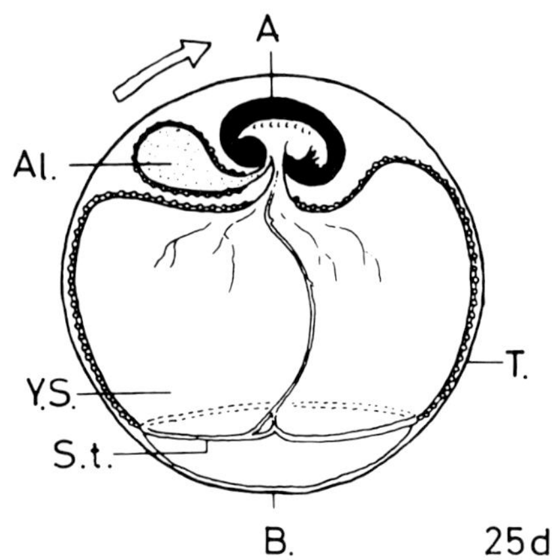

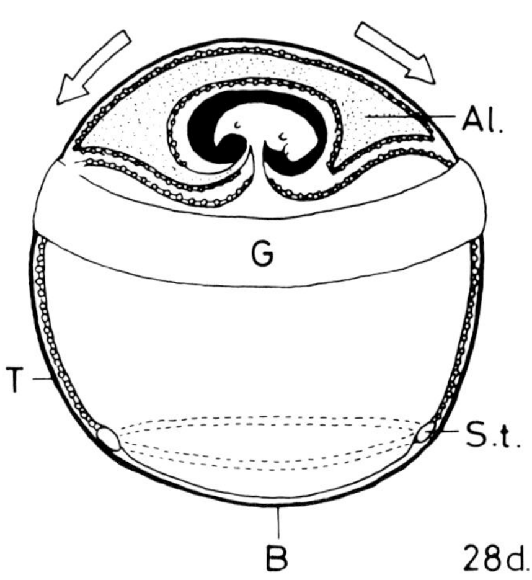

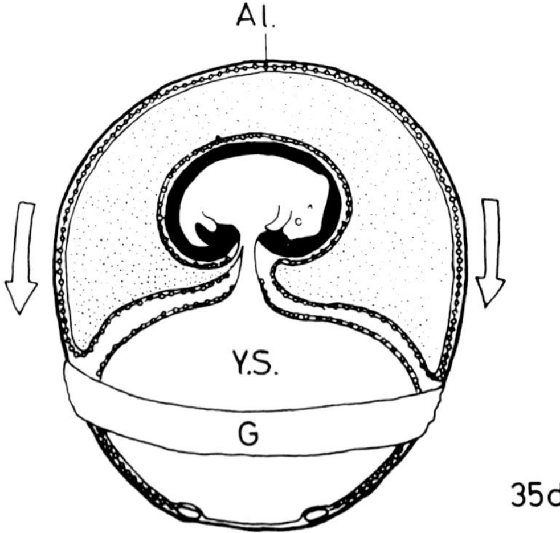

FIG. 9–3. Diagrammatic representation of the development and differentiation of the extraembryonic membranes of the equine conceptus between days 25 and 35 after ovulation. A, amnion; Al, allantois; B, nonvascular bilaminar omphalopleure; G, chorionic girdle; St, sinus terminalis; T, trophoblast of the chorion; YS, yolk sac. Open arrows show direction of growth of the allantois.

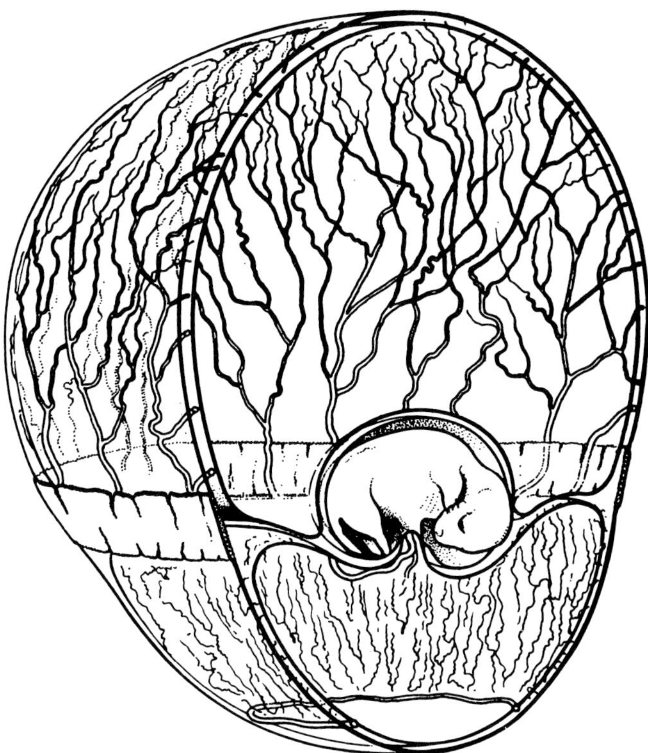

FIG. 9–4. Diagrammatic facsimile of a horse conceptus at day 36 after ovulation. The chorionic girdle is seen as a band-like thickening of the trophoblast surrounding the conceptus at the abutment of the enlarging allantochorionic and regressing choriovitelline membranes. The sinus terminalis and persisting circle of nonvascularized bilaminar omphalopleure are situated at the abembryonic pole.

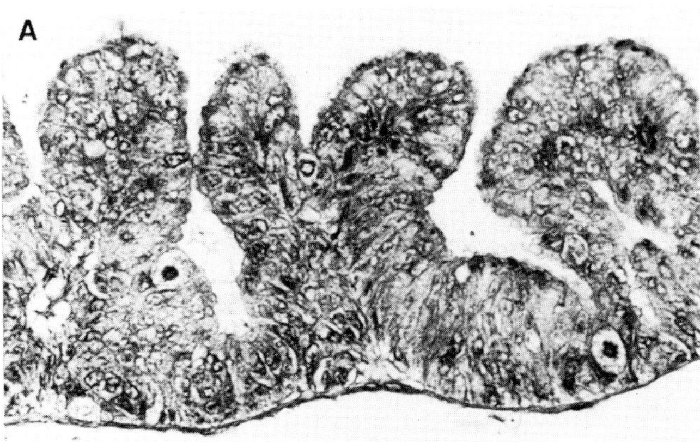

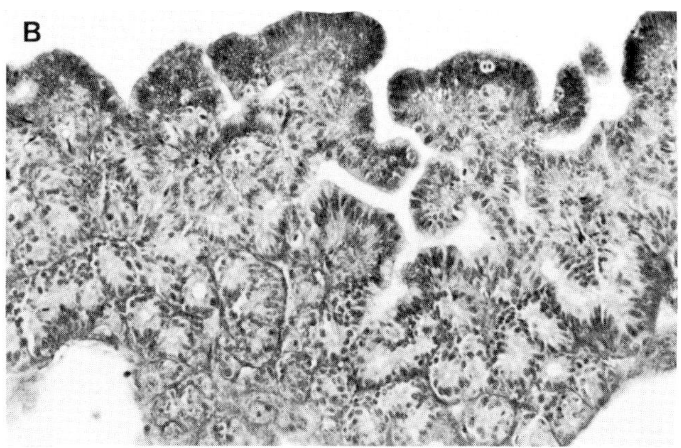

FIG. 9–5. Histologic sections of the chorionic girdle (progenitor of the endometrial cups) at *(A)* day 28 (× 180) and *(B)* day 36 (× 120) after ovulation.

ated trophoblast cells that remain behind and form confluence with the rest of the normal chorion.

DEVELOPMENT AND REGRESSION OF THE ENDOMETRIAL CUPS

The young endometrial cup at day 45 of gestation consists of a densely packed mass of large trophoblast-derived cup cells. Little stroma is left between adjacent cup cells and only occasional blood and lymph vessels exist. The apical portions of many of the endometrial glands have been obliterated during the original invasion of the chorionic girdle, but the fundic regions remain intact and become increasingly distended throughout the lifespan of the cup (Fig. 9-7B). This glandular enlargement seems to occur both as a result of blockage of the apical outlets and some form of hyperstimulation of secretory epithelium. Large quantities of carbohydrate-rich PAS-positive material accumulate within the gland lumena before being released onto the surface of the cup when the latter begins to degenerate beyond about day 70 of gestation (Fig. 9-7C and D).

At the time of maximum growth and hormone output (days 55 to 70), endometrial cups appear grossly as a circle or horseshoe-shaped area of pale, raised plaques on the surface of the endometrium at the base of the gravid uterine horn. Only a slight indentation in the lumenal surface of the cups exists at this stage and little, if any, exocrine secretion is accumulated in the depression. Individual cups may vary tremendously in size, ranging from small isolated mounds measuring as little as 1.0 cm in diameter to long, unbroken "ribbons" of tissue measuring 1.0 to 1.5 cm in width and greater than 10 cm in length (Figs. 9-8A and B). This great variability in size occurs within and between mares and it seems to have two interacting causes. First, there is appreciable variation between individual conceptuses in the width and overall development of the progenitor chorionic girdle, which directly affects the breadth and overall sizes of the endometrial cups that develop following invasion of the endometrium at days 36 to 38.[87] These differences in girdle dimensions are most marked when mating across the equine species to produce interspecific conceptuses and when using embryo transfer to create extraspecific pregnancies[88] (see Chapter 63). However, there is also circumstantial evidence of genetic factors influencing chorionic girdle development and the size of the resulting endometrial cups within normal intraspecific horse matings.[89]

The second factor influencing endometrial cup size, and hence the amount of eCG secreted into maternal blood, is the surface architecture and tone of the mater-

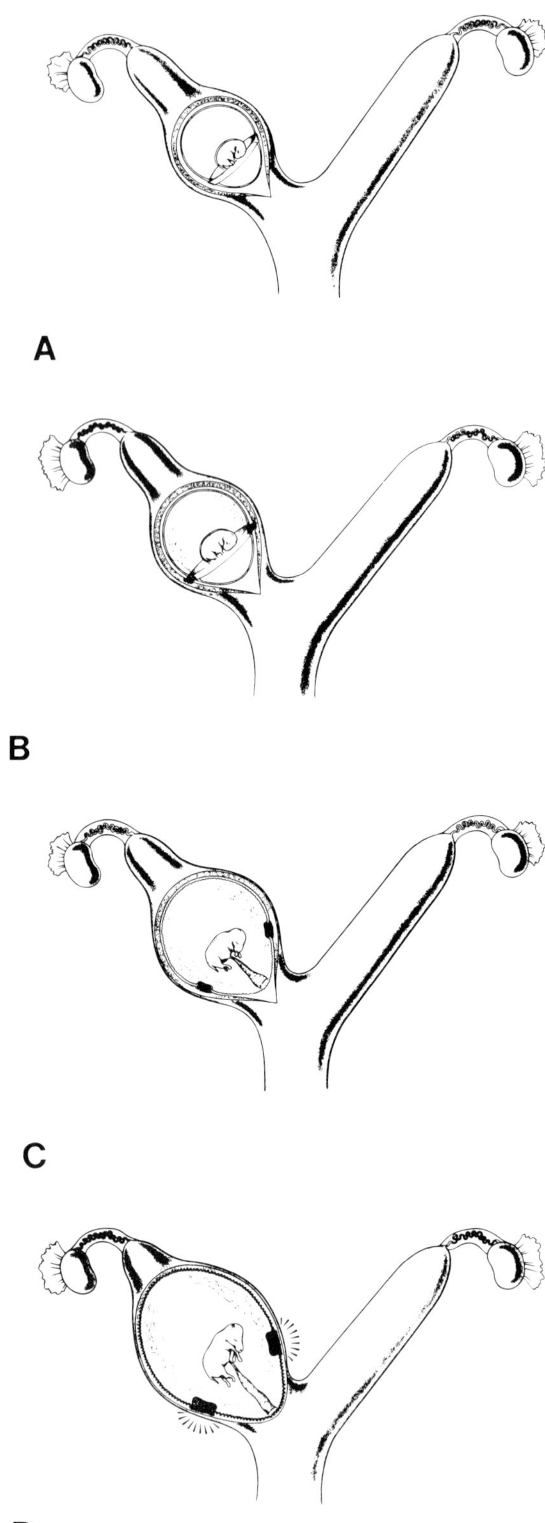

FIG. 9–6. Diagrammatic representation of endometrial cup development in the mare. *A*, Day 35, the intact chorionic girdle surrounds the conceptus situated at the base of the gravid uterine horn. *B*, Day 37, the chorionic girdle cells are actively invading the maternal endometrium. *C*, Day 40, the invaded girdle cells are transforming into large eCG-secreting endometrial cup cells. *D*, Day 50, the mature endometrial cup is eliciting a cell-mediated response from the maternal immune system.

nal endometrium at the time of girdle invasion. The preinvaded chorionic girdle is held closely against the endometrium by the dual actions of increased uterine tone and expansion of the developing fluid-filled conceptus. But, as illustrated in Figure 9-8A and B, the surface of the endometrium to which the girdle becomes attached may vary from highly folded and ridged to flattened and almost smooth. Should the girdle lie apposed to the ridged surface at the time of invasion, it will only be able to gain access at the apices of the ridges, leaving the valleys between them untouched. Then as the uterus expands further with increasing gestation, the ridges will tend to flatten out and disappear, so leaving isolated, discrete cups. On the other hand, should the chorionic girdle invade an area of smooth endometrium at day 36, unbroken lengths of girdle will invade giving rise to the continuous ribbons of endometrial cup tissue sometimes seen later in gestation (Fig. 9-8A).[88]

In the mature endometrial cup at days 60 to 70, the transformed eCG-secreting trophoblast cells have many unusual features: they are large compared to other cell types in the uterus, are essentially round, and are almost always binucelated (Fig. 9-7D). The nuclei are large euchromatic bodies that contain dense, characteristic nucleoli. The cytoplasm is filled with short profiles of endoplasmic reticulum that resemble granules, some lipid droplets are present and a few mitochondria are scattered throughout the cell. The Golgi apparatus is a significant structure, and many smooth-surfaced Golgi-associated vesicles are evident. Nonetheless, the cup cells contain no obvious dense secretory granules, and secretion, therefore, appears to be constitutive rather than regulated like the pituitary gonadotrophins. It is of interest that chorionic girdle cells recovered from mares prior to their invasion of the endometrium at day 36 and cultured in vitro appear to undergo the same transformation processes as in vivo. They form monolayer colonies of binucleated cells, which show the same morphologic features as mature endometrial cup cells in the mare.[86,90] With increasing time in culture the binucleate cells tend to coalesce to form a type of multinucleated syncitium.[80]

A striking feature of the endometrial cup reaction is the associated maternal cellular response. At the time of the initial invasion of the chorionic girdle at days 36 to 38, significant numbers of lymphocytes are already accumulated in the subepithelial endometrial stroma beneath the migrating girdle cells (Fig. 9-7A). These lymphocytes seem to disappear from the tissues during the next few days as the girdle cells are transforming into endometrial cup cells, but they begin to reappear again in increasing numbers from around day 50 onward (Fig. 9-7B). During most of the 60- to 80-day lifespan of the cups, the accumulating mononuclear cells—initially composed almost entirely of T-lineage small lymphocytes and isolated macrophages, but being joined as gestation advances by increasing numbers of B-lymphocytes, plasma cells, and eosinophils[91]—remain clustered in the endometrial stroma at the periphery of the cup tissue[13,78] (Fig. 9-7C and D). But beyond days

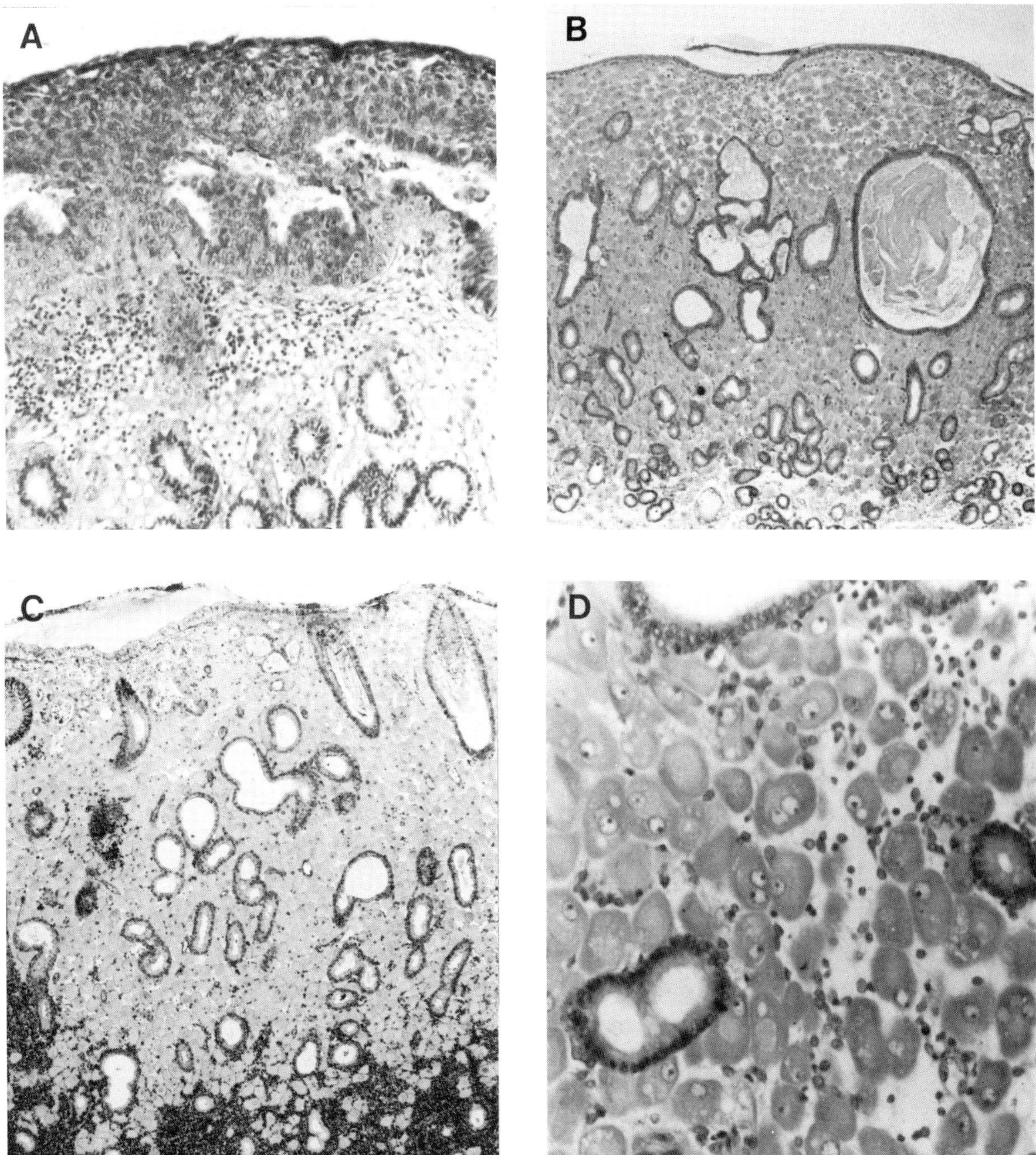

FIG. 9–7. Histologic sections of endometrial cups at different stages of development. *A,* At day 37, showing the chorionic girdle attached to, and beginning to invade, the endometrium. The lumenal epithelium and the epithelium of some glands have been dislodged and are replaced by invading girdle cells. Note the accumulation of lymphocytes in the subepithelial stroma (× 100). *B,* At day 45 after ovulation. The young cup is a solid mass of large, eCG-secreting cells and the lumenal surface is already covered by a regenerated layer of endometrial epithelium. The basal portions of some endometrial glands are grossly distended with accumulated exocrine secretion. Relatively few lymphocytes are visible in the stroma beneath the cup (× 100). *C,* At day 71. Some degeneration of endometrial cup cells is commencing at the lumenal surface of the cup where a small amount of exocrine secretion is trapped beneath the overlying allantochorion. A dense band of lymphocytes and plasma cells is accumulated at the periphery of the cup where they are attacking and destroying cup cells (× 100). *D,* Higher magnification at the lateral border of the endometrial cup in *C,* showing the large binucleated cup cells and invading maternal leucocytes (× 230).

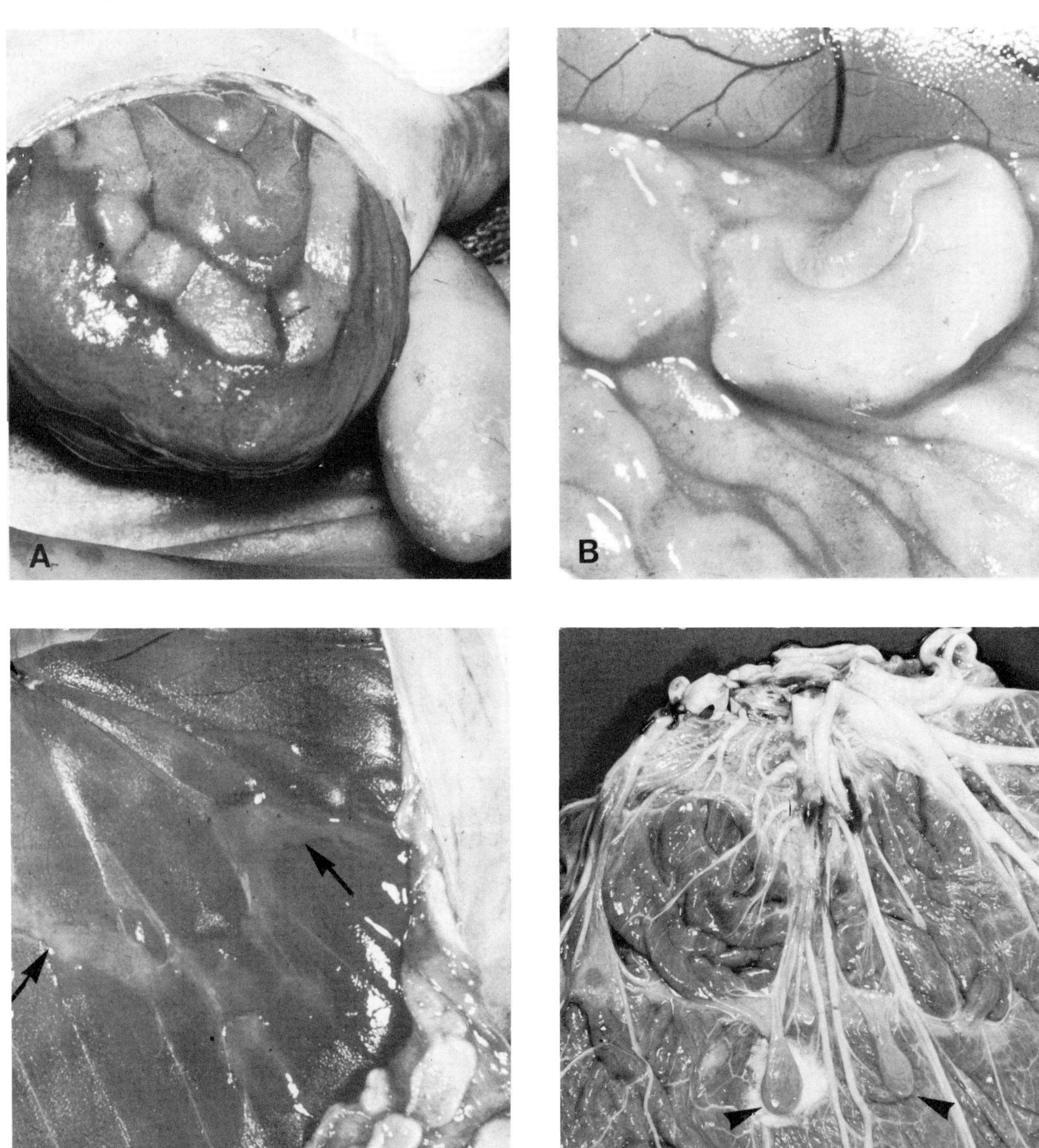

FIG. 9–8. *A,* A continuous band of young endometrial cup in the gravid uterine horn of a pony mare at day 45 of gestation. The cups appear as pale, raised plaques on the surface of the endometrium. *B,* Mature endometrial cup at day 81 of gestation. The allantochorion is pulled back to expose the saucer-shaped cup. The depression in the center of the cup is caused by commencing necrosis and sloughing of the cup cells in this region. *C,* Degenerating endometrial cups at day 95 of gestation. The cups are becoming pale and "cheesy" in appearance and significant quantities of sticky, honey-colored, eCG-rich exocrine secretion are adhered to the underlying allantochorion (arrow). *D,* Fetal surface of the placenta of a mare at term showing two pendulous allantochorionic pouches (arrows) filled with necrotic endometrial cup and inspissated endometrial cup secretion.

70 to 80, as the large cup cells at the lumenal surface of the cup begin to degenerate and slough off, the accumulated leucocytes begin to invade the tissue and appear to destroy the cup cells at the base and periphery[88] (Fig. 9-7C).

As the combination of degenerative changes progresses, sloughing of necrotic cells from the surface of the cup increasingly unblocks the outlets of distended endometrial glands. The accumulated secretion begins to exude from the glands and, mixing with the contents of the disintegrating cup cells, becomes increasingly rich in eCG activity and progressively more inspissated, glutinous, and sticky. It fills the central depression on the surface of the cup and adheres to the overlying allantochorion (Fig. 9-8C). A distinct line of separation forms between the periphery of the cup tissue and the endometrial stroma packed with accumulated leucocytes. Eventually, between days 100 and 140, but with considerable variation between mares and individual endometrial cups within the same mare, the necrotic lump of cup debris and admixed glutinous cup secretion is sloughed completely from the endometrial surface. In areas of the uterine horn where the dehisced material is above the conceptus, the lump may invaginate into the allantochorion via the action of gravity thereby giving rise to pedunculated structures, which hang within the allantoic cavity (Fig. 9-8D). These were termed allantochorionic pouches by Clegg et al.[31]

In summary, the equine endometrial cups comprise, in effect, a carefully timed injection of specialized trophoblast cells into the maternal endometrium. The migrating cells undergo a major transformation in structure and function when they reach the endometrial stroma, where they remain in tightly packed clusters for the following 60 to 80 days. They secrete large quantities of eCG, which is released initially into the maternal circulation via the lymphatic system draining the uterus and later accumulates in the exocrine secretion of the endometrial glands via release of the contents of the degenerating cup cells. The invading chorionic girdle cells express high concentrations of paternally derived class I MHC antigens,[86] which stimulate a strong maternal humoral immune response in all mares carrying fetuses that are not histocompatible with the mare at the class I MHC barrier.[13,92] These paternal class I MHC antigens and, as yet unidentified, tissue-specific antigens expressed by the fetal cup cells, also elicit a strong cell-mediated maternal immune response which hastens the death and eventual desquamation of the cups from the endometrium before midgestation. Yet, despite this strong sensitization of the mare to foreign antigens expressed by this invasive component of the fetal placenta, no similar response is generated against the remaining majority of the noninvasive epitheliochorial placenta, and the conceptus is carried safely to term.[93]

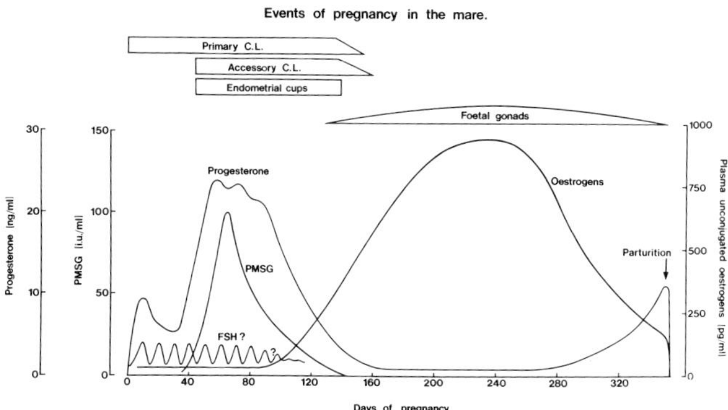

FIG. 9–9. Diagrammatic representation of the main endocrinologic changes and associated morphologic events during pregnancy in the mare.

FUNCTIONS OF eCG IN THE MARE

Soon after their discovery of eCG in 1930, Cole and his colleagues drew attention to the close relationship that exists between the secretion of gonadotropic hormone and the considerable degree of secondary luteal development that occurs in the mare's ovaries.[26] They noted that on or soon after the first appearance of eCG in maternal blood around day 40 one or more accessory ovulations occurred in the maternal ovaries, with further secondary luteal structures appearing in an accumulative fashion during the next 100 or more days of gestation. Amoroso et al.[94] described the same phenomenon, and Allen[79] counted as many as 35 distinct luteal structures in the ovaries of one mare at day 140 of pregnancy. This coincidental development, persistence, and regression of endometrial cups and secondary corpora lutea in mares between 40 and 150 days of gestation, together with the known dual biologic activities of eCG, led to the general assumption that eCG provided both the gonadotropic and the luteotrophic stimuli for these accessory luteal structures (Fig. 9-9); however, several

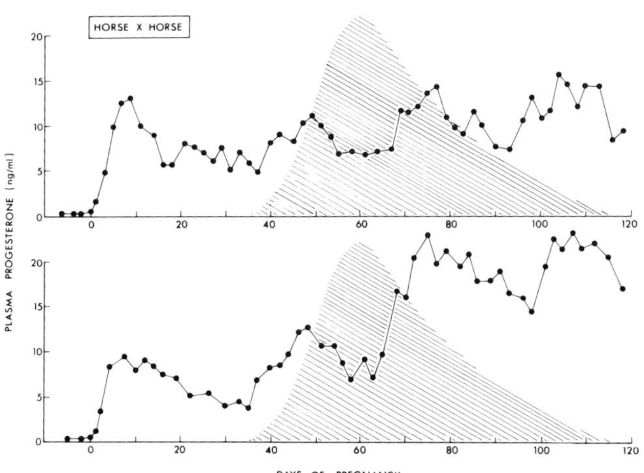

FIG. 9–10. Peripheral plasma progesterone concentrations measured in two pony mares during the first 120 days of gestation. The period of eCG secretion is shown diagrammatically in hatched profile. Note the accumulative rises in progesterone levels that begin around day 40 with successive development of secondary corpora lutea.

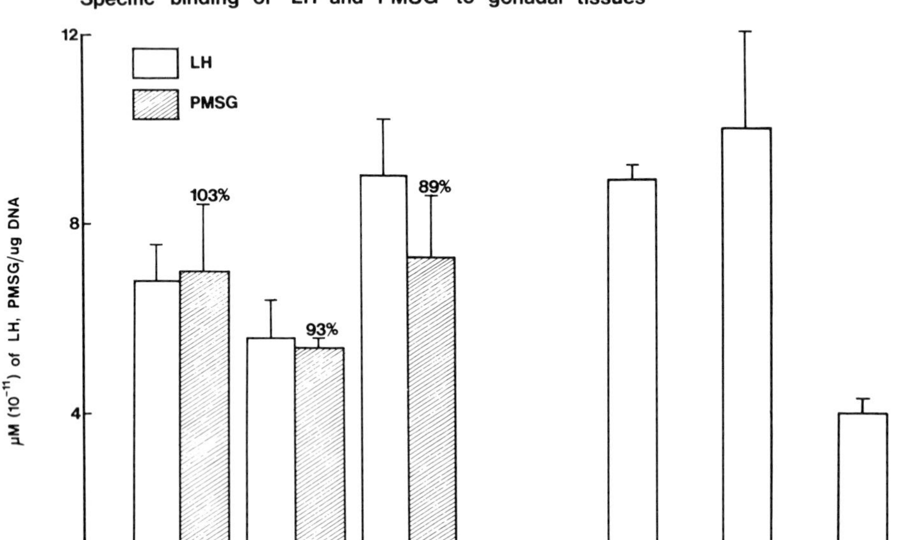

FIG. 9–11. The binding of ^{125}I-human LH (open bars) and ^{125}I-PMSG (eCG; hatched bars), expressed as μM hormone bound per μg DNA, to rat, pig, cow, and horse gonadal tissues. In the rat testis, boar testis, and cow CL the binding of PMSG per μg DNA is very similar to that of LH (103%, 93%, and 89%, respectively). However, in all the horse tissues, the binding of PMSG is extremely low and is equivalent to only 2 to 7% of the LH binding in each case.

more recent studies have shed fresh light on the phenomenon.

Serial measurements of the concentrations of pituitary FSH and LH in the serum of cycling and pregnant mares showed that throughout the spring and summer months of the physiologic breeding season FSH is released from the pituitary gland in mares at intervals of approximately 10 to 12 days.[95,96] The rhythmic pattern of release is controlled essentially by day length and the secretion of follicular inhibin and/or estradiol, but it is not influenced by negative feedback effects of progesterone. Thus the releases of pituitary FSH continue unchanged during early pregnancy just as in the estrous cycle (Fig. 9-9). This finding coincides well with the earlier observations of Bain,[97] van Rensburg and van Niekerk,[98] and others that considerable follicular growth occurs in the mare's ovaries around days 18 to 23 of gestation and hence at the time the mare could have been expected to have returned to estrus and reovulate had she not been pregnant. However, these large follicles do not ovulate, and they tend to regress and make way for a further wave of follicular growth some 10 to 12 days later. This normally coincides with the initial onset of eCG secretion between days 36 and 40 when two significant changes in ovarian steroid hormone production occur. First, as demonstrated originally by Terqui and Palmer[99] and confirmed by Jeffcott et al.[100] and others, there is a sharp and pronounced rise in plasma estrogen concentrations; as shown by ovariectomy studies, this increased production of estrogen is ovarian in origin.[99] Second, in most but not all mares, a pronounced rise in plasma progesterone concentrations is observed as a result of the first secondary ovulation.[13]

As illustrated in Figure 9-10, further and usually quite distinct rises in plasma progesterone concentrations occur during the following 80 to 100 days of gestation, each rise signaling the development of another secondary luteal structure, formed either by ovulation or by luteinization without rupture of a mature follicle. Clearly, the continuing secretion of pituitary FSH, not eCG, stimulates the waves of follicular growth in the pregnant mare. The LH-like component of eCG, in the absence of pituitary LH, merely acts to induce final maturation of the dominant follicle in the wave and to either ovulate or luteinize it. Such a concept is also supported by the finding of that mares which conceive late in the breeding season, so that they pass through early pregnancy in the short-day (winter) period of ovarian inactivity, show normal concentrations of eCG in their serum but have many fewer secondary ovulations than those which conceive earlier in the year.[13]

It has been shown that eCG stimulates progesterone secretion by slices of horse luteal tissue maintained in vitro,[101] and the hormone must therefore be considered as having some luteotrophic properties. However, this appears to be at a relatively low level in vivo, which may be important to prevent the mare's ovaries becoming hyperstimulated each time she becomes pregnant. Horse CG exhibits a much lower capacity to bind to horse gonadal receptors ($< 2\%$) than does either horse or human pituitary FSH and LH, although it binds with

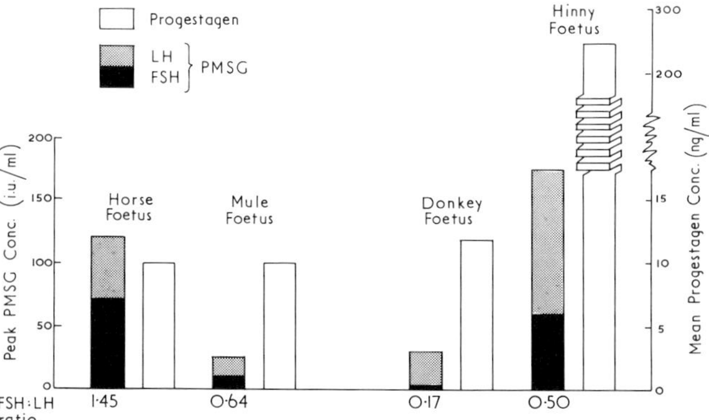

FIG. 9–12. Comparison of the mean plasma progestagen concentrations during the period of eCG (PMSG) production (open bars), the mean peak PMSG concentrations measured by hemagglutination-inhibition (H-I) assay (shaded bars), the FSH (solid shading) and LH (stippled shading) content of PMSG measured by radioreceptor assays and the calculated FSH to LH ratios of the PMSG in each case, in mares carrying intraspecies horse ($n = 9$) and interspecies mule ($n = 3$) fetuses, and in jenny donkeys carrying intraspecies donkey ($n = 3$) and interspecies hinny ($n = 3$) fetuses.

equal avidity as these and other pituitary gonadotrophins to the gonadal tissues of other species[102] (Fig. 9-11). Thus, instead of gross stimulation occurring around day 60 of pregnancy when eCG levels are at a peak, only the single ovulations described above that result essentially from the pituitary FSH-stimulated waves of follicular growth continue to occur.

A noteworthy exception to the relative lack of ovarian responsiveness to eCG in the mare, is the situation that pertains in the jenny when it carries either an interspecies hinny conceptus or a transferred extraspecies donkey-in-horse conceptus. Here, endometrial cup size, eCG secretion rate, secondary luteal development in the ovaries, and plasma progesterone concentrations between days 40 and 120 of gestation are all much higher than in donkeys carrying normal intraspecific donkey conceptuses.[13,88,103–105] However, this breakthrough in ovarian responsiveness is explained not just by the increased amounts of gonadotropin produced by the larger-than-normal endometrial cups (see Chapter 63). Rather, it is more likely to be caused by the previously mentioned higher FSH to LH ratio of the CG produced by the hinny conceptus (Fig. 9-12). Thus when the female donkey, whose ovaries are prepared genetically to encounter low levels of a CG containing very little FSH-like activity, encounters increased levels of CG with a much higher FSH content produced by the other types of conceptus, the normal protective barrier in the ovaries is overcome.[17]

One further question about the need for any luteotrophic role for eCG in equine pregnancy comes from recent studies on extraspecific equine pregnancies created by embryo transfer. As described in more detail in Chapter 63, in horse mares ($2n = 64$) carrying transferred donkey ($2n = 62$) conceptuses, the donkey chorionic girdle fails to invade the surrogate horse endometrium at days 36 to 38, with the results that no endometrial cups develop and eCG remains completely absent from maternal blood.[88] Although the majority of these donkey-in-horse pregnancies are aborted at days 80 to 90 of gestation, approximately 30% of them do manage to implant normally and are carried to term in the complete absence of eCG and without the development of any secondary corpora lutea beyond day 40; the primary corpus luteum persists and continues to secrete low, but adequate, amounts of progesterone to maintain pregnancy until the placenta is sufficiently well developed to assume this role around days 90 to 100.[106]

One final point in relation to the function of eCG in the pregnant mare is its possible role in stimulating growth and steroid production by the fetal gonads. As highlighted originally by Cole et al.[27] and studied by many others[107] since then, the gonads of both male and female equine fetuses undergo tremendous hypertrophy between days 100 and 240 of gestation, followed by regression and shrinkage to normal size at birth. This is mirrored by an equally striking increase and subsequent decline in the concentrations of both phenolic (estrone and estradiol) and ring B unsaturated (equilin and equilenin) estrogen concentrations in maternal blood and urine,[108–110] and firm evidence now exists that the enlarged gonads secrete 19-carbon steroid precursors such as dehydroepiandrosterone (DHEA) and $^7\Delta$-OH-DHEA, which are then aromatized to estrogens by the placenta.[111–113] It would be easy to assume that eCG might be the essential gonadotropic stimulus for this enormous development of the fetal gonads, but limited evidence suggests this is unlikely to be the case. The gonads only really begin to enlarge significantly from days 100 to 120, when eCG levels in maternal blood have already fallen dramatically and have, in some mares, disappeared altogether. High concentrations of eCG persist in the inspissated exocrine secretion and endometrial cup debris attached to the allantochorion and occasionally forming the allantochorionic pouches described by Clegg et al.[31] As shown originally by Cole and Saunders[114] and confirmed by others,[115] however, eCG is selectively excluded from placental absorption and eCG activity remains undetectable or at low concentrations in fetal blood and fluids compared with the levels in maternal blood.

REFERENCES

1. Cole, H.H., and Hart, G.H.: The potency of blood serum of mares in progressive stages of pregnancy in effecting the sexual maturity of the immature rat. Am. J. Physiol., *83*:57–68, 1930.
2. Aschheim, S., and Zondek, B.: Die Schwangerschaftsdiagnose aus dem Harn durch Nachweis des Hypophysenvordeslapperhormons. Klin. Wochenschr., 7:1404–1411, 1928.
3. Phillip, E.: Hypophysenvorderlappen und Placenta. Zentralbl. Gynakol., *54*:450–453, 1930.

4. Collip, J.B.: Placental hormones. Br. Med. J., *2*:1080–1081, 1930.
5. Smith, B.E., and Engle, E.T.: Experimental evidence regarding the role of the anterior pituitary in the development and regulation of the genital system. Am. J. Anat., *40*:159–215, 1927.
6. Day, F.T., and Rowlands, I.W.: The time and rate of appearance of gonadotrophin in the serum of pregnant mares. J. Endocrinol., *2*:255–261, 1940.
7. Day, F.T., and Rowlands, I.W.: Serum gonadotrophin in Welsh and Shetland ponies. J. Endocrinol., *5*:108–115, 1947.
8. Aylward, F., and Ottaway, C.W.: The collection and examination of plasma from pregnant mares for gonadotrophic hormone. J. Comp. Pathol., *55*:159–167, 1947.
9. Bielanski, W., Ewy, Z., and Pigoniowa, H.: Differences in endocrine secretion of mares pregnant with stallion or jack. Bull. Acad. Pol. Sci. Vol. II Ser. Sci. Biol., *3*:37–39, 1955.
10. Bell, E.T., Loraine, J.A., Jennings, S., and Weaver, A.D.: Serum and urinary gonadotrophin levels in pregnant ponies and donkeys. J. Exp. Physiol., *52*:68–75, 1967.
11. Wide, M., and Wide, L.: Diagnosis of pregnancy in mares by an immunological method. Nature, *198*: 1017–1018, 1964.
12. Allen, W.R.: The immunological measurement of pregnant mare serum gonadotrophin. J. Endocrinol., *32*:593–598, 1969.
13. Allen, W.R.: Maternal recognition of pregnancy and immunological implications of trophoblast-endometrium interactions in equids. *In* Maternal Recognition of Pregnancy. CIBA Foundation Symposium. No. 64. Amsterdam, Excerpta Medica, 1979, pp. 323–352.
14. Nett, T.M., and Pickett, B.W.: Effect of diethyl-stilboestrol on the relationship between LH, PMSG and progesterone during pregnancy in the mare. J. Reprod. Fertil. Suppl., *27*:465–470, 1979.
15. Kindahl, H., Knudsen, O., Madej, A., and Edqvist, L.-E.: Progesterone, prostaglandin $F_2\alpha$, PMSG and oestrone sulphate during early pregnancy in the mare. J. Reprod. Fertil. Suppl., *32*:353–359, 1982.
16. Stewart, F., Allen, W.R. and Moor, R.M.: Pregnant mare serum gonadotrophin: Ratio of follicle stimulating hormone and luteinizing hormone activities measured by radioreceptor assay. J. Endocrinol., *71*:371–382, 1976.
17. Stewart, F., Allen, W.R., and Moor, R.M.: Influence of foetal genotype on the follicle stimulating hormone luteinizing hormone ratio of pregnant mare serum gonadotrophin. J. Endocrinol., *73*:419–425, 1977.
18. Saunders, F.J., and Cole, H.H.: Two gonadotropic substances in mare serum. Proc. Soc. Exp. Biol. Med., *32*:1476–1478, 1935.
19. Saunders, F.J., and Cole, H.H.: Means of augmenting the ovarian response to gonadotropic substances. Proc. Soc. Exp. Biol. Med., *33*:505–508, 1936.
20. Cole, H.H., and Erway, J.: 48-hour test for equine gonadotropin with results expressed in international units. Endocrinology, *29*:514–519, 1941.
21. Goss, H. and Cole, H.H.: Sex hormones in the blood of mares. III. Some chemical properties of the ovary-stimulating principle. Endocrinology, *15*:214–224, 1931.
22. Cole, H.H., Guilbert, H.R., and Goss, H.: Further considerations of the properties of the gonad-stimulating principle of mare serum. Am. J. Physiol., *102*:227–240, 1932.
23. Goss, H., and Cole, H.H.: Further studies on the purification of mares gonadotropic hormone. Endocrinology, *26*:244–249, 1940.
24. Cole, H.H.: On the biological properties of mare gonadotropic hormone. Am. J. Anat., *59*: 299–332, 1936.
25. Cole, H.H., Pencharz, H.I., and Goss, H.: On the biological properties of highly purified gonadotropin from pregnant mare serum. Endocrinology, *27*:548–553, 1940.
26. Cole, H.H., Howell, C.F., and Hart, G.H.: The changes occurring in the ovary of the mare during pregnancy. Anat. Rec., *49*:199–209, 1931.
27. Cole, H.H., Hart, G.H., Lyons, W.R., and Catchpole, H.R.: The development and hormonal content of fetal horse gonads. Anat. Rec., *56*:275–293, 1933.
28. Cole, H.H., and Hart, G.H.: Concerning gonadotropic substances in mare serum. Proc. Soc. Exp. Biol. Med., *32*:370–373, 1934.
29. Catchpole, H.R., and Lyons, W.R.: The gonad stimulating hormone of pregnant mares. Am. J. Anat., *55*:167–227, 1934.
30. Cole, H.H., and Goss, H.: The source of equine gonadotropin. *In* Essays in Honor of Herbert M. Evans. Berkeley, University of California Press, 1943, pp. 107–119.
31. Clegg, M.T., Boda, J.M., and Cole, H.H.: The endometrial cups and allantochorionic pouches in the mare with emphasis on the source of equine gonadotrophin. Endocrinology, *54*:448–463, 1954.
32. Catchpole, H.R., Cole, H.H., and Pearson, P.B.: Studies on the rate of disappearance and fate of mare gonadotropic hormone following intravenous injection. Am. J. Physiol., *112*:21–26, 1935.
33. Cole, H.H., Bigelow, M., Finkel, J., and Rupp, G.R.: Biological half-life of endogenous PMS following hysterectomy and studies on levels in urine and milk. Endocrinology, *81*:929–930, 1967.
34. Bielanski, W., Ewy, Z., and Pigoniowa, H.: Differences in the level of gonadotrophin in the serum of pregnant mares. Proceedings of the Third International Congress on Animal Reproduction and Artificial Insemination. Cambridge. 1956, pp. 110–11.
35. Clegg, M.T., Cole, H.H., Howard, C.B., and Pigon, H.: The influence of foetal genotype on equine gonadotrophin secretion. J. Endocrinol., *25*:245–248, 1962.
36. Rimington, C., and Rowlands, I.W.: Serum gonadotrophin. 1. Preparation of a stable concentrate from pregnant mare's serum. Biochem. J., *35*:736–748, 1941.
37. Rimington, C., and Rowlands, I.W.: Serum gonadotrophin. 2. Further purification of the active material. Biochem. J., *38*:54–60, 1944.
38. Gospodarowicz, D.: Purification and physico-chemical properties of the pregnant mare serum gonadotrophin (PMSG). Endocrinology, *91*:101–106, 1971.
39. Papkoff, H., Bewley, T.A., and Ramachardran, J.: Physicochemical and biological characterisations of pregnant mare serum gonadotropin and its subunits. Biochim. Biophys. Acta, *532*:185–194, 1978.
40. Christakos, S., and Bahl, O.P.: Pregnant mare serum gonadotropin purification and physicochemical, biological and immunological characterisation. J. Biol. Chem., *254*:4253–4258, 1979.
41. Farmer, S.W., and Papkoff, H.: Immunochemical studies with pregnant mare serum gonadotropin. Biol. Reprod., *21*:425–431, 1979.
42. Aggarwal, B.B., and Papkoff, H.: Relationship of sialic acid residues to in vitro biological and immunological activities of equine gonadotrophins. Biol. Reprod., *24*:1082–1087, 1981.

43. Raacke, I.D., Lostroh, A.J., Boda, J.M., and Li, C.H.: Some aspects of the characterization of pregnant mare serum gonadotrophin. Acta Endocrinol. (Copenh.), *26*:377–387, 1957.

44. Gospodarowicz, D., and Papkoff, H.: A simple method for the isolation of pregnant mare serum gonadotropin. Endocrinology, *80*:699–708, 1967.

45. Moore, W.T., and Ward, D.N.: Pregnant mare serum gonadotropin: Rapid chromatographic procedures for the purification of intact hormone and isolation of subunits. J. Biol. Chem., *255*:6923–6929, 1980.

46. Bangham, D.R., and Woodward, P.M.: The second international standard for serum gonadotrophin. Bull. World Health Organ., *35*:761–773, 1966.

47. Papkoff, H.: Chemical and biological properties of the subunits of pregnant mare serum gonadotropin. Biochem. Biophys. Res. Commun., *58*:397–404, 1974.

48. Stewart, F., Thompson, J.A., Leigh, S.A., and Warwick, J.M.: Nucleotide (cDNA) sequence encoding the horse gonadotrophin α-subunit. J. Endocrinol., *115*:341–346, 1987.

49. Moore, W.T., Burleigh, B.D., and Ward, D.N.: Chorionic gonadotrophins: Comparative studies and comments on relationships to other glycoprotein hormones. *In* Chorionic Gonadotrophins. Edited by S. Segal. New York, Plenum Press, 1980, pp. 89–126.

50. Talmadge, K., Vamvakopoulos, N.C., and Fiddes, J.C.: Evolution of the genes for the β-subunits of human chorionic gonadotropin and luteinizing hormone. Nature, *307*:37–40, 1984.

51. Policastro, P.F., Daniels-McQueeh, S., Carle, G., and Boime, I.: A map of hCG-β-LHβ gene cluster. J. Biol. Chem., *261*:5907–5916, 1986.

52. Crawford, R.J., Tregear, G.W., and Niall, H.D.: The nucleotide sequences of baboon chorionic gonadotropin β-subunit genes have diverged from the human. Gene, *46*:161–169, 1986.

53. Bousfield, G.R., Sugino, H., and Ward, D.N.: Demonstration of a COOH-terminal extension on equine lutropin by means of a common acid-labile bond in equine lutropin and equine chorionic gonadotropin. J. Biol. Chem., *260*:9531–9533, 1985.

54. Bousfield, G.R., Liu, W.-K., Sugino, H., and Ward, D.N.: Structural studies on equine glycoprotein hormones. Amino acid sequence of equine lutropin B-subunit. J. Biol. Chem., *262*:8610–8620, 1987.

55. Sugino, H., Bousfield, G.R., Moore, W.T., and Ward, D.N.: Structural studies on equine glycoprotein hormones. Amino acid sequence of equine chorionic gonadotropin β-subunit. J. Biol. Chem., *262*:8603–8609, 1987.

56. Mougdal, N.R., and Papkoff, H.: Equine luteinizing hormone possesses follicle stimulating hormone activity in hypophysectomized female rats. Biol. Reprod., *26*:935–952, 1982.

57. Combarnous, Y., Guillame, F., and Martinet, N.: Comparison of in vitro follicle stimulating hormone (FSH) activity of equine gonadotropins (luteinizing hormone, FSH and chorionic gonadotropin) in male and female rats. Endocrinology, *115*:1821–1827, 1984.

58. Stewart, F., and Maher, J.K.: Analysis of horse and donkey gonadotrophin genes using Southern blotting and DNA hybridization techniques. J. Reprod. Fertil. Suppl., *44*:19–26, 1991.

59. Fiddes, J.C., and Goodman, H.M.: The cDNA for the β-subunit of human chorionic gonadotropin suggests evolution of a gene by read-through into the 3;-untranslated region. Nature, *286*:684–687, 1980.

60. Leigh, S.E.A., and Stewart, F.: Partial cDNA sequence for the donkey chorionic gonadotrophin-β subunit suggests evolution from an ancestral LH-β gene. J. Mol. Endocrinol., *4*:143–150, 1990.

61. Damm, J.B.L., et al.: Structure determination of the major N- and O-linked carbohydrate chains of the β subunit from equine chorionic gonadotropin. Eur. J. Biochem., *189*:175–182, 1990.

62. Bahl, O.P., Thotakura, N.R., and Anumula, K.R.: Biological role of carbohydrates in gonadotropins. *In* Hormone Receptors in Growth and Reproduction. Edited by B.B. Saxena. New York, Raven Press, 1984, pp. 165–182.

63. Bahl, O.P., and Waugh, P.V.: Characterization of glycoproteins: Carbohydrate structures of glycoprotein hormones. Adv. Exp. Med. Biol., *206*:381–388, 1986.

64. Catchpole, H.R.: Physiology of the gonadotropic hormones. *In* Gonadotropins: Their Chemical and Biological Properties and Secretory Control. Edited by H.H. Cole, San Francisco, W.H. Freeman, 1963, pp. 40–70.

65. Butt, W.R., Crook, A.C., and Cunningham, F.J.: Studies on human urinary and pituitary gonadotrophins. Biochem. J., *81*:596–605, 1961.

66. Aggarwal, B.B., et al.: Purification and characterization of donkey chorionic gonadotrophin. J. Endocrinol., *85*:449–454, 1980.

67. Roser, J.F., et al.: Chemical, biological and immunological properties of pituitary gonadotropins from the donkey (Equus asinus): comparison with the horse (Equus caballus). Biol. Reprod., *30*:1253–1258, 1984.

68. Rowson, L.E.A.: The role of research in animal reproduction. Vet. Rec., *95*:276–296, 1974.

69. Saumande, J., and Chupin, D.: Superovulation: A limit to egg transfer in cattle. Theriogenology, *7*:141–148, 1977.

70. Christie, W.B., Newcomb, R., and Rowson, L.E.A.: Ovulation rate and egg recovery in cattle treated repeatedly with pregnant mare serum gonadotrophin and prostaglandin. Vet. Rec., *104*:281–284, 1979.

71. Elsden, R.P., Nelson, L.D., and Seidel, G.E.: Superovulation of cows with follicle stimulating hormone and pregnant mare's serum gonadotropin. Theriogenology, *9*:17–25, 1978.

72. Gordon, I.: Synchronization of estrus and superovulation in cattle. *In* Mammalian Egg Transfer. Edited by C.F. Adams. Boca Raton, CRC Press, 1982, pp. 63–80.

73. Zondek, B.: Hormonelle Schwangerschaftstreaktion aus dem Harn bei Mensch und Tier. Klin. Wochenschr., *9*:2285–2289, 1930.

74. Schauder, W.: Untersuchungen über die Eihäute und Embryotrophe des Pferdes. Arch. Anat. Physiol., *1912*:259–302, 1912.

75. Mossman, H.W.: Comparative morphogenesis of the fetal membranes and accessory uterine structures. Contrib. Embryol. Carneg. Inst., *26*:129–246, 1937.

76. Kirby, D.R.S.: Immunological aspects of pregnancy. *In* Advances in Reproductive Physiology. Vol. 3. Edited by A. McLaren. London, Logos Press Ltd., 1968, pp. 33–79.

77. McManus, J.F.A.: Histological demonstration of mucin after periodic acid. Nature, *158*:202–203, 1946.

78. Amoroso, E.C.: Endocrinology of pregnancy. Br. Med. Bull., *11*:117–125, 1955.

79. Allen, W.R.: Equine gonadotrophins. Ph.D. thesis, University of Cambridge, 1970.

80. Allen, W.R., and Moor, R.M.: The origin of the equine endometrial cups. I. Production of PMSG by fetal trophoblast cells. J. Reprod. Fertil., *29*:313–316, 1972.
81. Allen, W.R., Hamilton, D.W., and Moor, R.M.: The origin of the equine endometrial cups: II. Invasion of the endometrium by trophoblast. Anat. Rec., *177*:475–501, 1973.
82. Ewart, J.C.: A Critical Period in the Development of the Horse. London, Adam & Charles Black, 1897.
83. Van Niekerk, C.H.: The early diagnosis of pregnancy, the development of the foetal membranes and nidation in the mare. J. S. Afr. Vet. Med. Assoc., *36*:483–488, 1965.
84. Van Niekerk, C.H. and Allen, W.R.: Early embryonic development in the horse. J. Reprod. Fertil. Suppl., *23*:495–498, 1975.
85. Crump, A., et al.: Expression of major histocompatibility complex (MHC) antigens on horse trophoblast. J. Reprod. Fertil. Suppl., *35*:379–388, 1987.
86. Donaldson, W.L., Zhang, C.H., Oriol, J.G., and Antczak, D.F.: Invasive equine trophoblast expresses conventional class I Major Histocompatibility Complex antigens. Development, *110*:63–71, 1990.
87. Allen, W.E.: Ovarian changes during early pregnancy in pony mares in relation to PMSG production. J. Reprod. Fertil. Suppl., *23*:425–428, 1975.
88. Allen, W.R.: Immunological aspects of the endometrial cup reaction and the effect of xenogeneic pregnancy in horses and donkeys. J. Reprod. Fertil. Suppl., *31*:57–94, 1982.
89. Martinek, S.D., Bristol, F., and Murphy, B.D.: Effects of the dam on equine chorionic gonadotropin concentrations during pregnancy. Domest. Anim. Endocrinol., *7*:551–562, 1990.
90. Moor, R.M., Allen, W.R., and Hamilton, D.W.: Origin and histogenesis of equine endometrial cups. J. Reprod. Fertil. Suppl., *23*:391–396, 1975.
91. Kydd, J.H., Butcher, G.W., Antczak, D.F., and Allen, W.R.: Expression of Major Histocompatibility Complex (MHC) class 1 molecules on early trophoblast. J. Reprod. Fertil. Suppl., *44*:463–477, 1991.
92. Antczak, D.F., Bright, S.M., Remick, C.N., and Bauman, B.E.: Lymphocyte alloantigens of the horse. Serologic and genetic studies. Tissue Antigens, *20*:172–187, 1982.
93. Antczak, D.F., and Allen, W.R.: Invasive trophoblast of the genus Equus. Ann. Inst. Pasteur, *135*:325–331, 1984.
94. Amoroso, E.C., Hancock, J.L., and Rowlands, I.W.: Ovarian activity in the pregnant mare. Nature, *161*:353–356, 1948.
95. Evans, M.J., and Irvine, C.H.G.: Serum concentrations of FSH, LH and progesterone during the oestrous cycle and early pregnancy in the mare. J. Reprod. Fertil. Suppl., *23*:293–300, 1975.
96. Urwin, V.E., and Allen, W.R.: Pituitary and chorionic gonadotrophin control of ovarian function during early pregnancy in equids. J. Reprod. Fertil. Suppl., *32*:371–381, 1982.
97. Bain, A.M.: The ovaries of the mare during early pregnancy. Vet. Rec., *80*:229–231, 1967.
98. Van Rensburg, S.J., and van Niekerk, C.H.: Ovarian function, follicular oestradiol-17β and luteal progesterone and 20α-hydroxy-pregn-en-one in cycling and pregnant equines. Onderstepoort J. Vet. Res., *35*:301–318, 1968.
99. Terqui, M., and Palmer, E.: Oestrogen pattern during early pregnancy in the mare. J. Reprod. Fertil. Suppl., *27*:441–446, 1979.
100. Jeffcott, L.B., et al.: Changes in maternal hormone concentrations associated with induction of fetal death at day 45 of gestation in mares. J. Reprod. Fertil. Suppl., *35*:461–467, 1987.
101. Squires, E.L., Stevens, W.B., Pickett, B.W., and Nett, T.M.: Role of Pregnant Mare Serum Gonadotrophin in luteal function of pregnant mares. Am. J. Vet. Res., *40*:589–591, 1979.
102. Stewart, F., and Allen, W.R.: The binding of FSH, LH and PMSG to equine gonadal tissues. J. Reprod. Fertil. Suppl., *27*:431–440, 1979.
103. Allen, W.R.: Factors influencing pregnant mare serum gonadotrophin production. Nature, *223*:64–66, 1969.
104. Sheldrick, E.L., Wright, P.J., Allen, W.R., and Heap, R.B.: Metabolic clearance rate, production rate and source of progesterone in donkeys with fetuses of different genotypes. J. Reprod. Fertil., *51*:473–476, 1977.
105. Stewart, F., and Allen, W.R.: Biological functions and receptor binding activities of equine chorionic gonadotrophins. J. Reprod. Fertil., *62*:527–536, 1981.
106. Allen, W.R., Kydd, J.H., and Antczak, D.F.: Xenogeneic donkey-in-horse pregnancy created by embryo transfer: Immunological aspects of a model of early abortion. *In* Immunology of the Fetus. Edited by G. Chauoat. Boca Raton, CRC Press, 1990, pp. 267–283.
107. Hay, M.F., and Allen, W.R.: An ultrastructural and histochemical study of the interstitial cells in the gonads of the fetal horse. J. Reprod. Fertil. Suppl., *23*:557–561, 1975.
108. Cox, J.E.: Oestrone and equilin in the plasma of the pregnant mare. J. Reprod. Fertil. Suppl., *23*:463–468, 1975.
109. Raeside, J.I., and Liptrap, R.M.: Patterns of urinary oestrogen excretion in individual pregnant mares. J. Reprod. Fertil. Suppl., *23*:469–475, 1975.
110. Pashen, R.L., and Allen, W.R.: The role of the fetal gonads and placenta in steroid production, maintenance of pregnancy and parturition in the mare. J. Reprod. Fertil. Suppl., *27*:499–509, 1979.
111. Bhavnani, B.R.: Oestrogen biosynthesis in the pregnant mare. J. Endocrinol., *89*:19–32, 1981.
112. Pashen, R.L., Sheldrick, E.L., Allen, W.R., and Flint, A.P.F.: Dehydroepiandrosterone synthesis by the fetal foal and its importance as an oestrogen precursor. J. Reprod. Fertil. Suppl., *32*:389–397, 1982.
113. Tait, A.D., Hodge, L.C., and Allen, W.R.: The biosynthesis of the 3β-hydroxy-5,7-androstadien-17-one by the horse fetal gonad. FEBS Lett., *182*:107–110, 1985.
114. Cole, H.H., and Saunders, F.J.: The concentration of gonad-stimulating hormone in blood serum and of oestrin in the urine throughout pregnancy in the mare. Endocrinology, *19*:199–208, 1935.
115. Rowlands, I.W.: Levels of gonadotropins in tissues and fluids with emphasis on domestic animals. *In* Gonadotropins: Their Chemical and Biological Properties and Secretory Control. Edited by H.H. Cole. San Francisco, W.H. Freeman, 1963, pp. 75–107.

CHAPTER 10

ADRENAL STEROIDS

T.M. Nett

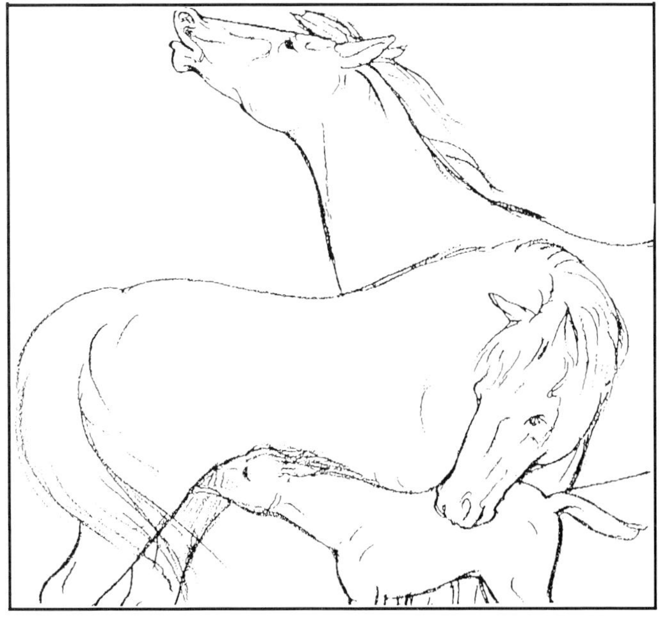

The adrenal cortex is site of synthesis of several steroid hormones. These can be categorized as glucocorticoids or mineralocorticoids, depending on their biologic activities. The most prevalent of the glucocorticoids present in the circulation of horses is cortisol.[1] Other glucocorticoids (corticosterone, cortisone, and deoxycorticosterone) have also been identified as secretory products of the equine adrenal cortex[2] but are present in much smaller quantities than cortisol. The adrenal cortex also secretes the mineralocorticoid aldosterone, but in much smaller quantities than glucocorticoids. Blood concentrations of glucocorticoids increase after administration of adrenocorticotropic hormone (ACTH).[3,4] In contrast, blood concentrations of aldosterone do not vary in concert with cortisol.[5] Therefore, secretion of aldosterone does not appear to be under direct regulation of adrenocorticotropic hormone.

As in other species, a diurnal variation in the secretion of glucocorticoids seems to exist in the horse. Minimum concentrations of cortisol appear to occur during late afternoon or early evening, and maximum concentrations are observed at midmorning.[6–9] In addition to the diurnal variation in concentrations of cortisol in horses, there appears to be an episodic secretion of cortisol in horses with a mean interpulse interval of approximately 2.5 h.[9] Such rhythms should be considered when collecting samples for determining concentrations of cortisol in horses for clinical evaluation.

BIOSYNTHESIS OF ADRENAL STEROIDS

Little information is available concerning the biosynthesis of steroids in the adrenal gland in the horse. Therefore, the following has been adapted from information available about other species.[10] The biosynthetic pathway and the structures of steroids produced by the adrenal gland are depicted in Figure 10-1. Cholesterol serves as the precursor for adrenal steroids. Although the adrenal cortex is capable of synthesizing cholesterol from acetate, it appears that most of the cholesterol used for biosynthesis of adrenal steroids is sequestered from the circulation. Normally, the rate-limiting step in biosynthesis of adrenal steroids is the conversion of cholesterol to pregnenolone. Upon stimulation of the adrenal cortex by ACTH, the conversion of cholesterol to pregnenolone is accelerated. Once pregnenolone is formed, it is readily converted to cortisol, corticosterone, or aldosterone by the pathways indicated in Figure 10-1. Glucocorticoids are produced in the zona glomerulosa of the adrenal cortex, whereas aldosterone is produced in the zona reticularis. The equine adrenal cortex also contains these zones,[11] so it is assumed that the glucocorticoids and aldosterone are biosynthesized in the same zones as in other species.

It should be noted from Figure 10-1 that the adrenal gland also has the ability to produce sex steroids (estrogens, androgens, and progestins). Therefore, it is possible for the adrenal gland to produce these steroids in sufficient quantities to have biologic effects, particularly in the case of an overactive adrenal gland. If the adrenal

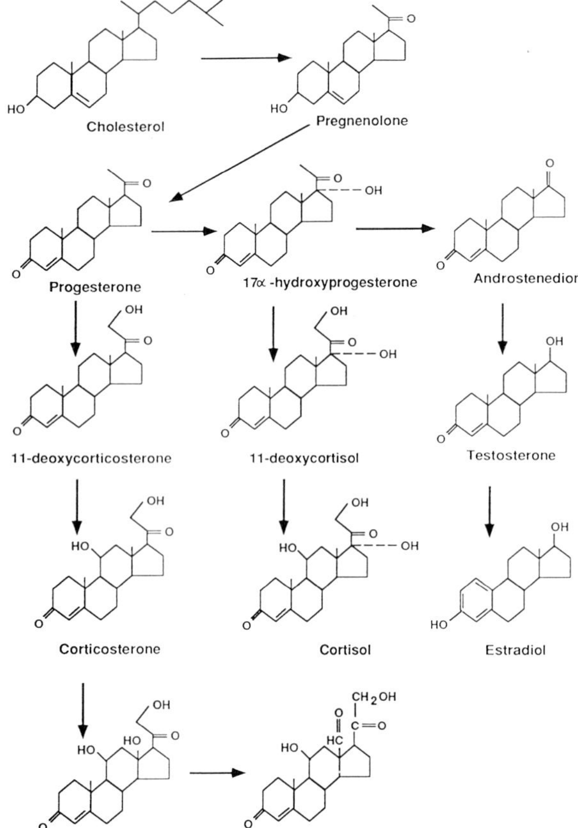

FIG. 10–1. Assumed pathway for biosynthesis of adrenal steroids in the horse.

cortex does produce sex steroids in quantities sufficient to have biologic effects, such effects will almost always be detrimental to normal reproductive processes, because sex steroids inhibit secretion of gonadotropins. The inhibition of gonadotropin secretion would, in turn, reduce gonadal activity and disrupt normal production of gametes.

BIOLOGIC FUNCTIONS OF ADRENAL STEROIDS

The primary function of aldosterone is to increase resorption of sodium in the distal convoluted tubule of the kidney. It also appears to cause sodium retention in sweat glands and glands of the alimentary canal. In cases of adrenal insufficiency, a sodium diuresis occurs that can be life threatening.

Glucocorticoids (cortisol and corticosterone), as the name implies, have effects on carbohydrate metabolism. These effects include promotion of gluconeogenesis and liver glycogen deposition and elevation of blood glucose. Glucocorticoids also inhibit uptake of amino acids and synthesis of proteins in tissues other than liver. Uptake of amino acids by the liver is actually accelerated where they are deaminated and used as substrates for energy metabolism (gluconeogenesis). Because of the reduction in protein synthesis, chronic elevation of glucocorticoids, as occurs in some disease states, may have a protein-wasting effect. Glucocorticoids also have anti-inflammatory and immunosuppressive actions. These actions have lead to the wide-spread use of synthetic glucocorticosteroids in clinical practice.

With respect to reproduction, administration of the synthetic glucocorticoid dexamethasone to mares has been shown to inhibit ovulation, apparently by decreasing secretion of luteinizing hormone (LH).[12] Glucocorticosteroids also have been implicated in the inhibition of LH secretion in primates[13] and cows,[14,15] possibly by reducing sensitivity of the anterior pituitary gland to gonadotropin-releasing hormone. However, whether physiologic concentrations of cortisol are capable of inhibiting secretion of LH in horses is still open to question. Serum concentrations of cortisol are lower during estrus than during diestrus in cycling mares,[16] suggesting that a decline in serum cortisol may be associated with increased secretion of LH and ovulation. In contrast, increased serum concentrations of cortisol were induced in mares on the first day of estrus by loading the animals into a trailer and hauling them for 12 h.[17] Compared to control mares (not transported), increased concentrations of cortisol resulting from transportation had no effect on serum concentrations of LH or estradiol, estrous behavior, ovulation, duration of the estrous cycle, or pregnancy rates. Thus supraphysiologic concentrations of cortisol may be necessary to induce adverse effects on reproduction in mares.

Administration of adrenocorticotropin to stallions increased serum concentrations of cortisol and decreased serum concentrations of testosterone but did not affect serum concentrations of LH.[4] This suggests that increased concentrations of cortisol may have a direct testicular effect to reduce secretion of testosterone.

In cattle and sheep, the hypothalamic-pituitary-adrenal axis is involved in the initiation of parturition. In these species, there is an increase in the secretion of cortisol by the fetal adrenal glands 2 to 3 days prior to parturition. Destruction of the fetal pituitary during gestation eliminates the rise in cortisol and prolongs gestation, whereas administration of glucocorticoids will induce early parturition in these species.[18] In contrast, the role of cortisol in parturition in mares appears to be of less importance. The circulating concentration of cortisol in the mare does not increase prior to parturition.[19] Moreover, large amounts of dexamethasone were required to induce parturition in mares (100 mg/day for each of four successive days).[20] Owing to the large quantity of dexamethasone required for induction of parturition in mares compared to other species, it seems likely that the results may be attributable to a pharmacologic effect. Thus the role of glucocorticoids in parturition in mares remains to be determined.

REFERENCES

1. James, V.H.T., Horner, M.W., Moss, M.S., and Rippon, A.V.: Adrenal cortical function in the horse. J. Endocrinol., *48*:319–335, 1970.
2. Zolovick, A., Upson, D.W., and Eleftheriou, B.E.: Diurnal

variation in plasma glucocorticosteroid levels in the horse (Equus caballus). J. Endocrinol., *35*:249–253, 1966.

3. MacHarg, M.A., Bottoms, G.D., Carter, G.K., and Johnson, M.A.: Effects of multiple intramuscular injections and doses of dexamethasone on plasma cortisol concentration and adrenal responses to ACTH in horses. Am. J. Vet. Res., *46*:2285–2287, 1985.
4. Wiest, J.J., et al.: Effect of administration of adrenocorticotropic hormone on plasma concentrations of testosterone, luteinizing hormone, follicle stimulating hormone and cortisol in stallions. Equine Vet. Sci., *8*:168–170, 1988.
5. Guthrie, G.P., Jr., Cecil, S.G., and Kotchen, T.A.: Renin, aldosterone and cortisol in the Thoroughbred horse. J. Endocrinol., *85*:49–53, 1980.
6. Bottoms, G.D., Roesel, O.F., Rausch, F.D., and Akins, A.L.: Circadian variation in plasma cortisol and corticosterone in pigs and mares. Am. J. Vet. Res., *33*:785–790, 1972.
7. Kumar, M.S.A., Liao, T.F., and Chen, C.L.: Diurnal variation in serum cortisol in ponies. J. Anim. Sci., *42*:1360, 1976.
8. Larsson, M., Edqvist, L.E., Ekman, L., and Persson, S.: Plasma cortisol in the horse, diurnal rhythm and effects of exogenous ACTH. Acta Vet. Scand., *20*:16–24, 1979.
9. Toutain, P.L., Oukessou, M., Autefage, A., and Alvinerie, M.: Diurnal and episodic variation of plasma hydrocortisone concentrations in horses. Domest. Anim. Endocrinol., *5*:55–59, 1988.
10. Liddle, G.W.: The adrenals. *In* Textbook of Endocrinology. 6th ed. Edited by R.H. Williams. Philadelphia, W.B. Saunders, 1981, pp. 249–292.
11. Cameron, E.H.D., and Grant, J.K.: Biochemistry of histologically defined zones in the adrenal cortex: cortisol synthesis in the horse. J. Endocrinol., *37*:413–420, 1967.
12. Asa, C.S., and Ginther, O.J.: Glucocorticoid suppression of oestrus, follicles, LH and ovulation in the mare. J. Reprod. Fertil. Suppl., *32*:247–251, 1982.
13. Dubey, A.K., and Plant, T.M.: A suppression of gonadotropin secretion by cortisol in castrated male rhesus monkeys (Maccaca mulatta) mediated by interruption of hypothalamic gonadotropin-releasing hormone release. Biol. Reprod., *33*:423–431, 1985.
14. Li, P.S., and Wagner, W.C.: In vivo and in vitro studies on the effect of adrenocorticotropic hormone or cortisol on the pituitary response to gonadotropin-releasing hormone. Biol. Reprod., *29*:25–37, 1983.
15. Padmanabhan, V., Keech, C., and Convey, E.M.: Cortisol inhibits and adrenocorticotropin has no effect on luteinizing hormone-releasing hormone-induced release of luteinizing hormone from bovine pituitary cells in vitro. Endocrinology, *112*:1782–1787, 1983.
16. Asa, C.S., Robinson, J.A., and Ginther, O.J.: Changes in plasma cortisol concentrations during the ovulatory cycle of the mare. J. Endocrinol., *99*:329–334, 1983.
17. Baucus, K.L., et al.: Effect of transportation on the estrous cycle and concentrations of hormones in mares. J. Anim. Sci., *68*:419–426, 1990.
18. Adams, W.M., and Wagner, W.C.: The role of corticoids in parturition. Biol. Reprod., *3*:223–228, 1970.
19. Nathanielsz, P.W., Rossdale, P.D., Silver, M., and Comline, R.S.: Studies on fetal, neonatal and maternal cortisol metabolism in the mare. J. Reprod. Fertil. Suppl., *23*:625–630, 1975.
20. Alm, C.C., Sullivan, J.J., and First, N.L.: Induction of premature parturition by parenteral administration of dexamethasone in the mare. J. Am. Vet. Med. Assoc., *165*:721–722, 1974.

CHAPTER 11

MELATONIN

D.C. Sharp
B.D. Cleaver

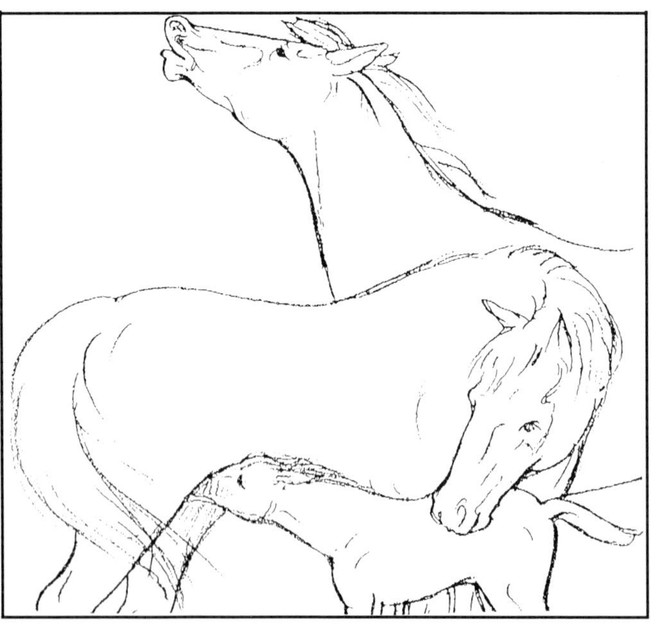

HISTORY OF THE PINEAL AND DISCOVERY OF MELATONIN

The pineal gland, main source of the indole amine melatonin, was recognized by early Greek anatomists who were struck by that fact that the pineal is unpaired and is situated close to the fourth ventricle through which cerebrospinal fluid (CSF) flows. These Greek philosophers attributed to the pineal the role of a valve, controlling the flow of thought. Rene Descartes, expanded on this idea by proposing that the pineal translated messages coming into the brain into direct musculoskeletal actions.[1] In other words, he had described the function of a neuroendocrine transducer, a description that turned out to be entirely prescient.

Centuries passed with little further elaboration on Descarte's quaint concept of pineal function until 1917, when McCord and Allen observed that extracts from bovine pineals caused blanching of the skin of tadpoles when injected.[2] In 1958, a dermatologist and biochemist interested in pigmentation isolated the factor that caused blanching of the melanocytes in frog skin, and it was reported that the substance was 5-methoxy-*N*-acetyl tryptamine, or melatonin.[3] The name is somewhat unfortunate, because current understanding of melatonin function suggests that blanching of melanocytes is far from its physiologic raison d'être. In addition, the name melatonin is treacherously close to the name of a completely different hormone, melanocyte-stimulating hormone (MSH), and care should be taken not to confuse the two. Current appreciation of the role of melatonin is that it may be involved in several components of the endocrine system, but of greatest importance to this volume is its potential role as a regulator or signaler of seasonal reproductive changes.

Although the action of melatonin on pigmentation changes in frogs was of scientific interest, involvement of the pineal in reproductive function was first noted in clinical cases of precocious puberty that were associated with pineal tumors.[4–6] Tumors in the pineal area have also been associated with delayed puberty. This apparent dichotomy has been explained by the hypothesis that some tumors secrete excess melatonin, and hence suppress normal reproductive development, whereas other tumors in the pineal area actually result in the destruction of the normally inhibitory effects of the pineal, thus enabling premature gonadal reproductive development. It has been reported that such tumorous growths extend over a considerable portion of the diencephalon, involving the hypothalamus and pituitary, and the direct involvement of the pineal in stimulating precocious reproductive function does not seem likely.[6]

If the pineal plays some role in regulation of the onset of puberty, then one could argue that changes in circulating melatonin concentrations or patterns should be measurable. The evidence for that, however, is mixed. Arendt estimated serum melatonin at midday and at midnight in six prepubertal and three pubertal children.[7] Melatonin concentrations at the midday sample were about 14 pg/mL whereas melatonin concentrations in the midnight samples were 128 and 162 pg/mL in postpubertal and prepubertal children, respectively. In contrast, Silman et al. measured circulating melatonin in normal schoolchildren and found a marked decline in serum melatonin in boys in Tanner stage II puberty.[8] They hypothesized that the decrease in circulating melatonin was causally related to the onset of puberty. Although the data are not unequivocal, they do point to a general decline in melatonin concentrations at the time of puberty. Regardless of the real role played by the pineal in precocious puberty, the pineal was to be inexorably linked to reproductive function from the time of its first clinical association with reproductive dysfunction.

BIOSYNTHETIC PATHWAY

Elucidation of the structure of melatonin as an indole amine (5-methoxy-*N*-acetyl tryptamine)[3] (Fig. 11-1) attracted the interest of many researchers, including Axelrod who was interested in indole metabolism as well as transmethylation reactions. Axelrod and Weissbach reported the isolation and purification of an enzyme from bovine pineals which *O*-methylated several indoles.[9] However, of all the hydroxy indoles that served as substrate for the enzyme, *N*-acetylserotonin was by far the best substrate, and the enzyme was named hydroxyindole-*O*-methyltransferase (HIOMT).[9] This latter enzyme was found to be highly localized in the pineals of mammals, birds, and amphibians, leading these scientists to speculate that synthesis of melatonin was essentially unique to the pineal. In the course of their studies another enzyme was isolated from pineal tissues, which converted serotonin to *N*-acetylserotonin, the substrate for hydroxyindole-*O*-methyltransferase.[9] The discovery of this second important enzyme led Axelrod and colleagues to propose a biosynthetic pathway for melatonin originating with the amino acid tryptophan (Fig. 11-1).

An association between pineal function and environmental lighting had long been suspected, based on diverse observations. Holmgren had reported that amphibian pineals were equipped with photoreceptors that were capable of responding to light.[10] In fact, the parietal eye or so-called third eye, as the pineal was sometimes referred to in lower vertebrates, has recently been shown to have many functions in common with the retina. Exposure of rats to constant light resulted in changes both to the gonads[11] (increased weight) and to the pineal[12] (reduced weight). Furthermore, administration of pineal extracts was shown to decrease the constant light-induced, ovarian hypertrophy and persistent estrus in rats.[13] Therefore, with this background of postulated pineal-light interaction, Wurtman et al. exposed rats to constant light or constant darkness and found that the concentration of HIOMT was markedly suppressed in rats exposed to light compared with rats exposed to darkness.[13] This indicated that melatonin synthesis would be reduced in the pineals of animals exposed to constant light, and the gonad-inhibiting role of melatonin would then be reduced, leading to the observed ovarian hypertrophy. A similar result was ob-

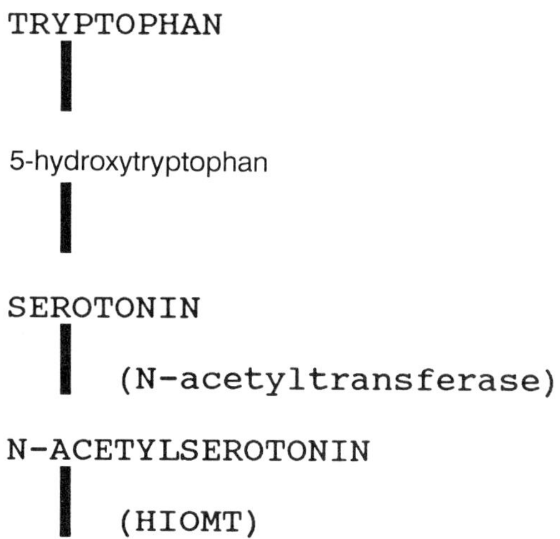

FIG. 11–1. Melatonin biosynthetic pathway. The enzyme, *N*-acetyltransferase (NAT) is the rate-limiting step in the synthesis.

served when pony mares were exposed to constant light, except that gonadotropin-releasing hormone (GnRH) was the end point, not gonadal weight.[14]

The mechanism by which the pineal, located between the two cerebral hemispheres, could respond to changes in environmental lighting, however, was unclear. Ariens-Kappers[15] had shown that the pineal was richly innervated by sympathetic fibers arising from the superior cervical ganglia, and Wurtman et al.[16] performed a series of experiments in which the effects of constant light were compared in intact rats and rats with some portion of the sympathetic path from the retina of the eye to the pineal ablated. They found that removal of the eyes prevented the light-mediated decrease in HIOMT, as did removal of the superior cervical ganglia, section of the preganglionic fibers, and section of the postganglionic fibers. They interpreted these observations to mean that information about environmental lighting reaches the pineal via the retina, midbrain pathways, preganglionic fibers, superior cervical ganglia, and postganglionic fibers which terminate directly in the pinealocytes. Wurtman et al. further proposed that this transformation of neuronal signals to a humoral response (melatonin) indicated that the pineal is a neuroendocrine transducer, essentially the definition that Descartes had envisioned, although not in those words.[16]

These studies with constant light or dark were, of course, extreme conditions, but reports of measurable effects on pineal indole metabolism with normal day/night (nyctohemeral) changes were also beginning to surface. Quay reported that serotonin levels were considerably higher in the pineal during the day than in the night.[17] However, the assumption that the environmental light mediation of pineal biochemistry was a direct signal-response function was to prove naive. Snyder et al. demonstrated that when rats were maintained in darkness, the rhythm in pineal serotonin production persisted, whereas in rats maintained in constant light,

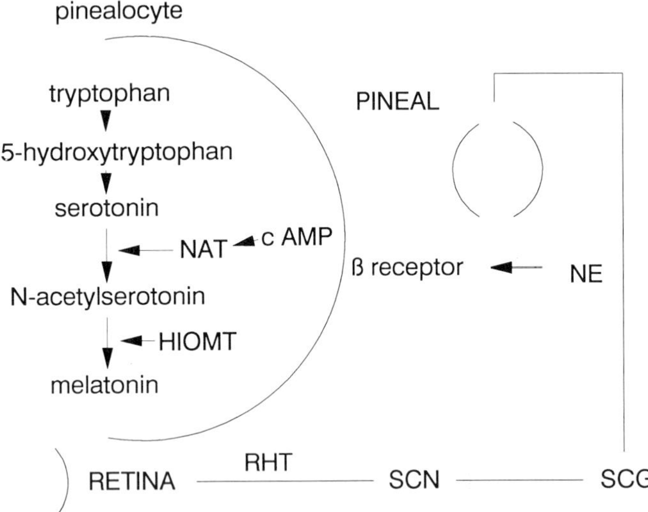

FIG. 11–2. Adrenergic regulation of melatonin synthesis by the pineal gland. Norepinephrine (NE) released from postganglionic sympathetic fibers from the superior cervical ganglia (SCG) during darkness stimulate cyclic adenosine monophosphate (cAMP) which, in turn, leads to synthesis of the rate-limiting enzyme in the biosynthetic path, *N*-acetyltransferase (NAT). RHT, retinohypothalamic tract; SCN, suprachiasmatic nucleus.

the rhythm in serotonin production was essentially abolished.[18] These observations as well as many subsequent experiments by a variety of workers has established that secretion of pineal components is regulated by the circadian time-keeping system, as opposed to a direct photic response.[19–21]

Klein and Weller[20] reported a rhythm in *N*-acetyltransferase (NAT), the enzyme that converts serotonin to *N*-acetylserotonin, that was 180° out of phase with the rhythm in serotonin reported by Quay[17] and Snyder et al.[18] and interpreted this observation to indicate that the synthesis of NAT was the rate-limiting step in the biosynthetic pathway to melatonin. They also showed that this rhythm was abolished by interruption of the sympathetic pathway, similar to the observations of Wurtman et al.[16] At the same time, Klein et al.[21] demonstrated a marked stimulation of NAT by norepinephrine in pineal organ cultures, as well as a marked increase in cyclic adenosine monophosphate (cAMP) after the addition of norepinephrine to the cultures. The evidence for adrenergic regulation of the NAT rhythm was enhanced by Degouchi and Axelrod[22] when they demonstrated that the effect of noradrenergic agents on pineal NAT synthesis could be blocked by addition of β-adrenergic blockers, such as propranolol. Current understanding of the adrenergic regulation of melatonin synthesis by the pineal gland is outlined in Figure 11-2.

ANATOMIC PATHWAY

An understanding of the anatomic pathway by which light reaches the pineal is important to the discussion of regulation of melatonin synthesis and the circadian time-keeping system. The retina is the primary photoreceptor of the circadian system of mammals, although the pineal may respond directly to light in some birds and lower vertebrates. Electrical activity resulting from retinal stimulation is conducted along a specialized projection of fibers that passes directly to the suprachiasmatic nucleus (SCN) from the retina.[23] This retinohypothalamic projection (RHP) exists in all mammalian species so far studied, including the horse. Sharp et al. demonstrated the existence of a RHP in horses by anterograde flow of tracer (horseradish peroxidase) administered into the aqueous humor of three horses.[24] The horses were killed 48 h later, and the brain was fixed in Mesulam fixative. Sections of hypothalamus, which included the area of the SCN were incubated using the tetramethylbenzidene procedure to generate a color reaction to the horseradish peroxidase (HRP). In all cases, the SCN on the hemisphere opposite to the side of administration of the HRP was markedly stained by the color reaction product. The opposite SCN was marked because visual fibers in the horse undergo complete decussation at the optic chiasm. The presence of color reaction in the SCN indicates that in the horse as in other mammals there is a direct retinal projection to the suprachiasmatic nuclei of the hypothalamus. The significance of this pathway is severalfold. First, it permits interpretation, and perhaps adjustment, of incoming photic signals before they are sent to the pineal, or other parts of the brain. Second, if the SCN serve as the regulators of biologic time, this would enable the SCN to keep apprised of any changes in photic input. Third, this separate pathway permits the apparently paradoxical situation in which an animal can be completely visually impaired, from the standpoint of not being able to perceive and interpret light impulses as objects, yet still be completely competent in their ability to perceive and respond to the entraining effects of photoperiod. Thus the fact that an animal is visually blind does not necessarily mean that photic messages do not reach the brain as usual. It may depend on the location of the lesion that causes the blindness. Obviously, lesions to the eye, optic nerve, and SCN would abrogate any entraining effects of photoperiod. However, lesions posterior to the SCN would not likely interfere with the circadian time-keeping system, and care should be taken in predicting the effects of blindness on reproductive competence until the location of the lesion is known.

After electrical impulses reach the SCN, they traverse the hypothalamus and midbrain by pathways still unidentified in the horse. In rodents, where the pathways have been extensively worked out, it is known that efferent fibers exit the SCN dorsoventrad, passing through the paraventricular nuclei[25] then through the midbrain bundle to the anteriomedial-lateral cell column of the spinal cord to the superior cervical ganglia where they terminate in preganglionic, sympathetic fibers. From the superior cervical ganglia, postganglionic axons travel back up into the brain, passing down the nervi conarii to the pineal where they terminate as terminal axons closely associated with pinealocytes.[25] Interruption of this pathway anywhere along its somewhat convoluted path results in aberrant pineal function.

Development of sensitive radioimmunoassay (RIA) systems which could measure circulating or urinary melatonin concentrations in a variety of mammalian species has helped further the understanding of this complex photically regulated neuroendocrine system. Rollag and Niswender published one of the first RIA systems for measuring melatonin in the peripheral circulation and reported the presence of nyctohemeral rhythms in melatonin in sheep.[26] The daytime (photophase) concentrations of melatonin were essentially nondetectable, whereas the nighttime (scotophase) melatonin concentrations often exceeded 200 or 300 pg/mL, a robust rhythm which has made the sheep a useful research animal with which to study pineal rhythms and their influence on reproduction. Other species do not demonstrate such a robust rhythm; however, melatonin is usually elevated during the scotophase, relative to the photophase (sheep,[26] human,[27,28] and horse,[29]). In one study, sheep were also exposed to constant light or constant darkness to test the effects of these lighting regimes on melatonin rhythms.[26] When sheep were exposed to constant light, melatonin rhythms were essentially abolished, but appeared to persist in sheep maintained in constant darkness.[26] This latter observation is somewhat contrary to circadian theory, which predicts that under conditions of constant darkness, the melatonin rhythm, if truly circadian, should "free run." That is, should continue to demonstrate rhythmic fluctuations, but with a new period that reflects an inherent, endogenous component. However, Rollag and Niswender maintained the sheep in constant darkness for only 4 days, possibly insufficient time for the expression of endogenous rhythms.[26] In similar studies, circulating melatonin concentrations were measured in pony mares under normal light and dark conditions for 3 weeks, then the photoperiod was switched to constant darkness, and the mares were monitored for an additional 3 weeks.[30] An attempt was made to monitor other circadian rhythms as evidence of a circadian shift, such as locomotor activity (measured with hiking pedometers), body temperature, and water intake. There was a clear rhythm in secretion of melatonin, with daytime concentrations of 20 to 40 pg/mL and nighttime concentrations of 100 to 150 pg/mL. Furthermore, locomotor activity and water intake demonstrated distinct rhythms. For the first 3 days of constant darkness, however, there was no apparent difference in the rhythms of melatonin, locomotor activity, or water intake. When sampled again over the last 3 days of the 3-week constant-dark period, the patterns of melatonin secretion, locomotor activity, and water intake were all severely disturbed, with little agreement with the previously regular rhythms in these end points. Furthermore, during the light:dark 12:12 period, there was good agreement among the four mares with respect to the phase angle of the respective rhythms. After 3 weeks of constant darkness, however, there was little agreement among mares as to the phase of the rhythms, suggesting that they were in free run.[30] A typical 24-h pattern of melatonin secretion in pony mares is presented in Figure 11-3.

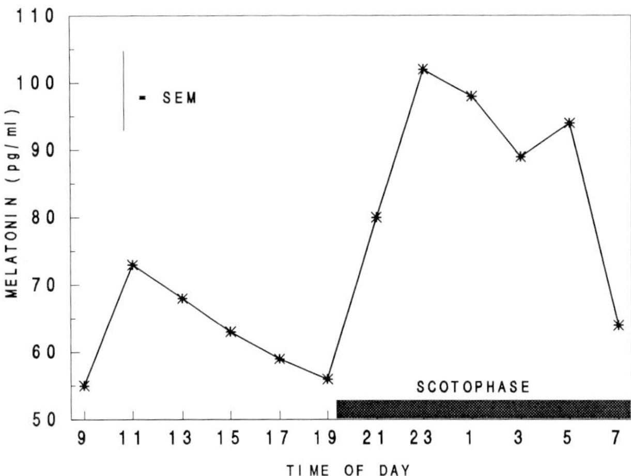

FIG. 11–3. Circulating melatonin concentrations in six pony mares under ambient lighting conditions. Note the prominent increase at the time of first darkness. SEM, standard error of mean.

In further studies of melatonin secretion, Sharp and Grubaugh demonstrated that the rhythm of melatonin in the peripheral circulation was entrainable to different photoperiods.[31] Because of high variability experienced in sampling mares at 1-h intervals, jugular vein samples were collected at 10-min intervals for 30 h from pony mares under L:D 16:8 or L:D 8:16 and showed that the secretion of melatonin was highly episodic.[31] The term *episodic* is defined as "a noteworthy happening, for which the time can usually be fixed, occurring in the course of ordinary events." In contrast, *pulsatile* is defined as "characterized by a rhythmic pulsation, as in the heart beat." The difference is not trivial, as underlying mechanisms of secretion regulation may be different. The irregularly occurring episodes, or events, of melatonin secretion seem a poor biologic signal, because reliability is lacking. Episodes of melatonin were short lived, often confined to one sample, and were represented in equal numbers during the photophase and scotophase, but were not necessarily regular in frequency (i.e., were not pulsatile). High-pressure liquid chromatography was used to isolate fractions in several of the episodic samples which comigrated with authentic melatonin. The fractions were subsequently reassayed using the same RIA, with the same results, so it seems likely that the episodes represent melatonin. Despite these curious episodes, there was a distinct difference in mean melatonin concentrations between photophase and scotophase, regardless of the photoperiod to which the mares were exposed. The significance, if any, of these episodes of melatonin is unknown. These observations indicate that the secretion of melatonin from the pineal is a highly complex process, which likely involves direct photic stimuli, as well as a training component of photoperiod.

CIRCADIAN TIME-KEEPING SYSTEM

In order to understand the role of melatonin in reproductive function, as well as the regulation of melatonin secretion, it is necessary to understand the circadian time-keeping system. The term *circadian* comes from the latin *circa* meaning "about," and *dies,* meaning "a day." Therefore, the term circadian describes events that take place with a periodicity of about 24 h. Two stipulations must be met before a rhythmic occurrence can be accurately described as being circadian: (1) under constant conditions, such as constant darkness, the rhythm must be expressed with a period (tau) that is close to, but not necessarily exactly, 24 h and represents the expression of a genetically inherent rhythm; and (2) under conditions of entrainment, such as a normal light to dark photoperiod, the rhythm must be entrained precisely to the photoperiod (usually exactly 24 h). Care should be taken in referring to events that occur in a quotidian (everyday) fashion, because they may not be derived from the circadian system, even though they appear to occur regularly. The circadian time-keeping system is an important synchronizer of a great variety of physiologic events in the interest of maintaining homeostasis, and a role of the circadian system in regulating reproduction is no less important. For instance, in rodents, the time of ovulation is very precisely regulated to occur at night. These animals are nocturnal, therefore, this is a critical consideration, because ovulation occurring during the day would be unaccompanied by breeding. Likewise, the growing field of chronopharmacology indicates the importance of the circadian system: the efficacy of many drugs has been shown to depend on the (circadian) time of administration. In the latter regard, this is often no small matter with a range in efficacy from insignificant to life-threatening.

The existence of a biologic time-keeping system is the real-life version of the quackery-induced "biorhythm" charts that readily predict your moods, intelligence, sexual prowess, and emotional status, all for only a quarter. Because the circadian system is inherent, each of us with a unique rhythm, the source of the timer is of fundamental importance. Although not all the answers are available yet, a consensus of researchers identifies the SCN as the potential source of the clock, or oscillator. Studies in a variety of species have shown that most circadian rhythms are abolished by ablation of the SCN, making the paired nuclei prime suspects for the role of central oscillator.

EFFECTS OF MELATONIN ADMINISTRATION

If melatonin plays such an important role in reproduction one might ask why a practical way of manipulating it for breeding purposes has not yet been developed for the horse industry. There are many answers to that question, but two remain the greatest obstacle to the use of melatonin practically in a horse breeding program. (1) Despite all that is known about melatonin synthesis and secretion, the target tissue is still not known, and hence the necessary experiments to determine alternate ways of influencing the reproductive system cannot be conducted. Melatonin is unique among endocrine hormones in that we know where it comes from and why, but we do not know where it works. (2) The problem with using melatonin in a practical breeding system is that its action is counter to the results desired. As will be shown below, administration of melatonin can indeed mediate reproductive events, but negatively. At the moment, what is desired is a way of removing melatonin or neutralizing its action.

For all the potent antireproduction effect melatonin has been shown to exhibit, there is little known about its site of action. The potential role of melatonin in timing central neuroendocrine events associated with reproduction can be inferred from the fact that under certain conditions, melatonin administration is inhibitory to gonadal function and, under different conditions, can be positive.[32]

Administration of melatonin directly into the portal vessels of the pituitary or into the median eminence reduced pituitary LH in rats.[33,34] Thus implantation of melatonin into the hypothalamus in a variety of species (rat,[32,33] white-footed mouse,[35] and golden hamster[36,37]) has been shown to reduce pituitary and circulating LH concentrations. More recently, Reppert et al. have demonstrated specific melatonin receptors in the suprachiasmatic nuclei, adding support for the concept that melatonin exerts an action on the central oscillator of the biologic clock.[38] Such a concept is consonant with the idea of the pineal as a mediator of solar time.

In agreement with this concept, Strauss et al. reported that administration of melatonin via subcutaneous beeswax implants in ovariectomized pony mares during the summer resulted in significantly reduced hypothalamic GnRH content, suggesting a central action for melatonin.[39] Likewise, Cleaver et al. reported that exposure of mares to constant light resulted in a marked decrease in circulating melatonin concentrations and an increase in hypothalamic GnRH content.[14] These data seem to suggest that circulating melatonin concentrations and hypothalamic GnRH content are inversely related and emphasize the practical need for melatonin-secretion and/or receptor-binding antagonists (Fig. 11-4).

EXPERIMENTAL MODELS

Another difficulty in studying the effects of melatonin administration has been choosing an experimental model. Because the effects of the pineal are subtle and often prolonged in their time course, researchers have sought unique models with which to investigate the effects of the potential pineal hormone melatonin. Blockade of compensatory ovarian hypertrophy (COH) was such a model.[40] It was known that removal of one ovary in litter-bearing species such as rats and hamsters, resulted in an increase in the number of follicles developing and ovulating on the remaining ovary. This compensatory ovarian hypertrophy is sensitive to antigonadotropin stimuli and, therefore, turned out to be a sensitive test system for melatonin. However, little use of COH has been made in studies of

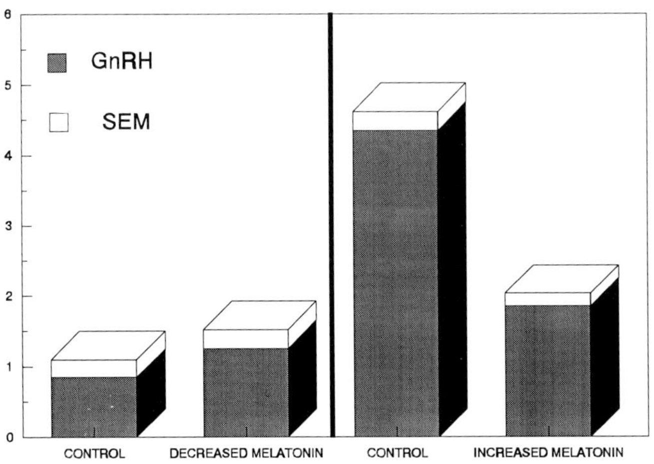

FIG. 11–4. Hypothalamic GnRH following either increased or decreased melatonin secretion via implant or constant light exposure, respectively. SEM, standard error of mean. Adapted from Cleaver, B.D., et al.: Effect of constant light exposure on circulating gonadotropin levels and hypothalamic gonadotropin-releasing hormone (GnRH) content in the ovariectomized pony mare. J. Reprod. Fertil. Suppl., *44*:259–266, 1991.; and Strauss, S.S., Chen, C.L., Kalra, S.P., and Sharp, D.C.: Localization of gonadotropin releasing hormone in the hypothalamus of ovariectomized pony mares. J. Reprod. Fertil. Suppl., *27*:123–129, 1979.)

melatonin on reproductive function in domestic livestock.

Perhaps the most widely used, and the most appropriate, model system with which to test the effects of melatonin is the inhibition of sexual recrudescence in seasonal animals. The golden hamster has been a useful research animal for these studies, as it is a highly photoperiodic species and undergoes extensive gonadal regression in the winter (short day).[41] The male hamster is especially useful because the testes are normally quite large; it is easy to monitor gonadal regression by measuring testicular diameter noninvasively. However, after about 20 weeks of short day, gonadotropins begin to be secreted, and complete reproductive function is reestablished (sexual recrudescence). Melatonin implants in beeswax implanted in the SCN of golden hamsters caused testicular regression in animals exposed to long day and blocked testicular regression in animals transferred to short day. The return to sexual competence in anestrous hamsters can be accelerated by switching the photoperiod from short day (L:D 8:16) to long day (L:D 16:8).[41]

A similar experiment has been conducted in horses with similar results. Anestrous pony mares were used to test the hypothesis that melatonin administration would block the stimulatory effects of long-day photoperiod on date of the first ovulation of the year.[42] Four experimental groups were established, with five mares in each group: Group A, short-day control (ambient light, about L:D 9:15); Group B, short-day melatonin administration; Group C, long-day melatonin administration, and Group D, long-day control (long day was an additional 2.5 h of artificial light beginning at sunset); Studies from our laboratory have indicated that the nocturnal rise in melatonin in horses was closely coupled to first darkness;[31] therefore, we reasoned that the 2.5 h of artificial light would delay the secretion of melatonin by a like amount. Melatonin administration was timed to provide elevated circulating melatonin concentrations during the 2.5 h that the mares in Group C and D were exposed to artificial light. Melatonin (25 mg/animal) was administered orally, in a small bolus of grain feed 4 h before the time that elevated concentrations were desired. The dates of the first ovulation of the year were similar for Groups A, B, and C. The date of the first ovulation of the year for mares in Group D was significantly earlier (Fig. 11-5). These data indicate that the stimulatory effect of long day (Group D) was blocked by the administration of melatonin (Group C), and the mare is, in some respects, similar to other long-day breeders such as hamsters.[21]

On the other hand, administration of melatonin to sheep prior to the onset of the natural breeding season has been shown to advance its onset.[43,44] In these studies, melatonin was administered either orally or vaginally. This concept has obvious practical value to sheep breeders and is currently in field testing for that purpose. Furthermore, administration of melatonin late in the breeding season in sheep extended reproductive function,[45] lending credence to the idea that melatonin serves primarily to set the clock for inherent, endogenous neuroendocrine functions. Administration of melatonin at unphysiologic times, or in unphysiologic modes, such as constant administration via implants, may reset the biologic clock 180°.

Another model that has been useful in studies of melatonin secretion is the ovariectomized, estrogen-primed ewe. Legan et al. demonstrated that gonadotropin secretion in ovariectomized ewes remains elevated throughout the year, unless there is a low concentration of circulating estrogens (3 to 5 pg/mL).[46] In the latter case, gonadotropins decrease under the influence of long day and increase again under short day. It was hypothesized that the hypothalamus becomes sensitized to the negative feedback effects of estradiol under the influence of long day and leads to reduced LH secretion.[46] Bittman used this model to test the effects of melatonin on LH secretion.[45] Two groups of pinealectomized, ovariectomized, estradiol-treated ewes were used in this experiment. Both groups were exposed to melatonin administered as square-wave infusions to mimic the pattern of melatonin secretion during short day. Gonadotropin concentrations were elevated in both groups. After 8 weeks, the melatonin infusion was changed in one group of ewes to mimic the pattern expected during long day, and gonadotropin concentrations fell within 3 to 4 weeks. This experiment, as well as the one by Cheves and Sharp,[42] indicated that melatonin patterns of secretion can affect LH secretion. Furthermore, their experiment indicated that faced with conflicting photoperiodic and melatonin signals (i.e., stimulatory photoperiod, inhibitory melatonin secretion) mares (and likely ewes) preferentially respond to the melatonin signals.[42]

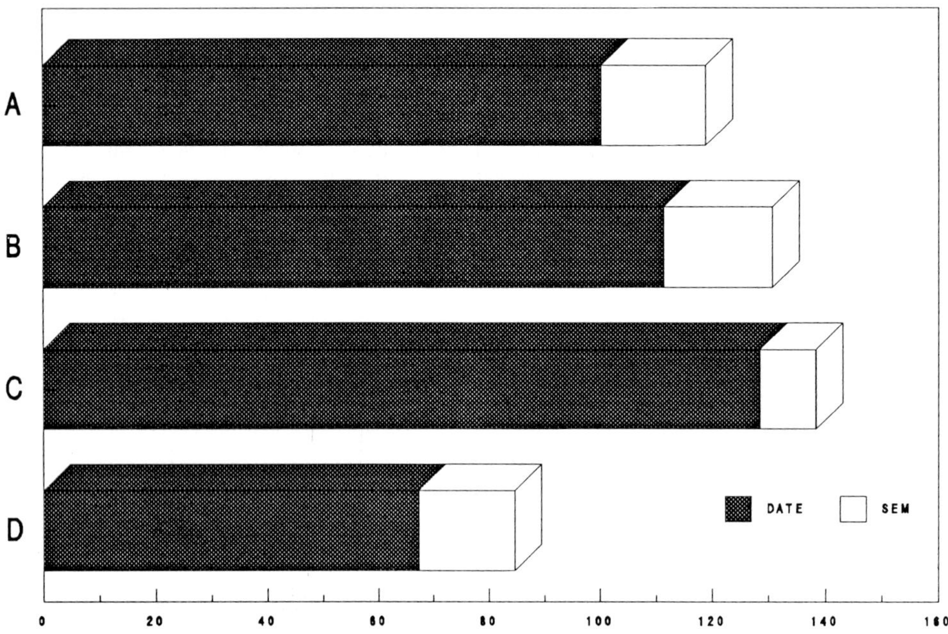

FIG. 11–5. Date of first ovulation of the year in light-exposed and melatonin-treated anestrous pony mares. Groups A, B, C, and D are nonlighted and nonmelatonin treated, nonlighted and melatonin treated, lighted and melatonin treated, and lighted and nonmelatonin treated, respectively. SEM, standard error of mean.

THE MELATONIN SIGNAL

The nature of the melatonin signal remains enigmatic and the source of much heated debate. The argument is not unique to melatonin action and relates to the question of many circadian-based functions. The question is whether melatonin acts by virtue of the timing of its secretion (relative to circadian time) or whether the duration of the nocturnal surge is important in conveying seasonal photoperiodic information to the central nervous system. The former is known as the coincidence theory because it argues that melatonin secretion affects an action only when it is coincident with some, as yet unknown, circadian-based event. The latter argument is known as the hourglass theory because it states that the total cumulative secretion of melatonin is important in conveying photoperiodic information. Unfortunately, there is evidence in support of both concepts, and the argument will not likely be resolved until a better understanding of the target tissue, and the action of melatonin at that tissue, is obtained.

In support of the coincidence theory, Tamarkin et al. administered melatonin twice daily to pinealectomized hamsters exposed to long day and reported that gonadal regression was induced only when the injections occurred at specific times of the day (4:00 p.m.).[47] Injections of identical concentration but at other times of the day (9:00 a.m. or 1:30 p.m.) were ineffective in inducing gonadal regression. On the other hand, Goldman reported that multiple injections of melatonin were effective in inducing gonadal regression in hamsters, and he concluded that the timing of the injections was not as important as the cumulative dose.[19] The argument will not likely be easily solved, but it seems clear that melatonin administered in continuous form, as with implants, represents a different, probably pharmacologic, physiologic treatment compared with periodic or circadian-timed modes of administration.

PRACTICAL CONSIDERATIONS

Melatonin implants are already being given serious consideration in inducing early breeding onset in sheep, but so far there has been little promise of a practical application in horses. At first glance, the difference appears to reflect the difference in short-day versus long-day breeders (sheep versus horses). However, it is interesting that both species appear to use melatonin to inform them of changes in the photoperiod. Because the onset of long days results in a reduction in melatonin secretion (shorter duration, later onset of nocturnal surge, and lower amplitude nocturnal surge[31]), it is perhaps understandable that administration of melatonin holds little promise, at least in a regime similar to that of sheep. If there were a pharmacologic treatment that would reduce or neutralize the effects of melatonin, perhaps, in theory, it might prove to be useful, but no such treatment is available currently.

Conversely, a treatment is readily available that serves to reduce melatonin secretion, delay the nocturnal surge, and reduce the amplitude of the nocturnal surge. That treatment is photoperiod, and it still represents the best way to induce an early onset of the breeding season in horses. That exposing mares to artificially lengthened day works through altering melatonin secretion was demonstrated by Cheves, and Sharp, when the effects of long day were blocked by administration of melatonin.[42] Similarly, it has been demonstrated that pinealectomized, anestrous mares do not respond to stimulatory photoperiod as do pineal-intact mares, suggesting that artificial light works by altering melatonin secretion.[31] Therefore, artificial photoperiod is perhaps the best way to use melatonin to advance the onset of the breeding season.

REFERENCES

1. Wurtman, R.J., and Axelrod, J.: The Pineal Gland. Sci. Am., *213*:50–60, 1965.
2. McCord, C.P., and Allen, F.P.: Evidences associating pineal gland function with alterations in pigmentation. J. Exp. Zool., *23*:207–224, 1917.
3. Lerner, A.B., et al.: Isolation of melatonin, the pineal factor that lightens melanocytes. J. Am. Chem. Soc., *80*:2587, 1958.
4. Heubner, O.: Tumor der glandula pinealis. Dtsch. Med. Wochenschr., *24*:214, 1898.
5. Kitay, J.: Pineal lesions and precocious puberty: A review. J. Clin. Endocrinol. Metab., *14*:622–625, 1954.
6. Borit, A., and Schmidek, H.H.: Pineal tumors and their treatment. *In* The Pineal Gland. Edited by R.J. Reiter. New York, Raven Press, 1984, pp. 323–344.
7. Arendt, J.: Melatonin assays in body fluids. J. Neural Transm. Suppl., *13*:265–278, 1978.
8. Silman, R.E., Leone, R.M., Hooper, R.J.L., and Preece, M.A.: Melatonin, the pineal gland and human puberty. Nature, *282*:301–303, 1979.
9. Axelrod, J., and Weissbach, H.: Enzymatic *O*-methylation of *N*-acetylserotonin to melatonin. Science, *131*:1312, 1961.
10. Holmgren, N.: Ark. Zool., *11*:1–13, 1918.
11. Fiske, V.M.: Effect of light on sexual maturation, estrous cycles, and anterior pituitary of the rat. Endocrinology, *29*:187–196, 1941.
12. Fiske, V.M., Pound, J., and Putnam, J.: Effect of light on the weight of the pineal in the rat. Endocrinology, *66*:489–491, 1960.
13. Wurtman, R.J., Roth, W., Altschule, M.D., and Wurtman, R.J.: Interactions of the pineal and exposure to continuous light on organ weights of female rats. Acta Endocrinol. (Copenh.), *36*:617–624, 1961.
14. Cleaver, B.D., et al.: Effect of constant light exposure on circulating gonadotropin levels and hypothalamic gonadotropin-releasing hormone (GnRH) content in the ovariectomized pony mare. J. Reprod. Fertil. Suppl., *44*:259–266, 1991.
15. Ariens-Kappers, J.: Innervation of the epiphysis cerebri in the albino rat. Anat. Rec., *136*:220–227, 1960.
16. Wurtman, R.J., Axelrod, J., and Fischer, J.E.: Melatonin synthesis in the pineal gland: Effect of light mediated by the sympathetic nervous system. Science, *143*:1328–1330, 1964.
17. Quay, W.B.: Circadian rhythms in rat pineal serotonin and its modification by estrous cycle and photoperiod. Gen. Comp. Endocrinol., *3*:473–479, 1963.
18. Snyder, S.H., Zweig, M., Axelrod, J., and Fischer, J.E.: Control of the circadian rhythm in serotonin content of the rat pineal gland. Proc. Natl. Acad. Sci. U.S.A., *53*:301–305, 1965.
19. Goldman, B.D.: The physiology of melatonin in mammals. *In* The Pineal Gland. Edited by R.J. Reiter. New York, Raven Press, 1984, pp. 145–182.
20. Klein, D.C., and Weller, J.: Indole metabolism in the pineal gland: A circadian rhythm in *N*-acetyltransferase. Science, *169*:1093–1095, 1970.
21. Klein, D.C., Berg, G.R., and Weller, J.: Melatonin synthesis: Adenosine 3′5′-monophosphate and norepinephrine stimulate *N*-acetyltransferase. Science, *168*:979–980, 1970.
22. Degouchi, T., and Axelrod, J.: Control of circadian change in serotonin-*N*-acetyltransferase in the pineal organ by the β-adrenergic receptor. Proc. Natl. Acad. Sci. U. S. A., *69*:2547–2550, 1972.
23. Moore, R.Y.: The innervation of the pineal gland. Prog. Reprod. Biol., *4*:1–29, 1978.
24. Sharp, D.C., Grubaugh, W.R., Gum, G.G., and Wirsig, C.R.: Demonstration of a direct retino-hypothalamic projection in the mare. Biol. Reprod. Suppl. 1, *30*:156, 1984.
25. Inouye, S., and Turek, F.W.: Horizontal knife cuts either ventral or dorsal to the hypothalamic paraventricular nucleus block testicular regression in golden hamsters maintained in short days. Biol. Reprod. Suppl. 1, *32*:56, 1985.
26. Rollag, M.D., and Niswender, G.D.: Radioimmunoassay of serum concentrations of melatonin in sheep exposed to different lighting regimes. Endocrinology, *98*:482–489, 1976.
27. Waldhauser, F., Lynch, H.J., and Wurtman, R.J.: Melatonin in human body fluids: Clinical significance. *In* The Pineal Gland. Edited by R.J. Reiter. New York, Raven Press, 1984, pp. 345–370.
28. Arendt, J., Wirz-Justice, A, and Bradtke, J.: Annual rhythm of serum melatonin in man. Neurosci. Lett., *7*:327–330, 1977.
29. Grubaugh, W.R., et al.: The effects of pinealectomy in pony mares. J. Reprod. Fertil. Suppl., *32*:293–295, 1982.
30. Berglund, L.A., Sharp, D.C., and Grubaugh, W.R.: Effects of constant darkness on melatonin rhythms in pony mares. Biol. Reprod. Suppl. 1, *24*:71, 1981.
31. Sharp, D.C., and Grubaugh, W.R.: Pulsatile secretion of melatonin during the scotophase in mares. Biol. Reprod. Suppl., *128*:100, 1983.
32. Cardinali, D.P.: Molecular mechanisms of neuroendocrine integration in the central nervous system: An approach through the study of the pineal gland and its innervating sympathetic pathway. Psychoneuroendocrinology, *8*:3–30, 1982.
33. Fraschini, F., Collu, R., and Martini, L.: Mechanisms of inhibitory action of pineal principles on gonadotropin secretion. *In* The Pineal Gland. Edited by G.E.W. Wolstenholme and J. Knight. London, Churchill Livingstone, 1971, pp. 259–273.
34. Cardinali, D.P.: Melatonin. A mammalian pineal hormone. Endocr. Rev., *2*:327–346, 1981.
35. Glass, J.D., and Lynch, G.R.: Evidence for a brain site of melatonin action in the white-footed mouse, Peromyscus leucopus. Neuroendocrinology, *34*:1–6, 1982.
36. Reiter, R.J.: Seasonal aspects of reproduction in a hibernating rodent: Photoperiodic and pineal effects. *In* Survival in the Cold. Edited by X.J. Mussachia and L. Jansky. Amsterdam, Elsevier, 1981, pp. 1–11.
37. Rusak, B.: Suprachiasmatic lesions prevent an antigonadal effect of melatonin. Biol. Reprod., *22*:148–154, 1980.
38. Reppert, S.M., Weaver, D.F.R., Rivkees, S.A., and Stopa, E.G.: Putative receptors in a human biological clock. Science, *242*:7813, 1988.
39. Strauss, S.S., Chen, C.L., Kalra, S.P., and Sharp, D.C.: Lo-

calization of gonadotropin releasing hormone in the hypothalamus of ovariectomized pony mares. J. Reprod. Fertil. Suppl., *27*:123–129, 1979.

40. Vaughan, M.K., et al.: Inhibition of compensatory hypertrophy in the mouse and vole: A comparison of Altschule's extract, pineal indoles, vasopressin, and oxytocin. Gen. Comp. Endocrinol., *18*:372–377, 1972.

41. Reiter, R.J.: Interaction of photoperiod, pineal and seasonal reproduction as exemplified by findings in the hamster. *In* Progress in Reproductive Biology. Edited by R.J. Reiter. Basel, Karger, 1978, pp. 169–190.

42. Cheves, L.L., and Sharp, D.C.: The effects of oral melatonin on the onset of the breeding season of pony mares under artificially lengthened photoperiod. Proceedings of the Fifth Florida Neuroendocrine Symposium, Tallahassee, FL, 1985.

43. Arendt, J., Symons, A.M., Laud, C.A., and Pryde, S.J.: Melatonin can induce early onset of the breeding season in ewes. J. Endocrinol., *97*:395–400, 1983.

44. Nowak, R., and Rodway, R.G.: Effect of intravaginal implants of melatonin on the onset of ovarian activity in adult and prepubertal ewes. J. Reprod. Fertil., *74*:287–293, 1986.

45. Bittman, E.L.: Melatonin and photoperiodic time measurement: Evidence from rodents and ruminants. *In* The Pineal Gland. Edited by R.J. Reiter. New York, Raven Press, 1984, pp. 155–192.

46. Legan, S.J., Karsch, F.J., and Foster, D.L.: The endocrine control of seasonal reproductive function in the ewe: A marked change in response to negative feedback action of estradiol on luteinizing hormone secretion. Endocrinology, *101*:818–824, 1973.

47. Tamarkin, L., Westrom, W.K., Hamill, A.I., and Goldman, B.D.: Effect of melatonin on the reproductive systems of male and female Syrian hamsters: A diurnal rhythm in sensitivity to melatonin. Endocrinology, *99*:1534–1541, 1976.

CHAPTER 12

REPRODUCTIVE PEPTIDE AND PROTEIN HORMONES

T.M. Nett

In addition to the hormones discussed in preceding chapters, there are several other peptide and protein hormones that have effects on the reproductive system in both males and females. These include oxytocin, prolactin, relaxin, inhibin, and activin. Data regarding the roles and relative importance of these hormones in equids are meager. Therefore, much of the information presented in the following discussion has been adapted from knowledge gained from other species.

OXYTOCIN

Oxytocin is a neuropeptide synthesized as part of a large precursor molecule, neurophysin, in the magnocellular neurons of the hypothalamus. Cell bodies containing oxytocin have been observed in the supraoptic, paraventricular, and surprisingly, the arcuate nuclei of the horse.[1] The gene encoding oxytocin and its associated neurophysin (OT-NP) has been sequenced in several species.[2] The structure of the gene appears to be highly conserved across species and contains three exons and two introns. To date, little information is available regarding the regulation of this gene. When the gene is expressed, mRNA is produced and subsequently translated into OT-NP (a 106–amino acid protein) on ribosomes attached to the rough endoplasmic reticulum in neurons. Subsequent to translation, the protein is transported to the Golgi apparatus for glycosylation of the mature peptide and then packaged into membrane-bound secretory vesicles. The 9 amino acids that comprise oxytocin appear to be enzymatically cleaved from neurophysin (the 93 carboxy terminal amino acids) as the secretory vesicles are being transported from the cell bodies in hypothalamic nuclei to nerve terminals in the posterior pituitary.[3] When oxytocin is released from the posterior pituitary, the cleaved neurophysin is also released in equimolar amounts. To date, no biologic function has been ascribed to neurophysin secreted from the posterior pituitary.

Both oxytocin and OT-NP have been found in other tissues, including the adrenal gland,[4] testis,[4] and corpus luteum.[5] The function of oxytocin produced by these tissues has not yet been elucidated, but there is speculation that it may participate in regulation of steroidogenesis.

Release of oxytocin from nerve terminals in the posterior pituitary occurs as a result of stimulation of oxytocin neurons in the hypothalamus. The most studied stimulus for release of oxytocin in vivo is suckling. In mares, suckling causes an increase in plasma concentrations of oxytocin which, in turn, is associated with an increase in intramammary pressure and milk ejection.[6] Increased secretion of oxytocin also occurs during delivery. The first notable increase in plasma concentrations of oxytocin occurs during the expulsive stage of labor[7] and just prior to rupture of the placental membranes.[8] Concentrations of oxytocin remain elevated through delivery of the fetus and the placenta and then return to baseline within an hour.

Circulating concentrations of oxytocin also vary dur-

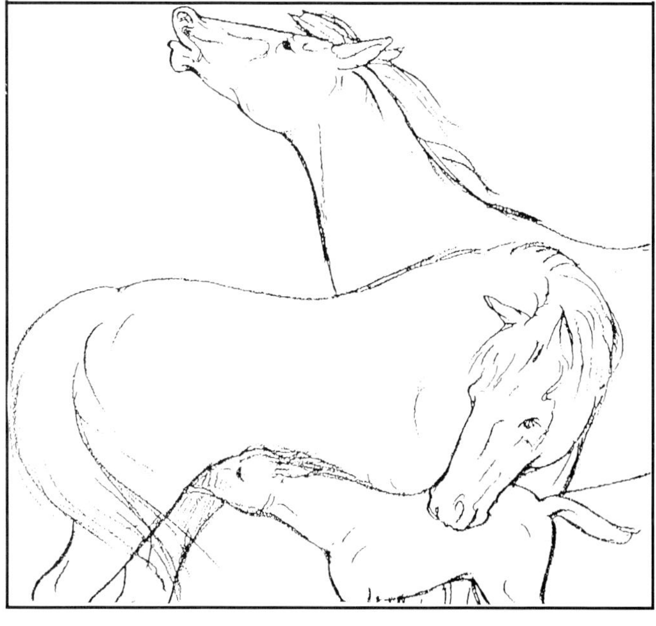

ing the estrous cycle in mares. The highest concentration appears to occur late in diestrus just prior to regression of the corpus luteum.[9] As indicated above, the corpus luteum can serve as a source of oxytocin. Although it remains to be proven in mares, the corpus luteum is likely to be the source of the increased circulating concentrations of oxytocin in late diestrus. Oxytocin may increase secretion of prostaglandin $F_2\alpha$ by the uterus to stimulate regression of the corpus luteum at the end of the estrous cycle. Moreover, the presence of an embryo may prevent oxytocin from stimulating the secretion of prostaglandin $F_2\alpha$ from the uterus during early pregnancy.[10]

The major clinical use of oxytocin is for induction of parturition. Oxytocin causes a rapid and predictable onset of labor, and parturition usually occurs within 90 min.[11] Prostaglandin $F_2\alpha$ increases sharply after treatment with oxytocin, which mimics the pattern of secretion observed during the second stage of labor.

PROLACTIN

Equine prolactin is a single-chain protein composed of 199 amino acids.[12] Development of specific and sensitive radioimmunoassays[13,14] has led to the characterization of the secretory patterns of this hormone in both stallions and mares. Administration of dopamine-receptor–blocking agents to horses results in a rapid increase in circulating concentrations of prolactin. Likewise, treatment of horses with bromocriptine, a dopamine agonist, decreases circulating concentrations of prolactin.[15] Therefore, as in other species, secretion of prolactin from the anterior pituitary of the horse appears to be under the negative regulation of dopamine from the hypothalamus. Thyrotropin-releasing hormone, another hypothalamic peptide, has been shown to induce secretion of prolactin in horses,[13,16] but its importance in the physiologic regulation of prolactin secretion in this species remains to be determined.

In mares, circulating concentrations of prolactin are greater in the summer than in the winter.[13] Likewise, pituitary concentrations of prolactin are highest during the summer and lowest during the winter.[17] The lower concentrations of prolactin in the winter appear to be the result of reduced day length. Exposure of mares to 16 h of light during the fall or winter months increases secretion of prolactin.[16] Despite the presence of an annual cycle of prolactin secretion, there does not appear to be any changes in circulating concentrations of prolactin related to stage of the estrous cycle in mares.[18,19]

An increase in secretion of prolactin seems to occur during the last few days of pregnancy in mares.[20,21] The event that triggers this release of prolactin has not been identified, but it is speculated that the increase is associated with declining concentrations of estradiol and progesterone that occur at that time. In other species, the large prepartum increase in concentrations of prolactin is necessary for completion of mammary development and initiation of milk secretion.[22,23] Considering that circulating concentrations of prolactin increase in the mare at a similar time, it seems likely that these functions may also hold true for the horse. In fact, the rise in prolactin concentrations appears to occur concomitantly with a rapid increase in the quantity of milk constituents produced by the mare.[24]

Circulating concentrations of prolactin remain high and variable for the first several weeks after parturition in mares that are nursing foals.[20,25] In other species, continued postpartum secretion of prolactin depends on stimuli provided by the young when nursing.[26–28] Although only limited data are available, a similar situation appears to exist in the mare. The role of prolactin in maintaining lactation is yet to be defined. In rodents, high levels of prolactin are essential for maintenance of lactation, whereas in ruminants secretion of prolactin can be completely suppressed with little effect on milk production.[29] The requirement of prolactin for galactopoiesis in the mare has not been examined; however, because circulating concentrations of prolactin decrease to basal levels by 1 to 2 months after parturition,[20] even though suckling and lactation continue, it seems likely that prolactin is not required for maintenance of lactation in the mare.

In stallions, as in mares, circulating concentrations of prolactin vary with season and are higher in the summer than in winter.[30] Also as in mares, concentrations of prolactin in serum reflect changes that occur in the anterior pituitary gland.[17] Similar seasonal changes in circulating concentrations of prolactin were also observed in geldings, suggesting that testicular hormones are not involved in the regulation of prolactin secretion in stallions. There is also an effect of age on concentrations of prolactin in stallions. Levels of prolactin increase with age for approximately 5 yr.[30] Sexual stimulation results in an immediate increase in secretion of prolactin in stallions.[31] The increase in prolactin after sexual stimulation is not correlated with a change in any of the reproductive hormones, but is temporally related to an increase in circulating concentrations of cortisol. To date, a physiologic function has not been ascribed to prolactin in stallions.

RELAXIN

Relaxin is a protein hormone normally associated with pregnancy. Relaxin is a member of the insulin family of peptides and is similar in size to insulin, having a molecular weight of approximately 6000. As for insulin, relaxin is synthesized as a single polypeptide chain that is modified by proteolytic cleavage to form the mature protein.[32] The biologically active protein is composed of two peptide chains, designated A and B, connected by disulfide bonds. The amino acid sequence of relaxin has been reported for several species,[33] but not for the horse. However, equine relaxin has been purified and has a molecular weight similar to relaxins from other species.[34]

Relaxin is produced by the corpus luteum, uterus, and/or placenta, depending on the species.[33] In the horse, the placenta appears to be the primary, and possibly the sole, source of relaxin.[35] The placenta appears to begin secreting relaxin about day 80 of pregnancy with an initial peak in circulating concentrations occurring about day 175. Levels of relaxin then decrease slightly until about day 225 of gestation, after which they increase gradually until parturition.[36,37] Unlike other species, the horse does not appear to have a large prepartum rise in circulating concentrations of relaxin. After parturition, levels of relaxin rapidly return to baseline once the placenta has been expelled.

Biologically, relaxin functions to alter connective tissue structure in the pubic symphysis and cervix and to inhibit uterine contractility. Estrogen enhances the ability of relaxin to act on each of these tissues, presumably by increasing the number of receptors for relaxin in the target tissues.[33] In fact, relaxin has little, if any effect on these tissues unless the animal has been exposed to estrogen. Alterations in connective tissue structure attributable to relaxin are a decrease in size and number of collagen bundles in the extracellular matrix of the pubic symphysis[38] and cervix.[39] This results in a "softening" of these tissues and increases their distensibility. The effect of relaxin on the uterus is to reduce the frequency of uterine contractions during pregnancy.[33] However, near the end of gestation stimulating agents such as oxytocin and prostaglandin appear to override the effects of relaxin on the uterus and thus stimulate highly coordinated uterine contractions and delivery of the fetus.[40] In addition to its effects on the reproductive tract, relaxin may also influence the mammary gland by stimulating growth of mammary parenchymal tissue during late gestation.[41]

The preceding discussion on the biologic effects of relaxin is an integration of information concerning known actions of relaxin in several mammalian species. To date, no reports on the biologic effects of relaxin in the horse are available. Therefore, although it seems likely that relaxin does have the same effects in the horse as in other mammalian species, this remains to be proven.

INHIBIN AND ACTIVIN

In 1932, McCullagh coined the term inhibin for a water-soluble substance isolated from bull testes that prevented pituitary hypertrophy after castration.[42] In 1976, a compound with similar biologic activity was found to be present in bovine follicular fluid.[43] However, it was 1985 before four separate laboratories successfully isolated and characterized inhibin from porcine or bovine follicular fluid.[44–47] More recently, the genes for inhibin from several species have been cloned, and recombinant inhibin has been produced.[48]

Inhibin has a molecular weight of 32,000 and is composed of two subunits designated α and β. There appears to be only one α-subunit for inhibin within a species, but there are two different β-subunits termed βA and βB. Combination of the α-subunit with either β-subunit produces a biologically active inhibin (inhibin A or inhibin B) (Fig. 12-1). The primary sites of production of these molecules appear to be Sertoli's cells and granulosa cells.[49] However, extragonadal expression of these proteins does occur, suggesting that they may have functions in addition to regulating secretion of follicle-stimulating hormone (FSH).[50]

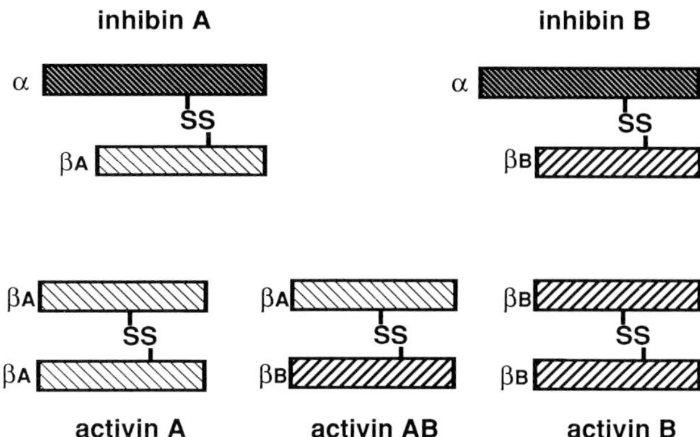

FIG. 12–1. Structures of the various forms of inhibin and activin. Inhibin A and B have a common α-subunit and similar, but not identical, β-subunits. The subunits are connected by disulfide bonds (SS). Activin is a dimer of the β-subunits of inhibin; therefore, there are three forms of activin, depending on the combination of subunits.

Biologically, inhibin acts to decrease synthesis and release of FSH. Treatment with inhibin prompts a rapid and dramatic decrease in the amount of mRNA encoded for FSH β-subunit.[51,52] In contrast, the effect of inhibin on secretion of FSH is relatively slow. About 24 h of exposure of pituitary cells to inhibin in vitro is required to produce a significant suppression in basal or gonadotropin-releasing hormone (GnRH) stimulated secretion of FSH, and the degree of suppression increases with additional time of exposure. The rapid effect of inhibin on synthesis of FSH compared to its relatively slow effect on secretion has led to speculation that the mechanism by which inhibin decreases secretion of FSH is by reducing synthesis of FSH and thereby decreasing the amount of hormone available for release.[53]

In some instances, inhibin also appears to influence secretion of luteinizing hormone (LH); however, this appears to be a result of the ability of inhibin to alter the number of GnRH receptors on gonadotrophs rather than by a direct effect on release of LH. In rats, inhibin decreases the number of GnRH receptors and thereby decreases the ability of GnRH to stimulate LH release.[54] In contrast, inhibin increases the number of GnRH receptors and enhances GnRH-induced release of LH in sheep.[55,56] Unlike its influence on FSH, inhibin does not alter synthesis of LH by gonadotrophs.

During the purification and characterization of inhibin, compounds in follicular fluid having biologic activities opposite to that of inhibin were found. These compounds have been termed activin.[57] Activins are dimers of the β-subunits of inhibin and, therefore, can exist in three forms. Activin A is a homodimer of inhibin βA subunits, activin B is a homodimer of inhibin βB subunits and activin AB is a heterodimer composed of an inhibin βA and an inhibin βB subunit (Fig. 12-1).

Each of these compounds has FSH-stimulating activity. As for inhibin, the effect of activin on secretion of FSH is relatively slow, requiring several hours to induce an increase in basal release of FSH in cultured pituitary cells,[58] whereas its effect on synthesis of FSH occurs much more rapidly.[59] Therefore, the principal effect of activin in regulating circulating concentrations of FSH may be to increase the quantity of FSH in the anterior pituitary available for release.

As indicated above, there is extragonadal expression of the subunits for inhibin and activin. In fact, expression of the mRNAs encoding the α- and βB-subunits of inhibin occurs in pituitary gonadotrophs of rats.[60] Recently, evidence was presented that activin B, produced by homodimer formation of βB-subunits in pituitary cells, selectively modulates synthesis and release of FSH in cultured anterior pituitary cells.[61] Such autocrine regulation of FSH may well account for the divergent secretory patterns of LH and FSH often observed physiologically.

Unfortunately, little is known regarding either inhibins or activins in the horse. We have no reason to assume that either the chemistry or biology of these compounds in the horse would be substantially different from that in other species. A recent report indicates that granulosa-theca cell tumors obtained from mares produce subunits of inhibin.[62] Such tumors could secrete biologically active inhibin, which may affect gonadotropin production in afflicted mares. In support of this hypothesis, in mares bearing a granulosa-theca cell tumor the contralateral ovary is usually atrophied.[63,64]

Clearly, much remains to be determined about the biology of inhibin and activin in equids. The potential pharmacologic uses of these compounds for manipulating circulating concentrations of FSH, and ultimately ovarian and testicular function, are great. Future research in this area will be beneficial to the equine industry.

REFERENCES

1. Melrose, P.A., and Knigge, K.M.: Topography of oxytocin and vasopressin neurons in the forebrain of Equus caballus: Further support of proposed evolutionary relationships for proopiomelanocortin, oxytocin and vasopressin neurons. Brain Behav. Evol., *33*:193–204, 1989.
2. Gainer, H., Alstein, M., Whitnall, M.H., and Wray, S.: The biosynthesis and secretion of oxytocin and vasopressin. *In* The Physiology of Reproduction. Edited by E. Knobil and J.D. Neill. New York, Raven Press, 1988, pp. 2265–2282.
3. Gainer, H., Russell, J.T., and Loh, Y.P.: The enzymology and intracellular organization of peptide precursor processing: The secretory vesicle hypothesis. Neuroendocrinology, *40*:171–184, 1985.
4. Nicholson, H.D., et al.: Identification of oxytocin and vasopressin in the testis and adrenal tissue. Regul. Pept., *8*:141–146, 1984.
5. Ivell, R., and Richter, D.: The gene for the hypothalamic peptide hormone oxytocin is highly expressed in the bovine corpus luteum: Biosynthesis, structure and sequence analysis. EMBO J., *3*:2351–2354, 1984.
6. Ellendorf, F., and Schams, D.: Characteristics of milk ejection, associated intramammary pressure changes and oxytocin release in the mare. J. Endocrinol., *119*:219–227, 1988.
7. Haluska, G.J., and Currie, W.B.: Variation in plasma concentrations of oestradiol-17β and their relationship to those of progesterone, 13,14-dihydro-15-keto-prostaglandin $F_2\alpha$ and oxytocin across pregnancy and at parturition in pony mares. J. Reprod. Fertil., *84*:635–646, 1988.
8. Haluska, G.J.: Trachtigkeit und geburt bei der stute: Uterin aktivitat und endokrinologie. Tierarztl. Prax. Suppl., *4*:56–62, 1989.
9. Tetzke, T.A., Ismail, S., Mikuckis, G., and Evan, J.W.: Patterns of oxytocin secretion during the oestrous cycle of the mare. J. Reprod. Fertil. Suppl., *35*:245–252, 1987.
10. Goff, A.K., Pontbriand, D., and Sirios, J.: Oxytocin stimulation of plasma 15-keto-13,14-dihydro prostaglandin $F_2\alpha$ during the oestrus cycle and early pregnancy in the mare. J. Reprod. Fertil. Suppl., *35*:253–260, 1987.
11. Pashen, R.L.: Oxytocin—The induction agent of choice in the mare? J. Reprod. Fertil. Suppl., *32*:645, 1982.
12. Lehrman, S.R., et al.: Primary structure of equine prolactin. Int. J. Pept. Protein Res., *31*:544–554, 1988.
13. Roser, J.F., Chang, Y.S., Papkoff, H., and Li, C.H.: Development and characterization of a homologous radioimmunoassay for equine prolactin. Proc. Soc. Exp. Biol. Med., *174*:510–517, 1984.
14. Thompson, D.L., Jr., Weist, J.J., and Nett, T.M.: Measurement of equine prolactin with an equine-canine radioimmunoassay: Seasonal effects on the prolactin response to thyrotropin releasing hormone. Domest. Anim. Endocrinol., *3*:247–252, 1986.
15. Johnson, A.L., and Becker, S.E.: Effects of physiologic and pharmacologic agents on serum prolactin concentrations in the nonpregnant mare. J. Anim. Sci., *65*:1292–1297, 1987.
16. Johnson, A.L.: Seasonal and photoperiod-induced changes in serum prolactin and pituitary responsiveness to thyrotropin-releasing hormone in the mare. Proc. Soc. Exp. Biol. Med., *184*:118–122, 1987.
17. Thompson, D.L., Jr., and Johnson, L.: Concentrations of prolactin, luteinizing hormone and follicle stimulating hormone in pituitary and serum of horses: Effect of sex season and reproductive state. J. Anim. Sci., *63*:854–860, 1986.
18. Johnson, A.L.: Serum concentrations of prolactin, thyroxine and triiodothyronine relative to season and the estrous cycle in the mare. J. Anim. Sci., *62*:1012–1020, 1986.
19. Worthy, K., et al.: Plasma prolactin concentrations in non-pregnant mares at different times of the year and in relation to events in the cycle. J. Reprod. Fertil. Suppl., *35*:269–276, 1987.
20. Worthy, K., et al.: Plasma prolactin concentrations and cyclic activity in pony mares during parturition and early lactation. J. Reprod. Fertil., *77*:569–574, 1986.
21. Roser, J.F., et al.: Plasma prolactin concentrations in mares and their neonates after oxytocin induction of parturition. Domest. Anim. Endocrinol., *6*:101–110, 1989.
22. Schams, D., Reinhardt, V., and Karg, H.: Effects of 2-Br-α-ergokryptine on plasma prolactin levels during parturition and onset of lactation in cows. Experientia, *28*:697–699, 1972.
23. Kann, G.: Influence of the suppression of the prepartum surge of prolactin by ergocryptine on the milk yield and

on the post-partum anoestrus of the nursing ewe. Ann. Biol. Anim. Biochim. Biophys., *16*:163–170, 1976.

24. Forsyth, I.A., Rossdale, P.D., and Thomas, C.R.: Studies on milk composition and lactogenic hormones in the mare. J. Reprod. Fertil. Suppl., *23*:631–635, 1975.

25. Nett, T.M., Holtan, D.W., and Estergreen, V.L.: Levels of LH, prolactin and oestrogens in the serum of post-partum mares. J. Reprod. Fertil. Suppl., *23*:201–206, 1975.

26. Grosvenor, C.E., Whitworth, N., and Mena, F.: Milk secretory response of the conscious lactating rat following intravenous injections of rat prolactin. J. Dairy Sci., *58*:1803–1807, 1975.

27. Concannon, P.W., et al.: Parturition and lactation in the bitch: Serum progesterone, cortisol and prolactin. Biol. Reprod., *19*:1113–1118, 1978.

28. McNeilly, A.S., and Friesen, H.G.: Prolactin during pregnancy and lactation in the rabbit. Endocrinology, *102*:1548–1554, 1978.

29. Tucker, H.A.: Lactation and its hormonal control. *In* The Physiology of Reproduction. Edited by E. Knobil and J.D. Neill. New York, Raven Press, 1988, pp. 2235–2263.

30. Thompson, D.L., Jr., and Johnson, L.: Effects of age, season and active immunization against estrogen on serum prolactin concentrations in stallions. Domest. Anim. Endocrinol., *4*:17–22, 1987.

31. Rabb, M.H., et al.: Effects of sexual stimulation, with and without ejaculation, on serum concentrations of LH, FSH, testosterone, cortisol and prolactin in stallions. J. Anim. Sci., *67*:2724–2729, 1989.

32. Kemp, B.E., and Niall, H.D.: Relaxin. Vitam. Horm., *41*:70–115, 1984.

33. Sherwood, O.D.: Relaxin. *In* The Physiology of Reproduction. Edited by E. Knobil and J.D. Neill. New York, Raven Press, 1988, pp. 585–673.

34. Stewart, D.R., and Papkoff, H.: Purification and characterization of equine relaxin. Endocrinology, *119*:1093–1099, 1986.

35. Stewart, D.R., Stabenfeldt, G.H., Hughes, J.P., and Meagher, D.M.: Determination of the source of equine relaxin. Biol. Reprod., *27*:17–24, 1982.

36. Stewart, D.R., and Stabenfeldt, G.: Relaxin activity in the pregnant mare. Biol. Reprod., *25*:281–289, 1981.

37. Stewart, D.R.: Development of a homologous equine relaxin radioimmunoassay. Endocrinology, *119*:1100–1104, 1986.

38. Chihal, H.J., and Espey, L.L.: Utilization of the relaxed symphysis pubis of guinea pigs for clues to the mechanism of ovulation. Endocrinology, *93*:1441–1445, 1973.

39. Leppi, T.J., and Kinnison, P.A.: The connective tissue ground substance in the mouse uterine cervix: An electron microscopic histochemical study. Anat. Rec., *170*:97–118, 1971.

40. Porter, D.C.: The myometrium and the relaxin enigma. Anim. Reprod. Sci., *2*:77–96, 1979.

41. Hurley, W.L., et al.: Effect of relaxin on mammary development in ovariectomized pregnant gilts. Endocrinology, *128*:1285–1290, 1991.

42. McCullagh, D.R.: Dual endocrine activity of the testes. Science, *76*:19–20, 1932.

43. De Jong, F.S., and Sharpe, R.M.: Evidence of inhibin-like activity in bovine follicular fluid. Nature, *263*:71–72, 1976.

44. Robertson, D.M., et al.: Isolation of inhibin from bovine follicular fluid. Biochem. Biophys. Res. Commun., *126*:220–226, 1985.

45. Miyamoto, K., et al.: Isolation of porcine follicular fluid inhibin of 32 K daltons. Biochem. Biophys. Res. Commun., *129*:396–403, 1985.

46. Ling, N., et al.: Isolation and partial characterization of Mr 32,000 protein with inhibin activity from porcine follicular fluid. Proc. Natl. Acad. Sci., U.S.A., *82*:4041–4044, 1985.

47. Rivier, J., Spiess, J., Vaughan, J., and Vale, W.: Purification and partial characterization of inhibin from porcine follicular fluid. Biochem. Biophys. Res. Commun., *133*:120–127, 1985.

48. Tierney, M.L., et al.: Physiochemical and biological characterization of recombinant human inhibin. Endocrinology, *126*:3268–3270, 1990.

49. Cuevas, P., et al.: Immunohistochemical detection of inhibin in the gonad. Biochem. Biophys. Res. Commun., *142*:23–30, 1987.

50. Munier, H., Rivier, C., Evans, R.M., and Vale, W.: Gonadal and extragonadal expression of inhibin α, βA and βB subunits in various tissues predicts diverse functions. Proc. Natl. Acad. Sci., U. S. A., *85*:247–251, 1988.

51. Mercer, J.E., Clements, J.A., Funder, J.W., and Clarke, I.J.: Rapid and specific lowering of pituitary FSHβ mRNA levels by inhibin. Mol. Cell. Endocrinol., *53*:251–254, 1987.

52. Attardi, B., et al.: Rapid and profound suppression of messenger ribonucleic acid encoding follicle-stimulating hormone β by inhibin from primate Sertoli cells. Mol. Endocrinol., *3*:280–287, 1989.

53. Jakubowiak, A., Janecki, A., and Steinberger, A.: Similar effects of inhibin and cycloheximide on gonadotropin release in superfused pituitary cell cultures. Biol. Reprod., *41*:454–463, 1989.

54. Wang, O.F., Farnworth, P.G., Findlay, J.K., and Burger, H.G.: Effects of 31 K bovine inhibin on specific binding of gonadotropin-releasing hormone to rat anterior pituitary cells in culture. Endocrinology, *123*:2161–2166, 1988.

55. Laws, S.C., Beggs, M.J., Webster, J.C., and Miller, W.L.: Inhibin increases and progesterone decreases receptors for gonadotropin-releasing hormone in ovine anterior pituitary culture. Endocrinology, *127*:373–380, 1990.

56. Gregg, D.W., Schwall, R.H., and Nett, T.M.: Regulation of gonadotropin secretion and number of gonadotropin-releasing hormone receptors by inhibin, activin A, and estradiol. Biol. Reprod., *44*:725–732, 1991.

57. Ling, N., et al.: A homodimer of the beta-subunits of inhibin A stimulates secretion of pituitary follicle stimulating hormone. Biochem. Biophys. Res. Commun., *138*:1129–1137, 1986.

58. Schwall, R.H., et al.: Recombinant expression and characterization of human activin-A. Mol. Endocrinol., *2*:1237–1242, 1988.

59. Attardi, B., and Miklos, J.: Rapid stimulatory effect of activin-A on messenger RNA encoding the follicle-stimulating hormone β-subunit in rat pituitary cell cultures. Mol. Endocrinol., *4*:721–726, 1990.

60. Roberts, V., et al.: Production and regulation of inhibin subunits in pituitary gonadotropes. Endocrinology, *124*:552–554, 1988.

61. Corrigan, A.Z., et al.: Evidence for an autocrine role of activin B with rat anterior pituitary culture. Endocrinology, *128*:1682–1684, 1991.

62. Piquette, G.N., et al.: Equine granulosa-theca cell tumors express inhibin α- and βA-subunit messenger ribonucleic acids and proteins. Biol. Reprod., *43*:1050–1057, 1990.

63. Bergeron, H., Crouch, G.M., and Bowen, J.M.: Granulosa theca cell tumor in a mare. Compend. Contin. Educ. Practicing Vet., *5*:S141–S145, 1983.

64. Jubb, K.V.F., Kennedy, P.C., and Palmer, N.: Pathology of Domestic Animals. Vol. 3. 3rd ed. San Diego, Academic Press, 1985, pp. 306–407.

CHAPTER 13

PUBERTY

E.L. Squires

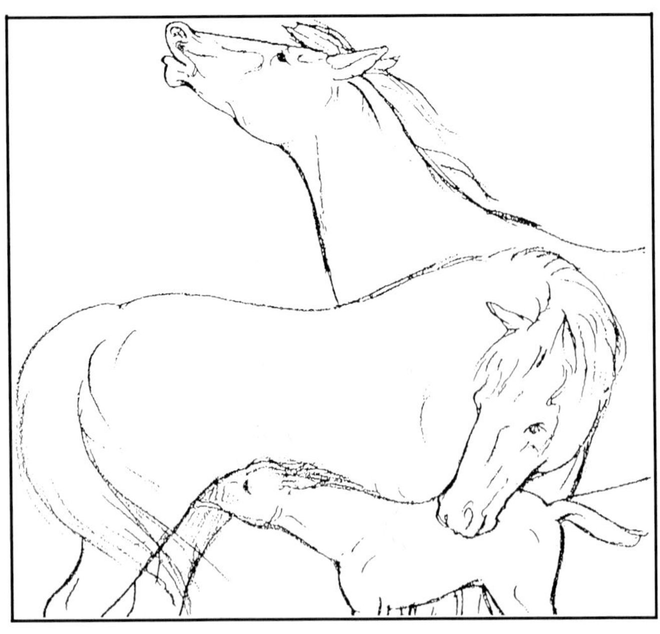

The one or more factors that determine onset of puberty in female horses are poorly understood because of a limited number of studies. Because the horse is considered a non–food-producing animal in most of the world, little emphasis is placed on hastening onset of puberty. Most breeders are content to allow puberty to occur spontaneously, and in general, fillies are not bred until they are 3 yr of age, even though puberty is generally accepted to occur between 12 and 24 months.[1,2] Therefore, most of the information in this chapter stems from studies done in sheep, a seasonal breeder that has been extensively studied. Attainment of puberty in a seasonal breeder is complicated. Any reproductive strategy must allow puberty to occur during a certain season of the year so that offspring are born in a favorable environmental season. The season of conception varies with the duration of pregnancy. Typically, species in which gestation is very long, such as the mare, ovulate during the spring and summer, whereas those species with gestation of intermittent durations (sheep) mate in the fall, such that birth coincides with a suitable environment. Several factors will be reviewed that have been shown to influence onset of puberty, such as age, weight, body composition, energy intake, pheromones, and season. In addition, this chapter deals with the maturation of the hypothalamic-pituitary-ovarian axis in the prepubertal animal and presents a conceptual model of how puberty is initiated.

NUTRITION

Apparently, no studies are available on growth-related cues influencing onset of puberty in fillies. However, data are available to demonstrate a delay in onset of puberty in ewe lambs and heifers exposed to low nutritional intake. The exact mechanism for nutritionally delayed onset of puberty is unknown, but investigators provided evidence that restricted energy intake prevents or slows the maturational process at the hypothalamic-pituitary level.[3,4] Both frequency and amplitude of pulses of LH were suppressed in heifers fed restricted levels of dietary energy, as compared to heifers that were fed a diet adequate in energy.[3] In addition, the magnitude of the luteinizing hormone (LH) peak after administration of gonadotropin-releasing hormone (GnRH) was less in heifers fed a restricted energy diet. In a series of experiments, Foster and colleagues investigated how nutritional factors influence the onset of puberty in lambs.[5] Lambs raised on low nutrition remained anovulatory during the first breeding season because growth was retarded. Thus, even though the lambs were at the appropriate age for puberty, estrus and ovulation did not occur because of undernutrition. Kirkwood and Aherne studied the relationship between age, weight, and puberty in a nonseasonal breeding animal, the gilt.[6] They concluded that neither age nor weight is a reliable indicator of reproductive development but that minimum threshold values for these characteristics must be achieved before puberty can occur. In addition, they suggested that a minimum adipose to lean tissue ratio was a prerequisite for puberty in gilts and that this may be a more superior measure of reproductive development than either age or weight. Unfortunately, no study that examines the effect of body composition and/or growth rate on the onset of puberty in fillies is known. Obviously, this is an area that should receive additional attention.

SEASON

One factor that has received some attention is the effect of the season of birth on the onset of puberty. The timing of puberty by photoperiod has been studied extensively in the female sheep. In a classic study by Foster and Ryan, the reversal of the annual photoperiod in autumn-born lambs was demonstrated to prevent the delay in puberty that occurs in autumn-born lambs in a natural photoperiod.[7] Although artificial light is commonly used to hasten onset of breeding season in adult mares,[8] only limited studies have been conducted on the influence of photoperiod on puberty in female horses. One project was designed to determine the effect of photoperiod on the onset of puberty in female ponies.[9] Thirteen, 6- to 8- month-old fillies were randomly assigned to three treatment groups. Group 1 received 16 h of fixed daily photoperiod (light), group 2 received a daily photoperiod equivalent to the ambient day length, and group 3 was exposed to a 9-h fixed daily photoperiod. This study was conducted from December to August. Hair shedding, which is common under long photoperiod, occurred first in group 1, followed by group 2, then group 3. The incidence of puberty was defined as one or more ovulations. The proportion of fillies ovulating by the end of the project were: two of four, five of five, and two of four, for groups 1, 2, and 3, respectively. The study concluded that a 16-h fixed photoperiod would not hasten puberty but, instead, interfered with the attainment of puberty. Puberty also appeared to be retarded in the group exposed to a 9-h fixed photoperiod, but the results were less pronounced for those in the 16-h group. Unfortunately, these conclusions were based on a relatively small number of animals per treatment. However, the results were similar to the failure of a short, fixed photoperiod (stimulatory) to hasten the onset of puberty in sheep. The female horse may require an alternating short and long photoperiod in order to be stimulatory.

Although other external determinates of puberty, such as pheromones,[10] male effects, such as the ram effect in sheep,[11] and nutrient intake[12] have been shown to affect the onset of puberty in several species, these factors have apparently not been evaluated in the horse.

HYPOTHALAMIC-PITUITARY AXIS

Wesson and Ginther conducted a series of studies in which plasma gonadotropin levels were determined in prepubertal ponies.[13–16] In the first study, blood samples were taken biweekly from four spring-born fillies, from approximately 3 weeks to 4 months of age.[13] Plasma concentrations of LH and follicle-stimulating hormone (FSH) were determined. Concentrations of LH remained low and constant, whereas FSH increased from a low in May and early June to a high in late June through July (Fig. 13-1). In the second experiment, nine spring-born foals were assigned to either an ovarian-intact or ovariectomy group.[14] Ovariectomies were performed on August 16 when ponies were 4 months old. Concentrations of LH and FSH were determined in samples collected every other day in August. From September through December, blood was collected at least biweekly, and from January to February blood was collected every other day. There was no effect of ovariectomy on concentrations of either FSH or LH. In both groups, LH remained low and constant throughout this period. In contrast, mean concentrations of FSH decreased from a high in the summer and early fall, to a low during late fall, but concentrations increased again during January to February (Fig. 13-1). In the third experiment, concentrations of LH and FSH were examined for five late-born (summer) fillies. Mean plasma LH was higher on day of birth than any other day. Throughout the sampling period for this group, LH remained low. Concentrations of FSH for these late-born fillies was extremely variable, although some of the profiles were similar to spring-born fillies. The fact that the pattern of LH and FSH secretion in the prepubertal filly were quite different suggested separate regulatory mechanisms for these two gonadotropins. In addition, the absence of an immediate rise in gonadotropins following ovariectomy indicated the absence of a negative-feedback relationship between the ovary and the hypothalamic-hypophysial unit at this age.

A subsequent study by these same investigators examined the gonadotropin patterns in prepubertal fillies.[15] Eight female pony foals were used in that study. The female foals were divided into five spring-born (April to May) foals and three foals born in mid-June. As in the previous study, the mean concentration of LH on the day of birth was higher for LH than for all other days. From 1 month to approximately 8 months of age, concentrations

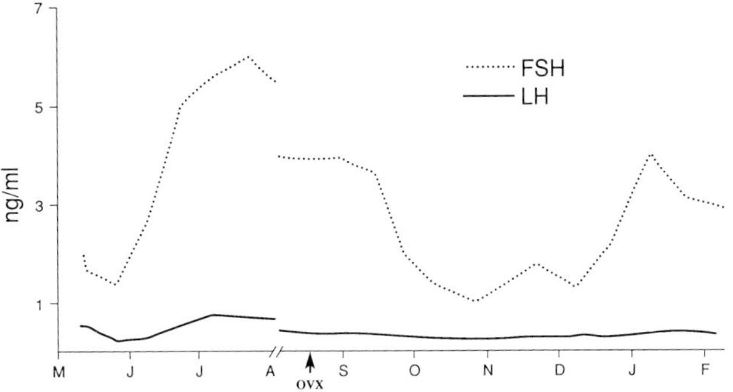

FIG. 13–1. Concentrations of LH (—) and FSH (----) in prepubertal fillies from 3 weeks to 9 months. Ovaries were removed from fillies at 4 months. (From Wesson, J.A., and Ginther, O.J.: Plasma gonadotropin levels in intact and ovariectomized prepubertal ponies. Biol. Reprod., *20*:1099–1104, 1979.)

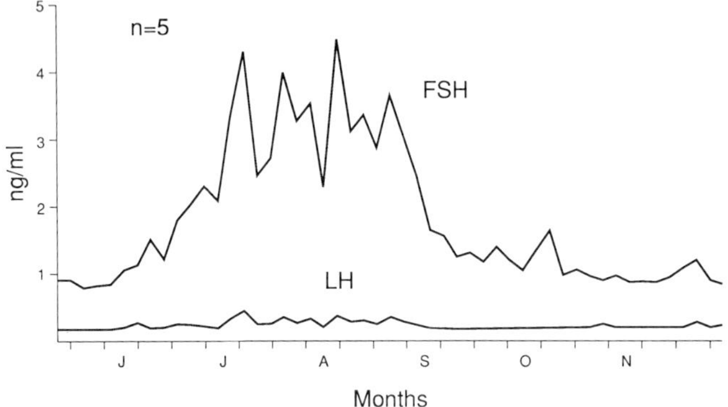

FIG. 13–2. Concentrations of gonadotropins at 4-day intervals in five spring-born fillies from 1 to 8 months of age. (From Wesson, J.A., and Ginther, O.J.: Plasma gonadotropin concentrations in intact female and intact and castrated male prepubertal ponies. Biol. Reprod., *22*:541–549, 1980.)

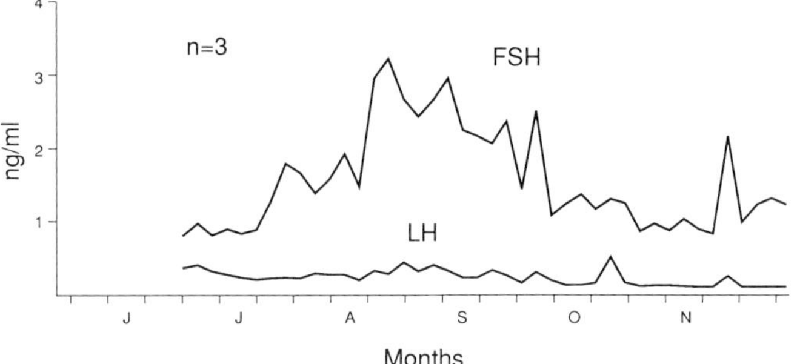

FIG. 13–3. Concentrations of gonadotropins at 4-day intervals for three, mid-June–born fillies from 2 weeks to 6 months of age. (From Wesson, J.A., and Ginther, O.J.: Plasma gonadotropin concentrations in intact female and intact and castrated male prepubertal ponies. Biol. Reprod., *22*:541–549, 1980.)

of LH remained low and constant. Concentrations of FSH, in contrast, increased from a low in early June to a high from mid-July through early September. Thereafter, concentrations of LH decreased by late September and remained relatively low and relatively constant until the end of the project (Figs. 13-2 and 13-3). Patterns of gonadotropins for fillies born in June (Fig. 13-3) were similar to those born in April and May (Fig. 13-2).

Another investigation, which included some of the same mares from previous studies, examined the reproductive behavior and concentrations of gonadotropins in 14 female ponies during the period from 10 to 21 months of age (February 1978 to January 1979). Eleven fillies had intact ovaries and three had been ovariectomized at 4 months of age. The fillies were further classified as spring born or late born. Fillies were teased for estrous behavior individually by a stallion every 8 days from mid-February through March, every 4 days from April 1 until the first filly was observed to show estrous behavior and every 2 days from May 19 until September 1, or 30 days after the last day that estrous behavior was observed, whichever came later. The occurrence of ovulation was determined by concentrations of LH and progesterone. Blood samples were taken once every 4 days from February until May, every 2 days from May until September, and every 4 days thereafter. All samples were assayed for LH and FSH. The first ovulation (puberty) for all ponies born during the spring occurred during late spring or early summer of the following year. This was in agreement with a slaughterhouse survey where puberty was estimated to occur at 12 to 15 months of age.[16] Only 3 of the 35 ovulations were not associated with estrus, and two of these occurred in one animal. This is in contrast with the lack of estrus in the majority of ewe lambs experiencing their first ovulation.[5] Three ponies that were born during June or July also ovulated the following year, whereas two that were born in August or September did not. However, body weight was not different at the time of puberty. In addition, the time of onset of the breeding season (month of first ovulatory estrus) was similar for the spring-born group of fillies to that reported for older adult ponies. All intact, spring-born fillies ovulated during late spring when they were 12 to 15 months old. Two of five late-born fillies did not ovulate, and fewer ovulations and a shorter breeding season were observed in late-born than in spring-born fillies. This emphasizes the effect of season on the onset of puberty of fillies. In the two late-born fillies that were said not to have ovulated, several LH and progesterone surges occurred, which were similar to the surges associated with ovulation in the remaining fillies. Changes in plasma concentrations of FSH and LH preceding, during, and immediately after the first ovulatory period were similar to that reported for adult ponies (Fig. 13-4). Estrous behavior accompanied 90% of the ovulations, and plasma concentrations of FSH and LH followed a seasonal pattern in the ovariectomized fillies, with the highest levels occurring during the summer.

More recently, a study was conducted to evaluate further the maturation of the hypothalamic-pituitary-ovarian axis of the filly.[17] This study involved 15 light-horse fillies born during July and August. The dams of these fillies had been administered either 2 mL of Neobee oil per 50 kg of body weight or 2 mL of Altrenogest per 50 kg of body weight from day 20 to 320 of gestation. The study represents 11 fillies from dams treated with Altrenogest and 4 control fillies. The objectives of this study were to assess (1) clitoral size, (2) age-associated changes in LH and FSH, (3) GnRH-induced LH and FSH release from 32 to 96 weeks of age, (4) changes in LH and FSH during transition into the breeding season and during the first two estrous cycles, (5) age of puberty and characterization of first estrous cycles, (6) pregnancy rate, and (7) effect of maternal treatment with Altrenogest on reproductive parameters. Nine fillies (treated, $n = 5$; control, $n = 4$) were selected to monitor hormonal changes in prepubertal and pubertal mares. Age-associated changes in LH and FSH were monitored from 4 to 68 weeks of age by collecting seven blood samples (one every 4 days) at 8-week intervals; thus six "windows" were examined and each window contained seven blood samples. Beginning at

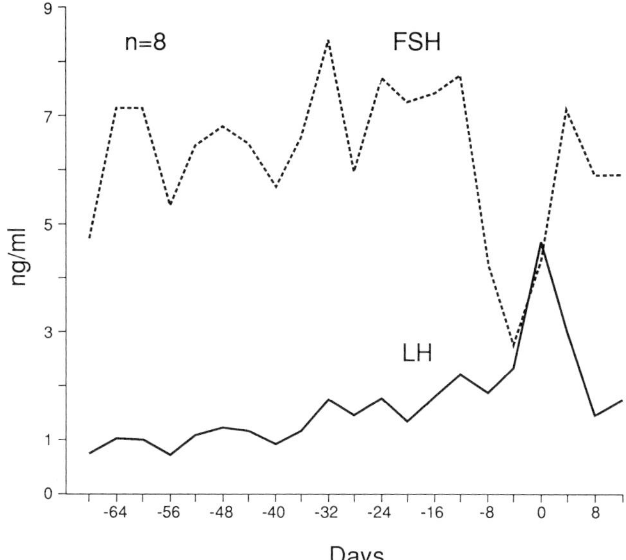

FIG. 13–4. Concentrations of gonadotropins at 4-day intervals for 68 days through 12 days after first ovulatory LH surge in eight yearling fillies. (From Wesson, J.A., and Ginther, O.J.: Plasma gonadotropin concentrations in intact female and intact and castrated male prepubertal ponies. Biol. Reprod., *22*:541–549, 1980.)

72 weeks of age, blood samples were collected every 4 days until first estrus. Samples were collected daily during estrus and on days 4, 6, 10, and 14 after ovulation for the first two estrous cycles. "Challenges" with GnRH were administered every 8 weeks from 32 to 96 weeks of age to assess maturation of the hypothalamic-pituitary axis. Blood was collected at 20-min intervals, before and after GnRH administration. Three dependent variables were assayed for each of the nine GnRH challenges: baseline hormonal concentrations, highest concentrations after GnRH minus the baseline concentration, and minutes from GnRH administration to the highest concentration of gonadotropins achieved. Puberty was defined as the age when the first ovulation accompanied by behavioral estrus occurred. Beginning in February, all fillies were teased daily with a stallion to determine behavioral estrus and ovaries were examined every 3 days by ultrasonography. Once a 35-mm follicle was detected, ovaries were examined every other day or daily if the follicle was advancing rapidly in size. Ovulation was detected by ultrasonography and ovaries were examined every 3 days during diestrus. Once mares had established a normal cycle, they were inseminated every other day during estrus with 500 million progressively motile spermatozoa from one stallion. Pregnancy diagnosis was made by ultrasonography. The infantile period, which was marked by low gonadotropin concentrations, appeared to be from birth to 8 months. The beginning of the prepubertal period was marked by increased concentrations of LH and FSH between 8 and 14 months of age. Serum concentrations of LH were then depressed to lower levels after 56 weeks, presumably due to the negative feedback effect of estradiol on the hypothalamus. Concentrations of LH

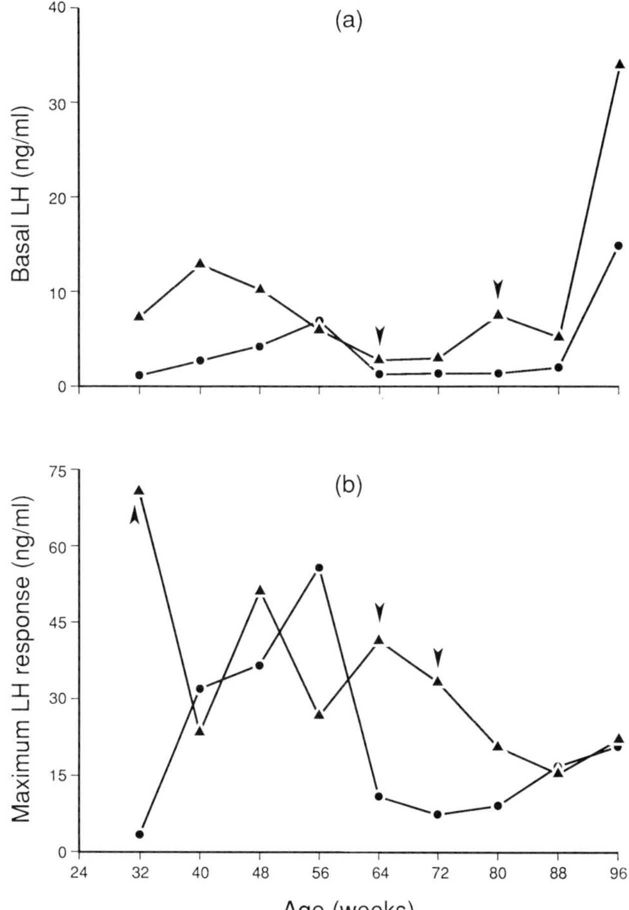

FIG. 13–5. *(A)* Basal concentrations of LH and *(B)* maximum release of LH after GnRH administration in Altrenogest-treated (▲) fillies (n = 5) and control (●) fillies (n = 4). Arrows indicate significant difference between groups. (From Naden, J., Squires, E.L., and Nett, T.M.: Effect of maternal treatment with Altrenogest on age at puberty, hormone concentrations, pituitary response to exogenous GnRH, oestrous cycle characteristics and fertility of fillies. J. Reprod. Fertil., *88*:185–195, 1990.)

remained suppressed until 88 weeks of age. This long period of LH suppression was attributed to a seasonal effect. Concentrations of FSH were erratic from 56 to 88 weeks, with no obvious seasonal effect. The low concentration of LH from 1 to 8 months of age was similar to previous reports.[13,14] The higher concentrations of LH and FSH in fillies from dams treated with Altrenogest was unexpected, because maternal treatment of mares with Altrenogest had no effect on gonadotropin concentration in colts.[18] This pattern of LH secretion in control fillies was similar to that reported for prepubertal ewes[5,7] and gilts.[19] The LH response to GnRH administration in fillies was similar to the pattern reported for prepubertal colts.[20] The amount of LH released in response to GnRH was greatest at 40 to 60 weeks of age. The decrease in LH response after 64 weeks of age may have been due to season, because this represented October. By February or March, the LH response to GnRH was once again increased (Fig. 13-5). This re-

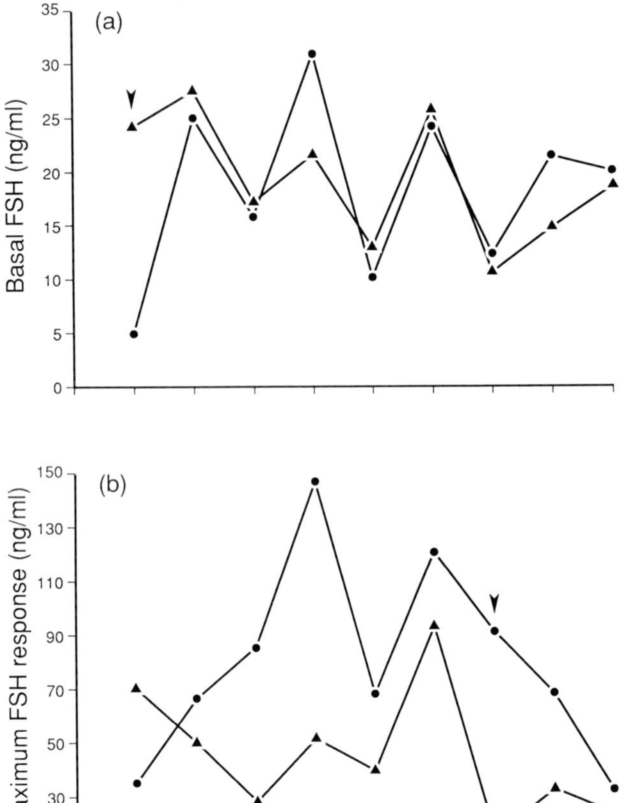

FIG. 13-6. *(A)* Basal concentrations of FSH and *(B)* maximum release of FSH after GnRH administration every 8 weeks from 24 to 96 weeks in five treated (▲) and four control (●) fillies. Arrows indicate significant difference between groups. (From Naden, J., Squires, E.L., and Nett, T.M.: Effect of maternal treatment with Altrenogest on age at puberty, hormone concentrations, pituitary response to exogenous GnRH, oestrous cycle characteristics and fertility of fillies. J. Reprod. Fertil., *88*:185–195, 1990.)

duced LH response to GnRH during the nonbreeding season was similar to that reported for adult mares.[21] The increased LH response to GnRH and the decreased FSH response in both groups of fillies after 80 weeks (Fig. 13-6) was similar to that reported for adult mares as the first ovulation of the breeding season approached.

A MODEL FOR ONSET OF PUBERTY

There are two schools of thought regarding the mechanism for initiation of puberty. One possibility is that at least one component of the endocrine system is incapable of functioning in an adult fashion until at or near the time of puberty. An alternative view is that all components of the endocrine system of the prepubertal female are mature but one or more specific components are inhibited from functioning in an adult fashion. Because the administration of GnRH has been shown to result in LH and FSH release in a variety of species prior to the time of puberty, it would appear that the pituitary is able to synthesize and secrete gonadotropins during the prepubertal period. Increasing levels of estradiol during the follicular phase of the estrous cycle are thought to induce a preovulatory surge of LH; thus the preovulatory gonadotropin surge by estradiol is a component of the endocrine system that is essential for puberty to occur. Surges in LH secretion similar to those present before ovulation in mature cows have been induced in prepubertal heifers by the administration of estradiol.[22] This component of the endocrine system appears to be functional in the prepubertal period. Apparently, estradiol has not been injected into prepubertal mares to determine the LH response. However, in a study in our laboratory, estradiol 17β was injected during the transitional period to determine the acute and long-term response to this steroid.[23] Treatment (1 mg estradiol 17β per day) was administered for 7 days during early transition, (approximately 60 days prior to ovulation) and late transition (approximately 30 days prior to ovulation). Blood samples were collected frequently on day 1 of treatment and daily for 8 days. Administration of estradiol during early and late transitions suppressed both LH and FSH secretion for 8 h after injection. Estradiol also suppressed number of LH and FSH pulses within 12 h after initial injection.

The gradual increase in LH prior to onset of puberty would appear to be common in the heifer, ewe, and filly. The exact mechanism for increased concentrations of LH prior to onset of puberty in the mare has not been determined. In the heifer, frequency of LH pulses was shown to be the best predictor of age at puberty.[3] Correlation coefficient of the regression of frequency of LH pulses on days before puberty was 0.88. Increased pulse frequency of LH has also been associated with the onset of puberty in ewes.[5] It would appear that the hypothalamic pulse generator that regulates the pulsatile secretion of gonadotropins is suppressed in the prepubertal ewe, lamb, heifer, and possibly, filly. Apparently this GnRH pulse generator is extremely sensitive to estradiol, and therefore, pulses of LH are maintained at low levels during the prepubertal state. This phenomenon has been coined the "gonadostat hypothesis." As sexual maturation occurs, responsiveness to steroid-negative feedback decreases and secretion of LH increases to a point at which follicular growth is stimulated. Estrogen secretion is enhanced and, in turn, the preovulatory surge of gonadotropins is induced by increasing estrogen. This process culminates in ovulation.

The mechanism whereby the negative effect of estradiol is diminished as puberty approaches has not been clearly delineated. A decrease in concentration of cytosolic receptors for estradiol in the anterior medial basal hypothalamus and in the anterior pituitary has been shown to occur during the period of sexual maturation in heifers. This decline in receptors coincides with the decline in estradiol negative feedback and an increase in LH secretion. The negative-feedback action of estra-

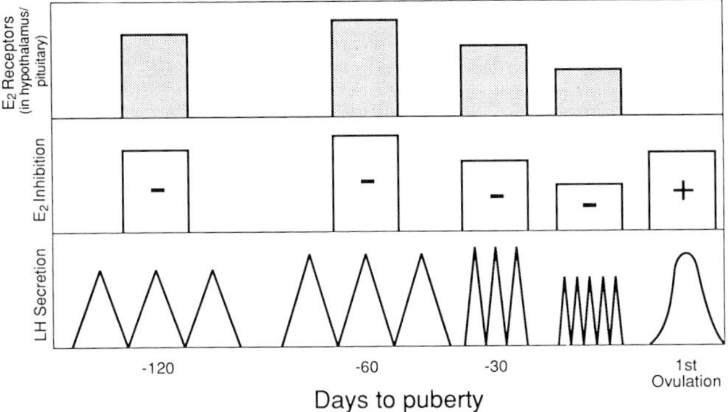

FIG. 13–7. Model for endocrine control of puberty. Minus sign (−) indicates inhibitory effects of estradiol and positive sign (+) signifies positive effect.

diol on secretion of LH can be altered by growth rate. That is, when growth rate was retarded in ewes, the negative-feedback action of estradiol on LH was continued, and thus the pulses of LH were slower in ewe lambs that were given restricted amounts of food.[3] Both frequency and amplitude of pulses of LH were suppressed in heifers fed restricted levels of dietary energy compared with heifers that were fed a diet adequate in energy.[3] Therefore, results of studies in ewe lambs and heifers both indicate that pituitary responsiveness to exogenous stimuli is depressed when quantities of food intake are restricted.

In summary, the low-frequency endogenous pulses of LH in prepubertal sheep, cattle, and possibly fillies are not capable of stimulating follicular growth to the preovulatory stage. Ovarian estradiol acts on the hypothalamus to suppress the generation of pulses of GnRH that maintain the secretion of LH at low levels and, in turn, prevent growth of ovarian follicles to the point at which ovulation occurs. As the concentrations of estradiol receptors in the medial basal hypothalamus decline, the frequency with which pulses of LH are generated increases. Follicles can develop to a more advanced stage, as frequency of pulses of LH increase and produce concentrations of estrogens that stimulate uterine growth and development. At the point at which pulses of LH occur at one per hour, concentrations of LH are obtained that drive ovarian follicular growth to the preovulatory stage, estradiol induces a preovulatory surge of gonadotropins, and ovulation occurs as the result of gonadotropins acting on the mature follicle (Fig. 13-7). Further studies are needed in the horse to determine if the gonadostat theory explains the mechanism for onset of puberty.

REFERENCES

1. Mitchell, D., and Allen W.R.: Observations on reproductive performance in the yearling mare. J. Reprod. Fertil. Suppl., *23*:531–536, 1975.
2. Nishikawa, Y., and Hafez, E.S.E.: Horses. *In* Reproduction in Farm Animals. Edited by E.S.E. Hafez. Philadelphia, Lea & Febiger, 1975, pp. 288–300.
3. Kinder, J.E., Day, M.L., and Kittok, R.J.: Endocrine regulation of puberty in cows and ewes. J. Reprod. Fertil. Suppl., *34*:167–186, 1987.
4. Short, R.E., and Adams, D.C.: Nutritional and hormonal interrelationships in beef cattle reproduction. Can. J. Anim. Sci., *68*:29–39, 1989.
5. Foster, D.L., et al.: Determinants of puberty in a seasonal breeder. Recent Prog. Horm. Res., *42*:331–384, 1986.
6. Kirkwood, R.N., and Aherne, F.X.: Energy intake, body composition and reproductive performance of the gilt. J. Anim. Sci., *60*:1518–1529, 1985.
7. Foster, D.L., and Ryan, K.D.: Endocrine mechanisms governing transition into adulthood in female sheep. J. Reprod. Fertil. Suppl., *30*:75–90, 1981.
8. Kooistra, L.H., and Ginther, O.J.: Effect of photoperiod on reproductive activity and hair in mares. Am. J. Vet. Res., *36*:1413–1419, 1975.
9. Wesson, J.A., and Ginther, O.J.: Influence of photoperiod on puberty in the female pony. J. Reprod. Fertil. Suppl., *32*:269–274, 1982.
10. Vandenbergh, J.G.: Pheromones and Reproduction in Mammals. New York, Academic Press, 1983, pp. 95–110.
11. Dyrmundsson, O.R.: Advancement of puberty in male and female sheep. *In* New Techniques in Sheep Production. Edited by F.M. Marai and J.B. Owen. London, Butterworth, 1987, pp. 65–76.
12. Kirkwood, R.N., Cumming, D.C., and Aherne, F.X.: Nutrition and puberty in the female. Proc. Nutr. Soc., *46*:177–192, 1987.
13. Wesson, J.A., and Ginther, O.J.: Plasma gonadotropin levels in intact and ovariectomized prepubertal ponies. Biol. Reprod., *20*:1099–1104, 1979.
14. Wesson, J.A., and Ginther, O.J.: Plasma gonadotropin concentrations in intact female and intact and castrated male prepubertal ponies. Biol. Reprod., *22*:541–549, 1980.
15. Wesson, J.A., and Ginther, O.J.: Puberty in the female pony: Reproductive behavior, ovulation and plasma gonadotropin concentrations. Biol. Reprod., *24*:977–986, 1981.
16. Wesson, J.A., and Ginther, O.J.: Influence of season and age on reproductive activity in pony mares based on a slaughterhouse survey. J. Anim. Sci., *52*:119–129, 1981.
17. Naden, J., Squires, E.L., and Nett, T.M.: Effect of maternal treatment with Altrenogest on age at puberty, hormone concentrations, pituitary response to exogenous GnRH, oestrous cycle characteristics and fertility of fillies. J. Reprod. Fertil., *88*:185–195, 1990.
18. Naden, J., Amann, R.P., and Squires, E.L.: Testicular growth, hormone concentrations, seminal characteristics and sexual behavior in stallions. J. Reprod. Fertil., *88*:167–176, 1990.
19. Diekman, M.A., Trout, W.E., and Anderson, L.L.: Serum profiles of LH, FSH and prolactin from 10 weeks of age until puberty in gilts. J. Anim. Sci., *56*:139–145, 1983.
20. Naden, J., Squires, E.L., Nett, T.M., and Amann, R.P.: Effect of maternal treatment with Altrenogest on pituitary response to exogenous GnRH in prepubertal stallions. J. Reprod. Fertil., *88*:177–183, 1990.
21. Silva, P.J., Squires, E.L., and Nett, T.M.: Pituitary respon-

siveness of mares challenged with GnRH at various stages of the transition into the breeding season. J. Anim. Sci., *64*:790–796, 1987.

22. Schillo, K.K., Dierschke, D.J., and Hauser, E.R.: Regulation of luteinizing hormone secretion in prepubertal heifers: Increased threshold to negative feedback action of estradiol. J. Anim. Sci., *54*:325–336, 1982.

23. Wiepz, G.J.: The effect of estradiol-17 β and(or) progestins on reproductive patterns of transitional mares. M.S. thesis, Colorado State University, 1987.

CHAPTER 14

THE NORMAL ESTROUS CYCLE

P.F. Daels
J.P. Hughes

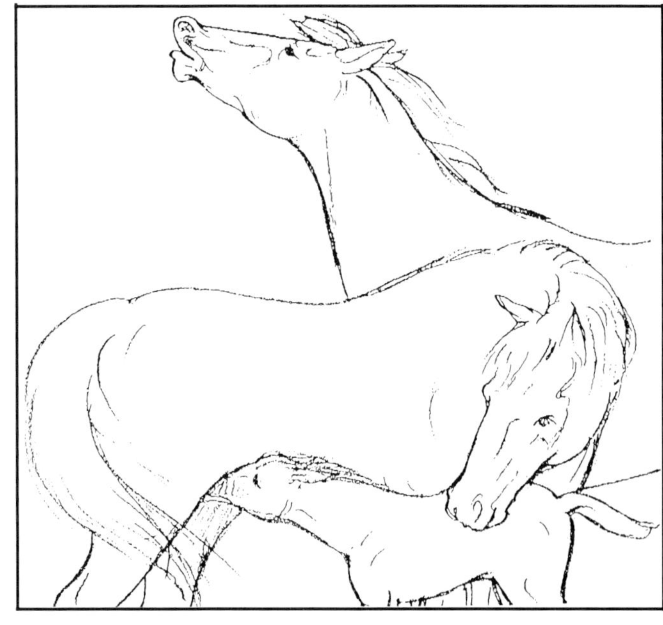

The mare is a seasonal polyestrous animal. Reproductive activity is regulated primarily by photoperiod but also by nutrition and climate (principally temperature).[1–10] In the temperate climate zones around the world, the majority of the mares undergo cyclic sexual activity during the spring and summer (breeding season), and only a few mares are reproductively active during the late fall and winter (anestrous season). With the increase in day length in early spring, ovarian activity is gradually stimulated. During the spring transition from anestrus to the breeding season, follicular development may be irregular with follicles developing and regressing for some time (weeks to months).[10] Eventually, follicular development culminates in the first ovulation of the season. Following this, mares generally continue to have regular ovulatory cycles. The percentage of mares that ovulate decreases gradually during the fall and only a small percentage of mares will continue to ovulate throughout the winter.

In this chapter, the behavioral, morphologic, and endocrinologic changes that occur during the normal estrous cycle are reviewed. Variations in cyclic patterns including failure to ovulate, failure of follicles to develop, erratic cycle duration, erratic estrous behavior, and spontaneous prolongation of the lifespan of the corpus luteum (CL) are discussed elsewhere (see Chapters 15 and 16).

DEFINITIONS AND TERMS

The estrous cycle is defined as the repetitive sequence of events that prepares the mare for conception. It may be conveniently divided into estrus (follicular phase) and diestrus (luteal phase). Estrus is the period during which the mare is sexually receptive to the stallion, the genital tract is prepared to accept and transport spermatozoa, and ovulation occurs. During estrus, the dominant follicle(s) develops and secretes estrogen, which induces sexual receptivity. Ovulation, the release of the oocyte, occurs approximately 24 to 48 h before the end of sexual receptivity. Diestrus is the period during which the mare is not receptive to the stallion and the genital tract is prepared to accept and nurture the conceptus. After ovulation, the ruptured follicle develops into a CL, which secretes progesterone. Increasing progesterone secretion causes the mare to reject the stallion's sexual advances. The period during which the CL secretes progesterone is termed the luteal or diestrous phase of the cycle. The end of the luteal phase is marked by regression of the CL (luteolysis) 14 to 15 days after ovulation and the onset of estrus 1 or 2 days later (Fig. 14-1).

DURATION OF THE CYCLE

The classic definition of the estrous cycle is the cyclic interval from the beginning of one estrus to the beginning of the next. A more precise definition of the mare's estrous cycle is the period between two ovulations that

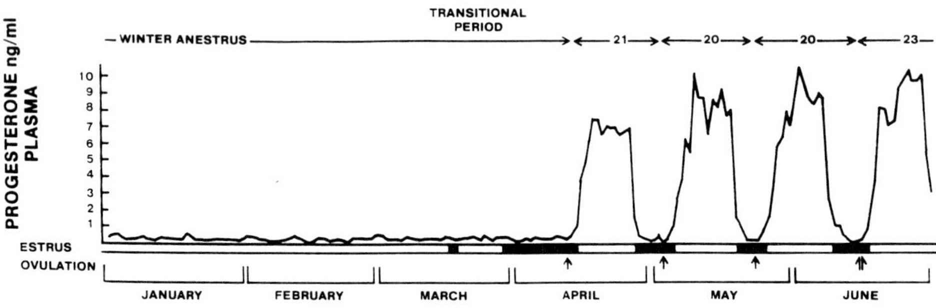

FIG. 14–1. Daily plasma progesterone concentrations of a seasonally polyestrous mare in the Northern Hemisphere. Estrous cycle durations are indicated at the top of the figures. The dark horizontal bars represent sexual receptivity, and the vertical arrows represent ovulations. Winter anestrus with inactive ovaries occurred from December through March. A prolonged split estrus associated with increased follicular activity occurred during the transitional period (March and April). Normal 20- to 23-day estrous cycles occurred from April through November. A diestrous ovulation occurred in July. (From Neely, D.P.: Studies on the control of luteal function and prostaglandin release in the mare. Ph.D. thesis. University of California, Davis, 1979.)

coincide with estrus and/or low progesterone concentration (< 1 ng/mL).[6,7] Unlike estrous behavior, which can occur as a gradual change over days, ovulation is a very specific event that occurs in a short time (minutes) which can be detected objectively using rectal palpation, ultrasonography, or progesterone analysis.[11] Estrous behavior and progesterone concentration are included in this definition because ovulation occasionally occurs during diestrus, when progesterone concentration is elevated and signs of estrous behavior are absent.[12–15] Diestrous ovulations do not represent the end point of the cycle (Chapter 16). In addition, mares that cycle regularly but do not display the typical behavior associated with estrus ("silent heat") can be included in this definition because they have progesterone concentrations less than 1 ng/mL at the time of ovulation. Based on this definition, the average estrous cycle duration is 21 days.[12] The average duration of the estrous cycle reported in the literature ranges from 19 to 22 days, diestrus and estrus average 14 to 15 days and 5 to 7 days, respectively.[2,5–7,12,16–23] The literature reports a considerable variety in both average and range of estrous cycle duration. If the occasional shortened and prolonged diestrus periods are considered to be abnormal and are excluded from calculation, the luteal phase duration appears to be fairly constant with no detectable seasonal variation.[2,5,12,22,24]

Deviations of the duration of the luteal phase are usually several days and are generally associated with uterine disorders, causing premature regression of the CL, through the secretion of prostaglandin $F_2\alpha$ ($PGF_2\alpha$), or are associated with persistence of the CL (Chapter 16). The duration of follicular phase is primarily influenced by season but also by individual variation, breed, and follicular status at the onset of estrus.[1,3,12,22,25] Duration of estrus typically decreases as the season progresses, with the shortest estrus duration observed during the summer[1,7,12] (Table 14-1). This shortening of estrus most likely represents an acceleration of folliculogenesis prior to ovulation with increasingly favorable photoperiod.

The average duration of estrus for individual mares ranges from 2 to 12 days and appears fairly repeatable within individual mares.[7,22,25] The diameter of the largest follicle at the time of luteolysis influences the time from onset of estrus to ovulation and diestrus. The larger the follicular diameter on the first day of estrus, the sooner the follicle will ovulate and the shorter the estrous period will be.[23,26,27] Estrous duration has also been correlated with the time of recruitment of the ovu-

TABLE 14–1. EFFECT OF SEASON ON DURATION OF ESTRUS IN 10 MARES OVER A 2-YR PERIOD*

MONTH	NUMBER OF ESTRUS PERIODS	MEAN DURATION OF ESTRUS (DAYS)	NUMBER OF CYCLES OBSERVED	MEAN CYCLE DURATION (DAYS)
January	18	5.06	22	32.2
February	13	6.69	20	34.4
March	26	8.38	25	26.1
April	29	7.76	28	21.9
May	28	5.72	39	19.5
June	28	4.47	31	21.1
July	20	4.70	28	24.6
August	24	4.75	27	20.4
September	27	4.44	32	20.6
October	31	4.53	35	20.4
November	27	5.20	25	24.8
December	22	7.23	21	30.4

*Adapted from Hughes, J.P., Stabenfeldt, G.H., and Evans, J.W.: Clinical and endocrine aspects of the estrous cycle of the mare. Proc. Am. Assoc. Equine Pract.,119–148, 1972.

latory follicle. Sirois et al. reported that mares that recruited a follicle early in diestrus typically had a larger size follicle on day 1 of estrus and had a shorter estrous cycle than mares that recruited the ovulatory follicle later in the luteal phase.[27] Measurement of estrogen concentration during estrus suggested that neither the shape nor the magnitude of the estrogen rise correlated with the duration of estrus. However, short estrous cycles were associated with an early onset of the estrogen surge, which occurred before luteolysis.[26] This observation again suggests that follicular size on day 1 of estrus plays a critical role in time of ovulation.

Ponies have a longer estrous cycle than horses. The estrous cycle of ponies averages 25 days, with diestrus and estrus averaging 16 and 8 days, respectively.[22] The average duration of the estrous cycle in the donkey (Equus asinus) is 25 to 26 days, and duration of diestrus and estrus are 18 to 19 and 6 to 8 days, respectively.[28–30] Nonconception estrous cycles in zebras and Przewalski's horses (Equus przewalskii) have been reported to be 20 to 26 and 24 days, respectively.[31,32]

OVARIAN DYNAMICS

FOLLICLE GROWTH PATTERN

Mares are exceptional in that they can have considerable follicular growth during the luteal phase. It appears as though follicular development occurs continuously throughout the estrous cycle and development of large antral follicles (> 30 mm diameter) can occur at any time during the luteal phase of the cycle. The majority of follicles that develop during the luteal phase will regress during or at the end of the luteal phase. Occasionally, a large antral follicle will reach preovulatory size and ovulate during diestrus without any signs of estrus. These diestrous ovulations are believed to be normal fertile ovulations.[14,15,17]

Time of the estrous cycle at which the ovulatory follicle is recruited has been under debate for many years. Ultrasonography has allowed researchers to characterize the dynamic changes in ovarian follicular populations during the estrous cycle.[10,11,23,27,33–36] Follicles tend to grow in waves, either one or two waves per cycle.[23,27,34,35] Around ovulation, a crop of small follicles (2 to 5 mm) become identifiable within the ovaries. Several small follicles continue to grow at steady rate (2.5 to 3.0 mm/day) during the luteal phase and reach a diameter of about 25 to 30 mm near the time of luteolysis.[34] At that time, one or two follicles become the dominant follicles and continue to grow while the remaining follicles become atretic.[23,34] Sirois et al. were able to identify individual follicles and follow their development throughout the estrous cycle.[27] In their studies, the most common pattern of follicular growth consisted of one follicular wave per estrous cycle. The ovulatory follicle was identified as an antral follicle within days after ovulation and was the largest follicle for approximately 10 days before ovulation. An alternative pattern was observed in which two follicular waves occurred. The second follicular wave appears in midluteal phase following regression or diestrous ovulation of the follicle which had developed during the first follicular wave (Fig. 14-2).

At the onset of luteolysis, the largest follicle usually continues to enlarge and eventually becomes the primary ovulatory follicle. In one study, involving 241 ovulatory cycles, 226 ovulations involved the primary follicle and only 15 ovulations involved a second and smaller follicle that was present at the onset of estrus.[12] Some follicles soften within 24 h prior to ovulation, others soften and become turgid again before ovulation, and others remain turgid prior to ovulation.[7,36] Sensitivity of the ovary to palpation shortly before and after

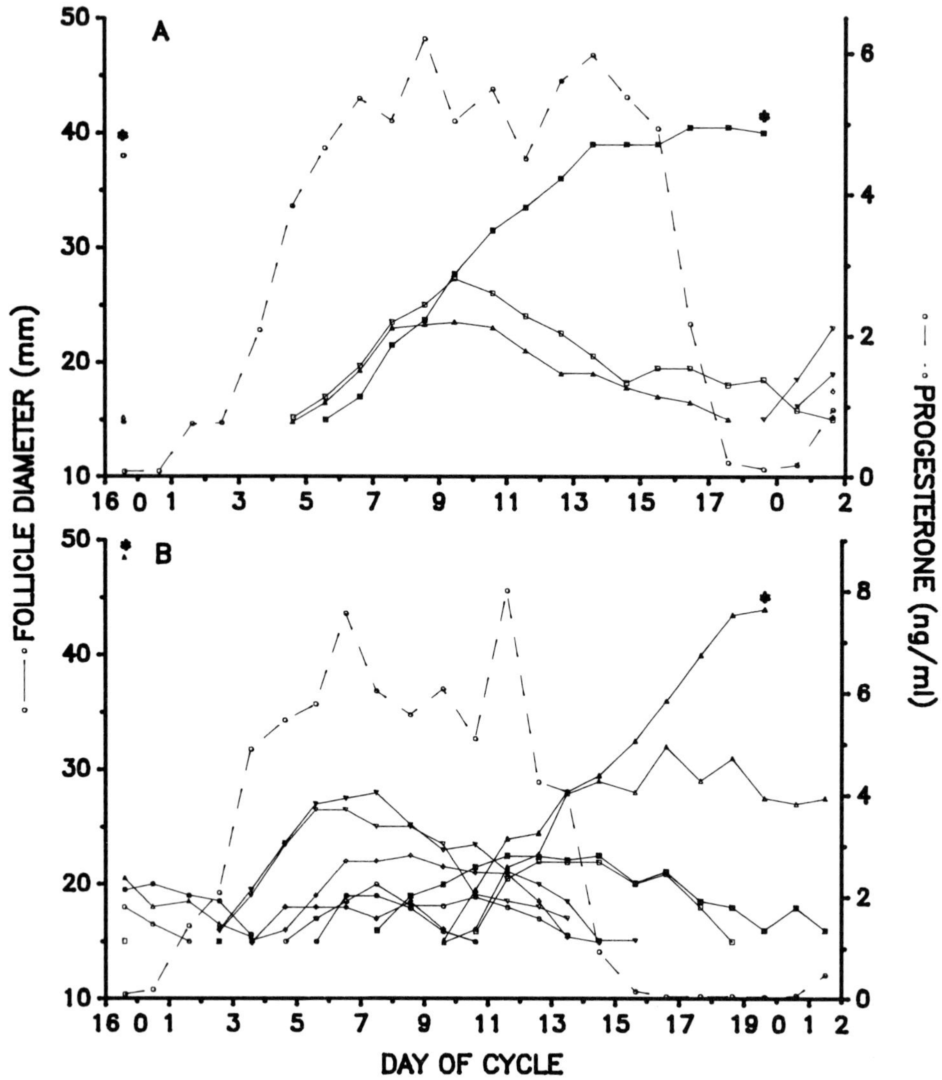

FIG. 14–2. Examples of the patterns of growth and regression of individual follicles (solid lines represent individual follicles in both ovaries) and plasma progesterone (dotted lines). *A*, A complete estrous cycle in a mare with one follicular wave. *B*, A complete estrous cycle in a mare with two follicular waves. The asterisk denotes an ovulatory follicle 1 day prior to ovulation. (Adapted from Sirois, J., Ball, B.A., and Fortune, J.E.: Patterns of growth and regression of ovarian follicles during the oestrous cycle and after hemiovariectomy in mares. Equine Vet. J. Suppl., *8*:43–48, 1989.)

ovulation may occur but is variable between mares.[12] The ovulatory follicle increases from an average size of 30 mm, 6 days prior to ovulation to ≥ 45 mm less than 24 h before ovulation[7,10,23,34,36,37] (Fig. 14-3). Ovulation of follicles as small as 30 mm and as large as 60 mm measured the day before ovulation has been reported. The preovulatory size of the follicle is influenced by season. In one study, the diameter of the follicle on the day before ovulation was significantly larger in April (46 mm) and May (48 mm) than in July (40 mm) (Fig. 14-4).[38] During the height of the breeding season, when the duration of estrus is shortest, it is not unusual for a mare in estrus for 3 to 4 days to ovulate a follicle less than 35 mm in diameter. More recently, these observations have been confirmed with ultrasonography.[11,23,34–36,39–43]

OVULATION

The evacuation of the follicle is a rapid process.[11,44] Ultrasonographic characterization of the ovulatory process suggests that the major portion of the follicular fluid disappears in less than 2 min.[11] Following ovulation, the cavity of the follicle begins to fill with blood and is usually easily palpable in 12 h as a soft, mushy structure termed the corpus hemorrhagicum. Usually within 2 to 2.5 days this structure has reached its maximum size. Its consistency changes from soft and spongy to rubbery and then becomes more liver-like with age. On occasion, the follicular cavity fills with blood to its preovulatory size and is indistinguishable from the original follicle by rectal palpation. This is the exception, however; most are distinguishable as corpora lutea. With

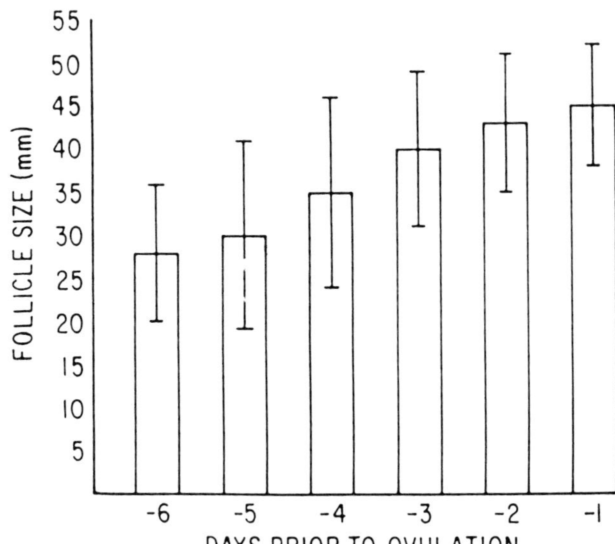

FIG. 14–3. Progressive change in the size of ovulatory follicles during the 6 days immediately prior to ovulation. (From Hughes, J.P., Stabenfeldt, G.H., and Evans, J.W.: Clinical and endocrine aspects of the estrous cycle of the mare. Proc. Am. Assoc. Equine Pract., 119–148, 1972.)

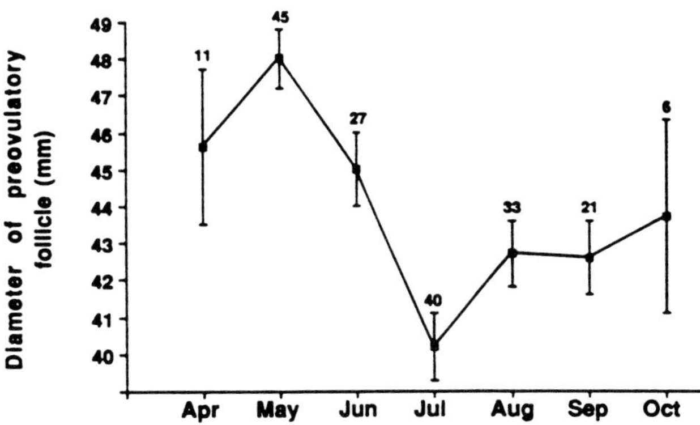

FIG. 14–4. Mean diameter of preovulatory follicle on day before ovulation for April through October. Number of observations is shown at the upper limit of each bar depicting the standard error of the mean (SEM). Diameters were significantly greater in May than in June, July, August, and September. (From Ginther, O.J., and Pierson, R.A.: Regular and irregular characteristics of ovulation and the interovulatory interval in mares. J. Equine Vet. Sci., *9*:4–12, 1989.)

the introduction of ultrasonography, the differentiation between follicle and corpus hemorrhagicum has become much easier (Chapter 31). Two morphologic types of corpora lutea, fluid-filled and non–fluid-filled, have been described using ultrasonography and occur with the same frequency.[45] Fluid-filled corpora lutea have a central nonechogenic cavity, but both types appear to have the same size luteal area and progesterone secretion is similar.[46]

Time of Ovulation

Ovulation is much more reliably associated with the end of behavioral estrus than with the beginning.[12] In one report, 78% of mares ovulated within 48 h before the end of estrus, 12% ovulated more than 48 h before the end of estrus, and 10% ovulated after the end of estrous behavior[12] (Table 14-2).

Ovulation appears to occur more frequently during the night. According to one study,[47] 23 out of 25 ovulations occurred between 11:00 p.m. and 7:00 a.m. In another study,[12] of 46 ovulations 39% occurred between 4:00 p.m. and 12:00 a.m., 37% between 12:00 a.m. and 8:00 a.m., and 24% between 8:00 a.m. and 4:00 p.m. (Fig. 14-5). However, in an experiment reported by Ginther et al., 17 ovulations occurred during the day and 13 during the night.[1]

Multiple Ovulation

The occurrence of double ovulations has been reported to vary from 4 to 44% and probably averages around 16% in mares.[17,22,38] The incidence of triple ovulations is small (< 1%).[22] Various factors such as, breed, genetic predisposition, and reproductive status have been reported to influence the incidence of multiple ovulation.[48] Thoroughbred, European Warmblood, and Draft mares have the highest incidence of multiple ovulations; Quarter Horse, Appaloosa, and pony mares have the lowest incidence; and Standardbred mares are in between.[48] There appears to be a tendency for multiple ovulation in some mares or family lines with some mares having double ovulations in more than 70% of their estrous cycles.[12,48] The incidence appears to increase with age and is influenced by season (highest incidence during March through May).[12,49] Double ovulations occur as frequently from the same as from opposite ovaries, and the preovulatory follicular size is similar for double ovulations that occur on the same or opposite ovaries.[48] However, Squires et al. reported a higher embryo recovery rate following bilateral ovulation compared with unilateral ovulations.[50] The average interval between double ovulations averages 1 day, with a range from 0 to 5 days.[7,12] Multiple ovulations do not appear to affect duration of the estrous cycle, estrus, or diestrus (Table 14-3), and progesterone concentrations are similar in mares with one or two corpora lutea.[12]

CYCLIC CHANGES IN THE TUBULAR GENITALIA

With the exception of the ovary, which is controlled by gonadotropins, changes in the remainder of the genital tract (oviduct, uterus, cervix, vagina, and vulva) are predominantly controlled by two classes of ovarian steroids: progesterone and estrogen.

UTERUS

Palpable changes in uterine tone are used clinically to determine the stage of the estrous cycle. During estrus, high estrogen concentrations in the absence of proges-

TABLE 14–2. DAY OF OVULATION IN RELATIONSHIP TO ESTRUS

DAY OF OVULATION FROM END OF ESTRUS	NUMBER OF OBSERVATIONS	PERCENT OF OVULATIONS
−3	42	11.9
−2	113	32.0
−1	162	45.9
0*	31	8.7
+1	4	1.1
+2	1	0.3
+3	0	0

*0 = First day of no sexual receptivity following estrus. Adapted from Hughes, J.P., Stabenfeldt, G.H., and Evans, J.W.: Clinical and endocrine aspects of the estrous cycle of the mare. Proc. Am. Assoc. Equine Pract., 119–148, 1972.

terone secretion cause the uterus to have only slight tone and tubularity. Edema of the uterus during estrus imparts a heavier feeling at that time.[5] Uterine, cervical, and vaginal secretions are abundant and watery. Within 1 to 3 days following ovulation, tone and tubularity increase to a stage interpreted as moderate tone and tubularity and the edema disappears. This is sometimes maintained until the next estrus, whereas in other mares it diminishes and then increases again just before estrus. Some mares develop a high degree of turgidity during diestrus, but this is usually only observed in pregnant mares. In other diestrous mares that still have ovarian activity (without ovulation) or that have a persistent CL, the uterus may maintain slight to moderate uterine tubularity and tone. Progesterone alone or in combination with estrogen causes the increase in uterine tone and decreases uterine edema.[51] Uterine, cervical, and vaginal secretions are scant and pasty when the mare is under progesterone influence. These gross changes are accompanied by histologic changes in the endometrium (Chapter 26).[52] During anestrus with little or no ovarian activity or in the absence of ovarian steroids as a result of ovariectomy the uterus loses its muscular tone and becomes nonedematous and flaccid.

CERVIX

Characteristic changes occur in the cervix during the estrous cycle.[5,7] Although there is considerable variation in the degree of change between mares, individual mares are fairly consistent. Just before or with the onset of estrus, the cervix begins a progressive softening and relaxation. As estrus progresses, the vaginal mucosa around the cervix becomes more hyperemic (pink), edema of the cervix increases, and the secretions passing through the cervix become more abundant and fluid in consistency. The greatest degree of cervical changes (in color, edema, and relaxation) occurs around ovulation, but because of variation between mares, these characteristics are unreliable as predictors of ovulation. Cervical relaxation and other cervical changes are induced by the presence of increasing con-

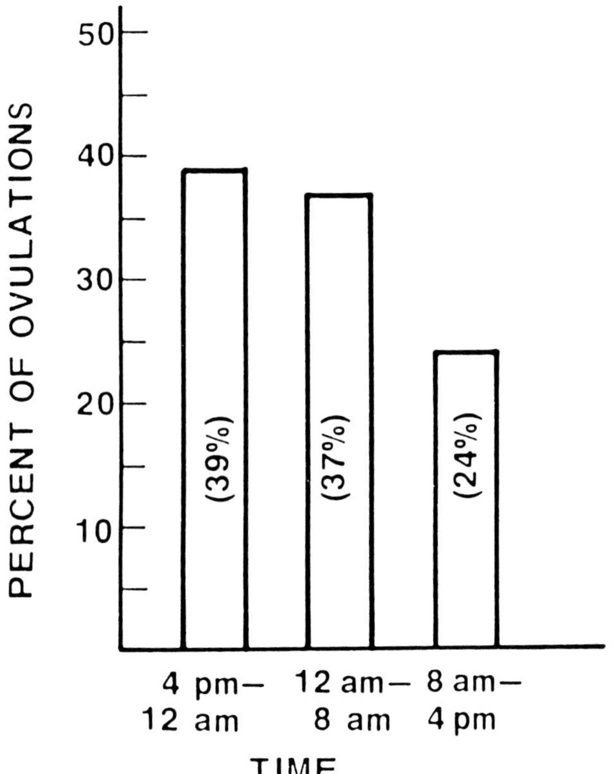

FIG. 14–5. The distribution of time of ovulation in mares as determined by rectal palpation at 8:00 a.m., 4:00 p.m., and 12:00 p.m. (n = 46). (Adapted from Hughes, J.P., Stabenfeldt, G.H., and Evans, J.W.: Estrous cycle and ovulation in the mare. J. Am. Vet. Med. Assoc., *161*:1367–1374, 1972.)

centrations of estrogen in the absence of progesterone. During diestrus, elevated progesterone levels cause the cervix to be tightly closed, paler in color with no edema, and covered with only a scant amount of viscous mucus. Similar to the uterus, anestrous mares with little or no ovarian activity (no active luteal tissue) may develop a flaccid cervix. On visual examination, the cervix may be closed or covered by the dorsal folds, but in some instances the cervix may be fully dilated allowing free access to the uterine lumen. Most mares in anestrus, however, have a tight cervix.

VAGINA AND VULVA

Changes observed in the vagina and vulva are consistent with those seen in the cervix and uterus. During estrus, the vagina becomes more relaxed and flaccid. The vulva is variable in its degree of relaxation and softening. Mares that suffer from moderate to severe pneumovagina are likely to have more pronounced signs during estrus. The vulva tends to become more edematous, and the ventral aspect can drop as much as 2.5 cm. Clear, stringy fluid lubricates the vagina, and sometimes excess fluid pools in its cranial vault. During diestrus, the vagina feels sticky and dry and the vulva is small and tightly closed. Vaginal mucosa is pale during diestrus and anestrus.

TABLE 14–3. ESTROUS CYCLE DATA ON MARES WITH ONE OR TWO OVULATIONS PER CYCLE

NUMBER OF OVULATIONS/ ESTROUS CYCLE	ESTROUS CYCLE DURATION (DAYS)	DURATION OF ESTRUS (DAYS)	CORPUS LUTEUM LIFE SPAN (DAYS)
1	18.7 ± 3.4* (12)	5.1 ± 1.9 (22)	12.6 ± 2.9 (18)
2	19.0 ± 3.0 (15)	6.0 ± 1.2 (10)	12.2 ± 3.3 (17)

*Mean ± standard deviation; number of observed cycles is in parentheses. (Adapted from Stabenfeldt, G.H., Hughes, J.P., and Evans, J.W.: Ovarian activity during the estrous cycle of the mare. Endocrinology, *90*:1379–1384, 1972.)

ENDOCRINE ASPECTS OF THE ESTROUS CYCLE

Hormones from the hypothalamus, pituitary, ovary, and uterus control the dynamic changes in the genital tract and sexual behavior through complex interactions. These include gonadotropin-releasing hormone (GnRH) from the hypothalamus, gonadotropins (follicle-stimulating hormone and luteinizing hormones) from the anterior pituitary, steroids (progesterone and estradiol) as well as peptide hormones (inhibin) from the ovary, and $PGF_2\alpha$ from the endometrium. The nature, source, and effect of these hormones have been discussed in detail in previous chapters.

GONADOTROPIN-RELEASING HORMONE

Modulation of reproductive activity by changing photoperiod is achieved through the regulation of gonadotropin-releasing hormone (GnRH) secretion. The pineal gland is thought to play an important role in bringing changing photoperiod information to the hypothalamus. The signal sent from the pineal gland involves the secretion of the pineal hormone melatonin (Chapter 11).[9,53] Although the link between increased photoperiod and GnRH secretion is still under speculation, it is clear that GnRH is the key stimulator of ovarian function. Gonadotropin-releasing hormone reaches the anterior pituitary via the hypothalamo-pituitary portal system and stimulates the synthesis and secretion of gonadotropins (luteinizing hormone and follicle-stimulating hormone), which in turn reach the ovary through the systemic circulation[54] (Fig. 14-6).

LUTEINIZING HORMONE

Concentrations of luteinizing hormone (LH) are persistently low from days 5 to 16 of the cycle (ovulation = day 0) and LH is believed to be the main luteotropic agent in the mare (Fig. 14-7). After luteolysis, levels increase slowly but progressively to reach maximum levels 2 days after ovulation and then decline progressively over the next 4 or 5 days to low diestrus values.[21,55–58] During diestrus, luteal progesterone secretion is maintained by basal LH concentrations. After luteolysis, the negative feedback of progesterone on pituitary LH secretion is removed and estrogen, secreted by the large follicles, preferentially stimulates LH secretion. In turn, LH stimulates development and maturation of the primary follicle and follicular estrogen secretion, thus creating a closed positive-feedback loop (Fig. 14-6).

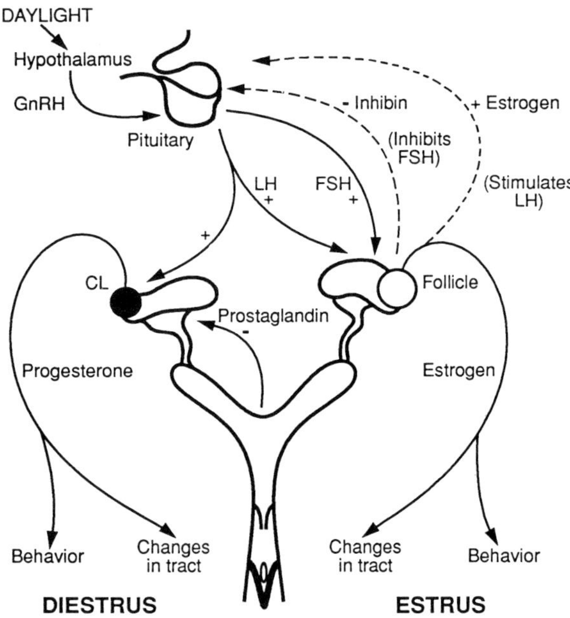

FIG. 14–6. Summary of the endocrinology of the estrous cycle. (Adapted from Rossdale, P.D., and Ricketts, S.W.: Equine Stud Farm Medicine. 2nd ed. Philadelphia, Lea & Febiger, 1980.)

The mare, in contrast to most other species investigated, does not show an acute preovulatory LH peak, resulting from a rapid surge in LH release. No obvious explanation exists for the duration of the LH rise in the mare. The persistence of high LH levels into the postovulatory period is believed to account for the relatively high incidence of double ovulations, with the second ovulation occurring as long as 4 days after the first.[17,57] Preovulatory growth and ovulation can occur in the presence of relatively low LH concentrations, i.e., diestrous levels.[57,59] This brings into question the exact role of LH during ovulation in the mare. It is likely that LH is important for ovulation in the mare but may be with a less-precise relationship than is usually observed in other domestic animals.[59] However, Alexander and Irvine reported that the levels of bioactive LH peak be-

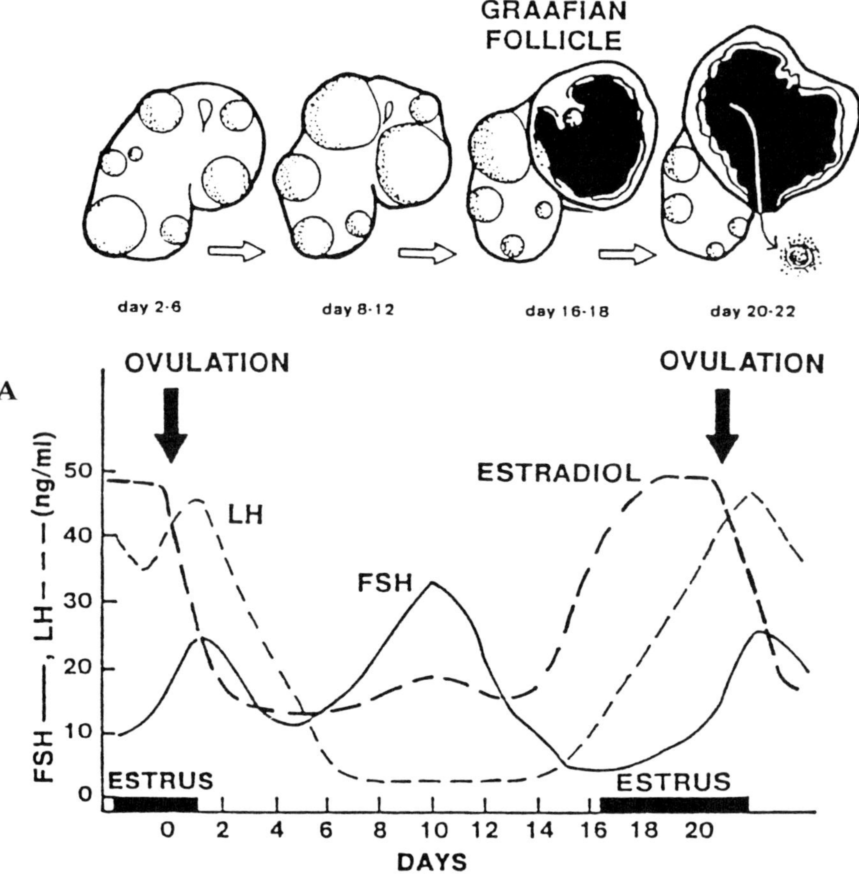

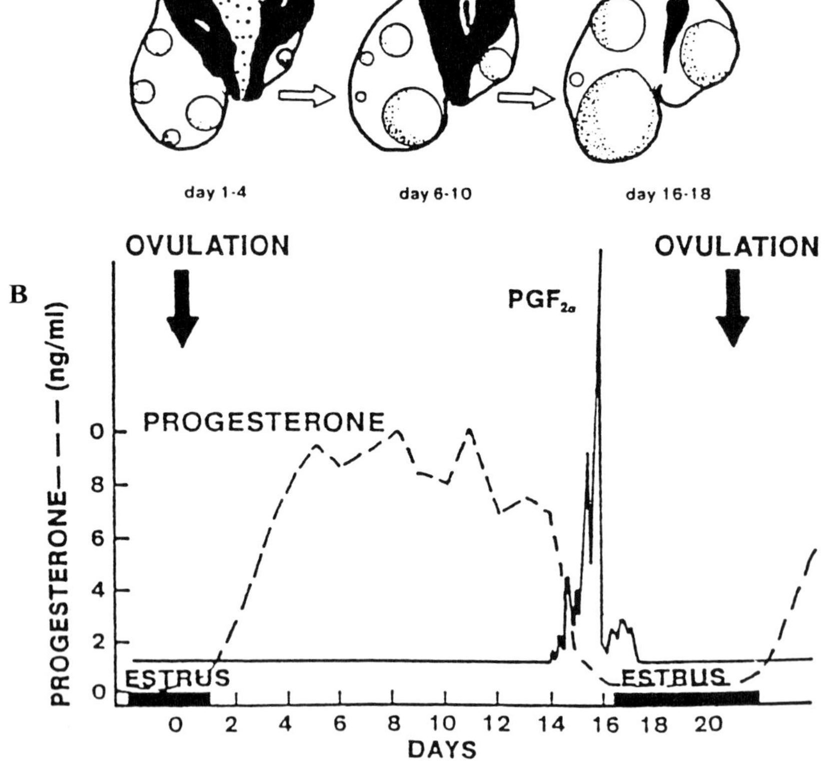

(Legend appears on facing page)

fore ovulation.[60] They suggested that changes in specific activity in the secreted LH, rather than concentrations of the immunoreactive LH, are the important criteria (Chapter 5).

FOLLICLE-STIMULATING HORMONE

The secretion of follicle-stimulating hormone (FSH) during the estrous cycle is biphasic with surges at 10- to 12-day intervals (Chapter 5). Peak values are reached at the end of estrus, just after ovulation and during the mid- to late luteal phase, approximately 10 days before the next ovulation[56] (Fig. 14-7). FSH supports the continued growth of small follicles and stimulates follicular estrogen secretion. Secretion of FSH is lowest during early estrus because of the secretion of inhibin-like proteins by the graafian follicle, which inhibits the secretion of FSH but not LH (Chapter 5).[61] Progesterone has a negative-feedback effect on LH, but not on FSH, secretion. Increasing FSH secretion during late diestrus is the main stimulus for follicular development. As the growing follicle reaches the preovulatory stage it produces protein hormones (presumably inhibin) that inhibit pituitary FSH secretion (Fig. 14-6). The inhibitory action on FSH combined with the stimulatory effect of estrogen on LH secretion creates the environment required for the final maturation of the graafian follicle (high LH secretion) and prevents further development of immature follicles (low FSH secretion).

ESTROGEN

Follicular estrogen secretion reaches a peak 1 or 2 days before ovulation.[2,20,24,26,58,62–66] After ovulation, estrogen concentration decreases to reach baseline diestrous levels within 2 days. Similar to other species, the horse experiences a surge of estrogen of follicular origin, which seems to initiate the LH release that leads to ovulation. When using conjugated estrogens in urine as a parameter for ovarian estrogen secretion, a second surge in estrogen secretion may occur during diestrus.[26,63,67] The many midsize follicles that are present during the luteal phase may contribute to the rise of the total estrogen pool during diestrus. At the end of diestrus, these follicles undergo atresia, which could account for the decrease in estrogen levels at the time of luteolysis.[63,67] Recent studies suggest that the CL may also be a (minor) contributor to the diestrus estrogen rise.[59,63,68]

Estrogen concentrations, during estrus, have been shown to correlate well with ovarian activity, sexual receptivity, and grossly observable changes in the reproductive tract. In the absence of progesterone (concentrations < 1 ng/mL), estrogen secreted by the preovulatory follicle induces sexual receptivity; induces relaxation of the cervix and vulva; stimulates secretions from the uterus, cervix, and vagina; allows passage and transport of semen; and plays a role in follicular maturation and ovulation.

PROGESTERONE

During estrus, progesterone concentrations in plasma are below 1 ng/mL. After ovulation, progesterone concentration increases rapidly to maximal values within 6 days, remains high during the luteal phase (6 to 10 ng/mL), and declines rapidly following regression of the CL around day 14 or 15[7,17,69,70] (Figs. 14-7B and 14-8). Progesterone inhibits estrous behavior, brings about closure of the cervix, and prepares the uterus for support of pregnancy. The effects of progesterone on behavior and morphologic characteristics of the cervix and uterus are dominant over the effects of estrogen. As discussed earlier, progesterone inhibits the preovulatory LH surge. However, in contrast to many other species, in the mare progesterone does not completely inhibit folliculogenesis and ovulation. Thus, during the luteal phase, follicles may continue to grow and ovulate in the face of elevated progesterone concentrations (Chapter 16).

FIG. 14–7. Summary of hormonal and ovarian changes throughout the estrous cycle of the mare. *A*, Diagram of follicular development and ovulation in the mare in relationship to peripheral concentrations of FSH, LH, and estradiol during the normal 21-day estrous cycle. *B*, Diagram of CL development and regression in relationship to peripheral concentrations of progesterone and $PGF_{2}\alpha$ during the normal 21-day estrous cycle. The vertical arrows represent ovulation and the horizontal bars indicate estrous behavior. Day 0 is the day of ovulation. The concentrations of estradiol and $PGF_{2}\alpha$ are not given, because significant variation in concentrations exists in the literature. CH = corpus hemorrhagicum, CL = corpus luteum, CA = corpus albicans (or regressing CL). (Adapted from Noden, P.A., Oxender, W.D., and Hafs, H.D.: The cycle of oestrus, ovulation and plasma levels of hormones in the mare. J. Reprod. Fertil. Suppl., 23:189–192, 1975; Oxender, W.D., Noden, P.A., Hafs, H.D.: Estrus, ovulation, and serum progesterone, estradiol and LH concentrations in mares after increased photoperiod during winter. Am. J. Vet. Res., *38*:203–207, 1977; Irvine, C.H.G.: Endocrinology of the estrous cycle of the mare: Applications to embryo transfer. Theriogenology, *15*:85–104, 1981; Neely, D.P.:Studies on the control of luteal function and prostaglandin release in the mare. Ph.D. thesis. University of California, Davis, 1979; and Neely, D.P., et al.: Prostaglandin release patterns in the mare: Physiological, pathophysiological, and therapeutic responses. J. Reprod. Fertil. Suppl., 27:181–189, 1979.)

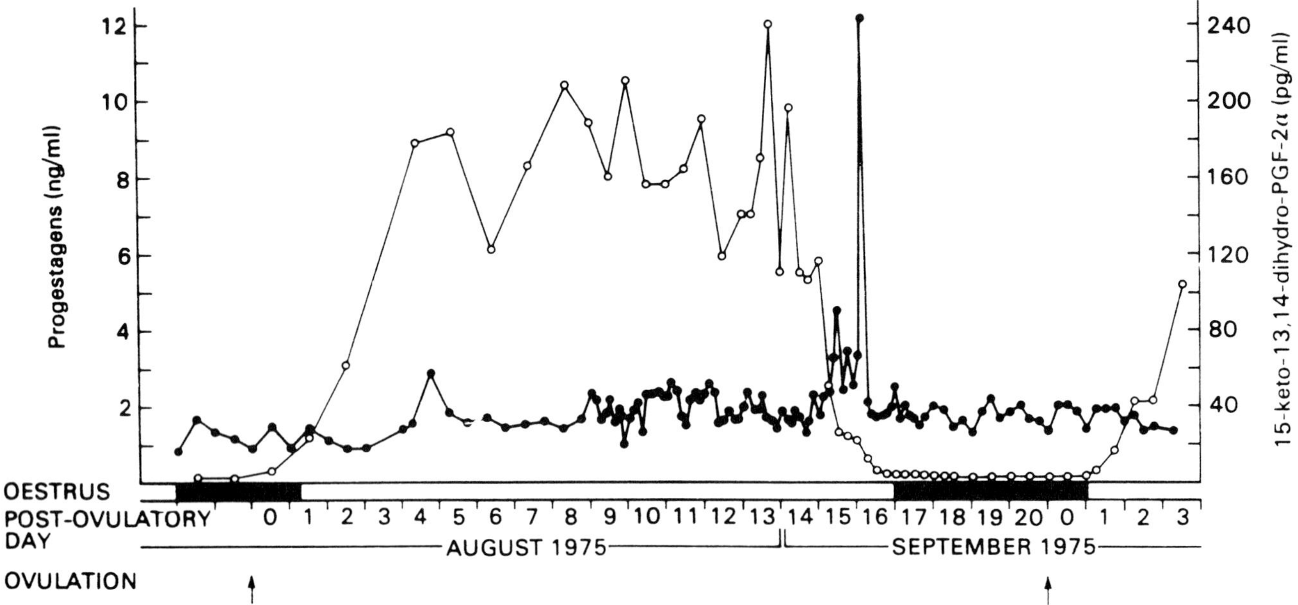

FIG. 14–8. Peripheral plasma concentrations of 13, 14-dihydro-15-keto-$PGF_2\alpha$ (filled circle) and progestagens (open circle) during a normal estrous cycle. Vertical arrows indicate ovulation and horizontal bars mark estrus. (Adapted from Neely, D.P. et al.: Prostaglandin release patterns in the mare: Physiological, pathophysiological, and therapeutic responses. J. Reprod. Fertil. Suppl., *27*:181–189, 1979).

PROSTAGLANDIN

Prostaglandin $F_2\alpha$ is recognized as the primary luteolytic agent in the mare.[5,71–77] In nonpregnant mares, the life span of the CL is controlled by release of $PGF_2\alpha$ from the uterus between days 13 and 16 after ovulation. Functional luteolysis measured by a decline of progesterone concentration, occurs over approximately 40 h. The first release of $PGF_2\alpha$ precedes the first decline in progesterone concentrations by about 4 h and is followed by additional more-substantial releases of $PGF_2\alpha$ during and following luteolysis[71,74] (Fig. 14-8).

REFERENCES

1. Ginther, O.J., Whitmore, H.L., and Squires, E.L.: Characteristics of estrus, diestrus, and ovulation in mares and effects of season and nursing. Am. J. Vet. Res., *33*:1935–1939, 1972.
2. Hughes, J.P., Stabenfeldt, G.H., and Evans, J.W.: Estrous cycle and ovulation in the mare. J. Am. Vet. Med. Assoc., *161*:1367–1374, 1972.
3. Ginther, O.J.: Occurrence of anestrous, estrus, diestrus, and ovulation over a twelve-month period in mares. Am. J. Vet. Res., *35*:1173–1179, 1974.
4. Belonje, P.C. and van Niekerk, C.H.: A review of the influence of nutrition upon the oestrous cycle and early pregnancy in the mare. J. Reprod. Fertil. Suppl., *23*:167–169, 1975.
5. Hughes, J.P., Stabenfeldt, G.H., and Evans, J.W.: The oestrous cycle of the mare and its uterine control. Aust. Vet. J., *53*:415–419, 1977.
6. Hughes, J.P., Stabenfeldt, G.H., and Evans, J.W.: The oestrous cycle of the mare. J. Reprod. Fertil. Suppl., *23*:161–166, 1975.
7. Hughes, J.P., Stabenfeldt, G.H., and Kennedy, P.C.: The estrous cycle and selected functional and pathologic ovarian abnormalities in the mare. Vet. Clin. North Am., *2*:225–239, 1980.
8. Colquhoun, K.M., Eckersall, P.D., Renton, J.P., and Douglas, T.A.: Control of breeding in the mare. Equine Vet. J., *19*:138–142, 1987.
9. Sharp, D.C.: Transition into the breeding season: Clues to the mechanisms of seasonality. Equine Vet. J., *20*: 159–161, 1988.
10. Ginther, O.J.: Folliculogenesis during the transitional period and early ovulatory season in mares. J. Reprod. Fertil. Suppl., *90*:311–320, 1990.
11. Townson, D.H., and Ginther, O.J.: Ultrasonic characterization of follicular evacuation during ovulation and fate of the discharged follicular fluid in mares. Anim. Reprod. Sci., *20*:131–141, 1989.
12. Hughes, J.P., Stabenfeldt, G.H., and Evans, J.W.:Clinical and endocrine aspects of the estrous cycle of the mare. Proc. Am. Assoc. Equine Pract., 119–148, 1972.
13. Hughes, J.P., Couto, M.A., and Stabenfeldt, G.H.: Luteal phase ovulations: What are the options? Proc. Soc. Theriogenol., pp. 123–125, 1985.
14. Hughes, J.P., and Stabenfeldt, G.H.: Conception in a mare with an active corpus luteum. J. Am. Vet. Med. Assoc., *170*:733–734, 1977.
15. Vandeplassche, M., Henry, M., and Coryn, M.: The mature mid-cycle follicle in the mare. J. Reprod. Fertil. Suppl., *27*:157–162, 1979.
16. Andrews, F.M., and McKenzie, F.F.: Estrus, ovulation and related phenomena in the mare. Univ. Missouri Res. Bull., p. 329, 1941.
17. Stabenfeldt, G.H., Hughes, J.P., and Evans, J.W.: Ovarian

activity during the estrous cycle of the mare. Endocrinology, *90*:1379–1384, 1972.

18. Back, D.G., Pickett, B.W., Voss, J.L., and Seidel, G.E., Jr.: Observations on the sexual behavior of nonlactating mares. J. Am. Vet. Med. Assoc., *165*:717–720, 1974.

19. Stabenfeldt, G.H., Hughes, J.P., Evans, J.W., and Geschwind, I.I.: Unique aspects of the reproductive cycle of the mare. J. Reprod. Fertil. Suppl., *23*:155–160, 1975.

20. Hillman, R.B., and Loy, R.G.: Oestrogen excretion in mares in relation to various reproductive states. J. Reprod. Fertil. Suppl., *23*:223–230, 1975.

21. Noden, P.A., Oxender, W.D., and Hafs, H.D.: The cycle of oestrus, ovulation and plasma levels of hormones in the mare. J. Reprod. Fertil. Suppl., *23*:189–192, 1975.

22. Ginther, O.J.: Reproductive Biology of the Mare: Basic and Applied Aspects. Ann Arbor, McNaughton, Gunn, 1979.

23. Pierson, R.A., and Ginther, O.J.: Follicular population dynamics during the estrous cycle of the mare. Anim. Reprod. Sci., *14*:219–231, 1987.

24. Palmer, E., and Jousset, B.: Urinary oestrogen and plasma progesterone levels in non-pregnant mares. J. Reprod. Fertil. Suppl., *23*:213–221, 1975.

25. Satoh, S., and Hoshi, S.: Studies on the reproduction in the mare. III The oestrous duration and oestrous cycle. J. Jpn. Soc. Vet. Sci., *12*:237–250, 1934.

26. Palmer, E., and Terqui, M.: The measurement of total plasma oestrogens during the follicular phase of the mare's oestrous cycle. Theriogenology, *7*:331–338, 1977.

27. Sirois, J., Ball, B.A., and Fortune, J.E.: Patterns of growth and regression of ovarian follicles during the oestrous cycle and after hemiovariectomy in mares. Equine Vet. J. Suppl., *8*:43–48, 1989.

28. Vandeplassche, G., Wesson, J.A., and Ginther, O.J.: Behavioral, follicular and gonadotropin changes during the estrous cycle in donkeys. Theriogenology, *16*:239–249, 1981.

29. Ginther, O.J., Scraba, S.T., and Bergfelt, D.R.: Reproductive seasonality of the jenney. Theriogenology, *27*:587–592, 1987.

30. Henry, M., Figueiredo, A.E.F., Palhares, M.S., and Coryn, M.: Clinical and endocrine aspects of the oestrus cycle in donkeys (Equus asinus). J. Reprod. Fertil. Suppl., *35*:297–303, 1987.

31. King, J.M.: A field guide to reproduction of the Grant's zebra and Grevy's zebra. East Afr. Wildlife J., *3*99–117, 1961.

32. Monfort, S.L., Arthur, N.P., and Wildt, D.E.: Monitoring ovarian function and pregnancy by evaluating excretion of urinary oestrogen conjugates in semi-free-ranging Przewalski's horses (Equus przewalskii). J. Reprod. Fertil., *91*:155–164, 1991.

33. Fortune, J.E., and Sirois, J.: Ovarian follicular dynamics during the estrous cycle in heifers monitored by real-time ultrasonography. Biol. Reprod., *39*:308–317, 1988.

34. Palmer, E.: New results on follicular growth and ovulation in the mare. *In* Follicular Growth and Ovulation Rate in Farm Animals. Edited by J.F. Roche and D. O'Callaghan. Dordrecht, Martinus Nijhoff, 237–255, 1987.

35. Ginther, O.J.: Follicular dynamics in heifers and mares. Proc. Soc. Theriogenol., pp. 2–12, 1989.

36. Townson, D.H., and Ginther, O.J.: Size and shape changes in the preovulatory follicle in mares based on the digital analysis of ultrasonic images. Anim. Reprod. Sci., *21*:63–71, 1989.

37. Pierson, R.A., and Ginther, O.J.: Ultrasonic evaluation of the preovulatory follicle in the mare. Theriogenology, *24*:359–368, 1985.

38. Ginther, O.J., and Pierson, R.A.: Regular and irregular characteristics of ovulation and the interovulatory interval in mares. J. Equine. Vet. Sci., *9*:4–12, 1989.

39. McKinnon, A.O., Squires, E.L., and Voss, J.L.: Ultrasonic evaluation of the mare's reproductive tract. I. Compend. Contin. Education Practicing Vet., *9*:336–345, 1987.

40. Kahn, W., and Leidl, W.: Sonography of ovarian activity in mares. Gynakol. Tierklinik. Koniginstr., *42*:257–266, 1987.

41. Squires, E.L., McKinnon, A.O., and Shideler, R.K.: Use of ultrasonography in reproductive management of mares. Theriogenology, *29*:55–70, 1988.

42. McKinnon, A.O., Squires, E.L., and Shideler, R.K.: Diagnostic ultrasonography of the mare's reproductive tract. J. Equine. Vet. Sci., *8*:329–333, 1988.

43. Ginther, O.J.: Ultrasonic imaging of equine ovarian follicles and corpora lutea. Vet. Clin. North Am. Equine Pract., *4*:197–213, 1988.

44. Carnevale, E.M., McKinnon, A.O., Squires, E.L., and Voss, J.L.: Ultrasonographic characteristics of the preovulatory follicle preceding and during ovulation in mares. J. Equine. Vet. Sci., *8*:428–431, 1988.

45. Townson, D.H., and Ginther, O.J.: Ultrasonic echogenicity of developing corpora lutea in pony mares. Anim. Reprod. Sci., *20*:143–153, 1989.

46. Townson, D.H., Pierson, R.A., and Ginther, O.J.: Characterization of plasma progesterone concentrations for two distinct luteal morphologies in mares. Theriogenology, *32*:197–204, 1989.

47. Witherspoon, D.M., and Talbot, R.B.: Nocturnal ovulation in the equine animal. Vet. Rec., *87*:302–304, 1970.

48. Ginther, O.J., Douglas, R.H., and Lawrence, J.R.: Twinning in mares: A survey of veterinarians and analyses of theriogenology records. Theriogenology, *18*:333–347, 1982.

49. Squires, E.L., Stevens, W.B., Pickett, B.W., and Nett, T.M.: Role of pregnant mare serum gonadotropin in luteal function of pregnant mares. Am. J. Vet. Res., *40*:889–891, 1979.

50. Squires, E.L., McClain, M.G., Ginther, O.J., and McKinnon, A.O.: Spontaneous multiple ovulation in the mare and its effect on the incidence of twin embryo collections. Theriogenology, *28*:609–613, 1987.

51. Hayes, K.E.N., and Ginther, O.J.: Role of progesterone and estrogen in development of uterine tone in mares. Theriogenology, *25*:581–589, 1985.

52. Kenney, R.M.: Cyclic and pathologic changes of the mare endometrium as detected by biopsy, with a note on early embyronic death. J. Am. Vet. Med. Assoc., *172*:241–262, 1978.

53. Kilmer, D.M., et al.: Melatonin rhythms in pony mares and foals. J. Reprod. Fertil. Suppl., *32*:303–307, 1982.

54. Evans, M.J., and Irvine, C.H.G.: Measurement of equine follicle stimulating hormone and luteinizing hormone: Response of anestrous mares to gonadotropin releasing hormone. Biol. Reprod., *15*:477–484, 1976.

55. Oxender, W.D., Noden, P.A., and Hafs, H.D.: Estrus, ovulation, and serum progesterone, estradiol and LH concentrations in mares after increased photoperiod during winter. Am. J. Vet. Res., *38*:203–207, 1977.

56. Evans, M.J., and Irvine, C.H.G.: Serum concentrations of FSH, LH and progesterone during the oestrous cycle and early pregnancy in a mare. J. Reprod. Fertil. Suppl., *23*:193–200, 1975.

57. Geschwind, I.I., et al.: Plasma LH levels in the mare during the oestrous cycle. J. Reprod. Fertil. Suppl., *23*:207–212, 1975.

58. Pattison, M.L., Chen, C.L., Kelley, S.T., and Brandt, G.W.: Luteinizing hormone and estradiol in peripheral blood of mares during estrous cycle. Biol. Reprod., *11*:245–250, 1974.
59. Montavon, S.M., et al.: The effect of a potent GnRH agonist on gonadal and sexual activity in the horse. Theriogenology, *33*:1305–1321, 1990.
60. Alexander, S., and Irvine, C.H.G.: Radioimmunoassay and in-vitro bioassay of serum LH throughout the equine oestrous cycle. J. Reprod. Fertil. Suppl., *32*:253–260, 1982.
61. Bergfelt, D.R., and Ginther, O.J.: Delayed follicular development and ovulation following inhibition of FSH with equine follicular fluid in the mare. Theriogenology, *24*:99–108, 1985.
62. Pattison, M.L., Chen, C.L., and King, S.L.:Determination of LH and estradiol-17β surge with reference to the time of ovulation in mares. Biol. Reprod., *7*:136, 1972.
63. Daels, P.F., et al.: Urinary and plasma estrogen conjugates, estradiol and estrone concentrations in nonpregnant and early pregnant mares. Theriogenology, *35*:1001–1017, 1991.
64. Knudsen, O. and Velle, W.: Ovarian estrogen levels in the nonpregnant mare: Relationship to histological appearance of the uterus and to clinical status. J. Reprod. Fertil., *2*:130–137, 1961.
65. Terqui, M., and Palmer, E.: Oestrogen pattern during early pregnancy in the mare. J. Reprod. Fertil. Suppl., *27*:441–446, 1979.
66. Plotka, E.D., et al.: Periovulatory changes in peripheral plasma progesterone and estrogen concentrations in the mare. Am. J. Vet. Res., *36*:1359–1362, 1975.
67. Lasley, B., et al.: Estrogen conjugate concentrations in plasma and urine reflect estrogen secretion in the nonpregnant and pregnant mare: A review. J. Equine. Vet. Sci., *10*:444–448, 1990.
68. Daels, P.F., et al.: The corpus luteum: Source of oestrogen during early pregnancy in the mare. J. Reprod. Fertil., Suppl., *44*:501–508, 1991.
69. Plotka, E.D., Witherspoon, D.M., and Foley, C.W.: Luteal function in the mare as reflected by progesterone concentrations in peripheral blood plasma. Am. J. Vet. Res., *33*:917–920, 1972.
70. Stabenfeldt, G.H., et al.: Endogenous and exogenous manipulation of the corpus luteum of the mare. In Twenty-eighth International Congress of Physiological Sciences. Edited by G. Pethes and V.L. Frenyo. Budapest, Pergamon Press, pp. 133–139, 1981.
71. Neely, D.P., et al.: Prostaglandin release patterns in the mare: Physiological, pathophysiological, and therapeutic responses. J. Reprod. Fertil. Suppl., *27*:181–189, 1979.
72. Stabenfeldt, G.H., et al.: The role of the uterus in ovarian control in the mare. J. Reprod. Fertil., *37*:343–351, 1974.
73. Stabenfeldt, G.H., et al.: Physiologic and pathophysiologic aspects of Prostaglandin $F_2\alpha$ during the reproductive cycle. J. Am. Vet. Med. Assoc., *176*:1187–1194, 1980.
74. Stabenfeldt, G.H., et al.: Control of luteolysis in the mare. Acta Vet. Scand. Suppl., *77*:159–170, 1981.
75. Daels, P.F., Stabenfeldt, G.H., Kindahl, H., and Hughes, J.P.: Prostaglandin release and luteolysis associated with physiological and pathological conditions of the reproductive tract in the mare: A review. Equine Vet. J. Suppl., *8*:29–34, 1989.
76. Douglas, R.H., and Ginther, O.J.: Concentration of prostaglandin F in uterine venous plasma of anesthesized mares during estrous cycle and early pregnancy. Prostaglandins, *11*:251–260, 1976.
77. Ginther, O.J., and First, N.L.: Maintenance of the corpus luteum in hysterectomized mares. Am. J. Vet. Res., *32*:1687–1691, 1971.

CHAPTER 15

VERNAL TRANSITION

D.C. Sharp
S.D. Davis

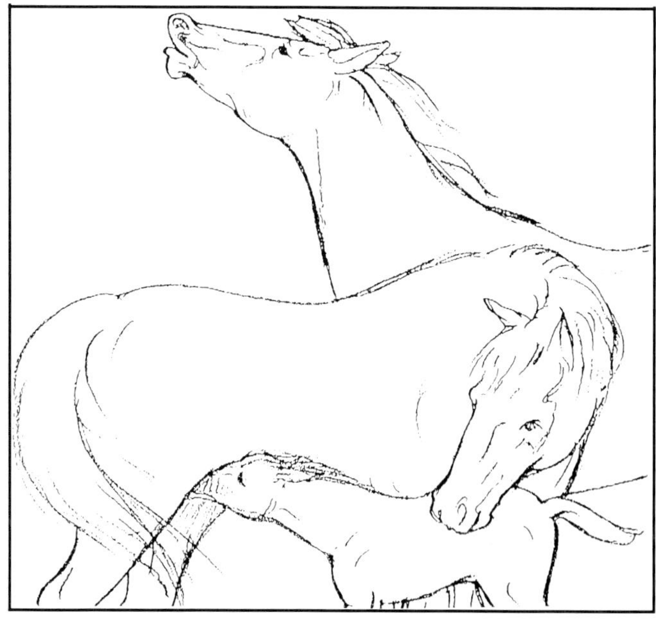

ANNUAL REPRODUCTIVE CYCLE

BREEDING SEASON

The breeding season, which runs from approximately April through October, in the Northern hemisphere, is the time of year characterized by sexual competence in mares and stallions. The relatively long period of sexual competence often surprises breeders who are used to thinking of the breeding season ending in June, but it must be remembered that that date is an artificial one, created by humans. Mares are "polyestrous" during the breeding season, meaning that they display repeated periods of estrus and diestrus if not bred, and this period is characterized by all the behavioral, hormonal, and morphologic changes described in this book.

AUTUMNAL TRANSITION INTO ANESTRUS

Although the autumnal transition period of the annual reproductive cycle is less well defined, it may be thought of as the time between complete sexual competence and anestrus. During that time, mares may undergo some follicular development, but the follicles do not ovulate. Ginther reported that mares during transition into anestrus may have fluctuations in follicle-stimulating hormone (FSH) but that the ovulatory surge of luteinizing hormone (LH) is absent, likely accounting for the ovulatory failure.[1] This transitional period is poorly understood for two reasons: (1) there has been little research done on that time of the annual reproductive cycle and (2) it is more difficult to study mechanisms regulating the phenomenon because transition into anestrus appears to be less rigidly controlled than the vernal transition and the time course of events shows greater variation among mares when compared with events of the vernal transition. Thus the standard deviation about the date of the last ovulation of the year is considerably greater than the standard deviation about the date of the first ovulation of the year, a situation that complicates research because changes within individual mares are potentially confounded in time when compared with other mares in an experiment. That caveat notwithstanding, however, the apparent failure of LH secretion is in agreement with the hypothesis that seasonal factors act to diminish gonadotropin-releasing hormone (GnRH) secretion, LH synthesis and secretion, or a combination of the two. The result is the beginning of the functional hypothalamic-pituitary decline that characterizes the anestrous period.

ANESTRUS

Anestrus is the period of sexual incompetence, indeed of sexual indifference, within the annual reproductive cycle and occurs during winter months (November to January) in the Northern Hemisphere. During anestrus, the hypothalamic-pituitary axis becomes essentially nonfunctional, with hypothalamic GnRH content and secretory rate declining to near zero.[2–4] Sharp and Grubaugh[4] measured GnRH secretion using push-pull perfusion, a technique in which GnRH can be assessed directly in the hypothalamus, or in the pituitary.[5] Using this technique during the months of November and December, the majority of pony mares tested did not have detectable GnRH secretion.[4] These results agreed well with the observations of reduced hypothalamic GnRH[2,3]and strongly suggest that the primary failure within the hypothalamic-pituitary axis is failure of GnRH secretion. Perhaps, as a result of reduced GnRH secretion, pituitary LH content declines during anestrus,[6] although the cause of reduced pituitary LH content is not yet established. Because of the reduced pituitary LH stores, a single challenge dose of GnRH administered during anestrus results in a greatly reduced LH response when compared with similar doses administered during vernal transition or during the breeding season.[7,8] On the other hand, pituitary FSH content does not change throughout the year suggesting that mechanisms regulating LH and FSH synthesis and storage are different.[3] Although during anestrus pituitary LH content is reduced and FSH content is not, neither hormone is secreted into the peripheral circulation, most likely because of the lack of GnRH secretion.

In concert with the reduced circulating gonadotropins, ovarian activity declines and folliculogenesis is essentially arrested. Ultrasonographic examination of mares in deep winter anestrus reveals only one or two follicles with a diameter of 10 to 15 mm. In addition to the relative absence of follicles, measurements of ovarian dimensions grossly at rectal palpation suggest that the ovaries become smaller during anestrus. As would be expected, attempts to measure peripherally circulating estrogens or progesterone are usually met with non-detectable levels.[9–11]

Behaviorally, anestrous mares range from positive to indifferent to negative in regard to a stallion, all of which suggests that the broad range of behaviors is indicative of a lack of hormone stimulus. Ginther described an objective method of observing sexual behavior in mares in which an operator records actual behaviors (such as raising the tail, kicking, etc.).[1] One of the behavioral signs reported was the relative tolerance of a mare to being mounted by a stallion, but still refusing intromission by clamping the tail tightly down. He labeled this behavior "down," and as can be seen in Figure 15-1, anestrous mares displayed this behavioral sign with the greatest frequency during anestrus and vernal transition (Sharp, D.C.: Unpublished observations). Because mares displaying this sign do little else to object to the stallion's presence, it is a sign of passivity, and its greater frequency during anestrus points out the relative lack of strongly motivated behaviors, such as active acceptance of the stallion or active rejection. Although it is not clear that sexual behavior in mares emanates solely from circulating steroid hormones, it seems reasonable to speculate that the relatively passive behavior of anestrous mares reflects the absence of hormonal guidelines. The relatively passive sign (indifferent) occurs with greater frequency during anestrus and vernal transition, whereas two signs that appear to reflect a more active role on the part of the mare appear with greater frequency during the vernal transition and breeding season.

Pelage changes during the annual reproductive cycle are of interest, in addition to the changes in behavior, hormonal concentrations, and structure during the annual reproductive cycle. During anestrus, the coat becomes long and shaggy. Measurements of hair length in pony mares indicate that the hair coat may reach an average length of 30 mm.[12] In addition to the length of hair, it is firmly attached. It may come as a surprise to some that these changes in hair coat are mediated by changes in day length, not temperature, as are the reproductive changes (chapter 19). In addition, nutritional status can influence onset of the breeding season to some extent, primarily acceleration of the time of onset in mares that are gaining weight during the late winter and spring,[1] but this serves only as a moderation of the major impeller of seasonal rhythms: photoperiod.

VERNAL TRANSITION

Of the four phases of the annual reproductive cycle of mares, vernal transition may be the most significant, for several reasons. Vernal transition from anestrus into the breeding season is a time of highly ambiguous signals from mares. This fact combined with the pressure on breeders and veterinary practitioners to get mares in foal early in the year results in reproductive inefficiency as well as great frustration. However, vernal transition need not be so frustrating or inefficient, because it proceeds through a series of events that are reasonably consistent and reliable, and the practitioner or breeder who takes time to monitor mares in vernal transition closely will have more success.

The vernal transition is a time of renewed sexual function, characterized by renewed follicular development on the ovaries, onset of estrous behavior, and renewed secretion of pituitary gonadotropins and ovarian hormones. Throughout most of the transition phase, as will be pointed out in the following section, mares remain anovulatory, despite consecutive development of several large ($>$ 30 mm) follicles. The presence of large, albeit anovulatory, follicles and strong estrous behavior are ambiguous signs that can confuse and confound the breeder and veterinarian alike. Furthermore, to add to the confusion, not all horse mares become anestrous during the winter, although the majority (80%) of them do so.[12] Most pony mares, on the other hand, undergo a complete winter anestrus.[12] Therefore, the breeder faced with a mare in estrus and presenting a large follicle on one ovary must first know whether the mare has indeed been cycling (ovulating) previously and, therefore, might ovulate, or whether it is in the transitional phase and not likely to ovulate spontaneously.

Of critical importance to the breeder and scientist is the observation that the time course of the transition into the breeding season is remarkably consistent, per-

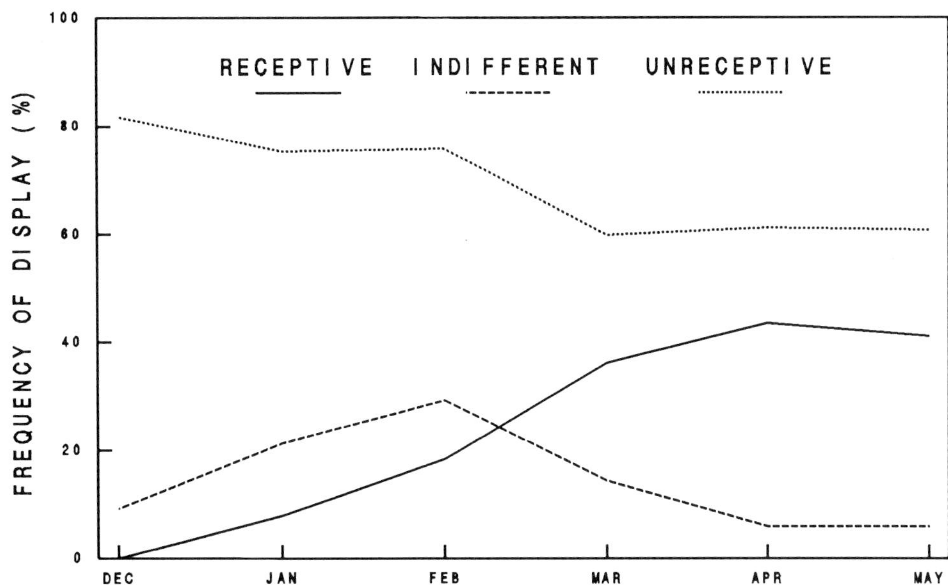

FIG. 15–1. Behavioral patterns of mares throughout the year. Frequency of occurrence of three major behavioral signs in response to teasing by a stallion—receptive (elevated tail while being mounted by a stallion), indifferent (acceptance of stallion mounting, but with tail clamped down to prevent intromission), and nonreceptive (active rejection of stallion's advances)—are shown by month. The relatively passive sign (indifferent) occurs with greater frequency during anestrus and vernal transition, whereas two signs which appear to reflect a more active role on the part of the mare appear with greater frequency during the vernal transition and breeding season.

haps the most consistent of the four phases of the annual reproductive cycle. Dates of the first ovulation of the year in pony mares did not vary over a 5-yr period, regardless of indigenous weather over the observation period.[12] Breeding records from a major Thoroughbred farm in the Ocala, FL area were examined over a 14-yr period. It was apparent, based on retrospective examination of dates of foaling, that the majority of mares were not bred until early April. This coincides well with research in Florida with Thoroughbred and Quarter Horse mares, in which the mean (± SEM) date of the first ovulation of the year was April 7 ± 9.1. This supports the idea that date of first ovulation of the year is highly regulated in mares, by some presumably external factor that varies little from year to year.

This fact is useful in two practical ways. (1) In the situation described above, where a mare in transition is in estrus and has a large follicle on one ovary, chances of her ovulating are far greater the closer it is to April. By the same token, complaints by breeders of mares that are in estrus all the time and do not seem to ovulate can often be understood with a glance at the calendar. (2) On breeding farms where frequent monitoring of ovarian status by palpation and/or ultrasonography is not possible or feasible, it may be advisable to wait until April. This may seem like cold comfort to a breeder anxious to get a mare in foal, but it is considerably more efficient than spending time and money on a mare that is not yet ready to ovulate. Fortunately, there are some practical methods that can be considered, as discussed below.

EVENTS ASSOCIATED WITH SEXUAL RECRUDESCENCE DURING VERNAL TRANSITION

INCREASED GnRH SECRETION

As pointed out above, GnRH secretion declines during anestrus, and re-establishment of GnRH secretion is among the first events of vernal transition. Sharp and Grubaugh[4] demonstrated that GnRH secretion was virtually undetectable in most mares during November and December (in the Northern Hemisphere), but that by February, all mares tested had detectable GnRH concentrations and elevated secretion rates relative to mares in November and December (Fig. 15-2). Furthermore, increased GnRH secretion precedes any major changes in circulating FSH, LH, estrogen, or progesterone. These data indicate, therefore, that one of the first changes in the hypothalamic-pituitary-ovarian axis in vernal transition is re-establishment of GnRH secretion. Whether this increase is a direct effect of increasing photoperiod after the winter solstice or whether it reflects a more complex organization, as in a circannual rhythm, remains to be understood.

INCREASED FSH SECRETION

With frequent monitoring of mares during vernal transition, the next obvious change is an increase in circulating FSH concentrations.[6,8] In pony mares at a lati-

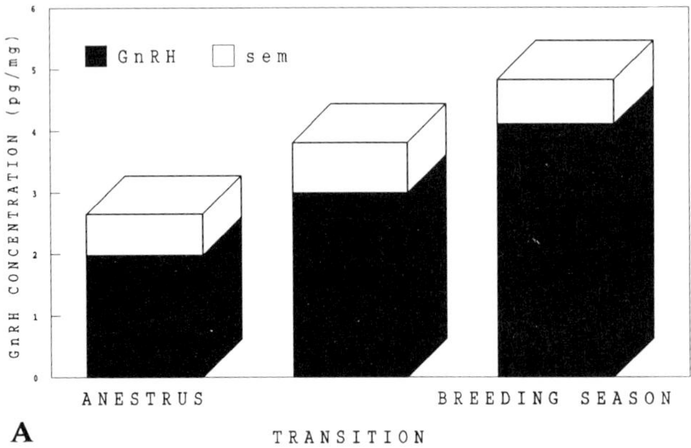

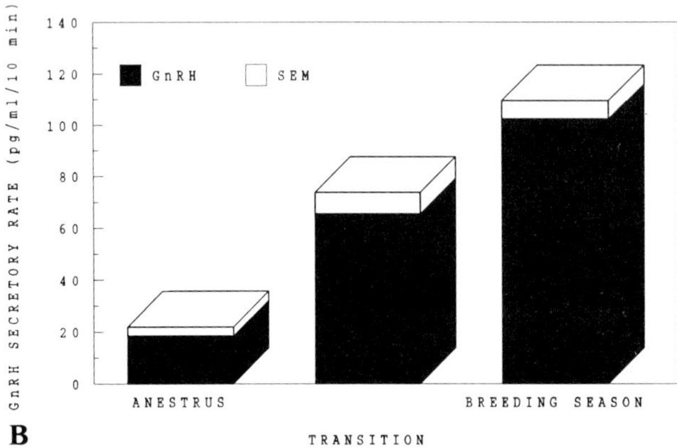

FIG. 15–2. *A*, Hypothalamic GnRH content (pg/mL). *B*, GnRH secretory rate (pg/mL/10 min). SEM, standard error of the mean. (Data from Strauss, S.S., Chen, C.L., Kalra, S.P., and Sharp, D.C.: Localization of gonadotropin-releasing hormone (GnRH) in the hypothalamus of ovariectomized pony mares by season. J. Reprod. Fertil. Suppl., *27*:123–129, 1979; and from Sharp, D.C., and Grubaugh, W.R.: Use of push-pull perfusion techniques in studies of gonadotropin-releasing hormone secretion in mares. J. Reprod. Fertil. Suppl., *35*:293–300, 1987.)

tude of approximately 30° north (Gainesville, FL) the increase in circulating FSH can often be detected as early as late January or early February. It is important to note that the increase in circulating FSH does not necessarily indicate establishment of complete reproductive function, because time from first significant increase in FSH to time of first ovulation of the year may be quite lengthy (> 60 days).[10] It seems reasonable to speculate that the increase in circulating FSH reflects increased GnRH secretion, because pituitary FSH stores do not change throughout the year[3] and FSH is available for release. However, at that time circulating LH, as monitored daily, remains essentially baseline, likely reflecting the reduced pituitary LH stores of anestrus.[13] In this regard, Fitzgerald et al. reported a change in pattern of LH secretion during vernal transition in horse mares.[14,15] When blood samples were collected frequently (15-min intervals) for 8 or 24 h, these workers reported a gradual increase in the number of secretory events, which they called "pulses."[14,15] Their choice of the term *pulsatile* is perhaps unfortunate, because the secretory events they reported were irregular in timing and low in frequency (maximum of just over three pulses per 12-h period). Thus the term pulsatile may mislead one to compare mechanisms of gonadotropin secretory regulation in the mare with other species in which a pulse generator is thought to regulate GnRH output and, hence, gonadotropin output. Whether such a pulse generator exists in mares, has yet to be demonstrated. Studies of GnRH secretion from the hypothalamus of pony mares,[2] by push-pull perfusion,[4] and by measurement of GnRH in pituitary venous effluent of horses (McDowell, personal communication) have not unequivocably demonstrated evidence for the presence of highly regular, high-frequency GnRH pulses during vernal transition. The point is not a trivial one, if the evolutionary advantage of pulsatile secretion is considered. Such a secretory pattern is thought to convey more information than a secretory pattern with only low versus high concentrations (or "on" versus "off" in terms of tissue response). A pulsatile secretory pattern can theoretically convey four possible messages: (1) low frequency, low amplitude; (2) low frequency, high amplitude; (3) high frequency, low amplitude; and (4) high frequency, high amplitude. However, it is difficult to understand, in terms of current knowledge of pituitary and ovarian function, the nature of the message conveyed (from hypothalamus to pituitary, or from pituitary to ovary) by a pattern of secretion characterized by only a few increases in circulating hormone per 12-h (i.e., three per 12-h) period. Doubtless, this information suggests that the hypothalamic-pituitary axis is slowly reawakening during vernal transition, but caution should be advised in overinterpreting the role of a pulse generator in horses until further information is available.

FOLLICULAR DEVELOPMENT

At about the time increased FSH is detected in the circulation, palpation and/or ultrasonographic examination of the ovaries reveals an increase in follicular development. Sharp and Ginther first described the pattern of follicular development of mares during vernal transition as a sigmoidal-shaped curve with an initial slow increase in number and size of ovarian follicles, a steeply sloped portion of the growth curve as both size and number of follicles increase markedly, followed by a plateau shortly before the date of the first ovulation of the season.[16] The average follicle size is a useful end point, because it incorporates both size and number of follicles; a typical pattern of increase in average follicular size, as determined by ultrasonography, is shown in Figure 15-3.

During the period of rapid and extensive follicular development, ovulation does not occur, as assessed by the lack of significant circulating progesterone and by frequent ultrasonographic scanning of the ovaries to detect potential ovulation and/or luteal structures. Pony mares develop an average of 3.7 ± 0.9 consecutive anovula-

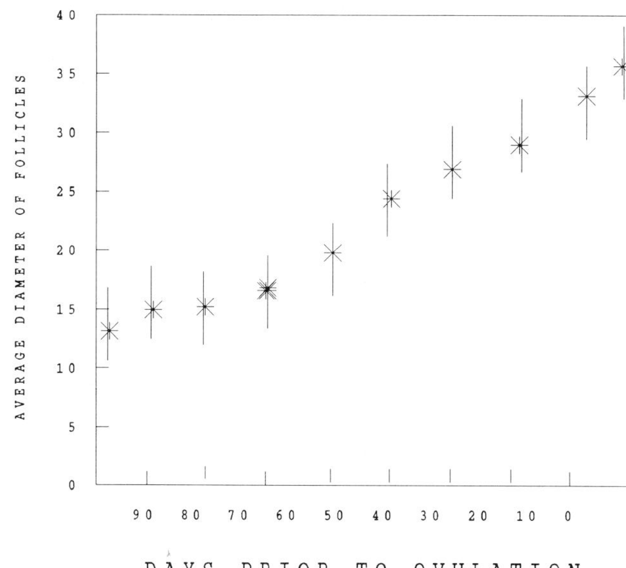

FIG. 15–3. Changes in mean size of follicles in mares during vernal transition, in millimeters. Data have been standardized to the day of the first ovulation of the year.

tory 30-mm follicles during vernal transition.[10] The follicles enlarge, fail to ovulate, and remain at or about 30 mm for approximately a week, then subsequently regress, still fluid filled as assessed by ultrasonography. As a major follicle is in the progress of regressing after failing to ovulate, another follicle develops. Although it is difficult to determine a time course of follicular development precisely, the total time course for the process of renewed folliculogenesis, from first detection of follicle growth to first ovulation is about 55 to 60 days. Because the average number of major follicles detected is 3.7, it follows that the interval between 30-mm follicles is about 12 to 14 days. The development of large, anovulatory follicles is one of the sources of frustration and indecision to practitioners and breeders during the vernal transition, because palpation and ultrasonography do not provide sufficient information to predict whether or not the follicle will ovulate. Therefore, large anovulatory follicles of vernal transition are a source of reproductive inefficiency, primarily because of the inability to discern which follicle will be the ovulatory one. With nearly four such follicles developing consecutively, at an average interval of 12 to 14 days, it is easy to see how much time can be lost.

To confound the situation even further, mares often display sexual receptivity during much of the prolonged vernal transition. Thus, one can appreciate the breeder's dilemma when faced with pressure to begin breeding mares as early in the year as possible and presented with mares that are, by all measures, fully sexually receptive and have large (> 30 mm) follicles. Yet, until a given mare has gone through the entire course of transitional events (Table 15-1) it is likely that breeding will be a waste of time, unless the horse has been monitored extensively and it is certain that the first ovulation of the year has already been experienced.

TABLE 15–1. COURSE OF EVENTS IN VERNAL TRANSITION

1. Increased GnRH secretion from the hypothalamus
   ↓
2. Increased FSH secretion, but not LH secretion
   ↓
3. Initiation of folliculodysgenesis
   3.7 consecutive 30-mm anovulatory follicles
   Lack of estrogen secretion
4. Onset of estrous behavior
   ↓
5. Development of steroidogenically competent follicle
   ↓
6. Renewed LH synthesis and secretion
   ↓
7. Ovulation

It is of interest that circulating estrogen (estradiol and estrone) concentrations remain relatively low throughout the period of marked folliculogenesis, suggesting that the developing follicles are not competent steroidogenically.[9,10] Furthermore, follicular fluid estrogen and androgen concentrations are both significantly lower in the first two or three anovulatory transitional follicles.[17] Therefore, it seems likely that the first several follicles that develop in vernal transition are not capable of complete steroidogenesis, although the site of such a synthetic defect is not yet known.

ONSET OF ESTROUS BEHAVIOR

It is somewhat puzzling why mares in vernal transition begin to exhibit estrous behavior when changes in circulating estrogens, at first, are minor. Caution should be exercised in interpreting this fact, however, because it has been reported that mares in frank anestrus and, indeed, even ovariectomized mares often fulfill all the criteria of complete estrous behavior.[1] The former displays, however, are usually less than 3 days in duration, whereas estrous behavior during vernal transition is usually prolonged, lasting as long as 40 or 50 days.[12] The adrenal gland may be a source of steroid signal stimulating sexual behavior in ovariectomized or anestrous mares, as suggested by researchers who monitored sexual behavior in ovariectomized mares administered dexamethasone to reduce adrenal steroid production.[18] They reported suppression of sexual behavior in dexamethasone-treated, ovariectomized mares compared with ovariectomized control mares.[18] Another possible explanation for estrous display during vernal transition is that mares having experienced little or no circulating estrogen throughout anestrus may become sensitive to small changes in the hormone. In that regard, Nishikawa reported that anestrous mares were more sensitive to small doses of synthetic and natural estrogens than were mares during diestrus.[19] Another explanation may lie in the report of McCue et al. that conjugated estrogens increase in the peripheral circulation of mares in vernal transition as early as 7 weeks prior to the first ovulation of the year.[20] Seamans and Sharp showed a high percentage of tritium label appearing in the water-soluble fraction when follicle tissues (granulosa and theca; harvested from early- and late-transition mares) were incubated with radiolabeled progesterone or androstenedione percursor.[9] Thus incorporation of these precursors into free estrogens was limited in the early stages of transition, but, apparently, production of conjugated estrogens is favored during the early transition stages and may reflect the unique steroidogenic function of the anovulatory follicles developing at that time. It is not known whether conjugated estrogens are unconjugated in the brain to elicit sexual behavior, but that possibility should be explored. Regardless of the cause of the profound estrous display during vernal transition, it remains a major source of frustration to the breeder and practitioner who are in need of reliable indicators for breeding.

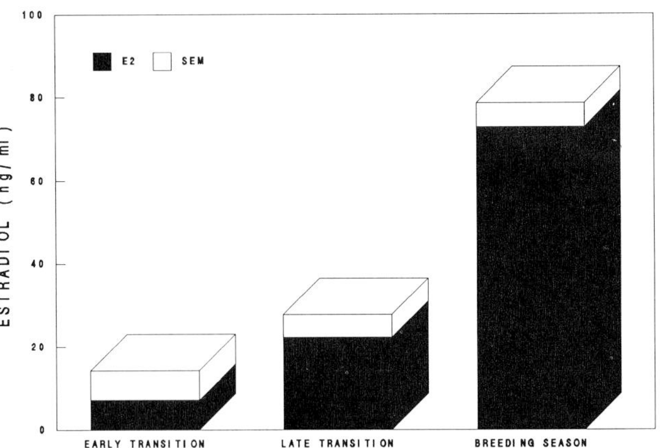

FIG. 15–4. Estrogen production (ng/mL incubation medium) by follicular tissues (granulosa alone, theca alone, and granulosa and theca combined) collected in early transition (first 30-mm follicle) late in transition (average follicle diameter 28 mm and at least three previous anovulatory follicles), and during the breeding season (second ovulation of the year). E2, estradiol concentration; SEM, standard error of the mean.

DEVELOPMENT OF STEROIDOGENICALLY COMPETENT FOLLICLE

Estrogen concentrations change little in early transition, despite the presence of large, anovulatory follicles on the ovaries. Davis et al. reported that circulating estradiol concentrations remained below the sensitivity of the assay (5 to 6 pg/mL) until about 1 week prior to the first ovulation of the year.[10] Seamans and Sharp incubated theca, granulosa, and combined theca and granulosa cells with radioactive precursors (progesterone and/or androgen) to study the ability of transitional follicles to aromatize androgens to estrogens.[9] Although late transitional and cyclic follicles had a tendency to aromatize androgens to estrogens more efficiently than early transitional follicles, this difference was not significant. In addition, the pattern of androgen secretion, primarily androstenedione, in the peripheral plasma of mares during vernal transition was essentially parallel to the pattern of estradiol, with a significant elevation in circulating concentrations shortly before the first ovulation of the year. The failure to demonstrate an aromatase shortage as well as similarly timed increases in estradiol and androstenedione suggest that the steroidogenic defect in early transition follicles lies earlier in the biosynthetic path than conversion of androgens to estrogens. Similarly, estrogen concentrations were significantly lower in follicular fluid collected from the first three consecutive large follicles of the year when compared with estrogen concentrations in follicular fluid collected from the fourth or fifth consecutive large follicles[17] (Fig. 15-4). Furthermore, in vitro incubation of theca cells or granulosa cells recovered from these same follicles indicated that the production of androgens and estrogens increased with progression through the transition and consecutive follicle formation.[17]

It has been documented that the early follicles could be distinguished at gross examination, by their relative avascularity.[9,17] Furthermore, centrifuging the follicular fluid from early transitional follicles yielded considerably fewer (twofold to fourfold) granulosa cells when compared with follicles near the expected time of ovulation or during the breeding season. These data are in agreement with the report of Kenney et al. that described physical, histologic, and hormonal aspects of follicles, which were defined as atretic.[21] These authors observed that relatively avascular follicles contained significantly lower estradiol and prostaglandin (PGE) concentrations than follicles judged to be normal preovulatory follicles based on histologic criteria.

Thus the foregoing data suggest that early transitional follicles may not be fully functional steroidogenically and, therefore may not contribute substantially to ovarian-hypothalamic-pituitary feedback relationships necessary for complete sexual function. Regardless of location of the defect, it is clear that as long as there is a need to breed mares early in the spring, there will be a need to distinguish early, steroidogenically incompetent follicles from preovulatory, steroidogenically competent follicles.

RENEWED LH SYNTHESIS

The last event of the vernal transition is increased LH secretion, which is followed shortly by the first ovulation of the year. Throughout vernal transition, FSH secretion is elevated, although highly variable, but LH concentrations, when monitored with samples collected once or twice daily, remain baseline throughout.[1,10,12] From February through May, measurements of GnRH secretion in pony mares via push-pull perfusion revealed elevated GnRH secretion relative to the time of deep anestrus (November and December), but there was no indication of changing trends in GnRH secretion.[4] That is, no evidence existed for an increasing secretory rate as transition progressed, or for a change in the pattern of episodes of GnRH secretion. Indeed, little evidence was found for episodic-type secretion of GnRH at all. These data agree with the measurement of GnRH in cavernous sinus plasma by McDowell (personal communication) in horse mares during vernal transition. It may be that the modest, but significant, increase in GnRH secretion from anestrus to the transitional phase, stimulates available pituitary FSH stores, but is ineffective given the relatively paltry amount of available pituitary LH in eliciting an LH response. In that regard, it has been shown that the LH response to administration of GnRH is considerably lower in anestrous mares than in mares during the breeding season. Furthermore, the response increased little, if any, until near the time of the first ovulation of the year.[7,10] Estrogen secretion may be an important signal in the regulation of LH synthesis and secretion, (either directly or indirectly through increased GnRH secretion), because the surge in estradiol (and androstenedione) precede the secretion of substantial amounts of LH by a matter of a few days.

Further support for the idea that estrogen secretion precedes LH secretion in a causal fashion was offered by the report of Sharp et al. who administered estrogen, progesterone, or a combination to ovariectomized pony mares during the equivalent time of vernal transition.[22] Circulating LH was monitored, as was the response to administered GnRH. After 16 days of treatment, the mares were killed and pituitary gonadotropin content assessed by radioimmunoassay. In two separate experiments, conducted over 2 yr, estrogen administration was associated with significantly elevated LH concentrations in the peripheral circulation after approximately 1 week of treatment.[22] Furthermore, at the end of both experiments, pituitary LH content was significantly higher than control mares, progesterone-treated mares, or estradiol plus progesterone–treated mares. The response to GnRH administration was not significantly altered, except by the combination treatment, which markedly suppressed LH concentrations prior to GnRH as well as eliminating the GnRH response entirely. Therefore, these data indicate that administration of estradiol to ovariectomized mares at the equivalent time of vernal transition resulted in increased pituitary content and peripherally circulating concentrations of LH. It is reasonable to propose that in ovarian-intact mares, secretion of estrogen from the first steroidogenically competent follicle of the year is instrumental in stimulating LH synthesis and secretion.

SITE OF ESTROGEN ACTION

It would be useful to know the site of action of the estrogen. In this regard, data from our laboratory have suggested that estrogen administration to anestrous mares exposed to long day for 4 weeks resulted in greatly increased GnRH secretion as assessed by push-pull perfusion. Although the number of animals was small (three treated, one control) the large increase in GnRH in the three estrogen-treated, long-day exposed mares was in stark contrast to the unchanging GnRH secretion in the control mare (vehicle administered, short-day exposed). These data suggest that at least one site of action of estrogen is at the hypothalamus, stimulating increased GnRH secretion. GnRH has been shown to stimulate increased mRNA for the LH β-subunit in sheep.[23,24] Likewise, these researchers reported that pulsatile GnRH administration to hypothalamic-disconnected sheep resulted in increased pituitary mRNA for the LH β-subunit, lending credence to the idea that estrogen could affect pituitary LH subunit synthesis through enhanced GnRH secretion.[24]

Therefore, the crux of the vernal transition appears to be the reinitiation of LH synthesis and secretion, and it seems a reasonable hypothesis that this is accomplished by an estrogen-stimulated increase in GnRH secretion. This hypothesis does not rule out, however, a direct effect of estrogen on the pituitary as well.

With development of a steroidogenically competent follicle and reestablishment of LH synthesis and secretion, the stage is fully set for the first ovulation of the year. Once this has occurred, vernal transition, by definition, has ended and the breeding season has begun (Fig. 15-5).

PRACTICAL CONSIDERATIONS

Because it is likely that the horse industry will continue to prefer early-born foals for some time to come, the breeding problems associated with vernal transition will likely continue. Two main strategies should be considered in the efforts to breed mares as early in the spring as possible. These are (1) nonintervention, but vigorous monitoring of the naturally occurring transitional events so that breeding can be effected at the appropriate time and (2) intervention so as to truncate the transitional phase, or to initiate it earlier, with the result of eliciting ovulation earlier in the year. Of the two strategies, the former will most likely appeal to purists—and can certainly be said to be the most effective at this time—but it fails to satisfy the criterion of accelerating the process. On the other hand, many of the schemes for stimulating an early onset of the breeding season show great promise but have yet to provide convincing and repeatable results, the use of artificial lighting excepted. The latter is probably the most successful way to stimulate earlier onset of the breeding season (Chapter 19).

It is up to the management, of course, to choose what approach to take in attempting to breed mares early in the spring, and it is hoped that the following will provide a glimpse of the array of methods currently being tested or proposed. In the end, economics will likely dictate what course of action to take. On one hand, frequent monitoring of vernal transition events can be time-consuming and expensive and, as pointed out, does not gain much time. On the other hand, monitoring the events of transition is essential whether waiting for the naturally occurring ovulation or attempting to induce it earlier. In addition, it may not be cost effective to spend time and money on a treatment that does not

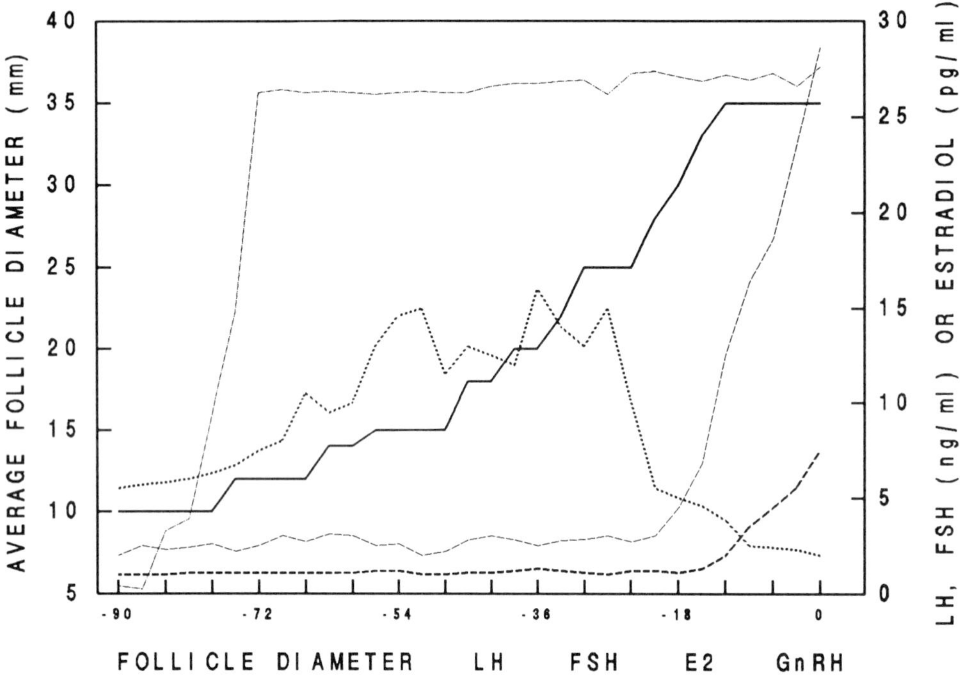

FIG. 15–5. Pattern of major hormonal and ovarian events in days throughout the vernal transition.

work. In the end, the latter may result in breeding dates that are no earlier, and may in fact be later, than the natural breeding date.

One further note of caution seems indicated, because the following discussion addresses methods for anticipating or stimulating the first ovulation of the year. That is, are the efforts and expense to breed mares at the first ovulation of the year justified? What is known of the quality of the first oocyte produced, and what is the quality of the uterine environment to which the resulting zygote will be exposed? The former question has not been answered as far as can be determined, but should be addressed in a carefully controlled manner. The latter also remains unanswered, but evidence indicates that the total amount of protein, as well as the amount of a uterine-specific protein (uteroferrin), is significantly lower in diestrus of mares after the first ovulation of the year compared with subsequent diestrus periods. Similarly, it has been shown that the circulating concentration of LH is significantly lower at the time of the first ovulation of the year compared with subsequent ovulatory estrous periods.[11,15] These observations do not necessarily indicate that breeding at the first ovulation of the year should not be attempted, but they raise questions that should be borne in mind when considering the following sections.

MONITORING EVENTS OF VERNAL TRANSITION

As mentioned above, one approach to the problem of determining first ovulation is to be patient and to monitor mares carefully for signs of impending ovulation, rather than attempt to change the pattern of vernal transition.

Follicular Development

One of the characteristic changes of the vernal transition that is most accessible to the average breeder or veterinary practitioner is the pattern of follicular development, which can be monitored by transrectal palpation or by transrectal ultrasonography of the ovaries. Because one of the frustrating ambiguities of the vernal transition is the presence of large, anovulatory follicles, frequent monitoring of follicular development is an important way of assessing a given mare's progress along the continuum of events in vernal transition. For instance, palpating or scanning a mare once (and observing a large follicle on one ovary) does not give sufficient information to make a breeding decision. Most mares undergo development of three to four consecutive anovulatory follicles before the first ovulation of the year, and it is important to know if a given follicle is early or late in this progression, because early follicles are likely doomed to atresia whereas later developing follicles may possibly be preovulatory. Admittedly, there is no guarantee of ovulation associated with the knowledge that a follicle is the fourth or even the fifth consecutive follicle, but the odds that it will be ovulatory are greatly increased.

As vernal transition proceeds, the total number of follicles on both ovaries increases from less than one to an average of eight to ten, and this multiple follicle, or "grape cluster," appearance is especially apparent with ultrasonography. Care should be taken not to confuse this physiologic state with growth of multiple accessory follicles during early pregnancy.

Gonadotropin Secretion

Monitoring gonadotropin secretion as a means of monitoring progress in vernal transition and/or predicting ovulation date shows little promise. Secretion of FSH, as pointed out previously, is highly variable, making it of little value in attempts to predict impending events. The LH surge that precedes first ovulation of the year might prove to be of some value; however, two criteria would first have to be met. (1) Such a test would have to be simplified to be run under field conditions, because most LH assays currently being run in research laboratories are double-antibody assays that require 5 to 7 days to run. "Dipstick" and other quick assays have been proposed,[25] but have been slow to develop. (2) Because of the variation in LH concentrations among mares and among assay systems, a single test at the time of manual examination would be inadequate, and repeated tests over a period of days to observe the upward swing of LH concentrations would have to be done.

Although the idea of monitoring estrogens to identify the potential preovulatory state of vernal transition follicles is not tested, it seems reasonable to do so. Davis et al.[10] and Seamans and Sharp[9] reported that there was a relatively sharp rise in circulating estrogen concentration that preceded the first ovulation of the year by about 7 to 10 days, presumably accompanying formation of the first steroidogenically competent follicle of the year. The former authors used a commercially available assay system (Diagnostic Products Corp., estradiol double antibody assay) with a sensitivity of about 6 pg/mL. Essentially nondetectable estrogen concentrations were reported throughout most of the vernal transition in pony mares, with concentrations rising to more than 30 pg/mL 7 to 10 days prior to first ovulation of the year and about 5 days prior to a significant elevation in circulating LH concentrations.[10] This report is encouraging because it suggests that the increase in estrogens is sharp enough to be practically detectable. However, development of "barnside" type of assay systems would be desirable for practical breeding application.

POTENTIAL METHODS FOR ACCELERATING THE ONSET OF THE BREEDING SEASON

Artificial Lighting

The use of artificial lighting to advance the onset of the breeding season is still the most reliable way to accelerate the onset of the breeding season (Chapter 19). First proposed by Burkhart, this method uses artificially lengthened day to trick the mare's endocrine system into beginning vernal transition early.[26] It is important to point out that the use of artificial lighting does not truncate the transition, it moves the entire process, intact, earlier in the year. The significance of this is that the transition is a lengthy process lasting 6 to 8 weeks or more.[12] Therefore, the breeder who wishes to take advantage of this system and have mares ready for breeding by February or so will not gain anything by turning the lights on in January. To be effective in advancing the transition, breeders should begin the artificial lighting program no later than the first of December, and November is even better.[12]

Gonadotropin Administration

Because failure of gonadotropin secretion is really the basic reason for sexual dysfunction in the winter, it would seem logical that administration of gonadotropins to anestrous mares would reinitiate reproductive capacity. Indeed, that is the case. Lapin and Ginther[27] and Douglas et al.[28] reported that administration of pituitary extracts to anestrous pony mares resulted in follicular development and ovulation within 3 weeks. Unfortunately, such pituitary extracts are not available commercially and would be extremely costly. Furthermore, the pituitary preparations available to veterinarians currently are from porcine or bovine pituitaries and have little effect in stimulating equine ovarian activity. Therefore, the idea of administering pituitary gonadotropins and stimulating ovarian activity is sound from the physiologic standpoint but is not yet available clinically. With the rapid biotechnologic advances being made, it may be only a matter of time before equine gonadotropin DNA is cloned and expressed in vitro, making it available in large quantities.

An alternative to the direct administration of gonadotropin would be to administer GnRH and let the mare release its own gonadotropin. Such an approach has been attempted experimentally by several workers and shows some promise.[29–31] This work was slow to develop initially, because of the belief that GnRH would have to be administered in a pulsatile fashion, with doses administered every hour or so. Indeed, such a protocol seems to work,[29] but suffers from a lack of clinical practicality. Promise of clinical applicability came from the reports of researchers who demonstrated that subcutaneous implants,[30,31] or once daily administration of long-acting GnRH analogues[8] stimulated gonadotropin release and led to an earlier onset of the breeding season (i.e., earlier date of first ovulation). The efficacy of using GnRH analogue to stimulate gonadotropin synthesis and/or release may depend on the particular analogue used, and this area is ripe for further investigation. Davis et al. used the native hormone itself and two substituted molecules, [D-Ala^6] LH-RH, and des-Gly^{10} LH-RH, (D-Ala^6, and des-Gly, respectively) administered at doses of 400 μg, twice daily, IV (GnRH), 9 μg once daily IV (des-Gly), or 3 μg, twice daily IV (D-Ala^6), to pony mares in frank anestrus (beginning date of the experiment was January 20).[8] It is interesting that FSH secretion and follicular development were stimulated in all three groups, but LH secretion was not stimulated. Consequently, treated mares underwent anovulatory follicular development for a longer period than did control mares. Mares administered D-Ala[6] developed an average of 10 consecutive anovulatory follicles (> 30 mm; mean interval between follicles was 12 days) prior to development of the first ovulatory follicle. Whether the failure to stimulate LH synthesis and/or release was a direct function of the analogues used, or the fact that these were pony mares and in deep anestrus cannot be stated.

Thus the administration of GnRH to anestrous mares with the idea of stimulating synthesis and/or release of endogenous gonadotropins is a promising technique that may aid breeders and veterinarians by truncating the vernal transition period and thus causing an earlier first ovulation of the year.

As has been discussed, secretion of estrogen from a steroidogenically competent follicle may be an important last step in re-establishment of a functional hypothalamic-pituitary-ovarian axis in mares in vernal transition. From that concept, it would seem that administration of estrogen to mares in early transition might be of benefit in stimulating an earlier onset of the breeding season. This concept has not been tested extensively as yet, and current knowledge of the endocrine patterns during vernal transition would predict that estrogen administration would have to be well timed if it were to be successful. That is, circulating FSH declines as estrogen rises near the time of the first ovulation of the year.[1,8] Furthermore, stimulation of LH synthesis and/or secretion by estrogen administration simultaneously results in a decrease in circulating FSH.[22] Therefore, improperly timed estrogen administration, relative to the cycle of follicular formation, could lead to LH release, but diminished FSH release, hence cessation of follicular development. Clearly more work is needed to determine whether estrogen administration could be used practically as an alternative method of truncating the vernal transition and accelerating the date of the first ovulation of the year.

Several reports have appeared that describe the efficacy of administering progesterone for accelerating the date of the first ovulation of the year.[32–34] It is not clear how this might work to re-establish a functional hypothalamic-pituitary-ovarian axis, because in mares undergoing vernal transition naturally, little evidence exists of an increase in progesterone concentrations until after the first ovulation of the year.[11,13] Progesterone administration could act to increase the precursor pool for formation of estrogens, but no evidence is known for this in mares. Finally, the researchers administering progesterone have largely used mares of relatively unknown status (i.e., did not know how far along the continuum of events they were) or were known to be in late transition. Therefore, this method should be given a more circumspect examination before practical acceptance.

REFERENCES

1. Ginther, O.J.: Reproductive Biology of the Mare. Ann Arbor, McNaughton, Gunn, 1979, pp. 83–108.
2. Strauss, S.S., Chen, C.L., Kalra, S.P., and Sharp, D.C.: Localization of gonadotropin-releasing hormone (GnRH) in the hypothalamus of ovariectomized pony mares by season. J. Reprod. Fertil. Suppl., *27*:123–129, 1979.
3. Hart, P.J., Squires, E.L., Imel, K.J., and Nett, T.M.: Seasonal variation in hypothalamic content of gonadotropin-releasing hormone (GnRH), pituitary receptors for GnRH, and pituitary content of luteinizing hormone and follicle stimulating hormone in the mare. Biol. Reprod., *30*:1055–1062, 1984.
4. Sharp, D.C., and Grubaugh, W.R.: Use of push-pull perfusion techniques in studies of gonadotropin-releasing hormone secretion in mares. J. Reprod. Fertil. Suppl., *35*:293–300, 1987.
5. Levine, J.E., and Ramirez, V.D.: Luteinizing hormone-releasing hormone release during the rat estrous cycle and after ovariectomy, as estimated with push-pull cannulae. Endocrinology, *111*:1439–1455, 1982.
6. Silvia, P.J., Squires, E.L., and Nett, T.M.: Changes in the hypothalamic-hypophyseal axis of mares associated with seasonal reproductive recrudescence. Biol. Reprod., *35*:897–905, 1986.
7. Silvia, P.J., Squires, E.L., and Nett, E.L.: Pituitary responsiveness of mares challenged with GnRH at various stages of the transition into the breeding season. J. Anim. Sci., *64*:790–796, 1987.
8. Davis, S.D., Sharp, D.C., and Grubaugh, W.R.: Stimulation of LH by LHRH analogs in anestrous pony mares. Biol. Reprod. Suppl. 1, *34*:143, 1986.
9. Seamans, K.W., and Sharp, D.C.: Changes in equine follicular aromatase activity during sexual recrudescence. J. Reprod. Fertil. Suppl., *32*:225–233, 1982.
10. Davis, S.D., Grubaugh, W.R., and Weithenauer, J.: Follicle integrity and serum estradiol 17β patterns during sexual recrudescence in the mare. Biol. Reprod. Suppl. 1, *36*:121, 1987.
11. Oxender, W.D., Noden, P.A., and Hafs, H.D.: Estrus, ovulation and serum progesterone, estradiol and LH concentrations in mares after an increased photoperiod during winter. Am. J. Vet. Res., *398*:230–207, 1977.
12. Sharp, D.C.: Environmental influences on reproduction in horses. *In* Veterinary Clinics of North America: Large Animal Practice. Edited by J. Hughes. Philadelphia, W.B. Saunders, 1980. pp. 207–273.
13. Sharp, D.C., Garcia, M.C., and Ginther, O.J.: Luteinizing hormone during sexual maturation in pony mares. Am. J. Vet. Res., *38*:548–550, 1979.
14. Fitzgerald, B.P., I'Anson, H., Loy, R.G., and Legan, S.J.: Evidence that changes in LH pulse frequency may regulate the seasonal modulation of LH secretion in ovariectomized mares. J. Reprod. Fertil., *69*:685–692, 1983.
15. Fitzgerald, B.P., et al.: Changes in pulse frequency and amplitude in intact mares during the transition into the breeding season. J. Reprod. Fertil., *79*:485–493, 1987.
16. Sharp, D.C., and Ginther, O.J.: Induction of ovarian activity and estrous behavior in anestrous mares with light and temperature. J. Anim. Sci., *41*:1368–1372, 1975.
17. Davis, S.D., and Sharp, D.C.: Intra-follicular and peripheral steroid characteristics during vernal transition in the pony mare. J. Reprod. Fertil. Suppl., *44*:333–340, 1991.
18. Asa, C., and Ginther, O.J.: Glucocorticoid suppression of oestrus, follicles, LH and ovulation in the mare. J. Reprod. Fertil. Suppl., *32*:247–251, 1982.
19. Nishikawa, Y.: Studies on Reproduction in Horses. Tokyo, Japan Racing Association, 1959.
20. McCue, P.M., et al.: Follicular and endocrine responses of anoestrous mares to administration of native GnRH or a GnRH agonist. J. Reprod. Fertil. Suppl., *44*:227–233, 1991.

21. Kenney, R.M., Condon, W., Ganhjam, V.K., and Channing, C.: Morphological and biochemical correlates of equine ovarian follicles as a function of their state of viability of atresia. J. Reprod. Fertil. Suppl., *27*:163–171, 1979.

22. Sharp, D.C., et al.: Effects of steroid administration on luteinizing hormone and follicle stimulating hormone in ovariectomized pony mares in the springtime: Pituitary responsiveness to gonadotropin-releasing hormone (GnRH), circulating gonadotropin concentrations and pituitary gonadotropin content. Biol. Reprod., in press.

23. Hamernik, D.L., and Nett, T.M.: Gonadotropin-releasing hormone increases the amount of messenger ribonucleic acid for gonadotropins in ovariectomized ewes after hypothalamic-pituitary disconnection. Endocrinology, *122*:959–960, 1988.

24. Mercer, J.E., Clements, J., Funder, J.W., and Clarke, I.J.: LHβ mRNA levels are regulated primarily by GnRH and not by negative estrogen feedback on the pituitary. Neuroendocrinology, *47*:563–566, 1988.

25. Campbell, K.L.: Solid state assays: Reagents and film technology for dipstick assays. *In* Non-Radiometric Assays: Technology and Application in Polypeptide and Steroid Hormone Detection. Edited by B.D. Albertson and F.P. Haseltine. New York, A.R. Liss, 1988, pp. 237–287.

26. Burkhart, J.: Transition from anoestrus in the mare and the effects of artificial lighting. J. Agric. Sci. Cambridge, *37*:64–68, 1947.

27. Lapin, D.R., and Ginther, O.J.: Induction of ovulation and multiple ovulations in seasonally anovulatory and ovulatory mares with an equine pituitary extract. J. Anim. Sci., *44*:834–842, 1977.

28. Douglas, R.H., Nuti, L., and Ginther, O.J.: Induction of ovulation and multiple ovulations in seasonally-anovulatory mares with equine pituitary fractions. Theriogenology, *2*:133–142, 1974.

29. Johnson, A.L.: Pulsatile administration of gonadotropin-releasing hormone advances ovulation in cycling mares. Biol. Reprod., *35*:1123–1130, 1986.

30. Hyland, J.H. et al.: Infusion of gonadotropin-releasing hormone (GnRH) induces ovulation and fertile oestrus in mares during seasonal anoestrus. J. Reprod. Fertil. Suppl., *35*:211–220, 1987.

31. Allen, W.R., et al.: Induction of ovulation in anoestrous mares with a slow-release implant of a GnRH analogue (ICI 118-630). J. Reprod. Fertil. Suppl., *35*:469–478, 1987.

32. Taylor, T.B., Pemstein, R., and Loy, R.G.: Control of ovulation in mares in the early breeding season with ovarian steroids and prostaglandin. J. Reprod. Fertil. Suppl., *32*:219–224, 1982.

33. Evans, M.J., and Irvine, C.H.G.: Induction of follicular development and ovulation in seasonally acyclic mares using gonadotropin-releasing hormone and progesterone. J. Reprod. Fertil. Suppl., *27*:113–121, 1979.

34. Squires, E.L., et al.: Relationship of altrenogest to ovarian activity, hormone concentrations and fertility of mares. J. Anim. Sci. *56*:901–910, 1983.

CHAPTER 16

THE ABNORMAL ESTROUS CYCLE

P.F. Daels
J.P. Hughes

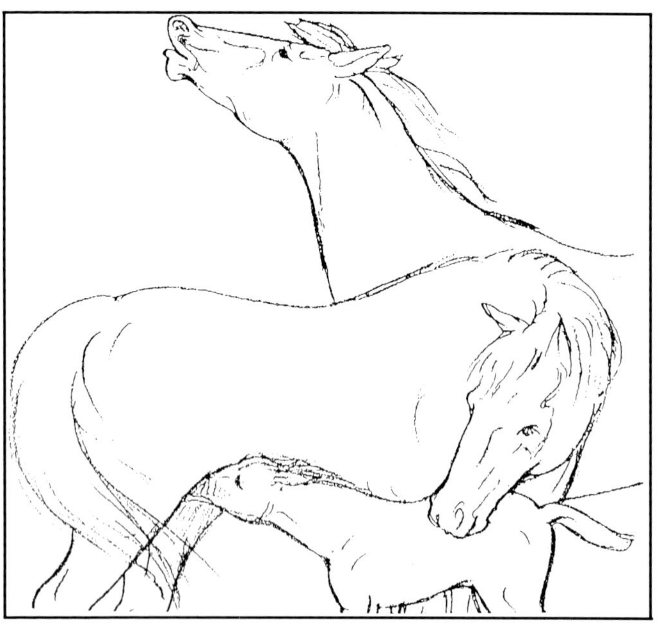

Mares are seasonal breeders and most irregularities in their estrous cycles are related to the transition from winter anestrus into the breeding season and the transition from cyclic reproductive activity to winter anestrus. However, abnormal follicular development, ovulation, and behavioral patterns are also observed during the breeding season when most mares have normal estrous cycles. The irregularities in the reproductive pattern of mares can be classified based on the pattern of estrous behavior. On this basis, we distinguish anestrus or absence of estrous behavior for a prolonged period (i.e., longer than the average duration of diestrus), shortened interval between estrous periods or shortened luteal phase ("short cycle"), and irregular and prolonged estrus. The underlying reasons for the observed irregularities in the reproductive pattern are diverse and are summarized in Table 16–1.

In general, "anestrus" is defined as a period of reproductive quiescence between two estrous cycles or quiescence of the ovary and hence the entire reproductive tract.[1] In the mare, this definition does not exactly fit all clinical syndromes of reproductive inactivity, and therefore, the term is used to indicate a prolonged period without signs of estrous behavior (sexual receptivity). Anestrus can be the result of a variety of aberrations of the normal cyclic pattern (Table 16–1). In the absence of follicular development, estrogen secretion remains low and fails to stimulate estrous behavior. Prolongation of the life span of the corpus luteum (CL) with continued secretion of progesterone will inhibit expression of estrous behavior even when estrogen secretion is elevated. Finally, mares may fail to exhibit signs of estrous behavior even though they have normal cyclic ovarian activity, including regression of the CL and ovulation. The absence of expression of normal estrous behavior despite normal cyclic ovarian activity is commonly referred to as silent heat.

During the breeding season, estrous periods are separated by periods of diestrus. Occasionally, a shortened diestrous period marks the period between two distinct estrous periods. Whereas the duration of estrus is influenced by many factors including season, the duration of diestrus is fairly constant and averages approximately 14 to 15 days (Chapter 14). As will be explained later in this chapter, premature regression of the CL is the result of premature endometrial prostaglandin release stimulated by uterine inflammation and manipulation or systemic prostaglandin release as a result of systemic illness.

Excessively short or long periods of estrous behavior are common during the transition from winter anestrus to active reproductive function. Intermittent estrus in early spring reflects inadequate gonadotropin support, resulting in partial development of follicles followed by regression without ovulation and cessation of estrous behavior. Regression of follicles may be followed by development of a new wave of follicles and estrous behavior at short intervals. Excessively long periods of estrus during the physiologic breeding season reflect either abnormal gonadotropin secretion or dysfunction of the gonads (e.g., ovarian neoplasia).

TABLE 16–1. DIFFERENTIAL DIAGNOSIS OF ABNORMAL REPRODUCTIVE FUNCTION

I. ANESTRUS: NO SIGNS OF ESTROUS BEHAVIOR	
A. Anestrus caused by ovarian quiescence:	
Winter anestrus	Ovarian inactivity or depressed follicular activity without ovulation
Postpartum anestrus	Ovarian inactivity in the postpartum period
Anestrus	Ovarian inactivity as a result of body condition (age, debility, undernourishment)
Chromosomal abnormalities	Absence of functional ovarian tissue caused by gonadal dysgenesis
Pituitary abnormalities	Ovarian inactivity owing to adenomatous hyperplasia of the intermediate, pituitary (Cushing's syndrome)
Ovarian tumors	Granulosa-theca cell tumor, cystadenoma
B. Anestrus caused by prolonged luteal phase	
Persistent corpus luteum	Failure of CL to regress
Diestrus ovulation	Formation of another CL late in the luteal phase that is nonresponsive to $PGF_2\alpha$ at the time of initial luteolysis
Pyometra	Inadequate uterine $PGF_2\alpha$ secretion because of severe endometrial destruction
Pregnancy	Continued luteal function as a result of the presence of a conceptus
Pseudopregnancy	Continued luteal function caused by the presence of a conceptus at the time of expected luteolysis
Iatrogenic	Progesterone and progestin, nonsteroidal anti-inflammatory drugs
C. Anestrus caused by abnormal behavior:	
Silent heat	Normal cyclic ovarian activity and ovulation without signs of estrous behavior, anabolic steroid administration
II. SHORTENED LUTEAL PHASE	
Endometritis	Regression of the CL caused by premature uterine $PGF_2\alpha$ secretion in response to uterine inflammation
Pyometra	Regression of the CL because of premature uterine $PGF_2\alpha$ secretion as a result of endometritis
Systemic illness	Regression of the CL caused by endotoxin-induced systemic $PGF_2\alpha$ secretion
Iatrogenic	Regression of the CL caused by administration of $PGF_2\alpha$ or its analogue, uterine manipulation, uterine infusion, or trauma of the uterus (biopsy)
III. IRREGULAR OR PROLONGED ESTRUS	
Anestrus	Mares in winter anestrus may occasionally display estrous behavior in the absence of detectable ovarian activity, fresh sweet clover (high content of estrogenic compounds) will occasionally induce estrous behavior despite totally inactive ovaries
Transitional period	Follicular development without ovulation at the start and end of the physiological breeding season
Tumor	Granulosa-theca cell tumor
Chromosomal abnormalities	XO mares

The duration of the estrous cycle may be altered in different ways by the same condition. For example, pyometra may be associated with either a shortened or prolonged luteal phase. To avoid repetition, we have chosen to describe each condition and its effect(s) on the estrous cycle separately. An overview of how these conditions fit in the observed aberrations of the normal cyclic pattern is shown in Table 16–1.

PHOTOPERIOD

WINTER ANESTRUS

Mares are seasonal polyestrous. The majority of mares, in temperate climate zones, undergo cyclic sexual activity during spring and summer and very few mares are reproductively active in the late fall and winter months. While there are areas of the world where a large proportion of the mares cycle the year around, the farther north or south from the equator, the more pronounced the occurrence of an anovulatory period during the winter[2–4] (Chapter 19). In a California study, only 20 to 25% of mares came into estrus and ovulated in January and February, whereas 75 to 85% developed signs of estrus and ovulated during April through June.[5,6] In another study, in South Africa, 85% of the mares were anovulatory during winter and early spring.[7,8] Similarly, in Australia, a study of slaughter specimens indicated 18% of mares ovulated during the winter, whereas a high of 91% ovulated during the summer.[4] The duration of winter anestrus is typically 2 to 6 months and is influenced by changes in photoperiod (determined by latitude) and possibly also by climate (temperature) and nutrition (body condition). During winter anestrus, a large proportion of mares have little or no ovarian activity and have follicles smaller than 20 mm (deep anestrus). The uterus and cervix in those mares often feel flaccid and thin on rectal palpation, and the uterus has low endometrial gland density on histologic examination (Chapter 26). Some mares will have significant ovarian activity with follicles increasing to 35 mm in size and then regressing without ovulation.[9] Depending on the time of the year, those mares are described as being in shallow (winter) or transitional (early spring) anestrus.

SPRING TRANSITION

In the spring, the mare responds to increased day length with an increase in follicular development and establishment of cyclic ovarian activity. The duration of transition from winter anestrus to cyclic ovarian activity and the onset of ovarian activity can be quite variable (Chapter 15). Some mares develop a wave of follicles, come into estrus, and ovulate. Other mares develop waves of follicles, which subsequently undergo atresia without ovulation (Fig. 16–1). Several waves of follicles may occur before gonadotropin secretion is adequate to support final maturation of a dominant follicle and ovulation.[10,11] The first ovulation of the season is generally followed by normal, cyclic activity. Clusters of large follicles (> 30 mm) on the ovaries of transitional mares are commonly found before the first ovulation. Most of these large follicles are atretic, and their presence merely reflects the fact that regression of atretic follicles is about twice as long as their development.[12] Some of these large follicles, however, appear to be in a state of suspended maturation, awaiting an LH surge to initiate ovulation. This is supported by the fact that transitional mares that have a large follicle will ovulate in response to human chorionic gonadotropin (hCG) administration.[13] Estrous behavior may be observed intermittently, most likely at the peak of follicular waves, or continuously for several weeks. During the transition period, estrous behavior may vary from interest in the stallion without allowing breeding to standing heat for weeks at a time, without ovulation.

Ovulation and cyclic ovarian activity in anestrous or transitional mares can be achieved through various means, including manipulation of the photoperiod and/or pharmacologic means (progestin, gonadotropin-releasing hormone, and hCG). For a detailed discussion of these treatment protocols refer to other chapters of this volume.

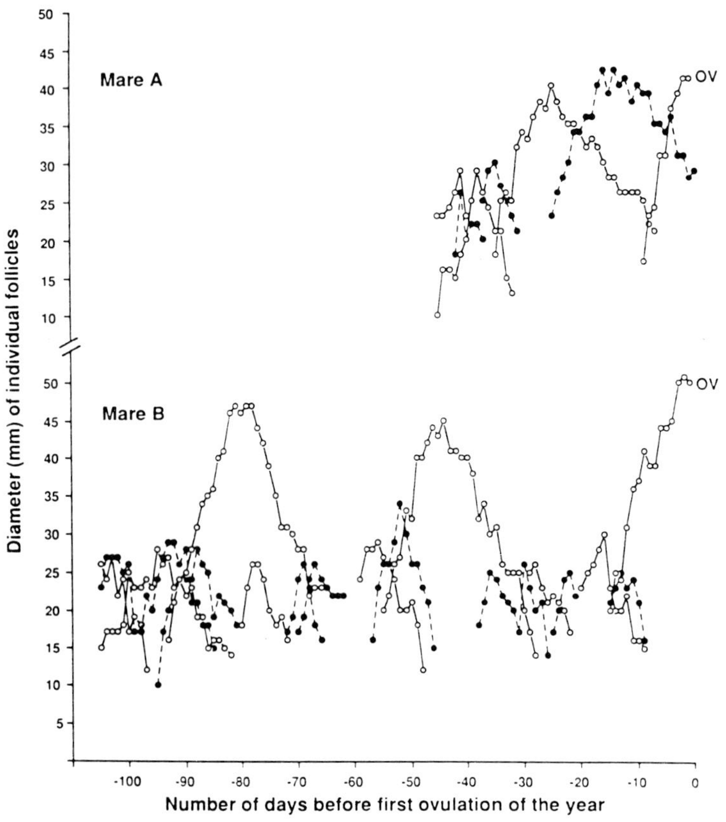

FIG. 16–1. Diameter profiles of individual follicles in two mares during the transitional period before the first ovulation of the year. OV, ovulation from the indicated follicle. (From Ginther, O.J.: Follicular dynamics in heifers and mares. Proc. Soc. Theriogenol., 2–12, 1989.)

FALL TRANSITION

The response to decreasing photoperiod is often slow in that cyclic ovarian activity may not be terminated until October or November (Northern Hemisphere). Mares enter winter anestrus by either failing to develop a follicle or failing to ovulate a developing follicle after regression of the corpus luteum.

PREGNANCY AND PSEUDOPREGNANCY

In the pregnant mare, the presence of the conceptus extends the life span of the CL. Observations indicate that the embryo may begin its luteostatic effect as early as days 11 and 13 after ovulation, allowing continued secretion of progesterone by the CL.[14,15] If embryonic loss occurs after day 13 or 14 of pregnancy but before development of endometrial cups, the CL may persist for a variable period of 35 to 90 days following conception. In these mares, regression of the active CL and reestablishment of normal estrous cycles can be achieved by administration of prostaglandin $F_2\alpha$ ($PGF_2\alpha$) or its analogue (Chapter 34). If the fetus is lost in the presence of functional endometrial cups (between days 35 and 150 days of gestation), death of the fetus will not result in simultaneous destruction of endometrial cups; rather, they will continue to secrete equine chorionic gonadotropin (eCG) for a period similar to that in the pregnant mare, up to 150 days after conception[16–18] (Chapters 9 and 58). In these "pseudopregnant" mares, functional luteal tissue persists and more secondary CL may develop during the period of chorionic gonadotropin secretion. However, in some mares the primary and secondary CL regress within 20 days after loss of the conceptus despite the high concentrations of eCG in blood.[19–21] Regression of the CL and return to estrus may be achieved by multiple injections of prostaglandin.[22–24] In general, these mares may return to estrus and ovulate but their fertility is low, although fertile ovulations have been observed in the presence of elevated levels of chorionic gonadotropin.[19–21,24] The formation of a CL during the endometrial cup phase often occurs as a result of luteinization of anovulatory follicles. Normal cyclic activity is reestablished after regression of the endometrial cups and disappearance of eCG from the blood.[24,25] On occasion, mares are presented for persistent anestrus during the breeding season. Before initiating treatment to induce estrus in such mares, it is imperative to first examine the reproductive tract for pregnancy.

POSTPARTUM PERIOD

More than 95% of the mares will ovulate and resume cyclic reproductive activity within 20 days after foaling. Occasionally, mares fail to re-establish a normal cyclic reproductive pattern after parturition, commonly referred to as lactational anestrus or postpartum anestrus. This condition can be the result of (1) prolongation of the luteal phase following ovulation during foal heat (most common); (2) ovulation at foal heat and development of CL, followed by ovarian inactivity; or (3) ovarian inactivity following parturition without ovulation at foal heat. Postpartum anestrus caused by persistence of the luteal phase should not be confused with anestrus as a result of ovarian quiescence and it can be corrected successfully by $PGF_2\alpha$ administration (Chapter 34). Postpartum anestrus caused by ovarian inactivity can last 1 to 3 months. The ovarian activity in these mares ranges from complete ovarian inactivity and absence of estrous behavior following parturition to estrous behavior and follicular activity with or without ovulation at foal heat followed by a period of decreased ovarian activity without ovulation. There appears to be a strong seasonal effect on the incidence of postpartum anestrus. Anestrus following parturition occurs more often in January, February, and March rather than later in the breeding season.[26] Anestrus following parturition is also more frequent in older mares with fair to poor body condition but even in these mares the incidence of anestrus following parturition is low (less than 5% of the total population). Researchers have been unable to demonstrate a clear link between lactation and postpartum anestrus. Anestrus during the postpartum period is more likely the result of unfavorable photoperiod and poor body condition exacerbated by the stress of lactation. Foaling mares on a weight-losing diet had a significantly longer interval to first and second postpartum ovulation.[27] Postpartum anestrus in the early breeding season may be prevented by maintaining mares in good body condition and exposing them to 16 h of light per day starting 2 months before foaling. Because the effect of season, age, and body condition seems to be stronger than that of lactation, the term lactational anestrus seems inappropriate and postpartum anestrus appears to be a more accurate term.[26,28]

BEHAVIORAL ANESTRUS (SILENT HEAT)

Behavioral anestrus is a psychic disorder of mares characterized by the absence of receptivity to the stallion during the reproductive cycle. A small percent of mares fail to show estrus, even though normal ovarian cyclicity with regression of the CL, follicle growth, and ovulation occur.[29–31] In a study by Hughes et al., one mare came into estrus only twice during a 2-yr study and one failed to come into estrus during the first 5 months of the study, although rectal palpation of the ovaries and plasma progestin concentrations indicated normal cyclic ovarian activity in both mares.[5] Mares are particularly prone to manifest psychologic anestrus for several months after foaling.[29] Highly nervous mares who are anxious about their foals seem to be most affected. Maiden mares and nervous, shy mares also are prone to silent heat. As discussed later in this chapter, mares treated with anabolic steroids often display abnormal sexual behavior, which may persist for months following treatment, even though they have normal ovarian activity. The incidence of behavioral anestrus varies with teasing efficiency but may be as high as 15% on well-managed farms.[29,32]

When dealing with behavioral anestrus it is important to establish if the mare has cyclic ovarian activity. Rectal palpation and ultrasonography of the genital tract, together with visual examination of vagina and cervix on a repeated basis, every 2 to 3 days, will determine the stage of the cycle. In addition to the examination of the genital tract, repeated progesterone analysis and administration of $PGF_2\alpha$ or its analogue followed by close monitoring and administration of hCG can be used to time insemination in mares with silent heat. When it is established that a mare has normal ovarian cycles but fails to demonstrate estrous behavior at the appropriate time, careful observation and detailed records are essential to determine when the mare is in estrus. The method of teasing can have a profound effect on a mare's behavior.[31] A standard teasing procedure should be followed, allowing mares to become accustomed to the routine and thus minimize nervous suppression of normal estrous behavior (Chapter 20).[29,31] Maiden and nursing mares should be handled carefully and given ample time to become familiar with the procedure. Some maiden mares feel threatened by an aggressive stallion and become defensive. Some foaling mares will only display estrous behavior when the foal is absent and others only when the foal is very close. Most mares when teased intensively during estrus will show some signs of estrus to the observant handler. A few will continue to be nonreceptive even under optimal conditions.[31] The majority of these mares will stand for natural cover when properly restrained (Chapter 85). Rarely, a mare may resist all attempts at breeding even though all physical characteristics suggest that the mare is in estrus. In such instances, artificial insemination, if allowed, is the solution.

PYOMETRA

The term pyometra in the mare has, for clinical convenience, been used to describe the accumulation of excessive amounts of abnormal fluid in the uterus. The accumulation of purulent material in the uterus is accompanied by severe inflammation and destruction of the endometrium. Depending on the degree of inflammation and destruction of the endometrium, the life span of the CL may be normal, shortened, or prolonged. In cases of endometritis with an intact endometrium, premature release of prostaglandin as a result of uterine inflammation and regression of the CL will result in a shortened luteal phase (Table 16–2). In mares with chronic pyometra, destruction of the endometrium may be so extensive that it can no longer secrete sufficient amounts of prostaglandin, resulting in a prolonged luteal phase.[33] In one study, mares with shortened estrous cycles had the least endometrial damage.[33] More severe endometrial damage was associated with a lengthening of the estrous cycle caused by persistence of the corpus luteum. In a few mares, a complete loss of cyclic luteal function was observed. Ovulation occurred at infrequent intervals, resulting in the constant presence of functional luteal tissue; the longest continuous luteal phase observed was 613 days. No cyclic $PGF_2\alpha$ release patterns were observed in these mares (Fig. 16–2).

TABLE 16–2. DURATION OF LUTEAL ACTIVITY (PLASMA PROGESTERONE > 1 NG/ML) AND OVULATORY INTERVALS (PLASMA PROGESTERONE < 1 NG/ML) IN 16 MARES WITH PYOMETRA

MARE ID NUMBER	DURATION OF LUTEAL ACTIVITY (DAYS)	OVULATORY INTERVALS (DAYS)
18	12, 9, 18, 29*	24, 18, 22
21	422*	—
30	9, 157	20
32	5, 6, 5	17, 15, 13
34	5, 5, 9, 12	16, 13, 20, 19
50	152	—
53	Progesterone < 0.1 ng/mL for 14 months	—
54	11, (124†), 13, 14, 8, 7, 12, 28*	20, 23, 16, 18, 14
55	12, 29, 7, 12, 69, 10, (169†)	28, 41, 12, 41, 75
57	(98†), 613	—
76	17, 49, 17, (112†), 49, 16	25, 59, 53, 18
85	7, 12, 89*	21, 21
93	58, 32, 23, 36	64, 38, 29, 45
98	22*	—
127	139*	—
244	16, 12	29, 23

*Destroyed when active corpus luteum was still present.
†Winter anestrus.
(Adapted from Hughes, J.P., et al.: Pyometra in the mare. J. Reprod. Fertil. Suppl., *27*:321–329, 1979.)

DIESTROUS OVULATIONS

The mare is rather unique among domestic species in her ability to develop and ovulate large follicles during diestrus, when circulating progesterone concentrations are elevated (>1 ng/mL).[5,6,34–36] Diestrous ovulation can occur between days 2 and 15 of the luteal phase in the face of progesterone concentrations as high as 8 ng/mL.[5,6] Ovulation during diestrus is not accompanied by signs of estrus. The cervix is pale, dry, and tight on visual examination; cervical mucus is viscous and sticky; and the mare remains nonreceptive to the stallion.[6]

If ovulation occurs before day 10 of diestrus, both CL respond to $PGF_2\alpha$ and the duration of the estrous cycle is normal. When ovulation occurs late in the luteal phase near or during the time of normal $PGF_2\alpha$ release from the uterus, the mature CL resulting from ovulation at the previous estrus will respond to the luteolytic effects of the $PGF_2\alpha$ release. However, the newly formed CL from the diestrous ovulation will lack the 4- to 5-

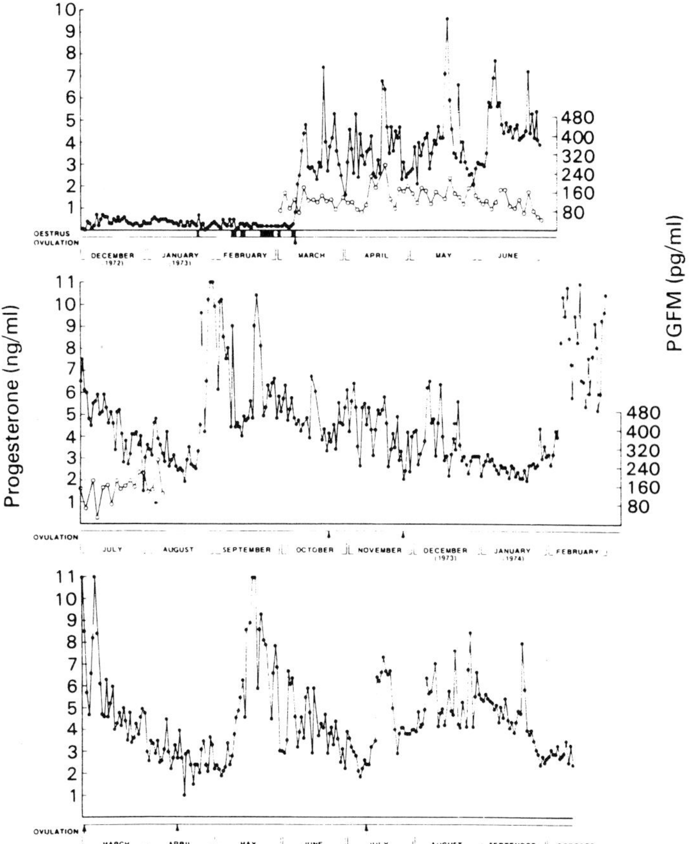

FIG. 16–2. Plasma progesterone (●) and $PGF_2\alpha$ metabolite (13,14-dihydro-15-keto metabolite) (○) concentrations in a mare with pyometra. Continual luteal activity was observed over a period of 613 days. No significant changes in 13,14-dihydro-15-keto metabolite were noted over a 5-month period at the beginning of the observational period. (From Hughes, J.P., et al.: Pyometra in the mare. J. Reprod. Fertil. Suppl., *27:*321–329, 1979.)

day period of maturation and will not respond to the luteolytic effect of $PGF_2\alpha$, resulting in persistence of this CL for a variable period[37–39] (Fig. 16–3).

Even though diestrous ovulations are generally not accompanied by changes in the tubular genital tract, these are fertile ovulations, and conception following artificial insemination has been reported.[40,41] In addition, a CL formed during diestrus appears to have the same steroidogenic potential and produces progesterone equally as well as those formed during estrus.[42]

PERSISTENCE OF THE LUTEAL PHASE

Prolongation of luteal activity in the nonpregnant mare is one of the most important causes of infertility in the mare.[39,43] The luteal phase can be prolonged because of a variety of causes, some of which have been discussed elsewhere in this chapter. Causes for persistence of the luteal phase can be summarized as (1) failure of the CL to respond to $PGF_2\alpha$ because of development of CL in late diestrus (diestrous ovulation),[5,6,34–36] (2) fetal or pharmacologic inhibition of uterine $PGF_2\alpha$ secretion (pregnancy and pseudopregnancy, nonsteroidal anti-inflammatory drugs), (3) inability of the uterus to secrete $PGF_2\alpha$ owing to extensive destruction of the endometrium (pyometra),[33] (4) disruption of uterine function resulting in failure of $PGF_2\alpha$ secretion at the proper time (manipulation of the genital tract,[14] including embryo flushing, intrauterine infusion of penicillin,[44] and repeated oxytocin administration[15] and (5) idiopathic persistence of the CL. A schematic overview of the causes is shown in Table 16–3. The first four causes are discussed elsewhere in this chapter. Idiopathic persistence of the CL refers to those mares that have a prolonged luteal phase as a result of the persistence of the primary CL (CL that developed at the end of preceding estrus) and do not have a diestrous ovulation or a uterine condition (no embryo or embryonic loss, and have no recognized uterine pathology). Spontaneous or idiopathic persistence of the CL that originates from an estrous-phase ovulation has been accepted as a clinical

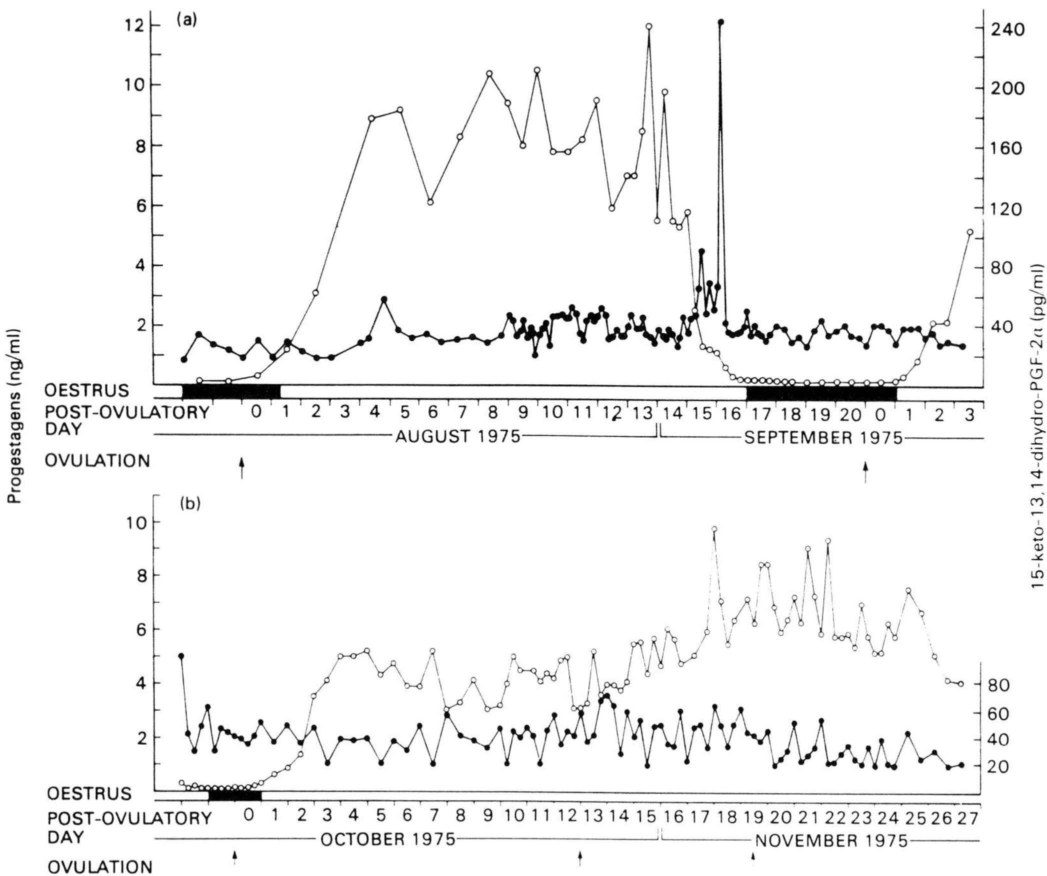

FIG. 16–3. Peripheral plasma concentrations of $PGF_2\alpha$ metabolite (14-dihydro-15-keto metabolite) (●) and progestagens (○) during (A) a normal estrous cycle and (B) the same mare when failure to release $PGF_2\alpha$ resulted in a persistent luteal phase. Diestrous ovulation occurred on days 13 and 19. (From Neely, D.P., et al.: Prostaglandin release patterns in the mare: Physiological, pathophysiological, and therapeutic responses. J. Reprod. Fertil. Suppl., *27:*181–189, 1979.)

entity by many reviewers.[45–50] However, some controversy is found concerning the existence of this type of anomaly, and some researchers have argued that this condition may have been confused with prolongation of the luteal phase caused by ovulation late in the luteal phase.[45] Many of these studies predated the use of ultrasonography to monitor the presence of a CL and, in some instances, the detection of ovulation subsequent to estrous phase ovulation was unreliable.[51] Hypothetical examples of dysfunctions that could cause the spontaneous prolongation of the luteal phase include failure of the CL to respond to $PGF_2\alpha$, failure of uterine $PGF_2\alpha$ to reach the CL, and failure of the uterus to synthesize and/or release prostaglandin $F_2\alpha$.[45]

OVARIAN DISEASE

Ovarian disease may be suspected in ovaries that are larger than 10 to 12 cm in diameter and in which the ovulation fossa is obliterated. However, physiologic enlargement of ovaries may occur in mares that develop several large follicles (up to 10 cm in diameter), in mares during the transitional period when several large follicles develop but fail to ovulate, and during pregnancy when eCG stimulates the development of multiple large follicles and secondary corpora lutea. Ultrasonography may be particularly useful in differentiating these conditions (Chapter 31).

HEMATOMA

Hematomas of the ovary may be confused with ovarian tumors, but are rarely pathologic. Hemorrhage into the follicular lumen occurs regularly during ovulation. The amount of hemorrhage varies considerably. On occasion, hemorrhage continues to distend the former cavity of the follicle, resulting in a hematoma of variable size that persists for a variable period, often past the following ovulation. The functional life span of the luteal tissue that develops in the hematoma is normal and ovarian activity is unaffected.[5,9] A hematoma may become so large that it remains within the ovary for several cy-

TABLE 16–3. SCHEMATIC OVERVIEW OF DIFFERENT CONDITIONS THAT MAY ALTER THE ESTROUS CYCLE*

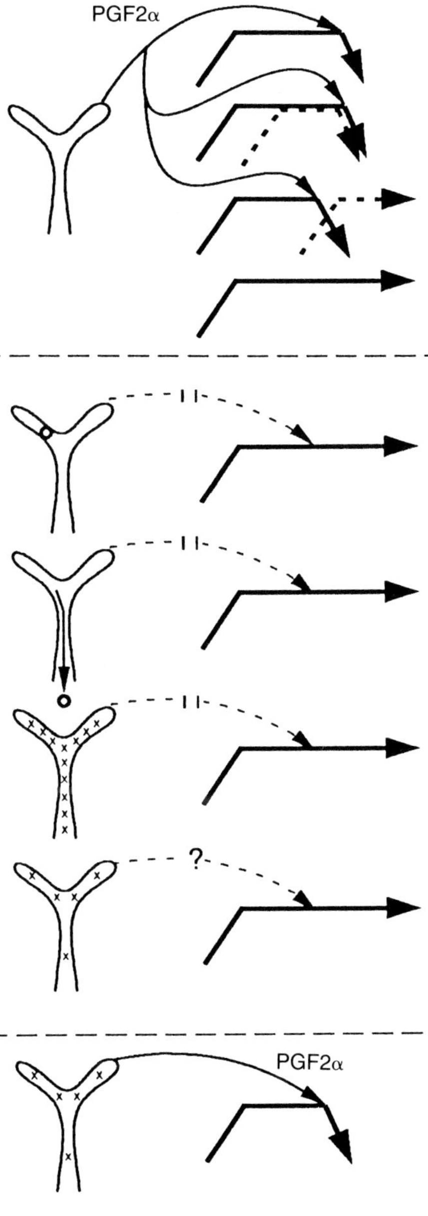

Condition of Uterus	Luteal or Progesterone Profile	Length of Luteal Activity	
Normal estrous cycle	PGF2α	Normal (14 days)	Regression of primary corpus luteum at expected time
Ovulation in early diestrus		Normal (14 days)	Secondary corpus luteum mature and responsive to PGF
Ovulation in late diestrus		Prolonged (length unknown)	Secondary corpus luteum mature and unresponsive to PGF
Idiopathic prolongation of luteal phase		Prolonged	Persistence of primary corpus luteum without known pathological conditions
Pregnancy		Prolonged	Normal maintenance of primary corpus luteum
Embryo lost after critical period		Prolonged	Persistence of primary corpus luteum after embryonic loss
Severe uterine pathology		Prolonged	Uteropathic persistence of primary corpus luteum
Intrauterine intervention with minimal uterine irritation	?	Prolonged	Interference with normal PGF2α dynamics resulting in persistence of primary corpus luteum
Inflammation with intrauterine irritant	PGF2α	Shortened	Uteropathic early regression of primary corpus luteum

*Solid arrow, development and regression of the primary CL; broken-line arrow, development of CL from a diestrous ovulation. (Adapted from Ginther, O.J.: Prolonged luteal activity in mares—A semantic quagmire. Equine Vet. J., *22*:152–156, 1990.)

cles before it is reabsorbed, leaving a firm, calcified area. On occasion the hematoma persists resulting in destruction of ovarian germinal tissue, because of pressure, and leaving a large encapsulated fluid-filled cavity or clotted residue. If the affected ovary becomes nonfunctional, the contralateral ovary normally continues its cyclic activity.

NEOPLASIA

Cystadenoma

Few cases of cystadenoma have been observed in the mare.[52–56] In two mares with cystadenoma, plasma testosterone concentrations were elevated.[52,55] In one jenny, testosterone values appeared normal but decreased significantly after removal of the tumor.[54] In another mare, testosterone was undetectable in cyst fluid.[53] No changes in behavior have been reported and small follicles and luteal tissue have been observed on the contralateral ovary.[52,53] All reported cases were presented because of infertility, and although the mares may have had normal estrous cycles at the initial stages of the development of the tumor, it is not clear if mares with cystadenoma continue to have normal estrous cycles.

GRANULOSA-THECA CELL TUMOR

Granulosa-theca cell tumors, while rare, are the most common ovarian tumors followed by cyst adenomas. Granulosa-theca cell tumors result in the destruction of the affected ovary, rendering it nonfunctional and are most often associated with complete atrophy of the contralateral ovary.[55,57,58] Exceptionally, mares with granulosa-theca cell tumors will continue to have normal ovarian activity on the contralateral ovary.[58,59]

Mares with granulosa-theca cell tumors often have elevated plasma testosterone or estrogen concentrations and demonstrate three main types of behavioral patterns: (1) anestrus, (2) continuous or intermittent estrous behavior, and (3) stallion-like behavior, which includes teasing and mounting other mares and aggressiveness[6,55,57,58,60,61] (Table 16–4). Stallion-like behavior is generally associated with high testosterone concentrations (i.e., > 100 pg/mL plasma).[55] The reason for intermittent to continuous estrous behavior seems less obvious. Estrogen concentrations are similar in mares displaying anestrus or estrous behavior. Individual differences in sensitivity to estrogen in the absence of progesterone, rather than estrogen concentrations per se, may be responsible for the inconsistent behavioral pattern.

Why the contralateral ovary of mares with a granulosa-theca cell tumor is completely inactive is not clear. In contrast, mares with cystadenoma also have elevated testosterone secretion, but the activity of the contralateral ovary does not seem to be completely inhibited, and we have observed at least one mare that conceived while a cystadenoma was present. In view of the total lack of follicular development on the contralateral ovary in mares with granulosa-theca cell tumor, that ovarian activity persists in the presence of elevated testosterone concentrations in mares with cystadenoma seems surprising. However, testosterone may not be the reason for the ovarian activity observed in mares with granulosa-theca cell tumors. Testosterone concentrations are not elevated in 10 to 50% of mares with granulosa-theca cell tumor, and yet most have an inactive, contralateral ovary. New data indicate that secretion of high amounts of inhibin by the neoplastic granulosa cells which inhibit pituitary follicle-stimulating hormone (FSH) secretion may be the reason for atrophy of the contralateral ovary. Piquette et al. have demonstrated that the equine granulosa-theca cell tumors express the mRNA for inhibin and also secrete inhibin subunits.[62] The interplay of inhibin and ovarian steroids with pituitary gonadotropin secretion may be responsible for the inactivity observed in the contralateral ovary.

TABLE 16–4. SEXUAL BEHAVIOR BEFORE AND AFTER SURGICAL REMOVAL OF GRANULOSA-THECA CELL TUMORS IN 78 MARES

PRESURGICAL		POSTSURGICAL	
Anestrus	20*	Normal	58
Continuous estrus	14	Mild stallion-like behavior	7
Stallion-like behavior	29	No information	5
Not recorded	15		
Total	78	Total	70†

OCCURRENCE OF ESTROUS CYCLES AND FERTILITY AFTER SURGICAL REMOVAL OF GRANULOSA-THECA CELL TUMOR IN 70 MARES

Regular estrous cycles	42	Bred postsurgically (30 produced livefoals)	39
Irregular sexual behavior longer than 12 months after surgery	7	Not bred postsurgically	13
		Both ovaries removed	2
Remained anestrous longer than 12 months postsurgically	8	No report	16
Both ovaries removed	2		
No report	11		
Total	70	Total	70

*Number of mares expressing specific behavior

†Eight cases did not survive long enough for postsurgical observations.

(Adapted from Meagher, D.M., et al.: Granulosa cell tumors in mares—A review of 78 cases. Proc. Am. Assoc. Equine Pract., 133–142, 1977.)

Surgical removal of the affected ovary results in the reestablishment of normal estrous cycles in most mares.[57] The reproductive performance after surgical removal of the neoplastic ovary in 70 mares is summarized in Table 16–4. Time from hemiovariectomy to resumption of normal estrous cycles depends on the individual mare and time of year surgery is performed and ranged from 2 to 16 months.[57,63] In a study done by Meagher et al., 12 mares were examined daily, and the interval from surgery to first ovulation for 10 of those mares ranged from 83 to 392 days (mean 209 days).[57] The other two mares failed to ovulate in 225 and 524 days, respectively. Mares that are operated late in the breeding season may not return to cyclic ovarian activity until the following spring.[55] The occurrence of winter anestrus with its suppressive effects on gonadotropin secretion undoubtedly influences the time of return to ovarian cyclicity. Normal fertility can be expected following surgery, providing that the rest of the genital organs were normal at the time of surgery (Table 16–4).[57,63]

GERM CELL TUMORS

Most germ cell tumors in the mare are benign cystic teratomas which are hormonally inactive. Affected mares have normal estrous cycles.[6] Arrhenoblastoma has been reported in one mare and was associated with aggressive, stallion-like behavior.[64] After surgical removal of the affected ovary, normal estrous cycles were observed in the following breeding season, and the mare conceived 2 yr after surgery.

ENDOMETRITIS

During mating or insemination, the uterus is commonly contaminated with bacteria and other irritants which induce a transient uterine inflammation. The inflammation may induce uterine secretion of $PGF_2\alpha$; however, the CL formed during or immediately following estrus is immature and does not respond to the potentially luteolytic amounts of $PGF_2\alpha$. If endometritis occurs after day 5 to 6 of diestrus, inflammation of the uterus induces a surge of $PGF_2\alpha$ secretion, which results in a rapid decline of progesterone and complete luteolysis (Fig. 16–4).[37,65] Experimental inoculation of the uterus with Streptococcus zooepidemicus during diestrus resulted in a reduction of the interval between ovulations.[66,67] Inoculation during estrus does not affect the interovulatory interval. As with bacterial endometritis, endometritis caused by intrauterine infusion[68–71] or endometrial biopsy[72,73] can trigger the release of $PGF_2\alpha$ from the uterus and result in luteolysis.

IATROGENIC FACTORS

INTRAUTERINE INFUSION

Intrauterine infusion for the induction of estrus in the mare was used as early as 1935.[74,75] Infusion of acidic saline, or any other irritant, in the diestrous uterus causes $PGF_2\alpha$ release, within 5 min, which often results in regression of the mature CL and shortening of the diestrus period (Fig. 16–5).[76] Occasionally, infusion of physiologic saline during the luteal phase does not elicit $PGF_2\alpha$ secretion. Pascoe et al. found that the acidity of saline was critical to $PGF_2\alpha$ secretion.[68] Infusion of acidic saline, as opposed to saline with a neutral pH, consistently initiated $PGF_2\alpha$ secretion within minutes. Pascoe proposed that if fluids are close to the physiologic state (physiologic saline with neutral pH or phosphate buffered solutions), little or no secretion of $PGF_2\alpha$ will occur. Sometimes the secretion of $PGF_2\alpha$ occurs 48 to 72 h after the infusion of physiologic saline with neutral pH. This delayed release is probably the result of a slow developing endometritis caused by bacterial contamination at the time of infusion. This agrees with the observation that intrauterine infusion of physiologic saline containing antibiotics did not cause immediate or delayed release of $PGF_2\alpha$.[77]

MANIPULATION OF THE GENITAL TRACT

It is clear that manipulation of the genital tract, including palpation and manipulation of the uterus,[77] cervical dilatation,[73,78,79] embryo flushing, and embryo transfer[14] can induce the release of $PGF_2\alpha$.[14] However, the extent of $PGF_2\alpha$ release and the impact on luteal function are quite variable and are impossible to predict. Bowen et al. observed no change in mean estrous cycle length following nonsurgical embryo collection and autotransfer in mares and concluded $PGF_2\alpha$ release, if present, was insufficient to induce luteolysis.[80] Betteridge et al. monitored $PGF_2\alpha$ secretion during embryo recovery and embryo insertion and found that several components of the procedure caused $PGF_2\alpha$ release.[14] Prostaglandin release was observed in 75% of the mares during cervical dilatation and uterine manipulation and less frequently during vaginal distention and infusion of phosphate buffered saline. Sirois et al. reported that, during similar procedures, sig-

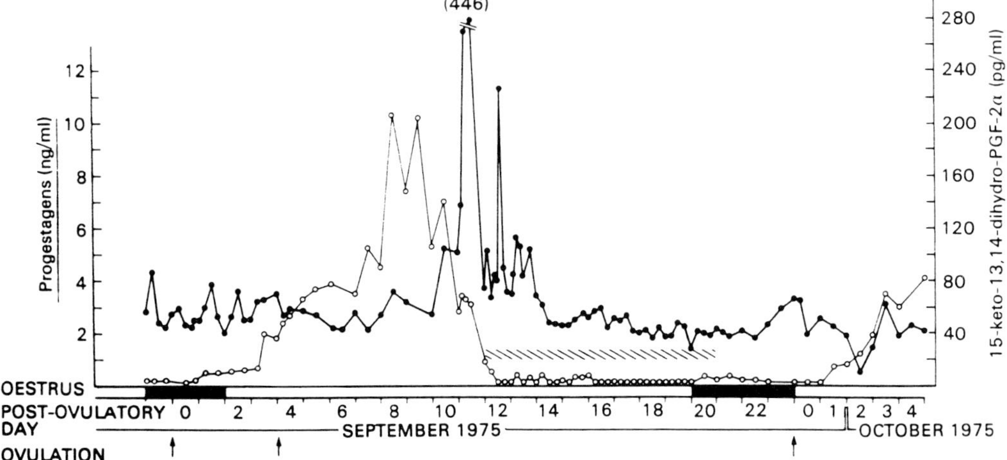

FIG. 16–4. Plasma concentrations of 13,14-dihydro-15-keto metabolite (●) and progesterone (○) of a mare with an endometrial infection which caused premature $PGF_2\alpha$ release and luteolysis. A diestrous ovulation occurred on day 4. The hatched bar indicates the presence of a cervicovaginal exudative discharge, which correlates closely with the major surge release of prostaglandin $F_2\alpha$. (Adapted from Neely, D.P., et al.: Prostaglandin release patterns in the mare: Physiological, pathophysiological, and therapeutic responses. J. Reprod. Fertil. Suppl., *27*:181–189, 1979.)

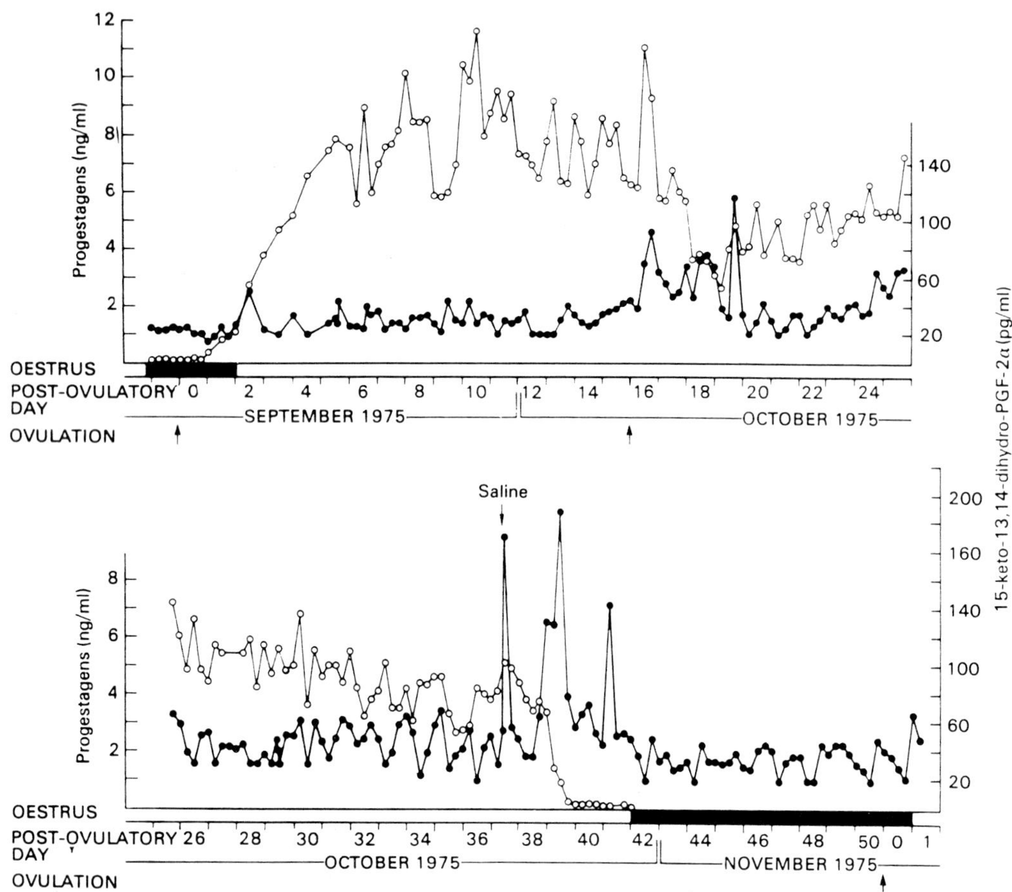

FIG. 16–5. Plasma concentrations of 13,14-dihydro-15-keto metabolite (●) and progesterone (○) of a mare, with a persistent luteal phase, which was given an intrauterine infusion of sterile physiological saline on day 37 of the prolonged luteal phase. A diestrous ovulation occurred on day 16 and likely resulted in prolongation of the luteal phase. (Adapted from Neely, D.P., et al.: Prostaglandin release patterns in the mare: Physiological, pathophysiological, and therapeutic responses. J. Reprod. Fertil. Suppl., *27:*181–189, 1979.)

nificant increases in $PGF_2\alpha$ secretion occurred in some but not all mares and only in one mare was the $PGF_2\alpha$ secretion associated with luteolysis.[81]

Although embryo flushing is likely to shorten the luteal phase, the relative frequent occurrence of prolonged luteal phases following embryo collection may be associated with pregnancy (i.e., the embryo remained in the uterus despite the uterine lavage) but it may also suggest that intrauterine intervention during the luteal phase may interfere with physiologic $PGF_2\alpha$ dynamics and result in prolongation of the cycle.[14] Likewise, intrauterine infusion of a 15 mL penicillin solution has been reported to prolong the luteal phase.[44]

ENDOMETRIAL BIOPSY

Obtaining an endometrial biopsy in the midluteal phase (day 4 to 10 after ovulation) can, but does not consistently, cause premature regression of the CL and return to estrus.[73,82,83] As suggested earlier, cervical and uterine manipulation and uterine trauma associated with taking an endometrial biopsy may induce an immediate release of $PGF_2\alpha$, resulting in luteolysis. The reported time course of decline in progesterone secretion and return to estrus suggests that obtaining a biopsy induces an immediate release of $PGF_2\alpha$ release (Fig. 16–6).[73] According to one source, the acute release of $PGF_2\alpha$ from the uterus and luteolysis can be blocked by concurrent treatment with phenylbutazone.[72] This suggests that the trauma inflicted by taking the biopsy is the trigger for uterine $PGF_2\alpha$. Alternatively, some researchers have suggested that the luteolytic effect of the endometrial biopsy is mediated through bacterial endometritis as a result of uterine contamination during the procedure. When mares received an intrauterine antibiotic infusion following biopsy, progesterone concentrations remained elevated and mares did not return to estrus prematurely, suggesting that bacterial contamination was a factor in inducing luteolysis (Table 16–5).[83]

ANABOLIC STEROIDS

The effect of anabolic steroids on reproductive function and estrous behavior varies among preparations and depends on their androgenic characteristics. Anabolic steroids, derivatives of testosterone, have generally high

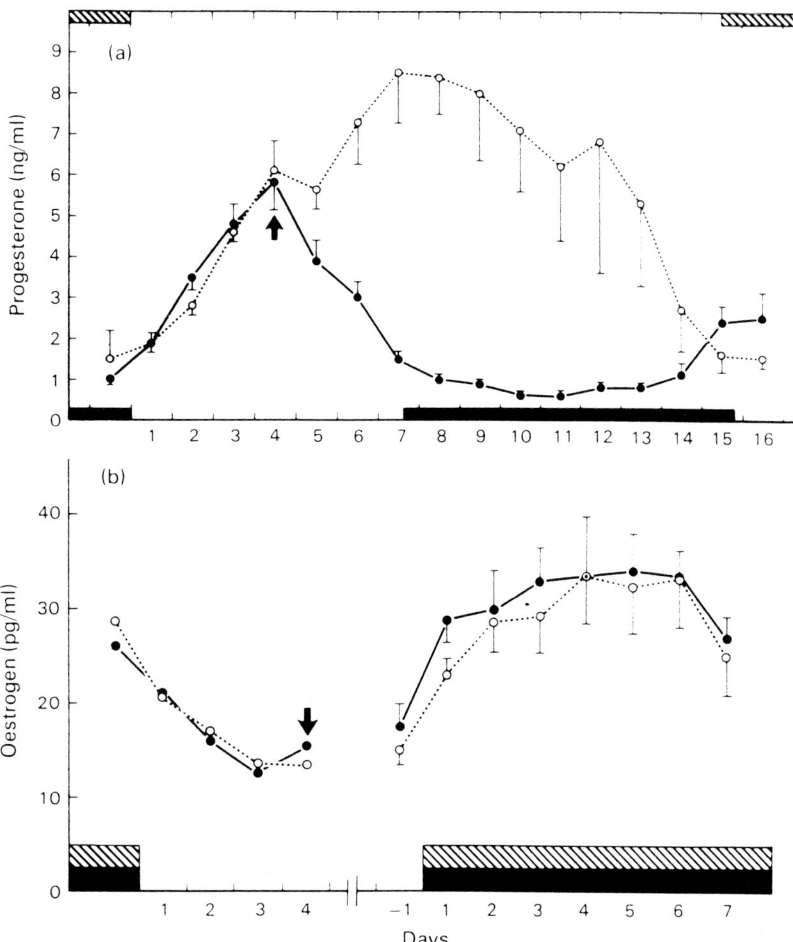

FIG. 16–6. Mean serum progesterone concentrations for five paired estrous cycles in mares that were biopsied (arrow) 6 or 7 days after ovulation (●) and respective control cycles (○). Estrus is indicated by the solid horizontal bars for treatment cycles and broken horizontal bars for control cycles. (Adapted from Hurtgen, J.P., and Ganjam, V.K.: The effect of intrauterine and cervical manipulation on the equine oestrous cycle and hormone profiles. J. Reprod. Fertil. Suppl., *27:*191–197, 1979.)

anabolic potency and minimal, but variable, androgenic potency. Several studies have shown a dose- and drug-dependent suppression of estrous behavior and ovarian function.[84–92] In general, at lower doses, anabolic steroids cause abnormal sexual activity, characterized by stallion-like behavior, mounting of mares in estrus, and aggressiveness toward other horses.[85,87,93–95] Treated mares failed to exhibit normal estrous behavior and did not allow mating, even though they had normal, cyclic ovarian activity.[87,88,90] At higher doses, ovarian activity is inhibited and ovulation is erratic or absent. The effects of steroid administration persist following the end of treatment.[85] When prepuberal mares are treated for a prolonged period, clitoral hypertrophy occurs and persists after the end of treatment.[85,87] In a group of 2-yr-old mares, the detrimental effect of steroid treatment on internal genitalia appeared to be reversed within a few months.[90] Abnormal behavior, however, including absence of signs of estrus, violent rejection of the stallion, and stallion-like behavior toward other mares persisted into the following breeding season. The steroid-treated mares required a management program involving daily palpation and artificial insemination if fertilization was to be achieved, because of the lack of normal estrous behavior.

PROGESTERONE AND PROGESTIN

In nonpregnant mares, progestins are used for the suppression of undesirable estrous behavior or for synchronization of ovulation in cycling mares (Chapters 33 and 39). Progestin, in adequate dosage, effectively inhibits the expression of estrous behavior at all stages of the estrous cycle. The synchronization of estrus is based on the inhibitory effect of progestin on pituitary gonadotropin secretion and subsequent delay of ovulation. However, mares may ovulate in spite of progestin treatment, particularly when treatment is started late in the luteal phase. We have observed a high incidence of persistence of the luteal phase subsequent to ovulation during progestin treatment. In 11 of 12 mares that ovu-

TABLE 16–5. DURATION OF DIESTRUS AND CONCENTRATION OF PROGESTERONE AT THE TIME OF BIOPSY (DAY 0) AND 4 DAYS LATER (DAY 4) IN FOUR MARES DURING THREE CONSECUTIVE ESTROUS CYCLES

ESTROUS CYCLE	TREATMENT	DIESTRUS (DAYS)	SERUM PROGESTERONE CONCENTRATIONS	
			Day 0 (ng/mL)	Day 4 (ng/mL)
1	Control	15.8 ± 0.8*	5.8 ± 0.9	9.8 ± 0.8
2	Biopsy†	8.3 ± 0.6	9.2 ± 1.0	1.4 ± 0.5
3	Biopsy† and antibiotic‡	22.3 ± 5.2	8.1 ± 1.5	10.2 ± 1.4

*Values are expressed as means plus or minus the standard error of the mean.
†Biopsy was taken 4 days after ovulation.
‡Gentamicin sulfate (500 mg) was infused immediately after biopsy.
(Adapted from Baker, C.B., Newton, D.I., Mather, E.C., and Oxender, W.D.: Luteolysis in mares after endometrial biopsy. Am. J. Vet. Res., *42*:1816–1818, 1981.)

lated while being treated with altrenogest, a synthetic progestin, the resulting CL persisted for more than 20 days (maximum observed 54 days). When those mares were treated with prostaglandin, they returned to estrus and ovulated within the expected time.

NONSTEROIDAL ANTI-INFLAMMATORY DRUGS

Pascoe studied the inhibitory effect of phenylbutazone, flunixin meglumine, naproxen, and meclofenamic acid on endometrial $PGF_2\alpha$ synthesis after intrauterine infusion of sterile acidic saline and concluded that administration of a pharmacologic dose of nonsteroidal anti-inflammatory drugs (NSAIDs) effectively inhibited the release of $PGF_2\alpha$ from the uterus for up to 10 h.[77,96] Other studies indicate that phenylbutazone administration prevents luteolysis following uterine biopsy on day 4 after ovulation and flunixin meglumine administration reduces intraluminal $PGF_2\alpha$ concentrations in the nonpregnant mare.[72,79] However, daily administration of phenylbutazone (2 gm IV) did not prevent spontaneous luteolysis during normal estrous cycles.[97] Similarly, administration of flunixin meglumine (500 mg at 8-h interval IV) starting on day 12 after ovulation failed to prevent consistent regression of the CL (D. Appel, personal communication). The available information indicates that NSAIDs can acutely inhibit endometrial $PGF_2\alpha$ secretion induced by iatrogenic stimulation of the uterus (saline infusion, biopsy, embryo flushing). However, chronic treatment with NSAIDs at current clinical dosage does not appear to inhibit the spontaneous release of $PGF_2\alpha$ associated with luteolysis.

PROSTAGLANDIN $F_2\alpha$

The administration of $PGF_2\alpha$ or its analogue between day 5 of diestrus and spontaneous luteolysis results in the immediate regression of the CL and return to estrus within a few days (Chapters 8 and 34).

SYSTEMIC ILLNESS

ENDOTOXEMIA

Endotoxin has long been known to cause abortion in women as well as in other species.[98] Early studies in mice implicate $PGF_2\alpha$ as the mediator of the abortifacient action of endotoxin.[99] More recently the involvement of $PGF_2\alpha$ in endotoxin-induced abortion has been shown in pigs,[100] goats,[101] cows,[102] and horses.[103] In the horse, the immediate and pronounced release of $PGF_2\alpha$ during endotoxemia can result in regression of the CL. In the nonpregnant diestrous mare, experimentally induced endotoxemia stimulated a surge of $PGF_2\alpha$, luteolysis, and premature return to estrus.[104,105] The rate of decline in progesterone secretion and the time to estrus were similar to those observed following intramuscular administration of $PGF_2\alpha$ or its analogue. The effect of endotoxemia on the reproductive cycle can be blocked by timely administration of NSAIDs;[106] however, NSAIDs need to be administered early in the disease process. Administration of the NSAID flunixin meglumine before systemic endotoxin injection successfully prevents luteolysis normally associated with endotoxemia.[106] Flunixin meglumine administered 2 h after endotoxin injection failed to prevent luteolysis because of the rapid onset of $PGF_2\alpha$ secretion.

OTHER AILMENTS

Cushing's syndrome caused by adenomatous hyperplasia of the intermediate pituitary has been associated with anestrus in aged mares.[107] Persistent anestrus has also been diagnosed in older mares which did not show obvious clinical signs of Cushing's disease but were later diagnosed as affected with the disease. The exact cause of anestrus in these mares is unclear, but several mechanisms have been suggested. Severe compression of the pars distalis of the pituitary resulting in destruction of the luteinizing hormone (LH) and FSH-secreting cells has been observed (P. Kennedy, personal communication). In women, secondary amenorrhea is commonly observed in naturally occurring forms of hypercortisolism. Endogenous overproduction of glucocorticoids is accompanied by increases in secretion of adrenal androgens, some of which may serve as precursors of extraovarian estrogens. These steroids may have an inhibitory effect on the hypothalamo-pituitary-gonadal axis and disrupt the menstrual cycle in women. A similar mechanism may apply in the mare.

NUTRITION AND BODY CONDITION

The effect of nutrition needs further investigation to understand its effect on reproductive function. Cyclic, ovarian activity has been shown to start earlier in the spring in mares on a higher plane of nutrition than those fed maintenance rations.[8] Furthermore, onset of estrus and ovulation appeared to be delayed in barren and maiden mares entering the breeding season in thin condition.[27] Mares fed dried feed have a dramatic increase in ovulatory activity and ovulation when they are turned out on fresh grass in the spring.[6]

CHROMOSOMAL ABNORMALITIES

The most common chromosomal abnormalities are the 63 XO and the 64 XY sex reversal (phenotypic female) (Chapter 30). Mares with these types of chromosomal abnormalities have hypoplastic ovaries, fail to develop follicles, and do not cycle normally. These mares may exhibit estrous behavior occasionally, but generally any cyclic behavioral pattern is absent.

REFERENCES

1. Swenson, M.J.: Dukes' Physiology of Domestic Animals. 10th ed. Ithaca, Cornell University Press, 1984.
2. Saltiel, A., Calderon, A., Garcia, N., and Hurley, D.P.: Ovarian activity in the mare between latitude 15° and 22°N. J. Reprod. Fertil. Suppl., *32:*261–267, 1982.
3. Evans, J.W., Hughes, J.P., and Stabenfeldt, G.H.: The effect of season on the equine estrous cycle. J. Anim. Sci., *33:*253–257, 1971.
4. Osborne, V.E.: An analysis of the pattern of ovulation as it occurs in the annual reproductive cycle of the mare in Australia. Aust. Vet. J., *42:*149–154, 1966.
5. Hughes, J.P., Stabenfeldt, G.H., and Evans, J.W.: Clinical and endocrine aspects of the estrous cycle of the mare. Proc. Am. Assoc. Equine Pract., 119–148, 1972.
6. Hughes, J.P., Stabenfeldt, G.H., and Kennedy, P.C.: The estrous cycle and selected functional and pathologic ovarian abnormalities in the mare. Vet. Clin. North Am. Large Anim. Pract., *2:*225–239, 1980.
7. Van Niekerk, C.H.: Patterns of the oestrus cycle of mares. J. S. Afr. Vet. Med. Assoc., *38:*295–298, 1967.
8. Belonje, P.C., and van Niekerk, C.H.: A review of the influence of nutrition upon the oestrous cycle and early pregnancy in the mare. J. Reprod. Fertil. Suppl., *23:*167–169, 1975.
9. Hughes, J.P., Stabenfeldt, G.H., and Evans, J.W.: Estrous cycle and ovulation in the mare. J. Am. Vet. Med. Assoc., *161:*1367–1374, 1972.
10. Ginther, O.J.: Folliculogenesis during the transitional period and early ovulatory season in mares. J. Reprod. Fertil., *90:*311–320, 1990.
11. Ginther, O.J.: Follicular dynamics in heifers and mares. Proc. Ann. Meet. Soc. Theriogenol., 2–12, 1989.
12. Palmer, E.: New results on follicular growth and ovulation in the mare. *In* Follicular Growth and Ovulation Rate in Farm Animals. Edited by J.F. Roche and D. O'Callaghan. Dordrecht, Martinus Nijhoff, 1987, p. 237–255.
13. Carnevale, E.M., Squires, E.L., McKinnon, A.O., and Harrison, L.A.: Effect of human chorionic gonadotropin on time to ovulation and luteal function in transitional mares. J. Equine. Vet. Sci., *9:*27–29, 1989.
14. Betteridge, K.J., Renard, A., and Goff, A.K.: Uterine prostaglandin release relative to embryo collection, transfer procedure and maintenance of the corpus luteum. Equine Vet. J. Suppl., *3:*25–33, 1985.
15. Goff, A.K., Pontbriand, D., and Sirois, J.: Oxytocin stimulation of plasma 15-keto-13,14-dihydro prostaglandin $F_2\alpha$ during the oestrous cycle and early pregnancy in the mare. J. Reprod. Fertil. Suppl., *35:*253–260, 1987.
16. Squires, E.L., and Ginther, O.J.: Follicular and luteal development in pregnant mares. J. Reprod. Fertil. Suppl., *23:*429–433, 1975.
17. Squires, E.L., Douglas, R.H., Steffenhagen, W.P., and Ginther, O.J.: Ovarian changes during the estrous cycle and pregnancy in the mare. J. Anim. Sci., *38:*330–338, 1974.
18. Squires, E.L., Garcia, M.C., and Ginther, O.J.: Effects of pregnancy and hysterectomy on the ovaries of pony mares. J. Anim. Sci., *38:*823–830, 1974.
19. Allen, W.R.: Hormonal control of early pregnancy in the mare. Vet. Clin. North Am. Large Anim. Pract., *2:*291–302, 1980.
20. Allen, W.R.: Factors influencing pregnant mare serum gonadotropin production. Nature, *223:*64–66, 1969.
21. Mitchell, D., and Allen, W.R.: Observations on reproductive performance in the yearling mare. J. Reprod. Fertil. Suppl., *23:*531–536, 1975.
22. Rathwell, A.C., Asbury, A.C., Hansen, P.J., and Archbald, L.F.: Reproductive function of mares given $PGF_2\alpha$ daily from day 42 of pregnancy. J. Reprod. Fertil. Suppl., *35:*507–508, 1987.
23. Varner, D.D., et al.: Effect of equine abortifacients on fetal viability and post-abortion reproductive performance. Proceedings of the International Congress on Animal Reproduction and Artificial Insemination, 1988, p. 130.
24. Penzhorn, B.L., Bertschinger, H.J., and Coubrough, R.I.: Reconception of mares following termination of pregnancy with prostaglandin $F_2\alpha$ before and after day 35 of pregnancy. Equine Vet. J., *18:*215–217, 1986.
25. Ginther, O.J.: Ultrasonic Imaging and Reproductive Events in the Mare. Cross Piains, WI, Equiservices, 1986.
26. Loy, R.G.: Characteristics of postpartum reproduction in mares. Vet. Clin. North Am. Large Anim. Pract., *2:*345–359, 1980.
27. Henneke, D.R., Potter, G.D., and Kreider, J.L.: Body condition during pregnancy and lactation and reproduc-

tive efficiency of mares. Theriogenology, *21:*897–909, 1984.

28. Neuschaefer, A., Bracher, V., and Allen, W.R.: Prolactin secretion in lactating mares before and after treatment with bromocryptine. J. Reprod. Fertil. Suppl., *44:*551–559, 1991.

29. Hughes, J.P., and Stabenfeldt, G.H.: Anestrus in the mare. Proc. Am. Assoc. Equine Pract., 89–96, 1977.

30. Hughes, J.P., Stabenfeldt, G.H., and Evans, J.W.: Clinical and endocrine aspects of the estrous cycle of the mare. Proc. Am. Assoc. Equine Pract., 119–125, 1973.

31. Grimmett, J.B.: Behavioral anestrus. *In* Current Therapy in Equine Medicine. Edited by N.E. Robinson. Philadelphia, W.B. Saunders, 1983, pp. 400–401.

32. Irvine, C.H.G.: The abnormal estrous cycle. *In* Post-Graduate Course on Equine Reproduction. Massey University, 1976.

33. Hughes, J.P., et al.: Pyometra in the mare. J. Reprod. Fertil. Suppl., *27:*321–329, 1979.

34. Stabenfeldt, G.H., Hughes, J.P., and Evans, J.W.: Ovarian activity during the estrous cycle of the mare. Endocrinology, *90:*1379–1384, 1972.

35. Henry, M., Coryn, M., and Vandeplassche, M.: Multiple ovulation in the mare. Zbl. Vet. Med. A., *29:*170–184, 1982.

36. Vandeplassche, M., Henry, M., and Coryn, M.: The mature mid-cycle follicle in the mare. J. Reprod. Fertil. Suppl., *27:*157–162, 1979.

37. Neely, D.P., et al: Prostaglandin release patterns in the mare: Physiological, pathophysiological, and therapeutic responses. J. Reprod. Fertil. Suppl., *27:*181–189 1979.

38. Neely, P., Hughes, J.P., Stabenfeldt, G.H., and Evans, J.W.: The influence of intrauterine saline infusion on luteal function and cyclic ovarian activity in the mare. Equine Vet. J., *6:*150–158, 1974.

39. Stabenfeldt, G.H., Hughes, J.P., Evans, J.W., and Neely, D.P.: Spontaneous prolongation of luteal activity in the mare. Equine Vet. J., *6:*158–163, 1974.

40. Hughes, J.P., Couto, M.A., and Stabenfeldt, G.H.: Luteal phase ovulations: What are the options? Proc. Ann. Meet. Soc. Theriogenol., 123–125, 1985.

41. Hughes, J.P., and Stabenfeldt, G.H.: Conception in a mare with an active corpus luteum. J. Am. Vet. Med. Assoc., *170:*733–734, 1977.

42. Hughes, J.P., et al.: Production of corpora lutea formed by ovulation during the luteal phase of the estrous cycle (diestrous ovulation). Vlaams Diergeneesk. Tijdschr. *53:*191–196, 1984.

43. Stabenfeldt, G.H., et al.: Physiologic and pathophysiologic aspects of prostaglandin $F_2\alpha$ during the reproductive cycle. J. Am. Vet. Med. Assoc., *176:*1187–1194, 1980.

44. Allen, W.E.: Effect of intrauterine infusion of penicillin solution on luteal function in pony mares. Vet. Rec., *109:*216–217, 1981.

45. Ginther, O.J.: Prolonged luteal activity in the mare—A semantic quagmire. Equine Vet. J., *22:*152–156, 1990.

46. Ginther, O.J.: Reproductive Biology of the Mare—Basic and Applied Aspects. Cross Plains, WI, published by the author, 1979.

47. Henry, M., Coryn, M., Spincemaille, J., and Vandeplassche, M.: Prolonged luteal activity in the mare. Zuchthyg, *16:*145–153, 1981.

48. Lauderdale, J.W.: A review of patterns of change in luteal function. J. Anim. Sci. Suppl. 2, *62:*79–91, 1986.

49. Roberts, S.J.: Veterinary Obstetrics and Genital Diseases (Theriogenology). 3rd ed. Woodstock, VT, published by the author, 1986.

50. Lofstedt, R.M.: Physiology of the equine estrous cycle. Vet. Med. Small Anim. Clin., *74:*1441–1450, 1979.

51. Allen, W.E.: Abnormalities in the oestrous cycle in the mare. Vet. Rec., *104:*166–167, 1979.

52. Hinrichs, K., et al.: Serous cystadenoma in a normally cyclic mare with high plasma testosterone values. J. Am. Vet. Med. Assoc., *194:*381–382, 1989.

53. Held, J.P., Buergelt, C., and Colahan, P.: Serous cystadenoma in a mare. J. Am. Vet. Med. Assoc., *181:*496–498, 1982.

54. Taylor, T.S., Bowen, J.M., and Montgomery, D.L.: Cystadenoma of the ovary in a jennet. Compend. Contin. Educ. Practicing Vet., *5:*S677–S679, 1983.

55. Stabenfeldt, G.H., et al.: Clinical findings, pathological changes and endocrinological secretory patterns in mares with ovarian tumours. J. Reprod. Fertil. Suppl., *27:*277–285, 1979.

56. Hughes, J.P., Kennedy, P.C., and Stabenfeldt, G.H.: Pathology of the ovary and ovarian disorders in the mare. Proceedings of the International Congress on Animal Reproduction and Artificial Insemination, 1980, pp. 203–222.

57. Meagher, D.M., et al.: Granulosa cell tumors in mares—A review of 78 cases. Proc. Am. Assoc. Equine Pract., 133–143, 1977.

58. Hinrichs, K., and Hunt, P.R.: Ultrasound as an aid to diagnosis of granulosa cell tumor in the mare. Equine Vet. J., *22:*99–103, 1990.

59. Hinrichs, K., Watson, E.D., and Kenney, R.M.: Granulosa cell tumor in a mare with functional contralateral ovary. J. Am. Vet. Med. Assoc., *197:*1037–1038, 1990.

60. Frazer, G.S., and Threlfall, W.R.: Differential diagnosis of enlarged ovary in the mare. Proc. Am. Assoc. Equine Pract., 21–28, 1986.

61. Pugh, D.G., Bowen, J.M., and Gaughan, E.M.: Equine ovarian tumors. Compend. Contin. Educ. Practicing Vet., *7:*S710–S716, 1985.

62. Piquette, G.N., et al.: Equine granulosa-theca cell tumors express inhibin α- and βA-subunit messenger ribonucleic acids and proteins. Biol. Reprod., *43:*1050–1057, 1990.

63. Clark, T.L.: Clinical management of equine ovarian neoplasms. J. Reprod. Fertil. Suppl., *23:*331–334, 1975.

64. Mills, J.H.L., Fretz, P.B., Clark, E.G., and Ganjam, V.K.: Arrhenoblastoma in a mare. J. Am. Vet. Med. Assoc., *171:*754–757, 1977.

65. Stabenfeldt, G.H., et al.: The influence of chronic uterine infection on luteal activity in the mare. Proceedings of the Eighth International Congress on Animal Reproduction and Artificial Insemination. Kracow, 1976.

66. Hughes, J.P., and Loy, R.G.: Investigations on the effect of intrauterine inoculations of Streptococcus zooepidemicus in the mare. Proc. Am. Assoc. Equine Pract., 289–292, 1969.

67. Hughes, J.P., Stabenfeldt, G.H., and Evans, J.W.: The oestrous cycle of the mare and its uterine control. Aust. Vet. J., *53:*415–419, 1977.

68. Pascoe, D.R., Stabenfeldt, G.H., Hughes, J.P., and Kindahl, H.: Endogenous prostaglandin $F_2\alpha$ release induced by physiologic saline solution infusion in utero in the mare: Effect of temperature, osmolarity, and pH. Am. J. Vet. Res., *50:*1080–1083, 1989.

69. Stabenfeldt, G.H., et al.: Endogenous and exogenous

manipulation of the corpus luteum of the mare. Proceedings of the Twenty-eighth International Congress of Physiological Sciences. Edited by G. Pethes and V.L. Frenyo. Budapest, Pergamon Press, 1981, p. 133–139.

70. Neely, D.P., Hughes, J.P., and Stabenfeldt, G.H.: The effect of intrauterine saline infusion on luteal function and cyclic activity in the mare. J. Reprod. Fertil. Suppl., *23:*235–239, 1975.

71. Couto, M.A., and Hughes, J.P.: Intrauterine inoculation of a bacteria-free filtrate of streptococcus zooepidemicus in clinically normal and infected mares. J. Equine Vet. Sci., *5:*81–86, 1985.

72. Ellsworth-Swihart, M., Archbald, L.F., Ingraham, R.H., and Godke, R.A.: Effect of phenylbutazone (PBZ) on luteolysis in the mare induced by uterine biopsy. Theriogenology, *23:*381–387, 1985.

73. Hurtgen, J.P., and Ganjam, V.K.: The effect of intrauterine and cervical manipulation on the equine oestrous cycle and hormone profiles. J. Reprod. Fertil. Suppl., *27:*191–197, 1979.

74. Vandeplassche, M.: Some aspects of equine infertility. Proceedings of the Second Annual Congress of the British Equine Veterinarian Association. 1963, pp. 54–63.

75. Zwaenepoel, H., and Royer, A.: Technique de l'Elevage du Poulain. Brussels, Tychon, 1935.

76. Neely, D.P., et al.: Effect of intrauterine saline infusion during the late luteal phase on the estrous cycle and luteal function of the mare. Am. J. Vet. Res., *40:*665–668, 1979.

77. Pascoe, D.R.: Single embryonic reduction in the mare with twin conceptuses: Studies of hormone profiles and drug therapies using a physiological model, and manual and surgical reduction technique in vivo. Ph.D. dissertation. Davis, University of California, 1986.

78. Pieterse, M.C., et al.: Transvaginal ultrasound guided follicular aspiration of bovine oocytes. Theriogenology, *35:*19–24, 1991.

79. Berglund, L.A., Sharp, D.C., Vernon, M.W., and Thatcher, W.W.: Effect of pregnancy and collection techniques on prostaglandin F in the uterine lumen of pony mares. J. Reprod. Fertil. Suppl., *32:*335–341, 1982.

80. Bowen, M.J., Salsbury, J.M., Bowen, J.M., and Kraemer, D.C.: Non-surgical embryo auto-transfer in the mare. Equine Vet. J. Suppl., *3:*100–102, 1985.

81. Sirois, J., Betteridge, K.J., and Goff, A.K.: $PGF_2\alpha$ release, progesterone secretion and conceptus growth associated with successful and unsuccessful transcervical embryo transfer and reinsertion in the mare. J. Reprod. Fertil. Suppl., *35:*419–427, 1987.

82. Hurtgen, J.P., and Whitmore, H.L.: Induction of estrus and ovulation by endometrial biopsy in mares with prolonged diestrus. J. Am. Vet. Med. Assoc., *175:*1196–1197, 1979.

83. Baker, C.B., Newton, D.I., Mather, E.C., and Oxender, W.D.: Luteolysis in mares after endometrial biopsy. Am. J. Vet. Res., *42:*1816–1818, 1981.

84. Upjohn Co.: Winstrol-V: Anabolic Steroid without Side Effects on Reproductive Behavior. Kalamazoo, MI, 1990.

85. Squires, E.L., Voss, J.L., Maher, J.M., and Shideler, R.K.: Fertility of young mares after long-term anabolic steroid treatment. J. Am. Vet. Med. Assoc., *186:*92–95, 1985.

86. Turner, J.E., and Irvine, C.H.G.: Effect of prolonged administration of anabolic and androgenic steroids on reproductive function in the mare. J. Reprod. Fertil. Suppl., *32:*213–218, 1982.

87. Maher, J.M., Squires, E.L., Voss, J.L., and Shideler, R.K.: Effect of anabolic steroids on reproductive function in young mares. J. Am. Vet. Med. Assoc., *183:*519–524, 1983.

88. Pickett, B.W., et al.: Anabolic steroids in mares. *In* Management of the Mare for Maximum Reproductive Efficiency. Fort Collins, Animal Reproduction Laboratory, Colorado State University, 1989, pp. 29–38.

89. Bourke, J.M.: Anabolic steroids and fertility in Thoroughbred mares. J. Reprod. Fertil. Suppl., *32:*623–624, 1982.

90. Skelton, K.V., Dowsett, K.F., and McMeniman, N.P.: Ovarian activity in pubertal fillies treated with anabolic steroids. J. Reprod. Fertil. Suppl., 1991.

91. Squires, E.L., Todter, G.E., Berndtson, W.E., and Pickett, B.W.: Effect of anabolic steroids on reproductive function of young stallions. J. Anim. Sci., *54:*576–582, 1982.

92. Steele, D.P.: Effect of methanedienone on plasma FSH, LH, progesterone and oestrogen levels, heamatology, serum biochemistry and reproductive function in yearling fillies. J. Reprod. Fertil. Suppl., *32:*630, 1982.

93. McDonnell, S.M., Hinrichs, K., Cooper, W.L., and Kenney, R.M.: Use of an androgenized mare as an aid in detection of estrus in mares. Theriogenology, *30:*547–553, 1988.

94. McDonnell, S.M., Garcia, M.C., Blanchard, T.L., and Kenney, R.M.: Evaluation of androgenized mares as an estrus detection aid. Theriogenology, *26:*261–266, 1986.

95. Schumacher, E.M.A., Blackshaw, J.K., and Skelton, K.V.: The behavioral outcomes of anabolic steroid administration to female horses. Equine Pract., *9:*11–15, 1987.

96. Pascoe, D.R., et al.: Management of twin conceptuses by manual embryonic reduction: Comparison of two techniques and three hormone treatments. Am. J. Vet. Res., *48:*1594–1599, 1987.

97. Archbald, D.F., Olsen, L.M., Ingraham, R.H., and Godke, R.A.: Inability of phenylbutazone to alter the function of the corpus luteum in the mare. Equine Vet. J., *15:*275–282, 1983.

98. Roberts, J.S., et al.: Hormonal and related factors affecting the release of prostaglandin $F_2\alpha$ from the uterus. J. Steroid Biochem., *6:*1091–1097, 1975.

99. Skarnes, R.C., and Harper, M.J.K.: Relationship between endotoxin-induced abortion and the synthesis of prostaglandin F. Prostaglandins, *1:*191–203, 1972.

100. Wrathall, A.E., Wray, C., Bailey, J., and Wells, D.E.: Experimentally induced bacterial endotoxaemia and abortion in pigs. Br. Vet. J., *134:*225–230, 1978.

101. Fredriksson, G., Kindahl, H., and Edqvist, L.-E.: Endotoxin-induced prostaglandin release and corpus luteum function in goats. Anim. Reprod. Sci., *8:*109–121, 1985.

102. Giri, S.N., et al.: Effect of endotoxin infusion on circulating levels of eicosanoids, progesterone, cortisol, glucose and lactic acid, and abortion in pregnant cows. Vet. Microbiol., *21:*211–231, 1990.

103. Daels, P.F., Stabenfeldt, G.H., Kindahl, H., and Hughes, J.P.: Prostaglandin release and luteolysis associated with physiological and pathological conditions of the reproductive tract in the mare: A review. Equine Vet. J. Suppl., *8*:29–34, 1989.

104. Fredriksson, G., Kindahl, H., and Stabenfeldt, G.: Endotoxin-induced and prostaglandin-mediated effects on corpus luteum function in the mare. Theriogenology, *25*:309–316, 1986.

105. Daels, P.F., et al.: Effect of Salmonella typhimurium endotoxin on $PGF_2\alpha$ release and fetal death in the mare. J. Reprod. Fertil. Suppl., *35*:485–492, 1987.

106. Daels, P.F., et al.: Effects of flunixin meglumine on endotoxin-induced prostaglandin $F_2\alpha$ secretion during early pregnancy in the mare. Am. J. Vet. Res., *52*:276–281, 1991.

107. Beech, J.: Tumors of pituitary gland (pars intermedia). *In* Current Therapy in Equine Medicine 2. Edited by N.E. Robinson. Philadelphia, W.B. Saunders, 1987, p. 182–185.

CHAPTER 17

FOLLICULOGENESIS AND OVULATION

R.A. Pierson

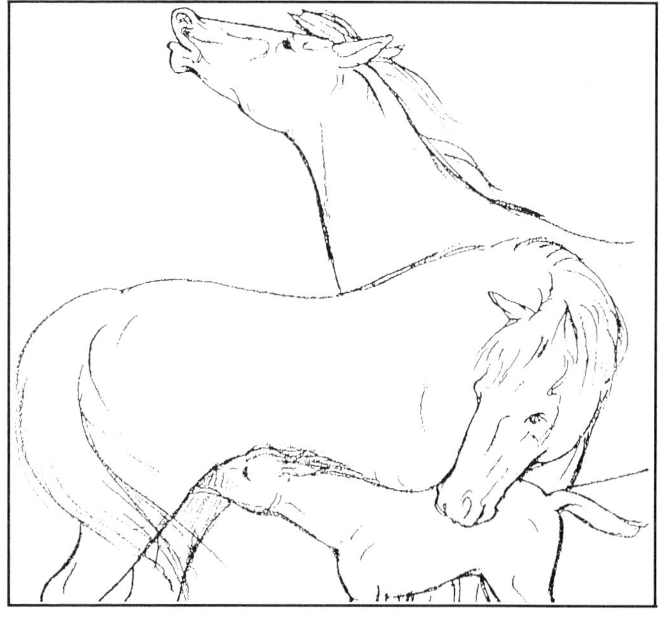

The study of folliculogenesis and ovulation is, and will remain, one of the most fascinating aspects of reproductive biology. The fundamental mechanisms of initiation of follicular growth and development, selection of the follicle destined to ovulate, and the final phases of follicular maturation remain largely unknown. Understanding and control of the cycles of follicular development with the goal of establishing a pregnancy remain of paramount importance in brood mare practice. Specific details of endocrinologic mechanisms and transition from the anovulatory to ovulatory seasons of the year are addressed in other chapters. The goal of this chapter is to provide a synopsis of fundamental aspects of folliculogenesis and ovulation which may be integrated into both basic and clinical frameworks with which to better understand ovarian function in mares.

OOGENESIS

Oogenesis is simply the formation and development of ova (oocytes), or female gametes. The process of oogenesis during early embryonic development provides the basis for the conceptual understanding of folliculogenesis and ovulation in the adult mare. Primordial germ cells, from which ova will eventually arise, differentiate from the epithelium of the yolk sac early on during embryonic development. The primordial germ cells migrate though the developing mesentery of the embryo and colonize the primitive gonadal ridge (ovarian analge). Oogonial multiplication by cellular mitosis apparently begins on approximately day 50 of gestation and may continue until approximately days 150 to 160.[1–3]

During the early fetal period of development, primordial germ cells proliferate by both mitosis and meiosis within the cortex of the developing ovary. At approximately days 70 to 80 of gestation, meiotic cell divisions begin. Eventually, mitotic divisions are halted and meiotic divisions are predominant. The oocytes enter the first meiotic division and are arrested in meiotic prophase.[3] Meioses occur from approximately days 75 to 160. Few germ cell divisions are observed after day 180. No further development occurs for the vast majority of oocytes. Substantial atresia of oocytes occurs during fetal life. Peak levels of atretic follicles are observed at approximately day 100. Meiosis resumes only following the luteinizing hormone (LH) surge for the selected few oocyte/follicle complexes which attain preovulatory status during adult life. The current general understanding is that the number of oocytes in the ovaries present at birth represents the total complement of oocytes available to the mare throughout her reproductive life.

As embryonic development and differentiation ensues, primordial follicles are formed when the oocytes become encased with surrounding cells. Primordial follicles are found within the ovaries from early fetal life though ovarian senescence. The processes of oogenesis and folliculogenesis thus represent a continuum rather than separate and distinct events. The fates of the oocytes and follicles are inextricably intertwined throughout a mare's reproductive lifetime.

FOLLICULOGENESIS

The follicle is the fundamental structural and functional unit of the ovary. Our understanding of the mechanisms involved in transformation of primordial follicles from a static state into the growing pool of active follicles is fragmentary at best. However, once a follicle enters the growing, or active, pool of follicles it progresses through a series of developmental changes that may be identified on the basis of physiologic and morphologic criteria. The entry of a primordial follicle into the growth and differentiation processes of folliculogenesis represents an irreversible commitment to one of two fates: atresia or ovulation. Atresia is the fate of all but a small percentage of all follicles. The cycles of development of follicles have been divided into functional divisions for the purposes of describing the events which occur during folliculogenesis. They are the selection phase, during which many follicles develop and subsequently undergo atresia; the dominance phase, during which one follicle becomes larger than all of the others; and the phase of ovulation or atresia, during which the dominant follicle either proceeds to ovulate or undergoes atresia. The ovarian follicle has both endocrine (production of estrogens and nonsteroid hormones) and exocrine (nurture and release of the oocyte) functions. The primary function of the follicle may be considered to be ovulation of an oocyte capable of being fertilized and subsequent structural and functional transformation into a luteal gland capable of adequate progesterone production. It must be considered that follicular development is a concomitant, concerted development of all of the components of the follicle. The following discussion is based on the commonly used descriptions in the literature and reflects a concise description of the morphology of the follicle from primordial through preovulatory development and emphasizes structural and functional aspects of ovarian follicular development that occur after the entry of follicles into the active, growing pool.

MORPHOLOGY OF OVARIAN FOLLICLES

The ovarian follicle consists of the oocyte enveloped within a supportive epithelium stratum granulosum (granulosa cells) and surrounded by an adjacent stromal connecting tissue theca folliculi (thecal cells) with subdivisions tunica interna (theca interna) and tunica externa (theca externa). The structure of ovarian follicles in mares is essentially the same as that described for mice, rabbits, humans, and other species.[3,4] Follicles undergo a series of developmental stages. Briefly, a primordial follicle is defined as the oocyte surrounded by a single, flattened layer of presumptive granulosa cells. The follicle is delineated by an intact basal lamina. The transition to a primary follicle marks the entry of the follicle into the growing pool of follicles and is represented by growth of the oocyte, formation of the zona pellucida surrounding the oocyte, and differentiation and mitotic division of the granulosa cells to form a single layer of cuboidal epithelium. The theca interna becomes more developed and the cells are transformed from flattened to cuboidal or polyhedral shape. The differentiation of one to several additional layers of granulosa cells represents transformation of a primary to a secondary follicle. Primary and secondary follicles are collectively described as preantral follicles.

Coalescence of small pockets of fluid exudate from the granulosa cells marks the formation of an antrum and the transition from secondary follicle to tertiary follicle. The follicle wall consists of the granulosa and thecal layers. The granulosa cells are separated from the theca interna by a basal lamina. Ovarian follicles in mares develop an antrum at approximately 300 μm.[5] Further development of the follicles is marked by a dramatic increase in volume of the antrum and differentiation and thickening of the follicular wall. The antrum may attain a diameter of 35 to 50 mm and the wall may attain thickness of 5 mm to 6 mm.[3,6]

Atresia, as it applies to ovarian follicles, is by definition, failure of the follicle to penetrate the ovarian surface and release the oocyte. The stages of atresia are well described across species and some aspects of atresia specific to the mare have been reported.[5,7,8] Atresia is the fate of the vast majority ($>$ 99% in monovular species) of follicles and represents the loss of follicles as a result of a natural selection process. Atresia is regarded as a committed, irreversible process; that is, once a follicle begins to undergo atresia the process may not be reversed.[7,8] The morphologic stages associated with atresia occur in both the oocyte and the follicular epithelium as the follicle regresses. The events that lead to follicular atresia are specific to the stage of development of the follicle; however, a brief description of some of the generalizations that may be made regarding atresia follow. The first detectable signs of atresia are the appearance of pyknotic nuclei in the granulosa cells followed by degeneration of the oocyte and breakdown of the granulosa cells. Cleavage of the oocyte also may be observed. The steroidogenic cells of the theca interna atrophy and estradiol production is decreased. The vascularity in the theca interna decreases markedly. Biochemical markers of atresia are increased lysosomal activity and decreased protein and nucleic acid synthesis.[5,7,8] Future research into the mechanisms of atresia may be a key area in the development of new hypotheses regarding requirements of follicular growth.

ENDOCRINE ASPECTS OF FOLLICULOGENESIS

The activity of the ovaries is regulated by hormones released into the systemic circulation (endocrine regulation), local intercellular diffusion of substances (paracrine regulation), and autoregulation by release of substances which bind to the cell's own receptors (autocrine regulation). The pituitary gonadotropins, follicle-stimulating hormone (FSH) and luteinizing hormone (LH), are the major components of the endocrine control of follicular growth. Other hormones such as inhibin, activin, prolactin, and insulin also make important contributions. Steroid hormones apparently are involved in folliculogenesis at all levels of regulation: endocrine, paracrine, and autocrine. However, the mechanisms which initiate and control early follicular growth and development remain largely unknown, especially in regard to entry of follicles into the actively growing pool.

Follicles develop to the antral stage in the absence of the main reproductively active gonadotropic hormones FSH and LH.[9–11] Some evidence exists, however, that the rate of preantral follicle growth may be accelerated by gonadotropins.[11] Thereafter, the gonadotropins are required for continued development. In mares, it has been hypothesized that follicles may grow as large as 2 mm without gonadotropic support.[12] Inhibition of circulating FSH levels in pony mares with a nonsteroidal, inhibin-like fraction of equine follicular fluid reduced follicular development and suppressed the physiologic mechanism for selection of the ovulatory follicle.

Growth of large follicles in mares during the later portion of diestrus has been attributed to high circulating concentrations of FSH.[3,13] The concentrations of FSH and LH tend to be reciprocally related during the estrous cycle. The roles of FSH and LH in the development of growing antral follicles are thought to be as follows: preantral follicles acquire receptors for LH in the thecal cell membranes and for FSH in the granulosa cell membranes, the thecal cells produce androgens under the influence of LH, androgens then pass across the basal lamina into the follicle proper, and aromatization of androgens into estrogen occurs under the influence of FSH as the androgens pass into the granulosa cells.[14,15] A critical point in the life of the follicle is the acquisition of membrane receptors for LH by the granulosa cells.[16] Luteinizing hormone acts to induce greater estrogen synthesis under FSH influence. It is this capacity to secrete large amounts of estrogen which induces synthesis of LH receptors in granulosa cells and facilitates transition of the follicle from the small antral stage to the preovulatory stage. Thus both FSH and LH are required for the production of follicles that are capable of ovulating. Estrogen induces LH receptors in granulosa cells and prepares the follicle to be competent to respond to preovulatory increases in gonadotropin secretion which bring about the final phases of preovulatory follicular maturation.

Early in the ovulatory season, the pattern of circulating FSH secretion during the estrous cycle is bimodal with the first peak observed approximately between days 3 to 5 and the second peak from days 11 to 13 postovulation. Later in the ovulatory season the pattern of FSH secretion is unimodal with peak concentrations reached between days 11 to 13 later in the ovulatory season.[3,13,17,18] The bimodal FSH profiles observed early in the ovulatory season led to the development of a two-wave theory of follicular development during the estrous cycle.[13] Waves of follicular growth were thought to correspond with the unimodal and bimodal FSH profiles early and late in the ovulatory season and were based apparently on a theoretical positive association between FSH concentrations and increased follicular activity during diestrus.

In summary, follicular growth during the estrous cycle of the mare is a dynamic process. Gonadotropins are the primary regulators of follicular growth; however, gonadotropins alone cannot account for all of the events of follicular growth. The responsiveness of follicles to the gonadotropins is modulated by other ovarian factors. Estrogen is also a key modulator in that it enhances the responsiveness of granulosa cells to basal concentrations of gonadotropins and enhances the development of LH receptors. Furthermore, estrogen induces the preovulatory LH surge. Progestins and androgens play an important role in follicular development as do recently identified nonsteroidal factors such as inhibins, follicle regulatory protein, and substance P, although definitive roles for those compounds remain to be elucidated.

MORPHOLOGIC ASPECTS OF FOLLICULOGENESIS

The factor or factors which stimulate reinitiation of development of the primordial follicle to the further stages of follicular evolution remain obscure. Several observations have been made which may be interpreted to mean that the process may not depend on gonadotropic hormones and that follicles may develop to the small antral stage in the absence of gonadotropic stimulation. A recent study of porcine follicular development suggested that an intact pituitary is necessary for antral development beyond the 1- to 2-mm stage. However, the number of follicles which mature is highly dependent on the presence of gonadotropin.[9,10,16,19,20]

The time required for follicular development has been investigated in laboratory animals and cows using measurements of follicular volume and mitotic indices.[21,22] In rats, the rate of development varied among stages of folliculogenesis with the slowest rate of change occurring while follicles were growing from 0.1 to 0.5 mm in diameter. Maximum growth rate can be found in follicles through the range of 1 to 2 mm. Slower but consistent growth characterizes development from 2 to 10 mm. The time required for development from 0.4 to 1 mm was estimated to be 22.1 days, spanning more than one estrous cycle.[23] Follicular growth rates have been studied in cattle using mitotic indexes. On the basis of these studies, it was concluded that approximately two estrous cycles are required for a follicle to grow from 0.13 mm to preovulatory diameter.[22] The entire process of development from primary to preovulatory follicle in the cow was estimated to require approximately 60 days. Similar preliminary studies have been done in mares.[24] It appears to take approximately two estrous cycles for follicles to grow from 100 μm to 1000 μm. Further data on growth rates for larger follicles were not reported. Recall that antral follicles exist in the equine ovary within a range of diameters from approximately 0.3 mm to 50 mm. Because there are substantial species differences to consider, direct comparison of data between mares and cows is difficult. The assumption that the time course followed for follicular development may be similar is purely speculative.

PATTERNS OF FOLLICULAR DEVELOPMENT DURING THE OVULATORY CYCLE

Follicular changes during the estrous cycle of the mare have been studied since the early 1920s.[25] Early research done in this area has been reviewed.[26,27] An extensive review and compilation of the literature on follicular dynamics in mares was done approximately a decade ago.[3] More recently, the incorporation of ultrasonographic imaging into equine ovarian research has led to a dramatic increase in the understanding of ovarian follicular development in mares.[19,28] This noninvasive imaging technology has provided the ability to monitor sequentially the ovarian follicular population, including follicles as small as 2 mm. Investigations of the basic and applied mechanisms of ovarian follicular development, physiologic selection of the ovulatory follicle, and ovulation in mares are currently active research areas.

During the course of several studies based on ultrasonographic examination of the ovaries, the numbers of follicles have been counted and classified into various diameter categories.[19,28] Initial studies following the fates of individually identified follicles also have been reported.[29,30] It must be remembered that in ultrasonographically based studies, ovarian cyclicity may be described more accurately in terms of interovulatory intervals rather than the behaviorally based estrous cycle. Therefore, care is required in comparing the results of various studies. Numbers of follicles have been grouped into categories based on 5-mm increments of diameter. The number of small follicles (2 to 5 mm) decreased during the preovulatory period (late diestrus to early estrus) and increased during the postovulatory period (estrus to early diestrus). The mean number of medium-size follicles (6 to 10 mm and 11 to 15 mm) remained approximately constant over the interovulatory interval. This observation was attributable to growth of newly recruited follicles entering into the medium size diameter classifications, where they either became atretic or continued to grow into the larger-diameter categories, and concomitant regression of follicles from the cohort recruited during the previous ovarian cycle. In the large-follicle categories (16 to 20 mm and >20 mm), a wave of increased follicular activity was observed, which began in mid-diestrus and ended just before ovulation. The wave of activity in these large-follicle categories was most probably the result of a mid- or late diestrus surge of FSH, which initiated growth of small- and medium-size follicles into large follicles. This supposition is supported by the temporal association between circulating FSH concentrations and increased follicle numbers. The number of follicles 16 to 20 mm and > 20 mm reached a maximum 5 to 7 days before ovulation and then declined markedly. The decline in follicles apparently represented regression of the follicles in the cohort from which the ovulatory follicle arose. The days on which peak numbers of follicles in the larger categories were attained corresponded with declining FSH concentrations and increasing LH concentrations. Luteal regression, declining progesterone concentrations, and peak concentrations of prostaglandin $F_2\alpha$ ($PGF_2\alpha$) reportedly occur approximately 2 days earlier.[3] Waves of follicular development following similar time courses were observed during studies using ultrasonography to identify sequentially individual large follicles.[29,30] Individual mares have differing levels of follicular development during the interovulatory interval; that is, some mares had more follicles of a given size. However, the patterns created by the follicular growth curves were similar. To date, data from the ultrasonographic studies have supported the hypothesis that one wave, as opposed to two waves, of follicular growth occur during the equine estrous cycle.[13,19,28–30]

PHYSIOLOGIC SELECTION OF THE OVULATORY FOLLICLE

The follicle destined to ovulate is somehow physiologically selected for continued development and eventual ovulation. The processes by which the selection mechanism occurs have not been determined and remain among the great mysteries in reproductive biology. Current concepts of selection of the dominant follicle in women and nonhuman primates have been critically evaluated, and it has been determined, in primates, that the selection process is completed only during the cycle in which the individual ovulation occurs.[10,22,31–33] This concept is consistent with studies of the patterns of follicular development observed in mares and with the time required for ovulation following injection of a luteolytic dose of $PGF_2\alpha$ and with the patterns of follicular growth following surgical ablation of the dominant follicle.[28–30,34–36] Whether selection is a random event or a process in which the selected follicles are individually chosen has not been determined. The time of follicular recruitment and follicular dynamics before antrum formation are not known.

The hypothesis that selection of the follicle destined to ovulate must have occurred by the time that the diameters of the two largest follicles in ovaries begin to diverge has been recently developed.[28] With this rationale, the selection mechanism occurs approximately 6 days before ovulation. A cohort of similar-size follicles may grow together until the time of physiologic selection, when the ovulatory follicle is selected for or other follicles are selected against.[28] The selected follicle undergoes favored growth and the other follicles in the cohort become atretic and decrease in diameter, as indicated by the dramatic decrease in the numbers of large follicles approximately 5 to 6 days preceding ovulation.[3,28–30,37] The timing of that important event during the interovulatory interval is also consistent with division of the interovulatory interval into follicular and luteal phases, based on ultrasonographically detectable characteristics.[19]

The selection process in mares may involve both FSH and LH, because LH concentrations increase at approximately the same time as selective growth of the ovulatory follicle and rise concurrently with the increasing diameter of the ovulatory follicle.[3,38] Luteinizing hormone concentrations begin to increase approximately 2 days before the time when the preovulatory follicle may be ultrasonographically identified.[6,39] This point in the ovulatory cycle occurs at the same time that FSH concentrations begin to decline.[3] Increasing LH concentrations also occur concurrently with the ultrasonographically detectable increases in the thickness of the wall of the preovulatory follicle, which may be the result of LH-dependent development and hypertrophy of the theca interna.[6] In rats, FSH alone apparently is responsible for selection of follicles which will ovulate during the following estrus.[23] Intraovarian factors such as follicular estrogen levels, inhibins, prostaglandins, and glycosaminoglycans may also play roles in the processes of follicular growth and development.[31,33,39–41] Angiogenesis, or the generation of new capillaries, around the follicle coincides with the development of follicles.[42] Proximity to the intraovarian vasculature may also be involved in selection. Follicles with greater access to nutrients and circulating hormones may be able to subjugate other follicles farther from the vascular supply. Atresia has been associated with thecal ischemia.[43] Therefore, greater blood flow to the selected follicle and the selected follicle's own estrogen production are almost certainly involved in maintaining the dominant stature of the selected follicle.[40,44]

Preovulatory follicles have a more extensive and permeable capillary network than other follicles.[44] The considerable vascularity which exists around the dominant follicle may allow it to accumulate more of the circulating gonadotropins and thus survive while the other members of its cohort undergo atresia. However, enhanced vascularity may be either a cause or reflection of selection. Selection and final growth and maturation of the ovulatory follicle have been postulated to be simply the result of chance development of a follicle coincidentally with luteal regression and a preovulatory gonadotropin surge.[11]

Studies addressing follicular status at various times during the estrous cycle in mares have demonstrated that all follicles greater than 10 mm, except the preovulatory follicle, were in early atresia on day 17 postovulation.[45] The observation has been made that the largest nonatretic follicle underwent selected growth between days 14 and 17 postovulation and more follicles were in early atresia on day 17. Follicular recruitment of the pool of follicles from which the preovulatory follicle arises apparently occurred 12 to 14 days preceding ovulation and involved follicles 5 to 15 mm in diameter. In addition, before the selection process, the selected follicle and follicles which became subordinate to the dominant follicle grew on parallel courses to similar stages of development in the presence of an active corpus luteum.[37]

THE FOLLICULAR PHASE AND PREOVULATORY FOLLICLES

The ovaries of mares in the follicular phase of the estrous cycle are characterized by the presence, and apparently selected growth, of a large (> 25 mm) follicle. The dominant follicle persists to produce large amounts of estrogen, approximately 500- to 1000-fold more than smaller follicles.[46] Other follicles in the cohort from which the preovulatory follicle arose enter the sequence of events leading to atresia and regression. Mares which will spontaneously ovulate multiple follicles may exhibit more than one large follicle during this time. In a recent review of estrous cycles in mares studied by ultrasonography, the mean duration of the follicular phase was 7.7 days (±1.8 SD).[19] Thus the follicular phase of most mares is consistent with the period of behavioral estrus.[3,19]

The dominant preovulatory follicle is the most steroidogenically active follicle and is also the most responsive to gonadotropin stimulation. Increased responsiveness to LH is partially due to an increase in the number of LH receptors in the thecal cells. Increased responsiveness to FSH is most probably the result of the increased number of granulosa cells and increased intracellular responsiveness to FSH stimulation. These effects are induced or amplified by estradiol.[9,47] The dominant follicle exhibits the greatest estrogen biosynthetic activity and appears to inhibit the development of subordinate follicles. The inhibition appears to be exerted at the local (paracrine) as well as systemic (endocrine) level.[10] Many theories have been proposed and many factors implicated in the paracrine inhibition of smaller follicles by the dominant follicle. A systemic factor must also be involved, because the dominant follicle is able to inhibit follicles in the ovary in which it is located as well as the contralateral ovary. Most experimental work on the characteristics of follicular dominance has been done in cattle or in humans as part of clinical embryo transfer or in vitro fertilization programs. In cattle, ablation of the dominant follicle leads to compensatory development of medium-size follicles within 4 days.[10] The primary candidates for regulation of follicular growth are inhibin and follicular regulatory protein (FRP). Follicle regulatory protein is apparently released by the dominant follicles of women, pigs, and rats and acts to inhibit FSH stimulated follicular growth and aromatase activity.[48]

The diameter of the ovulatory follicle in mares on the day before ovulation is approximately 45 mm.[3,19,37] Ultrasonographically based measurements typically have used the average of two linear measurements of the follicle taken at the follicular fluid-follicle interface at the longest and widest dimensions of the follicle. The ultrasonographic measuring technique reflects only the diameter of the follicular antrum. Measurements from studies based on transrectal palpation include the follicular wall and, to some extent, the surrounding ovarian stroma. Therefore, technique of measurement is important to consider when comparing the results of studies from various laboratories.

The ability to estimate the interval from examination of an individual follicle to ovulation is of tremendous practical importance. Two studies designed to investigate this question have failed to provide precise indicators of the interval to ovulation, although crude estimates are possible. In a study to evaluate the palpable turgidity of preovulatory follicles, it was determined that approximately 90% of follicles exhibited a change from turgid to soft immediately before ovulation.[49] In a study of ultrasonographically detectable attributes of preovulatory follicles in mares, the follicle which ovulated became the largest follicle in either ovary by approximately 6 days before ovulation, could be identified on a day to day basis, and increased in diameter at approximately 2.5 mm per day until ovulation occurred.[6] Preovulatory follicles in mares have also been shown to undergo pronounced changes in shape as ovulation approaches.[6] Preovulatory follicles typically developed a pear-shaped or conical appearance with the apex of the follicle pointing to the ovulation fossa. The changes in shape observed in the ultrasonographically based study were likely related to the relative turgidity of the follicles in the study, based on transrectal palpation. Other ultrasonographically detectable attributes of the preovulatory follicles have been evaluated, such as changes in the gray-scale values, thickness of the follicular wall, and changes in the follicular fluid. However, a reliable means of precisely predicting when ovulation will occur has not yet been determined. Assessment of the diameter of the preovulatory follicles appeared to be as reliable an indication of impending ovulation as any other. This particular aspect of preovulatory follicle evaluation by ultrasonography is currently the topic of intensive investigation in several laboratories.

The average diameter of the preovulatory follicle in mares also appears to vary according to month of the ovulatory season.[19] In mares with single ovulations, preovulatory follicle diameters ranged from means of approximately 48 mm in May to approximately 40 mm in July. This observation may be of importance in determining appropriate breeding dates, if ultrasonographic examinations are incorporated into an overall brood mare management program. When potential double ovulations were considered, bilateral double ovulations occurred at mean preovulatory follicle diameters of approximately 40 mm. Unilateral double ovulations occurred at approximately 35 mm.[19] Approximately 50% of double ovulations reviewed were synchronous. Mean preovulatory follicular diameters were the same in synchronous (approximately 36 mm) and asynchronous (approximately 40 mm) ovulations. However, for unilateral synchronous double ovulations, the first follicle to ovulate was larger (approximately 39 mm) than the second follicle to ovulate (approximately 34 mm). Preovulatory follicular diameters for bilateral double ovulations were the same for the first and second ovulations. As a practical consideration in brood mare management, double ovulations appear to occur at slightly smaller diameters (approximately 4 to 5 mm) than single ovulations.[19]

IRREGULARITIES IN FOLLICULAR DEVELOPMENT DURING THE OVULATORY CYCLE

Ovulations occur during the luteal phase of the estrous cycle in mares; however, the incidence of diestrus ovulations is somewhat open to interpretation.[3,19,41,50–53] Reports based on progesterone profiles and sexual behavior may be interpreted to mean that ovulations occurred in approximately 21% of diestrous periods on days 2 to 15.[34,41] In studies based on ultrasonography, diestrous ovulations were observed in 9% of the cycles.[19] Of 69 mares studied for complete ovulatory cycles, 6 had secondary ovulations 3, 3, 5, 7, 9, and 11 days, respectively, after the primary follicular phase ovulation. The 3 mares for which secondary ovulations were 3, 3 and 5 days apart had inconclusive uterine echotexture and estrous behavior during the interim between ovulations. The following luteal phases for these mares were of apparently normal duration. The 3 mares for which ovulations were 7, 9, and 11 days apart exhibited luteal phase uterine echotexture and sexual behavior at the time of the secondary ovulation. Mares which had luteal phase ovulations on days 7 and 9, respectively, exhibited apparently normal interovulatory intervals based on the primary ovulation. Regression of the luteal glands formed following the primary and secondary ovulations occurred at the same time. One mare which exhibited diestrous ovulation on day 11 had a prolonged luteal phase of 36 days. The primary luteal gland regressed, based on ultrasonographic appearance, at the expected time. The prolonged luteal phase was apparently caused by the luteal gland, which resulted from the diestrous ovulation. In this regard, it has been postulated that luteal glands formed after late diestrous ovulations are not able to respond to the $PGF_2\alpha$ release by the uterus, thus their life span may be prolonged. Luteal glands resulting from earlier diestrous ovulations may be mature enough to respond to the luteolytic signal.

OVULATION

Ovulation is the culmination of a complex series of events which is set into motion with elevated LH concentrations and results in the collapse of the preovulatory follicle and expulsion of the oocyte from the follicle.[54] In most species, the primary stimulus for ovulation is a sudden, very brief rise in peripheral LH concentrations. In mares, however, the physiologic trigger for ovulation may simply be increased LH concentration past an as yet undetermined threshold. A unique aspect of LH secretion in mares is that LH concentrations do not "surge" as in other mammals, but rather exhibit a continuous increase, beginning approximately 6 to 7 days before ovulation.[3,38] Peak LH concentrations are not reached until approximately 1 to 3 days following follicular rupture. Disintegration of the apex of the follicle, final maturation of the oocyte, and evacuation of the follicular fluid must be coordinated for successful ovulation. Subsequent functional and morphologic changes in the cells comprising the follicular epithelium and theca interna must be completed to form the luteal gland. While the direct observation of ovulation by laparoscopy or ultrasonography may be quite dramatic, remember that the event of ovulation is the result of a long series of biochemical, physiologic, and morphologic changes in the tissues of the follicle.

The mechanism of ovulation has been the subject of several reviews.[55–59] Most of the fundamental experimental work regarding mammalian ovulation has been done in animals and more recently in humans. The concepts presented herein have been developed from the original literature and recent reviews with the inclusion of information specific to the mare.

Ovulation in mares is distinctive because of the anatomic organization of the equine ovary. The corticomedullary reversal which occurs during embryonic development leaves the ovulation fossa as the only location on the ovary that is covered with germinal epithelium and from which ovulation may occur.[3,60,61] The exact effects of this anatomic reorganization on the events of ovulation may only be speculated on at the present time. However, the results of laparoscopic and ultrasonographic investigations of ovulation in the mare appear to indicate that the formation of pronounced stigma which protrudes from the surface of the ovary before follicular rupture does not occur.[60,62–64]

BIOCHEMICAL ASPECTS OF OVULATION

Luteinizing hormone radically alters the structure and activity of the preovulatory follicle. Luteinizing hormone effects are apparently effected via the cAMP mediated protein kinase system which influences the follicle in a series of distinct steps.[56–58] The biochemical changes in the follicle following LH stimulation are increased progesterone production, activation of proteolytic enzymes, increased prostaglandin E_2 and $F_2\alpha$ synthesis, increased prostacyclin (PGI_2) synthesis, and decreased glycosaminoglycan production. Although LH is released from the pituitary in a pulsatile manner, the role of LH pulsatility in ovulation has not been determined. Roles for luteinizing hormone-releasing hormone (LHRH), progesterone, oxytocin, catecholamines, noradrenaline, and serotonin have also been postulated; however, exact mechanisms are not clear.[56,58]

Hyperemia of the preovulatory follicle and increased blood flow to the follicle are apparently the result of increased prostaglandin E_2 (PGE_2), although histamine and bradykinins have also been implicated.[56,58] An increase in mast cell infiltration of the tissues surrounding the follicle before ovulation has been noticed. Edema of the theca interna is induced by dramatically increased fenestration of capillaries.

The vasoconstriction and reduced blood flow which occurs at the apex of the follicle as rupture of the follicle approaches are apparently mediated by $PGF_2\alpha$. The LH trigger is followed by increased prorenin concentration in the preovulatory follicle. Thus the prorenin-renin-angiotensin system has also been implicated in the final aspects of vasoconstriction. Ovulation has also been compared with an inflammatory response in an interesting hypothesis.[65] Many of the similarities between ovulation and inflammation are profound; however, further exploration of those ideas is beyond the scope of this brief synopsis.

Proteolytic enzymes play a major role in follicular rupture.[56–58,66] The increased secretion of plasminogen activator converts plasminogen in the follicular fluid to plasmin in response to LH stimulation. Plasmin then acts directly on latent collagen. Collagenolyases and serine proteases complete the proteolysis of collagen. The net effect is decreased tensile strength of the follicular wall to a point at which rupture occurs.

The walls of preovulatory follicles also contain noteworthy amounts of smooth muscle cells. Laparoscopic investigations of ovulation in laboratory animals and ultrasonographic studies in mares and women seem to show noticeable contractions of the follicle during ovulation, especially at the base of the follicle.[60,62,63,67] Adrenergic, norandrenergic, and dopaminergic nerve fibers all have been demonstrated in the deep layers of smooth muscle cells around the follicle; however, the results of pharmacologic studies in this area are confusing. Adrenergic neurons in the follicle wall may possibly be activated by LH and secrete norepinephrine, which may in turn interact with, or stimulate, release of histamine from surrounding mast cells. In addition, α-adrenergic agonists appear to enhance follicular hyperemia by affecting the contractility of the vascular endothelial cells.

MORPHOLOGIC ASPECTS OF OVULATION

Ovulation is the result of cytologic and biochemical changes in the follicular wall. For successful ovulation to occur, follicular fluid containing the oocyte must pass through the follicular epithelium, basal lamina, theca interna, theca externa, ovarian stroma, tunica albuginea, and germinal epithelium. Typically, by the time a follicle receives the LH stimulus it has grown large enough that it is bulging from the surface of the ovary, so the ovarian stroma probably offers little or no resistance to ovulation.[56] However, because of the unique anatomic configuration of the ovary in mares, this may not be as true in the equid compared with other species, which may ovulate from any surface of the ovary. Obviously, the constraints of the connective tissue surrounding the ovary play a profound role in determining the shape of the preovulatory follicle; however, any impediment to ovulation by stromal elements between the developing follicle and the ovulation fossa or unique aspects of biochemical degradation of stromal tissues have not been critically examined.

Following the physiologic trigger of increased LH, the first noticeable morphologic alteration is that the capillaries which surround the preovulatory follicle become increasingly fenestrated and the theca interna becomes edematous because of plasma effusion from the newly fenestrated vasculature. The collagen comprising the theca externa and tunica albuginea dissociates as the result of increased plasmin released by plasminogen activator from the granulosa cells and increased collagenase activity originating from the fibroblasts of the albuginea. Weakening of the follicular wall occurs over the entire wall; however, rupture is localized to the apex. The wall of the follicle is not destroyed, but reorganized, thus facilitating transformation to the corpus luteum.[55–59]

At the apex of the follicle the cells of the germinal epithelium lose microvilli, the nuclei become pyknotic, and they loosen from the tunica albuginea. Immediately below the apex, the granulosa cells are lost; however, the thecal cells remain. Granulosa cells which have been fixed to the basal lamina at the apex of the follicle lose their columnar appearance at approximately the same time as dissociation of the basal lamina. Hydrolases from the degenerating cells on either side contribute to the localized destruction of the thecal cells and remaining layers. As thinning of the apical follicular wall occurs in association with dissociation and fragmentation of the collagen, collagen fibrils separate allowing formation of a stigma. Following stigma formation, hydrostatic pressure from the follicular fluid overcomes the resistance of the remaining tissue and follicular rupture results.[55–59]

The idea that increased intrafollicular pressure is a cause of ovulation has been largely discredited. Accumulation of follicular fluid during growth of the follicle does not result in increased follicular pressure. Hydrostatic pressure in the follicle appears to remain consistent with that of the surrounding capillaries. In the species studied thus far, no increases in intrafollicular pressure have been observed before ovulation.[56]

FOLLICULAR RUPTURE IN MARES

Ovulation may be detected by transrectal palpation, progesterone assay, or ultrasonography. The site of a recent ovulation may be detected by digital palpation of a depression on the surface of the ovary which marks the location of the former ovulatory follicle.[3] Increased plasma progesterone concentrations indicate that ovulation has occurred and that the corpus luteum is functional. Ultrasonographic detection of the site of ovulation in mares is peculiar in that the walls of the collapsed former follicle appear hyperechoic (brighter) for 1 to 4 days following ovulation.[6] The unusual ultrasonographic appearance of the early corpus luteum may aid in identification of the site of ovulation in clinical reproduction programs.

Details of the timing of the process of ovulation are available in mares. In initial studies of the ultrasonographic morphology of the ovaries, ovulation occurred in two mares while ultrasound examinations were being conducted for other studies.[68] Both follicles appeared to collapse over a few seconds, although no specific measurements were made. More recently, transrectal ultrasonography has been used to study the ovulatory process in a small group of mares using frequent or continuous observation.[62–64] The duration and pattern of follicular evacuation has been studied using continuous observation.[63,64] Two distinct patterns of fluid loss were observed. The first pattern occurred in three of five mares and was described as a rapid evacuation of the follicular fluid with decrease of the antrum to less than 10% of the original antral area within 60 s of the onset of follicular rupture. The second pattern was observed in two of five mares and was characterized by a gradual decrease in the area of the antrum over approximately 6 to 7 m. Approximately 50% of the original antral area remained in the follicle 60 s following initiation of ovulation. In another study, the range of duration of ovulation in mares was described as 5 to 90 s with little to no residual fluid following follicular evacuation.[64] Observations of ovulations in mares appear to be consistent with incidental observations and other studies directed at specific portions of the ovulatory process in other species.[69]

Evacuation of all follicular fluid apparently does not occur immediately following the initial loss of the majority of follicular fluid. Residual fluid was observed in the antra of approximately 80% of recently evacuated follicles in two recent ultrasonographically based studies of equine ovulation. The time required for complete apposition of the follicular walls ranged from 0.5 to 5 h.[62,63] Thus, the sites of ovulation will probably be observed to contain variable amounts of fluid for a period of time following ovulation. To determine whether the fluid is residual from ovulation or represents infiltration of blood from capillaries in the internal aspect of the follicular wall or is the result of rupture of the follicle across an arteriole or venule during ovulation may be difficult.

In one mare, a small echoic spot was visualized during follicular evacuation.[62] The spot was floated freely in the follicular antrum and was approximately 2 mm in diameter. The small echo was interpreted to represent the cumulus/oocyte complex and was visualized only for 10 s. The oocyte/cumulus complex has been ultrasonographically detected in the follicles of sheep and is routinely evaluated in human ultrasonography.[67,69] However, over the course of thousands of examinations of preovulatory follicles in mares by the author, echoes interpreted as the cumulus/oocyte complex have been observed only twice. This may be a reflection of a closely adherent relationship between the oocyte and the follicular wall in mares or differences in the image quality and resolving power between veterinary and human ultrasonographic instruments.

The fate of the fluid discharged during ovulation has been the subject of further investigation.[64] Fluid from the ovulating follicle could not be detected in the oviduct ipsilateral to the ovulation. It has not been possible consistently to identify the oviduct in mares with ultrasonography; however, the location of a fluid-filled area greater than 2 mm in diameter should be possible. Fluid collections in the area of the ovulation fossa and oviducts were observed, although they were small and transient. Therefore, most of the follicular fluid was likely filtered by the oviductal fimbria into the abdominal cavity and only a small volume of follicular fluid appears to accompany the oocyte/cumulus complex into the oviduct. These observations are consistent with the observation of ovulation in women, in whom the oviduct is ultrasonographically identifiable.[67,69] Following a series of ovulations, no fluid was detected in the oviduct and large volumes of fluid not detected before ovulation were observed in the posterior pelvic cul-de-sac.[67,69]

OVULATORY DYSFUNCTION

Mares apparently do not exhibit all of the types of ovulatory failure observed in other species. Cystic follicles, as described in cows and other species, have not been demonstrated in mare.[3] Follicles which attain preovulatory diameter at the appropriate time of the cycle and do not ovulate but undergo atresia and regress have been described in women and appear to be a cause of infertility. In addition, the formation of luteinized, unruptured follicles (LUF) has been described in humans and other species.[70] In this type of ovulatory failure, LUF, the follicle attains preovulatory diameter and then the wall of the follicle begins to acquire the appearance associated with luteinization; however, rupture of the follicle does not occur. Echoes interpreted as the cumulus/oocyte complex have been ultrasonographically demonstrated within the lumen of the structure.

The most common form of ovulation failure in mares apparently is the hemorrhagic anovulatory follicle syndrome ("autumn follicle") in which a follicle fails to rupture and fills with blood.[3] These unruptured follicles may reach a large diameter. The progression of events presented herein is based on a composite of several hemorrhagic follicles followed during the course of other studies.[19] Initially, free-floating echogenic spots are seen within otherwise anechoic follicular fluid. The spots may swirl if ballotted, indicating that the fluid is liquid. Over a period of days the hemorrhagic follicle increases in diameter (e.g., 60 to 90 mm) and the density of the spots increases. Then growth of the follicles ceases and the echogenic spots coalesce and become organized into apparently fibrinous bands which traverse the follicle. Interconnected bands may form a network within the follicle. The follicular contents appear gelatinous, and the echoic areas only quiver on ballottment. The outer walls of the structures appear thick (approximately 4 to 7 mm) and the echotexture is consistent with that of luteinized tissue. The hemorrhagic follicles gradually regress and are usually no longer detected after approximately 1 month. Uterine morphology associated with hemorrhagic follicles usually has a progestational appearance.[19] That is, the estrogenic uterine morphology characteristic of the follicular phase did not develop. Although critical experiments have not been done, follicles which become hemorrhagic may be deficient in estrogen.

SPECIAL TECHNIQUES

The recent interest in and prospects for in vitro fertilization in mares necessitates the development of specialized techniques for obtaining oocytes.[71–75] Follicular oocytes have been collected from mares using in situ aspiration of the follicular contents with a needle and syringe apparatus. A similar apparatus connected to a continuous irrigation system and vacuum pump was used in a subsequent study to evacuate follicles exteriorized at laparotomy.[74] Equine oocytes may be recovered by follicular puncture and evacuation.[75] Pretreatment with exogenous LH apparently did not increase the success rate of oocyte collection.[71] Oocytes may also be collected via transabdominal flank puncture and colpotomy.[74] A technique for transvaginal ultrasonographically guided follicular puncture and oocyte collection will probably soon be realized. Technically assisted follicular aspiration may have quite dramatic effects on the ultrasonographic appearance of the subsequent luteal gland although aspiration seems to have no effect on subsequent luteal function in the mare; however, the effects on other folliculogenesis during subsequent ovulatory cycles remains unknown.[76]

REFERENCES

1. Deansly, R.: Germ cell development and the meiotic prophase in the fetal horse ovary. J. Reprod. Fertil. Suppl., *23:*547–552, 1978.
2. Mauleon, P., and Mariana, J.C.: Oogenesis and folliculogenesis. *In* Reproduction in Domestic Animals. 3 ed. Edited by H.N. Cole and P.T. Cupps, New York, Academic Press, 1977, pp. 175–198.
3. Ginther, O.J.: Reproductive Biology of the Mare—Basic and Applied Aspects. Cross Plains, WI, published by the author, 1979, pp. 133–216, 255–320.
4. Centrola, G.M.: Structural changes: Follicular development and hormonal requirements. *In* The Ovary. Edited by G.B. Serra. New York, Raven Press, 1983, pp. 95–112.
5. Kenney, R.M., Condon, W., Ganjam, V.K., and Channing, C.P.: Morphological and biochemical correlates of equine ovarian follicles as a function of their state of viability or atresia. J. Reprod. Fertil. Suppl., *27:*163–171, 1979.
6. Pierson, R.A., and Ginther, O.J.: Ultrasonic evaluation of the preovulatory follicle in the mare. Theriogenology, *24:*359–368, 1985.
7. Centrola, G.M.: Structural changes: Atresia. *In* The Ovary. Edited by G.B. Serra. New York, Raven Press, 1983, pp. 113–122.
8. Ryan, R.J.: Follicular atresia: Some speculation of biochemical markers and mechanisms. *In* Dynamics of Ovarian Function. Edited by N.B. Schwartz and M. Hunzicker-Dunn. New York, Raven Press, 1981, pp. 1–11.
9. Richards, J.S.: Maturation of ovarian follicles: Actions and interactions of pituitary and ovarian hormones on follicular cell differentiation. Physiol. Rev., *60:*51–89, 1980.
10. Greenwald, G.S., and Terranova, P.F.: Follicular selection and its control. *In* The Physiology of Reproduction. Edited

by E. Knobil and J.D. Neill. New York, Raven Press, 1988, pp. 387–446.

11. Hansel, W., and Convey, E.M.: Physiology of the estrous cycle. J. Anim. Sci., Suppl. 2, *57*:404–424, 1983.
12. Bergfelt, D.R., and Ginther, O.J.: Delayed follicular development and ovulation following inhibition of FSH with equine follicular fluid in the mare. Theriogenology, *24*:99–108, 1985.
13. Irvine, C.H.G.: Endocrinology of the estrous cycle of the mare: Applications to embryo transfer. Theriogenology, *15*:85–104, 1981.
14. Moon, Y.S., Dorrington, J.H., and Armstrong, D.T.: Stimulation action of follicle stimulating hormone on estradiol-17β secretion by hypophysectomized rat ovaries in organ culture. Endocrinology, *97*:244–247, 1975.
15. Gore-Lagnton, R.E., and Armstrong, D.T.: Follicular steroidogenesis and its control. *In* The Physiology of Reproduction. Edited by E. Knobil and J.D. Neill. New York, Raven Press, 1988, pp. 331–386.
16. Richards, J.S.: Hormonal control of ovarian follicular development: A 1978 perspective. Recent Prog. Horm. Res., *35*:343–373, 1979.
17. Evans, M.J., and Irvine, C.H.G.: Serum concentrations of FSH, LH and progesterone during the oestrous cycle and early pregnancy in the mare. J. Reprod. Fertil. Suppl., *23*:193–200, 1973.
18. Turner, D.D., Garcia, M.C., and Ginther, O.J.: Follicular and gonadotrophin changes throughout the year in pony mares. Am. J. Vet. Res., *40*:1694–1700, 1979.
19. Ginther, O.J., and Pierson, R.A.: Regular and irregular characteristics of ovulation and the interovulatory interval in mares. J. Equine Vet. Sci., *9*:4–12, 1989.
20. Kraeling, R.R., Barb, C.R., and Rampacek, G.B.: Ovarian response of the hypophysial stalk-transected pig to pregnant mare serum gonadotrophin. Domest. Anim. Endocrinol., *3*:177–183, 1986.
21. Scaramuzzi, R.J., Turnbull, K.E., and Nancarrow, C.D.: Growth of graafian follicles in cows following luteolysis induced by prostaglandin $F_2\alpha$ analogue, cloprostenol. Aust. J. Biol. Sci., *33*:63–69, 1980.
22. Lussier, J.G., Matton, P., and Dufour, J.J.: Growth rates of follicles in the ovary of the cow. J. Reprod. Fertil., *81*:301–307, 1987.
23. Hirshfield, A.N., and Midgley, A.R.: The role of FSH in the selection of large ovarian follicles in the rat. Biol. Reprod., *19*:606–611, 1978.
24. Driancourt, M.A.: Follicular kinetics in the mare ovary. Ann. Biol. Anim. Biochim. Biophys., *19*:1443–1453, 1979.
25. Seaborne, E.: The oestrus cycle of the mare and some associated phenomena. Anat. Rec., *30*:277–286, 1925.
26. Andrews, F.N., and McKenzie, F.F.: Estrus, ovulation, and related phenomena in the mare. Agricultural Experimental Station, University of Missouri Research Bulletin No. 329. 1941, pp. 1–117.
27. Hammond, J., and Wodzicki, K.: Anatomical and histological changes during the estrous cycle of the mare. Proc. R. Soc. Lond. [Biol.], *120*:1–23, 1941.
28. Pierson, R.A., and Ginther, O.J.: Follicular population dynamics during the estrous cycle of the mare. Anim. Reprod. Sci., *14*:219–231, 1987.
29. Palmer, E.: New results on follicular growth and ovulation in the mare. *In* Follicular Growth and Ovulation Rate in Farm Animals. Edited by J.F. Roche and D. O'Callaghan. Dordecht, Martinus Nijhoff, 1987, pp. 237–255.
30. Sirois, J., Ball, B.A., and Fortune, J.E.: Patterns of growth and regression of ovarian follicles during the oestrous cycle and after hemiovariectomy in mares. Equine Vet. J. Suppl., *8*:43–48, 1989.
31. Hodgen, G.D.: The dominant ovarian follicle. Fertil. Steril., *38*:281–300, 1982.
32. Gougeon, A.: Dynamics of follicular growth in the human: A model from preliminary results. Hum. Reprod., *1*:81–87, 1986.
33. Baird, D.T.: A model for follicular selection and ovulation: Lessons from superovulation. J. Steroid Biochem., *27*:15–23, 1987.
34. Johnson, A.L., Becker, S.E., and Roma, M.L.: Effects of gonadotrophin-releasing hormone and prostaglandin $F_2\alpha$ on corpus luteum function and timing of the subsequent ovulation in the mare. J. Reprod. Fertil., *83*:545–551, 1988.
35. Loy, R.G., Buell, J.R., Stevenson, W., and Hamm, D.: Sources of variation in response intervals after prostaglandin treatment in mares with functional corpora lutea. J. Reprod. Fertil. Suppl., *27*:229–235, 1979.
36. Neely, D.P., et al.: Prostaglandins release patterns in the mare: Physiological, pathological and therapeutic responses. J. Reprod. Fertil. Suppl., *27*:181–189, 1979.
37. Driancourt, M.A., and Palmer, E.: Time of ovarian follicular recruitment in cyclic pony mares. Theriogenology, *21*:591–600, 1984.
38. Whitmore, H.L., Wentworth, B.C., and Ginther, O.J.: Circulating concentrations of luteinizing hormone during estrous cycle of mares as determined by radiommunoassay. Am. J. Vet. Res., *34*:631–636, 1973.
39. Hodgen, G.D., Kenigsburg, D. Collins, R.L., and Schenden, R.S.: Selection of the dominant ovarian follicle and hormonal enhancement of the natural cycle. Ann. N.Y. Acad. Sci., *442*:23–37, 1985.
40. Greenwald, G.S., and Terranova, P.F.: Follicular selection and its control. *In* The Physiology of Reproduction. Edited by E. Knobil and J. Neill. New York, Raven Press, 1988, pp. 387–446.
41. Ying, S.Y.: Inhibins, activins and follistatins. J. Steroid Biochem., *33*:705–713, 1989.
42. Richards, J.S.: Maturation of ovarian follicles: Actions and interactions of pituitary and ovarian hormones on follicular cell differentiation. Physiol. Rev., *60*:51–89, 1980.
43. Carson, R., Findlay, J., Mattner, P., and Brown, B.: Relative levels of thecal blood flow in atretic and non-atretic ovarian follicles of the conscious sheep. Aust. J. Exp. Biol. Med. Sci., *64*:381–387, 1986.
44. Moor, R.M., and Seamark, R.F.: Cell signalling, permeability, and microvascular changes during follicle development in mammals. J. Dairy Sci., *69*:927–943, 1986.
45. Driancourt, M.A., et al.: Ovarian follicular populations in pony and saddle-type mares. Reprod. Nutr. Dev., *22*:1035–1047, 1982.
46. Baird, D.T.: Factors regulating the growth of the preovulatory follicle in the sheep and human. J. Reprod. Fertil., *69*:343–352, 1983.
47. Peluso, J.J., Charlesworth, J., and England-Charlesworth, C.: Role of estrogen and androgen in maintaining the preovulatory follicle. Cell Tissue Res., *216*:615–624, 1981.
48. Tsafriri, A.: Local non-steroidal regulators of ovarian function. *In* The Physiology of Reproduction. Edited by E. Knobil and J.D. Neill. New York, Raven Press, 1988, pp. 527–566.
49. Parker, W.G.: Sequential changes of the ovulating follicle in the estrous mare as determined by rectal palpation.

Proceedings of the Annual Conference of Veterinarians. Fort Collins, Colorado State University, 1971, pp. 1–25.

50. Hughes, J.P., et al.: Production of progesterone by corpora lutea formed by ovulation during the luteal phase of the oestrus cycle (diestrous ovulations). Vlaams Diergeneesk. Tijdschr., *53:*191–196, 1984.

51. Stabenfeldt, G.H., Hughes, J.P., Evans, J.W., and Neely, D.P.: Spontaneous prolongation of luteal activity in the mare. Equine Vet. J., *6:*158–163, 1974.

52. Hughes, J.P., Stabenfeldt, G.H., and Evans, J.W.: Clinical and endocrine aspects of the estrous cycle of the mare. Proc. Am. Assoc. Equine Pract., 119–148, 1972.

53. Hughes, J.P., Couto, M.A., and Stabenfeldt, G.H.: Luteal phase ovulations: What are the options? Proc. Soc. Theriogenol., 123–125, 1985.

54. Mossman, H.W., and Duke, K.L.: Comparative Morphology of the Mammalian Ovary. Madison, University of Wisconsin Press, 1973.

55. Balboni, G.C.: Structural changes: Ovulation and luteal phase. *In* The Ovary: Comprehensive Endocrinology. Edited by G.B. Serra. Raven Press, New York, 1983, pp. 123–142.

56. Guraya, S.S.: Biology of Ovarian Follicles in Mammals. New York, Springer-Verlag, 1985, pp. 195–213.

57. Thibault, C., and Levasseur, M.C.: Ovulation. Hum. Reprod., *3:*513–523, 1988.

58. Lipner, H.: Mechanism of mammalian ovulation. *In* The Physiology of Reproduction, Edited by E. Knobil and J. Neil. New York, Raven Press, 1988, pp. 447–488.

59. Morioka, N., et al.: Mechanisms of mammalian ovulation. *In* Development of Preimplantation Embryos and Their Environment. Edited by K. Toshinoga and T. Mori. Wiley-Liss, New York, 1989, pp. 65–85.

60. Bergin, W.C., and Shipley, W.D.: Genital health in the mare. I. Ovulation fossa. Vet. Med. Small Anim. Clin., *63:*362–365, 1968.

61. Witherspoon, D.M., and Talbot, R.B.: Ovulation site in the mare. J. Am. Vet. Med. Assoc., *157:*1452–1459, 1970.

62. Townson, D.H., and Ginther, O.J.: Duration and pattern of follicular evacuation during ovulation in the mare. Anim. Reprod. Sci., *15:*131–138, 1987.

63. Carnevale, E.M., McKinnon, A.O., Squires, E.L., and Voss, J.L.: Ultrasonographic characteristics of the preovulatory follicle preceding and during ovulation in mares. J. Equine Vet. Sci., *8:*428–431, 1988.

64. Townson, D.H., and Ginther, O.J.: Ultrasonic characterization of follicular evacuation during ovulation and fate of the discharged follicular fluid in mares. Anim. Reprod. Sci., *20:*131–141, 1989.

65. Espey, L.L.: Ovulation as an inflammatory reaction-A hypothesis. Biol. Reprod., *22:*73–106, 1980.

66. Woessner, J.F., Jr., et al.: Connective tissue breakdown in ovulation. Steroids, *54:*491–499, 1989.

67. Pierson, R.A., Martinuk, S.D., Chizen, D.R., and Simpson, C.W.: Ultrasonographic visualization of human ovulation. *In* From Ovulation to Implantation. Edited by J.H.L. Evers and M.J. Heineman. Amsterdam, Excerpta Medica, 1990, pp. 73–79.

68. Ginther, O.J., and Pierson, R.A.: Ultrasonic anatomy of equine ovaries. Theriogenology, *21:*471–483, 1984.

69. Bomsel-Helmreich, O.: Ultrasound and the preovulatory human follicle. Oxf. Rev. Reprod. Biol., *7:*1–72, 1985.

70. Katz, E.: The luteinized unruptured follicle and other ovulatory dysfunctions. Fertil. Steril., *50:*839–850, 1988.

71. McKinnon, A.O., et al.: Heterogenous and xenogenous fertilization of in vivo matured equine oocytes. J. Equine Vet. Sci., *8:*143–147, 1988.

72. Zhang, J.J., Boyle, M.S., and Allen, W.R.: Recent studies on in vivo fertilization of in vitro matured horse oocytes. Equine Vet. J. Suppl., *8:*101–104, 1989.

73. Bezard, J., Magistrini, M., Duchamp, G., and Palmer, E.: Chronology of equine fertilization and early embryonic development in vivo and in vitro. Equine Vet. J. Suppl., *8:*105–110, 1989.

74. Vogelsang, M.M., et al.: Methods for collecting follicular oocytes from mares. Theriogenology, *29:*1007–1018, 1988.

75. Hinrichs, K., Kenney, D.F., and Kenney, R.M.: Aspiration of oocytes from mature and immature preovulatory follicles in the mare. Theriogenology, *34:*107–112, 1990.

76. Watson, E.D., and Sertich, P.L.: Effect of aspiration of follicular fluid on subsequent luteal function in the mare. Theriogenology, *33:*1263–1268, 1990.

CHAPTER 18

LUTEAL PHASE

D. Niswender
T.M. Nett

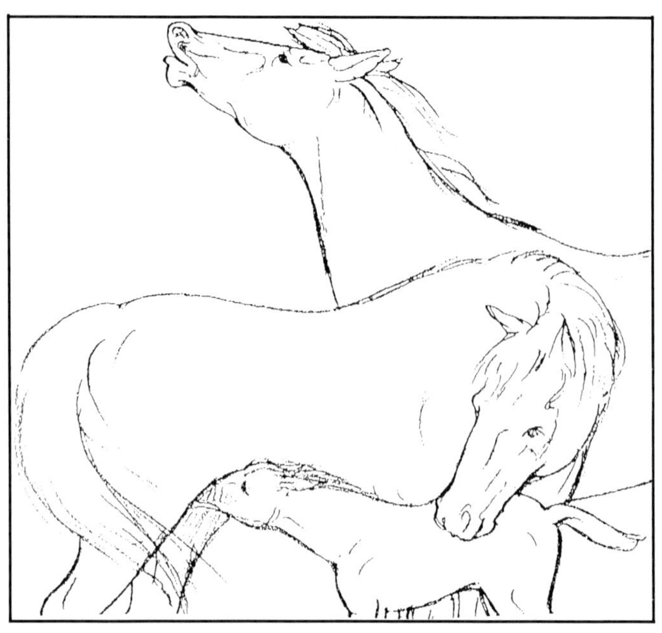

In mares, as in other mammalian species, ovulation of the ovarian follicle is followed by formation of the corpus luteum (CL). Normal secretion of progesterone from this gland is a requirement for maintenance of normal pregnancy. However, some aspects of this process are different in horses from other domestic animals.

Because of the unique structure of the equine ovary, ovulation can occur at only one site on the ovary, the ovulation fossa.[1] Essentially the entire structure of the corpus luteum is contained within the ovarian stroma as a result of this anatomic feature. Although the corpus luteum of the mare reaches it maximum diameter within approximately 3 days of ovulation[2] the maximum secretion of progesterone does not occur until about 9 days after ovulation.[3]

CELL TYPES IN THE EQUINE CORPUS LUTEUM

In domestic ruminants, rabbits, rats, and several primate species the CL appears to be derived from both steroidogenic cell types in the preovulatory follicle: the cells of the theca interna and granulosa cells.[4] In ruminants, small luteal cells are thought to originate from the theca interna with a diameter ranging from 12 to 20 μm and contain abundant mitochondria and lipid droplets but do not contain stacked, rough endoplasmic reticulum or protein-containing secretory granules. These cells contain receptors for luteinizing hormone (LH), which activate the protein kinase A second messenger system to stimulate synthesis and secretion of progesterone. Large luteal cells (20 to 45 μm in diameter), thought to originate from granulosa cells, also contain abundant mitochondria but do not have lipid droplets. These cells contain stacks of rough endoplasmic reticulum and abundant protein-containing secretory granules. Large cells are known to be the source of luteal oxytocin[5] and relaxin[6] in ruminants. These cells also contain receptors for prostaglandin (PG) E_2 and $PGF_2\alpha$ and most of the luteal receptors for estradiol.[7] Activation of the protein kinase C second messenger system, which is stimulated by $PGF_2\alpha$, inhibits the synthesis and secretion of progesterone. Prostaglandin $F_2\alpha$–stimulated calcium influx may cause cell death, because large luteal cells are ineffective in equilibrating intracellular free calcium levels.[8] Thus this cell type appears to play a critical role in mediating the luteolytic process in ruminants.

However, based on histologic studies,[9,10] the steroidogenic cells of the equine CL appear to be derived primarily, if not exclusively, from granulosa cells. Theca cells begin degenerating just prior to ovulation, and their degeneration is nearly complete by 24 h after ovulation. In contrast, granulosa cells, which are approximately 10 μm in diameter at ovulation, have enlarged to 15 μm by 24 h following ovulation and undergo cytologic changes characteristic of luteinization. Luteinization of the granulosa cells appears to be complete by 3 days postovulation, but cell growth continues until day 9 (average diameter, 37.5 μm), when maximal progesterone secretion occurs. On day 9, in addition to the large, light-staining luteal cells, approximately 15% of the luteal cells are small cells. These small cells are eosinophilic and are thought to represent a resting stage that can be converted to the large, light-staining luteal cells. If the mare does not become pregnant, the process of luteolysis begins by day 12 postovulation. The large luteal cells begin to decrease in diameter, and by day 16 their diameter averages 20 μm. This reduction in size is correlated with decreased circulating concentrations of progesterone. It seems clear that additional research needs to be conducted to elucidate precisely the cell types and their follicular source of origin in the equine corpus luteum. Future research also needs to address the biochemical characteristics of these cells.

TROPIC SUPPORT OF THE CORPUS LUTEUM

The CL of the mare appears to primarily depend on luteinizing hormone for trophic support. This conclusion is based on two kinds of evidence. First, antisera raised against the gonadotropin fraction of equine pituitary extracts will induce luteal regression.[11] On the other hand, administration of human chorionic gonadotropin (hCG) or equine pituitary extract can extend the life span of the CL in mares.[2] As in several other species, the concentration of receptors for LH in the CL of the mare parallels the circulating concentrations of progesterone. [12] Interestingly, the affinity of these receptors for LH also appears to increase when the secretion of progesterone is maximal. This phenomenon appears to be unique to the equine corpus luteum. In summary, the life span of the CL during the estrous cycle of the mare is clearly regulated by a pituitary gonadotropin, probably luteinizing hormone.

LH is apparently the gonadotropin that regulates luteal secretion of progesterone.[13] A dose-dependent increase in progesterone secretion from suspended luteal cells in vitro occurs following addition of equine LH or hCG. Serum concentrations of progesterone also increase following hCG treatment of mares during the early-luteal phase of the estrous cycle. Although Kelly et al. provided evidence for two types of equine luteal cells based on diameters,[13] data are lacking regarding the biochemical characterization of the two distinct cell types. In fact, morphologic evidence suggests that equine steroidogenic luteal cells are derived predominately from follicular granulosa cells.

LUTEAL REGRESSION DURING THE CYCLE

As in other species, $PGF_2\alpha$ appears to be responsible for regression of the CL at the end of the estrous cycle of the mare.[14] The concentration of PGF in the uterine venous blood is lower on days 10 and 14 of pregnancy than in nonpregnant mares.[15] A redirecting of the secretion of $PGF_2\alpha$ into the uterine lumen as noted in pigs[16] does not seem to occur and neither does a reduction in the sensitivity of the CL to $PGF_2\alpha$ during early pregnancy as noted in sheep.[17] On the contrary, the ability of the CL to bind $PGF_2\alpha$ increases rather than decreases during early pregnancy.[18] No unilateral effect of the uterus or embryo on luteal function exists as noted in most other domestic animals.

It is interesting that the CL of the horse appears to be composed predominately, if not exclusively, of cells of granulosa origin. In the sheep these luteal cells contain all of the receptors for $PGF_2\alpha$ and appear to mediate the luteolytic actions of this hormone. This may explain the observation that the equine CL is sensitive to $PGF_2\alpha$.[2]

There is evidence that oxytocin may play a role in regulating the secretion of prostaglandins from the uterus of nonpregnant mares.[19] Injections of oxytocin during the late-luteal phase of the estrous cycle resulted in enhanced blood concentrations of 13,14-dihydro,-15-keto $PGF_2\alpha$ (PGFM), the primary metabolite of $PGF_2\alpha$. The response to oxytocin was considerably reduced in pregnant mares. An increased secretion of oxytocin occurs during the late-luteal phase of the estrous cycle.[20] Thus evidence shows that oxytocin may lead to uterine secretion of $PGF_2\alpha$ and luteolysis in horses in a manner similar to that observed in other domestic species.[21]

MATERNAL RECOGNITION OF PREGNANCY

The mechanism(s) responsible for maintenance of the primary CL during early pregnancy in the mare is not well understood. The CL must continue to secrete progesterone for the first 50 to 70 days of gestation.[22] During that period, pregnancy can be maintained in mares after ovariectomy by treatment with progesterone.[23] Removal of the equine embryo on day 14 or thereafter results in extension of the life span of the corpus luteum.[23] Therefore, the signal from the pregnant uterus for maintenance of the CL must be given on or before day 16. The concentration of progesterone in serum from pregnant mares follows a temporal pattern similar to that of the nonpregnant mare through the first 12 days postestrus.[24,25] From that point, the concentration of progesterone falls rapidly for a 2-day period in cycling mares, whereas a gradual, partial decline in pregnant mares occurs until days 20 to 35.[26] The concentration of progesterone in serum then increases again, with maximal levels being achieved by day 100 of pregnancy. This is in contrast to the pattern observed in hysterectomized mares in which the gradual decline initiated on day 12 continues until luteal function is lost completely sometime between days 100 and 200.[24,27]

Certainly, the conceptus is involved in maternal recognition of pregnancy and the subsequent maintenance of the primary CL in mares. At least two different mechanisms seem to be involved. First, unfertilized ova are trapped in the oviduct of mares where they degenerate over a period of months.[28] In contrast, the fertilized ovum produces a substance that ensures its selective passage through the oviduct and into the uterus. Once in the uterus, the conceptus must come into contact with essentially the entire endometrial surface to prevent luteal regression. Because the equine conceptus does not elongate but rather remains spherical until well into the second month of gestation, endometrial contact is achieved by migration of the conceptus throughout the uterus. In fact, the equine conceptus appears to traverse the entire uterus about every 2 h during the critical period for recognition of pregnancy.[29]

Interaction of the conceptus with the endometrium is speculated to prevent production and secretion of $PGF_2\alpha$.[29] The nature of the substance produced by the conceptus to inhibit production of $PGF_2\alpha$ has not been identified but it is believed that it may be estrogen. The equine conceptus is capable of synthesizing estradiol in vitro[30] and small quantities of estrogen induce a uterine tone characteristic of pregnancy. Once the CL of pregnancy is established, the secretion of progesterone gradually decreases until secretion of equine chorionic gonadotropin begins on about day 35.[26]

In mares, increases in secretion of follicle-stimulating hormone occur at approximately 10-day intervals throughout early pregnancy,[31] and this results in waves of follicular activity.[32] Secretion of massive quantities of equine chorionic gonadotropin beginning around day 35 of gestation induces ovulation or luteinization of these follicles and formation of secondary corpora lutea.[33] Function of the primary CL is also stimulated by equine chorionic gonadotropin.[34] The secondary corpora lutea appear similar to the primary CL in structure and function and secrete progesterone until their trophic support (equine chorionic gonadotropin) disappears from the circulation at approximately day 150 of gestation, at which time they regress along with the primary corpus luteum. Progestational support for the remainder of pregnancy in the mare is provided by the fetal placenta.[35]

The mechanisms involved in maternal recognition of pregnancy in the mare are more like those in humans than in other domestic species. In cattle and sheep a trophoblastic protein[36] inhibits uterine secretion of $PGF_2\alpha$, and the embryo also secretes an additional protein that inhibits the actions of $PGF_2\alpha$ at the level of the luteal cell.[37] There is no evidence that similar proteins are secreted by the equine conceptus.

PSEUDOPREGNANCY

A condition termed pseudopregnancy occurs in both bred and nonbred mares and is characterized by a lack of estrus for 1 to 2 months; considerable follicular development; tense uterine tone; closed and firm cervix; and a pale, dry vagina.[2] In general, this condition has been attributed to death of the conceptus early in gestation.

In cases where the conceptus is removed, or dies, after the critical period for luteal maintenance (day 14), the CL is maintained for a period of 20 to 40 days. Experimentally, when loss of pregnancy is induced before day 36 by crushing the fetus, aspirating the placental fluid, or infusing intrauterine saline, the primary CL persisted for 1 to 3 weeks. Thus most cases of pseudopregnancy are probably a result of fetal death following the initial signal for maintenance of the CL of pregnancy. However, it has been carefully documented under research conditions that pseudopregnancy can also occur in nonbred pony, Thoroughbred, and Quarter Horse mares.[2] The causative factors that induce pseudopregnancy in nonbred mares are not understood.

REFERENCES

1. Mossman, M., and Duke, K.L.: Some comparative aspects of the mammalian ovary. *In* Handbook of Physiology. Vol. 2. Bethesda, American Physiological Society, 1973.
2. Ginther, O.J.: Reproductive Biology of the Mare. Basic and Applied Aspects. Ann Arbor, McNaughton, Gunn, 1979.
3. Nett, T.M., Pickett, B.W., Seidel, G.E., Jr., and Voss, J.L.: Levels of luteinizing hormone and progesterone during the estrous cycle and early pregnancy in mares. Biol. Reprod., *14*:412–415, 1976.
4. Niswender, G.D., et al.: Regulation of luteal function in domestic ruminants: New concepts. Recent Prog. Horm. Res., *41*:101–142, 1985.
5. Sawyer, H.R., Moeller, C.L., and Kozlowski, G.P.: Immunocytochemical localization of neurophysin and oxytocin in ovine corpora lutea. Biol. Reprod., *34*:543–548, 1986.
6. Fields, M.J., Fields, P.A., Castro-Hernandez, A., and Larkin, L.H.: Evidence for relaxin in corpora lutea of late pregnant cows. Endocrinology, *107*:869–876, 1980.
7. Fitz, T.A., Mayan, M.H., Sawyer, H.R., and Niswender, G.D.: Characterization of two steoridogenic cell types in the ovine corpus luteum. Biol. Reprod., *27*:703–711, 1982.
8. Wiltbank, M.C., Diskin, M.G., and Niswender, G.D.: Differential actions of second messenger systems in the corpus luteum. J. Reprod. Fertil. Suppl., *43*:65–75, 1991.
9. Van Niekerk, C.H., Morgenthal, J.C., and Gerneke, W.H.: Relationship between the morphology of and progesterone production by the corpus luteum of the mare. J. Reprod. Fertil. Suppl., *23*:171–175, 1975.
10. Harrison, R.J.: The early development of the corpus luteum of the mare. J. Anat., *80*:160–166, 1946.
11. Pineda, M.H., Ginther, O.J., and McShan, W.H.: Regression of the corpus luteum in mares treated with an antiserum against an equine pituitary fraction. Am. J. Vet. Res., *33*:1767–1773, 1972.
12. Roser, J.F., and Evans, J.W.: Luteal luteinizing hormone receptors during the postovulatory period in the mare. Biol. Reprod., *29*:499–510, 1983.
13. Kelly, C.M., Hoyer, P.B., and Wise, M.E.: In vitro and in vivo responsiveness of the corpus luteum of the mare to gonadotrophin stimulation. J. Reprod. Fertil., *84*:593–600, 1988.
14. Douglas, R.H., and Ginther, O.J.: Effect of prostaglandin $F_2\alpha$ on estrous cycles or corpus luteum in mares and gilts. J. Anim. Sci., *40*:518–522, 1975.
15. Douglas, R.H., and Ginther, O.J.: Concentrations of prostaglandin F in uterine venous plasma of anesthetized mares during the estrous cycle and early pregnancy. Prostaglandins, *11*:251–260, 1976.
16. Bazer, F.W., and Thatcher, W.W.: Theory of maternal recognition of pregnancy in swine based on estrogen con-

trolled endocrine versus exocrine secretion of prostaglandin $F_2\alpha$ by the uterine endometrium. Prostaglandins, *14:*397–399, 1977.

17. Silvia, W.J., and Niswender, G.D.: Maintenance of the corpus luteum of early pregnancy in the ewe. IV. Changes in luteal sensitivity to prostaglandin $F_2\alpha$ throughout early pregnancy. J. Anim. Sci., *63:*1201–1207, 1986.

18. Vernon, M.W., Zavy, M.T., Aisquith, R.L., and Sharp, D.C.: Prostaglandin $F_2\alpha$ in the equine endometrium: Steroid production and production capacities during the oestrous cycle and early pregnancy. Biol. Reprod., *25:*581–589, 1981.

19. Goff, A.K., Pontbriand, D., and Sirois, J.: Oxytocin stimulation of plasma 15-keto-13,14-dihydro prostaglandins F-2alpha during the oestrous cycle and early pregnancy in the mare. J. Reprod. Fertil. Suppl., *35:*253–260, 1987.

20. Tetzke, T.A., Ismail, S., Mikuckis, G., and Evans, J.W.: Patterns of oxytocin secretion during the oestrous cycle of the mare. J. Reprod. Fertil. Suppl., *35:*245–252, 1987.

21. Flint, A.P.F., and Sheldrick, E.L.: Ovarian peptides and luteolysis. *In* Implantation of the Human Embryo. Edited by R.G. Edwards, J.M. Purdy, and P.C. Steptoe. London, Academic Press, 1985, pp. 235–242.

22. Holtan, D.W., Squires, D.L., Lapin, D.R., and Ginther, O.J.: Effect of ovariectomy on pregnancy in mares. J. Reprod. Fertil. Suppl., *27:*457–463, 1979.

23. Hershman, L., and Douglas, R.H.: The critical period for the maternal recognition of pregnancy in pony mares. J. Reprod. Fertil. Suppl., *27:*395–401, 1979.

24. Squires, E.L., Wentworth, B.C., and Ginther, O.J.: Progesterone concentration in blood of mares during the estrous cycle, pregnancy and after hysterectomy. J. Anim. Sci., *39:*759–767, 1975.

25. Holtan, D.W., Nett, T.M., and Estergreen, V.L.: Plasma progestins in pregnant, postpartum and cycling mares. J. Anim. Sci., *40:*251–260, 1975.

26. Nett, T.M., and Pickett, B.W.: Effect of diethylstilbestrol on the relationship between LH, PMSG and progesterone during pregnancy in the mare. J. Reprod. Fertil. Suppl., *27:*465–470, 1979.

27. Stabenfeldt, G.H., et al.: The role of the uterus in ovarian control in the mare. J. Reprod. Fertil., *37:*343–351, 1974.

28. Van Niekerk, C.H., and Gerneke, W.H.: Persistence and pathogenetic cleavage of tubal ova in the mare. Onderstepoort J. Vet. Res., *31:*195–232, 1966.

29. Leith, G.S., and Ginther, O.J.: Characterization of intrauterine mobility of the early equine conceptus. Theriogeneology, *22:*401–408, 1984.

30. Mayer, R.E., et al.: Estrogen production by the early equine conceptus. Proceedings of the Sixty-ninth Annual Meeting of the American Society of Animal Science (abstr.). 1977, p. 186.

31. Evans, M.J., and Irvine, C.H.G.: Serum concentrations of FSH, LH and progesterone during the oestrous cycle and early pregnancy in the mare. J. Reprod. Fertil. Suppl., *23:*193–200, 1975.

32. Allen, W.E.: Ovarian changes during gestation in pony mares. Equine Vet. J., *6:*135–138, 1974.

33. Cole, H.H., Howell, C.E., and Hart, G.H.: Changes occurring in the ovary of the mare during pregnancy. Anat. Rec., *49:*199–209, 1931.

34. Squires, E.L., Stevens, W.B., Pickett, B.W., and Nett, T.M.: Role of pregnant mare serum gonadotropin in luteal function of pregnant mares. Am. J. Vet. Res., *40:*889–891, 1979.

35. Moss, G.E., Estergreen, V.L., Becker, S.R., and Grant, B.D.: The source of 5 α-pregnanes that occur during gestation in the mare. J. Reprod. Fertil. Suppl., *27:*511–519, 1979.

36. Roberts, R.M., et al: The polypeptides and genes for ovine and bovine trophoblast protein-1. J. Reprod. Fertil. Suppl., *43:*3–12, 1991.

37. Wiltbank, M.C., Knickerbocker, J.J., Wiepz, G.J., and Niswender, G.D.: Ovine conceptal protein blocks the action of prostaglandin $F_2\alpha$ ($PGF_2\alpha$) on large luteal cells. Biol. Reprod. Suppl. 1, *42:*77, 1991.

SECTION C

BREEDING MANAGEMENT

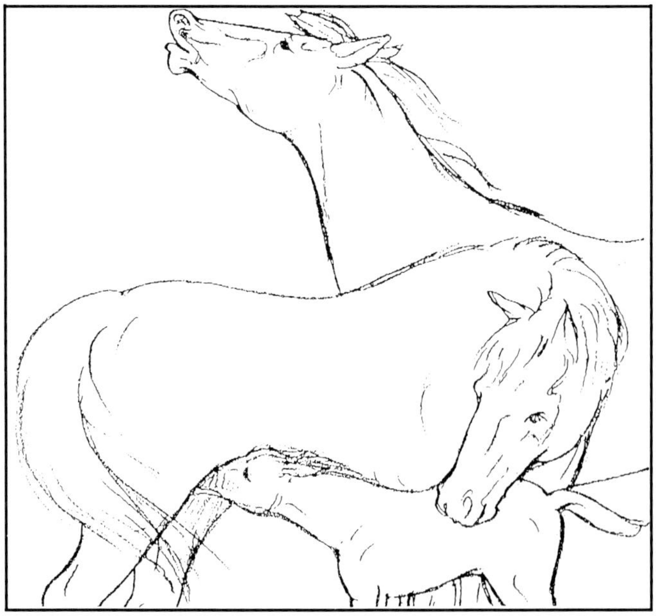

CHAPTER 19

PHOTOPERIOD

D.C. Sharp
B.D. Cleaver
S.D. Davis

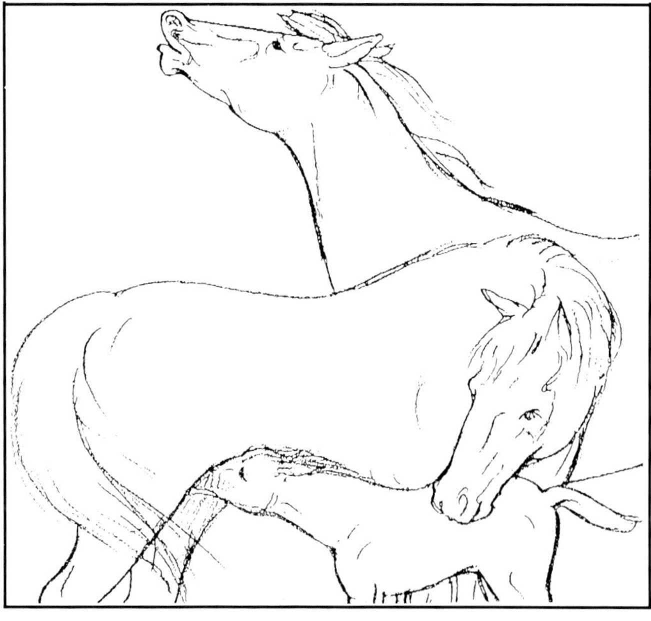

The world is filled with cyclic events, the result of the daily rotation of the earth and its annual revolution around the sun. Faced with such cyclic phenomena, the natural tendency for most living things to fit into their environments as efficiently and harmoniously as possible, led to the development of a temporal organization, or time-keeping system. Many naturally occurring events have clock-like regularity, such as the rising and setting of the sun, lunar cycles, and the annual change in seasons. The majority of plants and animals have evolved inherent oscillating systems with frequencies closely matching these natural rhythms.[1] Thus circadian rhythms take place with a frequency approximating 24 h, circalunar rhythms have a frequency approximating the lunar cycle (29 days), and circannual rhythms have a frequency approximating 1 yr. The advantage of these inherent rhythms is that they provide animals with the ability to function well in a changing environment. For instance, many of the body's functions, such as core temperature, respiratory rate, heart rate, blood pressure, secretion of certain hormones, etc. are reduced during night hours when the body is at rest. For that matter, the rhythm of sleeping and waking is a good example of daily oscillations that are inherent, yet subject to entrainment from outside influences. Most people are aware of the regularity with which they retire and wake again some time later, and many would admit to the superfluity of alarm clocks because they wake spontaneously at about the time the alarm rings. However, twice a year, that rhythm is disturbed by outside influences in that the clocks are set differently (back in the fall, ahead in the spring). At those times, many people experience some difficulty adjusting to the new time (entrainment); the adjustment usually takes place within 1 to 2 weeks. The point is that the sleep/wake cycle is a biologic rhythm that adheres to the strict definition of a circadian rhythm. To be considered circadian, a rhythmic phenomenon must satisfy the following criteria: (1) It must be inherent. It must persist in the absence of environmental periodicities, in a rhythm different from, but usually close to, the period of the solar day. This phenomenon is called free-running. (2) It must be entrainable to some exogenous rhythm, such as the solar day.

For a rhythm to occur every day does not necessarily mean that it is circadian, and care should be taken in describing a rhythm as circadian until it has been demonstrated to fit the above definition. Similarly, care should be taken in using the word *diurnal,* because that means simply "occurring *during* the day," and implies no circadian basis at all, although a diurnal rhythm may indeed be circadian. The term *quotidian* means, simply, occurring *every* day. For the purist, the term *nyctohemeral* is useful because it pertains to rhythms that occur during both night and day. The secretory pattern of melatonin is usually characterized as being nyctohemeral. Another important aspect of circadian rhythms is that once entrained by some environmental factor (day length, food intake, and temperature are among common Zeitgebers, or time givers) not only is the frequency of the environmental factor imposed on the internal clock but also the inherent rhythm is phased appropriately to local time.[2] Entrainment, therefore, involves control of both the period and the phase of the rhythm, and having achieved steady-state entrainment to an environmental Zeitgeber, an animal can count on performing certain behavioral and/or physiologic activities at "the right time of the day."

To understand the phenomenon of photoperiodism and, therefore, to utilize it practically, it is first helpful to understand the anatomic correlates of the system.

ANATOMICAL PATHWAY FOR PHOTOPERIODISM

Although in many lower animals it is possible for the influence of solar radiation to affect brain structures directly, in mammals, the majority of the evidence indicates that the retina of the eye is the primary photoreceptor. Photic information is then conveyed to brain structures by a complex nervous pathway. In all species so far studied, there is a projection of nerve fibers from the retina of the eye to the hypothalamus. This nerve projection is called the retinohypothalamic tract (RHT),[3] and its presence in the horse has been demonstrated.[4] Administration of horseradish peroxidase into the vitreous humor of the eye and subsequent staining of brain structures with tetramethyl benzidine (TMB) indicated the presence of color reaction in the contralateral suprachiasmatic nucleus (SCN). Absolute decussation of the optic nerves at the optic chiasm in the horse explains the appearance of the color reaction in only the contralateral suprachiasmatic nuclei. The importance of this feature of the photic pathway will become more clear in the discussion of the role of the SCN below. From the SCN, nerve fibers pass through the medial basal hypothalamus to the intermediolateral cell column of the spinal cord and exit the cranium. The nerve fibers terminate as preganglionic fibers in the superior cervical ganglia along the sympathetic chain. From the superior cervical ganglia, postganglionic, sympathetic fibers traverse back into the cranium where they enter the pineal through the nervii conarii.[3] In the pineal, the postganglionic fibers terminate directly on the pinealocytes.

The importance of this circuitous pathway by which the effects of light are conveyed to the pineal will be evident from discussion below. For the moment, it is sufficient to state that interruption of the photic pathway at any point along its continuum from retina to pinealocyte will interrupt the time-keeping process and result in abnormal seasonal reproductive patterns.[5]

FREE-RUNNING RHYTHMS

Rhythmic phenomena are perhaps best understood through analogy to physical oscillators, with which they have much in common. At least the terminology to describe circadian rhythms can be borrowed from oscillator theory. An oscillation is defined by its period. That is, the duration of time from one distinct phase of the rhythm to the time of reoccurrence of the same phase is called the period, or tau (τ). The period of the sleep/wake rhythm, for instance, would be from the time of rising in the morning of one day to the time of rising the following morning. When an arithmetic value can be expressed from a rhythm, such as concentration of a hormone in the peripheral circulation, the rhythm can also be described by its range of oscillation, i.e., the difference between the maximum and minimum values of the end point within one period and by the arithmetic mean. Extremes (minimum and maximum values) are often expressed as deviations from this arithmetic mean as a way of standardizing and comparing rhythms among different animals. Any given point in an oscillation may be different from previous and succeeding points, and thus it is important to define the moment-to-moment states of a rhythm. By convention, each instantaneous point of an oscillation is defined as a phase of the entire oscillation, and that particular point on the abcissa is referred to as the phase angle[2] (Fig. 19–1). The phase angle is measured in fractions of the entire oscillation, which is considered to be 360°. Therefore, if the rhythm has an easily detected and quantified point in time, such as an obvious nadir or zenith, it can arbitrarily be assigned a phase angle value (say 0°) and other points along the oscillation described relative to that point. For example, if an individual awakes precisely at 6:00 a.m., and begins to sleep at 6:00 p.m., the time of waking could be defined as 0° phase angle, and the time of sleep onset would then be defined as 180°.

Although the underlying mechanisms that drive the many inherent rhythms within mammals are not yet well understood, it is clear that many physiologic functions do in fact oscillate with a consistent period that is likely genetically derived. These self-sustaining oscillations are expressed with periods that reflect individual uniqueness in the absence of environmental factors. Well-known examples of such free-running rhythms are the sleep/wake rhythms of individuals existing, for the sake of research, in environmentally controlled chambers in which temperature, light, and other environmental inputs are essentially neutral. In such cases, the individuals are allowed to have lighting, but it is at their demand, not instituted through any external timing mechanisms. Television, radio, watches, and even newspapers, which might provide cues as to the time of

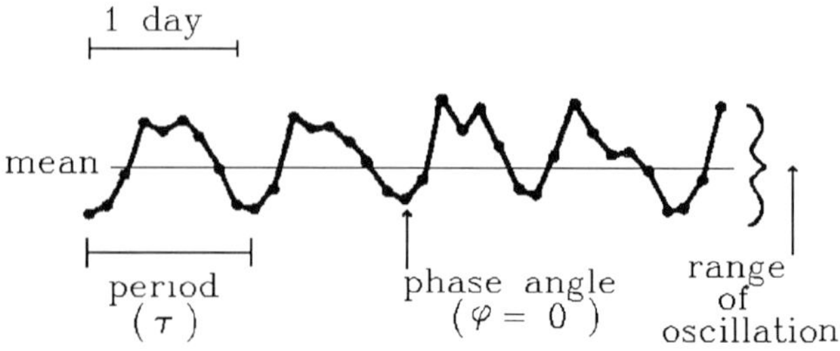

FIG. 19–1. Twenty-four-hour cortisol secretion pattern.

day, were not present in such experiments. Under such Zeitgeber-free conditions, the sleep/wake rhythm of individuals usually departs from the precise 24-h rhythm of those of us subjugated by alarm clocks and rigid schedules, usually expanding to a period of more than 24 h. It is not unusual for such an individual to establish a repeatable pattern (oscillation) of sleep and wakefulness with a period of 25 to 26 h. Similarly, hamsters who are habituated to running on an exercise wheel generally begin their locomotor activity precisely at the onset of darkness when subjected to a 24-h photoperiod. However, when subjected to constant conditions, such as constant darkness, the period from onset of exercise usually expands to slightly more than 24 h (hence the term free-running). The precision of the system is well illustrated by the fact that the period of the free-running rhythm of locomotion is often only a few minutes different from 24 h, but can be measured accurately[6] (Fig. 19–2)

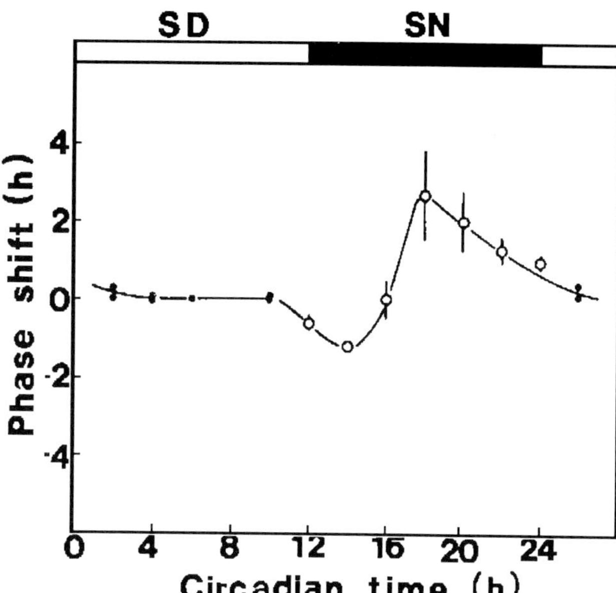

FIG. 19–3. Example of a phase response curve. The response is shifted only when a stimulus (light pulse) coincides with specific circadian times (i.e., 12 to 22 h). SD, subjective day; SN, subjective night; ●, subjective day; ○, subjective night.

ENTRAINMENT OF CIRCADIAN RHYTHMS

The chaos that might result if an organism were left with a variety of important physiologic functions expressing their own independent self-sustaining oscillations, with no regard for the consequences on other physiologic events, can be readily understood. What might be the outcome if such important physiologic functions as blood pressure, heart rate, and respiration rate were to be at their maxima during the time an individual were asleep at night, instead of during a time of greater physical activity? The consequences of ovulation occurring in the daytime, for a normally nocturnally active animal such as the rat, are immediately evident and predictable. Therefore, the coordination of

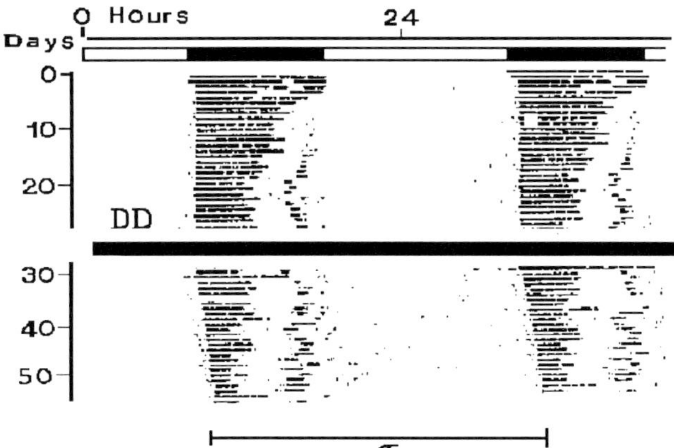

FIG. 19–2. Activity record of hamster wheel running. Each horizontal line represents 1 day. The hamster began to free run about day 30, when the photoperiod was changed to constant darkness (DD). (Adapted from Elliott, J.A.: Circadian rhythms, entrainment and photoperiodism in Syrian hamster. *In* Biological Clocks in Seasonal Reproductive Cycles. Edited by B.K. Follett and D.E. Follett. Bristol, Scientechnica, 1981, pp. 203–217.)

these self-sustaining rhythms through the process of entrainment is a necessary and critical part of homeostasis. Entrainment—the synchronization of an inherent self-sustaining rhythm by periodic factors in the environment, such as photoperiod—is achieved through phase control. Entrainment of a naturally occuring rhythm will not take place if the frequency of the Zeitgeber deviates too much from its own frequency, and the rhythm will continue to free run. To entrain a self-sustaining rhythm, the phase of the inherent rhythm must be adjusted, either advanced (positive sign) or delayed (negative sign) by the Zeitgeber, and once entrained, the phase of the entrained rhythm must be corrected frequently. In steady state systems, the phase angle of the entrained rhythm may be adjusted at least once during each period.[2] The amount of phase shift required to entrain a rhythm is a function of the phase angle of the inherent rhythm, and the degree of shift can be expressed graphically in comparison to the phase angle of the Zeitgeber. Such a graphic expression (Fig. 19–3) is called a phase response curve (PRC), and enables researchers to describe a variety of rhythms in relationship to each other, and to common environmental Zeitgebers.

As will be appreciated, this rather complex timekeeping system is an important modulator of homeostasis, and the consequences of disruption of the system are yet to be understood. Although the consequences of circadian desynchronization in mammals are not known, some reports note that ablation of a gland that coordinates many rhythms in cockroaches leads to a reduction in lifespan by about 20%.

THE SUPRACHIASMATIC NUCLEI AS BIOLOGIC CLOCK

The fact that there are many self-sustaining oscillations in the body, yet a single Zeitgeber, photoperiod, is capable of entraining the vast majority of them to a precise 24-h period implies the existence of a single "clearinghouse" or anatomic location in which the photic information is processed and passed on to the various organs or tissues regulating the rhythmic expression. Recent research has revealed exciting news about the suprachiasmatic nuclei as the anatomic location of the biologic clock.[7] For one, the suprachiasmatic nuclei are anatomically appropriate for such a function, because photic information can be conveyed directly to the SCN where such processing could be effected. Many experimental approaches have demonstrated that destruction of the SCN in a variety of mammalian species leads to loss of inherent rhythmicity of a large number of physiologic processes. However, caution is urged before making the assumption either that the SCN is the single major information processing center or that it is the sole information processing center. A clue to the biochemic mechanisms of the SCN was recently uncovered by researchers who showed that photoperiod signals that cause a phase shift in daily rhythms in rats and hamsters evoke the expression of a regulatory gene called *c-fos* in the SCN.[8] *C-fos* is one of a group of so-called immediate-early genes, which are among the first to be activated when a cell undergoes a change in transcription. These genes produce proteins that bind onto the DNA and regulate the expression of other genes during the process of transcribing genetic message from RNA. The proteins expressed by *c-fos* bind DNA and regulate the expression of other genes. It was shown that *c-fos* was expressed in hamsters exposed to entraining photoperiods, but only when the phase angle of the Zeitgeber matched the phase angle of receptivity. That is, *c-fos* was expressed in the SCN during the circadian continuum only at times when the light signal resulted in reentrainment of the animal's circadian clock. Thus the activation of genes within the SCN at particular times of the animal's circadian clock fits with predictions that the Zeitgeber must coincide with a particular phase angle of responsiveness. This glimpse into the molecular biologic aspects of circadian rhythms is only the beginning and promises to be a major step toward a better understanding of the biochemical processes that regulate this exotic branch of physiology. Such questions as how does light modulate the rhythm of the SCN and where does the pineal hormone melatonin work may now quickly fall to the probing inquiries of molecular biology.

NATURE OF THE PHOTOPERIODIC SIGNAL

One of the questions and, hence, arguments that remains is whether the photic signal is conveyed through the duration of light exposure (or conversely the duration of dark exposure) or whether the signal is conveyed by coincidence of the Zeitgeber (light or dark) with some photosensitive portion of the circadian clock. The former argument is referred to as the hourglass theory and states that the duration of light (or darkness), like a quantity of sand running through an hourglass, is sufficient to convey the signal of day length to the circadian system.[9] On the other hand, the latter argument is referred to as the external coincidence theory because it states that the information regarding duration of day is conveyed by the coincidence of light with a poorly understood phase of the circadian clock called the photosensitive phase.[10] The recent discovery of *c-fos* expression only when light exposure occurred at a specific circadian time provides a preliminary understanding of the way a photosensitive phase might work, although why the gene is expressed only at certain times is not yet understood.

The secretion of melatonin from the pineal is a hormonal reflection of the solar day. That is, melatonin is secreted primarily during the night, and in many species, represents the duration of darkness relatively faithfully. Furthermore, experimental manipulation of melatonin can be used to alter reproductive status of many species, and therefore, the administration of melatonin to pinealectomized animals has been used as a test system with which to study the relative importance of coincidence versus duration of a signal (melatonin) in eliciting a reproductive response.

Although the nature of the photoperiodic signal is not yet known, it is clear that horses are highly photoreceptive. Burkhardt was first to demonstrate stimulation of the reproductive system with artificial light in horses.[11] He reported an earlier onset of the breeding season in mares exposed to artificially lengthened day, when the length of day was increased at a rate twice as fast as naturally occurring day length. Since that first report, a variety of lighting regimes has been used to stimulate an earlier onset of the breeding season in anestrous mares.[5]

QUALITY AND QUANTITY OF LIGHT AND ITS INFLUENCE ON THE CIRCADIAN SYSTEM

LIGHT INTENSITY

One of the questions most asked by horse breeders when faced with the decision to use artificial lighting in their breeding program is how much light is enough. It is a fair question, and one that still has not been researched satisfactorily, yet some guidelines are available. Burkhardt used a simple incandescent light and was able to induce early sexual recrudescence in anestrous mares.[11] As a result of his work, and that of others, it has been widely accepted that a plain 100-W incandescent bulb in a 12- × 12-ft box stall is sufficient light to elicit a reproductive response. This information, however useful, does not fill the void of answers needed, as many questions remain. For instance, What role does bright moonlight play, if any? What affect, if any, might there be if a neighbor has an outside security light several hundred yards away? What is the minimum intensity of light required to elicit a reproductive response? The average intensity of light generated by Burkhardt's 100-W incandescent bulb was approximately 10 footcandles (107 lux).

Another question that many breeders face is how to measure the intensity of existing light systems. The best way to do this, of course, is to use a sensitive photometer. Fortunately, most single-lens reflex cameras have such a photometer and can be used in a crude way to test whether the intensity of light may be sufficient to elicit a reproductive effect. To use such a system, set the DIN (ASA) reading of the camera to 400 and the shutter speed to ¼ s. Because the metering system of most cameras is sensitive to a focal point of light, or an averaged area of light, it is important to diffuse the light entering the camera, so as to estimate the general illumination, not a point source of light. This can be done by holding a plain white Styrofoam cup over the lens. With this homemade diffuser in place, hold the camera as if to take a picture, at approximately mare's eye level, and set the aperture recommended for appropriate exposure. Table 19–1 illustrates the intensity, in footcandles or lux, associated with aperture reading. In all photoperiod experiments conducted by the authors, an average light intensity of 10 footcandles (107 lux) has been sufficient to cause photostimulation.

PRACTICAL MANAGEMENT SYSTEMS

When to Begin Lighting

One of the most important tenets of photostimulation of early sexual recrudescence is that it does not condense the vernal transition phase (Chapter 15). Rather, photostimulation of early sexual recrudescence results in a shift of the entire process earlier than would occur if mares were exposed only to natural conditions. Because the vernal transition is a relatively lengthy process (40 to 60 days or more) it is immediately apparent that little or no benefit will be derived from beginning an artificial lighting program a month before anticipated results. For instance, if it is desirable to begin breeding mares in February for an early foaling, beginning the lighting regime in January will not accomplish the goal, because the vernal transition alone may require 6 to 8 weeks. Therefore, it is recommended that a program of artificial lighting be initiated no later than December 1. Remember that many mares require a cycle or two to combat infections or sort out other difficulties, and it seems wise to have the opportunity to deal with such problems before breeding. Therefore, the wise breeder should plan to have the mares cycling in January so that their reproductive health can be ascertained before breeding. This means an even earlier start for the photostimulation regime, i.e., November. Although it is not known with certainty that exposure to short day is important to the annual reproductive pattern in mares, data from other species suggest that to be so. Therefore, exposure to short day may also be important in mares, and it is probably wise not to override this potentially important signal. That is, it may not be beneficial, and it could even be deleterious, to maintain mares on long day throughout the year. Further work is needed in this area.

TABLE 19–1. USE OF SINGLE-LENS REFLEX CAMERA TO ESTIMATE LIGHT INTENSITY*

APERTURE READING	INTENSITY (FOOTCANDLES)	INTENSITY (LUX)
f8	45	485
f5.6	12	129
f4	**10**	**108**
f3.5	5	54
f2	3	32

*With camera set at DIN (ASA) 400, shutter speed set at ¼ s, and a plain white Styrofoam cup placed over the lens, the aperture readings indicate the approximate light intensities indicated (in footcandles and lux). The figures in boldface represent the minimum light intensity used in most studies.

Lighting Systems

The decision to employ artificial lighting in a breeding program may involve some construction and changes in the physical plant of a farm and, therefore, requires some thought. The existing management system may be an important variable in such a decision. For instance, if it is the current management system to maintain barren mares in stalls overnight, then the lighting system will be relatively easy to install. In fact, the basis for the lighting system may well already be in place, and require only an inexpensive timing device to control the lights. The intensity of the light should be checked, as described above. As discussed above, either fluorescent or incandescent bulbs will likely suffice if the intensity is high enough. For those considering construction of new facilities, installation of both incandescent and fluorescent bulbs may be a consideration.

If current management does not include housing mares in stalls overnight, an outdoor lighting paddock may be an important consideration. Although construction of such a paddock is initially more expensive than retrofitting a series of box stalls, such a facility may be cheaper in the long run, because the labor of cleaning stalls daily is eliminated. It is a good idea to consult lighting specialists before constructing such a paddock, because they should be able to provide information about numbers and types of fixtures to provide even illumination at a given intensity. The size of the paddock and the number of mares to be exposed in any given area are variables that are best left to the breeder's judgment. It is probably wise not to crowd animals into too small an enclosure, not for any fault of the physiology but simply to avoid the potential for injury. As will be discussed below, one management system that works well involves exposure of the mares for a short time in the evening, then releasing them from the paddock to spend the balance of the night grazing. This accomplishes the required stimulation, avoids the necessity of costly feeding while in the paddock area, and saves wear and tear on the paddock itself (as well as on the animals).

REQUIRED LENGTH OF PHOTOSTIMULATION

The classic length of day required to elicit a reproductive response in anestrous mares is at least 14.5 h of light per day.[12] However, this axiom may not be entirely true. Consider, for example, mares exposed to natural conditions. The timing of the onset of the breeding season is reasonably consistent within a range of latitudes from 43° north to 18° north. This means that mares enter the breeding season at approximately the same time as far south as Mexico City[13] and as far north as Madison, Wisconsin,[14] but the day length at lower latitudes never reaches 14.5 h. In fact, at the authors' institute in Gainesville, Florida (29.6° north), the longest day of the year is only 14 h and 3 min, yet horses in Florida enter the breeding season at approximately the same time as their more northern counterparts.[5] What, then, is the signal for initiation of reproductive onset, and how can that signal be best duplicated in a management system? Unfortunately the answer to that question is not available, but several possibilities are open for consideration.

Evening Only

Sharp reported that an early onset of the breeding season could be stimulated by exposing anestrous mares to only 2 to 2.5 h of additional artificial light (at approximately 10- to 12-footcandle intensity).[5] The artificial lighting regime was begun at sunset every evening, and the time of "lights on" was updated every week or so to match the natural time of sunset as it changed. The beginning of photostimulation was in late October. Furthermore, Sharp reported that artificial light of similar duration (i.e., 2 to 2.5 h) was ineffective when applied prior to the time of sunrise, suggesting that evening light may be unique.

Night Interruption or "Pulse Lighting"

Palmer and Driancourt reported that early onset of the breeding season could also be stimulated by exposing anestrous mares to a 1-h pulse of artificial light, if the pulse were timed appropriately.[12] They reported that the pulse of light exposure was effective when it occurred 9.5 to 10.5 h after the onset of darkness.[12] This lighting regime also appears to have practical application, primarily in management systems in which mares are housed routinely in stalls overnight. The application of this lighting regime to outdoor paddocks, however is of lesser utility, because it eliminates one advantage of paddock exposure, the short time of confinement.

NATURE OF THE PHOTIC SIGNAL

One possibility is that the onset of the vernal transition occurs in response to changes in day length. In that case, the nature of the signal could include the absolute day length (i.e., requiring a certain minimum threshold), the rate of change of day length, or the change in sign (i.e., from decreasing day length to increasing day length). Of these possibilities, the requirement for an absolute day length is questionable in view of the observations mentioned above. The rate of change of day length also does not seem very likely; however, the experimental proofs that have addressed this end point may be flawed by virtue of the experimental intervention. That is, a variety of experimental regimes have been used to study stimulation of early sexual recrudescence, including turning additional artificial lighting on instantaneously,[15] adding the artificial lighting at a rate twice the rate of natural photoperiod,[11] and increasing the day length at the same rate as ambient day length, but at a time of year when natural light is decreasing.[16] Although these various lighting regimes have not been studied in a single experiment, the results generally agree well. Therefore, it does not seem likely that the rate of change of day length is especially critical, although more studies are necessary before accepting that conclusion completely. The possibility that animals sense only a change in sign, that is, a change from decreasing to increasing day length, also remains to be explored.

The onset of vernal transition in mares exposed to natural conditions may reflect one of two other possibilities. First, the onset of sexual recrudescence may be the expression of an endogenous circannual rhythm. Studies to confirm the existence of a circannual rhythm of reproductive function in horses have not been done, but several studies suggest that such a phenomenon may exist.[17] To demonstrate the existence of circannual rhythms of reproductive function, horses will have to be housed in constant conditions for a period of 3 yr or more to see if they begin to free run. In this regard, it would be of interest to study horses housed at the equator to learn whether they have discrete annual reproductive patterns. It seems reasonable to predict that each individual animal may have periods of reproductive competence and incompetence, but no longer coordinated among herd mates, or by month of the year.

The other possibility is that the return to sexual function in the springtime reflects development of refractoriness to inhibitory photoperiod. In this model, decreasing day length exerts an inhibitory effect on reproductive function, but mares eventually become refractory to the inhibitory effect of short day and resume reproductive function. The mechanisms by which animals become refractory to the inhibitory effects of photoperiod are not understood.

The naturally occurring onset of sexual recrudescence and photostimulated onset of sexual recrudescence may involve different mechanisms. For one thing, the presence or absence of the pineal gland affects the outcome of the two phenomena differently. Removal of the pineal, or severing the nervous pathway by which light reaches the pineal (i.e., superior cervical ganglionectomy), does not interfere with the timing of the onset of the breeding season during the first year postsurgery, however, the onset of the breeding season is delayed in the second year postsurgery.[18,19] This suggests that the pineal gland may participate in a process analogous to entrainment of a circadian rhythm. That is, the pineal may act to set the phase angle of some self-sustaining rhythm relative to environmental signals. In the absence of the pineal, entrainment to the environmental Zeitgeber does not occur, and the rhythm enters a free run. This is speculative, because the existence of circannual rhythms has not been established; however, the role of the pineal in regulating timing of the annual reproductive pattern has been established. On the other hand, the presence of the pineal appears to be a requisite for photoinduction of early sexual recrudescence. Grubaugh et al. demonstrated that pinealectomized mares did not respond to an artificial lighting regime that successfully induced early sexual recrudescence in pineal-intact mares.[19]

EFFECT OF PHOTOPERIOD ON GESTATION

The possibility that photoperiod can influence gestational length came from observations that mares bred early in the spring appeared to undergo longer gestations than did mares bred later in the year.[20] Hodge et al. demonstrated that exposure of bred mares to artificially lengthened day during the latter third of gestation resulted in shorter gestational length than observed in mares exposed to natural light.[21] Thus these data suggest that gestational length may have photoperiod-mediated influences, but the mechanisms of action remain poorly understood. It is not known, for instance, whether photoperiod information is somehow conveyed directly to the fetus to alter the timing of parturition induction or to alter the course of growth and development or whether photoperiod acts indirectly through the mares whose endocrine system then affects the fetus. This interesting, and potentially useful, phenomenon deserves further study however, before acceptance into practical application, because it is so poorly understood

The importance of understanding mechanisms of photoperiodic regulation of reproduction is that an incomplete understanding will lead to our inability to use this biologic control system for practical purposes. As with much of biology, practical alteration of function can be done only with complete understanding of the function.

REFERENCES

1. Saunders, D.S.: An Introduction to Biological Rhythms. New York, John Wiley, 1977.
2. Aschoff, J.: Circadian rhythms: General features and endocrinological aspects. *In* Endocrine Rhythms. Edited by D.T. Krieger. New York, Raven Press, 1979, pp. 1–61.
3. Moore, R.Y.: The anatomy of central neural mechanisms regulating endocrine rhythms. *In* Endocrine Rhythms. Edited by D.T. Krieger. New York, Raven Press, 1979, pp. 63–87.
4. Sharp, D.C., Grubaugh, W.R., Gum, G.G., and Wirsig, C.R.: Demonstration of a direct retinohypothalamic projection in the mare. Biol. Reprod. Suppl. 1, *30:*156, 1984.
5. Sharp, D.S.: Environmental influences on reproduction in horses. *In* Veterinary Clinics of North America: Large Animal Practice. Edited by J. Hughes. Philadelphia, W.B. Saunders, 1980, pp. 207–273.
6. Elliott, J.A.: Circadian rhythms, entrainment and photoperiodism in the Syrian hamster. *In* Biological Clocks in Seasonal Reproductive Cycles. Edited by B.K. Follett and D.E. Follett. Bristol, Scientechnica, 1981, pp. 203–217.
7. Rusak, B., Robertson, H., Wisden, W., and Hunt, S.: Light pulses that shift rhythms induce gene expression in the suprachiasmatic nucleus. Science, *248:*1237–1239, 1990.
8. Kornhauser, J., Nelson, D., Mayo, K., and Takahashi, J.: Photic and circadian regulation of c-fos gene expression in the hamster suprachiasmatic nucleus. Neuron, *5:*127–130, 1990.
9. Lees, A.D.: Photoperiodism in insects. *In* Photophysiology. Edited by A.C. Giese. New York, Academic Press, 1968, pp. 47–137.
10. Bunning, E.: The Physiological Clock. 3rd ed. New York, Springer Verlag, 1973.
11. Burkhardt, J.: Transition from anoestrus in the mare and the effects of artificial lighting. J. Agric. Sci., *37:*64–68, 1947.
12. Palmer, E., and Driancourt, M.A.: Photoperiodic stimulation of the winter anestrous mare: What is a long day? *In* Photoperiodism and Reproduction in Vertebrates. Edited by R. Ortavant, J. Peletier, and J.-P. Ravault. Nouzilly, Institut National de la Recherche Agronomique, 1981, pp. 67–82.
13. Saltiel, A., Calderon, A., Garcia, N., and Hurley, D.P.: Ovarian activity in the mare between latitude 15° and 22°N. J. Reprod. Fertil. Suppl., *32:*261–267, 1982.
14. Ginther, O.J.: Reproductive Biology of the Mare. Ann Arbor, McNaughton, Gunn, 1979.
15. Loy, R.G.: How the photoperiod affects reproductive activity in mares. Mod. Vet. Pract., pp 47–49, May 1967.
16. Sharp, D.C., and Ginther, O.J.: Induction of ovarian activity and estrous behavior in anestrous mares with light and temperature. J. Anim. Sci., *41:*1368–1372, 1975.
17. Clay, C.M., Squires, E.L., Amann, R.P., and Pickett, B.W.: Influences of season and artificial photoperiod on stallions: Testicular size, seminal characteristics and sexual behavior. J. Anim. Sci., *64:*517–525, 1987.
18. Sharp, D.C., Vernon, M.W., and Zavy, M.T.: Alteration of seasonal reproductive patterns in pony mares following superior cervical ganglionectomy. J. Reprod. Fertil. Suppl., *27:*87–93, 1979.
19. Grubaugh, W.R., et al.: The effects of pinealectomy in pony mares. J. Reprod. Fertil. Suppl., *32:*293–295, 1982.
20. Howell, C., and Rollins, W.: Environmental sources of gestation length of the horse. J. Anim. Sci., *10:*789–805, 1951.
21. Hodge S.L., et al.: Influence of photoperiod on the pregnant and postpartum mare. Am. J. Vet. Res., *43:*1752–1755, 1982.

CHAPTER 20

ESTROUS DETECTION

E.L. Squires

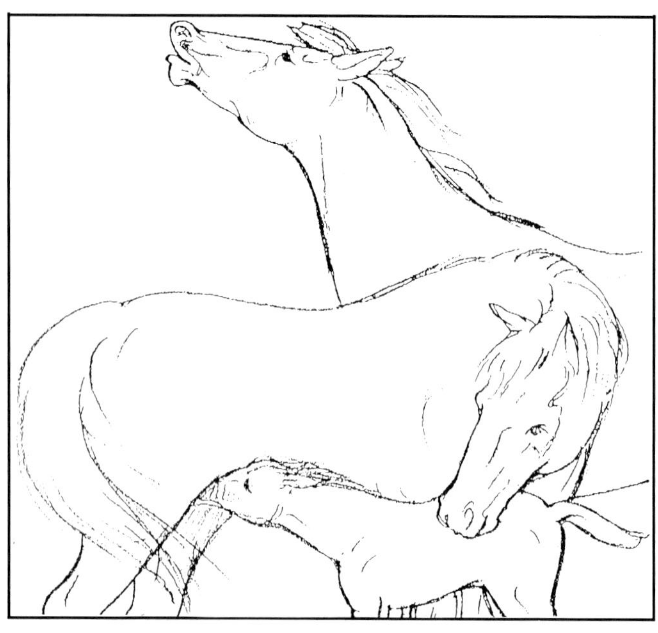

The ability to detect estrus and inseminate, or breed, mares at the time of ovulation is essential for a successful breeding program. Inadequate or improper teasing methods are one of the major causes of poor reproductive rates on farms. Detection of estrus (teasing) is a laborious, boring, time-consuming job that is seldom enjoyed by farm personnel. Those farms that relegate the task of teasing to the lowest paid or least-experienced personnel are most likely to have a lower pregnancy rate. The most skilled and interested person, generally the breeding manager, should be involved in estrous detection. Because of the subtle changes in the mare's behavior, it is important that the same individual observe the mare each day. Although alternative methods have been sought for estrous detection, the only accurate means of detecting estrus in a mare is by exposing each mare individually to a male horse, generally an active stallion.

When teasing a group of mares, two groups of mares should receive highest priority: (1) those that are currently in estrus and being bred and (2) those that have been bred and exhibited diestrus for approximately 14 days. The latter group should be observed closely to determine if they return to estrus. It has been shown that mares that have been bred and have not exhibited estrus for 20 consecutive days have a 92% chance of being pregnant.[1] Thus an accurate method of pregnancy diagnosis is estrous detection. Once mares are determined to be in estrus, management procedures for mating or insemination can be put in place.

BEHAVIORAL SIGNS OF ESTRUS AND DIESTRUS

Although homosexual behavior is common in cattle and is an aid in detection of estrus, this behavior is extremely rare in mares. In addition, mucus on the vulvar lips is not a common sign of estrus in the mare. If exudate is seen on the vulvar lips or on the inside of the buttocks, infection of the reproductive tract should be anticipated. In a study at our laboratory, a mare was considered to be cycling normally after it had exhibited at least 4 days of estrus followed by at least 8 days of diestrus.[1] The next estrous period was considered the beginning of normal cyclicity. Beginning on April 1, each mare was teased daily in the morning with two stallions until every mare was pregnant or the study was terminated. A mare was required to show positive signs of estrus to at least one of two stallions to be considered in estrus. The following criteria were recorded on a yes/no basis to determine the relationship of these responses to occurrence of estrus or diestrus of the mare: (1) ears back, (2) fence pushing, (3) tail raising, (4) kicking, (5) striking, (6) squatting, (7) squealing, (8) urinating, (9) winking (eversion of the vulvar lips). In the first study, 35 mares were teased at two tease rail locations, which were out of sight from each other.[1] Each mare was led to station one, and teased by the first stallion: first at the head, then buttocks, and finally external genitalia. Each mare was then led to station two and teased in a similar manner. The recorder at station two was unaware of the mare's reaction to the first stallion. In the second year, 54 mares were teased in a specially constructed teasing chute. The first stallion teased all mares from one direction. When the last mare was teased, a second stallion was used to tease the mares in reverse order. The term "indifferent" was added to the estrous/diestrous category for mares that exhibited neither a positive nor a negative response to the stallion. This condition was considered a diestrous response. When mares were cycling normally, the indifferent responses were generally shown by mares coming into or going out of estrus. All stallions were numbered and a record was kept to identify the stallion used to tease each mare. The relationship (coefficient of correlation) of the nine criteria of estrous behavior are presented in Table 20-1. Winking, with a coefficient of correlation of 0.84 in year 1 and 0.87 in year 2, was the most highly correlated ($p < 0.01$) response with estrus for both years. Thus 70 (year 1) to 76% (year 2) of the mares exhibited eversion of the vulva lips when in heat (Fig. 20–1). Numerous other responses were highly correlated with estrous behavior. However, as would be expected, winking, tail raising, squatting, and urinating were all highly correlated among themselves within each year. Because all of these responses were so closely related, tail raising and urination contributed very little additional information. It became clear that the most effective combination of responses for determining estrus was winking, tail raising, failure to kick, and squatting. This means that a mare that winked, squatted, and failed to kick had a 76% (year 1) to 84% (year 2) chance of being in heat. All responses included in the calculations gave multiple coefficient of correlations of 0.87 (year 1) and 0.92 (year 2). Squealing,

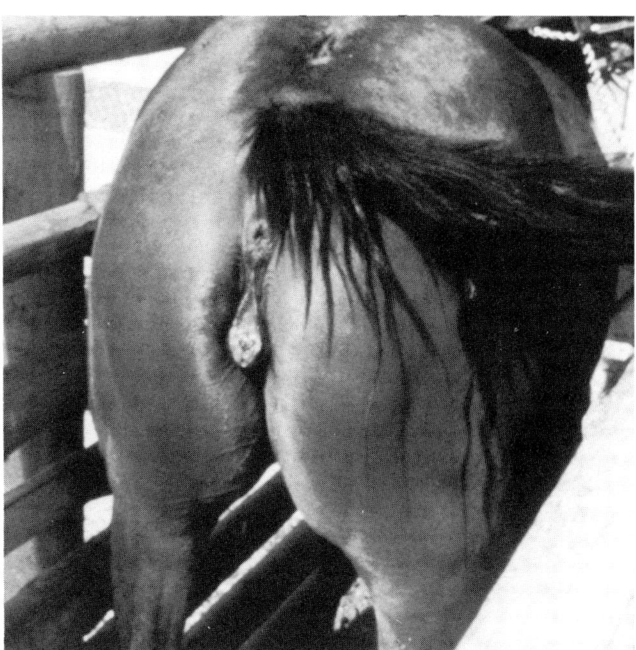

FIG. 20–1. Mare exhibiting winking of the vulvar lips.

fence pushing, and striking, with coefficient of correlations of 0.5 or less for both years, added little information for detecting estrus. The frequency of behavioral responses before and after ovulation are presented in Figure 20–2. Of all estrous signs observed, mares' reaction to the teaser stallion peak on the day of ovulation.[2] In contrast, the frequency of the diestrous signs—ears back and kicking—increased dramatically in the first 2 days after ovulation and by day 3 or 4 after ovulation, nearly 100% of the mares were exhibiting these diestrous signs. Similar studies have been conducted on sexual behavior of nonlactating mares.[3,4] One study defined estrus as standing firmly with the tail up while being mounted, plus at least one of the following: (1) urinating anytime during teasing, (2) winking anytime during teasing, or (3) tail raising before or after being mounted. Determination of not meeting these criteria was defined as nonestrus, i.e., diestrus, anestrus, and/or pregnancy. The behavioral signs occurring most frequently ($p < 0.05$) during estrus, in decreasing order, were tail raising, remaining calm, winking, posturing, urinating, and nuzzling. By definition, all mares in estrus stood with tail up while being mounted. The signs occurring most frequently during nonestrus, in decreasing order, were moving, ears back, switching tail, local response, kicking, raising in rear, biting, pawing, shaking head, and rearing.

TABLE 20–1. COEFFICIENTS OF CORRELATION OF MARE RESPONSES WITH CONDITION* OF MARES DURING TEASING

	COEFFICIENTS OF CORRELATION†	
	Year	
MARE RESPONSE(S) DURING TEASING	1	2
Eversion of vulvar labia (winking)	0.84	0.87
Squatting	0.81	0.78
Tail raising	0.81	0.70
Urinating	0.80	0.75
Kicking	−0.69	−0.78
Ears back	−0.64	−0.72
Squealing	−0.50	−0.49
Fence pushing	0.47	0.28
Striking	−0.38	0.31

*Estrus, diestrus.
†Significantly different ($p < 0.01$) if greater than 0.81.
(Adapted from Back, D.G., Pickett, B.W., Voss, J.L., and Seidel, G.E., Jr.: Observation on the sexual behavior of nonlactating mares. J. Am. Vet. Med. Assoc., *165*:717–720, 1974.)

ROLE OF THE STALLION

Few studies have been conducted to determine how aggressiveness of the stallion affects estrous behavior of the mare. It is generally assumed that a noisy, but gentle, stallion that nuzzles a mare from front to back is the

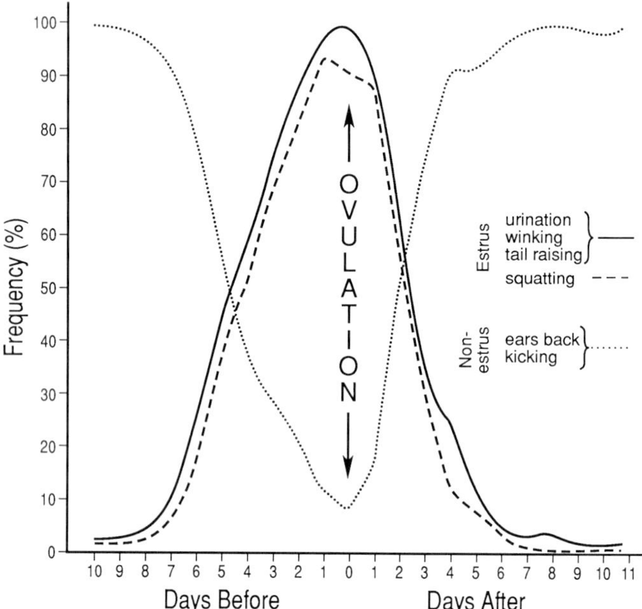

FIG. 20–2. Frequency of behavioral characteristics before and after ovulation. (From Artificial insemination (AI) of mares. *In* Technician's Manual for Artificial Insemination. American Breeders Service, Inc., 1972.)

best teaser; however, no controlled studies have been conducted to test this hypothesis. Needless to say, selection of a teaser stallion is an important, integral part of a teasing procedure. A "good teaser" should meet the following criteria: (1) be aggressive and enthusiastic, (2) be controllable, (3) tease the mare without excessive roughness, and (4) not give up too quickly. The ideal tease stallion is one that will "work" the mare from front to back, beginning with the nose, then flank area, and last, the buttock area. Excessive biting of the mare by the stallion during teasing can often lead to diestrous signs, such as moving, kicking, striking, and biting, even though the mare may be in estrus.

Curling of the upper lip is a frequent behavioral manifestation by the stallion demonstrated when teasing the mare. This is referred to as flehmen stance, or flehmen, coined in 1930.[5] Studies of olfaction in domestic horses are lacking. One study described the response of domestic horses to horse feces and a mixture of urine and vaginal secretion.[6] The differences in response of mares, geldings, and stallions to urine/vaginal secretions and fecal samples were studied. The ability of stallions to detect estrus in mares with odor cues from urine/vaginal secretions and ability of stallions to distinguish between individual mares from their urine/vaginal secretions was investigated. In all cases the odors were tested in absence of the donor animal. Stallions were significantly more responsive than mares and geldings. This was shown in both flehmen and sniffing behavior to urine/vaginal secretions and in sniffing behavior to fecal samples. However, stallions showed no significant differences in response to the odor of urine/vaginal secretions of an estrous mare from that same mare when not in estrus. Parameters evaluated were frequency, latency, and duration of flehmen as well as duration of responsiveness to samples. The stallions did, in fact, differentiate between samples from individual mares. The study suggested that the ability to discriminate between individual odors may be the mechanism whereby stallions identify "favorite" mares. The inability of stallions to show preference for urine samples from an estrous versus a diestrous mare is similar to the results of the study by Houpt and Guida.[7]

A series of studies was conducted to determine if mares respond similarly to two different stallions.[1] This involved 7,713 individual teasings to two stallions, including both normal and abnormal cycles. It was found that mares exhibited the same estrous behavior (estrus, diestrus) to both stallions in 94.9% of the observations (Table 20–2). The mares' responses were not the same to both stallions in 5.2% (398) of the teasings. Of that group, 308 of the mares (77.4%) were in diestrus to the first stallion, but in estrus to the second stallion. This was only 4% of the total teasings, but 12.9% of the times that mares were observed in estrus. Mares were cycling normally in only 28.6% of these teasings (88 of 308). Of these, 43.4% did not "show" on the first day of estrus, and 25.3% did not show on the last day of estrus. The authors concluded that for maximum reproductive efficiency, normal cycling mares should be teased daily with only one stallion. All abnormally cycling mares, mares previously bred and due to cycle, and mares exhibiting the first day of diestrus should be teased with a second stallion or perhaps by the same stallion at a second location if two stallions are not available.

As noted, there have been many clinical and research reports on estrous detection primarily involving teasing with a restrained or confined mare. However, little information is available on the sexual interplay when a stallion is introduced into a group of mares. One study tested whether the presence of a stallion had a stimula-

TABLE 20–2. RESPONSE OF MARES TEASED WITH TWO STALLIONS

MARE RESPONSE TO STALLION			
First Stallion	Second Stallion	*N**	Percent
Estrus	Estrus	1990	25.8
Diestrus	Diestrus	4987	64.7
Indifferent	Indifferent	91	1.2
Diestrus	Indifferent	102	1.3
Indifferent	Diestrus	145	1.9
Estrus	Diestrus	59	0.8
Estrus	Indifferent	31	0.4
Diestrus	Estrus	176	2.3
Indifferent	Estrus	132	1.7

*Number of observations (teasings).
(From Back, D.G., Pickett, B.W., Voss, J.L., and Seidel, G.E., Jr.: Observation on the sexual behavior of nonlactating mares. J. Am. Vet. Med. Assoc., *165*:717–720, 1974.)

tory effect on time of ovulation, whether a stallion is more likely to breed the same mare when more than one mare is in estrus, and whether breeding occurs preferentially in those estrous mares that are closest to ovulation.[8] A sexually rested stallion was introduced daily for 30 days into each of three herds of 20 mares. Observations of sexual and mating behavior were made for 1 h. The stallion remained with the herd until another stallion was introduced the following day. Other mares were isolated from stallions and were bred by artificial insemination. The diameter or growth of the preovulatory follicle for the 6 days preceding ovulation and the duration of the interovulatory interval for mares that did not become pregnant were not affected significantly by the presence of a stallion. The number of breedings per hour of observation and the duration of interval from introduction of a stallion into the herd of mares to first breeding were significantly different among stallions; interval between breedings was similar among stallions. Mean number of breedings per stallion per hour was not significantly affected by number of mares in estrus. The stallion did tend to rebreed the same mare more often than expected as a result of chance alone. The hypothesis that breeding occurs preferentially in those estrous mares that are closest to ovulation was not supported.

ALTERNATIVE METHODS FOR ESTROUS DETECTION

Although the ideal means of estrous detection is by exposing (where mare and stallion can have contact) each mare daily to a stallion, this requires that a teaser horse be maintained or that the breeding stallion be used. Maintenance of a teaser horse may be cost prohibitive for a small breeding farm. Alternatively, using the breeding stallion as a teaser may, in some cases, induce abnormal sexual behavior.[9] Some breeders have attempted to use pony stallions as teasers. The obvious advantage is pony stallions are generally more easily managed and the cost of maintenance is less. However, based on clinical impression, rarely is a pony stallion as effective as a horse stallion. Some mares are very aggressive toward the pony stallion, whereas other mares appear to be frightened.

Another alternative that has been investigated is the use of an androgen-treated mare. Some workers tested the hypothesis that testosterone propionate would induce male sexual behavior in pony mares.[10] Four pony mares of mixed breeds and one pony stallion were used in this study conducted in the fall. Two mares were administered 150 mg of testosterone propionate every other day for 20 days. Additional injections were administered every 10 days thereafter for 20 days. The other two mares and stallion served as controls. Tests for male sexual behavior were conducted 26 and 40 days after the first injection of testosterone propionate. The sexual behavior test consisted of placing testosterone propionate–treated mares, control mares, and the stallion individually in a pen with three cyclic mares for 10 min. At least one of the cyclic mares was in estrus and one in diestrus. Control mares exhibited little male sexual behavior. Both testosterone propionate–treated mares exhibited mounting, sniffing, flehmen, biting, and vocalization behavior in the presence of an estrous mare. The testosterone propionate–treated mares mounted and bit estrous mares more frequently than the stallion did, but exhibited less sniffing, flehmen, and vocalization behavior in the presence of an estrous mare than the stallion. Mares in estrus were mounted by the testosterone propionate–treated mares and the stallion an average of four times and one time, respectively, during the 10-min test. The researchers concluded that testosterone propionate–induced male sexual behavior in intact mares, and testosterone propionate–treated mares effectively detected estrous mares.

In a subsequent study teaser mares were administered the anabolic steroid boldenone undecylenate (500 mg IM every 1 to 2 weeks) and allowed to run loose with a group of mares.[11] Estrus was determined by observation of the group for a 30-min period. In the second month, the experimental marking harness was used on the androgenized mares to help detect mares mounted when in estrus. During the first month, the number of estrous periods detected by the stallion was 18 compared with 5 for androgenized mares. Data for the second month were 16 and 9, respectively. The study concluded that the androgenized mare was not an adequate estrous detection aid. In another study, various doses of anabolic steroids were administered to 2-yr-old fillies.[12] Although not critically tested, mounting behavior was observed in all anabolic steroid–treated fillies, as was male-like behavior toward estrous mares in the majority of steroid-treated fillies. However, only those fillies administered a higher-than-recommended dose of boldenone undecylenate were aggressive enough to be used as teasers. In addition, when the steroid-treated fillies were used to tease each mare individually, their effectiveness as teasers was minimal.

Other aids that have been tested as to their effectiveness for detection of estrus in mares have generally been shown to be of little value. For example, measurement of electrical resistance of the mucus of the vagina was shown to be an ineffective and unreliable means of estrus detection in cattle[13] and mares.[14] In a study conducted at our laboratory, a total of 61 normally cycling mares were teased daily by a stallion to detect estrus. The mares in estrus were palpated daily to determine ovulation. Immediately after palpation, the vulva was washed with soap and water and wiped with 2% tamed-iodine solution. A stainless steel probe containing two electrodes was then introduced into the vagina until it touched the external os of the cervix. It was then rotated twice around the lumen of the vagina and pressed down on the floor of the vagina. The ideal pattern consisted of a greater than 15% decrease in transmittal 24 to 48 h prior to ovulation. A total of 72 complete cycles was completed in one study, and 39 complete cycles, in a second study. Only 50% of the ovulations were accompanied by a single drop in resistance. Of those mares experiencing only a single decrease, the decrease in transmittal occurred only in 64 and 68% of the cases within 24 h before ovulation. The number of estrous cycles in which a single decrease in transmittal greater than 15% occurred was calculated, either −3, −2, −1, 0, or +1 days in relation to ovulation; this represented only 44 and 51% of the total estrous cycles examined. Thus the procedure is not a reliable means of estrous detection.

Body temperature has been studied and suggested as a possible predictor of ovulation in several domestic species and in the human. Rectal temperatures were taken four times daily with a high-speed digital thermometer in four nonpregnant mares from day 1 of estrus through 3 days after the end of the second estrus.[15] Mares were teased daily to determine the beginning and end of estrus and palpated every other day during estrus to determine the day of ovulation. No change in temperature occurred that could be used to predict estrus or ovulation.

Vagina and milk temperatures were measured at each milking in 15 postpartum cows.[16] The authors concluded that measurement of neither milk temperature nor vagina temperature was a useful aid in estrous detection. Thus, in summary, the most effective means of estrous detection in horses seems to be exposure of a mare daily to an aggressive, intact stallion.

METHODS OF ESTROUS DETECTION

Teasing techniques vary widely among farms, depending on conditions such as facilities, personnel (labor force), number of mares, and personal preference. The number of foaling mares compared to nonlactating mares also has a major impact on the teasing technique. It is common knowledge that lactating mares require more time and labor to tease than nonlactating mares, because maternal instinct interferes with the teasing procedure. A system of teasing should be used that protects the foal from injury.

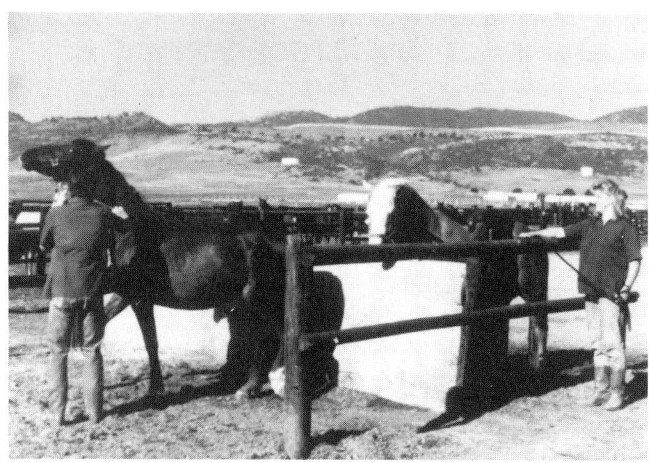

FIG. 20–4. Mare positioned at a tease rail for teasing with a stallion.

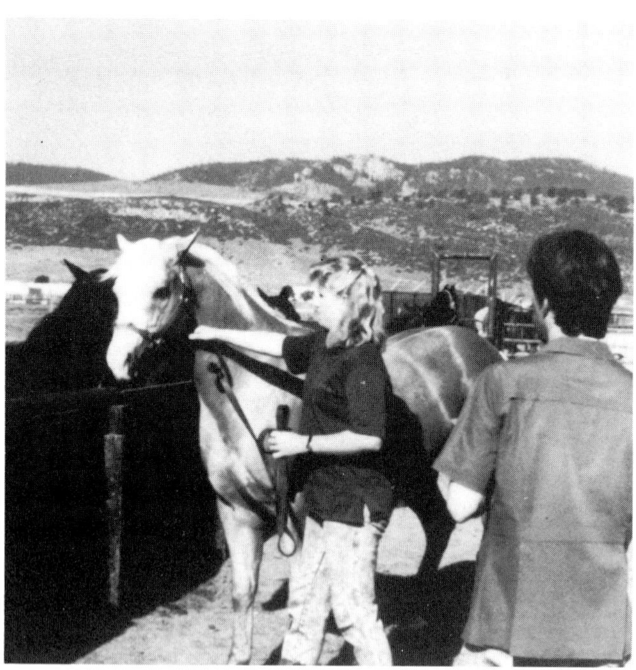

FIG. 20–3. Mares positioned in a chute and teased with a stallion for estrous detection.

The primary considerations in the teasing program include (1) safety of the handler, mare, and stallion; (2) accuracy; and (3) labor. There are two broad classifications of teasing techniques: individual and group. Presented below are some of the advantages and disadvantages of various teasing methods.

TEASE CHUTE

The tease chute (Fig. 20–3) has been used to tease research mares at Colorado State University since 1971 and works best for mares that are maintained in groups either in pastures or in large paddocks. The mares are brought in each day to a set of holding pens and then funneled down the chute. The chute is designed to hold 12 mares positioned 12 ft apart. They are restrained by a short nylon rope with a panic snap. The stallion is led from one end of the chute to the opposite end and each mare is teased individually. Several doors are located along the chute that allow mares in estrus to be removed, placed into holding pens, and later moved as one group to the palpation or breeding shed. Those mares not needed for further examination are released and returned to the pastures. This system has worked extremely well for thousands of experimental mares at Colorado State University, but has the disadvantage that only nonlactating mares can be teased in this fashion because mares must be haltered and tied for teasing. Although principally nonlactating experimental mares have been teased in this facility, no major injuries have occurred. On occasion, a mare will fall upside down in the chute, which requires considerable effort on the part of the personnel to reposition the mare. Perhaps if the chute were a three-rail pipe fence, struggling by the mares would be minimized and repositioning would be expedited. Another possible advantage of a three-rail pipe chute is that the stallion would have greater visibility and access to the mare. Regardless of construction, this system allows several mares to be observed at once. Thus the "shy" mare that may exhibit estrus only after the stallion has gone on to another mare will be more easily identified. In addition, many times mares will exhibit estrus in the chute before the stallion arrives at their position.

TEASE RAIL

The tease rail is generally the best for farms breeding less than 50 mares. A tease rail (Fig. 20–4) can be constructed inexpensively near the barn or pasture where the mares are housed. This system is accurate and safe; however, each mare must be individually led to the rail, which requires considerable time and labor. Tease rails can be easily positioned close to where mares are housed, thus minimizing handling time of mares. This also allows lactating mares to be separated from their foals for the short time needed for teasing.

STALL TEASING

It is a common procedure on many breeding farms to present the stallion to each mare in her stall. Depending on construction of the stall door, this may or may not be satisfactory. If Dutch doors are used, with the upper door open and the bottom door sufficiently low for the stallion to nuzzle the mare, this method may be satisfactory. However, if the doors are constructed like those in Figure 20–5, then accuracy and safety of this procedure is compromised. It is difficult to expose a stallion safely through this type of stall door.

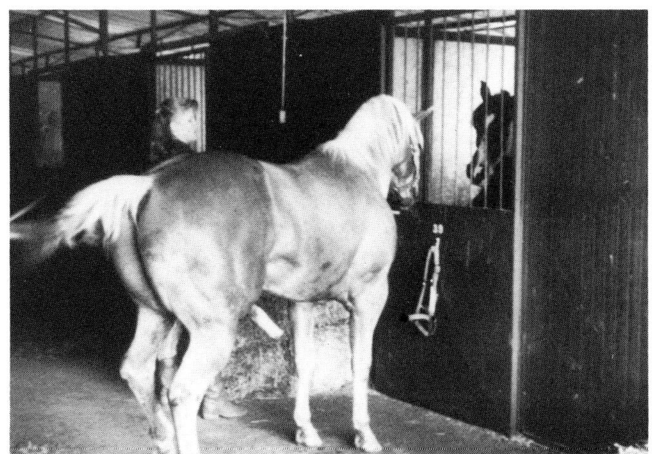

FIG. 20–5. Mare in a box stall teased with a stallion.

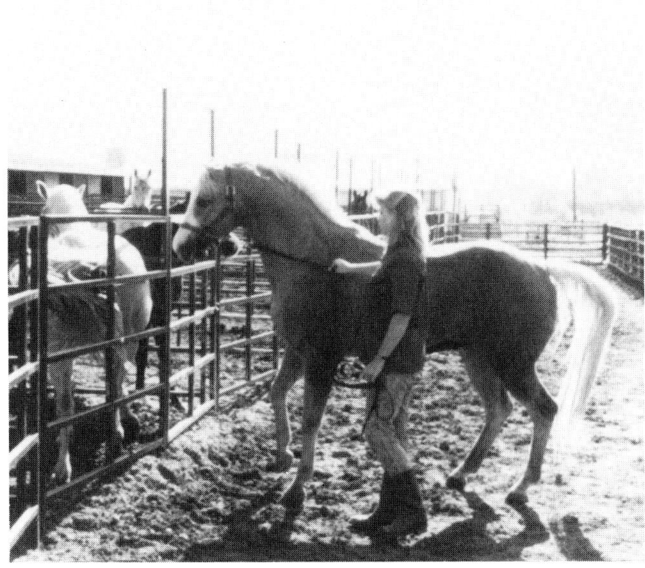

FIG. 20–6. Mares in metal pens being teased with a stallion.

PEN TEASING

The safety of pen teasing depends on the construction of the pens. For example, teasing mares in metal pens should be discouraged because the mare may injure her leg by kicking at the fence and hitting the metal rails (Fig. 20–6). Generally, mares can be safely teased in wooden pens without risk of injury (Fig. 20–7). In either of the pens, two people are required, a stallion handler and someone who directs the mare toward the stallion. Not every mare in estrus will approach a stallion. Certainly, this type of system requires minimal labor, but safety and accuracy are limiting factors.

PADDOCK TEASING

This is a common procedure for teasing, particularly on some Quarter Horse farms in the Southwest. This method allows teasing of a large number of mares at one time. Mares are placed in a paddock and the stallion is either led to the paddock and handled outside the pen (Fig. 20–8) or placed in the small enclosure adjacent to the paddock (Fig. 20–9). Two major disadvantages of this procedure exist. (1) Not every mare in estrus will voluntarily approach the stallion. In some studies, only 60% of mares that were in estrus voluntarily exposed themselves to the stallion.[4] (2) Some mares are aggressive and will occupy all the stallion's time so the remaining mares have no opportunity to be teased. A good breeding farm manager should be aware of these deficiencies and take mares out of the pens as they exhibit estrus and force other mares to be exposed to the stallion.

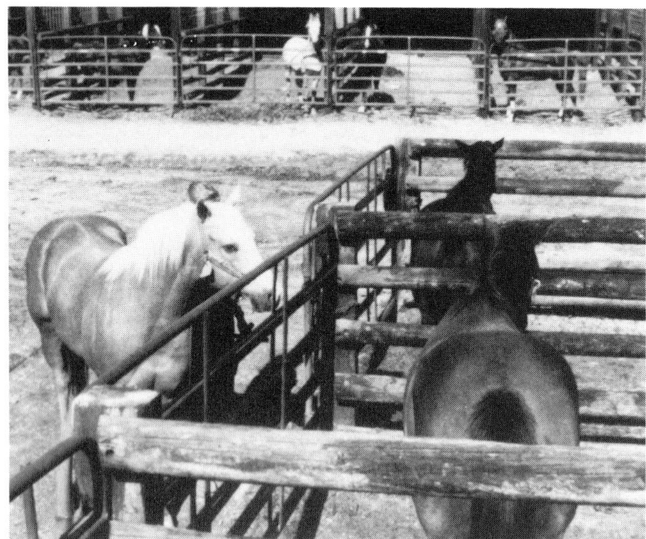

FIG. 20–7. Mares in wooden pens being teased with a stallion.

PASTURE TEASING

The procedure of taking the stallion directly into the pasture with a group of mares should be discouraged. Although many breeders have successfully used this procedure for years, it is extremely dangerous. Often a diestrous or pregnant mare, particularly a lactating mare, may attack the stallion, resulting in injury to animals and possibly personnel.

USE OF ANDROGEN-TREATED OR VASECTOMIZED ANIMALS

As discussed previously, androgen-treated animals have been used with limited success with cattle and sheep and are not an accepted method for detection of estrus in mares. Use of a marking harness fitted to a vasectomized stallion for detection of estrus in free-roaming mares has received only limited attention. There are problems of safety and spread of venereal disease when a vasectomized animal is used as a teaser.

In summary, each teasing method has advantages and disadvantages that should be recognized by the breeder and veterinarian. No one teasing method is necessarily better than another. The accuracy of a teasing method depends on the conscientiousness of the personnel involved in teasing and selection of a teaser. Although not included in the scope of this chapter, record keeping of days in estrus, time of ovulation, number of days in diestrus, and intervals between estrous periods and between ovulations are extremely important data that should be readily accessible to the stallion manager and veterinarian.

INTENSITY OF BEHAVIORAL SIGNS

Behavioral signs are generally categorized as receptive or nonreceptive toward the stallion, but some personnel have used gradation of these two classifications. Several investigators have reported that intensity of behavioral signs increases progressively during estrus, reaching maximal intensity as ovulation approaches.[2,17,18] Ginther conducted a study involving 70 estrous cycles.[4] Negative and positive values were assigned to estrous (+) and nonestrous values (−) as follows: +3, standing for mounting with tail raised; +1, urinating; +1, winking; +1, tail raising; 0, standing for mounting with tail down; −1, kicking; −1, switching; −1, ears back; −1, moving; and −3, not standing for mounting. Thus combinations of these values were used as an intensity index of estrous behavior. The results did not support the assumption that there was a gradual increase in intensity from beginning of estrus until ovulation. However, the transition from diestrus to estrus and from estrus to diestrus occurred gradually. In a "short" estrus of 3 or 4 days, intensity did increase until ovulation occurred. When estrus was longer, the increase in intensity in early estrus was followed by a prolonged plateau. Ginther concluded that the mare does not respond with increasing intensity of estrus except for the first 1 or 2 days of estrus. Wallach et al. reported a decreased time from the appearance of tail raising, urination, and squatting as the mare approached ovulation.[19] Latency to tail raising appeared to be associated with maturation of the ovulatory follicle, indicating a measurable increase in sexual receptivity as ovulation occurred. In another study, the frequency of mares displaying kicking and ears back, decreased as ovulation approached; whereas, the frequency of mares exhibiting tail raising, winking of the vulva lips, urination, and squatting was greatest around the time of ovulation.[2] Further studies are needed to determine if changes in intensity of behavioral signs can be used as an indication of impending ovulation. With the use of ultrasonography, ovula-

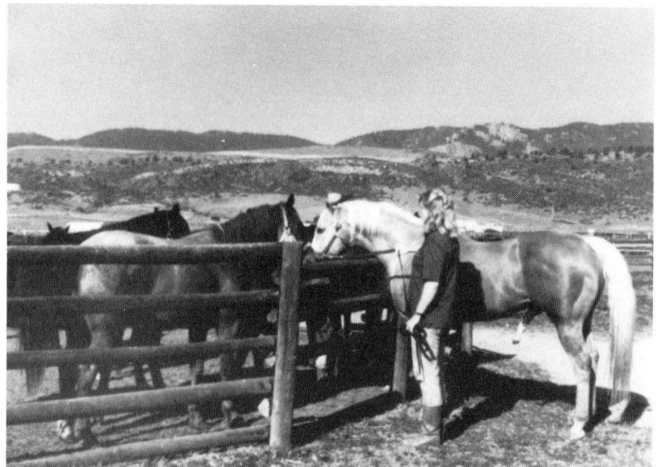

FIG. 20–8. Mares in a paddock being teased by leading a stallion outside the paddock.

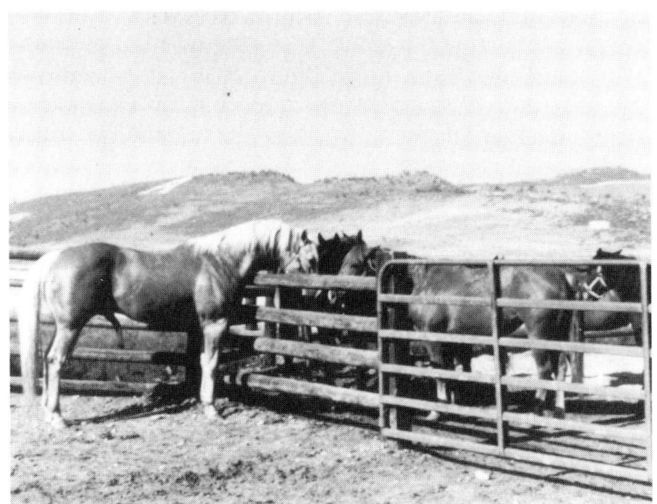

FIG. 20–9. Mares being teased with a stallion in an adjacent paddock.

tion can be more accurately detected; therefore, some of the earlier studies correlating behavioral signs with ovulation should be repeated.

IRREGULARITIES IN SEXUAL BEHAVIOR

Unfortunately, not all mares exhibit clear signs of estrus or diestrus. Some mares are quite indifferent to the stallion, and some become refractory to the teasing procedure. Mares that are indifferent to a stallion should be teased with a second stallion, preferably at another location. Some mares become conditioned to a certain teasing procedure and their cyclic patterns are difficult to discern. For example, mares that fail to exhibit estrus in a tease chute often show signs of estrus when teased in a paddock setting. It may be that placing a mare in a chute is enough of a stress to suppress cyclicity or to suppress behavioral signs. The best approach for a refractory mare is to change the teasing method.

One of the major causes of infertility in mares is cyclic irregularities. This may include subestrus, anovulatory estrous cycles, silent estrus, split estrus, diestrous ovulation, and multiple ovulations. Subestrus is defined as diminished signs of estrus, typical of the first or last day of estrus. Causes of diminished signs of estrus in mares are not known but may be hormonally related. Follicular development the day before ovulation in mares with subestrus was compared with that of mares showing distinct signs of estrus. There was no significant difference in development of the follicle in mares with normal versus abnormal estrus.[4] Mares in estrus for several days then in diestrus for 1 to 2 days, followed by several other days of estrus, are categorized as experiencing a split-estrous period. Generally, ovulation does not occur until the second part of this estrous period. Therefore, if one does not continue to breed through the second portion of the estrous period, conception will be highly unlikely. Split-estrous periods would appear to be more common early in the season. This is also true of anovulatory cycles. Mares in this category develop a large follicle, but the follicle fails to ovulate and the mare goes out of estrus. If these mares are not being examined by palpation per rectum and/or ultrasonography, the assumption would be made that ovulation had occurred. Failure of the follicle to ovulate appears to be common during the last estrous cycle of the year. This type of follicle has been termed an "autumn" follicle. Failure of the mare to exhibit estrus and not ovulate late in the year has been associated with low luteinizing hormone (LH) concentrations.[20] Mares may also ovulate on a regular basis but not exhibit estrus, i.e., silent heat. These mares can be a major problem in a breeding program, because frequent palpations and/or ultrasonographic examinations are needed to determine if the mare is physiologically cycling without showing behavioral signs of estrus. The incidence of silent heat is often greater in mares that are lactating.

PHYSIOLOGIC CONTROL OF SEXUAL BEHAVIOR

Very little is known about the physiologic control of sexual behavior in mares. Neuroendocrine mechanisms at the level of the brain are very likely involved. Studies to determine involvement of pheromones in sexual behavior of the mare and stallion apparently have not been conducted. In addition, studies to determine how important tactile and olfactory stimuli are on the mare's sexual behavior are lacking. It would seem as though this area of equine reproduction and research had been very badly neglected, even though it is a major component of a breeding farm operation. It is generally accepted that receptor sites for estrogen are present in the brain; thus estrogen acts directly on the brain. The rise in estrogen and/or the decline in progesterone results in the expression of estrus. In contrast, once progesterone rises above approximately 1 ng/mL of serum, mares exhibit diestrus; in fact the interval from day of ovulation to the first day of diestrus is consistently 1 to 2 days.

Similar periods of sexual receptivity in ovariectomized and seasonally, anovulatory mares have been reported.[20] Both groups of mares solicited and accepted copulation without exogenous steroid treatment. The number of days each mare was in estrus and the pattern of occurrence of estrus was extremely variable among animals. The intensity of estrus exhibited by ovariectomized and seasonally anovulatory mares was similar to the first or last day of estrus for mares during the middle of the breeding season. Administration of dexamethasone, an adrenal cortex suppressant, eliminated all signs of estrus in ovariectomized mares, providing evidence for adrenal steroid support of estrous behavior.[22]

A subsequent study evaluated in greater detail the ability of estradiol and progesterone to stimulate or inhibit the occurrence of sexual behavior or alter the estrous response of ovariectomized mares.[23] In the first experiment, mares were treated either with estrogen, progesterone, a combination of estrogen and progesterone, or no treatment. Daily treatment (5 days) with estradiol resulted in increased levels of receptive behavior in ovariectomized mares as compared to controls. The response was relatively rapid (4 h) and lasted throughout the treatment. Progesterone treatment resulted in an absence of sexual behavior except on day 1. The concurrent administration of estradiol and progesterone produced a biphasic effect on behavior. Initially, the combined estrogen-progesterone treatment was stimulatory but became inhibitory after the first day. In the second experiment, the same authors determined the time course of a single injection of either estradiol-17β or estradiol benzoate. Estradiol-17β appeared to augment receptivity sooner than estradiol benzoate. In the third experiment, the authors demonstrated that 0, 1, or 10 mg of progesterone had no inhibitory effect on estrous behavior, but 100 mg was inhibitory. The suppression of estrous behavior in ovariectomized mares occurred after 2 days of treatment with 100 mg of progesterone. The sensitivity of the behavior centers to estrogen probably varies with season. Only a small amount of estradiol seems to be necessary for expression of estrus in anovulatory mares, whereas a larger dose of estradiol may be needed for expression of estrus in cycling mares.

Because suppression of the adrenal cortex with dexamethasone inhibited manifestation of estrous behavior in ovariectomized and anovulatory mares,[22] a subsequent study was conducted to evaluate the effects of dexamethasone on sexual behavior and biologic function of the preovulatory mare.[24] The study examined 16 pony mares and 8 pony stallions. On the day of ovulation, mares were assigned alternatively to either a dexamethasone-treated group or a control group. Two injections each of 15 mg of dexamethasone were given at 8:00 a.m. and 6:00 p.m. beginning on day 10 after ovulation. Control mares were sham injected. Behavioral tests were conducted each afternoon. Tail raising near the stallion, urination, presentation, and walking away were scored for females. Precopulatory investigation, mounting, intromission, and ejaculation were scored for males, and approaching, following, threatening, and kicking were scored for both mares and stallions. All 8 control mares ovulated during the treatment period compared with only 1 of 8 treated mares. Follicular growth in the control mares appeared to be normal but follicles in the treated group were significantly smaller by day 19. Estrous behavior accompanied ovulation in 7 of 8 control mares. In the 1 treated mare that ovulated, normal estrous behavior occurred for 6 days. No estrous behavior was observed in the remaining treated mares. On day 6 of treatment with dexamethasone, mean plasma concentrations of LH were significantly lower than that on day 9 before treatment or on day 15 in control mares. During the treatment phase, mean concentrations of LH were less than that in controls. These results are similar to the suppression of estrus observed in ovariectomized mares administered dexamethasone. Ovulation in the dexamethasone-treated mares appeared to be blocked because of a suppression of LH secretion. The mechanism whereby estrous behavior was suppressed in intact, dexamethasone-treated mares was not determined. The authors suggested that dexamethasone decreased adrenocorticotropin hormone (ACTH), which decreased adrenal steroid production of androgens and estrogens. Further studies are needed to determine what factors are involved in controlling the expression of estrus or diestrus in the mare.

REFERENCES

1. Back, D.G., Pickett, B.W., Voss, J.L., and Seidel, G.E., Jr.: Observations on the sexual behavior of nonlactating mares. J. Am. Vet. Med. Assoc., *165:*717–720, 1974.
2. Artificial insemination (AI) of mares. *In* Technician's Manual for Artificial Insemination. American Breeders Service, DeForest, WI, 1972.
3. Hughes, J.P., Stabenfeldt, G.H., and Evans, J.W.: Estrous cycle and ovulation in the mare. J. Am. Vet. Med. Assoc., *161:*1367–1375, 1972.
4. Ginther, O.J.: Reproductive Biology of the Mare: Basic and Applied Aspects. Ann Arbor, McNaughton, Gunn, 1979, pp. 59–75.
5. Schneider, K.M.: Das flehmen. Zool. Garten., *4:*183–198, 1930.
6. Marinier, S.L., Alexander, A.J., and Waring, G.H.: Flehmen behavior in the domestic horse: Discrimination of nonspecific odours. Appl. Anim. Behav. Sci., *19:* 227–237, 1988.
7. Houpt, K.A., and Guida, L.: Flehmen. Equine Pract., *6:*32–35, 1984.
8. Ginther, O.J.: Sexual behavior following introduction of a stallion into a group of mares. Theriogenology, *19:*877–887, 1983.
9. Pickett, B.W., et al.: Management of the stallion for maximum reproductive efficiency II. *In* Colorado State University, Animal Reproduction Laboratory Bulletin No. 05. Fort Collins, CO, 1989, pp. 83–92.
10. Withrow, J.M., Sargent, G.F., Scheffrahn, N.S., and Kesler, D.J.: Induction of male sex behavior in pony mares with testosterone propionate. Theriogenology, *20:*485–490, 1983.
11. McDonnell, S.M., Hinrichs, K., Cooper W., and Kenney, R.M.: Use of an androgenized mare as an aid in detection of estrus in mares. Theriogenology, *30:*547–553, 1988.
12. Maher, J.M., Squires, E.L., Voss, J.L., and Shideler, R.K.: Effect of anabolic steroids on reproductive function of young mares. J. Am. Vet. Med. Assoc., *183:*519–524, 1983.
13. Edward, D.F., and Levin, R.J.: An electrical method of detecting optimum time to inseminate cattle, sheep and pigs. Vet. Rec., *95:*416–425, 1974.
14. Squires, E.L., Pickett, B.W., Shideler, R.K., and Voss, J.L.: Detection of ovulation and pregnancy using electrical conductivity and ultrasound. Proc. Am. Assoc. Equine Pract., 199–209, 1981.
15. Ammons, S.F., Threlfall, W.R., and Kline, R.C.: Equine body temperature and progesterone fluctuations during estrus and near parturition. Theriogenology, *31:* 1007–1019, 1989.
16. Fordham, D.P., McCarthy, T.T., and Rowlinson, P.: An

evaluation of milk temperature measurements for detecting oestrus in dairy cattle. Vet. Res. Comm., *11:*367–391, 1987.

17. Andrews, F.N., and McKenzie, F.F.: Estrus, ovulation and related phenomena in the mare. *In* University of Missouri Agricultural Experimental Station Research Bulletin No. 329. Columbia, MO, 1941.

18. Nishikawa, Y.: Studies on Reproduction in Horses. Tokyo, Japan Racing Association, 1959.

19. Wallach, S.J., Oxender, W.D., and Douglas, R.H.: Analysis of pre-ovulatory estrous behavior in horse and pony mares. Paper presented at the Annual Meeting of the American Society of Animal Science, Madison, WI, July 23–27, 1977.

20. Snyder, D.A., et al.: Follicular and gonadotrophic changes during transition from ovulatory to anovulatory season. J. Reprod. Fertil. Suppl., *27:*95–101, 1979.

21. Asa, C.S., Goldfoot, D.A., Garcia, M.C., and Ginther, O.J.: Sexual behavior in ovariectomized and seasonally anovulatory mares. Hormone Behav., *14:*46–54, 1980.

22. Asa, C.S., Goldfoot, D.A., Garcia, M.C., and Ginther, O.J.: Dexamethasone suppression of sexual behavior in ovariectomized mares. Horm. Behav., *14:*55–65, 1980.

23. Asa, C.S., Goldfoot, D.A., Garcia, M.C., and Ginther, O.J.: The effect of estradiol and progesterone on the sexual behavior of ovariectomized mares. Physiol. Behav., *33:*681–686, 1984.

24. Asa, C.S., and Ginther, O.J.: Glucocorticoid suppression of oestrus, follicles, LH and ovulation in the mare. J. Reprod. Fertil. Suppl., *32:*247–251, 1982.

REPRODUCTIVE EXAMINATION OF THE MARE

CHAPTER 21

HISTORY

R.K. Shideler

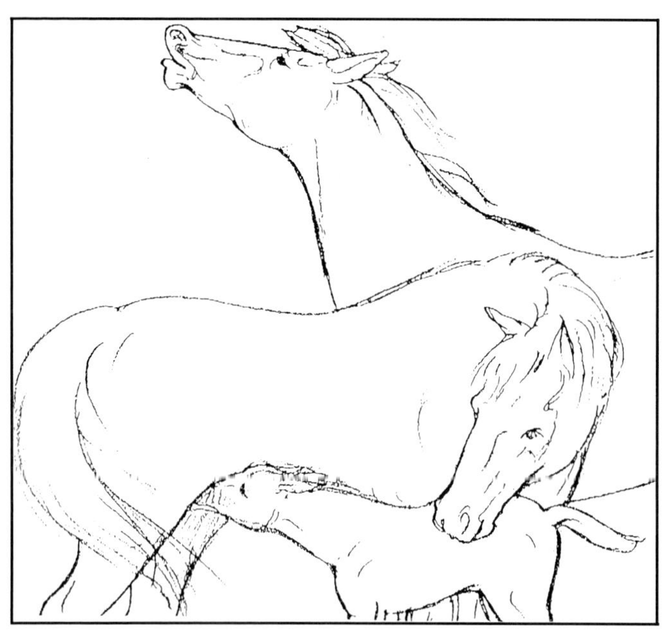

Historic information regarding the reproductive performance of the mare is essential to diagnosis, prognosis, and selection of therapy when presented with an individual case of infertility. Many cases may be evaluated for which repetitious events of abnormal cycling patterns, infection, ovulation failure, early embryonic death, twinning, and abortion will provide valuable insight into potential fertility or treatment regimens. Immediate past athletic performance or use and its attending management, including hormonal administration, may also be of anamnestic importance.

FACTORS THAT RELATE TO REPRODUCTIVE POTENTIAL

AGE

Age-related impact on the ability of a mare to conceive and carry a foal to term ranges from postpubertal to senescence. The 2- and 3-yr-old mare may experience abnormal cycling patterns and aberrant behavior attitudes. These can be related to postpubertal maturation, perhaps breed associated, and may also be affected by management factors and drug use associated with athletic performance. Pluripara mares are subjected to anatomic changes that tend to adversely affect reproductive performance. These would include lengthening of the vulvar labia and decreased function and response of the vestibular sphincter. Advanced age appears to be a contributing factor to the incidence of anatomic changes in vaginal contour and predisposition to pneumovagina and urine pooling.[1] Although there is a trend for older mares to have a decreased reproductive potential, uterine health in a consistently noninfected mare does not appear to be significantly compromised by age.[2]

BREED

Identification of breed in the process of acquiring historic data provides information that may indirectly influence examination findings. Breed organizations differ in policy on natural versus artificial insemination, semen preservation and transport, and embryo transfer. This factor may, on occasion, complement or decrease potential fertility. Generally, a healthy mare of any breed, bred to a normal stallion, does not experience reproductive failure. However, there is a tendency for greater incidence of reproductive failure and increased management effort in the miniature breeds and the very large draft breeds. Also, breed may have an effect on ovulatory rate. The importance of early foaling (and breeding) varies among breeds and this may also influence success rates on breeding farms. This latter relates to seasonality of the mare, the natural prime cycling periods, and the January 1 birth date for some breeds.

STATUS

The present state of reproductive status of a mare is also important. A barren mare is one that has been bred but is not pregnant at the time of examination. This implies failure of conception or pregnancy maintenance from the last breeding. An exception would be the individual successfully bred on previous years and intentionally not bred during the immediate preceding season. A maiden mare is one of any age that has never been bred. Obviously, the younger postpubertal mare would be expected to be normal. The older maiden mare (>5 yr) would have an increased potential over time for uterine infection, because vulvar conformation may change sufficiently to allow aspiration of air (pneumovagina). The term wet mare is applied to one having recently foaled that is nursing a foal. Within each of these categories is the potential for some adverse influence on reproductive efficiency; however, lower fertility is usually attained in barren mares. Therefore, accurately identifying the mare's status is useful historic information.

PAST BREEDING RECORDS

The value of past reproductive records depends on their accuracy and completeness. Well-documented previous performance examination findings are helpful when a mare is presented for reproductive evaluation. Some of the recorded parameters that may contribute to the overall evaluation of the mare are the following.

Previous Foaling Data

Information on number of foals delivered, gestational length, parturition abnormalities, retained placenta, and live foals produced may directly or indirectly have some influence on reproductive efficiency.

Cycling Patterns

The recorded data from previous year(s) give an indication of endocrine function and traditional patterns. Many mares tend to be repetitious in cyclic events, especially in the area of estrus duration, follicular maturation, and ovulation. Information on the number of cycles bred in the previous season is also valuable. Progression through anestrus and the transitional phase will often follow a similar pattern among individuals; however, response to seasonal influence in both barren and postfoaling mares can vary. The effect of abnormal cyclic patterns on reproductive efficiency is significant.

Previous Reproductive Surgery

Evidence of, or recorded data relating to, previous surgery of the reproductive tract is indicative of a need to correct some abnormality that can or may compromise conception or pregnancy maintenance. The conformational relationship of the vulva to the anus or the length and flaccidity of the vulvar labia would verify the need for a Caslick operation. Likewise, additional examination procedures will verify the need for episioplasty and/or urethroplasty (see Chapters 2 and 48 for details of abnormal perineal conformation).

Previous Indications of Uterine Infection and Treatment

Information about prior uterine infection and treatment will be most important when evaluating the mare. Previous, initial, and/or baseline data will be invaluable when compared with results of a subsequent examination of the reproductive tract. Improvement, degeneration, or failure to change will all be contributory to prognosis as well as evaluation of the efficacy of previous treatment.

Early Embryonic Death and Abortion

Evidence of early embryonic death during previous season(s) is suggestive of several possible causes.[3–7] Certain embryo losses are related to specific time periods, endocrine control, infection, genetics, and twinning.[8–10] Accurate history and records will often be beneficial to determine the exact cause. The reason for abortion or fetal loss after approximately 50 days of gestation also may be supported with accurate historic information, when correlated with other examination and diagnostic laboratory findings.

PREVIOUS ATHLETIC USE OR PERFORMANCE

Mares are often added to the breeding herd following an athletic career. The inherent hazards of athletic performance, transportation, drug therapy, and disease exposure may compromise reproductive performance. Injury with subsequent pain or severe disability may adversely affect cyclic patterns, behavior, or general body condition. Disease entities with varying degrees of debility may also alter cyclic patterns and lower conception rates. Horses in high-level performance events occasionally are injected with anabolic steroids. Aside from the intent of its original use, the side effects of decreased reproductive performance in young mares and stallions are significant.[11–13] Behavioral attitudes developed in training may also compromise reproductive performance of the young mare for several months after arrival at the breeding farm.

GENERAL HEALTH

A history of previous medical events can be beneficial when correlated with the prebreeding physical examination, because illness and stress may alter cyclic events. Pain from laminitis, severe navicular disease, fractures, and tendonitis are not conducive to the highest reproductive potential. Conditions such as chronic obstructive pulmonary disease (heaves) with its attending cough and expiratory dyspnea at the least, may pre-

REPRODUCTIVE PERFORMANCE HISTORY

1. Date ____________ 5. Mare name/no. ____________
2. Owner ____________ 6. Breed ____________
3. Address ____________ 7. Age ____________
____________ 8. Weight ____________
4. Phone ____________

9. Status
   a. Maiden ________ (M)
   b. Barren: 1 2 3 4 >5 yr (B)
      (1) Last foal: 1 2 3 4 >5 yr
   c. Wet ________ (W)
      (1) Foaling date ________
   d. Pregnant ________ (P)
   e. Unknown ________
10. Last breeding date ________
11. Method of service: Natural __ AI __
12. Cycles bred previous season: 1 2 3 4 or more
13. Cycle pattern: Normal __ Abnormal __
14. Previous foaling problems: Yes __ No __
15. Previous uterine infection: Yes __ No __
16. History of early embryonic loss: Yes __ No __
17. History of abortion: Yes __ No __
   a. Gestational stage _____ months

FIG. 21–1. Example of a suitable breeding history record.

dispose to pneumovagina. Vaginal prolapse has also been observed as a consequence of chronic cough and dyspnea. Management efforts to control this condition are often rewarding. Known cardiac disease, especially valvular insufficiencies, also may require management change or special attention. A prior knowledge of an existing debility or health hazard will provide management opportunity to compensate in an effort to increase reproductive potential. Prior knowledge and properly recorded examination findings may avoid future communication problems, should such disease entities result in death. History of general body condition change such as weight or hair coat could be helpful in management planning.

RECORD SYSTEM FOR TABULATING HISTORIC INFORMATION

Developing a record system for the acquisition of data that will relate to prior reproductive performance of the mare is of prime importance. The system should include all information relevant to the status of the mare and factors that will affect reproductive performance. The record should be conducive to data input and retrieval; Figure 21–1 is an example.

REFERENCES

1. Roberts, S.J.: Infertility in the mare. Veterinary Obstetrics and Genital Diseases. (Theriogenology). 3rd ed. Published by the author, Woodstock, 1986, pp. 599–600.
2. Shideler, R.K., et. al.: Endometrial biopsy in the mare. Proc. Am. Assoc. Equine Pract., pp. 97–104, 1977.
3. Ball, B.A., Little, T.V., Hillman, R.B., and Woods, R.L.: Pregnancy rates at days 2 and 14 and estimated embryonic loss rates prior to day 14 in normal and subfertile mares. Theriogenology, *26:*611–619, 1986.
4. Ball, B.A., and Woods, G.L.: Embryonic loss and early pregnancy loss in the mare. Compend. Contin. Educ. Practicing Vet., *9:*459–471, 1987.
5. Ginther, O.J., Bergfelt, D.R., Leith, G.S., and Scraba, S.T.: Embryonic loss in mares: Incidence and ultrasonic morphology. Theriogenology, *24:*73–86, 1985.
6. Villahoz, M.D., Squires, E.L., Voss, J.L., and Shideler, R.K.: Some observations on early embryonic death in mares. Theriogenology, *23:*915–924, 1985.
7. Woods, G.L.: Pregnancy loss: A major cause of infertility in the mare. Equine Pract., *11:*29–32, 1989.
8. Ginther, O.J.: Twinning in mares: A review of recent studies. J. Equine Vet. Sci., *2:*127–135, 1982.
9. Ginther, O.J., and Douglas, R.H.: The outcome of twin pregnancies in mares. Theriogenology, *18:*237–244, 1982.
10. Pickett, B.W., et. al.: Twinning and early embryonic death. Management of the Mare for Maximum Reproductive Efficiency. *In* Animal Reproduction and Biotechnology Laboratory Bulletin No. 6. Fort Collins, Colorado State University, 1989, pp. 115–120.
11. Pickett, B.W., et. al.: Anabolic steroids in horses. Management of the Mare for Maximum Reproductive Efficiency. Animal Reproduction and Biotechnology Laboratory Bulletin No. 6. Fort Collins, Colorado State University, 1989, pp. 29–45.
12. Shoemaker, C.F., Squires, E.L., and Shideler, R.K.: Safety of altrenogest in pregnant mares and on health and development of offspring. J. Equine Vet. Sci., *9:*67–72, 1989.
13. Squires, E.L., Shideler, R.K., and McKinnon, A.O.: Reproductive performance of offspring from mares administered altrenogest during gestation. J. Equine Vet. Sci., *9:*73–76, 1989.

CHAPTER 22

EXTERNAL EXAMINATION

R.K. Shideler

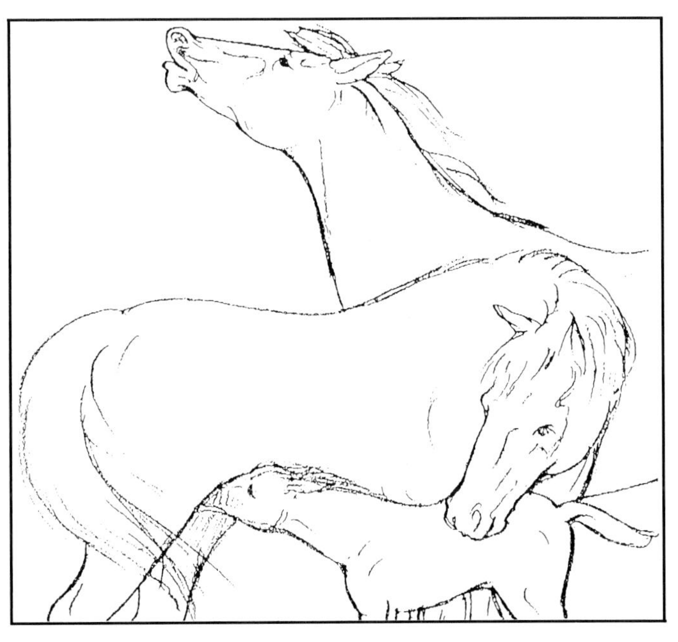

Clinical evaluation of the individual mare is essential to correlate physical findings with the potential for reproductive performance. Identification of the mare in the context of records, historic data retrieval, and future reference is mandatory. Identification can be verified by a registration certificate, recording the animal's markings, tattoo numbers, brands, and photographs. Legal as well as medical ramifications may occasionally be sufficient stimulus for establishing identity of each individual examined and subsequently treated. Factors that can affect behavior, cycling, conception, and ability to carry a foal to term may include the following.

GENERAL BODY CONDITION

Studies have been conducted to establish the relationship of body condition and fat covering to fertility. This evidence indicates that normal condition ranging from moderately thin to overweight did not appear to decrease pregnancy rates significantly,[1-3] while in fact, mares with higher body condition score achieved better pregnancy rates.[1] Therefore, only in those cases of extreme weight loss or obesity would reproductive potential be markedly affected, because flushing and supplemental feeding during early breeding season did not result in increased pregnancy rates.[4] Clinical impressions from farm managers, veterinarians, and nutritionists appear to substantiate that balanced nutritional intake and adequate body condition are positive factors in encouraging maximum fertility. A policy encouraged by some farms to enhance management-client relations is the arrival picture and recorded weight taken of each mare admitted to the farm. The presence of a scale can be invaluable in dealing with clients who believe their mare has lost weight. Several factors influence general body condition, in addition to nutrition.

DENTAL ABNORMALITIES

One of the primary considerations that can be associated with the weight-losing horse is inability to properly masticate food. All ages of horses have some predisposition to dental aberration.[5-7] The younger mare may exhibit chewing difficulty during the period of tooth eruption, retained deciduous teeth, and shedding of caps. Middle-age and older animals are potential candidates for "points" or sharp edges of upper and lower molars that may interfere with chewing. Malocclusion predisposes to abnormal growth rates of the second premolar with attending mastication problems. Missing teeth, wave mouth, root abscesses, and occasional trauma with fractures may also contribute to compromised dentition. Other disease or neoplasia may be contributory to weight loss, debility, and stress.

PARASITISM

Effects of excessive internal parasite burden have been frequently reported.[8–13] Mares in the age category to be presented for prebreeding examination are most likely susceptible to infection from, or would show the effects of, invasion by Strongylus vulgaris or Gastrophilus sp. During its migration, Strongylus vulgaris can create lesions within arteries that result in compromised blood supply or ischemia to the large intestine and subsequent colic. The gastrophilus or bot larvae select the stomach as a site for attachment and occasional penetration. Heavy burden or infection with these parasites is commonly associated with weight loss, poor body condition and occasionally more severe clinical symptoms.

NEOPLASIA

Several types of tumors that could potentially affect reproductive performance in the mare.

Granulosa Theca Cell Tumor

Granulosa theca cell tumor is ovarian in origin and is commonly associated with abnormal behavior, masculinity, and irregular cycles. Most cases are reported in middle-age and older mares, although in 78 mares the range was 2 to 20 yr.[14] Diagnosis is based on history, rectal examination, ultrasonographic scanning, and often assay of serum concentration of testosterone.[15,16] The neoplastic ovary is moderately to extremely enlarged and nodular on rectal palpation. On ultrasonographic scanning, multilobular "honeycomb" appearance is common.[14,15] Testosterone levels elevated greater than 50 pg/mL would be considered significant, although not specific, for diagnosis.[14–16]

Pituitary or β Cell Adenoma

Pituitary or β cell adenoma involves the pars intermedia of the pituitary gland. This syndrome is characterized by weight loss, muscle wasting, poor general body condition, and a long hair coat (often curly) that persists into the summer months. Excessive sweating, polyuria/polydipsia, hyperglycemia, and glycosuria are often accompanying symptoms. Elevated plasma concentrations of adrenocorticoids may also be associated with Cushing's syndrome.[17] Pituitary adenoma occurs in older mares, usually in excess of 13 yr and in most instances may be identified by correlating history, age, and clinical symptoms. Necropsy diagnosis is definitive.

Melanomas

Melanomas are tumors not uncommonly seen in older or aged gray/white horses. External evidence is most frequently observed around the anus, tail, and perineal region. Appearance in other locations on the body—such as the body wall, head, and neck—are frequently visible as extension, or metastasis, of the original site. Melanomas are less common than tumors of ı and uterus such as carcinomas, fibromas, and mas in relation to infertility in the mare.[17]

Hypothyroidism

Hypothyroidism, although common in dogs and reported as a cause of infertility in that species,[18] is less common in equids. Clinical symptoms associated with the disease include obesity and alopecia. Other than metabolic changes associated with thyroid deficiency, no adverse effect on reproductive efficiency is seen. Diagnosis may be confirmed with the thyroid-stimulating hormone (TSH) response test.[19]

Mammary Gland Abnormalities

Mastitis/mammitis is characterized by an enlarged, edematous, and painful udder. One-half or the entire gland may be involved. Incidence is highest at weaning time because of cessation of nursing, accumulation of milk in the gland, some degree of edema and inflammation, and a predisposition to ascending infection. A common sequela to mastitis is fibrosis of part or all of the gland. Unresolved inflammation, infection, and fibrosis frequently render the gland nonfunctional for milk production in subsequent foalings.

Puerperal edema and/or mammitis may be observed in the neonatal period and is usually associated with failure to nurse by the foal or possibly a systemic septicemia in the mare. A thorough examination of the udder is necessary to determine the capability of the mare to lactate normally.

Hermaphroditism (Intersex)

Intersexes are individuals in which the determination of primary sex is difficult because of congenital anatomic variations and abnormalities of the genital organs. It is uncommon in sheep, goats, and cattle and rare in the horse.[20] True hermaphrodites have both testis and ovaries or ovotestis. Male pseudohermaphrodites phenotypically resemble females but have testis and female hermaphrodites resemble males but have ovaries. Variations and degree of clinical change can occur (Fig. 22–1). In the mare, external intersex appearance is usually confined to the clitoral-vulvar area in which the clitoris may be enlarged or literally resemble the penis. The urethral opening may be located in the normal caudal vaginal location or in the penis-like structure. Anestrous and stallion-like behavior frequently accompany the clinical examination observations.

Amniocentesis to collect amniotic fluid and cells for diagnostic analysis has been commonly performed in humans early in gestation to detect suspected fetal aberrations or for sex determination. Only limited investigation has been done in animals.[21]

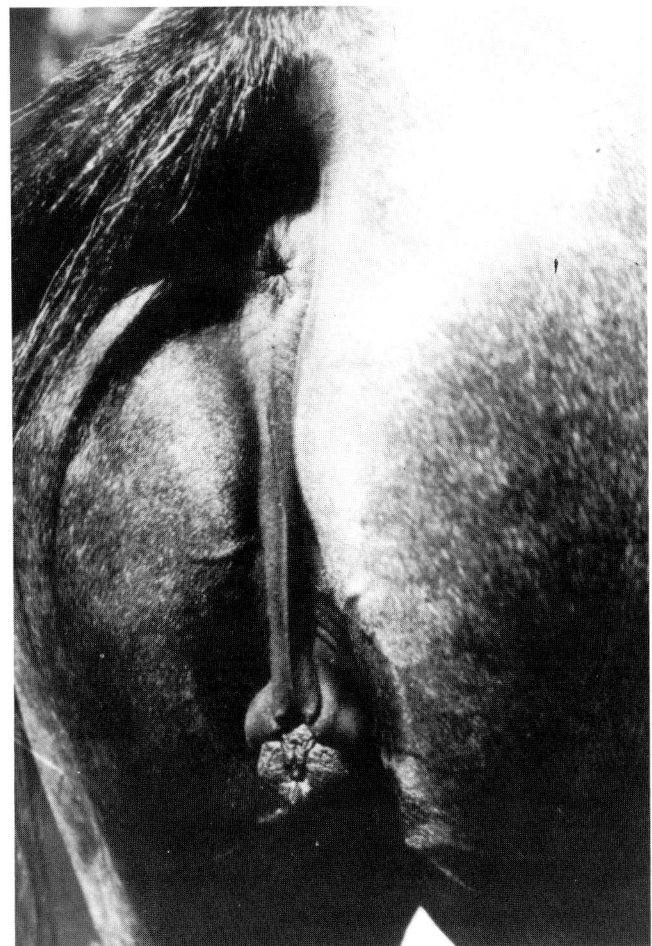

FIG. 22–1. Congenital anomaly of the external genitalia in a mare. The vulvar fissure is absent and the clitoris is enlarged and resembles a glans penis.

Clitoral Enlargement

Clitoral enlargement as a singular clinical entity, with or without behavioral changes, is most commonly associated with systemic administration of anabolic steroids (Fig. 22–2). Studies to determine the effect of anabolic steroids on reproductive function of young mares reported marked clitoral enlargement as a clinical sign, in addition to behavioral changes and reduced reproductive performance.[22–24] Enlargement of the clitoris at the time of external examination of the mare would be one indication of prior anabolic steroid therapy. This treatment regimen, under the assumption that it is helpful in increasing muscle mass and speed, is frequently used in high-athletic performance events. There is little evidence to support the use of anabolic steroids for this latter purpose in horses.

AGE CONFIRMATION

Reference has been made in other sections to the relationship of age to uterine biopsy grade and reproductive efficiency. Although no significant relationship between age and fertility in normal mares seems to exist, a trend toward decreased performance is evident in older mares as a result of a strong tendency to develop vulvar and perineal changes that predispose to ascending infection and endometritis.[25–27] Therefore, age identification by visual dental examination not only verifies the age but may present evidence of need for dentistry that would enhance body condition.

MUSCULOSKELETAL ABNORMALITIES

Although primary consideration is given to the normal reproductive tract when accepting a mare into the breeding herd, musculoskeletal abnormalities do pose problems and risk to conception and pregnancy maintenance. Pain and stress may adversely affect cycling and reproductive efficiency. Careers in athletic performance predispose the mare to fractures, tendinitis, arthritis, and other painful conditions. Chronic conditions, including laminitis and navicular disease, may also result in pain, debility, and anorexia. Each of these problems may be detrimental to reproductive efficiency. Advanced pregnancy normally involves greater weight in the mare, compounding painful effects of limb and joint disease. Maintenance of pregnancy may also be affected by abdominal adhesions resulting from previous surgery characterized by chronic or recurring colic. Additional musculoskeletal causes could include organ dysfunction and anemia factors. Clinical laboratory blood chemistry and profiles would be helpful in determining the cause and effect of these diseases.

The presence of abdominal wall defects also poses some potential hazard to the mare in pregnancy. Umbilical hernias are relatively common in the neonatal foal. Evidence is available to indicate this is hereditary.[28] Umbilical hernia is most commonly repaired and corrected at 1 to 6 months of age. Surgical correction ap-

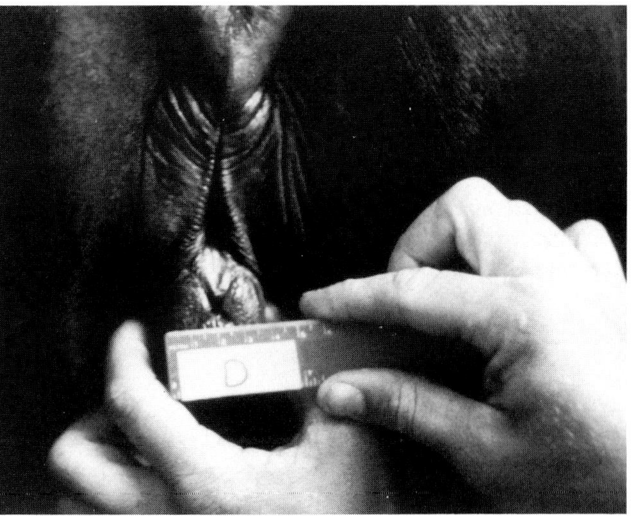

FIG. 22–2. Clitoral enlargement caused by administration of anabolic steroids.

pears to be the treatment of choice.[29] The potential for strangulation of a segment of intestine is always present; however, with increased abdominal mass and weight in advanced pregnancy, the protrusion of intestine through a ventral abdominal defect is intensified.

Ventral edema, often seen in advanced pregnancy and associated with confinement or lack of exercise, should not be confused with the much larger swelling associated with ruptured prepubic tendon. The latter may be life threatening and will always compromise the capability of the mare to expel the fetus at parturition.

Evidence of scars anywhere in the ventral abdominal area may be an indication of prior surgical intervention for colic. Occasionally, postoperative abdominal adhesions may form and could interfere with uterine enlargement and positioning in late pregnancy. An initial physical examination of the mare will usually identify the cause and allow a planned treatment regimen prior to expected reproductive performance.

CARDIOPULMONARY EXAMINATION

Chronic respiratory or cardiac disease can play a part in reproductive failure. Identifying these anomalies early will be helpful in eliminating time and economic loss incurred during the breeding season. Chronic obstructive pulmonary disease (COPD) is debilitating. When accompanied with dyspnea and cough, COPD, in addition to illness and stress, increases the potential for pneumovagina and subsequent genital tract infection. Cardiac disease, although relatively uncommon in the horse, may appear in some older mares. Auscultation as part of the physical examination will identify some of these abnormalities. No adverse short-term effect may be evident; however, over time a valvular insufficiency and congestive heart failure can terminate reproductive performance.

Edema of the ventral abdomen and lower limbs is an indication of potential cardiovascular abnormality. Vasculitis with increased capillary permeability produces edema that can be associated with equine purpura hemorrhagica (EPH) and equine infectious anemia (EIA).[30] Marked anemia is present in advanced cases of EIA. As each can have an adverse effect on reproductive efficiency, prompt diagnosis is essential. Laboratory confirmation with serology and the Coggin test (EIA) will positively identify this condition. Diagnosis of EPH is based on clinical symptoms of edema of the head and limbs and often a history of prior infection with Streptococcus equi.

PERINEAL CONFORMATION

The area involving the vulva and the anus may change anatomic relationships or show alterations from normal vulvar size and tone. The presence of abnormalities and their degree of change may predispose to pneumovagina and urine pooling.[25] Therefore, a clinical evaluation of this area is consistent with, and included in, the general physical examination. Details of conformational faults are covered in Chapter 2 and surgical procedures to correct these faults are found in Chapters 48 and 49.

Evidence of Caslick operation, episioplasty or perineal body resection, urethroplasty, or third-degree perineal laceration repair is beneficial historic data in determining past events and predicting future needs and potential for reproductive efficiency. The Caslick Index is a scoring system by which numerical values are assigned to degrees of variation from normal anovulvar relations. Pascoe reports in a study of 9020 mares that mares with a Caslick Index of <150 had a significantly higher pregnancy rate than those with a score of >150. Pregnancy rate was significantly lower in mares without a Caslick operation and with an index of >150 compared with mares with a score of <150. All mares showed a decrease in pregnancy rate with age. It is suggested that mares with Caslick Index of >100 be sutured.

ATTITUDE AND BEHAVIOR

Although behavioral patterns of the mare may not adversely affect reproductive performance, some management procedures may be altered. Attitude toward handlers and other horses and abnormal teasing behavior during estrus may compromise daily work schedules. Anticipation of these handling and schedule changes may reduce stress and complications at a later time.

Behavioral characteristics of the foal may be genetic, acquired, or a combination of both. Clinical impression tends to support the hypothesis that such foal traits, good or bad, mimic those of the dam to a greater degree than the sire.

Extreme changes in behavior in the mare, especially masculinization and stallion-like attitude, are suggestive of hormonal, neoplastic or therapeutic origin. The behavioral changes associated with granulosa cell tumors, intersex, and anabolic steroid therapy were discussed earlier in this chapter.[14–16]

REFERENCES

1. Henneke, D.R., Potter, G.D., and Kreider, J.L.: Body condition during pregnancy and lactation and reproductive efficiency in the mare. Theriogenology, *21*:897–909, 1984.
2. Kubiak, J.R., et al.: The difference of energy intake on the reproductive performance of nonpregnant mares. Theriogenology, *28*:587–598, 1987.
3. Morris, R.P., et al.: Follicular activity in transitional mares as affected by body condition and dietary energy. *In* Proceedings of the Equine Nutrition and Physiology Symposium. 1987, pp. 93–99.
4. Voss, J.L., and Pickett, B.W.: The effect of nutritional supplement on conception rate in mares. Proc. Am. Assoc. Equine Pract., pp. 49–54, 1973.
5. Uhlinger, C.A.: Disorders of the oral cavity. *In* Large Ani-

mal Internal Medicine. Edited by B.P. Smith. St. Louis, C.V. Mosby, 1990, pp. 624–631.

6. Shideler, R.K.: Dentistry for the snafflebit horse. Proc. Am. Assoc. Equine Pract., 301–312, 1983.
7. Baker, G.J.: Dental disorders in the horse. Compend. Contin. Educ. Practicing Vet., *4*:S507–S515, 1982.
8. Uhlinger, C.A.: Parasite control programs. *In* Large Animal Internal Medicine. Edited by B.P. Smith. St. Louis, C.V. Mosby, 1990, pp. 1513–1524.
9. Lyons, E.T.: Common internal parasites found in the stomach, large intestine and cranial mesenteric artery of Thoroughbreds in Kentucky at necropsy (1985–1986). Am. J. Vet. Res., *48*:268–271, 1987.
10. Klei, T.R.: Morphologic and clinicopathologic changes following *Strongylus vulgaris* infections of immune and nonimmune ponies. Am. J. Vet. Res., *93*:1300–1307, 1982.
11. Maas, J.: Alterations in body weight and size—Parasitism. *In* Large Animal Internal Medicine. Edited by B.P. Smith. St. Louis, C.V. Mosby, 1990, pp. 171–172.
12. Bello, T.R.: The control and treatment of internal parasites. Somerville, American Hoescht, Animal Health Division, 1981.
13. Uhlinger, C.A.: Ascarid infection in horses. *In* Large Animal Internal Medicine. Edited by B.P. Smith. St. Louis, C.V. Mosby, 1990, pp. 1523–1524.
14. Meagher, D.M., et al.: Granulosa cell tumors in mares, a review of 78 cases. Proc. Am. Assoc. Equine Pract., 133–143, 1977.
15. Hinrichs, K., and Hunt, P.R.: Ultrasound as an aid to diagnosis of granulosa cell tumor in the mare. Equine Vet. J., *22*:99–103, 1990.
16. Liu, I.K.M.: Ovarian abnormalities. *In* Current Therapy in Equine Medicine. 2nd ed. Edited by N.E. Robinson. Philadelphia, W.B. Saunders, 1987, pp. 500–503.
17. Roberts, S.J.: Pituitary adenoma. *In* Veterinary Obstetrics and Genital Diseases (Theriogenology), 3rd ed. Woodstock, VT, S.J. Roberts, 1986, pp. 620–621.
18. Goying, L.S., Reineke, E.P., and Schirmer, R.G.: Clinical diagnosis and therapy of hypothyroidism in dogs. J. Am. Vet. Med. Assoc., *141*:341–347, 1962.
19. Roberts, S.J.: Hypothyroidism. *In* Veterinary Obstetrics and Genital Diseases (Theriogenology), 3rd ed. Woodstock, VT, S.J. Roberts, 1986, pp. 718–719.
20. Roberts, S.J.: Hermaphrodism. *In* Veterinary Obstetrics and Genital Diseases (Theriogenology), 3rd ed. Woodstock, VT, S.J. Roberts, 1986, pp. 72–75.
21. Eaglesome, M.D., Mitchell, D., Singh, E., and Hare, W.C.D.: Collection and cytogenics of fetal fluids from heifers during third month of pregnancy. Theriogenology, *1*:195–214, 1977.
22. Maher, J.M., Squires, E.L., Voss, J.L., and Shideler, R.K.: Effect of anabolic steroids on reproductive function of young mares. J. Am. Vet. Med. Assoc., *186*:583–587, 1985.
23. Squires, E.L., Voss, J.L., Maher, J.M., and Shideler, R.K.: Fertility of young mares after long term anabolic steroid treatment. J. Am. Vet. Med. Assoc., *186*:583–587, 1985.
24. Pickett, B.W., et al.: Anabolic steroids in mares. Management of the mare for maximum reproductive efficiency. *In* Animal Reproduction and Biotechnology Laboratory Bulletin No. 06. Fort Collins, Colorado State University, 1989, pp. 29–36.
25. Pascoe, P.R.: Observations on length and angle of declination of the vulva and its relation to fertility in the mare. J. Reprod. Fertil. Suppl., *27*:299–305, 1979.
26. Roberts, S.J.: Pneumovagina. Infertility in the mare. *In* Veterinary Obstetrics and Genital Diseases (Theriogenology), 3rd ed. Woodstock, VT, S.J. Roberts, 1986, pp. 599–600.
27. Shideler, R.K., et al.: Endometrial biopsy in the mare. Proc. Am. Assoc. Equine Pract., 97–104, 1977.
28. Ralston, S.L., and Shideler, R.K.: Inheritance of umbilical hernias in horses. Tenth International Congress on Animal Reproduction and Artificial Insemination, 1984, p. 530.
29. Turner, A.S., and McIlwraith, C.W.: Umbilical herniorrhaphy in the foal. *In* Techniques in Large Animal Surgery. 2nd ed. Edited by A.S. Turner and C.W. McIlwraith. Philadelphia, Lea & Febiger, 1982, pp. 254–259.
30. Smith, B.P.: Diseases of the hematopoietic and hemolymphatic system. *In* Large Animal Internal Medicine. Edited by B.P. Smith. St. Louis, C.V. Mosby, 1990, pp. 1073–1074.

CHAPTER 23

RECTAL PALPATION

R.K. Shideler

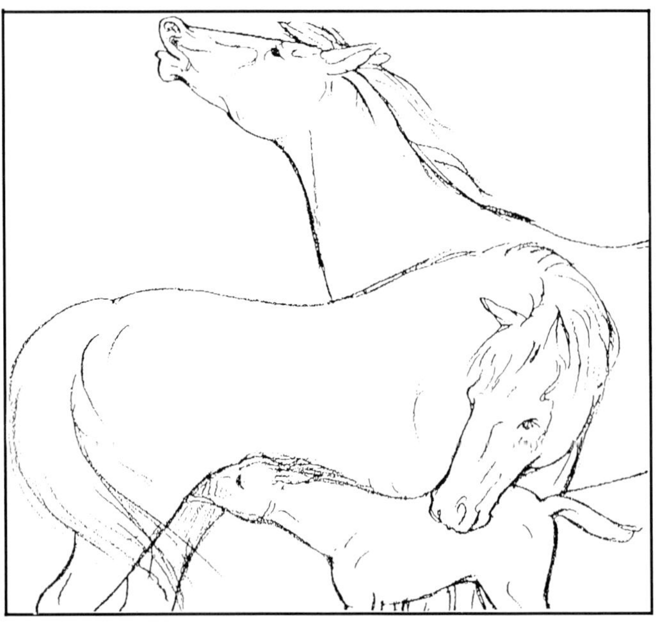

Rectal palpation is a valuable management procedure on many equine breeding farms. It is performed as part of a reproductive tract examination. The rectal palpation of the uterus, ovaries, and cervix has been the basic means by which diagnosis, prognosis and treatment selection have been made for more than 50 yr. While subsequent diagnostic technics have been developed to complement this procedure and significantly contribute to definitive information, rectal palpation remains a dependable and desirable examination procedure.

Advantages of direct palpation of the reproductive tract via the rectum are time required, relative safety, lack of discomfort to the mare, and general management efficiency. Palpator experience, restraint facilities, and farm management objectives obviously are influential in achieving these advantages. Irwin reported in a trial using 487 pregnant mares that early manual pregnancy testing does not increase the abortion rate if undertaken carefully.[1] Voss et al. conducted a trial to determine the effect of palpation on fertility.[2] Nonlactating mares were examined by an experienced palpator and followed by an inexperienced student. Mares were subsequently artificially inseminated on their first normal estrus. Mares were divided into three groups and palpated daily during estrus, daily until 50 days pregnant and a control group that was not palpated. Nonpalpated mares had fewer cycles per pregnancy and a higher percentage of pregnancy per cycle than palpated mares. Daily palpation through 50 days of pregnancy did not appear detrimental, as no early embryonic loss or abortion was noted during this period. Because that study did not reflect normal management procedures for a breeding farm, another experiment was designed. One group of mares was palpated every other day in estrus, and a second group was not palpated. Pregnancy rates following every-other-day insemination were higher in nonpalpated mares than in those palpated (91.7 vs. 83.3%, respectively). A later study used two palpators per mare in one group of mares and one palpator per mare in the second group.[3] Palpation was stopped in both groups when ovulation was detected. Analysis of these data showed no difference in pregnancy rates between one and two palpators (81 vs. 79%, respectively). Voss et al. hypothesized that the decrease in fertility because of excessive palpation may be caused by alteration in gamete transport, particularly the ovum, in the postovulation period.[2] Those reports relate to frequency of palpation, proximity to ovulation, and technician experience. When the management plan is based on known data, uses skilled and experienced palpators, and is correlated with specific individual mare needs for maximum reproductive efficiency, deleterious effects of rectal palpation appear to be minimal. Some reports do cite the occurrence of rectal tears during palpation.[4] This potential is inherent; however, it appears to be highly correlated to technical experience and restraint facilities. Insurance claims substantiate the potential for injury from this procedure.[5] Reports on surgical repair techniques also confirm the incidence of rectal lacerations.[6,7]

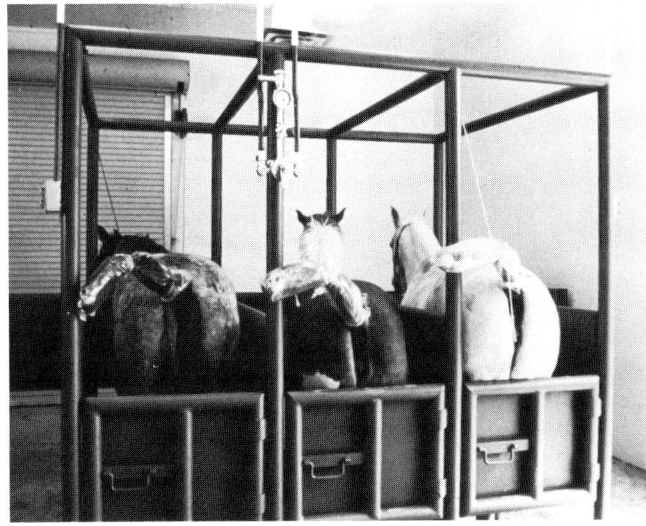

FIG. 23–1. Stocks for mare restraint.

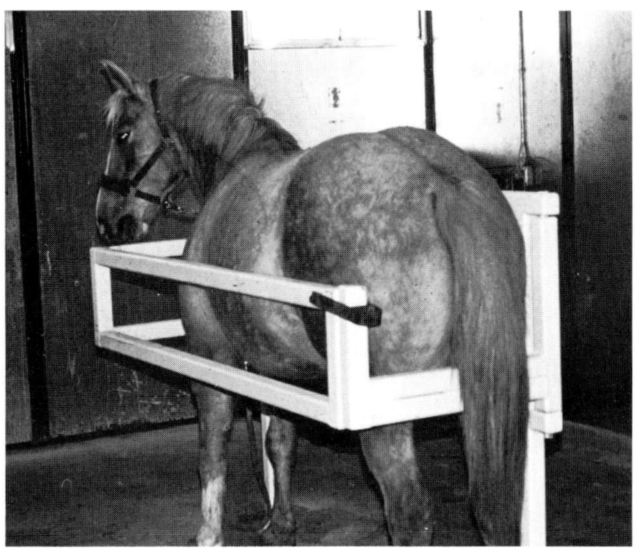

FIG. 23–2. Single stock for mare restraint.

Rectal palpation of the reproductive tract is a traditional and fundamental procedure used as a part of reproductive management. The procedure is used on many equine breeding farms for detection of follicular activity and ovulation, assessment of abnormalities of the genital tract, and diagnosis of pregnancy.[2] With experience and adequate restraint facilities, it is efficient, time-cost effective, and a complement for other diagnostic procedures. The advantages of this procedure far outweigh disadvantages and potential hazard.

PREPARATION FOR RECTAL EXAMINATION

Initial preparation for examination should include safety measures for the mare and veterinarian. Restraint mechanisms would appropriately include stocks. Well-made stocks provide the most effective means to control the individual horse and concurrently prevent injury to the mare during examination. Equally important is the safety provided to the palpator by preventing sudden or excessive movement by the mare. Three types of stock are shown in Figures 23–1, 23–2, and 23–3.

Additional means of restraint are available when needed in the absence of stocks or for the intractable individual. A variety of drugs for chemical restraint, sedation, and/or tranquilization is available. Drugs used for tranquilization change behavior and/or reduce anxiety, which in many cases is sufficient restraint for palpation. Sedatives and other central nervous depressants may be desirable in those individuals requiring a greater degree of control or whose behavioral characteristics so dictate. The nose twitch has long been a suitable method for short-term control and restraint and as such, is compatible with the needs of rectal palpation in many instances. Other procedures that may be helpful include the application of hobbles, picking up a foreleg, or lifting and forcefully bending the tail forward.

MATERIALS

Procedural preparation for rectal palpation includes plastic shoulder length obstetrical gloves and a lubricant. Some palpators prefer to wear a surgical glove pulled over the plastic glove. An inexpensive and suitable lubricant is carboxymethylcellulose. This chemical may be purchased in bulk form and mixed in quantities commensurate with need. Other packaged lubricant gels are suitable, convenient, more expensive, and may be purchased sterile, if desired. If straining on the part of the mare is excessive, topical anesthetics such as Xylocaine (lidocaine HCL, Lyphomed, Inc., Rosemont, IL) may be applied to the rectal mucosa.

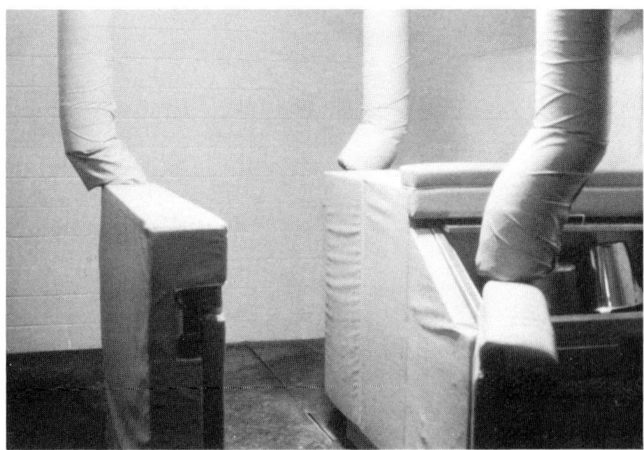

FIG. 23–3. Padded stock for mare restraint.

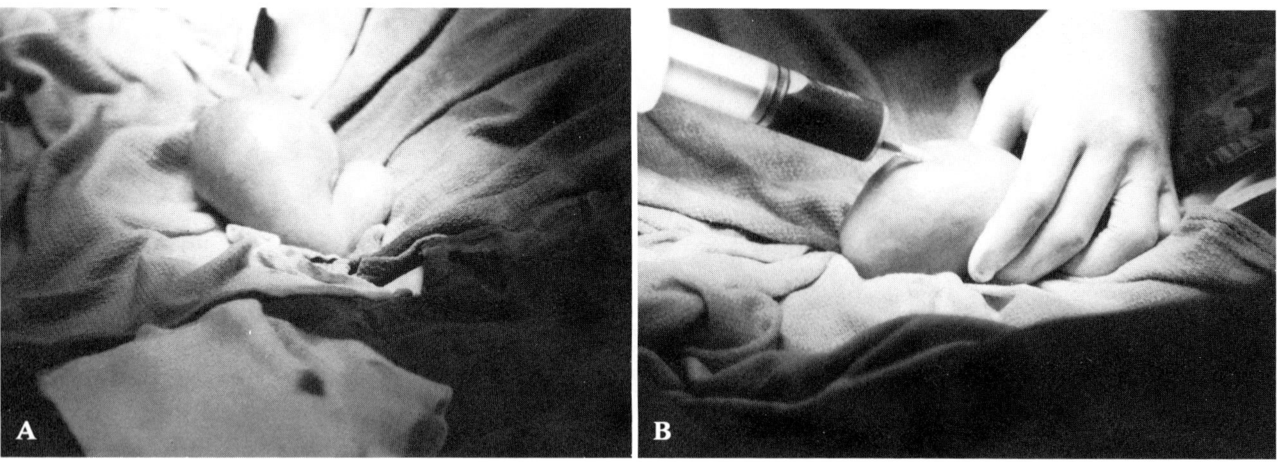

FIG. 23–4. *A*, Hematoma within uterine wall, detected on rectal palpation. *B*, Aspiration of hematoma within uterine wall before incision and drainage.

PURPOSE OF RECTAL PALPATION

Three major objectives are, in large part, ascertained by rectal palpation.

PHYSICAL ABNORMALITIES

Manual (digital) examination may determine the palpable presence of normal as well as abnormal physical features of the reproductive tract. The presence of normal ovaries, uterus, oviducts, and cervix are, of course, fundamental for fertility. Variations in size, location, and tone can be meaningful. Uterine enlargement with poor tone may be associated with luminal fluid, excessive endometrial or lymphatic cyst formation, inflammatory changes affecting the endometrium, pyometra, or simply age-related loss of tone. Position of the uterus may be influenced by pregnancy, postpartum period, age, fluid content, or adhesions associated with previous parturition/dystocia. Congenital defects and genetic abnormalities may also affect size and location of the ovaries, uterus, and cervix.

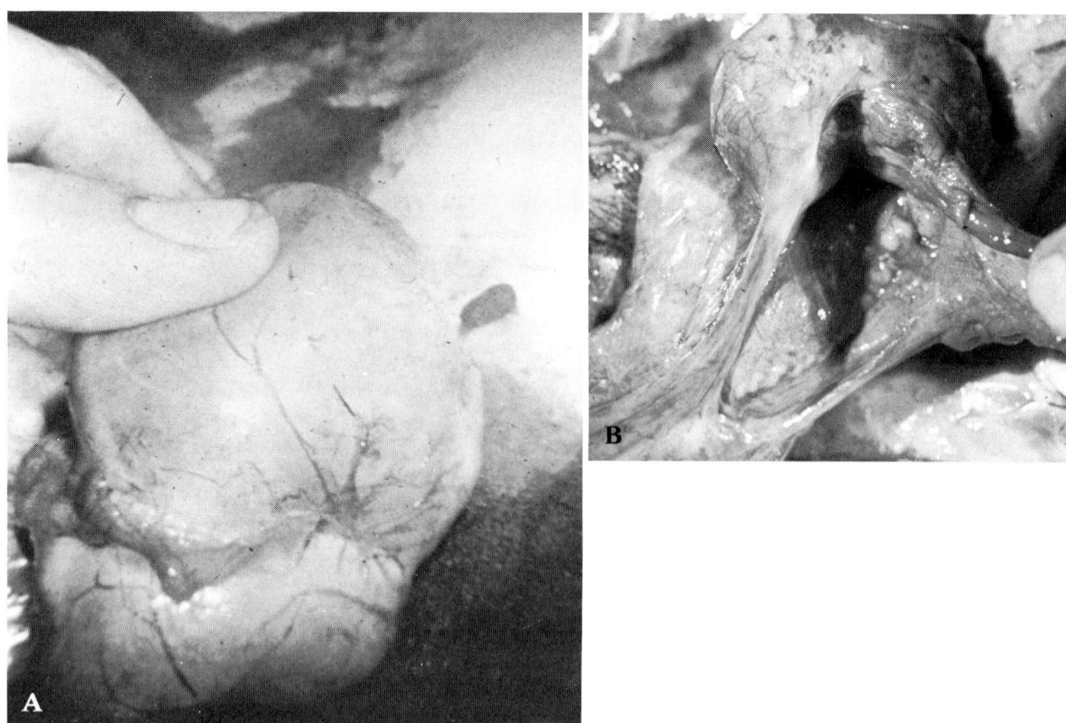

FIG. 23–5. *A*, Normal ovary with follicle. *B*, Ovary—ovulation fossa and ovarian ligament.

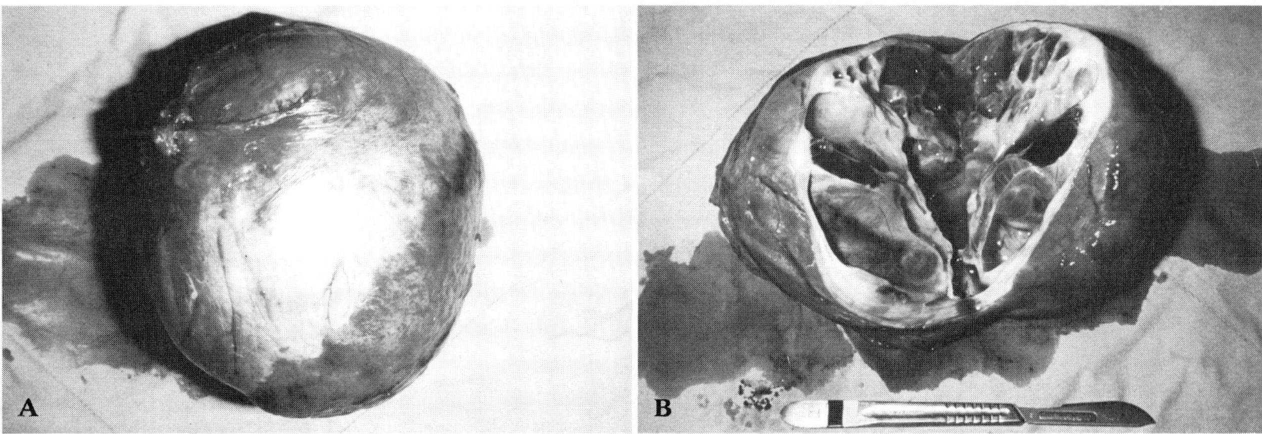

FIG. 23–6. *A*, Granulosa-theca cell tumor. *B*, Cut section, internal view, granulosa-theca cell tumor.

Basic criteria determined by palpation are size of the ovary, general consistency (structure), and follicular activity. Size is primarily related to season and stage of cycle. Ovaries are small and with little or no follicular activity during anestrus. Enlargement and progression in follicular development are noted as the mare progresses through the transitional period into normal cycling season. Excessively or persistently small ovaries are indicative of depressed or juvenile development. Abnormally large ovaries, with firm or nodular appearance can be related to neoplasia[8] (Chapter 45). Occasionally, an enlarged ovary may contain a nonovulatory follicle ranging from 80 to 150 mm in diameter. Examination of the uterus is made to determine the correlation of size, tone, and luminal content to stage of cycle, season of the year, age, puerperal period, and several potentially pathologic conditions that will be identified and/or confirmed with additional diagnostic techniques (Chapter 31). Among these uterine abnormalities can be cysts, abscesses, or hematomas[9] (Fig. 23–4) within the uterine wall. The cervix is palpable by pressing downward with fingertips toward the pelvic floor. At the caudal uterine body it is approximately 40 mm in diameter in the nonpregnant mare and is generally about 80 mm in length to the posterior os. Its length and width change in direct relation to stage of estrous cycle and pregnancy status with a soft, wide feel apparent in estrus and palpable firmness similar to that of an index finger during early pregnancy.

ENDOCRINE FUNCTION

Manual examination of the ovaries provides evidence of effect of circulating hormones and stage of cycle. The presence and size of follicles and size of the ovary should correlate with estrous behavior. Early estrus is indicated by 20- to 30-mm follicles accompanied by behavioral signs when teased by a stallion. Progressive enlargement of the follicle to ≥ 40 mm is commonly interpreted as nearing ovulation. Estrous behavioral signs and follicular development reflect a systemic release of estrogen, follicle-stimulating hormone (FSH), and ultimately luteinizing hormone (LH) (Fig 23–5). When examination of the mare is conducted at 1- or 2-day intervals, ovulation is readily recognized by the disappearance of the mature follicle. A depression on the surface of the ovary, previously identified as follicle site,

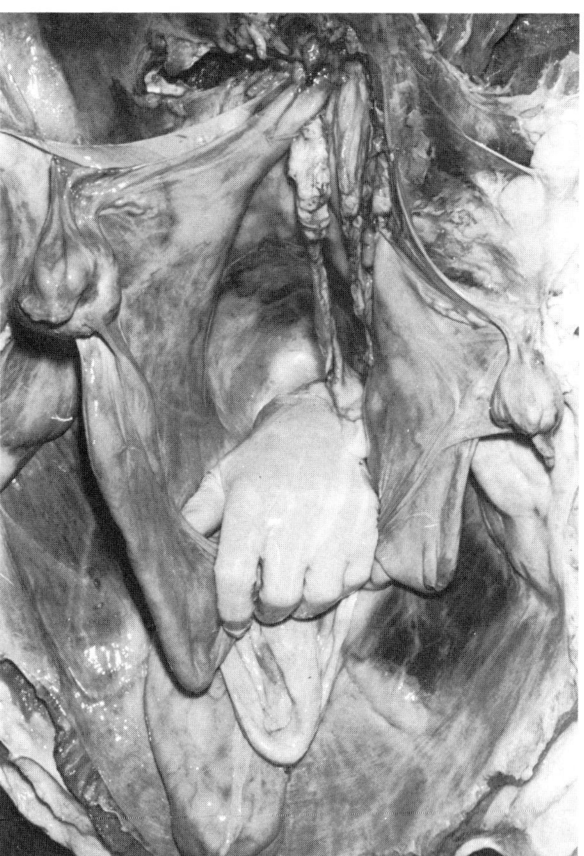

FIG. 23–7. Palpation of uterus.

is commonly palpated immediately after ovulation. Several hours to 1 day after ovulation, the ovulated follicle fills with blood (corpus hemorrhagicum) and regains tone and size similar to a follicle. An enlarged, firm ovary with characteristic mininodular surface, correlated with abnormal sexual behavior and supported with ultrasonographic scanning may suggest the presence of a granulosa cell tumor (Fig. 23–6). The contralateral ovary is often small and nonfunctional (Chapter 45).

The uterus, on rectal examination, may also reflect hormonal influence by changes in tone and thickness. The uterus of the estrous mare will normally have flaccid to moderate tone with some thickening of the walls. The thickened endometrium and edematous endometrial folds during estrus are sometimes palpable but easily confirmed by ultrasonography. Hormonal and receptor deficit may be reflected by atony, flaccidity, and a thin uterine wall, often typical of the anestrus and transitional mare. In contrast, the pregnant uterus is characterized by firm or good tone and is tubular in nature, representing the influence of progesterone and a presently unidentified fetal-maternal hormonal interaction.

The cervix is a sensitive organ in the reproductive tract; it will react to subtle and normal endocrine change. Estrogen influence tends to soften the cervix and increase its secretions. Progesterone tends to influence closure of the cervix, making its palpation character one of firmness and less pliability. Sudden declining changes in serum progesterone concentrations during pregnancy may be characterized by a progressing (cranially to caudally) softening of the cervix. This is often the first clinical alert to impending early embryonic death (EED). Most EED after 20 days seems to be associated with fetal death (loss of heartbeat) well before occurrence of (> 5 days) tone changes in either the cervix or the uterus.

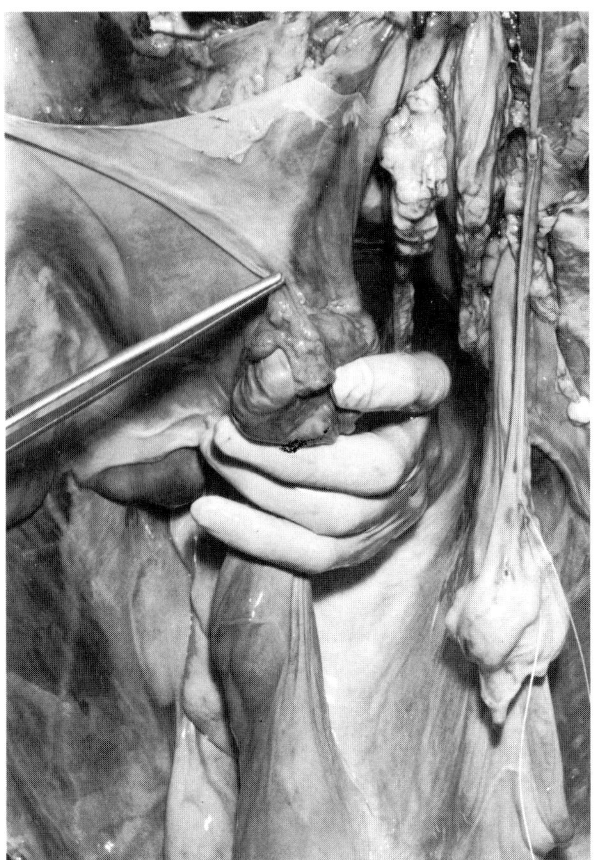

FIG. 23–9. Palpation of right ovary.

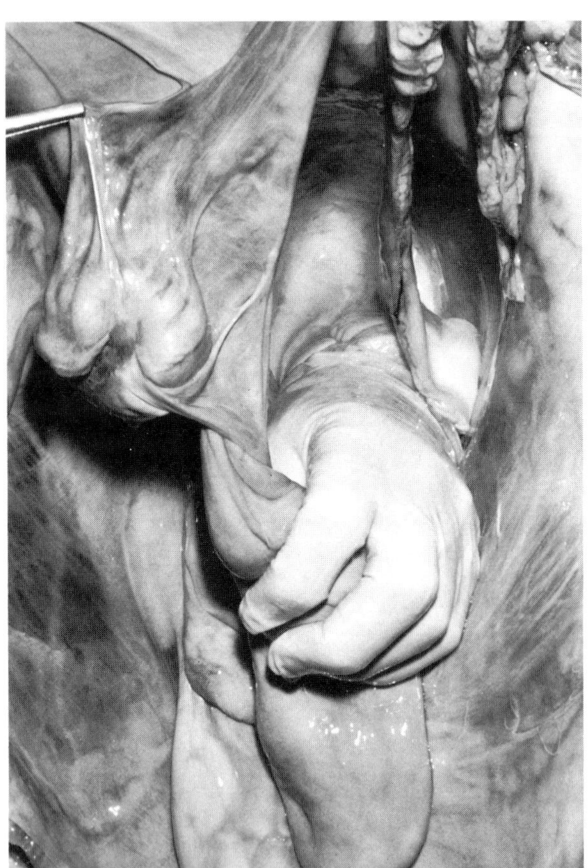

FIG. 23–8. Palpation of right uterine horn.

PREGNANCY DETERMINATION

The reflection of hormonal influence—in the form of a tight, closed cervix and excellent uterine tone—is the initial criterion needed for indication of pregnancy. The presence of a vesicle, usually first palpable between 17 and 22 days after ovulation, will confirm the status. A more detailed section on pregnancy diagnosis follows. Pregnancy determination is included as an important facet of rectal palpation, because knowledge of the status of the mare must always precede all other diagnostic and examination procedures.

PALPATION PROCEDURE

Whenever possible, a complete history of the mare's previous foaling, cycling, and/or breeding activities should be reviewed. Reproductive status and reason for rectal palpation need to be established. It is essential to confirm or rule out pregnancy before carrying out procedures used in the reproductive examination of the mare.

Preparation for rectal examination includes a shoulder-length obstetrical glove with adequate lubrication. Entrance through the anus into the rectum frequently identifies the need to evacuate manure from this region. This is accomplished carefully and slowly to prevent mucosal trauma and/or irritation to the rectum and caudal colon. Rectal tears involving mucosa, muscularis, and/or serosa are uncommon; however, an awareness of the potential is essential. The majority of tears observed have involved the dorsum of the rectum and are located 4 to 30 cm cranial to the anus. This might lead to the hypothesis that such lacerations occur when removing fecal material or entrance conditions might favor excessive stretching of the rectum such as gas accumulation. Caution should be observed in the presence of strong peristaltic waves.

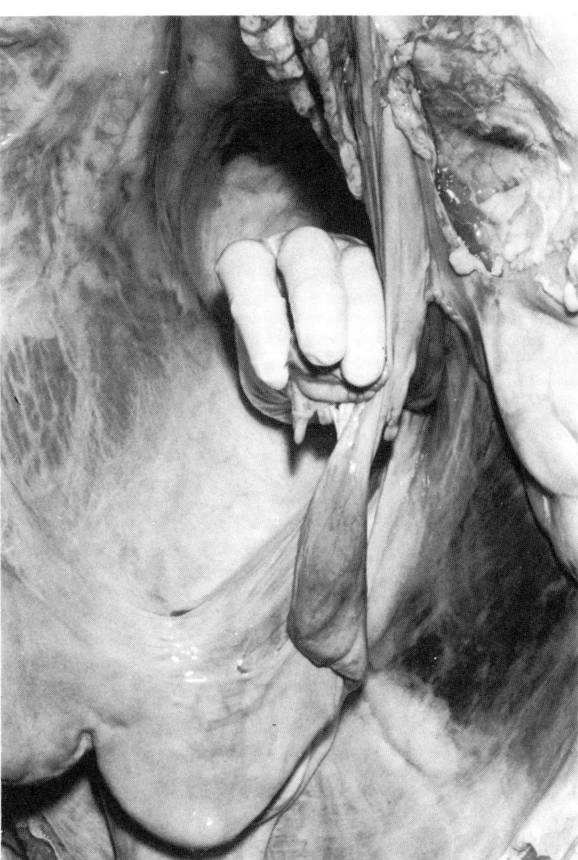

FIG. 23–11. Palpation of left ovary.

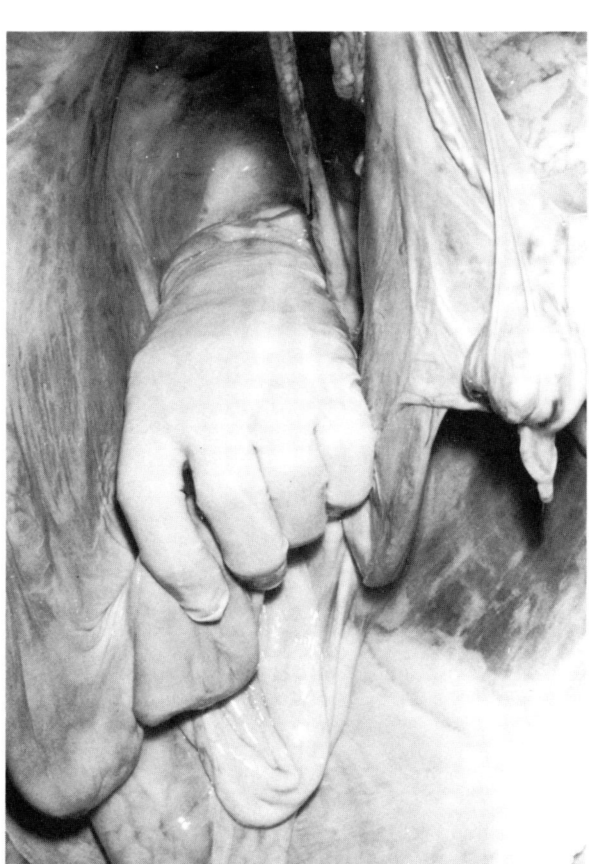

FIG. 23–10. Palpation of left uterine horn.

Once the hand and arm have been inserted into the rectum, orientation within the bony pelvis and identification of the cranial pelvic brim is helpful. The fingers may be cupped over the body of the uterus (Fig. 23–7), which lies just cranial to and often slightly ventral to the anterior brim of the pelvis in the normal nonpregnant mare. The uterus will be soft, pliable, relatively flat, and even flaccid. It is generally 4 to 7 cm wide and 2 to 5 cm thick.[4] Maiden and young mares' uteri may be smaller and carried higher. The postpartum mare will present a larger uterus carried lower and more cranially. The uterus gradually involutes, becomes smaller, and regains its previous nonpregnant position over a period of 2 to 4 weeks.

Having identified the uterus, the cupped hand may follow the organ laterally to the ovary (Fig. 23–8). Size and tone of the uterine body and horn are evaluated at this time. The ovary is identified as a round to kidney-shaped mass attached to the uterine horn by the utero-ovarian ligament and oviducts. It is suspended by the broad ligament of the uterus. The ovarian ligament is attached to the posterior pole of the ovary. The greater

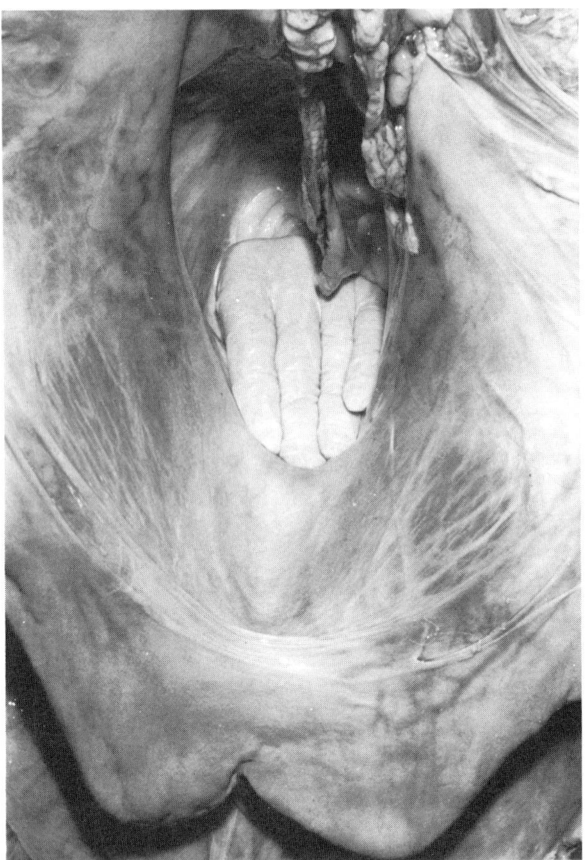

FIG. 23–12. Palpation of cervix.

curvature and anterior pole are round and essentially free of attachment. Opposite the greater curvature, or convex surface, will be the ovulation fossa. This is a palpable depression on the ventral or concave aspect of the ovary (Fig. 23–9). Raised, smooth fluctuant areas on the surface of the ovary are follicles. The size may range from 5 to 60 mm or larger, depending on stage of estrous cycle. Size, degree of maturation, and tone or fluctuance, especially when correlated with ultrasonographic scanning, are closely related to time of ovulation.[10–12] Abnormalities in size and texture of the ovary should be related to season and cycle stage to correctly determine their significance.

The hand may then follow the horn of the uterus across the body and traverse the opposite horn (Fig. 23–10), palpating carefully for normal or abnormal size, tone, or luminal content. The contralateral ovary is identified and examined (Fig. 23–11). The location of the ovaries is usually just cranial to the shaft of the ilium and at the 3 and 9 o'clock or 2 and 10 o'clock positions. Some palpators prefer to identify and examine the ovaries initially and follow this with the uterine examination. On completion of ovarian and uterine examination, the arm and hand are withdrawn to midpelvis. The tips of the fingers are pressed against the floor of the pelvis to identify the cervix, located caudal to the body of the uterus (Fig. 23–12). Its size and softness are indicators of hormonal influence and will correlate closely with behavioral patterns and utero-ovarian findings. The cervix responds rapidly to increasing estrogen release and is approximately 80 mm long, flattening out to 30 to 50 mm in width during estrus. The cervix will become firmer and will be 20 to 30 mm in width in diestrus and quite firm; it is closed and often 20 mm or less in diameter in early pregnancy. After 60 days of gestation, the cervix elongates and will be somewhat less firm than in early pregnancy.

A filled urinary bladder is often palpated ventral and/or cranial to the brim of the pelvis. Proper orientation and identification of the uterus and cervix will eliminate possible indecision or incorrect relationship to a pregnant uterus.

Rectal palpation of the reproductive tract, pelvis, and caudal abdomen provides the opportunity to achieve additional experience and knowledge. Special emphasis on learning normal intestinal, splenic, and kidney positions will prove beneficial in colic examination.

REFERENCES

1. Irwin, C.F.P.: Early pregnancy testing and its relationship to abortion. J. Reprod. Fertil. Suppl., *23:*485–488, 1975.
2. Voss, J.L., Pickett, B.W., Bach, D.G., and Burwash, L.D.: Effect of rectal palpation on pregnancy rate of nonlactating normally cycling mares. J. Anim. Sci., *41:* 829–834, 1975.
3. Heesemann, C.P.: Effect of ovarian activity and allyl trenbolone on the estrous cycle and fertility of mares. M.S. thesis. Colorado State University, 1981.
4. Roberts, S.J.: Internal examination for pregnancy in the mare. *In* Veterinary Obstetrics and Genital Diseases (Theriogenology). 3rd ed. Woodstock, VT, S.J. Roberts, 1986, pp. 25–26.
5. Stauffer, V.D.: Equine rectal tears—A malpractice problem. J. Am. Vet. Med. Assoc., *178:*798–799, 1981.
6. Arnold, J.S., and Meagher, D.M.: Management of rectal tears in the horse. J. Equine Med. Surg., *2:*64–71, 1978.
7. Rick, M.C.: Management of rectal injuries. Vet. Clin. North Am., Equine Pract., 5:407–428, 1989.
8. Meagher, D.M., et al.: Granulosa cell tumors in mares—A review of 78 cases. Proc. Am. Assn. Equine Pract., 133–143, 1977.
9. Shideler, R.K., Squires, E.L., Trotter, G., and Tarr, S.: Uterine hematoma in the mare. J. Equine Vet. Sci., *10:*187–193, 1990.
10. Carnevale, E.M., McKinnon, A.O., Squires, E.L., and Voss, J.L.: Ultrasonographic characteristics of the preovulatory follicle preceding and during ovulation in mares. Theriogenology, *29:*232, 1988.
11. McKinnon, A.O., Squires, E.L., and Pickett, B.W.: Follicular dynamics preceding and during ovulation. *In* Equine Reproductive Ultrasonography. Fort Collins, CO, Colorado State University, Animal Reproduction Laboratory Bulletin No. 04. 1988, pp. 41–49.
12. Pierson, R.A., and Ginther, O.J.: Ultrasonic evaluation of the preovulatory follicle in the mare. Theriogenology, *24:*359–368, 1985.

REPRODUCTIVE EXAMINATION OF THE MARE

CHAPTER 24

ULTRASONOGRAPHY

A.O. McKinnon
E.M. Carnevale

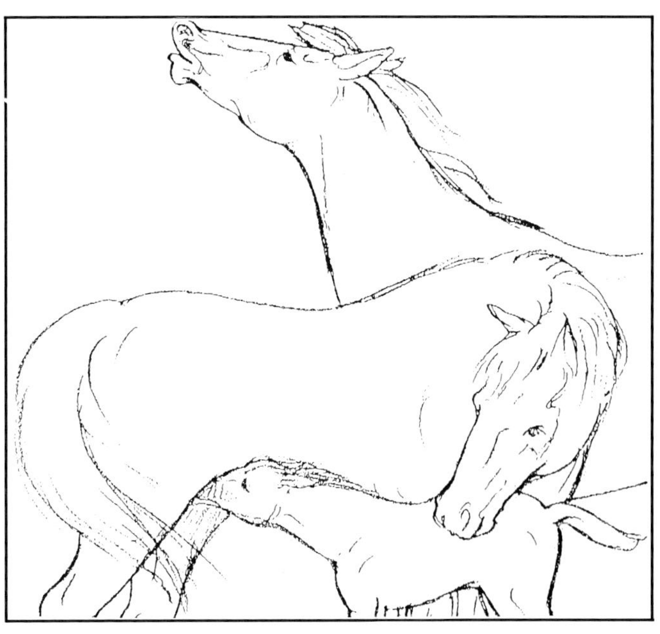

Ultrasonographic evaluation should be considered a routine part of reproductive examination of the mare. The ability to examine the uterus and ovaries noninvasively provides information on reproductive function that previously was not accurately available. Like other reproductive examination procedures, it should be used as a diagnostic aid to form an overall picture of reproductive health. Initially, costs to the client limit its application to pregnancy diagnosis, but once the full versatility of equipment was understood and accepted, ultrasonography became a routine part of reproductive examination on well-managed breeding farms.

Some of the applications of diagnostic ultrasonography of the mare's reproductive tract are listed below.

UTERUS

1. Pregnancy diagnosis.
2. Management of twins.
3. Diagnosis of normal fetal development and occasionally sex.
4. Diagnosis of impending or actual early embryonic death.
5. Stage of estrous cycle determination.
6. Diagnosis of uterine pathologic processes such as intrauterine fluid, uterine cysts, air, debris, and occasionally abscessation or neoplasia.

OVARIES

1. Stage of estrous cycle determination.
2. Assessment of status and number of preovulatory follicles.
3. Examination of development and morphology of the corpus luteum (CL).
4. Diagnosis of ovarian irregularities, neoplasia, and periovarian cysts.

These applications are discussed in detail in Chapter 31. This chapter presents information on principles, equipment, procedures, and recognition of artifacts associated with reproductive ultrasonography.

PRINCIPLES

Ultrasonography is based on the principle of high-frequency sound waves produced by electrical stimulation of piezoelectric crystals in a transducer. As sound waves are propagated through tissue, a proportion is reflected back to the transducer, converted to electrical impulses, and displayed on a screen. Thus, the transducer is alternately a transmitter and receiver of sound waves. The magnitude of reflected sound waves is directly proportional to the difference in density at the interface, or junction, of two tissues. As sound waves go deeper into the body, weakening or attenuation occurs. In general, the greater the density of tissues, such as muscle and bone, the greater the impedance to propagation of sonographic waves, and the greater the strength of the echo produced. Fluid is an excellent medium for transmission of ultrasonic waves because it provides little impedance until the signal encounters an interface with an adjacent tissue of different density. Fluid-filled structures appear black or anechoic on the ultrasonographic image. Both air and gas are poor propagators of ultrasonic signals and cause severe attenuation. For this reason, close contact of the transducer with tissue to be examined is essential. Dense tissue such as bone reflects most of the ultrasonic beam, and the image on the screen appears white. Other tissues are seen in various shades of gray, depending upon their ability to reflect sound waves. The ultrasonic beam passes through tissue as a narrow band and scans only a narrow section.

Most modern ultrasonographic instruments used for examination of the mare's reproductive tract are B-mode, real-time scanners. B-mode refers to brightness modality where the ultrasonographic image is a two-dimensional display of white dots produced on a screen. Brightness of dots is proportional to amplitude of returning echoes. When repeated signals are transmitted, received, and processed, a continual visual image of tissues is produced, which permits observation of their structure and motion in real time (B-mode, real-time).[1]

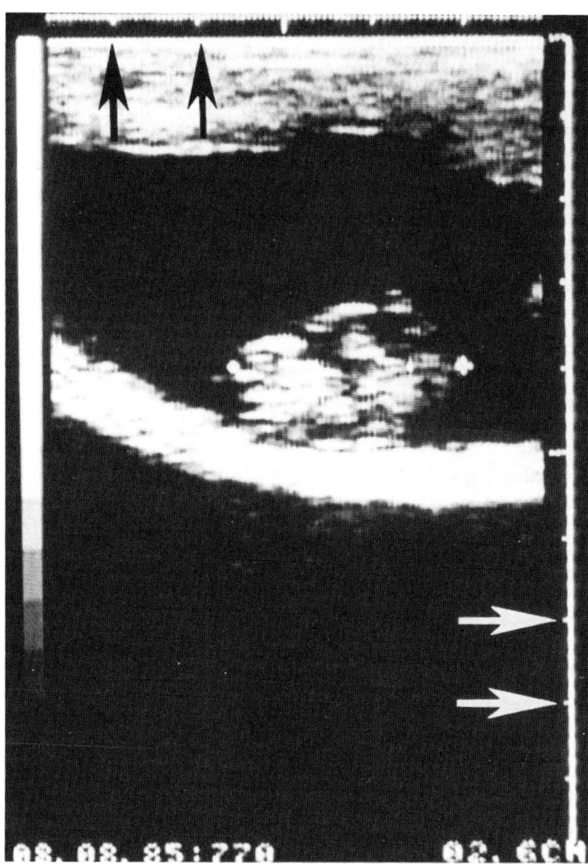

FIG. 24–2. Ultrasonographic image from a linear-array scanner. Arrows delineate 10-mm markers.

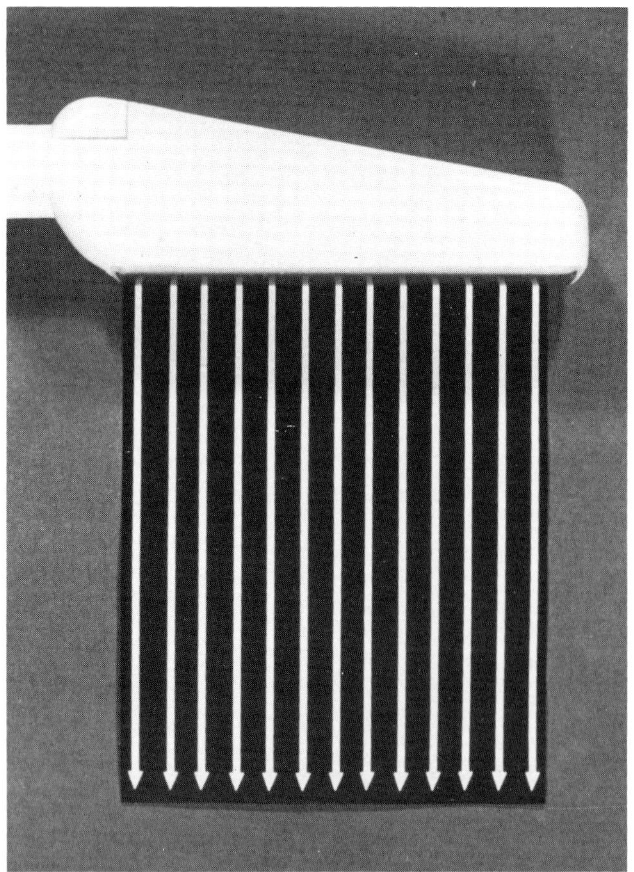

FIG. 24–1. A linear-array transducer. Width of the rectangular sound beam corresponds to length of the active or crystalized portion of the transducer.

EQUIPMENT

The two major types of real-time ultrasonographic transducers used for reproductive examination of the mare are linear and sectorial. Physical arrangement of the crystals within the transducer determines the pattern by which sound waves are propagated from the transducer. With linear-array scanners, the width of the rectangular ultrasonic beam corresponds to length of the active, crystallized portion of the transducer (Figs. 24–1 and 24–2). A linear-array transducer is oriented in the longitudinal plane with respect to the mare's body. Therefore, images of the cervix and uterine body are longitudinally oriented and those of the uterine horn are cross sectional. Images of tissues closest to the transducer are at the top of the screen. Sector scanners produce a beam that is triangular in shape, because sound waves radiate from a single point or source (Fig. 24–3). The sound beam generally travels transversely to the mare's body and consequently, images of the cervix and uterine body are cross sectional, whereas images of the horns are longitudinal or oblique.

Resolution, which is the ability to detect small differences in tissue density, depends on frequency of sound waves.[1] High frequency provides greater detail and lower frequency provides greater tissue penetration. Ultrasonographic frequencies are measured in megahertz (MHz; 1 hertz [Hz] = 1 sound wave/s). The lower-

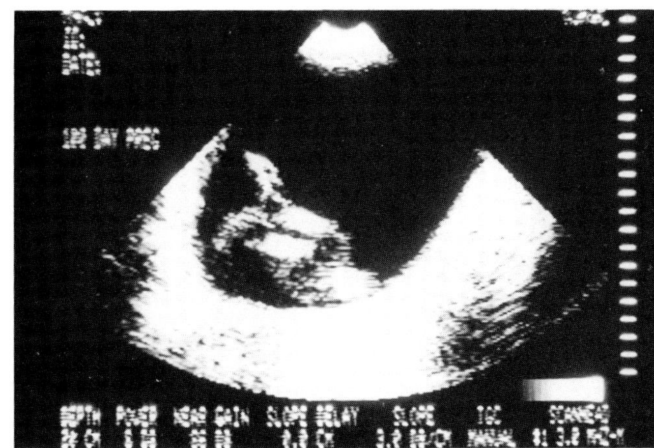

FIG. 24–3. Ultrasonographic image from a sector scanner. Sector scanners produce a sound beam that is triangular in shape because the sound waves radiate from a single point or source in the transducer.

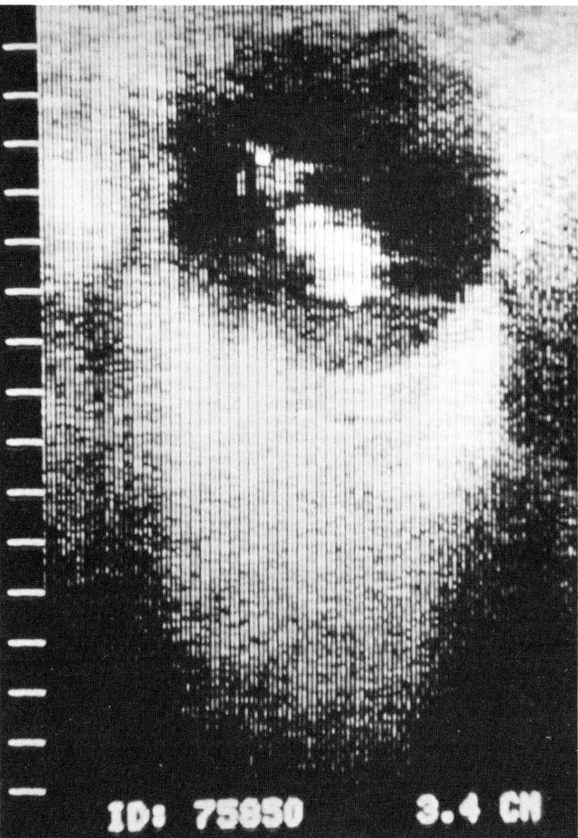

FIG. 24–4. Ultrasonographic image from a 3-MHz transducer. Lower-frequency transducers (3 MHz) have less tissue resolution but greater tissue penetration.

frequency transducers (3 and 3.5 MHz) are suited for viewing larger structures at a greater distance from the transducer (Fig. 24–4) than the 5- or 7.5-MHz transducers. Higher-frequency transducers (5 to 7.5 MHz) are most useful for detailed study of structures close to the transducer.[1] All photographs of ultrasonographic images in this chapter and Chapter 31, except Figures 24–3 and 24–4, were recorded using a 5-MHz transducer from either the Corometrics 210 DX or the Equisonics 300 (Table 24–1). Image size will vary with equipment. A 5-MHz transducer can be used to detect a conceptus on day 10, follicles as small as 3 mm,[1] and presence of a CL throughout most of diestrus.[2,3] In comparison, a 3- or 3.5-MHz transducer can be used to detect a conceptus at about days 13 to 15, follicles approximately 6 to 8 mm in diameter, and the presence of a CL for 5 to 6 days postovulation.[4] The principal uses of lower-frequency transducers are to study an older fetus, by either intrarectal or abdominal scanning, and pathologic conditions elsewhere in the body, such as liver or cardiac disease.

Most modern ultrasonographic equipment enables the operator to freeze and/or record images and automatically measure structures with a caliper-adjustment control. Some machines have split-frame capability with memory and various scanning frequencies (Table 24–1).

PROCEDURES

The procedure and precautions for intrarectal ultrasonographic examinations are similar to those for rectal palpation, and no additional restraint is required. The transducer should be well lubricated and protected by the examiner's hand to prevent trauma to the rectal wall. Care should be taken to prevent fecal material from attaching to the transducer. After evacuating fecal material from the rectum, the probe is introduced and moved across the reproductive tract in the following pattern: uterine body, right uterine horn, right ovary, right uterine horn, uterine body, left uterine horn, left ovary, left uterine horn, uterine body, and cervix. Good contact must exist between the transducer and rectal wall. Air in the rectum or a gas or fluid-filled loop of bowel will result in a distorted image. To minimize scanning errors, principally those of omission, conduct

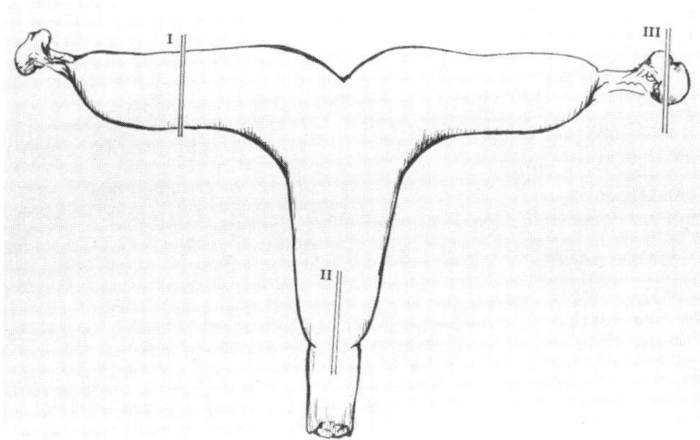

FIG. 24–5. Diagrammatic view of the mare's reproductive tract. I, cross section of uterine born; II, longitudinal section of uterine body and cervix; III, cross section of ovary.

TABLE 24–1. ULTRASONOGRAPHIC EQUIPMENT AVAILABLE IN THE UNITED STATES AS OF JANUARY 1992

	ALOKA			AUSONICS		DYNAMIC IMAGING	E.I. MEDICAL
	210 DX	260	500	Microimager 1000	Microimager 2000	Concept 2000	The Ultra-Vision
Price	$9,000–10,000 (transducer dependent)		$16,000 (transducer dependent)	$13,500	$16,500	$25,000	$9,800
Weight (lb)	18	37	22	22	22	30	8
Scanning method	Linear	Linear/sector	Linear/convex sector	Mechanical sector	Mechanical sector	Linear, sector convex, annular	Linear/sector
Frequencies (MHz)	3.0, 5.0, 7.5	Linear: 3.0, 3.5, 5.0, 7.5 Sector: 3.0, 3.5, 5.0, 7.5	2.5 to 10.0	2.5, 3.5, 5.0 (Reproductive 5.0)	2.5, 3.5, 5.0 (Reproductive 5.0)	2.5, 3.5, 5.0, 6.5, 7.5, 10.0	Linear: 3.5, 5.0, 7.5 Sector: 3.5, 5.0, 7.5
Gray levels	16	16	64	16	32	256	128
Frame rate/second	15/30	15/30	30	13–30	13–30	25–30	18/30
Video output	Yes	Yes	Yes	Yes	Yes	Yes	Yes
Monitor size (in.)	5.5	5.5	7.0	5.0	5.0	7	4
Alpha-numeric keyboard	Numeric	Yes	Yes	Yes	Yes	Yes	Yes
Calipers/area (circumference)	Yes/no	Yes/yes	Yes/yes	Yes/yes	Yes/yes	Yes	Yes/yes
Remote freeze	Yes	Yes	Yes	Yes	Yes	Yes	Yes
Approximate probe size (in.)	Variable: 5.0 MHz; 2.0 long, streamlined	Variable: sector small and in line	Variable	6.0 × 1.5 0°–90° transrectal transducer (5.0 MHz), longitudinal image in a forward direction	6.0 × 1.5 0°–90° transrectal transducer (5 MHz), longitudinal image in a forward direction	4.8 × 1 1.0 × 1.1	5.0 MHz, 2.5 × 5.0; 7.5 MHz, 1.5 × 2.5
Distributors	Corometrics Medical Systems, Inc., Wallingford, CT			E.I. Medical, Loveland, CO; Universal Medical Systems, Inc., Yonkers, NY		Classic Medical Supply, Inc., Tequesta, FL	E.I. Medical, Loveland, CO

the same scanning procedure during each examination.

A brief manual examination should precede all ultrasonographic procedures to facilitate proper orientation of the reproductive tract, to enable repositioning of intestinal contents that are occasionally interposed between the rectum and uterus, and to assess tone and size of various components of the reproductive tract. With practice, ultrasonographic examination is expedient; however, caution is advised when examining mares in suboptimal conditions such as mares straining or in conditions of too much external light interference, inadequate restraint, etc. so that all parts of the reproductive tract are adequately visualized.

NORMAL ANATOMY—UTERUS

A thorough knowledge of ultrasonographic anatomy and understanding of dynamic changes in the uterus are essential for ultrasonographic evaluation of the mare's reproductive tract. The dynamic changes visualized with ultrasonography mirror the ovarian hormonal influences and aid in estimating reproductive potential.

The relationship between orientation of a linear array transducer and orientation of the mare's reproductive tract is shown in Figures 24–5 to 24–8. Because the probe is generally held in a sagittal plane, images of the cervix and uterine body are longitudinally orientated

EQUISONICS	ESOATE BIOMEDICAL	PIE MEDICAL		SHIMADZU	TOKIMEC (TOKYO KEIKI)	WES MED
EQ 300	SIM 4000C	Scanner 450	Scanner 480	SDL-32B	LS1000	WIC 50
Currently not in production	$13,500	9,500	$15,000 (dual frequency, 5.0/7.5 MHz)	$8,500–10,000 (depends on transducer and accessories)	$12,900	3.2 MHz: $7,295 5.0 MHz: $8,295
38	28	20	25	15	30	40
Linear	Sector	Linear	Linear	Linear	Linear	Linear
3.5, 5.0, 7.5	2.25, 3.5, 5.0, 7.5	3.5, 5.0, 7.5	3.5/5.0 and 5.0/7.5	3.5, 5.0, 7.5	3.5, 5.0, 7.5	3.2, 5.0
64	16	32	64	32	64	64 (16 Levels of color)
24	25	30	28	30	24	15
Yes	Yes	Yes	Yes	Yes	Yes	Yes
9	8	7	7	5.5	7.0	7
Yes	Yes	Yes	Yes	Yes (numeric)	Yes/yes	Yes
Yes/yes	Yes	Yes	Yes	Yes/no	Yes	Yes/yes
Yes	Yes	Yes	Yes	Yes	No	Yes
5.0 and 7.5 MHz; 5.5 × 0.5–1 × 0.5; 3.5 MHz 5.0 × 1.0	5.0 × 1.5	4.5 × 0.8 × 0.9	4.5 × 0.8 × 0.9	6.0 × 1.0 × 0.75; 7.0 × 1.5 × 1.0; smaller probe available	5.0 and 7.5 MHz; 5.5 × 0.5 × 1.0 × 0.5; 3.5 MHZ, 5.0 × 1.0	6.0 × 0.5 × 0.5
Products Group International, Inc.; Boulder, CO	Classic Medical Supply, Inc., Tequesta, FL	Classic Medical Supply, Inc., Tequesta, FL		Precision Veterinary Instruments, Inc., Englewood, CO	Products Group International, Inc., Boulder, CO	Wes Med Medical Systems, Bothell, WA

with the cervix to the left of the ultrasonographic picture. The orientation of craniad on the right and caudad on the left of the image remains constant throughout this chapter and Chapter 31. Uterine horns are seen in cross section as the transducer is moved left or right. Depending on orientation of the horn at a given examination, manipulation of the uterus may be necessary to obtain a true cross section.

Ultrasonographic characteristics of the uterus during the anovulatory season, estrous cycle, and pregnancy may often be differentiated. During anestrus, the cross section of the uterine horns (Fig. 24–9) and the longitudinal section of the uterine body (Fig. 24–10) are often flat and irregular and may contour closely to surrounding abdominal organs. In estrus, uterine horns are well rounded and both horns and body commonly have an interdigitated pattern of alternating echogenic and nonechogenic areas[5] (Figs. 24–11 and 24–12). The areas of decreased echogenicity are the outer edematous portion of endometrial folds. The edema is caused by the effects of estrogen. This ultrasonographic pattern resembles the appearance of a sliced orange. Endometrial folds generally parallel estrogen production and are visible at the end of diestrus, become more prominent as estrus progresses, and decrease or disappear within 24 h before the time of ovulation.

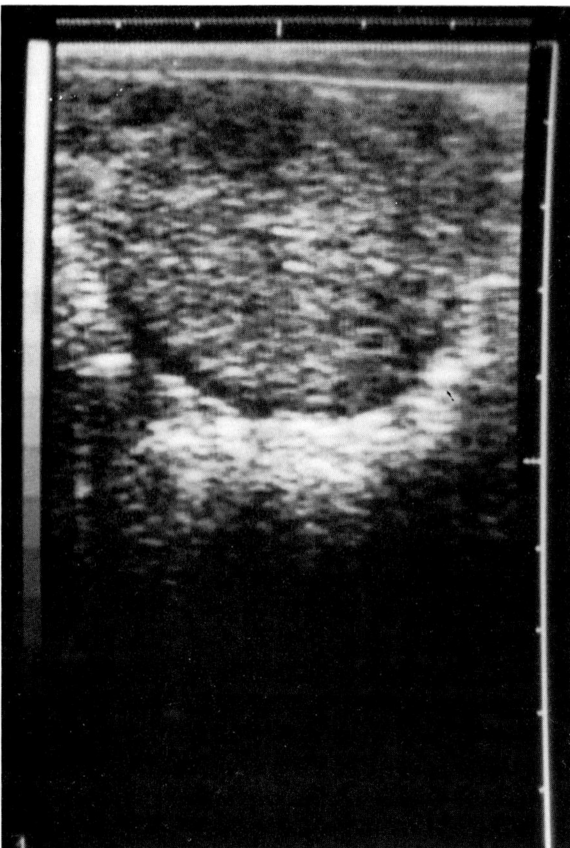

FIG. 24–6. Ultrasonographic image of a uterine horn (cross-sectional image from Fig. 24–5 located at I).

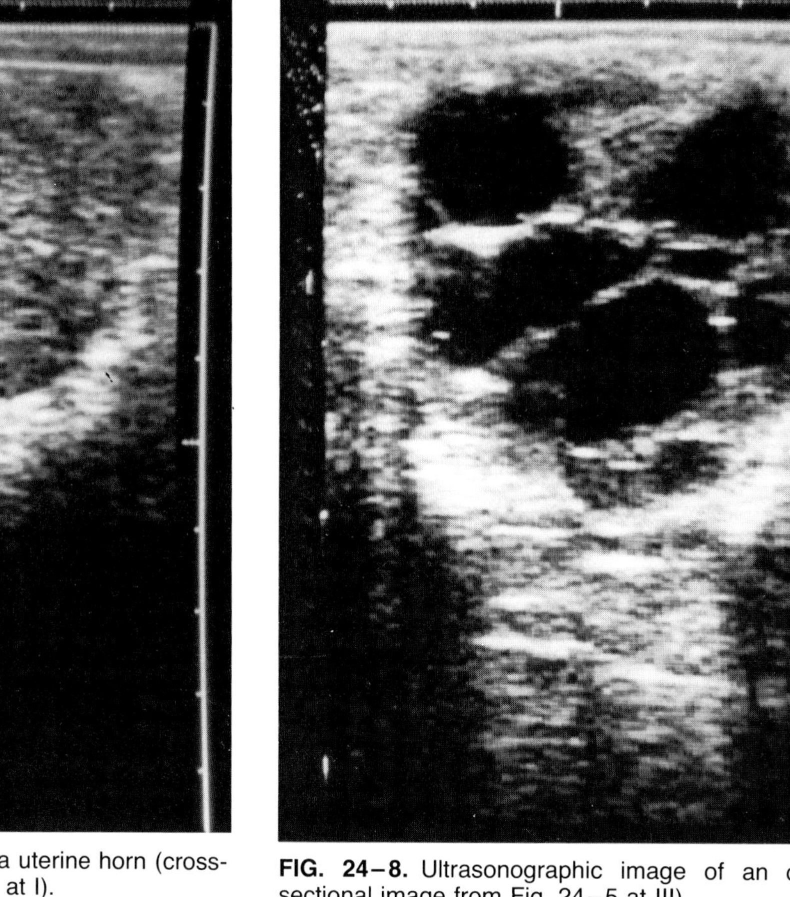

FIG. 24–8. Ultrasonographic image of an ovary (cross-sectional image from Fig. 24–5 at III).

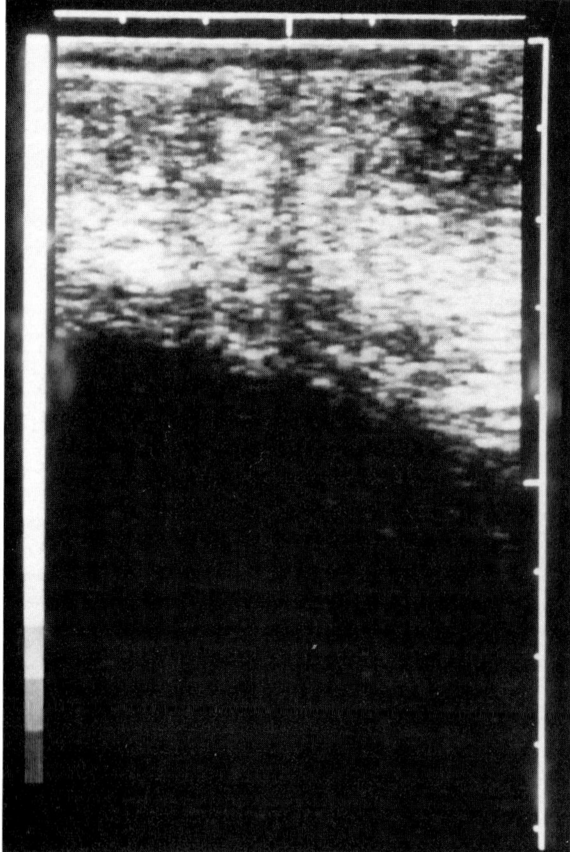

FIG. 24–7. Ultrasonographic image of mare's uterine body and cervix (longitudinal section located in Fig. 24–5 at II).

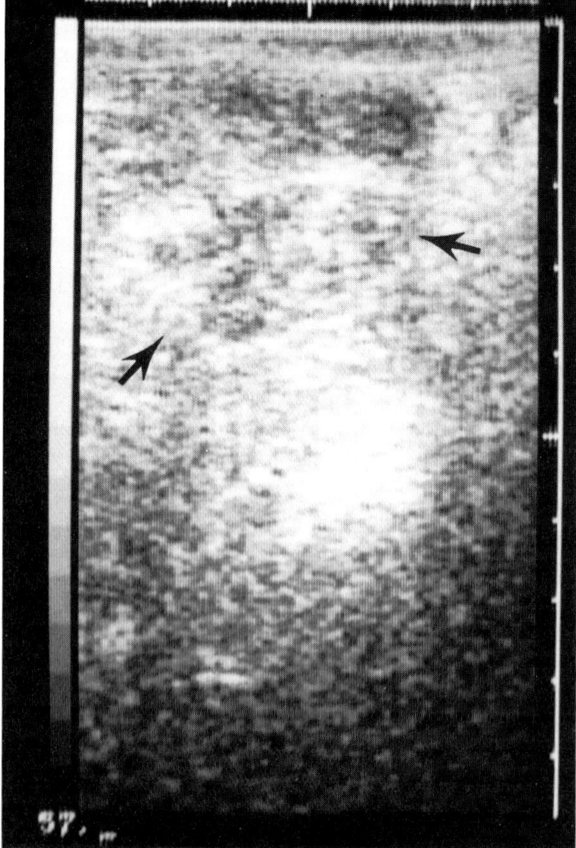

FIG. 24–9. Ultrasonographic image of a uterine horn (arrows) from a mare in anestrus. Notice flat and irregular outline and close contour to surrounding organs.

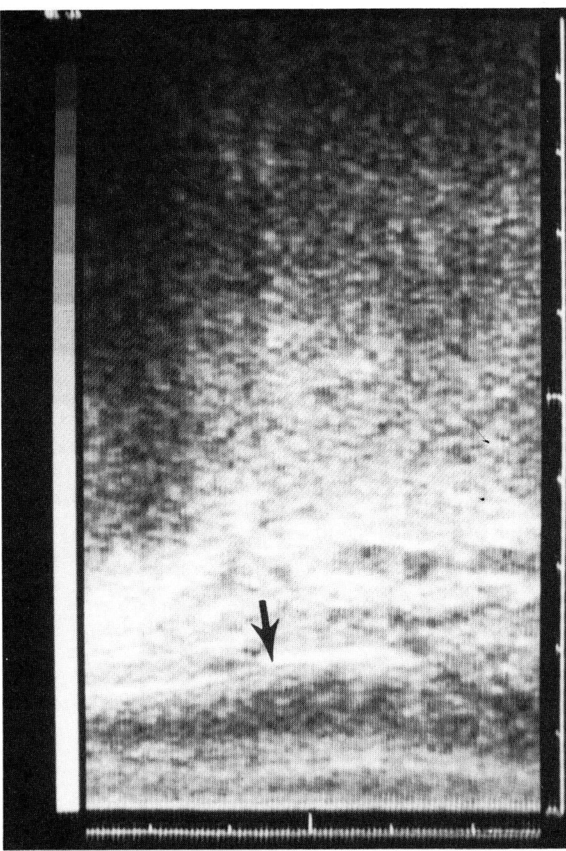

FIG. 24–10. Ultrasonographic image of a uterine body (arrow) from a mare in anestrus. Structure is flat.

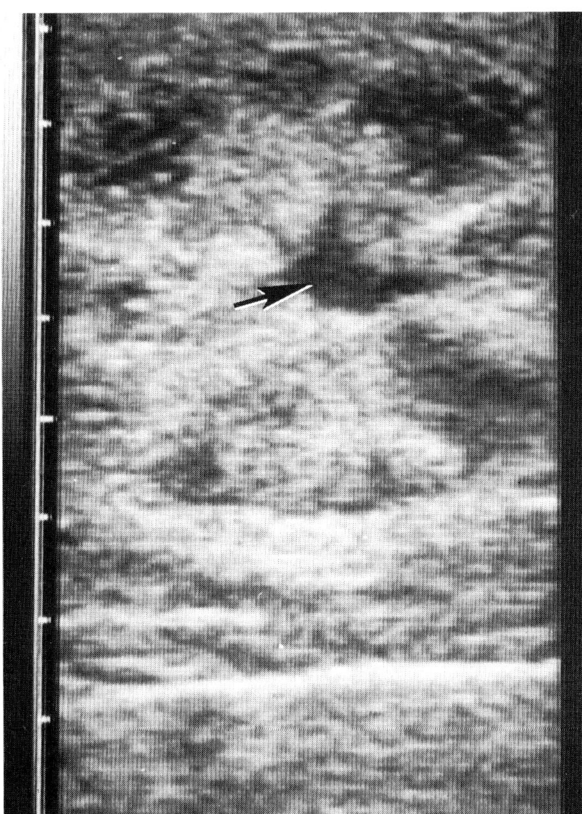

FIG. 24–11. Ultrasonographic image of a uterine horn from a mare in estrus. Presence of endometrial folds in this image is not an indication of endometritis. However, fluid (arrow) within the lumen may be a sign of uterine infection.

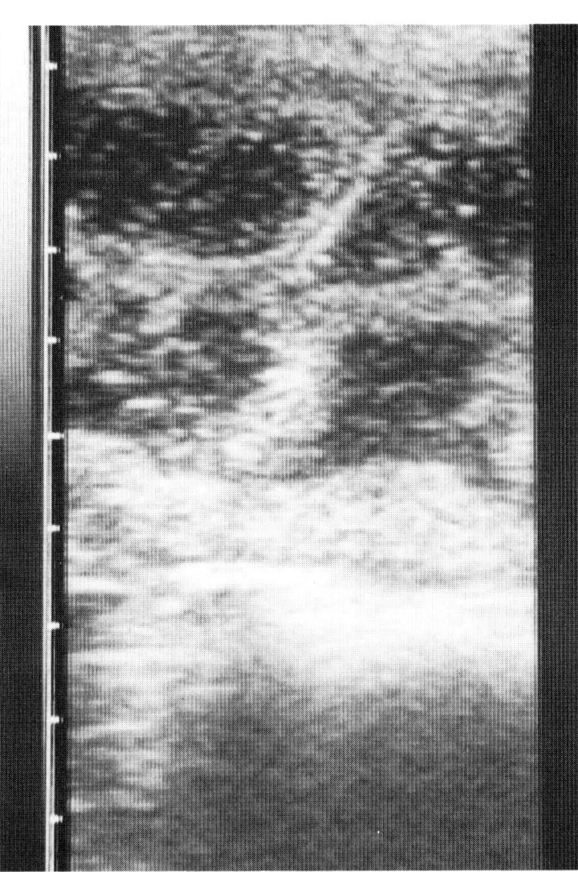

FIG. 24–12. Ultrasonographic image of the uterine body from a mare in estrus. Body of uterus is rounded and has an interdigitated pattern of alternating echogenic and nonechogenic areas.

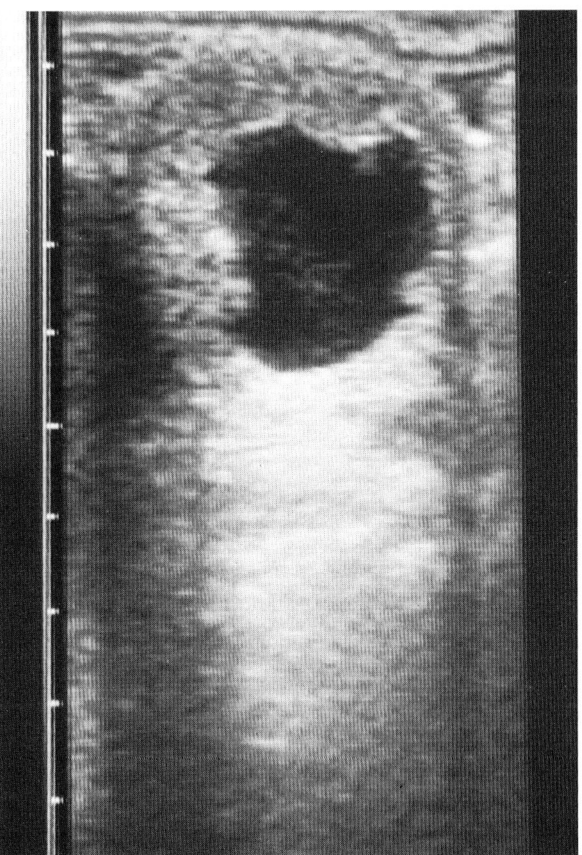

FIG. 24–13. Ultrasonographic image of a 20-day pregnancy with slight endometrial folding.

In one report, ultrasonographic properties of the uteri of 16 mares were determined each day of the cycle.[4] Endometrial folds were not distinguishable during diestrus and were most prominent during estrus. The number of mares with intermediate or images characteristic of estrus increased gradually from day −7 (2/14) (day of ovulation equals day 0) to day −3 (11/16), to day −2 (10/16), then declined between days −1 and +1 (0/12). From a preliminary study, involving 100 mare cycles, endometrial folds were graded from 0 (no folds) to 3 (prominent endometrial folds) and were most prominent 1 or 2 days before ovulation (Table 24–2).[6] A change to a lower grade could be used to predict ovulation. For example, a change from grade 3 to 0 was concomitant with ovulation. Practitioners should be aware of the extent of change in height of endometrial folds between diestrus and early estrus. Prominence of endometrial folds during estrus (Figs. 24–11 and 24–12) should not be considered pathologic. Before the observation became common knowledge, some veterinary practitioners mistook prominent endometrial folds for endometritis, and unnecessarily treated mares. Ability to clearly observe endometrial folds depends on transducer frequency and resolution of ultrasonographic equipment. On occasion, impending early embryonic death is suspected when during routine scanning for pregnancy, the embryonic vesicle is located in a uterus with prominent endometrial folds.

When a mare is in diestrus, individual endometrial folds are less distinct, or not discernible and the echo texture is more homogeneous (see Fig. 24–6). When scanning the uterine body, the uterine lumen is often identified by a hyperechogenic white line. This is the result of apposition of endometrial surfaces, and probably is caused by specular reflection.[4] In general, during diestrus the entire uterine portion of the reproductive tract is well circumscribed and defined.

Ultrasonographic images of the pregnant uterus are often identical to those of diestrus with the exception that after day 16, slight endometrial folds may again be visualized. However, endometrial folds (Fig. 24–13) are not as prominent as during estrus and may be associated with increasing uterine tone.

TABLE 24–2. NUMBER OF MARES DISPLAYING ENDOMETRIAL FOLDS IN RELATION TO DAY OF OVULATION

GRADE OF ENDOMETRIAL FOLDS	TIME FROM OVULATION (DAYS)*				
	−3	−2	−1	0	+2
0	73	27	33	64	95
1	3	17	24	24	4
2	18	35	27	12	1
3	6	21	16	0	0

*Day of ovulation = day 0.

(Adapted from McKinnon, A.O., et al.: Diagnostic ultrasonography of uterine pathology in the mare. Proc. Am. Assoc. Equine Pract., 605–622, 1987.)

ARTIFACTS

Certain types or formations of tissue may cause waves to bend (refract), bounce back and forth or re-echo (reverberate) or to become weakened or entirely blocked. These distortions may be mistaken for normal or pathologic structures or changes. Fluid-filled structures such as follicles, embryonic vesicles, and uterine cysts are common in the mare's reproductive tract and are responsible for causing the most notable artifacts. An intense echogenic formation beneath a fluid-filled structure is noted as an enhanced through-transmission artifact (Fig. 24–14). This artifact is common beneath images of follicles and embryonic vesicles. Sound waves passing through fluid are not as attenuated as waves passing through adjacent tissue. Therefore, a brighter echo exists beneath the fluid-filled structure when compared with echos of corresponding depth beneath adjacent tissues. Intensity of echos resulting from through-transmission can be reduced by proper adjustment of gain controls.[1]

When an ultrasonic beam strikes the side of a curved structural boundary at less than 90°, it may bend or refract, causing a shadowing or lack of echo formation beyond the site of refraction. Refraction artifacts are es-

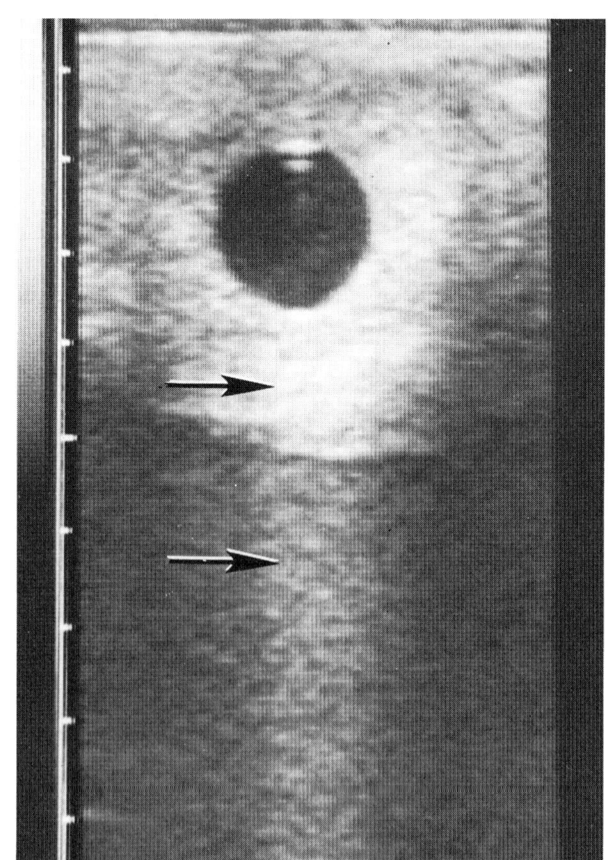

FIG. 24–14. Ultrasonographic image of enhanced through-transmission artifact (arrows) beneath the image of an embryonic vesicle.

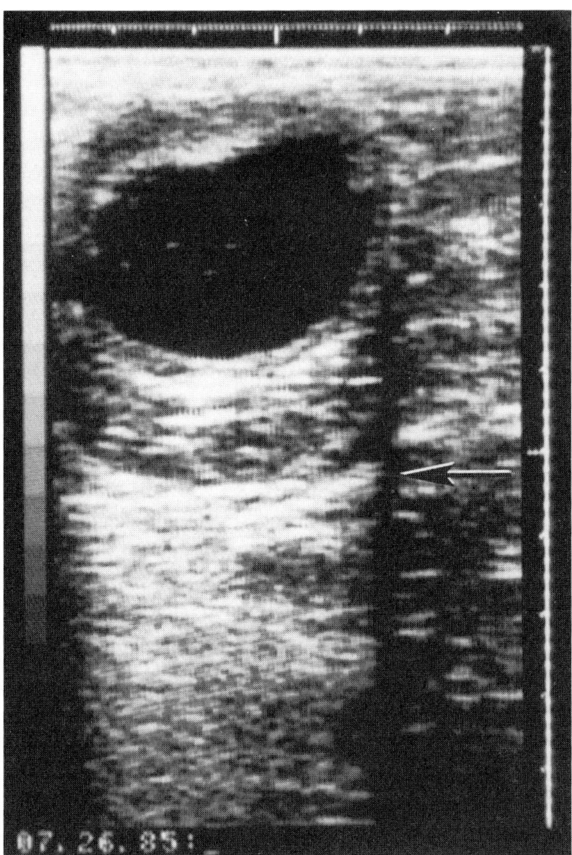

FIG. 24–15. Ultrasonographic refraction creating an artifact beneath the edges of an ovary (arrow).

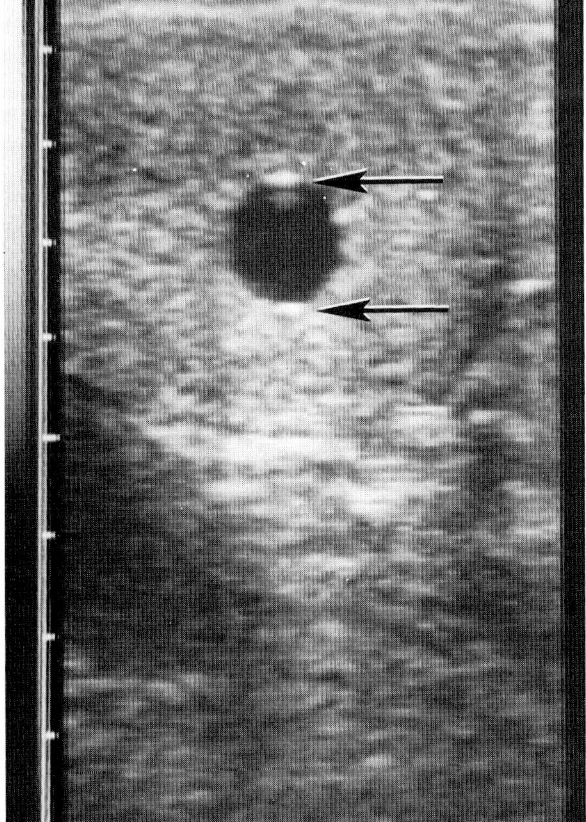

FIG. 24–16. Ultrasonographic image of specular reflection (arrows).

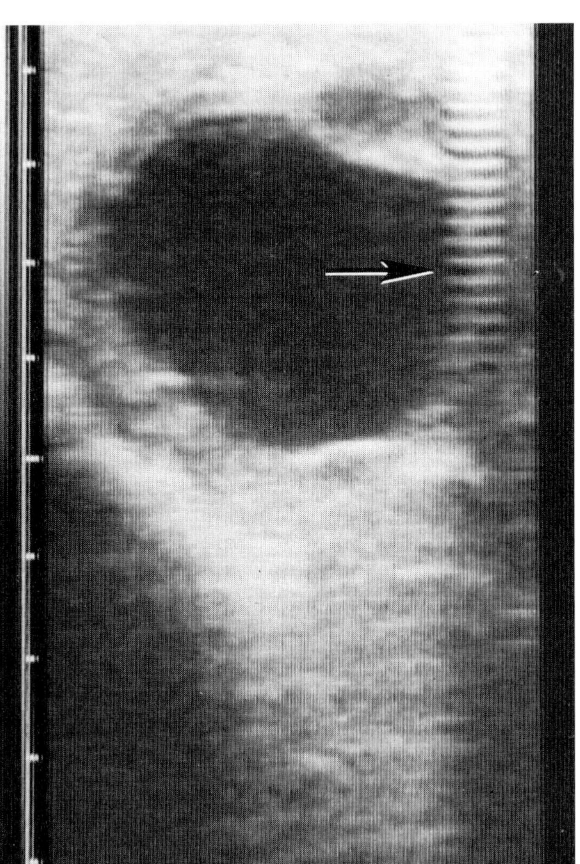

FIG. 24–17. Ultrasonographic image of reverberation artifact (arrow).

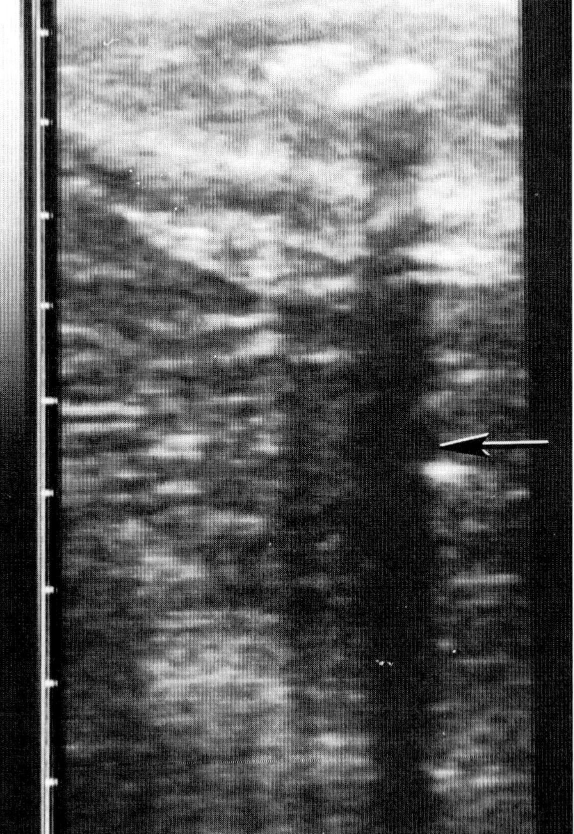

FIG. 24–18. Ultrasonographic image of shadowing (arrow) from a foreign body (tip of uterine culturette).

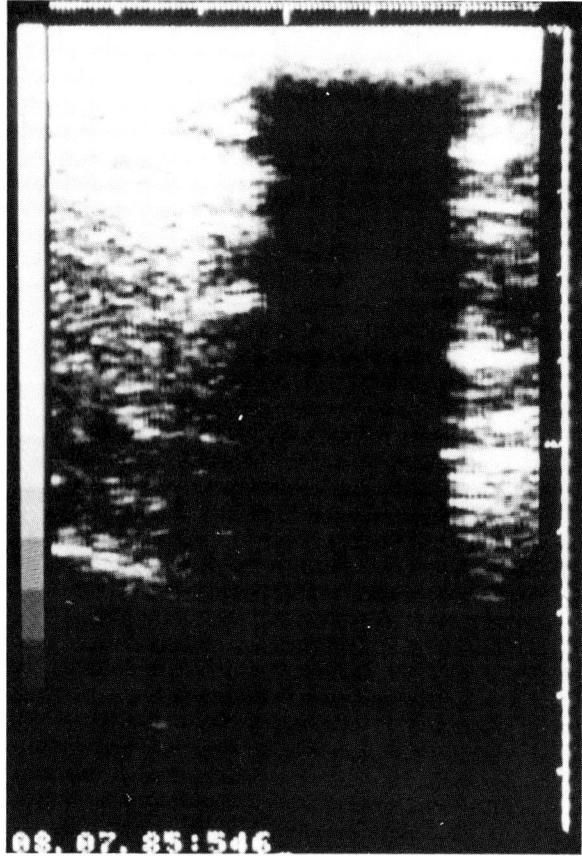

FIG. 24–19. Ultrasonographic image of shadowing caused by fecal material on the transducer.

pecially common with images associated with follicles (Fig. 24–15).

When an ultrasonic beam strikes the upper and lower surface of a fluid-filled, spherical structure, a highly echogenic reflection is produced on the screen. This is termed specular reflection (Fig. 24–16). Specular reflection was originally confused and incorrectly identified as being embryonic structure.

Reverberation artifacts (Fig. 24–17) are commonly seen during intrarectal examination of the mare's reproductive tract because of gas-filled intestines around the area of interest. Reverberation occurs when sound waves encounter a highly reflective, gas-filled structure and bounce back and forth between intestine and transducer. Because of the lag time of each returning echo as perceived by the transducer, bright echos are recorded on the screen at deeper and deeper, evenly spaced intervals.

Shadowing is an artifact characterized by lack of an echo beneath a dense structure and is caused by complete reflection or absorption of ultrasonographic waves. This artifact is uncommon in images of mares' reproductive system because of the relative lack of tissues with density comparable to bone. A notable exception is the occurrence of shadowing beneath fetal bone after death of the fetus, and occasionally from foreign bodies such as a tip of a uterine culturette (Fig. 24–18). The presence of fecal material on the transducer may also result in portions of the ultrasonographic image being obscured because of a shadowing artifact (Fig. 24–19).

REFERENCES

1. Ginther, O.J., and Pierson, R.A.: Ultrasonic evaluation of the reproductive tract of the mare; principles, equipment and techniques. J. Equine Vet. Sci., *3*:195–201, 1983.
2. Ginther, O.J., and Pierson, R.A.: Ultrasonic evaluation of the reproductive tract of the mare: Ovaries. J. Equine Vet. Sci., *4*:11–16, 1984.
3. McKinnon, A.O., Squires, E.L., and Voss, J.L.: Ultrasound evaluation of the mare's reproductive tract—Part I. Compend. Contin. Educ. Practicing Vet., *9*:336–349, 1987.
4. Ginther, O.J., and Pierson, R.A.: Ultrasonic anatomy and pathology of the equine uterus. Theriogenology, *21*:505–515, 1984.
5. McKinnon, A.O., Squires, E.L., and Voss, J.L.: Ultrasound evaluation of the mare's reproductive tract—Part II. Compend. Contin. Educ. Practicing Vet., *9*:472–482, 1987.
6. McKinnon, A.O., et al.: Diagnostic ultrasonography of uterine pathology in the mare. Proc. Am. Assoc. Equine Pract., 605–622, 1987.

CHAPTER 25

VAGINAL EXAMINATION

M.M. LeBlanc

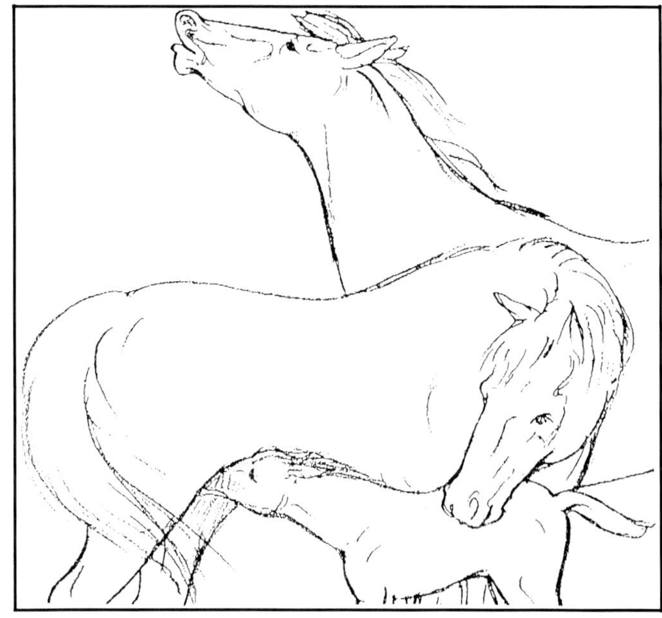

Vaginoscopic examination is an essential part of a reproductive evaluation. It is extremely helpful in identifying stage of the estrous cycle, pathologic changes, and anatomic variations. Inflammatory changes, such as mucosal hyperemia, vesicovaginal reflux (urine pooling), and suppurative exudates, often are discovered. In addition, persistent hymen, rectovaginal defects, and other conditions affecting fertility may be confirmed.

PREPARATION AND TECHNIQUE

Preparation of the mare for vaginal examination requires restraint, preferably in stocks or in a stall and out of direct sunlight. The tail should be wrapped and the perineal area washed carefully with a nonirritating soap. After ample rinsing, the labia should be blotted dry and clean, moist cotton used to wipe the inner edges of the labia and clitoral fossa. Scrubbing the perineal region reduces the number of bacteria present on the lips of the vulva; however, organisms including Streptococcus zooepidemicus and Escherichia coli, can reside in the clitoral fossa of normal mares. Low numbers of these bacteria have also been recovered from the vestibule.[1] Because these organisms may serve as a source of uterine inoculum during vaginal or uterine manipulations, the clitoral fossa should be avoided when passing a speculum into the vagina.

The speculum should be inserted into the vestibule at a craniodorsad directed 45° angle. The lips of the vulva need to be retracted manually at the time of insertion and the speculum eased into the vestibule by twisting it along the long axis. Once the speculum has been passed through the vestibular sphincter, it is directed horizontally (Fig. 25-1). Resistance will be encountered at the vulvovaginal fold (vestibulovaginal sphincter) in normal mares during estrus. In mares with poor perineal conformation, the speculum will fall easily into the anterior vagina. The vulvovaginal fold serves as a barrier to ascending bacterial invasion of the cranial tract (see Chapter 2). This seal is frequently incomplete or lost in older mares leading to pneumovagina and an increased susceptibility to endometritis. The integrity of the vulvovaginal fold is best evaluated during estrus using an unlubricated vaginal speculum. When performing a vaginal examination during a progesterone-dominant phase, sterile lubricant needs to be liberally applied to a speculum before insertion.

INSTRUMENTATION

Various types of speculum are available for vaginal examination (Fig. 25-2). Each has its advantages and disadvantages. The metal trivalve (Caslisk) speculum provides excellent visibility of the cervix and anterior vagina. It is used for evaluation of cervical tears, rectal-vaginal fistulas, and assessment of integrity of urethral extensions. It is, however, cumbersome to sterilize and relatively expensive. Disposable, sterile black plastic,

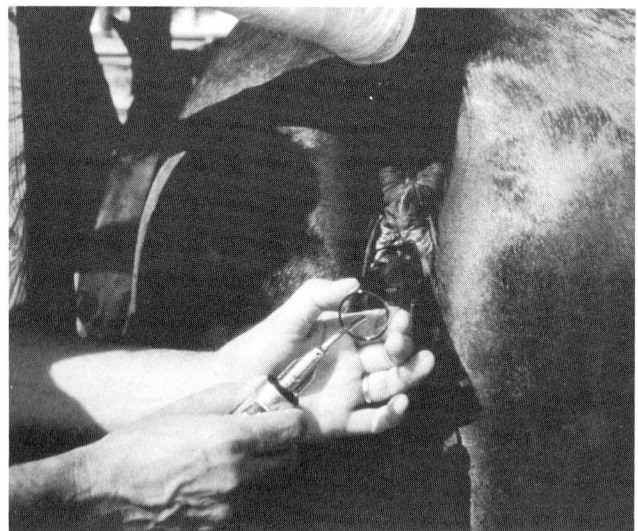

FIG. 25–1. Insertion of glass tube used as a vaginal speculum with mare in stocks.

white plastic, or cardboard specula provide excellent visibility of the cervical os, are inexpensive, and can be discarded after use. They do not provide good visualization of the vaginal mucosa nor can the competency of the vestibulovaginal sphincter be evaluated because these specula require an ample application of sterile lubricant to facilitate insertion. A glass tubular speculum for vaginal examination is preferred. It is readily and inexpensively made from heat-resistant glass tubing cut to 35- to 38-cm (14- to 15-in.) lengths and fire polished. These specula are easily cleaned, can be autoclaved individually, are easily passed into the cranial vagina, and permit maximum visualization. The major disadvantage is they shatter if dropped.

A bright beam of light focally directed is needed to assess the vaginal walls and cervix (Fig. 25–1). Light sources include penlights, halogen illuminators attached to either long- or short-handled transilluminators (Welsh Allyn Halogen Illuminator; Fig. 25–2), and flashlights. Penlights and ophthalmic light sources are considered superior to flashlights because they transmit a brighter and more focally directed light beam. Light sources need to be recharged or batteries need to be replaced frequently to maintain a bright light beam.

HORMONAL INFLUENCE ON VAGINAL AND CERVICAL APPEARANCE

Vaginoscopic examinations help determine stage of the estrous cycle.[2] In estrus, the cervix softens and drops toward the floor of the vagina. During maximal relaxation, 24 to 48 h before ovulation, the cervix of multiparous mares flattens on the vaginal floor and the opening of the os presents as a horizontal slit. Maiden and younger mares usually have a lesser degree of softening. This configuration has been referred to as a "wilted rose." Edema, mucus secretion, and hyperemia of both the cervical and vaginal mucosa are present and correlate with estrogen secretion by the developing follicle. Early in estrus, the external cervical os commonly has edematous folds of mucosa, which resolve as ovulation approaches. Mucus secretion appears as an increasing shine of the cervical and vaginal mucosal. Estrogens also enhance the blood supply to the reproductive tract causing hyperemia, which is manifested as a pink color of all visible surfaces. Inflammatory and physiologic changes of the cervix and vagina can be determined by evaluating the degree of hyperemia. Evaluations must be made shortly after dilation of the vagina because artifactual reddening can be produced quickly by air contact with the tissues.

In diestrus, the cervical and vaginal surfaces become pale and dry. The color of the membranes is typically gray or pale white with a yellowish cast. The external cervical os projects into the cranial vagina from high on the wall and is tightly contracted lending itself to the terms high, dry, and tight, or rose bud. The appearance of the cervix correlates well with the elongated, firm consistency felt on rectal palpation.

In pregnancy, the cervix may be intensely white and tightly closed. In late pregnancy, the mucosa of the vaginal wall is covered by a thick, sticky exudate, which prevents the usual ballooning effect caused by introducing a speculum.[3] It is sometimes difficult to visualize the cervical os late in pregnancy because it is pulled cranioventrad. The gonadal steroids estrogen and progesterone produce specific visual clues in the speculum examination. Total lack of steroid production likewise results in a typical picture. Inactive ovaries are

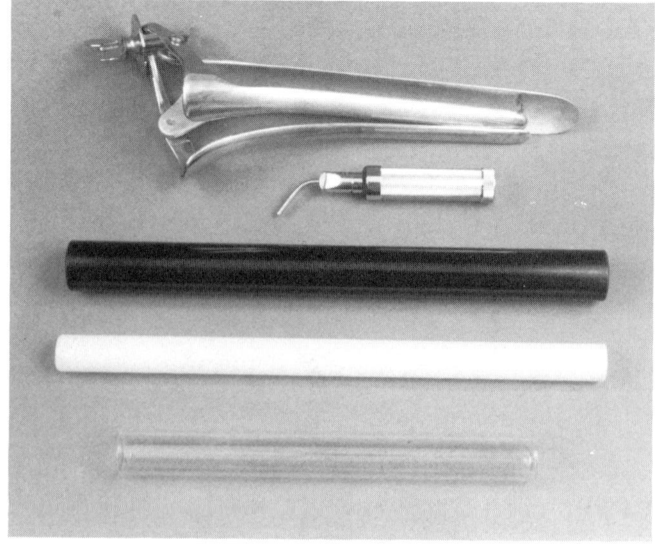

FIG. 25–2. Specula available for vaginoscopy in the mare. The Caslick speculum is at the top. Light source is a Welsh Allyn Halogen Illuminator.

commonly found in winter anestrus and in conditions of gonadal dysgenesis. Cervical and vaginal color in anestrus is blanched, almost white. The cervix becomes atonic and flaccid and often gapes open to reveal the uterine lumen. Blood vessels are scarce on the vaginal wall and little hyperemia occurs after exposure to air.

DIGITAL EXAMINATION OF THE VAGINA AND CERVIX

Evaluation of the mare's reproductive tract is incomplete without manually examining the vaginal and cervical lumen. Aseptic technique is essential, both in preparation of the mare and of the hand and arm of the examiner. A sterile shoulder-length glove is ideal, but a practical alternative is a clean plastic sleeve with a sterile surgeon's glove applied over it. Lubrication should be with a sterile, water-soluble product. When the gloved hand is introduced into the mare's vagina, the labia should be parted with the fingers of the other hand to reduce contamination. The vestibular-vaginal junction should be tight, making it difficult for the examiner to pass his or her hand. If the examiner's hand slips easily into the anterior vagina, the mare may be predisposed to pneumovagina. The hymen area should be palpated in maiden mares to ensure the absence of tissue bands formed by hymen remnants. These bands could later contribute to a rectovaginal perforation at parturition. Manual vaginal examination also aids in the assessment of small vaginal tears, vaginal adhesions, or minute rectovaginal fistulas, which may be felt more easily than seen.

The cervix should always be palpated directly if a complete reproductive examination is performed. By carefully dilating the external os and then palpating the entire cervical canal, it is possible to locate lacerations and adhesions not evident by vaginoscopy.

EXUDATES AND THEIR ORIGIN

The source of exudates seen at the lips of the vulva can usually be determined by vaginoscopy.[2,3] Inflammatory changes caused by endometritis are seen most frequently on the second or third day of estrus, after the perineum has relaxed under the influence of estrogens and prior to the flushing action of the increased secretions. On speculum examination, a grayish, watery to white, purulent exudate may be present on the vaginal floor. Exudate may be seen passing out of the cervical os from the uterus and the vaginal mucosa may be hyperemic. If pneumovagina is present, the mucus and exudate will often have a "foamy" appearance because air has mixed with the mucus.[4]

The pooling of urine (vesicovaginal reflux) in the cranial fornix of the vagina is seen in older, multiparous mares that have developed problems associated with pneumovagina, such as a pelvic canal that slopes cranioventrad. Many times it is observed in those mares only during estrus on the day before ovulation when estrogen levels and perineal relaxation are highest. It may be transient, as seen during the first postpartum estrus when the vaginal structures are stretched, relaxed, and pulled forward by the weight of the involuting uterus.[4] Fluid in the vaginal fornix may be confirmed to be urine by visual inspection of color, by smell, or biochemically (osmolality, urea content).[2] On speculum examination, the urine often covers at least a portion if not the entire cervix. Inflammatory cells are often mixed with the urine and its salt sediment. In severe cases, the urine flows into the uterus when the cervix is relaxed which causes cervicitis and endometritis.

Vaginal varicosities in the region of the perforated hymen are not uncommon.[4] These varicosities may rupture late in pregnancy leading to blood dripping from the vulvar lips. If observed at breeding, the bleeding must be differentiated from vaginal rupture. Varicose veins are detected by speculum examination of the hymen. They usually are 1 to 2 cm in diameter and the color of venous blood inside a bluish translucent vein wall (Chapter 70).

DELETERIOUS CONSEQUENCES FROM VAGINAL EXAMINATION

Once the health of the genital tract has been established, consistent routine vaginoscopic examinations may be deleterious. Repeated exposure of the vagina, cervix, and uterus to air, with its accompanying contaminants, may produce unnecessary irritation and inflammation. This is a major consideration in older mares with lowered resistance to contamination. Many mares with a relaxed cervix will experience distension of the uterus with air after speculum examination. This air should be expressed by rectal compression of the distended genital tract.

ENDOMETRIAL CULTURE THROUGH A SPECULUM

It may be beneficial in mares susceptible to endometritis to obtain endometrial swabs through a speculum placed in the vagina and avoid introducing a swab manually. If an endometrial swab is introduced manually, both the outside of the culture instrument and the finger used to cannulate the cervix are exposed to bacteria in the vulvar and vestibular area. If the culture instrument is introduced via the speculum, it is protected from the vulvar and vestibular area, and it is the only thing except air contacting the cervix and uterus.

REFERENCES

1. Hinrichs, K., Cummings, M.R., Sertech, P.L., and Kenney, R.M.: Clinical significance of aerobic bacterial flora of the uterus, vagina, vestibule, and clitoral fossa of clinically normal mares. J. Am. Vet. Med. Assoc., *193*:72–75, 1988.
2. Asbury, A.C.: Examination of the mare. *In* Equine Medicine and Surgery. Edited by P. Colahan, I. Mayhew, A. Merritt, and J. Moore. Goleta, American Veterinary Publishers, 1991, pp. 954–955.
3. Rossdale, P.D., and Ricketts, S.W.: Equine Stud Farm Medicine. Philadelphia, Lea & Febiger, 1980, pp. 51–52.
4. Neely, D.P., Liu, I.K.M., and Hillman, R.B.: Evaluation and therapy of genital disease in the mare. *In* Equine Reproduction. Edited by J.P. Hughes. Princeton Junction, Veterinary Learning Systems, 1983, pp. 53–55.

CHAPTER 26

ENDOMETRIAL BIOPSY

P.A. Doig
R.O. Waelchli

Endometrial biopsy is an integral part of breeding soundness evaluation of brood mares. The main value of the technique has been to provide a basis for predicting future ability of the uterus to carry a foal to term. The technique is also useful in detecting changes associated with reduced fertility that are not easily diagnosed by other methods and for monitoring response to specific uterine therapy. Although not foolproof or the final answer to fertility assessment, it is valuable when used in conjunction with detailed reproductive examination to increase accuracy of both diagnosis and prognosis.

INDICATIONS

Endometrial biopsy is indicated in any nonpregnant mare in which uterine disease is suspected. The only known contraindication is pregnancy.[1] The following conditions warrant the use of endometrial biopsy.[1]

1. *Barren Mares.* Maiden mares or mares that have previously foaled and are presently not pregnant, although they have been bred during the most recent breeding season, using good breeding management practices.
2. *Repeat Breeder Mares during the Physiologic Breeding Season.* These mares may be defined as nonpregnant mares that have been bred within 48 h before ovulation in three or more cycles with semen of normal fertility.
3. *Mares with a History of Early Embryonic Death or Abortion.*
4. *Behaviorally Anestrous Nonpregnant Mares during the Physiologic Breeding Season.* Includes mares in which behavioral signs of estrus do not occur at the same time as physiologic changes and in mares with hypoplasia of ovaries and tubular genitalia. Other causes include prolonged diestrus, debilitation, disease of the hypothalamus or pituitary gland, or granulosa cell tumour.
5. *Mares Requiring Genital Surgery.* The endometrium of mares with a surgical problem involving the vulva, vagina, cervix, uterus, or ovary (pneumovagina, urovagina, rectovaginal lacerations or fistulas, cervical adhesions and tears, granulosa cell tumor, uterine leiomyoma) may not be capable of supporting a pregnancy to term. The probability of the mare carrying a foal to term should obviously be determined before any surgical intervention.
6. *Pyometra and Mucometra.* Generally, mares with pyometra have a poor chance of conceiving and carrying a foal to term. Endometrial biopsy should be performed after the uterus has involuted and the uterine contents removed.
7. *Fertility Evaluation.* An endometrial biopsy is indicated in cases of a prepurchase examination of a brood mare or in other cases where a written certificate relating to reproductive potential is required.

The usual time for evaluating endometrial biopsies is just before or during the physiologic breeding season, when mares are presented for prebreeding evaluation.

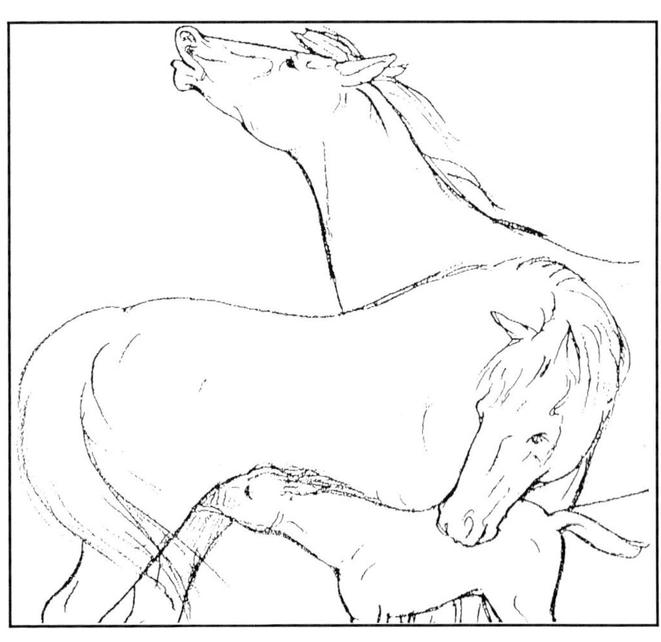

However, sampling at that time may not allow sufficient time for recovery in mares needing treatment. Mares found barren when examined in the fall should be biopsied at that time. This allows for sufficient time to carry out treatment and mares can be reassessed early in the spring when cycles have recommenced. Samples in the spring, during the transition phase from winter anestrus, can also be useful to detect mares that may be cycling, but have not yet recovered endometrially from seasonal atrophy. Many of those mares are unlikely to be ready for breeding during the following 30 to 60 days,[2] and their identification can be valuable on busy breeding farms.

TECHNIQUE

A variety of instruments has been used to obtain acceptable endometrial samples. Either a trocar cannula type (Equibov Veterinary Specialty Equipment, Campbellville, Ontario, Canada) or a larger alligator jaw (Pilling Surgical Instrument Co., Fort Washington, PA) instrument has been used. For proper interpretation, specimens should be of sufficient size to provide at least 1 to 2 cm of endometrium on the histologic section.[3]

In the absence of palpable uterine abnormalities, one sample is essentially representative of the endometrium as a whole.[3–7] When palpably variable areas are detected, a sample should be obtained from each as well as from the uniform area.

Because the equine cervix is easily dilated, samples may be obtained at any stage of the estrous cycle. The endometrial architecture changes with the stage of the cycle and the season of the year.[3,8] For this reason, the person evaluating the biopsy should be informed of the stage of cycle and physical findings at the time the sample was taken.

Detailed descriptions of the sampling technique are available.[2,3,5] Fixatives most commonly used are 10% formalin and Bouin's solution. Bouin's solution tends to produce a firmer specimen than formalin with less tissue distortion on sectioning. Following 2 to 4 h in Bouin's solution, the tissues should be transferred to 10% formalin before being transported to the laboratory. Excessive fixation in Bouin's solution may result in dense specimens, which do not stain well with hematoxylin. Routine histologic procedures are followed and the sections are stained with hematoxylin and eosin (H&E).

NORMAL ENDOMETRIAL ANATOMY

Histologic characteristics observed in endometrial biopsy specimens may be physiologic (cyclic or seasonal), pathologic, or artifactual. [3,5] A knowledge of normal cyclic and seasonal changes is critical for the assessment and interpretation of pathologic changes. Numerous reports have described the normal structure of the endometrium and only most relevant features will be discussed in this section.[3,5,9–11]

Characteristics that should be noted include height of luminal epithelium, configuration of glands, and amount of edema in the lamina propria. These characteristics may vary with seasonal and cyclic changes. Endometrial biopsy, as a part of fertility examination, may be performed during any season and often the clinician is not aware of the actual stage of cycle. Although typical characteristics can be seen in many mares at known stages of the cycle, a correct estimation of stage of cycle based on histologic features alone, may not be possible in every mare. Considerable variations can occur among individual mares and also among different sections of a biopsy specimen.

During anestrus, endometrial glands are inactive (Fig. 26–1). Luminal and glandular epithelial cells may be either cuboidal or squamous. Epithelial cells have increased basophilia of cytoplasm. Individual gland branches have a small cross-sectional diameter, and in longitudinal section, glands appear as thin, straight tubes. Edema of the lamina propria, other than artifactual, is uncommon. Glandular atrophy of the anestrous endometrium may not be uniform. Scattered nonatrophic glands with low columnar epithelium may occur. Glandular atrophy is generally more pronounced in areas distant from the lumen. Epithelium of glandular ducts is often low columnar with paler-staining cytoplasm than that of deeper glands. Groups of closely associated glands in cross section, resulting from coiling of gland branches, are common in deep areas of anestrous endometrium.

Histologic characteristics of transitional endometrium are not clearly defined. Correct interpretation may be further complicated by erratic estrous behavior of the mare and variable ovarian findings during rectal palpation. During transition from winter anestrus to the period of cyclicity, the endometrium gradually resumes its activity. Luminal and glandular epithelial cells often reflect different degrees of activity. Luminal and upper glandular epithelial cells are the first to become active and may be columnar, while deep gland sections remain inactive with low epithelial cells. The reverse may

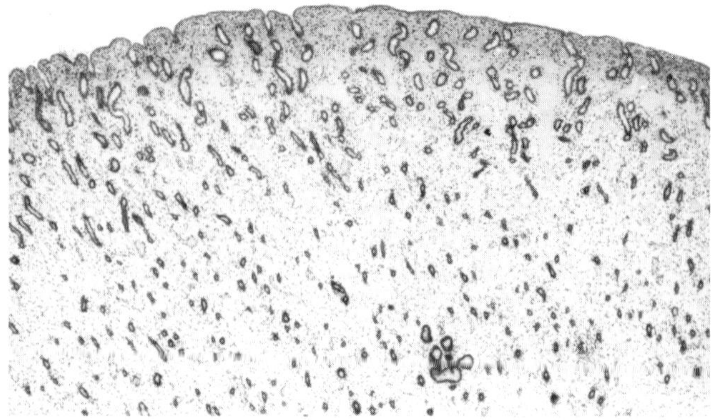

FIG. 26–1. Endometrial section from a seasonally anestrous mare. Luminal and glandular epithelial cells are mostly cuboidal, and the inactive glands have contracted lumina (× 82).

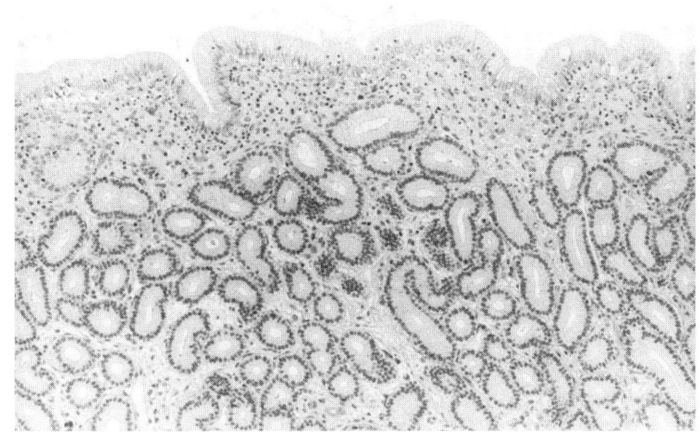

FIG. 26–2. Endometrial section from an estrous mare. Luminal and glandular epithelial cells are tall columnar. Mild acute endometritis is reflected by polymorphonuclear leukocytes scattered in the stratum compactum and migrating through the luminal epithelium (× 205).

be observed in other parts of the same specimen where the glandular epithelium may appear more active than the luminal epithelium.

During estrus, luminal and glandular epithelial cells are usually columnar to tall columnar (Fig. 26–2). Cells are pale staining, and vacuoles in the basal portion of luminal epithelium are common. However, variations often occur, and in some estrous mares or in certain sections of a specimen, these characteristics may not be as pronounced as in others. Polymorphonuclear leukocytes (PMNs) are often located in capillaries under the epithelium and along margins of venules in the lamina propria. During estrus, considerable edema of the lamina propria may exist, which must be differentiated from artifactual edema caused by the biopsy procedure. Because of tall epithelial cells, glandular branches in cross section have a large diameter, and on longitudinal section, glands appear relatively straight and nontortuous.

During diestrus, epithelial cells can vary from columnar to cuboidal, depending on stage relative to preceding or subsequent estrous periods. Glandular branches in diestrus are often tortuous, and on longitudinal section, they may adopt what has been described as a "string of pearls" appearance[3] (Fig. 26–3).

HISTOLOGIC CHANGES

Endometrial lesions observed on histologic examination include glandular degeneration, lymphatic lacunae, endometrial atrophy, and cellular infiltrations.[2,3,5,11,12]

GLANDULAR DEGENERATION

Degenerative changes include periglandular fibrosis, cystic dilation of glands, and glandular necrosis. Fibrosis most commonly occurs around glands or in association with the basement membrane of the luminal epithelium. When convoluted gland branches are involved, fibrotic glandular nests are formed, which vary in size depending on the number of branches involved (Fig. 26–4). Number of layers of fibrosis around gland branches or nests can vary from 2 or 3 in mild cases, to more than 10 when fibrosis is severe.[13] Widespread fibrosis, regardless of severity, has a more detrimental effect than localized changes on ability of the uterus to carry a foal to term.[3] For this reason, frequency with which fibrosed nests occur (number per linear field) is a critical component of the classification system.

Fibrosed nests should not be confused with the clustering or bunching of glandular branches, which commonly occurs during seasonal anestrus and the transition period. In those cases, although distinct separation from other glands is observed, no layers of fibrosis surrounding the tightly coiled clusters of gland branches occurs.

Cystic distention of glands is common in fibrosed nests (Fig. 26–5). Widespread mild glandular distention, usually with inspissated secretion, is frequently seen during anestrus and the transitional stage. In some cases, the number of distended glands during transition can be quite high, giving a "Swiss cheese" type appearance to the endometrium. In the majority of cases, transitional glandular distention disappears when the mare enters the physiologic breeding season. When widespread, nonfibrosed glandular distention, usually without inspissated material, persists into the physiologic breeding season, an associated decrease in fertility seems to occur.[3]

Glandular necrosis and destruction is a less common finding, but dramatic, especially when monitored by serial sampling. Although not pathognomonic, glandular necrosis occurring in association with an intense cellular response should alert the clinician to the possibility of a fungal infection.[14]

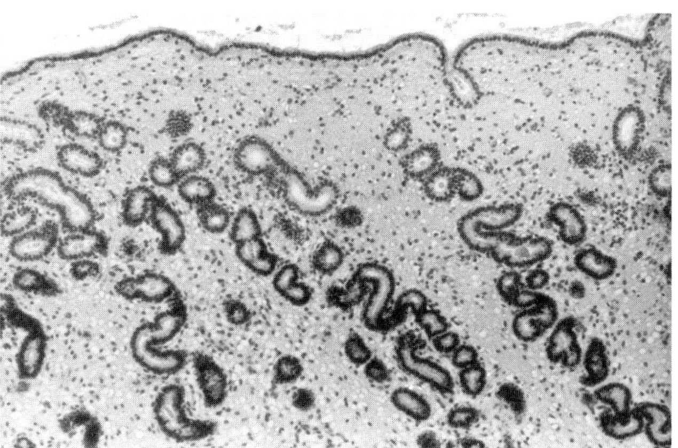

FIG. 26–3. Endometrial section from a diestrous mare. Luminal and glandular epithelial cells are mostly low columnar. Maximum tortuosity of glands is causing a typical "string of pearls" appearance (× 205).

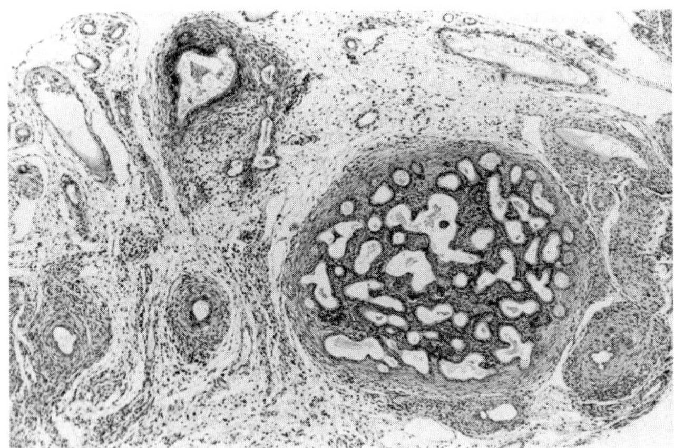

FIG. 26–4. Endometrial section with a fibrotic glandular nest and individual gland branches with severe fibrotic degeneration (× 82).

LYMPHATIC LACUNAE

Derived from dilated lymphatics, lacunae are irregularly shaped areas containing lightly stained eosinophilic material and are surrounded by a thin endothelial margin.[3] Artifactually induced edema can be differentiated because it lacks a regular margin.

ENDOMETRIAL ATROPHY

Characterized by inactive cuboidal luminal and glandular epithelial cells and contraction of the lumen of glands, endometrial atrophy is a typical feature of seasonal anestrus. It is considered abnormal when observed during the physiologic breeding season. Widespread atrophy is caused by a lack of ovarian steroids and is most often seen in aged mares with poor ovarian activity. Endometrial hypoplasia that occurs in mares with gonadal dysgenesis resulting from chromosomal abnormalities, particularly Turner's syndrome (XO), presents similar findings. Senile gland atrophy with apparent reduction of gland numbers, which may be more severe in localized areas, may also be seen in aged mares.

CELLULAR INFILTRATIONS

Cellular infiltrations consist of PMNs, lymphocytes, plasma cells, eosinophils, hemosiderin-laden macrophages, and mast cells. Polymorphonuclear leukocytes are indicative of acute endometritis. In biopsy specimens from mares with acute inflammation of the endometrium, PMNs are usually found in the stratum compactum and between luminal epithelial cells migrating into the uterine lumen (Fig. 26–6). Even in severe cases, a large number of PMNs is not usually seen in the lumen, presumably because the leukocytes are lost during processing. In severe cases, PMNs may be found in deeper layers of the lamina propria. Dilated glands containing degenerated PMNs may be seen in acute endometritis of any degree of severity.

Chronic inflammation is characterized predominantly by infiltrations of lymphocytes and plasma cells and less commonly by eosinophils and mast cells. Like PMNs, chronic infiltrations are most common in the stratum compactum and acute and chronic reactions may be seen together. Chronic reactions are also common deeper in the lamina propria, usually in the form of discrete foci, which may be widely or frequently scattered or may have a diffuse distribution. Chronic inflammation, especially involving plasma cells or when seen in mares after a period of sexual rest, indicates continuing antigenic stimulation and the possibility of an ongoing infectious process.

Eosinophils have been found infrequently in cases of fungal endometritis[14] and are a common component of acute inflammation associated with pneumouterus (wind sucking).[15] Hemosiderin-laden macrophages are commonly seen in biopsy specimens of mares that have recently foaled or aborted.[3]

CORRELATION BETWEEN BIOPSY FINDINGS AND CULTURE RESULTS

Inflammatory lesions of the endometrium are not necessarily associated with the recovery of aerobic bacteria. Association between histologic lesions and uterine infection is especially poor in cases of chronic inflammation.[16] The presence of PMNs is more highly correlated with recovery of bacteria and appears to have an important influence on the breeding outcome.[17]

A recent study compared the value of histologic, cytologic, and bacteriologic examinations in assessing acute inflammation and infection, respectively, and determined subsequent effect on fertility.[18] Samples from

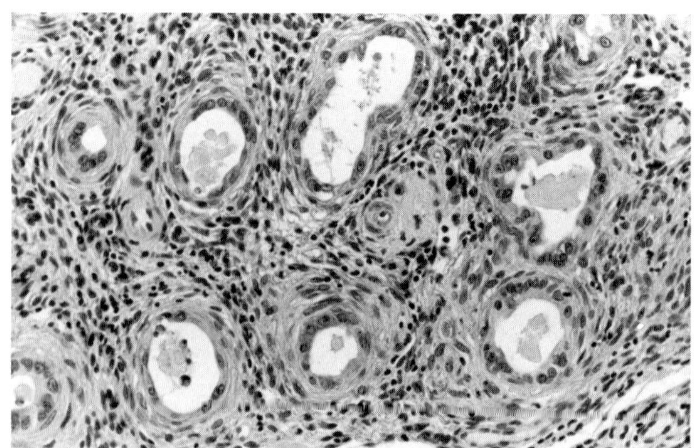

FIG. 26–5. Endometrial section with diffuse fibrosis of individual gland branches. Epithelial cells are atrophied. There is also diffuse infiltration with mononuclear cells (× 410).

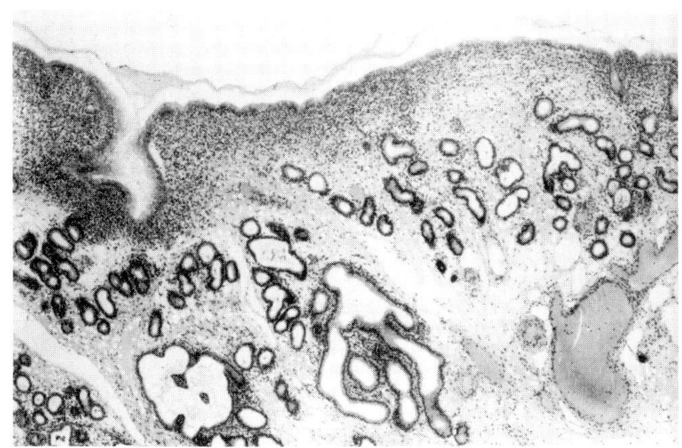

FIG. 26–6. Endometrial section with severe diffuse infiltration of the stratum compactum with polymorphonuclear and mononuclear leukocytes and nonuniform cystic glandular degeneration (× 82).

201 mares were evaluated for the presence of PMNs in the endometrium. Cell numbers were classified as absent, small (widely scattered), or large (frequently scattered to diffuse). Aerobic bacterial culture and cytologic examinations were carried out using standard techniques.[19] Culture results were classified as significant (pure cultures of known pathogens), insignificant (mixed cultures or contaminants), or negative. Conventional uterine therapy was carried out when indicated, based on clinical and laboratory findings and all mares were bred by natural cover. Polymorphonuclear leukocytes were detected in 43 (21%) biopsy specimens and in 26 (13%) cytologic smears. Culture results were considered significant in 18 (9%) cases. Polymorphonuclear leukocytes were present (biopsy and/or cytologic specimens) in all cases where culture results were considered significant. No difference in occurrence of PMNs was observed in cases where culture results were considered insignificant or negative (Table 26–1). Each of the parameters evaluated (recovery of significant bacteria and presence of PMNs in cytologic and histologic samples) was associated with a decrease in subsequent fertility, based on one breeding season, despite various treatments having been carried out (Table 26–2). Minimum contamination breeding techniques, however, were not employed at the time of breeding. The study showed that the presence of large numbers of PMNs in biopsy specimens has a high correlation with the recovery of bacteria considered to be pathogenic, but not those that commonly occur as commensals. Presence of PMNs in large numbers is also associated with poor fertility if the mare is bred by natural cover without steps being taken to minimize bacterial exposure.

Diagnosis of acute endometritis is most reliable using endometrial biopsy, but cytologic examination of an endometrial smear can provide a valuable diagnostic alternative when biopsy results are not available or when an immediate diagnosis is needed. The best approach is to use multiple diagnostic techniques concurrently in the diagnosis of uterine abnormalities.

CATEGORIZATION

Kenney originally proposed a classification system that was based on three categories: an essentially normal group (category I), a severely affected group (category III), and an in-between group (category II).[1] Foaling rates of category I mares were considered to reflect overall breeding management, whereas foaling rates in category III were considered to reflect the severe changes in the endometrium. Foaling rates in category II were considered to reflect endometrial changes, but they may be improved with good management, including veterinary care.

Other researches have used similar grading systems involving three or four categories.[20–26] When foaling rates for each category were determined, a good correlation existed, on a group basis, between the severity of endometrial lesions and the mares' subsequent ability to carry a foal to term (Table 26–3). Ability to carry a foal to term is the best prognostic end point, rather than pregnancy, because pregnant mares may lose the conceptus, as a result of microscopic change in the endometrium.[3,26]

Using the system originally proposed by Kenney as a basis, one study subsequently found that extent of fibrosis could be divided into four categories—absent, mild, moderate, and severe—to allow a more precise prediction of foaling probability.[21] Both rating systems, however, used the same criteria for the most severe group to identify those endometria with extremely poor chance of carrying to term. This is perhaps the most critical feature for any rating system. Any system used must identify a well-defined group of endometria that have an extremely poor potential for carrying a foal to term, because mares with those uteri represent a con-

TABLE 26–1. CORRELATIONS BETWEEN CULTURE RESULTS AND THE OCCURRENCE OF POLYMORPHONUCLEAR LEUKOCYTES IN 201 HISTOLOGIC (H) AND CYTOLOGIC (C) SPECIMENS

CULTURE	*N*	PARAMETERS	*N*	PERCENT*
Significant†	18	H and/or C+	18	100
		H and C−	0	0[ab]
Insignificant‡	62	H and/or C+	14	23
		H and C−	48	77[a]
Negative§	121	H and/or C+	22	18
		H and C−	99	82[b]

*Ratios (H and/or C+ vs. H and C−) with identical superscripts are significantly different ($p < 0.001$).

†Pure cultures of β-hemolytic streptococci, Escherichia coli, Staphylococcus aureus, Klebsiella pneumoniae, and Pseudomonas aeruginosa.

‡Mixed cultures of α-hemolytic streptococci, Actinomyces spp., nonspecified coliforms (lactose positive enterbacteria other than E. coli), aerobe sporing rods, Neisseria spp., nonhemolytic Staphylococcus spp., and plus or minus growth of any type of bacteria.

§No bacterial colonies on primary plate.

(From Waelchli, R.O., Corboz, L., and Winder, N.C.: Comparison of histological, cytological and bacteriological findings in the endometrium of the mare. J. Vet. Med. Assoc., *35*:442–449, 1988.)

TABLE 26–2. CORRELATION BETWEEN HISTOLOGIC AND CYTOLOGIC POLYMORPHONUCLEAR LEUKOCYTES AND BACTERIOLOGIC RESULTS WITH SUBSEQUENT PREGNANCY AND FOALING RATES

	NUMBER BRED	NUMBER PREGNANT	PERCENT	NUMBER FOALING	PERCENT
Histology Negative*	176	113	64	94	55
Histology Positive†	12	0	0‡	0	0‡
Cytology Negative§	170	107	63	91	54
Cytology Positive‖	18	6	33‡	3	17‡
Culture Negative#	115	77	67	61	53
Culture Insignificant#	58	34	59	32	55
Culture Significant#	15	2	13‡	1	7‡

*An average of less than two neutrophilic leukocytes per × 200 field.
†An average of less than or equal to two neutrophilic leukocytes per × 200 field.
‡Chi-square analysis for association: $p < 0.05$.
§No neutrophilic leukocytes observed.
‖Any number of neutrophilic leukocytes observed.
#Definitions pertaining to types of cultures as in Table 26–1.
(Waelchli, R.O.: The diagnostic and prognostic value of endometrial biopsy in the mare under non-uniform breeding management conditions. Habilitationsschrift, Univ. of Zurich, 1990.)

tinuing economic loss to the owner and are unlikely to be improved with treatment.[27] Although those mares are not sterile, they are very poor risks as brood mares, and their identification is a major objective of the biopsy procedure. A synthesis of the original three-category system and the modified four-category system was proposed in 1986.[2]

CATEGORIES

CATEGORY I—NORMAL ENDOMETRIUM

No atrophy is present during the physiologic breeding season and no hypoplasia of glands is observed. Pathologic changes involving inflammation or fibrosis are slight and sparsely scattered.

CATEGORY IIA—MILD ENDOMETRIAL HISTOLOGIC CHANGES

Inflammatory changes are characterized by slight to moderate, diffuse infiltration of the stratum compactum with inflammatory cells or scattered, but frequent, foci in the stratum compactum and stratum spongiosum. Fibrotic changes are frequent and scattered, involving individual glandular branches of any degree of severity (usually one to three layers) or fibrotic nests of glandular branches averaging less than two per 5-mm linear field in at least four fields.

Frequent, scattered glandular branches with moderate cystic distention associated with glandular atrophy or lymphatic lacunae that is so extensive it produces palpable localized changes in the endometrial folds also qualifies for this category. These changes are additive, thus if both inflammatory and fibrotic changes are observed, each of which qualify the endometrium for category IIA, the category is lowered to IIB.

CATEGORY IIB—MODERATE ENDOMETRIAL HISTOLOGIC CHANGES

Inflammation is characterized by widespread, moderate, diffuse infiltration of the stratum compactum with inflammatory cells or moderately severe foci. Fibrosis is widespread and moderate, usually involving four or more layers around individual glandular branches. The number of fibrotic nests of glandular branches averages two to four per 5-mm linear field.

Widespread, but nonuniform, moderate, cystic gland degeneration associated with gland atrophy also qualifies for category IIB. These changes are also additive, and endometria with both inflammatory and fibrotic lesions qualifying for category IIB are lowered to category III.

CATEGORY III—SEVERE ENDOMETRIAL HISTOLOGIC CHANGES

Inflammation characterized by widespread, diffuse, severe infiltration of the stratum compactum with inflammatory cells or uniform widespread fibrosis of individ-

TABLE 26–3. COMPARISON OF CATEGORY FOALING RATES IN STUDIES USING SIMILAR THREE-CATEGORY RATING SYSTEMS

RESEARCHER	FOALING RATE (%)			
	Category I	Category II	Category III	Reference
Kenney*	68	51	11	3
Kenney†	92	67	5	3
Doig	88	64	8	
Ashbury	81	24	6	22
Shideler et al.	61	48	35	24
de la Concha-Bermejillo and Kennedy‡	78	55	36	23
Waelchli	70	34	0	18

*Biopsies performed by 28 veterinary practitioners; breeding management, including stallions, heterogeneous.
†Similar protocol but management less heterogeneous than in series A.
‡Relative to a 2-yr period.

ual glandular branches or fibrotic nests averaging five or more per 5-mm linear field qualify for category III. Widespread, but nonuniform, severe cystic glandular degeneration associated with glandular atrophy, severe glandular atrophy during the physiologic breeding season, or lymphatic lacunae so severe that they produce a palpable "jelly-like" texture of the endometrial folds, also qualify for this category.

Two studies, using similar categorization systems involving four categories, have reported extremely poor foaling rates of category III mares and excellent foaling rates in category I. Categories IIA and IIB had foaling rates that were intermediate in each study, but variable between studies (Table 26–4).[21,26] The variability between studies may have been the result of differences in the interpretation of lesions or other management factors that appear to influence category IIA and IIB foaling rates.

TABLE 26–4. FOALING RATES (PERCENT FOALING) FROM TWO STUDIES USING SIMILAR FOUR-CATEGORY RATING SYSTEMS

CATEGORY	NUMBER FOALING/NUMBER BRED (%)	
	Doig et al.*	Waelchli†
I	47/57 (82)	70/100 (70)
IIA	155/209 (74)	24/57 (42)
IIB	59/129 (46)	5/27 (18)
III	0/8 (0)	0/8 (0)
Overall	261/403 (65)	99/192 (52)

*Doig, P.A., McKnight, J.D., and Miller, R.B.: The use of endometrial biopsy in the infertile mare. Can. Vet. J., *22*:72–76, 1981.
†Waelchli, R.O.: Endometrial biopsy in mares under non-uniform breeding management conditions: Prognostic value and relationship with age. Can. Vet. J., *31*:379–384, 1990.

OTHER FACTORS INFLUENCING PROGNOSIS

AGE

Increased age is associated with a decrease in fertility. Part of the decrease in fertility in older mares is undoubtedly the result of increased severity of endometrial fibrosis. An association has been made between increased severity of fibrosis and an increase in mean age of mares in each category.[21] However, an adverse effect of age that is not related to endometrial changes seems to exist. In one study, mares younger than the median age had foaling rates of 62%, versus only 39% for mares older than the median age.[26] This difference was statistically significant. Within categories, foaling rates for the younger mares were numerically higher than those for older mares, but the difference was only significant in category I mares, which had no endometrial lesions (Table 26–5). More studies are needed to determine if there is a definable point at which age should be considered when predicting foaling probabilities in mares within each endometrial category.

YEARS BARREN

Number of years barren has been shown to have a significant effect on foaling probability of mares with mild (category IIA), or moderate fibrosis (category IIB).[21] Category IIA mares barren 1 yr had foaling rates of 82%, compared with 53% for those barren 2 yr or more. In category IIB, the difference between mares barren 1 yr (62%) and those barren 2 yr or more (28%) was even more dramatic.

Differences were believed to be caused by a reduction or gradual impairment in the ability to clear bacteria from the uterus following breeding, because the years barren effect was diminished through minimum-contamination breeding.[21]

A recent study, which compared fewer mares in each

TABLE 26–5. BREEDING PERFORMANCE OF 192 MARES RELATIVE TO ENDOMETRIAL HISTOLOGIC CATEGORY SUBDIVIDED BY THE CATEGORY MEDIAN AGE

CATEGORY	AGE	NUMBER BRED	NUMBER PREGNANT (%)	NUMBER FOALING (%)	PREGNANCY LOSS (%)
I	4–9	52	47 (90)*	42 (81)*	5 (11)
	10–21	48	32 (67)*	28 (58)*	4 (12)
IIA	5–13	28	16 (57)	13 (46)	3 (19)
	14–22	29	12 (41)	11 (38)	1 (8)
IIB	7–16	15	6 (40)	4 (27)	2 (33)
	17–24	12	3 (25)	1 (8)	2 (67)
III	5–10	4	0 (0)	0 (0)	— —
	11–20	4	0 (0)	0 (0)	— —

*Within category I pregnancy rates ($p < 0.01$) and foaling rates ($p < 0.05$) were different.

category, showed a numerical overall reduction ($p = 0.1$) in foaling rates for mares barren 2 yr or more compared with mares barren 1 yr (58% vs. 43%).[18]

BREEDING MANAGEMENT

Minimizing bacterial contamination of the uterus at the time of breeding through a minimum-contamination technique[28] can have a critical effect on foaling rates. The technique reduces the adverse effect of fibrosis and years barren in mares with mild or moderate fibrosis.[21] In mares where there is moderate fibrosis, coupled with inflammation, minimum contamination breeding has virtually doubled the foaling rate.[21]

PROGNOSIS

Because a number of factors, other than endometrial change can influence the breeding outcome, any probable foaling rate index should use a range, especially for categories IIA and IIB to account for these effects[2,3,25,26,27] (Table 26–6). Young mares barren only 1 yr and bred using minimum-contamination techniques have a much better prognosis than older mares barren 2 yr or more and bred by natural cover.

TABLE 26–6. PROBABLE FOALING RATE INDEX OF MARES ACCORDING TO ENDOMETRIAL CATEGORY

CATEGORY	DEGREE OF ENDOMETRIAL CHANGE	EXPECTED FOALING RATE (%)
I	Absent	>80
IIA	Mild	50–80
IIB	Moderate	10–50
III	Severe	<10

REFERENCES

1. Kenney, R.M.: Clinical aspects of endometrial biopsy in fertility evaluation of the mare. Proc. Am. Assoc. Equine Pract., pp. 105–122, 1977.
2. Kenney, R.M., and Doig, P.A.: Equine endometrial biopsy. *In* Current Therapy in Theriogenology 2. Edited by D.A. Morrow. Philadelphia, W.B. Saunders, 1986, pp. 723–729.
3. Kenney, R.M.: Cyclic and pathologic changes of the mare endometrium as detected by biopsy, with a note on early embryonic death. J. Am. Vet. Med. Assoc., *172:*241–262, 1978.
4. Bergman, R.V., and Kenney, R.M.: Representativeness of a uterine biopsy in the mare. Proc. Am. Assoc. Equine Pract., 355–361, 1975.
5. Ricketts, S.W.: The technique and clinical application of endometrial biopsy in the mare. Equine Vet. J., *7:*102–108, 1975.
6. Waelchli, R.O., and Winder, N.C.: Distribution of histological lesions in the equine endometrium. Vet. Rec., *124:*274–276, 1989
7. Blanchard, T.L., Garcia, M.C., Kintner, L.D., and Kenney, R.M.: Investigation of the representativeness of a single endometrial sample and the use of trichrome staining to aid in the detection of endometrial fibrosis in the mare. Theriogenology, *28:*445–450, 1987.
8. Gross, T.L., and LeBlanc, M.M.: Seasonal variation of histomorphologic features of equine endometrium. J. Am. Vet. Med. Assoc., *184:*1379–1382, 1984.
9. Brandt, G.W.: The significance and interpretation of uterine biopsy in the mare. Proc. Am. Assoc. Equine Pract., pp. 279–294, 1970.
10. Hammond, J., and Wodzicky, K.: Anatomical and histological changes during the oestrous cycle in the mare. Proc. R. Soc. London [Biol.], *130:*1–23 1941.
11. Leishman, D., Miller, R.B., and Doig, P.A.: A quantitative study of the histological morphology of the endometrium of normal and barren mares. Can. J. Comp. Med., *46:*17–20, 1982.
12. Ricketts, S.W.: Endometrial biopsy as a guide to diagnosis of endometrial pathology in the mare. J. Reprod. Fertil. Suppl., *23:*341–345, 1975.

13. Kenney, R.M.: Prognostic value of endometrial biopsy of the mare. J. Reprod. Fertil. Suppl., *23:*347–348, 1975.
14. Hurtgen, J.P., and Cummings, B.A.: Diagnosis and treatment of fungal endometritis in mares. Proc. Theriogenology, pp. 18–22, 1982.
15. Slusher, S.H., Freeman, K.P., and Roszel, J.F.: Eosinophils in equine uterine cytology and histology specimens. J. Am. Vet. Med. Assoc., *184:*665–670, 1984.
16. Henry, M., Vandeplassche, M., and Bouters, R.: A comparison of the bacteriological, cytological and histological findings for evaluating endometritis in the mare. Vlaams Diergeneesk. Tijdschr., *51:*498–512, 1982.
17. Shideler, R.K., et al.: Endometrial biopsy in the mare. Proc. Am. Assoc. Equine Pract., pp. 97–104, 1977.
18. Waelchli, R.O.: The diagnostic and prognostic value of endometrial biopsy in the mare under non-uniform breeding management conditions. Habilitationsschrift, University of Zurich, 1990.
19. Waelchli, R.O., Corboz, L., and Winder, N.C.: Comparison of histological, cytological and bacteriological findings in the endometrium of the mare. J. Am. Vet. Med. Assoc., *35:*442–449, 1988.
20. Gordon, L.R., and Sartin, E.M.: Endometrial biopsy as an aid to diagnosis and prognosis in equine infertility. J. Equine Med. Surg., *2:*328–336, 1978.
21. Doig, P.A., McKnight, J.D., and Miller, R.B.: The use of endometrial biopsy in the infertile mare. Can. Vet. J., *22:*72–76, 1981.
22. Asbury, A.C.: Some observations on the relationship of histologic inflammation in the endometrium of mares to fertility. Proc. Am. Assoc. Equine Pract., pp. 401–404, 1982.
23. de la Concha-Bermejillo, A., and Kennedy, P.C.: Prognostic value of endometrial biopsy in the mare: A retrospective analysis. J. Am. Vet. Med. Assoc., *181:*680–681, 1982.
24. Shideler, R.K., McChesney, A.E., Voss, V.L., and Squires, E.L.: Relationship of endometrial biopsy and other management factors on fertility of broodmares. J. Equine Vet. Sci., *2:*5–10, 1982.
25. Neely, D.P.: Evaluation and therapy of genital disease in the mare. *In* Equine Reproduction. Edited by D.P. Neely, I.K.M. Liu, and R.B. Hillman. Lawrenceville, Veterinary Learning Systems, 1983, pp. 39–56.
26. Waelchli, R.O.: Endometrial biopsy in mares under non-uniform breeding management conditions: Prognostic value and relationship with age. Can. Vet. J., *31:*379–384, 1990.
27. Kenney, R.M.: The role of endometrial biopsy in fertility evaluation. Proc. Am. Assoc. Equine Pract., pp. 177–201, 1978.
28. Kenney, R.M., Bergman, R.V., Cooper, W.L., and Morse, G.W.: Minimal contamination techniques for breeding mares: technique and preliminary findings. Proc. Am. Assoc. Equine Pract., pp. 327–336, 1975.

CHAPTER 27

UTERINE AND CLITORAL CULTURES

S.W. Ricketts
A. Young
E.B. Medici

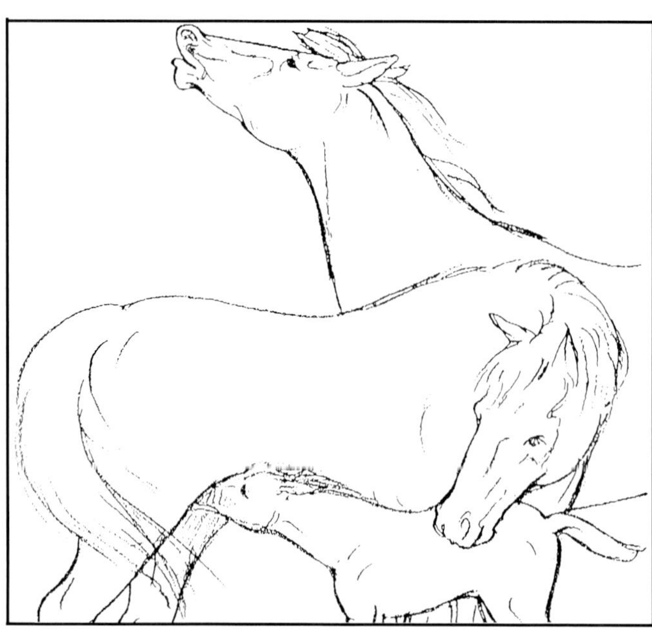

Dimock and Snyder[1] and Dimock and Edwards[2] concluded that, if correctly performed during estrus, bacteriologic examination of the mare's cervix is a reliable method of detecting uterine infection. They found a good correlation between presence of uterine infection and infertility. These authors and Lord Porchester's committee[3] drew attention to Klebsiella pneumoniae as a potential cause of equine venereal disease.

Both studies concluded that bacteriologic examinations of the cervix should be routine aids to equine stud farm preventive medicine, and surveys of equine cervical bacteriologic examinations were published from all over the world.[4–8] Nevertheless, these recommendations were not universally accepted until the outbreak of contagious equine metritis (CEM), which was first reported in Newmarket during 1977, highlighted the effect that epidemic venereal disease could have on the Thoroughbred breeding industry.[9,10] Simpson and Eaton-Evans[11,12] defined the clitoral fossa and sinuses as potential areas of chronic symptomless CEM carrier status and clitoral swabbing became incorporated into routine stud farm preventive medicine programs.[10] Horse breeding industries around the world formulated "codes of practice," primarily for control of CEM. Where applied quickly and rigorously, these have been highly successful. In the UK, the Horserace Betting Levy Board's "Code of Practice for the Control of Contagious Equine Metritis and Other Equine Reproductive Diseases" has

1. Eradicated CEM (Taylorella equigenitalis has not been isolated in the UK Thoroughbred horse population since January 1986).[13]
2. Reduced the incidence of venereal disease caused by K. pneumoniae and Pseudomonas aeruginosa.
3. Resulted in improved management and communications within the horse breeding industry.

In some continental European countries where similar control measures were not applied in time, CEM remains endemic, now apparently in a more insidious form.

Debate has continued regarding use of uterine swab screening techniques for the premating diagnosis of nonvenereal acute endometritis.[14,15] It is now recognized that

1. Swabs must be taken from the endometrium, through the open estrous cervix, for results to be meaningful.[16]
2. Guarded swabs collect fewer insignificant contaminant organisms.[17]
3. Concurrent cytologic examinations markedly improve diagnostic accuracy.[18]
4. Anaerobic bacteria can play an important role.[19]

OBJECTIVES

Genital swab samples are collected from mares, for microbiologic examinations, for the following important reasons.

VENEREAL DISEASE SCREENING

Before the start of breeding operations, swab samples are collected from the vestibule, clitoral fossa, and sinuses[20] at any stage of the estrous cycle, and from the endometrium[21] during early estrus. These swab samples are cultured aerobically to screen for presence of Ps. aeruginosa and K. pneumoniae and microaerophilically for presence of T. equigenitalis.[22] If these organisms are isolated, the mare is not presented to the stallion until it has been specifically treated and a series of repeat swab samples (usually three sets taken at appropriate intervals, i.e., 7 days apart for clitoral swabs and during three estrous periods for endometrial swabs) have suggested successful elimination.

The objective of these screening cultures is to prevent contamination of the stallion's genitalia by mares who are either symptomless carriers of, or acutely infected with, potential venereal disease organisms.

ACUTE ENDOMETRITIS SCREENING

Samples are collected before start of breeding operations and subsequently if and each time the mare returns to estrus after mating. Concurrent endometrial swab and smear samples are collected during early estrus,[23] for bacteriologic culture[21] and cytologic examination, screening for the presence (>± polymorphonuclear leucocytes (PMN) or absence (<± PMN) of acute endometritis.[18,19,23] In addition to routine venereal disease screening, as described above, the swab samples are cultured aerobically to screen for the presence of other potential nonvenereal acute endometritis producers (see below). If there are cytologic signs of acute endometritis then the bacteriologic isolates are examined and appropriate antibiotic treatment is applied.[19,24] The mare is re-examined at the next estrus with repeat smear and swab examinations to prove successful resolution. If potential venereal disease–producing organisms are isolated, the mare is managed and treated as described above, irrespective of the cytologic results.

The objectives of these procedures are (1) to prevent potential venereal disease carrier mares, or mares with acute infections, from contaminating the stallion's genitalia and (2) routinely to identify mares with nonvenereal acute endometritis so that this can be resolved before mating and chances for successful conception and gestation can be maximized.

EXAMINATION/INVESTIGATION OF GENITAL ABNORMALITIES

Bacteriologic examinations are an essential part of the complete gynecologic examination of a mare and should be performed in mares who fail to conceive, suffer early fetal death or abortion, show signs of genital abnormality, or are being routinely examined as barren mares after the end of the mating season.[24,25] Swab samples are collected from the vestibule, clitoral fossa, and sinuses at any stage of the estrous cycle and from the endometrium during estrus. If the mare is not in estrus, a uterine aspirate, washing, and/or endometrial biopsy specimen may be collected and cultured. In addition to routine venereal disease screening, as described above, endometrial swab samples are cultured aerobically and anaerobically to screen for presence of other potential nonvenereal acute endometritis producers (see below).[19] At the same time, complete gynecologic examinations are performed, including collection of endometrial biopsy specimens. If there are histologic signs of acute endometritis, the bacteriologic isolates are examined to make sure appropriate antibiotic treatment is applied. A followup examination is made to assess the response to treatment at the next estrus or if performed after the mating season, following an appropriate period of rest. If potential venereal disease–producing organisms are isolated then the mare is managed and treated as described above, irrespective of the histologic results.

The objectives of these procedures are (1) to prevent potential venereal disease carrier mares, or mares with acute infections, from contaminating the stallion's genitalia and (2) to identify mares with acute endometritis so that this can be resolved to improve chances for successful conception and gestation, either before the next estrus or, for routine barren mare examinations, before the next mating season.

TECHNIQUES

PREPARATION OF THE MARE

For all gynecologic examinations, the mare should be bridled and restrained with her hindquarters at a door frame or, ideally, in stocks, in a manner that facilitates a safe, thorough, and relaxed examination.[26] For fractious mares, a twitch or sedation may be required. The tail should be bandaged and held to one side. The perineum should be washed with warm, clean water. Disinfectants should not be used before taking clitoral/vestibular swabs.[20] Before collection of endometrial swab samples, the perineum is again thoroughly washed with warm, clean water. Disinfectants are unnecessary and, if used regularly and excessively, may encourage the colonization of the clitoral fossa with resistant organisms such as Ps. aeruginosa and K. pneumoniae.[27]

COLLECTION OF SAMPLES

Laboratory results are only as good as the samples examined allow them to be.[28] Swab samples should be collected with appropriate and careful technique, using suitable equipment.

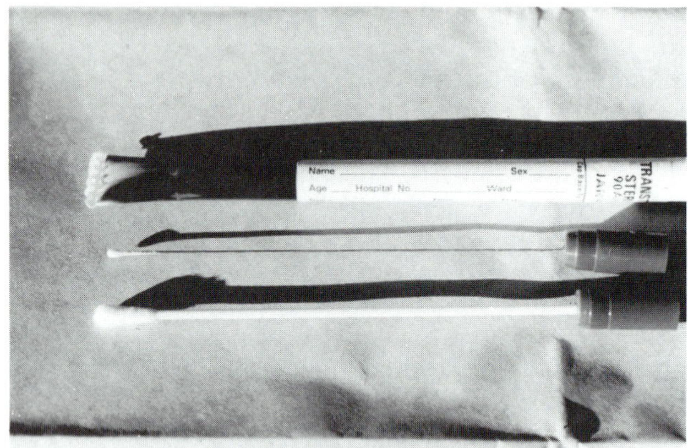

FIG. 27–1. Standard hospital-type swabs with Amies charcoal transport medium. Standard-tipped swab (below) for swabbing the vestibule and the clitoral fossa. Narrow-tipped swab (above) for swabbing the clitoral sinuses.

Clitoral/Vestibular Swabs

Standard hospital-type swabs with Amies charcoal transport medium (Medical Wire and Equipment Co., Ltd., Corsham, Wiltshire, UK) may be used for this purpose (Fig. 27–1). With a gloved hand, using the thumb and index finger either side of the ventral commisure of the vulva and with the second finger under the base of the vulva, the vulval lips are parted and the clitoris is everted. A sterile swab is placed in the ventral aspect of the vestibule to pick up material before thoroughly swabbing all areas of the clitoral fossa (Fig. 27–2). A narrow-tipped (pediatric-type) sterile swab is then placed in the central clitoral sinus (Fig. 27–3) and, if present, the lateral sinuses and rotated to pick up smegma. The swabs are immediately placed into the transport medium and clearly labeled with the name of the mare and the date and site of swabbing. It is of note that a recent report has suggested that the lateral sinuses may be too shallow to support growth of T. equigenitalis.[29]

Nonguarded Endometrial Swabs

Extended standard hospital-type swabs (Fig. 27–4) with Amies charcoal transport medium may be used for nonguarded endometrial swabs. A sterile, preferably disposable, speculum is passed into the vagina and the cervix is viewed using a penlight. If the cervix is sufficiently relaxed, i.e., the mare is in estrus, the extended swab may be carefully passed through the sterile speculum (Fig. 27–5) and through the relaxed cervix into the uterine body, where it is rotated to pick up secretions.[21] The swab is then carefully removed from the uterus, through the cervix and the sterile speculum, and placed immediately into the transport medium. The swabs must be clearly labeled with the mare's name and the date and site of swabbing.

Another swab is taken immediately, in a similar manner, but is not placed into transport medium. This swab is used for making an endometrial smear for cytologic examination (Chapter 28).

Guarded/Semiguarded Swabs

A number of specially designed swabs (e.g., Kallajan Industries Inc., Long Beach, CA) (Fig. 27–6), using a variety of guarding techniques, are available commercially. These are passed through the relaxed estrous cervix into the uterine lumen, either via a sterile vaginal speculum as described above or manually, guarded in a sterile gloved hand. Double-gloving and double-guarded techniques have been described.[17] Specific technical details depend on the swab used and preferences for speculum or manual passage. The objective is to obtain a true endometrial sample, without contamination by vaginal or cervical material, by exposing the swab tip only when it is inside the uterine lumen. The swab is retracted into its sterile sheath before careful removal from the uterus and placed immediately into transport medium. The swabs must be clearly labeled with the mare's name and the date and site of swabbing.

Another swab is taken immediately, in a similar manner, but is not placed into transport medium. This swab is used for making an endometrial smear for cytologic examination (Chapter 28). Cytologic examinations may be performed on material harvested by special brushes incorporated in dual-system devices, in or on the cap (Fig. 27–6) or swab sheath of some guarded swabs.

Uterine Aspirations and Washings

If the uterine lumen contains fluid or purulent material, a sample may be aspirated using a sterile insemination pipette, via a sterile vaginal speculum or by manual

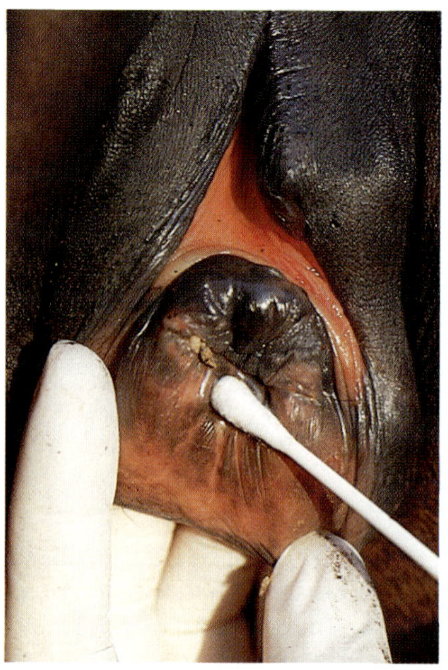

FIG. 27–2. A sterile swab is used to thoroughly swab all areas of the clitoral fossa.

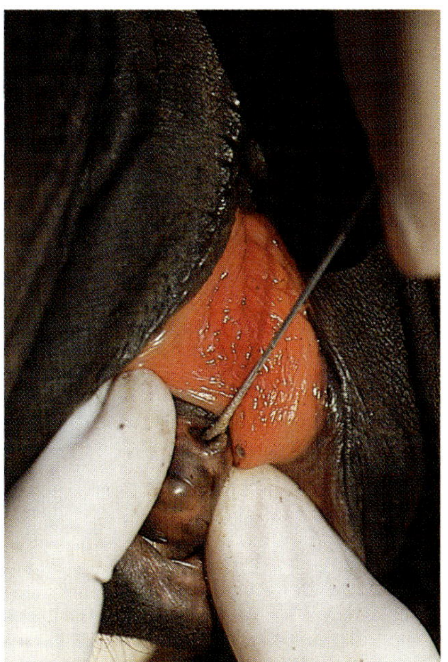

FIG. 27–3. A narrow-tipped (pediatric-type) sterile swab is placed in the central clitoral sinus and rotated to pick up smegma.

manipulation, guided if necessary by ultrasonography. Alternatively, and if the uterus does not contain fluid or pus, a uterine washing may be performed. Sterile saline (20 to 50 mL) may be introduced into the uterus via an insemination pipette, and the end of the pipette may be used to gently dislodge epithelial cells into the lumen before aspirating the fluid.[30] Another technique is to place a sterile Foley-type egg flushing catheter (Sherwood Medical, St. Louis, MO) through the cervix and to inflate its bulb just inside the uterine lumen. A 250-mL pack of sterile saline solution is then connected to the catheter and the fluid is passed into the uterus by gravity flow. While maintaining the airtight connection between the empty saline bag and the catheter, the uterus may be massaged per rectum and as the bag is lowered the saline refills the bag which is then sealed with a clamp. The sedimented washings may be examined bacteriologically and cytologically. A Cytospin centrifuge (Cytospin 2, Shandon Scientific Ltd., Cheshire, UK) provides an excellent sample for cytologic staining. If there is to be a delay in processing, the fluid should be swabbed in an aseptic manner and placed into bacteriologic transport medium and another portion should be fixed in Cytospin fixing fluid (Shandon Scientific Ltd.) (50:50) for cytologic preservation.

Endometrial Biopsy

Using aseptic techniques, tissue samples may be retrieved from the jaws of biopsy punches, following endometrial biopsy. If there is to be a delay in processing, the tissue should be carefully swabbed and placed into bacteriologic transport medium (Chapter 26).

HANDLING OF SAMPLES

The most meticulously collected samples can be rendered useless by improper handling.

Transport Media

If there is any delay between swab collection and processing, the use of bacteriologic transport medium is essential. In 1977, studies clearly demonstrated that bacteriologic transport medium was required to prevent T. equigenitalis from becoming nonviable during transit to the laboratory and providing false-negative results.[9,10] This organism was also found to be sensitive to light, and thus Amies transport medium, with added charcoal, became the standard all-purpose bacteriologic transport medium for equine gynecologic practice.

Transport to the Laboratory

Ideally, there should be minimal delay between swab collection and laboratory processing. In practice, arrangements should be made so that swabs, in transport medium, reach the laboratory within 48 h of collection, even though studies suggest that longer viability is possible.[31] During transport, swab samples should not be subjected to extremes of temperature and should be shielded from direct sunlight. Packaging should be safe and secure to prevent breakages and to satisfy postal regulations.

Laboratory Techniques

Equine gynecologic bacteriology is a specialized and demanding subject, which requires experience, care, and attention to detail.[22] Important clinical decisions may be made directly on the basis of results, significance of which should be fully understood by laboratory personnel. The standard of facilities and technical staff must be sufficient to allow accuracy and efficiency, which are essential to provide the clinician with useful results.

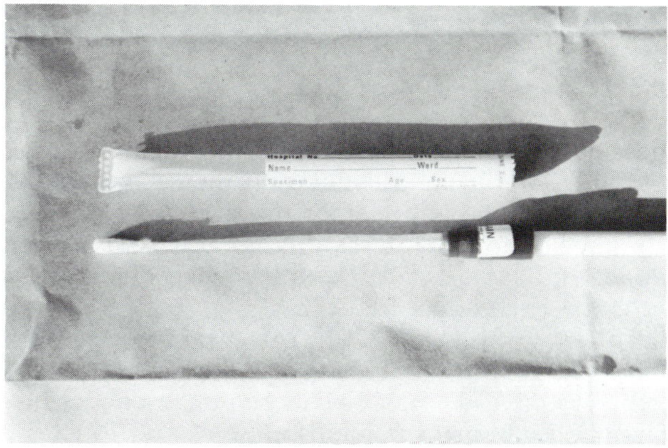

FIG. 27–4. A standard hospital-type swab, extended with a sterilizable plastic rod in order to allow passage through a speculum.

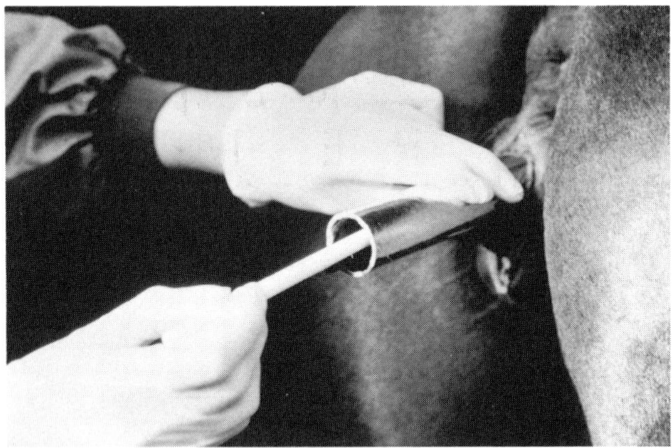

FIG. 27–5. An extended swab is carefully passed through a sterile speculum and through the relaxed cervix into the uterine body, where it is rotated to pick up secretions.

A plentiful and reliable supply of fresh, good-quality agar plates is essential. Media may be purchased in dehydrated form and made up as required, or as prepoured plates. Agar plates have a limited shelf life and should be used when as fresh as possible or only stored for short periods. If they are to be stored before use they should be refrigerated and tightly sealed in plastic to prevent drying out. Incubators must be reliable and functioning at the required temperature and atmospheric conditions.

Swabs should be inoculated onto agar plates in an environment that is clean and free from sources of plate contamination, using careful standard plating techniques.[32]

Aerobic Culture

For all routine equine gynecologic bacteriologic examinations, we recommend that swabs are directly inoculated onto two plates: (1) a rich peptone-based blood agar medium (Oxoid Ltd., Basingstoke, Hampshire, UK) and (2) a MacConkey agar medium (Oxoid Ltd.). Both are incubated under humid, but otherwise normal, atmospheric (aerobic) conditions at 37° C for up to 48 h. Cultures are examined at 24 and 48 h.

Microaerophilic Culture

For all routine equine gynecologic cultures, we recommend that swabs are directly inoculated onto two plates, both containing a specialized heated (chocolated) blood agar medium, specifically designed for the isolation of T. equigenitalis[33] and incubated under conditions of 5 to 10% carbon dioxide and increased humidity at 37° C for up to 6 days. This medium should be a rich peptone-based, glucose-free, agar medium to which L-cystine (300 mg/L) or the soluble L-cystine hydrochloride (100 mg/L), sodium sulfite (200 mg/L), 2 to 5% heated horse or sheep blood, and amphotericin B (5 mg/L) has been added. Streptomycin sulfate (200 mg/L) should be added to one of the agar plates. Cultures are examined at 2, 3, 4, and 6 days. A control strain of T. equigenitalis (National Collection of Type Cultures, Central Public Health Laboratory, Colindale, London, UK) should be cultured in parallel with each batch of swabs to ensure satisfactory media and incubation conditions.

Anaerobic Culture

For anaerobic culture, we recommend that swabs are directly inoculated onto two plates of Wilkins-Chalgren anaerobe agar (Oxoid Ltd.) containing 5% horse blood and incubated in an atmosphere of 10% hydrogen, 10% carbon dioxide, and 80% nitrogen at 37° C for 48 h. One plate contains 100 mg/mL neomycin. A disk containing 5 mg/mL metronidazole is placed on each plate in the area of heavy inoculum. Cultures are examined at 24 and 48 h.

Swabs may be incubated anaerobically in an enrichment medium of Robertson's meat granules (Lab M, Amersham International, Lancashire, UK) rehydrated in gas-liquid chromatography (GLC) broth (Lab M) for 24 h before innoculation onto Wilkins-Chalgren anaerobe agar as described above.

Fungal Culture

Pathogenic fungi such as Candida spp. and Aspergillus spp. will often grow on blood agar incubated under aerobic conditions. For specific fungal culture, we recommend that swabs are directly inoculated onto plates containing Sabouraud dextrose agar (Oxoid Ltd.) and incubated under normal atmospheric conditions at 37° C for up to 4 days.

Identification

Using the cultural conditions recommended above, an experienced technician should be able to identify the majority of equine aerobic pathogens by their colonial

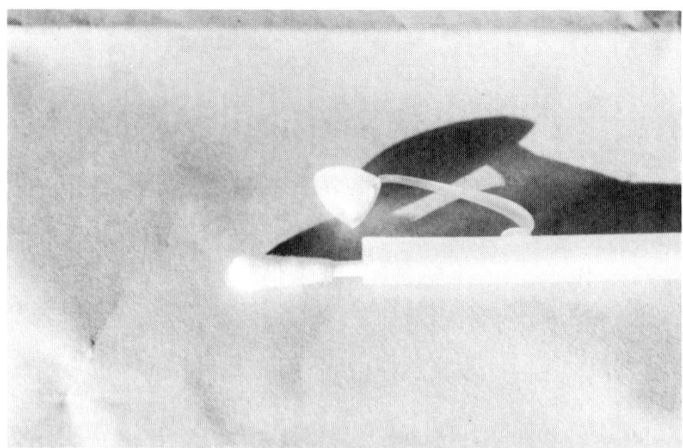

FIG. 27–6. A specially designed guarded swab, which may be used to collect uterine samples for bacteriological and cytological (cellular material retrieved from the cap) examinations.

appearance on blood and McConkey agar. To facilitate this, good inoculation technique is required to allow adequate colony separation. For well-collected endometrial swabs, visual identification from the primary inoculum is usually straightfoward, but for clitoral swabs, which often grow luxuriant mixed cultures, more detailed investigation is required.

Aerobic Pathogens. Pseudomonas aeruginosa produces nonhemolytic, greenish, characteristic smelling colonies on blood agar after 24 h aerobic culture. It grows readily and luxuriantly on McConkey agar, and being a lactose fermenter, it produces pink colonies. Gram's stain reveals gram-negative rods. It must be differentiated from Ps. fluorescens and the other pseudomonads by growth ability at 41 to 42° C (only Ps. aeruginosa is able to grow at this temperature) and oxidation of potassium gluconate (all pyocyanogenic and the rare apyocyanogenic strains of Ps. aeruginosa give positive reactions). Some isolates take 48 h to grow on blood agar at 37° C, only producing small colonies; therefore, all aerobic culture plates should be examined again at 48 h.

Klebsiella pneumoniae produces large, nonhemolytic, mucoid colonies on blood agar after 24 h aerobic culture. It grows readily and luxuriantly on McConkey agar (Fig. 27–7), and being a lactose fermenter, it produces pink colonies that are mucoid. Gram's stain reveals gram-negative rods. Isolates should be confirmed by biochemical typing (see below) before being further differentiated by immunofluorescent capsular typing (see below).

Streptococcus zooepidemicus produces pinpoint colonies, with a clear zone of β hemolysis, on blood agar after 24 h aerobic culture. It does not grow on McConkey agar. Gram's stain reveals gram-positive cocci. Staphylococcus aureus produces cream, yellow, to gold colonies, sometimes with a clear zone of β hemolysis, on blood agar after 24 h aerobic culture. It does not grow on McConkey agar. Gram's stain reveals gram-positive cocci. Escherichia coli produces creamy colonies, sometimes with a clear zone of β hemolysis, on blood agar after 24 h aerobic culture. It grows readily on McConkey agar, and being a lactose fermenter, it produces pink colonies. Gram's stain reveals gram-negative rods.

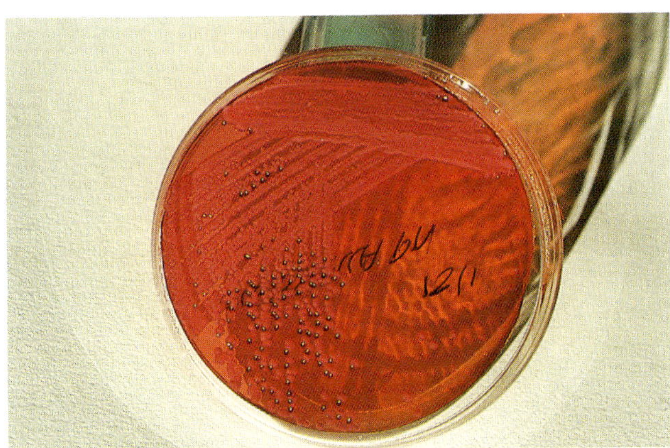

FIG. 27–7. Klebsiella pneumoniae growing readily and luxuriantly on McConkey agar, producing large, mucoid, pink (nonlactose fermenting) colonies after 24 h aerobic culture.

Microaerophilic Pathogens. All small, pale, translucent colonies are investigated first for their oxidase and catalase activities. Taylorella equigenitalis will give a fast (< 10 s) positive oxidase and a positive catalase reaction. If both are positive, a Gram's stain is performed. If this reveals a small gram-negative coccobacillus, a phosphatase test is performed to look for a positive reaction. A slide agglutination test is then performed, using specific rabbit T. equigenitalis antiserum (Mono-Tayl, Bionor, Skien, Norway). If T. equigenitalis is confirmed in the UK, the isolate is legally notifiable[13] and must be reported and referred to the local divisional veterinary officer of the Ministry of Agriculture Veterinary Services who will investigate both the isolate and, if reconfirmed to be T. equigenitalis, clinical circumstances further. Occasionally, aerobic pathogens, such as Ps. aeruginosa, will grow under microaerophilic conditions, providing a useful additional "screen."

Anaerobic Pathogens. Obligate anaerobes are differentiated from facultative anaerobes by their growth inhibition around the metronidazole disk. Isolates are purified and identified using standard methods.[34]

Fungal Pathogens. Candida spp. produce gray to white, raised, glistening, soft and creamy colonies within 48 h incubation on blood or Sabouraud agar at 37° C. Aspergillus spp. grow on Sabouraud agar. These fungi can be confirmed by examining colony smears mounted in lactophenol cotton blue and species differentiation can be made using standard methods.[35]

Subculture

Where identification from the primary inoculation is not straightforward, often because mixed cultures or overgrowth of a contaminant nonpathogen has occurred, purification by subculture is essential. A single well-isolated colony should be transferred onto a solid nonselective medium identical to that on which the original isolation was made and culture should be performed under identical temperature and atmospheric conditions.

Gram's Stain

Gram's stain is performed using standard methods.[35] For reliable results, the culture smear must not be too thick and the gram-positive organisms must not be overdecolorized with acetone.

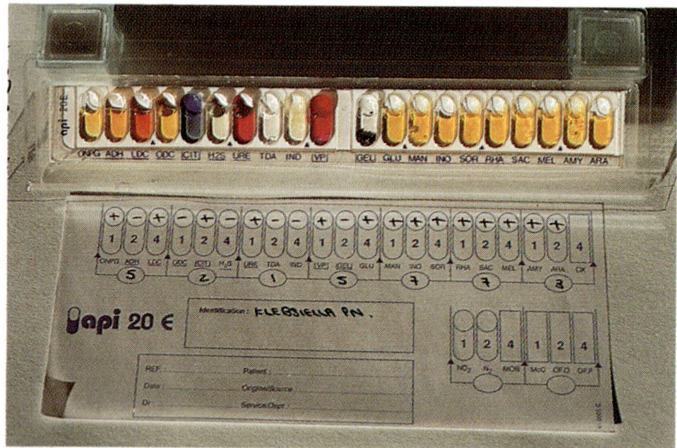

FIG. 27–8. Klebsiella pneumoniae confirmed by the commercially available, prepacked biochemical reaction system API 20E.

Biochemical Tests

Commercially available, prepacked biochemical reaction systems have revolutionized clinical bacteriology in accuracy, ease, and convenience of use (Fig. 27–8). Systems are available for differentiation of gram-negative rods (API 20E, API Bio Mérieux, Vercieu, France), streptococci (Streptococcal Grouping Kit, Oxoid Ltd.) and staphylococci (API Staph, API Bio Mérieux). These systems are simple to use and provide excellent results if manufacturers' instructions are followed meticulously. Clearly, it is essential that only single colonies or pure cultures are used to inoculate reaction compartments or spurious results will be produced. The API 20E system is designed for results to be interpreted with the aid of an "API Quick Index," which lists over 900 profiles and which is sufficient for most cases. It differentiates some 51 bacteria on a plus/minus scoring system. When this is insufficient, users have free telephone access to the API 20E computer service.

Capsule/Serotyping

Klebsiella pneumoniae capsule types may be differentiated by immunofluorescent staining with specific fluorescein isothiocyanate (FITC) labeled antisera.[36] First, the isolate must be subcultured for purity and then grown on Worfel-Ferguson medium (Oxoid Ltd.) to swell the capsules. Capsular types 1, 2, 5, 7, and 68 are most commonly isolated from equine genital swab samples[37] and only types 1, 2, and 5 have been isolated in association with outbreaks of true venereal disease (see below). Pseudomonas aeruginosa serotypes may be differentiated but no correlation has been found between serotype and potential venereal pathogenicity.[38]

Antibiotic Sensitivity Tests

Specialized agar medium (Sensitest Agar, Oxoid Ltd.) should be used routinely to overcome sulfonamide and trimethoprim antagonists and fresh blood need only be added for particularly fastidious organisms. Selective media should not be used for antibiotic sensitivity tests.

One medium-size colony should be emulsified in 5 mL sterile medium, distilled water, or nutrient broth; a swab is dipped into this and drained before being evenly spread over the agar plate. Tests run on direct inoculums may give next-day, but spurious, results, unless the culture is pure and the inoculum size is satisfactory.

Standard or personalized antibiotic impregnated disks can be used; the choice depends on clinical preferences and antibiotic availability. Although eight disks are commonly used per plate, six may be preferable to avoid close proximity interactions between antibiotic diffusion in agar leading to misinterpretation. These tests are qualitative and not quantitative and zone sizes cannot be correlated with degree of sensitivity or insensitivity. Disk sensitivity tests run on organisms that require more than 48 h for visible growth, e.g., T. equigenitalis, are not practical.

INTERPRETATION OF RESULTS

It is the clinician's responsibility to interpret the results provided. Interpretation is based not only on the organisms isolated but on clinical history of the mare and results of other gynecologic examinations. A major advance during the last 12 yr has been the routine use of concurrent endometrial cytologic examinations, which have markedly improved the accuracy of interpretation of routine premating endometrial bacteriologic results.[23,18]

SPECIES ISOLATION FREQUENCY

Tables 27–1 and 27–2 present the frequency with which commonly identified aerobic and microaerophilic bacterial species have been isolated, in the authors' practice laboratory, from routine clitoral and endometrial swab samples, using the techniques described above (nonguarded endometrial swabbing techniques). Table 27–1 shows that normal microflora of the equine clitorial area most frequently includes E. coli, Streptococcus faecalis, Corynebacterium spp., Staph. aureus, Streptococcus spp. (β-hemolytic), and Staphylococcus albus. Pseudomonas aeruginosa, isolated in 1% of these clitoral swab samples, was the most frequently isolated potential venereal disease producer. Table 27–2 shows that using nonguarded swabbing techniques, 39% "no growths" can be expected. The most frequent aerobic species isolated from these endometrial swab samples were Streptococcus spp. (β hemolytic), E. coli, Staph. albus, and Staph. aureus.

CLASSIFICATION OF SIGNIFICANCE OF ISOLATES

Bacteriologic examinations of endometrial swab samples, taken with whatever equipment and by whatever techniques, cannot be accurately interpreted without

TABLE 27–1. AEROBIC AND MICROAEROPHILIC BACTERIAL SPECIES ISOLATED FROM 1000 ROUTINE EQUINE CLITORAL SWABS IN THE AUTHORS' PRACTICE LABORATORY (1990)

BACTERIA ISOLATED	NUMBER OF ISOLATES	PERCENT ISOLATION*
Taylorella equigenitalis	0	0.0
Klebsiella pneumoniae	6	0.6
Pseudomonas aeruginosa	10	1.0
Escherichia coli	724	72.4
Streptococcus faecalis	318	31.8
Corynebacterium spp.	228	22.8
Staphylococcus aureus	202	20.2
Streptococcus (β hemolytic)	172	17.2
Staphylococcus albus	106	10.6
Acinetobacter spp.	86	8.6
Bacillus spp.	30	3.0
Enterobacter aerogenes	7	0.7
Pasteurella spp.	6	0.6
Proteus spp.	6	0.6
Streptococcus spp. (α hemolytic)	6	0.6
Streptococcus spp. (nonhemolytic)	6	0.6
Citrobacter spp.	1	0.1

*Each expressed as percentage of total isolates.

concurrent endometrial cytologic data.[19] Table 27–3 correlates 16,386 bacterial species isolates, obtained from 24,913 routine concurrent endometrial swab and smear examinations performed in the authors' practice laboratory over an 11-yr period, with their concurrent cytologic results. Acute endometritis was diagnosed with 21% of the isolates. Pseudomonas aeruginosa (46%), Proteus spp. (34%), K. oxytoca (34%), Enterobacter aerogenes (30%), Streptococcus spp. (β hemolytic) (29%), K. pneumoniae (29%), Pasteurella spp. (27%), E. coli (23%), Streptococcus faecalis, and Staph. aureus (20%) were isolated with concurrent cytologic signs of acute endometritis in more than 20% frequency. Any bacterial species may be isolated in association with acute endometritis in individual mares but, in general terms, they may be classified according to their primary potential.

Potential Venereal Disease Producing Organisms

Only T. equigenitalis, Ps. aeruginosa, and K. pneumoniae have been isolated as causes of true venereal disease in mares. True equine venereal disease is defined by infection of the stallion with a specific pathogen by an infected or carrier mare, followed by production of epidemic acute endometritis caused by the same pathogen in subsequent mares mated. Infected mares are those who have normal as well as those who have abnormal local uterine immunologic defense mechanisms. If potential venereal disease–producing bacteria are isolated from either vestibular/clitoral swabs or from endometrial swabs, with or without concurrent cytologic evidence of acute endometritis, the mare in question should be identified as being unsuitable for natural mating until successfully treated.

Two strains of T. equigenitalis, i.e., streptomycin-sensitive and -insensitive strains, have been isolated from mares with venereal acute endometritis. The sensitive strain was first isolated in Newmarket in 1977. The insensitive strain was subsequently isolated in Kentucky but has yet to be seen in the UK. Both strains appear capable of producing epidemic venereal disease in mares. When first diagnosed, the organism produced severe acute endometritis with most mares developing copious vaginal discharge. It is now reported that the disease, which is apparently still present in parts of continental Europe, is much more insidious, producing minimal clinical signs, although the organism itself is indistinguishable from that originally isolated. All strains of T. equigenitalis should be considered potential venereal pathogens, and if isolated, the following standard procedures should be adopted:

1. Isolation and should be notified to the Ministry of Agriculture (UK).
2. All sexual contacts should be traced and investigated.
3. Mares with isolates should be treated and proven to be clear from both infection and a symptomless carrier state before they are presented again for mating.

TABLE 27–2. AEROBIC AND MICROAEROPHILIC BACTERIAL SPECIES ISOLATED FROM 34,272 EQUINE ENDOMETRIAL SWABS CULTURED IN THE AUTHORS' PRACTICE LABORATORY (1973–1989)

BACTERIA ISOLATED	NUMBER OF ISOLATES	PERCENT ISOLATION*
No growth	13,431	39
Pure growth	12,025	35
Mixed growth	8,816	26
Taylorella equigenitalis	28	0.08
Klebsiella pneumoniae	192	0.6
Pseudomonas aeruginosa	99	0.3
Streptococcus (β hemolytic)	6,213	18.1
Escherichia coli	5,077	14.8
Staphylococcus albus	4,584	13.4
Staphylococcus aureus	3,132	9.1
Streptococcus spp. (nonhemolytic)	2,025	5.9
Corynebacterium spp.	1,645	4.8
Streptococcus spp. (α hemolytic)	1,384	4.0
Streptococcus faecalis	580	1.7
Bacillus spp.	518	1.5
Coliforms	221	0.6
Proteus spp.	178	0.5
Enterobacter aerogenes	98	0.3
Acinetobacter spp.	59	0.2
Neisseria spp.	39	0.1
Pasteurella spp.	12	0.03

*Each expressed as percentage of total isolates.

TABLE 27–3. AEROBIC AND MICROAEROPHILIC BACTERIAL SPECIES ISOLATED IN THE AUTHOR'S PRACTICE LABORATORY (1978–1989) CORRELATED WITH CONCURRENT ENDOMETRIAL CYTOLOGIC RESULTS

		CYTOLOGIC FINDINGS				
		PMN +ve*		PMN −ve†		
Bacteria Isolated		Pure Culture	Mixed Culture	Pure Culture	Mixed Culture	Total Isolates
Taylorella equigenitalis	Number	0	0	0	0	0
	Percent	0	0	0	0	0.0
Klebsiella pneumoniae	Number	15	12	37	32	96
	Percent	16	13	38	33	0.6
Pseudomonas aeruginosa	Number	3	7	6	6	22
	Percent	14	32	27	27	0.13
Streptococcus spp. (β hemolytic)	Number	645	638	1,209	1,961	4,453
	Percent	15	14	27	54	27.2
Staphylococcus albus	Number	163	280	1,091	1,102	2,636
	Percent	6	11	41	42	16
Staphylococcus aureus	Number	109	364	764	1,214	2,451
	Percent	5	15	31	49	15
Escherischia coli (nonhemolytic)	Number	184	338	681	338	2,230
	Percent	8	15	31	15	13.6
Corynebacterium spp.	Number	60	146	570	811	1,587
	Percent	4	9	36	51	9.7
Streptococcus spp. (α hemolytic)	Number	29	130	286	662	1,107
	Percent	3	12	26	59	6.8
Streptococcus spp. (nonhemolytic)	Number	57	99	385	491	1,032
	Percent	6	10	37	47	6.3
Anthracoides sp.	Number	14	24	109	126	273
	Percent	5	9	40	46	1.7
Streptococcus faecalis	Number	3	43	13	151	210
	Percent	1	20	6	73	1.3
Proteus spp.	Number	7	20	13	40	80
	Percent	9	25	16	50	0.5
Escherichia coli (hemolytic)	Number	11	5	35	22	73
	Percent	15	7	48	30	0.4
Acinetobacter spp.	Number	3	1	31	17	52
	Percent	6	2	59	33	0.3
Enterobacter aerogenes	Number	8	7	19	16	50
	Percent	16	14	38	32	0.3
Pasteurella spp.	Number	4	0	5	6	15
	Percent	27	0	33	40	0.09
Neisseria spp.	Number	0	1	10	2	13
	Percent	0	8	76	16	0.08
Klebsiella oxytoca	Number	0	1	2	0	3
	Percent	0	34	66	0	0.02
Moraxella spp.	Number	0	0	0	1	1
	Percent	0	0	0	100	0.005
Total Isolates	Number	1,315	2,116	5,266	7,689	16,386
	Percent	8	13	32	47	100

*Pmn +ve indicates ≥0.5% polymorphonuclear leucocytes on endometrial smear.
†Pmn −ve indicates <0.5% polymorphonuclear leucocytes on endometrial smear.

Different serotypes of Ps. aeruginosa have been isolated from horses but no reliable association with venereal pathogenicity has been identified.[38] Although it is recognized that some isolates may not behave as true venereal pathogens, mechanical contamination of the stallion's penile and preputial smegma may lead to administrative problems and treatment can be difficult, owing to the resistance of this organism to antimicrobial drugs and to its ability to reappear following apparent clearance. Therefore, no alternative exists but to consider all isolates potential venereal pathogens and to take appropriate action, as described above. Experience suggests that small, slow-growing colonies (see above) are not isolated under circumstances where true venereal disease occurs, but this is not recommended as a prognostically reliable characteristic.

Different capsular types of K. pneumoniae have been isolated from horses and have been correlated with potential venereal pathogenicity.[37] Capsular types 1, 2, and 5 have been isolated in association with true epidemic venereal disease in horses; therefore, these capsular types should be considered potential venereal pathogens, and appropriate action taken, as described above. Capsular types 7, 68, and others are occasionally isolated from penile, clitoral, and fecal swabs but have not been isolated in association with true epidemic venereal disease in horses and, therefore, should not be considered potential venereal pathogens

Nonvenereal Acute Endometritis–Producing Organisms

The external genitalia of the normal mare, including the vestibular and clitoral areas, irrespective of age and reproductive status, possess a mixed aerobic (Table 27–1) and obligate anaerobic microflora.[19] Isolation of bacteria, other than the potential venereal disease–producing bacteria discussed above, from these sites is, therefore, of no significance.

It has been stated the normal equine uterus is bacteriologically sterile or has a temporary, nonresident, rather than a resident microflora.[39] Studies have since shown that even in maiden mares with no cytologic evidence of acute endometritis, obligate anaerobic bacteria can inhabit the uterus as surface commensals.[19] Even using double-guarded, occluded swabs, following repeated external genital scrubbing with disinfectants, bacteria were isolated from 15 out of 48 (31%) endometrial swabs taken from mares with no evidence of acute endometritis.[40] During the breeding season, parturition and then natural mating results in repeated contamination of the uterine lumen with environmental and external genital microflora. Transient endometritis is, therefore, an inevitable sequel to parturition and coitus, and at those times the normal, genitally healthy mare produces an efficient transient acute endometritis, which resolves within 48 to 72 h.[14,15] Mares with genital abnormality, e.g., pneumovagina, vulval, rectovaginal, or cervical injury or mares that have impaired local immune mechanisms, produce an inefficient, persistent acute endometritis. Thus endometritis is more a reflection of the individual mare's genital abnormalities than the microbial organisms isolated. Virtually any bacterial species may be involved but experience suggests that the aerobes Streptococcus spp. (β hemolytic), E. coli, Staph. aureus, and Staph. albus (Table 27–3) and the anaerobe Bacteroides fragilis[19] are the most commonly isolated species, both in pure and mixed cultures, from acute endometritis cases. Enterobacter aerogenes, Pasteurella spp., and K. oxytoca are infrequently isolated, in general terms, but are relatively often isolated in cases of acute endometritis (Table 27–3). All these species may be isolated from endometrial swab samples either as significant acute endometritis producers or as insignificant contaminants or epithelial surface commensals. Thus for accurate interpretation, clinical (vaginal discharge, cervicitis, uterine fluid pooling, pyometritis) and/or concurrent endometrial cytologic data (active PMN with endometrial epithelial cells) must be used to determine significance.

Contaminant/Commensal Organisms

Contaminant/commensal organisms are the normal microflora of the external genitalia and perineal skin. They are, therefore, of no significance when isolated from clitoral/vestibular swab samples.

The organisms that are seldom isolated, in pure culture, from acute endometritis cases are the aerobes Moraxella spp., Neisseria spp., Streptococcus spp. (α hemolytic), Corynebacterium spp., Anthracoides spp., Acinetobacter spp., Streptococcus spp. (nonhemolytic), and Staph. albus, and the anaerobes Fusobacterium spp., Peptostreptococcus anaerobius, Peptococcus spp., Clostridium spp., Bacteroides melaninogenicus, and Veillonella spp. Nevertheless, for accurate interpretation, clinical and/or concurrent endometrial cytologic data must be be used to determine significance.

CORRELATION WITH CONCURRENT ENDOMETRIAL CYTOLOGIC EXAMINATIONS

A survey of concurrent endometrial cytologic and aerobic bacteriologic examinations performed on mares under routine stud farm practice conditions during the course of four breeding seasons[18] showed that bacteria were isolated from 65% of the (nonguarded) swabs examined. A total of 18% of mares had cytologic evidence of acute endometritis, comprising 10% who had bacteriologic isolates that would have traditionally been interpreted as significant (on the basis of growth purity, intensity, and species isolated), 4% who had nonsignificant bacteriologic isolates, and 4% who yielded no bacterial growth. Without concurrent cytologic data, the latter 4% would have gone undetected. Conversely, 13% of the mares would have been falsely interpreted as having significant bacterial isolates when concurrent cytologic results revealed no evidence of acute endometritis. Another, smaller, survey that included anaerobic bacterial cultures performed on mares under similar conditions isolated bacteria from 61% of the swabs examined. In that study, 20% of mares had cytologic evidence of acure endometritis, comprising 8% who had mixed aerobic and anaerobic isolates, 5% who had aerobic isolates only, 5% who had anaerobic isolates alone, and 2% who yielded no bacterial growth. These findings and subsequent experience using these techniques in practice have confirmed that for diagnosis of nonvenereal acute endometritis in mares, cytologic rather than bacteriologic data are of primary importance.

CONCLUSIONS

Routine bacteriologic examinations should be performed as follows.

Vestibular/clitoral swabs should be collected before

breeding commences at the start of each season to screen for potential venereal disease carrier status with aerobic and microaerophilic cultures, screening specifically for Ps. aeruginosa, K. pneumoniae, and T. equigenitalis, in order that such cases are not presented to the stallion for natural mating. Vestibular/clitoral swabs should also be taken from sexual contacts if any of these organisms are subsequently isolated from mares after breeding has commenced or if there is clinical evidence of epidemic acute endometritis and as part of the complete gynecologic examination of a barren mare after the end of the breeding season. Although CEM has been eradicated in most countries, the organism is still found in some horse populations and vigilant screening must be maintained internationally to protect equine fertility and export/import trade.

Concurrent endometrial swabs and smears should be collected during estrus before breeding commences and at each subsequent estrous period where conception has not occurred to screen for acute endometritis, in order that such cases can be treated and resolved before mating to maximize chances for conception and normal pregnancy. Diagnosis of acute endometritis should be made on cytologic evidence and not bacterial isolates (with the exception of Ps. aeruginosa, K. pneumoniae, and T. equigenitalis). Bacterial isolates should be used to maintain screening for the potential venereal disease–producing organisms and to make sure that when acute endometritis is diagnosed, appropriate treatment is applied.

Endometrial aspirates, flushings, and/or biopsies should be collected and cultured under aerobic, microaerophilic, and anaerobic conditions and examined mycologically, in addition to being examined cytologically and/or histologically, in cases of diagnosed uterine abnormality (rectal palpation, ultrasonography) and as part of the complete gynecologic examination of a barren mare after the end of the breeding season.

Stallion managers should require negative clitoral and endometrial cultures for Ps. aeruginosa, K. pneumoniae, and T. equigenitalis before they initially accept a mare for natural mating. These organisms excluded, "clean smears" should satisfy their requirement for "clean swabs."[40]

REFERENCES

1. Dimmock, W.W., and Snyder, E.M.: Bacteria of the genital tract of mares and the semen of stallions and their relation to breeding efficiency. J. Am. Vet. Med. Assoc., *64:*288–298, 1923.
2. Dimock, W.W., and Edwards, P.R.: Pathology and bacteriology of the reproductive organs of mares in relation to sterility. *In* Research Bulletin of the Kentucky Agricultural Experimental Station, Lexington. No. 286. 1928.
3. Porchester, Lord: Uterine infections in mares. Vet. Rec., *77:*110–111, 1965.
4. Farrely, B.Y., and Mullaney, P.E.: Cervical and uterine infections in Thoroughbred mares. Ir. Vet. J., *18:*201–212, 1964.
5. Collins, S.M.: A study of the incidence of uterine infections in Thoroughbred mares in Ireland. Vet. Rec., *76:*673–676, 1964.
6. Bain, A.M.: The role of infection in fertility in the Thoroughbred mare. Vet. Rec., *78:*168–175, 1966.
7. Elliott, R.E.W., Callaghan, E.J., and Smith, B.L.: The microflora of the cervix of the Thoroughbred mare: A clinical and bacteriologic survey in a large practice in Hastings. N. Z. Vet. J., *19:*291–302, 1971.
8. Scott, P., et al.: The aerobic bacterial flora of the reproductive tract of the mare. Vet. Rec., *88:*58–61, 1971.
9. Platt, H., et al.: Genital infections in mares. Vet. Rec., *101:*20, 1977.
10. David., J.S.E., Frank, C.J., and Powell, D.G.: Contagious metritis 1977. Vet. Rec., *101:*189–190, 1977.
11. Simpson, D.J., and Eaton-Evans, W.E.: Developments in contagious equine metritis. Vet. Rec., *102:*19–20, 1978.
12. Simpson, D.J., and Eaton-Evans, W.E.: Sites of CEM infection. Vet. Rec., *102:*488, 1978.
13. Meldrum, K.C.: The UK Contagious Equine Metritis (C.E.M.). Ministry of Agriculture, Fisheries and Food, Tolworth, UK. Crown Copyright BL 5888, 1989.
14. Peterson, F.B., McFeely, R.A., and David, J.S.E.: Studies on the pathogenesis of endometritis in the mare. Proc. Am. Assoc. Equine Pract., pp. 279–282, 1969.
15. Hughes, J.P., and Loy, R.G.: The relation of infection to infertility in the mare and stallion. Equine Vet. J., *7:* 155–159, 1974.
16. Greenhof, G.R., and Kenney, R.M.: Evaluation of reproductive status of nonpregnant mares. J. Am. Vet. Med. Assoc., *167:*449–458, 1975.
17. Blanchard, T.L., et al.: Comparison of two techniques for obtaining endometrial bacteriologic cultures in the mare. Theriogenology, *16:*85–93, 1981.
18. Wingfield Digby, N.J., and Ricketts, S.W.: Results of concurrent bacteriologic and cytologic examinations of the endometrium of mares in routine stud farm practice 1978–1981. J. Reprod. Fertil. Suppl., *32:*181–185, 1982.
19. Ricketts, S.W., and Mackintosh, M.E.: Role of anaerobic bacteria in equine endometritis. J. Reprod. Fertil. Suppl., *35:*343–351, 1987.
20. Powell, D.G., David, J.S.E., and Frank, C.J.: Contagious equine metritis. The present situation reviewed and a revised code of practice for control. Vet. Rec., *103:*399–402, 1978.
21. Ricketts, S.W.: Bacteriological examinations of the mare's cervix: Techniques and interpretation of results. Vet. Rec., *108:*46–51, 1981.
22. Mackintosh, M.E.: Bacteriological techniques in the diagnosis of equine genital infections. Vet. Rec., *108:*52–55, 1981.
23. Wingfield Digby, N.J.: Studies of endometrial cytology in mares. Equine Vet. J., *10:*167–170, 1978.
24. Ricketts, S.W.: The barren mare. Diagnosis, prognosis, prophylaxis and treatment for genital abnormality. Part 1., In Practice, *11:*119–125, 1989.
25. Ricketts, S.W.: The barren mare. Diagnosis, prognosis, prophylaxis and treatment for genital abnormality. Part 2., In Practice, *11:*156–164, 1989.
26. Rossdale, P.D., and Ricketts, S.W.. Equine Studfarm Medicine. 2nd ed. London, Bailliere Tindall, 1980.
27. Ricketts, S.W.: Klebsiella aerogenes in mares. Vet. Rec., *99:*489–490, 1976.
28. Ricketts, S.W.: The laboratory as an aid to clinical diag-

nosis. Vet. Clin. North Am. Equine Pract., *3:*445–460, 1987.

29. McAllister, R.A., and Sack, W.O.: Identification of anatomical features of the equine clitoris as potential growth sites for Taylorella equigenitalis. J. Am. Vet. Med. Assoc., *196:*1965–1966, 1990.

30. Freeman, K.P., and Johnston, J.M.: Collaboration of a cytopathologist and practitioner using equine endometrial cytology in a private broodmare practice. Proc. Am. Assoc. Equine Pract., 629–639, 1987

31. Atherton, J.G.: Isolation of the C.E.M. organism. Vet. Rec., *102:*67, 1978.

32. Cowan, S.T., and Steel, K.J.: Manual for the Identification of Medical Bacteria. 2nd ed. Cambridge, Cambridge University Press, 1974.

33. Taylor, C.E.D., et al.: The causative organism of contagious equine metritis, 1977—Proposal for a new species to be known as Haemophilus equigenitalis. Equine Vet. J., *10:*136–144, 1978.

34. Willis, A.T.: Anaerobic Bacteriology: Clinical and Laboratory Practice. 3rd ed. London, Butterworths, 1977.

35. Cottral, G.E. (Ed.): Manual of Standardized Methods for Veterinary Microbiology. Ithaca, Cornell University Press, 1978, pp. 583–587.

36. Riser, E., Noone, P., and Bonnet, M.L.: A new serotyping method for Klebsiella species: Development of the technique. J. Clin. Pathol., *29:*305–308, 1976.

37. Platt, H., Atherton, J.G., and Orskov, I.: Klebsiella and Enterobacter organisms isolated from horses. J. Hyg. Camb., *77:*401–408, 1977.

38. Atherton, J.G., and Pitt, T.L.: Types of Pseudomonas aeruginosa isolated from horses. Equine Vet. J., *14:*329–332, 1982.

39. Woolcock, J.B.: Equine bacterial endometritis. Vet. Clin. North Am. Large Anim. Pract., *2:*241–251, 1980.

40. Hinrichs, K., et al.: Bacteria recovered from the reproductive tracts of normal mares. Proc. Am. Assoc. Equine Pract., pp. 11–16, 1989.

CHAPTER 28

UTERINE CYTOLOGY

Derek Brook

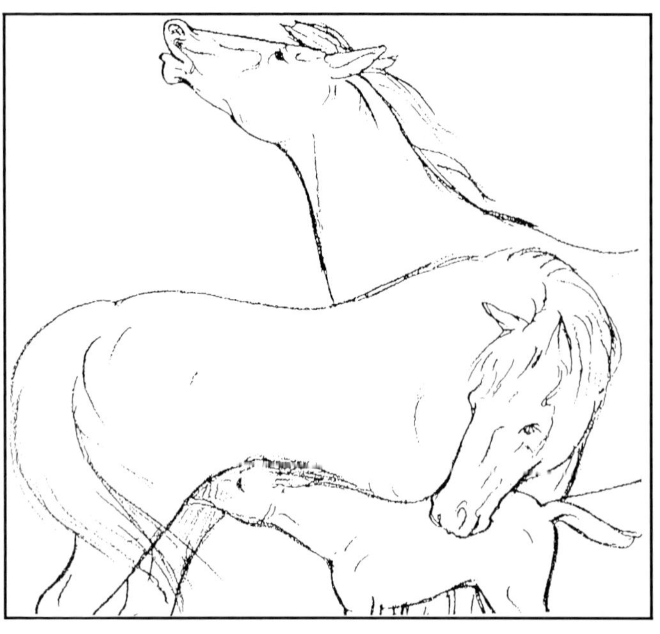

Since isolation of bacteria from the mare's reproductive tract in the 1920s,[1,2] much debate and controversy has arisen over interpretation of these findings. It has been stated that "probably no procedure in reproductive practice stirs such a divergence of opinion and is accomplished under such a broad spectrum of techniques than culture of the mare's genital tract."[3] Originally it was thought that bacteria in any part of the reproductive tract was cause for concern.[4–7] Cervical and vaginal samples were obtained,[2,4,8] and if any organisms were cultured, the mare was subsequently treated, even if it had no history of reproductive problems.[9] This practice began to change as further research showed that normal mares could have a resident bacterial population in certain parts of the reproductive tract, especially the vagina.[10,11] One study of postmortem specimens showed that of 100 normal mares, each having culture material taken from various places, the numbers showing bacterial growth were as follows: 95 from the vagina, 75 from the external uterine os, 45 from the cervical canal, and 33 from the uterus.[12] Bacteria, therefore, can often be found in the more caudal parts of the tract and is not necessarily a cause for concern.

This view has been subsequently reiterated many times.[13–26] Hemophilus equigenitalis and certain strains of Pseudomonas and Klebsiella are exceptions to this.[15,27] Once it was established that bacteria in the caudal part of the tract need not affect fertility, the dilemma of their presence in various parts of the uterus had to be resolved. Some studies show that the normal uterus should be essentially free from bacteria.[16,23,28,29] More recent research using flush techniques, with sophisticated guarded equipment (Fig. 28–1), has shown that the normal mare may have a small number of bacteria even in the uterine horns.[30] The transient forward migration of bacteria usually occurs during coitus and foaling,[11,13] and this contamination is quickly eliminated by the normal, healthy endometrium. Conflicting evidence, however, exists concerning the significance of the continued presence of bacteria in the uterus. Apparently, some mares will conceive while infected,[12,31] but many of these will subsequently abort or produce septicemic foals.[31] Surprisingly, some mares with grossly infected fetal fluids and placentas produce live, healthy foals. Identification of these mares (schematically represented in Fig. 28–2) is often difficult.

A tremendous range of cause and effect apparently exists when dealing with bacteria and equine endometria. The virulence of the organism and the "reactability" of the tissues bring about many different syndromes ranging from nonsignificant surface contamination to severe acute endometritis. A further complicating factor is variability of the endometrium to resist infection.[32] Unfortunately, with presently available knowledge we are unable to adequately assess virulence of a particular pathogen or the way in which the mare will respond to its presence. Certain procedures, however, can assist in enhancing the level of diagnostic accuracy. The use of endometrial cytology smears has proved to be beneficial in this respect. By examining

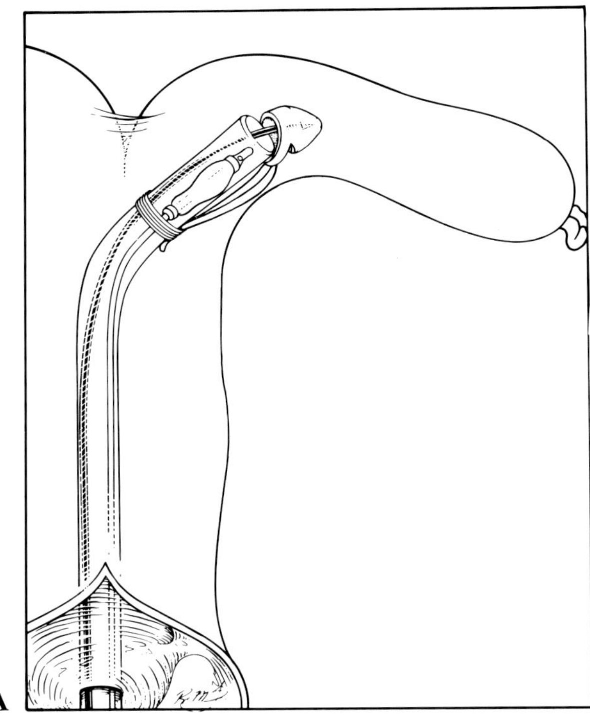

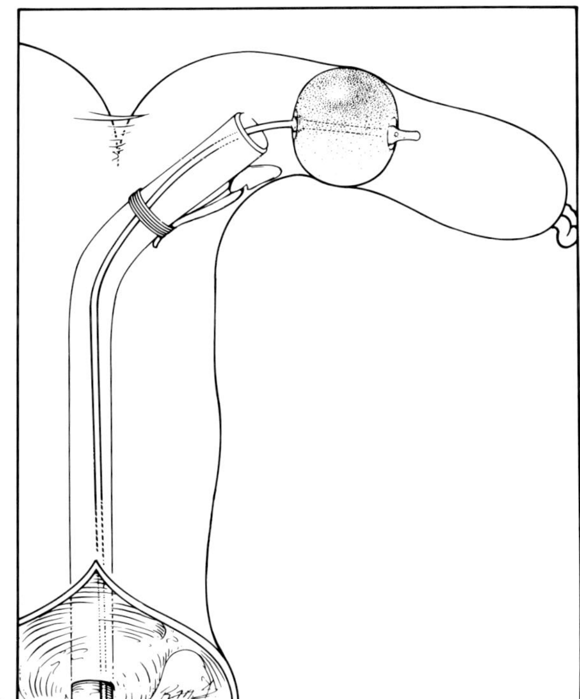

FIG. 28–1. *A*, Guarded uterine lavage system, showing device in uterus with guard cap dislodged before advancement of balloon-tipped catheter. *B*, Balloon catheter inflated in uterine horn ready for lavage of the distal part of that horn. (Courtesy of Dr. A.R. Schmidt).

the reproductive tract for neutrophils, innocuous superficial contamination can be distinguished from significant endometritis.[33–36]

Early studies performed by Knudsen first indicated the value of endometrial cytology.[28] Good correlation existed between the presence of neutrophils and the isolation of bacteria. In the last decade many papers have confirmed these initial findings.[37–53] Reports, however, continue to be published on the results of studies using unguarded or partially guarded techniques. Generally they show poor correlation between the presence of neutrophils and bacteria,[36,54] which is almost always caused by the isolation of vaginal or cervical contaminants. Figures 28–2 to 28–4 schematically represent the range of conditions that can exist.

COLLECTION OF SAMPLES FOR ANALYSIS

STAGE OF CYCLE

Many different opinions have been offered concerning the ideal time to obtain material for culture and cytology examination although some degree of consistency is now emerging. A survey of reports indicated that anestrus sampling can be unreliable.[22] Occasionally diestrus is advocated, but others have specified late diestrus or early estrus,[25] and others suggest the time when the cervix first begins to relax.[10,13–15,55] The majority opinion appears to be to perform the examination only when the mare is in midestrus.[4,8,20,48,56–59] Uterine defenses are believed to be maximal at that time,[60] so that if bacteria and neutrophils are present, a significant problem is likely to exist. Evidence shows that false negatives can occur if cultures are taken only in diestrus or even during a prolonged transitional estrus.[8,32,56,58] The possibility of iatrogenic infection, especially if the uterine defense mechanisms are compromised, exists if diestrous cultures are performed. Chronically infected mares can have negative cultures if they are not in

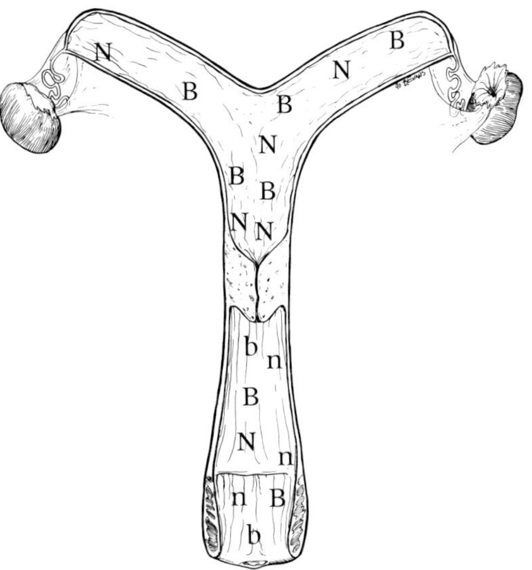

FIG. 28–2. Schematic representation of mare with bacterial endometritis (Category 3). n, few neutrophils; N, high concentration of neutrophils; b, few bacteria; B, high concentration of bacteria.

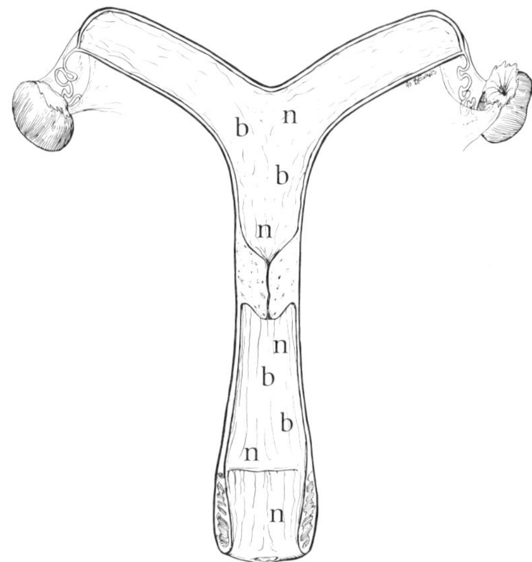

FIG. 28–3. Schematic representation of number of bacteria and neutrophils in the normal mare (category 1). n, few neutrophils; b, few bacteria.

midestrus when the sample is taken.[33] Therefore, the recommendation is that the tests should be performed only when the mare is fully in estrus.

COLLECTION METHODS

The use of some kind of guarded culture device is essential. Because the cervix and vagina are in direct communication with the perineal area, they are constantly challenged by mirco-organisms and foreign material.[30] Figure 28–3 represents the normal mare, and the degree to which this occurs depends on perineal conformation. The use of unguarded instruments will cause the collection of material only representative of the first mucous membrane contacted. If this happens to be the external cervical os, it is pointless to then advance the instrument into the uterus.

Guarded culture rods are now readily available and the ones most commonly used are either the Kalayjian (Kalayjian Industries Inc., Long Beach, CA), McCullough (McCullough Cartwright, Barrington, IL), modified Tiegland (Haver-Lockhart, Kansas City, KS), or Accu-CulShure (Accu-med Corp., Pleasantville, NY). All comprise outer guarded tubes with an inner rod holding a calcium alginate swab. After routine washing of the perineal area, the device is introduced into the vagina by means of either a speculum or lubricated gloved hand. The author prefers the manual technique as the introduction of air via the speculum method is thought undesirable.[14,25,61] The index finger is used to locate the external cervical os and the instrument is then guided through the cervix. Once inside the uterus, the inner plastic rod is advanced and the tip rubbed along the surface of the endometrium. If only material for the cytologic examination is to be collected, the swab is pulled back into the guard tube and the instrument is then immediately withdrawn and the swab tip rolled back and forth on a clean microscope slide. If a concomitant bacterial examination is being performed, the swab should remain in contact with the endometrial surface for approximately 30 s to allow time for adequate adsorption of any organisms.[30] Some clinicians prefer to use two swabs, an initial one for the bacteriologic examination and a second one for the cytologic examination.[39] Others, including the author, find the use of one swab satisfactory. It is essential if one swab is used that on withdrawal from the uterus it be stroked immediately onto an agar plate so that a quantitative as well as a qualitative examination of bacteria can be made.[13] One advantage of using two swabs is that the second one can be premoistened with saline, allowing better preservation of cellular integrity.[42,47] This is not necessary, however, when performing rapid screening tests for the presence or absence of neutrophils. Once the material has been rolled onto the microscope slide, it should be rapidly fixed using a commercial aerosol fixative (Spray-cyte, Clay-Adams, Parsippany, NJ). Air drying of specimens is not advised, as severe cellular distortion can occur.[41]

Research has shown there are certain drawbacks in obtaining samples for cytologic examination using the above-described technique. These include the possibility of causing cellular distortion and the collection of material only from a localized area of the endometrium.[50] A debate exists as to how significant these drawbacks are. If a detailed examination of fine structures within the cells is being performed, then the technique is not adequate. If the clinician is simply looking for the presence

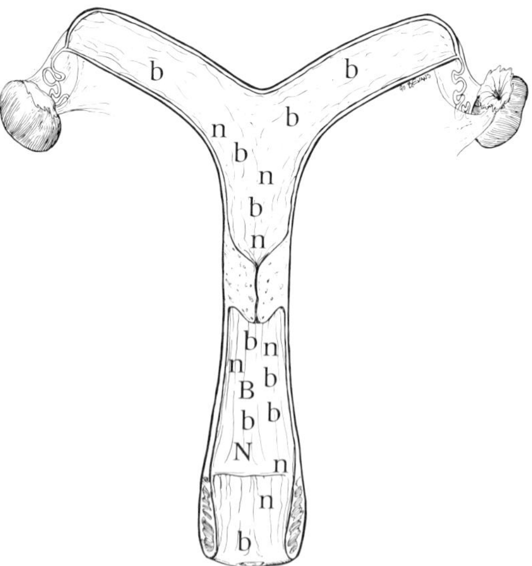

FIG. 28–4. Schematic representation of mare with slightly more bacteria and neutrophils than normal (category 2). This may or may not be significant. n, few neutrophils; N, high concentration of neutrophils; b, few bacteria; B, high concentration of bacteria.

or absence of neutrophils, it is perfectly satisfactory. With reference to the collection of material only from the specific area contacted by the swab, this could be significant, although some research has shown that the majority of problems that occur within the uterus are generalized. The use of uterine lavage has become more popular recently in an attempt to avoid the drawbacks of the swab method and to assess if a more accurate diagnosis can be made. Some of the initial techniques used relatively unguarded systems and probably resulted in contamination by cervical or vaginal organisms.[39,51,62] A flushing catheter (Fig. 28–1) is an exception and does allow the collection of strictly uterine horn material.[30] It is, however, not commercially available at this time. From a practical viewpoint, the use of a guarded culture instrument seems to be presently adequate for routine brood mare practice.[33,40,42,44–46] In addition, attempts to flush uteri may actually create more irritation and result in inappropriate use of clinician's time, particularly if the diagnostic aim is the presence or absence of neutrophils.

STAINING METHODS

The generally accepted staining method is the "Diff-Quik" (American Scientific Products, McGaw Park, IL).[3,33,35,40–42,47,63] That test is easy to perform, gives rapid results, and provides adequate cellular differentiation. For more detailed examination of cellular structures Sano's modification of Pollack's trichrome method is advocated.[35,64] That test takes approximately 40 min and the advantages do not warrant its use except for research purposes.

Occasionally, specialized staining methods performed on a second slide are advantageous.[42,47] The methods include Gram's stain for the demonstration of bacteria and fungi[41,54] and the new methylene blue stain for the demonstration of bacterial capsules.[46]

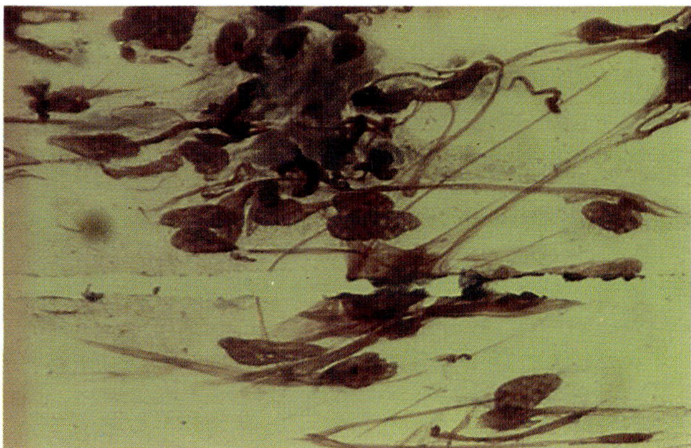

FIG. 28–5. Endometrial smear of normal uterus showing epithelial cells and mucus.

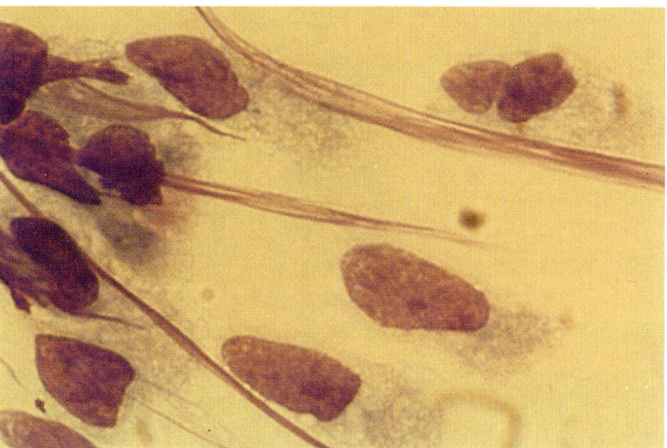

FIG. 28–6. Higher magnification of epithelial cells showing distortion caused by swab collection procedure.

RECOGNITION OF VARIOUS CELL TYPES

EPITHELIAL CELLS

Epithelial cells are by far the most commonly seen cells in the normal uterine smear. They are usually nonciliated. However, especially in diestrus, they are occasionally ciliated.[41] They range from being cuboidal in anestrus to tall columnar in the normally cycling mare.[33,59,64] When collected in estrus, epithelial cells usually appear with mucus extending from the cytoplasm (Figs. 28–5 and 28–6). Mucus is not apparent if the collection method is uterine lavage[30] (Fig. 28–7). Nuclei stain basophilically, showing large pink to violet reaction. The cytoplasm is often vacuolated in its basal third and light blue in color[40] (Fig. 28–7). The rare columnar ciliated cells often have faintly eosinophilic cytoplasm.[41,64] Distortion is often apparent in cells collected by swab: the rolling out process can cause elongation (Fig. 28–6). Maiden and younger mares will produce smears containing large numbers of epi-

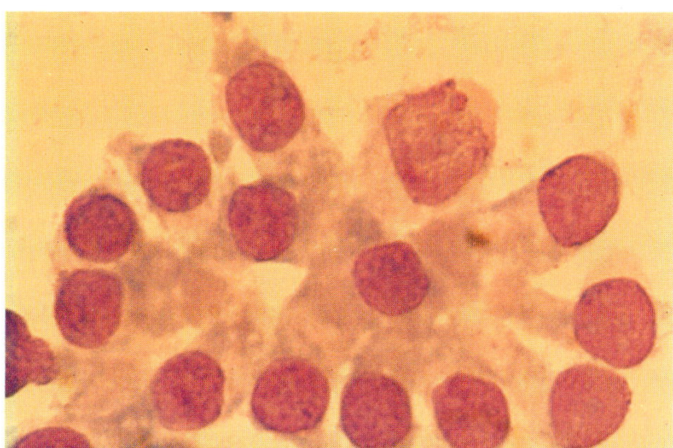

FIG. 28–7. Epithelial cells from uterine smear of mare in estrus. Collection method was uterine lavage, hence no mucus or cellular distortion.

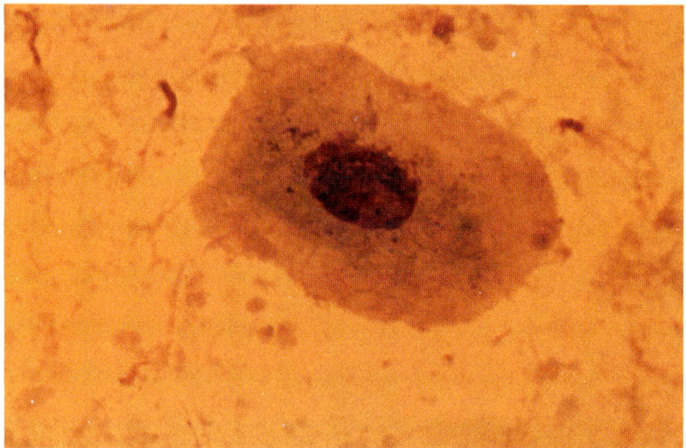

FIG. 28–8. Squamous epithelial cell from uterine smear, indicating vaginal contamination.

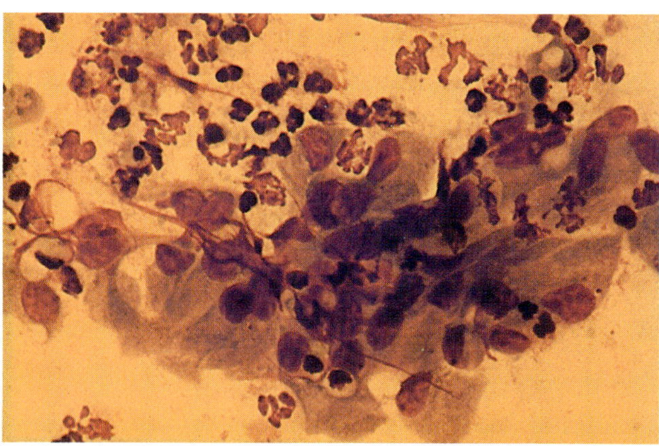

FIG. 28–9. Uterine smear of mare with endometritis, showing epithelial cells and neutrophils.

thelial cells with overlapping cytoplasm and mucus, resembling a "honeycomb" pattern.[40] Mares in anestrus typically have cuboidal or low columnar epithelial cells, little cytoplasmic vacuolation, and no attached mucus.[32]

Squamous epithelial cells are rare and usually represent either cervical or vaginal contamination during the collection procedure or urine pooling[33,41,50,51,64] (Fig. 28–8). They have also been occasionally identified in early postpartum smears.[33] Degenerate epithelial cells, often lacking cytoplasm, are frequently seen in poorly fixed or air-dried smears.[22,41] Early researchers attributed the presence of these to reduced fertility,[22] but more recent studies have not confirmed that.[33] For detailed descriptions of epithelial cell structure and its relationship to different stages of the estrous cycle, refer to other published work.[41,50,64]

NEUTROPHILS

Neutrophils are the predominant cell types in mares with bacterial evidence of infection[28,36,52,65] (Figs. 28–9 to 28–11). Correctly prepared smears from normal mares rarely contain neutrophils, although they will appear transiently after breeding, foaling, and uterine lavage.[52,66]

Experiments have shown that the normal mare's endometrium will react to bacterial inoculation by producing an intense infiltration of neutrophils, which subsides within 72 h or less.[23,65] This reaction will last longer in barren mares as will the inflammatory reaction to natural breeding or artificial insemination.[33] Mature hypersegmented neutrophils have been said to be indicative of nonseptic inflammation, whereas those involved in the septic process are pyknotic and karyolytic[45] (Fig. 28–11).

Attempts were made during the 1980s to quantitate the neutrophils isolated and to assign varying degrees of significance to these numbers (Table 28–1). The quantitative estimation proved difficult, because it depends on the collection method. Clearly, if vast numbers of neutrophils are present, a significant problem exists, and conversely, if none is found, the mare has no inflammation of the endometrium. Difficulty arises when "several" neurophils are present and other diagnostic procedures, such as quantitative and qualitative bacteriologic culture, must be used to arrive at a diagnosis or recommendation.

OTHER INFLAMMATORY CELLS

Large macrophages have only been reported in the early postpartum period and are usually present with red blood cells and neutrophils[33,35,40] (Figs. 28–11 and 28–12). They are often multinucleated and vacuolated (Fig. 28–12).

Lymphocytes are relatively rare[52] and sometimes difficult to distinguish from immature neutrophils. They have been associated with chronic endometritis[46] and lymphatic stasis of the endometrium.[28] Other authors have indicated that their presense is not significant.[45] Eosinophils are also a rare finding and in most instances have been associated with vaginal wind sucking[51] (Fig. 28–13).

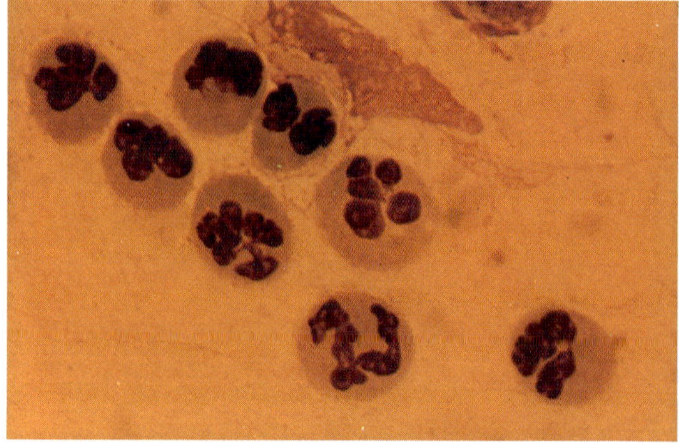

FIG. 28–10. Endometrial smear from mare with endometritis, showing neutrophils at various stages of maturity.

TABLE 28–1. QUANTITATIVE ESTIMATION OF NEUTROPHILS IN ENDOMETRIAL SMEARS

AUTHORITY	YEAR	METHOD OF QUANITATION
Knudsen	1964	Positive if > 1 neutrophil in 5 fields (× 240)
Wingfield-Digby	1978	Estimates ratio of neutrophils to epithelial cells
Asbury	1982	Positive if ratio of epithelial cells to neutrophils > 10:1
Asbury	1984	Positive if more than 1 neutrophil in 5 high-powered fields
Couto and Hughes	1984	Graded according to ratio of neutrophils to epithelial cells in 8 fields (× 100)
Brook	1985	Negative if no PNMs in 10 fields (× 400) Doubtful if 1 to 5 PMNs* in 10 fields Positive if > 5 PMNs in 10 fields
la Cour and Sprinkle	1986	Used a 0 to 5 grading method, depending on ratio of PMNs to epithelial cells
Ball et al.	1988	Positive if > 2% of cells were neutrophils
Purswell et al.	1989	Positive if ≥ 1 neutrophil per field (× 400)
Ricketts and Mackintosh	1989	Negative 0% neutrophils +/− less than 0.5% PMNs + 0.5 to 5% PMNs 2+ 5 to 30% PMNs 3+ > 30% PMNs

*PMNs, polymorphonuclear leukocytes.

RED BLOOD CELLS

Red blood cells are not commonly seen but will occasionally occur in postfoaling smears and in cases of severe acute endometritis[33,40,52] (Fig. 28–11). They have been reported in normal mares caused by physiologic hyperemia,[41] in cases associated with trauma as a result of cytologic sampling techniques, and obviously, after collection of biopsy specimens.[52]

CALCIUM CARBONATE CRYSTALS

Calcium carbonate crystals are occasionally seen in mares that have a tendency to pool urine.[50] However, this is not sufficient evidence to confirm the condition as being a problem, as it may be transient. A confirmatory diagnosis can only be made if repeat smears show a similar picture and include squamous epithelial cells and if clinical findings substantiate it.

BACTERIA, YEASTS, AND FUNGI

Bacteria are only rarely visible in smears stained by the Diff-Quik method[33] (Fig. 28–11), even if a culture is positive. They can be made more readily visible by the use of Gram's stain. Occasionally, the methylene blue stain is used when a suspicion of Klebsiella sp. infection exists.[67] The capsule of the organism is made visible by this stain. Gram's stain has been suggested as a reasonable procedure to hasten the initiation of antibacterial therapy while waiting for culture results.[4,42,54] Fungal elements, including branching hyphae and conid-

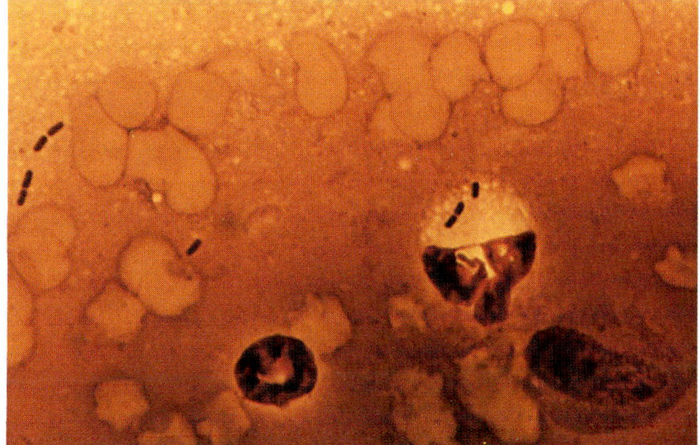

FIG. 28–11. Postfoaling smear showing bacteria, degenerate neutrophils, and red blood cells.

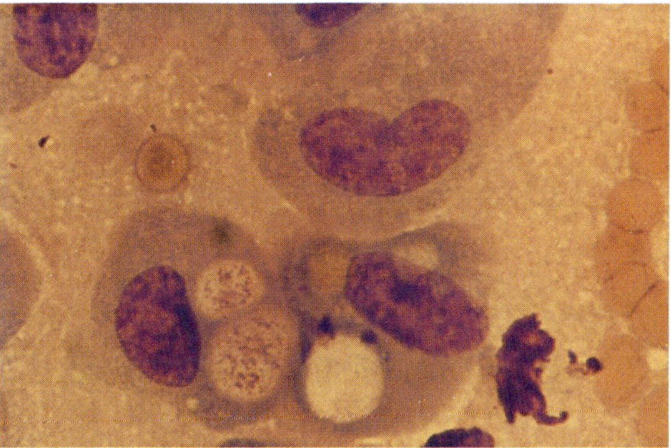

FIG. 28–12. Smear showing large vacuolated macrophages, typical of the immediate postpartum period.

iophores, are readily visible with the Diff-Quick stain[33,40,47,50,68–70] (Fig. 28–14).

INTERPRETATION OF UTERINE SMEARS

The schematic representations in Figures 28–2 to 28–4 cover the majority of mares encountered by the practitioner. In order to determine into which category the mare fits, it is essential to do a quantitative as well as a qualitative examination of any bacteria and or neutrophils present. These findings should also be evaluated in conjunction with the reproductive history of the mare.

Fortunately, during the 1980s clinicians had, by and large, moved away from the use of unguarded culturing instruments. Furthermore, the tendency to use broth to potentiate the growth of every single organism present has declined. Likewise, the blanket swabbing of every mare, even maidens, is no longer in vogue. Many normal mares were subjected to intrauterine treatment because the isolation of a single bacterial contaminant from the vagina subsequently yielded a heavy growth of that particular organism after broth incubation.

Presently available equipment used correctly can identify mares in categories 1 and 3 (Figs. 28–2 and 28–3). A smear producing only healthy epithelial cells combined with a negative culture result is easy to interpret as a clean, healthy mare (Fig. 28–3). Alternatively, a smear containing more neutrophils than epithelial cells, combined with a pure, heavy bacterial growth of any organism, is adequate proof of significant endometritis (Fig. 28–2).

A mare in category 2 (Fig. 28–4) with only a few neutrophils and a few colonies of bacteria is difficult and sometimes challenging to interpret. Likewise, the mare may show inconsistent results such as the false negative when no bacteria are obtained but lots of neutrophils exist or the false positive when a large amount of bacteria exist but no neutrophils are found. Because

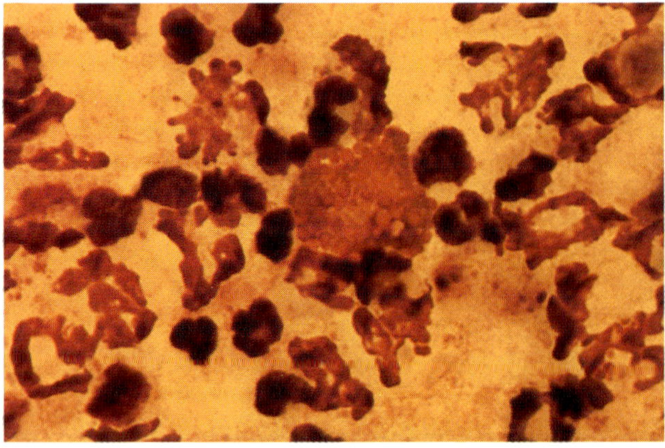

FIG. 28–13. Smear from endometrium of mare prone to wind sucking. A large eosinophil is present in the center of the smear.

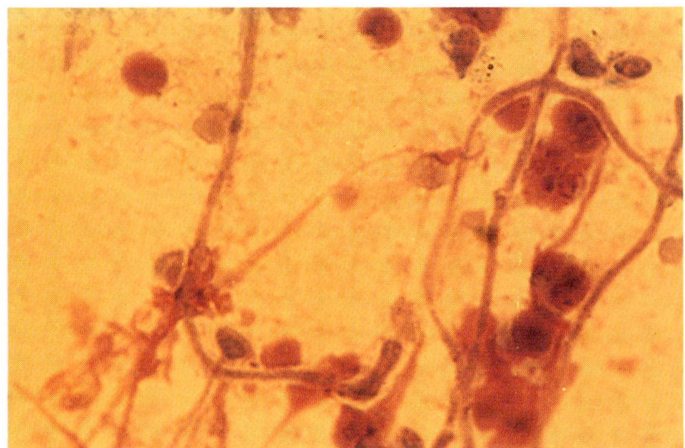

FIG. 28–14. Smear from mare with fungal endometritis, showing branching hyphae.

no set guidelines are used at present to accurately quantitate both colony-forming units (CFUs) and neutrophils, the practitioner must rely on using all the available information to arrive at a diagnosis. Table 28–1 shows the different methods that have been used to quantitate the neutrophils present, but until a totally standardized method of collection of the sample is developed, categorical diagnosis is impossible.

False positives (positive bacteriologically and negative cytologically) can occur with either surface contamination or contamination of the swab during the collection procedure by bacteria in the posterior part of the reproductive tract. Chronically infected mares may also produce false positive results in diestrus and only show a neutrophil response when in estrus.[33] False negatives can occur in several situations.[52]

1. Presence of antibiotics in the uterus.
2. Deep-seated infections.[35]
3. Presence of anerobes, micoplasma, etc. or other organisms not detectable by conventional or routine culture methods.
4. Noninfectious irritation, e.g., foreign body in the uterus.
5. Postfoaling and postnatural service.

SUMMARY

The examination of endometrial smears is relatively easy to perform and produces rapid results. By using this technique, uterine inflammation can be diagnosed and a decision as to whether or not to cover a mare can be quickly made without having to wait for culture results. It should also be a part of any breeding soundness examination.[45] Correct technique is essential, and the practitioner is encouraged to do the entire procedure within his or her own facility. On occasions, when quantitative results are doubtful, the entire clinical picture must be assessed before arriving at any conclusions.

REFERENCES

1. Schiebell, G.: Untersuchunden über die bakterienflora im uterus sterilen stuten (Dissertation). Hanover, Chr Jessen und Sohn, 1920, pp. 47–56.
2. Dimock, W.W., and Edwards, P.R.: The pathology and bacteriology of the reproductive organs of mares in relation to sterility. *In* Bulletin of the Kentucky Agricultural Experimental Station, Lexington. No. 286, 1928, pp. 157–163.
3. Asbury, A.C.: The reproductive system. *In* Equine Medicine and Surgery. Vol 2. 3rd ed. Edited by R.A. Mansmann and E.S. McAllister. Santa Barbara, American Veterinary Publications, 1982, pp. 1312–1336.
4. Collins, S.M.: A study of the cervical and uterine infection in thoroughbred mares in Ireland. Vet. Rec., *76*:673–677, 1964.
5. Day, F.T.: The veterinary clinicians' approach to breeding problems in mares. Vet. Rec., *69*:1258–1265, 1957.
6. Millar, W.C., and Barnett, G.: Twenty years of equine research. Veterinarian, *5*:51–64, 1968.
7. Millar, R., and Francis, J.: The relation of clinical and bacteriologic findings to fertility in Thoroughbred mares. Aust. Vet. J., *50*:351–354, 1974.
8. Gadd, J.D.: The relationship of bacterial cultures, microscopic smear examination and medical treatment to surgical correction of barren mares. Proc. Am. Assoc. Equine Pract., 362–368, 1975.
9. Ommert, W.: Discussion panel on brood mare problems. Proc. Am. Assoc. Equine Pract., 99–104, 1964.
10. O'Briain, C.: Clinical aspects of the bacteriology of the reproductive tract of the Thoroughbred mare. Ir. Vet. J., *16*:181–194, 1962.
11. Farrelly, B.T., and Mullaney, M.A.: Cervical and uterine infection in Thoroughbred mares. Ir. Vet. J., *18*:201–212, 1964.
12. Scott, P., et al.: The aerobic bacterial flora of the reproductive tract of the mare. Vet Rec., *88*:58–61, 1971.
13. Asbury, A.C.: Bacterial endometritis. *In* Current Therapy in Equine Medicine. Edited by N.E. Robinson. Philadelphia, W.B. Saunders, 1983, pp. 410–414.
14. Allen, W.E., and Newcombe, J.R.: Aspects of genital infection and swabbing techniques in the mare. Vet. Rec., *104*:228–231, 1979.
15. Woolcock, J.B.: Equine bacterial endometritis. *In* Veterinary Clinics of North America: Large Animal Practice. Edited by J.P. Hughes. Philadelphia, W.B. Saunders, 1980, pp. 241–251.
16. Conboy, H.S.: Diagnosis and therapy of equine endometritis. Proc. Am. Assoc. Equine Pract., 165–171, 1978.
17. Hughes, J.P., Loy, R.G., Asbury, A.C., and Burd, H.E.: The occurrence of Pseudomonas in the reproductive tract of mares and its effect on fertility. Cornell Vet., *56*:595–610, 1966.
18. Crouch, J.F., et al.: Venereal transmission of Klebsiella aerogenes in a Thoroughbred stud from a persistently infected stallion. Vet. Rec., *90*:21–25, 1972.
19. Ellsworth, K.C.: The significance and interpretation of cervical cultures in the mare. Proc Am. Assoc. Equine Pract., 129–132, 1966.
20. Brandt, G.W.: The significance and interpretation of uterine biopsy in the mare. Proc. Am. Assoc. Equine Pract., 279–283, 1970.
21. Newcombe, J.R., and Allen, W.E.: Proceedings Colloques de la Societé national pour l'étude de la sterilité et de la fecondité. Masson, pp. 289–303, 1977.
22. Solomon, W.J., Schultz, R.H., and Fahning, M.L.: A study of chronic infertility in the mare utilizing uterine biopsy, cytology and cultural methods. Proc. Am. Assoc. Equine Pract., 55–68, 1972.
23. Peterson, F.B., McFeely, R.A., and David, J.S.E.: Studies on the pathogenesis of endometritis in the mare. Proc. Am. Assoc. Equine Pract., 279–287, 1969.
24. Witherspoon, D.M., Goldston, R.T., and Adsits, M.E.: Uterine culture and biopsy in the mare. J. Am. Vet. Med. Assoc., *161*:1365–1366, 1972.
25. Nyborg, R.G.: Uterininfektioners udbredelse art ag betydning hos hopper i et tilfaeldigt ialgt afsnit af den danske landayl. Dansk Maanedsskr. Dyrlaeg, *63*:205–208, 1954.
26. Elliot, R.E.W., Calaghan. E.J., and Smith, B.L.: The microflora of the cervix of the Thoroughbred mare. A clinical and bacteriological survey in a large animal practice in Hastings. N.Z. Vet. J., *19*:291–302, 1971.
27. Ricketts, S.W.: Bacteriological examinations of the mare's cervix: Techniques and interpretation of results. Vet. Rec., *108*:46–51, 1981.
28. Knudsen, O.: Endometrial cytology as a diagnostic aid in mares. Cornell Vet., *54*:415–422, 1964.
29. Roberts, S.J.: Veterinary Obstetrics and Genital Diseases. Ann Arbor, Edwards Brothers, 1971.
30. Schmidt, A.R.: Guarded right uterine horn lavage in the mare for bacteriology and cytology. Masters thesis. Michigan State University, 1988.
31. Hoppe, R., Domanski, E., and Dobrowolska, A. (eds.): Causes and treatment of inflammation of the genital tract in the mare with special reference to the process caused by hemolytic cocci. *In* Third International Congress of Animal Reproduction and Artificial Insemination. Vol. 2. 1956, pp. 83–85. Cambridge, 1956, pp. 83–85.
32. Liu, I.K.M.: Uterine defense mechanisms in the mare. Vet. Clin. North Am. Large Anim. Pract., *4*:221–228, 1988.
33. Brook, D.: Exfoliative endometrial cytology in the mare. Master's thesis. Stellenbosch, South Africa, 1983.
34. Brook, D.: Diagnosis of equine endometrial candidiasis by direct smear and successful treatment with amphotericin B and oxytetracycline. J. S. Afr. Vet. Assoc., *53*:261–263, 1982.
35. Brook, D.: The diagnosis of equine bacterial endometritis. Compend. Contin. Ed. Practicing Vet., *6*:S300–S306, 1984.
36. Wingfield Digby, N.J., and Ricketts, S.W.: Results of concurrent bacteriological and cytological examinations of the endometrium of mares in routine stud farm practice. J. Reprod. Fertil. Suppl., *32*:181–185, 1982.
37. Asbury, A.C.: Pathogenesis and diagnosis of uterine infection in mares. *In* Proceedings of the Western States Veterinary Conference. Vol. 13. Edited by K.D. Weide. Intermountain Veterinary Medical Association, Las Vegas, 1984, pp. 9–14.
38. Asbury, A.C.: Endometritis diagnosis in the mare. Equine Vet. Data, *5*:166, 1984.
39. Ball, B.A., et al.: Use of a low-volume uterine flush for microbiologic and cytologic examination of the mare's endometrium. Theriogenology, *29*:1269–1283, 1988.
40. Brook, D.: Cytological and bacteriological examination of the mare's endometrium. Equine Vet. Sci., *5*:16–22, 1985.
41. Couto, M.S., and Hughes, J.P.: Technique and interpretation of cervical and endometrial cytology in the mare. Equine Vet. Sci., *4*:265–273, 1984.

42. Crickmann, J.A., and Pugh, D.G.: Equine cytology: A review of techniques and interpretations. Vet. Med., pp. 650–656, 1986.
43. Gross, T.L., and LeBlanc, M.M.: Seasonal variation of histomorphological features of equine endometrium. J. Am. Vet. Med. Assoc., *184*:1379–1382, 1984.
44. Knudsen, O.: A combined cytologic and bacteriologic endometrial examination in the mare. Proc Am. Assoc. Equine Pract., pp. 431–433, 1982.
45. La Cour, A., and Sprinkle, T.A.: Relationship of endometrial cytology and fertility in the broodmare. Equine Pract., 7:28–36, 1985.
46. Neely, D.: Equine Reproduction, Somerville, Veterinary Learning Systems, 1983.
47. Pugh, D.G., Bowen, J.M., Kloppe, L.H., and Simpson, R.B.: Fungal endometritis in mares. Compend. Contin. Educ. Practicing Vet., *8*:S173–S181, 1986.
48. Ricketts, S.W., and Mackintosh, M.E.: Role of anaerobic bacteria in equine endometritis. J. Reprod. Fertil. Suppl., *35*:343–351, 1987.
49. Rossdale, P.D., and Ricketts, S.W.: The Practice of Equine Stud Farm Medicine. 2nd ed. Philadelphia, Lea & Febiger, 1980.
50. Roszel, J.F., and Freeman, K.P.: Equine endometrial cytology. Vet Clin North Am. Large Anim. Pract., *4*:247–262, 1988.
51. Slusher, S.H., Freeman, K.P., and Reszel, J.F.: Eosinophils in equine uterine cytology and histology specimens. J. Am. Vet. Med. Assoc., *184*:665–670, 1984.
52. Wingfield Digby, N.J.: Studies of endometrial cytology in mares. Equine Vet. J., *10*:167–170, 1978.
53. Blanchard, T.L., Garcia, M.C., Hurtgen, J.P., and Kenney R.M.: Comparison of two techniques for obtaining endometrial bacteriologic cultures in the mare. Theriogenology, *16*:85–93, 1981.
54. Shin, S.J., Lein, D.H., Aronson, A.L., and Nusbaum, S.R. The bacteriological culture of equine uterine contents: In-vitro sensitivity of organisms isolated and interpretation. J. Reprod. Fertil. Suppl., *27*:307–315, 1979.
55. Hughes, J.P.: Reproductive panel discussion. Proc. Am. Assoc. Equine Pract., 188–201, 1978.
56. Rasbech, N.O.: Effects of equine genital infections on reproduction. Nord. Vet. Med., *17*:305–317, 1965.
57. Bain, A.M.: The role of infection in infertility in the Thoroughbred mare. Vet. Rec., *78*:168–171, 1966.
58. Bruner, D.W.: Notes on genital infection in the mare. Cornell Vet., *41*:247–250, 1951.
59. David, J.B.S., et al.: Contagious metritis. Vet. Rec., *101*:189–190, 1977.
60. Ganjam, V.K., et al.: Effects of ovarian hormones on the phagocytic response of ovariectomized mares. J. Reprod. Fertil. Suppl., *32*:169–174, 1982.
61. Newcombe, J.R.: Comparison of the bacterial flora of three sites in the genital tract of the mare. Vet. Rec., *102*:169–170, 1978.
62. Zavy, M.T., Blazer, F.W., and Sharp, D.C.: A non-surgical technique for the collection of uterine fluid from the mare. J. Anim. Sci., *47*:672–676, 1978.
63. Purswell, B.J., Ley, W.B., Sriranganathan, N., and Bowen, J.M.: Aerobic and anaerobic bacterial flora in the postpartum mare. Equine Vet. Sci., *9*:141–144, 1989.
64. Freeman, K.P., Roszel, J.F., and Slusher, S.H.: Equine endometrial cytologic smear patterns. Compend. Contin. Educ. Practicing Vet., *8*:349–360, 1986.
65. Hughes, J.P., and Loy, R.G.: Investigation of the effect of intrauterine innoculation of Streptococcus zooepidemicus in the mare. Proc. Am. Assoc. Equine Pract., 289–292, 1969.
66. Bennett, D.G., et al.: Reaction of the equine endometrium to intrauterine infusion. Proc. Am. Assoc. Equine Pract., 135–139, 1980.
67. Platt, H., Atherton, J.G., and Orskov, I.: Klebsiella and Enterobacter organisms isolated from horses. J. Hyg. Camb., *77*:41–44, 1976.
68. Hurtgen, J.P.: Fungal metritis. Equine Vet. Data, *5*:20–21, 1984.
69. Blue, M.G.: Myotic invasion of the mare's uterus. Vet. Rec., *113*:131–132, 1983.
70. Blue, M.G., and Hannwacker, M.A.: Endometritis in the mare caused by a coryneform organism, a case report and experimental studies. Cornell Vet., *74*:331–134, 1984.

CHAPTER 29

ENDOSCOPY

M.M. LeBlanc

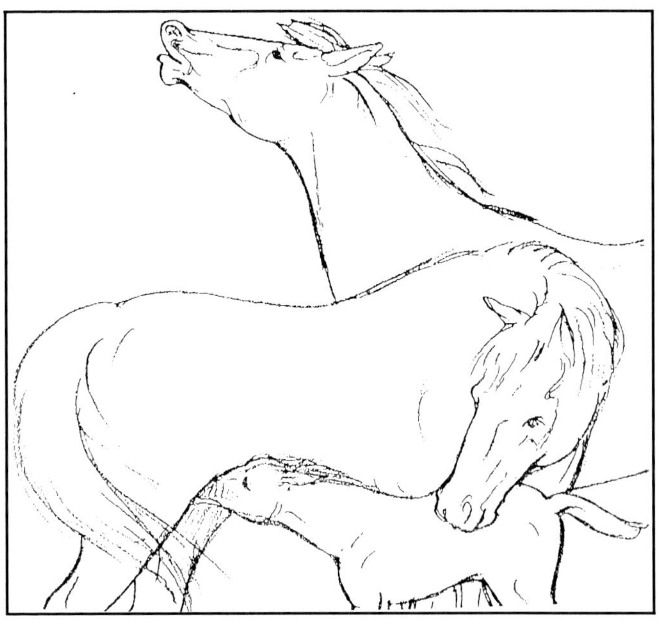

Examination of the uterine lumen through a flexible fiberoptic instrument or video endoscope can be a valuable diagnostic procedure. Endoscopic examination should be considered when uterine abnormalities detected by rectal palpation or ultrasonography need further identification or when the cause of infertility cannot be determined by other diagnostic procedures. For instance, endoscopy was helpful in determining the cause of infertility in 26 of 40 problem mares (65%).[1] Adhesions, intrauterine synechia, areas of discoloration, and enlargements at the uterotubal junction are identified only by endoscopy. Structural enlargements on the surface of the endometrium such as lymphatic cysts or polyps are identified easily with ultrasonography. Removal of these structures, however, is best performed through an endoscope.

TIMING OF PROCEDURE

Before endoscopy, mares should have a complete reproductive examination—including digital or manual palpation, ultrasonographic, cytologic, bacteriologic, and histologic studies—of the uterus. These diagnostic procedures are helpful in determining the presence or absence of lesions within the uterine lumen. Endoscopy may be performed during estrus or diestrus, although diestrus is preferred. During diestrus, the uterus distends more readily and less medium is spilled because the cervix is tightly closed. During estrus, the uterus distends with difficulty because medium escapes through the relaxed, open cervix.

When the uterus is under influence of progesterone, bactericidal activity and neutrophil phagocytosis are decreased.[2] Mares undergoing endoscopic examinations during diestrus may, therefore, experience greater endometrial inflammation than mares having endoscopy performed during estrus. Because many mares that are examined have endometritis or are prone to endometritis, prophylactic antibiotics are warranted.

PREPARATION OF MARE

Preparation of the mare for endoscopy is similar to that for any gynecologic procedure. Mares should be restrained in stocks. The tail should be wrapped and the perineal area washed carefully with a nonirritating soap. The labia should be blotted dry and clean, moist cotton used to wipe the inner edges of the labia and clitoral fossa. A clean plastic sleeve with a sterile surgeon's glove applied over it or a sterile shoulder-length glove is placed over the examiner's arm. Because the procedure is usually performed in infertile mares aseptic technique is essential.

INSTRUMENTATION

Endoscopic examination of the uterine lumen is best performed with a fiberoptic endoscope designed for gastrointestinal or colonic examination, for example, gastrointestinal fiberscope type 2T flexible esophagealscope and colonoscope Model CF-MB2 (Olympus Corp. of America, New Hyde Park, NY).[3] The fiberscope needs to be at least 1 m in length with an outer diameter of 12.6 mm or greater. Ancillary instruments such as cannulas, flexible biopsy forceps or scissors, small tissue forceps, and small suction tubes can be passed through channels within the endoscope. These instruments are helpful in aspirating fluid in lymphatic cysts but they are not of adequate size to obtain an endometrial sample (biopsy) large enough for meaningful evaluation.

Because of the large size of the uterine lumen, a strong bright beam of light is needed to see the endometrium. The majority of light sources are fitted with halogen or xenon lamps and produce between 100 and 300 w. High-intensity (300-w), cold-light supply (xenon, short-arc lamp) offers excellent light for still photography and videotaping.[3] Light sources of lower wattage (150 w) may not provide sufficient light, especially if a second eyepiece or videocamera is attached to the scope.

DISINFECTION

Ideally, the fiberoptic instrument should be sterilized with ethylene oxide prior to intrauterine use. A practical alternative is to thoroughly clean the working end of the instrument in either an iodophor or a glutaraldehyde solution.[3] Fiberoptic endoscopes are easily damaged because they are made of synthetic resin materials and special rubbers. Only disinfectants approved by the manufacturer should be used to clean them. Fiberoptic endoscopes can be immersed in a large pan filled with disinfectant solution either repeatedly or for the time prescribed by the manufacturer, usually no longer than 20 min. Prolonged immersion may damage instruments with failing seals. Before introducing it into the uterus, the fiberscope should be wiped clean with alcohol and allowed to dry.

DISTENTION OF THE UTERINE LUMEN

The uterine lumen should be distended before endoscopy with either fluid, such as sterile physiologic saline, or an inert gas, such as carbon dioxide. Both media allow an adequate view of the uterine body and horns. Sterile water is nonirritating, economical, and has excellent optical qualities as a distention medium. It is difficult to see the endometrium, however, if there are large quantities of exudate floating in the solution. Carbon dioxide allows excellent viewing, high-quality photography, and is readily available.[3] Carbon dioxide must be delivered under pressure and, therefore, may cause significant endometrial damage and abdominal discomfort.

Distention media can be either infused through a channel in the fiberscope or through a catheter placed in the uterine lumen. The author prefers passing a uterine flushing tube, such as the equine uterine flushing catheter #EUF-80 (Bivona Inc., Gary, IN), through the cervix prior to introduction of the fiberoptic endoscope. Then as the tip of the endoscope passes into the cervix, small volumes of fluid are introduced to fill the uterine body and horns. Fluid delivery is controlled by gravity flow and the amount used depends on the degree of distension of the uterine lumen. In older mares 1 to 2 L of fluid can be infused into the uterus without discomfort to the mare.

APPEARANCE OF NORMAL ENDOMETRIUM

With the tip of the endoscope placed in the uterine lumen, the body of the uterus and bifurcation of the two horns can be identified. The latter appears as a vertical pillar especially evident as inflation of the horns commences and should not be confused with an intraluminal adhesion. The normal uterine mucosa has a glistening pink appearance and no exudate present on its surface. The endoscope is then advanced down each uterine horn to systematically observe all of the endometrium. The horns should distend easily and uniformly. The diameter of the uterine horns should be greatest at their junction with the uterine body.

PATHOLOGIC CHANGES

Typical lesions observed are cystic structures, adhesions, and textural and color changes of the endometrium. Areas of discoloration may vary from localized hyperemic areas that suggest inflammatory changes to areas of pale, blanched tissue that suggest decreased vascularity.[1] Exudate may be firmly attached to the endometrium or floating freely within the lumen. Adhesions can vary from thin, elongated synechia to short, thick bands of endometrial tissue. Adhesions may form following infusion of irritating compounds such as Lugol's solution into the uterus,[1] or as an aftermath of severe dystocia, retained placenta, or postpartum metritis.

Endometrial cysts, originating from lymphatic or glandular tissue, are frequently seen. Lymphatic cysts are thought to develop from obstructed lymphatic channels and are seen most commonly in multiparous mares with uteri that have undergone fibrotic changes.[4] Lymphatic cysts may appear as spheroidal or cylindrical structures that are either pedunculated or sessile.[5] They range from 1 to 20 cm in diameter and differ markedly from the surrounding endometrium. Most lymphatic cysts are situated in the mid to distal portion of a horn or at the bifurcation of the uterine body and often are divided by septa.[5] Lymphatic cysts can be drained by advancing a biopsy forceps through the operating channel of the fiberoptic scope, grasping the cyst, aspirating the lymphatic fluid, and lavaging the cyst cavity.

Endometrial glandular cysts, thought to result from hormonal changes, are small (<1 cm in diameter) and are embedded within the endometrium.[6] They are usually smooth, round, and firm and are similar to endometrial tissue, and because they are embedded, they do not move with flushing or probing. Attempts at their removal have been unsuccessful.[5]

The relationship between intrauterine cysts and infertility is not clear. Large lymphatic cysts may impede motility of the early conceptus, restricting the ability of the vesicle to prevent luteolysis after day 10. Later in pregnancy, contact between the cyst wall and the yolk sac or allantois may prevent absorption of nutrients. In one report, only older mares with either five or more cysts or cysts $\geq$10 mm in diameter had an increased embryonic loss rate to day 40. Those with a lower number of cysts or cysts $\leq$10 mm in diameter did not have increased embryonic loss.[7] Uterine cysts have also been seen in conjunction with chronic infiltrative lymphocytic endometritis.[8]

Whether removal of lymphatic cysts improves fertility remains conjectural. Many large lymphatic cysts are removed but there are no data supporting or disproving the influence of the procedure on future fertility.

AFTERCARE OF MARE

As noted, endoscopy of the uterus results in some degree of inflammation to the endometrium. The degree of inflammation depends on when the procedure is conducted during the estrous cycle, the distention medium used, and the status of uterine defense mechanisms of the mare. It is advisable to administer systemic antibiotics immediately before and for 48 h after uterine endoscopy. Breeding mares during the estrus immediately following endoscopic examination should be avoided if the endometrium becomes greatly inflamed following endoscopy. When aseptic technique is followed, no long-term adverse effects on endometrial integrity should occur.

REFERENCES

1. Mather, E.C., et al.: The use of fiber-optic techniques in clinical diagnosis and visual assessment of experimental intrauterine therapy in mares. J. Reprod. Fertil. Suppl., *25:*293–297, 1979.
2. Watson, E.D., et al.: Effect of ovarian hormones on promotion of bactericidal activity by uterine secretions of ovariectomized mares. J. Reprod. Fertil., *79:*531–537, 1987.
3. Wilson, G.L.: Equine hysteroscopy: Equipment for diagnostic endoscopy and photography. Vet. Med., *80:*76–88, 1985.
4. Hughes, J.P.: Clinical examination and abnormalities in the mare. *In* Current Therapy in Theriogenology. Edited by D.A. Morrow. Philadelphia, W.B. Saunders, 1980, p. 706–719.
5. Wilson, G.L.: Diagnostic and therapeutic hysteroscopy for endometrial cysts in mares. Vet. Med., *80:*59–63, 1985.
6. Kenney, R.M.: Cyclic and pathologic changes of the mare endometrium as detected by biopsy, with a note on early embryonic death. J. Am. Vet. Med. Assoc., *172:*241–262, 1978.
7. Adams, G.P., et. al.: Effect of uterine inflammation and ultrasonically-detected uterine pathology on fertility in the mare. J. Repro. Fertil. Suppl., *35:*445–454, 1987.
8. McKinnon, A.O., et al.: Diagnostic ultrasonography of uterine pathology in the mare. Proc. Am. Assoc. Equine Pract., 605–622, 1987.

CHAPTER 30

CYTOGENETIC ABNORMALITIES

A.T. Bowling
J.P. Hughes

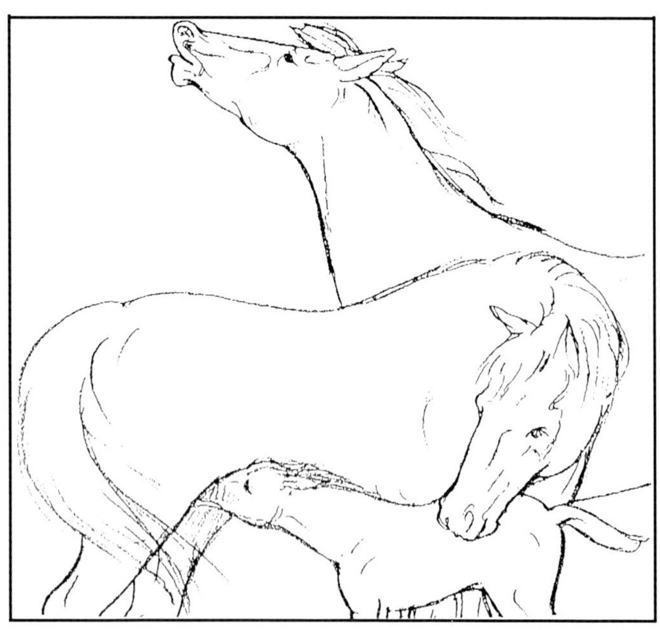

Human clinical research has shown that abortion, infertility, and syndromes of multiple congenital defects are highly correlated with chromosomal abnormalities. Significant chromosomal defects occur in about 5 cases per 1000 newborn babies.[1] Equine clinical cases have shown that chromosomal disorders can affect horses as well as humans, but the incidence of chromosomal abnormalities is not known. This chapter surveys published reports from the clinical perspective to help veterinarians and horse breeders identify horses with problems that are likely to be related to chromosomal disease.

USES OF KARYOTYPING

The primary use of karyotyping in horses is as a tool to evaluate breeding candidates with clinical abnormalities or history of infertility. The most commonly reported karyotypic abnormalities are errors in number or structure of the sex-determining chromosomes in infertile mares. Horses with chromosomal disease can be directed to performance careers before undue time, money, and emotional energy have been invested in the animals as breeding candidates. Most chromosomal abnormalities occur spontaneously and cannot be transmitted to offspring because the conditions cause sterility. An inherited condition may be present when chromosomal sex does not match gonadal or phenotypic sex, and the breeding program that produced the affected animal may want to be alerted to that potential.

Karyotyping may also be useful to define the basis for defects in sporadic cases of young horses with multiple congenital abnormalities. Sex chromosomal errors can cause growth deficits, and breeders with keen observation skills may identify fillies as potential candidates for chromosomal disease. Changes in other chromosomes may cause unthrifty appearance, slow growth, and gait or behavior abnormalities in young horses of either sex. Because of the extreme rarity of chromosomal disease and the current lack of definition of phenotypes produced by chromosomal disease in young horses, it is not anticipated that large numbers of young horses will be candidates for karyotyping based on physical criteria but the possibility should be kept in mind.

CHROMOSOMES DIRECT DEVELOPMENT FROM CONCEPTION TO BIRTH

Normal development is directed by gene products, which are assembled using linear DNA sequences (genes) found in chromosomes.

GENETIC MATERIAL

Genetic material is DNA precisely packaged in chromosomes. The diploid chromosome number of the domestic horse is 64 ($2n = 64$). The entire strict arrangement of DNA sequences in chromosomes is necessary for normal growth, development, and sexual maturity, because genes are the templates for production of structural proteins and for enzymes and hormones. A few slight deviations in the DNA array are compatible with life, but usually result in phenotypic abnormality.

NORMAL SEXUAL DEVELOPMENT

Normal sexual development proceeds in systematic manner. The normal karyotype of the female domestic horse is designated as 64,XX and the male as 64,XY. Chromosomal sex (either XX or XY) is determined at time of fertilization, depending on whether the male gamete (spermatozoan) that fertilizes the X-bearing female gamete (ovum) contains an X or a Y chromosome. Chromosomal sex of the zygote determines gonadal sex during the complex process of early embryonic development. In the presence of genetic information borne on the Y chromosome, the XY embryo becomes male with the conversion of the indifferent gonad to a testis, inhibition of Mullerian duct development, and stimulation of Wolffian ducts to form vasa deferentia and epididymides. The XX embryo becomes female, continuing differentiation of the gonad into ovaries and Mullerian ducts into oviducts, uterus, and vagina. Phenotypic sex is determined by chromosomal and gonadal sex. Chromosomal errors that interfere with any part of the chain of events can lead to abnormal development and infertility.

CHROMOSOMAL DEFECTS

Chromosomal defects interrupt the orderly progression. Chromosomes are exactly replicated during meiosis and subsequently packaged into gametes. Occasionally during gamete formation a spontaneous error (mutation) occurs in the duplication of the precise DNA sequence. A change even as small as a single nucleotide can lead to gametic, zygotic, or embryonic loss. Viable gene changes occur infrequently. Identification of carriers with single gene alterations is not achieved by karyotyping, but with protein electrophoresis or with the emergent technology using complementary DNA probes.

Karyotyping is used to detect extensive alterations in DNA sequences. Karyotypic changes may be produced (1) when chromosomes fail to separate from each other in meiotic division (nondisjunction), resulting in daughter cells with incorrect numbers of chromosomes, or (2) when chromosomes break, resulting in loss or gain of genetic material or a new arrangement, such as inversion of a segment within a single chromosome or translocation of a segment to another chromosome. Large-scale changes are likely to result in gametic or early embryonic loss, with the exception of some that involve sex chromosomes that have less potential than autosomal errors to involve genes directing essential development, growth, and metabolism processes. Variations in the X chromosome might be compatible with viability in females because their second X chromosome could direct production of the normal protein products, but be lethal in males, which do not have another X chromosome. Sex chromosome abnormalities are not generally compatible with fertility.

KARYOTYPING STANDARDS, PROCEDURES, AND TERMINOLOGY

In the horse karyotype, chromosomes are arranged as 32 pairs according to size, centromere position (site of spindle fiber attachment), and band patterns.

STANDARDS

The current standard species karyotype for the horse was established at the Second International Conference for Standardization of Domestic Animal Karyotypes, INRA, Jouyen Josas, France, 1989.[2] In the sex chromosome pair, the X is a large metacentric (biarmed) and the Y is an acrocentric. Among the 31 autosomal pairs, 13 are metacentric or submetacentric and 18 are acrocentric (Fig. 30–1). Assignment of chromosome pairs is aided by chemical or enzymatic treatments, which induce banding patterns reflecting variations in chromosome structure among chromosomes of similar size but different constituency. Four banding techniques used to define the unique identity of each chromosomal pair are provided in the 1989 standard: (1) trypsin treatment followed by Giemsa staining, or Giemsa (G) banding, which defines regions of high concentration of base sequences containing adenine and thymidine;[3,4] (2) barium hydroxide treatment followed by giemsa staining or centromeric (C) banding, which identifies constitutive heterochromatin,[4,5] (3) 5-Bromodeoxyuridine (BUDR) incubation followed by Giemsa staining, or reverse (R) banding, which produces reversed banding patterns compared to G banding;[6] and (4) silver staining, which identifies nucleolar organizer regions (Ag-NOR).[7]

PROCEDURES

A karyotype can be obtained from any tissue with cells in division. Practically speaking, this criterion of actively dividing cells eliminates autolyzed tissues, conventionally frozen tissues, and probably even refrigerated tissues as a source of material for karyotype analysis. A karyotype could be obtained directly from fixing and staining cells of any rapidly dividing tissue, such as an early embryo or bone marrow. Alternatively, a karyotype can be obtained from a tissue biopsy that has been stimulated to divide under conditions of laboratory culture.

Convention has been to use peripheral blood lymphocytes, which are easy to obtain and relatively reliably and rapidly lead to establishment of a karyotype. Samples for karyotyping of horses should be obtained

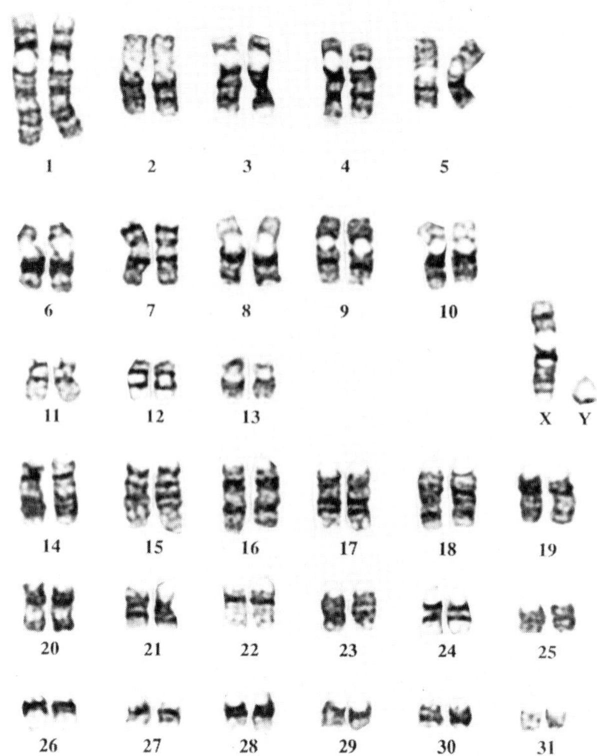

FIG. 30–1. Karyotype of a normal male horse, G banding, with chromosome pairs numbered and arranged corresponding to the 1989 standard. Pairs are ordered according to descending size in three groups: sex chromosomes on the third line at the right edge; metacentric or submetacentric autosomal pairs numbered 1 to 13 on lines one to three; and acrocentric autosomal pairs numbered 14 to 31 on lines four to six.

in acid citrate dextrose (ACD) or heparin, and unrefrigerated samples should be sent by rapid courier to the laboratory. Lymphocytes are cultured asceptically for 64 to 72 h under conditions that stimulate them to divide and then harvested and fixed. Differential banding and staining treatments are applied to fixed cells on slides, then cells in which the chromosomes are suitably spread for analysis are photographed. A karyotype is prepared by cutting out the chromosomes from a photographic print and arranging the pairs according to the standard. In conventionally stained, unbanded preparations, horse chromosomes are easy to count, but unequivocal identification of each pair and the critical determination of the sex chromosome constitution may be difficult. The X chromosome is similar in size and shape to the second largest metacentric. The Y chromosome is similar in size to the smallest autosome. The C banding treatment provides clear identification of sex chromosomes; Y is unique within the karyotype as being entirely heterochromatic and X is the only large metacentric with an interstitial heterochromatic band. In XX females, one X shows the interstitial band less distinctly (as a result of the normal process of inactivation of one X chromosome from early in embryo development), which may make the second X difficult to discern unless care is taken. Discrimination of sex chromosomes from autosomes can be achieved with G banding, which also provides markers for correctly identifying homologous autosomal pairs and the composition of structural changes. A second tissue may be used for karyotyping to confirm or enhance the diagnosis based on peripheral blood, particularly for cases in which more than one cell line is detected, but is not necessary in most cases.

VARIATION

No obvious differences in karyotype have been described that distinguish either breeds of horses or single genes such as those producing coat color differences. Variations that can be visualized in karyotypes include changes in chromosome number (aneuploidy) and structure. Among aneuploid changes, monosomy is found only for sex chromosomes and trisomy is found only for sex chromosomes and smaller autosomes. Structural changes may involve deletion, duplication, insertion, inversion, or translocation. A coded notation using conventions established for the human karyotype is generally used to describe the abnormalities.[8] Occasionally chimerism or mosaicism is encountered in which abnormalities are found in some, but not all, cells of the tissue sample. Peripheral blood chimerism occurs when two populations of circulating blood cells from different zygotes are joined following placental anastomosis in twin pregnancies. In chimeric twins of unlike sex, a mixed karyotype of two cell lines would be obtained from lymphocytes, although solid tissues from such animals would demonstrate only a single karyotype. More than one cell line could also be the result of mosaicism in which a chromosomal error occurring during cell division in a single zygote was maintained in a clonal cell line. Sufficient numbers of cells need to be analyzed to distinguish chimerism/mosaicism from technical errors occurring during the karyotyping process.

REPORTING

A karyotype report should contain the following information: identification of animal (name, age, sex, breed, owner, referring veterinarian), tissue used, number of cells for which chromosome number was determined, number of cells karyotyped, banding techniques used, and description of any abnormalities and significance, if known.

CLINICAL CASES INVOLVING INFERTILITY OR SUBFERTILITY

An earlier report pointed out that about half of breeding age mares with primary infertility and gonadal hypoplasia had detectable chromosomal abnormality.[9] Type of chromosomal disease can only be differentiated with karyotyping, because various abnormal karyotypes may not produce phenotypes distinguishable from each other. Occasional cases of subfertility in which infectious agents can be clearly ruled out are also candidates for karyotyping.

MARES WITH NORMAL EXTERNAL GENITALIA, HYPOPLASTIC INTERNAL GONADS, AND PRIMARY INFERTILITY

Mares presenting with chronic and primary infertility, failure to cycle regularly or at all, small ovaries (0.5 × 0.5 × 1.0 cm) lacking follicular activity, flaccid uterus and cervix, hypoplastic endometrium, and elevated levels of plasma luteinizing hormone (LH) are prime candidates for chromosomal disease.

63,X Gonadal Dysgenesis

The most commonly observed and reported karyotypic abnormality is X monosomy, an aneuploid defect of sex chromosomes probably first reported in 1968, but the unbanded chromosome preparations were inadequate to identify chromosomes unambiguously.[10] In 1975, Chandley et al.[11] and Hughes et al.[12] provided clear examples of X monosomy in infertile mares. The karyotype is analogous to that found in human female gonadal dysgenesis known as Turner's syndrome. X monosomy is the leading identified cause of first trimester abortion in human pregnancy, but has not yet been documented as a cause of early fetal or embryonic loss in horses. The condition appears to occur sporadically, probably from nondisjunction during meiosis, and no compelling evidence in humans or horses has been found to indicate an inherited tendency. Among mares with detectable X monosomy and gonadal dysgenesis, Bowling et al. estimated that about 15% demonstrated a second cell line with structurally normal sex chromosomes, either 63,X/64,XX or 63,X/64,XY, probably the result of chromosome loss in a clonal cell line during early embryonic development.[9]

Congenital heart disease and bony anomalies, characteristic of Turner's, have not been reported in the 63,X horse. Affected foals tend to be small and weak at birth and at maturity are small compared with the breed standard. Suspected chromosomal disease in two small yearling fillies was subsequently verified as 63,X in one case and 63,X/64,XX in the other.[9] Based on examination of reproductive structures and case reports to date, mares with X monosomy and gonadal hypoplasia should be considered effectively sterile. One alleged fertile 63,X mare was shown by analysis of blood genetic markers to have been fraudulently assigned as the dam of foals.[13]

64,XY Sex Reversal

The second most commonly observed karyotypic abnormality in the horse is found in infertile mares for which phenotypic sex does not match chromosomal sex.[9] In 1975, Chandley et al. reported an infertile Thoroughbred mare with the karyotype of a normal equine male.[11] The condition subsequently has been diagnosed in additional Thoroughbreds as well in the Shetland, Arabian, Quarter Horse, Appaloosa, and Morgan.[9,14,15] Characteristics are similar to 63,X gonadal dysgenesis, but phenotype is more variable and may include more than one genetic entity (e.g., XY gonadal dysgenesis; X-linked testicular feminization). In XY gonadal dysgenesis, ovaries of phenotypic females are small and inactive, and the cervix and uterus are flaccid. In testicular feminization, external genitalia are female but the cervix and uterus may be lacking; histologic examination of gonads may disclose characteristics of both ovaries and testes, and masculine behavior may be observed. Stature is not usually reported as small; race winners and show champion mares are among cases identified. One XY mare eventually produced a foal despite an early presentation of infertility.[16] Analysis of family data has provided evidence that XY sex reversal may be caused by genetic (single-gene) defects transmitted either through males or females.[9,14,15]

Other X Chromosome Defects

The classic syndrome of primary infertility with gonadal dysgenesis has also been associated with at least two other abnormal karyotypes.

64,XX,delXp. In three mares phenotypically indistinguishable from X monosomy, a short-arm (p) deletion in one of the pair of X chromosomes has been identified.[9] One of the mares was identified as a small, unthrifty yearling, reportedly born with hind legs so weak that splints were applied to assist the foal to rise. This mare twice developed follicles at age four, was mated and ovulated, but failed to conceive. A second mare has produced two fillies (parentage verified) after pasture exposure to a stallion, despite failure to detect estrus or follicle development with intensive examination in two prior breeding seasons. The dam's abnormal X chromosome was transmitted to one foal; the other foal received the normal X.

65,XXX. X trisomy was first reported in an infertile Thoroughbred mare[11] and subsequently documented in five additional cases.[9] This is a fertile karyotype in humans, generally without a recognizable phenotype, but as yet no evidence of fertility for this karyotype in horses has been reported.

MARES WITH NORMAL EXTERNAL GENITALIA AND GONADS AND POOR PRODUCTION RECORD

While chromosome abnormalities are not as likely to be found among mares that appear normal and have produced a foal, if other causes of infertility can be effectively ruled out, then chromosomal disease should be considered as a possibility in barren mares with repeated failure to conceive and bear a foal.

Balanced Translocation Heterozygote

Complete but rearranged genetic material, such as centric fusions between pairs of chromosomes that are normally separate, would not be expected to affect phenotype, but could potentially be a source of lowered fertility (in either sex), as demonstrated in cattle and pigs. Long has published an excellent review on the effects of chromosomal translocation in domestic animals.[17] The effect is related to the production of chromosomally unbalanced gametes during meiosis and results in lowered fertility, not infertility. The rarity of balanced translocation heterozygotes among reports of chromosomal disease in horses may reflect that this problem is more difficult to recognize clinically in horses than in animals with litters or intensively managed for reproduction, such as cattle.

64,XX,t(1q,2q). An 11-yr-old Thoroughbred mare with only two foals in 8 yr at stud was found to have an abnormal karyotype consisting of heterozygosity for a balanced reciprocal translocation between the two largest autosomes.[18] This case illustrates the role that chromosomal disease may play in subfertility, as well as the more dramatic examples of infertility.

65,(Balanced Translocation). In 17 Caspian ponies from Iran, an autosomal numerical polymorphism was observed among both males and females with normal sex chromosomes. Six animals had 65 chromosomes rather than the 64 expected in domestic horse.[19] Presumably horses with $2n = 66$ could occur as well, although none was reported. The findings could be explained as centric fission of a metacentric chromosome into two acrocentrics as compared with other domestic horses, although the authors suggested the origin followed natural hybridization between domestic horses and Przewalski's horse (Equus przewalskii). Assignment of the chromosomes involved per the 1989 standard could be not determined from the published figure. Low fertility reported in these horses could be the result of production of chromosomally unbalanced gametes by either sex, corresponding to the situation documented in cattle and pigs, but no direct correlation evidence was provided.

Other Structural Abnormalities

Single examples of other abnormalities involving the X chromosome provide additional cases to illustrate effects of chromosomal disease on female reproduction.

64,X,−X,+der(X),t(Xp;15q). An unbalanced X-autosome translocation was found in a Thoroughbred mare with normal internal and external genitalia and regular estrous cycles that was investigated because of infertility.[20] Physically, the mare was small and thin, walked with a stiff gait, and showed little interest in her surroundings. Both parents had normal chromosome complements. Functionally, the karyotype had a deletion for the p arms of one X chromosome and was trisomic for chromosome 15. The effect of trisomy for this large autosome may have been mitigated by X-inactivation. This mare was a half-sibling of a colt with trisomy for chromosome 28.

64,XX,delXq/64,XY. Halnan et al. reported a chimeric/mosaic karyotype in a 4-yr-old Standardbred mare with a good track record, which was barren at end of the first season of breeding, had clinically normal external genitalia and normal cycles, but showed extremely aggressive behavior.[21] The mare subsequently produced a foal.[22]

63,X/64,XY/65,XXY. Halnan and Irwin evaluated a 7-yr-old Thoroughbred mare after being barren for 3 yr at stud.[23] The mare had a poor racetrack performance record, was of small stature, was docile to handle, showed regular cycles, and had no palpable anatomic abnormalities. At laparotomy, she showed hypoplasia of uterine tubes, endometrium, and myometrium. The authors hypothesized that the male genotype in mosaic form suppressed maturation of paramesonephric ducts.

STALLION INFERTILITY

Although rare variants have been reported, application of karyotyping to problems of stallion infertility has not been a productive area of clinical importance. McIlwraith et al. detected XX/XY whole-body chimerism in a cryptorchid Arabian cross 3-yr-old colt with both testes undescended and not palpable in the inguinal canal, but fertility would not have been anticipated in any case.[24] Balanced translocation heterozygotes with the potential for producing unbalanced gametes through meiotic nondisjunction, such as reported among phenotypically normal Caspian ponies, could lead to lowered male fertility.[19] Another example of potential infertility would be the phenotypically normal stallion with the 4/14 (1989 standard) balanced translocation first described by Quéinnec et al.[25] (Willer et al.[26] noted that the analysis was revised), who was gelded before breeding so the effect on fertility is unknown. Halnan and Watson reported an infertile Standardbred stallion with abnormal spermatozoa and poor motility with a 64,XY,del13q karyotype and an infertile stock horse stallion with 63,X/64,XY.[27]

AMBIGUOUS EXTERNAL GENITALIA

Ambiguity of phenotypic sex appears to be associated with a variety of karyotype abnormalities in the horse. Many reports were made before the use of banding techniques, so chromosome identification may be inadequate. Among the variants reported are perineal structure mostly female, but a long anogenital distance, vulvar fold, (usually) blind vagina, a hypospadias penis in place of a clitoris, gonads as intrabdominal testicles, male libido, and XX sex chromosome constitution, such as the case described in an Arabian filly.[28] This phenotype resembles the inherited XX sex reversal syndrome seen in various breeds of dogs. Such cases in horses could also be associated with an inherited abnormality, but no data specific to that point have yet been presented in horses.

Other cases of intersexuality in the horse appear to be associated with more than one cell line and may best be explained as double fertilization or whole-body chimerism arising from fusion of early embryos. A colt with a vulvar opening, right testis without germ cells, and XX and XY cells in karyotypes of lymphocytes and fibrous tissue was most likely a whole-body chimera resulting from fusion of dizygotic twins in early embryogenesis.[29] Two intersex cases described by Dunn et al.—one 64,XX/64,XY and one 63,X/64,XY—each had an underdeveloped penis, bilateral seminal vesicles, uterine tissue, and bilateral ovotestes; chimerism and the subsequent phenotypic effect could have resulted either from double fertilization or fusion of blastocysts.[30]

CHROMOSOMAL DEFECTS IN ABORTION AND MISCARRIAGE

Blue attempted to establish tissue cultures of equine abortus material to obtain evidence for the frequencies and types of chromosomal abnormalities associated with equine abortion but failed to establish a single culture, probably reflecting the generally poor condition of such material when received.[31] Among 12 aborted fetuses successfully cultured by Haynes and Reisner, no major structural or numerical abnormalities were found, but C-band polymorphisms were observed in two cases.[32] The polymorphisms were also present in the normal parents.

CHIMERISM IN TWIN BORN FEMALES

Freemartinism in cattle, sheep, and goats leads to masculinization and infertility in females born twin to males. No reports have yet documented a freemartin effect in horses. Podliachouk et al. found XX/XY chimerism in six out of seven heterosexual horse twins, but no abnormalities of the reproductive tract in 14 females twin to males.[33] Using studbook information from the Arabian Horse Registry of America, production of registered foals from mares born cotwin to males and to females were compared. Among 35 male-female pairs through registration number 200,000 (about 1978), 24 females had registered foals and 11 had none. Among 19 female-female pairs (38 mares) in the same interval, 30 had registered foals and 8 had none. The difference between these groups is not statistically significant. Thus studbook evidence in Arabian horses also fails to provide evidence to support the presence of a freemartin effect which limits fertility in the mare.

MULTIPLE PHENOTYPIC ABNORMALITIES AND GROWTH DEFICITS

Chromosomal errors of either sex chromosomes or autosomes are likely to be associated with abnormalities in growth patterns. It is more usual to find deficits involving sex chromosomes, because autosomal imbalances are not as likely to be compatible with life as those involving the sex chromosomes, except perhaps for trisomies of the smallest chromosomes.

AUTOSOMAL TRISOMY

Among human infants, the most familiar example of autosomal trisomy is trisomy 21 (Down syndrome), the incidence of which is highly correlated with increased maternal age. Affected cases show mental retardation, physical abnormalities, and health deficits. Four cases of autosomal trisomy have been found in horses, each involving a different chromosome and manifested sufficiently to be evident in yearlings.

65,XY,+23

A yearling Standardbred male, described as thin, with a rough hair coat, pronounced facial asymmetry, dysmetric gait, and small testicles, was found to be trisomic for chromosome 23.[34] Neither the age of the parents nor the relative size of animal was given.

64,XX,−26,+t(26q26q)

A yearling Thoroughbred female of top-class racing pedigree was evaluated by karyotyping because of multiple abnormalities including rough coat, dull mental attitude, stiff gait, small size for age, and poor conformation. At her birth, the dam was 5 yr old and the sire was 6 yr. Neither parent was karyotyped, but both were assumed to be normal from available breeding records. Karyotyping proved chromosome 26 to be present in triplicate, two of the homologues united at a single centromere to produce a metacentric chromosome.[9,35] At age 5, the mare produced a colt with a normal chromosome complement.

65,XY,+28

A small (1.25 m at 2 yr) cryptorchid male who constantly walked in small circles was found to be trisomic for chromosome 28.[20] His chromosomally normal Thoroughbred dam was 14 yr old when he was born, but his sire was unknown.

65,XX,+30

A small (1.29 m at 2 yr) Arabian female with severe angular deviation of the front legs and mild polydactyly born to a 23-yr-old mare and a 4-yr-old stallion was found to be trisomic for chromosome 30.[35] Both parents were chromosomally normal and neither had the conformational defects of the offspring. The affected filly was active and had a bright attitude.

CHANGES IN GROWTH PATTERNS

Sex chromosomal abnormalities may cause alteration in growth patterns. Both 63,X and 64,XXdelXp are associated with small mature stature and have been diagnosed in yearling fillies referred because of small size and unthrifty appearance.[9] Obviously, nutritional status could also cause such phenotypic effects, but on farms with excellent foal management, these characteristics might be unusual enough to warrant karyotyping rare cases in which these traits were observed.

STRUCTURAL POLYMORPHISMS, NO KNOWN ASSOCIATED DEFECTS

Familiarity with the normal variation (heteromorphisms) that may occur in the equine karyotype without apparent phenotypic effect on health or fertility is critical in evaluating clinical cases so that unwarranted conclusions as a result of inexperience with equine chromosomes may be avoided.

C BANDING

Chromosome 13 was noted by Buckland et al. to be heteromorphic in four of nine normal animals for size of the centromeric heterochromatin block.[4] Ryder et al. confirmed polymorphism among normal animals and also noted polymorphism in the homologous chromosome 12 of Przewalski's horses.[36]

Y CHROMOSOME SIZE

Power reported greater size variability exists in the horse Y chromosome than has been reported for the human chromosome.[37] Comparing a group of 11 males with clinical abnormalities (e.g., XY sex reversal, infertility, congenital abnormalities, and trisomy 28) to 20 clinically normal males, no apparent association of Y chromosome size with disease was found.

NUCLEOLAR ORGANIZER REGIONS

The site of RNA synthesis is localized in specific silver-staining nucleolar organizer regions (NORs), which occur on chromosomes 1, 28, and 31 (nomenclature per 1989 standard). Kopp et al. studied the variability of Ag-NOR expression within and between individuals and found a maximum of six NORs (range three to six).[7] In 19 horses (Lippizan, Hanoverian, and Shetland), both homologues of 1 and at least one 31 were always present.

RARE FEMALE FERTILITY IN MULES AND HINNIES

Most female horse/donkey hybrids have atrophic ovaries and males are azoospermic. Occasional female hybrids exhibit estrous cycles and ovulate, but production of viable gametes, let alone zygotes, is so infrequent as to have been extremely difficult to document. The donkey differs in chromosome number from the horse by one fewer pair ($2n = 62$), but significant differences in morphology show multiple rearrangements have occurred in evolution so that hybrids would only rarely be expected to produce genetically balanced gametes. At last scientific technology has crossed paths with examples of the rare occurrence of fertile hybrids between the donkey and the horse in both reciprocal crosses (mule or hinny) and has verified with karyotyping and blood typing that hybrid females can be fertile.[38,39] Scientific reports verify fertility only in female hybrids. The lack of evidence for male fertility may reflect lack of opportunity but is more likely to be an example of Haldane's law, which predicts male sterility in species hybrids. Offspring of female hybrids have had chromosome numbers ranging from 60 to 64, showing that an effective gametic chromosomal combination is not uniquely defined as consisting only of horse or donkey chromosomes.[40] The possibility of genetic imbalance, especially trisomy, is not ruled out by the viability of the offspring. None of the offspring of the hybrids has been documented to have reproduced, but it is anticipated that once the initial barrier to hybrid fertility has been breached, in ensuing generations the likelihood of fertility becomes more probable. Until such time as the hybrid-derived karyotype comes to consist of simple pairs of homologous chromosomes, infertility is likely to be an ongoing problem.

CONCLUSION

Chronic primary infertility in the mare can often be related to chromosomal disease and karyotyping such cases would be likely to establish a cause for the infertility. Routine postnatal cytogenetic screening of foals has been advocated but it would be costly compared to the number of poor breeding risks found and the long-term prognosis for many of the abnormalities is presently unknown.[41,42] Fertile horses are seldom karyotyped, thus the incidence of chromosomal abnormalities among them is unknown. Research progress in cytogenetics of the horse has relied on clinicians to identify relevant cases and significant findings are still anticipated from this collaboration.

ACKNOWLEDGMENTS

The authors gratefully acknowledge the superb technical expertise of Lee Millon, including careful tending of cultures, analysis of slides, photography, and preparation of karyotypes and figures.

REFERENCES

1. Milunsky, A.: The Prevention of Genetic Disease and Mental Retardation. Philadelphia, W.B. Saunders, 1975.
2. Richer, C.L., et al.: Standard karyotype of the domestic horse (Equus caballus). Hereditas, *112:*289–293, 1990.
3. Seabright, M.: A rapid banding technique for human chromosomes. Lancet, *2:*971–972, 1971.
4. Buckland, R.A., Fletcher, J.M., and Chandley, A.C.: Characterization of the domestic horse (Equus caballus) karyotype using G- and C-banding techniques. Experientia, *32:*1146–1149, 1976.
5. Sumner, A.T.: A simple technique for demonstrating centromeric heterochromatin. Exp. Cell Res., *75:*304–306, 1972.
6. Romagnano, A., and Richer, C.-L.: R-banding of horse chromosomes. J. Hered., *75:*269–272, 1984.
7. Kopp, E., Mayr, B., Kalat, M., and Schleger, W.: Polymorphisms of NORs and heterochromatin in the horse and donkey. J. Hered., *79:*332–337, 1988.
8. Harnden, D.G., and Klinger, H.P., eds.: ISCN 1985: An International System for Human Cytogenetic Nomenclature. Basel, Karger, 1985.
9. Bowling, A.T., Millon, L., and Hughes, J.P.: An update of chromosomal abnormalities in mares. J. Reprod. Fertil. Suppl., *35:*149–155, 1987.
10. Payne, H.W., Ellsworth, K., and DeGroot, A.: Aneuploidy in an infertile mare. J. Am. Vet. Med. Assoc., *158:*1293–1299, 1968.
11. Chandley, A.C., et al.: Chromosome abnormalities as a cause of infertility in mares. J. Reprod. Fertil. Suppl., *23:*377–383, 1975.
12. Hughes, J.P., Benirschke, K., Kennedy, P.C., and Trommershausen-Smith, A.: Gonadal dysgenesis in the mare. J. Reprod. Fertil. Suppl., *23:*385–390, 1975.
13. Bowling, A.T.: Blood typing invalidates alleged evidence of fertility of XO mare. Theriogenology, *24:*203–210, 1985.
14. Kieffer, N.M., Burns, S.J., and Judge, N.G.: Male pseudohermaphroditism of the testicular feminizing type in a horse. Equine Vet. J., *8:*38–41, 1976.
15. Kent, M.G., Shoffner, R.N., Buoen, L., and Weber, A.F.: XY sex-reversal syndrome in the domestic horse. Cytogenet. Cell Genet., *42:*8–18, 1986.
16. Sharp, A.J., Wachtel, S.S., and Benirschke, K.: H-Y antigen in a fertile XY female horse. J. Reprod. Fertil., *58:*157–160, 1980.
17. Long, S.E.: Segregation patterns and fertility of domestic mammals with chromosome translocations. *In* The Cytogenetics of Mammalian Autosomal Rearrangements. Edited by A. Daniel. New York, Liss, 1988, pp. 383–396.
18. Power, M.M.: The effects of a balanced reciprocal translocation t(1q:2q) on the reproductive performance of a mare. Paper presented at the Sixth North American Colloquium on Cytogenetics of Domestic Animals, West Lafayette, IN, July 23–27, 1989.
19. Hatami-Monazah, H. and Pandit, R.V.: A cytogenetic study of the Caspian pony. J. Reprod. Fertil., *57:*331–333, 1979.
20. Power, M.M.: Equine half sibs with an unbalanced X;15 translocation or trisomy 28. Cytogenet. Cell Genet., *45:*163–168, 1987.
21. Halnan, C.R.E., Hutchins, D.R., and Brownlow, M.: Failure to conceive in a standardbred mare: Karyotype 64,XX:64,XY. Equine Vet. Sci., *5:*161–162, 1985.
22. Halnan, C.R.E.: Cytogenetics of Animals. Wallinford, CAB, 1989.
23. Halnan, C.R.E., and Irwin, C.F.P.: Dysgenesis of the tubal system in an infertile mare karyotype 63,X:64,XY:65, XXY. Equine Vet. Sci., *5:*328–329, 1982.
24. McIlwraith, C.W., Owen, R., and Basrur, P.K.: An equine cryptorchid with testicular and ovarian tissues. Equine Vet. J., *8:*156–160, 1976.
25. Quéinnec, G., Berland, H.M., Darré, R., and Carlotti, D.: Anomalie chromosomique chez un cheval. Rev. Med. Vet., *38:*323–327, 1975.
26. Willer, S., Willer, H., and Wiesner, E.: Chromosomenaberrationen beim Pferd. Mh. Vet. Med., *36:*386–394, 1981.
27. Halnan, C.R.E., and Watson, J.I.: Detection by G- and C-band karyotyping of gonosome anomalies in horses of different breeds. J. Reprod. Fertil. Suppl., *32:*626–627, 1982.
28. Gerneke, W.H., and Coubrough, R.I.: Intersexuality in the horse. Onderstepoort J. Vet. Res., *37:*211–216, 1970.
29. Basrur, P.K., Kanagawa, H., and Gilman, J.P.W.: Further studies on the cell populations of an intersex horse. J. Comp. Med., *34:*294–298, 1970.
30. Dunn, H.O., Smiley, D., and McEntee, K.: Two equine true hermaphrodites with 64,XX/64,XY and 63,X/64,XY chimerism. Cornell Vet., *71:*123–135, 1981.
31. Blue, M.G.: A cytogenetical study of prenatal loss in the mare. Theriogenology, *15:*295–309, 1981.
32. Haynes, S.E., and Reisner, A.H.: Cytogenetic and DNA analyses of equine abortion. Cytogenet. Cell Genet., *34:*204–214, 1982.
33. Podliachouk, L., Vandeplassche, M., and Bouters, R.: Gestation gémellaire, chimérisme et freemartinisme chez le cheval. Acta Zool. Pathol. Antverp., *58:*13–28, 1974.
34. Klunder, L.R., et al.: Autosomal trisomy in a Standardbred colt. Equine Vet. J., *21:*69–70, 1989.
35. Bowling, A.T., and Millon, L.V.: Two autosomal trisomies in the horse: 64,XX,26,+t(26q26q) and 65,XX,+30. Genome, *33:*679–682, 1990.
36. Ryder, O.A., Epel, N.C., and Benirschke, K.: Chromosome banding studies of the Equidae. Cytogenet. Cell Genet., *20:*323–350, 1978.
37. Power, M.M.: Y chromosome length variation and its significance in the horse. J. Hered., *79:*311–313, 1988.
38. Ryder, O.A., Chemnick, L.G., Bowling, A.T., and Benirschke, K.: Male mule foal qualifies as the offspring of a female mule and jack donkey. J. Hered., *76:*379–381, 1985.
39. Rong, R., et al.: A fertile mule and hinny in China. Cytogenet. Cell Genet., *47:*134–139, 1988.
40. Zong, E., and Fan, G.: The variety of sterility and gradual progression to fertility in hybrids of the horse and donkey. Heredity, *62:*393–406, 1989.
41. Halnan, C.R.E.: Sex chromosome mosaicism and infertility in mares. Vet. Rec., *116:*542–543, 1985.
42. Long, S.E.: Chromosome anomalies and infertility in the mare. Equine Vet. J., *20:*89–93, 1988.

REPRODUCTIVE EXAMINATION OF THE MARE

CHAPTER 31

DIAGNOSTIC ULTRASONOGRAPHY

A.O. McKinnon
J.L. Voss
E.L. Squires
E.M. Carnevale

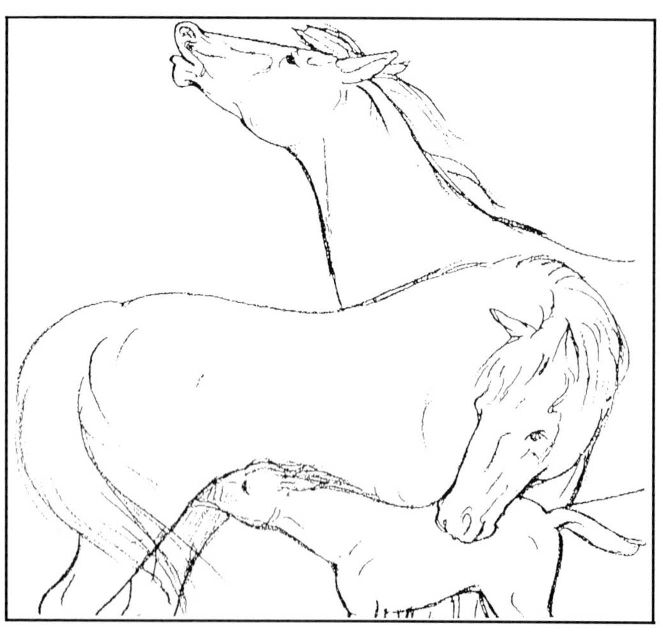

Few people predicted the impact that ultrasonography would have on equine reproductive management and understanding of reproductive physiology. The ability to examine a mare's reproductive tract noninvasively with ultrasonography provided the opportunity to diagnose pregnancy earlier than by rectal palpation, effectively manage twins, and detect impending early embryonic death (EED). However, ultrasonography should not be limited to these areas. It can be used to diagnose uterine disease, such as intrauterine fluid, air, debris, cysts, and occasionally abscessation and neoplasia. In addition, ultrasonographic examination of the ovaries may aid in determining stage of estrous cycle, status of preovulatory follicles, development and morphologic assessment of the corpus luteum (CL), and in interpreting ovarian irregularities, such as anovulatory or hemorrhagic follicles, neoplasia, and periovarian cysts.

The costs of equipment initially resulted in a rather limited application of reproductive ultrasonography. Clients enthusiastically support use of ultrasonography to detect pregnancy. However, the same fee schedules for routine examination before and/or after breeding are not as easily accepted. Perhaps another approach for practitioners involved with large numbers of brood mares would be a single fee per year per mare for use of equipment and a smaller fee per examination, whether the examination involved ultrasonography, rectal palpation, or both. If this philosophy were adopted, then a more logical and thus practical approach to diagnosis and treatment of physiologic and anatomic abnormalities of the mare's reproductive tract would be forthcoming. In addition, valuable information would be available from correlation of fertility data with normal and abnormal ultrasonographic observations. Regardless, informed clientele prefer routine ultrasonography, and its use results in a more interactive approach to farm management with an increased awareness of the events associated with breeding, ovulation, and early fetal development. If the use of ultrasonography has a drawback, it is that some clients want to purchase their own equipment and pursue their own diagnoses.

GROWTH AND DEVELOPMENT OF THE NORMAL FETUS

Fertilization occurs at the ampullary/isthmus junction of the oviduct and requires a viable oocyte and spermatozoon.[1] The first maternal recognition of pregnancy may be as early as 48 h postovulation in mares and is associated with production of an immunosuppressive agent, a pregnancy-specific protein called early pregnancy factor (EPF). Early pregnancy factor has been detected in mice, sheep, humans,[2] and mares[3] and may have promise for future early detection of pregnancy and EED.

Another event in maternal recognition of pregnancy occurs on or before 6 days postovulation. Fertilized ova are transported from the oviduct through the uterotubule junction and into the uterus by 5 to 6 days postovulation,[4] while unfertilized ova (UFO) are generally retained in the oviduct.[5] After fertilization (day 0) and initial cleavage, each equine blastomere (cells produced by cleavage) divides approximately every 24 h. Based on oviductal flushes, clinicians commonly collect 4- to 8-cell embryos on day 2 postovulation and 8- to 16-cell embryos on day 3.[6] A 32- to 64-cell embryo is classified as a morula (Fig. 31–1) and is the youngest developmental stage of embryo that can be harvested from the uterus. Generally, 6-day embryos are late morulas or early blastocysts (Fig. 31–2). A blastocyst is recognized by development of a blastocele cavity within the embryo. The blastocele cavity, or yolk sac, is fluid filled, and continued expansion of the blastocele allows ultrasonographic determination of pregnancy as early as 10 days postovulation. Day-7 embryos (Fig. 31–3) are generally expanded blastocysts. Embryos are generally visible to the naked eye by 7 to 8 days postovulation.

A third event in maternal recognition of pregnancy occurs between 12 and 16 days. During this time the conceptus is extremely mobile, and the conceptus probably prevents the release of or inhibits the function of prostaglandin $F_2\alpha$ ($PGF_2\alpha$) that would normally destroy the CL, resulting in a return to estrus.[7,8] The conceptus may also produce substances that are luteotropic. For diagnosis of pregnancy at 10 to 12 days, a 5- or 7.5-MHz transducer is necessary. However, because of embryonic loss in early pregnancy, discontinuation of the teasing program after initial examination for pregnancy is inappropriate. From a practical standpoint, the first examination could be postponed until approximately 18 to 20 days postovulation, thus eliminating scanning of mares that are destined to return to estrus. One exception would be scanning of breeds that have a history of twinning or multiple ovulations (i.e., Thoroughbreds). These mares should be examined at days 12 to 15 postovulation to most effectively manage manual embryonic reduction. Frequency of subsequent scans depends on such factors as presence of twins, size and quality of the vesicle and embryo, reproductive history, availability of the mare, and economics. Timing of the initial pregnancy examination depends on factors such as breed, economics, and client education.

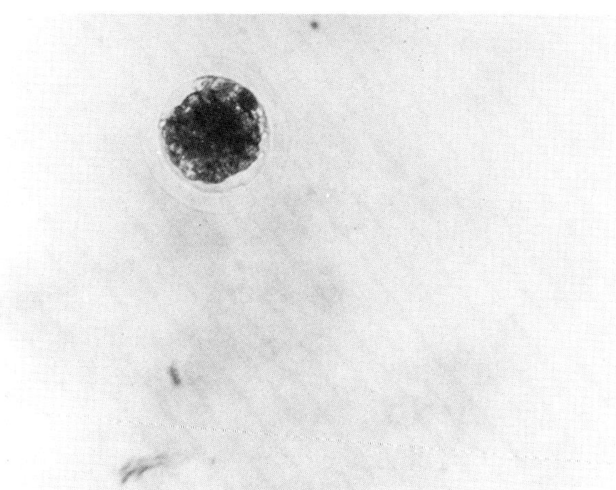

FIG. 31–1. An early equine morula.

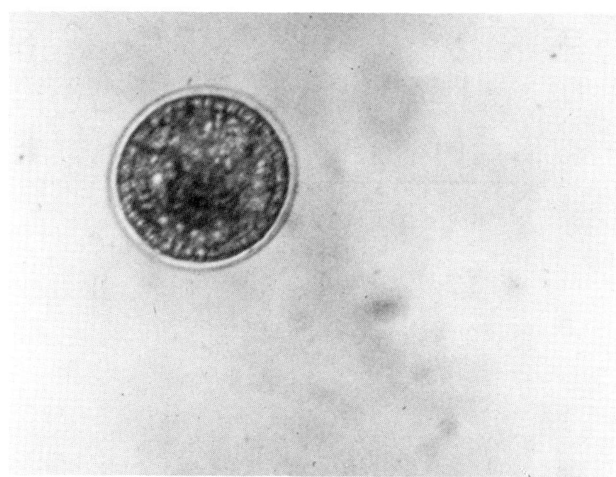

FIG. 31–2. An early equine blastocyst.

CHARACTERISTICS OF THE CONCEPTUS

Days 10 to 17

Ultrasonographic scanning has resulted in an increase in our knowledge of the dynamics of early pregnancy. Ultrasonographic images of the conceptus at various stages have been grouped together for convenience (Figs. 31–4 to 31–15). Researchers have shown that the early equine conceptus is highly mobile within the uterine lumen.[9] Regardless of the side of entry into the uterus, the equine conceptus moves between the uterine horns and uterine body. Small vesicles (day 10) are spherical (Fig. 31–4) and found most frequently in the uterine body (Fig. 31–16). Transuterine movement occurs at intervals of less than 2 to 4 h.[9] Mobility begins to decrease by day 15, and after day 17 transuterine migration can no longer be detected.[9,10] Thereafter, the

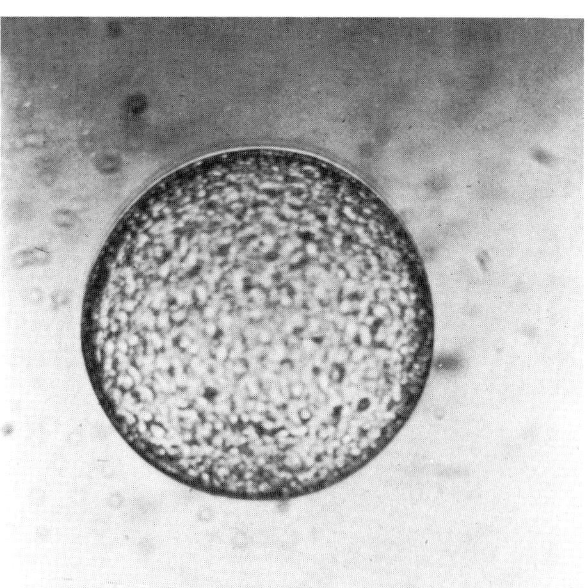

FIG. 31–3. An expanded equine blastocyst.

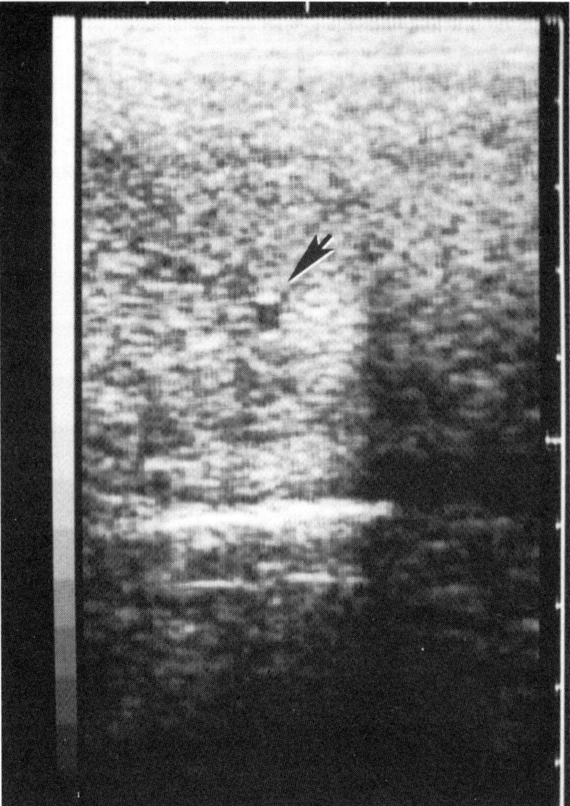

FIG. 31–4. Ultrasonographic image of a 10-day-old embryonic vesicle (arrow).

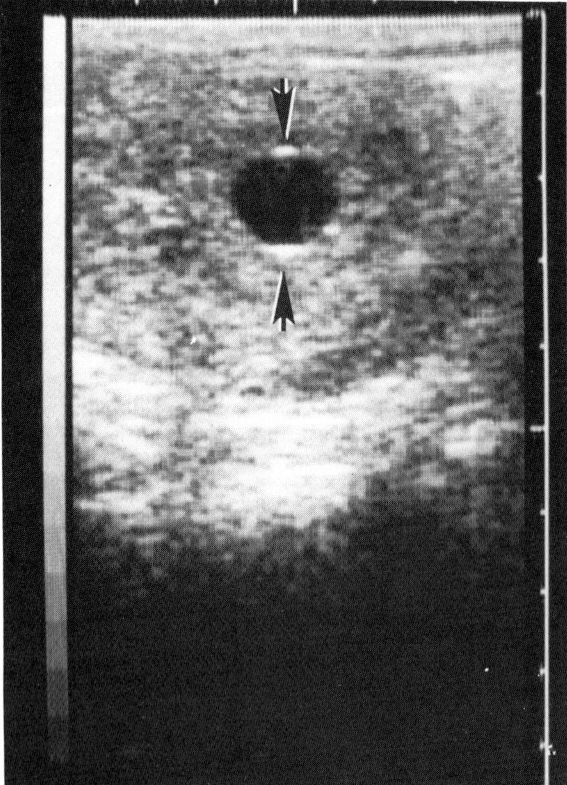

FIG. 31–5. Ultrasonographic image of a 12-day-old embryonic vesicle. Note the presence of dorsal and ventral specular reflection, which is artifactual (arrows).

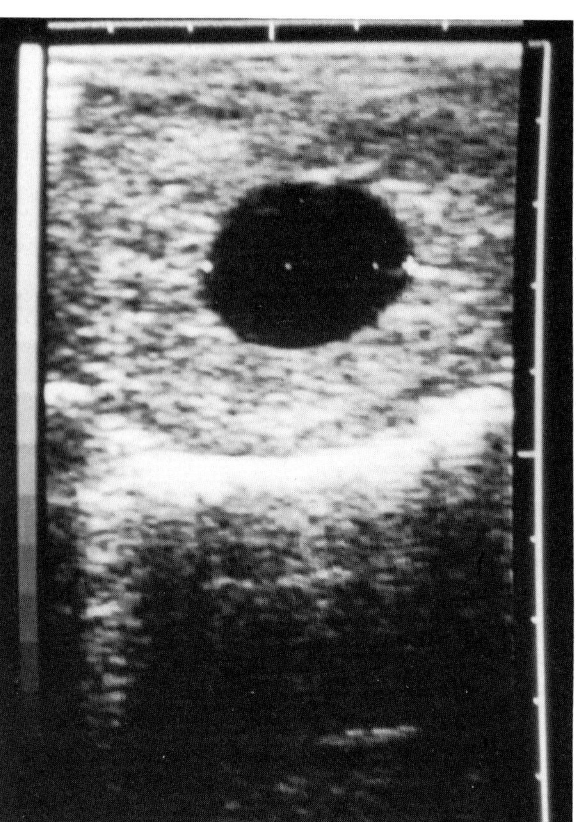

FIG. 31–6. Ultrasonographic image of a 15-day-old embryonic vesicle. The vesicle is still round.

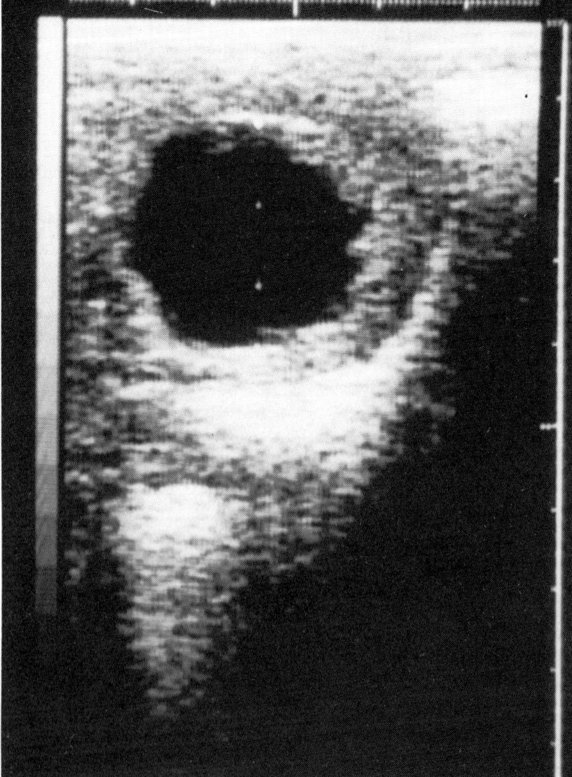

FIG. 31–7. Ultrasonographic image of an 18-day-old embryonic vesicle. The embryonic vesicle has stopped moving (fixed) and becomes quite irregular.

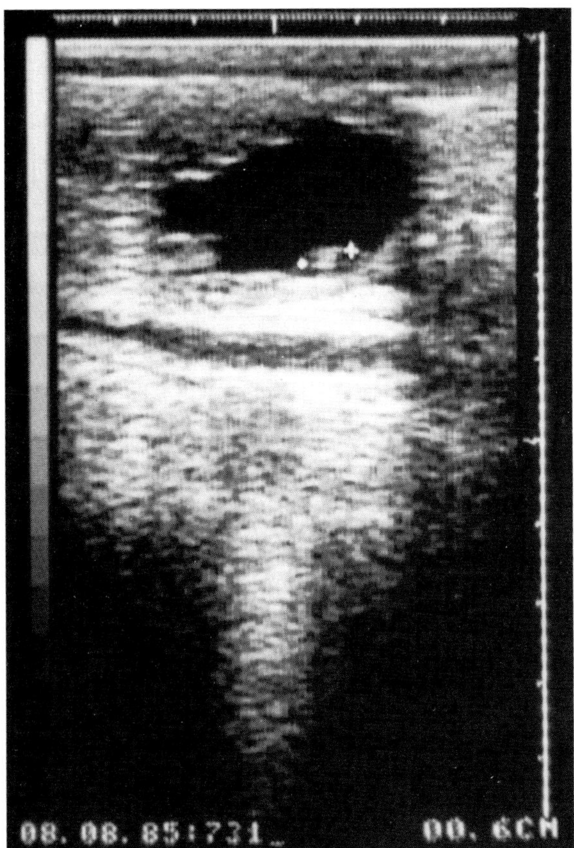

FIG. 31–8. Ultrasonographic image of a 22-day-old fetus (delineated by electronic calipers). The heartbeat is commonly detectable about this time.

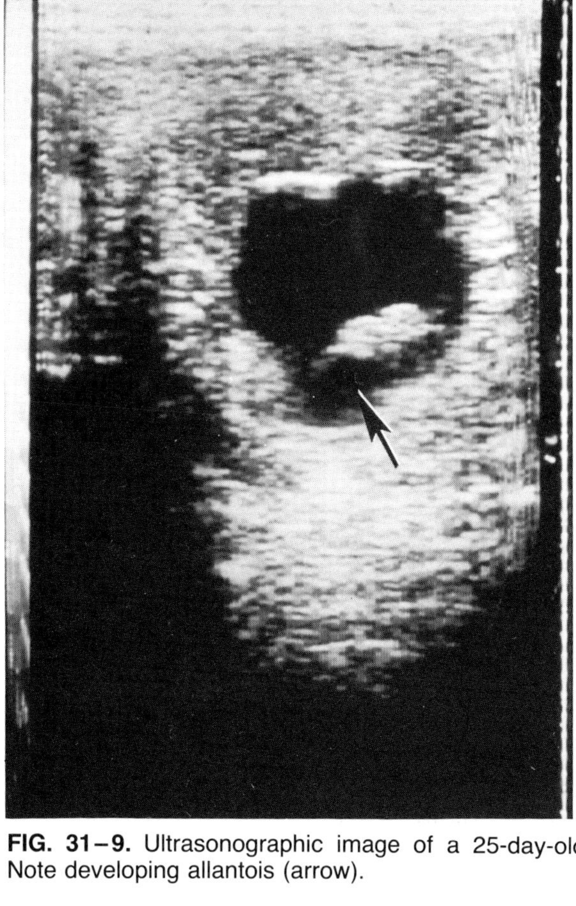

FIG. 31–9. Ultrasonographic image of a 25-day-old fetus. Note developing allantois (arrow).

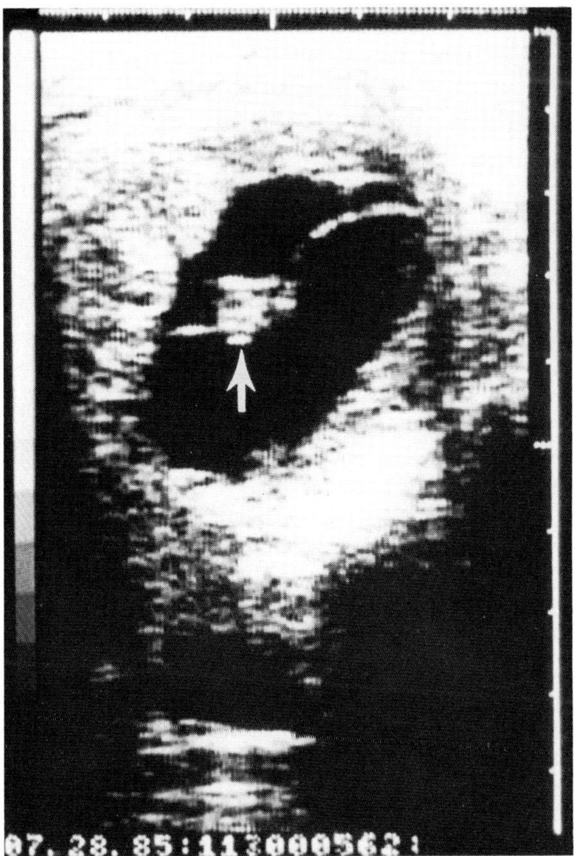

FIG. 31–10. Ultrasonographic image of a 29-day-old fetus. Note the developing allantois has pushed the embryo (arrow) dorsad and note the regression of the yolk sac.

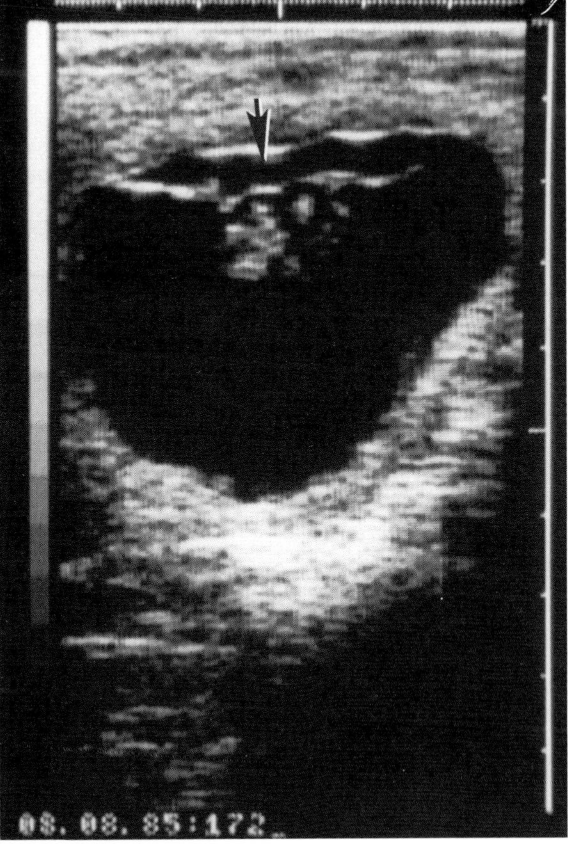

FIG. 31–11. Ultrasonographic image of a 38-day-old fetus. The yolk sac has almost regressed (arrow).

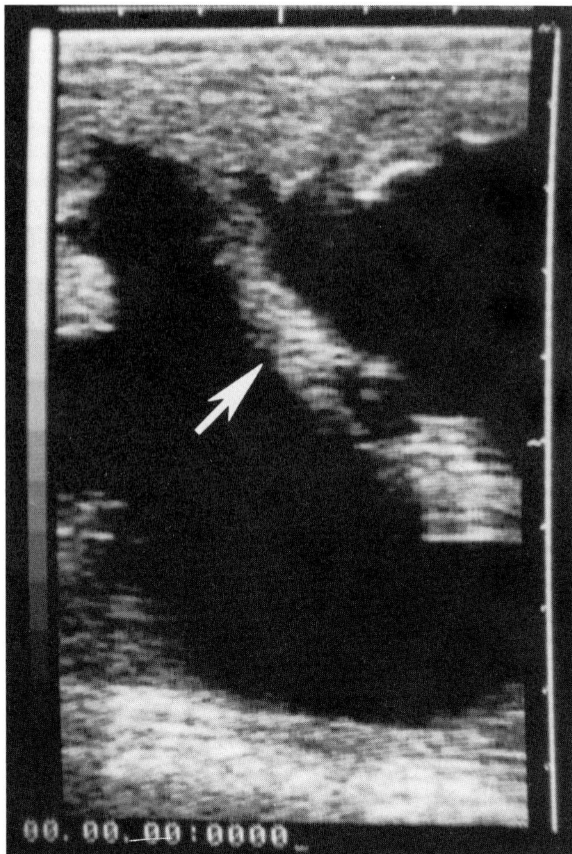

FIG. 31–12. Ultrasonographic image of a 45-day-old fetus. Note developing umbilical cord (arrow).

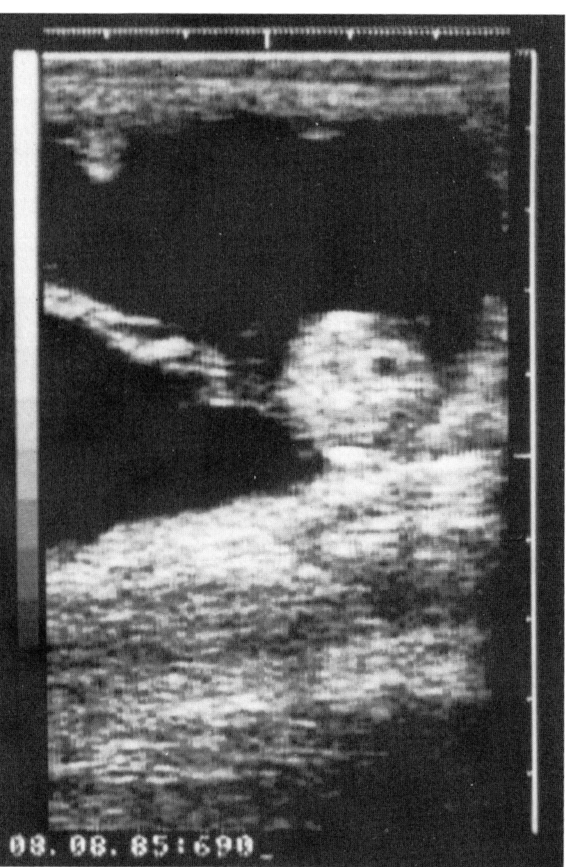

FIG. 31–13. Ultrasonographic image of a 55-day-old fetus in dorsal recumbency on the ventral uterine floor.

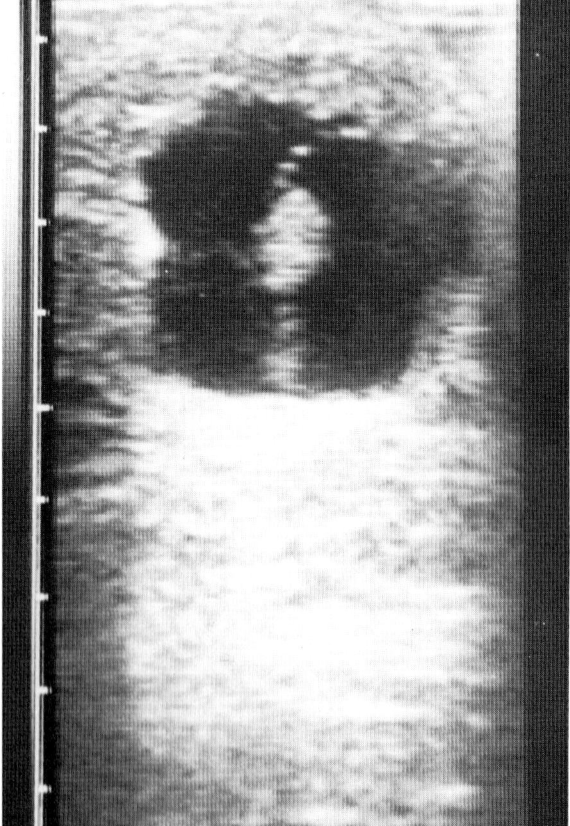

FIG. 31–14. Ultrasonographic image of a 30-day-old fetus with apposition of yolk sac and allantois giving the impression of a vertically orientated line.

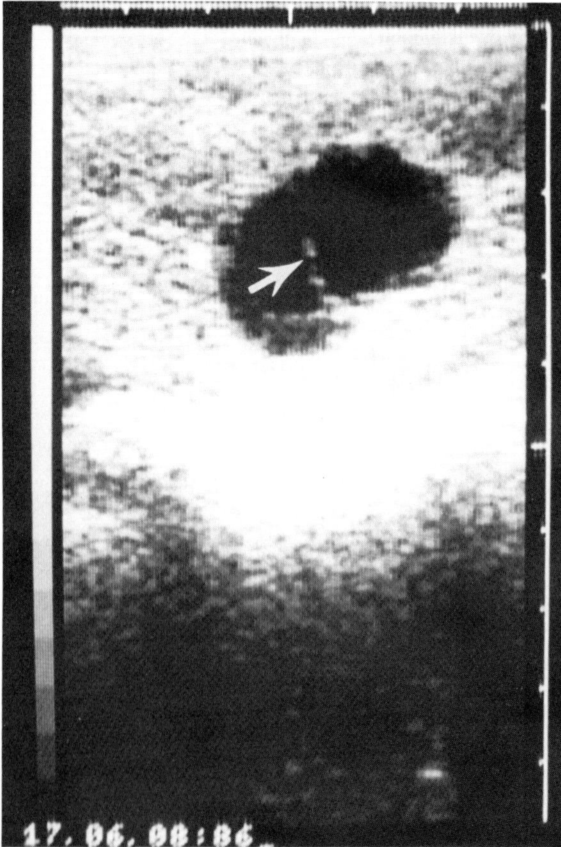

FIG. 31–15. Ultrasonographic image of twin 14-day-old conceptuses in apposition. Note: vertically orientated line (arrow).

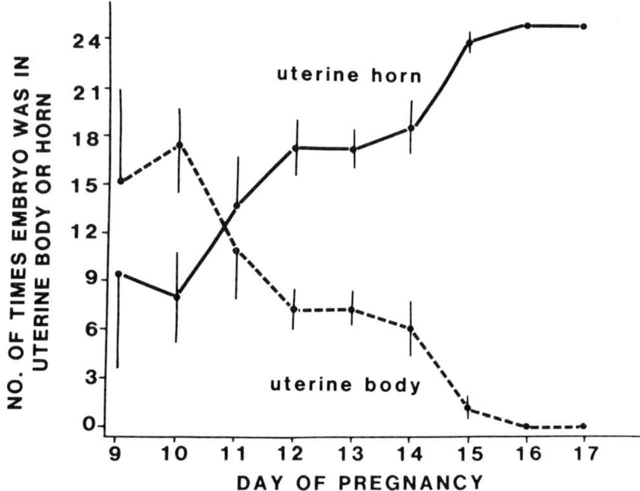

FIG. 31–16. Location of vesicle in the uterus in relation to gestation. Solid line, uterine horn; dashed line, uterine body. (Adapted from Ginther, O.J.: Ultrasonographic Imaging and Reproductive Events in the Mare. Cross Plains, WI, Equiservices, 1986.)

vesicle is fixed at the caudal portion of one of the uterine horns. Extensive mobility of the early conceptus may be caused by the spherical form and turgidity of the vesicle and longitudinal arrangements of endometrial folds. Researchers have demonstrated that restriction of embryonal movement resulted in pregnancy failure.[8] These investigators suggested that pregnancy failure was caused by inability of the conceptus to reduce uterine secretion of $PGF_2\alpha$.

When scanning for an early vesicle, the investigator should move the transducer slowly so the image or tissue slice visualized (2 to 3 mm wide) is not passed over the vesicle too rapidly. A systematic technique should be developed to avoid omitting or scanning too rapidly a portion of the reproductive tract. Because the vesicle is moving, it may be found anywhere within the uterine lumen from the tip of a uterine horn to the cranial aspect of the cervix (Fig. 31–16). Early detection of an embryonic vesicle requires a high-frequency transducer (5 MHz) and a high-quality screen. Frequently, ultrasonographic images of a 10- to 14-day vesicle has a bright echogenic line (specular reflection) on the dorsal and ventral poles with respect to the transducer (Figs. 31–4 and 31–5). These are not associated with the embryonic disk or other structures of the developing conceptus. A water-filled balloon (1.5 cm in diameter) placed in the uterus will have similar, if not identical, ultrasonographic characteristics.

TABLE 31–1. SIZE OF VESICLE DURING EARLY GESTATION

	STAGE OF GESTATION (DAYS)						
	15	20	25	30	35	40	50
Mean size (cm)*	1.96	2.73	3.22	3.62	4.42	5.94	8.84
± Standard deviation	0.50	0.36	0.31	0.27	0.12	0.16	0.11

*Recorded with a 3-MHz transducer.

(Adapted from Squires, E.L., Voss, J.L., Villahoz, M.D., and Shideler, R.K.: Use of ultrasound in broodmare reproduction. Proc. Am. Assoc. Equine Pract., 27–43, 1983.)

TABLE 31–2. SIZE OF EMBRYO DURING EARLY GESTATION

	STAGE OF GESTATION (DAYS)				
	25	30	35	40	50
Mean size (cm)*	1.76	1.95	2.15	2.78	3.49
± Standard deviation	0.59	0.51	0.46	0.36	0.28

*Recorded with a 3-MHz transducer.

(Adapted from Squires, E.L., Voss, J.L., Villahoz, M.D., and Shideler, R.K.: Use of ultrasound in broodmare reproduction. Proc. Am. Assoc. Equine Pract., 27–43, 1983.)

Days 17 to 22

The vesicle is spherical in shape before day 17 (Fig. 31–6). The increase in size of vesicle and embryo is presented in Tables 31–1 and 31–2, respectively.[11] Others have reported similar data for the equine conceptus[12–14] (Fig. 31–17). The vesicle has a growth

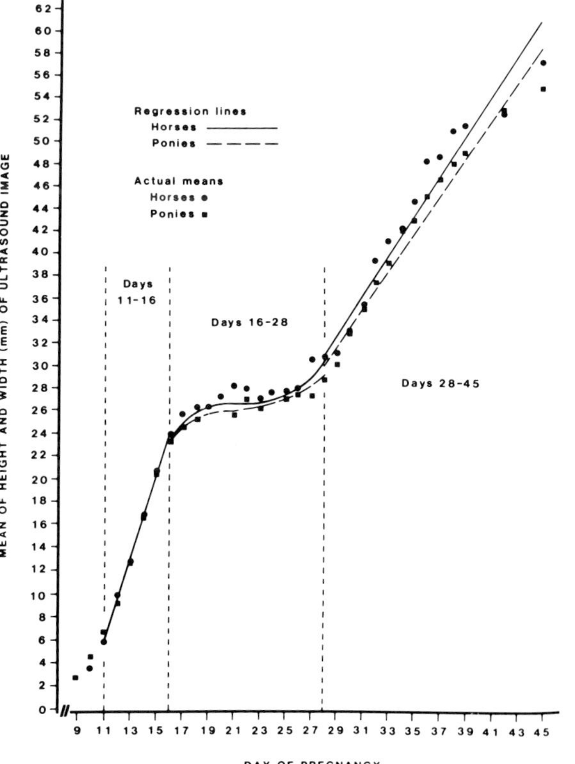

FIG. 31–17. Growth characteristics of the conceptus. Regression lines: solid line, horses; dashed line, ponies. Actual means: circles, horses; squares, ponies. (Adapted from Ginther, O.J.: Ultrasonographic Imaging and Reproductive Events in the Mare. Cross Plains, WI, Equiservices, 1986.)

plateau between days 17 to 26, then growth resumes at a slightly slower rate.[12,13] After day 17, the vesicle is often irregular in shape (Figs. 31–7 and 31–8).[13]

Fixation of the early conceptus on days 16 to 17 apparently is caused by the uterine tone and thickening of the uterine wall as well as rapid growth of the conceptus.[10] Increasing uterine tone may explain why the vesicle changes shape as pregnancy advances. Fixation generally occurs in the caudal portion of the uterine horn near the bifurcation (corpus cornual junction). In postpartum mares, the previously gravid horn provides less restriction, and thus the conceptus generally fixes in the opposite uterine horn. Fixation occurs with greater frequency in the right horn in maiden and barren mares.[9]

Orientation is defined as rotation of the embryonic vesicle so the embryo proper is on the ventral aspect of the yolk sac.[10] On day 14, the vesicle is highly mobile and the embryo is probably not orientated. Shortly after the end of the mobility phase (days 15 to 17), the dorsal uterine wall begins to enlarge and encroach on the yolk sac. Encroachment is enhanced by increasing uterine tone. The disproportionate thickening and encroachment of the uterine wall on the vesicle, in addition to the massaging action of uterine contractions, cause the vesicle to rotate so the thickest portion of the yolk sac (embryonic pole) assumes a ventral position.[10] Hypertrophy of the uterine wall is especially prominent on each side of the dorsal midline. This probably accounts for the midline location of the apex of the triangular-shaped vesicle and the thinness of the uterine wall ventrally. The embryo is first detected ultrasonographically within the vesicle at days 20 to 25 and is most commonly observed in the ventral position (Fig. 31–8). The heartbeat is commonly detected about day 22 and is an important indicator of the embryo's well-being.

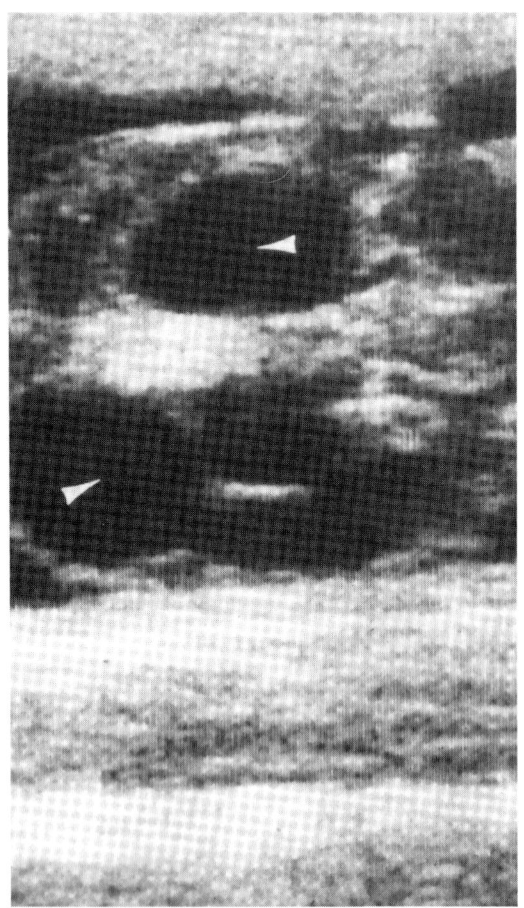

FIG. 31–18. Ultrasonographic image of an abnormally developing fetal monster, day 65 postovulation. Note fluid accumulation within the head region (arrows).

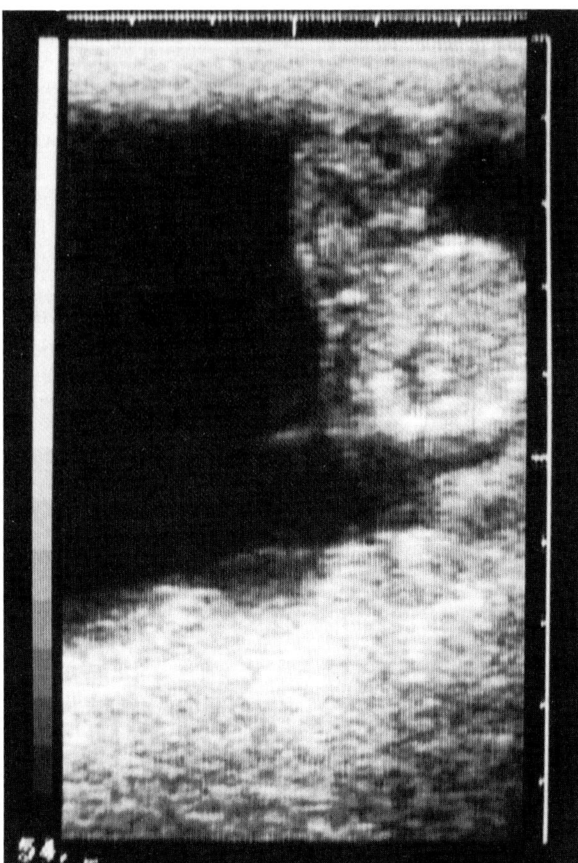

FIG. 31–19. Ultrasonographic image of a fetus the same age of gestation as Figure 31–18. This fetus is believed to be developing normally. Both were flushed as 7-day embryos (from the same donor mare) and transferred into separate recipient mares.

Days 22 to 55

The ultrasonographer must understand and interpret clinically the growth of the allantois, which is initially recognized on day 24 (Fig. 31–9), and concurrent with its expansion, the contraction of the yolk sac. The interplay of growth between these two fluid-filled structures result in the embryo moving from the ventral (day 22; Fig. 31–8) to dorsal (day 40; Fig. 31–11) aspect of the vesicle. After day 40 (Fig. 31–12), the yolk sac degenerates, and the umbilical cord elongates from the dorsal pole, permitting the fetus to gravitate to the ventral floor where it is seen in dorsal recumbency from day 50 onward (Fig. 31–13). Apposition of yolk sac and allantois results in an ultrasonographically visible line normally oriented horizontally (Fig. 31–10). On occasion, we have identified this junction in a vertical configuration (Fig. 31–14) and believe it has no deleterious effect on continuing pregnancy. Twin vesicle walls, when in contact, generally appear as an ultrasonographically visible, vertically oriented line (Fig. 31–15). With knowledge of the approximate stage of gestation and growth characteristics of the conceptus, the clinician can differentiate between presence of an abnormally orientated singleton (Fig. 31–14) or of two apposed yolk sacs (twins; Fig. 31–15).

Developmental abnormalities are more easily detected with ultrasonography than rectal palpation. On one occasion, ultrasonography was used to detect an abnormally developing fetal monster (Figs. 31–18 and 31–19), with excessive fluid in the cranium.

Obviously, with the appropriate equipment, accurate aging of the young fetus is possible by ultrasonography. No reliable method for accurately determining fetal age late in gestation has been developed. However, fetal eye size (Figs. 31–20 and 31–21) determined by ultrasonography, has been correlated ($r = 0.92$) with fetal

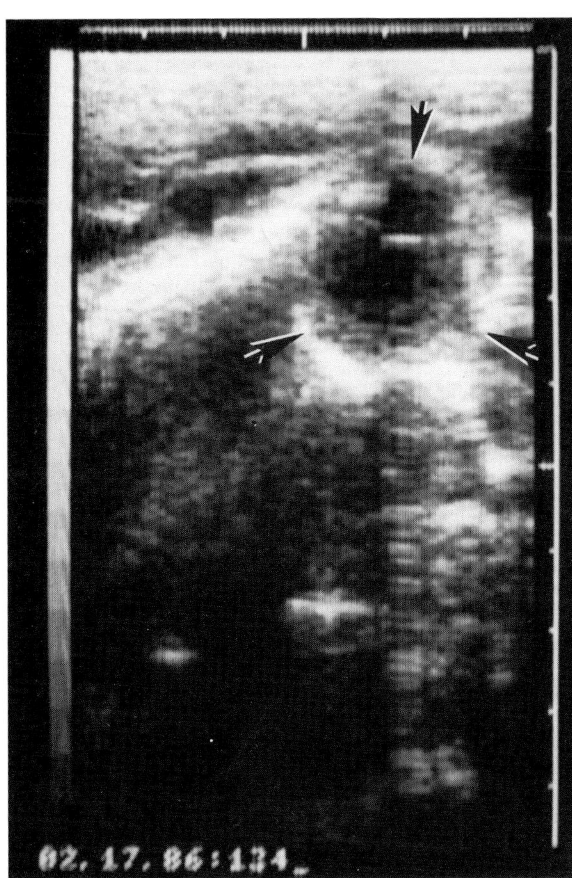

FIG. 31–20. Ultrasonographic measurement of fetal eye size to estimate fetal age. Note characteristics of the eye from a 180-day developing fetus (arrows).

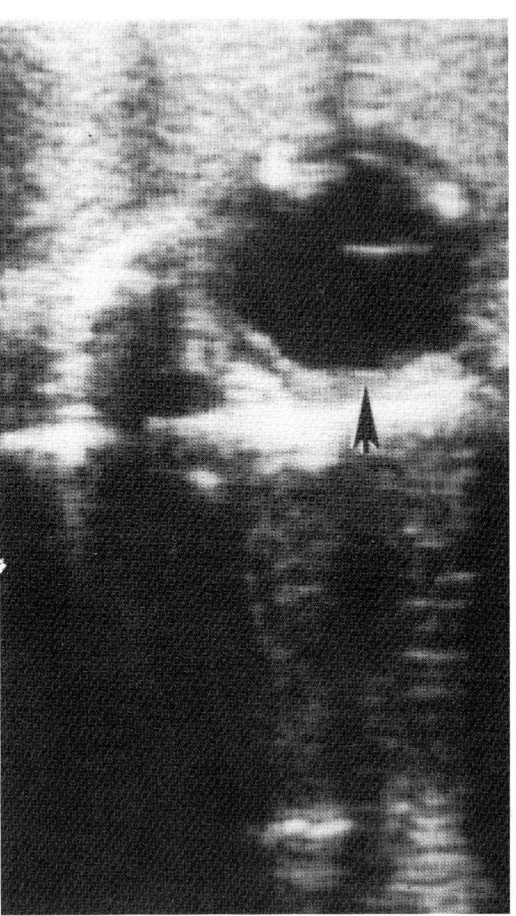

FIG. 31–21. Ultrasonographic measurement of fetal eye size to estimate fetal age. Note characteristics of the eye from a 230-day developing fetus (arrow).

age.[15] Presented in Figure 31–22 is a graph that can be used to predict age of the fetus after 100 days of gestation. Measurement of fetal eye size was made with a 5-MHz transducer in mares of known gestational age. Eye size was calculated from the sum of width plus length. Identification of the eye was not difficult because of dorsopubic positioning of the fetus after day 90.

Early studies on the efficacy of ultrasonography for pregnancy diagnosis have demonstrated extreme accuracy after day 15 (> 97.4%).[11,16,17] False-positive diagnoses were related to misinterpretation of uterine cysts and false negatives were attributed to operator inexperience and scanning too rapidly.[11] These studies were performed with 3-MHz transducers and ability to diagnose pregnancy have further improved with the advent of 5-MHz transducers, better image quality, more information on early conceptal development, and increased operator experience. Experience has taught that the following factors are important in accurate identification of an early pregnancy.

1. Equipment quality and transducer frequency.
2. Mare restraint and examination environment.
3. Age of the conceptus at the time of examination and interval between multiple ovulations.

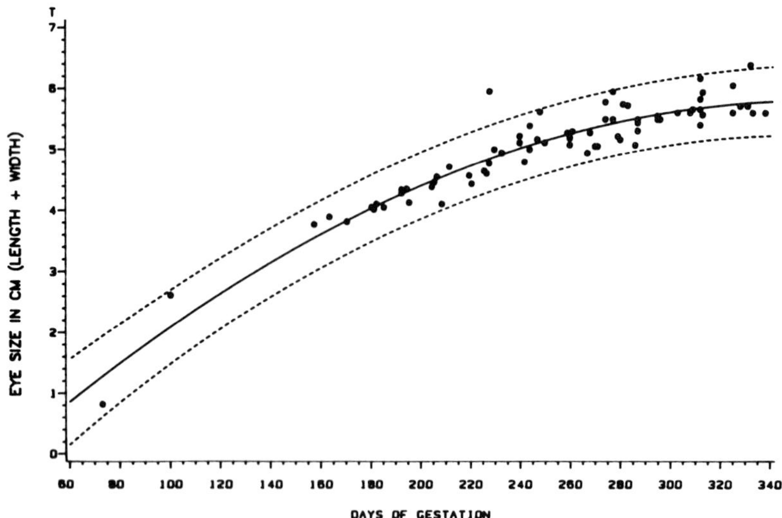

FIG. 31–22. The relationship between day of gestation and size of fetal eye (length plus width in centimeters) with 95% confidence intervals for measurements (r = 0.92). (Adapted from McKinnon, A.O., Squires, E.L., and Pickett, B.W.: Equine reproductive ultrasonography. Animal Reproduction Laboratory Bulletin No. 04. Fort Collins, Colorado State University, 1988.)

4. Operator experience.
5. Opportunity to re-examine the mare.

In humans, no deleterious effects of ultrasonography have been reported.[18] Frequent manipulation with the transducer within the mare's rectum or sound waves at a frequency of 3 MHz have been determined not to be detrimental to continuing pregnancy.[11]

DETECTION AND MANAGEMENT OF TWINS

Multiple pregnancy (twins) in the mare is undesirable, because only approximately 60% of mares with twin embryos deliver live, single foals; while 31% lose both pregnancies[19] and 9% carry both foals to term. In addition, of the 9% of twin foals carried to term, both foals are born dead 64.5% of the time, one foal is born alive 21% of the time, and live twins occur 14.5% of the time.[20] Twinning is second only to endometritis as the leading cause of abortion in mares. Mares carrying twins to term often require assistance at birth, and surviving foals are usually weaker, more susceptible to infection, and develop more slowly. When twin foals are born alive, one foal is generally weaker and often dies within 3 to 4 days. Mares that abort twin pregnancies often have a higher incidence of retained fetal membranes, may not recycle, and may be difficult to impregnate during the same or subsequent breeding season.[19,21] This results in reduction of reproduction efficiency.

A variety of breeding strategies and postconception treatments have been developed to reduce or prevent twinning in mares. However, until recently most have been unsuccessful. When the likelihood of twinning is high, breeding may be withheld and the mare recycled with prostaglandins. When twin conception occurs, treatment such as crushing of one vesicle[22] and abortion with prostaglandins or saline[23,24] have been reported as means of managing twin pregnancies.

Twins in most species arise either by division of a fertilized ovum or multiple ovulations resulting in multiple ova. The possibility of twins occurring from release of a single, fertilized ovum can probably be discounted in mares because twins are almost always dizygotic, i.e., derived from two ova.[25] For horse embryos, the "capsule" (see Chapter 56) may be important in preventing the "pinching effect" of the zona pellucida on hatching embryos seen occasionally in other species that do not have a capsule.[6] This pinching effect now is believed to be the mechanism for a single ovum dividing into twins (A. Trounson, personal communication).

Two patterns of double ovulation are recognized: (1) synchronous ovulations may occur from either ovary, but are separated by no more than one day, and (2) asynchronous ovulations which occur from 2 to 10 days apart during the same estrous period. In the latter case, progesterone levels do not rise until after the second ovulation.[26] The pattern of ovulation was originally reported to have a dramatic influence on twinning as determined by rectal palpation. The mare has a natural biologic mechanism for elimination of twins.[27] This mechanism has been reported to operate less efficiently when twin embryos arose from asynchronous ovulation.[28] Furthermore, twin fetuses were rare in association with synchronous ovulation.[21] However, from results of more recent research, using ultrasonography for pregnancy detection, twins were as likely to occur from synchronous as from asynchronous ovulation.[29] Recovery of twin embryos from the uterus 6 to 7 days post-

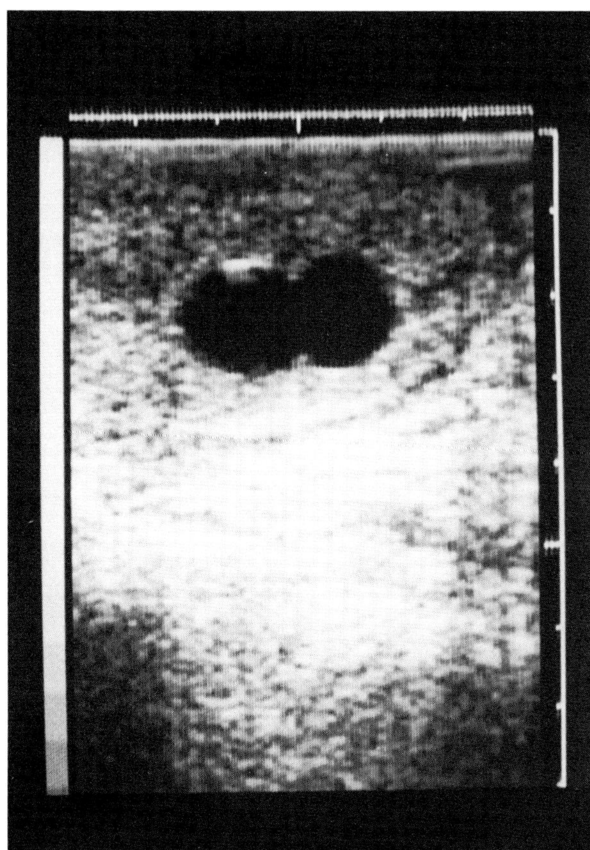

FIG. 31–23. Two 12-day embryonic vesicles before separation.

ovulation was not different for synchronous and asynchronous ovulations. In addition, transfer of these embryos into separate recipients usually resulted in two pregnancies with survival rates similar to normal, single embryo transfers.[30,31] Therefore, the embryo reduction mechanism does not seem to become effective until after the embryo enters the uterus and, most commonly, is coincident with cessation of the mobility phase (days 16 to 17).

The exact mechanism for elimination of one of the embryonic vesicles has not been elucidated, but researchers believe its success is largely related to how the twin vesicles become fixed in the uterus. Twin vesicles fixed together at one corpus cornual junction approximately 70% of the time.[29] When this occurs, successful reduction to a single pregnancy is common. Embryonic reduction may be facilitated by competition for available nutrients. When twin pregnancies fix at opposite corpus cornual junctions, embryonic reduction is much less frequent.[32]

Manual crushing of one twin vesicle between 12 and 30 days of pregnancy resulted in an extremely high (96%) rate of single, embryonic reduction.[33] Frequent scanning or minor manipulation is necessary to identify good separation of the vesicles (Figs. 31–23 and 31–24). The smaller vesicle should be manipulated into and crushed at the tip of one uterine horn. Frequently a distinct popping sensation is recognized when the vesicle is ruptured. After day 16, the vesicles are likely to be fixed at the corpus cornual junction and manual reduction may be more difficult, if both are fixed on the same side (Fig. 31–25). Crushing of one vesicle is then performed in situ.[33] The ability to gently and accurately separate twins and manipulate one into the extremity of a uterine horn is greatly facilitated by monitoring with ultrasonography. The uterine horn is forced against the cranial and lateral margin of the pelvis and pressure increased by forcing the transducer down onto the vesicle (Fig. 31–26) until the vesicle is destroyed.

Monitoring with ultrasonography and nonintervention until day 30 is another accepted method of treatment. If a mare has not adjusted to one pregnancy by day 30, prostaglandins can be administered to terminate the pregnancy or the crushing of one can be attempted. Prostaglandins should be given before formation of endometrial cups (days 35 to 40). If rebreeding is not desired or practical, induction of abortion can be delayed for as much as 70 to 80 days. When twins are diagnosed after formation of endometrial cups (Fig. 31–27), surgical intervention to remove one conceptus has been advocated (D.R. Pascoe, personal communication). The technique was most successful when twins became fixed in opposite corpus cornual junctions (8 single foals from 10 twin pregnancies) compared with

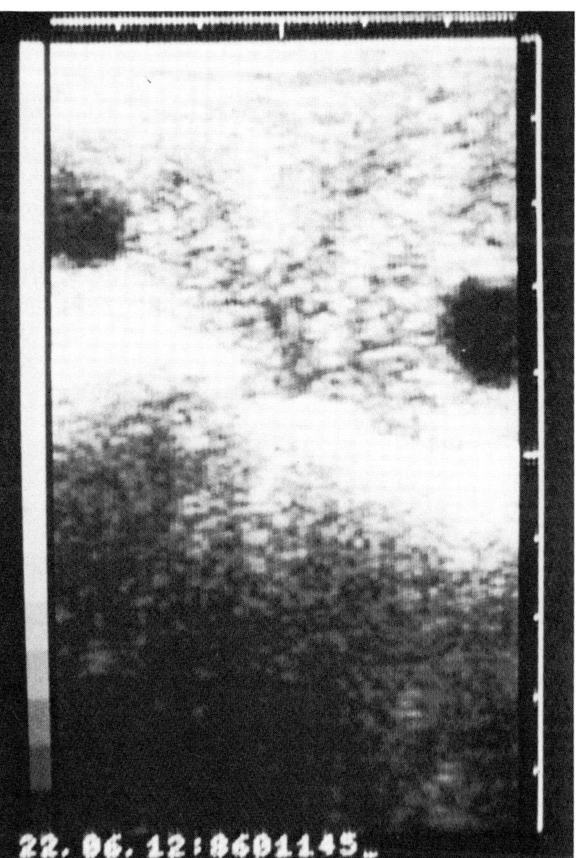

FIG. 31–24. Separation of the vesicles in Figure 31–23 before crushing.

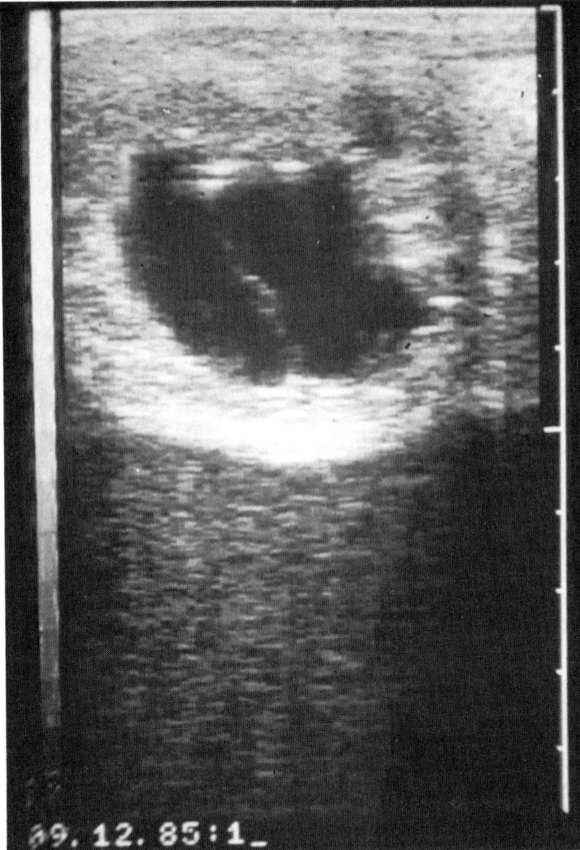

FIG. 31–25. Two 20-day embryonic vesicles fixed together at one corpus cornual junction.

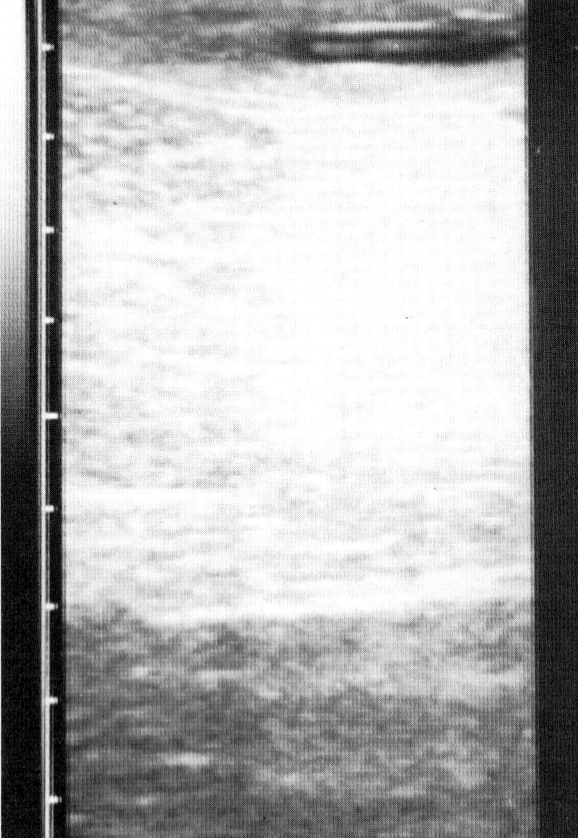

FIG. 31–26. Destruction of one twin vesicle with pressure from a transducer.

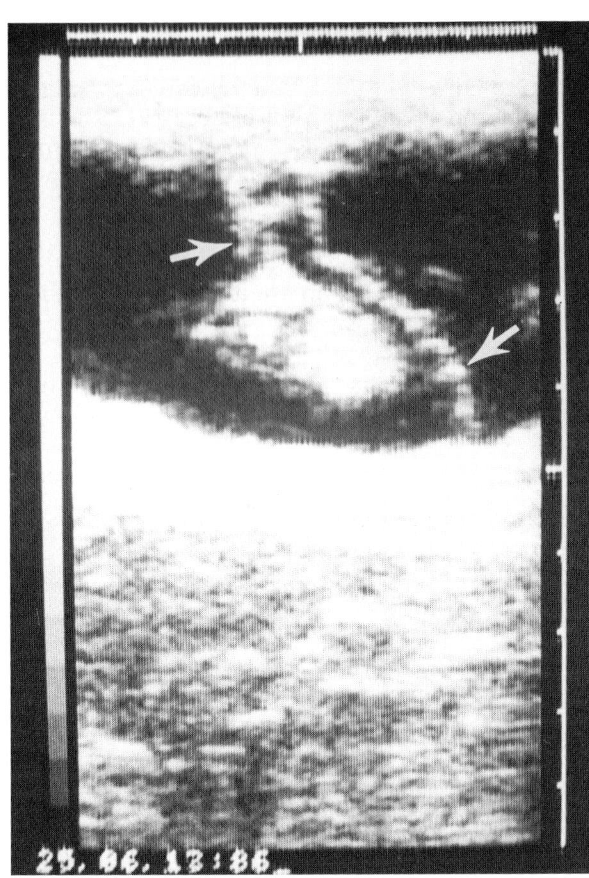

FIG. 31–27. Twin 45-day pregnancies. Note presence of two umbilical cords (arrows).

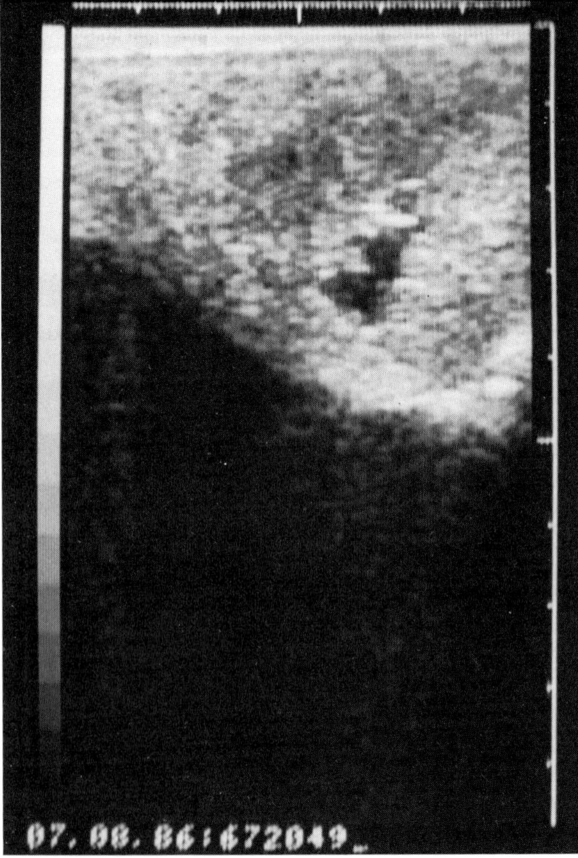

FIG. 31–28. Small amount of fluid remaining at the corpus cornual junction after EED.

twins that fixed together (0 foals from 8 twin pregnancies).

A sophisticated technique involving cardiac puncture of one cotwin and lethal injection of potassium chloride is currently being used.[34] This procedure is performed with either a 3- or 5-MHz sector transducer with a biopsy needle guide attached. After tranquilization of the mare, the fetus is identified by ventral abdominal transcutaneous ultrasonography. After confirming that the mare has twin pregnancies, an attempt is made to identify a discrepancy in size between the pregnancies. If a size difference exists, fetal reduction may have already been initiated by the mare. A 6-in., 18-gauge needle is inserted into the heart of the chosen fetus, while monitoring directly with ultrasonography through the abdominal wall, and potassium chloride is injected until cessation of heartbeat. This procedure has been performed in over 30 mares, with the earliest pregnancy being 54 days and the latest 168 days. However, twin pregnancies between 70 and 110 days of gestation are preferred.[34] Approximately 50% of the cases treated have resulted in mummification of one fetus, while the other proceeded to term. Unfortunately, the other sequel is death and abortion of both fetuses within 30 days of the procedure. It was difficult to determine whether these abortions were the natural tendency of mares to eliminate twins or a result of intrauterine invasion. However, this is not a stage of gestation when a large percentage of abortions are expected from mares carrying twin pregnancies. No adverse effects on the health of the mares were reported. Our experiences with the technique have not been as encouraging. The method is not technically difficult; however, most mares failed to produce live foals at term. Our success has apparently improved by replacing potassium chloride with 10 to 15 mL penicillin/streptomycin aqueous suspension.

Methods may be developed that will allow one fetus to be carried successfully to term despite twin pregnancy determined late in gestation. On three occasions, when premature lactation began at approximately 8 months of gestation and supplemental progesterone was initiated and continued up to 2 weeks before expected delivery, a live foal was delivered concurrent with a mummified fetus.[35] Although the live foals were small, each nursed and continued to develop normally. However, further research is needed before a recommendation of widespread supplementation of progesterone to mares with twin pregnancies can be made.

EARLY EMBRYONIC DEATH

Early embryonic death (EED) results in low reproductive performance of mares.[36] Notifying the client that a valuable mare has undergone embryonic loss is a distressing experience for a breeding manager or veterinarian. Clients enthusiastically support use of ultrasonography for early pregnancy detection. However, not all pregnancies continue to survive, even in normal mares. Improvement in ultrasonographic equipment has permitted investigation of early embryonic losses between days 10 and 20 of gestation.[37] This technique, combined with embryo recovery, permits investigation of embryo losses between day 6, which is the first time an embryo can be routinely recovered from the uterus, and day 11, which is the first time the vesicle can be consistently detected by ultrasonography. The incidence of EED before day 6 is unknown. However, Ball et al. suggested that a major proportion of EED in infertile mares occurred in the oviduct.[38] The incidence of EED has been reported to be between 5 and 30% of established pregnancies.[39–42] In other studies using ultrasonography, EED seemed to occur in mares much earlier than previously reported.[37,43] Various causes and factors responsible for EED in mares, apart from presence of twins, have been suggested, including nutrition,[44–46] plant estrogens and photoperiod,[47] seminal treatments,[48] lactational stress and foal heat breedings,[49] genital infections,[39,41,49,50] chromosomal abnormalities,[51] hormonal deficiencies,[45] anabolic steroids,[37] stress,[45,52] failure of maternal recognition, and deficiency of pregnant mare serum gonadotropin (PMSG) production.[53,54]

Migration of the conceptus was originally believed to be a contributing factor in early embryonic death;[55] however, it is now known to be a normal characteristic of the horse conceptus.[9] Lactating mares and mares bred during foal heat have been reported to have a higher incidence of EED than nonlactating mares.[49,56,57] However, in a survey of 2562 pregnancies in lactating and nonlactating mares, the incidence of EED was similar.[58]

Before the advent of ultrasonography, recognition and timing of EED was difficult. From data collected at Colorado State University over 2 breeding seasons involving 356 mares diagnosed pregnant using ultrasonography, the overall incidence of EED through day 50 postovulation was 17.3%.[37] The majority (77.1%) of EED occurred before day 35 postovulation. During the period 15 to 35 days postovulation, a greater ($p < 0.05$) incidence of EED occurred between days 15 to 20 (26.2%) and 30 to 35 (29.5%) postovulation compared with other time periods. Maternal recognition of pregnancy has been reported to occur between 14 and 16 days postovulation.[7,8] In the study at our laboratory, 13.3% of mares pregnant at day 15 lost their pregnancies by day 35.[37] Formation of endometrial cups occurs on approximately day 35.

Early embryonic death is diagnosed when an embryonic vesicle seen previously is not observed on two consecutive ultrasonographic scans and/or when only remnants of a vesicle are observed (Fig. 31–28). Ultrasonographic criteria for impending EED are an irregular and indented vesicle (depending on age), fluid in the uterine lumen, and vesicular fluid that contains echogenic spots (Fig. 31–29). Early embryonic death is suspected, particularly after day 30, when no fetal heartbeat is observed, poor definition of fetal structure exists, fetal fluids are echogenic, or the largest diameter of the fetal vesicle is two standard deviations smaller than the mean established for that specific day of age.

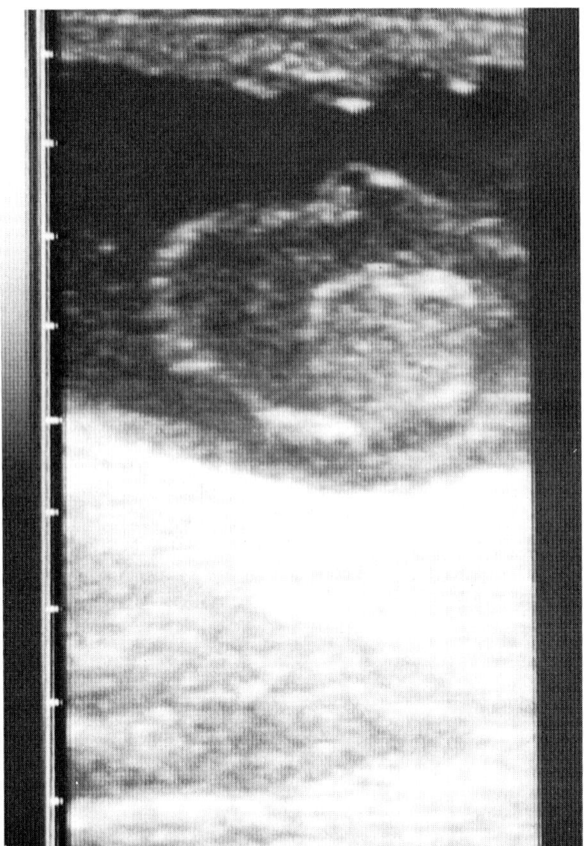

FIG. 31–29. Early embryonic death. Note disruption of placental membranes and increased echogenicity of fetal fluid.

Vesicles increasing in size more slowly than normal may also be characteristic of early embryonic death.[43] Indications obtained by ultrasonographic scanning of impending loss at later stages include failure of fixation, an echogenic ring within the vesicle, a mass floating in a collection of fluid, and a gradual decrease in volume of placental fluid with disorganization of placental membranes[43] (Figs. 31–30 to 31–34).

Ultrasonographic scanning during early pregnancy is an extremely useful management tool for pregnancy detection and determination of EED. However, if pregnancy rates are not reported until day 50, the discrepancy between pregnancy and foaling rates decreases.

Few, if any, treatments exist to consistently decrease incidence of EED, but artificial insemination can limit bacterial challenge to a mare's uterus, thus reducing potential losses from endometritis. In addition, any new information on causes and treatment of endometritis should result in increased breeding efficiency. The transfer of embryos from mares with poor uterine-biopsy grades into normal recipient mares is recommended to provide an environment more conductive to pregnancy maintenance.[42] Unfortunately, recovery of embryos from infertile mares is low. Supplementation with progesterone to habitually aborting mares or mares with primary luteal inadequacy has been advocated.[59] However, little experimental evidence supports the efficacy of this procedure.[54] One report suggests genetic abnormalities would not appear to be a major cause of EED in mares.[60] Perhaps the changes most likely to result in a decrease in incidence of EED is improving management factors related to nutrition, environmental temperature, infectious diseases, and other stresses.

UTERINE DISEASE

With ultrasonography the uterus can be examined noninvasively to determine pathologic changes and to monitor therapeutic regimen(s). The three most common forms of uterine disease detected by ultrasonography are accumulations of intrauterine fluid, air, and cysts. Less commonly, fetal remnants, debris, abscessation, and neoplastic conditions are observed.

INTRAUTERINE FLUID

Ultrasonography is extremely valuable for estimating quantity and quality of fluid in the uterine lumen. Rectal palpation is only accurate when the quality of intrauterine fluid is large (> 100 mL) and/or when uterine tonicity changes. Confirmation of intrauterine fluid,

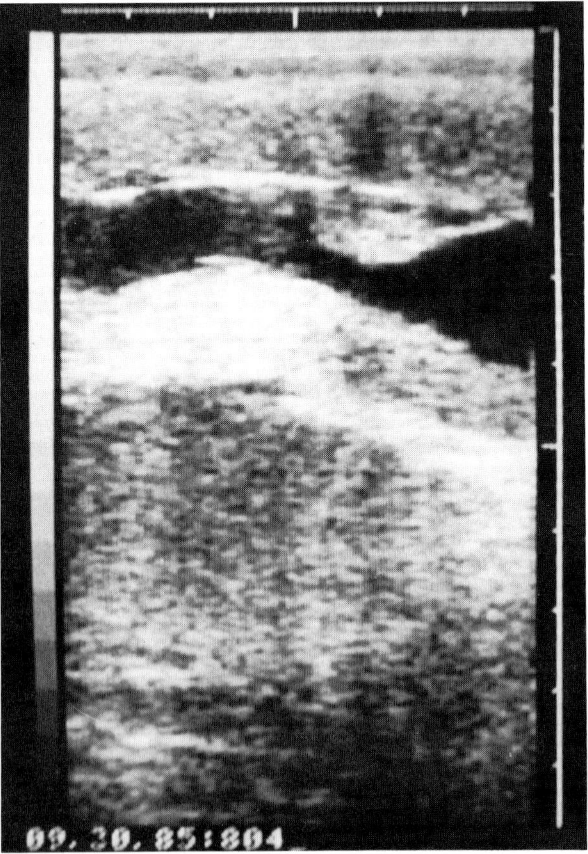

FIG. 31–30. Early embryonic death. The fetus is being expelled through the cervix.

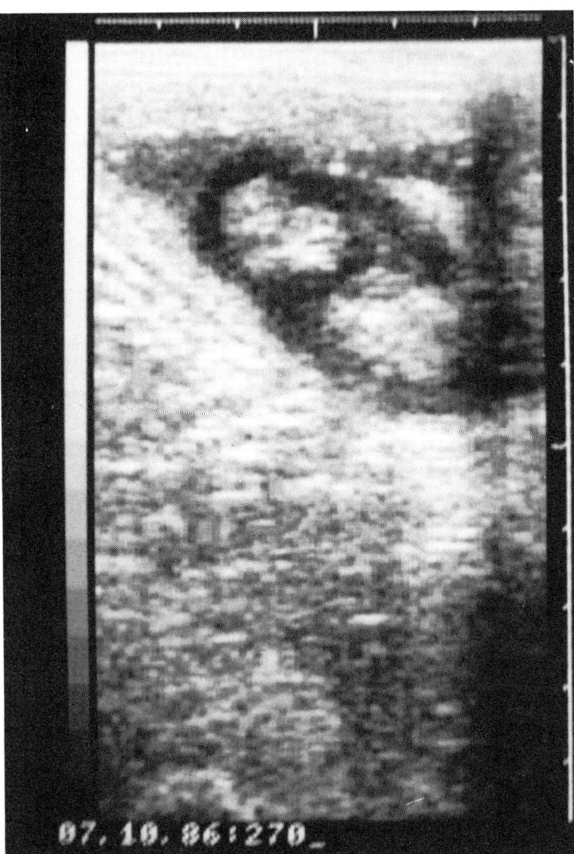

FIG. 31–31. Early embryonic death. Note resorption of fetal fluids.

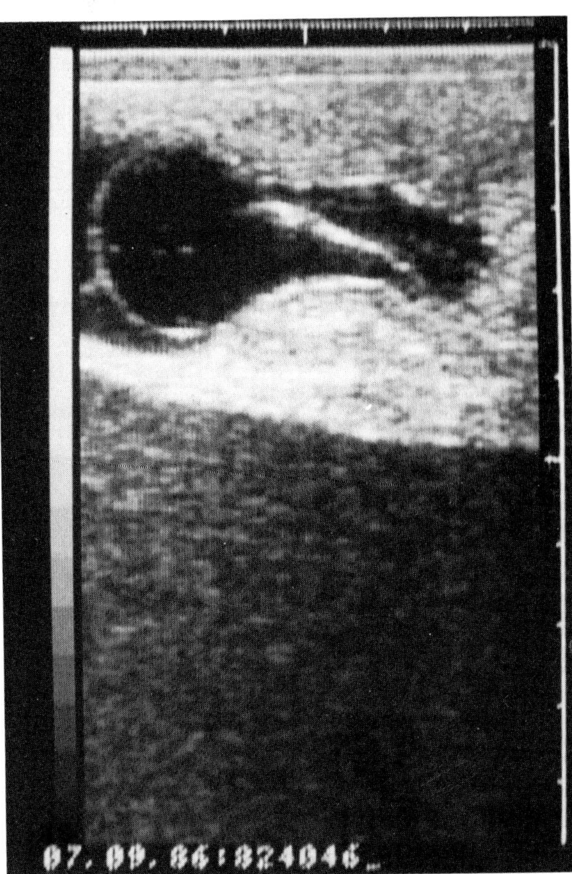

FIG. 31–32. Apparent increase in size of the amnionic cavity and loss of fetal outline.

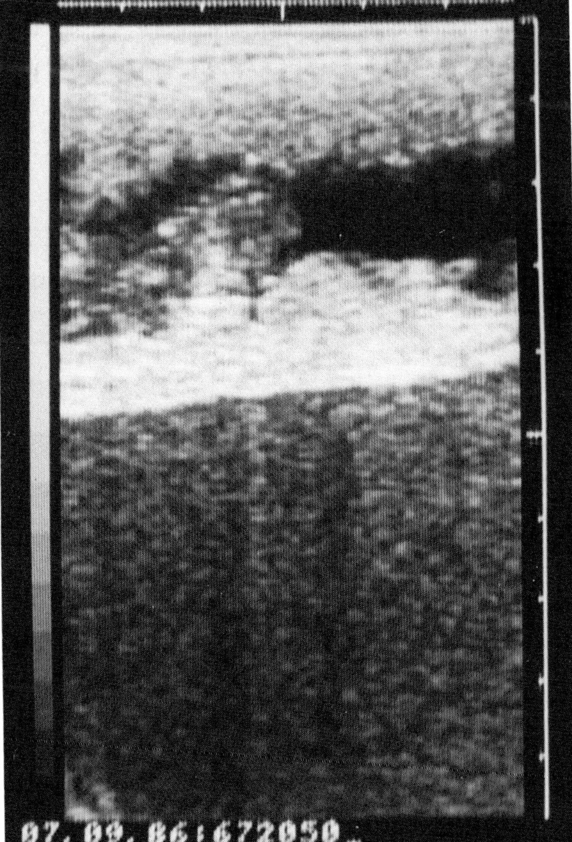

FIG. 31–33. Decreased fetal fluids. Fetus is in the uterine body instead of at the corpus cornual junction.

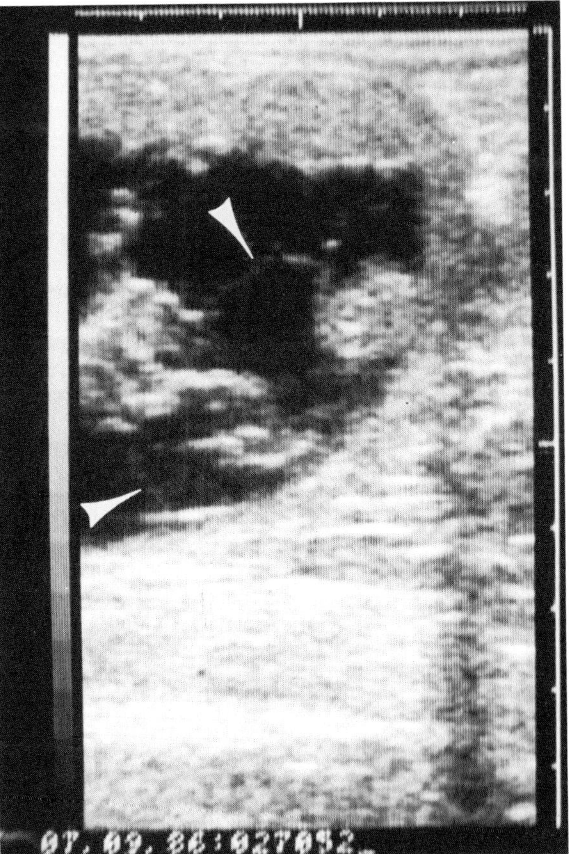

FIG. 31–34. Disrupted placental membranes (arrows).

TABLE 31–3. ULTRASONOGRAPHIC EVALUATION OF INTRAUTERINE FLUID

ULTRASONOGRAPHIC GRADE OF UTERINE FLUID	ULTRASONOGRAPHIC CHARACTERISTICS OF UTERINE FLUID	GROSS CHARACTERISTICS OF UTERINE FLUID
Grade I* (Fig. 31–35)	White (strongly echogenic or hyperechoic)	Thick and creamy
Grade II (Fig. 31–36)	Light gray (semiechogenic or hyperechoic)	Milky
Grade III (Fig. 31–37)	Dark gray (hypoechoic—few hyperechoic foci suspended in anechoic medium)	Obvious turbidity and sedimentation
Grade IV (Fig. 31–38)	Black (anechoic)	Clear

*The degree of echogenicity is related to debris and inflammatory material in uterine fluid.

(Adapted from McKinnon, A.O., Squires, E.L., and Pickett, B.W.: Equine reproductive ultrasonography. Animal Reproduction Laboratory Bulletin No. 04. Fort Collins, Colorado State University, 1988; and McKinnon, A.O., et al.: Ultrasonographic studies on the reproductive tract of postpartum mares: Effect of involution and uterine fluid on pregnancy rates in mares with normal and delayed first postpartum ovulatory cycles. J. Am. Vet. Med. Assoc., *192*:350–353, 1988.)

without invasive techniques such as lavage and cytologic analysis, was difficult until direct, noninvasive visualization was made possible with ultrasonography.

Volumes of fluid within the uterine lumen are estimated with ultrasonography and quality is graded from I to IV according to degree of echogenicity[15,61] (Table 31–3; Figs. 31–35 to 31–38). Degree of echogenicity is related to amount of debris or white blood cell infiltration into the fluid. Grade I fluid has large numbers of neutrophils and grade IV has very few neutrophils. Observations on quality and quantity of uterine fluid have been used to assess efficacy of various therapeutic procedures on individual animals treated for naturally occurring endometritis. Experiments have been conducted to determine the relationship of intrauterine fluid to fertility.[61–63]

Ultrasonographic Studies of the Uterus after Parturition

In the equine industry, economic incentives influence breeders to attempt a foaling interval of 12 months or less. This commonly necessitates breeding of mares during the first postpartum ovulation. However, fertility has been reported to be lower in mares bred during the first postpartum ovulatory period compared with mares bred during subsequent cycles,[49,64–66] and EED has been reported to be higher for mares bred at this time.[49,57,67] This decreased fertility may be caused by failure of elimination of microbes during uterine involution[49,67,68] or their introduction at breeding.[69] In addition, presence of uterine fluid during estrus[61] and diestrus[62,63] has been shown to reduce fertility of mares.

A study was conducted to evaluate two hypotheses: (1) uterine involution and fluid accumulation could be effectively monitored with ultrasonography and used to predict the fertility of mares bred during the first postpartum ovulatory cycle and (2) delaying ovulation with a progestin would result in improved pregnancy rates in mares bred during the first postpartum ovulatory period.[61] The previously gravid horn was larger than the nongravid horn for a mean of 21 days (range 15 to 25) after parturition. Uterine involution was most obvious at the corpus cornual junction. When the results of three ultrasonographic scans were similar, over a 5-day period, the uterus was considered to be involuted. On the average, uterine involution was completed by day 23 (range 13 to 29).

Quantity and quality of uterine fluid were not affected by progestin treatment. The number of mares with detectable uterine fluid decreased after day 5 postpartum (Table 31–4). Uterine fluid generally decreased in quantity and improved in quality between days 3 and day 15.

Fewer ($p < 0.005$) mares became pregnant when uterine fluid was present during the first postpartum ovulatory period (3 of 9, 33%), compared with mares that had no detectable fluid (26 of 31, 84%). Mares with uterine fluid during breeding did not have appre-

TABLE 31–4. ULTRASONOGRAPHIC ASSESSMENT OF INTRAUTERINE FLUID QUANTITY AND QUALITY FROM 45 MARES AFTER PARTURITION

POSTPARTUM DAYS	NUMBER OF MARES WITH DETECTABLE UTERINE FLUID	MEAN UTERINE FLUID QUALITY (GRADES I–IV)
3	34	2.1
5	37	2.8
7	28	3.2
9	11	2.7
11	6	3.3
13	7	3.4
15	2	3.0

(Adapted from McKinnon, A.O. et al.: Ultrasonographic studies on the reproductive tract of postpartum mares: effect of involution and uterine fluid on pregnancy rates in mares with normal and delayed first postpartum ovulatory cycles. J. Am. Vet. Med. Assoc., *192*:350–353, 1988.)

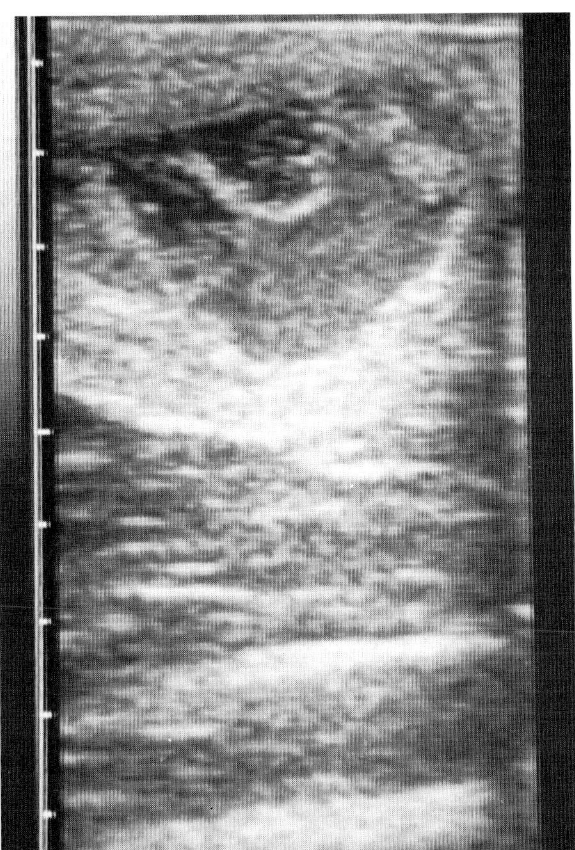

FIG. 31–35. Grade I intrauterine fluid—white is strongly echogenic.

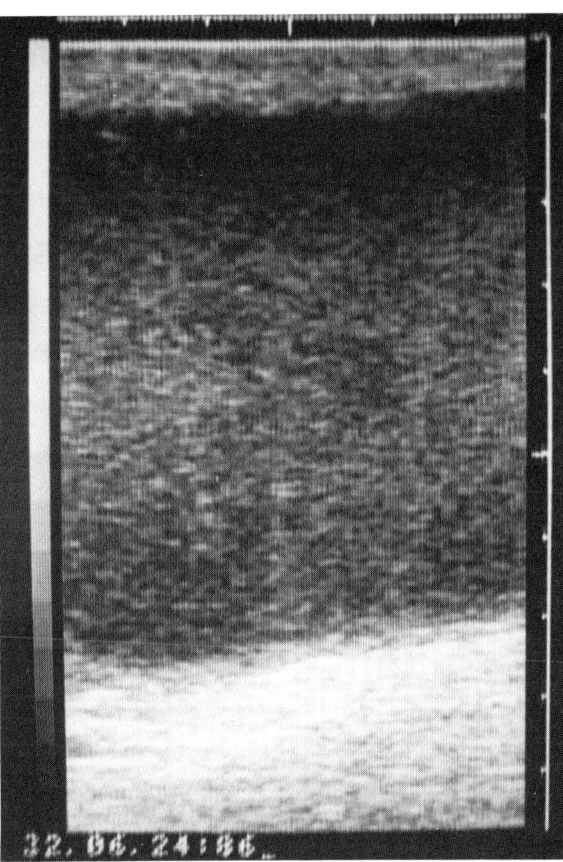

FIG. 31–36. Grade II intrauterine fluid—light gray is semiechogenic or hyperechogenic.

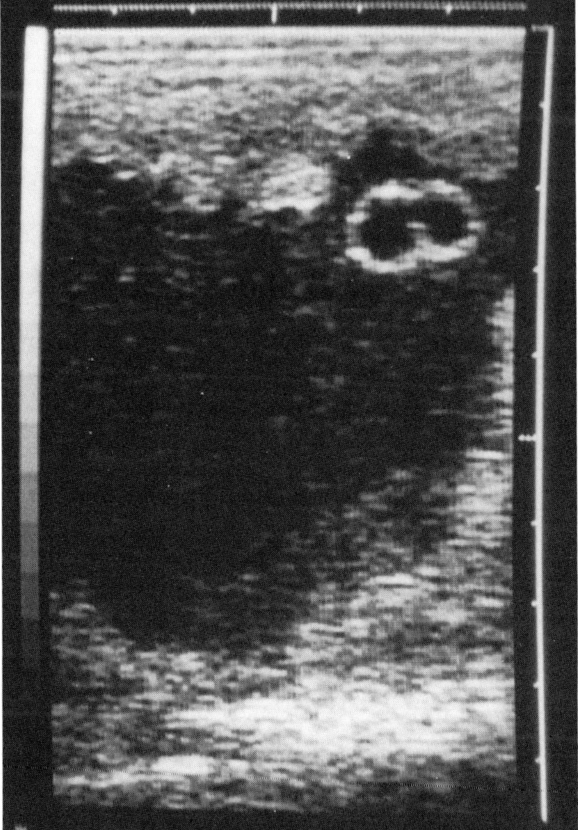

FIG. 31–37. Grade III, intrauterine fluid—dark gray is hypoechogenic, and a few hyperechoic foci are suspended in an anechoic medium.

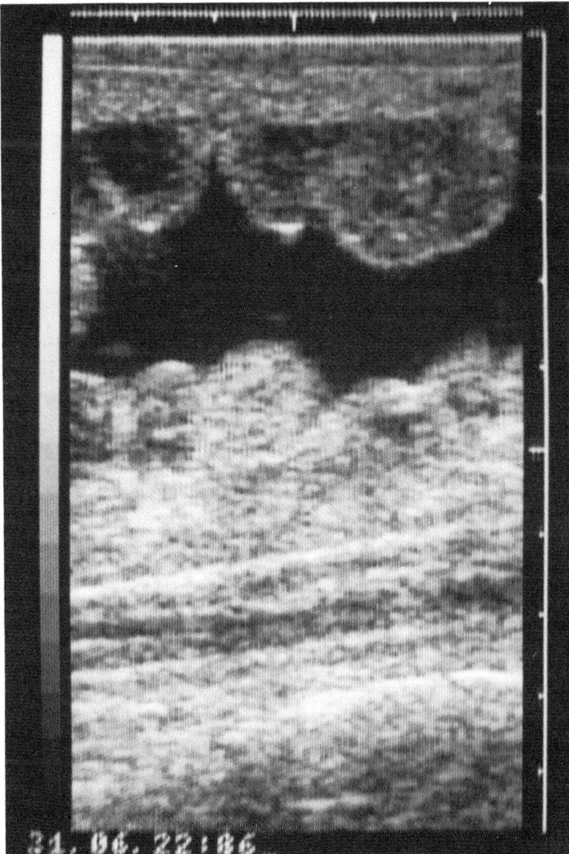

FIG. 31–38. Grade IV, intrauterine fluid—black is anechoic.

ciably larger uterine dimensions compared with those mares that did not have fluid. No relationship between uterine size on day of ovulation and pregnancy rate was found. Ovulations were delayed and pregnancy rates improved in progestin-treated mares. More ($p < 0.05$) mares became pregnant (23/28, 82%) when they ovulated after day 15, in the first postpartum ovulatory period than mares that ovulated before day 15 (6/12, 50%).

Ultrasonography has been proven useful in detecting mares with postpartum uterine fluid.[61] Furthermore, it could be used to aid in determining whether a mare should be bred, treated, or not bred during the first postpartum ovulatory period. During estrus, uterine fluid may be spermicidal and/or an excellent medium to support bacterial proliferation. When fluid is present during diestrus, it may cause premature luteolysis or EED.[63] The quantity of uterine fluid during the first postpartum ovulatory period appeared to be related to the stage of uterine involution and was reduced or eliminated by delaying the ovulatory period with progestins.

Progestin treatment not only allowed time for elimination of uterine fluid before the first postpartum ovulation but also significantly delayed the first postpartum ovulation. Results of this study concurred with those of others that concluded that progestin treatment delayed the onset of the first postpartum ovulatory period but did not affect rate of uterine involution.[70–73] Long-term progestin administration to normal, cycling mares has not been shown to affect fertility adversely.[74] However, treatment with progestins will affect uterine defense mechanisms,[75,76] and thus care is recommended before prolonged progestin treatment is administered to postpartum mares or mares susceptible to infection.

Because decreased pregnancy rates were associated with uterine fluid and pregnancy rates increased as ovulation was delayed, we suggest both techniques could be used to manipulate breeding strategies and improve pregnancy rates from normal mares bred during the first postpartum ovulatory period.

Effect of Intrauterine Fluid on Pregnancy Rate and Early Embryonic Death

A study was designed to determine the influence of intrauterine fluid on pregnancy rate and EED.[62] It was concluded from this study that (1) the presence of small amounts of intrauterine fluid during estrus in cycling mares did not affect pregnancy rates at either day 11 or 50; (2) intrauterine fluid, detected 1 or 2 days after ovulation, did not affect day-11 pregnancy rates, but was associated with a significant increase in EED and reduced day-50 pregnancy rates; and (3) the presence of intrauterine fluid during diestrus (days 1 to 20 post-ovulation) was associated with a significant decrease in day-50 pregnancy rates.

Diagnosis of Endometritis

Numerous techniques are available to diagnose endometritis. However, no technique is completely reliable. The common, currently accepted techniques are (1) rectal palpation, (2) vaginal-speculum examination, (3) bacterial culture of uterine contents, (4) cytological examination of uterine contents, (5) endometrial biopsy, and (6) ultrasonography. A study was conducted to examine the efficacy of individual diagnostic techniques to predict endometritis. This study demonstrated that ultrasonography was as accurate as all the other diagnostic tests of endometritis.[62] In addition, the study determined that in progesterone-dominated mares, multiple invasive procedures (i.e., culture, biopsy, vaginal-specular examination, and cytologic specimen collection) resulted in persistent endometritis, thus highlighting the usefulness of a noninvasive diagnostic test such as ultrasonography.[62]

UTERINE CYSTS

Before ultrasonography, uterine cysts were most commonly diagnosed from postmortem examination[77] and occasionally by rectal palpation.[78] More recently they have been diagnosed by hysteroscopy[79] and ultrasonography.[62,80,81]

Cysts in the uterus are fluid filled and apparently have two origins. The histologic structures of uterine cysts have been described.[77,78] Endometrial cysts arise from endometrial glands and are usually ≤ 10 mm in

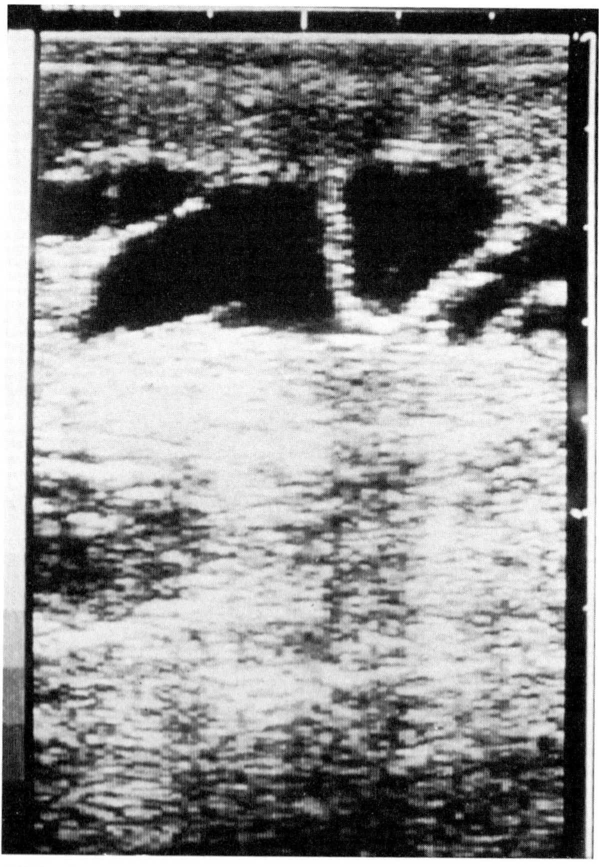

FIG. 31–39. Multiple uterine cysts at the corpus cornual junction.

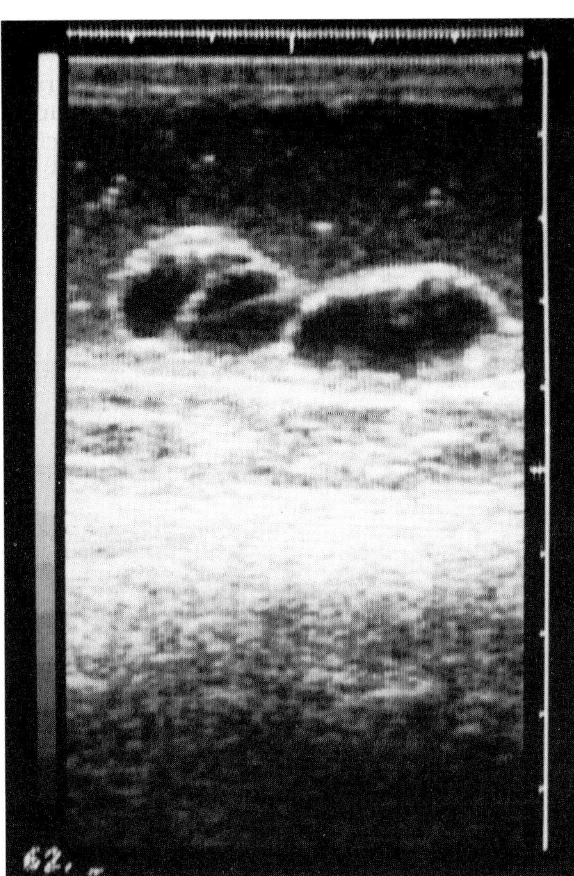

FIG. 31–40. Multiple, apparently compartmentalized, cysts in the uterine body surrounded by grade II intrauterine fluid.

diameter.[78] Their incidence and significance is largely unknown. The second form of uterine cysts are lymphatic in origin and generally are larger than endometrial cysts (Fig. 31–39 and 31–40). They are common in older mares[63] and have been associated with both normal and abnormal uterine biopsies.[78] Size of uterine cysts may be indicative of origin. In one study, large, endometrial, glandular cysts were suspected but were not substantiated with histologic examination.[79]

No data have been reported on the growth rate of uterine cysts. Despite the occasional large cysts reported,[79] they probably do not grow at a similar rate as the early embryonic vesicle (days 10 to 20). When visualized with ultrasonography, cysts are usually rounded, with irregular borders, and are occasionally multiple or compartmentalized. Movement of the early equine conceptus (days 10 to 16), presence of specular reflection, spherical appearance, and growth rate of the embryo may aid in its differentiation from uterine cysts.

The relationship between infertility and uterine cysts is axiomatic. Cysts may impede movement of the early conceptus, restricting the reported ability of the vesicle to prevent luteolysis after day 10.[8] Later in pregnancy, contact between the cyst wall and yolk sac or allantois may prevent absorption of nutrients. This may be more important when considering the report that large uterine cysts are more commonly located at the junction of the uterine horn and body,[79,82] the most common site of vesicle fixation.[10] Finally, cysts are often indicative of uterine disease. They may reflect senility or be associated with endometritis. Adams et al. report an association between number of uterine cysts, age of mare, and endometrial biopsy.[63]

The number of treatments proposed for uterine cysts probably reflects the inability of any individual treatment to be consistently useful. Rupture of the fluid-filled structures has been attempted via uterine-biopsy forceps,[78,83] surgery,[41] fine-needle aspiration,[84] and via hysteroscopy.[79,84] Electrocoagulative removal of cysts has been described.[79,82] Although the number of treated mares was extremely low (n = 6) and the mares were rigorously selected for treatment, this technique may have future application for individuals.[82] Endometrial curettage[41] and repeated lavage with warm saline (40 to 45° C) have also been advocated.[79] Although no reports exist on respective efficiency of the treatments, endometrial curettage and saline lavage are frequently applied to treat the primary problem, which would appear to be lymphatic blockage.

The conclusions from one study suggested that (1) uterine cysts, when detected by ultrasonography, were lymphatic in origin; (2) uterine cysts did not change rapidly in size or shape, although they were more diffi-

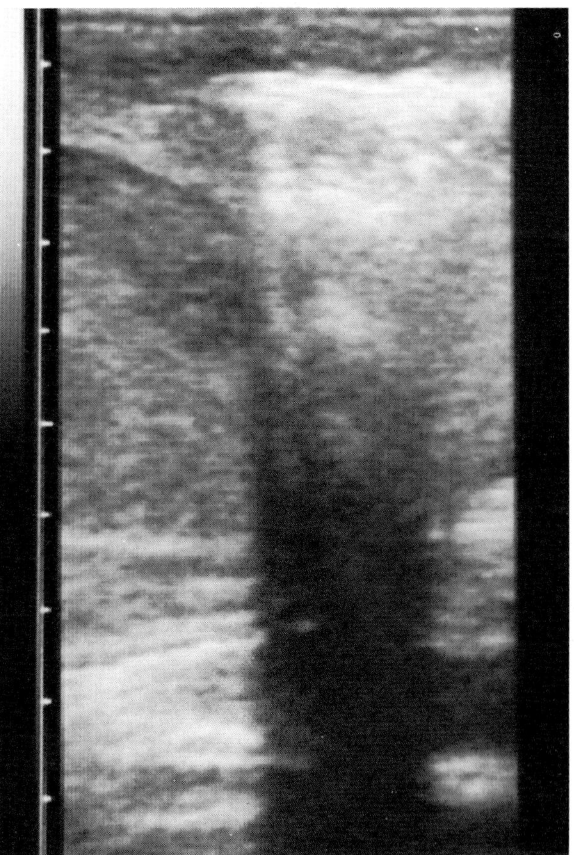

FIG. 31–41. Hyperechogenic reflections slightly cranial to the cervix, characteristic of air.

cult to detect during estrus; (3) treatment with infrared radiation was not effective; (4) no consistent location for uterine cysts existed; and (5) uterine cysts were usually associated with chronic, infiltrative, lymphocytic endometritis.[62]

MISCELLANEOUS UTERINE DISEASES

Recently less commonly recognized forms of uterine disease have been identified, the most common of which was air in the uterus.[15] Air is recognized as multiple, hyperechogenic reflections (occasionally a ventral reverberation artifact is present), and it appears to be more prevalent slightly cranial to the cervix (Fig. 31–41), although it can be present in the cranial body or uterine horns (Fig. 31–42). Air, when present < 24 h after artificial insemination, is considered normal. However, air should not be found in normal mares $\geq$ 48 h after breeding. The observation of air in the uterus of mares that have not been bred recently is an indication of pneumouterus and reflects failure of the competency of the vaginal labia, vestibulovaginal sphincter, and/or cervix.[62]

On occasion, strongly echogenic areas in the uterine lumen are observed with a concomitant echo shadow, such as is seen with dense tissue like fetal bone, which

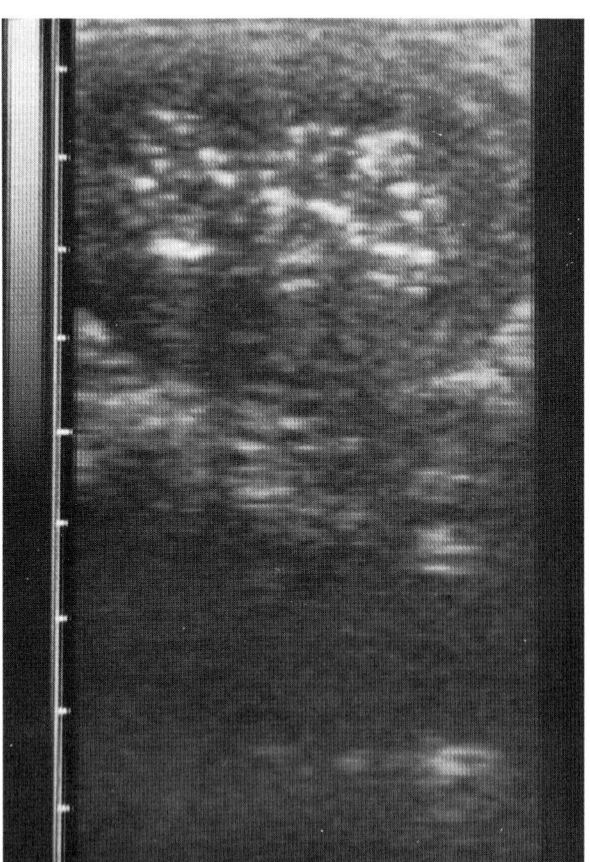

FIG. 31–42. Hyperechogenic reflections caused by air in the uterine horn.

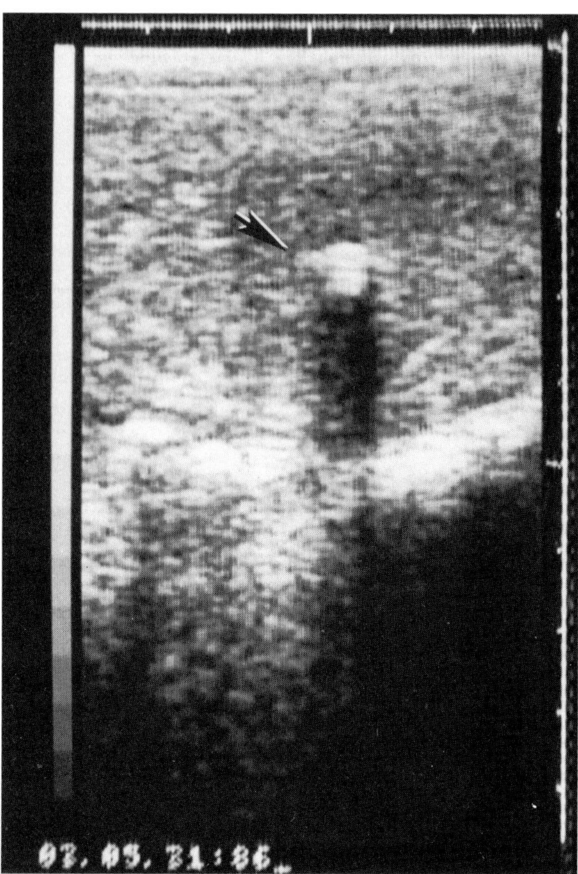

FIG. 31–43. Ultrasonographic image of a hyperechogenic body in a mare's uterus (arrow) that was confirmed subsequently as the tip of a uterine culturette.

might be expected after mummification.[80] The authors have also identified a similar ultrasonographic image (Fig. 31–43) that was confirmed subsequently as the tip of a uterine culturette.

Undoubtedly many other forms of less commonly recognized uterine diseases such as uterine neoplasia, abscesses, and hematomas will be recognized as ultrasonography of the uterus becomes more routine.

FOLLICULAR DYNAMICS PRECEDING AND DURING OVULATION

Ultrasonography is useful for monitoring dynamic follicular and luteal changes of equine ovaries, because it permits rapid, visual, noninvasive access to the reproductive tract. A 5-MHz transducer has greater resolution and is more suitable for evaluation of ovaries than a 3- or 3.5-MHz transducer. Follicles as small as 2 to 3 mm can be seen,[85,86] and the CL can usually be identified throughout its functional life.[87] Potential applications of ultrasonographic examination of the ovaries include (1) estimating stage of the estrous cycle, (2) assessing preovulatory follicles, (3) determining ovula-

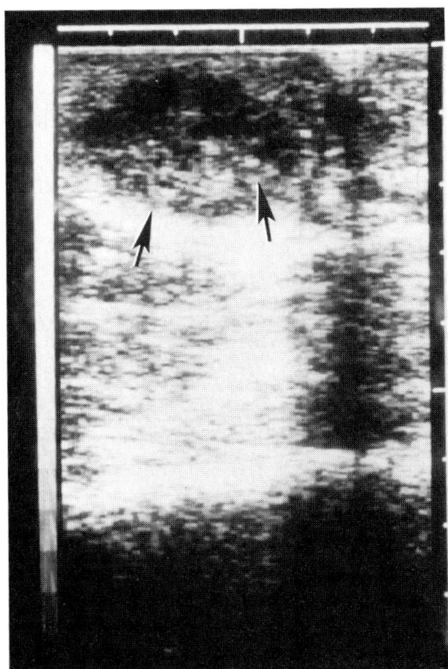

FIG. 31–44. Ultrasonographic characteristics of an anestrous ovary (ovary delineated by arrows).

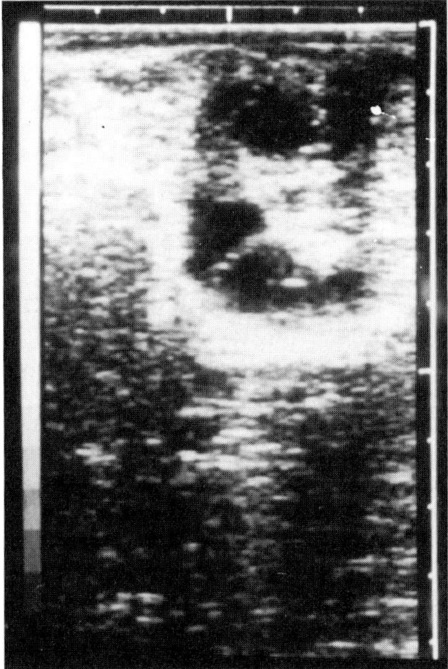

FIG. 31–46. Ultrasonographic characteristics of small follicles in an ovary of a mare in early diestrus.

tion, (4) examining the CL, and (5) diagnosing ovarian abnormalities and disease.

STAGE OF THE ESTROUS CYCLE

Follicles, like other fluid-filled structures, are nonechogenic and appear as black, roughly circumscribed ultrasonographic images (Figs. 31–44 to 31–48). Compression by adjacent follicles, luteal structures, or ovarian stroma occasionally can result in irregular-shaped follicles. The apposed walls of adjacent follicles are often straight. The diameter can be estimated by adjusting an irregular-shaped follicle to an approximately equivalent circular form.

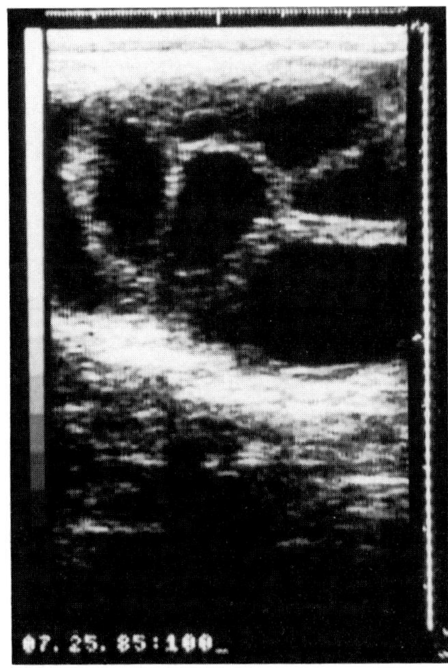

FIG. 31–45. Ultrasonographic characteristics of multiple follicles in an ovary of a mare in transitional estrus.

Sequential monitoring of dynamic changes in a follicular population during the estrous cycle has been made possible by ultrasonography.[15] During anestrus, inactive ovaries are readily differentiated from functional ovaries with ultrasonography. Occasional small follicles (2 to 5 mm) may be present, but absence of an ultrasonographically visible CL is characteristic of anestrus (Fig. 31–44).

Multiple, large follicles (Fig. 31–45), characteristic of transitional mares before their first ovulation of the year, are particularly frustrating to practitioners and researchers. Generally, follicular atresia and subsequent growth occurs until one follicle becomes dominant and ovulates. During transition, some ovulations are difficult to detect by palpation, and in these cases ultrasonographic observation of a CL may confirm whether the mare has entered the ovulatory season. With the use of a 5-MHz transducer, the CL should be ultrasonographically visible for approximately 14 days after ovulating.[87]

Examination with ultrasonography has resulted in the confirmation of the presence of many 5- to 10-mm follicles during early diestrus (Fig. 31–46); growth of larger follicles at midcycle; observation of selective, accelerated growth of an ovulatory follicle beginning 6 days before ovulation; and regression of larger nonovulatory follicles a few days before ovulation.[88,89] Ultrasonographic examination of the ovaries should not replace sound management techniques such as regular teasing and rectal palpation to determine stage of the

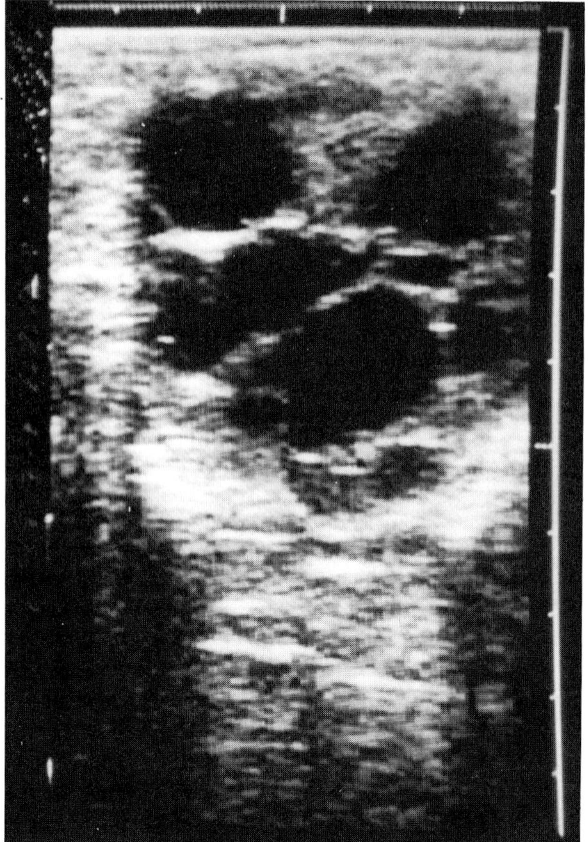

FIG. 31–47. Ultrasonographic characteristics of follicles in an ovary of a mare during late diestrus.

estrous cycle; rather, it should be used as a powerful ancillary aid.

PREOVULATORY FOLLICLES

The ability to detect time of ovulation accurately has significant practical application. Selective growth of a single preovulatory follicle is initiated about 6 days before ovulation.[89] Various characteristics can be used, within certain limitations, to predict time of ovulation. Softening of the follicle commonly occurs within 24 h of ovulation in approximately 70% of mares.[90] Ultrasonographically, this is frequently associated with a change in follicular shape (Fig. 31–49) from spherical to pear or irregular shapes,[89] which may be caused by disruption of ovarian stroma as the follicle progresses toward the fossa in preparation for ovulation.

The mare's ovary is structurally inverted in comparison with most species, with the exception of the ovulation fossa, which is a 0.5- to 1-cm depression on the lesser curvature.[91] The tunica albuginea and mesovarium forms a thick serosal coating covering the ovarian surface. Connective-tissue tracts extend from the ovulation fossa to the periphery, which forces the follicle to grow centrally toward the fossa.[92] These structural arrangements restrict ovulation to the ovulation fossa. Cinematographic and histologic studies have been used to determine the exact location of follicular rupture.[93,94] However, the time sequence and follicular changes during ovulation are not well characterized.

Although stallion semen has been reported to survive for up to 5 days or longer in the mare's reproductive tract,[84,95] a lapse before ovulation of > 48 h between breeding is generally believed to result in decreased numbers of viable spermatozoa and reduced fertility.[95] Use of frozen, cooled, or poor-quality semen may markedly hinder the life span of spermatozoa after insemination. Although no critical studies have been performed, the mare's oocyte probably begins to lose viability within 12 to 24 h after ovulation.[84,95,96] In addition, semen deposited in the uterus after ovulation requires time to reach the oviduct (site of fertilization) and for capacitation. Breeding or insemination, particularly with semen of reduced longevity, just before ovulation would maximize pregnancy rates and prevent overuse of an individual stallion.

Accurate prediction of impending ovulation would allow for collection of mature equine oocytes for in vitro fertilization or for gamete transfer from infertile mares.[97–99] In addition, recently ovulated oocytes or

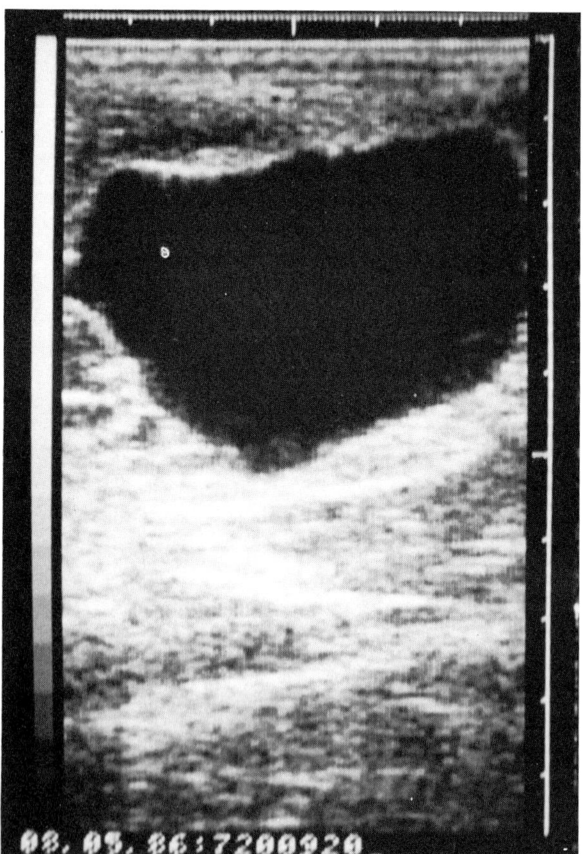

FIG. 31–48. Ultrasonographic characteristics of a large preovulatory follicle.

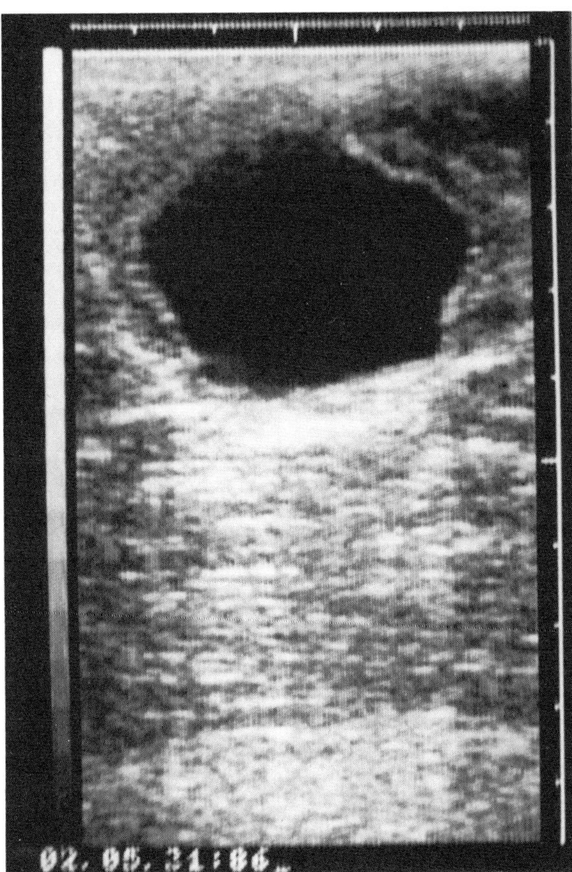

FIG. 31–49. Ultrasonographic characteristics of an irregular-shaped preovulatory follicle.

early cleavage embryos could be recovered from the oviduct at specific times postovulation.

In one study, various criteria such as percentage change in shape, size of follicle, echogenicity of follicular fluid and wall, and thickness of follicular wall were evaluated for their ability to predict time of ovulation.[89] Size of the preovulatory follicle was as accurate as any method in determining ovulation time. Generally, double, preovulatory follicles ovulated after attaining a smaller maximum diameter than single, preovulatory follicles.

Thickening of the follicle wall occurs in most preovulatory follicles before ovulation (Fig. 31–50). However, it generally occurs too early to be an adjunct to predicting ovulation. Increased echogenicity of follicular fluid is sometimes seen before ovulation (Fig. 31–51), perhaps because of degeneration and subsequent shedding of granulosa cells from the follicular wall. This can be an indicator of impending ovulation, although it is neither common or consistent enough to be particularly diagnostic.

In general, the combination of softening of a large follicle, particularly when associated with pain as determined by rectal palpation, and a substantial change in shape of the follicle, as detected with ultrasonography, can be used to predict ovulation within a 24-h period for most mares.

CHARACTERISTICS OF OVULATION

A study was performed to determine ultrasonographic characteristics of ovulation.[100] A total of 15 light horse mares were assigned to the experiment on acquiring the following preovulatory, follicular parameters: (1) diameter of ≥ 40 mm, (2) marked softening on palpation per rectum, (3) pain on palpation, and (4) a change in shape from round to irregular. Preovulatory follicles were observed at < 1-h intervals for 12 h or continually when signs of impending ovulation existed. Ovulation was defined as a rapid decrease in follicular size characterized by disappearance of the large, fluid-filled, nonechogenic structure. A B-mode, real-time linear array scanner with a 5-MHz transducer was used for ultrasonographic examinations.

A total of 13 of 15 mares ovulated within the 12-h examination period (mean = 85 min; range 15 min to 3 h 37 min after beginning of observation). As ovulation approached, flattened or irregular images (Figs. 31–49, 31–50, and 31–51) of the follicles were noted, concomitant with reduced follicular tone. The reduced tone was likely caused by diminished tensile strength of the follicular wall or perhaps a slow release of fluid from the follicle, although no fluid was visualized outside the follicle as ovulation approached. An echogenic nodule (approximately 5 to 10 mm) was noted within the follicles of two mares before ovulation (Fig. 31–52). These may have represented the cumulus oophorous, which has previously been visualized in women.[101]

Before ovulation, 10 of 13 follicles developed a tear in the follicular wall, which was characterized by a jagged protrusion of the follicular border toward the ovulation fossa (Fig. 31–53). In 7 mares, the tear or point was first observed an average of 41 min (range 15 to 77) before ovulation and was a consistent indicator of impending ovulation. A tear or pointed appearance observed with ultrasonography just before ovulation is likely caused by the breakdown of ovarian stroma and protrusion of the follicle toward the ovulation fossa. These observations probably parallel deterioration of the follicular wall, stigma formation and protrusion of the basement membrane just before ovulation, as observed in other species.[102] Witherspoon and Talbot observed the rupture of deep layers of ovarian connective tissue, as well as surface cuboidal and columnar cells in the area of the ovulation fossa.[94] When the ovary was exposed by laparotomy, just before ovulation, tearing of a few strands of tissue on the external surface and protrusion of the follicle into the fossa was occasionally visualized.[93,94]

Ovulation, defined as a rapid decrease in follicular size (Fig. 31–54), occurred in an average of 42 s (range 5 to 90). Little or no follicular fluid remained in the follicle after ovulation. Two mares failed to ovulate within 12 h after initiation of scanning and subsequently

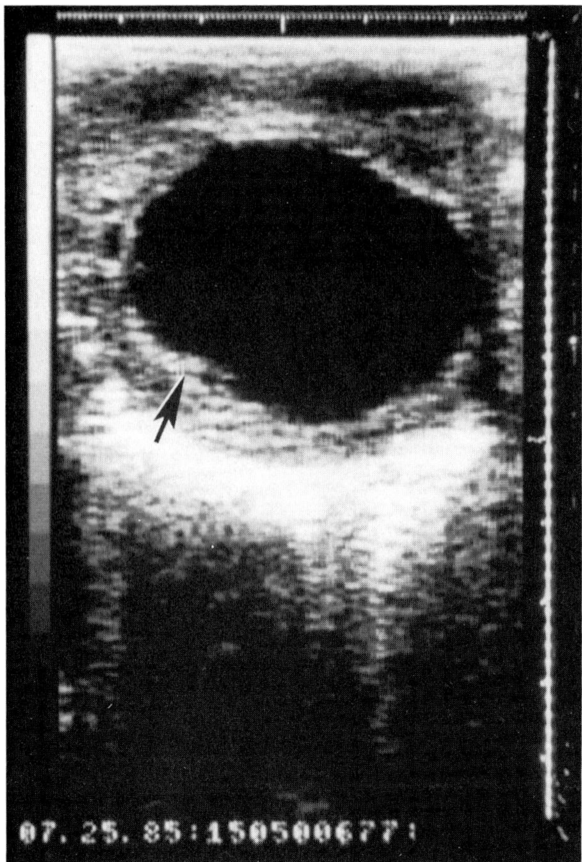

FIG. 31–50. Ultrasonographic characteristics of thickening of the follicular wall (arrow) as sometimes seen before ovulation.

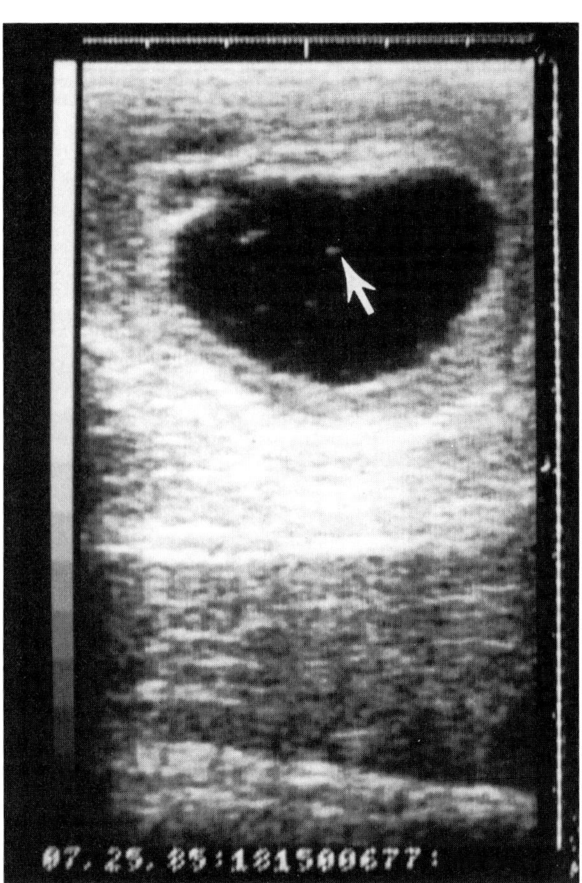

FIG. 31–51. Echogenic (arrow) debris in follicular fluid.

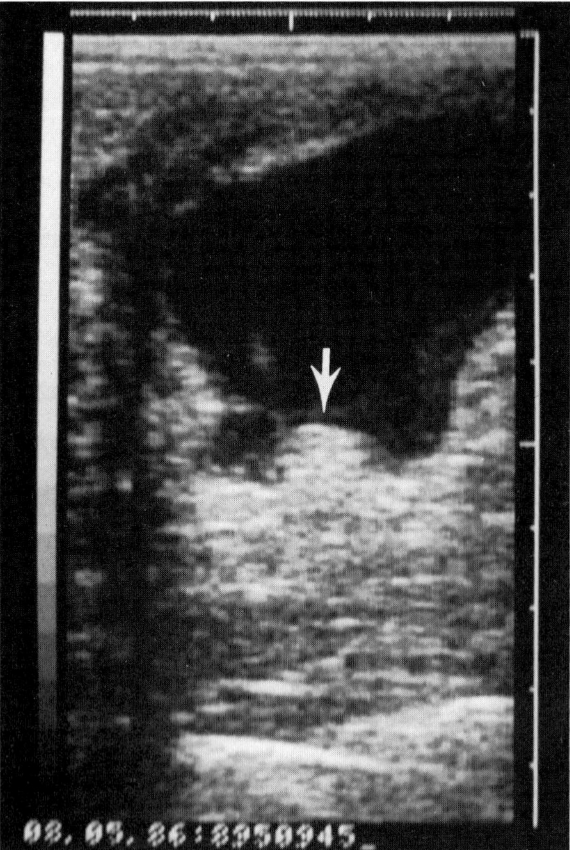

FIG. 31–52. An echogenic nodule that is presumed to be the cumulus oophorous (arrow), which is occasionally detected on the follicular wall before ovulation.

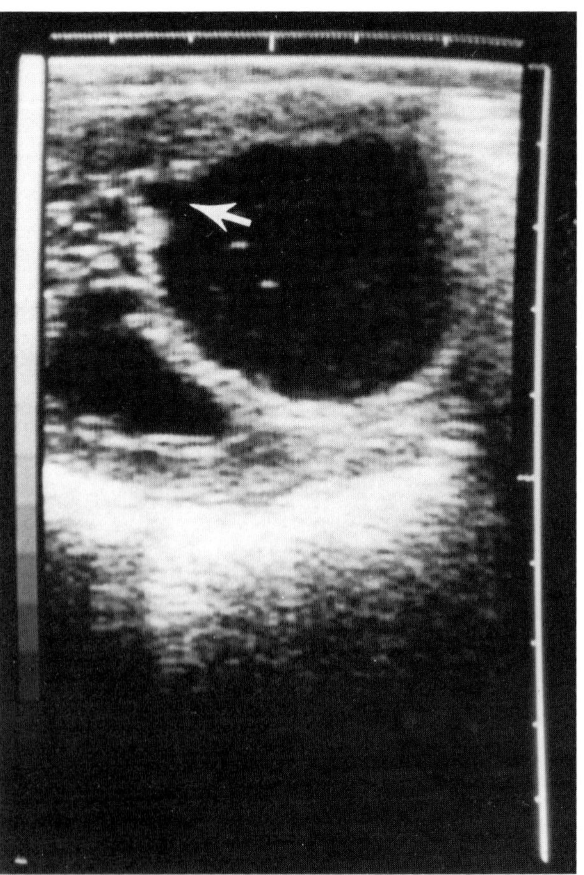

FIG. 31–53. A follicle just before ovulation. Note the presence of a pronounced neck-like process of the follicular wall (arrow), and increased echogenicity of follicular fluid.

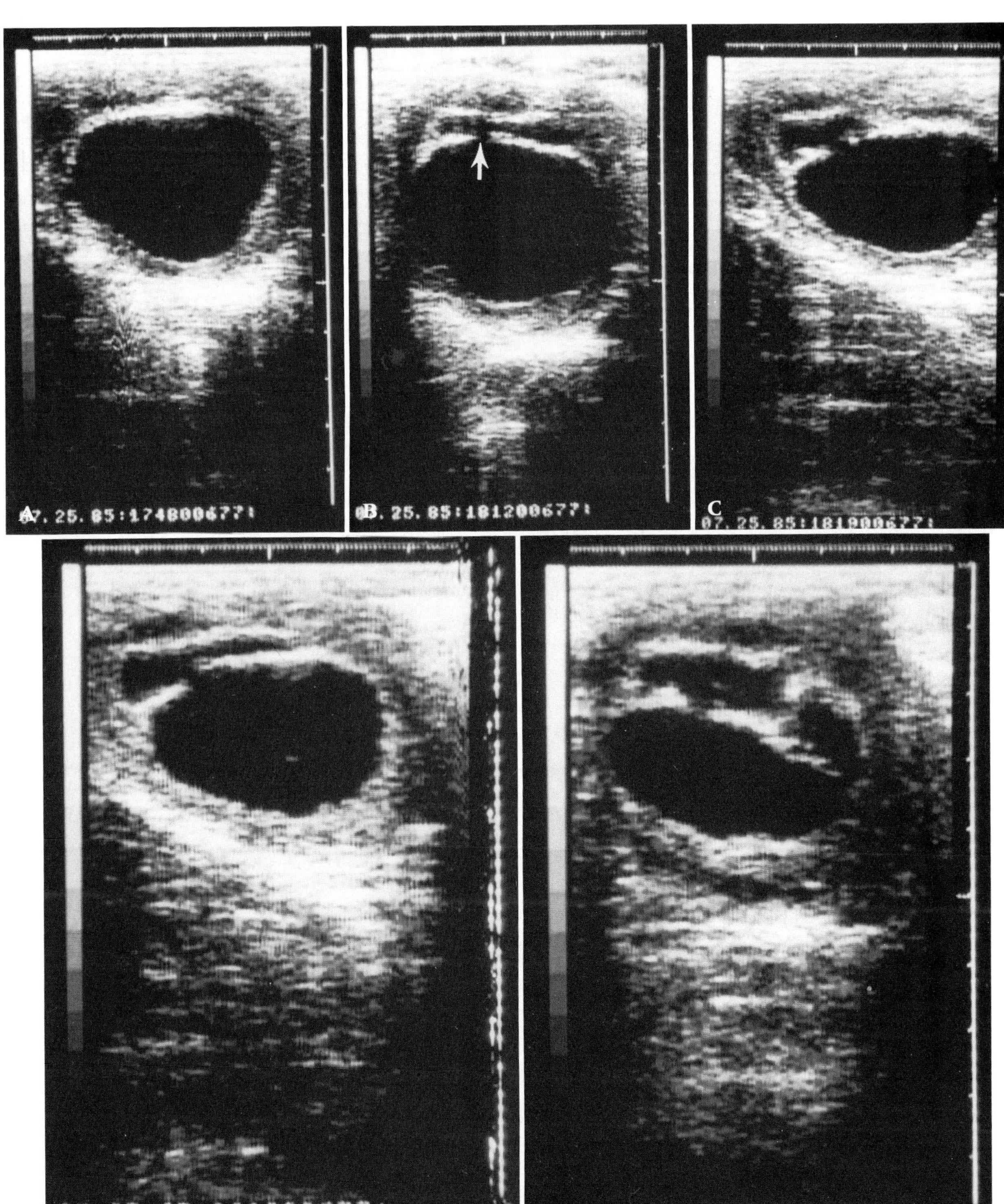

FIG. 31–54. *A,* The process of ovulation recorded by ultrasonography. Preovulatory follicle 50 min before the beginning of ovulation. *B,* Preovulatory follicle 30 min before the beginning of ovulation. Note rent in dorsal follicular wall (arrow). *C,* Preovulatory follicle 20 min before the beginning of ovulation. Note decrease in follicular size. *D,* Preovulatory follicle 15 min before the beginning of ovulation. *E,* The beginning of ovulation. Ovulation has been defined as a rapid decrease in follicular size.

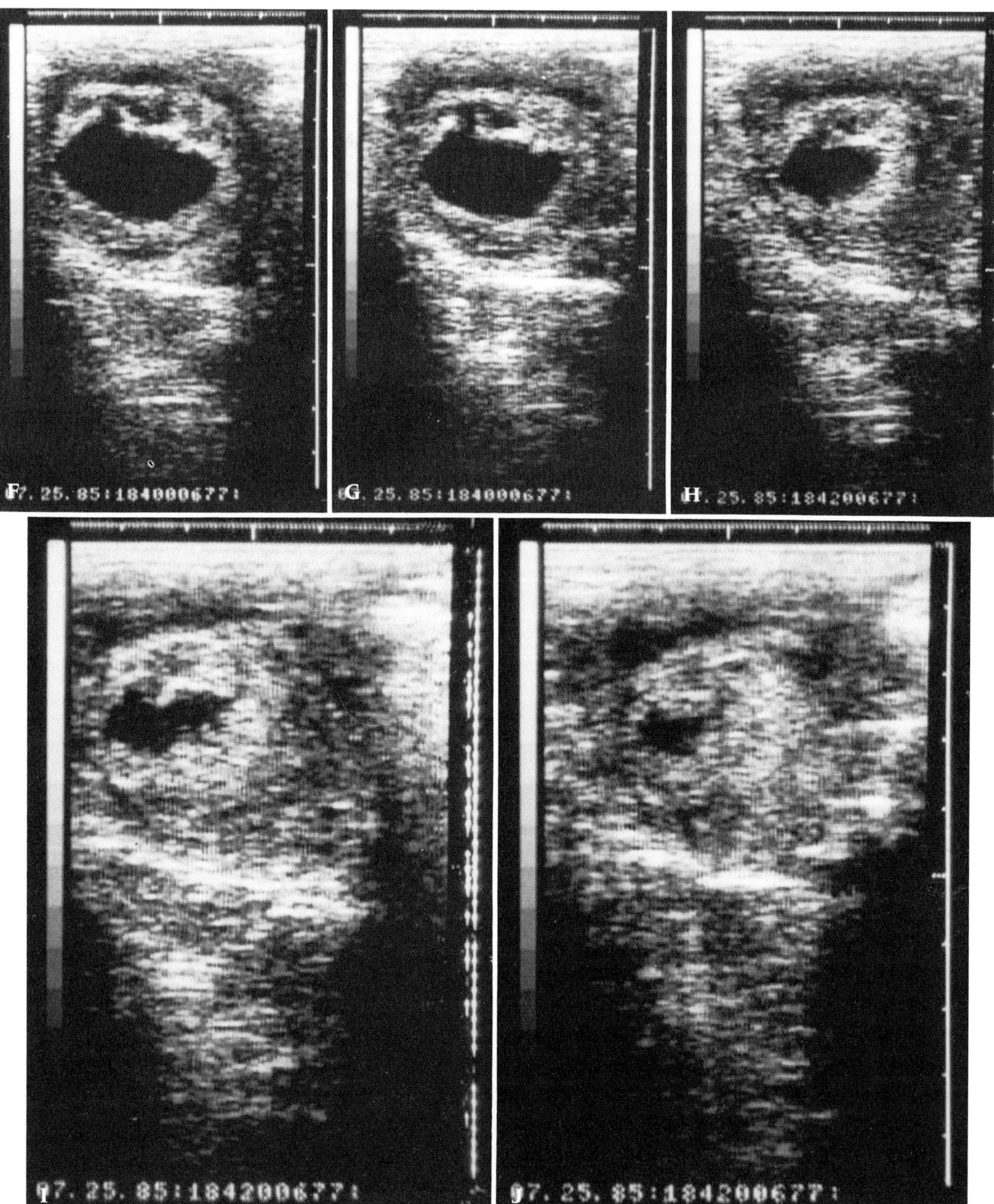

FIG. 31–54 *(continued)*. *F–J*, The process of ovulation occurred over approximately 60 s.

formed anovulatory hemorrhagic follicles (AHFs). This occurrence was possibly the result of the season.[103] Abnormal ovulations such as AHFs and luteinized, unruptured follicles may initially display a similar sequence of events as normal, preovulatory follicles without ovulation.[15]

Increased echogenicity of the follicular wall was visualized in all follicles before ovulation (Figs. 31–50 and 31–51). Appearance of echogenic "spots" within the follicular fluid, probably caused by the dispersal of granulosa cells, was noted in 7 of 13 (54%) follicles (Fig. 31–51). However, echogenic spots within follicular fluid, or a bright, echogenic follicular border, were not consistently useful in predicting time of ovulation.

A bright echogenic border, an irregular shape, and a tear in the follicular wall was predictive of imminent ovulation.

EFFICACY OF ULTRASONOGRAPHY FOR DETERMINING OVULATION

In one study, the accuracy of rectal palpation and ultrasonography for detection of ovulation was compared.[11] A total of 34 normally cycling, nonlactating mares of light horse breeds were used. Data collection began on day 2 of estrus or when a ≥ 35-mm follicle was detected by palpation. The mares were palpated rectally and scanned every 12 h. Rectal palpation was performed by one investigator and ultrasonographic scanning by a second. Each was unaware of the diagnosis made by the other. A 3-MHz, linear-array, real-time ultrasonographic scanner was used in the study. Mares that ovulated, based on palpation, but had a second ovulatory-size follicle continued to be palpated until a second ovulation occurred or the mare returned to estrus. The technician utilizing rectal palpation defined ovulation as absence of the follicle and a soft, sometimes painful indentation. Ovulation based on ultrasonography was defined as a change in the echogenic pattern characterized by disappearance of the large, black, fluid-filled, nonechogenic structure and the presence of an echogenic area.

In 24 of 34 mares, ovulation was detected at the same time by both methods. Three ovulations were detected by ultrasonography 12 h before detection by palpation and five ovulations were detected with ultrasonography 12 h after detection by palpation. Thus, within 12 h, ovulation was detected by both methods in 32 of 34 mares. In 1 mare, detection of ovulation by ultrasonography occurred 36 h before detection by palpation. In addition, ovulation was detected by ultrasonography in 1 mare, but the technician failed to detect ovulation in the same mare by palpation.

Double ovulations were detected by ultrasonography in 3 of 34 mares. The ovulations occurred on the same ovary within 12 h. The double ovulations were not diagnosed by rectal palpation. Close apposition of two follicles on one ovary may have been responsible for failure of the palpator to recognize both structures. The recognition of double ovulation is important to prevent twin pregnancies and in an embryo transfer program for correct scheduling of recipient mares.

Although ultrasonographic scanning of mares' ovaries should not be used as a replacement for rectal palpation, occasions obviously occur when the technique may be more accurate. Even with daily, manual ovarian examination, ovulation(s) may not always be accurately determined. Use of ultrasonography in these circumstances allows the clinician to make a more accurate determination concerning ovulation. In cases for which ovulation is detected by ultrasonography and not by palpation, it is usually associated with a well-circumscribed developing corpus hemorrhagicum which, although smaller, has palpation characteristics similar to that of a fluid-filled follicle. These structures either collapse and refill with blood or apparently fail to collapse completely.[103]

FORMATION AND DEVELOPMENT OF THE CORPUS LUTEUM

The CL is present during two-thirds of the mare's estrous cycle, and for the first 6 months of pregnancy.[104] Progesterone, a primary hormonal product from the CL, has a multitude of functions, including initiation and maintenance of pregnancy. Therefore, methods to evaluate the CL are extremely important. Because of the position of the CL within the ovary, palpation per rectum is of little value for identification and evaluation. However, ultrasonography has been shown to be an effective and accurate means of identifying this structure. Some of the reasons for ultrasonographic evaluation of corpora lutea are to (1) detect ovulation; (2) evaluate CL formation; (3) determine size and characteristics of the CL; (4) determine if failure of a mare to display estrus is caused by prolonged maintenance of a CL or absence of a CL and follicular activity; (5) distinguish between anovulatory hemorrhagic follicles, luteinized unruptured follicles, and CL; and (6) determine if a mare has ovulated more than one follicle.

After rupture of the follicle, a corpus hemorrhagicum is formed as a transient phenomenon in the development of the CL in the mare.[14] However, an ultrasonographic study demonstrated that the equine luteal gland may involve two ultrasonically distinct luteal structures.[87,93] Both types of luteal structure are uniformly echogenic on day 1. One type, classified as uniformly echogenic, is seen in approximately 50% of the CL and the percent of echogenicity remains constant for the duration of diestrus (Figs. 31–55 to 31–58). The other, classified as centrally nonechogenic (corpus hemorrhagicum) develops a nonechogenic center on day 0 or day 1 (Figs. 31–59 to 31–61). The percentage of CL considered echogenic was lowest on day 3, and increased linearly throughout diestrus. In a subsequent study, the time required for accumulation of fluid and formation of central clots (nonechogenic areas) were studied by ultrasonography.[105] Examinations were conducted at 15-min intervals for the first 2 h after ovulation, again at 8 h, and thereafter at 12 h intervals for 5 days. In 2 of 10 mares, a nonechogenic area did not develop within the luteal gland, and in 1 mare only a small central area (0.5 cm^2) was detected at 20 and 32 h, and not thereafter. In 5 mares, a nonechogenic central area developed within the luteal gland after expulsion of follicular fluid. Size of the nonechogenic area varied from 0.5 to 11.6 cm.[2] For those mares with central nonechogenic areas, echogenic lines within the central area were detected. These were attributed to clotting and fibrinization of the contents. From the results of another study, when CL evaluations were made on days 5 to 7 postovulation, the number of centrally nonechogenic CL seemed to be lower (9.2%, n = 192 cycles)[103] than that reported previously.[87] In addition, the

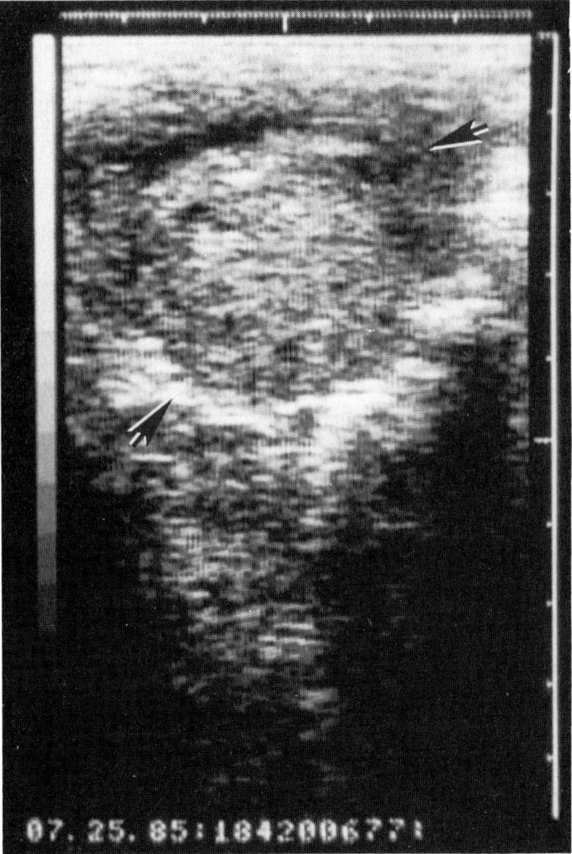

FIG. 31–55. Uniformly echogenic CL (arrows) on day of ovulation (day 0).

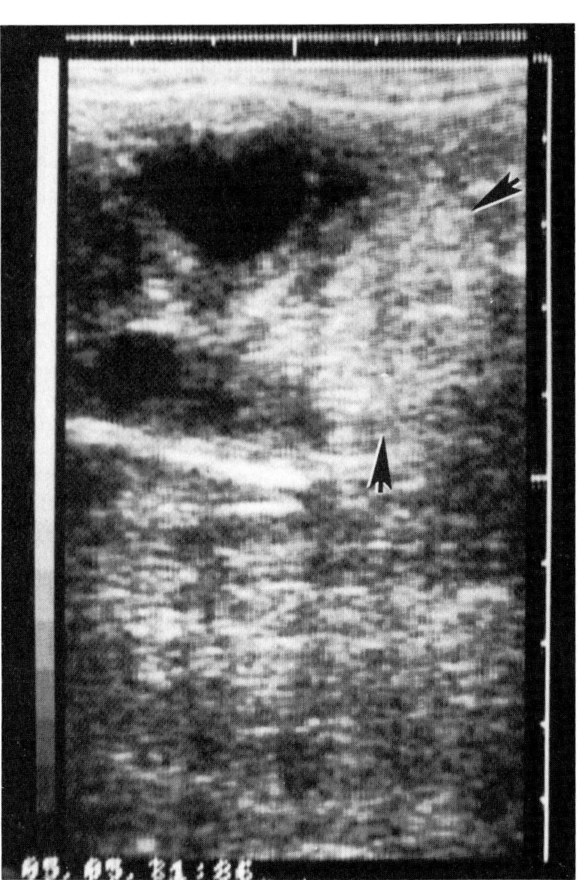

FIG. 31–56. Uniformly echogenic CL on day 7 (arrows).

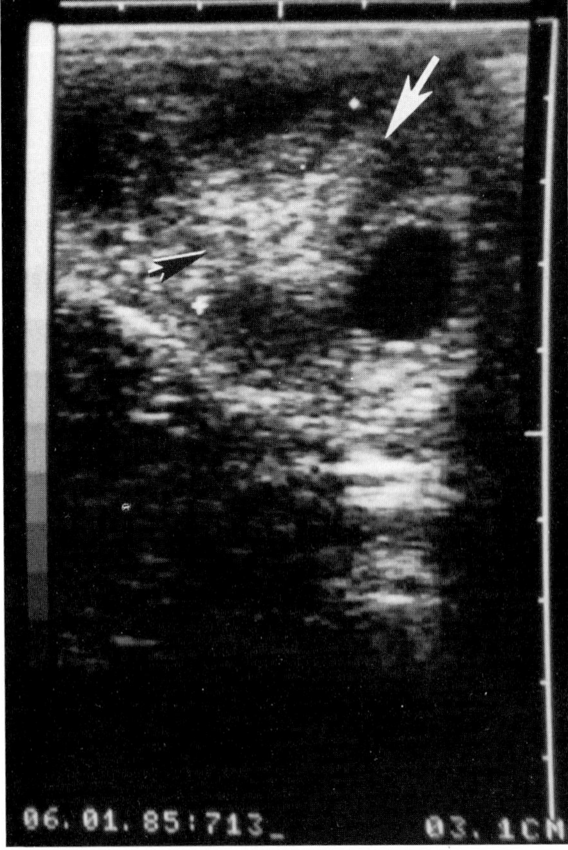

FIG. 31–57. Uniformly echogenic CL on day 14 (arrows).

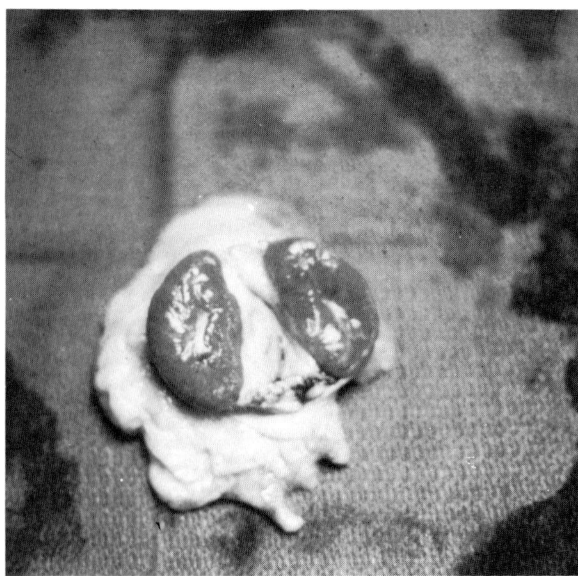

FIG. 31–58. Gross characteristics of a CL that would be uniformly echogenic when visualized with ultrasonography.

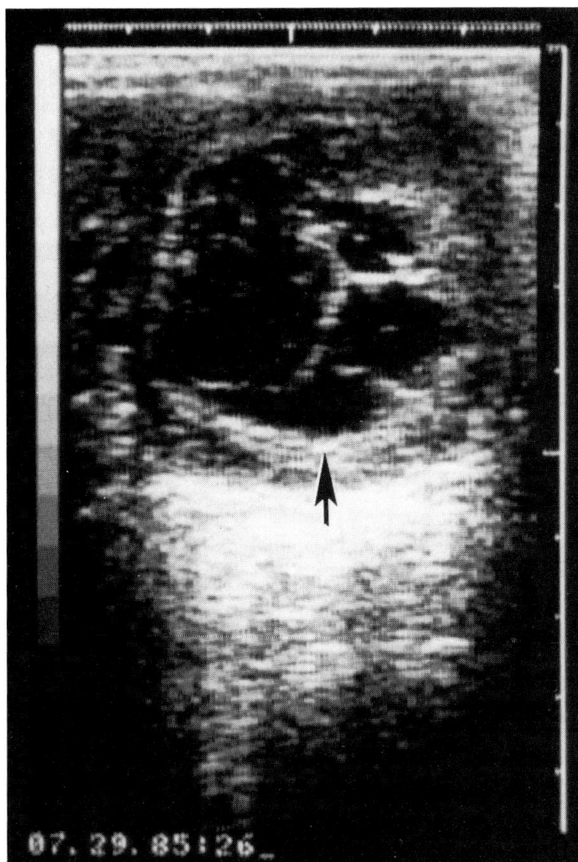

FIG. 31–59. Corpus hemorrhagicum or central nonechogenic (arrow) CL on day 1 postovulation.

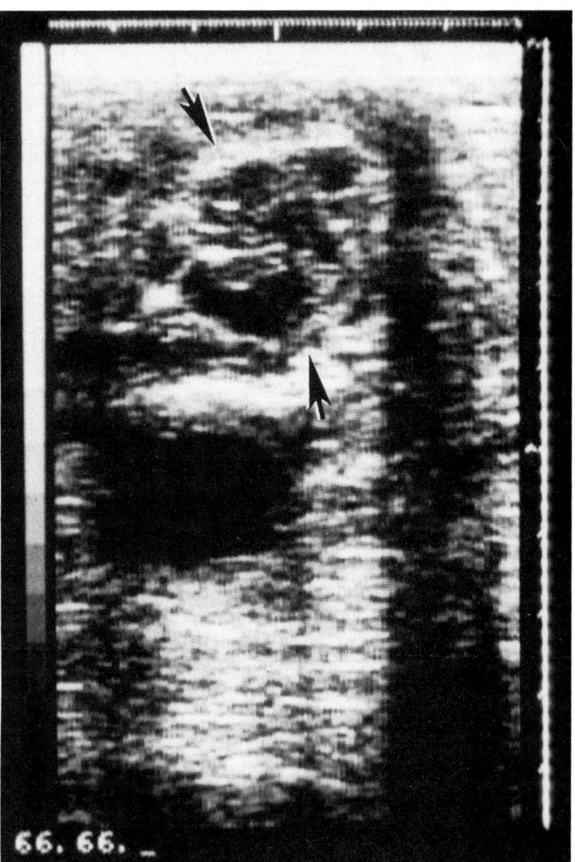

FIG. 31–60. Corpus hemorrhagicum on day 9 postovulation. The borders of the luteal structure are designated by arrows.

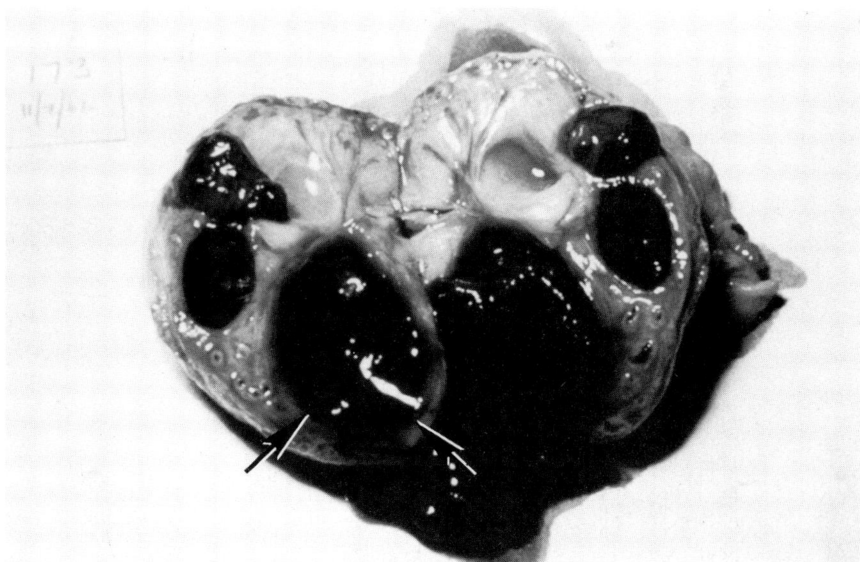

FIG. 31–61. Gross characteristics of a developing corpus hemorrhagicum, which would appear as a centrally, nonechogenic CL when visualized with ultrasonography.

incidence of at least one centrally nonechogenic CL increased with double ovulations (36%, n = 23). However, from the results of more recent data, a higher percentage of centrally nonechogenic CL was observed.[15] This depends, to some extent, on days postovulation (Table 31–5). Comparative studies on duration of diestrus, concentrations of progesterone, and fertility data should be conducted to determine categorically if both morphologic types of CL are normal.

Ginther reported on the accuracy of detecting a CL with ultrasonography.[14] Location of the CL was established by daily palpation per rectum. Ultrasonographic examinations were done by another technician unaware of the site of ovulation. The ultrasonographer recorded location of the CL, indicated that one was not found, or noted uncertainty about identification. The ultrasonographer was correct in 88% of the examinations conducted on days 0 to 14 postovulation. In the remaining 12%, the ultrasonographer recorded the locations as uncertain. In addition, in all 12 mares that were in estrus, the location of the CL was recorded as uncertain. From these results, ultrasonography apparently can be used to visualize a CL, even if the site of ovulation is unknown. Therefore, ultrasonography is an extremely valuable diagnostic tool for determining the presence or absence of the CL.

Presented in Figures 31–55 to 31–61 is a series of ultrasonographic images and gross characteristics of CL at various stages of development. The ultrasonographic image is affected by amount of blood or serum within the CL. Blood is nonechogenic, whereas luteal cells are echogenic. Generally, luteinization begins on the periphery of the structure and migrates medially. Normally, as the CL ages, blood is resorbed and a uniformly echogenic, luteal structure develops. Fibrin-like material can separate the blood clot into areas of dark, nonechogenic sections containing red blood cells, serum, and/or perhaps follicular fluid. Lighter areas may be indicative of fibrin strands or developing luteal tissue. Although the ultrasonographic properties of the mature CL are similar to ovarian stroma, a CL can be distinguished by its defined borders. Ginther found that the ultrasonographic texture of the luteal gland was characterized by an echo pattern indicative of loosely organized, well-vascularized tissue, whereas ovarian stroma generally yielded brighter echoes in a pattern representative of dense tissue.[14] Also, the majority of CL had a distinct mushroom or gourd shape.

In glands classified as centrally nonechogenic, the nonechogenic area was first visible on day 0 or 1 postovulation. These types of luteal structures were at their greatest echogenicity on the day of ovulation (75 to 100% of the gland). This was probably the result of the ultrasonographic properties of collapsed follicular walls. The nonechogenic area, which was the central cavity, enlarged over days 1 to 3 because of the enlargement of the blood clot (Fig. 31–59). As the blood clot resorbed, that portion of the structure that was echogenic increased throughout the remaining portion of the cycle (Fig. 31–60). In contrast, luteal glands that were characterized as uniformly echogenic did not change (Fig. 31–57) throughout the cycle, except the brightness (gray scale) changed throughout the life of the corpus luteum.

Ginther demonstrated that both types of glands change in echogenicity throughout the diestrous period.[14] Initially, the CL is highly echogenic on the day of ovulation (Fig. 31–55). At this time it is easiest to identify. The echogenicity decreases over the first 6 days of diestrus, remains at a minimum level for several days during the middle of diestrus, then increases over days 12 to 16. The bright hyperechogenic echoes on day 0 may be caused by apposition of collapsed follicular walls. An increase in brightness of the CL during the time of CL regression was also observed. The ultrasonographic changes are apparently indicative of changes in luteal hemodynamics and may be indicative of changes in patterns of blood flow within the CL as well as changes in tissue density.

With experience, the practitioner can become accurate at using ultrasonography to confirm ovulation and to detect the presence of a CL. Ultrasonography can also be used to diagnose pseudopregnant mares. A persistent CL and absence of an embryonic vesicle are evidence of a pseudopregnancy. Once these mares are identified, prostaglandins can be safely given to induce estrus. Echogenicity of this structure can be used to determine, to some extent, the age of the CL. Hyperechogenicity is

TABLE 31–5. PERCENTAGE OF ECHOGENIC AND NONECHOGENIC CL VISUALIZED WITH ULTRASONOGRAPHY

	DAY POSTOVULATION*								
Characteristic	0	1	2	3	4	5	6	7	8
Echogenic	76	63	54	46	64	71	75	56	100
Nonechogenic	24	37	46	54	36	29	25	44	0
Number of mares observed	62	16	69	13	22	93	12	16	6

*Ovulation is defined as day 0.

(Adapted from McKinnon, A.O., Squires, E.L., and Pickett, B.W.: Equine reproductive ultrasonography. Animal Reproduction Laboratory Bulletin No. 04. Fort Collins, Colorado State University, 1988.)

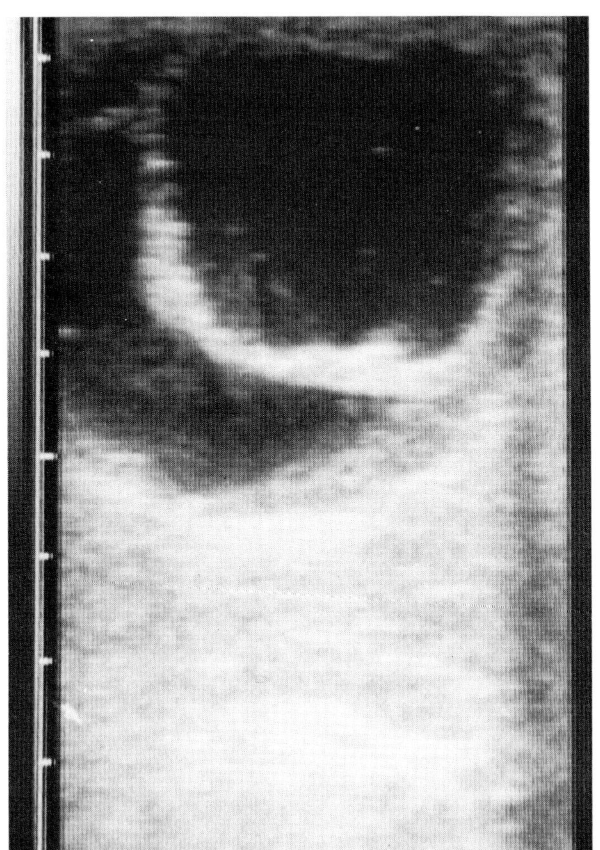

FIG. 31–62. Ultrasonographic image of double preovulatory follicles.

typical of the first few days after ovulation or during CL regression. The first few days usually can be distinguished from the last few days on the basis of gland size. In the middle of diestrus, the CL will be lower on the gray scale than either at the beginning or the end. However, the structure will be at maximal size during the middle of diestrus. If the CL contains a central nonechogenic cavity, the ratio of luteal tissue to blood clot and degree of organization of the clot can be of assistance in estimating age of the gland. The blood clot develops during the first few days, then progressively becomes more organized and proportionally smaller.

OVARIAN ABNORMALITIES

The ability to noninvasively examine the mare's ovaries permits diagnosis of various forms of ovarian abnormalities and disease. Some ovarian abnormalities that have been recognized with ultrasonography are (1) multiple preovulatory follicles, (2) AHF, (3) luteinized unruptured follicles, (4) persistent CL, and (5) various ovarian tumors and periovarian cysts.

MULTIPLE PREOVULATORY FOLLICLES

Because the mare normally ovulates only one follicle during each estrous cycle, multiple ovulations may be considered an abnormality.[106] Breed influences the incidence of multiple ovulation. For example, Thoroughbreds, warm bloods, and draft mares have been shown to have the highest incidence of multiple ovulation, whereas Quarter Horses, Appaloosas, and ponies have the lowest incidence; Standardbreds are intermittent.[20] Multiple preovulatory follicles (Fig. 31–62) or ovulations (Fig. 31–63) may be particularly difficult to detect by rectal examination, especially when they are in close apposition on one ovary. In one study, more embryos were obtained from multiple ovulating mares that bilaterally ovulated than from those in which multiple ovulations were unilateral.[31] Multiple ovulations should be encouraged when ultrasonography is available to eliminate one of two developing vesicles at 14 days, because multiple ovulation increases the probability of conception.

The ability to collect and transfer multiple embryos from a donor mare has the potential of improving efficiency of an equine embryo transfer program. The viability of embryos collected from naturally and induced

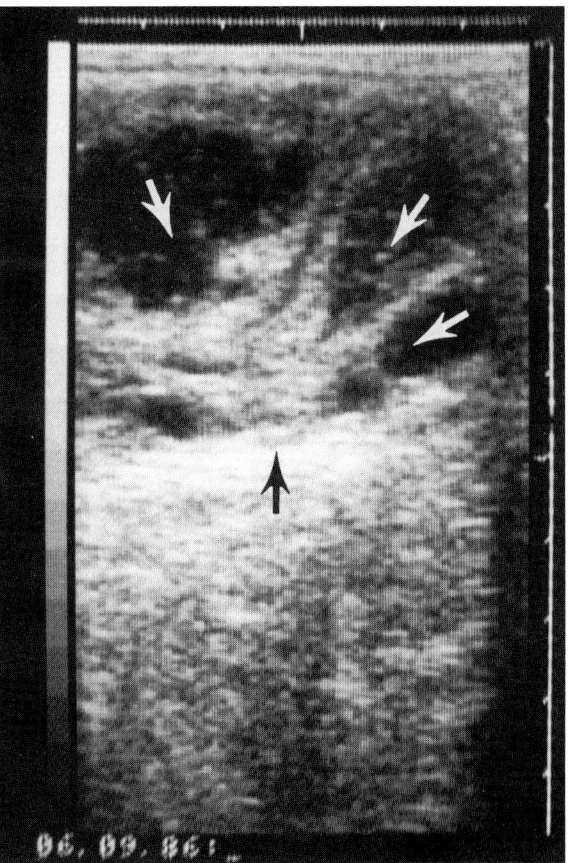

FIG. 31–63. Ultrasonographic image of a triple ovulation (white arrows). All ovulations have tracts to the ovulation fossa (black arrow).

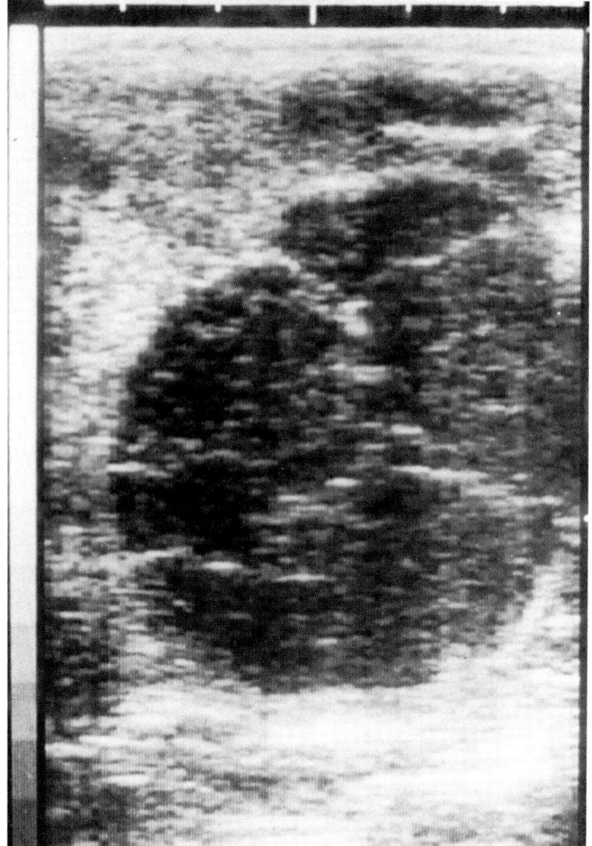

FIG. 31–64. Ultrasonographic image of an anovulatory, hemorrhagic follicle.

multiply ovulating versus singly, naturally ovulating mares is similar.[31] Recovery of embryos from singly ovulating mares was 53% compared with 106% for naturally doubly ovulating mares; pregnancy rates 50 days after surgical transfer were 68 and 129%, respectively. Treatment of singly ovulating mares with equine pituitary extract resulted in two embryos recovered per donor compared with 0.65 for control mares.[31] Nonsurgical pregnancy rates for embryos collected from superovulated mares were identical to those obtained from untreated controls.[31]

ANOVULATORY HEMORRHAGIC FOLLICLES

Anovulatory hemorrhagic follicles are the result of preovulatory follicles growing to an unusually large size (70 to 100 mm), failing to ovulate, filling with blood, and gradually receding (Figs. 31–64 and 31–65). Ultrasonography has been used to confirm this condition in mares when it was first identified as an abnormality by rectal palpation. This phenomenon may be recognized as an entity distinct from a corpus hemorrhagicum by its size and by ultrasonographic characteristics. The blood in an AHF is distinctly echogenic, whereas normal development of the corpus hemorrhagicum results in a generally nonechogenic central blood clot (15 to 35 mm in diameter). However, both may have criss-crossing fibrin-like strands. The formation of luteal tissue around the periphery of an AHF follicle is rare or minimal. We have noted in some mares, development and subsequent ovulation during the same estrous cycle of another follicle after formation of an anovulatory hemorrhagic follicle. In these mares, behavioral signs of estrus persisted throughout an unusually long cycle of approximately 12 days, or 5 days after recognition of an anovulatory hemorrhagic follicle. Unfortunately, serum progesterone has not been measured in these animals. AHFs may possibly be the previously reported "autumn" follicles,[106] because most have occurred toward the end of the ovulatory season. Perhaps AHFs develop because of insufficient stimulus for ovulation from gonadotropic-releasing hormones. After the last ovulation of the year, mares may develop a large follicle at the expected time, but the follicle does not ovulate and the mare enters the anovulatory season.[106]

LUTEINIZED UNRUPTURED FOLLICLES

Although anovulatory estrous periods are common during the anovulatory season, they are rare during the ovulatory season.[106] An incidence of 3.1% was reported in Thoroughbreds and Quarter Horses,[26] and even these may have been misdiagnosed because palpation was used.

Luteinized unruptured follicles have been reported in women[107] and mice, but not in nonpregnant mares. The phenomenon is thought to be associated with reproductive senility. One study was initiated to recover embryos from oviducts of old, infertile mares.[15] On some occasions when the oviducts were flushed 2 days postovulation, no embryos or unfertilized ova were recovered, and from close examination of the ovulation fossa recent ovulation did not appear to have occurred. Surgical removal of two ovaries from two mares confirmed that ovulation into the ovulation fossa had not occurred, and from prior ultrasonographic examination

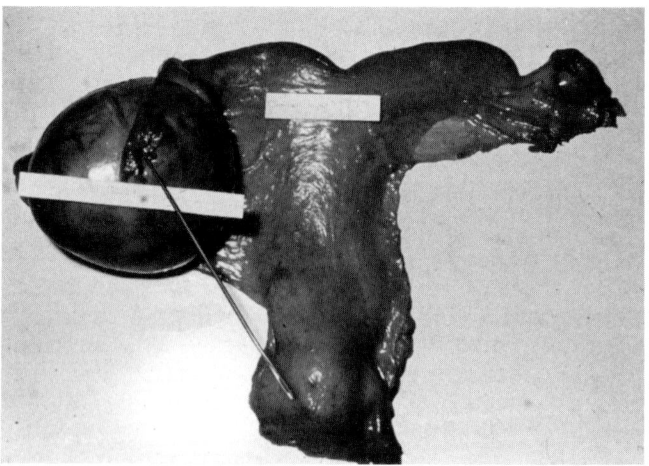

FIG. 31–65. Gross postmortem characteristics of an anovulatory, hemorrhagic follicle. (Courtesy of Dr. V. E. Osborne).

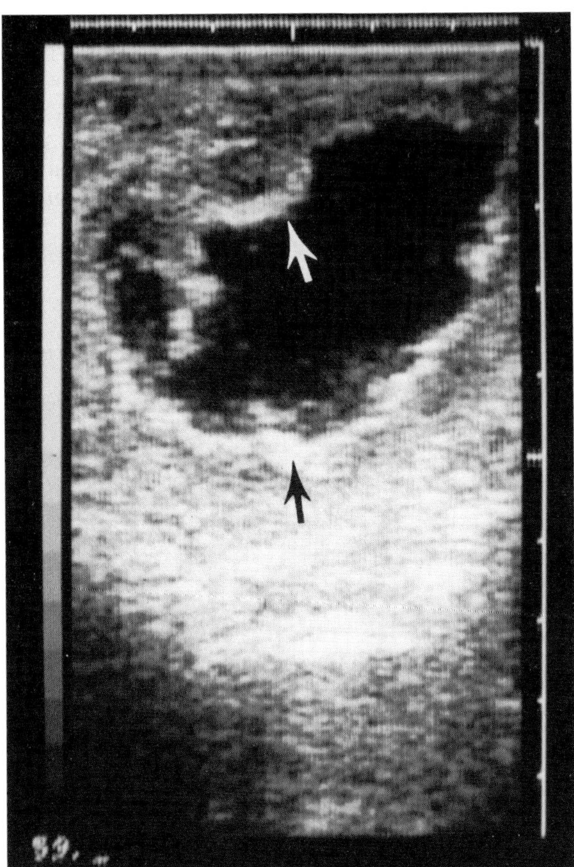

FIG. 31–66. Ultrasonographic image of a luteinized, unruptured follicle. Note extreme irregularity and thickening of the follicular wall indicative of luteal tissue (arrows).

an atypical corpus hemorrhagicum seemed to have been formed (Fig. 31–66). Both mares ceased displaying signs of estrus within 1 day of the suspected ovulation. Concentrations of progesterone levels were not available. These structures may have been luteinized unruptured follicles similar to those in women and mice and may be associated with senility. Luteinization without ovulation occurs quite commonly in pregnant mares in association with formation of secondary CL.[104]

PROLONGED MAINTENANCE OF THE CORPUS LUTEUM

Rectal palpation of the CL, although possible on occasion,[90] is generally unrewarding. Prolonged maintenance of the CL, resulting in pseudopregnancy[108] can be differentiated from an anovulatory or anestrous condition by ultrasonography. The CL is first visible on the day of ovulation (day 0) as a strongly echogenic, circumscribed mass of tissue.[87] The echogenicity gradually decreases throughout diestrus. However, just before regression of the CL, echogenicity increases. This may reflect changes in luteal hemodynamics. In one study, the CL could be observed for a mean of 17 days ($n = 55$).[87] On occasion, the presence of a CL may be seen as a circumscribed, highly echogenic area of tissue in the ovary in mares that failed to return to estrus at the expected time. Prolonged maintenance of the CL is more usually recognized in normally cycling mares that have been bred. Generally, the mare fails to return to estrus at the expected time, even though she is not pregnant. Perhaps pregnancy is initiated and the embryo prevents secretion of prostaglandin $F_2\alpha$ before undergoing early embryonic death. In another study, removal of the conceptus early in pregnancy (days 7 to 11) resulted in return to estrus at the expected time or slightly earlier, whereas removal later (days 14 to 16) resulted in prolonged maintenance of the CL, or pseudopregnancy.[7]

OVARIAN NEOPLASIA

The incidence of ovarian tumors is relatively common in mares when compared with other domestic species. The incidence of ovarian tumors in horses has been reported to be as high as 5.6% of all neoplasms.[109] By far the two most common tumors are granulosa-thecal cell tumors (Figs. 31–67 and 31–68) and teratomas.[110] Granulosa-theca cell tumors are usually large, benign steroid-producing tumors, often associated with behavioral changes and poor reproductive performance. The most common history is a barren, anestrous mare. Other clinical signs are intermittent or continuous estrus, nymphomania, and stallion-like behavior.[109] The ultrasonographic characteristics of granulosa-thecal cell tumors will vary. Gross characteristics may be solid or cystic. Palpation may reveal a smooth surface; a knobby, hard surface; or sometimes a soft surface with obvious follicular development. The unaffected ovary is usually small and inactive. Surgical excision is the treatment of choice, and most mares will return to normal

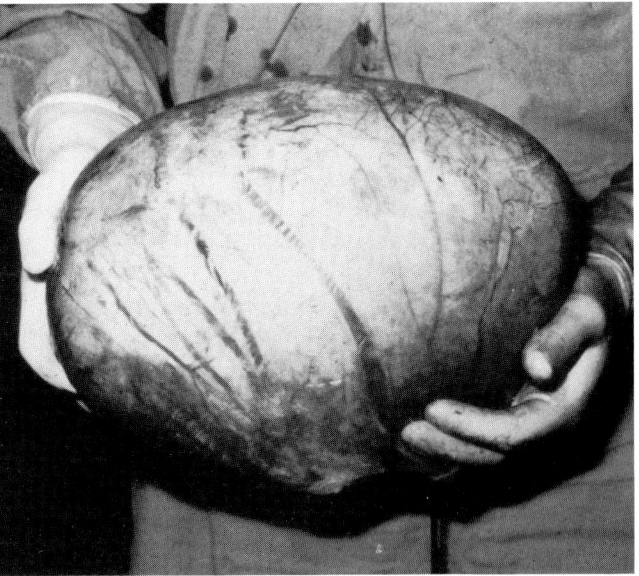

FIG. 31–67. Gross characteristics of a granulosa-theca cell tumor.

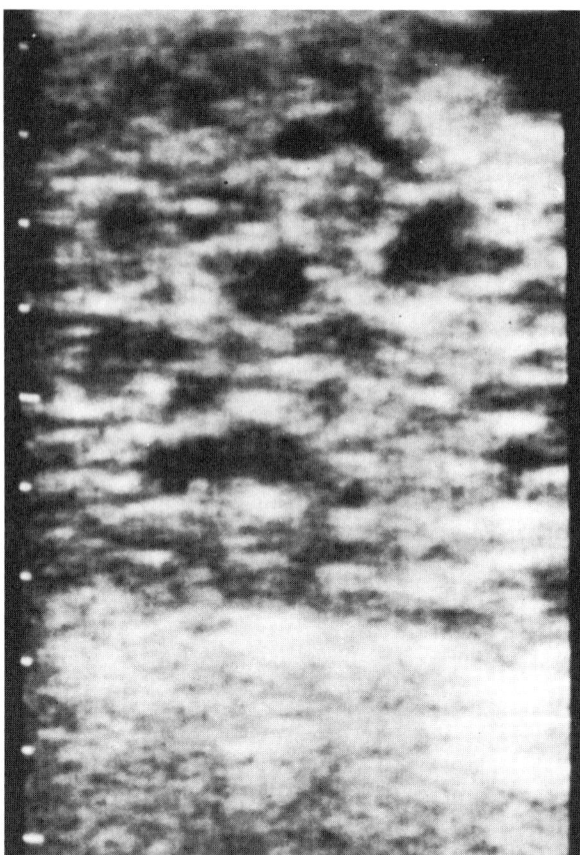

FIG. 31–68. Ultrasonographic image of a granulosa-theca cell tumor.

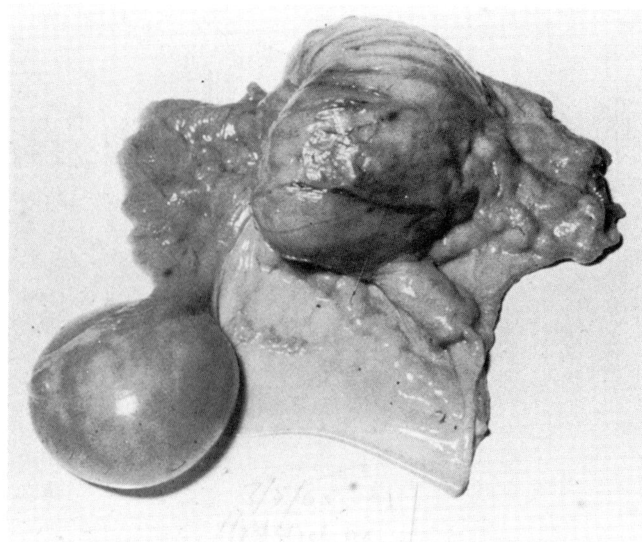

FIG. 31–69. Gross characteristics of a cyst or Hydatid of Morgagni. (Courtesy of Dr. V. E. Osborne).

reproductive performance within 2 to 16 months after surgery.

Ovarian teratomas are benign and nonsecretory. The tumors arise from germ cells and are usually nondescript epithelial tissue, but may contain cartilage, skin, bone, hair, nerves, sebaceous material, and even teeth. They may be solid or cystic. They generally do not interfere with fertility and are most commonly discovered during routine rectal palpation, unless they become extremely large and affect other organs.

Ultrasonographic examination may help differentiate between neoplasia and other large nonneoplastic structures, such as anovulatory hemorrhagic follicles or an ovary during the transitional period with multiple, nondominant follicles. However, in general, definite diagnosis will rely on histologic or gross examination of the affected ovary.

PERIOVARIAN CYSTS

Embryonic vestiges and cystic accessory structures associated with the ovary and oviduct are quite common in mares. These cysts, although often small, may occasionally be confused with an ovarian follicle. Rectal palpation in these circumstances is generally more accurate than ultrasonography in determining whether the struc-

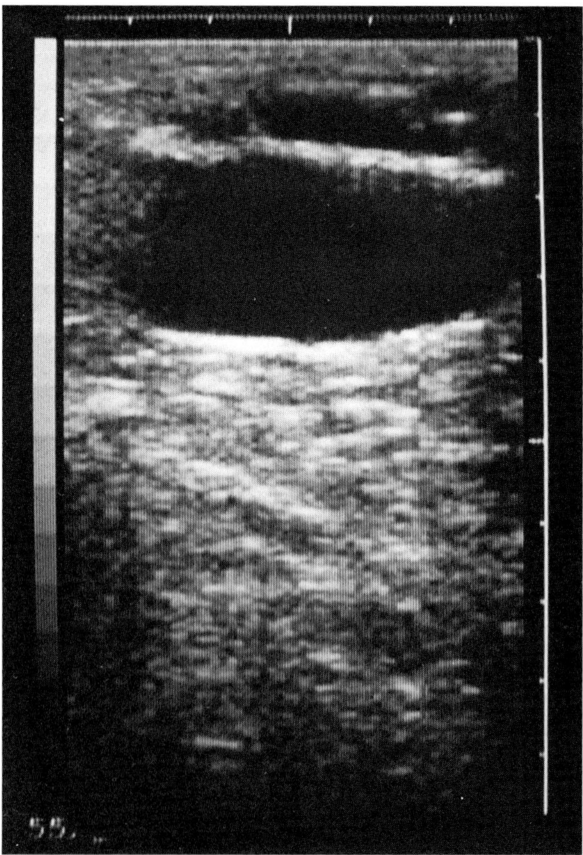

FIG. 31–70. Ultrasonographic image of a Hydatid of Morgagni.

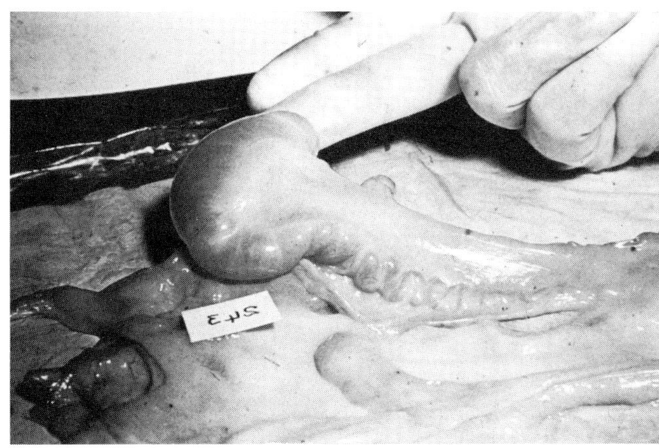

FIG. 31–71. Gross characteristics of a hydrosalpinx. (Courtesy of Dr. V. E. Osborne).

ture is part of the ovary. Small fimbrial cysts (< 10 mm) probably do not cause infertility; however, on occasion, cystic remnants of the mesonephric tubules and ducts may grow quite large (30 to 40 mm in length and 10 to 15 mm in diameter). One such recognized cyst is the hydatid of Morgagni (Figs. 31–69 and 31–70). This type of cyst has been diagnosed with ultrasonography, although it is sometimes difficult to distinguish between ovarian follicles and periovarian cysts.

MISCELLANEOUS OVARIAN ABNORMALITIES

Hydrosalpinx is not common in mares,[14] but because it is a fluid-filled structure (Fig. 31–71), it may be detected with ultrasonography. Definitive diagnosis will probably require laparoscopy or exploratory surgery.

Information about other types of ovarian abnormalities is just beginning to be obtained. We have identified cystic follicular structures that have not ovulated. Some have regressed and others have persisted. Only careful documentation and hormonal analyses will determine the causes of and treatments for many of the previously unidentified abnormalities.

REFERENCES

1. Austin, C.R., and Short, R.V.: Reproduction in mammals. *In* Germ Cells and Fertilization. Book 1. Edited by C.R. Austin and R.V. Short. London, Cambridge University Press, 1973.
2. Rolfe, B.E.: Detection of fetal wastage. Fertil. Steril., *37:*655–660, 1982.
3. Gidley-Baird, A.A., and O'Neil, C.: Early pregnancy detection in the mare. Equine Vet. Data, *3:*42, 1982.
4. Oguri, N., and Tsutsumi, Y.: Non-surgical egg transfer in mares. J. Reprod. Fertil., *41:*313–320, 1982.
5. Van Niekerk, C.H., and Gerneke, W.H.: Persistence and parthenogenetic cleavage of tubal ova in the mare. Onderstepoort J. Vet. Res., *31:*195–232, 1966.
6. McKinnon, A.O., and Squires, E.L.: Morphologic assessment of the equine embryo. J. Am. Vet. Med. Assoc., *192:*401–406, 1988.
7. Hershman, L., and Douglas, R.H.: The critical period for the maternal recognition of pregnancy in pony mares. J. Reprod. Fertil. Suppl., *27:*395–401, 1979.
8. McDowell, K.J., Sharp, D.C., Peck, L.S., and Cheves, L.L.: Effect of restricted conceptus mobility on maternal recognition of pregnancy in mares. Equine Vet. J. Suppl., *3:*23–24, 1985.
9. Ginther, O.J.: Mobility of the early equine conceptus. Theriogenology, *19:*603–611, 1983.
10. Ginther, O.J.: Fixation and orientation of the early equine conceptus. Theriogenology, *19:*613–623, 1983.
11. Squires, E.L., Voss, J.L., Villahoz, M.D., and Shideler, R.K.: Use of ultrasound in broodmare reproduction. Proc. Am. Assoc. Equine Pract., 27–43, 1983.
12. Ginther, O.J.: Ultrasonic evaluation of the reproductive tract of the mare: The single embryo. J. Equine Vet. Sci., *4:*75–81, 1984.
13. Ginther, O.J.: Ultrasonic anatomy and pathology of the reproductive tract. Proceedings of the Equine Ultrasound Short Course. Fort Collins, Colorado State University, 1984, pp. 16–25.
14. Ginther, O.J.: Ultrasonographic Imaging and Reproductive Events in the Mare. Cross Plains, WI, Equiservices, 1986.
15. McKinnon, A.O., Squires, E.L., and Pickett, B.W.: Equine reproductive ultrasonography. Animal Reproduction Laboratory, Bulletin No. 04. Fort Collins, Colorado State University, 1988.
16. Palmer, E., and Draincourt, M.: Use of ultrasonic echography in equine gynecology. Theriogenology, *13:*203–216, 1980.
17. Simpson, D.J., et al.: Use of ultrasound echography for early diagnosis of single and twin pregnancy in the mare. J. Reprod. Fertil. Suppl., *32:*431–439, 1982.
18. Sikov, M.R., and Hildebrand, B.P.: Advances in the study of birth defects. *In* Teratological Testing. Vol. 2. Edited by T.V.N. Persaud. Baltimore, University Park Press, Baltimore, 1979.
19. Ginther, O.J., and Douglas, R.H.: The outcome of twin pregnancies in mares. Theriogenology, *18:*237–244, 1982.
20. Ginther, O.J.: Twinning in mares: a review of recent studies. J. Equine Vet. Sci., *2:*127–135, 1982.
21. Ginther, O.J., Douglas, R.H., and Lawrence, J.R.: Twinning in mares: A survey of veterinarians and analyses of theriogenology records. Theriogenology, *18:*333–347, 1982.
22. Pascoe, R.R.: A possible new treatment for twin pregnancy in the mare. Equine Vet. J., *11:*64–65, 1979.
23. Kooistra, L.H., and Ginther, O.J.: Termination of pseudopregnancy by administration of prostaglandin $F_2\alpha$ and termination of early pregnancy by administration of prostaglandin $F_2\alpha$ or colchicine or by removal of the embryo in mares. Am. J. Vet. Res., *37:*35–39, 1976.
24. Pascoe, R.R.: Methods for the treatment of twin pregnancy in the mare. Equine Vet. J., *15:*40–42, 1983.
25. Jeffcott, L.B., and Whitwell, K.E.: Twinning as a cause of foetal and neonatal loss in the Thoroughbred mare. J. Comp. Pathol., *83:*91–106, 1973.
26. Hughes, J.P., Stabenfeldt, G.H., and Evans, J.W.: Clinical and endocrine aspects of the estrous cycle of the mare. Proc. Am. Assoc. Equine Pract., 119–151, 1972.
27. Ginther, O.J., Douglas, R.H., and Woods, G.L.: A biological embryo-reduction mechanism for the elimination

of excess embryos in mares. Theriogenology, *18:*475–485, 1982.
28. Ginther, O.J.: Effect of reproductive status on twinning and on side of ovulation and embryo attachment in mares. Theriogenology, *20:*383–395, 1983.
29. Ginther, O.J.: Relationships among number of days between multiple ovulations, number of embryos, and type of embryo fixation in mares. Theriogenology, *7:*82–88, 1987.
30. Squires, E.L., Garcia, R.H., and Ginther, O.J.: Factors affecting success of equine embryo transfer. Equine Vet. J. Suppl., *3:*92–95, 1985.
31. Squires, E.L., et al.: Reproductive characteristics of spontaneous single and double ovulating mares and superovulated mares. J. Reprod. Fertil. Suppl., *35:*399–403, 1987.
32. Ginther, O.J.: Using a twinning tree for designing equine twin-prevention programs. J. Equine Vet. Sci., *8:*101–107, 1988.
33. Pascoe, D.R., et al.: Comparison of two techniques and three hormone therapies for management of twin conceptuses by manual embryonic reduction. J. Reprod. Fertil. Suppl., *35:*701–702, 1987.
34. Rantanen, N.W., and Kincaid, B.: Ultrasound guided fetal cardiac puncture: A method of twin reduction in the mare. Proc. Am. Assoc. Equine Pract., 173–179, 1988.
35. Roberts, S.J., and Myhre, G.: A review of twinning in horses and the possible therapeutic value of supplemental progesterone to prevent abortion of equine twin fetuses the latter half of the gestation period. Cornell Vet., *73:*257–264, 1983.
36. Ball, B.A., and Woods, G.L.: Embryonic loss and early pregnancy loss in the mare. Compend. Contin. Educ. Practicing Vet., *9:*459–471, 1987.
37. Villahoz, M.D., Squires, E.L., Voss, J.L., and Shideler, R.K.: Some observations on early embryonic death in mares. Theriogenology, *23:*915–924, 1985.
38. Ball, B.A., Little, T.V., Hillman, R.B., and Woods, G.L.: Pregnancy rates at days 2 and 14 and estimated embryonic loss rates prior to day 14 in normal and subfertile mares. Theriogenology, *26:*611–619, 1986.
39. Day, F.T.: Clinical and experimental observations on reproduction in the mare. J. Agri. Sci., *30:*244–261, 1940.
40. Kenney, R.M.: Cyclic and pathologic changes of the mare endometrium as detected by biopsy, with a note on early embryonic death. J. Am. Vet. Med. Assoc., *172:*241–262, 1978.
41. Rossdale, P.D., and Ricketts, S.W.: Equine Stud Farm Medicine. 2nd ed. Philadelphia, Lea & Febiger, 1980.
42. Shideler, R.K., McChesney, A.E., Voss, J.L., and Squires, E.L.: Relationship of endometrial biopsy and other management factors on fertility of broodmares. J. Equine Vet. Sci., *2:*5–10, 1982.
43. Ginther, O.J., Bergfelt, D.R., Leith, G.S., and Scraba, S.T.: Embryonic loss in mares: Incidence and ultrasonic morphology. Theriogenology, *24:*73–86, 1985.
44. Belonje, P.C., and van Niekerk, C.H.: A review of the influence of nutrition upon the oestrous cycle and early pregnancy in the mare. J. Reprod. Fertil. Suppl., *23:*167–169, 1975.
45. Van Niekerk, C.H., and Morgenthal, J.C.: Fetal loss and the effect of stress on plasma progestagen levels in pregnant Thoroughbred mares. J. Reprod. Fertil. Suppl., *32:*453–457, 1982.
46. Van Niekerk, C.H., and van Heerdon, J.S.: Nutrition and ovarian activity of mares early in the breeding season. J. S. Afr. Vet. Assoc., *43:*351–360, 1972.
47. Swerczek, T.W.: Early fetal death and infectious placental diseases in the mare. Proc. Am. Assoc. Equine Pract., 173–179, 1980.
48. Moberg, R.: The occurrence of early embryonic death in the mare in relation to natural service and artificial insemination with fresh or deep-frozen semen. J. Reprod. Fertil. Suppl., *23:*537–539, 1975.
49. Merkt, H., and Gunzel, A.R.: A survey of early pregnancy losses in West German Thoroughbred mares. Equine Vet. J., *11:*256–258, 1979.
50. Hoppe, R.: The embryonic mortality in the mare. Proceedings of the International Congress on Animal Reproduction and Artificial Insemination, 1968, pp. 1573–1576.
51. Bishop, M.W.H.: Paternal contribution to embryonic death. J. Reprod. Fertil., *7:*383–396, 1964.
52. Van Niekerk, C.H.: Early embryonic resorption in mares. J. S. Afr. Vet. Assoc., *36:*61–69, 1965.
53. Allen, W.R.: Maternal recognition of pregnancy and immunological implications of trophoblast-endometrium interactions in equids. *In* Maternal Recognition of Pregnancy. Ciba Foundation Symposium No. 64. New York, Excerpta Medica, 1979.
54. Allen, W.R.: Is your progesterone therapy really necessary? Equine Vet. J., *16:*496–498, 1984.
55. Moberg, R.: The possible influence of site of pregnancy compared with site of ovulation on the incidence of early embryonic death in the mare. Proceedings of the International Congress on Animal Reproduction and Artificial Insemination, 1976, pp. 610–612.
56. Fiolka, V.G., Kuller, H.J., and Lender, S.: Embryonale Mortalitat beim Pferd. Mh. Vet. Med., *40:*835–838, 1985.
57. Lieux, P.: Comparative results of breeding on first and second post-foaling heat periods. Proc. Am. Assoc. Equine Pract., *26:*129–132, 1980.
58. Bain, A.M.: Foetal losses during pregnancy in the Thoroughbred mare: A record of 2,562 pregnancies. N. Z. Vet. J., *17:*155–158, 1969.
59. Douglas, R.H., Burns, P.J., and Hershman, L.: Physiological and commercial parameters for producing progeny from subfertile mares by embryo transfer. Equine Vet. J. Suppl., *3:*111–114, 1985.
60. Romagnano, A., Richer, C.L., King, W.A., and Betteridge, K.J.: Analysis of X-chromosome inactivation in horse embryos. J. Reprod. Fertil. Suppl., *35:*353–361, 1987.
61. McKinnon, A.O., et al.: Ultrasonographic studies on the reproductive tract of postpartum mares: Effect of involution and uterine fluid on pregnancy rates in mares with normal and delayed first postpartum ovulatory cycles. J. Am. Vet. Med. Assoc., *192:*350–353, 1988.
62. McKinnon, A.O., et al.: Diagnostic ultrasonography of uterine pathology in the mare. Proc. Am. Assoc. Equine Pract., 605–622, 1987.
63. Adams, G.P., Kastelic, J.P., Bergfelt, D.R., and Ginther, O.J.: Effect of uterine inflammation and ultrasonically-detected uterine pathology on fertility in the mare. J. Reprod. Fertil. Suppl., *35:*445–454, 1987.
64. Bain, A.M.: Estrus and infertility of the Thoroughbred mare in Australasia. J. Am. Vet. Med. Assoc., *131:*179–185, 1957.
65. Caslick, E.A.: The sexual cycle and its relation to ovulation with breeding records of the Thoroughbred mare. Cornell Vet., *27:*187–206, 1937.
66. Jennings, W.E.: Some common problems in horse breeding. Cornell Vet., *31:*197–216, 1941.

67. Platt, H.: Aetiological aspects of abortion in the Thoroughbred mare. J. Compar. Pathol., *83:*199–205, 1973.
68. Andrews, F.N., and McKenzie, F.F.: Estrus, ovulation and related Phenomenon in the mare. University of Missouri Research Bulletin No. 329. 1941.
69. Bruner, D.W.: Notes on genital infection in the mare. Cornell Vet., *41:*247–250, 1951.
70. Loy, R.G., Pemstein, R., and Taylor, T.B.: Effects of injected ovarian steroids on reproductive patterns and performance in post-partum mares. J. Reprod. Fertil. Suppl., *32:*199–204, 1982.
71. Loy, R.G., Hughes, J.P., Richards, W.P.C., and Swan, S.M.: Effects of progesterone on reproductive function in mares after parturition. J. Reprod. Fertil. Suppl., *23:*291–295, 1975.
72. Pope, A.M., Campbell, D.L., and Davidson, J.P.: Endometrial histology of post-partum mares treated with progesterone and a synthetic GnRH (AY–24,031). J. Reprod. Fertil. Suppl., *27:*587–591, 1979.
73. Sexton, P.E., and Bristol, F.M.: Uterine involution in mares treated with progesterone and estradiol 17-β. J. Am. Vet. Med. Assoc., *186:*252–256, 1985.
74. Squires, E.L., Shideler, R.K., Voss, J.L., and Webel, S.K.: Clinical applications of progestins in mares. Compend. Contin. Educ. Practicing Vet., *5:*S16–S22, 1983.
75. Evans, M.J., et al.: Clearance of bacteria and non-antigenic markers following intra-uterine inoculation into maiden mares: Effect of steroid hormone environment. Theriogenology, *26:*37–50, 1986.
76. Winter, A.J.: Microbial immunity in the reproductive tract. J. Am. Vet. Med. Assoc., *181:*1069–1073, 1982.
77. Arthur, G.H.: An analysis of the reproductive function of mares based on post-mortem examination. Vet. Rec., *70:*682–686, 1958.
78. Kenney, R.M., and Ganjam, V.K.: Selected pathological changes of the mare uterus and ovary. J. Reprod. Fertil. Suppl., *23:*335–339, 1975.
79. Wilson, G.L.: Diagnostic and therapeutic hysteroscopy for endometrial cysts in mares. Vet. Med., *80:*59–63, 1985.
80. Ginther, O.J., and Pierson, R.A.: Ultrasonic anatomy and pathology of the equine uterus. Theriogenology, *21:*505–515, 1984.
81. McKinnon, A.O., Squires, E.L., and Voss, J.L.: Ultrasound evaluation of the mare's reproductive tract—Part II. Compend. Contin. Educ. Practicing Vet., *9:*472–482, 1987.
82. Brook, D., and Frankel, K.: Electrocoagulative removal of endometrial cysts in the mare. J. Equine Vet. Sci., *7:*77–81, 1987.
83. Baker, C.B., and Kenney, R.M.: Systemic approach to the diagnosis of the infertile or subfertile mare. *In* Current Therapy in Theriogenology. Edited by D.A. Morrow. Philadelphia, W.B. Saunders, 1980, pp. 721–736.
84. Neely, D.P.: Equine gestation. *In* Equine Reproduction. Edited by D.P. Neely, I.K.M. Liu, and R.B. Hillman. Princeton Junction, Veterinary Learning Systems, 1983.
85. Ginther, O.J., and Pierson, R.A.: Ultrasonic evaluation of the reproductive tract of the mare; principles, equipment and techniques. J. Equine Vet. Sci., *3:*195–201, 1983.
86. Ginther, O.J., and Pierson, R.A.: Ultrasonic evaluation of the reproductive tract of the mare: Ovaries. J. Equine Vet. Sci., *4:*11–16, 1984.
87. Pierson, R.A., and Ginther, O.J.: Ultrasonic evaluation of the corpus luteum of the mare. Theriogenology, *23:*795–806, 1985.
88. Ginther, O.J., and Pierson, R.A.: Ultrasonic anatomy of equine ovaries. Theriogenology, *21:*471–483, 1984.
89. Pierson, R.A., and Ginther, O.J.: Ultrasonic evaluation of the preovulatory follicle in the mare. Theriogenology, *24:*359–368, 1985.
90. Parker, W.A.: Sequential changes of the ovulating follicle in the estrous mare as determined by rectal palpation. Proceedings of the Annual Conference of the College of Veterinary Medicine and Biomedical Sciences. Fort Collins, Colorado State University, 1971.
91. Bergin, W.C., and Shipley, W.D.: Genital health in the mare: Observations concerning the ovulation fossa. Vet. Med. Small Anim. Clin., *63:*362–365, 1968.
92. Prickett, M.E.: Pathology of the equine ovary. Proc. Am. Assoc. Equine Pract., 145–154, 1966.
93. Witherspoon, D.M.: The site of ovulation in the mare. J. Reprod. Fertil. Suppl., *23:*329–330, 1975.
94. Witherspoon, D.M., and Talbot, R.B.: Ovulation site in the mare. J. Am. Vet. Med. Assoc., *157:*1452–1459, 1970.
95. Pickett, B.W., Squires, E.L., and McKinnon, A.O.: Procedures for collection, evaluation and utilization of stallion semen for artificial insemination. Animal Reproduction Laboratory Bulletin No. 03. Fort Collins, Colorado State University, 1987.
96. Woods, J., Bergfelt, D.R., and Ginther, O.J.: Effects of time of insemination relative to ovulation on pregnancy rate and embryonic loss rate in mares. Equine Vet. J., *22:*410–415, 1990.
97. Carnevale, E.M., McKinnon, A.O., and Squires, E.L.: Effect of preovulatory follicular fluid aspiration upon luteal function in the mare. Theriogenology, *29:*231, 1988.
98. McKinnon, A.O., et al.: Heterogenous and xenogenous fertilization of in vivo matured equine oocytes. J. Equine Vet. Sci., *8:*143–147, 1988.
99. McKinnon, A.O., Wheeler, M.B., Carnevale, E.M., and Squires, E.L.: Oocyte transfer in the mare: Preliminary observations. J. Equine Vet. Sci., *6:*306–309, 1987.
100. Carnevale, E.M., McKinnon, A.O., Squires, E.L., and Voss, J.L.: Ultrasonographic characteristics of the preovulatory follicle preceding and during ovulation in mares. J. Equine Vet. Sci., *8:*428–431, 1988.
101. Hill, L.M., Breckle, R., and Coulam, C.B.: Assessment of human follicular development by ultrasound. Mayo Clin. Proc., *57:*176–180, 1982.
102. Espey, L.L.: Ovulation. *In* The Vertebrate Ovary: Comparative Biology and Evolution. Edited by R.E. Jones. New York, Plenum Press, 1978.
103. McKinnon, A.O., Squires, E.L., and Voss, J.L.: Ultrasonic evaluation of the mare's reproductive tract—Part I. Compend. Contin. Educ. Practicing Vet., *9:*336–345, 1987.
104. Squires, E.L., Douglas, R.H., Steffenhagen, W.P., and Ginther, O.J.: Changes during the estrous cycle and pregnancy in mares. J. Anim. Sci., *38:*330–338, 1974.
105. Townson, D.H., and Ginther, O.J.: The development of fluid-filled luteal glands in mares. Anim. Reprod. Sci., *17:*155–163, 1988.
106. Ginther, O.J.: Reproductive Biology of the Mare—Basic and Applied Aspects. Cross Plains, WI, published by the author, 1979.
107. Holtz, G., et al.: Luteinized unruptured follicle syndrome

in mild endometriosis. Assessment with biochemical parameters. J. Reprod. Med., *30*:643–645, 1985.

108. Roberts, S.J.: Veterinary Obstetrics and Genital Diseases (Theriogenology). 2nd ed. Ithaca, NY, published by the author, 1971.

109. Pugh, D.G., Bowen, J.M., and Gaughan, E.M.: Equine ovarian tumors. Compend. Contin. Educ. Practicing Vet., *7*:S710–S716, 1985.

110. Jubb, K.V.F., and Kennedy, P.C.: The female genital system. *In* Pathology of Domestic Animals. Vol. 1. 2nd ed. Edited by K.V.F. Jubb and P.C. Kennedy. New York, Academic Press, 1970, pp. 502–507.

CHAPTER 32

REPRODUCTIVE ENDOCRINE FUNCTION TESTING IN MARES

R.F. Nachreiner
J.H. Hyland

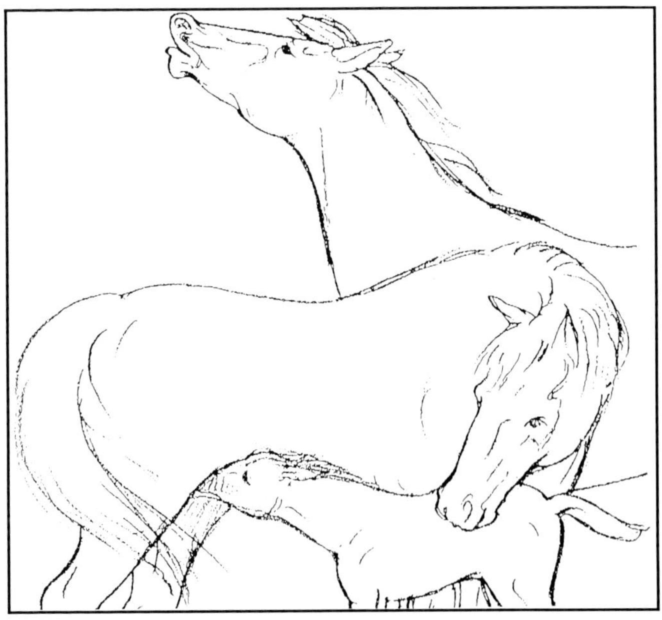

MEASUREMENT OF HORMONES IN BIOLOGIC FLUIDS

Until the early 1960s, measurement of hormones in blood and urine was only possible using chemical or biologic techniques. These methods required large amounts of sample and were time consuming and expensive. When Rosalyn Yalow and the late Solomon Berson in the United States and Roger Ekins in England accidentally discovered the principle of radioimmunoassay (RIA), the science of endocrinology was revolutionized.

Radioimmunoassay is based on the production of a specific antibody directed against the hormone to be measured. It also requires an antigen (hormone) to which a radioactive label is attached. As shown in the following equation, addition of a sample containing the hormone (Ag) to the antibody (Ab) and labeled antigen (Ag*) results in competition between labeled and unlabeled hormone for the antibody:

$$Ag^* + Ab + Ag \leftrightharpoons Ag^*{-}Ab + Ag{-}Ab + Ag^* + Ag$$

The higher the concentration of hormone in the sample, the lower the amount of radioactive hormone that is bound to the antibody. Thus, if it is known how much labeled antigen is added to the mixture, it is possible to quantify the amount of hormone in the sample by counting the radioactivity in the antigen-antibody complex. However, to do this one first has to separate bound and unbound antigen. This can be done using a second antibody directed against the first or absorption of unbound antigen with dextran-coated charcoal.

The RIA is extraordinarily sensitive: it is possible to measure one trillionth of a gram of some substances in blood and urine. Although this degree of sensitivity is useful, few RIA experts would use the technique for absolute measurements, especially in reproductive endocrinology. It is generally more important to characterize hormone profiles over time, which reflect effectiveness of mechanisms controlling secretion.

Although RIA has contributed greatly to the rapid growth of knowledge in endocrinology, the repeatability of results among laboratories measuring the same hormone is often poor because of different antibodies and reagents and different methods of separation of bound and free hormones. Another disadvantage is the use of radioactive materials, which require special facilities for handling and expensive equipment for measuring activity. The use of enzyme labels has improved safety and has facilitated hormone measurement in less sophisticated facilities. The repeatability of the assay kits based on enzyme labels is excellent, and results seem to correlate well with RIA run in parallel.

Assays using an enzyme label are called enzyme-linked immunosorbent assays (ELISA) and are now widely used in diagnostic medicine. The principle of ELISA is similar to that of RIA, although many variations of the basic method exist (Fig. 32–1). In most ELISA, the antibody directed against the hormone or antigen is bound to the bottom of a well in a plastic plate called a multiwell plate. The sample is added to

Progesterone antibodies attached to plastic well.

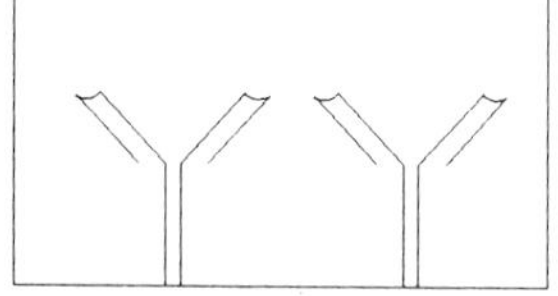

Addition of sample containing progesterone and enzyme-labelled progesterone supplied by the manufacturer.

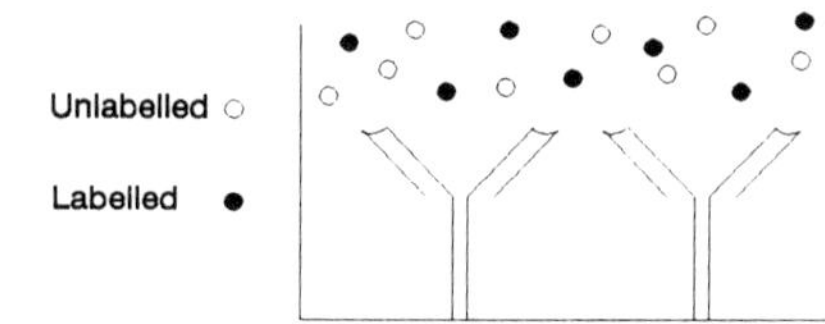

Labelled and unlabelled progesterone molecules compete for antibody.

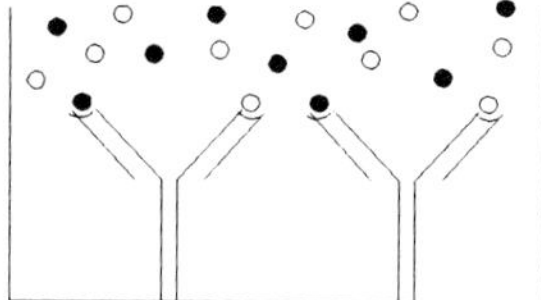

Wash to remove unbound progesterone.

Add substrate which reacts with enzyme causing a colour change.

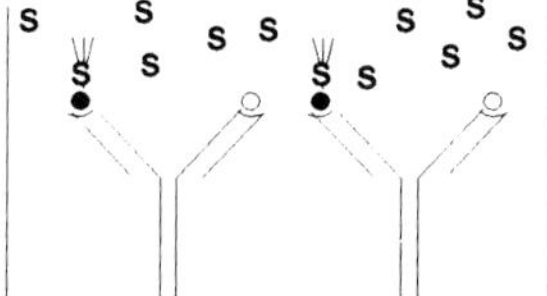

Addition of amplifier intensifies colour and improves readability. Intensity of colour is inversely proportional to the concentration of progesterone in sample.

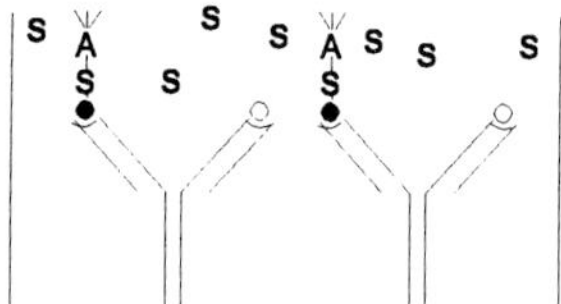

FIG. 32–1. The principle of enzyme linked immunosorbent assay (ELISA), which is used in a number of practical hormone assay kits. S, Substrate; A, amplifier.

the well and the antigen binds to the antibody. The excess antigen is washed off and enzyme-labeled antigen is added. The labeled and unlabeled antigens are allowed to compete for the antibody for several minutes and the free antigens are then washed out of the well. Addition of a substrate which is acted on by the enzyme attached to the antigen results in a color change. The intensity of the color depends on the amount of enzyme attached to the wells. Therefore, the higher the concentration of hormone in the sample, the weaker the color in the well. The difference in the intensity of color of samples containing high or low hormone concentrations can usually be easily distinguished with the naked eye. If a more quantitative measurement is required, a plate scanner can be used. This expensive piece of equipment is not necessary for most clinical work.

The RIA, enzyme immunoassay (EIA), and related techniques hold much promise in diagnosing endocrine disorders in mares. These procedures are sensitive, specific, and precise. Although few reagents have been developed specifically for diagnosing equine disorders, those designed for human diagnostics are often valid when slightly modified. They have been commonly used for reproductive endocrinology research in large and small animals, but few reports are available on their usefulness in equine clinical practice. Perhaps few reproduction related endocrinopathies occur, because infertility results in fewer offspring carrying the genes which promote endocrine infertilities.

The RIA has been used extensively for the assessment of serum hormones. "Turnaround time" is slow as most RIAs take 3 to 6 h of laboratory time. The use of radioactive substances in the assay has precluded it from "horse-side" on-farm applications. The addition of 3 to 6 days in the mail for delivery of sample and result makes the procedure impractical for careful reproductive monitoring. EIA procedures which use a color change as the end point are being developed for on-farm use.[1] Some of these assays can be run in 5 to 10 min and give a qualitative rather than a quantitative result; however, these kit assays are satisfactory for most hormone measurements on the farm. Further technologic advances should provide more quantitative "on-farm procedures" and objective means by which to determine end points.

SAMPLE HANDLING

Most laboratory procedures use serum for hormonal analyses. Progesterone and other steroids may be absorbed or enzymatically altered by red blood cells. Loss of progesterone is a problem in cows but not in mares.[2] Protein hormones may be affected by enzymatic degradation by proteases found in serum.[3] Hence false-positive and false-negative results can occur in diagnostic procedures from improper sample handling. It is best to work closely with a laboratory that has determined the effects of various sample handling procedures. If you are not sure, call the laboratory to find out whether there are specific suggestions for transporting a valid sample from the mare to the laboratory. For on-farm EIA kits, follow the instructions carefully. It makes a difference in the accuracy of the diagnosis.

HORMONE ASSAY KITS AVAILABLE FOR HORSES

Although these types of assay kits are extremely useful for assisting busy practitioners in "getting a handle" on mares under their care, they have yet to be widely accepted by veterinarians. At the time of writing, kits are available to measure progesterone, estrone sulfate, and equine chorionic gonadotropin (eCG/PMSG). All except the Rapi Tex agglutination test for eCG (discussed later in this chapter) are based on the ELISA and rely on a color change for determining the concentration of hormone present in the sample.

PROGESTERONE ASSESSMENT IN MARES

Progesterone is an excellent monitor of ovarian function. It has been used extensively for research in many species to determine ovarian cycles and to evaluate objectively constraints to reproductive efficiency.[4] Analysis of serial samples from female animals can objectively determine seasonal, lactational, and postpartum anestrous periods, inadequate estrus detection, artificial insemination (AI) at inappropriate times (luteal phase), prolonged luteal activity resulting in anestrous conditions (pseudopregnancy), successful corpus luteum (CL) regression after prostaglandin (PG) therapy, apparent early pregnancy (high concentrations 21 to 24 days after ovulation), and early embryonic death. Progesterone analyses may not be as useful in the mare for diagnosing abortion. Placental tissue may continue to produce eCG and may support luteal maintenance when fetal death or abortion occurs after day 38.[5] Progesterone as an indicator of ovarian cycles may be less useful on a practical basis in mares because estrus is more prolonged and a decrease in progesterone results in less predictable timing of estrus and ovulation than in many other species.[6]

Anestrous Conditions

Progesterone concentrations are useful in determining whether anestrous conditions are due to a lack of ovarian activity (low progesterone, <1 ng/ml) or retained or prolonged CL function[7,8] (generally considered >2 ng/ml[8]). When higher (i.e., luteal) progesterone concentrations are found, one must determine that the mare is not pregnant because pregnancy is the most common cause of luteal maintenance. Prolonged luteal activity can be a serious detriment to efficient reproduction, often resulting in the mare's barrenness for the duration of the current breeding season.[9] If the mare is not pregnant, PG therapy is often used therapeutically to cause regression of the CL and to initiate ovarian cycles. Low (nonluteal) progesterone concentrations which persist for prolonged periods are also associated with anestrous periods. This occurs naturally during seasonal anestrus and can occur during the breeding season when abnormal conditions exist, such as nutritional deficiencies.

Aid to Estrous Detection

Most mares show adequate estrous behavior, and progesterone assays are not needed to help in objectively determining ovarian cycles. Some mares are a problem, however, and an additional objective end point is beneficial.[8] Some of the rapid mare-side assays may be useful for this purpose. Commercial laboratories are usually too slow in their turnaround time to give clinically useful information on these mares. Samples can be obtained every other day and the estimated progesterone concentrations plotted to show the cycle. Some mare-side assays are difficult to read, but continued practice with them or the use of reading devices tend to make the results more reliable. When progesterone concentrations are found to decrease sharply, more intensive observations and clinical examinations may help to determine estrus and optimal breeding times.

Inappropriate Timing of Artificial Insemination or Breeding

A rapid mare-side progesterone assay can be useful in determining that AI would be inappropriate. Finding significant luteal activity (>1 ng/ml) indicates that the mare is past the optimal time for breeding.[8] In addition, low serum progesterone concentrations (<1 ng/ml) help to confirm estrous observations.

Effectiveness of Prostaglandin Therapy

Prostaglandins are not always completely effective in causing CL regression in mares, although mares are more sensitive to PG than cattle.[10] Most problems seem to arise when PG are given to mares with young (less than 5 days old) CL which are resistant to treatment. In these cases, partial regression of the CL occurs with a transient fall in progesterone concentrations. Progesterone concentrations then rebound to normal diestrous concentrations within 2 or 3 days. The post-treatment fall in progesterone concentrations is sufficient to promote gonadotropin release, which stimulates growth of a follicle or follicles. The mare shows estrus for the period of the progesterone decline, during which time the follicle may undergo ovulation. As a result, another CL is produced several days after the first and the mare appears not to have responded to the PG injection. If another PG injection is given within the resistant period of the second CL, the whole cycle of events is repeated, leading to the assumption that the PG injection has not worked. It is therefore advisable not to give PG injections more frequently than every 10 to 12 days if the age of the CL is not known. Breeding programs using PG could be more successful if progesterone assays are used to confirm the regression of the CL and to intensify estrus observations in those mares.

Pregnancy Diagnosis

Progesterone is not a hormone specific for pregnancy, so it is a poor indicator to use for pregnancy diagnosis.[9] A 15 to 20% false-positive error rate for pregnancy diagnosis has been predicted. Although serum concentrations >2 ng/ml around day 20 or 21 after ovulation are suggestive of pregnancy, factors such as persistent luteal-phase diestrous ovulation and fetal wastage may also result in similar concentrations. Serum progesterone analyses could be a helpful adjunct to other diagnostic procedures, such as transrectal palpation and teasing. Lack of progesterone is an excellent indicator of the absence of pregnancy. Progesterone concentrations <1 ng/ml are rare in serum of a pregnant mare.[11]

Assessment of Adequate Progesterone to Support Pregnancy Maintenance

Because progesterone is needed to maintain pregnancy, it seems logical to monitor concentrations in habitually aborting mares to determine whether inadequate luteal function may be a contributing factor. In some cases, a compromised progesterone concentration may be suspected. Less than 1 ng/ml is generally agreed to be a level which will not adequately support pregnancy.[11] Hence, at some level above 1 ng/ml, therapy should begin to maintain pregnancy. Although some workers have found that concentrations between 1 and 2 ng/ml have maintained pregnancy, most prefer to begin progesterone supplementation when concentrations drop below 2 ng/ml.

PROGESTERONE KITS

Progesterone kits have been primarily developed for pregnancy detection in cows with later adaptation of the tests for mares.[12,13] Three commercial mare-side progesterone kits were compared with RIA and were found to be accurate and reliable.[1] Of the three kits, tested, none are available under the original trade names. This situation indicates the difficulties manufacturers' experience in having these types of management aids accepted by the veterinary profession. Four progesterone ELISA tests are available at the time of writing this chapter, although only two of these (Target and CITE, described later in this chapter) are truly "mare-side" kits.

Mare Progesterone Assay Kit (Novo Nordisk, Cambridge, England) and Enzygnost Serum Progesterone Test Kit Vet (Behring Diagnostics, Sydney, Australia).

This is the same kit, distributed by two different companies. It is a quantitative or semiquantitative test and is a 96-well plate with 5 standards and costs approximately $140. Serum or plasma can be used. The test takes approximately 1 h to run and involves 5 steps. A 100-μl pipette and distilled water are necessary extras. If 1 sample and 5 standards are used each time, a total of 16 samples per kit could be assayed, at $8.75 per sample. In reality, 1 or 2 standards and several test samples are included in each run, at a cost of $3 to $5 per sample. To make the assay quantitative requires a microtiter plate reader.

Target Equine Progesterone Assay Kit (BioMetallics, Princeton, NJ).

This semiquantitative test can be used with whole blood, milk, serum, or plasma. There are 20 cups per kit, which costs $120, or $6 per test. No extras are required and it takes approximately 15 min for a result. After addition of reagents, progesterone concentrations are estimated by reading the color: bright blue, <1 ng/ml; light blue, 1-5 ng/ml; and white, >5 ng/ml.

CITE Semi-Quant Progesterone Assay (IDEXX Corp., Portland, ME).

This is a semiquantitative, self-contained test for whole blood, serum, or plasma. A kit costs $79 for 10 tests, or $7.90 per test, and takes about 10 min to run. The test is based on the immobilization of different concentrations of antiprogesterone monoclonal antibody in two spots on a fiber membrane. Addition of sample, enzyme-conjugated progesterone, and substrate results in production of color, the intensity of which is inversely proportional to the concentration of progesterone in the sample. The result is read as progesterone concentrations of <1 ng/ml, 1 to 4 ng/ml, or >4 ng/ml.

Bioresearch Ireland Progesterone Assay Kit (Wien Laboratories, Inc., Succasunna, NJ).

This kit is a sandwich-type ELISA, which involves an extra step in comparison to the other tests. The test takes 2½ to 3 h to run and requires a plate reader. In addition, bovine serum albumin needs to be added to the solutions in the United States because of the prohibition on importation of bovine products into the United States from the United Kingdom, as a result of bovine spongiform encephalopathy (BSE). The kit contains 96 wells and costs approximately $210. The maximum and minimum number of tests that can be run is similar to the Novo Nordisk and Behring tests. That is, the cost per test ranges from $2.30 to $13.00. This kit does not appear to be useful for the busy veterinarian.

USING MARE-SIDE ASSAY KITS

The only practical mare-side assay kits available at the time of writing are those that measure progesterone. They can be used to determine the reproductive status of mares at the beginning of the breeding season or to assess the adequacy of progesterone production in pregnant mares.[14] Studs attended by the University of Melbourne (Australia) Veterinary Clinic are recommended to commence teasing at the beginning of August (January in the Northern Hemisphere). Mares showing regular estrus (approximately 15 days between the end of one estrus and the beginning of the next) are separated and are served at the appropriate time. Mares which exhibit prolonged or intermittent estrus are submitted to rectal palpation and ultrasonography. Those with ovarian follicles around 2 cm in diameter are placed on altrenogest (Regumate). The remainder can be treated with gonadotropin-releasing hormone (GnRH), either by injection or infusion, or allowed to settle into regular cyclicity with time. A blood sample is taken from mares which have not shown estrus by late August. Plasma progesterone concentrations are measured using RIA or a progesterone kit. Mares with plasma progesterone concentrations >1 ng/ml are treated with $PGF_2\alpha$, are treated as cycling mares, and are served at the appropriate time. If progesterone concentrations are <1 ng/ml and the ovaries contain follicles less than 2 cm in diameter, the mares are treated with GnRH infusions, delivered by osmotic minipump.[15] Mares with ovarian follicles greater than 2 cm in diameter are usually treated with altrenogest.

The foregoing treatment regimen can be used in mares under ambient conditions or in those held under artificial lighting to stimulate cyclicity. Measurement of plasma progesterone concentrations allows the veterinarian to identify mares which contain a functional CL and are likely to respond to $PFG_2\alpha$. Identification of these mares is a great advantage during the early breeding season because their reproductive behavior can be predicted. The use of progesterone measurements for assessing luteal adequacy is a dubious practice. There appears to be great variation among mares in the concentrations of progesterone necessary to carry a foal to term.[16] Moreover, in an unpublished experiment conducted on commercial Thoroughbred stud farms in Victoria (Australia), embryo death preceded luteolysis. Under these circumstances, measurement of plasma progesterone concentrations would be useless for predicting whether a mare is likely to carry a pregnancy to term.

MEASUREMENT OF PITUITARY FUNCTION

The pituitary gland is responsible for the release, under control of the hypothalamus, of appropriate amounts of the gonadotropins, luteinizing hormone (LH), and follicle-stimulating hormone (FSH). Pituitary dysfunction is apparently rare, although adenomas involving the tissues of the sella turcica have been recorded.[17] These tumors usually occur in aged mares and are associated with inappropriate hair growth, polydipsia, polyuria, and infertility. Pregnant mares may have a lengthened gestation and cushingoid symptoms requiring induction of parturition to alleviate damage to the abdominal musculature and to prevent the onset of foot problems.

Published data on the use of gonadotropin assays for assessing pituitary function in mares appear to be scant. Most stud farms appear to have one or two mares which fail to undergo regular cyclicity and ovulation during the breeding season. These mares appear to be slower to respond to increasing photoperiod, either natural or artificial. This situation is probably not pathologic but reflects a difference in the rate of transition into the breeding season. It is generally accepted that transition into the breeding season which culminates in fertile estrus is associated with increased GnRH production and release by the hypothalamus.[18,19] Because assays are too insensitive to allow measurement of peripheral GnRH concentrations, LH responses are used indirectly to measure GnRH release. In mares under natural photoperiod, the ability to respond to GnRH was demonstrated to be a function of pituitary LH content.[20] Furthermore, by treating mares with GnRH at various times of transition into the breeding season, LH release was greater in mares kept under a stimulatory photoperiod than in mares in natural lighting.[21]

Presumably, GnRH-stimulated LH release could be used to measure pituitary responsiveness early in the breeding season and to assess the effect of artificial lighting programs or the likely response to other treatments such as GnRH infusion. This is not likely to be useful, however, because ovarian estrogens may be involved in the onset of cyclicity in mares.[22] The excitatory amino acids, aspartate and glutamate, have been implicated in the control of GnRH secretion. Use of an analogue, N-methyl-D-aspartate (NMDA) in hamsters,[23] as well as in sheep,[24,25] showed that this substance was a potent releaser of GnRH and suggests that NMDA may be useful in assessing the depth of anestrus in seasonally breeding animals. It has potential use in the mare. By measuring the LH response to NMDA prior to the breeding season, it may be possible to predict mares which will respond to treatments for advancing the breeding season.

ESTRONE SULFATE MEASUREMENT

Estrone sulfate is a metabolite of estrone which is produced in the fetoplacental unit and the ovaries. Plasma and urine estrone sulfate concentrations in the pregnant mare increase from around day 35 of gestation.[26,27] A second, more dramatic rise occurs from day 60 as a result of fetal and placental contribution to the estrone sulfate pool. At least part of the initial estrone sulfate rise comes from the CL.[28] Whether the developing embryo contributes to this rise is not clear, although the yolk sac contains large concentrations of estrone sulfate from day 40 of pregnancy.[29]

Measurement of plasma or urine estrone sulfate concentrations therefore has the potential for being a sensitive indicator of fetal viability. This is certainly true from around day 60 of pregnancy, when the fetoplacental unit is functional.

MARE-SIDE ESTRONE SULFATE KIT

The only ELISA kit commercially available for estrone sulfate analysis is Bioresearch Ireland Equine Oestrone Sulphate EIA (Wien Laboratories, Inc., Succasunna, NJ). The principle of this assay is the same as the sandwich ELISA for progesterone and eCG. Its use is limited by the necessity to have a plate reader for obtaining results. The busy practitioner is more likely to send samples to laboratories with established estrone sulfate assays. Although ultrasound echography is the most immediate method for assessing fetal viability, at times its use is unwanted or impractical. At these times, hormonal tests for fetal viability are useful.

TESTOSTERONE MEASUREMENT

Testosterone is usually low in mare serum (<60 pg/ml).[30] However, disorders of steroid-producing tissues can result in increased testosterone concentrations. Mares with large ovarian tumors, usually of granulosa-theca cell origin, often have serum testosterone concentrations over 150 pg/ml.[9] In these mares, the negative feedback usually causes gonadotropin suppression and the opposite ovary becomes small over time. Because normal basal concentrations in stallions are 200 to 1000 pg/ml, the disorder results in levels which approach male concentrations. It is not surprising that anestrus, clitoral enlargement, and some stallion-like characteristics can occur in these mares.

MEASUREMENT OF EQUINE CHORIONIC GONADOTROPIN (PREGNANT MARE SERUM GONADOTROPIN)

Equine chorionic gonadotropin (eCG), also known as pregnant mare serum gonadotropin (PMSG), has been used for many years as a diagnostic indicator of pregnancy.[5,9] Early tests were bioassays which used laboratory animals to determine the presence of the gonadotropin in serum between days 40 to 100 of gestation.[11] In the 1960s, a hemagglutination-inhibition procedure was developed as a field procedure to detect the hormone.[31] More recently, several companies have shown interest in adapting it to the EIA for analysis. The onset of early pregnancy diagnosis using ultrasonographic imaging has considerably delayed development by the commercial companies because much of this market has been lost. Problems in performing ultrasonographic imaging on miniature horses and ponies, fractious mares, those with previous rectal tears, and those needing confirmation of transrectal palpation findings are all justifications for using the eCG laboratory technique. The presence of eCG does not ensure pregnancy and/or fetal viability. Embryonic death can occur, but the endometrial cups remain active and continue to produce eCG.[5] Hence the test will not be 100% accurate for diagnosing pregnancy if the fetus is lost after formation of the endometrial cups, around day 40 of gestation.

Confirmation of pregnancy, especially after day 60, is more accurate using plasma estrone sulfate concentrations.

MARE-SIDE KITS

Withdrawal of the popular mare immunologic pregnancy (MIP) test from the market has left two kits available for eCG/PMSG measurement.

Bioresearch Ireland Equine eCG/PMSG EIA (Wien Laboratories, Inc., Succasunna, NJ).

This sandwich-type ELISA kit costs \$275 for 96 wells. The cost per test therefore ranges from \$3.00 to \$17.00 per sample. It takes 2½ to 3 hours to obtain results, and necessary extras are micropipettes to deliver 20 to 50 μl of solution and a plate reader. This kit is not practical for normal clinical veterinary practice.

Rapi Tex PMSG (Behring Diagnostics, Sydney, Australia).

This test is based on the agglutination of polystyrene particles sensitized with antibodies to eCG. The addition of a sample containing eCG causes the particles to agglutinate. This is read by eye after mixing on a special plate (supplied). The test costs \$300 and contains ingredients sufficient for approximately 20 samples.

MEASUREMENT OF FECAL STEROIDS

Fecal steroids are studied in several laboratories. Conjugated steroids are present in feces, serum, and urine in many species, including the mare.[32] Estrogens and progestins found in feces may be useful for monitoring estrous cycles and pregnancy at some time in the future, but they are not currently available for routine clinical use.

EQUINE FETAL PROTEIN MEASUREMENT

α-Fetoprotein is a glycoprotein found in high concentrations in fetal serum. Data have shown that equine fetal protein (EQFP) may be an assay which will benefit clinical reproductive practice.[33] The protein appears to increase throughout normal pregnancy. EQFP concentrations in mares with pregnancy failures have been outside the reported reference values, although some have been higher than normal, perhaps from absorption of fetal material after fetal death. Twin pregnancies and impending abortion have also been associated with elevated concentrations of EQFP. Low concentrations may be a result of conception failure. The assay is not currently available, and further data will be needed to determine the clinical usefulness of the procedure.

THYROID GLAND AND INFERTILITY

Many reports correlate hypothyroidism with infertility in humans. Reproductive abnormalities were not reported in thyroidectomized mares,[34] however, leading one to question the relationship of the mare's thyroid with infertility. It is hard to argue with clinical success, however, and many practitioners have reported clinical surmise of improvements in fertility after thyroid hormone supplementation. No well-controlled experiments have been reported which test the diagnostic and therapeutic approach to infertility caused by thyroid disease.

Without clinical data to the contrary, using baseline total thyroxine (TT_4) and total triiodothyronine (TT_3) assessment, appears to be the most economical and practical diagnostic approach at this time. New assays for free T_4 (FT_4) and free T_3 (FT_3) are also used in some laboratories, but they appear to offer little improvement in the diagnostic assessment of thyroid function. A common approach is to check baseline concentrations and, finding low levels, to give the animal a therapeutic trial if concentrations are low enough to warrant one. Nonthyroid-related illnesses and many drugs secondarily depress serum thyroid hormone concentrations and give a false indication of hypothyroidism. A rule of thumb is to avoid testing horses that are receiving phenylbutazone[35] or glucocorticoids, have chronic debilitating disease, or are anorectic. Ideally, they should receive no medications for 1 month before testing, to allow thyroid hormones to reach homeostasis. When baseline concentrations are low, a therapeutic trial is performed. The end point of a therapeutic trial (clinical improvement) may slowly occur when infertility is the major clinical problem. False-positive results may occur when the mare improves spontaneously, giving a false indication of therapeutic success. The diagnosis of hypothyroidism in a mare should not be taken lightly because of the expense of a therapeutic trial and prolonged therapy.

The hormone concentrations reported for normal thyroid function in a mare differ greatly from laboratory to laboratory. Part of the problem is that many different units (ng/dl, ng/ml, nmol/L, etc.) are used to report the normal ranges. Normal ranges are: TT_4, 6 to 32 nmol/L; TT_3, 0.4 to 1.5 nmol/L; FT_4, 8 to 21 pmol/L; and FT_3, 0.8 to 4.6 pmol/L. Few infertile mares have been found with T_4 and T_3 concentrations below these normal ranges.

If thyroid replacement therapy is initiated, 5 to 10 mg L-thyroxine per 500 kg body weight per day is a good starting dose. The mare should be tested again in 4 to 6 weeks to determine the adequacy of replacement therapy, and the dosage should be adjusted appropriately. As with most species, if therapy is discontinued, the mare should be weaned off the drug slowly. A sudden stoppage of exogenous therapy, even in a euthyroid mare, would leave the mare with an atrophied thyroid and low blood concentrations, a result of disuse atrophy. This is especially critical during gestation and lactation because inadequate thyroid function at critical periods may interfere with normal fetal function and lactation.[36] Stepwise reduction allows the thyroid to recover slowly over a 6- or 8-week period.

REFERENCES

1. Elmore, R.G.: Rapid progesterone assays: The latest in kit technology. Vet. Med., *80:*659–662, 1986.
2. Wiseman, B.S., et al.: Changes in procine, ovine, bovine and equine blood progesterone concentrations between collection and centrifugation. Ann. Reprod. Sci., *5:* 157–165, 1982.
3. Torrance, A.G., and Nachreiner, R.: Human-parathormone assay for use in dogs: Validation, sample handling studies and parathyroid function testing. Am. J. Vet. Res., *50:*1133–1177, 1989.
4. Oltner, R., and Edqvist, L.E.: Progesterone in defatted milk: Its relation to insemination and pregnancy in normal cows as compared with cows on problem farms and individual problem animals. Br. Vet. J., *137:*78–87, 1981.
5. Allen, W.R.: Hormonal control of early pregnancy in the mare. *In* Symposium on Equine Reproduction. Vet. Clin. North Am.: Large Anim. Pract., *2:*291–302, 1980.
6. Holtan, D.W., Nett, T.M., and Estergreen, V.L.: Plasma progestins in pregnant, postpartum and cycling mares. J. Anim. Sci., *40:*251–260, 1975.
7. Ginther, O.J.: Prolonged luteal activity in mares: A semantic quagmire. Equine Vet. J., *22:*152–156, 1990.
8. Hunt, B., Lein, D.H., and Foote, R.H.: Monitoring of plasma and milk progesterone for evaluation of postpartum estrous cycles and early pregnancy in mares. J. Am. Vet. Med. Assoc., *172:*1298–1302, 1978.
9. Stabenfeldt, G.H., and Hughes, J.P.: Diagnostic endocrinology of the horse. *In* Symposium on Equine Reproduction. Vet. Clin. North Am.: Large Anim. Pract., *2:*291–302, 1980.
10. Lauderdale, J.W., and Miller, P.A.: Regulation of reproduction in mares with prostaglandins. Proc. Am. Assoc. Equine Pract., 263–276, 1975.
11. Hyland, J.H.: Reproductive endocrinology: Its role in fertility and infertility in the horse. Br. Vet. J., *146:*1–16, 1990.
12. Sauer, M.J., Foulkes, J.A., Worsfold, A., and Morris, B.A.: Use of progesterone 110 glucuronide-alkaline phosphatase conjugate in a sensitive microtitre-plate enzyme immunoassay of progesterone in milk and its application to pregnancy testing in dairy cattle. J. Reprod. Fertil., *76:*375–391, 1986.
13. Stanley, C.J., et al.: Use of a new and rapid milk progesterone assay to monitor reproductive activity in the cow. Vet. Rec., *118:*664–667, 1986.
14. Rodger, J.: The Thoroughbred breeding season and the value of early foals. Aust. Equine Vet., *8:*37, 1990.
15. Hyland, J.H., and Jeffcott, L.B.: Control of transitional anoestrus in mares by infusion of gonadotrophin releasing hormone. Theriogenology, *29:*1383–1391, 1988.
16. Darenius, K., Einarsson, S., and Kindahl, H.: Endocrine studies of early pregnancy loss in the mare: comparison within mares between pregnancy loss and consecutive pregnancy. J. Reprod. Fertil. Suppl., *44:*726–727, 1992.
17. Beech, J.: Tumours of the pituitary gland. *In* Current Therapy in Equine Medicine 2. Edited by N.E. Robinson. Philadelphia, W.B. Saunders, 1987, pp. 182–187.
18. Strauss, S.S., Chen, C.L., Kalra, S.P., and Sharp, D.S.: Localization of gonadotrophin releasing hormone (GnRH) in the hypothalamus of ovariectomized pony mares by season. J. Reprod. Fertil. Suppl., *27:*123–129, 1979.
19. Thompson, D.L., et al.: Secretion of luteinizing hormone and follicle stimulating hormone in intact and ovariectomized mares in summer and winter. J. Anim. Sci., *64:*247–253, 1987.
20. Silvia, P.J., Squires, E.L., and Nett, T.M.: Pituitary responsiveness of mares challenged with GnRH at various stages of the transition into the breeding season. J. Anim. Sci., *64:*790–796, 1987.
21. Nequin, L.G., King, S.S., Matt, K.S., and Jursk, R.C.: The influence of photoperiod on gonadotrophin-releasing hormone stimulated luteinizing hormone release in the anoestrous mare. Equine Vet. J., *22:*356–358, 1989.
22. Sharp, D.C.: Transition into the breeding season: Clues to the mechanisms of seasonality. Equine Vet. J., *20:* 159–161, 1988.
23. Urbanski, H.F.: A role for N-methyl-D aspartate receptors in the control of seasonal breeding. Endocrinology, *127:*2223–2228, 1990.
24. Estienne, M.J., et al.: Effect of N-methyl-D, i-aspartate on luteinizing hormone secretion in ovariectomized ewes in the absence and presence of estradiol. Biol. Reprod., *42:*126–130, 1990.
25. Lincoln, G.A.: Luteinizing hormone responses to N-methyl-D, L-asparatate during a photoperiodically-induced reproductive cycle in the ram. J. Neuroendocrinol., *3:*309–317, 1991.
26. Kindahl, H., Knudsen, O., Madej, A., and Edqvist, L.-E.: Progesterone, prostaglandin F-2α, PMSG and oestrone sulphate during early pregnancy in mare. J. Reprod. Fertil. Suppl., *32:*353–359, 1982.
27. Evans, K.L., et al: Pregnancy diagnosis in the domestic horse through direct urinary estrone conjugate analysis. Theriogenology, *22:*615–620, 1984.
28. Daels, P.F., et al.: The corpus luteum: Source of oestrogen during early pregnancy in the mare. J. Reprod. Fertil. Suppl., *44:*501–508, 1992.
29. Heap, R.B., Hamon, M., and Allen, W.R.: Studies on oestrogen synthesis by the preimplantation equine conceptus. J. Reprod. Fertil. Suppl., *32:*343–352, 1982.
30. Silberzahn, P., Quincey, D., Rosier, C., and Leymarie, P.: Testosterone and progesterone in peripheral plasma during the oestrous cycle of the mare. J. Reprod. Fertil., *53:*1–5, 1978.
31. Allen, W.R.: A quantitative immunological assay for pregnant mare serum gonadotrophin. J. Endocrinol., *43:* 581–591, 1969.
32. Bamberg, E., et al.: Enzymatic determination of unconjugated oestrogens in faeces for pregnancy diagnosis in mares. Equine Vet. J., *16:*537–539, 1984.
33. Sorensen, K., et al.: Measurement and clinical significance of equine fetal protein in pregnant mares serum. Equine Vet. Sci., *10:*417–421, 1990.
34. Lowe, J.E., et al.: Equine hypothyroidism: The long term effects of thyroidectomy on metabolism and growth in mares and stallions. Cornell Vet., *64:*276–295, 1974.
35. Morris, D.D., and Garcia, M.C.: Thyroid stimulating hormone: Response test in healthy horses and effect of phenylbutazone on equine thyroid hormones. Am. J. Vet. Res., *44:*503–507, 1983.
36. Thompson, F.N., et al.: Thyroidal and prolactin secretion in agalactic mares. Theriogenology, *25:*575–580, 1986.

PHARMACOLOGIC MANIPULATION OF THE REPRODUCTIVE CYCLE

CHAPTER 33

PROGESTIN

E.L. Squires

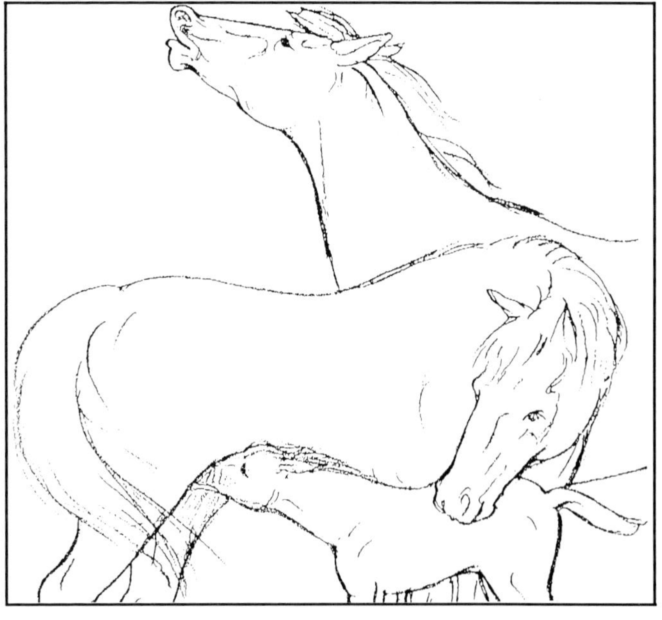

Administration of progesterone or progestin to mares is a common practice and has tremendous applicability for controlling the reproductive cycle of the mare. Clinical uses of progestin have included regulation of estrus in transitional mares; controlling estrus in cycling, nonlactating, and lactating mares; long-term suppression of estrus in show and race mares; improvement in uterine tone; and maintenance of pregnancy. The influence of progesterone on physiologic, endocrinologic, and behavioral responses has been discussed in previous chapters.

TYPES OF PROGESTIN

The types of progestin used by breeders and practitioners has been reviewed.[1] Table 33–1 presents a partial list of various progestin compounds used in brood mare reproduction. Progesterone in oil is commonly administered at a dosage of 150 to 300 mg IM daily. Some investigators administered doses of 50, 100, or 200 mg of progesterone in oil and reported peak concentrations at 6 h after injections of 1.6, 3.4 and 8.1 ng/mL, respectively.[2] Administration of 50, 100, 200, or 300 mg of progesterone in oil daily to ovariectomized embryo recipient mares maintained endogenous progesterone levels at 24 h of 0.46, 1.1, 2.6, and 4.8 ng/mL, respectively. Thus the present recommended dose of progesterone in oil is 150 to 300 mg administered IM daily. Estradiol (10 mg) has also been added to progesterone in oil as a combination treatment for suppression of estrus[3] and pregnancy maintenance.[4] No commercial preparations of progesterone plus estradiol are available, and those preparations are generally made by practitioners or private laboratories.[5]

The slow disappearance of progesterone in a proplene glycol base (repositol progesterone) from the bloodstream accounted for the popularity of its use. However, repositol progesterone is no longer available to the practitioner.[1] Recently, an orally active synthetic progestin (altrenogest, Regu-Mate) was developed for controlling estrus in mares. This appears to be the only orally active progestin effective in horses, although use of other orally active progestin has been advocated. These include melgestrol acetate (MGA) (Ovaban). When MGA was fed at a dosage of 10 or 20 mg/day for 9 to 15 days, it failed to inhibit estrus and ovulation.[6] Neely indicated that higher doses (> 100 mg) of MGA may be more effective in suppressing estrus.[1] Chlormadinone acetate (CAP), although not available in the United States, has been fed to horses in Europe. Unfortunately, CAP failed to suppress estrus and ovulation.[7] Another progestin compound reportedly used in Europe is proligestone (Delvosteron), a long-acting injectable progestin. Results of studies evaluating the effectiveness of proligestone have been equivocal.[1]

Medroxyprogesterone acetate (MPA) (Depo-Provera) has been suggested by practitioners to be an effective treatment for maintenance of pregnancy. This is supposedly a long-acting injectable progestin that is given every 8 to 14 days at a dose of 200 to 250 mg. How-

TABLE 33–1. TYPES OF PROGESTIN USED IN BROOD MARE REPRODUCTION

TYPE	TRADE NAME	COMMON DOSAGE	SOURCE
Injectable in oil	Progesterone	150 mg/day	Steris Labs, Inc., Phoenix, AZ
Injectable in water	Progesterone	150 mg/day	Lannet Co., Inc., Philadelphia, PA
Repositol progesterone	Reprogest	1000 to 2000 mg every 7 days	Not available
Oral	Regu-Mate	0.044 mg/kg	Hoechst-Roussel Agri-Vet, Somerville, NJ
Oral	Ovaban	10 to 20 mg/day	Schering Corp., Kenilworth, NJ
Oral	Chlormadinone acetate (CAP)	40 to 60 mg/day	Unknown
Injectable	Delvosteron	150 mg	Gist-brocades Animal Health, DeBilt, Holland
Injectable	Depo-Provera	200 to 250 mg every 8 to 14 days	Upjohn Co., Kalamazoo, MI
Injectable	Hyproval	500 mg/mare every other day	Wintec Pharmaceuticals Inc., Ellisville, MO
Implant	Synchro-Mate B	Unknown	CEVA Lab, Kansas City, KS

ever, no control studies have been conducted to evaluate the usefulness of this progestin.[8]

A similar product to MPA, hydroxyprogesterone caproate (Hyproval), was also introduced as a long-acting progestin. Unfortunately, this progestin was ineffective in preventing pregnancy loss and affecting sexual behavior.[1] Thus at present no long-acting injectable progestin is effective in suppressing estrus and maintaining pregnancy.

Another means of providing progestin over relatively long periods of time is via progestin implants[9,10] or sponges.[11] Bristol reported that a 6-mg implant of norgestomet (Synchro-mate B) was ineffective in controlling estrus.[9] Other studies demonstrated that norgestomet at a dosage of 3.0 mg/day had no affect on follicular activity, estrous behavior, or serum concentrations of luteinizing hormone (LH) in late transitional mares.[12] Norgestomet was found to be ineffective in suppressing estrus.[10] In contrast, sponges impregnated with 0.5 and 1.0 g altrenogest (Regu-Mate) and placed in the vagina for 7 days resulted in a high degree of synchronization of estrus and ovulation.[11] However, vaginal sponges did induce inflammation with adherence to vaginal mucosa.

INDICATIONS

REGULATION OF ESTRUS IN TRANSITIONAL MARES

One use of exogenous progesterone is to regulate estrus early in the breeding season. Transition from anestrus to the physiologic breeding season is characterized by erratic, long estrous periods, irregular estrous periods, and estrous periods not accompanied by ovulation. Studies have shown that a hormonal imbalance occurs during the transitional period, with high follicle-stimulating hormone (FSH) secretion and low LH secretion.[13] During winter, pituitary stores of LH and hypothalamic stores of gonadotropin-releasing hormone (GnRH) are extremely depressed. Concentrations of GnRH in the hypothalamus are readily replenished after the winter solstice, whereas pituitary stores of LH increase more slowly. This hormonal environment results in follicular development without ovulation. Typically, during February, March, and early April, in the Northern Hemisphere, mares develop several follicles greater than 30 mm before the time that one of these follicles becomes preovulatory in size and eventually ovulates. It is not unusual for mares to experience 10 to 20 days of estrus during the transitional period. Thus the goal of any hormonal treatment during the transitional period is to hasten the initial ovulation of the breeding season and to suppress the long, erratic estrous periods. Webel was the first to report on the use of an oral synthetic progestin for estrus and ovulation control in mares.[14] Since that time there have been numerous reports on the use of the oral progestin altrenogest for estrus regulation in the mare.[1,12,15–20] These studies have demonstrated that prerequisites must be met before mares are responsive to exogenous progesterone during the transition period. That is, the mare must be in mid- to late transition, have at least one follicle greater than 20 mm in size, and preferably be in estrus for an extended time, i.e., greater than 10 days. Initial studies demonstrated altrenogest was ineffective for inducing estrus and ovulation in mares in deep anestrus.[17] However, if mares were treated for a 2-week period during mid- to late transition, a greater number of treated mares exhibited estrus and ovulated, compared to untreated controls.[17–19] Follicular growth is inhibited during treatment with progestin, and it is thought that LH content in the pituitary is increased, resulting in a "rebound" of secretion of gonadotropins after cessation of treatment. Upon cessation of treatment, only one preovulatory follicle develops and ovulation occurs as a result of endogenous LH secretion.

A subsequent study was conducted in which the combined effects of artificial light and progestin were evaluated.[17] Mares were exposed to a 16-h photoperiod for 60 days before treatment with altrenogest for 12 days. Within treatment groups, one-half of the mares received human chorionic gonadotropin (hCG) on day 2 of estrus, and the other half received saline. All progestin-treated mares exhibited estrus within 12 days of the end of treatment; the average interval to estrus was 3.4 days. Administration of hCG on day 2 of estrus, shortened duration of estrus in both progestin-treated and control mares. However, more progestin-treated mares ovulated within 12 days after treatment than controls. It was concluded that treatment with altrenogest in combination with an artificial photoperiod was effective in regulation of estrus and ovulation and assisted in establishment of a normal estrous cycle early in the year. This combination of artificial photoperiod, progestin treatment, and hCG appeared to be one of the most effective regimes for induction of estrus and ovulation in the mare early in the year. Fertility of mares bred after progestin treatment did not appear to be altered.

Based on the success of altrenogest for regulation of estrus in transitional mares under controlled conditions, a clinical field trial was conducted involving 441 mature brood mares at 17 different locations.[18] Altrenogest was administered at the recommended dose of 0.044 mg/kg for 14 days during the months of January to May, which represented the period from winter anestrus to the natural breeding season. During treatment, estrus was suppressed in 262 of 278 mares (94%). Mares were divided into two groups according to the date of treatment, i.e., before or after mid-March. Those mares that were treated before mid-March did not exhibit estrus or ovulate sooner than untreated controls. However, treatment with altrenogest during the late-transition phase (after mid-March) resulted in shorter post-treatment estrus and a shorter interval to conception for treated versus control mares. These data further suggested that altrenogest assisted in normalizing the estrous cycle during late-transitional phase. Mares with active ovaries (diameter of the largest follicle greater than 20 mm) responded with shorter post-treatment estrous periods than those with inactive ovaries. Mares with active ovaries which were treated late in the transitional period responded with the highest percentage of normal cycles post-treatment. Mares in this category should be considered excellent candidates for treatment with progesterone or progestin. Squires et al. reported that the larger the follicle before treatment, the shorter the post-treatment estrus and the more favorable the post-treatment response.[19] Therefore, mares should be examined by rectal palpation and preferably ultrasonography to determine sizes of follicles on the ovaries before treatment. Only those mares with multiple follicles greater than 20 mm should be selected for treatment. In addition, mares with active ovaries that have been in estrus 10 days or longer appear to be excellent candidates for progestin treatment. Pregnancy rates of mares treated with altrenogest were similar to those of controls on each of the 17 locations.

Other workers have reported on use of injectable progesterone for estrus control in transitional mares.[21,22] They administered 150 mg IM of progesterone daily plus 10 mg of estradiol in combination with progesterone. Treated mares were also administered 10 mg of prostaglandin $F_2\alpha$ ($PGF_2\alpha$) on the last day of steroid treatment. The authors concluded that combined steroid-prostaglandin regime provided a satisfactory control of ovulation in mares early in the breeding season. More recently, Wiepz et al. conducted a trial to investigate the effect of altrenogest alone or in combination with estradiol on induction of estrus and ovulation in late transitional mares.[12] Treatments were initiated during the months of April and May and were given for 15 days. Both altrenogest treatments suppressed estrous behavior and follicular growth compared to controls. However, suppression of follicular activity was significantly greater for the combined steroid treatment. Unfortunately, the interval to estrus and ovulation was longer for mares given altrenogest plus estradiol compared with altrenogest treatment alone. These authors concluded that the greater suppression of follicular activity with combined steroids was of no advantage over altrenogest alone for induction of estrus and ovulation in late-transitional mares.

SYNCHRONIZATION OF ESTRUS IN CYCLING MARES

There are several situations where use of progestin in normally cycling mares may aid in more effective reproductive management. For example, if a stallion is scheduled to be gone to shows for part of the breeding season, progestin can be used to suppress estrus in mares until the stallion is available. In addition, estrus synchronization with progestin might be useful for situations where semen from the stallion is difficult to collect because of poor sexual behavior. Generally, the best treatment for this condition is sexual rest. Therefore, progestin can be used to suppress estrus while the stallion is being sexually rested. Mares could be placed on altrenogest treatment and taken off treatment when the stallion is mentally and physically able to ejaculate. Synchronization of estrus and ovulation may also be beneficial in maximizing the use of a stallion in an artificial insemination program and in cases where transported semen is being used for breeding. For example, in an artificial insemination (AI) program, the average ejaculate has sufficient spermatozoa to inseminate 15 to 20 mares. Therefore, in order to obtain pregnancies in a large number of mares in a short time, synchronization treatments are an important tool. In fact, the breeding season can be shortened so that the stallion can be used for alternative purposes. Another purpose is to synchronize ovulation in donors and recipients as part of an embryo-transfer program. In general, interval to estrus and ovulation after progestin treatment has been shown to be more consistent and less variable in normally cycling mares compared with transitional mares. However, the long follicular phase in the mare makes ovulation control more difficult when compared with other farm animals.

Essentially, there are three major approaches to estrous synchronization using progestin in cycling mares: (1) 14-day progestin treatment, (2) 7- or 8-day progestin treatment with prostaglandin $F_2\alpha$ given the last day, and (3) progesterone and estradiol for 7 or 8 days with prostaglandins given the last day of treatment. Squires et al. reported on use of the oral progestin altrenogest for estrous cycle control in cycling mares.[17] Once mares had established a normal cycle, they were assigned to one of the following groups: (1) controls, (2) altrenogest for 12 days beginning on day 3 of estrus (group 2), (3) altrenogest for 12 days beginning on day 5 of diestrus (group 3), and (4) day 10 of diestrus (group 4). Estrous behavior was suppressed within 2 days after initiation of treatment in the 10 mares in which treatment was begun during estrus. Of these 10 mares, 7 ovulated during treatment.

The interval from treatment to estrus was shorter for mares treated during diestrus versus those treated during estrus. In addition, interval from treatment to ovulation was shorter for mares treated during diestrus than for those treated during estrus. Webel reported an interval to estrus of 3.5 days for mares previously treated with altrenogest for 18 days.[14] In a subsequent study, mares were treated with altrenogest for 12 days after having previously been exposed to 16 h of photoperiod from December 1 until January 26.[17] On the first day of altrenogest treatment, 10 of 17 mares in the treated group were in estrus. Estrous behavior ceased in all mares by day 3 of treatment and continued to be inhibited for the duration of the treatment period. Mean interval from the end of altrenogest treatment to estrus was 3.4 days. The number of treated mares exhibiting first day of estrus within 12 days after treatment (17 of 17) was greater than that for controls (7 of 17). From those studies, the authors concluded that a short-term treatment with altrenogest was effective in controlling the long, erratic estrous periods frequently encountered at the onset of the breeding season and for synchronization of estrus in normally cycling mares or in mares previously exposed to an artificial photoperiod. In addition, altrenogest treatment had no detrimental effect on fertility, thus this approach could be used to effectively manage the estrous cycle of the mare.

Loy et al. have stated that progestin therapy alone does not uniformly inhibit follicular development in cycling mares.[21] Therefore, when progestin treatment is withdrawn, the ovulation pattern is variable. They advocated the combination of estradiol and progestin for controlling estrus and ovulation in cycling mares.

An experiment was conducted to provide more information on effects of steroid treatment started early in estrus when a follicle was present.[22] Treatment consisted of an injection of 200 mg IM of progesterone and 13.2 mg of estradiol-17β for 5 days beginning on the day of estrus when a follicle 25 mm or larger was first palpated. Treatment began on day 1 or 2 of estrus in 12 estrous periods and on day 3 of estrus in one mare. On treatment days 6 through 10, the dose was reduced to 150 mg of progesterone and 10 mg of estradiol. The treatment imposed in this study prevented ovulation of follicles present at the start of treatment in only 5 of 13 mares. In the five mares, ovulation of new follicles occurred 11 days after treatment in three mares, and 12 days after treatment in the others. In six of eight mares ovulating during treatment, intervals from end of treatment to ovulation ranged from 9 to 16 days, whereas two mares did not ovulate again during the experimental period. The effect of exogenous steroid treatment at the time of ovulation, and for variable times afterward, had inconsistent effects on corpus luteum (CL) function. Although those authors did not compare progesterone alone versus a combined steroid treatment, they concluded the combined steroid treatment provided a more precise control of ovulation, provided (1) no ovulation occurred during treatment and (2) CLs were not functional past the end of treatment. The interval over which post-treatment ovulations occurred under those conditions was 5 days, with 18 of 20 ovulations occurring on days 10, 11, and 12. They suggested that the poor response when treatment was initiated early in estrus might be overcome by extending the steroid treatment for 15 days before prostaglandin is given. Recently Squires conducted a study to compare progesterone versus progesterone plus estradiol. Addition of estradiol provided no additional beneficial affect on controlling estrus or ovulation.

DELAYING POSTPARTUM ESTRUS/OVULATION

Because of lowered fertility for mares bred on foal heat compared to second postpartum heat, attempts have been made to improve fertility of postpartum mares by delaying ovulation thus allowing more time for the uterus to involute. Early attempts to delay uniformly the first ovulation postpartum with exogenous progesterone were only partially successful. A bimodal response resulted when mares were given 100 or 200 mg of progesterone in oil per day from the day of foaling through day 10 postpartum.[21] The variable response was attributed to failure of progesterone treatment to inhibit follicular development early in the treatment period even though ovulation was prevented. A combined treatment of 200 mg of progesterone in oil plus 10 mg estradiol-17β appeared to result in greater suppression of ovarian activity than progesterone alone.[21] Distribution of ovulations from the last day of treatment appeared to be normal and were similar to that for intervals from parturition to first ovulation in untreated mares. Therefore, the authors conducted a further trial to evaluate the combined progesterone–estradiol-17β treatment.[22] Following the establishment of normal estrous cycles, mares were randomly assigned to one of three treatments: (1) controls—3 mL cottonseed oil daily for 10 days, (2) 150 mg progesterone plus 10 mg estradiol-17β daily for 10 days, and (3) same steroid treatment as group 2 but 10 mg of $PGF_2\alpha$ on day 1 and day 10. Ovarian follicular activity was inhibited during the 10-day steroid treatment in 14 of 16 mares in groups 2 and 3. After a 10-day treatment with combined progesterone-estradiol, seven of eight mares in group 2 returned to estrus within 6 days and ovulated within 12 days. After treatment, all group 3 mares returned to estrus within 8 days and ovulated within 13 days. No differences among group means for intervals from last injection to estrus or ovulation, or duration of post-treatment estrus were noted. The small range in days on which ovulation occurred post-treatment for groups 2 and 3 suggested a better synchrony of ovulation for treated mares versus controls.

Another series of experiments was conducted in which the effect of injected ovarian steroids on reproductive patterns and fertility of postpartum mares was studied.[3] A total of 41 mares was given 200 mg of progesterone and 10 mg of estradiol-17β in oil solution daily for 6 days, beginning within 12 h after parturition to 5 days postpartum and mated at the first ovulation feasible after treatment. These treatments were administered during the middle of the breeding season, i.e., mid-March to mid-May. Of the 41 mares, 36 were mated at the delayed first ovulation. Of the 116 untreated control mares, 66 were mated at the first and 50 at the second, or later, ovulation. Daily plasma samples were taken from the day of parturition until 6 days after the first ovulation postpartum for 29 steroid-treated mares and 13 untreated mares and were assayed for FSH and LH by radioimmunoassay. Conception rate at the delayed first ovulation postpartum was higher (58.5%) than in mares mated at the first normal ovulation (53%) but not as high as the mares mated at second or later ovulations postpartum (66.0%). The number of estrous periods per conception, the cumulative seasonal conception rate, and the interval from foaling to conception were not different between the experimentally delayed first ovulation and untreated mares. In addition, the concentrations of gonadotropins between steroid-treated and control mares were similar when normalized to the day of ovulation. The authors stated the steroid treatment was started within 12 h of parturition because the delay in start of treatment to 24 h or more resulted in progressively less control of follicular development and consequent ovulation time. That study indicated there was no advantage in breeding performance by delaying first ovulation postpartum over more conventional management systems. Although the steroid treatment inhibited both gonadotropins during treatment, there was no classic rebound of gonadotropins above that detected in untreated controls.

Studies were conducted in our laboratory to determine if delay in ovulation with the oral progestin altrenogest would result in improved pregnancy rates in mares bred during the first postpartum, ovulatory period.[23] A total of 45 mares were randomly assigned as they foaled to one of three treatment groups: (1) controls, (2) daily oral treatment with 0.044 mg/kg of altrenogest for 8 days beginning the day after parturition and injection of 10 mg of prostaglandin $F_2\alpha$ on day 9, and (3) daily oral treatment with 0.044 mg/kg of altrenogest for 15 days beginning the day after parturition. Ultrasonographic examination of each mare's reproductive tract was performed every other day beginning on day 3 and continued until day 31 after parturition. Measurements were taken for diameter at the tip and middle of each uterine horn and at the corpus corneal junction; quality and quantity of uterine fluid were also estimated. Follicular growth and ovulation were monitored by ultrasonography. Control mares were inseminated every other day with 500 million progressively motile spermatozoa, once a 35-mm follicle was detected. After withdrawal of altrenogest treatment, treated mares were inseminated, using identical criteria. Ovulations were delayed and pregnancy rates improved in progesterone-treated mares. In the untreated control group, 9 of 15 mares became pregnant on cycle 1 versus 11 of 12 mares (92%) in the short-term progestin-treated group and 9 of 13 (69%) mares given altrenogest for 15 days. Thus in that study treatment of mares with altrenogest for 8 days plus prostaglandin on day 9 improved fertility over untreated controls. When investigators categorized mares into those that ovulated after 15 days and those that ovulated before 15 days, pregnancy rates were higher for those that ovulated after 15 days (82% versus 50%). Results of that study concurred with those of others in which progestin treatment delayed onset of the first postpartum ovulatory period.

LONG-TERM SUPPRESSION OF ESTRUS

Practitioners are often asked to provide a treatment regime that will prevent the expression of estrus in show or race mares. This may require that estrus be suppressed for 1 month to several months. Two studies have been conducted in our laboratory to evaluate the long-term treatment with altrenogest on various hematologic and biochemical parameters in the mare and the effect on reproductive performance. In the first study, 20 mares were assigned to receive one of four levels of altrenogest: (1) control, (2) 0.044 mg/kg body weight, (3) 0.132 mg/kg body weight, and (4) 0.22 mg/kg body weight.[24] The drug was administered as a topdressing to grain daily beginning in August and continuing for 88 days. Mares were observed daily for signs of illness, dyspnea, inappetence, lethargy, and toxicity. Blood samples were obtained before and during treatment and were evaluated for various biochemical parameters using automated blood chemistry analysis or conventional laboratory methods. No signs of illness could be attributed to the feeding of altrenogest during this trial. The various parameters were well within the normal, established ranges. Thus the researchers concluded that long-term treatment with altrenogest did not have adverse or toxic effects on normal function of the mare.

Because that study was conducted during the nonbreeding season, a second study was conducted during the breeding season to evaluate reproductive performance of mares after long-term treatment.[20] Before February 1, 64 mares were assigned to one of four treatments: group 1, no treatment; or groups 2, 3, and 4 fed 0.044 mg altrenogest for 15, 30, and 60 days, respectively. Treatment for each group was initiated so that all mares received their final treatment on the same day (March 31). Altrenogest was dissolved in neobee oil at a concentration of 2.2 mg/mL and was applied in the morning's grain ration. Control mares received grain only. Progesterone treatment blocked estrous behavior within 3 days of the initiation of treatment and continued to suppress estrus for the duration of treatment. Fewer ($p < 0.05$) control than treated mares exhibited estrus within 12 days after treatment (1 of 16 vs. 30 of 50). The number of mares that exhibited estrus was similar for those treated with altrenogest for 15, 30, and 60 days. All of the mares were typical of mares early in the transition phase, and thus the treatment was not effective in establishing normal cycles. However, mares treated for 60 days had a shorter ($p < 0.05$) interval from January 1 to the end of the first posttreatment estrus (134 days) than control mares (154 days). A total of 31 of 46 (67.4%) altrenogest-treated mares were inseminated within 15 days after treatment compared with only 5 of 14 (36%) control mares. By 30 days after treatment, comparable values were 37 of 46 treated mares and 6 of 14 control mares. The number of mares that became pregnant within 45 days after treatment was higher ($p < 0.05$) for treated mares than for controls (37 vs. 14%, respectively). Mean date of conception was June 4, May 20, May 29, and May 15 for the four groups, respectively. First-cycle pregnancy rates and overall pregnancy rates were similar for all four groups.

Thus altrenogest used for extended periods appears to be effective in suppressing estrus and does not affect subsequent fertility. In fact, mares that were treated the longest became pregnant sooner than the control mares.

PREGNANCY MAINTENANCE

Progesterone supplementation to pregnant mares with a history of habitually aborting is a common practice. Low concentrations of progesterone in early gestation have been implicated as one of the signs associated with embryonic loss.[25,26] Douglas et al. compared concentrations of progesterone on days 5, 8, and 12 postovulation in mares that were pregnant on day 30 with those in mares that were not pregnant on day 30.[25] A greater number of mares that were nonpregnant had levels at day 12 less than 2.5 ng/mL compared with pregnant mares. A value of less than 2.5 ng/mL on day 12 was used as the critical value to identify mares that were considered to be exhibiting "luteal dysfunction." In a subsequent study by these same authors, 90 Thoroughbred mares sampled over 119 estrous cycles for concentrations of progesterone, displayed luteal dysfunction in 27 cycles. In addition, progesterone assays performed on blood samples from 32 mares, identified by clinicians as being subfertile, revealed 11 had luteal dysfunction (< 2.5 ng/mL) 12 days after ovulation. Controversy exists as to whether the CL is malfunctioning or if low concentrations of progesterone are caused by premature luteolysis as a result of endometrial irritants.[27,28] Thus whether because of luteal dysfunction or premature regression of the CL, low concentrations of progesterone is a cause of early embryonic loss. Other evidence for the role of ovarian progesterone in maintenance of pregnancy is the loss of pregnancy that occurs after ovariectomy. Removal of the mare's ovary during early gestation (prior to day 70) resulted in lowered concentrations of progesterone and loss of pregnancy.[29,30]

Unfortunately, controlled studies demonstrating the efficacy of exogenous progesterone for pregnancy maintenance in mares with a history of infertility are lacking. This is, in part, because of the difficulty of identifying and assembling large numbers of mares that habitually abort. Generally, the assay procedures for measuring concentrations of progesterone are too slow to be used as a screening procedure and mares are selected for progesterone therapy based on prior reproductive history. Enzyme assays or radioimmunoassay can, however, be used to monitor effects of exogenous progesterone on endogenous levels.[31] Therefore, most of the studies demonstrating the usefulness of exogenous progesterone/progestin for pregnancy maintenance have been with ovariectomized mares. In one study, workers ovariectomized 48 mares at 34 or 35 days of gestation and evaluated various dosages of progestin for their ability to maintain pregnancy. Mares were assigned to one of six groups: (1) controls, (2) 250 mg progesterone in oil every other day, (3) 500 mg repositol progesterone every 4 days, (4) 1000 mg repositol progesterone every 4 days, (5) 22 mg altrenogest daily, and (6) 44 mg altrenogest daily. Mares were treated from day 29 or 30 to day 100 unless abortion occurred. Maintenance of pregnancy in groups 1 through 6, respectively, were 0 of 8, 5 of 8, 1 of 8, 8 of 8, 7 of 8, and 7 of 8. Thus 500 mg of repositol was inadequate to maintain pregnancy, at least when given once every 4 days. Mean serum concentrations of progesterone for mares that maintained pregnancy consistently remained above 4 ng/mL after ovariectomy. Several other studies have demonstrated that ovariectomized mares administered 300 mg of progesterone[4,32] or 22 mg altrenogest[4,33] daily for 5 to 9 days will maintain pregnancy after embryo transfer. Progestin treatment is continued until day 100, the time at which secretion of progesterone from the placenta is adequate for pregnancy maintenance.[34] Generally, progestin therapy to either ovariectomized or intact pregnant mares is discontinued at the time of initial placenta progesterone production (day 100 to 120).

Currently, several schemes are used for exogenous progestin treatment of pregnant mares. Both injectable progesterone and altrenogest appear to be equally effective in maintaining pregnancy. A total of 14 of 20 ovariectomized embryo transfer recipients given 22 mg altrenogest maintained pregnancy compared with 14 of 20 pregnancies for recipients given 300 mg injectable progesterone daily.[4] Therefore, two recommended schemes are 0.044 mg/kg BW of altrenogest daily and 150 mg to 300 mg of injectable progesterone IM, daily. Generally, treatments are initiated 15 to 20 days after ovulation (first pregnancy exam) and continued until day 100 to 120. Mares suspected of early embryonic loss (before day 15) may benefit from treatments initiated 5 or 6 days after ovulation.[25] Clinicians often continue progestin supplementation longer in gestation, even in some cases to day 325. This is more than likely unnecessary. One alternative is to monitor serum progesterone and only continue progesterone supplementation in those mares with less than 4 ng/mL. This is more easily done when administering altrenogest, because its presence in the peripheral blood does not interfere with measurement of endogenous progesterone.[31]

Other indications for supplementation of progesterone include those mares under stress of colic[35] or transportation[36,37] and those under endotoxin influence.[38]

Apparently the effect of prolonged treatment of pregnant mares with injectable progesterone on reproductive performance of offspring has not been studied. However, administration of 44 mg of altrenogest to pregnant mares from day 20 to 325 of gestation had no significant effects on reproductive performance of fillies or stallions[39] or on subsequent reproductive performance of the dams.[40]

CONTRAINDICATIONS

The studies discussed previously on the safety of altrenogest for pregnant mares were based on reproductively normal, healthy young mares. The practitioner must be aware that no type of progestin should be administered to mares with a history of uterine infection. Washburn et al. observed that ovariectomized mares treated with progesterone had depressed phagocytic response.[41] Colbern et al. demonstrated that ovariectomized or intact mares exposed to intrauterine bacteria developed and maintained uterine infection as long as progesterone treatment was continued.[42] More recently, Alexander et al. conducted a study to determine the effect of progesterone treatment on susceptibility to uterine infection.[43] They selected 32 mares at a commercial stud farm as being transitional, and uterine swabs were taken for all mares before 16 mares were randomly selected for progesterone treatment (150 mg per day for 12 days). When mares exhibited estrus, a second swab was taken. All mares had "clean" uterine swabs before treatment. However, 56% of progesterone-treated mares returned bacteria-contaminated swabs, compared with 25% on controls. They concluded progesterone "can be detrimental to uterine health, particularly in older mares." However, based on other studies[14,15,17–20] and clinical findings, there is no evidence that progestin treatment for 12 to 15 days alters fertility of reproductively normal mares.

REFERENCES

1. Neely, D.P.: Progesterone/progestin therapy in the broodmare. Proc. Am. Assoc. Equine Pract., pp. 203–218, 1988.
2. Hawkins, D.L., Neely, D.P., and Stabenfeldt, G.H.: Plasma progesterone concentrations derived from the administration of exogenous progesterone to ovariectomized mares. J. Reprod. Fertil. Suppl., *27:*211–216, 1979.
3. Loy, R.G., Evans, M.J., Pemstein, R., and Taylor, T.B.: Effect of injected ovarian steroids on reproductive patterns and performance in postpartum mares. J. Reprod. Fertil. Suppl., *32:*199–204, 1982.
4. McKinnon, A.O., Squires, E.L., Carnevale, E.M., and Hermenet, M.S.: Ovariectomized steroid-treated mares as embryo transfer recipients and as a model to study the role of progestin in pregnancy maintenance. Theriogenology, *29:*1055–1063, 1988.
5. Lofstedt, R.M.: Some aspects of manipulation and diagnostic endocrinology of the broodmare. Proc. Soc. Theriogenol. pp. 67–72, 1986.
6. Loy, R.G., and Swan, S.M.: Effect of exogenous progestogens on reproductive phenomena in mares. J. Anim. Sci., *25:*821–879, 1966.
7. Arthur, G.H., and Allen, W.E.: Clinical observations on reproduction in a pony study. Equine Vet. J., *4:*109–117, 1972.
8. Neely, D.P.: Hormone therapy in mares. *In* Equine Reproduction. Edited by D. Neely, I.K.M. Liu, R.B. Hillman, and J.P. Hughes, Lawrenceville, NJ, Veterinary Learning Systems, 1983, p. 23.
9. Bristol, F.: Studies on estrous synchronization in mares. Proc. Soc. Theriogenology, 258–264, 1981.
10. Scheffrahn, N.S., et al.: Reproductive hormone secretions in pony mares subsequent to ovulation control during late winter. Theriogenology, *17:*571–585, 1982.
11. Palmer, E.: Recent attempts to improve synchronization of ovulation and to induce superovulation in the mare. Equine Vet. J. Suppl., *3:*11–18, 1985.
12. Wiepz, G.J., Squires, E.L., and Chapman, P.L.: Effects of norgestomet, altrenogest and/or estradiol on follicular and hormonal characteristics of late transitional mares. Theriogenology, *30:*181–193, 1988.
13. Silvia, P.J., Squires, E.L., and Nett, T.M.: Changes in the hypothalamic-hypophyseal axis of mares associated with seasonal reproductive recrudescence. Biol. Reprod., *35:*897–905, 1986.
14. Webel, S.K.: Estrous control in horses with a progestin. J. Anim. Sci., *41:*385, 1975.
15. Allen, W.R., et al.: Preliminary studies on the use of oral progestogen to induce oestrus and ovulation in seasonally anoestrous Thoroughbred mares. Equine Vet. J., *12:* 141–145, 1980.
16. Palmer, E.: Reproductive management of mares without detection of oestrus. J. Reprod. Fertil. Suppl., *27:* 263–270, 1979.
17. Squires, E.L., Stevens, W.B., McGlothlin, D.E., and Pickett, B.W.: Effect of an oral progestin on the estrous cycle and fertility of mares. J. Anim. Sci., *49:*729–735, 1979.
18. Webel, S.K., and Squires, E.L.: Control of the oestrous cy-

cle in mares with altrenogest. J. Reprod. Fertil. Suppl., *32:*193–198, 1982.

19. Squires, E.L., et al.: Relationship of altrenogest to ovarian activity, hormone concentrations and fertility of mares. J. Anim. Sci., *56:*901–910, 1983.
20. Squires, E.L., Shideler, R.K., Voss, J.L., and Webel, S.K.: Clinical applications of progestin in mares. Compend. Contin. Educ. Practicing Vet., *5:*516–522, 1983.
21. Loy, R.G., Pemstein, R., O'Canna, D., and Douglas, R.H.: Control of ovulation in cycling mares with ovarian steroids and prostaglandin. Theriogenology, *15:*191–200, 1981.
22. Taylor, T.B., Pemstein, R., and Loy, R.G.: Control of ovulation in mares in the early breeding season with ovarian steroids and prostaglandin. J. Reprod. Fertil. Suppl., *32:*219–224, 1982.
23. McKinnon, A.O., et al.: Ultrasonographic studies on the reproductive tract of postpartum mares: Effect of involution and uterine fluid on pregnancy rates in mares with normal and delayed first postpartum ovulatory cycles. J. Am. Vet. Med. Assoc., *192:*350–353, 1988.
24. Shideler, R.K., et al.: The effect of altrenogest, an oral progestin, on hematologic and biochemical parameters in mares. Vet. Hum. Toxicol., *25:*250–252, 1983.
25. Douglas, R.H., Burns, P.J., and Hershman, L.: Physiological and commercial parameters for producing progeny for subfertile mares by embryo transfer. Equine Vet. J. Suppl., *3:*111–114, 1985.
26. Ginther, O.J.: Embryonic loss in mares: Incidence, time of occurrence and hormonal involvement. Theriogenology, *23:*77–83, 1985.
27. Adams, G.P., Kastelic, J.P., Bergfelt, D.R., and Ginther, O.J.: Effect of uterine inflammation and ultrasonically-detected uterine pathology on fertility in the mare. J. Reprod. Fertil. Suppl., *35:*445–454, 1987.
28. McKinnon, A.O., et al.: Diagnostic ultrasonography of uterine pathology in the mare. Proc. Am. Assoc. Equine Pract., pp. 605–622, 1987.
29. Holtan, D.W., Squires, E.L., Lapin, D.R., and Ginther, O.J.: Effect of ovariectomy on pregnancy in mares. J. Reprod. Fertil. Suppl. *27:*457–463, 1979.
30. Shideler, R.K., et al.: Progestogen therapy of ovariectomized pregnant mares. J. Reprod. Fertil. Suppl., *32:*459–464, 1982.
31. Squires, E.L., Nett, T.M., Wiepz, G.J., and Mock, E.J.: Use of an enzyme assay for determination of progesterone in broodmares. Proc. Am. Assoc. Equine Pract., pp. 565–570, 1985.
32. Hinrichs, K., Sertich, P.L., Cummings, M.R., and Kenney, R.M.: Pregnancy in ovariectomized mares achieved by embryo transfer. Equine Vet. J. Suppl., *3:*74–75, 1985.
33. Parry-Weeks, L.C., and Holtan, D.W.: Effect of altrenogest on pregnancy maintenance in unsynchronized equine embryo recipients. J. Reprod. Fertil. Suppl., *35:*433–438, 1987.
34. Squires, E.L., and Ginther, O.J.: Collection technique and progesterone concentration of ovarian and uterine venous blood in mares. J. Anim. Sci., *40:*275–281, 1975.
35. Van Niekerk, C.H., and Morgenthal, J.C.: Fetal loss and stress on plasma progestogen levels in pregnant Thoroughbred mares. J. Reprod. Fertil. Suppl., *32:*453–457, 1982.
36. Baucus, K.L., et al.: Effect of transportation on early embryonic death in mares. J. Anim. Sci., *68:*345–351, 1990.
37. Baucus, K.L., et al.: Effect of transportation on the estrous cycle and concentrations of hormones in mares. J. Anim. Sci., *68:*419–426, 1990.
38. Daels, P.F., et al.: Effect of Salmonella typhimurium endotoxin on PFG-2 alpha release and fetal death in the mare. J. Reprod. Fertil. Suppl., *35:*485–492, 1987.
39. Squires, E.L., Shideler, R.K., and McKinnon, A.O.: Reproductive performance of offspring from mares administered altrenogest during gestation. J. Equine Vet. Sci., *9:*73–76, 1989.
40. Shoemaker, C.F., Squires, E.L., and Shideler, R.K.: Safety of altrenogest in pregnant mares and on health and development of offspring. J. Equine Vet. Sci., *9:*69–72, 1989.
41. Washburn, S.M., Klesius, P.H., Ganjam, V.K., and Brown, B.G.: Effect of estrogen and progesterone on the phagocytic response of ovariectomized mares infected in utero with B-hemolytic Streptococci. Am. J. Vet. Res., *43:*1367–1375, 1982.
42. Colbern, G.T., et al.: Development of a model to study endometritis in mares. J. Equine Vet. Sci., *7:*73–76, 1987.
43. Alexander, S.L., and Irvine, C.H.G.: Control of onset of breeding season in the mare and its artificial regulation by progesterone treatment. J. Reprod. Fertil. Suppl., *44:*307–319, 1991.

Prostaglandin $F_2\alpha$ ($PGF_2\alpha$) was first used to influence the estrous cycle of the mare by Douglas and Ginther in 1972.[1] A single injection of $PGF_2\alpha$ to diestrous mares caused rapid luteolysis and return to estrus in approximately 3 days. Because of the undesirable side effects of unmodified $PGF_2\alpha$, less toxic analogues were soon developed. The first such analogue to be widely used was fluprostenol, which was successful in inducing luteolysis in a number of situations in extensive field trials.[2,3] Subsequently several other analogues have been developed and used extensively. $PGF_2\alpha$ is probably the most widely used treatment for control of the cycle of the mare.

PHARMACOLOGIC MANIPULATION OF THE REPRODUCTIVE CYCLE

CHAPTER 34

PROSTAGLANDINS

C.H.G. Irvine

ADMINISTRATION

Early workers soon realized that the corpus luteum (CL) was not susceptible to $PGF_2\alpha$ until day 5 after ovulation, presumably because $PGF_2\alpha$ receptors which mediate its action are not present earlier.[4] However, after day 4, luteolysis can be induced in the mare with small doses of $PGF_2\alpha$, approximately 8 μg/kg compared with 144 μg/kg for the ewe.[5] Administration is equally effective by the intramuscular, intravenous, intrauterine, or intraluteal routes,[6] although the intramuscular route is usually used because of simplicity and less acute side effects. The equal effectiveness by any route of administration, as well as the small doses required, are probably caused by the slower peripheral degradation of $PGF_2\alpha$ in the tissues of the horse, especially in the lungs, which permits systemic distribution and recirculation.

Even when relatively nontoxic analogues are given by intramuscular injection some side effects such as sweating, diarrhea, or abdominal discomfort occur for up to 20 min in about 10% of horses. Intravenous injection often causes incoordination and dragging of the hind feet. Serious side effects are rare.

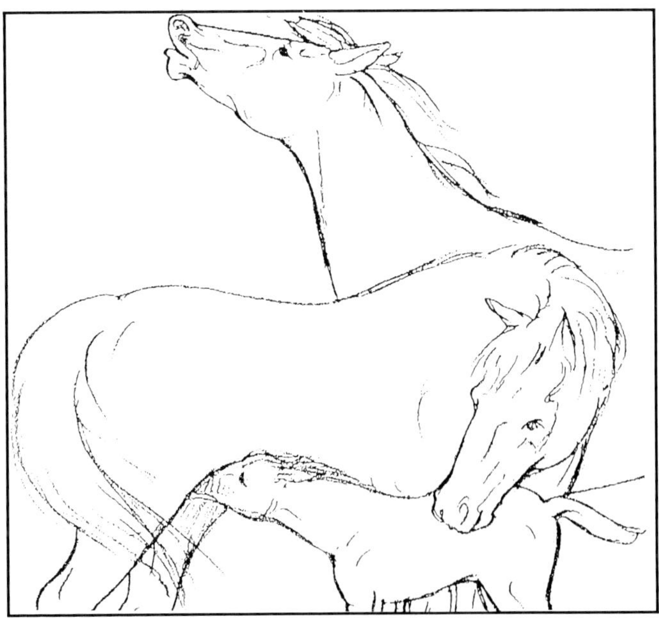

INDICATIONS

Listed below are some of the potentially useful applications of $PGF_2\alpha$ in manipulation of the mare's estrous cycle. Most of these depend on its luteolytic capabilities, although a direct effect on other tissues could play an important role, at least in some situations. These applications are (1) to terminate a persistent luteal state, (2) to ensure termination of the normal luteal phase, (3) to shorten the luteal phase, (4) to control the time of ovulation, (5) to induce gonadotropin secretion, and (6) to treat uterine infection.

TERMINATION OF A PERSISTENT LUTEAL STATE

A persistent luteal state (prolonged diestrus) may be caused by failure to lyse the CL. Luteolysis is caused by pulses of $PGF_2\alpha$ released by the nonpregnant uterus on days 13 to 15 after ovulation,[7] so failure of the endometrium to release adequate prostaglandin has been considered a possible cause of luteal persistence. While this is consistent with the frequent concurrence of prolonged luteal phase and endometritis, no causal link between them has been shown. Although persistence of a corpus luteum has been a widely accepted phenomenon[8] some recent work suggests that it is a rare event and that prolonged diestrus is most often the result of events described in the next section.[9]

Prolonged diestrus may be the result of luteinization, with or without preceding ovulation, of a diestrous follicle so that the new CL formed is 1 to 4 days old when the normal luteolytic episode of $PGF_2\alpha$ on day 13 to 15 of the original cycle occurs. Therefore, although the original CL is lysed, the new CL is refractory.[8] The decline in the plasma progesterone concentration may be so brief that estrus is not observed.[10] This may be a recurring event, leading to a prolonged period of diestrus.

Another cause of prolonged diestrus may be pseudopregnancy, as defined by Ginther, in which the physical and psychologic state of the mare mimics that of early pregnancy, but no fetus is present.[5]

Lactational mares occasionally exhibit prolonged diestrus after postpartum ovulation. It arises, presumably, from the causes described above and is responsive to $PGF_2\alpha$.[3] This should be distinguished from lactation-associated anestrus in which the ovaries are inactive and progesterone is low. The cause of lactation-associated anestrous is unclear, but the condition does not respond to $PGF_2\alpha$, nor does it appear to be the result of an elevated prolactin concentration.[11]

Irrespective of the cause of the persistent luteal state, $PGF_2\alpha$ is effective in lysing the CL in more than 80% of cases and in some reports over 98%.[12] Estrus appears in 2 to 3 days, provided follicles are present that are capable of generating estradiol. The interval to ovulation is highly variable, because it depends mainly on the stage of development of the largest follicle. Even when follicular development is active, a large follicle may have been arrested before the preovulatory stage. This is because luteal progesterone will have been slowing gonadotropin-releasing hormone (GnRH) pulse frequency and thus inhibiting the ovulatory luteinizing hormone (LH) surge (see Chapter 5 and Fig. 34-1). Luteolysis induced by exogenous $PGF_2\alpha$ at that time "removes the brakes" on the GnRH pulse generator, and the accelerated pulse frequency rapidly induces an LH surge, which may cause ovulation within 2 days. Estrus may be immediate and brief, occasionally so brief that it passes unobserved as a silent estrus;[10] the next observed estrus is after approximately 15 days, and ovulation is 21 days later. In one report, silent estrus occurred in over 50% of mares receiving $PGF_2\alpha$.[10] In about 33% of cases when a large follicle was present, it

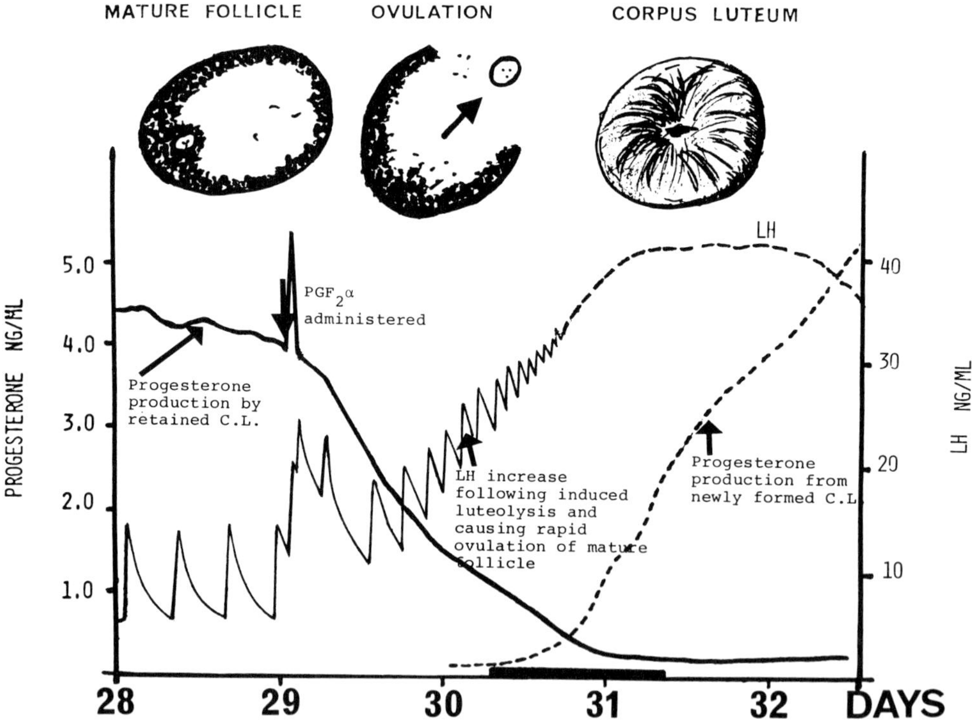

FIG. 34–1. Effects of administration of $PGF_2\alpha$ on a diestrous mare with a large follicle. Note LH pulse frequency of three per day typical of diestrus; an immediate, brief increase in LH caused by a direct effect effect of $PGF_2\alpha$ on the pituitary; and a delayed, prolonged increase in LH caused by the removal of the inhibitory effect of progesterone on the frequency of release of pulses of GnRH from the hypothalamus. The duration of estrus is represented by the black bar on the horizontal axis.

regressed and was replaced by another which ovulated approximately 9 days after treatment.[12] Conversely, if only small follicles are present when $PGF_2\alpha$ is given, follicular development and estrus may be prolonged and ovulation may occur in up to 10 days. Not surprisingly, during the anovulatory season, $PGF_2\alpha$ is usually ineffective in inducing estrus even though there may be luteal tissue present which is lysed by treatment.

The definition and cause of pseudopregnancy[5] is not firmly established. It is often associated with early embryonic death, after which a high plasma progesterone concentration is maintained for several weeks.[13] In pseudopregnancy, $PGF_2\alpha$ is likely to induce estrus followed by ovulation only if (1) the suspension of cyclicity has been caused by an active corpus luteum, (2) sufficient ovarian activity exists to generate an ovulatory follicle, and (3) the plasma concentration of a luteotropin is not so high that it antagonizes the luteolytic effects of $PGF_2\alpha$. In this regard, experiments have shown that in the ewe continuous infusion of ovine LH prevents luteolysis by endogenous $PGF_2\alpha$,[14] whereas administration of $PGF_2\alpha$ suppresses induction of progesterone secretion by the CL.[15] This reciprocal physiologic antagonism between $PGF_2\alpha$ and luteotropic hormones has been investigated by several groups. Their findings will be discussed in some detail, because they are of considerable practical relevance to reinitiation of cyclicity by $PGF_2\alpha$ following early embryonic death or induced abortion.

When a single dose of $PGF_2\alpha$ was given on day 32 of pregnancy all of 4 mares aborted, but only 2 returned to estrus and ovulated.[16] On day 35 of pregnancy, a single dose was sufficient to induce luteolysis, abortion, estrus, and ovulation in 7 of 8 mares.[17] All 5 mares given daily injections for 3 days commencing on day 42 underwent luteolysis, abortion, and an apparently normal ovulatory estrus but failed to conceive.[18] Abortion was induced by a single injection of $PGF_2\alpha$ in 4 of 6 mares between days 40 and 60 and in 2 of 4 mares on days 70 to 90.[19] In later work, single injections at day 70 were ineffective in all 8 mares, and although once or twice daily injections for 4 days induced abortion in all 16 mares, plasma progesterone levels did not fall below 1.4 ng/mL, and folliculogenesis was arrested.[17]

Because pregnancy is maintained in approximately 60% of mares ovariectomized at day 70,[20] luteolysis would not likely be the cause of the 100% abortion rate; the direct abortifacient effect of $PGF_2\alpha$ on the uterus probably plays a major role at that time. In all the above experiments, equine chorionic gonadotropin (eCG) secretion continued to increase to a normal peak around day 60; eCG is strongly luteotropic[21] and can induce final follicular maturation, ovulation, and corpus luteum establishment. When the plasma eCG concentration attains day-42 levels or higher, repeated injections of $PGF_2\alpha$ are required to induce luteolysis. Also such eCG concentrations, or the mechanism that generates them, interfere with subsequent conception or early pregnancy. If human chorionic gonadotropin (hCG) is administered repeatedly to pregnant mares before eCG reaches readily detectible levels, pregnancy is terminated;[22] this suggests that a continuous high level of occupancy of LH receptors by either eCG or hCG in early pregnancy is prejudicial.

TERMINATION OF A NORMAL LUTEAL PHASE

Common stud practice is to examine mares for pregnancy with ultrasonography on days 15 to 18 after ovulation. Although most nonpregnant mares will return to estrus soon after this time, the administration of $PGF_2\alpha$ as soon as a mare has been found to be nonpregnant ensures that it will come into estrus soon enough to be mated without missing a cycle, i.e., approximately 22 days after the previous ovulation. This procedure also ensures mating of nonpregnant mares that develop preovulatory follicles a little earlier than expected. This procedure is worthwhile late in the season and especially in breeds in which studbook authorities adopt a calendar which imposes a short breeding season.

SHORTENING THE LUTEAL PHASE

If for some reason a mare is not mated at a normal ovulation, the clinician may want to shorten the time to the next ovulation, particularly if it is near the end of the breeding season. Administration of $PGF_2\alpha$ on day 5 after ovulation will usually shorten the luteal phase considerably.

In many mares the reproductive tract is often in an unsuitable state for establishment of pregnancy at the time of the first postpartum ovulation at approximately 10 days. For this reason, many breeding farms do not mate mares until the second postpartum estrus approximately 31 days after parturition. If conception occurs at this ovulation, because of the 11-month plus 1-week gestation of the mare, the interval between foalings is likely to exceed 12 months. As a compromise, administration of $PGF_2\alpha$ during the first diestrus, i.e., at approximately 17 days postpartum, was introduced by Tolksdorff et al. in 1976 and has become widely practiced.[23] The relative merits of mating at the postpartum estrus, at a shortened second cycle, or at a normal second cycle have been widely debated without any consensus being reached, and the type of breeding operation apparently determines which method is most appropriate. In the author's experience at a stud in which foaling problems were rare and antibiotic-treated semen could be used, conception rates at the first postpartum estrus were as high as at any other time.[24] In any event, provided some selection of mares is made on the basis of uterine health, little or no benefit exists in postponing the first mating until a $PGF_2\alpha$-induced estrus at around 20 days postpartum (see Chapter 73 for a discussion on postpartum breeding strategies).

CONTROLLING THE TIME OF OVULATION

Control of ovulation could be useful for "appointment breeding," for synchronization, or as an alternative to hCG in advancing the time of ovulation. For reasons stated above, $PGF_2\alpha$ is much less successful in controlling the time of ovulation in the mare than in other species. While $PGF_2\alpha$ can terminate the luteal phase, it has not been shown to affect the uniquely long and variable follicular phase. A second injection of $PGF_2\alpha$ can improve control, although alternative treatments such as hCG and GnRH that directly affect follicular maturation are preferred. However, protocols employing $PGF_2\alpha$ for appointment breeding have been described.[25]

Synchronization of ovulation has much more limited application in horses than in other species. Also, although some complex protocols have been used, a useful degree of synchronization using $PGF_2\alpha$ alone is proving much more difficult to achieve[26] (see Chapters 38 and 39).

As an alternative to hCG in shortening the time to ovulation, $PGF_2\alpha$ analogue given 60 h after the onset of estrus induced ovulation in 81% of mares compared with 31% of controls;[27] conversely, a thesis report states that a $PGF_2\alpha$ analogue given on days 2 or 3 of estrus has no effect on interval to ovulation.[28] Responses were apparently not the result of direct or indirect stimulation of LH release, because LH concentrations did not differ from controls when $PGF_2\alpha$ was given 48 h after the onset of estrus.[29] This result differs from the marked increase in LH shown when anestrous or diestrous mares are injected with $PGF_2\alpha$ (see the next section).

INDUCTION OF GONADOTROPIN SECRETION

The administration of $PGF_2\alpha$ to diestrous mares is followed by an increase in LH.[30] Increased secretion of LH after $PGF_2\alpha$ has been attributed to a direct effect of $PGF_2\alpha$ on GnRH secretion[31] or indirectly via progesterone withdrawal, which permits an increase in GnRH pulse frequency.[32] However, experiments have shown that in transitional-phase mares in which progesterone is low, $PGF_2\alpha$ analogue administration induced immediate secretion of FSH and LH, although GnRH was elevated consistently only after FSH and LH had reached peak levels (Fig. 34–2).[33] Similarly, in diestrous mares, intravenous $PGF_2\alpha$ analogue caused an immediate marked increase in FSH and LH secretion, which lasted 1 to 2 h and was not associated with any increase in GnRH (Fig. 34–3). Again, that effect is not likely to be caused by progesterone removal because gonadotropins and progesterone rose concurrently for the first 30 min after $PGF_2\alpha$, before progesterone started to decline. Therefore, in diestrous and transitional mares, $PGF_2\alpha$ appears directly to stimulate gonadotropin secretion. This may be the basis of the successful induction by $PGF_2\alpha$ of estrus and fertile ovulation in acyclic mares showing baseline progesterone levels.[33]

TREATMENT OF UTERINE INFECTIONS

Infections of the uterus are a major cause of infertility in mares. Research has shown that progesterone predisposes the uterus to infection by constricting the cervix and inhibiting uterine contractions whereas estradiol has the opposite effect on the uterus and also stimulates the local immune system.[34] Administration of $PGF_2\alpha$ to diestrous mares lowers progesterone allowing LH and thus estradiol to increase. Furthermore, $PGF_2\alpha$ has a direct effect on the myometrium, where it induces high amplitude contractions.[35] This effect on uterine drainage does not solely depend on release from progesterone inhibition, because it occurs in ovariectomized[35] and anestrous[34] mares. Because clearance of bacteria, toxins, and debris is an important aspect of the first-line defence against infection, the administration of two or three injections of $PGF_2\alpha$ at 4-day intervals ensures that the hormonal environment is optimum for control of infection.

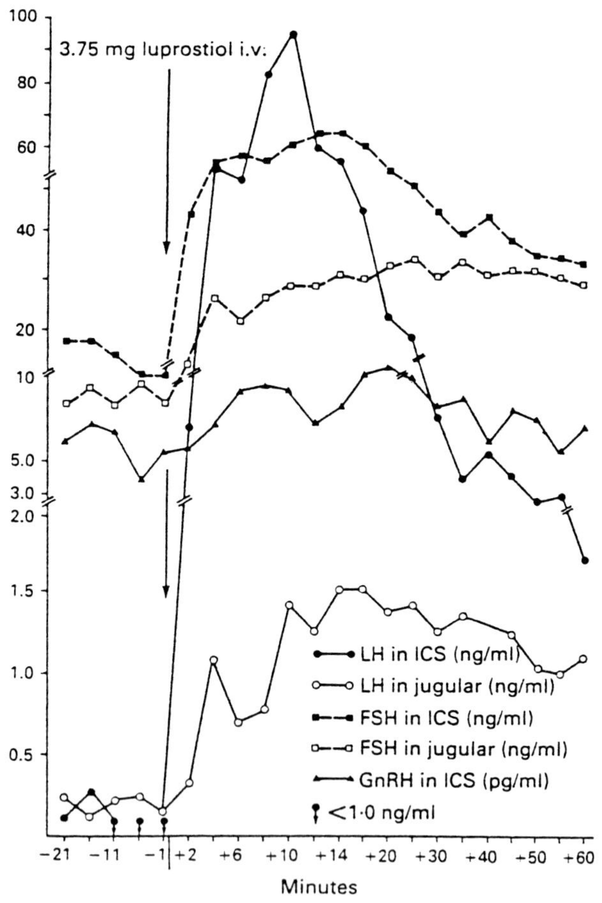

FIG. 34–2. Effects of treatment with 3.75 mg luprositol IV on LH, FSH, and GnRH concentrations in pituitary venous blood (ICS) and in the jugular vein of a mare in the transition phase. (From Jochle, W., Irvine, C.H.G., Alexander, S.L., and Newby, T.J.: Release of LH, FSH, and GnRH into pituitary venous blood in mares treated with the PGF analogue, luprositol during the transition period. J. Reprod. Fertil. Suppl., *35*:327–334, 1987.)

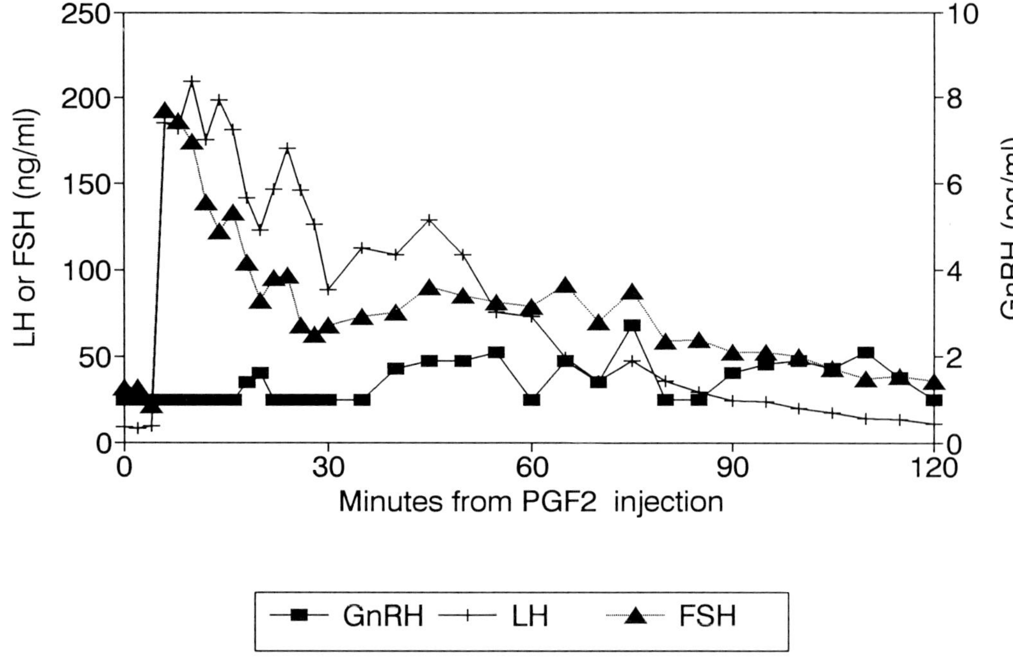

FIG. 34–3. Effects of treatment with 0.25 mg cloprostenol IM on LH, FSH, and GnRH concentrations in pituitary venous blood (ICS) of a mare in early diestrus.

RESULTS OF PGF$_2\alpha$ THERAPY

The major indication for PGF$_2\alpha$ treatment, luteolysis, is accomplished in more than 80% of cases. Reasons for failure of luteolysis are not clear, although some explanations are advanced for failure to induce estrus and ovulation. The estrus and ovulation which follow are normal, as are conception rates. Dose rates vary according to the preparation. Serious side effects are rare, if the agent is used in accordance with the manufacturers' recommendations.

REFERENCES

1. Douglas, R.H., and Ginther, O.J.: Effect of prostaglandin F$_2\alpha$ on length of diestrus in mares. Prostaglandins, *2:*265–268, 1972.
2. Allen, W.R., et al.: Further studies on the use of synthetic prostaglandin analogues for inducing luteolysis in mares. Equine Vet. J., *6:*31–35, 1974.
3. Berwyn-Jones, M.W., and Irvine, C.H.G.: Induction of luteolysis and oestrus in mares with a synthetic prostaglandin analogue (ICI 81008). N. Z. Vet. J., *22:*107–110, 1974.
4. Hafs, H.D., Louis, T.M., Noden, P.A., and Oxender, W.D.: Control of the estrous cycle with prostaglandin F$_2\alpha$ in cattle and horses. J. Anim. Sci. Suppl. 1, *38:*10, 1974.
5. Ginther, O.J.: Reproductive Biology of the Mare—Basic and Applied Aspects. Cross Plains, WI, published by the author, 1979.
6. Douglas, R.H., and Ginther, O.J.: Route of prostaglandin F$_2\alpha$ injection and luteolysis in mares. Proc. Soc. Exp. Biol. Med., *148:*263–269, 1975.
7. Neely, D.P., et al.: Prostaglandin release patterns in the mare: Physiological, pathophysiological and therapeutic responses. J. Reprod. Fertil. Suppl., *27:*181–189, 1979.
8. Stabenfeldt, G.H., Hughes, J.P., Evans, J.W., and Neely, D.P.: Spontaneous prolongation of luteal activity in the mare. Equine Vet. J., *6:*158–163, 1974.
9. Ginther, O.J., and Pierson, R.A.: Regular and irregular characteristics of ovulation and the interovulatory interval in mares. J. Equine Vet. Sci., *9:*4–12, 1989.
10. Nelson, E.M., Kiefer, B.L., Roser, J.F., and Evans, J.W.: Serum estradiol-17 concentrations during spontaneous silent estrus and after prostaglandin treatment in the mare. Theriogenology, *23:*241–250, 1985.
11. Neuschaefer, A., Bracher, V., and Allen, W.R.: Prolactin secretion in lactating mares before and after treatment with bromocryptine. J. Reprod. Fertil. Suppl., *44:*551–559, 1991.
12. Loy, R.G., Buell, J.R., Stevenson, W., and Hamm, D.: Sources of variation in response intervals after prostaglandin treatment in mares with functional corpora lutea. J. Reprod. Fertil. Suppl., *27:*229–235, 1979.
13. Irvine, C.H.G., Sutton, P., Turner, J.E., and Mennick, P.E.: Changes in plasma progesterone concentrations from days 17 to 42 of gestation in mares maintaining or losing pregnancy. Equine Vet. J., *22:*104–106, 1990.
14. Karsch, F.J., et al.: Maintenance of corpus luteum of the ewe by continuous infusion of LH. Biol. Reprod., *4:*129–136, 1971.
15. Behrman, H.R.: Prostaglandins in hypothalamo-pituitary and ovarian function, Ann. Rev. Physiol., *41:*687–700, 1979.
16. Kooistra, L., and Ginther, O.J.: Termination of pseudopregnancy by administration of prostaglandin F$_2$ and termination of early pregnancy by administration of prostaglandin F$_2$ or colchicine or by removal of embryos in mares. Am. J. Vet. Res., *37:*35–39, 1976.
17. Squires, E.L., Hillman, R.B., Pickett, B.W., and Nett,

T.M.: Induction of abortion in mares with Equimate: Effect of secretion of progesterone, PMSG and reproductive performance. J. Anim. Sci., *50:*490–495, 1980.

18. Rathwell, A.C., Asbury, A.C., Hansen, P.J., and Archbald, L.F.: Reproductive function of mares given PGF_2 daily from day 42 of pregnancy. J. Reprod. Fertil. Suppl., *35:*507–508, 1987.

19. Douglas, R.H., Squires, E.L., and Ginther, O.J.: Induction of abortion in mares with prostaglandin F_2. J. Anim. Sci., *39:*404–407, 1974.

20. Holtan, D.W., Squires, E.L., and Ginther, O.J.: Effect of ovariectomy on pregnancy in mares. J. Anim. Sci., *41:*359–360, 1975.

21. Bergfeldt, D.R., Pierson, R.A., and Ginther, O.J.: Resurgence of the corpus luteum during pregnancy in the mare. Anim. Reprod. Sci., *21:*261–270, 1989.

22. Allen, W.E.: Pregnancy failure induced by human chorionic gonadotrophin in pony mares. Vet. Rec., *96:*88–90, 1975.

23. Tolksdorff, E., et al.: Induction of ovulation during the postpartum period in the Thoroughbred mare with a prostaglandin analogue, Synchrocept(TM). Theriogenology, *6:*403–412, 1976.

24. Burns, S.J., Irvine, C.H.G., and Amoss, M.S.: Fertility of a prostaglandin-induced oestrus compared to normal postpartum oestrus. J. Reprod. Fertil., Suppl., *27:*245–250, 1979.

25. Squires, E.L., et al.: The effectiveness of PGF_2, hCG and GnRH for appointment breeding of mares. J. Equine. Vet. Sci., *1:*57–64, 1981.

26. Palmer, E., and Jousset, B.: Synchronization of oestrus and ovulation in the mare with a two PG-HCG sequences treatment. Ann. Biol. Anim. Biochim. Biophys., *15:* 471–480, 1975.

27. Savage, N.C., and Liptrap, R.M.: Induction of ovulation in cyclic mares by administration of a synthetic prostaglandin, fenprostalene, during oestrus. J. Reprod. Fertil. Suppl., *35:*239–243, 1987.

28. Hackmann, F.: Effect of PGF_2 analogue and palpation of clinically important parameters of reproduction in the mare. Masters' Thesis, Tierarztliche Hochschule Hannover, 1982.

29. Crickman, J.A., Momont, H.W., and Al-Hassam, M.J.: Plasma LH concentrations in the mare following administration of alfaprostol during oestrus. J. Reprod. Fertil. Suppl., *44:*686–688, 1991.

30. Noden, P.A., Oxender, W.D., and Hafs, H.D.: Early changes in serum progesterone, estradiol and LH during prostaglandin F_2 induced luteolysis in mares. J. Anim. Sci., *47:*666–671, 1978.

31. Haynes, N.B., Kiset, T.E., Hafs, H., and Marks, J.D.: Prostaglandin $F_2\alpha$ overcomes blockade of episodic LH secretion with testosterone, melenestrol acetate or aspirin in bulls. Biol. Reprod., *17:*723–728, 1977.

32. Leipheimer, R.E., Bona-Gallo, A., and Gallo, R.V.: Ovarian steroid regulation of basal pulsatile LH release between the morning of proestrus and estrus in the rat. Endocrinology, *118:*2083–2090, 1986.

33. Jochle, W., Irvine, C.H.G., Alexander, S.L., and Newby, T.J.: Release of LH, FSH and GnRH into pituitary venous blood in mares treated with the PGF analogue, luprositol during the transition period. J. Reprod. Fertil. Suppl., *38:*261–267, 1987.

34. Evans, M.J., Hamer, J.M., Gason, L.M., and Irvine, C.H.G.: Factors affecting uterine clearance of inoculated materials in mares. J. Reprod. Fertil. Suppl., *35:*327–334, 1987.

35. Capraro, D.L., Vernon, M.W., Abrams, R.M., and Sharp, D.C.: Effects of oxytocin and $PGF_2\alpha$ on mare uterine motility. J. Anim. Sci., *43:*277, 1976.

PHARMACOLOGIC MANIPULATION OF THE REPRODUCTIVE CYCLE

CHAPTER 35

HUMAN CHORIONIC GONADOTROPIN

J.L. Voss

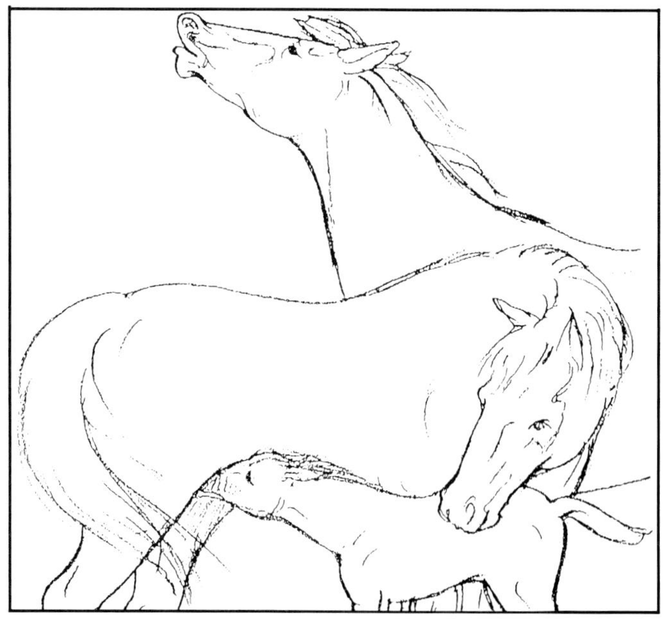

Human chorionic gonadotropin (hCG) is a protein consisting of two peptide chains containing galactose and hexosamine with a molecular weight of 30,000 and a half-life of 8 to 12 h.[1] The hormone is chemically different from pituitary luteinizing hormone (LH) but its biologic activity is primarily LH-like with some effects similar to those caused by follicle-stimulating hormone (FSH). The hormone is produced by cytotrophoblasts of the chorionic villi of the human placenta. It appears in the urine a few weeks after conception and reaches a peak at approximately 50 days of pregnancy and decreases thereafter to negligible quantities.[1]

When injected into mares, hCG has been shown to reduce the duration of estrus and increase the number of ovulations occurring within 48 h after injection.[2–11] The hormone is widely used by equine practitioners in management schemes to decrease the number of inseminations or matings per estrus and to synchronize more closely ovulation with mating or insemination. Synchronization of ovulation is more predictable when hCG is given after a follicle reaches 30 to 35 mm in diameter. Rcsults are less predictable during the transitional period[11] or in the presence of an atretic, regressing follicle.

SYNCHRONIZATION OF OVULATION

The use of gonadotropic hormones to induce ovulation in mares was first reported by Day in 1939.[2] From that beginning, the use of hCG as an ovulatory agent has been widely investigated and is used frequently in clinical practice. The dose to induce ovulation varies from 1500 to 4000 IU given intravenously or intramuscularly.

To assist synchronization schemes, hCG is frequently used in combination with luteolytic agents or products that stimulate follicular activity such as gonadotropin-releasing hormone (GnRH) and its analogues (see Chapters 38 and 39 for a detailed discussion of synchronization schemes). Although seasonally acyclic mares can be induced to develop preovulatory follicles by twice-daily administration of a crude pituitary extract containing equine FSH and LH, hCG alone is ineffective.[12] Therefore, timing of the administration of hCG in relation to follicular development is important. To determine time of ovulation more accurately, it is recommended that hCG be given when a follicle in excess of 30 mm in diameter is detected either by palpation or ultrasonography. The use of ultrasonography, along with clinical signs of estrus, provides an excellent management procedure to help determine when in the cycle to administer hCG.[13] When hCG is given to mares early in estrus (days 1, 2, or 3), it generally provides less predictable (lower percentage) synchronization of ovulation within a prescribed time.

Timing of mating or insemination with ovulation is important to conception. Pace and Sullivan demonstrated that fertilization rate was highest in mares inseminated with frozen semen within 12 h of ovulation.[14] Woods et al. reported that pregnancy rates were highest when mares were inseminated from 3 days before ovulation to 6 h after ovulation with no pregnancies occurring in mares inseminated after 30 h or more from ovulation.[15] A progressive decrease in pregnancy rates was noted until 30 h postovulation. They also observed a higher percentage of mares undergoing early embryonic death when inseminated more than 6 h after ovulation.

There are conflicting reports on the efficiency of postovulatory mating or insemination. The success of postovulatory insemination or mating obviously depends on the life span of the ovum and spermatozoa within the female tract. Thus the use of hCG in breeding programs can have a significant effect on reproductive efficiency. Numerous researchers have shown or suggested satisfactory fertility in mares bred or inseminated after ovulation.[14–21] In contrast, others have reported low or decreased pregnancy rates when mares were bred or inseminated after ovulation.[15,22–27]

Although many reports suggest hCG administration enhances fertility,[2,5,28] other evidence indicates that fertility is not enhanced in normally cycling mares or when ovulation is induced by hCG in synchronized mares.[8,9,15,29–35]

Synchronization of ovulation obviously has many advantages in a breeding program. Because ovulation can be predetermined, mares can be mated at a more precise time, perhaps increasing their chances of becoming pregnant and experiencing lower embryonic loss. This would be particularly of value in managing heavily booked stallions and stallions entered in athletic or show events and in the timing of shipping frozen or extended semen. The number of matings per mare in a natural breeding program can be reduced, minimizing the number of repeat breedings for nonovulating mares and increasing the book of valuable stallions.

REDUCING DURATION OF ESTRUS

Administration of hCG has been shown to reduce the duration of estrus in normally cycling mares.[5,8,9] Other workers have shown that hCG did not reduce duration of estrus when given later in the year (natural breeding season) when the follicular phase of the estrous cycle is shortest.[35–37] Another study found variation in duration of estrus and hCG treatment.[11] A shorter duration of estrus has also been reported when hCG was used in conjunction with prostaglandins or one of its synthetic analogues or other ovulation-synchronizing agents.[30,31,34,38]

After hCG administration and ovulation, a corpus luteum (CL) should form and the mares should go out of estrus sooner than untreated mares. Duration can be shortened 2 to 4 days with this management procedure. Less effect on duration of estrus will be noted the later during estrus that hCG is administered. Although a lower percentage of mares might respond early in the season, those that do might have more cycles per year and fewer matings or inseminations, and require less palpation and ultrasonography. Consequently, more mares could be bred to a given stallion. One report indicated that mares treated with hCG on their first cycle, but that failed to settle, became pregnant at a higher rate (without hCG treatment) during cycles two and three than did untreated mares.[9] It was speculated that the administration of hCG during the previous cycle may have helped establish better hormonal relationships for subsequent cycles.

EFFECT OF HCG ON CORPUS LUTEUM DEVELOPMENT AND PROGESTERONE PRODUCTION

It has been questioned whether hCG administration would establish a CL that would produce more progesterone and consequently maintain a higher percentage of pregnancies than untreated mares. Kelly et al. dispersed horse luteal cells to determine the effect of hCG on progesterone secretion in vitro.[39] In those luteal cells, equine LH and hCG stimulated progesterone production at all levels of treatment; hCG caused greater progesterone secretion than horse LH over the range of concentrations used. When seven mares received an intramuscular injection of 1000 IU of hCG on days 3, 4, and 5 after the end of estrus, there was an increase in peripheral progesterone concentrations beginning on day 7 and continuing until day 14 compared with untreated control mares.[39] The authors concluded that the mare CL was responsive to gonadotropins in vitro and that exogenous hCG can enhance serum progesterone concentrations throughout the estrous cycle and early pregnancy. Carnevale et al. found that hCG did not affect formation or function of the CL in mares in early transition.[40] However, hCG was not given until a follicle of 40 mm or larger was identified by ultrasonography and time to ovulation was decreased. Watson and Hinrichs aspirated preovulatory follicles of mares when the follicle grew to 32 to 34 mm in diameter.[41] They found that when the preovulatory follicle reached 35 mm in diameter in mares receiving hCG and follicular fluid was aspirated 28 to 32 h after treatment progesterone concentrations were significantly higher in follicular fluid from treated than in untreated mares. Michel et al. reported that 81.5% of mares injected with hCG showed increases (1 ng/mL) of progesterone by 72 h after injection compared with 65% for mares injected with GnRH or saline.[28] Synchronization of insemination or mating with ovulation may be more significant regarding pregnancy and fetal wastage than attempts to improve the function of the CL by increasing progesterone concentrations. Time of fertilization after ovulation may have a greater effect on embryonic loss.[15]

Allen reported that pregnant pony mares receiving hCG injections (2000 IU) had a reduction of peripheral progesterone concentrations.[42] He later reported that when pregnant pony mares were each given a series of three intravenous injections of 2000 IU of hCG on alternate days before day 39 of pregnancy, conceptual loss occurred.[43] Pregnant mares that received progesterone before or simultaneously with hCG maintained their pregnancies after hCG injection, but blood progestagen concentrations fell, suggesting partial lysis of the CL occurred.[44] After day 38 of gestation, repeated doses of hCG had no effect on plasma progestagen concentrations. Consequently, hCG may be contraindicated to mares during the first 38 days of gestation because of potential luteolysis.

ANTIBODY FORMATION

Because hCG is a protein, its administration will stimulate production of hCG antibody. Sullivan et al. were the first to suspect a potentially detrimental antibody problem in a study in which mares were given successive doses of hCG on each of three cycles.[8] A higher percentage of mares ovulated within 24 to 48 h and estrus was shortened during cycle 1. However, on cycle 2, no effect of hCG was noted, and by cycle 3, a reversal of the expected effects of hCG was reported. Although antibodies to hCG were not determined, it was theorized that anti-hCG antibody could have been responsible for this observation. Other researchers injected 12 mares with hCG on the appearance of a palpable 35-mm follicle during estrus on each cycle during the natural breeding season (March through October).[45] A total of 5 of the 12 mares developed significant levels of antibodies to hCG after two to five injections. The half-life of antibodies in individual mares ranged from 30 days to several months. However, in vivo antibodies to hCG did not cause ovulatory refractiveness and it was calculated that the total amount of antibody in any one mare could precipitate approximately 2 to 10 times the amount of hCG injected per cycle. Cross-reactivity of antibodies to equine chorionic gonadotropin (eCG) and endogenous LH seemed improbable. In another study using 30 reproductively sound mares over a 2-yr period, repeated injections of hCG over five successive cycles resulted in significant concentrations of anti-hCG antibodies in all treated mares after one to three injections.[46] However, no correlation was observed between magnitude of the immune response and duration of ovulation time or pregnancy rate. Mares continued to ovulate, conceive, and foal in the presence of significant concentrations of anti-hCG antibodies. No significant binding of anti-hCG antibodies to either eLH or eCG in vitro occurred. Furthermore, in that study, an inconsistent response to hCG in treated mares existed, regarding duration of estrus, duration of ovulation time, and number of inseminations per cycle.

Others found that mares immunized against hCG did not respond by ovulating within a prescribed time.[10] They tried to reduce the immune response to repeated injections of hCG by giving corticosteroids at the same time. However, the immune response could not be blocked by injection of the corticosteroids. Because of its immunogenicity, it has been suggested that no more than two injections be given during the same breeding season (see Chapter 38).

CONCLUSIONS

Human chorionic gonadotropin is a valuable armament to control the mare's estrous cycle pharmacologically. It is extremely valuable in synchronizing ovulation with mating and/or insemination. However, for its most dramatic effect in this regard, it should be given on day 2 or 3 of estrus after the development of a 30- to 35-mm follicle has been identified either by rectal palpation or, more preferably, by ultrasonography. When given early in the cycle or season, it may reduce the duration of estrus, and although a higher percentage of mares will ovulate in a prescribed time, the results are variable (see Chapters 38 and 39 for more detail). Because ovulation can be synchronized and the duration of estrus shortened, management programs can be developed to result in fewer matings or inseminations per cycle, less palpation and ultrasonography, breeding more mares to a given stallion, synchronizing shipment of frozen or diluted semen to mares, increasing the number of mares to a stallion's book, allowing use of a stallion for breeding that is entered in shows or athletic events, reducing costs of teasing, palpation and ultrasonography, and other management procedures.

REFERENCES

1. McDonald, L.E.: Hormones of the pituitary gland. *In* Veterinary Pharmacology and Therapeutics. 6th ed. Edited by N.H. Booth and L.E. McDonald. Ames, Iowa State University Press, 1988, pp. 590.
2. Day, F.T.: Ovulation and decent of the ovum in the fallopian tube of the mare after treatment with gonadotropic hormones. J. Agric. Sci. Camb., *29:*459–469, 1939.
3. Mirskaja, L.M., and Petropavlovskii, V.V.: The reduction of normal duration of heat in the mare by the administration of prolan. Probl. Zivotn., *4:*22–29, 1937.
4. Davisson, W.F.: The control of ovulation in the mare with reference to insemination with stored sperm. J. Agric. Sci., *37:*287–290, 1947.
5. Loy, R.G., and Hughes, J.P.: The effects of human chorionic gonadotropin on ovulation, length of estrus and fertility in the mare. Cornell Vet., *56:*41–50, 1966.
6. Ginther, O.J., Whitmore, H.L., and Squires, E.L.: Characteristics of estrus, diestrus and ovulation in mares and effects of season and nursing. Am. J. Vet. Res., *33:*1935–1939, 1972.
7. Nishikawa, Y., Kuroda, N., and Yamazaki, Y.: Studies on artificial induction of ovulation in mares. II. Effects of increased doses of prolan and copper sulfate. *In* Studies on Reproduction in Horses. Tokyo, Japan Racing Association, 1959, pp. 181–186.
8. Sullivan, J.J., Parker, W.G., and Larson, L.L.: Duration of estrus and ovulation time in nonlactating mares given human chorionic gonadotropin during three successive estrous periods. J. Am. Vet. Med. Assoc., *162:*895–898, 1973.
9. Voss, J.L., Pickett, B.W., Burwash, L.D., and Daniels, W.H.: Effect of human chorionic gonadotropin on duration of estrous cycle and fertility of normally cycling, nonlactating mares. J. Am. Vet. Med. Assoc., *165:*704–706, 1974.

10. Duchamp, G., Bour, B., Combarnous, Y., and Palmer, E.: Alternative solutions to hCG induction of ovulation in the mare. J. Reprod. Fertil. Suppl., *35:*221–228, 1987.
11. Webel, S.K., Franklin, V., Harland, B., and Dziuk, P.J.: Fertility, ovulation and maturation of eggs in mares injected with HCG. J. Reprod. Fertil., *51:*337–341, 1977.
12. Lappin, D.R., and Ginther, O.J.: Induction of ovulation and multiple ovulations in seasonally anovulatory and ovulatory mares with an equine pituitary extract. J. Anim. Sci., *44:*834–842, 1977.
13. McKinnon, A.O., Squires, E.L., and Pickett, B.W.: Equine reproductive ultrasonography. Animal Reproduction Laboratory Bulletin No. 04. Fort Collins, Colorado State University, 1988, pp. 41–49.
14. Pace, M.M., and Sullivan, J.J.: Effect of timing of insemination, numbers of spermatozoa and extender components on the pregnancy rate in mares inseminated with frozen stallion semen. J. Reprod. Fertil. Suppl., *23:*115–121, 1975.
15. Woods, J., Bergfelt, D.R., and Ginther, O.J.: Effects of time of insemination relative to ovulation on pregnancy rate and embryonic-loss rate in mares. Equine Vet. J., *22:*410–415, 1990.
16. Saltzman, A.A.: Insemination of mares after ovulation. Anim. Breed., *8:*16, 1940.
17. Cheng, P.L.: The present situation of artificial insemination of horses in China and some investigations on increasing conception rate of mare and breeding efficiency of stallion. Acta Vet. Zoo. Tech. Seneca, *5:*29–34, 1962.
18. Hughes, J.P., and Loy, R.G.: Artificial insemination in the equine. Cornell Vet., *60:*463–475, 1970.
19. Aliev, A., and Ochkin, D.: The optimum time of insemination. Anim. Breed. *47:*5273, 1979.
20. Allen, W.E.: Fertility in pony mares after post ovulation service. Equine Vet. J., *13:*134–135, 1981.
21. Belling, T.H., Jr.: Post ovulation breeding and related reproductive phenomena in the mare. Equine Pract., *6:*12–19, 1984.
22. Kamhi, S., and Varadin, M.: Time of breeding and ovulation in relationship with conception rate in mares. Proceedings of the International Congress on Animal Reproduction and Artificial Insemination, 1964, pp. 274–277.
23. Katila, T., Koskinen, E., Kuntsi, H., and Lindberg, H.: Fertility after post ovulatory insemination in mares. Proceedings of the International Congress on Animal Reproduction and Artificial Insemination, 1988, p. 96.
24. Cristanelli, M.J., Squires, E.L., Amann, R.P., and Pickett, B.W.: Fertility of stallion semen processed, frozen and thawed by a new procedure. Theriogenology, *22:*39–45, 1983.
25. Salazar-Valencia, F.: Embryo recovery rates in mares of the Pasofino Colombiano breed and deep freezing stallion semen in the tropics. Theriogenology, *19:*146, 1983.
26. Kloppe, L.H., et al.: Effect of insemination timing on the fertilizing capacity of frozen/thawed equine spermatozoa. Theriogenology, *29:*429–439, 1988.
27. Palmer, E.: Factors affecting stallion semen survival and fertility. Proceedings of the International Congress of Animal Reproduction and Artificial Insemination, 1984, pp. 377–379.
28. Michel, T.H., Rossdale, P.D., and Cash, R.S.G.: Efficacy of human chorionic gonadotrophin and gonadotrophin-releasing hormone for hastening ovulation in Thoroughbred mares. Equine Vet. J., *18:*438–442, 1986.
29. Hyland, J.H., and Bristol, F.: Synchronization of oestrus and timed insemination of mares. J. Reprod. Fertil. Suppl., *27:*251–255, 1979.
30. Squires, E.L., Stevens, W.B., McGlothlin, D.E., and Pickett, B.W.: Effect of an oral progestin on the estrous cycle and fertility of mares. J. Anim. Sci., *49:*729–735, 1979.
31. Holtan, D.W., Douglas, R.H., and Ginther, O.J.: Estrus, ovulation and conception following synchronization with progesterone, prostaglandin F2 alpha and human chorionic gonadotropin in pony mares. J. Anim. Sci., *44:*431–437, 1977.
32. Shilova, A.V., Platov, E.M., and Lebedev, S.G.: The use of human chorionic gonadotropin for ovulation date regulation in mares. Proceedings of the International Congress on Animal Reproduction and Artificial Insemination, 1976, p. 331.
33. Palmer, E., and Jousset, B.: Synchronization of oestrus in mares with a prostaglandin analogue and hCG. J. Reprod. Fertil. Suppl., *23:*269–274, 1975.
34. First, N.L.: Synchronization of estrus and ovulation in the mare with methallibure. J. Anim. Sci., *36:*1143–1148, 1973.
35. Squires, E.L., et al.: The effectiveness of $PGF_2\alpha$ HCG and GnRH for appointment breeding of mares. J. Equine Vet. Sci., *1:*5–9, 1981.
36. Bristol, F.: Studies on estrous synchronization in mares. Proc. Soc. Theriogenol., 258–264, 1981.
37. Palmer, E.: Control of the oestrous cycle of the mare. J. Reprod. Fertil., *54:*495–505, 1978.
38. Woods, G.L.: Ovarian response, embryo development, and reduction of excess (1) embryos in mares treated with an equine pituitary extract. Diss. Abst. Int. B Sci. Eng., *44:*3326, 1984.
39. Kelly, C.M., Hoyer, P.B., and Wise, M.E.: In-vitro and in-vivo responsiveness of the corpus luteum of the mare to gonadotrophin stimulation. J. Reprod. Fertil., *84:*593–600, 1988.
40. Carnevale, E.M., Squires, E.L., McKinnon, A.O., and Harrison, L.A.: Effect of human chorionic gonadotropin on time to ovulation and luteal function in transitional mares. J. Equine Vet. Sci., *9:*27–29, 1989.
41. Watson, E.D., and Hinrichs, K.: Changes in the concentrations of steroids and prostaglandin F in preovulatory follicles of the mare after administration of hCG. J. Reprod. Fertil., *84:*557–561, 1988.
42. Allen, W.E.: Administration of human chorionic gonadotropins (HCG) to pregnant pony mares. Vet. Rec., *94:*505, 1974.
43. Allen, W.E.: Pregnancy failure induced by human chorionic gonadotrophin in pony mares. Vet. Rec., *96:*88–90, 1975.
44. Allen, W.E.: The effect of human chorionic gonadotrophin and exogenous progesterone on luteal function during early pregnancy in pony mares. Anim. Reprod. Sci., *6:*223–228, 1983.
45. Roser, J.F., et al.: The development of antibodies to human chorionic gonadotrophin following its repeated injection in the cyclic mare. J. Reprod. Fertil. Suppl., *27:*173–179, 1979.
46. Wilson, C.G., Craig, R.D., Hughes, J.P., and Roser, J.F.: Effects of repeated hCG injections on reproductive efficiency in mares. J. Equine Vet. Sci., *10:*301–308, 1990.

PHARMACOLOGIC MANIPULATION OF THE REPRODUCTIVE CYCLE

CHAPTER 36

GnRH CLINICAL APPLICATION

C.H.G. Irvine

Gonadotropin-releasing hormone (GnRH) is rapidly becoming one of the most widely used drugs in therapy of the reproductive system. As Ziporyn observed, "There is no subspeciality of medicine that will be left untouched by the advances associated with GnRH or its analogs."[1] In the 16 yr since the structure of GnRH was announced, thousands of analogues have been prepared and over 100 have been used to promote or inhibit fertility; to treat neoplasia and cryptorchism; and to regulate reproductive cycles of domestic animals, birds, and fish. The rate of this research has intensified recently, and any review of clinical applications of GnRH is incomplete soon after it is written. For example, at the 1990 International Symposium on Equine Reproduction 9 of the 77 presentations related to GnRH, several of them using analogues that had not previously been reported in horses. As a result of this research activity the clinician has available GnRH analogue preparations which exert useful pharmacologic activity, either stimulatory (agonistic) or inhibitory (antagonistic), for any interval ranging from 10 min to 1 month.

The mechanism by which GnRH acts has been described in Chapter 4. This chapter will be restricted to clinical applications of GnRH and its analogues in manipulation of the mare's estrous cycle.

The major role of GnRH is to stimulate secretion of follicle-stimulating hormone (FSH) and luteinizing hormone (LH) so its administration is justified whenever extra secretion of FSH or LH is required. Thus it is commonly used to initiate follicular growth by induction of FSH release either in anestrous mares or in mares who fail to develop follicles during the breeding season. Another use is in induction of ovulation of preovulatory follicles via stimulation of LH release.

EARLY STUDIES ON THE CLINICAL APPLICATION OF GnRH

In 1974, GnRH was first given to anestrous and estrous mares by Ginther and Wentworth, who reported plasma LH concentrations doubling after GnRH administration.[2] The use of GnRH in manipulation of reproduction in the mare was first reported by Irvine et al. and Heinz and Klug in 1975.[3,4] Those workers gave repeated doses of 2 mg or single doses of 4 mg, and their results are difficult to relate to current concepts on gonadotropin regulation in which much smaller doses at frequent intervals are used to simulate the endogenous pattern.[5,6] In 1976, Evans and Irvine showed that GnRH induced FSH and LH release in the anestrous mare.[7] Subsequently, they devised a protocol of repeated injections of 1 mg GnRH designed to induce in the anestrous mare the FSH and LH profile they had observed in the cyclic mare. Follicular development, ovulation, and corpus luteum (CL) establishment occurred.[8] Subsequently, Bosu et al. confirmed the results using the same regimen.[9]

The protocols of earlier workers were cumbersome and were not uniformly successful. They were largely

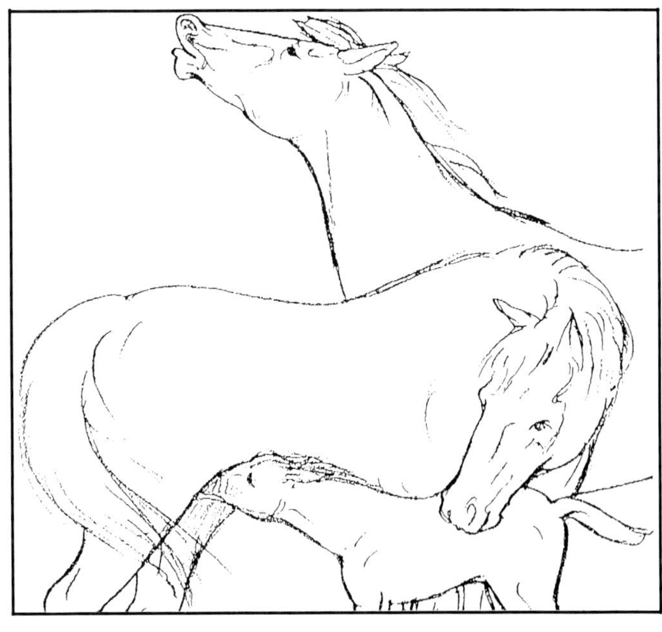

empiric, and although Knobil had shown in 1980 that in the monkey follicular development and ovulation could be induced only by hourly pulses of 6 μg GnRH,[10] the frequency and amplitude of GnRH pulses in the mare were unknown. In a series of studies, Alexander and Irvine showed LH pulses occurred 2 to 3 times daily during diestrus and approximately 30 times a day during estrus and could be generated by IV injection of 7 μg and 4 μg of GnRH, respectively.[5,6,11] The latter observations were largely confirmed by direct measurement of GnRH in pituitary venous blood.[11]

CURRENT STATUS OF THE USE OF GnRH

Because the breeding season imposed by the racing calendar is much earlier than the natural breeding season, hormonal manipulation to advance the mare's breeding season has received considerable attention. Gonadotropin-releasing hormone induces FSH and LH release in different ratios under different conditions. It is widely accepted that FSH induces follicular growth in the mare,[12] as in most other species, whereas human chorionic gonadotropin (hCG)[13] and equine chorionic gonadotropin (eCG),[14] which have high LH potency but no FSH potency in the horse, do not. Therefore, LH is assumed to play no role in early follicular development.

After the pattern of GnRH in blood bathing the pituitary of cyclic and acyclic mares became known,[6] treatment regimens were aimed at simulating that pattern. Recently, several novel methods have been used successfully.

PULSATILE INJECTION OF GnRH

Availability of small, portable, programmable, battery-driven pumps has made it possible to simulate the natural mode of GnRH delivery to the pituitary, although cost of such pumps restricts their use. Johnson induced follicular development, ovulation, and corpus luteum establishment in all mares treated with hourly IV injections of 2 or 20 μg GnRH; the mean day of ovulation was 11 and 13 days, respectively, after start of treatment, and the mean ovulation rates were 1.2 and 3, respectively.[15] Similarly Turner and Irvine injected 25 μg three times daily to a group of mares for 28 days.[16] Although preovulatory follicles had developed in 11 of 12 mares by day 21, no ovulations occurred in the mares; however, a subgroup of mares who were transferred to hourly injections on day 21 all ovulated within 6 days. In both experiments no controls ovulated. The experiments confirmed that relatively low doses of GnRH given either hourly or every 8 h can induce development of preovulatory follicles, but more hourly injections are required to induce ovulation.

CONTINUOUS ADMINISTRATION OF GnRH OR ANALOGUES

Although continuous administration of GnRH induces refractoriness of gonadotropes in many species (see Chapter 4), several experiments suggest that extremely high doses are required to induce this in the mare. For example, Garcia and Ginther showed that constant infusion of GnRH (2.37 μg/kg for 24 h) induced a steady rise in LH in the periovulatory mare.[17] This is consistent with prolonged elevation of GnRH reported throughout natural periovulatory LH surge[11] and may be related to raised estradiol concentrations at this time. In deeply anestrous mares, constant infusion of GnRH from minipumps induced ovulations in 50%.[16,18] In a simple protocol Allen et al. induced ovulation within 18 days in 15 of 20 anestrous mares with a single subcutaneous insertion of copolymer implants, which continually released the GnRH analogue, gosarelin (ICI 118 360) at a rate of 30 μg/day for 28 days.[19] Using implants which released the analogue buserelin (100 μg/24 h), Harrison et al. induced ovulation in 56% of late anestrous mares in 28 days compared with 0% of controls.[20]

While the latter experiments demonstrated the therapeutic potential of GnRH agonist implants, they also illustrated difficulties in determining a safe and effective dose. The analogue ICI 118 360 is stated as having a potency of 100 times that of GnRH itself[21] and so could be calculated as releasing the equivalent of 125 μg GnRH/h, which is approximately 40 times the effective dosage.[15] Although they believe that their response was "clearly insufficient," Allen et al. caution that because of the refractoriness which occurs with high doses increasing the dose may have a suppressive, rather than desired stimulatory, action on gonadotropin release in some animals (see Chapter 4). Nevertheless, in a subsequent study with gosarelin, Turner and Irvine found that a release rate of 180 μg/day induced a high rate of follicular development and a 50 to 75% ovulation rate with no adverse long- or short-term effects on the reproductive axis.[16] A comparable dose per kg body weight given to humans completely shuts off the reproductive axis and is, therefore, a useful treatment for prostatic or mammary carcinoma and polycystic ovarian disease.

This dose rate dilemma illustrates difficulty of rational use of analogues whose potency, mode, and duration of action in target tissues of the recipient are unknown. Potency estimates of GnRH and its analogues are based on the dose required to induce (or inhibit, in the case of antagonists) ovulation in the rat.[21] It is quite possible the gonadotrope receptor and the mechanism in the pituitary and ovary for regulating the response differ considerably between the horse and rat. Until these properties are better understood, the dose of various GnRH analogues will depend on direct experiment with each analogue in the horse, bearing in mind that the horse seems unusually resistant to the development of refractoriness.[22]

INTERMITTENT ADMINISTRATION OF GnRH OR AGONIST

A brief, preliminary report credited twice daily IV injection of 100 μg of a GnRH agonist (structure not given) with induction of follicular development and ovulation in all mares treated compared with 20% of controls.[23] Buserelin given similarly was effective in 44% of mares compared with 0% in controls.[23] GnRH itself (200 μg twice daily) was less effective. Ginther and Bergfeldt reported that twice daily IM injections of 100 to 400 μg of a GnRH analogue with a substitution of alanine in the 6 position and amidation of 9-proline induced ovulation within 21 days in 57% of deeply anestrous mares.[24] The multiple ovulation rate was greater for treated (27/86) than control (2/35) mares.

Once daily subcutaneous injection of a crude gonatropin extract induces follicular development and ovulation in deeply anestrous mares.[25] Thus release of a comparable amount of gonadotropin by a single large daily dose of GnRH or analogue should have a similar effect. However, the dose-response curve to GnRH in the anestrous mare is hyperbolic, flattens off after relatively small responses,[5] and lessens with successive days treatment.[8] A single daily dose regimen requires development of an agonist with a suitable duration of action to provide medium-term FSH responses.

Comparison of efficacy of the several methods of GnRH administration should take into account state of ovaries at time the experiments were done, because time to induced ovulation is directly related to amount of follicular development when treatment was commenced.[24] Of the treatments available in 1991, the use of long-acting implants provides reasonable efficacy with ease of treatment and minimal animal handling. When conception rates to the induced ovulations have been determined, they have been normal.[16,18,19,23]

USE OF GnRH DURING THE BREEDING SEASON TO ADVANCE OVULATION

The ability of GnRH to induce LH secretion[2] has led to its use as a nonantigenic substitute for hCG to advance ovulation in the mare for management purposes. In 1979, Ginther reviewed rather mixed responses obtained and commented that a long-acting form of GnRH was needed.[26] Although a range of analogues has subsequently become available, none has proved ideal, and induction of ovulation has been most consistently achieved by hourly injections (but not every 4 h), of GnRH itself.[27] However, it seems highly likely that a suitable single-dose analogue will be developed which could offer a useful alternative to hCG on the basis of cost and absence of antigenicity attributed to hCG.[28]

It may be relevant that a prolonged, ovulatory-type LH surge in the mare is most readily induced when GnRH is given at least 24 h after the peak of an endogenous or exogenous estradiol surge.[29,30]

USE OF GnRH IN MARES WITH ABSENT OR ABNORMAL CYCLICITY DURING BREEDING SEASON

GnRH has been used to induce ovulation in mares which fail to cycle during normal breeding season.[23] While this may be a logical use for GnRH, it is likely to be effective only if the acyclicity is the result of either insufficient GnRH stimulation of the pituitary or an inappropriate time course of GnRH secretion. A presumptive diagnosis may be made from either (1) inadequate follicular development, associated with low FSH levels in several blood samples, or (2) development of preovulatory follicles which fail to ovulate, associated with low LH levels in several blood samples. The low gonadotropin concentrations may be caused by defects at either the hypothalamus or pituitary. The location of the defect must be determined in order that logical therapy may be used. Differentiation between a hypothalamic or pituitary defect is usually done on the basis of the response to a provocative test in which the competence of the pituitary is assessed by the size of the response to GnRH. As with any provocative test, the size of the stimulus should be aimed at inducing hormone levels in the upper physiologic range. Giving excessive doses that are many times higher than those the gonadotropes are ever exposed to, provides only misleading information about the normal functioning of the system.[5] Ideally, blood samples should be collected at −30 and 0 min, then 10 μg GnRH IV is given and samples collected at +10, 20, 30, and 45 min, and the serum stored in the refrigerator until measured for LH or FSH, depending on which function is defective.

Interpretation of the test is best done on the basis of peak fractional increase in gonadotropin. A threefold to sixfold increase in FSH in anestrus or diestrus or a 25 to 60% increase in LH in estrus is a normal response. Gonadotropins are pulsatile in anestrus or diestrus and if the pre-GnRH concentrations are unusually high it is likely that the samples were taken during a pulse and the results would not be meaningful. If the mare shows a normal response to GnRH, it suggests the pituitary is able to respond to GnRH so that the inadequate basal gonadotropin concentrations would likely have been caused by inadequate GnRH. Therefore, GnRH, therapy is likely to be effective. However, if the gonadotropin response is subnormal the pituitary is likely to be inadequate and gonadotropin administration is the most logical treatment. Nevertheless, the pituitary insufficiency may be the result of a relatively long period of inadequate GnRH stimulation, which results in a reduced functional and storage capacity of the gonadotrope. In such cases, the pituitary insufficiency is secondary to hypothalamic insufficiency and should be treated as such.

If these tests indicate that inadequate GnRH stimulation is the cause of inadequate follicular development during the breeding season, the therapy used should be identical to that used to stimulate cyclicity during the nonbreeding season, as discussed. However, if the problem is failure of final follicular maturation and ovulation, at our present state of knowledge, hCG administration offers the simplest solution, although GnRH administration would be preferable when an effective delivery system becomes available.

GnRH therapy may be useful in a variety of circumstances. Development of new agonist GnRH formulations with controlled release has made it possible to program GnRH action at the pituitary. Furthermore, because requirements for GnRH, in terms of dosage and timing, are probably not as stringent in the horse as in the human or other species, GnRH does have considerable potential for regulation of reproduction in the mare. Nevertheless, because GnRH secretion directly reflects environmental influences it is probably more logical to search for management factors that suppress, or fail to stimulate, GnRH secretion. Inadequate nutrition, environmental stress, and lack of exposure to stallions have already been shown to reduce GnRH or LH secretion, and many other management factors are likely to be involved (see Chapter 4). Although the studmaster is often gratified by the immediate response which may be achieved with GnRH therapy, interests are often best served if management is critically examined and corrected when possible.

REFERENCES

1. Conn, P.M., McArdle, C.A., Andrews, W.V., and Huckle, W.R.: The molecular basis of gonadotropin-releasing hormone (GnRH) action in the pituitary gonadotrope. Biol. Reprod., *36:*17–35, 1987.
2. Ginther, O.J., and Wentworth, B.C.: Effect of a synthetic gonadotropin-releasing hormone on plasma concentrations of luteinizing hormone in ponies. Am. J. Vet. Res., *35:*79–81, 1974.
3. Irvine, D.S., Downey, B.R., Parker, W.G., and Sullivan, J.J.: Duration of oestrus and time of ovulation in mares treated with synthetic GnRH (AY-24,031). J. Reprod. Fertil. Suppl., *23:*279–283, 1975.
4. Heinz, H., and Klug, E.: The use of GnRH for controlling the oestrous cycle of the mare (preliminary report). J. Reprod. Fertil. Suppl., *23:*275–277, 1975.
5. Alexander, S.L., and Irvine, C.H.G.: Effect of graded doses of gonadotropin-releasing hormone on serum LH in mares in various reproductive states: Comparison with endogenously generated pulses. J. Endocrinol., *110:* 19–26, 1986.
6. Irvine, C.H.G., and Alexander, S.L.: A novel technique for measuring hypothalamic and pituitary hormone secretion rates from collection of pituitary venous effluent in the horse. J. Endocrinol., *113:*183–192, 1987.
7. Evans, M.J., and Irvine, C.H.G.: Measurement of equine follicle stimulating hormone and luteinizing hormone: response of anestrous mares to gonadotropin releasing hormone. Biol. Reprod., *15:*477–484, 1976.
8. Evans, M.J., and Irvine, C.H.G.: Induction of follicular development, maturation and ovulation by gonadotropin releasing hormone to acyclic mares. Biol. Reprod., *16:*452–456, 1977.
9. Bosu, W.T.K., Waelchli-suter, R.O., and Vasey, J.: Induction of ovulation with gonadotrophin releasing hormone and progesterone in seasonally anestrous mares. Can. Vet. J., *23:*332–336, 1982.
10. Knobil, E.: The neuroendocrine control of the menstrual cycle. Recent Progr. Horm. Res., *36:*53–88, 1980.
11. Alexander, S.L., and Irvine, C.H.G.: Secretion rates and short term patterns of GnRH, FSH and LH throughout the periovulatory period in the mare. J. Endocrinol., *114:*351–362, 1987.
12. Irvine, C.H.G.: Endocrinology of the estrous cycle of the mare: Application to embryo transfer. Theriogenology, *15:*85–104, 1981.
13. Palmer, E.: Control of the oestrous cycle of the mare. J. Reprod. Fertil., *54:*495–505, 1978.
14. Allen, W.E.: Ovarian changes during early pregnancy in pony mares in relation to PMSG production. J. Reprod. Fertil. Suppl., *23:*425–428, 1975.
15. Johnson, A.L.: Gonadotropin-releasing hormone treatment induces follicular growth and ovulation in seasonally anestrous mares. Biol. Reprod., *36:*1199–1206, 1987.
16. Turner, J.E., and Irvine, C.H.G.: The effect of various gonadotrophin-releasing hormone regimens on gonadotrophins, follicular growth and ovulation in deeply anoestrous mares. J. Reprod. Fertil. Suppl., *44:*213–225, 1991.
17. Garcia, M.C., and Ginther, O.J.: Plasma luteinizing hormone concentration in mares treated with gonadotropin-releasing hormone and estradiol. Am. J. Vet. Res., *36:*1581–1584, 1975.
18. Hyland, J.H., et al.: Infusion of gonadotrophin-releasing hormone (GnRH) induces ovulation and fertile oestrus in mares during seasonal anoestrus. J. Reprod. Fertil. Suppl., *35:*211–220, 1987.
19. Allen, W.R., et al.: Induction of ovulation in seasonally anoestrous mares with a slow-release implant of a GnRH analogue (ICI 118 630). J. Reprod. Fertil. Suppl., *35:*469–478, 1987.
20. Harrison, L.A., Squires, E.L., Nett, T.M., and McKinnon, A.O.: Use of gonadotropin-releasing hormone for hastening ovulation in transitional mares. J. Anim. Sci., *68:*690–699, 1990.
21. Dutta, L., et al.: Potent agonist and antagonist analogues of luliberin containing an asaglycine residue in position 10. Biochem. Biophys. Res. Commun., *81:*382–390, 1978.
22. Montovan, S.M., et al.: The effect of a potent GnRH agonist on gonadal and sexual activity in the horse. Theriogenology, *33:*1305–1321, 1990.
23. Fitzgerald, B.P., Affleck, K.J., and Loy, R.G.: Investigation of the potential of LHRH or an agonist to induce ovulation in seasonally anoestrous mares with observations on the use of the agonist in problem acyclic mares. J. Reprod. Fertil. Suppl., *35:*683–684, 1987.
24. Ginther, O.J., and Bergfeldt, D.R.: Effect of GnRH treatment during the anovulatory season on multiple ovulation rate and on follicular development during the existing pregnancy in mares. J. Reprod. Fertil., *88:*119–126, 1990.
25. Lapin, D.R., and Ginther, O.J.: Induction of ovulation and multiple ovulations in seasonally anovulatory and ovulatory mares with an equine pituitary extract. J. Anim. Sci., *44:*832–842, 1977.
26. Ginther, O.J.: Reproductive Biology of the Mare—Basic and Applied Aspects. Cross Plains, WI, published by the author, 1979.
27. Johnson, A.L.: Pulsatile administration of gonadotropin-

releasing hormone advances ovulation in cycling mares. Biol. Reprod., *35:*1123–1130, 1986.

28. Roser, J.F., et al.: Reproductive efficiency in mares with anti-hCG antibodies. Proceedings of the Ninth International Congress on Animal Reproduction and Artificial Insemination, 1980, pp. 627–630.

29. Vivrette, S.L., and Irvine, C.H.G.: Interaction of oestradiol and gonadotrophin-releasing hormone on LH release in the mare. J. Reprod. Fertil. Suppl., *27:*151–155, 1979.

30. Evans, M.J., and Irvine, C.H.G.: Induction of follicular development and ovulation in seasonally acyclic mares using gonadotrophin-releasing hormone and progesterone. J. Reprod. Fertil. Suppl., *27:*113–121, 1979.

PHARMACOLOGIC MANIPULATION OF THE REPRODUCTIVE CYCLE

CHAPTER 37

ESTROGENS, OXYTOCIN, AND ERGOT ALKALOIDS

S.P. Brinsko
D.D. Varner
T.L. Blanchard

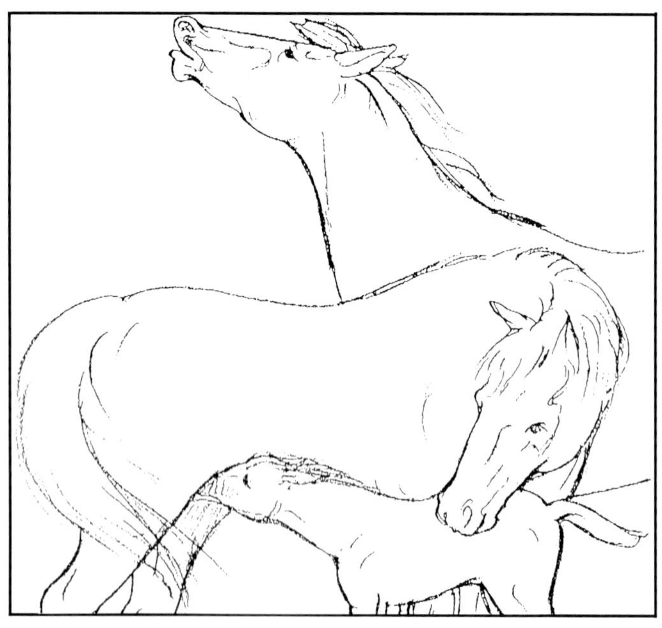

ESTROGENS

Estrogens are steroidal hormones produced primarily by ovarian follicles and the fetoplacental unit, although small amounts of estrogens are also produced in other areas of the body such as adipose tissue, skin, and the adrenal gland.[1,2] The fetoplacental unit secretes estrogens throughout gestation. Estrogens secreted by the developing conceptus may play an important role in maternal recognition of pregnancy and nutritional support of the embryo and fetus.[3]

The physiologic actions of estrogens in the mare include maturation of the reproductive tract and mammary glands as well as the modulation of gonadotropin secretion.[4] In the absence of progesterone, estrogens augment the expression of behavioral estrus. Elevated estrogen levels associated with physiologic estrus results in enhanced uterine resistance to infection.[5] Estrogens are thought to be involved in gestational support by the mechanisms mentioned above and, at least in the rat, by stimulating the synthesis of progesterone in response to lutineizing hormone (LH) by a yet unidentified step in steroidogenesis.[6] At parturition, estrogens are involved in modulation of uterine contractions and cervical relaxation.

Principal estrogens in the nonpregnant mare are estrone and estradiol-17β.[7] Estradiol-17β, secreted by the ovarian follicle, is the most potent naturally occurring estrogen. A large percentage of this hormone is presumed to be converted to estrone by liver metabolism before its elimination in the urine. Naturally occurring estrogens are rapidly excreted by the mare. Exogenous administration of up to 5 mg of estradiol-17β to ovariectomized mares results in peak serum levels by 6 h postinjection, with a return to preinjection serum levels within 48 h.[8] The predominant estrogens produced by the equine fetoplacental unit are estrone and equilin. Equilin and equilinin, another estrogen, are unique to the mare.[7]

AVAILABLE PREPARATIONS

No estrogenic preparations are currently approved for use in equids. Estradiol-17β, conjugated estrogens (e.g., salts of the sulfate esters of estrone, equilin, and equilinin) and esterified estrogens (e.g., estradiol cypionate, estradiol benzoate, and estradiol valerate) are approved for use in humans. Estradiol cypionate and estradiol benzoate are commercially available for use in cattle. Compared to free estradiol-17β, esterified estrogens are more potent and have a longer half-life. The synthetic nonsteroidal estrogen diethylstilbestrol is labeled for use in humans, but not for use in domestic animals. The reluctance to approve these products for use in the horse and other animals may be because of the increased risk of carcinoma development, a side effect which has been associated with their use in humans and laboratory animals.[9,10]

Several chemical companies produce estradiol-17β in a nonesterified, nonsulfated, crystalline form, which can be prepared for use in horses (usually in combination with progesterone).[11] However, because estradiol-17β is not currently approved for use in horses by the Food and Drug Administration (FDA), authorized use requires an investigational exemption.

ESTABLISHED USES

Enhancement of Sexual Receptivity

Ovariectomized and seasonally anovulatory mares may commonly exhibit persistent or erratic estrous behavior. This is the result of a low concentration (<1 ng/mL plasma) of circulating progesterone, because a low circulating progesterone concentration is more critical to sexual receptivity in the mare than increased circulating concentrations of estrogen. Compared with mares in physiologic estrus, especially near the time of ovulation, the intensity of behavioral estrus is not as strong in ovariectomized and seasonally anovulatory mares.[12] Although estrous behavior prevails in these mares, periods exist in which they are intolerant to the sexual advances of the stallion.

Exogenous estrogens, even when administered at low doses, will induce or augment receptive sexual behavior in ovariectomized or seasonally anovulatory mares. Intensified estrous behavior was observed within 4 h after intramuscular injection of 1 mg estradiol-17β to ovariectomized pony mares.[13] When an esterified estrogen was used at the same dose, onset of action was delayed but intensity of behavioral estrus exhibited was similar. Seasonally anestrous mares demonstrate similar responses to exogenous estrogens, because their ovaries are essentially inactive.

Ovariectomized or seasonally anovulatory mares are often given estrogens to provide a reliably receptive mare for stallions to mount during seminal collection. This is not recommended with mares in diestrus, because exogenous administration of even large doses of estrogen (e.g., 20 to 25 mg estradiol-17β) to mares with high circulating concentrations of progesterone will not induce sexual receptivity.[14] Although exogenous estrogen administration produces or intensifies psychic estrus in seasonally anovulatory mares, this estrous behavior is not accompanied by follicular maturation or ovulation.

Synchronization of Estrus/Ovulation

Variability in the duration of estrus makes synchronization of ovulation in mares more difficult than in cattle. Synchronization of ovulation is improved in randomly cycling mares when they are administered a combination of progesterone and estrogen rather than progesterone by itself.[15,16] The combined action of the two hormones provides a more profound negative feedback on gonadotropin release than does progesterone alone, which results in a more uniform inhibition of follicular development.[15–17] When the exogenous progesterone/estrogen therapy is discontinued, less diversity in follicular maturation and the date ovulation occurs. Fertility of mares undergoing this method of ovulation synchronization is normal.[15,16,18]

The recommended protocol involves intramuscular injections of progesterone (150 mg) combined with estradiol-17β (10 mg) in oil for 10 consecutive days with a single injection of prostaglandin $F_2\alpha$ also given on the last day of progesterone/estradiol injection.[15,16] After the steroid treatment regimen is discontinued, administering human chorionic gonadotropin (2500 IU) when a 35-mm follicle is detected may further improve ovulation synchrony.

Research using esterified estrogens rather than free estradiol-17β in the foregoing ovulation-synchronization protocol has not been reported. It is likely the effects of such products would be less predictable and less desirable because of their prolonged action.

Acceleration of the Ovulatory Season

Most mares are seasonally polyestrous, having a period of ovarian inactivity during winter months associated with short day length followed by a return to reproductive function with increasing day length in the spring. During the transition from ovarian quiescence to return of the ovulatory season, mares often display erratic patterns of estrous behavior that can last for several weeks. This transitional period is characterized by recruitment and atresia of multiple small anovulatory follicles. As the transition period progresses, follicles tend to become larger until a follicle matures, ovulates, and forms a corpus luteum thereby re-establishing normal cyclicity.

The progesterone/estradiol-17β protocol described above can be used to shorten the transitional period.[16] If mares are truly in the period of seasonal transition, prostaglandins are not needed at the end of the steroid injection series, because ovulation has not yet occurred and a corpus luteum is not present. The degree of ovarian follicular activity present at initiation of treatment greatly influences response. Mares must be in mid to late transition with ovarian follicles measuring 20 to 25 mm present in order for this protocol to be successful; therefore, proper candidate selection is critical.

Postponement of the First Postpartum Ovulation

The average interval from parturition to the first postpartum ovulation in mares is 10.2 days but can range from 5 to greater than 30 days.[19] This wide variability appears to be at least partially affected by the month of foaling, with the longest intervals in the northern hemisphere occurring in January to February and the shortest intervals occurring in May.[19] Proper management protocol to maximize the mare's reproductive efficiency during this time period has long been a subject of considerable controversy and has yet to be resolved.

The mare's endometrium is capable of involuting rapidly and is usually complete by 14 days following parturition.[20] The lower pregnancy rate associated with breeding during the first postpartum ovulation has been attributed to failure of the endometrium to be completely involuted when the embryo enters the uterus. Pregnancy rate at the first postpartum estrus would likely be improved if the timing of ovulation would ensure that the embryo entered the uterus after the endometrium had re-established its normal nonpregnant state. Attempts at enhancing uterine involution in normal mares before the first postpartum ovulation with uterine lavage[21,22] or myotonic agents[23] have thus far not proven to be successful. Following ovulation, a 5-day interval is required before the embryo enters the uterus; therefore, ovulation after day 10 postpartum would help to ensure that the endometrium has returned to normal before entry of the embryo. Loy and co-workers have demonstrated an improvement in pregnancy rate in mares ovulating after day 10 postpartum versus those ovulating on or before day 10 postpartum.[19]

The first postpartum ovulation can be delayed by treating mares with progesterone and estradiol-17β beginning within 12 to 24 h following parturition. Mares treated for 6 consecutive days (beginning within 12 h after parturition) with progesterone (150 mg) and estradiol-17β (10 mg) in oil experienced a 5.3-day delay in the interval from parturition to first postpartum ovulation (15.6 ± 2.6 days) when compared with untreated (control) mares (10.3 ± 2.4 days).[24] However, pregnancy rates were not improved when these mares were bred at this time compared with the control group. Bell and Bristol treated mares with the same hormonal regimen, but for only 5 days beginning the day of parturition, and reported a 5-day delay in the interval from parturition to first postpartum ovulation.[25] In this study, conception rate at the first postpartum estrus was 72% (42/58) in treated mares versus 59% (34/58) in control mares; however, control mares that ovulated after 10 days postpartum had a pregnancy rate of 69%, thus supporting the theory that additional time allotment for endometrial repair before the first postpartum ovulation will improve fertility of mares bred at the first postpartum estrus. This hormonal protocol seems to permit additional time for uterine involution.

Another plausible use of exogenous progesterone/estradiol-17β in postpartum mares is synchronization of the first postpartum estrus.[26] In one study, mares were treated with the steroid regimen described above, beginning within 18 h following parturition and continuing for 1 to 10 consecutive days. The duration of treatment varied among mares because of different foaling dates, but treatments ceased on the same day for all mares. Ovulation was effectively synchronized in these mares, because 92% (33/36) ovulated 10 to 16 days following the cessation of treatment. Pregnancy rate of mares bred at the delayed estrus was 81% (29/36).

UNESTABLISHED USES

Expression of Behavioral Estrus

A poorly understood phenomenon, which is occasionally observed in mares, is silent estrus. Despite having normal physiologic estrous cycles, some mares do not display behavioral estrus and often reject the stallion's sexual advances. If mares are artificially inseminated, this problem can be easily overcome; however, silent estrus is a real hindrance to natural breeding programs.

A relationship between progesterone/estrogen secretory patterns during the periovulatory period and expression of behavioral estrus in the mare has been reported.[27] Maximum circulating estradiol-17β concentrations were significantly lower in mares with silent estrus than in mares with normal estrous behavior. Silent estrous mares also had a significantly longer interval between maximum circulating estradiol-17β concentration and ovulation compared with mares exhibiting normal estrous behavior. Mares treated during diestrus with prostaglandins to induce regression of a functional corpus luteum tend to have a higher incidence of silent estrus. This may be related to a shorter interval from luteal regression to ovulation than occurs with natural luteolysis.[27,28]

Exogenous estrogen has occasionally been used before mating in mares experiencing silent estrus to help elicit estrous behavior, primarily to prevent injury to the stallion during natural service. No controlled studies regarding this use of exogenous estrogens have been reported; therefore, the success of such a practice is undocumented. It must be kept in mind that using exogenous estrogens in this manner may have undesirable side effects. Administering estrogens either before or after mating has been associated with both delayed and accelerated ovum/embryo transit time through the oviduct, which are reported to interfere with conceptus maintenance in a variety of animal species.[29–32] Exogenous estrogens may also have direct inhibitory effects on the ovum/embryo or cause alterations in the endometrium, which could interrupt pregnancy.[33,34] However, exogenous estrogen administration near the time of mating has also been shown to increase spermatozoal numbers in the oviducts of ewes and rabbits.[35–37] At this time, the state of our knowledge regarding the effects of estrogen administration near the time of mating on mare fertility is too deficient to recommend its use.

Treatment of Uterine Infection

Whether or not the use of exogenous estrogens offers any advantages to the treatment of endometritis in the mare has long been a subject of debate. Several animal species are more susceptible to uterine infections during the luteal phase than in the follicular phase, suggesting a hormonal influence on the susceptibility to genital infection.[38] Bacteria have been shown to be more adherent to the endometrium of ovariectomized mares administered progesterone than those under the influence of estrogen.[39] The precise mechanism(s) by which estrogens modulate uterine resistance to infection are not clearly understood.

Although estrogens appear to enhance uterine defense mechanisms, the usefulness of exogenously administered estrogens in the treatment of uterine infections remains questionable. Intrauterine infusion of estrogens alone does not appear to curtail uterine infection.[40] The use of estrogens locally or systemically, in conjunction with local antibiotic therapy, has not yet proven to be more effective than the use of antibiotics alone.

Induction of Parturition

Estrogen probably plays an important role in the initiation of parturition in mares. Studies in numerous species indicate that estradiol-17β induces formation of myometrial gap junctions (cell to cell contacts or nexuses), which facilitate myometrial electrical activity and coordinate the synchronized myometrial contractions at parturition.[41–44] In the rat and ewe, estrogen has been shown to increase uterine sensitivity to oxytocin and prostaglandin, probably by increasing the number of oxytocin and prostaglandin receptors in the myometrium.[45] This phenomenon may also occur in the mare, because maternal estradiol-17β concentrations increase slightly before parturition, despite declining concentrations of estrone and equilin.[46]

Some clinicians advocate the use of exogenous estrogens (estradiol cypionate, 3 mg, or diethylstilbestrol, 12 to 30 mg) 1 to 24 h before oxytocin administration for induction of parturition in the mare, especially if the cervix is not dilated or softening at the time of proposed parturition induction. Although exogenous estrogens have been reported to be helpful in this regard, we have used oxytocin alone to induce parturition in full-term mares having tight cervices without any resulting complications. In addition, placing estrogen in the vaginal fornix around the cervix and intramuscular injection of estrogen 24 h before parturition induction failed to produce relaxation or softening of the cervix in two preterm (10 to 11 months) mares.

Maintenance of Pregnancy

Estrogen concentrations increase dramatically in the uterine and blastocyst fluids of pregnant mares beginning after day 12 of gestation.[3] The heightened uterine tone detected early in gestation results from these estrogens, which are predominantly of conceptus origin.[3,47] These estrogens are also thought to provide a special milieu for the developing conceptus that is essential for its growth and well-being.[3,48] McDowell and colleagues detected more total protein and uteroferin in the uterine secretions of ovariectomized mares receiving exogenous estradiol and progesterone than in mares receiving progesterone alone.[49] These investigators proposed that early embryonic death may stem from deficient uterine secretions, which results in inadequate nourishment of the conceptus, thereby leading to its eventual loss of viability. Provided this is true, and exogenously administered estrogens are not detrimental to the mare or the developing conceptus, estrogen therapy may be useful (possibly more useful than progesterone) for deterring loss of the conceptus early in gestation. However, McKinnon and coworkers reported that pregnancy rates did not differ between ovariectomized embryo-recipient mares treated with progestogin alone or in combination with estradiol.[50]

OXYTOCIN

Oxytocin is a peptide synthesized in the hypothalamus and stored in the posterior pituitary gland. Release of oxytocin into the circulation precipitates contraction of smooth muscle in the uterus and oviducts as well as the myoepithelial cells of the mammary glands.[51,52]

AVAILABLE PREPARATIONS

Oxytocin is available as a clear injectable solution labeled as either oxytocin or posterior pituitary extract. Posterior pituitary extract is obtained from the posterior pituitary lobe of animals and contains both oxytocin and vasopressin. Anaphylaxis may occur in mares given the crude extract intravenously. Oxytocin synthesized for commercial use is pure, containing no vasopressin, so it is unlikely to produce anaphylaxis. Oxytocin should be kept refrigerated when not in use to maintain potency.[51,52]

ESTABLISHED USES

Induction of Parturition

Indications for inducing parturition in the mare should be limited to scheduling foaling for medical reasons to ensure that a veterinarian is present to provide assistance to the mare and/or foal when the health or life of either may be in danger and to teaching and research purposes. Elective induction of parturition for the sake of convenience alone is not recommended.

Fetal maturity is critical to its survival; therefore, whenever possible, the mare must show signs of imminent parturition before elective induction is undertaken.[53,54] A number of guidelines have been given [52,55] and include a minimum of 330 days of gestation or a mare which is within a few days of, or beyond, her expected foaling date. Significant development of the dam's udder and filling of the teats with thick, sticky colostrum is probably the best clinical indicator of fetal maturity. Relaxation of the sacrosciatic ligaments and the vulva are additional indicators of approaching parturition; however, these signs are not consistently evident, especially in primiparous mares. Ideally the mare's cervix should be softening and the sticky cervical mucus of pregnancy should be liquefying, but these are not critical parameters. Fetal maturity may also be estimated by quantification of the cation content in the dam's udder secretions.[56]

Corticosteroids, prostaglandins, and oxytocin have all been used to induce parturition in full-term mares. Oxytocin remains the most popular and, apparently, the most predictable drug used for this purpose in a variety of clinical situations.[52,55]

Early reports recommended administering 100 to 140 units of oxytocin to a 450-kg mare in a single intramuscular injection. With this method, mares show signs of marked discomfort and sweating in 10 to 15 min, and most deliver the foal within 30 min of injection. The speed of onset and severity of abdominal discomfort as well as other signs of labor are correlated with the dose of oxytocin.[55,57] It is likely that large doses of oxytocin may result in complications such as premature placental separation and fetal hypoxia. In pregnant ewes, oxytocin has been shown to provoke dose-related increases in intrauterine pressure with corresponding decreases in fetal Po_2, as well as dose-related inhibition of uterine activity corresponding to uterine spasm.[58,59] Complications associated with excessive oxytocin administration in women include contractile abnormalities of the myometrium, premature placental separation, and fetal malpresentation.[60] Slow-rate intravenous infusions of oxytocin are preferred to intravenous bolus administration in human medicine.[61]

Oxytocin can be administered by slow intravenous infusion (60 to 120 units in 1 L of normal saline until labor commences) to induce parturition in the mare.[62] This method is somewhat awkward and may inhibit the normal parturient behavior (e.g., restlessness, walking, and rolling) in some mares. A simpler, less awkward method is to give small (2.5 to 15 units) boluses at 15- to 20-min intervals until labor commences.[63] In our experience, 10 to 15 units administered every 15 to 20 min until stage II parturition produces satisfactory, predictable results. Three to four injections are usually given, and the foal is delivered within 1 h in most instances. Circulating concentrations of prostaglandin $F_{2}\alpha$ metabolites rise rapidly (peaking in 15 to 37 min) in mares administered small doses of oxytocin. Patterns of prostaglandin $F_{2}\alpha$ release appear to be similar to those observed with spontaneous foaling. Therefore, some investigators suggest little is gained by using higher doses of 40 to 120 units.[64,65] Apparently, if 40 units are used, repeated injections do not appear to be beneficial.[66]

Treatment of Retained Placenta

Fetal membranes are normally expelled within 30 min to 3 h in the mare.[52] However, it is not uncommon for the fetal membranes to remain in the mare for up to 12 to 16 h without clinical signs of illness.[52,67] Although no exact figures are available, the incidence of retained placenta in the mare is thought to vary from 2 to 10%.[52,68]

Dystocia increases the incidence of retained placenta in the mare[25,52,69] and may result from trauma to the uterus and delayed involution. Other factors may be mechanical interferences, hormonal imbalances, endometritis, and placentitis during pregnancy.[52,70,71] Disturbances of normal uterine contraction at parturition, not necessarily uterine inertia, and perhaps during the postpartum period is a likely cause.[71] This may result from maternal-fetal endocrine dysfunction, failure to release adequate oxytocin, or failure of the myometrium to respond to oxytocin. Reports of prompt placental expulsion following oxytocin-induced parturition, along with the failure of some mares with retained placenta to exhibit the characteristic abdominal discomfort associated with uterine contractions and placental expulsion attest to oxytocin's role in passage of the fetal membranes.[52,57,71,72] Administration of oxytocin for the treatment of retained placenta is supported by the favorable response to therapy.

Oxytocin used alone or in combination with other treatments, is the most common therapy for retained placenta in the mare and appears to be the most beneficial.[73] Recommended doses range from 20 to 120 units given intravenously, subcutaneously, or intramuscularly which may be repeated every few hours if the placenta is not passed.[52,74] Small doses (e.g., 20 units) may be given repeatedly at 30- to 60-min intervals if necessary. Signs of abdominal discomfort may appear within a few minutes of injection and are generally followed by straining. The degree of abdominal discomfort appears to be dose related and may be the result of intense, perhaps spasmodic, uterine contractions, as discussed earlier. A more physiologic response to treatment is thought to occur with a slow intravenous infusion of 30 to 60 units of oxytocin in 1 to 2 L of normal saline over 30 to 60 min, with 60 units administered over a 1-h period giving the best results.[71] The slow intravenous method is reported to be approximately 75% effective. If the fetal membranes are not expelled shortly after treatment, they are usually passed within 1 to 2 h or can often be removed with gentle traction on the exposed portion protruding from the mare's vulva. Mares that have experienced severe dystocia or abortion are less likely to respond. Although uterine response to oxytocin tends to decrease as the postpartum period progresses, the uterus of the mare will continue to contract in response to oxytocin injections.

A popular method for removal of retained fetal membranes in the mare is to distend the chorioallantoic cavity with 9 to 12 L of warm normal saline, with or without dilute (< 2%) povidone-iodine solution.[72] The opening of the placenta is held closed at the level of the vestibule or vulva to retain the fluid as it is infused. Stretch receptors are activated and endogenous oxytocin is released. Providing the uterus something to contract against seems to aid in separating the chorionic villi from the endometrial crypts. Membranes are usually expelled within 5 to 30 min. Combining this treatment with intravenous administration of 20 units of oxytocin as the mare begins to strain is often helpful. Other treatments that may be combined with oxytocin therapy include systemic and local antibiotic therapy, uterine lavage, exercise, and flunixin meglumine or phenylbutazone as prophylactic therapy to prevent the metritis-septicemia-laminitis complex.

UNESTABLISHED USES

Promoting Uterine Involution

Delayed uterine involution often follows prolonged dystocia and retention of fetal membranes. After the membranes have been expelled, administration of oxytocin can be continued in doses of 20 to 50 units, intramuscularly or subcutaneously, one to several times daily for several days in an effort to stimulate uterine contraction and reduction in uterine size. This therapy is useful following caesarean section and in postpartum mares that are not being nursed as a result of a compromised or dead foal. In these instances, oxytocin is best used in conjunction with medical therapy to control infection. Uterine lavage with warm (42° C) saline followed by 10 to 20 units of oxytocin aids in the removal of fluid and debris that have not been expelled. This technique must be used with caution in mares recovering from caesarean section. Whether daily injections of oxytocin hastens uterine involution has not been documented, but appears to benefit mares with postpartum complications in our experience. Although not adequately studied in the mare, refractoriness to oxytocin may occur, perhaps because uterine oxytocin receptors become refractory to high doses of exogenous oxytocin (i.e., down regulation) or a decrease in enzyme activity or precursors necessary for prostaglandin synthesis occurs.[75]

Uterine prolapse rarely occurs in the mare, but it occasionally follows severe dystocia and retained fetal membranes. The weight of the fetal membranes remaining attached to the tip of the uterine horn(s) may precipitate inversion, which may progress to uterine prolapse if left unattended. Immediate replacement of the uterus is necessary to avoid severe injury. Once the uterus has been replaced and the horns completely everted, institution of oxytocin therapy (20 to 50 units, intramuscularly) for 1 to 2 days should stimulate sufficient uterine contraction to reduce the chance of recurrence. Oxytocin should not be administered before returning the uterus to its normal position, because uterine contraction may make replacement difficult or impossible.[52] Therapy for the management of shock and sepsis is also indicated.

Uterine hemorrhage can be treated by repeatedly administering oxytocin in 20- to 50-unit boluses at 30- to 60-min intervals to aid uterine contraction and constriction of blood vessels. However, ergonovine may be the preferred drug to use for this condition because of its more prolonged contractile effects on the uterus and vasculature (see ergonovine discussion). Oxytocin may be contraindicated if a uterine blood vessel is bleeding into the broad ligament (uterine hematoma), because the broad ligament may tear as a result of the stimulated contractions allowing excessive bleeding into the abdomen.

Uterine rupture is usually discovered in the postpartum period after the mare develops peritonitis. If identified early, while relatively fresh, emergency surgery should be performed to repair the rent. Medical management for prevention and/or treatment of peritonitis is indicated along with repeated injections (20 to 50 units) of oxytocin to stimulate uterine contraction, as discussed above. Oxytocin injections can be administered over several days in an attempt to hasten reduction in uterine size and speed uterine healing. This treatment is most effective if the rent in the uterine wall is dorsally located and of small size.[52] For cases not detected soon after parturition, the prognosis is poor because microbial contamination of the peritoneal cavity is usually overwhelming.

The use of oxytocin may also be of benefit in conjunction with uterine lavage or flushing, such as in embryo recovery or, more commonly, lavage as adjunctive treatment for endometritis. While fluid return is not usually a problem, occasionally mares will pool fluid in the uterine horns, presumably caused by lack of uterine contraction. Intravenous injection of 20 to 40 units of oxytocin seems to improve evacuation of fluid in such mares. The authors routinely use oxytocin in conjunction with uterine lavage for treatment of endometritis. The effect of oxytocin treatment on fluid or embryo recovery rates has not been reported.

Milk Letdown

Both endogenous and exogenous oxytocin cause the myoepithelial cells surrounding the alveoli and lactiferous ducts of the mammary gland to contract, resulting in the ejection of milk ("milk letdown"). In some nervous mares, particularly primiparous mares, milk letdown may be inadequate for the foal's needs. In these situations, injection of 10 to 20 units of oxytocin intravenously may stimulate mares to release their milk for nursing; however, phenothiazine tranquilizers may be of more benefit.[76] As little as 0.5 unit of oxytocin has been demonstrated to cause a sufficient increase in intramammary pressure for milk letdown in cows; therefore, large doses of oxytocin are probably not indicated. Studies in the rat have shown endogenous and exogenous oxytocin stimulates prolactin release from the pituitary; oxytocin apparently plays a physiologic role in the hypothalamic control of prolactin secretion.[77] Despite these findings and the possibility that prolactin deficiency may underlie agalactia.[78] (T.F. Loch, personal communication), oxytocin has not been beneficial in stimulating milk flow in mares with true agalactia.

Improvement of Maternal Behavior

The role oxytocin plays in modifying maternal behavior remains to be elucidated, but it may be significant. Direct intracerebroventricular injection of oxytocin after estradiol priming improved maternal behavior in ewes. However, intravenous injection of oxytocin, with or without estradiol priming, did not affect maternal behavior.[79,80]

ERGOT ALKALOIDS

Mature parasitic fungi of the genus Claviceps contain various combinations of ergot alkaloids. The most common ergot mold, C. purpurea, parasitizes several types of grains and grasses. Ingestion of contaminated grains has caused outbreaks of ergotism in both man and animals but is infrequently encountered today. Ergot is a mixture of different types of alkaloids possessing a variety of biologic effects, the most important of which for this discussion are vasoconstriction and inhibition of prolactin/serotonin release. Ergot alkaloids are considered to be α-adrenergic antagonists and dopamine agonists; however, because they affect a variety of organs at concentrations less than those required for α-blockade, they are not used pharmacologically for their α-blocking properties.[81,82] Two ergot alkaloids, ergonovine and the semisynthetic bromocriptine, have had limited applications in equine reproductive therapeutics.

ERGONOVINE

Available Preparations

Ergonovine maleate is supplied as a clear injectable solution at a concentration of 0.2 mg/mL. It should be kept refrigerated and protected from light when not in use to ensure potency.

Possible Indications

Ergonovine maleate affects the uterus to a greater extent than other ergot alkaloids[83] and is used in veterinary medicine for its potent oxytocic activity. Also in contrast to other ergot alkaloids, ergonovine does not cause α-blockade; its vasoconstrictive effects are instead the result of direct stimulation of the vascular smooth muscle.[81] During pregnancy and immediately postpartum, the uterus is especially sensitive to the direct stimulatory effects of ergonovine on the myometrium; lesser effects are exhibited on vascular smooth muscle. Administering small doses of ergonovine will increase the force and frequency of myometrial contractions. More prolonged and forceful contractions, with increased resting tonus occur with large doses.[83]

Control of Postpartum Uterine Hemorrhage

In contrast to the prolonged and forceful uterine contractions resulting from administration of ergonovine maleate, oxytocin exerts a more dose-dependent response with wave-like uterine contractions; therefore, oxytocin rather than ergonovine is preferable for induction of parturition in the mare. However, ergonovine may be more useful in the control of postpartum hemorrhage where its contractile effect on the myometrium combined with its vasomotor properties should act synergistically to arrest uterine hemorrhage. Following intramuscular injection of 1 to 3 mg ergonovine maleate, the latency to onset of action is ≥ 15 min with a duration of 2 to 4 h.[83]

Promoting Passage of the Placenta

In species other than the mare, particularly the cow and the bitch, ergonovine maleate has been used in the management of retained fetal membranes and postpartum metritis, but its use is usually reserved for those instances when oxytocin therapy fails to elicit the desired response.[84] The use of ergonovine in the cow has traditionally been reserved for treatment of fetal membranes retained for greater than 48 h postpartum, because the bovine uterus appears to be much less responsive to oxytocin administration after this time. The mare's uterus, however, does not appear to become as refractive to the effects of oxytocin and is favored over ergonovine as an ecbolic agent because of its more physiologic action. Ergonovine is not used routinely for fear that the stimulation of a more intense response and much longer half-life than that of oxytocin may increase the chance of uterine rupture.

BROMOCRIPTINE

Bromocriptine is a semisynthetic ergot alkaloid whose structural conformation resembles dopamine.[78] Dopamine appears to be the major activator of the hypothalamic prolactin inhibitory factors which exhibits tonic inhibitory control of prolactin secretion from the anterior pituitary gland.[78,85] Bromocriptine, by virtue of its potent dopamine agonist properties, also inhibits prolactin secretion.[86]

During the middle ages, physicians observed that infants born to women suffering from gangrenous ergotism died because their mothers failed to lactate.[87] In these women, the use of rye flour contaminated with the ergot-producing fungus C. purpurea explains the phenomenon. In addition to the intense vasoconstriction which occurred as a result of ingesting ergot contaminants with the rye flour, prolactin was inhibited, which led to a cessation of lactation.[78] Early-twentieth-century obstetricians noted that some women treated with large doses of ergot for postpartum hemorrhage also had difficulty lactating.[78] These observations along with Shelesnyak's investigations[88,89] provided the impetus for the development of bromocriptine, which significantly suppresses prolactin secretion but has minimal vascular and uterotonic effects.[78] Bromocriptine has become an important drug in the treatment of prolactin-secreting tumors and for inducing lactational arrest in humans. Its use for these purposes has recently been employed in equine patients.[90] (T.F. Loch, personal communication).

Available Preparations

Bromocriptine is not labeled for use in horses but is available for use in humans as bromocriptine mesylate (2.5- or 5.0-mg capsules). It is also available through chemical supply companies as bromocriptine mesylate in crystalline salt form.

Possible Indications

Spurious Lactation in Nongravid Mares. Spurious lactation or galactorrhea in nongravid mares is uncommon, but can be a frustrating phenomenon. Because prolactin is the primary stimulus for mammary development and milk production, the use of bromocriptine for this condition would be a logical therapeutic choice. Preliminary studies using bromocriptine to cause cessation of lactation in mares have provided promising results (T.F. Loch, personal communication). The drug was administered by intramuscular injection at a dose of 0.08 mg/kg$^{0.75}$ (i.e., metabolic body weight) divided bid. Interestingly, other investigators found the inhibitory effect of bromocriptine occurred in the horse only when basal concentrations of prolactin were highest (in May) and that no effect was observed on serum prolactin concentrations or prolactin secretion in November when basal concentrations were low in normal mares.[91]

Premature Lactation in Pregnant Mares. Failure of passive transfer in foals commonly results from colostral loss owing to premature lactation in older, multiparous mares. Although it seems plausible that bromocriptine might be beneficial in alleviating this problem, its use for this condition cannot be advocated without further investigation. Bromocriptine crosses the placenta and can suppress fetal prolactin.[92] If administered during development of the fetal hypothalamic-pituitary axis, bromocriptine may induce subtle neuroendocrine changes that are not readily detectable.[78] In addition, administration of bromocriptine during pregnancy may jeopardize milk production after parturition. One method of preventing failure of passive transfer in foals whose dams prematurely lactate is to harvest the prematurely secreted colostrum and store it frozen until parturition occurs. Maintaining frozen "colostrum banks" on brood mare farms for this and other problems such as agalactia is highly advisable.

Lactational Anestrus. A small percentage of lactating mares fail to exhibit estrus in the postpartum period, and this can sometimes be corrected by early weaning of the foal. These mares are generally in good body condition, which distinguishes this disturbance from that associated with nutritional deprivation. It is suspected that lactation contributes to the disruption of reproductive cyclicity, possibly through increased prolactin production, and if so, bromocriptine may be a useful product to control this problem. A dose which would reestablish cyclicity yet maintain sufficient milk production for the nursing foal is likely to be difficult to acquire. Although high prolactin levels have been shown to suppress prolactin secretion during lactation in rats and women, these results have not been duplicated in domestic animals, including the mare.[93]

Miscellaneous Information. The majority of human patients receiving bromocriptine experience dose-related side effects, especially at the initiation of therapy. Side effects include postrual hypotension, hallucinations, erythromelalgia, digital vasospasm, and sphincter disturbances. Syncopal episodes occur in approximately 0.2% of human patients receiving their first dose of bromocriptine.[78] These side effects have not been reported in the horse.

REFERENCES

1. Mendelson, C.R., et al.: Use of a molecular probe to study regulation of aromatase cytochrome p-450. Biol. Reprod., *42:*1–10, 1990.
2. Siiteri, P.K.: Extraglandular oestrogen formation and serum binding of oestradiol: Relationship to cancer. J. Endocrinol., *89:*119p–129p, 1981.
3. Zavy, M.T., Vernon, M.W., Sharp, D.C., and Bazer F.W.: Endocrine aspects of early pregnancy in pony mares: A comparison of uterine luminal and peripheral plasma levels of steroids during the estrous cycle and early pregnancy. Endocrinology, *115:*214–219, 1984.
4. Reeves, J.J.:Endocrinology of Reproduction. *In* Reproduction in Farm Animals. 5th ed. Edited by E.S.E. Hafez. Philadelphia, Lea & Febiger, 1987, pp. 85–106.
5. Varner, D.D., and Blanchard, T.L.: An update on uterine defense mechanisms in the mare. J. Equine Vet. Sci., *10:*169–175, 1990.
6. Heap, R.B., and Flint, H.P.: Pregnancy. *In* Reproduction in Mammals, 2nd ed. Edited by C.R. Austin and R.V. Short. London, Cambridge University Press, 1982, pp. 153–194.
7. Ginther, O.J.: Reproductive Biology of the Mare—Basic and Applied Aspects. Cross Plains, WI, published by the author, 1979, pp. 47–50.
8. Hillman, R.B., and Loy, R.G.: Oestrogen excretion in mares in relation to various reproductive states. J. Reprod. Fertil. Suppl., *23:*223–230, 1975.
9. Booth, N.H., and McDonald, L.E. (eds.): Veterinary Pharmacology and Therapeutics. 5th ed. Ames, Iowa State University Press, 1982.
10. Physicians' Desk Reference. Oradell, NJ, Medical Economics, 1988.
11. Lofstedt, R.M.: Some aspects of manipulation and diagnostic endocrinology of the broodmare. Proc. Soc. Theriogenology, 67–93, 1986.
12. Asa, C.S., Goldfoot, D.A., Garcia, M.C., and Ginther, O.J.: Sexual behavior in ovariectomized and seasonally anovulatory pony mares (Equus caballus). Horm. Behav., *14:*46–54, 1980.
13. Asa, C.S., Goldfoot, D.A., Garcia, M.C., and Ginther, O.J.: The effect of estradiol and progesterone on the sexual behavior of ovariectomized mares. Physiol. Behav., *33:*681–686, 1984.
14. Neely, D.P.: Hormone therapy in mares. *In* Equine Reproduction. Edited by D.P. Neeley, I.K.M. Liu, and R.B. Hillman. Trenton, Veterinary Learning Systems, 1983, pp. 23–37.
15. Loy, R.G., Pemstein, P., O'Canna, D., and Douglas, R.H.: Control of ovulation in cycling mares with ovarian steroids and prostaglandin. Theriogenology, *15:*191–200, 1981.

16. Taylor, T.B., Pemstein, R., and Loy, R.G.: Control of ovulation in mares in the early breeding season with ovarian steroids and prostaglandin. J. Reprod. Fertil. Suppl., *32:*219–224, 1982.
17. Garcia, M.C., and Ginther, O.J.: Regulation of plasma LH by estradiol and progesterone in ovariectomized mares. Biol. Reprod., *19:*447–453, 1978.
18. Varner, D.D., Blanchard, T.L., and Brinsko, S.P.: Estrogens, oxytocin and ergot alkaloids—Uses in reproductive management of mares. Proc. Am. Assoc. Equine Pract., 219–241, 1988.
19. Loy, R.C.: Characteristics of postpartum reproduction in mares. Vet. Clin. North Am. Large Anim. Pract. *2:*345–359, 1980.
20. Gygax, A.P., Ganjam, V.K., and Kenney, R.M.: Clinical, microbiological and histological changes associated with uterine involution in the mare. J. Reprod. Fertil. Suppl., *27:*571–578, 1979.
21. Blanchard, T.L., et al.: Effects of postparturient uterine lavage on uterine involution in the mare. Theriogenology, *32:*527–535, 1989.
22. Shideler, R.K., McChesney, A.E., Squires, E.L., and Osborne, M.: Effect of uterine lavage on clinical and laboratory parameters in postpartum mares. Equine Pract., *9:*20–26, 1987.
23. Blanchard, T.L., et al.: Effects of myotonic agents on uterine involution in the mare. Abstract presented at the Seventieth Annual Meeting of the Conference of Research Workers in Animal Disease, Chicago, Nov. 6–7, 1989.
24. Loy, R.G., Evans, M.J., Pemstein, R., and Taylor, T.B.: Effects of injected ovarian steroids on reproductive patterns and performance in post-partum mares. J. Reprod. Fertil. Suppl., *32:*199–204, 1982.
25. Bell, R.J., and Bristol, F.: Fertility and pregnancy loss after delay of foal oestrus with progesterone and oestradiol-17β. J. Reprod. Fertil. Suppl., *35:*667–668, 1987.
26. Bristol, F., Jacobs, K.A., and Pawlyshyn, V.: Synchronization of estrus in post-partum mares with progesterone and estradiol 17β. Theriogenology, *19:*779–785, 1983.
27. Nelson, E.M., Kiefer, B.L., Roser, J.F., and Evans, J.W.: Serum estradiol-17β concentrations during spontaneous silent estrus and after prostaglandin treatment in the mare. Theriogenology, *23:*241–262, 1985.
28. Kiefer, B.L., et al.: Progesterone patterns observed with multiple injections of PGF analogue in the cyclic mare. J. Reprod. Fertil. Suppl., *27:*237–244, 1979.
29. Greenwald, G.S.: Species differences in egg transport in response to exogenous estrogen. Anat. Rec., *157:* 163–172, 1967.
30. Maia, H., Jr., Salinas, L.A., Fernandez, E.O., and Pauerstein, C.J.: Pharmacologic modification of the time course of ovum transport in guinea pigs. Fertil. Steril., *28:*1361–1364, 1977.
31. Pauerstein, C.J., Anderson, B.S., Chatkoff, M.L., and Hodgson, B.J.: Effect of estrogen and progesterone on the time-course of tubal ovum transport in rabbits. Am. J. Obstet. Gynecol., *120:*299–308, 1974.
32. Saksena, S.K., and Harper, M.J.K.: Relationship between concentration of prostaglandin F (PGF) in the oviduct and egg transport in rabbits. Biol. Reprod., *13:*68–76, 1975.
33. Herron, M.A., and Sis, R.F.: Ovum transport in the cat and the effect of estrogen administration. Am. J. Vet. Res., *35:*1277–1279, 1974.
34. Kennelly, J.J.: The effect of mestranol on canine reproduction. Biol. Reprod., *1:*282–288, 1969.
35. Hawk, H.W., and Cooper, B.S.: Improvement of sperm transport in estrous rabbits by exogenous estradiol. Biol. Reprod., *15:*402–405, 1976.
36. Hawk, H.W., and Cooper, B.S.: Improvement of sperm transport by the administration of estradiol to estrous ewes. J. Anim. Sci., *41:*1400–1406, 1975.
37. Rexroad, C.E., Jr., Cooper, B.S., and Hawk, H.W.: Relationship of estradiol and prostaglandins in sperm retention in the mated rabbit. Theriogenology, *12:*237–243, 1979.
38. Nishikawa, Y., Kamata, Y., and Baba, T.: Preventive effect of estradiol on manifestation of purulent endometritis in rat uteri infected with Escherichia coli: With special reference to morphological changes of the endometrial epithelium. Jpn. J. Vet. Sci., *49:*313–321, 1987.
39. Watson, E.D. Stokes, C.R., and Bourne F.J.: Influence of ovarian steroids on adherence (in vitro) of Streptococcus zooepidemicus to endometrial epithelial cell. Equine Vet. J., *20:*371–372, 1988.
40. Hamer, J.M., et al.: Effect of administration of estradiol and progesterone, and bacterial contamination, on endometrial morphology of acyclic mares. Anim. Reprod. Sci., *9:*317–322, 1985.
41. Garfield, R.E., Kannan, M.S., and Daniel, E.E.: Gap junction formation in myometrium: Control by estrogens, progesterone, and prostaglandins. Am. J. Physiol., *238:*C81–C89, 1980.
42. Garfield, R.E., Sims, S.M., Kannan, M.S., and Daniel, E.E.: Possible role of gap junctions in activation of myometrium during parturition. Am. J. Physiol., *235:* C168–C179, 1978.
43. Verhoeff, A., Garfield, R.E., Ramondt, J., and Wallenburg, H.C.S.: Electrical and mechanical uterine activity and gap junctions in estrogen-treated oophorectomized sheep. Am. J. Obstet. Gynecol., *155:*1192–1196, 1986.
44. Verhoeff, A., Garfield, R.E., Ramondt, J., and Wallenburg, H.C.S.: Myometrial activity related to gap junction area in periparturient and in ovariectomized oestrogen treated sheep. Acta Physiol. Hung., *67:*117–129, 1986.
45. Windmoller, R., Lye, S.J., and Challis, J.R.G.: Estradiol modulation of ovine uterine activity. Can. J. Physiol. Pharmacol., *61:*722–728, 1983.
46. Pashen, R.L.: Maternal and foetal endocrinology during late pregnancy and parturition in the mare. Equine Vet. J., *16:*233–238, 1984.
47. Hayes, K.E.N., and Ginther, O.J.: Role of progesterone and estrogen in development of uterine tone in mares. Theriogenology, *25:*581–590, 1986.
48. Weithenauer, J., McDowell, K.J., Davis, S.D., and Rothman, T.K.: Effect of exogenous progesterone and estrogen on early embryonic growth in pony mares. Biol. Reprod. Suppl. 1, *34:*102, 1986.
49. McDowell, K.J., Sharp, D.C., and Grubaugh W.: Comparison of progesterone and progesterone + estrogen on total and specific uterine proteins in pony mares. J. Reprod. Fertil. Suppl., *35:*335–342, 1987.
50. McKinnon, A.O., Squires, E.L., Carnevale, E.M., and Hermenet, M.J.: Ovariectomized steroid-treated mares as embryo transfer recipients and as a model to study the role of progestins in pregnancy maintenance. Theriogenology, *29:*1055–1063, 1988.
51. McDonald, L.E.: Veterinary Endocrinology and Reproduction. 3rd ed. Philadelphia, Lea & Febiger, 1980.
52. Roberts, S.J.: Veterinary Obstetrics and Genital Diseases (Theriogenology). 3rd ed. Woodstock, VT, published by the author, 1986.
53. Leadon, D.P., Jeffcott, L.B., and Rossdale, P.D.: Behavior

and viability of the premature neonatal foal after induced parturition. Am. J. Vet. Res., *47:*1870–1873, 1986.

54. Townsend, H.G.G., Tabel, H., and Bristol, F.M.: Induction of parturition in mares: Effect on passive transfer of immunity to foals. J. Am. Vet. Med. Assoc., *182:*255–257, 1983.

55. Hillman, R.B.: Equine parturition, *In* Equine Reproduction. Edited by D.P. Neely, J.K.M. Liu, and R.B. Hillman. Trenton, Veterinary Learning Systems Co., Inc., 1983, pp. 80–90.

56. Ousey, J.C., Dudan, F., and Rossdale, P.D.: Preliminary studies of mammary secretions in the mare to assess foetal readiness for birth. Equine Vet. J., *16:*259–263, 1984.

57. Hillman, R.B.: Induction of parturition in mares. J. Reprod. Fertil. Suppl., *23:*641–644, 1975.

58. Lye, S.J., Wlocek, M.E., and Challis, J.R.G.: Relation between fetal arterial pO_2 and oxytocin-induced uterine contractions in pregnant sheep. Can. J. Physiol. Pharmacol., *62:*1337–1340, 1984.

59. Marnet, P.G., Laurentie, M., Garcia-Villar, R., and Toutain, P.L.: Route of administration and uterine response to oxytocin in the ewe. J. Vet. Pharmacol. Ther., *9:*439–441, 1986.

60. Boyd, I.E.: The active management of labor. *In* Contemporary Obstetrics and Gynaecology. Edited by G.V.P. Chamberlain. London, Northwood Publications, 1977.

61. Marnet, P.G., Laurentie, M., Garcia-Villar, R., and Toutain, P.L.: Effects de doses excessives d'ocytocine sur la contractilite uterine chez la brebis. Revue Med. Vet., *136:*315–320, 1985.

62. Asbury, A.C.: The reproductive system. *In* Equine Medicine and Surgery. 3rd ed. Edited by R.A. Mannsmann, E.S. McAllister, and P.W. Pratt. Santa Barbara, American Veterinary Publications, 1982, pp. 1355–1356.

63. Pashen, R.L.: Low doses of oxytocin can induce foaling at term. Equine Vet. J., *12:*85–87, 1980.

64. Barnes, R.J., et al.: Foetal and maternal plasma concentrations of 13,14-dihydro-15-oxoprostaglandin F in the mare during late pregnancy and at parturition. J. Endocrinol., *78:*201–215, 1978.

65. Jeffcott, L.B., and Rossdale, P.D.: A critical review of current methods for induction of parturition in the mare. Equine Vet. J., *9:*208–215, 1977.

66. Stewart, D.R., Kindahl, H., Stabenfeldt, G.H., and Hughes, J.P.: Concentrations of 15-keto-13, 14-dihydroprostaglandin F2α in the mare during spontaneous and oxytocin induced foaling. Equine Vet. J., *16:*270–274, 1984.

67. Wright, J.G.: Parturition in the mare. J. Comp. Pathol., *53:*212–219, 1943.

68. Strzemienski, P.J., Dyer, R.M., Sertich, P.L., and Kenney, R.M.: Bactericidal activity of mare neutrophils in cycling and pregnant mares. J. Reprod. Fertil., *80:*289–293, 1987.

69. Rossdale, P.D., and Ricketts, S.W.: Equine Stud Farm Medicine. Philadelphia, Lea & Febiger, 1980.

70. Smith, J.M.: Hydrallantois in the Mare. Mod. Equine Med., March/April 7–12, 1983.

71. Vandeplassche, M., Spincemaille, J., and Bouters, R.: Aetiology, pathogenesis and treatment of retained placenta in the mare. Equine Vet. J., *3:*144–147, 1971.

72. Burns, S.J., Judge, N.G., Martin, J.E., and Adams, L.G.: Management of retained placenta in mares. Proc. Am. Assoc. Equine Pract., 381–390, 1977.

73. Threlfall, W.R., Provencher, R., and Carleton, C.L.: Retained fetal membranes in the mare. Proc. Am. Assoc. Equine Pract., 649–656, 1987.

74. Cox, J.E.: Excessive retainment of the placenta in a mare. Vet. Rec., *89:*252–253, 1971.

75. Goff, A.K., Pontbriand, D., and Sirois J.: Oxytocin stimulation of plasma 15-keto-13, 14-dihydro prostaglandin F2α during the oestrous cycle and early pregnancy in the mare. J. Reprod. Fertil. Suppl., *35:*253–260, 1987.

76. Cowels, R.R.: Lactation failure in the mare. Proc. Soc. Theriogenology, 222–233, 1983.

77. Samson, W.K., Lumpkin, M.D., and McCann, S.M.: Evidence for a physiologic role of oxytocin in the control of prolactin secretion. Endocrinology, *119:*554–560, 1986.

78. Barbieri, R.L., and Ryan, K.J.: Bromocriptine: endocrine pharmacology and therapeutic applications. Fertil. Steril., *39:*727–741, 1983.

79. Baldwin, B.A., Kendrick, K.M., and Keverne, E.B.: Intracerebroventricular oxytocin stimulates maternal behavior in sheep. J. Physiol., *381:*80P 1986.

80. Kendrick, K.M., Keverne, E.B., and Baldwin, B.A.: Intracerebroventricular oxytocin stimulates maternal behaviour in the sheep. Neuroendocrinology, *46:*56–61, 1987.

81. Adams, H.R.: Adrenergic and Antiadrenergic Drugs. *In* Veterinary Pharmacology and Therapeutics. 5th ed. Edited by N.H. Booth and L.E. McDonald. Ames, Iowa State University Press, 1982, pp. 89–112.

82. Henton, J.E.: Agalactia in the mare—A review and some new insights. Proc. Soc. Theriogenology, 203–221, 1983.

83. McDonald, L.E.: Hormones affecting reproduction. *In* Veterinary Pharmacology and Therapeutics. 5th ed. Edited by N.H. Booth and L.E. McDonald. Ames, Iowa State University Press, 1982, pp. 530–552.

84. Magne, M.L.: Acute Metritis in the Bitch. *In* Current Therapy in Theriogenology 2. Edited by D.A. Morrow. Philadelphia, W.B. Saunders, 1986, pp. 505–506.

85. Janssens, L.A.A.: Treatment of pseudopregnancy with bromocriptine an ergot alkaloid. Vet. Rec., *119:*172–174, 1986.

86. Caron, G.M., et al.: Dopaminergic receptors in the anterior pituitary gland. J. Biol. Chem., *253:*2244–2253, 1978.

87. Barger, G.: Ergot and Ergotism. London, Gurneney and Jackson, 1931.

88. Shelesnyak, M.C.: Ergotoxine inhibition of deciduoma formation and its reversal by progesterone. Am. J. Physiol., *179:*301–304, 1954.

89. Shelesnyak, M.C.: Maintenance of gestation in ergotoxine-treated pregnant rats by exogenous prolactin. Acta Endocrinol. (Copenh.), *27:*99, 1958.

90. Beech, J.: Tumors of the pituitary gland (pars intermedia). *In* Current Therapy in Equine Medicine 2. Edited by N.E. Robinson. Philadelphia, W.B. Saunders, 1987, pp. 182–185.

91. Johnson, A.L., and Becker, S.E.: Effects of physiological and pharmacological agents on serum prolactin concentrations in the nonpregnant mare. J. Anim. Sci., *65:*1292–1297, 1987.

92. Lowe, K.C., et al.: Effect of long-term bromocriptine infusion on plasma prolactin and ovine chorionic somatomammotropin in the pregnant ewe and fetal sheep. Am. J. Obstet. Gynecol., *135:*733–777, 1979.

93. Jainudeen, M.R., and Hafez, E.S.E.: Reproductive failure in females. *In* Reproduction in Farm Animals. 5th ed. Edited by E.S.E. Hafez. Philadelphia, Lea & Febiger, 1983, pp. 399–422.

CHAPTER 38

INDUCTION OF OVULATION

E. Palmer

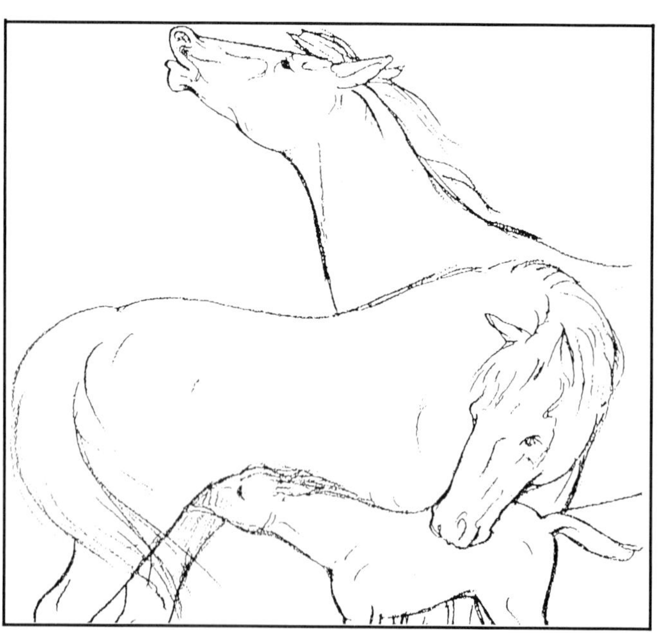

This chapter discusses induction of ovulation when the mare spontaneously presents a growth of follicle(s) up to a preovulatory size. In most cases, the mare is cyclic and will ovulate spontaneously but at an unpredictable time. In the transitional period or in some pathologic conditions, mares may present normal follicular growth but fail to ovulate. Our objective is to provide or induce the luteinizing hormone (LH) stimulus, which constitutes the natural signal for the follicle to ovulate.

INDICATIONS FOR INDUCED OVULATION

In cyclic mares, the purpose of induction of ovulation is generally to improve breeding management and synchronize ovulation more closely with mating or insemination or upon convenience. When the mare must be transported for mating or when special shipment is needed for fresh or cooled semen, the use of only one breeding per cycle is often mandated. When fresh semen or mating is used, an interval from insemination to ovulation of 0 to 48 h is acceptable, indicating the precision needed in timing of ovulation. When frozen semen is used, an interval shorter than 24 h from insemination to ovulation is necessary and more precision is needed. Recent research concerning in vitro fertilization indicates that the preovulatory follicle should be punctured a few hours before ovulation and requires a high accuracy of prediction of ovulation time.

In the transitional period, estrus may last 2 to 3 weeks, and the mare must be inseminated repeatedly, unless a strategy of assessment of the follicular growth and induction of ovulation is used. Furthermore, the need of induction is evident in the case of pathologic failure of ovulation, although the frequency and genesis of such an abnormality is not well documented.

TIMING OF INDUCTION

Initial research on induction of ovulation of mares used a fixed time during estrus; generally mares were treated on day 2 of estrus, and the effect of treatment was judged by the significant reduction of duration of estrus or of the interval from beginning of estrus to ovulation. However, variability of follicular development at this stage of the cycle may explain some of the differences in results (caused by insufficient size of the follicle at treatment). A more appropriate method consists of detecting the growth and size of the follicle by rectal palpation or, preferably, by ultrasonography and inducing ovulation when a developing follicle reaches a specific size.

Although the minimum size for a follicle to respond by ovulation from a luteinizing hormone (LH) stimulus has not been critically tested, the author has been highly successful when using a minimal size of 33 mm in pony mares and 35 mm in large mares.

In the transitional period or cases of pathologic anovulation, the growth of the follicle must be accurately followed to avoid treatment of an old atretic regressing follicle, which is obviously no longer capable of ovulating. After cessation of growth, regression of follicles is much slower than the growth, and they remain palpable or visible via ultrasonography for several days. Induction of ovulation following a single examination without verification that the follicle is in its growing period is, therefore, likely to fail in many cases.

INDUCING AGENTS

HUMAN CHORIONIC GONADOTROPIN

The use of human chorionic gonadotropin (hCG) for induction of ovulation has a long history. Day first administered 1000 "mares units" of hCG when the follicle was mature enough and induced ovulation.[1] Since Day's pioneering work in 1939, Davidson, in 1947, showed that ovulation was induced between 24 and 48 h after hCG injection.[2] Nishikawa, in 1959, gave hCG on day 1 of estrus and induced ovulation within 3 days in seven of nine mares.[3] Butterfield et al. reported that fertility was normal following systemic injection of 2500 IU of the hormone.[4] Loy and Hughes, using 2500 IU hCG intravenously on day 2 of estrus, reported ovulation 4.09 days after treatment, whereas control mares ovulated 6.53 days after treatment.[5] Webel et al. studied the precise timing of maturation of oocytes following hCG injection.[6]

Sullivan et al. first reported adverse effects of hCG administration; they found a reduction in the percentage of mares responding favorably during successive cycles.[7] Complete failure of expected induction was found on the third cycle. An immunologic cause was suspected. Roser et al. confirmed the hypothesis that mares develop antibodies after two to five injections when given on successive cycles. These antibodies did not cross-react with equine LH and natural cycles were not disturbed by anti-hCG immunization.[8] Duchamp et al. showed that mares immunized against hCG did not respond to hCG treatment by ovulating at a prescribed time.[9] They tried to reduce the immune response to repeated injections of hCG by giving corticoids at the same time but had no success. Seven of eight mares had high anti-hCG antibody titers after four injections of 2000 IU of hCG intravenously and this proportion was identical in animals given a long-acting corticoid injection at the same time.

Injection of 2000 to 2500 IU hCG is a well-documented method for induction of ovulation between 24 and 48 h after administration. However, because of its immunogenicity, no more than two injections should be given during the same year.

EQUINE PITUITARY EXTRACTS

The first step in the preparation of purified LH and follicle-stimulating hormone (FSH) is extraction with 40% ethanol, followed by reprecipitation with acetone or 80% ethanol.[10,11] The extract crude equine gonadotropin (CEG) contains 8 to 10% LH and 4 to 6% FSH. The FSH content has been used successfully for induction of follicular growth in anestrous mares and induction of multiple follicles in anestrous and cyclic mares.[12,13] Its LH content is also suitable to induce ovulation. Duchamp et al. showed that a single intravenous dose of 25 mg of CEG (equivalent to 2 mg LH), given when the growing follicle was 35 mm in diameter, induced ovulation between 24 and 48 h in 75% of treated mares, whereas only 40% of control mares ovulated in the same interval.[9] Bézard et al. also evaluated the time of ovulation following CEG administration in pony mares and found that at least 65% of ovulations occurred in the period from 34 to 40 h postinjection.[14] Fertility following such treatment appeared normal. Equine pituitary extracts, contrary to hCG, should not lead to formation of antibodies. However, this must be more carefully evaluated because gonadotropin preparations always show some heterogeneity and some of the isoforms might be read as foreign compounds when injected (IM or IV).

The greatest problems in the use of pituitary extract are its availability and its expense. Presently it is not on the market in any country, and only experimental preparations are available. The future of this method depends on the interest of the horse market and industry. In the future, equine LH made by recombinant biotechnologic techniques will probably be developed to replace that extracted from slaughter material.

In all the cases of use of hCG and CEG, the presence of a growing follicle ($\geq$ 35 mm) is essential for the precise timing of ovulation (34 to 40 h postinjection) after administration.

GONADOTROPIN-RELEASING HORMONE AND ANALOGUES

Since the identification and isolation of luteinizing hormone-releasing hormone (LH-RH) in 1971,[15] numerous studies have used the molecule to control ovarian activity. However, because the pulsatile release of gonadotropin-releasing hormone (GnRH) and LH was not taken into consideration in early studies, a rational use of LH-RH has not been developed. Many peptides have been synthesized which have agonist or antagonist effects and different half-lives, allowing various ways to control pituitary and ovarian activities.[16] The use of these products only for induction of ovulation in the cyclic mare will be discussed. At first, researchers used LH-RH to replace hCG administration for induction of ovulation during estrus. Reports from early trials were optimistic, because the interval from onset of estrus to ovulation found by Irvine et al. was shorter following daily injections of 2 mg GnRH (4.6 ± 0.8 days) or a single dose of 2 mg (7.3 ± 2.1 days) than in nontreated animals (10.3 ± 2.0 days).[17] Similar results were reported by Kreider et al.[18]

In spite of these encouraging results, further studies found much less efficiency of GnRH as an inducer of ovulation. A single injection or once daily injections of high doses (up to 5 mg) have been used with no effect on the interval to ovulation after treatment.[19–22] Duchamp et al. reported that after treatment with 2 mg LH-RH, when a follicle reached 35 mm, ovulation occurred between 24 and 48 h in only 40% (n = 30) of mares, a percentage not different from that in control mares (18%, n = 32) but significantly less than in mares treated with 2500 IU hCG (84%, n = 31).[9]

Johnson found that pulsatile administration of low doses of LH-RH (20 μg hourly) to cyclic mares beginning day 16 after ovulation induced ovulation in 2.9 ± 0.6 days (n = 7), whereas saline-treated mares ovulated in 5.9 ± 0.3 days (n = 7).[23] This study confirmed that pulsatile administration of low doses of LH-RH can be effective in inducing ovulation, but LH-RH is not easy to use in practice. Squires et al. tried repeated injections of a potent analogue of GnRH (buserelin) every 12 h and this was as successful as hCG (interval from treatment to ovulation 45.6 ± 15.2 h and 52.0 ± 23.9 h) when compared with an untreated group (76.0 ± 28.9 h).[24] Humke and Beaupoil used only one injection of buserelin, 20 or 40 μg, and induced 73% (n = 53) or 86% (n = 42) ovulation within 48 h, whereas only 42% (n = 48) control mares ovulated in the same interval.[25] These results need to be confirmed before LH-RH can be used as a simple, reliable alternative to hCG administration to induce ovulation.

PROSTAGLANDINS

The role of prostaglandins in the process of ovulation is well known and was reviewed by Armstrong.[26] A preovulatory rise is seen in prostaglandin $F_2\alpha$ ($PGF_2\alpha$) and prostaglandin E_2 (PGE_2) concentrations in follicular fluid, whereas inhibitors of prostaglandin synthesis block the ovulation process in various species. Savage and Liptrap induced ovulation by injecting one dose of 250 μg of an analogue of $PGF_2\alpha$ (fenprostalene) to mares 60 h after onset of estrus.[27] They found a significant reduction in the interval to ovulation in treated mares (41 ± 21 h, n = 16) when compared with control mares (73 ± 30 h, n = 16). Vidament (personal communication) tried to reproduce the results using the same dose and product injected to mares when the follicle reached 35 mm, but failed to show any difference in the interval from treatment to ovulation between treated (3.9 ± 1.5 days, n = 15) and control (3.1 ± 1.1 days, n = 17) mares. Squires et al. used another analogue of $PGF_2\alpha$ (luprostiol) and also failed to induce ovulation.[24]

Further studies are necessary before the use of prostaglandins for induction of ovulation in the mare can be proposed, and at present its use appears to be questionable.

REFERENCES

1. Day, F.T.: Ovulation and the descent of the ovum in the fallopian tube of the mare after treatment with gonadotrophic hormones. J. Agric. Sci. Camb., *29*:459–469, 1939.
2. Davison, D.F.: The control of ovulation in the mare with reference to insemination with stored sperm. J. Agric. Sci., *37*:287–290, 1947.
3. Nishikawa, Y.: Studies on Reproduction in Horses. Tokyo, Japan Racing Assoc., 1959.
4. Butterfield, R.M., Matthews, R.G., and Rophia, R.T.: Observations of the fertility of Thoroughbred mares. Aust. Vet. J., *40*:415–417, 1964.
5. Loy, R.G., and Hughes, J.P.: The effects of human chorionic gonadotropin on ovulation, length of estrus and fertility in the mare. Cornell Vet., *56*:41–50, 1966.
6. Webel, S., Franklin, V., Harland, B., and Dziuk, P.J.: Fertility, ovulation, and maturation of eggs in mares injected with hCG. J. Reprod. Fertil., *51*:337–341, 1977.
7. Sullivan, J.J., Parker, W.G., and Larson, L.L.: Duration of estrus and ovulation time in nonlactating mares given human chorionic gonadotropin during three successive estrous periods. J. Am. Vet. Med. Assoc., *162*:895–898, 1973.
8. Roser, J.F., et al.: The development of antibodies to human chorionic gonadotrophin following its repeated injection in the cyclic mare. J. Reprod. Fertil. Suppl., *27*:173–179, 1979.
9. Duchamp, G., Bour, B., Combarnous, Y., and Palmer, E.: Alternative solutions to hCG induction of ovulation in the mare. Reprod. Fertil. Suppl., *35*:221–228, 1987.
10. Brasselton, W.E., and McShan, W.H.: Purification and properties of FSH and LH from horse pituitary glands. Arch. Biochem. Biophys., *139*:45–58, 1970.
11. Guillou, F., and Combarnous, Y.: Purification of equine gonadotropins and comparative study of their acid dissociation and receptor-binding specificity. Biochim. Biophys. Acta, *755*:229–236, 1983.
12. Lapin, D.R., and Ginther, O.J.: Induction of ovulation and multiple ovulations in seasonally anovulatory and ovulatory mares with an equine pituitary extract. J. Anim. Sci., *44*:834–842, 1977.
13. Palmer, E.: Recent attempts to improve synchronization of ovulation and to induce superovulation in the mare. Equine Vet. J. Suppl., *3*:11–18, 1985.
14. Bézard, J., Magistrini, M., Duchamp, G., and Palmer, E.: Chronology of equine fertilization and embryonic development in vivo and in vitro. Equine Vet. J. Suppl., *8*:105–110, 1989.
15. Matsuo, H., et al.: Structure of the porcine LH and FSH. Releasing hormone I. The proposed amino acid sequence. Biochem. Biophys. Res. Commun., *43*:1334–1339, 1971.
16. Corbin, A., Bex, F.J., and Jones, R.C.: LH RH and analogs: contraceptive and therapeutic considerations. Int. J. Fertil., *30*:57–65, 1985.
17. Irvine, D.S., Downey, B.R., Parker, W.G., and Sullivan, J.J.: Duration of oestrus and time of ovulation in mares treated with synthetic GnRH (AY 24,031). J. Reprod. Fertil. Suppl., *23*:279–283, 1975.
18. Kreider, J.L., Cornwell, J.C., and Godke, R.A.: Effect of GnRH on estrus, ovulation and fertility in the mare. J. Anim. Sci., *42*:263–264, 1975.
19. Oxender, W.D., Noden, P.A., and Pratt, M.C.: Serum luteinizing hormone, estrus and ovulation in mares following treatment with protaglandin F2α and gonadotrophin releasing hormone. Am. J. Vet. Res., *38*:649–653, 1977.
20. Garcia, M.C., and Ginther, O.J.: Plasma LH concentration in mares treated with GnRH and estradiol. Am. J. Vet. Res., *36*:1581–1584, 1975.

21. Ginther, O.J., and Wentnorth, B.C.: Effect of a synthetic GnRH on plasma concentrations of LH in ponies. Am. J. Vet. Res., *35:*79–81, 1974.

22. Wallace, R.A., Squires, E.L., Voss, J.L., and Pickett, B.W.: Effectiveness of GnRH or GnRH analog in inducing ovulation and shortening estrus in mares. Am. Soc. Anim. Sci., Abstracts, 69th Annual Meeting, p. 215, 1977.

23. Johnson, A.L.: Pulsatile administration of gonadotropin-releasing hormone advances ovulation in cycling mares. Biol. Reprod., *35:*1123–1130, 1986.

24. Squires, E.L., Harrisson, L.A., McKinnon, A.O., and Voss, J.L.: Use of hCG, GnRH agonist or prostaglandin analog for induction of ovulation in mares. Proceedings of the International Congress on Animal Reproduction and Artificial Insemination, Dublin, 1988, p. 460–462.

25. Humke, R., and Beaupoil, J.: Trials to induce ovulation in the mare with a synthetic releasing hormone analogue. Berl. Munch. Tierarztl. Wochenschr., *92:*152–155, 1979.

26. Armstrong, D.T.: Prostaglandins and follicular functions. J. Reprod. Fertil., *62:*283–291, 1981.

27. Savage, N.C., and Liptrap, R.M.: Induction of ovulation in cyclic mares by administration of a synthetic prostaglandin, fenprostalene, during oestrus. J. Reprod. Fertil. Suppl., *35:*239–243, 1987.

PHARMACOLOGIC MANIPULATION OF THE REPRODUCTIVE CYCLE

CHAPTER 39

SYNCHRONIZATION OF OVULATION

F. Bristol

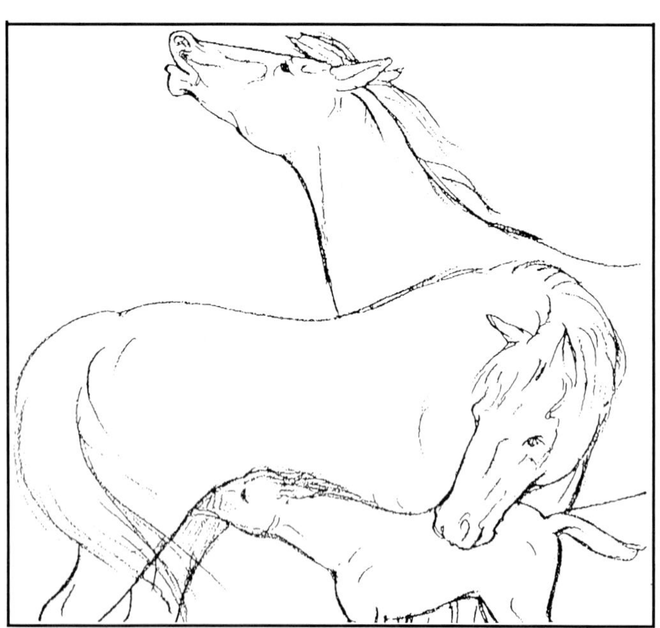

The relatively long and variable follicular phase of the estrous cycle and variation in time of ovulation in the mare result in labor-intensive breeding management. A great deal of time is spent on teasing unreceptive mares in diestrus and most stallions are reluctant to tease mares not showing estrus, especially if other mares in estrus are present. Mares showing signs of estrus are often examined repeatedly to try to predict time of ovulation to reduce the number of matings per estrus. A treatment regimen for synchronization of ovulation in cycling mares should be effective regardless of the stage of the estrous cycle.

Precise control of ovulation could be used to (1) reduce time devoted to estrous detection, (2) allow breeding of individual mares booked to a stallion that is only available at a specific time because of a heavy breeding schedule (heavy booking) or competitive events, (3) schedule mares for insemination with fresh transported semen, (4) synchronize donor and recipient mares in an embryo transfer program, and (5) allow insemination of groups of mares without detection of estrus to minimize labor and management costs.

In normally cycling mares, estrus can be synchronized by shortening or lengthening the diestrous phase of the cycle or with a combination of both these techniques. Although different techniques can be used to control the onset of the follicular phase, considerable variation in time from treatment to ovulation among mares exists, primarily because of inconsistent follicular development during estrus. This is further complicated because of seasonal variation. Almost all researchers have used human chorionic gonadotropin (hCG) in combination with the above techniques to control ovulation. An intramuscular injection of 1500 to 3300 IU of hCG on day 1 or 2 of estrus in normally cycling mares shortened the duration of estrus and hastened ovulation and most ovulated within 48 h of treatment.[1-4]

CYCLING MARES

PROSTAGLANDIN $F_2\alpha$ AND ANALOGUES

Many researchers have demonstrated the luteolytic effect of prostaglandin $F_2\alpha$ and its analogues.[5-8] The interval from a single prostaglandin treatment to onset of estrus and ovulation is variable in mares when compared with other species, and much of this variability depends on the stage of diestrus and follicular status of the ovary at time of treatment.[9,10] The greatest variation in response was observed in mares with large follicles (> 40 mm in diameter). Most of these ovulated shortly (5.1 ± 0.3 days) after treatment, while in some cases the follicles regressed and were replaced by another follicle that ovulated 9.0 ± 0.7 days after treatment.

Although prostaglandin $F_2\alpha$ and its analogues are effective luteolytic agents, the corpus luteum (CL) is refractory to them until approximately 5 days after ovulation. To synchronize estrus in a group of cycling mares at all stages of the estrous cycle, the double prostaglandin regimen, originally developed for cattle, has been adapted for mares. The interval between the two prostaglandin treatments varied between 14 and 15 days in most studies. Using this technique 77.8 to 92.0% of treated mares showed estrus within 6 days of the second prostaglandin treatment.[11–13] Because it is not possible to adequately synchronize ovulation with prostaglandin treatment alone, the double prostaglandin regimen was combined with hCG to reduce variability in the duration of estrus and time of ovulation (Fig. 39–1). Some researchers have given hCG 4 to 6 days after both of the prostaglandin treatments,[14–17] whereas others have treated mares only once with hCG, 5 to 6 days after the second prostaglandin treatment.[11–13,18,19] Palmer and Jousset reported that 75.8% (25 of 33) of mares ovulated 6 to 9 days after the second prostaglandin treatment or within 72 h of the hCG injection given 6 days after the second prostaglandin treatment.[14] In a similar trial, 78% ovulated in a 96-h period.[15] In a group of 13 pony mares that were synchronized for an embryo transfer trial, all mares ovulated between 7 and 10 days after the second prostaglandin treatment with 84.6% (11 of 13) ovulating within 48 h of hCG treatment.[16] The prostaglandin analogue cloprostenol was used in combination with hCG to synchronize a small group of mares and 5 of 8 ovulated within 48 h of the hCG treatment.[17]

Holtan et al. reported that only 26.1% (6 of 23) mares ovulated within 48 h of hCG treatment.[19] In this trial the two prostaglandin injections were given 18 days apart and hCG was given 6 days after the second prostaglandin only. In addition, this study was carried out during the months of June to August, and 26.1% of the mares ovulated before hCG was administered. Other workers have shown that hCG did not significantly reduce the duration of estrus when given during the middle of the natural breeding season when the follicular phase of the estrous cycle is shortest.[12,18,20] As the breeding season progresses, therefore, the interval between the second prostaglandin and the hCG injections should be reduced to induce a larger proportion of mares to ovulate within 48 h of hCG treatment.[20]

Gonadotropin-releasing hormone (GnRH) and its analogues are effective in causing release of luteinizing hormone (LH) when injected into cycling mares.[21] When GnRH was combined with prostaglandin in an attempt to hasten and synchronize ovulation, the time of ovulation was not significantly changed.[12,13,22]

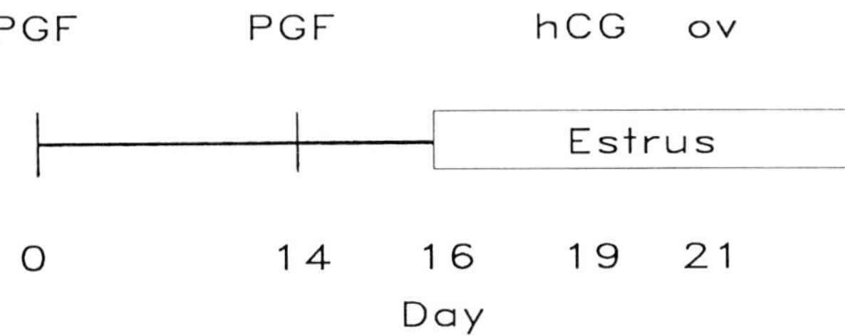

FIG. 39–1. Method for synchronization of ovulation in mares using prostaglandin $F_{2}\alpha$ (PGF) and human chorionic gonadotropin (hCG). ov, expected day of ovulation.

Squires et al. reported that a GnRH agonist given at 12-h intervals beginning on day 2 of estrus, or when the follicle reached a diameter of 35 mm, resulted in ovulation 45.6 h (± 15.2) after treatment, which was significantly shorter than 76.0 h (± 28.9) in control mares.[23] Mares required a mean of 3.8 injections before ovulation was induced. Although GnRH could be used as a substitute for hCG, it must be injected at least four times at 12-h intervals until other formulations or implants can be demonstrated efficacious.

PROGESTERONE AND PROGESTAGENS

Progesterone treatment must be administered long enough (15 to 18 days) to ensure that the CL will regress, and therefore, the only source of progesterone to suppress estrus is the exogenous progesterone. Unlike prostaglandins the response of mares to progesterone is not affected by stage of the estrous cycle at the beginning of treatment. Initially, a long-term treatment consisting of 20 daily progesterone injections was used.[15,24] Although this treatment suppressed signs of estrus, it did not always prevent ovulation during the course of treatment, hence synchronization of ovulation was inconsistent. Holtan et al. synchronized 21 pony mares with 18 daily injections of progesterone followed by hCG, 6 days after the last progesterone treatment.[19] A total of 11 (52.3%) of the mares ovulated within 48 h of hCG treatment however 4 (19.1%) ovulated before the hCG treatment. In addition to being a relatively poor method for synchronization of ovulation, this method of synchronization was time consuming and labor intensive.[15]

The progestagen altrenogest has been shown to suppress estrus in normally cycling mares.[25–28] Palmer impregnated intravaginal sponges with 0.5 or 1.0 g altrenogest and inserted them in mares for 20 days.[25] Mares were injected with prostaglandin 24 h after sponge insertion to eliminate any source of endogenous progesterone. The mares showed estrus 1.8 days (± 0.5) and 2.2 days (± 0.5), respectively, after the sponges were removed, and ovulation occurred 3.0 days (± 0.7) and 5.4 days (± 1.5) after the sponge removal. When altrenogest was administered orally to normally cycling mares at the recommended doses of 0.044 mg/kg for 15 days, the mares showed estrus in 3.4 days (± 1.9) and ovulated 8.8 days (± 2.2) after the end of treatment.[27] In a similar trial, Squires et al. reported an interval to estrus and ovulation of 5.0 days (± 2.4) and 10.2 days (± 3.6), respectively.[27] In summary, when normally cycling mares are treated with altrenogest for 15 days, they can be expected to show estrus 3 to 6 days after treatment withdrawal and to ovulate in 8 to 15 days.

To reduce time and cost incurred by long-term progestagen treatment, a short-term (8 days) regimen of altrenogest has been developed for synchronization of estrus[15,20,25] (Fig. 39–2). Because of the short duration of treatment and the possibility of ovulation during treatment, an injection of prostaglandin on the last day of

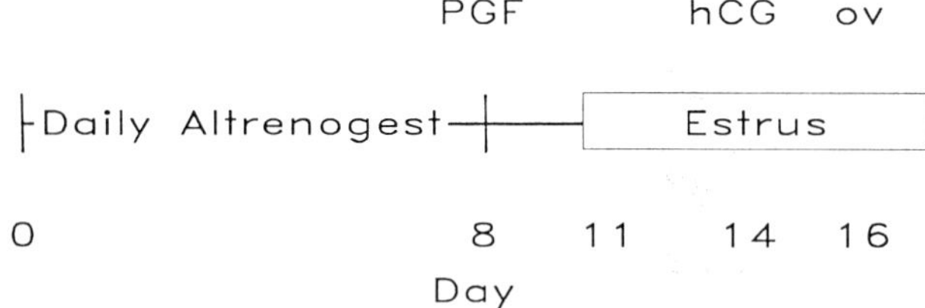

FIG. 39–2. Method for synchronization of ovulation in mares using altrenogest, prostaglandin $F_2\alpha$ (PGF), and human chorionic gonadotropin (hCG). ov, expected day of ovulation.

treatment is necessary to cause luteolysis of any CL that may be present. Intravaginal sponges impregnated with 0.5 g altrenogest were inserted in cycling mares for 8 days; the mares were treated with prostaglandin on the day of withdrawal.[25] The onset of estrus occurred in 3.8 days (± 1.0) after withdrawal; however, ovulation varied from 8 to 15 days after withdrawal. In a study using intravaginal sponges at various times during the breeding season, the mean interval to ovulation was 14.0, 10.1, 10.7, and 10.2 days, for treatments in April, May, July, and September, respectively, indicating seasonal variation in response to this synchronization regimen.[30] When altrenogest was fed to cycling mares for 8 days and combined with injections of prostaglandin on the last day of treatment and hCG 6 days later, 75% ovulated in a 96-h period.[15] However, in a similar trial, only 11 of 21 (52.3%) ovulated within 48 h of the hCG treatment.[25]

PROGESTERONE AND ESTRADIOL-17β

Short-term treatment with 10 daily intramuscular injections of 150 mg progesterone and 10 mg estradiol-17β and prostaglandin $F_2\alpha$ on the last day of the progesterone and estradiol treatment has been shown to be an effective method of synchronizing both estrus and ovulation[31] (Fig. 39–3). In one experiment, 13 of 16 (81.3%) mares ovulated 10 to 12 days after the last day of treatment. When those mares were combined with mares that did not receive prostaglandin but had no luteal function at the end of steroid treatment, 18 of 20 (90%) ovulated on days 10 to 12.[31] Varner et al. used the same treatment regimen in combination with an injection of hCG when a 35-mm follicle was detected in estrous mares.[32] In two trials, 73% (44 of 60) and 70% (33 of 47) of the mares ovulated between 10 and 12 days after the last steroid treatment. However, ovulations ranged from 8 to 17 days. Although this method results in relatively good synchronization of ovulation, it is time consuming because mares must be injected on a daily basis. The use of biodegradable microspheres for controlled release of progesterone and estradiol-17β may overcome this problem. In a preliminary study, Burns et al. injected 9 randomly cycling mares with 1.5 g progesterone and 100 mg estradiol that was microencapsulated.[33] All mares were treated with prostaglandin $F_2\alpha$ 14 days later. The mean interval from initial treatment to ovulation was 25.2 days (± 1.0).

EARLY POSTPARTUM MARES

In some instances it may be necessary to synchronize estrus and ovulation in mares that have recently foaled. Although some mares ovulate as early as 6 days after parturition, most mares do not have a mature CL until approximately 18 days after parturition. Therefore, prostaglandin $F_2\alpha$ and its analogues cannot be used in these mares. A series of daily progesterone injections,[34] or oral progestagens,[25] has been used to delay foal estrus. However, because progesterone does not consistently prevent ovulation in postpartum mares, the interval from the end of treatment to ovulation varied from 3 to 14 days. Daily injections of 200 mg progesterone and 10 mg estradiol-17β—provided the first injection is given on the day of parturition—delayed the onset of foal estrus and the first postpartum ovulation.[31,35] The duration of the delay is approximately equal to the number of days of treatment. Delay of foal estrus for 1 to 10 days was used to synchronize estrus and ovulation in postpartum mares.[36] As the mares foaled, they were given daily injections of progesterone (150 mg) and estradiol-17β (10 mg), beginning on the day of parturition. Because treatment for all mares ceased on the same day, individual mares received a varying number of injections. The mean interval from the end of treatment to the onset of estrus was 9.4 days (range 7 to 14); however, ovulations varied from 10 to 16 days after the last treatment.

ANESTROUS MARES

Estrus has been synchronized in anestrous mares during the winter using photoperiodic stimulation in conjunction with short-term altrenogest, prostaglandin, and hCG treatment.[25] Although cyclic activity was stimulated in all treated mares, ovulation was only synchronized to occur within 48 h of hCG treatment in a large proportion (> 75%) of the mares that were stimulated with light for at least 70 days before initiating the synchronization treatment. Taylor et al. used photoperiodic stimulation in conjunction with progesterone, estradiol-17β, and prostaglandin injections early in the breeding season.[37] Ovulations were widely distributed with 80%

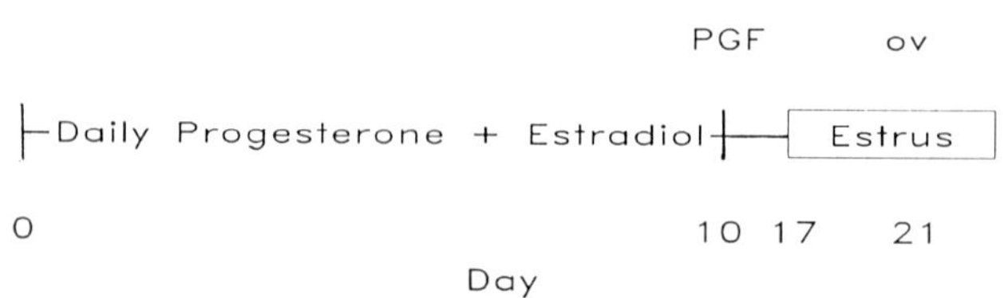

FIG. 39–3. Method for synchronization of ovulation in mares using progesterone and estradiol-17β. PGF, prostaglandin $F_2\alpha$; ov, expected day of ovulation.

occurring 9 to 16 days after the end of treatment, whereas only 54% occurred on days 11 to 13.

SUMMARY

Although estrus can be synchronized, at present no regimen is sufficiently precise so that the day of ovulation can be consistently predicted. The techniques reviewed above result in relatively good synchronization of ovulation within a 4-day period. For an embryo transfer program, it has been estimated that at least 10 potential recipient mares would be required to have an 80% probability of one's ovulating within 24 h of the donor; however, only 3 recipients would be required if recipients were to ovulate within 48 h of the donor.[38] Synchronization of ovulation during the middle of the natural breeding season has less variability than during the early part of the season or during an artificially advanced breeding season.[15,20,29,37]

The various methods for synchronization of ovulation that have been reviewed provide approximately the same degree of synchronization. The double injection of prostaglandin in conjunction with hCG requires the least labor input and the most labor-intensive procedure involves daily injections of progesterone and estradiol-17β for 10 days.

REFERENCES

1. Loy, R.G., and Hughes, J.P.: The effects of human chorionic gonadotrophin on ovulation, length of estrus, and fertility in the mare. Cornell Vet., *56:*41–50, 1966.
2. Sullivan, J.J., Parker, W.G., and Larson, L.L.: Duration of estrus and ovulation time in nonlactating mares given human chorionic gonadotropin during three successive estrous periods. J. Am. Vet. Med. Assoc., *162:*895–898, 1973.
3. Voss, J.L., Pickett, B.W., Burwash, L.D., and Daniels, W.H.: Effect of in human chorionic gonadotropin on duration of estrous cycle and fertility of normally cycling, nonlactating mares. J. Am. Vet. Med. Assoc., *165:* 704–706, 1974.
4. Voss, J.L., et al.: The effect of HCG on duration of oestrus, ovulation time and fertility in mares. J. Reprod. Fertil. Suppl., *23:*297–301, 1975.
5. Douglas, R.H., and Ginther, O.J.: Effect of prostaglandin $F_2\alpha$ on length of diestrus in mares. Prostaglandins, *2:* 265–268, 1972.
6. Douglas, R.H., and Ginther, O.J.: Effect of prostaglandin $F_2\alpha$ on estrus cycle or corpus luteum in mares and gilts. J. Anim. Sci., *40:*518–526, 1975.
7. Noden, P.A., Oxender, W.D., and Hafs, H.D.: Estrus, ovulation, progesterone and luteinizing hormone after prostaglandin $F_2\alpha$ in mares. Proc. Soc. Exp. Biol. Med., *145:*145–150, 1974.
8. Oxender, W.D., Noden, P.A., and Hafs, W.D.: Oestrus, ovulation and plasma hormones after prostaglandin $F_2\alpha$ in mares. J. Reprod. Fertil. Suppl., *23:*251–259, 1975.
9. Loy, R.G., Buell, J.R., Stevenson, W., and Hamm, D.: Sources of variation in response intervals after prostaglandin treatment in mares with functional corpora lutea. J. Reprod. Fertil. Suppl., *27:*531–537, 1979.
10. Hughes, J.P., and Loy, R.G.: Variations in ovulatory response associated with the use of prostaglandins to manipulate the lifespan of the normal diestrous corpus luteum or the prolonged corpus luteum of the mare. Proc. Am. Assoc. Equine Pract., 173–175, 1978.
11. Hyland, J.H., and Bristol, F.: Synchronization of oestrus and timed insemination of mares. J. Reprod. Fertil. Suppl., *27:*251–255, 1979.
12. Squires, E.L., et al.: The effectiveness of $PGF_2\alpha$, hCG and GnRH for appointment breeding of mares. J. Equine Vet. Sci., *1:*5–9, 1981.
13. Voss, J.L., et al.: Effects of synchronization and frequency of insemination on fertility. J. Reprod. Fertil. Suppl., *27:*257–261, 1979.
14. Palmer, E., and Jousset, B.: Synchronization of oestrus in mares with a prostaglandin analogue and hCG. J. Reprod. Fertil. Suppl., *23:*269–274, 1975.
15. Palmer, E.: Different techniques for synchronization of ovulation in the mare. Proceedings of the International Congress on Animal Reproduction and Artificial Insemination, Krakow, 1976, pp. 495–498.
16. Allen, W.R., et al.: Viability of horse embryos after storage and long distance transport in the rabbit. J. Reprod. Fertil., *47:*387–390, 1976.
17. Bosu, W.T.K., and Turner, L.: Changes in plasma progesterone concentrations in mares treated with cloprostenol and human chorionic gonadotrophin and inseminated during estrus. Can. Vet. J., *24:*253–257, 1983.
18. Bristol, F.: Studies on estrous synchronization in mares. Proc. Soc. Theriogenol., 258–264, 1981.
19. Holtan, D.W., Douglas, R.H., and Ginther, O.J.: Estrus, ovulation and conception following synchronization with progesterone, prostaglandin $F_2\alpha$ and human chorionic gonadotropin in pony mares. J. Anim. Sci., *44:*431–438, 1977.
20. Palmer, E.: Control of the oestrous cycle of the mare. J. Reprod. Fertil., *54:*495–505, 1978.
21. Ginther, O.J., and Wentworth, B.C.: Effect of asynthetic gonadotropin releasing hormone on plasma concentrations of luteinizing hormone in ponies. Am. J. Vet. Res., *55:*79–81, 1984.
22. Booth, L.C., Oxender, W.D., Douglas, T.H., and Woodley, S.L.: Estrus, ovulation, and serum hormones on mares given prostaglandin $F_2\alpha$, estradiol, and gonadotropin-releasing hormone. Am. J. Vet. Res., *41:*120–122, 1980.
23. Squires, E.L., Harrison, L.A., McKinnon, A.O., and Voss, J.L.: Use of hCG, GnRH agonist or prostaglandin analog for induction of ovulation in mares. Proceedings of the International Congress on Animal Reproduction and Artificial Insemination, Dublin, 1988, pp. 460–462.
24. Loy, R.G., and Swan, S.M.: Effects of exogenous progesterone on reproductive phenomena in mares. J. Anim. Sci., *25:*821–826, 1966.
25. Palmer, E.: Reproductive management of mares without detection of oestrus. J. Reprod. Fertil. Suppl., *27:* 263–270, 1979.
26. Squires, E.L., Stevens, W.B., McGlothlin, D.E., and Pickett, B.W.: Effect of an oral progestin on the estrous cycle and fertility of mares. J. Anim. Sci., *49:*729–735, 1979.
27. Squires, E.L., et al.: Relationship of altrenogest to ovarian activity, hormone concentrations and fertility of mares. J. Anim. Sci., *56:*901–910, 1983.
28. Webel, S.K.: Estrous control in horses with a progestin. J. Anim. Sci., *41:*385, 1975.
29. Squires, E.L., Webel, S.K., Shideler, R.K., and Voss, J.L.:

A review on the use of altrenogest for the broodmare. Proc. Am. Assoc. Equine Pract., 221–231, 1981.

30. Driancourt, M.A., and Palmer, E.: Seasonal and individual effects on ovarian and endocrine responses of mares to a synchronization treatment with progestagen-impregnated vaginal sponges. J. Reprod. Fertil. Suppl., *32:*283–291, 1982.

31. Loy, R.G., Pemstein, R., O'Canna, D., and Douglas, R.H.: Control of ovulation in cycling mares with ovarian steroids and prostaglandin. Theriogenology, *15:*191–197, 1981.

32. Varner, D.D., Blanchard, T.L., and Brinsko, S.P.: Estrogens, oxytocin and ergot alkaloids—Uses in reproductive management of mares. Proc. Am. Assoc. Equine Pract., 219–241, 1988.

33. Burns, P.J., et al.: A preliminary report on the efficacy of biodegradable microspheres for the controlled release of progesterone and estradiol for synchronization of ovulation in mares. Theriogenology, *33:*202, 1990.

34. Loy, R.G., Hughes, J.P., Richards, W.P.C., and Swan, S.M.: Effects of progesterone on reproductive function in mares after foaling. J. Reprod. Fertil. Suppl., *23:*291–295, 1975.

35. Bell, R.J., and Bristol, F.: Fertility and pregnancy loss after delay of foal oestrus with progesterone and oestradiol-17β. J. Reprod. Fertil. Suppl., *35:*667–668, 1987.

36. Bristol, F., Jacobs, K.A., and Pawlyshyn, V.: Synchronization of estrus on post-partum mares with progesterone and estradiol-17β. Theriogenology, *19:*779–785, 1983.

37. Taylor, T.B., Pemstein, R., and Loy, R.G.: Control of ovulation in mares in the early breeding season with ovarian steroids and prostaglandin. J. Reprod. Fertil. Suppl., *32:*219–224, 1982.

38. Irvine, C.H.G.: Endocrinology of the estrous cycle of the mare: Applications to embryo transfer. Theriogenology, *15:*85–104, 1981.

PHARMACOLOGIC MANIPULATION OF THE REPRODUCTIVE CYCLE

CHAPTER 40

CONTRACEPTION

J. F. Kirkpatrick
J. W. Turner, Jr.

Down regulation of fertility in the horse is a limited subject. Historically, equine fertility control has focused on castration of the stallion. Most often, this common procedure is carried out not only to limit reproduction but also to eliminate androgen production and accompanying aggressive behavior. Recently, interest in contraception of the horse has increased, largely because of uncontrolled populations of free-roaming feral horses.

CONTRACEPTION OF THE STALLION

Initial attempts at chemical contraception of feral horses focused on the stallion and attempted to exploit the harem-like social structure common to most equids. To test the concept, Kirkpatrick and Turner vasectomized two mature feral stallions inhabiting the Pryor Mountain National Wild Horse Range, in Montana, and studied their bands for the following two years. No foals appeared among accompanying mares, and stallions exhibited normal sexual behaviors. This experiment was later repeated with a larger number of feral stallions in Nevada and the results were much the same (Cheryl Asa, St. Louis Zoo, personal communication).

Several potential contraceptive compounds, including testosterone cypionate, testosterone propionate, quinestrol (17α-ethinylestradiol 3-cyclopentyl ether), estradiol-17β, and α-chlorohydrin (3-chloro-1,2-propanediol) have been tested in domestic pony stallions. The α-chlorohydrin led to neurological disorders and tests were discontinued. Repeated intramuscular injections of the two androgens and quinestrol (1.7 g/100 kg, monthly × 6) resulted in significant oligospermia and impairment of sperm motility, but Silastic implants containing estradiol failed to achieve significant reductions in sperm numbers, probably because of poor release rates.[1,2]

A microencapsulated form of testosterone propionate (mTP) was selected for field tests of contraceptive effectiveness in feral horses in Challis, Idaho. The microencapsulation polymer (D,L-lactide) coating (Southern Research Institute, Birmingham, AL) permitted a sustained release, after intramuscular injection, for up to 6 months. On contact with intercellular water, the lactide coating erodes and releases the active steroid inside. The actual coating is converted to carbon dioxide and lactic acid. A total of 7 experimental and 8 control stallions were located by helicopter and darted in December with approximately 300 mg succinylcholine and after immobilization stallions received injections of 5.0, 7.5, or 10 g IM mTP in the hip. Stallion libido and quantitative aspects of sexual behavior, based on elimination marking behavior,[3] were unaffected and breeding took place, but there was an 83% reduction in foal production compared with mares bred by control stallions (2 foals vs. 13, respectively), with no differences between fertility and the doses of mTP administered.[2,4]

Concerns for safety of stallions, dangers of immobilization, and high cost of immobilizers (approximately $50 per dose of etorphine and reversal agent for an equid) led to an attempt to deliver 3.0 g mTP remotely,

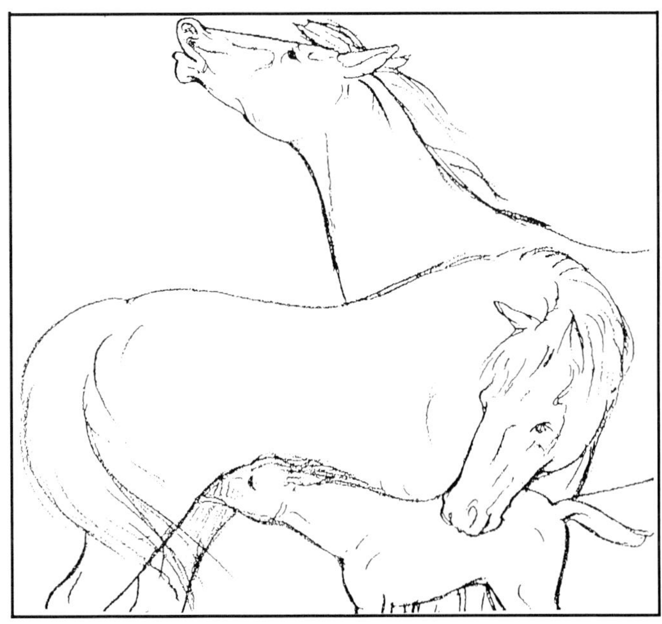

to feral harem stallions on Assateague Island National Seashore, by means of barbless darts. In this study, the stallions were located and darted from the ground, without capture or immobilization. The pharmacologic success of mTP contraception was evident, with a 28.9% fertility rate for the mares accompanying treated stallions and an approximate 45% fertility rate among control mares, but the logistics of delivering 3.0 g microcapsules in four separate doses to each stallion was discouraging.[5]

CONTRACEPTION OF THE MARE

STEROIDS

Difficulty of darting a stallion up to four times, plus concerns over band infidelity by mares, turned the focus of contraception in horses to the mare. Based on experience with persistent corpora lutea[6] and data which indicated that plasma progesterone concentrations in excess of 0.5 to 1.0 ng/mL inhibited ovulation in mares,[7–9] attempts were made to administer contraceptive doses of progestins to feral horses. Kirkpatrick and Turner, using remotely delivered darts, administered the microencapsulated synthetic progestin norethisterone (norethindrone, mNET) to six feral mares on Assateague Island.[5] This progestin, which has been used so successfully to inhibit fertility in women was given in a dose of approximately 2.0 g, in microcapsules similar to those used in previous studies with testosterone propionate. All six mares receiving the mNET produced a foal a year later, a highly improbable event among Assateague mares, where annual foaling rates seldom exceed 55%.[10]

In another experiment, groups of 30 captive feral mares in Nevada were each implanted with Silastic rods containing 8.0 g estradiol (E), 24 g progesterone (P), 8 g E plus 8 g P, 4 g E plus 12 g P, 12gE plus 12 g P, or no hormone.[11] Fewer mares receiving 8 g E, 12 g P plus 4 g E, or 8 g E plus 8 g P displayed estrus, but all animals displaying estrus, treated or control, ovulated. These data indicated a rapid decline in plasma steroid concentrations within 5 weeks of implantation and suggested increased metabolic clearance of the steroid. Because of the rapid decline in estradiol and progesterone concentrations, Silastic implants containing the synthetic estrogen ethinylestradiol (EE_2) or EE_2 plus P were placed in captive feral mares.[12] Animals pregnant at time of implantation delivered healthy foals, and contraceptive efficacy ranged from 88 to 100% through two breeding seasons and was approximately 75% for three seasons. Endocrine studies of these mares suggested that contraception was affected by blocking ovulation and/or implantation. In a similar study, intraperitoneal implants of 1.5, 3.0, or 8.0 g EE_2 alone also resulted in contraceptive efficacy of 75 to 100% through two breeding seasons, and rates of EE_2 decline in the plasma suggest a contraceptive life of 16, 26, and 48 to 60 months for the 1.5 g, 3.0 g, and 8.0 g, respectively.[13]

Results achieved with estradiol, progesterone, and ethinylestradiol in mares bring to focus advantages and disadvantages of natural versus synthetic steroids for contraceptive purposes in the horse. Steroids native to the mare, such as estradiol and progesterone are recognized by the mares' metabolic enzymes and degraded so rapidly that contraceptive doses must be so large that they are difficult or impossible to administer. The use of some synthetic steroids, such as ethinylestradiol, may delay metabolic degradation and permit sustained contraceptive effects and provide useful down regulation in certain instances. Any risk, however small, of the passage of these synthetic steroids to humans or wildlife may make registration by regulatory agencies such as the Food and Drug Administration (FDA), the United States Department of Agriculture (USDA), or the Environmental Protection Agency (EPA) unlikely.

IMMUNOCONTRACEPTION

Because of difficulties associated with delivering large masses of microencapsulated steroids, dangers associated with capture and restraint of horses, surgical procedures associated with intraperitoneal implants, concern over long-term effects of steroid contraception, and passage of synthetic steroids through the food chain, attention has turned to immunocontraception. One immunologically based contraceptive strategy involves blocking the release of gonadotropin-releasing hormone (GnRH), thereby preventing pituitary secretion of follicle-stimulating hormone (FSH) and luteinizing hormone (LH) and their subsequent tropic actions on the ovary or testes.[14] Immunization of domestic mares against GnRH blocked ovulation in three of five mares for 4 months.[15] Each mare was inoculated with 2.0 mg GnRH conjugated to human serum albumin emulsified in Freund's complete adjuvant (FCA). Analysis of plasma LH revealed a lack of pulsatile secretion, which was correlated to antibody titers. The high variability in the mares' response to the antigen and the subsequent variabilities in antibody titers suggested this approach was unreliable.

In a study to immunize captive mares with GnRH conjugated to ketolymphohemocyanin (KLH), either aluminum hydroxide (alum) or monophosphoryl lipid A/trehalose 6,6-dimycolate/BCG cell wall skeleton (triple adjuvant, TA) was used as the adjuvant.[16] Those mares immunized with GnRH plus TA had higher antibody titers and significantly less ovarian follicular activity. The vaccine was field tested on 29 feral mares on Cumberland Island National Seashore. The vaccine was freeze-dried and administered as a solid biodegradable 0.25-caliber bullet by means of an air-powered gun (Ballistivet, Inc., White Bear Lake, MN). After imbedding in the tissue of the target mare, the compressed compound forming the biobullet degrades over 24 h, releasing the antigen. A total of 25 treated mares survived and 17 (68%) produced foals, which was not significantly different from control foaling rates.

Immunization against GnRH has also been attempted in the stallion.[17] Four weanling colts were passively immunized, either intramuscularly or subcutaneously, with an anti-GnRH antibody (Peptide Technology. Ltd., Sydney, Australia), and given booster inoculations approximately 75 days later. Colts immunized intramuscularly maintained plasma testosterone concentrations of < 0.15 ng/mL, equivalent to concentrations in geldings, for 5 months following the booster inoculation after which testosterone concentrations rose to control levels for yearlings. Colts immunized subcutaneously had small increases in plasma testosterone concentrations, up to 0.37 ng/mL, between the two immunizations but decreases similar to those seen in the intramuscular group after the second inoculation. Antibody titers were generally higher in the colts immunized intramuscularly, although sexual development was effectively delayed for 12 months in both groups of colts.

A second immunocontraception strategy for horses is based on the identification of antibodies directed against the zona pellucida of the ovum in naturally infertile mares[18] and immunological cross-reactivity of equine zona-positive antisera and porcine sperm binding.[19] Liu et al. immunized 10 captive feral mares and 4 domestic mares with the protein equivalent of 2000 to 5000 porcine zonae pellucidae (PZP).[20] Freund's complete adjuvant was used for the first inoculation and Freund's incomplete adjuvant (FIA) for the three monthly booster inoculations which followed. Of the 14 treated mares 13 failed to conceive during the first year. The 4 domestic mares all conceived during the second year, after antibody titers had decreased.

A field test of the PZP vaccine was carried out on Assateague Island National Seashore.[21] For the test, 26 feral mares were remotely inoculated with approximately 5000 PZP (65 μg protein) and FCA in March 1988 by means of barbless darts. The mares received a second inoculation, with FIA, 2 weeks later, and some mares received a third inoculation with FIA 1 month later. Only a single foal was produced by the treated mares whereas 50% of the 6 sham-injected controls produced foals, and 45% of 11 untreated mares produced foals. Of the 26 PZP-treated mares, 14 were pregnant at the time of inoculation and all 14 produced healthy foals, thus the PZP vaccine had no effect on pregnancies in progress. Once antigen recognition has taken place, a single annual booster inoculation is sufficient to maintain contraceptive levels of antibodies,[22] and animals that do not receive booster inoculations return to normal fertility.[20,22] Trials are currently under way with PZP contraception in feral burros inhabiting the Virgin Islands National Park and captive Przewalski's horses in the Cologne Zoo.

The mechanism of action of PZP-induced contraception in mares is thought to be a block to fertilization.[20] One of the three major proteins of the noncellular zona pellucida ZP3 is the receptor molecule for sperm surface molecules.[23] The role of the ZP3 receptor in the horse has been confirmed in vitro as a zona pellucida–induced acrosome reaction with horse sperm.[24]

Despite return of normal fertility among PZP-treated mares, the long-term effects of continuous PZP immunocontraception have not been described. In the domestic rabbit,[25] the domestic dog,[26] and the baboon[27] evidence suggests the antibody response of the treated animal attacks not only the zona pellucida of the mature ovum but oocytes and other ovarian tissues, with resulting changes in estradiol and progesterone secretion. These effects have not been demonstrated thus far in the horse. Plasma progesterone concentrations from PZP-treated mares indicated that ovulations and luteal formation occurred during the period of infertility, and no evidence of histologic changes in the ovary was found.[20] Work in progress indicates that three consecutive years of treatment of feral mares have no effect on sexual behavior or ovarian endocrine profiles.

PZP-induced contraception in the mare may be useful to prevent untimely or undesirable breedings and anti-GnRH contraception may be useful for the same purpose in the stallion and at the same time eliminate the aggressive behaviors associated with intact stallions. In the case of captive exotic equids, such as Przewalski's horse and zebras, contraception may be useful to prevent the expression of undesirable genetic traits ("floppy mane," for example) or merely to prevent the production of surplus animals, without the need to remove animals and disrupt the well-defined equid social structure. Finally, contraception may represent a publicly acceptable approach to the management of feral horses and burros inhabiting public lands.

REFERENCES

1. Kirkpatrick, J.F.: Reproductive Biology and Chemical Fertility Control in Wild Horses. Contract YA-512-CT, Final Report. Washington, D.C., Bureau of Land Management, U.S. Department of Interior, 1982.
2. Turner, J.W., Jr., and Kirkpatrick, J.F.: Steroids, behaviour and fertility control in feral stallions in the field. J. Reprod. Fertil. Suppl., *32:*79–87, 1982.
3. Turner, J.W., Jr., Perkins, A., and Kirkpatrick, J.F.: Elimination marking behavior in feral horses. Can. J. Zool., *59:*1561–1566, 1981.
4. Kirkpatrick, J.F., Turner, J.W., Jr., and Perkins, A.: Reversible fertility control in feral horses. J. Equine Vet. Sci., *2:*114–118, 1982.
5. Kirkpatrick, J.F., and Turner, J.W., Jr.: Chemical fertility control and the management of the Assateague feral ponies. National Park Service Contract CA 1600-3-0005, Final Report. National Park Service, Assateague Island National Seashore, 1987.
6. Stabenfeldt, G.H., Hughes, J.P., Evans, J.W., and Neely, D.P.: Spontaneous prolongation of luteal activity in the mare. Equine Vet. J., *6:*158–163, 1974.
7. Squires, E.L., Wentworth, B.C., and Ginther, O.J.: Progesterone concentration in blood of mares during the estrous cycle, pregnancy and after hysterectomy. J. Anim. Sci., *39:*759–767, 1974.
8. Noden, P.A., Oxender, W.D., and Hafs, H.D.: Early changes in serum progesterone, estradiol, and LH during prostaglandin F2α-induced luteolysis in mares. J. Anim. Sci., *47:*666–671, 1978.
9. Palmer, E., and Jousset, B.: Urinary oestrogen and plasma

progesterone levels in non-pregnant mares. J. Reprod. Fertil. Suppl., *23:*213–221, 1975.

10. Keiper, R., and Houpt, K.: Reproduction in feral horses: An eight-year study. Am. J. Vet. Res., *45:*991–995, 1984.

11. Vevea, D.N., et al.: Effects of hormone implants on estrus and ovulation in feral mares. Biol. Reprod. Suppl. 1, *36:*146, 1987.

12. Plotka, E.D., et al.: Effective contraception of feral horses using homogenous silastic implants containing ethinylestradiol (EE2) or EE2 plus progesterone. Biol. Reprod. Suppl. 1, *40:*169, 1989.

13. Plotka, E.D., and Vevea, D.N.: Serum ethinylestradiol (EE2) concentrations in feral mares following hormonal contraception with homogenous silastic implants. Biol. Reprod. Suppl. 1, *42:*43, 1990.

14. Schanbacher, B.D.: Active immunization against LH-RH in the male. *In* Immunological Aspects of Reproduction in Mammals. Edited by D.B. Crighton. London, Butterworths, 1984, pp. 345–362.

15. Safir, J.M., Loy, R.G., and Fitzgerald, B.P.: Inhibition of ovulation in the mare by active immunization against LHRH. J. Reprod. Fertil. Suppl., *35:*229–237, 1987.

16. Goodloe, R., Warren, R.J., and Sharp, D.C.: Sterilization of feral horses by immunization against LHRH. Proc. Wildl. Dis. Assoc., *37:*25, 1988.

17. Dowsett, K.F., et al.: A preliminary study of immunological castration in colts. J. Reprod. Fert. Suppl., *44:* 183–190, 1991.

18. Liu, I.K.M., and Shivers, C.A.: Antibodies to the zona pellucida in mares. J. Reprod. Fertil. Suppl., *32:*309–313, 1982.

19. Shivers, C.A., and Liu, I.K.M.: Inhibition of sperm binding to porcine ova by antibodies to equine zonae pellucidae. J. Reprod. Fertil. Suppl., *32:*315–318, 1982.

20. Liu, I.K.M., Bernoco, M., and Feldman, M.: Contraception in mares heteroimmunized with porcine zonae pellucidae. J. Reprod. Fertil., *85:*19–29, 1989.

21. Kirkpatrick, J.F., Liu, I.K.M., and Turner, J.W., Jr.: Remotely-delivered immunocontraception in feral horses. Wildl. Soc. Bull., *18:*326–330, 1990.

22. Kirkpatrick, J.F., Liu, I.K.M., Turner, J.W., Jr., and Bernoco, M.: J.W., Jr.: Antigen recognition in feral mares previously immunized with porcine zonae pellucidae. J. Reprod. Fertil. Suppl., *44:*321–325, 1991.

23. Florman, P.M., and Wassarman, H.M.: O-linked oligosaccharides of mouse egg ZP3 account for its sperm receptor activity. Cell, *41:*313–324, 1985.

24. Arns, M.J., et al.: Zona pellucida-induced acrosome reactions in equine spermatozoa. Proceedings of the Fifth International Symposium on Equine Reproduction, Deauville, July 1–7, 1990, pp. 70–71.

25. Wood, D.M., Liu, C., and Dunbar, B.S.: Effect of alloimmunization and heteroimmunization with zona pellucida on fertility in rabbits. Biol. Reprod., *25:*439–450, 1981.

26. Mahi-Brown, C.A., Yanagimachi, R., Hoffman, J.C., and Huang, T.T.F., Jr.: Fertility control in the bitch by active immunization with porcine zonae pellucidae: Use of different adjuvants and patterns of estradiol and progesterone levels in estrous cycles. Biol. Reprod., *32:*761–772, 1985.

27. Dunbar, B.S., Lo, C., Powell, J., and Stevens, J.C.: Use of a synthetic peptide adjuvant for the immunization of baboons with denatured and deglycosylated pig zona pellucida protein. Fertil. Steril., *52:*311–318, 1989.

CHAPTER 41

EMBRYO TRANSFER

E.L. Squires

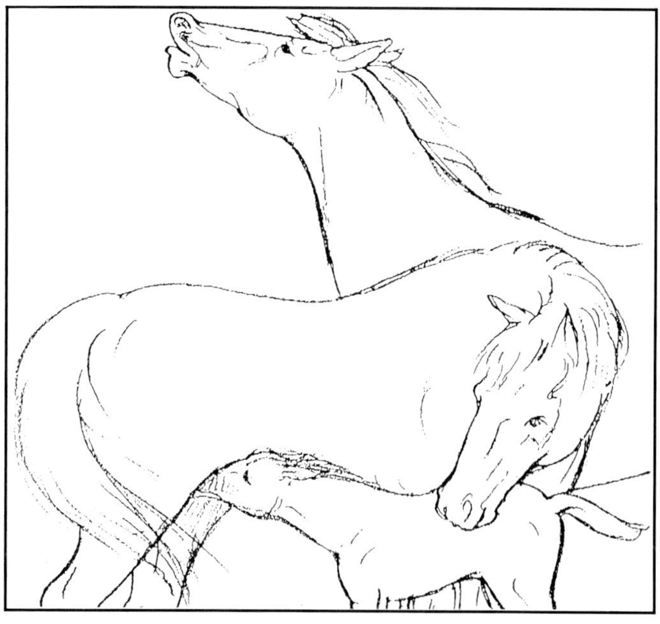

Acceptance of embryo transfer (ET) by the majority of the horse registries has stimulated use of this technique during the last decade. Some advantages of embryo transfer are that it allows one to (1) obtain foals from older, problem mares; (2) increase production from genetically superior mares; (3) obtain embryos from mares that foal late in the breeding season; and (4) produce foals from 2-yr-old mares.

In this chapter, the current procedures used at Colorado State University (CSU) for embryo recovery and transfer are reviewed and factors affecting the success of embryo recovery and transfer are discussed.

EMBRYO TRANSFER PROCEDURES

The technique used for embryo recovery has changed little over the last decade. Donor mares are bred or inseminated during estrus and embryo recovery attempted 7 days after ovulation (day 0 = day of ovulation). A catheter with a 75 mL cuff is introduced through the cervix and the cuff inflated with air. The catheter is then drawn back against the internal opening of the cervix to ensure a tight seal (Fig. 41–1). A liter of modified Dulbecco's phosphate-buffered saline (DPBS) with 1% fetal calf serum (FCS) is infused into the uterus by gravity flow and immediately drained out of the uterus and into a filter cup (Fig. 41–2). This process is repeated at least twice per recovery attempt. Expulsion of the second and third liter of fluid is assisted by massage of the uterus per rectum. After the majority of fluid is recovered (> 90%), the cuff on the catheter is deflated, the catheter withdrawn, and the fluid within the catheter and outlet tubing drained into the filter cup. The fluid within the filter cup is poured into a search dish, and the cup rinsed and the contents collected into the same search dish (Fig. 41–3). Medium contained in the search dish is then examined under × 10 magnification with a sterodissection microscope. Upon identification, embryos are given a quality score of 1 to 5, developmental stage is assessed, and the embryos are measured.[1] After location of the embryo, a fire-polished glass pipette attached to a 1 mL syringe is used to wash the embryo through 3 drops of DPBS plus 10% FCS. The embryo is maintained at room temperature in DPBS plus 10% FCS until transferred to a recipient.

Embryos collected and transferred on the same premises are generally maintained in culture for less than 1 h. Recipient mares used for transfer are normally cycling, 3 to 10 yr of age, and of Quarter Horse or Appaloosa types. Recipient mares are examined daily during estrus with ultrasonography to determine follicular size and ovulation.[2] Recipients are also examined 5 days after ovulation with ultrasonography for presence or absence of uterine folds and fluid and the structure and size of corpus luteum (CL) is noted. Those mares without fluid in the uterus or evidence of endometrial folds, having a tightly closed cervix, tubular uterus, and a CL greater than 30 mm were "passed" as potential recipients. On the day of transfer, a recipient is selected

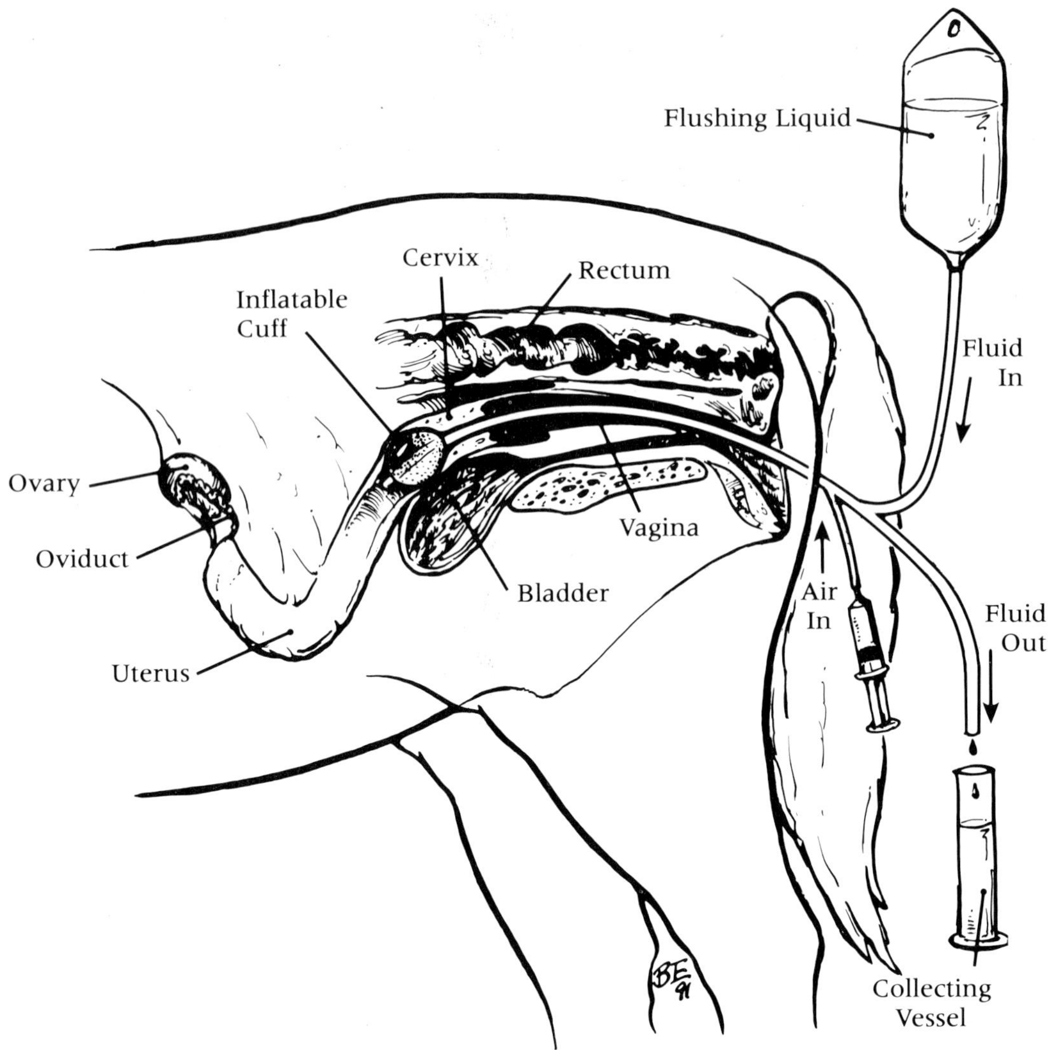

FIG. 41–1. A catheter positioned in the mare's uterus for embryo recovery.

that has ovulated 1 day prior (+1) to 3 days after the donor (−3). Recipients are placed in a stock and sedated with a mixture of 25 mg acepromazine maleate (Prom ACE, Fort Dodge Laboratory, Fort Dodge, IA), 250 mg xylazine hydrochloride (Rompun, Haver, Mobay Corp., Shawnee, KS), and 10 mg butophanol tartrate (Torbugesic, Fort Dodge Laboratory). An area of the paralumbar fossa, approximately 35 by 45 cm is clipped and scrubbed. Approximately 70 mL of 2% lidocaine hydrochloride is injected to provide a line block along the proposed site of incision. The area is then scrubbed again and draped for aseptic surgery. The skin is incised vertically and the musculature bluntly dissected and the peritoneum penetrated with index finger. The uterine horn is then exteriorized and penetrated at a point approximately 40 mm from the tip of the uterine horn. The embryo is aspirated with 0.5 mL of DPBS into a fire-polished pipette and transferred into the uterine horn adjacent to the corpus luteum. Muscle groups are reconstructed with a single continuous suture and the subcutaneous tissue and skin sutured separately. Alternatively, embryos are transferred nonsurgically with a modified ET pipette.

FACTORS AFFECTING EMBRYO RECOVERY

SEMINAL TREATMENT

Three major factors that affect embryo recovery are (1) day of embryo recovery, (2) seminal treatment, and (3) reproductive history of the mare. Recovery of equine embryos has been attempted as early as 5 days after ovulation, but recovery rate was < 10%. During the last 10 yr, embryo recovery attempts have been performed in experimental mares in our laboratory 6, 7, 8, or 9 days after ovulation. Recovery rates on days 7, 8, and 9 (Table 41–1) were similar (76%, 74%, and 81%) and were slightly higher than recovery rates on day 6 (62%). On a commercial basis mares are routinely "flushed" for embryos on day 7 after ovulation. Larger

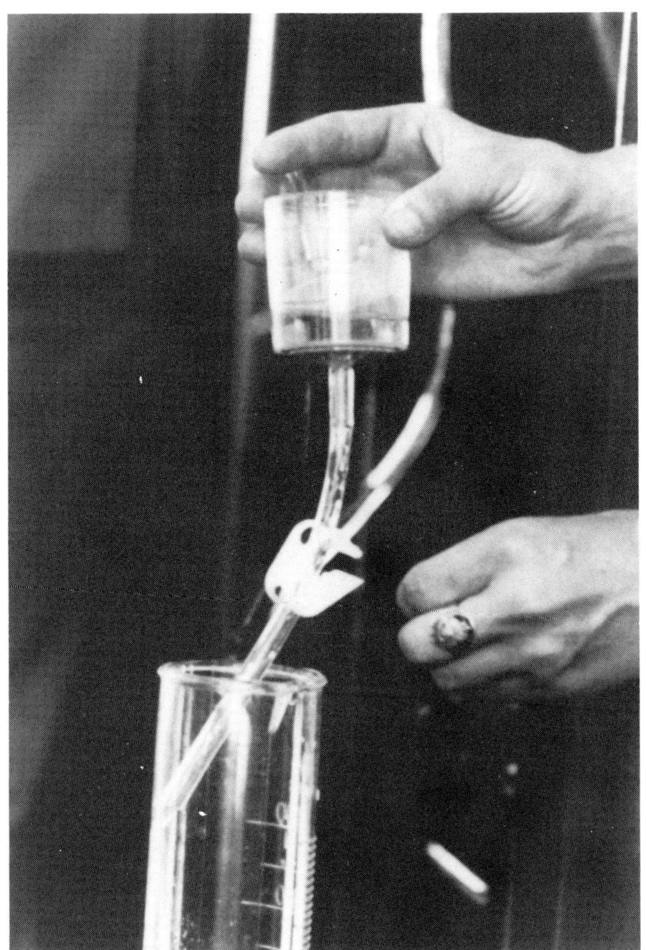

FIG. 41–2. Fluid draining out of the mare's uterus and into an embryo filter cup.

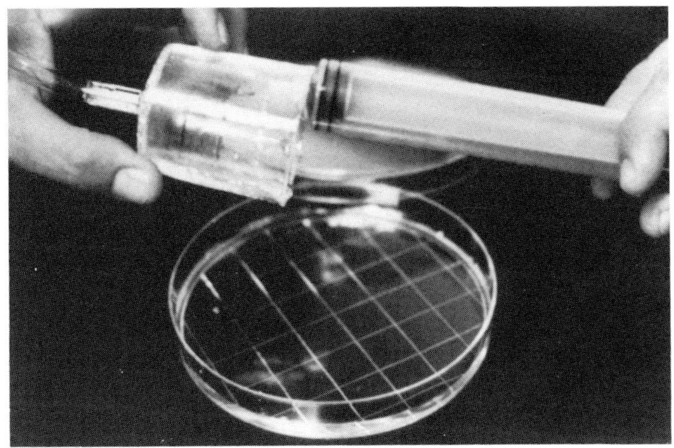

FIG. 41–3. Fluid in the filter cup being poured into the search dish and the cup rinsed with medium.

day-9 embryos are less viable for transfer, whereas small day-6 embryos are more appropriate for freezing.[3] Lower embryo recovery rate on day 6 results from failure of some embryos to enter the uterus by day 6. The 83 mares that failed to provide an embryo on day 6 were "flushed" again on day 7. An additional 18 embryos were obtained on day 7, of which the size and stage of development were similar to day-6 embryos. This suggested that failure of recovery on day 6 was the result of delayed oviductal transport.

Both the fertility of the oocyte and spermatozoa affect success of embryo recovery. Douglas reported an embryo recovery rate of 36% for mares bred to one stallion and 72% for a second stallion.[4] Recovery rates of embryos from donor mares inseminated at CSU have also varied with stallions. Embryo recovery has been used as a diagnostic tool to evaluate the fertility of stallions or to assess various seminal treatments such as type of extender and cooled and frozen semen.[5] Squires et al. reported a higher embryo recovery rate from mares inseminated with raw semen (78%) or spermatozoa extended in skim milk (62 and 78%) compared with those inseminated with spermatozoa in EDTA-lactose extender (48%).[6] More recently, Francl reported on the effects of seminal storage temperature and extender on recovery of embryos.[7] Storage of spermatozoa in E-Z Mixin (Animal Reproduction Systems, Chino, CA) extender at 20° C for 12 h or 5° C for 24 h had no affect on embryo recovery. However, storage of spermatozoa in E-Z Mixin for 48 h at 20° C resulted in 0% embryo recovery. Spermatozoa stored for 24 h in E-Z Mixin extender at 20 or 5° C resulted in embryo recovery rates of 50 and 59%, respectively, compared with 65% for mares inseminated with semen immediately after collection.

REPRODUCTIVE HISTORY

Numerous studies have demonstrated a significantly lower recovery of embryos from mares with a history of infertility compared with normal mares.[3,4,6,8–10] During the 1979 and 1980 season, only 10 of 36 (28%) embryos were recovered from infertile mares in our laboratory compared with 128 of 160 (80%) from normally cyclic mares.[6] A total of 60 donor mares owned by clients were presented for embryo transfer during the 1983 and 1984 breeding seasons.[3,11] In all, 89 embryos were recovered from 176 attempts (51%) compared with 92 embryos from 200 attempts (46%) in 1984. The lower recovery rate during 1984 was attributed to a greater number of attempts from older, barren mares. Douglas reported a 34.3% recovery from 35 barren mares.[12] Woods et al. compared embryo recovery rates from maiden and subfertile mares.[13] Only 19% of the flushes from subfertile mares resulted in a normal embryo, compared with 67% from maiden mares. In another study a total of 146 embryo recovery attempts performed on 34 subfertile donors yielded 41 transferable embryos (28%) from 27 mares.[14] A similar recov-

TABLE 41–1. EFFECT OF DAY ON EMBRYO RECOVERY RATES FROM EXPERIMENTAL MARES

DAY OF ATTEMPT	NUMBER OF ATTEMPTS	NUMBER OF EMBRYOS RECOVERED	PERCENT RECOVERY
6	137	86	62.0
7	96	73	76.0
8	293	218	74.4
9	53	43	81.1

ery rate (47%) was reported for a commercial embryo transfer station.[8] Recovery rate from commercial donors mated at clients' farms was lower than the recovery rates from commercial and experimental mares mated at our laboratory (27%, 59%, and 57%, respectively). Data from our laboratory were summarized for the 1990 breeding season into those recoveries performed at CSU from client mares (mostly subfertile) versus those client mares bred and flushed on the farm. Recovery rates were 40 of 97 (41%) and 56 of 166 (34%), respectively. Overall 37% of recovery attempts were successful. Recently, Vogelsang et al. presented a summary of embryo recovery rates from mares during 1985 to 1988.[9] Donor mares were categorized as maiden, having foaled within 2 yr (recent foal), and barren for > 2 yr (subfertile). Recovery rates for subfertile mares (29%) were less ($p < 0.05$) than that for foaling (53%) and maiden mares (61%). Mares that were barren for > 2 yr and 18 to 28 yr old provided embryos on only 44 of 192 attempts (23%). Thus the evidence is overwhelming that the success of recovering embryos from subfertile mares is < 30%.

Iuliano and Squires have also demonstrated that embryo recovery from 2-yr-old Arabian mares is depressed.[15] Only 40 of 110 attempts resulted in embryo recovery (36.3%). Steiner and Jordan reported a higher embryo recovery rate for mature Hanoverian mares compared with 2-yr-olds.[16] Lower recovery rate of embryos from 2-yr-old mares has been attributed to reproductive immaturity, because recovery rates tend to increase late in the breeding season.[15]

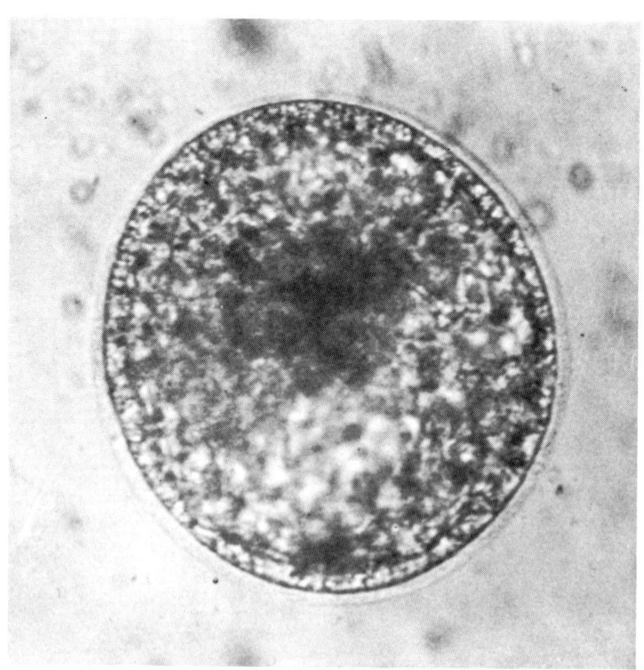

FIG. 41–4. Day-7 equine embryo, blastocyst stage.

EMBRYO SIZE AND MORPHOLOGY

Each embryo collected should be measured and graded and the developmental stage determined. Most of the embryos obtained commercially are 7 days old and are expanded blastocysts (Fig. 41–4). The average diameter for embryos collected 6, 7, and 8 days after ovulation are presented in Table 41–2. A rapid growth in the equine embryo occurs during each 24-h period. Thus only with frequent examination and determination of exact time of ovulation could one predict the size of equine embryos. McKinnon and Squires provided a detailed description of embryo evaluation. Briefly, embryos were assigned a quality score of 1 to 5: 1 = excellent, 5 = degenerated or dead (Table 41–3). Morphologic parameters evaluated were compactness of blastomeres, extruded and damaged blastomeres, color of embryo, embryo shape, size of perivitelline space, damage to zona pellucida, and developmental stage compared with embryo age. Fortunately, the majority of embryos obtained in our laboratory are grade 1 or 2 (Fig. 41–5). Although most embryos obtained are transferred, grade 3 and 4 embryos (Fig. 41–6) result in fewer pregnancies than grade 1 or 2.

The earliest developmental stage embryo harvested from the uterus is a morula. These are generally only collected on day 5 or 6 after ovulation. Their characteristic feature is a thick zona pellucida (Fig. 41–7). Transition from morula to early blastocyst results in formation of blastocoele cavity and thinning of the zona

TABLE 41–2. EFFECT OF DAY OF EMBRYO COLLECTION ON EMBRYO DIAMETER

DAY OF COLLECTION*	$\bar{X} \pm$ S.E.M. (MM)	RANGE (MM)
6	0.201 ± 0.003	0.132–0.380
7	0.488 ± 0.003	0.136–1.284
8	1.368 ± 0.015	0.369–3.980

*Day of ovulation = day 0.

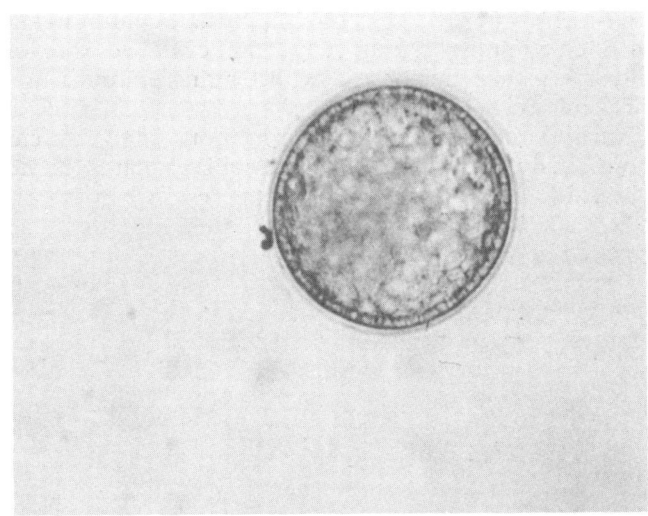

FIG. 41–5. Equine blastocyst, grade 1.

TABLE 41–3. CLASSIFICATION SYSTEM USED TO GRADE QUALITY OF EQUINE EMBRYOS

Grade 1	Excellent—An ideal embryo, spherical, with cells of uniform size, color, and texture
Grade 2	Good—minor imperfections such as a few extruded blastomeres, irregular shape, or trophoblastic separation
Grade 3	Fair—definite but not severe problems, presence of extruded blastomeres, degenerate cells, or collapsed blastocoele
Grade 4	Poor—severe problems, collapsed blastocoele, numerous extruded blastomeres, degenerate cells but with a viable appearing embryonic mass
Grade 5	Unfertilized or dead—unfertilized oocytes or total degenerate embryos

(Adapted from Slade, N.P., et al.: A new procedure for the cryopreservation of equine embryos. Theriogenology, *24*:45–58, 1985.)

pellucida. There is still some debate as to whether the zona is shed from the equine embryo. A capsule forms between the trophoblastic cells and the zona pellucida sometime between day 6 and 7.[17] The majority of day-7 and all of day-8 or -9 embryos are expanded blastocysts with no zona pellucida but an intact capsule. The spherical shape of the equine embryo during early gestation[1] apparently facilitates movement of the conceptus between uterine horns until day 16.[18] Unlike cattle, unfertilized equine embryos are generally not transported through the oviduct. Only in about 5% of the recovery attempts in mares are unfertilized ova obtained.[3] However, in some cases, distinguishing between an unfertilized ova and a morula or early blastocyst may be difficult.

FACTORS AFFECTING PREGNANCY RATES

RECIPIENTS

The reproductive health and synchrony of donor and recipients may be the leading factors affecting pregnancy rates after transfer. At CSU, recipients are used only if they have passed a reproductive exam, which includes palpation per rectum, ultrasonography of the genital tract, uterine culture, biopsy, and cytology. Mares are culled from the recipient herd if they (1) fail to ovulate or cycle regularly, (2) do not become pregnant after two embryo transfer attempts, and/or (3) have evidence of uterine disorder. Ideally, recipients should be 3 to 10 yr old, 450 to 500 kg, and of quarter horse or Appaloosa type.

SYNCHRONY OF DONOR AND RECIPIENT

Synchrony of ovulation between donor and recipient has been shown to affect pregnancy rates after surgical and nonsurgical transfer. During 1982 to 1987, embryos were transferred surgically into recipients that had ovulated +2 to −3 days in relation to the donor (day 0 = day of ovulation). Pregnancy rates in this study were similar for all days, except for lower pregnancy rates from transfer into recipients that had ovulated 2 days before (+2) the donor mare.[19,20] Oguri and Tsutsumi reported a 63% pregnancy rate for transfer into recipients that ovulated 48 h after the donor versus 0% for recipients ovulating 48 h before the donor.[21] In another study, no pregnancies resulted from transfers to recipients that ovulated 4 to 6 days after the donor, but pregnancy rates were similar for recipients ovulating 1, 2, and 3 days after the donor.[8] Thus, for maximum pregnancy rates, recipients should ovulate +1 to −2 days in relation to the donor. In general, recipients that have ovulated after the donor are better candidates than

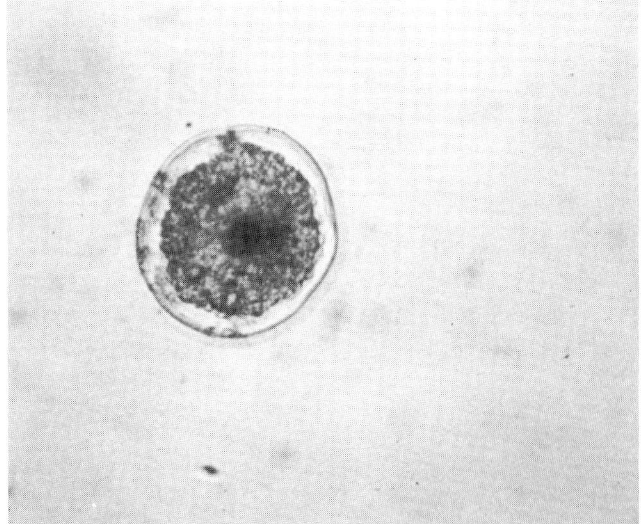

FIG. 41–6. Equine blastocyst, grade 3. Trophoblast is shrunken from the capsule and numerous extruded blastomeres.

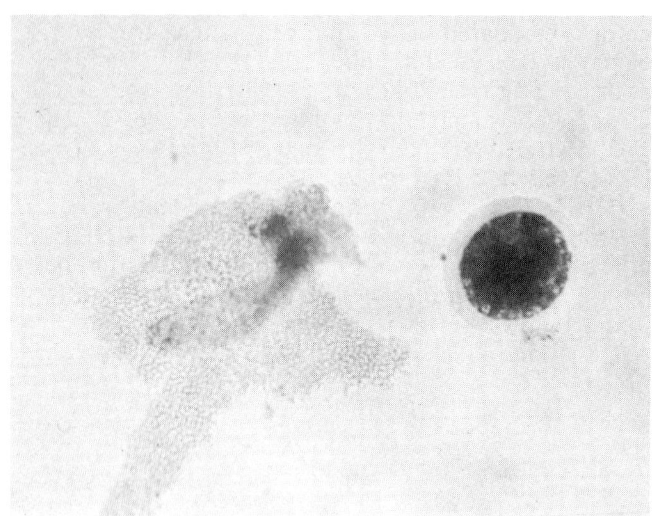

FIG. 41–7. Day-6 equine embryo with a thick zona pellucida, morula stage.

those that ovulate before the donor, particularly if the ovulation occurred 2 or more days before the donor.

OVARIECTOMIZED RECIPIENTS

Because ovulation control is somewhat difficult, generally two recipients are maintained for each donor to ensure proper synchrony between donor and recipient. One alternative to ovarian-intact mares is progestin-treated, ovariectomized mares. Hinrichs et al. administered 300 mg progesterone IM daily for 5 days before transfer into ovariectomized mares,[22] and 3 of 7 transfers resulted in pregnancies. In a subsequent study, three treatment regimens were used to prepare ovariectomized mares for embryo transfer: (1) 22 mg altrenogest daily starting 5 days before transfer, (2) 66 mg altrenogest daily starting 6 days before transfer, and (3) 300 mg injectable progesterone daily starting 5 days before transfer.[23] Intact, synchronized recipients were used as controls. Pregnancy rates were 1 of 6, 2 of 6, 2 of 5, and 13 of 19, respectively. The researchers concluded that 22 mg altrenogest was insufficient for pregnancy maintenance.

In contrast, McKinnon et al. reported similar pregnancy rates for embryos transferred into intact mares versus ovariectomized mares administered 300 mg injectable progesterone.[24] In addition, 14 of 20 transfers into ovariectomized mares receiving 22 mg altrenogest became pregnant compared with 14 of 20 transfers into recipients receiving 300 mg injectable progesterone. Initiation of progesterone treatment in ovariectomized mares corresponded to the day of donor ovulation. Others have reported a decrease in pregnancy rates if ovariectomized mares are administered progesterone for 10 or more days before transfer[23,25] or if intact mares are administered exogenous progestins for an extended time before transfer.[26–28] Periparturient events in ovariectomized progestin-treated mares were similar to that of intact mares.[29] Thus ovariectomized mares treated with either injectable progesterone (100 to 300 mg) or altrenogest (22 to 25 mg) for 5 to 7 days before transfer provide an alternative to ovarian intact recipients. Mares that remain pregnant after embryo transfer are continued on treatment until 120 to 150 days.

METHOD OF TRANSFER

Few studies have directly compared methods of embryo transfer. However, in studies in which comparisons were made, surgical transfer resulted in higher pregnancy rates than nonsurgical transfer.[6,30–32] Only 4 of 15 recipients that received embryos nonsurgically were pregnant at 50 days compared with 8 of 15 recipients with embryos that were transferred surgically.[30] In another study, surgical transfer resulted in higher ($p < 0.05$) pregnancy rates (31 of 43, 72%) than nonsurgical transfer (18 of 40, 45%).[32] In 1985, day-30 pregnancy rates from surgical transfer (115 of 175, 66%) were better than those from nonsurgical transfer (30 of 97, 39%).[20] Other studies have reported nonsurgical and surgical pregnancy rates, but no comparisons between the two methods were possible. Squires et al. reported on three methods of nonsurgical transfer: (1) unguarded pipette, (2) guarded pipette, and (3) Cassou gun.[3] Pregnancy rates were 11 of 56, 25 of 53, and 16 of 24, respectively. Averaged over several experiments in this same laboratory, a total of 44 day-8 embryos were transferred nonsurgically by the guarded pipette or Cassou gun method, and 21 pregnancies (47.8%) were obtained.

Flank incision has been used as the method of choice for transferring embryos from client mares in our laboratory since 1981. Table 41–4 presents the pregnancy rates for embryos transferred via flank incision from 1981 to 1990. Pregnancy rates after surgical transfer have varied little over this 9-yr period and averaged approximately 65%. In contrast, pregnancy rates at CSU with nonsurgical transfer have varied tremendously from year to year. Although statistical comparisons be-

TABLE 41–4. PREGNANCY RATES AFTER TRANSFER OF EMBRYOS VIA FLANK INCISION*

YEAR	NUMBER TRANSFERRED	NUMBER PREGNANT	PERCENT PREGNANT AT 50 DAYS
1981	5	4	80
1982	43	31	72
1983	89	61	69
1984	79	51	65
1985	175	111	63
1986	22	17	77
1987	17	11	65
1988	30	18	60
1989	25	17	71
1990	49	32	65

*Includes only embryos transferred within 1 h after collection.

tween nonsurgical and surgical transfer results could not be made, the surgical approach consistently gave 15 to 25% higher pregnancy rates.

Based on data from a commercial embryo transfer program, Vogelsang et al. reported 17 of 40 (43%) nonsurgical transfers resulted in a 50-day pregnancy.[8] Slightly higher nonsurgical pregnancy rates were reported by Douglas et al.: 22 of 41 (54%).[14] Others have reported nonsurgical pregnancy rates of 7 of 16;[33] 9 of 15;[34] 6 of 8, 11 of 22, 4 of 15, 6 of 11;[35] and 4 of 9.[36] Several reasons have been proposed for the lower pregnancy rates after nonsurgical transfer.[3] The introduction of low-grade infection as a result of penetration of the cervix in a diestrous mare appears to be the most likely cause of lowered fertility.[3,35]

AGE, SIZE, AND GRADE OF EMBRYO

The majority of embryo transfers have been done 6 to 9 days after ovulation. Limited studies are available that examined the effect of embryo age on pregnancy rate. Squires et al. compared results of embryo transfer with day-8 versus day-9 embryos.[31] When both surgical and nonsurgical methods were combined, more mares became pregnant with transfer of day-8 embryos (32%) than with day-9 embryos (4%). Vogelsang et al. reported no pregnancies after transfer of day-9 and day-10 embryos compared with 61%, 55%, and 25% pregnancy rates for 6-, 7-, and 8-day embryos.[8] In contrast, Fleury et al. reported 11 of 16 successful transfers with day-9 embryos.[36] The difference in results of those studies was not determined. Squires et al. suggested that the day-9 embryos, with their increased fluid volume-to-surface ratio may be more easily damaged during collection and transfer.[3] Subsequent studies in our laboratory have shown no difference in pregnancy rates for day-6, day-7, or day-8 embryos. Thus one has the flexibility of collecting embryos on either day 6, 7, or 8. Generally, only embryos for freezing are collected on day 6, and the majority of transfers are with day-7 embryos. One possible exception is the collection of embryos on day 6 from mares with a history of uterine infection. Size and age of embryo have been shown to be highly correlated.[32] Fewer pregnancies were obtained after nonsurgical transfer of embryos 1.25 to 2.83 mm in diameter compared with those of 0.4 to 1.24 mm. These same authors reported that size of embryo (mean 0.36 to 1.76 mm) did not influence pregnancy rate after surgical transfer unless the embryo was greater than 2.5 mm. However, in a more recent study, smaller embryos (< 250 μm) resulted in fewer pregnancies, and embryos greater than 500 μm resulted in more pregnancies after surgical transfer than those less than 500 μm.[37] Fleury et al. reported similar pregnancy rates for embryos 200 to 500 μm, 501 to 1000 μm, 1000 to 1700 μm, and 1.701 to 4.20 μm in diameter.[36]

Grade of an equine embryo before transfer dramatically affects pregnancy rates, which is similar to information reported with cattle.[38] Clark et al. reported 13 of 26 successful transfers with embryos of less than grade 2 compared with 1 of 6 pregnancies from transfer of grade 2 or greater (grade 1 = excellent, grade 4 = poor).[26] Pregnancy rates on day 50 after surgical transfer for embryos given a quality score of 1 or 2 (214 of 310, 69.0%) were better ($p < 0.05$) than those for embryos graded ≥ 3 (4 of 22, 18%).[20]

Carney et al. also reported higher pregnancy rates for grades 1 and 2 embryos compared with grades 3 and 4 embryos.[37] Woods et al. reported a higher number of abnormal embryos were obtained from infertile mares.[39] In contrast, Carney et al. reported a similar average grade of embryos for 2- to 6-yr-old, 7- to 12-yr-old, 13- to 18-yr-old and greater than 19-yr-old mares. Given the effect of size and grade of embryo on pregnancy rates, each embryo should be measured and graded before transfer.

Effect of age of donor on pregnancy rate after embryo transfer has been investigated.[9] Pregnancy rates were higher with embryos from 2- to 8-yr-olds (59 of 84; 70%) compared with 9- to 17-yr-olds (50 of 97, 52%) and 18- to 28-yr-olds (50 of 90, 56%). This is in contrast to a recent study in which pregnancy rates after surgical transfer of embryos from 2- to 6-yr-old, 7- to 12-yr-old, 13- to 18-yr-old, and greater than 19-yr-old mares were similar.[37] Age of donor mare also had no affect on early embryonic death. This is contrary to the reported high embryonic loss in early pregnancy of older, subfertile mares[40] and may aptly demonstrate the effect of removing an embryo from an unfavorable environment and transferring it into a more acceptable host.

EMBRYO CULTURE AND FREEZING

Culture systems have been devised that allow storage of equine embryos for 12 to 24 h,[41] which would permit movement of embryos within and between countries and eliminate the need for recipient and donor mares to be on the same premises. However, several studies were conducted before an appropriate medium was identified that maintained viability of equine embryos in culture. Storage of equine embryos in DPBS for 24 h at 37° C resulted in fewer pregnancies (3 of 15) compared with immediate transfer (8 of 17).[30] Douglas reported lower pregnancy rates for embryos stored > 6 h in DPBS plus 10% FCS, and 0 of 12 pregnancies for embryos recovered and stored in tissue culture medium (TCM)-199.[12] A preliminary trial demonstrated Ham's F10 was a better medium for maintaining viability of equine embryos than DPBS.[30] Subsequently, Slade et al. bisected equine embryos and stored one-half of each of five pairs in either Ham's F10 plus 10% FCS in 5% CO_2 in air at 37° C or DPBS plus 10% FCS in air at 37° C. Embryo quality for both whole and bisected embryos stored at 5° C in Ham's F10 plus 10% FCS, 5% CO_2, 5% O_2, and 90% N_2 was better at 24 h than for embryos stored in minimal essential medium (MEM) with Hank's balanced salt plus 10% FCS in air or DPBS plus 10% FCS. This preliminary study indicated that Ham's F10 was superior to DPBS in promoting growth and development while maintaining the quality of equine embryos. Further studies were conducted to evaluate various culture systems for maintaining viability of equine embryos for 12 to 24 h.[26,41] In one study, pregnancy rates for embryos stored for 12 h in Ham's F10 plus 10% FCS (8 of 16) were nearly identical to those transferred within 1 h of collection (7 of 16).[26] Because preparation of medium for cooling or transport of embryos under field conditions would be more practical with use of a nongassed medium, a study was designed to determine if Ham's F10 plus Hepes buffer would maintain embryo viability equal to Ham's F10 plus CO_2.[41] Unfortunately, pregnancy rates were lower ($p < 0.05$) for embryos stored in Ham's F10 plus Hepes buffer for 24 h at 5° C (4 of 20, 20%) than those cultured in Ham's F10 plus CO_2 (14 of 20, 70%) or DPBS and transferred ≤ 1 h (18 of 20, 90%). It was concluded that Ham's F10 plus CO_2 was superior to Ham's F10 plus Hepes for storage of embryos at 5° C for 24 h and that satisfactory pregnancy rates could be obtained from transfer of embryos stored in Ham's F10 plus CO_2 at 5° C for 24 h. The development of a system for maintenance of equine embryos in vitro for 24 h has resulted in widespread commercial application.[23,43]

Over three breeding seasons (1988 through 1990), embryos were collected on various breeding farms and transported to CSU for transfer.[37] Embryos were placed in a small culture tube (5 mL) containing Ham's F10 plus 10% FCS. A mixture of 5% CO_2, 5% O_2, and 90% N_2 was bubbled through the medium for 3 to 5 min. The medium was then filtered through a 22 μm millipore filter. The embryo was placed in a small culture tube filled with sterile medium and placed within a passive cooling unit (Equitainer, Hamilton-Thorn, Danvers, MA). The Equitainer cooled the embryo at 0.3° C/min to 5° C. The Equitainer was shipped by commercial airline and, upon arrival (< 24 h) at CSU, the embryo was removed from the container, placed in DPBS plus 10% FCS, and maintained at room temperature until transferred surgically into synchronized recipients. Donor mares at CSU provided 104 embryos for immediate transfer, which served as controls. A total of 136 embryos were transported (Table 41–5). Pregnancy rates at 50 days were similar for fresh (64%) and cooled, transported embryos (66%). Embryonic loss between days 12 and 50 was not altered by treatment (fresh vs. cooled, transported). In addition, pregnancy rates were similar for embryos with an interval between collection and transfer of ≤ 12 h versus ≥ 12 h to ≤ 24 h. Thus equine embryos can be cooled to 5° C and maintained in culture for up to 24 h without a decrease in fertility. Recently, a study was conducted to compare nonsurgical pregnancy rates of embryos stored in Ham's F10 plus 10% FCS at 5° C in an Equitainer for 18 or 36 h.[44] The longer storage time appeared to result in a decrease in embryo quality. However, pregnancy rates after nonsurgical transfer were similar for the two groups, 8 of 22 and 8 of 20 for 18- and 36-h storage, respectively. Thus transportation of cooled embryos requiring 36 h should not result in a decrease in fertility.

FREEZING EQUINE EMBRYOS

Cryopreservation of equine embryos at −196° C would allow more flexibility in import and export of equine embryos. Additional advantages are (1) genetic material can be stored indefinitely and (2) the number of recipients can be minimized. Cryopreservation of bovine embryos has become an integral part of the bovine embryo transfer industry, but relatively few equine embryos have been successfully transferred. Wilmut and Rowson reported the birth of the first calf from a frozen-thawed bovine embryo.[45] Since then, numerous studies have been conducted to determine optimal freezing and thawing procedures for bovine embryos. Other workers reported the birth of the first foal from a frozen-thawed day-6 embryo.[46] However, only 3 of 11 transfers resulted in pregnancies (27%) and 2 of 3 pregnant recipients subsequently aborted. A preliminary study was

TABLE 41–5. PREGNANCY RATES 50 DAYS AFTER SURGICAL TRANSFER OF FRESH AND OF COOLED, TRANSPORTED EQUINE EMBRYOS

TREATMENT	YEAR	NUMBER OF TRANSFERRED EMBRYOS	NUMBER OF PREGNANT RECIPIENTS	PERCENT OF PREGNANT RECIPIENTS
Fresh	1988	30	18	60
	1989	25	17	71
	1990	49	32	65
	All years	104	67	64
Cooled*	1988	24	17	71
	1989	55	32	58
	1990	57	41	72
	All years	136	90	66
Combined	1988–1990	240	156	65

*Placed in an Equitainer and cooled to 5° C then stored for 6 to 24 h.

(From Carney, N.J., et al.: Comparison of pregnancy rates from transfer of fresh versus cooled, transported equine embryos. Theriogenology, *36*:23–32, 1991.

conducted during the 1983 breeding season to evaluate 2 embryo freezing protocols.[47] Both day-6 and day-7 embryos were frozen in glass ampules with glycerol as a cryoprotectant. The results were consistent with those of other researchers in that smaller day-6 embryos withstood cryopreservation better than larger day-7 embryos. Four frozen-thawed, day-6 embryos transferred surgically into 3 recipients resulted in 2 live foals. Subsequently, a series of experiments were conducted to evaluate various freezing protocols for equine embryos.[48–50] Results of the first study demonstrated that freezing in 0.5 mL straws and plunging into liquid nitrogen at −33° C was superior to freezing in glass ampules and plunging at either −33 or 38° C.[48] In the second study, 23 embryos were packaged in straws and cooled from room temperature to −6° C at 4° C/min, −30° C at 0.3° C/min, and to −33° C at 0.1° C/min, then plunged into liquid nitrogen. Of the 17 embryos transferred surgically, 9 resulted in pregnancies.[48] Early blastocysts (mean diameter 173 μm) resulted in a higher ($p < 0.05$) pregnancy rate (8 of 10, 80%) than expanded blastocysts (1 of 7, 14%). Unfortunately, recovery of embryos less than 200 μm in diameter is difficult even at day 6. Therefore, recent efforts at CSU have been to develop techniques for freezing larger embryos. Seidel et al. hypothesized that the inability to freeze larger embryos may be the result of low permeability of cryoprotectants.[49] Thus a study was conducted to evaluate the use of propylene glycol as a cryoprotectant for equine embryos, 200 and 1000 μm in diameter. Two cooling rates from −6 to −33° C were evaluated (0.3° C/min, 0.8° C/min). Within each cooling treatment, straws were thawed either in a 37° C water bath for 20 s or at ambient temperature in air. The study included 4 embryos 130 to 175 μm, 23 embryos 200 to 945 μm, and 3 embryos > 1000 μm. All 4 of the small embryos had good structure after thawing and culture in Ham's F10 for 48 h; whereas, none of the large embryos survived. Post-treatment scores for the 23 embryos in the middle-size group ranged from excellent to dead. Rate of cooling had no effect on any response. A subsequent study[50] was designed to evaluate procedures for freezing day-7 embryos and to determine if ovariectomized-progestin treated mares could be used as recipients for frozen-thawed embryos. Excellent-quality embryos between 160 and 980 μm were recovered 6.5 to 7 days after ovulation. Embryos ≤ 200 μm were placed in 10% glycerol in DPBS and cooled from −6 to −30° C at 0.3° C/min, then to −33° C at 0.1° C/min. Embryos > 200 μm were frozen either in 10% glycerol plus 8.6% sucrose, cooled at 0.5° C/min from −6 to 25° C then plunged, or in 15% glycerol and 15% sucrose and embryos placed between gel-containing cold packs in a household freezer at −25° C for 30 min then plunged. Glycerol was removed in steps of 12%, 9%, 6%, 3%, and 0%, all with 10% sucrose, 6 min/step. A total of 4 of 8 recipients were pregnant after transferring embryos < 200 μm in diameter. However, only 2 of 24 larger embryos resulted in pregnancies. Thus pregnancies can be obtained from transfer of frozen-thawed equine embryos into either intact or ovariectomized mares. Unfortunately, more studies are needed before frozen-thawed day-7 embryos can be used to obtain acceptable pregnancy rates.

SUMMARY

The procedures for collection and transfer of equine embryos have become routine. Expanded use of equine embryo transfer depends on favorable changes in breed registry regulations as well as technologic advances. A 65% pregnancy rate is consistently obtained after surgical embryo transfer. It is unlikely that this pregnancy rate will be improved, because this percentage is quite similar to first-cycle pregnancy rates. Therefore, the greatest advances in embryo transfer will come in the area of embryo recovery. Superovulation has been used as a means of increasing recovery of multiple embryos.[51] However, further studies are needed to improve ovulation rates in response to superovulatory drugs and to determine why fertilization is lower in multiple-ovulating versus single-ovulating mares. Embryo recovery in old, infertile mares is generally less than 30%. This has been attributed, in part, to poor fertilization and/or oviductal transport. An alternative to the conventional embryo recovery methods is to aspirate oocytes directly from preovulatory follicles[52–54] and fertilize them in vitro[55–58] or in another mare.[55] Both fertilization methods have resulted in live foals. During the next decade, tremendous progress will most certainly be made in oocyte collection and in vivo and in vitro fertilizations.

REFERENCES

1. McKinnon, A.O., and Squires, E.L.: Morphological assessment of equine embryo. J. Am. Vet. Med. Assoc., *192*:401–406, 1988.
2. McKinnon, A.O., Squires, E.L., and Voss, J.L.: Ultrasound evaluation of the mare's reproductive tract: Part II. Compend. Contin. Educ. Practicing Vet., *9*:472–482, 1987.
3. Squires, E.L., Cook, V.M., and Voss, J.L.: Collection and transfer of equine embryos. Animal Reproduction Laboratory Bulletin No.-01. Fort Collins, Colorado State University, 1985.
4. Douglas, R.H.: Review of induction of superovulation and embryo transfer in the equine. Theriogenology, *11*:33–46, 1979.
5. Squires, E.L., Amann, R.P., McKinnon, A.O., and Pickett, B.W.: Fertility of equine spermatozoa cooled to 5 or 20° C. Proceedings of the International Congress on Animal Reproduction and Artificial Insemination, Dublin, 1988, pp. 297–300.
6. Squires, E.L., Imel, K.J., Iuliano, M.F., and Shideler, R.K.: Factors affecting reproductive efficiency in an equine embryo transfer programme. J. Reprod. Fertil. Suppl., *32*:409–414, 1982.
7. Francl, A.T., Amann, R.P., Squires, E.L., and Pickett, B.W.: Motility and fertility of equine spermatozoa in a milk extender after 2 or 24 hours at 20° C. Theriogenology, *27*:517–526, 1987.
8. Vogelsang, S.G., Bondioli, K.R., and Massey, J.M.: Com-

mercial application of equine embryo transfer. Equine Vet. J. Suppl., *3:*89–91, 1985.

9. Vogelsang, S.G., and Vogelsang, M.M.: Influence of donor parity and age on the success of commercial equine embryo transfer. Equine Vet. J. Suppl., *8:*71–72, 1989.
10. Ball, B.A., Little, T.V., Hillman, R.B., and Woods, G.L.: Pregnancy rates at days 2 and 14 and estimated embryonic loss rates prior to day 14 in normal and subfertile mares. Theriogenology, *26:*611–619, 1986.
11. Cook, V.C., and Squires, E.L.: Results from a commercial embryo transfer programme. Equine Vet. J. Suppl., *3:*103, 1985.
12. Douglas, R.H.: Some aspects of equine embryo transfer. J. Reprod. Fertil. Suppl., *32:*405–408, 1982.
13. Woods, G.L., Hillman, R.B., and Schlafer, D.H.: Recovery and evaluation of embryos from normal and infertile mares. Cornell Vet., *76:*386–394, 1986.
14. Douglas, R.H., Burns, P.J., and Hershman, L.: Physiological and commercial parameters for producing progeny from subfertile mares by embryo transfer. Equine Vet. J. Suppl., *3:*111–114, 1985.
15. Iuliano, M.F., and Squires, E.L.: Embryo transfer in two-year-old donor mares. Theriogenology, *24:*647–653, 1985.
16. Steiner, J.V., and Jordan, M.T.: Ovulation rates, embryo collection rates and embryo transfer rates for mature and two-year-old Hanoverian mares. Equine Pract., *10:*6–8, 1988.
17. Betteridge, K.J.: The structure and function of the equine capsule in relation to embryo manipulation and transfer. Equine Vet. J. Suppl., *8:*92–100, 1989.
18. Ginther, O.J.: Fixation and orientation of the early equine conceptus. Theriogenology, *19:*613–623, 1983.
19. McKinnon, A.O., and Squires, E.L.: Equine embryo transfer. Vet. Clin. North Am. Equine Pract., *4:*305–333, 1988.
20. McKinnon, A.O., Squires, E.L., and Voss, J.L.: Factors affecting equine embryo transfer pregnancy rates. Proceedings International Congress on Animal Reproduction and Artificial Insemination, Dublin, 1988, pp. 177–179.
21. Oguri, N., and Tsutsumi, Y.: Nonsurgical transfer of equine embryos. Arch. Androl., *5:*108, 1980.
22. Hinrichs, K., Sertich, P.L., Cummings, M.R., and Kenney, R.M.: Pregnancy in ovariectomized mares achieved by embryo transfer: A preliminary study. Equine Vet. J. Suppl., *3:*74–75, 1985.
23. Hinrichs, K., Sertich, P.L., and Kenney, R.M.: Use of altrenogest to prepare ovariectomized mares as embryo transfer recipients. Theriogenology, *26:*455–460, 1986.
24. McKinnon, A.O., Squires, E.L., Carnevale, E.M., and Hermenet, M.J.: Ovariectomized steroid-treated mares as embryo transfer recipients and as a model to study the role of progestins in pregnancy maintenance. Theriogenology, *29:*1055–1063, 1988.
25. Hinrichs, K., and Kenney, R.M.: Effect of timing of progesterone administration on pregnancy rate after embryo transfer in ovariectomized mares. J. Reprod. Fertil. Suppl., *35:*439–443, 1987.
26. Clark, K.E., Squires, E.L., McKinnon, A.O., and Seidel, G.E., Jr.: Viability of stored equine embryos. J. Anim. Sci., *65:*534–542, 1987.
27. Pool, K.F., et al.: Exogenous hormone regimens to utilize successfully mares in dioestrus (day 2-14 after ovulation) as embryo recipients. J. Reprod. Fertil. Suppl., *35:*429–432, 1987.
28. Parry-Weeks, L.C., and Holtan, D.W.: Effect of altrenogest on pregnancy maintenance in unsynchronized equine embryo recipients. J. Reprod. Fertil. Suppl., *35:*433–438, 1987.
29. Sertich, P.L., Hinrichs, K., and Kenney, R.M.: Histological aspects of uterine involution in the post parturient, ovariectomized embryo recipient mare: A model for the study of involution. J. Reprod. Fertil. Suppl., *35:*56–58, 1987.
30. Imel, K.J.: Recovery, culture and transfer of equine embryos. M.S. thesis. Fort Collins, Colorado State University, 1981.
31. Squires, E.L., Iuliano, M.F., and Shideler, R.K.: Factors affecting success of surgical and nonsurgical equine embryo transfer. Theriogenology, *17:*35–41, 1982.
32. Iuliano, M.F., Squires, E.L., and Cook, V.M.: Effect of age of embryo and method of transfer on pregnancy rate. J. Anim. Sci., *60:*258–263, 1985.
33. Allen, W.R., and Rowson, L.E.A.: Surgical and nonsurgical egg transfer in horses. J. Reprod. Fertil. Suppl., *23:*525–530, 1975.
34. Dowsett, K.F., Woodward, R.A., and Bodero, D.A.V.: A study of nonsurgical embryo transfer in the mare. Theriogenology, *31:*631–642, 1989.
35. Lagneaux, D., and Palmer, E.: Are pony and larger mares similar as recipients for non-surgical transfer of day 7 embryos. Equine Vet. J. Suppl., *8:*64–67, 1989.
36. Fleury, J.J., Costaneto, J.B.F., and Alvarenga, M.A.: Results from an embryo transfer programme with Mangalarga mares in Brazil. Equine Vet. J. Suppl., *8:*73–74, 1989.
37. Carney, N.J., et al.: Comparison of pregnancy rates from transfer of fresh versus cooled, transported equine embryos. Theriogenology, *36:*23–32, 1991.
38. Elsden, R.P., and Seidel, G.E., Jr.: Procedures for recovery, bisection, freezing and transfer of bovine embryos. Animal Reproduction Biotechnology Laboratory Bulletin No. 2. Fort Collins, Colorado State University, 1990. pp. 13–14.
39. Woods, G.L., Hillman, R.B., and Schlafer, D.H.: Recovery and evaluation of embryos from normal and infertile mares. Cornell Vet., *76:*386–394, 1986.
40. Ball, B.A., Little, T.V., Hillman, R.B., and Woods, G.L.: Pregnancy rates at day 2 and 14 and estimated embryonic loss rates prior to day 15 in normal and subfertile mares. Theriogenology, *26:*611–619, 1986.
41. Carnevale, E.M., Squires, E.L., and McKinnon, A.O.: Comparison of Ham's F10 with CO_2 or Hepes buffer for storage of equine embryos at 5C for 24 h. J. Anim. Sci., *65:*1775–1781, 1987.
42. Slade, N.P., Williams, T.J., Squires, E.L., and Seidel, G.E., Jr.: Production of identical twin pregnancies by microsurgical bisection of equine embryos. Proceedings of the International Congress on Animal Reproduction on Artificial Insemination. 1984, pp. 214.
43. Cook, V.M., et al.: Pregnancy rates of cooled, transported equine embryos. Equine Vet. J. Suppl., *8:*80–81, 1989.
44. Martin, J.M., Squires, E.L., Jasko, D.J., and Carney, N.J.: Effect of storage of equine embryos at 5° C for 18 and 36 hours. Theriogenology, *35:*238, 1991.
45. Wilmut, I., and Rowson, L.E.A.: Experiments on the low temperature preservation of cow embryos. Vet. Rec., *92:*686–688, 1973.
46. Yamamoto, Y., Oguri, N., Tsutsumi, Y., and Hachinohe, Y.: Experiments in freezing and storage of equine embryos. J. Reprod. Fertil. Suppl., *32:*399–403, 1982.
47. Takeda, T., Elsden, R.P., and Squires, E.L.: In vitro and in vivo development of frozen-thawed equine embryos. Proceedings of the International Congress on Animal Reproduction and Artificial Insemination. 1984, pp. 246–249.

48. Slade, N.P., et al.: A new procedure for cryopreservation of equine embryos. Theriogenology, *24:*45–58, 1985.
49. Seidel, G.E., Squires, E.L., McKinnon, A.O., and Long, P.L. Cryopreservation of equine embryos in 1,2-propanediol. Equine Vet. J. Suppl., *8:*87–88, 1989.
50. Squires, E.L., Seidel, G.E., Jr., and McKinnon, A.O.: Transfer of cryopreserved equine embryos to progestin-treated ovariectomized mares. Equine Vet. J. Suppl., *8:*89–91, 1989.
51. Squires, E.L., et al.: Reproductive characteristics of spontaneous single and double ovulating mares and superovulated mares. J. Reprod. Fertil. Suppl., *35:*399–403, 1987.
52. McKinnon, A.O., Wheeler, M.B., Carnevale, E.M., and Squires, E.L.: Oocyte transfer in the mare: Preliminary observations. J. Equine Vet. Sci., *6:*306–309, 1987.
53. Vogelsang, M.M., et al.: Method for collecting follicular oocytes from mares. Theriogenology, *29:*1007–1019, 1988.
54. Palmer, E., et al.: Non-surgical recovery of follicular fluid and oocytes of mares. J. Reprod. Fertil. Suppl., *35:*689–690, 1987.
55. McKinnon, A.O., et al.: Heterogenous and xenogenous fertilization of in vitro matured equine oocytes. J. Equine Vet. Sci., *8:*143–147, 1988.
56. Blue, B.J., et al.: Capacitation of stallion spermatozoa and in vitro fertilization of equine oocytes. Equine Vet. J. Suppl., *8:*111–116, 1989.
57. Del Campo, M.R., Donoso, M.X., Parrish, J.J., and Ginther, O.J.: In vitro fertilization of in vitro-matured equine oocytes. J. Equine Vet. Sci., *10:*18–22, 1990.
58. Palmer, E., Bezard, J., Magistrini, M., and Duchamp, G.: In vitro fertilization in the horse: A retrospective study. J. Reprod. Fertil. Suppl., *44:*375–384, 1991.

CHAPTER 42

BREEDING THE PROBLEM MARE

A.O. McKinnon
J.L. Voss

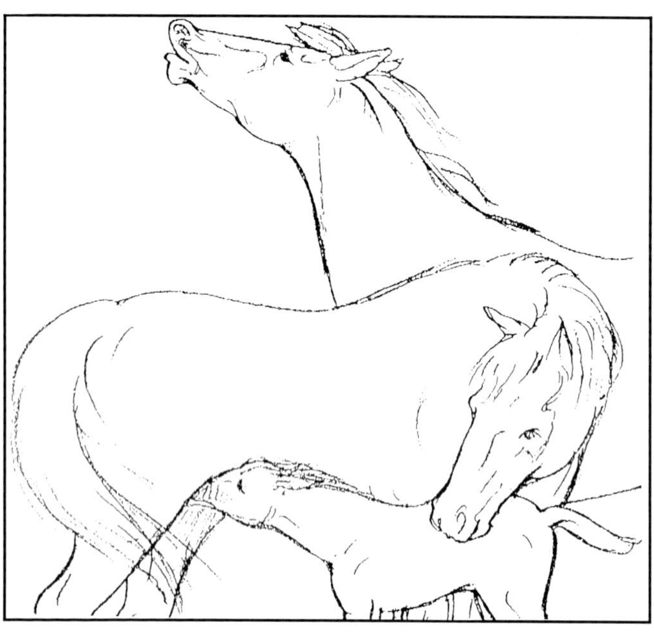

Management of the problem mare is one of the most challenging and potentially frustrating aspects of equine reproduction. No magical treatments exist despite anecdotal evidence of clients who each "once had a problem mare that remained barren until they either pasture mated her, infused her uterus with kerosene, supplemented her with vitamin E, took 10 L of blood from her, transported her after breeding, bred her to a pony teaser stallion, or fed her extracts from the local homeopath." The simple truth our clients need to understand is that apart from semen, it is hard work and persistent adherence to strict scientific principles and management techniques that result in conception and maintenance of pregnancy with problem mares. Many of the fundamentals of good breeding management are outlined in other chapters. This chapter will strive to amalgamate these principles into a practical approach.

People's attitudes and time constraints are major difficulties of successfully breeding the problem mare. Frequently, mares are on different breeding farms, and despite initial enthusiasm from all concerned, with each unsuccessful cycle a negative attitude engendered from the farm manager, veterinarian, and attendants becomes apparent. As the treatments change and the mare keeps returning to estrus, hidden pressures on the veterinarian to get to the next farm on time begin to influence judgment. Many veterinarians would gladly refer these cases to specialist facilities at the end of the season, but few think it necessary at the beginning.

This chapter outlines the philosophy and treatment of a problem mare program at the Goulburn Valley Equine Hospital (GVEH) in Shepparton, Victoria, Australia. However the approach, medical and surgical therapies, and management techniques should apply to any breeding establishment. This program has an annual enrollment of between 20 and 80 problem mares, boarded full-time on pasture at the hospital. The number of mares varies according to time of year, economic trends, and removal of pregnant mares and/or mares with hopeless prognoses. Facilities are designed to minimize handling time and maximize individual mare attention. An added benefit is that because most mares are bred at the hospital or transported to and immediately back from local farms for breeding they can be intensively managed and the psychologic oppression of mares returning to heat is generally only a local (hospital) phenomenon. The cost to the client is often greater because mares are able to be managed more intensively than on breeding farms. However, in our experience few people complain about billing once their mare is pregnant. Although a headache, constant owner communication and education reduces the number of dissatisfied clients when mares fail to become pregnant.

This represents one approach to breeding problem mares and is the combined opinions and experiences of the authors only. Many other philosophies and personal preferences exist that may not be addressed. Perhaps we should keep in mind that for any condition with so many different avenues of treatment (much of it anecdotal, undocumented, or not scientifically validated) and without an experimental model, to be dog-matic in recommendation for management is not only difficult, but inappropriate.

WHAT IS A PROBLEM MARE?

When a mare begins to be regarded as a problem breeder is at the discretion of the owner, veterinarian, or farm manager. Classically, a mare should be regarded as a potential problem if she fails to conceive to a fertile stallion on a well-managed breeding farm in three or more cycles in one season. We have seen instances of reproductively normal mares failing to conceive to a subfertile stallion for as long as three breeding seasons. Unfortunately, fertility of a stallion may not be common knowledge away from the breeding farm, particularly to the mare owner. In addition, improper handling and/or insemination techniques in an artificial insemination (AI) program are excellent methods for dramatically reducing pregnancy rates. Attention to pregnancy rate per cycle from maiden, dry, and wet mares may help determine if stallion fertility or management procedures should be questioned.

In evaluating a problem mare, all aspects of management should be examined. This might include nutrition, teasing techniques, parasite control, medical history, evaluation for chronic generalized disease (equine infectious anemia), and other management practices. Mares may become problems for many reasons. For example, mares failing to exhibit estrus in the breeding season may have a granulosa-theca cell tumor, gonadal dysgenesis, or pituitary adenoma or they may be pseudopregnant, unknowingly pregnant, or in anestrus. However, by far the most common type of problem mare presented is the one with persistent, unidentified, or inappropriately treated uterine infections. All mares presented to the GVEH have been barren two or more breeding seasons and most have received some treatment in the breeding seasons before referral. The following discussion relates only to mares with acute and/or chronic uterine inflammatory changes. Ovarian abnormalities and other forms of noninfectious infertility are reviewed elsewhere in this volume.

HOW THE PROBLEM OCCURS

Recognition of factors responsible for mares' susceptibility to uterine infection and persistent uterine inflammation or its sequelae should dramatically reduce the number of problem mares. However, the number of mares foaling each year has not appreciably improved in those breeds whose registries have kept accurate records for many years. This can be related partly to economic constraints and lack of genetic selection for fertility; however, extremely high (≥90%) pregnancy rates with only slightly lowered foaling rates consistently occur on some well-managed breeding farms. This fertility can be attributed partially to prebreeding selection of the most fertile mares and correcting faulty management procedures and noninfectious causes of infertility. However, careful management to ensure prompt treatment or prevention of uterine inflammation is most important.

Mares do not become problem breeders overnight. Susceptibility to infection is a graded condition and occurs primarily as a result of the effects of increasing age, reproductive tract damage, and bacterial challenge. Bacterial challenge is influenced by external conformation, breeding techniques, examination procedures, anatomic abnormalities, and postpartum events.

The physical barriers to infection are the external vaginal lips, the vestibular sphincter, and the cervix. The ability to isolate bacteria in normal mares decreases progressively from the clitoral fossa (94%) to the vestibule (69%), cranial vagina (42%), and uterus (31%).[1] In this study, no potential pathogens were isolated from vaginal or uterine cultures. Contamination of the uterus with bacteria is inevitable. Potentially pathogenic organisms are introduced at breeding, during and after parturition, during examination, and as a result of failure of physical barriers to infection (i.e., pneumovagina). When uterine defense mechanisms are functioning properly, massive challenges, either natural or experimental, fail to produce inflammation that lasts long enough to interfere with reproduction.[2–4] For embryo survival, mares must clear bacteria and inflammatory products from the uterus, as a result of breeding, by the time the embryo descends into the lumen about 5 to 6 days after ovulation.[5] Uterine defense mechanisms are mechanical and cellular. Mechanical contributions to uterine defense are myometrial contractions which assist in evacuation of uterine contents and a relaxed cervix during estrus. Physical clearance is more efficient during estrus.[6] Cellular responses are primarily phagocytosis. Efficient phagocytosis depends on (1) mobilization of an adequate number of neutrophils from the general circulation, with prompt migration of these cells through the endometrium and into the uterine lumen; (2) adequate chemotaxis of neutrophils to contaminating bacteria; (3) adherence of bacteria to the cellular membrane of the phagocyte (opsonization); and (4) ingestion and successful intracellular killing of bacteria by neutrophils.

While all causes for failure of uterine defense mechanisms have not been identified, some significant influences are well known. Repeated and overwhelming infections or contaminations, with predisposing factors such as perineal abnormalities and pneumovagina, are undoubtedly related to reduction in efficiency of the mare's defense mechanisms. Reduced efficiency of neutrophils to phagocytize bacteria and a defect in opsonization by complement and antibody have been identified in susceptible mares,[2,7–11] and this is not related to reduced or inadequate numbers of white blood cells.[8,12]

Failure of the uterus to evacuate mechanically contaminants and inflammatory products also appears to be important. Myometrial activity may be reduced in older multiparous mares,[6] and physical clearance of nonantigenic markers from the uterus of susceptible mares was delayed when compared with resistant

GOULBURN VALLEY EQUINE HOSPITAL

P.O. BOX 2020, SHEPPARTON, 3630 — TELEPHONE: (058) 299 566 — FAX: (058) 299 307

DR. J. R. VASEY, B.V.Sc., Dip.Vet.Surg., F.A.C.V.Sc.

SPECIALISTS IN EQUINE REPRODUCTION AND SURGERY

AND ASSOCIATES

DR. A. O. McKINNON, B.V.Sc., M.Sc., Dip. L.A. Med., Diplomate A.C.T.

Mare Fertility Evaluation

	Name	Address	Phone (work/home)
OWNER	....	....	........../..........
		....	
VETERINARIAN	....	....	........../..........
		....	

METHOD OF IDENTIFICATION .... **MARE NAME:** ....

DATE .... PLACE OF EXAMINATION ....

AGE .... BREED .... MARKINGS ....

....

Maiden .... Barren .... Foaling* .... EED* .... Abortion* .... *(Date ....
Day of gestation ....)

HISTORY OF REPRODUCTIVE PROBLEMS: ....

....

....

....

PREVIOUS REPRODUCTIVE EXAMINATION FINDINGS: ....

....

....

PREVIOUS REPRODUCTIVE SURGERIES, UTERINE TREATMENTS OR HORMONE TREATMENTS: ....

....

....

FERTILITY EVALUATION:

1. Physical Condition: ....
2. External Perineal Conformation: Normal .... Low Pelvis .... Tilted Vulva .... Sunken Anus ....
   Other ....
3. Rectal Examination: ....
   ....
4. Vaginal Examination: ....
   ....
5. Ultrasonographic Examination: ....
   ....
   ....
6. Uterine Culture: ....
   ....
7. Uterine Cytology: ....
   ....
8. Uterine Biopsy (see attached biopsy sheet): ....
   ....

INTERPRETIVE SUMMARY AND RECOMMENDATION: ....

....

....

....

....

....

....

....

....

....

....

....

....

....

FIG. 42–1. Reproductive examination form used at the Goulburn Valley Equine Hospital, Shepparton, Victoria, Australia.

mares.[13] If the cervix does not relax adequately or is compromised with adhesions or anatomic functional defects, evacuation may be impaired.

EXAMINATION PROCEDURES

Clients are encouraged to have a full reproductive examination performed on their mares to help decide on the probability of successful resolution of the problem. The exam is best performed while the mare is in estrus and definitely should be conducted before the mare enters anestrus. The reproductive examination form currently in use at the GVEH is presented in Figure 42–1. Clients are sent a copy of the evaluation as soon as possible and are then encouraged to discuss the prognosis. The reproductive examination procedures and interpretations are covered in detail elsewhere in this text (Chapters 21–30) and to avoid redundancy, only salient points relating to problem mares will be discussed here. The order of examination is always the same, and notes are written by an assistant at the time of examination to prevent accidental omission of data. Each year one or two mares presented will be pregnant, so invasive procedures such as culture and biopsy always follow rectal palpation and ultrasonographic examination. For daily examinations, mares are herded into a long chute system and are teased or can wait for admission into the palpation shed (Figs. 42–2 and 42–3). The system is designed to eliminate the need to catch any horse and is expedient and requires few personnel.

HISTORY

The prognosis for mares barren 3 yr or more is always guarded provided they come from well-managed breeding farms. Regardless of the number of years barren, we have more success in mares less than 18 yr old. Breed is important with relation to ability to use AI or embryo transfer. Access to old breeding records is desirable and may suggest where and why the problems began and why previous treatments were not successful.

PHYSICAL CONDITION

Body condition and estimated weight are recorded. Use of a scale or tape is preferable. Body condition, disease, and chronic pain may be related to timing of recrudescence to cyclicity. Hirsutism may be related to seasonal changes or a pituitary adenoma. Mares kept for an extended stay must always be sent home in better condition than when they arrived, although not overfat.

EXTERNAL CONFORMATION

Height of pelvis relative to anus; slope of vaginal lips; abnormalities of perineal body, clitoris, or labia; presence or need to modify a Caslick operation; and propensity to aspirate air or pool urine are all noted with suggestions for methods of improvement and necessity.

RECTAL EXAMINATION

Uterine tone and size and ovarian activity are assessed. Abnormalities such as sacculations and pyometra are also recorded. The main purpose of rectal examination is assessment of structure, tone, and form. To determine routinely the presence of uterine fluid with rectal palpation is not possible. Ovarian examination gives important information on cyclicity and ovarian abnormalities.

ULTRASONOGRAPHIC EXAMINATION

Quantity and quality of uterine fluid are related to degree of inflammation.[14] Uterine cysts are related to age and chronic endometritis.[14,15] Abnormalities detected and undetected by rectal examination are visualized.

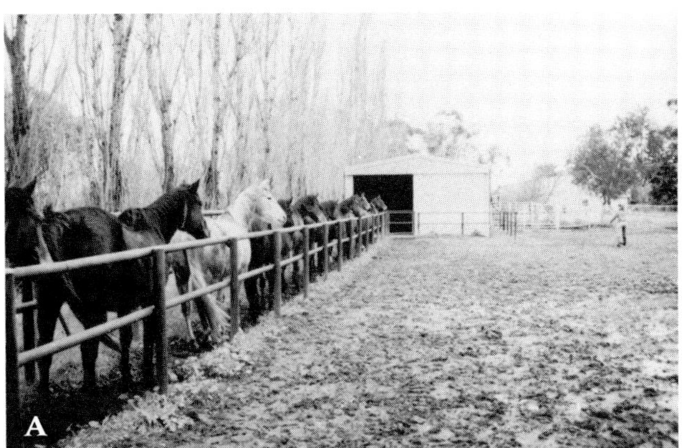

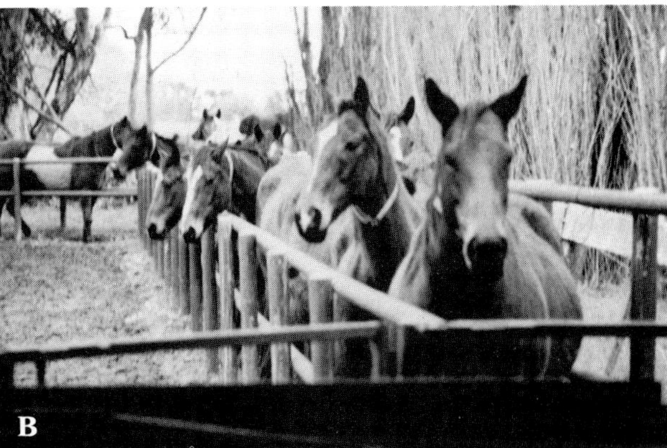

FIG. 42–2. *A*, Barren mares are processed through long holding races or chutes. *B*, Mares can be individually teased while in the chute system.

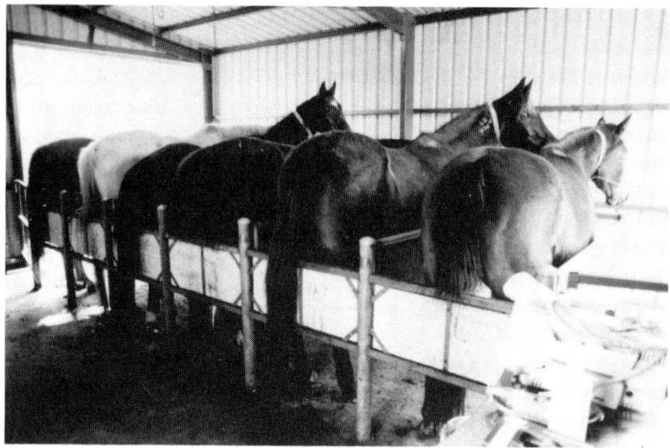

FIG. 42–3. Side-loading stocks or crushes are designed to hold six mares, open either way, and are able to be loaded by one person without catching the mare.

VAGINAL EXAMINATION

Manual examination is recommended. The vestibular sphincter and cervix are assessed for efficacy as barriers to infection. Cervical defects and adhesions are not uncommon. Many defects can be repaired surgically and some mares still can become pregnant despite absence of much of the cervix. If the cervix is relaxed, introduction of the whole hand into the uterus for manipulation is indicated. Small granulomatous lumps (2 to 4 mm) are occasionally identified and cysts and luminal adhesions can be removed or destroyed. Luminal adhesions imply a poor prognosis.

Recognition of problems such as vesicovaginal reflux may on occasion only be made during estrus when the reproductive tract is relaxed. However, some cervical defects are best recognized when the tone is increased as during diestrus.

CULTURE

Guarded culture techniques (Accu-Culshure specimen collection and transport system, Pleasantville, NY) are recommended. Samples are cultured aerobically for 48 h. Microaerophilic, anaerobic, and fungal culture techniques are used when indicated. Similarly, culture of uterine biopsy specimens may be necessary on occasion to detect causative agents of deep chronic endometritis.

CYTOLOGY

Results of uterine culture are best interpreted in relation to numbers of neutrophils detected from the endometrium by exfoliative cytology. However, mares with chronic endometritis may have little surface irritation.

UTERINE BIOPSY

A single biopsy may not always be totally representative of the uterus,[16,17] but a sample from the corpus cornual junction (site of embryonic fixation) is one of the most accurate determinants of inflammatory conditions and cellular infiltrates. Cell types and changes are classified to give an individual grading for acute, chronic, and fibrotic changes (0 to 3) (see Appendix I). The biopsy interpretation is one of the most important determinants of subsequent foaling rates,[18,19] and in addition, the degree of chronic versus acute inflammation helps decide therapy.

OTHER PROCEDURES

Examination for cytogenetic abnormalities and endoscopy for visualization of pathologic changes are performed as indicated.

MANAGEMENT PREBREEDING SEASON

Best results are achieved when we have the opportunity to assess and correct identified problems before the breeding season begins. Failure to treat an active chronic uterine infection during the nonbreeding season is one more insult to an already compromised reproductive tract.

The aim of prebreeding season management is to (1) eliminate uterine infection and inflammation and (2) prevent further contamination before and during the next breeding season. Economic considerations are highlighted during this time when mares are repeatedly treated and clients receive accounts, and yet no signs of success are evident, because it is too early to begin breeding.

CORRECTION OF PHYSICAL ABNORMALITIES

Many of the treatments during the nonbreeding season require multiple vaginal invasions to penetrate the cervix, thus a Caslick operation (see Chapter 48) or a breeding stitch may be damaged. Decisions on when to perform reconstructive surgery relative to treatment of infection or inflammation is generally obvious. Episioplasty and perineal body transection[20] are generally performed immediately, unless active inflammation is present, because once healed they provide little impedance to invasive treatment or examination procedures. Similarly, therapy for mares whose major inflammatory problem is related to vesicovaginal reflux is pointless until the primary problem has been treated.[21–23]

Surgery of cervical problems (Chapter 51) has often not been attempted because of difficulties of exposure and failure to identify the problem; furthermore occasionally mares successfully carry pregnancy despite cervical defects. We always attempt repair of major defects if possible and find that strong caudal traction of the cervix with two pairs of cervical forceps (Knowles forceps, Sontec Instruments, Englewood, CO) in mares heavily sedated and given epidural or local anesthesia often enables good visualization of and surgical access to the cervix in the caudal vagina or vestibule.

TREATMENT OF INFECTION AND INFLAMMATION

Frequently we have no choice as to what stage of the cycle mares are treated. Many mares (~ 70%) have entered anestrus during winter by the time they arrive for treatment. However, if possible, treatments are restricted during estrus to use the effects of increased drainage, contraction,[3,6] and increased efficiency of phagocytosis.[24,25]

Cervical adhesions are treated by local application of an oil-based corticosteroid and antibiotic creams (R.R. Pascoe, personal communication), and concurrent intrauterine elimination of infection. Treatment may involve daily topical application, disruption of adhesions, and massage for as long as 2 weeks. Although some mares will become pregnant by AI with adhesions of the cervix, these more frequently abort and the adhesions remain as a nidus of infection and should be eliminated.

Uterine infection with concomitant large amounts of debris and fluid are treated by voluminous saline lavage, 1 L at a time, until the effluent is grossly clear. Intrauterine antibiotics as determined by culture and sensitivity testing (Chapter 43) are administered after each daily lavage. When culture results are negative and active chronic infiltrative endometritis is identified from biopsy, a different and perplexing problem exists. Treatment of these mares may be inappropriate, because they possibly have already eliminated the infection and remain as mares susceptible to endometritis. However, our approach has been to attempt to reduce the inflammatory response, because many of these mares have small quantities of uterine fluid present. Therapy is prolonged (7 to 15 treatments) with administration of broad-spectrum intrauterine antibiotics performed daily or every other day. Concurrently, systemic estradiol esters are administered for 1 month. If uterine adhesions are present, local corticosteroid therapy is instituted. Currently, no reports assessing the efficacy of these treatments exist and extreme caution is advised. Immunosuppression from the corticosteroids, although reducing the lymphocytic infiltrate, may well result in establishment of an infection resistant to antibiotics. No estrogen preparations are approved for use in horses (Chapter 37). In addition, use of long-term estradiol therapy, although apparently beneficial on the local uterine environment, has in our experience and in the hands of others[26] resulted in long-term suppression of ovarian function. Some treated mares fail to cycle until well into the breeding season. Also, to date we know of no method to determine which mares with prolonged ovarian suppression will respond to estradiol therapy.

Regardless of the method of treatment, a reproductive evaluation is performed to assess efficacy at conclusion of therapy. At that time final reproductive surgeries (i.e., Caslick operation) may be completed. Local treatments after a Caslick operation can be administered by passing an infusion pipette into the vestibule, then guiding it through the cervix rectally, in a manner similar to, but with more difficulty than, intrauterine treatment in the cow.

PREBREEDING ASSESSMENT

Unfortunately, not all mares arrive for assessment and treatment during the nonbreeding season, and of those that do, not all respond to therapy enough to enable breeding to begin without added treatments.

The primary goal of the prebreeding assessment period is to have a uterine environment capable of supporting spermatozoa long enough so they can reach the oviduct in a condition capable of initiating fertilization. Only a few hours are necessary for spermatozoa to pass through the uterotubule junction and remain relatively free from toxic products in the uterus. However, fluid inflammatory products, when mixed with spermatozoa, cause an immediate decline in spermatozoal motility that is proportional to the amount of inflammatory products.[27] Also, addition of uterine fluid of grades 1 to 2[14] to spermatozoa before breeding mares by AI resulted in a decreased embryo recovery ($p < 0.05$).[27] Decline in spermatozoal motility in vitro can be arrested by addition of an extender to the uterine fluid before addition of spermatozoa.[27] However it appears that for best fertility, removal of inflammatory products from the uterus before introduction of spermatozoa is the most logical approach.

To meet these objectives, mares are examined in early estrus. Ultrasonographic identification of uterine fluid and culture and sensitivity results are used to determine whether uterine lavage, local antibiotics, or a combination of both are necessary to obtain a uterus free from inflammatory products at the time of breeding. To breed mares destined to return to estrus is an inappropriate use of time and finances, thus mares with abnormal uterine fluid accumulations detected at the time of breeding are often recycled as soon as prostaglandin $F_2\alpha$ ($PGF_2\alpha$) is capable of causing luteolysis.

BREEDING MANAGEMENT

If the uterine environment is prepared properly at the time of breeding, the next goal is to prevent contamination at, or immediately after, breeding. Clearly, breeding contamination is more easily controlled with AI than with natural service. However, both techniques result in introduction of bacteria. Research in this area was originally reported by Kenney et al. in 1975.[28] They demonstrated that hygienically collected semen from "noninfected" stallions contained numerous types of aerobic bacteria and fungi. The total number of aerobic microorganisms in each of eight ejaculations from five stallions collected ranged from 0.09 to 36 million.

However, addition of raw semen to nonfat dry milk seminal extenders containing either penicillin-streptomycin (1500 IU/mL and 1500 μg/mL, respectively) or gentamicin sulfate (1 mg/mL) resulted in no growth on any of the subcultures from treated samples, including 0 time, which was after about 5 minutes of exposure. Heavy growth was noted in all subcultures from raw semen.[28]

Aerobic bacteria commonly isolated from the urethra, semen, and prepuce of stallions are Escherichia coli and other coliforms, Pseudomonas aeruginosa, β hemolytic and nonhemolytic streptococci (Streptococcus zooepidemicus), Klebsiella spp., hemolytic and nonhemolytic staphylococci, Proteus spp., and Corynebacterium spp.

Further experimentation has demonstrated effective elimination of bacteria without affecting motility using seminal extenders containing either penicillin-gentamicin or polymyxin B sulfate (1000 IU/mL).[29] Thus the addition of raw semen to appropriate antibiotic-containing seminal extenders appears to be one method of ensuring minimal contamination at the time of breeding.[28,30] Some antibiotics affect spermatozoal motility at high concentrations and may adversely affect fertility.[30]

ARTIFICIAL INSEMINATION

If possible, mares are inseminated without disturbing reproductive surgeries such as the Caslick operation. The perineum is diligently cleaned and dried as previously described[30] and 500×10^6 progressively motile spermatozoa (PMS) mixed with appropriate antibiotic-containing extender are inseminated. Proper technique to ensure cleanliness of the stallion and collection equipment is important.[30] To ensure the antibiotics have had adequate time to eliminate bacterial growth, it is best to allow at least 15 min at 37° C before insemination. If a longer interval is required, extended semen may be cooled to 20° C and stored for at least 12 h[31] and often considerably longer at 4° C.[30,32] To reduce contaminating organisms to an absolute minimum, a method was devised[28] to "wash" spermatozoa by dilution with an antibiotic-containing extender, followed by centrifugation (300 g) to produce a "soft" pellet, decantation of the supernatant, and resuspension of the resulting pellet in fresh, warm extender. This technique has the added advantage of removing much of the seminal plasma, which reduces motility after prolonged incubation[30] with minimal damage to spermatozoa;[33] however, it is time-consuming and may not be necessary.

NATURAL SERVICE

Regardless of whether AI or natural service is used to breed mares, if a Caslick operation has to be opened, it should be immediately apposed after breeding. Temporary apposition may be achieved with Michelle clips; however, mares often become irritated by their continual reinsertion. Another technique is placement of breeding stitches that allow the penis or forearm to penetrate the vagina without damaging the labial commissures. Unfortunately, in many instances they are not effective because the vaginal lips are often not joined far enough ventrally to provide a good barrier to pneumovagina. Effective management often involves immediate replacement of stitches into the vulvar lips post-service. Mares and stallions to be bred by natural service should be well cleaned (Chapter 85). Strong disinfectants that may cause overgrowth of potentially pathogenic bacteria after prolonged use are avoided.

A technique of minimizing contamination by prebreeding infusion of 100 to 300 mL of antibiotic-enriched seminal extender has been described.[28] This technique has advantages; however, caution should be advised. For maximum reproductive efficiency, 500×10^6 PMS should be deposited into the reproductive tract.[34] However, lower spermatozoal numbers are quite effective in highly fertile stallions.[30] This information was derived from AI with small volumes of semen or semen plus extender. Recent information has indicated that spermatozoal concentration and volume of inseminate may be important factors in fertility. When mares were bred with 250×10^6 PMS in 100 mL of extender, embryo recovery rate was significantly depressed (13.6%; $p < 0.001$) compared with mares bred with these same spermatozoal numbers from the same ejaculates in 10 mL of extender (70.6%).[27] This finding becomes important when mares are bred to stallions naturally that, because of frequent breedings, may have low spermatozoal numbers in normal ejaculate volumes (30 to 150 mL).

Our approach for mares bred by natural service is to use ultrasonographic detection of quality and quantity of fluid combined with culture and sensitivity results to determine optimum treatments. For instance, if mares have a large volume of fluid detected, then voluminous lavage of the uterus with a physiologic solution (such as Dulbecco's phosphate buffered saline) that is not expected to be detrimental to spermatozoal survival is instituted immediately before breeding. Increased temperature (41° to 45° C) of infused fluids seems to aid in evacuation of uterine contents by increasing uterine tone. This procedure is slightly irritating; however, the aim is to clear the uterus of inflammatory products and enable spermatozoa to have a relatively safe passage into the oviduct before further inflammatory products are released. If small quantities of uterine fluid are detected, then intrauterine antibiotics are infused prebreeding ($\geq$ 12 h). If uterine fluid is detected at the time of scheduled breeding, depending on the type and volume of fluid, the mare is either recycled or a small volume of antibiotic-containing extender ($\leq$ 50 mL) is infused immediately prebreeding.

When organizing timing of breeding the problem mare, much effort is directed toward trying to breed only once, just before ovulation ($\leq$ 12 h). Induction of ovulation with human chorionic gonadotropin (hCG) is routine (Chapter 35), although difficulties are encountered with precise time of ovulation after the initial injection for the season. This is presumably mediated by antibody formation[35] and becomes important because many mares are bred on subsequent cycles. Mares are treated with hCG on days 2 and 3 of estrus when a follicle $\geq$ 30 and $\leq$ 40 mm is detected and when endometrial folds are prominent. Following this strict guideline for induction results in most of the mares ovulating between 36 and 48 h after treatment. In the near future, researchers expect that other drugs such as gonadotropin-releasing hormone (GnRH) analogues will be commercially available for routine induction of ovulation in cycling mares. Use of GnRH is expected to be associated with less immunogenicity because of its smaller molecular weight (Chapter 36), and could be used as a primary induction agent or between cycles when hCG was administered.

Mares are bred regardless of the number of preovulatory follicles and multiple ovulations are actively encouraged. Few effective, commercially available drugs are available to increase the number of ovulations per cycle. Follicle-stimulating hormone, although effective, is expensive for equine use, and crude pituitary extracts are not commercially available (Chapter 38). Recently, immunization against recombinant bovine inhibin α-subunit has been demonstrated effective in increasing ovulation rates in mares.[36] Conception rates are proportional to ovulation rates,[37] thus treatment by immunization against inhibin should improve pregnancy rates in normal and subfertile mares and in mares bred to subfertile stallions. With intensive reproductive management, multiple pregnancies when diagnosed early present little difficulty in reduction to a singleton.[38]

POSTBREEDING MANAGEMENT

The aim of therapies in the immediate period after breeding is to (1) reduce infection and inflammation to create a uterine environment capable of supporting pregnancy and (2) prevent further contamination.

Spermatozoa are safely in the oviduct within 4 h of breeding[39] and are protected from inflammatory products in the uterus and/or uterine treatments by the uterotubule junction. The embryo will not be released into the uterus until around 6 days after ovulation, however, because most intrauterine therapies have an attendant degree of inflammatory response; to allow time for foreign material to be expelled or absorbed, no treatments are administered from 4 days after ovulation. The cervix begins to exhibit increasing tone and improves as a barrier to infection within 2 days of ovulation, although it remains more relaxed when inflammation of the reproductive tract is present. In addition, the corpus luteum remains resistant to $PGF_2\alpha$ released from local inflammatory responses until at least day 5 after ovulation.

All mares are infused with 100 mL of plasma approximately 6 h after breeding. Plasma contains complement and is thought to increase the efficiency of the mare's cellular uterine defense mechanisms.[7] Broad-spectrum antibiotics may also be administered at that time (Chapter 43). Approximately 24 h after breeding, the uterine response to breeding and contamination is assessed by ultrasonography. If fluid is absent, then plasma and antibiotics (if indicated) are administered daily for an additional 2 days. If small amounts of fluid are detected, the same treatment is applied after first lavaging the uterus with buffered saline (pH $\sim$ 7.0). Saline is quite an irritant, especially with low pH.[40] Usually only 1 or 2 L are necessary to remove inflammatory products. When large amounts of fluid are detected, the fluid is recultured and removed by voluminous lavage until returning fluid is free from debris. Oxytocin is added (20 to 40 IU/L) to flushing solutions. Oxytocin increases myometrial contractions in estrogen-dominated reproductive tracts[41,42] and may aid in expulsion of material. Fluids warmed to above 40° C are *not* used at that time because the oviduct with gametes or early embryo is in close apposition to the uterus. Increased body temperature has been demonstrated to increase embryonic mortality.[43]

Final reproductive surgeries are completed on day 4 after ovulation (i.e., Caslick operation), and if further treatment is necessary, it is administered systemically. Some mares are maintained on systemic antibiotics and phenylbutazone until an early diagnosis of pregnancy is possible at day 11 to 13 after ovulation. Phenylbutazone (1 to 2 g daily) has been shown to prevent irritant $PGF_2\alpha$ release in mares subjected to uterine biopsy in diestrus.[44] Its use is discontinued if inflammatory uterine fluid is detected after day 7 or when a negative pregnancy diagnosis is confirmed (day 14). Because of potential toxicity of chronic phenylbutazone administration,[45] it is used sparingly and discontinued after a fetus is detected within a vesicle (day 20 to 22).

Mares that continue to produce large amounts of uterine fluid after ovulation, for multiple cycles, despite intensive management, are poor candidates for future reproductive performance. These mares often have mild acute and severe chronic endometritis with varying degrees of fibrosis. Although not commonly recommended, after discussion with the client, and with informed consent, irritant therapy may be used. Irritant therapy in the form of dilute disinfectants such as Lugol's iodine or chlorhexidine acetate have been advocated.[46] Some clinicians have used intrauterine infusion of kerosene as well. The response to irritant therapy is acute endometritis, which initiates stimulation of mechanical, cellular and humoral responses. However, extreme caution is advocated, because individual sensitivity sometimes results in irreversible degenerative changes with scarring and uterine adhesions.[47] A more logical approach is milder irritation with dilute povidone-iodine, hypertonic saline, or bacteria-free filtrates of streptococcal cultures.[48]

MANAGEMENT OF PREGNANCY AND PUERPERAL PERIOD

The incidence of early embryonic death and abortion is higher in mares that are difficult to get into foal. Pregnancy wastage is mediated by (1) luteolysis from $PGF_2\alpha$ release from an inflamed endometrium,[49] (2) absence of a pregnancy-specific factor secreted by a viable conceptus that functions to maintain ovarian steroid production,[50] and (3) failure of a damaged or compromised uterus to nourish or support fetal development adequately.[51,52] Genetic abnormalities would not appear to be a major factor contributing to equine early embryonic death after day 7.[53]

Despite the absence of any experimental evidence that a primary deficiency of progesterone production is a significant cause of equine pregnancy loss, many mares throughout the world are treated with natural progesterone or synthetic progestogens.[54] Much documented literature exists on doses needed to maintain pregnancy in mares ovariectomized between 20 and 80 days of pregnancy[55,56] Progesterone, which is the only maternal hormone needed to maintain early pregnancy[55,57] is primarily ovarian in origin until days 100 to 150. The placental unit begins to secrete progestins from around day 60; however, they are not capable of maintaining pregnancy in ovariectomized mares until after day 80.[57] Currently, when progestogen therapy is appropriate and, after initiation, when and how to withdraw it are difficult decisions. Exogenous progestogen therapy will maintain pregnancy when luteolysis is mediated by $PGF_2\alpha$ secretion from inadvertent iatrogenic administration,[58] administration of powerful endotoxins,[59] or failure of the conceptus to signal pregnancy associated with restriction of early conceptus mobility.[50] In these cases, supplemental therapy can be withdrawn after secondary corpora lutea formation or after the placenta is the primary source of progestins; however, therapy should begin before the expected decline in peripheral progesterone levels.

When problem mares are diagnosed pregnant at the GVEH, further therapy is determined by the amount of inflammation and infection at the time of breeding, presence or absence of uterine fluid at the initial pregnancy diagnosis, and previous history of early embryonic death or abortion. When uterine fluid is detected 1 or 2 days after ovulation, the incidence of early embryonic death (EED) is dramatically increased.[14] Similarly, luminal fluid with a positive early pregnancy diagnosis suggests a poor prognosis for embryonic survival.[14,15] These mares are treated with appropriately selected antibiotics and phenylbutazone for 5 to 7 days, then reevaluated. When pregnancy continues, antibiotics are administered for 5 consecutive days every month. As with many treatments for endometritis, no experimental data are available to document the efficacy of such treatments.

When a mare has a history of habitually aborting or experiencing EED, the decision of whether to supplement or not with progestins is largely at the discretion of the owners. Many owners, having invested so much time and money in getting the mare pregnant, will feel compelled to supplement, regardless of lack of documented efficacy and our discussions. In addition, most have friends that swear "that the only reason they ever saw a foal from their mare was . . . ."

Working with problem mares may be an enriching experience for the veterinarian. It certainly is an expensive experience for most clients. The lack of experimental evidence documenting efficacy of various intrauterine treatments is somewhat embarrassing and reflects the absence of an experimental model for susceptibility to infection. However, the pathophysiologic nature of various contributors to uterine defense in the mare appears to be gradually, albeit painfully, elucidated. The next decade holds exciting promise.

The preceding discussion represents *our views* only and, we hope, highlights areas where experimental evidence for treatments is sadly lacking.

REFERENCES

1. Hinrichs, K., Cummings, M.R., Sentich, P.L., and Kenney, R.M.: Bacteria recovered from the reproductive tracts of normal mares. Proc. Am. Assoc. Equine Pract., 11–16, 1989.
2. Asbury, A.C., Gorman, N.J., and Foster. G.W.: Uterine defense mechanisms in the mare: Serum opsonins affecting phagocytosis of Streptococcus zooepidemicus by equine neutrophils. Theriogenology, *27:*375–385, 1984.
3. Evans, M.J., et al.: Clearance of bacteria and nonantigenic markers following intrauterine inoculation into maiden mares: Effect of steroid hormone environment. Theriogenology, *26:*37–50, 1986.
4. Hughes, J.P., and Loy, R.G.: Investigations on the effect of intrauterine inoculations of Streptococcus zooepidemicus in the mare. Proc. Am. Assoc. Equine Pract., 289–292, 1969.
5. Oguri, N., and Tsutsumi, Y.: Nonsurgical recovery of equine eggs, and an attempt at nonsurgical egg transfer in horses. J. Reprod. Fertil., *31:*187–195, 1972.
6. Evans, M.J., Hamer, J.M., Grason, L.M., and Irvine, C.H.G.: Factors affecting uterine clearance of inoculated materials in mares. J. Reprod. Fertil. Suppl., *35:*327–334, 1987.
7. Asbury, A.C.: Uterine defense mechanisms in the mare: The use of intrauterine plasma in the management of endometritis. Theriogenology, *21:*387–393, 1984.
8. Lui, I.K.M., et al.: Comparison of peripheral blood and uterine-derived polymorphonuclear leukocytes from mares resistant and susceptible to chronic metritis: Chemotactic and cell elastimetry analysis. Am. J. Vet. Res. *46:*917–920, 1985.
9. Asbury, A.C., Halliwell, R.E.W., Foster, G.W., and Longino, S.J.: Immunoglobulins in uterine secretions of mares with differing resistance to endometritis. Theriogenology, *14:*299–304, 1980.
10. Watson, E.D., Stokes, C.R., and Bourne, F.J.: Uterine cellular and humoral defense mechanisms in mares susceptible and resistant to persistent endometritis. Immunol. Immunopathol., *16:*107–121, 1987.
11. Widders, P.R., Stokes, V.R., David, J.S.E., and Bourne, F.J.: Quantitation of the immunoglobulins in reproduc-

tive tract secretions of the mare. Res. Vet. Sci., *37:*324–330, 1984.

12. Liu, I.K.M., Cheung, A.T.W., Walsh, E.M., and Ayin, S.: The functional competence of uterine-derived polymorphonuclear neutrophils (PMN) from mares resistant and susceptible to chronic uterine infection: A sequential migration analysis. Biol. Reprod., *35:*1168–1176, 1986.

13. Troedsson, M.H.T., and Lui, I.K.M.: Uterine clearance of non-antigenic markers (^{51}Cr) in response to a bacterial challenge in mares potentially susceptible and resistant to chronic uterine infections. J. Reprod. Fertil. Suppl., *44:* 283–288, 1991.

14. McKinnon, A.O., et al.: Diagnostic ultrasonography of uterine pathology in the mare. Proc. Am. Assoc. Equine Pract., 605–622, 1987.

15. Adams, G.P., Kastelic, J.P., Bergfelt, D.R., and Ginther, O.J.: Effect of uterine inflammation and ultrasonically-detected uterine pathology on fertility in the mare. J. Reprod. Fertil. Suppl., *35:*445–454, 1987.

16. Blanchard, T.L., Garcia, M.C., Kintner, L.D., and Kenney, R.M.: Investigation of the representativeness of a single endometrial sample and the use of trichrome staining to aid in the detection of endometrial fibrosis in the mare. Theriogenology, *28:*445–450, 1987.

17. Dybdal, N.O., et al.: Investigation of the reliability of a single endometrial biopsy sample, with a note on the relation between uterine cysts on biopsy grade. J. Reprod. Fertil. Suppl., 44, 697, 1991.

18. Kenney, R.M.: Clinical aspects of endometrial biopsy in fertility evaluation of the mare. Proc. Am. Assoc. Equine Pract., 105–122, 1977.

19. Shideler, R.K., et al.: Endometrial biopsy in the mare. Proc. Am. Assoc. Equine Pract., 97–104, 1977.

20. Trotter, G.W., and McKinnon, A.O.: Surgery for abnormal vulvar and perineal conformation in the mare. Vet. Clin. North Am., *4:*389–405, 1988.

21. Brown, M.P.: Colahan, P.T., and Hawkins, D.L.: Urethral extension for treatment of urine pooling in mares. J. Am. Vet. Med. Assoc., *173:*1005–1007, 1978.

22. Monin, T.: Vaginoplasty: A surgical treatment for urine pooling in the mare. Proc. Am. Assoc. Equine Pract., 99–102, 1972.

23. McKinnon, A.O., and Belden, J.O.: A urethral extension technique to correct urine pooling (vesicovaginal reflux) in mares. J. Am. Vet. Med. Assoc., *192:*647–650, 1988.

24. Washburn, S.M., Klesivs, P.H., Ganjam, V.K., and Brown, B.G.: Effect of estrogen and progesterone on the phagocytic response of ovariectomized mares infected in utero with beta-hemolytic streptococci. Am. J. Vet. Res., *43:*1367–1370, 1982.

25. Asbury, A.C., and Hansen, P.J.: Effects of susceptibility of mares to endometritis and stage of cycle on phagocytic activity of uterine derived neutrophils. J. Reprod. Fertil. Suppl., *35:*311–316, 1987.

26. Nishikawa, Y.: Studies on Reproduction in Horses. Tokyo, Japan Racing Association, 1959.

27. Squires, E.L., et al.: Effect of uterine fluid and volume of extender on fertility. Proc. Am. Assoc. Equine Pract., 25–30, 1989.

28. Kenney, R.M., Bergman, R.V., Cooper, W.L., and Morse, G.W.: Minimal contamination techniques for breeding mares: Technique and preliminary findings. Proc. Am. Assoc. Equine Pract., 327–336, 1975.

29. Squires, E.L., et al.: Use of antibiotics in stallion semen for the control of Klebsiella pneumoniae and Pseudomonas aeruginosa. J. Equine Vet. Sci., *1:*43–48, 1981.

30. Pickett, B.W., Squires, E.L., and McKinnon, A.O.: Procedures for collection, evaluation and utilization of stallion semen for artificial insemination. Animal Reproduction Laboratory Bulletin No. 0-03, Fort Collins, Colorado State University, 1987.

31. Francel, A.T., Amann, E.L., Squires, E.L., and Pickett, B.W.: Motility and fertility of equine spermatozoa in a milk extender after 12 or 24 hours at 20° C. Theriogenology, *27:*517–525, 1987.

32. Douglas-Hamilton, D.H., et al.: A field study of the fertility of transported equine semen. Theriogenology, *22:* 291–304, 1984.

33. Pickett, B.W., et al.: Effect of centrifugation and seminal plasma on motility and fertility of stallion and bull spermatozoa. Fertil. Steril., *26:*167, 1975.

34. Pickett, G.W., Back, D.G., Burwash, L.D., and Voss, J.L.: The effect of extenders, spermatozoal numbers and rectal palpation on equine fertility. National Association of Animal Breeders Technical Conference on Artificial Insemination and Reproduction. 1974, pp. 47–58.

35. Roser, J.F., et al.: The development of antibodies to human chorionic gonadotropin following its repeated injection in the cyclic mare. J. Reprod. Fertil. Suppl., *27:*173–179, 1979.

36. McKinnon, A.O., et al.: Increased ovulation rates in mares after immunization against recombinant bovine inhibin alpha subunit. Equine Vet. J., *24:*144–146, 1992.

37. Squires, E.L., et al.: Reproductive characteristics of spontaneous single and double ovulating mares and superovulated mares. J. Reprod. Fertil. Suppl., *35:*399–403, 1987.

38. Pascoe, D.R., et al.: Comparison of two techniques and three hormonal therapies for management of twin conceptuses by manual embryonic reduction. J. Reprod. Fertil. Suppl., *35:*701–702, 1987.

39. Bader, H.: An investigation of sperm migration into the oviducts of the mare. J. Reprod. Fertil. Suppl., *32:*59–64, 1982.

40. Pascoe, D.R.: Single embryonic reduction in the mare with twin conceptuses: Studies of hormonal profiles and drug therapies using a physiological model and manual and surgical reduction technique in vivo. Ph.D. thesis. University of California, 1986.

41. Jones, D.M., Fielden, E.D., and Carr, D.H.: Some physiological and pharmacological factors affecting uterine motility as measured by electromyography in the mare. J. Reprod. Fertil. Suppl., *44:*357–368, 1991.

42. Lui, I.K.M., Troedsson, M.H.T., Williams, D.C., and Pascoe, J.R.: Electromyography of uterine activity in the mare: Comparison of single versus multiple recording sites. Proceedings of the Fifth International Symposium on Equine Reproduction, Deauville, July 1–7, 1990, pp. 120–121.

43. Thatcher, W.W., and Collier, R.J.: Effects of climate on bovine reproduction. *In* Current Therapy in Theriogenology. Edited by D.A. Morrow. Philadelphia, W.B. Saunders, 1986, pp. 301–309.

44. Ellsworth-Swihart, M., Archibald, L.F., Ingram, R.H., and Godke, R.A.: Effect of phenylbutazone on luteolysis in the mare induced by uterine biopsy. Theriogenology, *23:*381–387, 1985.

45. Snow, D.H., et al.: Phenylbutazone toxicoses in equidae: A biochemical and pathophysiologic study. Am. J. Vet. Res., *42:*1754–1759, 1981.

46. Threlfall, W.R.: Broodmare uterine therapy. Compend. Contin. Educ. Practicing Vet., *11:*246–254, 1980.

47. Mather, E.C., et al.: The use of fibre-optic techniques in clinical diagnosis and visual assessment of experimental intrauterine therapy in mares. J. Reprod. Fertil. Suppl., *27:*293–297, 1979.

48. Couto, M.A., and Hughes, J.P.: Intrauterine inoculation of a bacteria-free filtrate of Streptococcus zooepidemicus in clinically normal and infected mares. J. Equine Vet. Sci., *7:*265–273, 1985.

49. Neely, D.P., et al.: Prostaglandin release patterns in the mare: Physiological, pathophysiological, and therapeutic responses. J. Reprod. Fertil. Suppl., *27:*181–189, 1979.

50. McDowell, K.J., et al.: Restricted conceptus mobility results in failure of maternal recognition of pregnancy in mares. Biol. Reprod., *39:*340–349, 1988.

51. Kenney, R.M.: Clinical aspects of endometrial biopsy in fertility evaluation of the mare. Proc. Am. Assoc. Equine Pract., 105–122, 1977.

52. Kenney, R.M.: Cyclic and pathological changes of the mare endometrium as detected by biopsy, with a note on early embryonic death. J. Am. Vet. Med. Assoc., *172:*241–262, 1978.

53. Romagnono, A., Ricker, C.L., King, W.A., and Betteridge, K.: Analysis of X-chromosome inactivation in horse embryos. J. Reprod. Fertil. Suppl., *35:*353–361, 1987.

54. Allen, W.R.: Is your progesterone therapy really necessary? Equine Vet. J. *16:*496–498, 1984.

55. Shideler, R.K., Squires, E.L., Voss, J.L., and Eikenberry, D.J.: Exogenous progestin therapy for maintenance of pregnancy in ovariectomized mares. Proc. Am. Assoc. Equine Pract., 211–219, 1981.

56. Hinrichs, K., Sertich, P.L., Cummins, M.R., and Kenney, R.M.: Pregnancy in ovariectomized mares achieved by embryo transfer. Equine Vet. J. Suppl., *3:*74–75, 1985.

57. Holtan, D.W., Squires, E.L., Lapin, B.R., and Ginther, O.J.: Effect of ovariectomy on pregnancy in mares. J. Reprod. Fertil. Suppl., *27:*457–463, 1979.

58. Kastelic, J.P., Adams, G.P., and Ginther, O.J.: Role of progesterone in mobility, fixation, orientation and survival of 16 equine embryonic vesicles. Theriogenology, *27:*655–663, 1987.

59. Daels, P., et al: Effect of Salmonella typhimurium endotoxin on PGF-2 alpha release and fetal death in the mare. J. Reprod. Fertil. Suppl., *35:*485–492, 1987.

SECTION D

DISEASES OF THE MARE'S REPRODUCTIVE TRACT

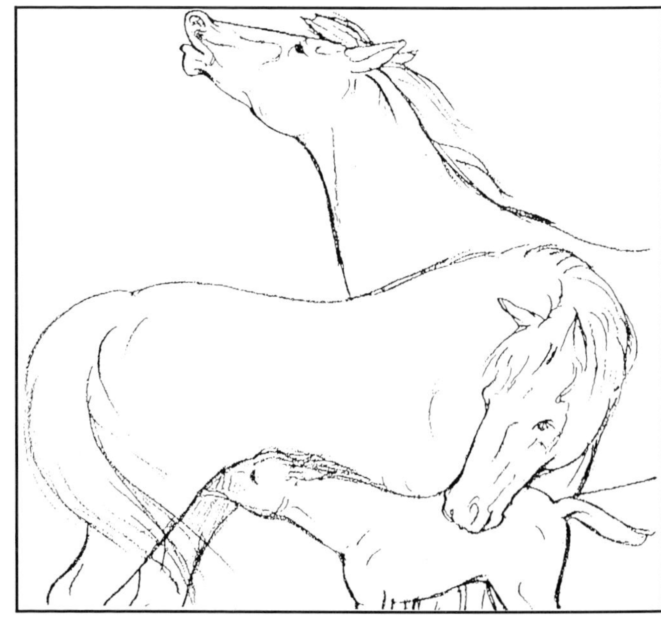

CHAPTER 43

INFECTIOUS CAUSES OF INFERTILITY

A.C. Asbury
S.K. Lyle

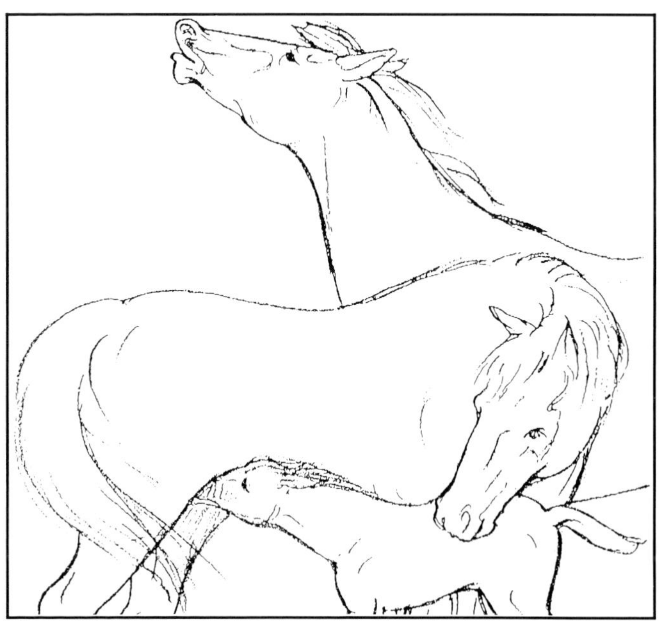

A major factor governing reproductive efficiency in mares is the ability to maintain an environment in the uterine lumen that is compatible with embryonic and fetal life. That environment is most easily disturbed by inflammatory processes that follow contamination of the uterus with micro-organisms introduced during ordinary reproductive events, such as breeding and parturition. Reproductive examinations and poor perineal conformation also contribute to contamination of the tract. The fertile mare copes with contamination by mounting an efficient defense, which quickly returns uterine environment to normal. Such mares are referred to as resistant to infection.

The susceptible mare, on the other hand, cannot respond as effectively and fails to clear inflammation from the lumen in time to provide an environment suitable for the descending embryo. When bred, the susceptible mare either fails to establish pregnancy or, in marginal cases, loses pregnancy because of low-grade endometrial inflammation. In general, loss of resistance to infection is associated with advancing age and multiparity, factors which are frequently associated with increasing value of mares.

Each missed opportunity for conception and each pregnancy loss becomes a major economic setback for the breeder, who is battling the season, life expectancy of the mare, stallion availability, rising costs of management, and interest on investment. Thus infectious infertility presents an enormous challenge to the economic stability of any breeding operation. Management to reduce the impact of uterine infections—either endometritis, acute metritis, or pyometra—on fertility is a clear goal of both breeders and veterinarians.

PATHOGENESIS OF ENDOMETRITIS

The pathogenesis of uterine infection is complex and poorly understood. Immunologic and physical factors must be considered important in uterine defense. Etiologic agents are those opportunists that survive as the defenses fail. This portion of the discussion is limited to endometritis; acute metritis and pyometra will be considered later in this chapter.

UTERINE DEFENSE MECHANISMS

The known major elements of uterine defense against contaminating microorganisms are neutrophil phagocytosis[1] and mechanical evacuation of the lumen.[2] The combination of rapid and efficient ingestion of bacteria and prompt expulsion of all cellular material and other inflammatory by-products through the cervix results in a return to a normal uterine environment in a matter of hours in normal mares.[1] The critical factor in the defense is time. Because the equine embryo descends from the isolated environment of the oviduct into the uterine lumen between 5 and 6 days after ovulation,[3] the uterus must be cleared of all embryo-toxic materials by that time if pregnancy is to be established. Active endometritis clearly is incompatible with embryonic health. In addition, an inflammatory process in the endometrium at 5 days postovulation, may disrupt the new corpus luteum through prostaglandin release.[1]

Susceptibility to uterine infection is, therefore, not an absolute state. Failure of the defense mechanisms only needs to be of the degree necessary to slow the process of clearance past a critical point. All mares experience endometritis following uterine contamination, but those that are resistant cope with the inflammation in a highly efficient manner.

During the past decade, considerable effort has been directed at definition of the process by which the mare's uterine defenses lose their efficiency. Studies have centered on the various components of the complex of phagocytosis and, more recently, on the mechanical aspects of uterine clearance. The results of these investigations have been reviewed by Watson.[4] Considerable difference of opinion is evident when these studies are compared, possibly caused by a wide variety in methods used.

Immediately following introduction of bacteria or other antigenic material into the mare's uterus, neutrophils and serum proteins begin a rapid migration toward the lumen.[5,6] At the same time, the uterus is stimulated to evacuate its contents out through the open cervix.[1,2] Myometrial contraction is more productive in the estrogen-dominated uterus.[2]

Chemotactic substances associated with bacteria[7] or uterine secretions[8] are important in recruiting neutrophils to the lumen. Migratory ability of neutrophils in mares with degenerative endometrial changes may be compromised.[9] Once in the lumen of susceptible mares, neutrophils either lose[10] or maintain[11] their ability to phagocytose bacteria.

Opsonins, specifically immunoglobulins and complement, are important in the phagocytic process, because they enhance adherence of organisms to the cell membrane of the phagocyte. A variety of studies on immunoglobulins (Ig) in uterine secretions of resistant and susceptible mares have been reported.[12–14] Concentrations of IgG, IgG(T), IgA, and IgM are described, with higher values consistently observed in the uterine flushings of susceptible mares. The principal immunoglobulin, IgG, involved in opsonization was predominant among the immunoglobulins. Uterine secretions from mares susceptible to endometritis were less effective in opsonizing bacteria than were those from resistant mares.[15,16]

Complement, an important nonspecific opsonin, was found in the inactive state in uterine secretions[15] and hemolytic complement was shown to be elevated in the secretions of mares with active endometritis.[16] The concept that complement depletion might explain reduced opsonization is the basis for treatment of susceptible mares with uterine infusions of plasma, an obvious source of all opsonins.[17]

Attempts to suggest a single or even multiple defect in the immunologic aspect of uterine defense that would explain reduction of resistance are not conclusive at this time. It is entirely possible that no such explanation is forthcoming and that another factor, not immunologically oriented, is the controlling variable. If that were the case, the evidence would support the mechanical evacuation of the uterus as the best candidate for that factor. A recent report indicates a significant delay in physical clearance of nonantigenic markers from the uterus of susceptible mares when compared with resistant mares.[18] In that study, the resistant mares cleared the markers in 24 h or less, while susceptible mares took more than 96 h. These data suggest that this ability may be a critical factor in the first line of defense against uterine infection. That same sentiment has been expressed by a noted investigator in the area.[19]

Reduction in ability to evacuate uterine contents mechanically fits the clinical picture of mares that lose their resistance to infection. The process tends to be a gradual one, increasing in severity after multiple foaling or after repeated insults to the uterus. An aged mare with a thickened and edematous uterus, with the degenerative changes of periglandular fibrosis and lymphatic stasis,[20] is the most likely candidate for reduced physical clearance and for susceptibility to endometritis.

ETIOLOGIC AGENTS

The causal organisms of endometritis are common surface soil, fecal bacteria, and yeasts. Streptococcus zooepidemicus is the agent most frequently isolated, particularly in the initial stages of uterine defense failure. The gram-negative bacteria Escherichia coli, Pseudomonas aeruginosa, and Klebsiella pneumoniae are the next most frequent recoveries. A 1928 survey of bacteria associated with uterine inflammation named the same four organisms, in order, as most important.[21] Because these organisms are readily available opportunists that are introduced to the uterus as contaminants, it follows that any bacterial, yeast, or fungal agent has the same potential. A study examining more than 1500 mares in a 4-yr period reported 19 different aerobic bacteria recovered from uterine swabs of 498 of those mares.[22] Most of the mares with positive cultures also exhibited signs of inflammation, indicating that endometritis was present.

Yeasts, especially Candida sp., and rarely fungi may become established in the mare uterus by virtue of reduced resistance and often as a result of antibiotic therapy.[23] Once well established in the endometrium, these organisms may be extremely difficult to treat and often produce significant damage to the endometrium and other parts of the tract.

Anaerobic bacteria have been recorded as isolates from the mare's uterus; Bacteroides fragilis is the most frequent organism recovered.[24] The importance of anaerobes in the disease process needs to be documented further.

Because all the foregoing organisms are potential pathogens that gain access to the tract by contamination, great care must be taken to evaluate their true role in the pathogenesis of endometritis. Culture techniques, to be most effective, should provide a guard to the swabs introduced through the vestibule, vagina, and cervix, so as to eliminate residents of the external portions of the tract. The diagnostic dilemma is further reviewed in the following section.

DIAGNOSIS

Because, by definition, endometritis is an inflammatory process, the diagnosis must be based on the presence of inflammation. This decision is often clouded by a history of infertility coupled with a positive uterine culture. The pitfall here is that the culture result, without evidence of inflammation, is likely the result of contamination in the culturing process. If treatment is instituted based on this incorrect diagnosis, there is a risk of compromising the fertility potential of the mare. An example would be the misinterpretation of a positive uterine culture of pseudomonas in a normal mare. Treatment with intrauterine aminoglycosides could result in chemical endometrial irritation, which could force a delay in breeding the mare or, worse, provide an opportunity for a real infectious agent to become established.

The key to the diagnosis, then, is to confirm or deny the presence of uterine inflammation. This process may be simple in cases where an obvious purulent exudate is present or may take all of the diagnostic skill and experience of the examiner, when the evidence is marginal. The most helpful aids in the diagnosis are physical examination of the external and internal aspects of the reproductive system, endometrial cytologic evaluation, demonstration of uterine fluid by ultrasonography, and inspection of recovered uterine flushes. Endometrial biopsy may be of use in difficult cases. These procedures have been described elsewhere in this volume. Only the interpretation will be reviewed here.

Any antigenic substance in the uterine lumen of the mare evokes a neutrophil response. These cells migrate from the superficial blood vessels, through the endometrial tissue, and into the lumen.[20] Continuing stimulus evokes continuing response until the source of the inflammation is removed and the process resolved. The presence of neutrophils in the lumen is, therefore, an absolute indicator of inflammation.[25] When the process is severe, the degree of cellularity is grossly visible as pus and when the process is subtle, the only evidence may be an increased number of cells seen on cytologic preparations of uterine secretions. Negative cytologic preparations, properly obtained from the uterus, are reliable indicators of endometrial health.

Positive signs of inflammation discovered on physical examination include the following:

Inspection	Exudate evident on external genitalia.
	Exudate evident in vagina per vaginoscopy.
	Hyperemia of cervix or vagina per vaginoscopy.
Palpation	Uterine fluid per rectal palpation.
	Cervical roughening per direct palpation.
Cytology	More than 1 neutrophil per 10 endometrial epithelial cells.
Uterine Flush	Any degree of cloudiness per visual inspection.
	Neutrophils in centrifuged sample.
Ultrasonography	Fluid layer in uterine lumen.
Endometrial Biopsy	Neutrophils migrating through tissue.

Evidence of inflammation in the reproductive tract must be correlated with cultural findings to complete the diagnostic process.[26] A suggested correlation of diagnostic criteria is presented in Table 43–1.

TREATMENT METHODS

Principal treatment for infertility of infectious causes can be directed at reducing the number of offending organisms by exposing them to chemotherapeutic agents by either local or systemic routes. Therapy may also involve methods that enhance natural defense mechanisms, as in uterine lavage to assist in the process of physical clearance of uterine contents. Active endometritis usually warrants therapy before breeding the mare, whereas more chronic, low-grade inflammations may best be managed by breeding and concentrating treatment after the mare is bred. In all cases, mares with documented susceptibility to infection must be managed differently from those that are resistant.

TABLE 43–1. DIAGNOSTIC CRITERIA FOR ENDOMETRITIS

PHYSICAL EXAM	CYTOLOGY	UTERINE FLUSH	ULTRASONOGRAPHY	CULTURE	DIAGNOSIS, COMMENTS
Discharge	Positive	Cloudy	Positive or negative	Organism repeatedly isolated	Acute endometritis
Normal or slightly positive	Positive	Cloudy or hazy	Positive or negative	Organism repeatedly isolated	Chronic (low-grade) endometritis
Inconclusive	Positive	Cloudy or hazy	Positive or negative	No growth	Endometritis; failed to isolate causal organism
Inconclusive	Negative	Clear	Negative	Organism isolated	Normal endometrium culture contaminated
Negative	Negative	Clear	Negative	No growth	Normal endometrium

(From Asbury, A.C.: The reproductive system. In Equine Medicine and Surgery. 3rd ed. Edited by R.A. Mansmann and E.S. McAllister. Santa Barbara, American Veterinary Publications, pp.1305–1402.).

LOCAL ANTIBIOTIC THERAPY

The infusion of various antibiotics, dissolved or suspended in water or saline, into the uterine lumen during estrus has been a traditional approach to treating endometritis. The objective of this therapy is to achieve high levels of drug at the site of inflammation, the surface, and the superficial aspects of the endometrium. Some data from pharmacokinetic studies and endometrial levels of antibiotics following both intrauterine and systemic administration have been published.[27–30] However, the basis for antibiotic therapy in management of uterine infections is largely empiric. Virtually all available antimicrobials have been evaluated by practitioners with purely clinical observation. Table 43–2 presents some drugs and doses that have been used with success for intrauterine infusion for bacterial endometritis.[31]

The efficacy of intrauterine antibiotics appears greater when specific bacteria, sensitive to the antibiotic used, are implicated as the cause of the inflammation. Strict adherence to aseptic techniques during infusion is important in excluding contaminants that may be resistant to the drugs in use. It is most logical to treat mares during estrus, when the cervix is relaxed and when natural defenses are more effective.[32,33] Daily infusion is the preferred schedule, ending when ovulation is detected or at the end of behavioral estrus.

Problems associated with local antibiotic therapy in mares include irritation by the drug itself, development of resistance in the causal organism, and promotion of superinfection by other organisms.

Irritation may be evident following use of the aminoglycosides without adequate dilution or buffering. Both gentamicin and amikacin are acidic and, if used full-strength, should be neutralized with an equal volume of 7.5% sodium bicarbonate. Anecdotal reports suggest that serious irritation to the reproductive tract may occur following the intrauterine use of various formulations of the tetracycline drugs.

Drug resistance may follow inadequate doses or insufficient repetition of treatments. Followup cultures during subsequent estrous periods yield the same causal agent with a change in antibiotic sensitivity. The possibility of repeated contamination from outside sources should be considered as well as changes in sensitivity in these instances. Repeated recovery of enteric organisms should prompt careful re-evaluation of perineal integrity and searches for fecal sources of the organisms.

In the so-called superinfection, treatment for one organism results in replacement of that bacteria with another, usually more stubborn to treat. A typical example is the mare with a positive Streptococcus zooepidemicus culture, treated with penicillin, that subsequently presents as a Pseudomonas aeruginosa problem. A possible source of this problem is contamination of the uterus by pseudomonas while treating the streptococci. A role for streptococci in promoting proliferation of other bacteria in the mare's uterus has been suggested.[34] Receptors for the bioactive sites of IgG are known to cause binding of complexes of the immunoglobulin to the cell wall of streptococci, resulting in complement depletion and compromised phagocytosis.

The ultimate superinfection problem is yeast or fungal overgrowth, which often follows protracted antibiotic therapy. These infections are difficult to treat, and may produce significant damage to the reproductive tract. Various antiseptic solutions, such as dilute povidone-iodine lavages, and specific antifungal compounds have been used with limited success. Treatment of yeast endometritis with vinegar or dilute acetic acid is favored by some clinicians.

We have found amphotericin B for injection useful, 50- to 100-mg doses infused daily, in a few cases. Other

TABLE 43–2. ANTIBIOTICS SUITABLE FOR INTRAUTERINE INFUSION IN MARES

DRUG	DOSE PER INFUSION	COMMENTS
Amikacin†	2 g	Excellent gram-negative spectrum
Ampicillin	3 g	Use only the soluble product
Carbenicillin	6 g	Broad spectrum, including active against some Pseudomonas
Gentamicin†	2 g	Excellent gram-negative spectrum plus some streptococci
Kanamycin	1–2 g	Most Escherichia coli are sensitive
Neomycin	4 g	Escherichia coli and some Klebsiella are sensitive
Penicillin	5 million units	Potassium penicillin G. primarily active against streptococci
Ticarcillin	6 g	Broad spectrum
Ticarcillin/clavulanic acid	6 g/200 mg	Broad spectrum

*Dissolve all drugs in 100 to 200 mL saline.
†Helpful to buffer with bicarbonate.
(From Asbury, A.C.: Infectious and immunologic considerations in mare infertility. Compend. Contin. Educ. Practicing Vet., 9:585–592, 1987.)

antiyeast or antifungal drugs used in human medicine have been tried in mares; clotrimazole currently shows some promise (J.P. Hurtgen, personal communication). Daily dosage with 500 mg of the drug, either in suspension or in the cream formulation, has been suggested.

SYSTEMIC ANTIBIOTIC THERAPY

Systemically administered antibiotics will produce tissue levels in the endometrium.[28–30] The clinical response to systemic treatment for endometritis has not been critically evaluated, and the basis for such an approach is again empiric. Until such time as a predictable, repeatable model of endometritis in cycling mares is developed, no controlled studies of any form of therapy for uterine infections will be conducted. Nonetheless, some practitioners have recorded impressive results using antibiotics systemically, alone, or in conjunction with local methods.

The antibiotics frequently used by systemic routes are penicillin G procaine, gentamicin sulfate, amikacin sulfate, ampicillin trihydrate, and trimethoprim and sulfamethoxazole combination. The dosages that have been used are those that would be indicated for any systemic infection.

The chief advantage of systemic antibiotics in these cases is the avoidance of reproductive tract contamination. When uterine defenses are seriously compromised, any iatrogenic source of pathogenic organisms is potentially damaging. Therapy during diestrus can be executed with little risk. Steady tissue levels achieved with systemic drugs may be more effective than intermittent high levels resulting from infusion. The chief disadvantage of such treatment schemes is cost.

UTERINE LAVAGE

Large-volume uterine lavage has become a popular treatment method for inflammatory disease of the mare's uterus over the past decade.[35] The original rationale for repeatedly irrigating the uterus was obviously to aid in the mechanical evacuation of uterine contents. Better understanding of the mechanisms of uterine defense leads to the suggestion of an additional benefit: the stimulation of the endometrium to recruit new neutrophils and serum proteins to the site of phagocytic activity.[31]

In addition to the enhancement of uterine defenses, lavage affords diagnostic advantages in the management of both endometritis and acute metritis. Inspection of the recovered fluids provides immediate information on the condition of the uterine lumen. The degree of cellularity and amount of other inflammatory components correlates well with the appearance of recovered fluid. This information provides both diagnostic and prognostic opportunity.[36]

The ideal technique for large-volume lavage in cycling mares involves a catheter that can be retained in the cervix by a cuff. An example is a large-bore (30 French), long (80-cm) catheter designed for equine embryo flushing (EUF-80, Bivona, Gary, IN). It is equipped with a 100-mL inflatable cuff and can be autoclaved.

The catheter should be introduced manually, passing the deflated cuff through the cervix with as little manipulation as possible. In estrous mares, excessive manipulation of the cervix results in rapid dilation, making retention of the catheter difficult. The cuff is then inflated and gentle back pressure is applied to the catheter to seat the cuff against the cervical os. During insertion, the outside end of the catheter should be clamped to prevent the aspiration of air into the uterus (Fig. 43–1). A closed system for administration of fluid is also necessary for the exclusion of air (Fig. 43–2). If air is allowed to enter the uterine lumen, recovery of fluid is more difficult.

Normal saline is the preferred fluid for lavage, because it is mildly irritating to the endometrium and clear, allowing easy inspection of the recovered material. Hypertonic saline may have an advantage of greater stimulation and resulting increases in cellular response. The fluid can be infused at room temperature or heated to 45 to 50° C. Warm fluid appears to enhance uterine contraction and may be an advantage in a mare with uterine edema or lymphatic stasis.[31]

A total of 1 to 2 L of fluid may be infused into the uterus of most multiparous mares without producing discomfort. A common approach to the technique of lavage is to infuse and then recover sequential liters of fluid as is indicated by the appearance of the recovered flush. In most cases fluid can be recovered by gravity, using the catheter to achieve a siphon effect. If air has been allowed to enter the uterus, gravity flow may not be possible, and manipulation of the uterus per rectum may be needed to achieve emptying. Fluid should be recovered in a clear container to aid in inspection. Graduations on the container are helpful to monitor the complete recovery of fluid.

In postpartum mares, uterine capacity and cervical

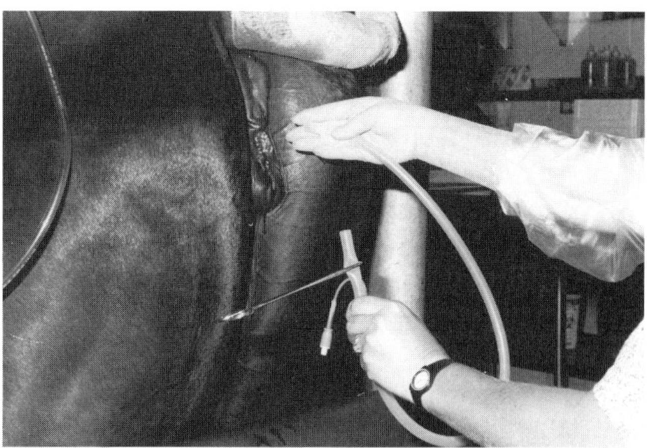

FIG. 43–1. Aseptic introduction of catheter with deflated cuff. Note clamp on outside end of catheter, preventing air aspiration.

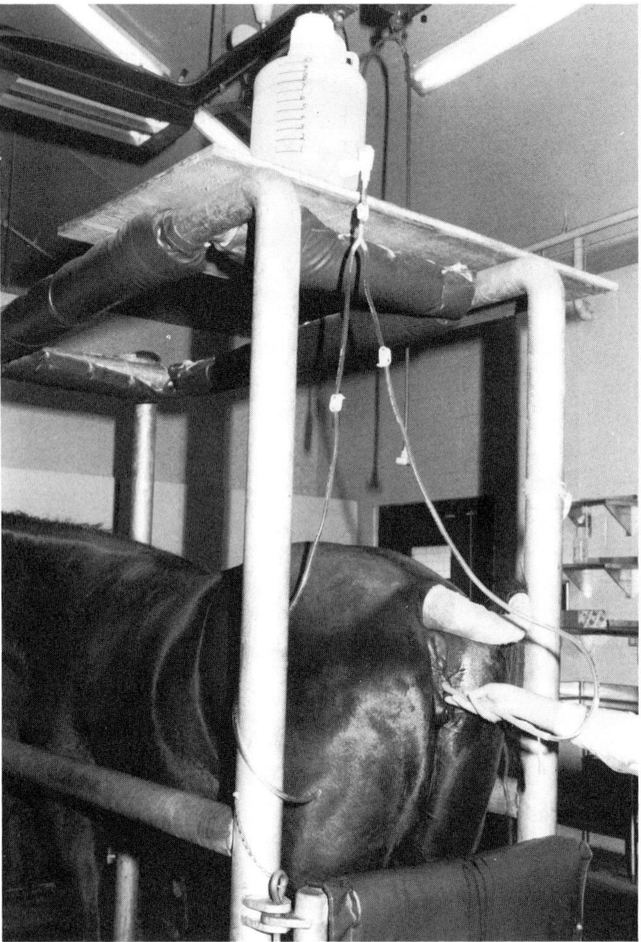

FIG. 43–2. Closed system of fluid infusion excludes air from uterine lumen.

size are much greater than in cycling mares, dictating a variation in approach. The principal indication for lavage in postpartum mares is acute metritis, which is characterized by large accumulations of fluid in the lumen. The objectives of lavage in these mares are rapid evacuation of the uterine contents and stimulation of uterine contraction.

An appropriate catheter for these cases is a neoprene or other plastic stomach tube with a lumen at least 15 to 20 mm in diameter. The tube is grasped near the end by a gloved hand, which is introduced into the mare's cervix. The hand is positioned in the cervical canal to occlude the lumen as much as possible, with the tip of the tube extending into the uterus no more than 4 or 5 cm.

Lavage is accomplished by rapidly filling the uterus to capacity (usually 10 to 15 L) with water or salt water at 45° C, and then siphoning the water back into another container. This is easily accomplished using a large funnel, pouring the water from a clean bucket (Fig. 43–3), elevating the funnel to fill the uterus (Fig. 43–4), and evacuating the fluid by a siphon effect created by lowering the funnel (Fig. 43–5). Repeated filling and emptying of the uterus may be indicated. Significant uterine contraction is usually evident following this technique.

OTHER TREATMENT METHODS

A list of treatments that have been used for infectious infertility would be exhaustive and indicative of the ingenuity of the veterinary profession. A wide variety of chemicals, both disinfectant and irritant, have been tried as well as natural substances such as plasma, colostrum, acidophilus cultures, buttermilk, and the like. A few of these approaches have merit in certain circumstances and deserve mention as possible adjuncts to treatment protocols or as primary treatment methods.

Because the mare's reproductive tract, including the uterus, cervix, and vagina, is highly sensitive to certain chemical irritants, great caution should be applied to any local treatment. Necrosis of tissue with subsequent adhesions are the consequences of inappropriate therapy. Chlorhexidine diacetate, an excellent disinfectant, has been known to destroy the reproductive tract of mares when applied in dilute solutions.[37]

One approach to intrauterine disinfectant therapy that has survived is infusion or lavage with dilute povidone iodine solutions. Stock solutions of the chemical should be diluted at least tenfold in water or saline before administration. Some mares appear to be highly sensitive to even dilute solutions. Any discomfort or physical signs of irritation after administration is an indication to discontinue treatment. An appropriate system for monitoring this reaction is the daily inspection of cervix and vagina through a vaginal speculum. Cervical edema or hyperemia is a sign of hypersensitivity.

Intrauterine plasma therapy, although controversial, has found acceptance by some practitioners since first reported.[17] Clinical indications are those cases for which no specific bacterial cause of the endometritis can be identified and in the prevention of recurrence of infection in highly susceptible mares. Success has been reported using both the mare's own plasma and that from heterologous sources.

Plasma for intrauterine use should be prepared in an aseptic manner, using either heparin or citrate solutions as anticoagulants. Because heat-sensitive complement may be an important factor in the function of intrauter-

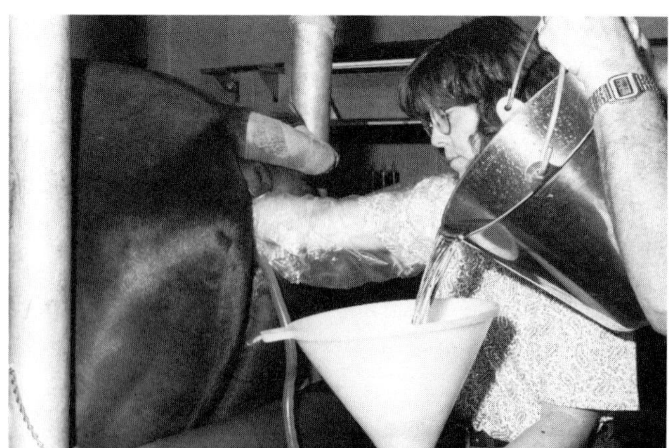

FIG. 43–3. Warm salt water is poured into clean funnel.

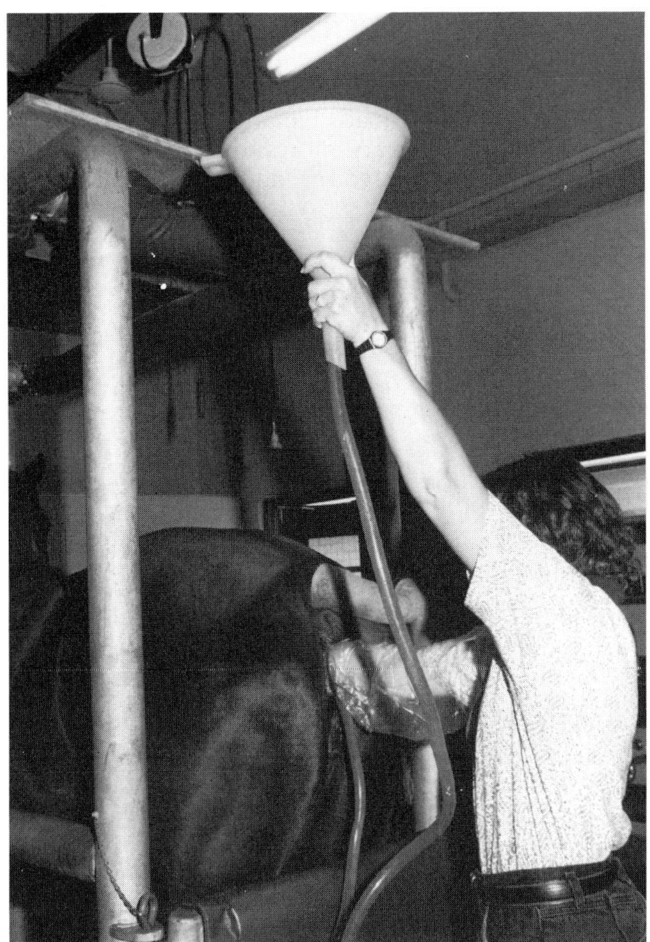

FIG. 43–4. Funnel is elevated to fill uterus.

ine plasma, it should be prepared without prolonged exposure to heat. Once prepared, it should be either infused within a few hours or frozen for subsequent use. The infusion dose recommended is 100 mL. Equine plasma retains its ability to opsonize bacteria for at least 100 days at household freezer temperatures.

An adjunct to other treatment systems for endometritis is management of the estrous cycle. Natural defenses against infection are most effective during estrus and depressed during diestrus.[32,33] Therefore, alteration of the cycle to provide frequent estrous periods may be helpful. This is best accomplished by inducing luteolysis with prostaglandins as soon as the corpus luteum will respond (5 to 6 days postovulation).[38] The frequency of estrus and the ability to use other means of treatment that are administered during estrus are thus maximized.

THERAPEUTIC APPLICATIONS

Treatment of infectious problems related to fertility will involve use of the therapeutic methods described, as they best relate to four major problems: acute endometritis, chronic endometritis, failure of uterine defenses, and acute (postpartum) metritis.

ACUTE ENDOMETRITIS

Active, or acute endometritis is characterized by the physical changes of cervical and vaginal hyperemia, discharge, or intrauterine fluid accumulation. Regardless of the intensity of the signs, cytologic evidence of luminal neutrophils should exist. When a specific causal agent is identified in conjunction with these findings, a combination of large-volume lavage and specific antibiotic therapy appears to be more beneficial than either treatment alone. In selected cases, the addition of systemic antibiotics to the regimen may improve results.

The addition of uterine lavage to the antimicrobial treatment does add time and expense to the approach. In our experience the extra time and cost is worth while. Mechanical evacuation of the uterine lumen allows the antibiotics to work without the same degree of interference from inflammatory debris. Inspection of the recovered flushing aids in evaluation of the treatment as it progresses. A scheme that has been successful is lavage on alternate days and local antibiotic therapy daily, during estrus. Thus a typical 5-day estrus would involve three uterine irrigations and five antibiotic administrations.

A similar scheme involving either dilute povidone-

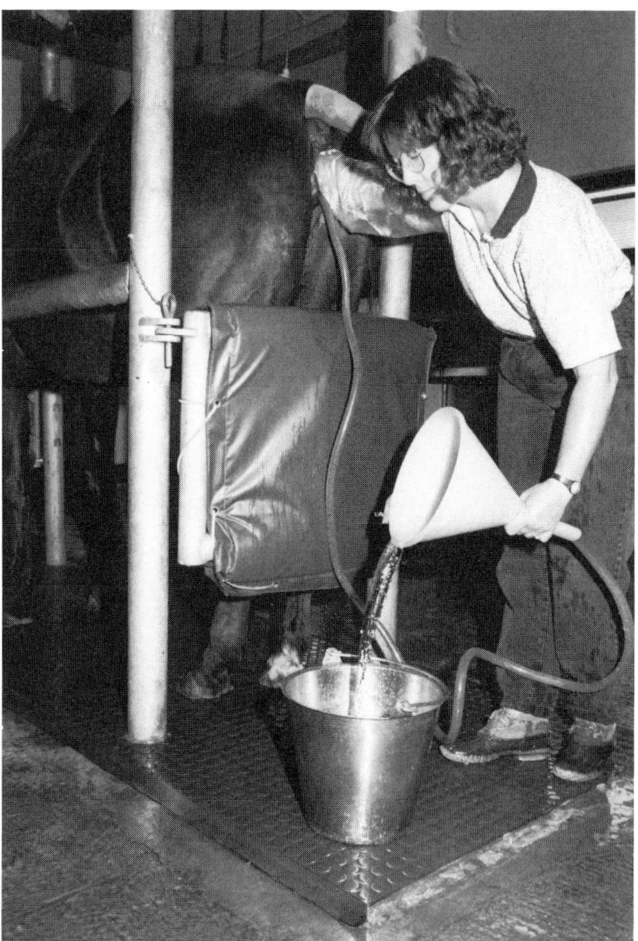

FIG. 43–5. Uterine contents evacuated by siphon effect.

iodine or plasma in combination with alternate-day lavage has been used. Indications for these nonantibiotic treatments are (1) when no specific causal organism can be identified, (2) when antibiotic sensitivity data suggest only impractical drugs, (3) when yeasts or fungi are incriminated in the cause, and (4) when prior antibiotic therapy has been unsuccessful.

A trend away from antibiotics in the treatment of endometritis is obvious in discussions with practitioners who are faced with many infectious infertility cases. Uterine lavage, with no concurrent therapy, has certainly been credited with improvement and or resolution of the problem in impressive numbers of cases. These impressions are purely subjective and are based on our numerous verbal consultations.

Once treatment of endometritis is successful, based on remission of inflammatory signs, both careful management and some consideration of postbreeding therapy will improve the fertility potential of these mares (see Failure of Uterine Defenses, later in this chapter).

CHRONIC ENDOMETRITIS

Diagnostic dilemmas associated with low-grade or chronic endometritis have been discussed. Frequently, the intensity of the inflammation in these cases is minimal and causal agents are not obvious. Treatment should be directed at reducing inflammation to the point at which fertility will not be compromised.

In addition to the approaches described for the acute form of endometritis, some consideration should be given to therapy that activates the inflammation, thereby stimulating new cellular and humoral responses. Irritation with dilute povidone-iodine or hypertonic salt solutions are examples. An interesting version of this approach is the inoculation of cell-free filtrates of streptococcal cultures to stimulate an inflammatory response without use of live bacteria.[39] In some chronic cases treated in this manner, the resulting acute flareup resulted in successful resolution of the endometritis.

All chronic endometritis cases are suspect for uterine defense failure and should be handled accordingly during subsequent attempts at breeding.

FAILURE OF UTERINE DEFENSES

Reduced uterine immunity in mares is manifested as a flareup of inflammation following any uterine contamination, especially breeding. Affected mares frequently appear clinically normal before breeding and then show positive signs for a brief time afterward. These cases represent significant frustration for the owner and practitioner. Either an inadequate prebreeding examination is suspected or the stallion is blamed for infecting the mare.

Management of these mares must include methods of reducing inflammation at the time of breeding (see below) and should probably focus on postbreeding treatment. In marginally affected mares one or two daily infusions of broad-spectrum antibiotics or plasma may resolve the postbreeding flareup successfully. In cases for which the inflammation is only marginally under control at breeding time, a more heroic approach is indicated. The following rationale is the basis for an extensive postbreeding program that has been a useful management tool at the University of Florida.[40]

Following mating, spermatozoa are transported rapidly through the uterus into the oviducts. Within 2 h of breeding all sperm cells capable of fertilization are safely in the oviduct.[41] After fertilization, the resulting embryo remains in the oviduct for about 5.5 days. Uterine treatments pose no threat to the embryo before day 5 postovulation, as long as treatments do not irritate the uterus for more than 24 h. The oviduct is protected from uterine infusion of fluids, even in high volume, by the valve at the uterotubal junction.

About 5 or 6 days are required for the newly formed corpus luteum to become responsive to prostaglandins. Thus diestrus will not be shortened or conception jeopardized by uterine infusions up to day 4 after ovulation, unless there is a residual irritation caused by the infusion.

For all of these reasons, mares may be safely treated with relatively nonirritating intrauterine therapy from 2 h after breeding through 4 to 5 days after ovulation. This concept is translated into the following protocol:

1. Within the first 24 h after breeding, successive lavages of the uterus with isotonic saline solution are made until the recovered fluid is clear.
2. When the uterus is completely emptied it is infused with either a relatively nonirritating broad-spectrum antibiotic (not one of the aminoglycosides), plasma, or both.
3. The procedure is repeated daily until all recovered fluid is clear or until the day 3 postovulation.
4. An additional treatment with antibiotic or plasma is infused on the day following the last lavage.

Ovulation time must be determined accurately in this system.

ACUTE METRITIS

Acute metritis as a postpartum entity is discussed elsewhere in this volume. The following therapeutic applications pertain only to the methods involved in this chapter. Postpartum metritis is triggered by massive contamination of the uterus alone or in conjunction with trauma associated with parturition. Bacterial growth, often involving a large gram-negative component of organisms, is usually rapid, with concurrent toxin production.

Acute metritis is an inflammation of the entire uterine wall, a condition which favors the passage of toxins from the uterine lumen into the general circulation. Treatment of the condition must be directed, in part, at removing the uterine contents repeatedly until bacterial growth and toxin formation is controlled. Large-volume lavage of the uterus, as described for the postpartum mare, is an ideal method for emptying the uterus and removing the offending sources of potential toxemia.

Lavage should continue until the recovered fluid is reasonably cleared. Until the infection is controlled, a tendency for more fluid to accumulate and further toxemia to develop exists. Therefore, close monitoring and repeated lavage, often several times daily, is indicated to control the condition. Following lavage there should be a noticeable improvement in the systemic signs (pulse rate, mucous membrane color, capillary refill time, etc.). Monitoring of these signs will give an excellent guide to the necessity for repeated flushing. Per rectum palpation of the uterus following lavage should indicate the contractile response to the treatment. If that response is not noted, water temperature may be increased to 50° C without concern for tissues. Obviously, systemic treatment plus monitoring and adjusting hydration are critical in these cases.

MANAGEMENT AND PREVENTION

The key component to successful management and prevention of infectious infertility is reducing uterine contamination. This can be done by limiting the number of breedings, by use of artificial insemination where permitted, and using antibiotic-containing semen extenders. The latter can be employed even in natural breeding programs by infusing mares with extender just before service.[42]

Serious attention must be paid to physical reasons for self-contamination. Because the integrity of the perineal area changes with aging and multiparity, each mare must be continually re-evaluated during her reproductive career. All foaling mares should be carefully examined for damage that might compromise the physical barriers to uterine contamination.

Reproductive examinations must be carried out as aseptically as possible in mares susceptible to endometritis. Air is an irritant and often a contaminant. Care in vaginoscopic procedures, including manual expression of air from the uterus per rectum after speculum examination, is warranted.

PYOMETRA

The accumulation of pus in the uterus is an infectious problem in mares that varies significantly from endometritis and metritis, and thus deserves special consideration. The underlying reasons for the failure of the uterus to drain are not well understood in many cases. Physical obstruction of the cervix as a result of trauma, with subsequent fibrosis, can be demonstrated in some instances. In others, a functional defect of the cervix is suspected, resulting in incomplete cervical dilation during estrus. In certain cases, no cervical lesions or dysfunction can be demonstrated, and the cause of the problem remains unexplained.

The clinical signs, clinical pathologic and pathologic aspects of a number of cases of pyometra have been described in detail.[43] In general, pyometra develops without concurrent clinical signs. As much as 60 L of exudate can collect in the uterus without producing signs of septicemia, depression, or anorexia. Rarely some suggestion of malaise is noted when the uterus becomes distended with pus.

External discharge may be noted intermittently, especially in those mares that continue to cycle and that still have some cervical patency. Cycle length is variable, with extended periods of diestrus recorded, similar to pyometra cases in cows. Other mares maintain regular cycles. Hematologic changes are minimal when noted. Pathologic findings include a wide range of endometrial inflammatory changes, but in prolonged cases endometrial atrophy is frequently noted.

The diagnosis of pyometra is confirmed by palpation of the uterus per rectum. It is often an incidental finding in routine reproductive evaluations, when no external discharge or systemic illness has called attention to the problem. In early stages, accumulated fluid can mimic pregnancy, but uterine wall consistency tends to be thicker and more meaty than in normal pregnancy. Ultrasonographic examination provides further confirmation, because the pus produces a homogeneous intermediate opacity typical of fluid. Confusing pyometra with a distended bladder can be avoided by confirming the locations of the ovaries, per rectum.

Often cases of pyometra are not brought to the attention of the practitioner until they are well established. The prognosis for remission with resumption of normal fertility in these mares is extremely poor. Chronic distension leads to permanent failure of the uterus to empty, and cervical dysfunction tends to persist. Even if pus accumulation can be controlled, endometrial changes, especially atrophy, may be permanent.

The logical approach to treatment of earlier cases is drainage through the cervix with subsequent, frequent warm water lavage of the uterine lumen. Fluid should be infused cautiously in cases for which the uterus is tightly distended, because rupture is a potential complication. Intrauterine antibiotics may be helpful in reversing accompanying endometritis. In all cases, endometrial biopsy will aid in making a prognosis before extended treatments produce economic concerns.

In those mares that are to be kept for purposes other than breeding, treatment options range from none in the majority of cases to hysterectomy in selected ones. If the owner can tolerate intermittent vaginal discharges and if the distended uterus causes no problem during athletic activities, no reason exists to treat the pyometra continuously. Discomfort during extreme exercise, such as jumping or speed events may dictate periodic draining and lavage of the uterus. Hysterectomy should not be undertaken without emptying the uterus as completely as possible. Surgical exposure required to remove the diseased uterus without contaminating the peritoneal cavity may be difficult to achieve.

REFERENCES

1. Hughes, J.P., and Loy, R.G.: Investigations on the effect of intrauterine inoculation of Streptococcus zooepidemicus in the mare. Proc. Am. Assoc. Equine. Pract., 289–292, 1969.
2. Evans, M.J., et al.: Clearance of bacteria and non-antigenic markers following intrauterine inoculation into maiden mares: Effect of steroid hormone environment. Theriogenology, *26:*37–50, 1986.
3. Hamilton, W.J., and Day, F.T.: Cleavage stages of the ova of the horse with notes on ovulation. J. Anat., *79:*127–130, 1945.
4. Watson, E.D.: Uterine defence mechanisms in mares resistant and susceptible to persistent endometritis: A review. Equine Vet. J., *20:*397–400, 1988.
5. Peterson, F.B., McFeely, R.A., and David, J.S.E.: Studies on the pathogenesis of endometritis in the mare. Proc. Am. Assoc. Equine Pract., 279–387, 1969.
6. Williamson, P., Penhale, W.J., Munyua, S., and Murray, J.: The acute reaction of the mare's uterus to bacterial infection. Proceedings of the International Congress on Animal Reproduction and Artificial Insemination. 1984.
7. Ward, P.A.: Bacterial factors chemotactic for polymorphonuclear leukocytes. Am. J. Pathol., *52:*725–736, 1968.
8. Blue, H.B., Blue, M.G., Kenney, R.M., and Merritt, T.L.: Chemotactic properties and protein of equine uterine fluid. Am. J. Vet. Res., *45:*1205–1208, 1984.
9. Liu, I.K.M., et al.: Comparison of peripheral blood and uterine-derived polymorphonuclear leukocytes from mares resistant and susceptible to chronic endometritis: Chemotactic and cell elastimetry analysis. Am. J. Vet. Res., *46:*917–920, 1985.
10. Liu, I.K.M., Cheung, A.T.W., Walsh, E.M., and Ayin, S.: The functional competence of uterine-derived polymorphonuclear neutrophils (PMN) from mares resistant and susceptible to chronic uterine infection: A sequential migration analysis. Biol. Reprod., *35:*1168–1174, 1986.
11. Asbury, A.C., and Hansen, P.J.: Effects of susceptibility of mares to endometritis and stage of cycle on phagocytic activity of uterine-derived neutrophils. J. Reprod. Fertil. Suppl., *35:*311–316, 1987.
12. Kenney, R.M., and Khaleel, S.A.: Bacteriostatic activity of the mare uterus: A progress report on immunoglobulins. J. Reprod. Fertil. Suppl., *23:*357–358, 1975.
13. Asbury, A.C., Halliwell, R.E.W., Foster, G.W., and Longino, S.J.: Immunoglobulins in uterine secretions of mares with differing resistance to endometritis. Theriogenology, *14:*299–304, 1980.
14. Widders, P.R., Stokes, V.R., David, J.S.E., and Bourne, F.J.: Quantitation of the immunoglobulins in reproductive tract secretions of the mare. Res. Vet. Sci., *37:*324–330, 1984.
15. Asbury, A.C., Gorman, N.T., and Foster, G.W.: Uterine defense mechanisms in the mare: Serum opsonins affecting phagocytosis of Streptococcus zooepidemicus by equine neutrophils. Theriogenology, *21:*375–385, 1984.
16. Watson, E.D., Stokes, C.R., and Bourne, F.J.: Uterine cellular and humoral defence mechanisms in mares susceptible and resistant to persistent endometritis. Immunol. Immunopathol., *16:*107–121, 1987.
17. Asbury, A.C.: Uterine defense mechanisms in the mare: The use of intrauterine plasma in the management of endometritis. Theriogenology, *21:*387–393, 1984.
18. Troedsson, M.H.T., and Liu, I.K.M.: Uterine clearance of non-antigenic markers (^{51}Cr) in response to a bacterial challenge in mares potentially susceptible and resistant to chronic uterine infections. J. Reprod. Fertil. Suppl., *44:* 283–288, 1991.
19. Allen, W.E., and Pycock, J.F.: Current views on the pathogenesis of bacterial endometritis in mares. Vet. Rec., *125:*298–301, 1989.
20. Kenney, R.M.: Cyclic and pathological changes of the mare endometrium as detected by biopsy, with a note on early embryonic death. J. Am. Vet. Med. Assoc., *172:*241–262, 1978.
21. Dimock, W.W., and Edwards, P.R.: The pathology and bacteriology of the reproductive organs of mares in relation to sterility. Agricultural Experimental Station Bulletin, Lexington, KY, 1928, p. 286.
22. Shin, S.J., Lein, D.H., Aronson, A.L., and Nusbaum, S.R.: The bacterial culture of equine uterine contents, in-vitro sensitivity of organisms isolated and interpretation. J. Reprod. Fertil. Suppl., *27:*307–315, 1979.
23. Farrely, B.T., and Mullaney, M.A.: Cervical and uterine infection in Thoroughbred mares. Irish Vet. J., *18:*201–212, 1964.
24. Ricketts, S.W., and Mackintosh, M.E.: Role of anaerobic bacteria in equine endometritis. J. Reprod. Fertil. Suppl., *35:*343–351, 1987.
25. Knudsen, O.: Endometrial cytology as a diagnostic aid in mares. Cornell Vet., *54:*415–422, 1964.
26. Asbury, A.C.: The reproductive system. *In* Equine Medicine and Surgery. 3rd ed. Edited by R.A. Mansmann and E.S. McAllister. Santa Barbara, American Veterinary Publications, 1982, pp. 1305–1402.
27. Allen, W.E.: Plasma concentrations of sodium benzylpenicillin after intrauterine infusion in pony mares. Equine Vet. J., *10:*171–173, 1978.
28. Caudle, A.B., et al.: Endometrial levels of amikacin in the mare after intrauterine infusion of amikacin sulfate. Theriogenology, *19:*433–439, 1983.
29. Brown, M.P., et al.: Amikacin sulfate in mares: Pharmacokinetics and body fluid and endometrial concentrations after repeated intramuscular administration. Am. J. Vet. Res., *45:*1610–1613, 1984.
30. Pedersoli, W.M., et al.: Endometrial and serum gentamicin concentrations in pony mares given repeated intrauterine infusions. Am. J. Vet. Res., *46:*1025–1028, 1985.
31. Asbury, A.C.: Infectious and immunologic considerations in mare infertility. Compend. Contin. Educ. Practicing Vet., *9:*585–592, 1987.
32. Winter, A.J., Broome, A.W.J., McNutt, A.H., and Casida, L.E.: Variations in uterine response to experimental infection due to the hormonal state of the ovaries. I. The role of cervical drainage, leukocytic numbers, and noncellular factors in uterine bactericidal activity. Am. J. Vet. Res., *21:*668–674, 1960.
33. Ganjam, V.K., et al.: Effect of ovarian hormones on the pathophysiological mechanisms involved in resistance vs. susceptibility to uterine infections in the mare. Proc. Am. Assoc. Equine Pract., 141–153, 1980.
34. Lyle, S.K.: Investigations on the uterine environment of the mare and its relationship to defense mechanisms. M.S. thesis. Gainesville, University of Florida, 1991.
35. Neely, D.P.: Evaluation and therapy of genital disease in the mare. *In* Equine Reproduction. Edited by D.P. Neely,

I.K.M. Liu, and R.B. Hillman. Lawrenceville, Veterinary Learning Systems, 1982, pp. 40–56.

36. Asbury, A.C.: Large-volume uterine lavage in the management of endometritis and acute metritis in mares. Comp. Contin. Educ. Practicing Vet., *12:*1477–1479, 1990.

37. Asbury, A.C.: Bacterial endometritis. *In* Current Therapy in Equine Medicine. Edited by N.E. Robinson. Philadelphia, W.B. Saunders, 1983.

38. Gustafsson, B.K., and Ott, R.S.: Current trends in the treatment of genital infections in large animals. Comp. Contin. Educ. Practicing Vet., *3:*S147–S152, 1981.

39. Couto, M.A., and Hughes, J.P.: Intra-uterine inoculation of a bacteria-free filtrate of Streptococcus zooepidemicus in clinically normal and infected mares. J. Equine Vet. Sci., *7:*265–273, 1985.

40. Asbury, A.C.: Post-breeding treatment of mares utilizing techniques that improve uterine defenses against bacteria. Proc. Am. Assoc. Equine Pract., 349–356, 1984.

41. Bader, H.: An investigation of sperm migration into the oviducts of the mare. J. Reprod. Fertil. Suppl., *32:*59–64, 1984.

42. Kenney, R.M., Bergman, R.V., Cooper, W.L., and Morse, G.W.: Minimal contamination techniques for breeding mares: techniques and preliminary findings. Proc. Am. Assoc. Equine. Pract., 327–336, 1975.

43. Hughes, J.P., et al.: Pyometra in the mare. J. Reprod. Fertil. Suppl., *27:*321–329, 1979.

CHAPTER 44

UTERINE ABNORMALITIES

S. D. Van Camp

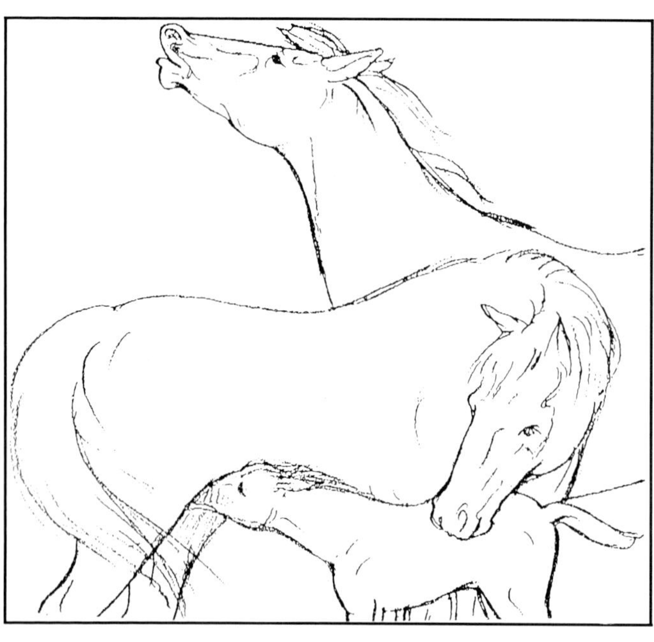

The causes of uterine disease associated with mare infertility can be subdivided into those of infectious and noninfectious origins. Infection is the most common cause of uterine infertility in the mare. Luckily, infection is also the most readily treated form of uterine disease. Diagnosis and management of infectious infertility have been discussed in other chapters of this volume. This chapter is limited to the topic of noninfectious uterine problems which cause infertility. These problems can occur in mares without a history of infection, although infection may be involved in the pathogenesis of these disorders.

For purposes of differential diagnosis, these abnormalities can be classified as follows:

1. Generalized abnormalities without discernible uterine enlargement, including endometrial gland hypoplasia and hyperplasia, endometrial atrophy, and endometrial fibrosis.
2. Generalized uterine enlargement, including pyometra, mucometra, and pneumouterus.
3. Discrete uterine abnormalities, including abscesses, cysts, sacculations, foreign bodies, and adhesions.
4. Parauterine abnormalities, including broad ligament hematomas and parauterine abscesses.

INAPPARENT GENERALIZED UTERINE ABNORMALITIES

Generalized uterine abnormalities without discernible uterine enlargement include (1) endometrial gland hyperplasia, (2) endometrial gland hypoplasia, (3) endometrial atrophy, and (4) endometrial fibrosis.

Endometrial gland hyperplasia occurs in endometria under strong hormonal influence. Pregnant and diestrous mares naturally show some degree of endometrial hyperplasia. The condition is observed subsequent to recent fetal resorption or abortion.[1] Endometrial gland hyperplasia is a frequent finding associated with hormone-secreting tumors such as ovarian sex-cord stromal cell tumors (granulosa cell tumors, thecal cell tumors, and luteomas). Treatment involves removing the underlying cause of hormonal influence or allowing the uterus to return to its nonpregnant state. Ovarian tumor-associated glandular hyperplasia is reversible. Fertility is usually restored with tumor removal.[2] Focal glandular hyperplasia can be seen in glandular nests surrounded by fibrosis.

Endometrial gland hypoplasia is occasionally seen in endometrial histologic specimens from mares with congenital infertility (for example, chromosomal intersex conditions). These mares usually have small hypoplastic ovaries. This is usually a permanent condition, and hormonal treatment is futile. Endometrial gland hypoplasia must be differentiated from seasonal endometrial atrophy that occurs during winter when the mare's ovaries are also small and inactive. Seasonal atrophy can be recognized by a low cuboidal epithelium and straight glands that occur throughout the nonedematous lamina propria. The glands frequently contain inspissated secretions.[3] If doubt remains about the diagnosis of endometrial gland hypoplasia, a second uterine biopsy specimen should be obtained during the natural breeding season.

Endometrial atrophy has been described by several authors.[3,4] It can occur in chromosomal intersex conditions, but it is also recognized in aged or debilitated mares. It is frequently associated with inactive ovaries, although it can also be seen in cyclic mares. Endometrial atrophy is a cause of repeat breeding usually associated with early embryonic death.

Endometrial atrophy should be suspected when the endometrial folds are not easily palpable through the uterine wall. This condition can be confirmed when a biopsy specimen is characterized by a "thinned endometrium with sparse, inactive glands often containing inspissated secretions."[3] Treatment is usually unrewarding unless the debilitation can be corrected.

Endometrial fibrosis is a degenerative uterine change. It is often diagnosed histologically in older, multiparous mares, but can also be identified in young mares. It may be a sequelae to multiple pregnancies or uterine infection and/or intrauterine therapy. The fibrotic changes may (1) surround the base of the endometrial glands, resulting in glandular nests; (2) encircle the neck of the glands, resulting in restriction of the glandular secretion outflow and leading to glandular dilatation and cyst formation; (3) localize beneath the basement membrane of the luminal epithelium; or (4) occur generally throughout the lamina propria of the endometrium. Fibrosis contributes to infertility by interfering with glandular and epithelial function. Conception occurs, but early embryonic death in the first 60 to 90 days of gestation usually results.

Interpretation of glandular nests must differentiate pathologic nests with fibrosis and the nonpathologic nests lacking periglandular fibrosis as seen in anestrous or transitional mares.[5] Masson stain or polarized light microscopy may help to determine the amount of fibrosis present. For further discussion of the appearance of endometrial fibrosis see Chapter 26.

Fibrosis of the endometrium is usually a permanent condition resulting in reduced or permanent infertility. Dimethyl sulfoxide (DMSO) therapy has been recommended in cases of uterine fibrosis, because DMSO causes changes in collagen and connective tissue.[6–8] However, its value in reducing fibrosis has not been tested scientifically. Treatment with DMSO alters neutrophil function, and its value in cases of uterine infection is still questionable.[9]

GENERALIZED UTERINE ENLARGEMENT

Gross enlargement of the uterus occurs in cases of pneumouterus, pyometra, and mucometra. Pneumouterus is associated with pneumovagina in mares with poor vulvar labial apposition or in mares with dorsocraniad sloped vulvas resulting in wind sucking. Poor tone of the vestibulovaginal sphincter allows air to reach the anterior vagina and penetrate the cervix. This condition is observed most frequently when the mare is in estrus and the cervix relaxed. It also may be seen in cases of cervical trauma and scarification that prevent closure of the cervix as well as cases of perineal body destruction. Occasionally, pneumouterus can be created iatrogenically by passage of a speculum into the vagina of the estral mare.

Chronic pneumouterus may lead to endometritis and infertility. It can usually be corrected by suturing of the vulvar lips with a Caslick operation.

Equine pyometra results in uterine enlargement. The uterus may contain from 0.5 to 60 L of exudate. In some cases, the material also may be present in the vagina if the cervix is patent. The uterine wall may be thick and fibrotic but is most often thin and friable. Obstruction of the cervical canal or uterine lumen is frequently present, resulting in accumulation of the pyometritic fluid. Externally, most pyometritic mares are asymptomatic. However, some mares with chronic pyometra may show a borderline normocytic, normochromic anemia.[10]

A retained corpus luteum and anestrus are not consistent signs in the mare with pyometra, unlike the cow. Pyometritic mares frequently continue to cycle regularly or experience short cycles. The degree of endometrial damage present determines whether or not prostaglandins are released from the uterus. If the damage is severe, prostaglandin synthesis and/or release may be prevented. In milder cases, prostaglandins may be released regularly or prematurely, resulting in normal or short interestrous intervals.[10]

Bacterial infection is frequently present in cases of equine pyometra; however, not all pyometras have bacteria present. In one study, Streptococcus zooepidemicus was the organism most frequently recovered.[10] Escherichia coli, Actinomyces sp., Pasteurella sp., Pseudomonas sp., and Propionibacterium sp. were also seen. In some cases more than one bacterium was present.

Therapeutic efforts are often unrewarding. If the mare with pyometra has not been cycling, prostaglandin therapy may help evacuate the uterus. Careful uterine lavage and intrauterine antibiotic therapy, based on bacterial culture and antibiotic sensitivity, are helpful. Any cervical or uterine adhesions present should be broken down if possible, or recurrence of pyometra is likely. Once evacuation is complete and the uterine wall has recovered, a biopsy is warranted to assess the degree of endometrial damage. Prognosis for fertility is poor in cases of equine pyometra, because the degree of endometrial damage is often severe.[11]

Mucometra is rare in the mare and can be confused with pyometra. McEntee reported on four cases in aged mares.[12] Cystic hyperplasia of the endometrium and lymphocytic infiltration of the endometrium were present in each case. Two of the cases were associated with endometrial atrophy. The age of these mares and the endometrial atrophy present make for a poor prognosis. Generalized uterine conditions usually result in a guarded to poor prognosis for fertility. The prognosis with discrete lesions may not be so severe.

DISCRETE UTERINE ABNORMALITIES

Discrete uterine abnormalities include (1) endometrial cysts, (2) ventral sacculations, (3) adhesions, (4) abscesses, (5) tumors, and (6) foreign bodies. These abnormalities are usually recognized initially on rectal palpation of the uterus or transrectal ultrasonography of the tract. Additional diagnostic efforts must be made to differentiate these abnormalities.

Endometrial cysts may be singular or multiple. These cysts originate from either uterine glands or lymphatic lacunae. The glandular cysts are usually the result of periglandular fibrosis and are too small to be detected by transrectal ultrasonography.[13,14] Their significance as a cause of infertility is unclear. The lymphatic lacunar cysts are actually areas of lymphangiectasia. These cysts can be several centimeters in diameter and may result in infertility or early abortion. They can be felt as discrete enlargements in the uterus and can occur anywhere in the uterus; they are most problematical when at the site of implantation in the junction of the uterine body and horns where they can be confused with a pregnancy. Care must be taken when twins are suspected ultrasonographically to be sure that one embryonic vesicle is not actually a cyst. The cysts are static or slow growing compared with an embryonic vesicle, and thus re-examination is prudent. Endoscopic examination of the uterine lumen is also helpful in diagnosing endometrial cysts. Endometrial fibrosis is frequently moderate to severe in mares with multiple endometrial cysts.

The importance of solitary cysts as a cause of infertility is unclear. Kenney feels that these result in infertility.[13] Ginther suggested that single cysts and groups of small cysts do not interfere with fertility.[15] However, in our clinic we recognize that mares with extensive or large cysts are frequently infertile.

The equine embryo is motile within the uterus during the first 16 to 17 days of gestation.[16] It must be motile during this time to prevent luteolysis and early embryonic death.[17] Cysts that are large enough to occlude the lumen and prevent migration of the embryo may lead to loss of the early pregnancy. On the other hand, embryos have been observed ultrasonographically being forced past endometrial cysts by uterine undulations.[15]

Treatment options for uterine cysts include mechanical curettage, hypertonic saline infusions, aspiration, or rupture with endoscopic biopsy instruments.[11] The value of these treatments in restoring fertility is unknown. In our clinic, endoscopic-guided laser photofulguration is effective in lysing the cysts. The cyst sites heal well after laser therapy and the formation of transluminal adhesions at the cyst site is minimal. Too few cases have been treated by laser to evaluate its effectiveness in restoring fertility at this time. Frequently, the endometrium over these cysts is atrophied and may not regenerate after removal of the cyst.[11]

Ventral uterine sacculations at the junction of the uterine horns and body are frequently seen in aged infertile mares.[13] These areas can be confused with early pregnancy by an inexperienced palpator. These sacculations are the result of focal myometrial atony and endometrial atrophy. Accumulation of lymphatic fluid in the myometrium is also frequently present as are endometrial cysts.[13]

Sacculations occur at the most dependent portion of the uterine horns where embryonic fixation and implantation occur. Bacteria, seminal fluid, and debris accumulate in these sacculations. Mares that fail to clear these substances within 24 h after breeding are susceptible to the establishment of chronic endometritis.[18] These sacculations are degenerative changes and response to therapy is poor. Repeated hot saline (40 to 45° C) uterine lavages and multiple oxytocin injections, administered to increase myometrial tone, have had questionable results.[11] Postcoital saline uterine lavage 1 or 2 days after breeding appears helpful in removing the seminal debris, although this is controversial.[19–22] For further information on this subject see Chapters 42 and 43.

Uterine adhesions are occasionally diagnosed on endoscopic evaluations of the uterus. They may develop subsequent to trauma associated with dystocia or intrauterine infusion, as a sequela to severe endometritis, or as the result of intrauterine therapy with caustic solutions. The adhesions may appear as single or multiple fine bands, thick bands, partial or complete sheets, or tunnels between adjacent endometrial folds.[23] The band type of adhesions may not significantly affect fertility. However, they may cause mechanical entrapment of the placenta after foaling. They can usually be broken down manually or with the use of an endoscope and a uterine biopsy forceps or electrocautery laser fiber. More extensive adhesions may result in infertility by causing pyometra or by restricting embryonic mobility within the uterus.[24]

Uterine abscesses occur infrequently in the mare but can be sequelae to uterine trauma from dystocia, artificial insemination, uterine therapy, or severe metritis or pyometra. Mares with acute abscessation may have evidence of neutrophilia, peritonitis, increased fibrinogen, recurrent febrile episodes, etc. If the abscesses are small and solitary it may be possible to drain them into the uterine lumen while the mare is in estrus. Systemic and intrauterine antibiotics and uterine lavages may be attempted to correct these. Often the abscesses reform and intraluminal adhesions develop. More often than not, the abscesses must be dissected out via an abdominal approach. The surgical site may represent a weakening in the uterine wall and uterine rupture may occur during the next pregnancy or at parturition. It is questionable whether these mares should be rebred. Embryo donation may be a viable option for these mares. Ovariohysterectomy is an option, but difficult in the mare.

Primary uterine neoplasia is extremely rare in the mare.[25] Solitary or multiple small leiomyomas 2.5 to 5.0 cm in diameter can be observed. Neeley reported that they are often pedunculated and can be removed with a surgical snare.[11] They can be felt by palpation as discrete nodules within the uterus. Larger leiomyomas are rare. Other tumors reported include rhabdomyosarcomas and carcinomas.[26]

Uterine foreign bodies are occasionally encountered.

They may be a nidus for establishment of chronic endometritis or pyometra. Usually these foreign bodies are fetal remnants remaining after fetal maceration or after dystocia and fetal emphysema or fetotomy. Intrauterine fetal remnants have been detected by rectal palpation, uterine endoscopy, endometrial cytology, and transrectal ultrasonography.[15,27,28]

Fetal remnants have been detected in endometrial cytologic specimens by detection of fetal muscle cells. (J.F. Rozel, personal communication). Calcified fetal bones appear as hyperechoic areas with underlying shadows on ultrasonography. The shadows are caused by the inability of the sound waves to traverse the bones. Porous or noncalcified bones may not cast a shadow. Ultrasonography can be used to aid removal of fetal bones from the uterus.[15,28]

PARAUTERINE ABNORMALITIES

Parauterine abnormalities encountered include hematomas and abscesses. Uterine hemorrhage may occur into the wall or lumen of the uterus or peritoneal cavity as a result of uterine trauma associated with dystocia or forced fetal extraction.[29] Only rarely does intrauterine hemorrhage result in death. The hemorrhage usually ceases as uterine involution progresses. However, fatal hemorrhage may occur as a result of blood vessel rupture at or near parturition. Middle-aged to old mares may rupture the middle uterine, internal iliac, or utero-ovarian arteries late in gestation or in association with parturition. If extramural rupture occurs, exsanguination into the peritoneal cavity can be expected.

Rupture of the vessels within the intact broad ligament results in a parauterine hematoma. These mares may appear colicky, sweaty, and in shock during the acute phase of the hemorrhage. However, they are often asymptomatic if the hematoma is small. Most of the hematomas are diagnosed later during a postpartum examination of the tract and usually occur in the right broad ligament.[30] They regress with time, and rebreeding is possible, although the vessels frequently rupture again at the same site during the next gestation, often with fatal results.[30]

Parauterine abscesses may result from bacterial colonization of a hematoma or be an extension of uterine wall trauma associated with dystocia or intrauterine therapy. Long-term antibiotic therapy may be helpful, but is often unrewarding because of the inability of the antibiotics to penetrate the abscesses. Surgical removal under general anesthesia is the preferred therapy if antibiotic therapy fails.

REFERENCES

1. Ricketts, S.W.: The techniques and clinical application of endometrial biopsy in the mare. Equine. Vet. J., *7:*102–108, 1975.
2. Bosu, W.T.K., Van Camp, S.D., Miller, R.B., and Owen, R ap R.: Ovarian disorders: Clinical and morphological observations in 30 mares. Can. Vet. J., *23:*6–14, 1982.
3. Kenney, R.M.: Cyclic and pathologic changes of the mare endometrium as detected by biopsy, with a note on early embryonic death. J. Am. Vet. Med. Assoc., *172:*241–262, 1978.
4. Greenhoff, G.R., and Kenney, R.M.: Evaluation of reproductive status of nonpregnant mares. J. Am. Vet. Med. Assoc., *167:*449–458, 1975.
5. Gross, T.L., and LeBlanc, M.M.: Seasonal variation of histomorphic features of equine endometrium. J. Am. Vet. Med. Assoc., *184:*1379–1382, 1984.
6. Ley, W.B., and Sponenberg, D.P.: Dimethyl sulfoxide (DMSO) intrauterine therapy in the mare. Proc. Soc. Theriogenology, 186–198, 1985.
7. Erk, Y., et al.: Dimethyl sulfoxide alteration of collagen. Ann. N. Y. Acad. Sci., *411:*364–368, 1983.
8. Gries, G., Bublitz, G., and Lindner, J.: The effect of dimethyl sulfoxide on the components of connective tissue (clinical and experimental investigations). Ann. N. Y. Acad. Sci., *141:*630–637, 1967.
9. Frazer, G.S., Rossol, T.J., Threlfall, W.R., and Weisbrode, S.E.: Histopathic effects of dimethyl sulfoxide on equine endometrium. Am. J. Vet. Res., *49:*1774–1781, 1988.
10. Hughes, J.P., et al.: Pyometra in the mare. J. Reprod. Fertil. Suppl., *27:*321–329, 1979.
11. Neeley, D.P.: Evaluation and therapy of genital disease in the mare. *In* Equine Reproduction. Edited by J.P. Hughes. Nutley, Hoffman-LaRoche, Inc., 1983, pp. 40–56.
12. McEntee, K.: The uterus: Atrophic, metaplastic, and proliferative lesions. *In* Reproductive Pathology of Domestic Mammals. New York, Academic Press, 1990, pp. 167–190.
13. Kenney, R.M., and Ganjam, V.K.: Selected pathological changes of the mare uterus and ovary. J. Reprod. Fertil. Suppl., *23:*335–339, 1975.
14. Adams, G.P., Kastelic, D.R., Bergfelt, D.R., and Ginther, O.J.: Effect of uterine inflammation and ultrasonography-detected uterine pathology on fertility in the mare. J. Reprod. Fertil. Suppl., *35:*445–454, 1987.
15. Ginther, O.J.: Embryo-uterine interactions. *In* Ultrasonic Imaging and Reproductive Events in the Mare. Cross Plains, WI, Equiservices, 1986, pp. 229–252.
16. Ginther, O.J.: Fixation and orientation of the early equine conceptus. Theriogenology, *19:*613–623, 1983.
17. McDowell, K.J., et al.: Restricted conceptus mobility results in failure of pregnancy maintenance in mares. Biol. Reprod., *39:*340–348, 1988.
18. Troedsson, M.H.T., and Lui, I.K.M.: Uterine clearance of non-antigenic markers (^{51}Cr) in response to a bacterial challenge in mares potentially susceptible and resistant to chronic uterine infections. J. Reprod. Fertil. Suppl., *44:* 282–288, 1991.
19. Brinsko, S.P., Varner, D.D., Blanchard, T.L., and Meyers, S.A.: The effect of postbreeding uterine lavage on pregnancy rate in mares. Theriogenology, *33:*465–475, 1990.
20. Asbury, A.C.: Large-volume uterine lavage in the management of endometritis and acute metritis in mares. Compend. Contin. Educ. Practicing Vet., *12:*1477–1479, 1990.
21. LeBlanc, M., and Asbury, A.C.: Rationale for uterine lavage after breeding in mares. Proc. Am. Assoc. Equine Pract., 623–628, 1987.
22. Adams, G.P., and Ginther, O.J.: Efficacy of intrauterine infusion of plasma for treatment of infertility and endo-

metritis in mares. J. Am. Vet. Med. Assoc., *194:*372–378, 1989.

23. Baker, C.B., and Kenney, R.M.: Systemic approach to the diagnosis of the infertile or subfertile mare. *In* Current Treatment in Theriogenology. Edited by D.A. Morrow, Philadelphia, 1980, pp. 721–736.
24. McKinnon, A.O., et al.: Diagnostic ultrasonography of uterine pathology in the mare. Proc. Am. Assoc. Equine Pract., 605–622, 1987.
25. Madwell, B.R., and Theilen, G.H.: Tumors of the urogenital tract. *In* Veterinary Cancer Medicine. 2nd ed. Edited by G.H. Theilen. Philadelphia, Lea & Febiger, 1987, pp. 583–600.
26. Roberts, S.J.: Infertility in the mare. *In* Veterinary Obstetrics and Genital Diseases (Theriogenology). 3rd ed. Woodstock, VT, published by the author, 1986, pp. 581–635.
27. Ginther, O.J., and Pierson, R.A.: Ultrasonographic anatomy and pathology of the equine uterus. Theriogenology, *21:*505–515, 1984.
28. Ginther, O.J.: Uterus. *In* Ultrasonic Imaging and Reproductive Events in the Mare. Cross Plains, WI, Equiservices, 1986, pp. 173–194.
29. Roberts, S.J.: Injuries and diseases of the puerperal period. *In* Veterinary Obstetrics and Genital Diseases (Theriogenology). 3rd ed. Woodstock, VT, published by the author, 1986, pp. 353–396.
30. Pascoe, R.R.: Rupture of the utero-ovarian or middle uterine artery in the mare at or near parturition. Vet. Rec., *104:*77, 1979.

CHAPTER 45

OVARIAN ABNORMALITIES

W.T.K. Bosu
C.A. Smith

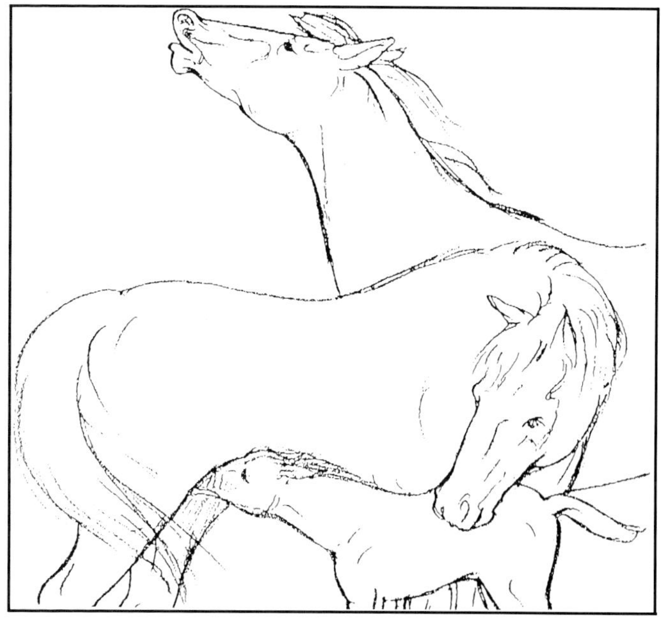

Several types of ovarian abnormalities occur in the mare (Table 45–1). These conditions usually result in either temporary infertility or render the animal infertile if not sterile. This chapter will review the types, diagnoses, and management of ovarian problems in mares.

CLINICAL HISTORIES ASSOCIATED WITH OVARIAN ABNORMALITIES

Mares with ovarian abnormalities may exhibit a wide spectrum of clinical signs. The most common complaints are abnormalities of the estrous cycle and behavioral changes. The behavioral changes include virilism with stallion-like behavior, characterized by mares acting like a stallion around other mares; aggressive behavior toward people and other horses; absence of estrus (anestrus); and prolonged or persistent estrus (nymphomania).[1,2] Some mares with ovarian abnormalities may have a history of normal reproductive events including pregnancy.

Mares with ovarian disease may also display evidence of abdominal or pelvic pain.[3,4] Therefore, ovarian abnormalities should be considered among differential diagnoses of the acute abdomen. Discomfort in some mares with abnormally enlarged ovaries has been noted in association with periods of exercise or athletic events. Lameness associated with large ovarian tumors has also been reported.[4] Clinical histories of mares with ovarian abnormalities may give no indication of the problem. The ovarian abnormalities in such cases may be detected serendipitously during prepurchase, prebreeding, pregnancy examinations or as incidental findings during postmortem examinations.

Ovarian abnormalities occur in mares of all ages, but are more commonly reported in mares 6 yr or older (which may partially represent lack of examination prior to breeding age). No breed predilection has been noted. Most mares will present during spring and summer, corresponding to the breeding season in temperate climates, when mares are commonly subjected to frequent clinical observations and examinations.

EXAMINATION PROCEDURES

INSPECTION

The first step in the examination of mares with suspected ovarian problems should include determination of behavior. If necessary, the mare should be teased by a stallion and her response recorded. Behavioral patterns associated with ovarian abnormalities in mares vary widely. Some mares with ovarian problems may be anestrous but anestrus caused by ovarian disease must be differentiated from physiologic anestrus. Cessation of estrous cycles is a normal reproductive event in 75 to 80% of mares in temperate climates and is termed seasonal anestrus.[5] Anestrus during the breeding season may be the result of pregnancy, planned or iatrogenic hormonal influence, or ovarian problems. Individual

TABLE 45–1. COMMON OVARIAN ABNORMALITIES IN THE MARE

- Ovarian neoplasms
  - Granulosa cell tumor
  - Teratoma
  - Dysgerminoma
  - Serous cystadenoma
- Anovulatory/atretic follicles
- Ovarian hematoma/hematocyst
- Ovarian abscessation
- Ovarian hypoplasia
  - Hypoplasia
  - Prepubertal ovaries
  - Seasonal anestrus
  - Malnutrition
  - Hypothalamic-anterior pituitary dysfunction
  - Diestrous phase ovaries
  - Gonadal dysgenesis

mares may display weak or silent estrus (especially during foal heat) and thus may not be detected by inattentive or uninformed owners.

Other mares with ovarian problems may exhibit nymphomania. These mares exhibit prolonged periods of estrous behavior or may display estrus at frequent, shortened interestrous intervals of 3 to 4 days. This behavior should be differentiated from prolonged periods of estrus commonly observed during the early spring transitional period when mares re-establish normal estrous cyclicity.[6]

Stallion-like or aggressive behavior in mares may be exhibited persistently or at intermittent intervals. Some mares may display abnormally aggressive behavior that is evident only during estrus. Changes of behavior may be the only and predominant sign in these mares. Thus mares that usually display docile temperament but become aggressive or vicious during estrus should be suspected of having ovarian problems. Many mares exhibiting virilism are difficult to restrain and resent examinations of the perineal region.

PHYSICAL EXAMINATION

Changes in physical appearance may be associated with some types of ovarian problems in mares. For example, mares displaying stallion-like behavior may develop the muscular conformation of males. In particular, the appearance of a crested neck has been noted in these mares. Precocious mammary gland development can also occur, but engorgement of the udder is usually moderate.[2] No secretions from the teats have been reported. The vulvar lips should be inspected for conformation, and any enlargement of the clitoris should be noticed. Some mares with ovarian problems may have poor body condition associated with anestrus. Poor nutrition will lead to weight loss, a condition that can also cause anestrus.[6]

REPRODUCTIVE SYSTEM EXAMINATION

Examination of the reproductive tract is the best means of identifying ovarian abnormalities. Affected mares may be unruly or aggressive, requiring tranquilization to perform a thorough and adequate examination safely. Nevertheless, adequate restraint should always be employed during examination of the reproductive system in mares. The examination should include the following procedures.

RECTAL PALPATION

Rectal palpation is the most commonly used and the simplest method for assessment of ovaries in mares. A systematic examination of the reproductive tract should include palpation per rectum of the cervix, uterine body, both uterine horns, and both ovaries. The ovaries must be examined for size, architecture, consistency, and position. The presence of an ovary smaller than 2 cm or larger than 8 to 10 cm in diameter should alert the examiner that the ovary may be abnormal. Usually only one ovary is enlarged or abnormal (Fig. 45–1) except in cases of ovarian hypoplasia for which both ovaries may be small. Ovarian problems characterized by enlargement usually result in loss of the common bean-shape appearance. Similarly, ovarian consistency may become hard or soft in some cases of ovarian hematoma. In some cases of granulosa cell tumors or ovarian abscess, large ovaries are found deeper in the abdominal cavity and place strain on the ipsilateral uterine horn. Ovarian problems should be differentiated from paraovarian cysts and remnants of the mesonephric duct, which can be found in mares varying in size from 0.5 to 5.5 cm.[5]

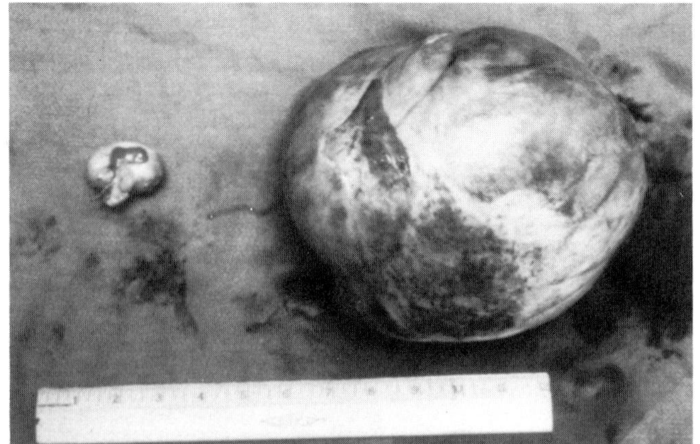

FIG. 45–1. Asymmetry in the size of ovaries of a mare. The left ovary is of normal size and shape. The right ovary is large and has lost the normal bean-shape appearance because of a granulosa cell tumor.

ULTRASONOGRAPHIC EXAMINATION OF THE REPRODUCTIVE TRACT

Ultrasonographic examination of the reproductive tract in mares is now routinely employed in equine reproduction and is useful to evaluate enlarged ovaries in mares.[7] Large follicular ovarian structures can often be differentiated on the basis of ultrasonographic findings.[8]

Ultrasonographic examination may prove most useful in detecting abnormalities in the internal structure of enlarged ovaries, which may aid diagnosis and assist in the choice of appropriate therapy or management. Some ovarian tumors can be differentiated by ultrasonography.[9,10] Whereas several examiners reported a characteristic honeycomb appearance of granulosa cell tumors caused by multilocular cysts, others have failed to identify a characteristic appearance that can be used to diagnose the presence of granulosa cell tumors accurately. Other uses of ultrasonography include the drainage of ovarian tumors with large cystic structures, and the decrease in size facilitates ease of surgical removal. Furthermore, repeated serial ultrasonographic examinations are useful to observe the progressive changes in large follicular structures.

Ultrasonography has also proven useful in establishing the functional status of animals with bilateral small ovaries associated with anestrus and follicular status of the unaffected ovary in cases of unilateral ovarian enlargement. In these cases, presence of significant follicular activity or luteal structures may indicate the ability of the ovary(s) to function normally.

VAGINOSCOPY

Vaginoscopic examination should always be included as a diagnostic procedure in any mare suspected of abnormal reproductive function. Examination of the vagina and cervix can yield valuable information concerning the reproductive status of the mare, especially the endocrine status (see Chapter 25). Characteristic changes occur in the color, tone, and location of the cervix during the various phases of the estrous cycle of the mare. Thus, vaginoscopic findings can be used in conjunction with history, results of rectal palpation, and ultrasonography to indicate accurately the reproductive and hormonal status of the mare. As in the use of rectal palpation and ultrasonography, serial vaginoscopic examinations may be most useful.

ENDOMETRIAL BIOPSY

Endometrial biopsy can be used to determine endocrine status of the mare and provide prognosis of future reproductive efficiency or fertility. The appearance of the endometrium reflects changes during the estrous cycle and seasonal anestrus (see Chapter 26). Endometrial biopsy is similar to vaginoscopic examination of the cervix, because they both reflect the hormonal environment present in the mare and can be used as adjuncts to the history, rectal palpation, and ultrasonography to diagnose accurately specific ovarian problems in mares.

HORMONE ASSAY

Hormonal profiles during winter anestrus, the transitional period, the estrous cycle, and pregnancy have been described in the mare.[6] Based on these patterns, it is clinically possible to use progesterone assays to determine presence of nonpalpable luteal tissue in small ovaries. For instance, demonstration of low concentrations in serum progesterone (< 1 ng/mL) in two samples collected 10 days apart is indicative of ovaries devoid of luteal tissue. However, if the serum progesterone of either of the samples collected at the 10-day interval is > 1 ng/mL, it is indicative of functional luteal tissue present within the ovary, regardless of the ovary's small size.

Similarly, some ovarian abnormalities are characterized by specific hormonal changes. Ovarian tumors in the mare are capable of producing progestins, androgens, estrogens, and proteins.[10] The diverse nature of steroid production may depend on the predominant secretory cell-type present in the tumor. Although progestin, androgen, and estrogen concentrations may be elevated in affected mares, only elevated serum testosterone concentrations appear consistently related to behavioral changes. Serum testosterone concentrations of > 100 pg/mL were noted in mares with stallion-like behavior.[11,12] Anestrous, irregular estrus, and persistent estrous behavior may be caused by an ovarian disease and manifested as infertility in the affected mare. However, definitive diagnosis cannot be reliably defined endocrinologically by any one steroid hormone. For final diagnosis, histopathologic examination of ovarian tissue and karyotype studies may be needed.

COMMON TYPES OF OVARIAN ABNORMALITIES AND CLINICAL FINDINGS

OVARIAN NEOPLASMS

Ovarian tumors are not uncommon in mares and the most prevalent are granulosa cell tumor, teratoma, dysgerminoma, and serous cystadenoma (Table 45–1).

Granulosa Cell Tumor

The most common ovarian tumor is the granulosa cell tumor (Fig. 45–2), which accounts for 2.5% of all equine neoplasms.[13] It arises from sex cord stromal tissue within the ovary, is usually benign, and is often hormonally active. Granulosa cell tumors occur in all breeds. It has been reported in mares of all ages, but the highest frequency is reported in mares between 5 and 9 yr of age. Reproductive behavior and endocrine patterns associated with the tumor vary. Stallion-like behavior is associated with serum testosterone concentra-

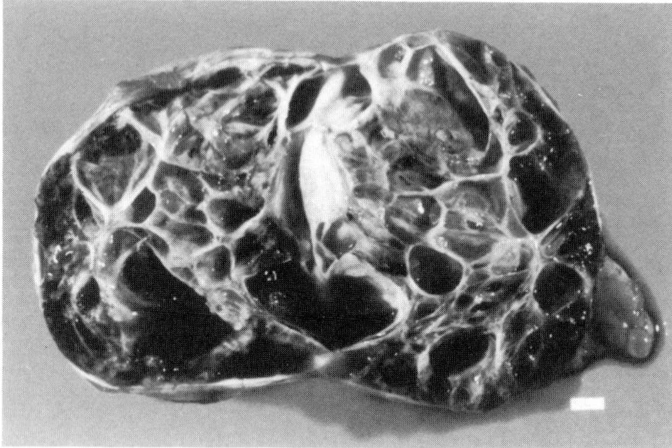

FIG. 45–2. Cut surface of a granulosa cell tumor removed from a mare. The multilocular cysts would result in a characteristic honeycomb appearance on ultrasonographic examination.

tions > 100 pg/mL,[11,12] but other hormonally linked behaviors are not readily apparent.

Rectal palpation in affected animals reveals the presence of one enlarged ovary which has lost the normal bean-shape structure and a contralateral ovary that is usually small, firm, and devoid of follicular activity. Occasionally, the affected ovary may be small and hard in consistency.[2] Ultrasonographic examination of the enlarged ovary may not yield a definitive diagnosis of granulosa cell tumor. However, combined with the history and rectal palpation findings, ultrasonographic findings are a useful adjunct for diagnosis of granulosa cell tumors. Affected ovaries vary in size and are spherical or lobulated. On cut surface, the tumor masses are either polycystic or solid grayish yellow with foci of hemorrhage or necrosis. The final diagnosis is obtained by histopathologic findings on examination of ovarian tissue.

Ovarian Teratoma

Ovarian teratomas are benign ovarian tumors that occur unilaterally and arise from germ cells. The affected ovarian mass may contain cysts, bone, cartilage, teeth, and hair (Fig. 45–3). Teratomas often have little effect on the other ovary, thus normal estrous cycles and pregnancy occur in their presence. They are usually "accidental" findings during routine examination of mares' reproductive tracts. Teratomas may cause pain and abdominal discomfort to the mare because of the tumors' size and weight.[6]

Dysgerminoma

Dysgerminomas are malignant ovarian tumors of germ cell origin that are rare. Rapid metastasis to the abdominal and thoracic cavities often occurs. The history may include chronic weight loss and abdominal discomfort. Rectal palpation reveals a unilaterally enlarged, multilobulated ovary or abdominal mass. Hormonal profiles may be abnormal but are not diagnostic. Hypertrophic osteopathy has been reported as sequellae to thoracic metastasis in the mare.[14] Because of the usually poor prognosis in these cases, it is recommended that thoracic radiographs and abdominocentesis be performed when dysgerminoma is suspected for assessment of metastasis.

Serous Cystadenoma

Serous cystadenoma is a benign primary epithelial ovarian tumor that arises from surface epithelium. The tumor has a reported gradual onset, and affected ovaries contain palpable cystic areas on the surface. Minimal effect on the function of the contralateral ovary is observed.[15]

ANOVULATORY/ATRETIC FOLLICLES

Structures termed persistent follicles and autumn follicles are large, tense, fluid-filled structures 10 to 15 cm in diameter found on ovaries of mares commonly during fall, but sometimes during the breeding season. They are nonpathologic structures indicative of the hormonal conditions present during seasonal transition in mares. These structures can persist for up to 60 days. They often contain blood and have a liquid to gelatinous consistency[16] (Fig. 45–4). The structures are apparently associated with declining gonadotropin output and inadequate concentrations of luteinizing hormone to either stimulate ovulation or maintain normal development of a corpus luteum in those cases in which ovulation occurs.[6] Large persistent follicular structures associated with persistent estrus or irregularities of the estrous cycle or infertility have been described in mares during the breeding season. These are sometimes referred to as anovulatory "cystic ovary" problems. Diagnosis of these structures is based on season and reproductive history of the mare.

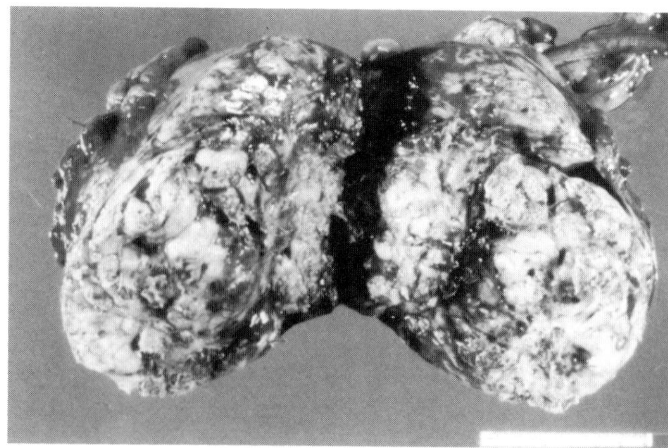

FIG. 45–3. Cut surface of ovarian teratoma removed from a mare. Note the presence of hair and cartilage in the ovarian mass.

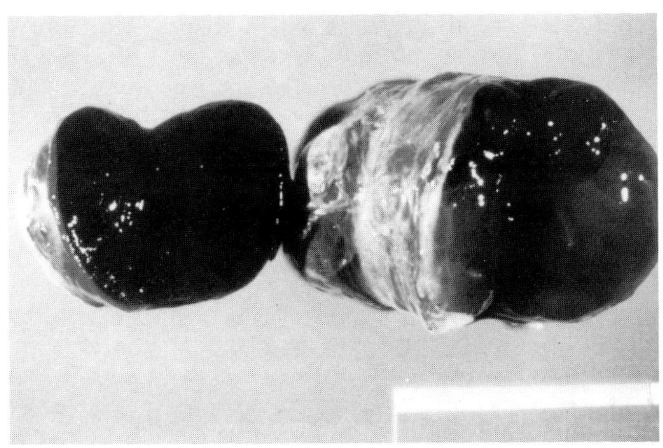

FIG. 45–4. Persistent follicles (autumn follicles) in the ovaries of a mare. The ovaries were filled with a gelatinous, hemorrhagic substance.

OVARIAN HEMATOMA/HEMATOCYST

Ovarian hematomas are characterized by enlarged blood-filled follicles, which are commonly found during routine examination of mares during the breeding season. A mechanism of formation of these structures has been described.[6] The follicular cavity overfills with blood following ovulation, causing formation of an ovarian hematoma (Fig. 45–5). These structures can become quite large (> 10 cm) and normally resolve over one to two estrous cycles. However, they may persist for 2 to 3 months. They usually do not interfere with normal estrous cycle activity.[2,8] Upon removal, these ovaries usually contain one large cyst filled with blood either freshly clotted or in various stages of hemolysis.

OVARIAN ABSCESSATION

Ovarian abscesses are rare. They generally occur as a result of needle aspiration of an enlarged, fluid-filled ovary. Ovariocentesis reportedly preceded an enlarged, hardened ovary with a thick, fibrous capsule encompassing a central core composed of thick, suppurative exudate (Fig. 45–6)[2] A history of ovariocentesis should alert examiners to consider ovarian abscessation as a diagnostic possibility.

OVARIAN HYPOPLASIA

Ovaries that are small (< 2 cm in diameter), firm, and hard may represent a hypoplastic condition. Small ovaries can occur during winter anestrus or may be the result of severe malnutrition or hypothalamic-anterior pituitary dysfunction. Ovaries of the mare during the diestrous phase (midluteal) of the estrous cycle can sometimes appear to be inactive. Ultrasonographic examination for presence of follicular activity or presence of a corpus luteum will rule out cessation or absence of estrous cycles. In addition, hormonal analysis for serum progesterone can be performed at 10-day intervals to assess presence of functional luteal tissue in the ovary.

Gonadal dysgenesis must be considered when other possible causes for small inactive ovaries have been excluded. In one report, mares with small ovaries were infertile because of chromosome abnormalities.[17] Turner's syndrome (63, XO genotype) was the most common chromosomal abnormality found in these mares. Affected animals were small for their age and did not exhibit normal estrous cycles, although some mares exhibited receptivity to the stallion at all times. Both ovaries were small and soft, and the rest of the reproductive tract was infantile. Other abnormal karyotypes reported to cause gonadal dysgenesis in the mare include 63X/64XX, 63X/64XY, 65XXX, and the 64XY sex-reversed condition.[6] Although a rapid screening test for XO karyotypic abnormalities is determination of sex chromatin appendages (drumsticks) present in polymorphic neutrophils (PMNs) of the mare, a final diagnosis is possible only after karyotypic analysis of fibroblasts or lymphocytes.

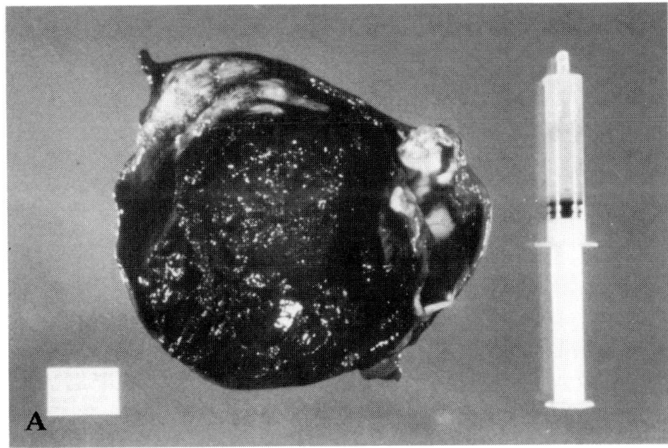

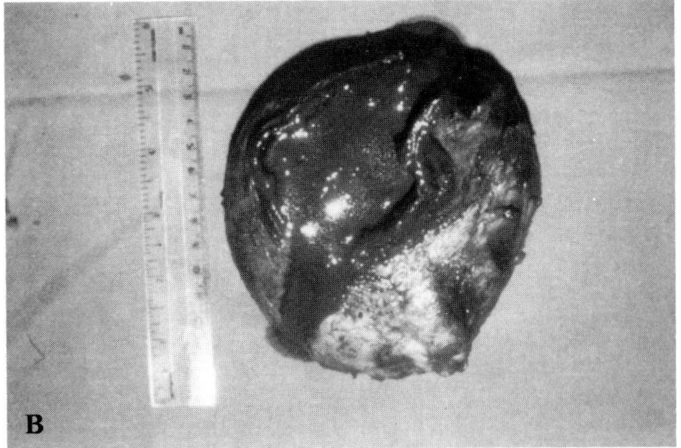

FIG. 45–5. *A* and *B*, Ovarian hematoma/hematocyst.

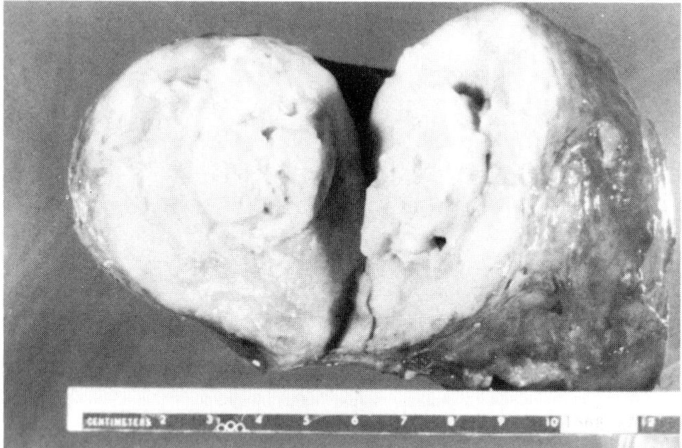

FIG. 45–6. Ovarian abscess; the central cavity is filled with purulent, caseous material.

DIFFERENTIAL DIAGNOSIS OF OVARIAN PROBLEMS IN MARES

The type of ovarian abnormality can be determined by history, palpation, ultrasonography, and hormonal analysis. In cases of an enlarged ovary, the examiner must consider the possibility of normal preovulatory follicles, ovarian neoplasms, anovulatory (autumn) follicles, postovulatory ovarian hematoma, and ovarian abscessation. The ovary contralateral to the enlarged ovary can be an important factor in differential diagnosis of ovarian tumors.[5] Because of their ability to produce and secrete hormones that are suppressive to hypothalamic function, granulosa cell tumors are accompanied by a small, inactive contralateral ovary. A mare with an opposite ovary that ovulates at regular intervals is much more likely to have an ovarian hematoma, teratoma, or cystadenoma than a granulosa cell tumor.

Small inactive ovaries may have several causes. Differential diagnoses include normal diestrous (midluteal) ovaries, seasonal anestrus, severe malnutrition, hypothalamic-anterior pituitary dysfunction, gonadal dysgenesis as a result of chromosomal aberrations, and prepubertal mares. A special situation that may result in small inactive ovaries is the mare placed on anabolic steroids during training to enhance performance. Suppressive effects of anabolic steroids on the reproductive system must be considered in any mare with a history of anabolic steroid treatment.

TREATMENT OF OVARIAN PROBLEMS

Choice of therapy depends on the condition, prognosis, and intended future use of the mare.

HORMONAL

Hormonal treatment is the method of choice for some types of ovarian problems. Persistent transitional follicles or persistent preovulatory follicles can be successfully treated by the administration (IM or IV) of 2000 to 3000 IU of human chorionic gonadotropin (hCG). Ovulation should occur within 48 h of treatment.[6] Similarly, hCG could be used in an attempt to induce ovulation of autumn follicles. However, successful use of hCG for the treatment of this condition has not been documented.

The use of progesterone has been employed for treatment of persistent follicles in transitional-phase mares. The use of 100 mg progesterone in oil administered by intramuscular injection for 7 days[18] or the oral administration of allyl trenbolone (Regumate, Hoechst Roussel, Sommerville, NJ) at a rate of 0.044 mg/kg of body weight for 12 to 15 days[19] suppresses estrous activity and decreases follicular activity within 2 days. Mares exhibit estrus within a few days after withdrawal of treatment. Hormonal therapies for enlarged ovaries caused by neoplasms, especially granulosa cell tumors, have been tried but the results have been poor.

Hormonal therapy for cases of bilateral small, firm ovaries depends on an accurate diagnosis and correct regimen. The use of prostaglandin $F_2\alpha$ to cause regression of an undetectable corpus luteum in diestrous (midluteal) mares causes a rapid drop in serum progesterone concentrations followed by estrus in 2 to 4 days.[20] This therapy will be ineffective on mares that do not have a functional corpus luteum present.

Hormonal treatment to stimulate follicular development and growth on inactive ovaries during the transition period or seasonal anestrus has proven costly and has been largely unsuccessful. Gonadotropin-releasing hormone (GnRH)[21] or GnRH combined with progesterone injections[22] can induce follicular development and ovulation in noncycling mares. However, requirement for multiple treatments and the poor response to therapy is a deterrent to its usage. Similarly, follicle-stimulating hormone (FSH) has proven to be of limited success[23] and pregnant mare serum gonadotropin (PMSG)[24] has proven largely unsuccessful in the stimulation of follicular growth in anestrous mares. Equine pituitary extracts have been used for induction of estrus and superovulation in experimental mares and ponies.[16]

In the cases of mares treated with anabolic steroids, cessation of hormonal therapy may allow small inactive ovaries to resume cyclicity. The use of anabolic steroids such as boldenone undecylenate and nandrolone decanoate in mares in training for athletic competition with the intent of increasing muscle mass and enhancing endurance inhibit hypothalamic and anterior pituitary function with a resultant decrease in gonadotropin secretion. Treated animals often have small, firm, inactive ovaries and exhibit stallion-like behavior. Following withdrawal of the steroids, at least 6 months may be required to regain normal ovarian activity.[6,25]

SURGICAL

Surgical correction is the method of choice for ovarian neoplasms. The surgical approach is most often via flank or ventral midline laparotomy. Pain, discomfort, and edema during the postoperative period were reportedly more severe in animals on which the flank approach was used compared with animals with ventral midline incisions.[1,2] Surgical removal via colpotomy is possible provided the affected ovary is not too large for removal through the vaginal incision. Drainage of fluid-filled cystic structures may enable the surgeon to reduce the size of the ovarian mass to facilitate its removal.

Bilateral ovariectomy is also indicated in the case of virilistic or vicious mares with bilateral ovarian hypoplasia caused by chromosomal abnormalities. Ovarian removal will often result in an improvement in temperament of the involved mare.

As with any surgical procedure, risks of anesthetic problems, intraoperative or postoperative hemorrhage, postoperative wound dehiscence, and postoperative infection are all possibilities that must be considered when arriving at a decision for surgical intervention. In few cases, ovariocentesis has been employed for the treatment of enlarged persistent follicular structures.[2]

The aim of successful treatment of ovarian conditions is return to normal estrous cycles and fertility in the affected animal. In most cases, speed of reversal of altered behavior and return of hormonal fertility depends on the type of ovarian problem and the duration. Hormonal induction of ovulation and hormonal therapy for conversion from the transitional phase results in the reestablishment of normal estrous cycles. Surgical removal of granulosa cell tumors allows the remaining ovary to return to normal activity within a few weeks to many months, depending on the duration of the neoplasm and the season of year when ovariectomy is performed. Mares suffering from bilateral ovarian hypoplasia owing to environmental or disease conditions can return to normal estrous patterns soon after correction of the underlying cause. However, mares suffering from gonadal dysgenesis as a result of chromosomal aberrations have a poor reproductive prognosis. Similarly, mares with dysgerminomas have a poor prognosis because of the metastatic nature of the neoplasm.

REFERENCES

1. Meagher, D.M., et al.: Granulosa cell tumors in mares—A review of 78 cases. Proc. Am. Assoc. Equine Pract., 133–143, 1977.
2. Bosu, W.T.K., Van Camp, S.C., Miller, R.B., and Owen, R.: Ovarian disorders: Clinical and morphological observations in 30 mares. Can. Vet. J., *23:*6–14, 1982.
3. Schmidt, G.R., Cowled, R.R., and Flynn, D.V.: Granulosa cell tumor in a broodmare. J. Am. Vet. Med. Assoc., *169:*635, 1976.
4. Scott, E.A., and Kunze, D.J.: Ovariectomy in the mare: Presurgical, surgical and post-surgical considerations. J. Equine Med. Surg., *1:*5–12, 1977.
5. Hughes, J.P., Stabenfeldt, G.H., and Kennedy, P.C.: The estrous cycle and selected functional and pathologic ovarian abnormalities in the mare. Vet. Clin. North Am. Large Anim. Pract., *2:*225–239, 1980.
6. Neely, D.P., Liu, I.K.M., and Hillman, R.B.: Equine Reproduction. Philadelphia, Veterinary Learning Systems, 1983.
7. Pierson, R.A., and Ginther, O.J.: Follicular population dynamics during the estrous cycle of the mare. Anim. Reprod. Sci., *14:*219–231, 1987.
8. Ginther, O.J.: Ultrasonic imaging of ovarian follicles and corpora lutea. Vet. Clin. North Am. Equine Pract., *4:*197–213, 1988.
9. Hinrichs, K., and Hunt, P.R.: Ultrasound as an aid to diagnosis of granulosa cell tumor in the mare. Equine Vet. J., *4:*99–103, 1990.
10. McKinnon, A.O., Squires, E.L., and Shideler, R.K.: Diagnostic ultrasonography of the mare's reproductive tract. J. Equine Vet. Sci., *8:*329–333, 1988.
11. Meinecke, B., and Gips, H.: Steroid hormone secretory patterns in mares with granulosa cell tumors. J. Vet. Med. Assoc., *34:*545–560, 1987.
12. Stabenfeldt, G.H., et al.: Clinical findings, pathological changes and endocrinological secretory patterns in mares with ovarian tumors. J. Reprod. Fertil. Suppl., *27:*277–285, 1979.
13. Sundberg, J.P., et al.: Neoplasms of Equidae. J. Am. Vet. Med. Assoc., *170:*150–151, 1977.
14. Meuten, D.J., and Rendano, V.: Hypertrophic osteopathy in a mare with a dysgerminoma. Equine Med. Surg., *2:*445–450, 1978.
15. Held, J.P., Buergelt, C., and Colahan, P.: Serous cystadenoma in a mare. J. Am. Vet. Med. Assoc., *181:*496–498, 1982.
16. Ginther, O.J.: Reproductive Biology of the Mare—Basic and Applied Aspects. Cross Plains, WI, published by the author, 1979.
17. Hughes, J.P., Benirschke, K., Kennedy, P.C., and Smith, A.T.: Gonadal dysgenesis in the mare. J. Reprod. Fertil. Suppl., *23:*385–390, 1975.
18. Van Niekerk, C.H., Coubrough, R.I., and Doms, W.H.: Progesterone treatment of mares with abnormal estrous cycles early in the breeding season. J. S. Afr. Vet. Assoc., *44:*37–45, 1973.
19. Squires, E.L., Webel, S.K., Shideler, R.K., and Voss, J.L.: A review on the use of altrenogest for the broodmare. Proc. Am. Assoc. Equine Pract., 221–231, 1981.
20. Allen, W.R., and Rowson, L.E.A.: Control of the mare's oestrous cycle by prostaglandins. J. Reprod. Fertil., *33:*539–543, 1973.
21. Evans, M.J., and Irvine, C.H.G.: Induction of follicular development, maturation and ovulation by gonadotrophin releasing hormone administration to acyclic mares. Biol. Reprod., *16:*452–462, 1977.
22. Evans, M.J., and Irvine, C.H.G.: Induction of follicular development and ovulation in seasonally acyclic mares using gonadotrophin releasing hormone and progesterone. J. Reprod. Fertil. Suppl., *27:*113–121, 1979.
23. Irvine, C.H.G.: Endocrinology of the estrous cycle of the mare: Applications to embryo transfer. Theriogenology, *15:*85–103, 1981.
24. Stewart, F., and Allen, W.R.: The binding of FSH, LH and PMSG to equine gonadal tissue. J. Reprod. Fertil. Suppl., *27:*431–440, 1979.
25. Squires, E.L., Voss, J.L., Maher, J.M., and Shideler, R.K.: Fertility of young mares after long term anabolic steroid treatment. J. Vet. Med. Assoc., *186:*583–587, 1985.

CHAPTER 46

CERVICAL PROBLEMS IN THE MARE

P.L. Sertich

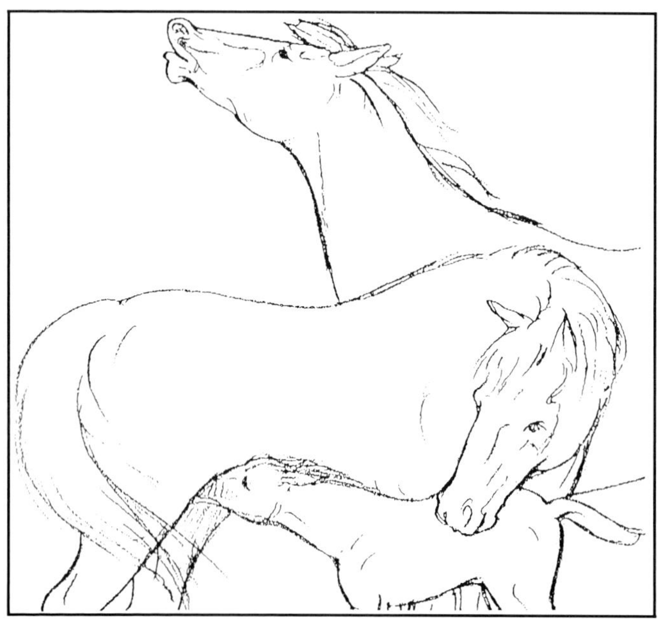

Preceded by the vulvar lips and transverse fold of the vagina, the cervix forms the third barrier between the uterus and the outside environment. The efficacy of these three barriers has been demonstrated.[1] To function normally, the cervix must relax during estrus to allow intrauterine deposition of semen and drainage of uterine secretions, close tightly so the uterus can provide a suitable environment for pregnancy, and dilate to allow passage of a foal at parturition. Mucus produced by the cervical mucosa aids in preventing infectious organisms from entering the uterus, especially when it becomes inspissated during pregnancy. Abnormalities that prevent the cervix from functioning normally may lead to infertility.

Normally, the size, shape, and consistency of the cervix relate to stage of the estrous cycle. Under the influence of progesterone, the cervix is closed, elongated, and tonic. During estrus, when plasma progesterone concentrations are low, the cervix will be relaxed and short; under the influence of estrogens, the cervix becomes edematous and moist. Unlike the cervix of the pluriparous mare, the cervix of a young maiden mare usually does not relax appreciably during estrus.[2] During pregnancy, the cervix elongates greatly and contracts. These pregnancy changes in cervical conformation are caused by luteal progesterone and, as has been shown in the uterus,[3] are probably mediated by a fetal/maternal hormonal interaction. During seasonal anestrus when both plasma estrogen and progesterone are low, the cervix may be closed but easily dilated or it may be short, thin, and open. If the character of the cervix does not relate to stage of the estrous cycle or reproductive status of the mare, the discrepancy must be investigated.

ANATOMY

The cranial paramesonephric or mullerian ducts give rise to the uterine horns. The caudal portion of the ducts fuse to form the uterine body, the cervix, and the cranial two-thirds of the vagina.[4]

The cervix is composed of mucosal and muscular layers. The caudal portion (portio vaginalis cervicis) of the cervix protrudes into the cranial vagina. The mucosa of the portio vaginalis is confluent with that of the vagina whereas the cranial luminal mucosa connects with longitudinal folds of the endometrium. The cervical mucosa is characterized by extensive crypts lined by goblet cells which produce mucus. A tubular, central layer is composed of smooth muscle. A fold of the mucosa may extend onto the wall of the vagina as a frenulum.[5] The average cervix of a nongravid mare is approximately 5 to 7 cm in length and 3 to 5 cm wide.[6]

EXAMINATION OF THE CERVIX

The cervix can be examined by palpation per rectum as well as direct visualization during speculum examination and palpation per vagina. On palpation per rectum, the cervix is compressed between the hand and the mare's pelvis so that the shape and degree of relaxation and edema of the cervix can be estimated and used to predict the state of the ovaries in regard to maturity of follicles and presence of a corpus luteum. Before speculum examination, the mare's perineum should be washed, rinsed, and dried. A sterile tube (approximately 3 × 45 cm) is passed through the retracted vulvar lips and the vestibule, over the transverse fold, and into the vagina. Visualization is accomplished with a light source. The character of the cervix is evaluated as well as the degree of relaxation as indicated by the location of the cervix in the vaginal vault. Thorough examination of the cervix requires direct manual palpation of all layers of the cervix, because some defects are not visible through a speculum. The perineum should be prepared as for a speculum exam and a sterile, gloved hand (lubricated with sterile water-soluble jelly) placed into the vagina. With the index finger or thumb placed into the lumen of the cervix, the entire circumference is carefully evaluated to ensure all layers of the cervix are intact.

PATHOLOGY

CERVICITIS

Inflammation of the cervix is usually associated with endometritis and/or vaginitis. The inflammation may be the result of irritation or infection (Fig. 46–1). Organisms that commonly cause endometritis, including β-hemolytic streptococci, Escherichia coli, Pseudomonas aeruginosa, and Klebsiella pneumoniae,[7] may also be responsible for cervicitis. Other noninfectious irritants such as aspirated air and urine (Fig. 46–2) as well as uterine medications, including antibiotics, antiseptics, and sclerosing medications (Fig. 46–3), can cause cervical inflammation. Removal of the offending organism or source of irritation will usually allow the cervicitis to resolve. Treatment of cervicitis is usually directed at resolving the accompanying endometritis and/or vaginitis.

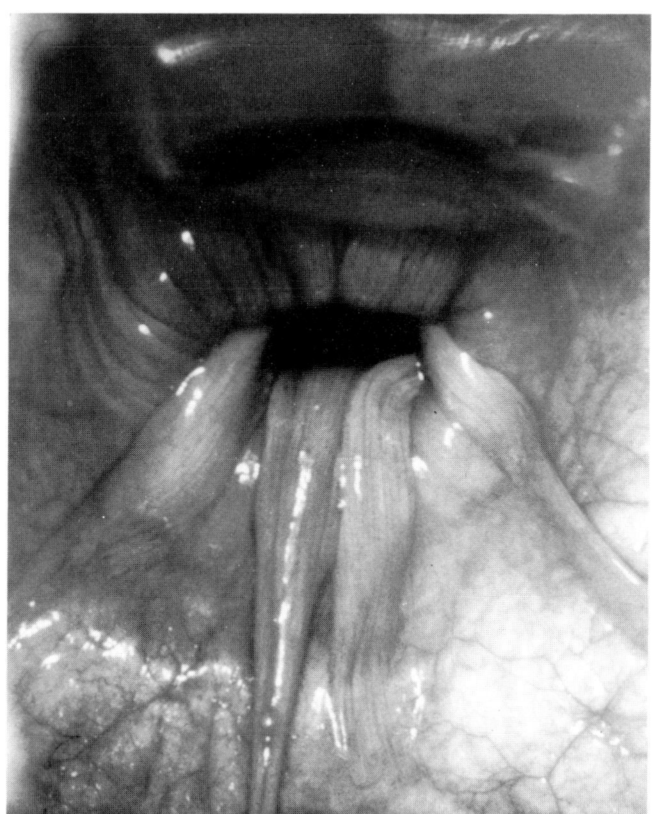

FIG. 46–1. Cervicitis is usually associated with endometritis or vaginitis.

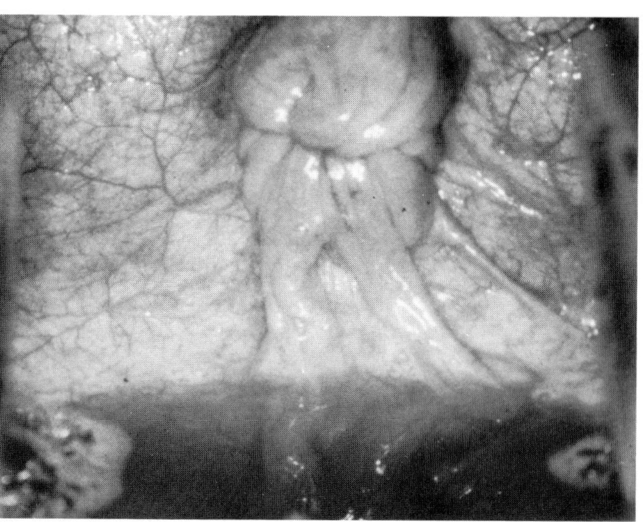

FIG. 46–2. Urovagina can lead to cervicitis because urine causes local irritation.

Infrequently, pregnant mares presented with a vulvar discharge may have cervicitis. The discharge may contain mucus produced by the cervical mucous glands. The infection may initially be localized to the cervix. If the mare is treated parenterally with appropriate antibiotics chosen on the basis of culture and sensitivity, the infection can be controlled with minimal involvement of the conceptus and the pregnancy can still result in a healthy foal.

CERVICAL LACERATIONS

Usually, cervical lacerations occur during parturition and thus are not often seen in maiden mares. Lacerations can occur during what appears to be an otherwise normal parturition. They can also occur during dystocia and subsequent forced extraction of a foal or fetotomy.

Cervical laceration, and particularly partial-thickness laceration, is frequently overlooked during routine breeding soundness examination, usually because of failure to manually examine the entire circumference of the cervix by direct digital palpation. Most lacerations cannot be adequately evaluated on speculum examination (Figs. 46–4 and 46–5). Because not all cervical lacerations will interfere with maintenance of pregnancy, the final decision regarding need for surgical

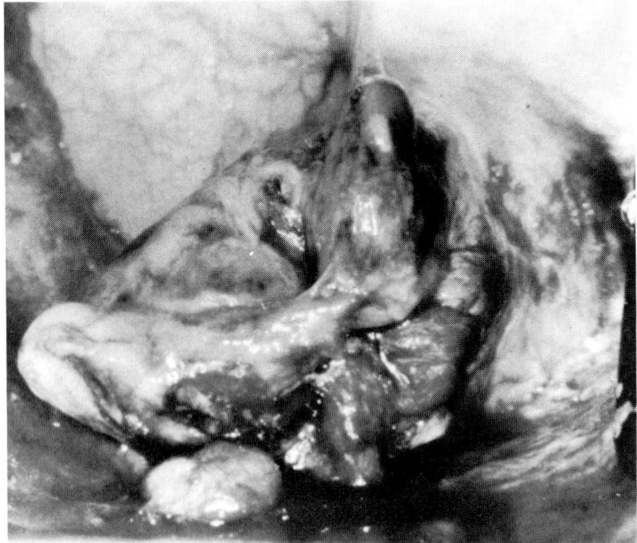

FIG. 46–3. Severe cervicitis after administration of uterine sulfa urea boluses containing acriflavin.

correction depends on the degree of competency of the cervical canal. Evaluation of the cervix must be performed while it is under the influence of either endogenous or exogenous progesterone to determine whether the cervix is able to close adequately.

Lacerations can be successfully corrected surgically with a high rate of subsequent pregnancy.[8] An endometrial biopsy is recommended before performing genital surgery to be sure the uterus does not have other abnormalities that may reduce the mare's chances of carrying a live foal to term. Surgical repair can be performed after foal heat when the cervix is under the influence of progesterone. The mare can generally be bred 30 days after repair and, ideally, should be bred by artificial insemination. If the mare is bred by natural service too soon after surgical repair, the sutured laceration may be torn. A breeding roll may help prevent deep penetration by the stallion during copulation. Pregnancy has also been established when the surgical repair is performed 2 to 3 days after breeding and ovulation. Repair of the cervix may have to be repeated after each subsequent foaling. The surgical procedures are discussed in Chapter 51.

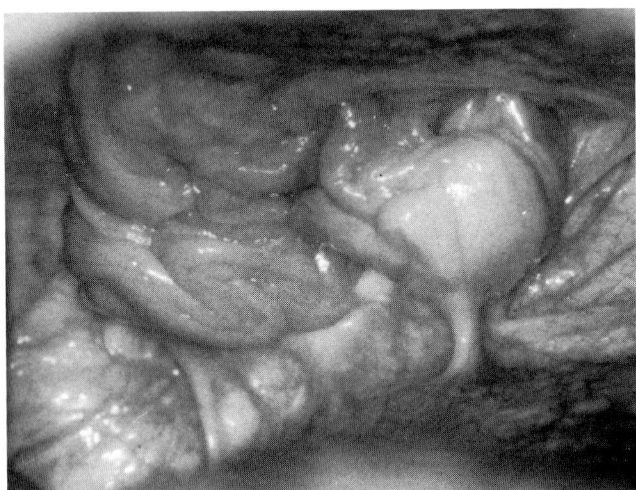

FIG. 46–4. Cervical lacerations at the 12 and 7 o'clock positions.

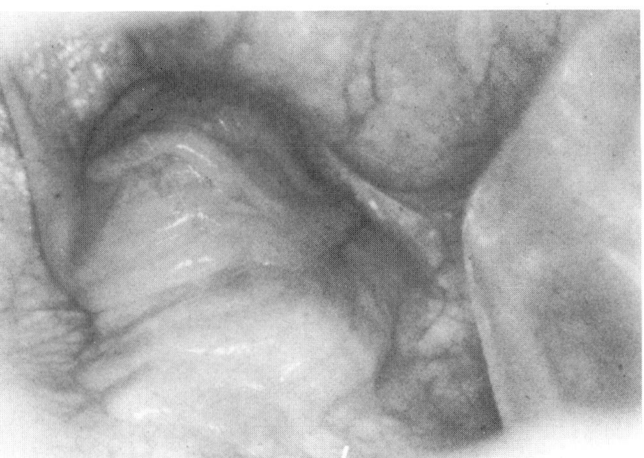

FIG. 46–5. Cervical lacerations at the 3 and 9 o'clock positions. Note the difficulty of visually assessing these defects.

CERVICAL ADHESIONS

The function of the cervix can be altered by cervical adhesions. Transluminal adhesions can prevent the cervix from opening as well as occlude the lumen (Fig. 46–6). This may result in excessive accumulation of fluid within the uterine lumen. Adhesions can also prevent the cervix from closing adequately to support pregnancy. This happens when the vaginal portion of the cervix is displaced and adheres to the vaginal wall. Adhesions may be thin and strand-like or thick.

Adhesions can form after trauma to the cervix during parturition and may be associated with a cervical laceration. They can also be of iatrogenic origin from overaggressive uterine therapy with caustic or irritating agents. Severe inflammation of the cervix and vagina with tissue sloughing can result in adhesions.

Diagnosis of cervical adhesions can be made by speculum examination, but accurate assessment of the lesion requires manual palpation per vagina of the cervix. Treatment of adhesions includes manual breaking down of the fibrous tissue by blunt dissection. Adhesions must be broken down daily because they regrow rapidly. Application of an antibiotic ointment containing corticosteroids will slow the regrowth of the adhesions. In some cases, soon after daily manipulation of the cervix is discontinued, the adhesions reoccur. An in-dwelling catheter through the cervix may help prevent transluminal adhesions from occluding the cervix. It may be necessary to cut extensive adhesions with long-handled scissors. The adhesions are more easily

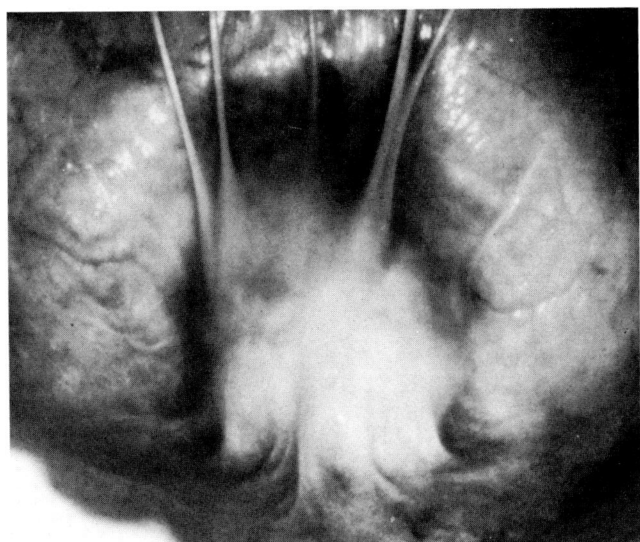

FIG. 46-6. Severe transluminal adhesions that completely occlude the cervix.

identified and cut if two traction sutures are placed through each side of the cervix.

DEVELOPMENTAL ANOMALIES—SEGMENTAL APLASIA, HYPOPLASIA, AND DOUBLE CERVIX

The absence of a cervix caused by segmental aplasia of the paramesonephric duct has been reported in a pony mare.[9] Hypoplasia of the cervix is rare in the mare. It has been seen in a mare with normal ovarian activity.[10] Pregnancy can be established and maintained with a retention suture being placed around the cervix to close it.[11] Mares with gonadal dysgenesis and 63 XO karyotype usually have a small, tubular, flaccid reproductive tract.[12,13] This is the result of a lack of ovarian hormones.[14,15] One horse with a 64 XY karyotype that was phenotypically female lacked a uterus and cervix.[13]

Four cases of double cervix caused by incomplete fusion of mullerian ducts are described in the literature.[16] Three of the four cases were in Clydesdale or Clydesdale-cross mares. Although one of the mares foaled normally, abortion and infertility also occurred. The relationship of this anomaly to fertility is unclear.

HYPERPLASIA AND NEOPLASIA

One case of cervical hyperplasia has been reported[17] in a 5-yr-old maiden mare. The mass was benign and no evidence of inflammation was present. It is not known whether this was a developmental or acquired problem. The mare had been hospitalized for suspected uterine prolapse.

Neoplasia of the cervix is rare in the mare. Recurrent uterocervical leiomyomas in two half-siblings have been reported.[18] The masses were removed surgically but recurred.

In a case presented to our clinic, a large (7 × 4 × 4 cm) fibroma of the cervix caused interference with the function of the cervix. The mass was surgically removed and the incision site repaired by three-layer closure. Sufficient normal cervix remained so that a competent cervical canal was formed.

REFERENCES

1. Hinrichs, K., Cummings, M.R., Sertich, P.L., and Kenney, R.M.: Clinical significance of aerobic bacterial flora of the uterus, vagina, vestibule, and clitoral fossa of clinically normal mares. J. Am. Vet. Med. Assoc., *193:*72–75, 1988.
2. Greenhoff, G.R., and Kenney, R.M.: Evaluation of reproductive status of nonpregnant mares. J. Am. Vet. Med. Assoc., *176:*449–458, 1975.
3. Hayes, K.E.N., and Ginther, O.J.: Role of progesterone and estrogen in development of uterine tone in mares. Theriogenology, *25:*581–590, 1986.
4. Roberts, S.J.: Veterinary Obstetrics and Genital Diseases (Theriogenology). 3rd ed. Woodstock, VT, published by the author, 1986.
5. Ginther, O.J.: Reproductive Biology of the Mare—Basic and Applied Aspects. Cross Plains, WI, published by the author, 1979.
6. Getty, R.: Sisson and Grossman's The Anatomy of the Domestic Animals. Philadelphia, W.B. Saunders, 1975.
7. Conboy, H.S.: Diagnosis and therapy of equine endometritis. Proc. Am. Assoc. Equine Pract., 165–171, 1978.
8. Brown, J.S., Varner, D.D., Hinrichs, K., and Kenney, R.M.: Surgical repair of the lacerated cervix in the mare. Theriogenology, *22:*351–359, 1984.
9. Schlotthauer, C.F., and Zollman, P.E.: The occurrence of so-called "white heifer disease" in a white Shetland Pony mare, J. Am. Vet. Med. Assoc., *129:*309–310, 1956.
10. Blanchard, T.L., et al.: Congenitally incompetent cervix in a mare. J. Am. Vet. Med. Assoc., *181:*266, 1982.
11. Evans, L.H., Tate, L.P., Cooper, W.L., and Robertson, J.T.: Surgical repair of cervical lacerations and the incompetent cervix. Proc. Am. Assoc. Equine Pract., 483–486, 1979.
12. Hughes, J.P., Benirschke, K., Kennedy, P.C., and Trommershausen-Smith, A.: Gonadal dysgenesis in the mare. J. Reprod. Fertil. Suppl., *23:*385–390, 1975.
13. Bowling, A.T., Millon, L., and Hughes, J.P.: An update of chromosomal abnormalities in mares. J. Reprod. Fertil. Suppl., *35:*149–155, 1987.
14. Pashen, R.L., Downie, C., and McCue, P.: An attempt to use progesterone treated XO mares as embryo recipients. Equine Vet. J. Suppl., *8:*59–61, 1989.
15. Hinrichs, K., Riera, F.L., and Klunder, L.R.: Establishment of pregnancy after embryo transfer in mares with gonadal dysgenesis. J. In Vitro Fertil. Embryo Transf., *6:*305–309, 1989.
16. Volkmann, D.H., and Gilbert, R.O.: Uterus bicollis in a Clydesdale mare. Equine Vet. J., *21:*71, 1989.
17. Riera, F.L., Hinrichs, K., Hunt, P.R., and Kenney, R.M.: Cervical hyperplasia with prolapse in a mare. J. Am. Vet. Med. Assoc., *195:*1393–1394, 1989.
18. Romagnoli, S.E., Momont, H.W., Hilbert, B.J., and Metz, A.: Multiple recurring uterocervical leiomyomas in two half-sibling Appaloosa fillies. J. Am. Vet. Med. Assoc., *191:*1449–1450, 1987.

CHAPTER 47

DEVELOPMENTAL ANOMALIES OF THE FEMALE REPRODUCTIVE TRACT

J.P. Hughes

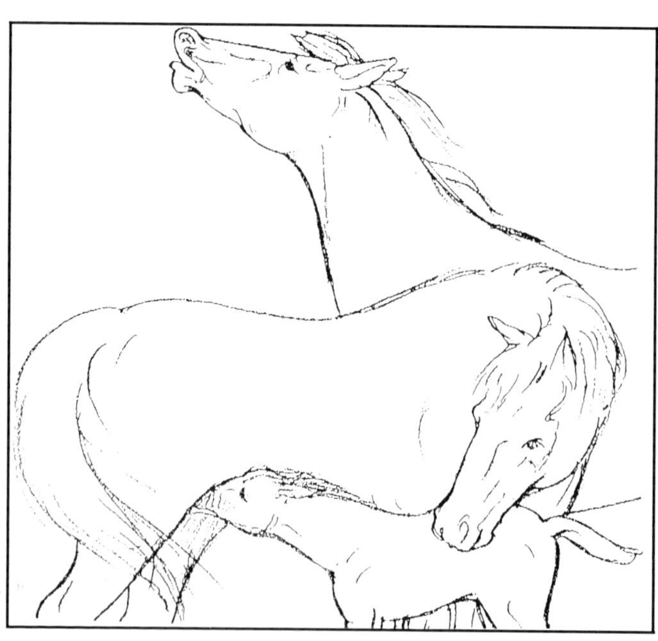

Chromosomal or genetic sex is established at time of fertilization; the heterogametic XY is male and homogametic XX is female. The sex chromosomes determine whether the indifferent gonad will develop into a testis or an ovary.[1] Genes associated with the Y chromosome initiate development of seminiferous tubules. H-Y antigen complex is responsible in some part for testicular differentiation.

Müllerian-inhibiting substance (MIS), produced by Sertoli's cells from the testes, suppresses müllerian duct development, and thus the uterus, fallopian tubes, and anterior vagina do not develop.[2] In the absence of MIS the müllerian ducts develop to form fallopian tubes, uterus, and anterior vagina. Thus adequate amounts of MIS must be secreted by the developing testes to inhibit development of internal female genitalia.[1,2]

Testosterone, secreted by the fetal testes, stimulates wolffian ducts to form into epididymides, vasa deferentia, and seminal vesicles. Testosterone is converted locally to dihydrotestosterone, which induces formation of the male external genitalia (penis, prepuce, and scrotum) and the prostate.[1,2] Thus chromosomal sex determines gonadal sex, and gonadal sex determines phenotypic sex.[2] In the absence of the testes, phenotypic development is female: The müllerian duct system develops, the wolffian duct system regresses, and the external genitalia (vulva, posterior vagina, and clitoris) develop as a phenotypic female.[2,3] The female tubular genitalia do not require hormones secreted by the fetal ovary to develop.

It can be appreciated that when there is disturbance in any part of this chain of events, abnormal development may occur. An animal with testes but ambiguous external genitalia may result from insufficient testosterone production, a deficiency in the enzyme (5α-reductase), which converts testosterone to dihydrotestosterone, or end organ insensitivity may exist with testicular feminization.[1]

Heredity and environment both play important roles in developmental anomalies. Some congenital malformations are undoubtedly the result of environmental factors such as progesterone, poisonous plants, and other agents to which the animal is exposed at a critical time. The embryo is susceptible to teratogenic stimuli during early development and the response to the teratogen is influenced by the genotype of the embryo.[4]

DEVELOPMENTAL DEFECTS

Ambiguous external genitalia and abnormalities of chromosomal and genital sex are discussed in Chapter 30.

VULVA

Pneumovagina associated with poor vulvar conformation is the most commonly encountered vulvar abnormality in the mare (Figs. 47–1 and 47–2). The problem has probably been accentuated by the selection of

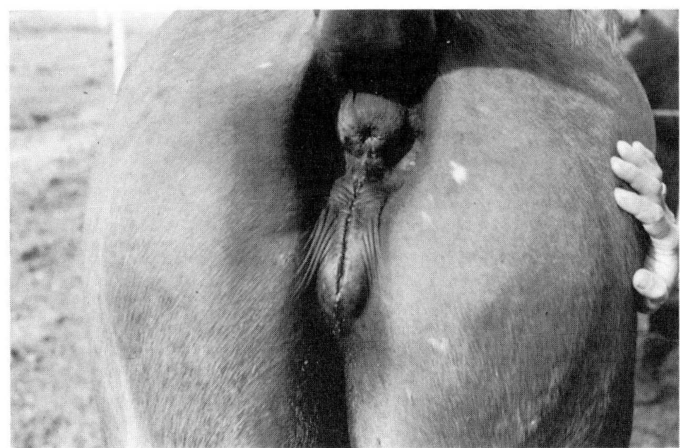

FIG. 47–1. Tilted vulva of a young mare, which will become more pronounced with age. The condition is associated with pneumovagina (wind sucking).

mares for speed, performance, and conformation without regard to reproductive health.

CLITORIS

Most cases of clitoral enlargement in the horse are associated with some form of hermaphroditism. The most common form encountered is the male pseudohermaphrodite with testes and a 64,XX karyotype. The vulva is often displaced ventrally with varying degrees of enlargement of the clitoris to one resembling a short penis[6] (Fig. 47–3). An occasional mare is encountered with an enlarged clitoris and failure to cycle caused by anabolic steroids administered during her training or racing career. These mares should be considered but not confused with the intersex animal described previously. The ovaries exhibit varying degrees of inactivity but are otherwise normal in size and shape. The internal and external genitalia are normal except for the somewhat enlarged clitoris.

Exogenous androgen therapy given to the pregnant

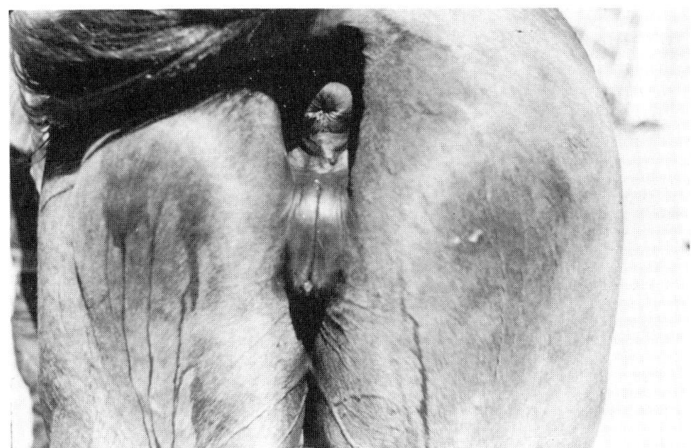

FIG. 47–2. External genitalia of a mare with a sunken anus creating a "shelf" with the dorsal vulvar lips horizontal.

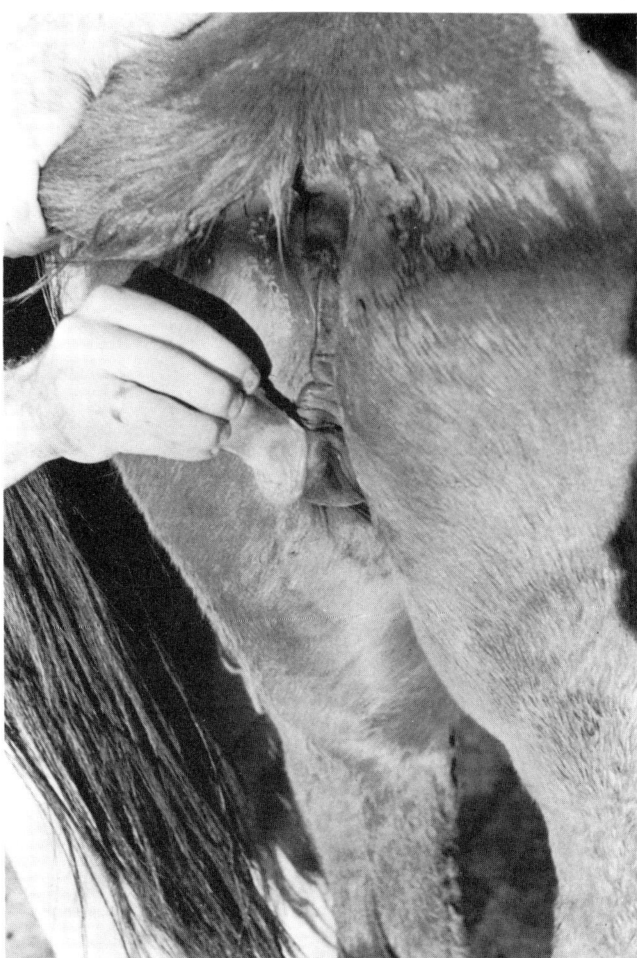

FIG. 47–3. Male pseudohermaphrodite with the clitoris resembling a short penis. The gonads were testes and the karyotype 64,XX.

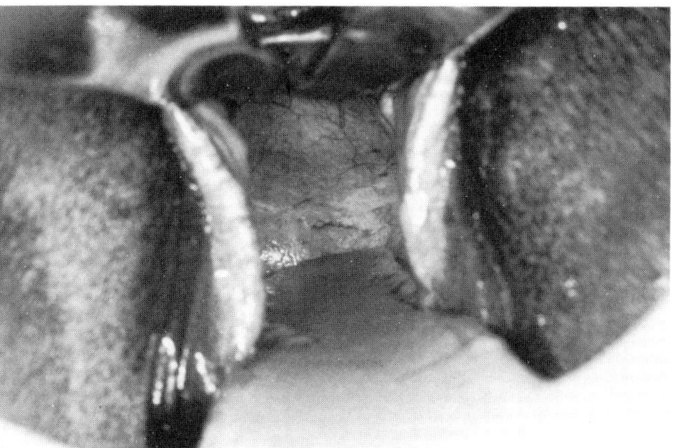

FIG. 47–4. Speculum view of the vagina ending in a blind pouch. This was a mare with testicular feminization. The cervix and uterus were absent, the gonads were testes, and the karyotype was 64,XY.

mare during organogenesis has the potential to result in clitoral enlargement. In a study in which altrenogest, a synthetic progestagen, was administered per os from day 20 to day 320 of gestation, the females born to the treated animals had clitori larger than normal from birth through 21 months (until the end of the test period).[5] However, no effect on fertility was noted.

ANTERIOR VAGINA, CERVIX, AND UTERUS

Developmental anomalies of the anterior vagina, cervix, and uterus of the mare are the result of partial or complete inhibition of müllerian ducts. These anomalies are rare in the mare, but appear to occur more frequently in the cervix than in the vagina or uterus[6] (Fig. 47–4).

One mare was reported to have a divided vagina with a separate cervix for each half.[7] A Clydesdale mare with a double cervix and a curtain of tissue dividing the anterior vagina has been described;[6] another Clydesdale mare was documented with a divided cervix and a uterine body divided by a complete wall;[8] and a third had a duplication of the caudal portion of the cervix.[9]

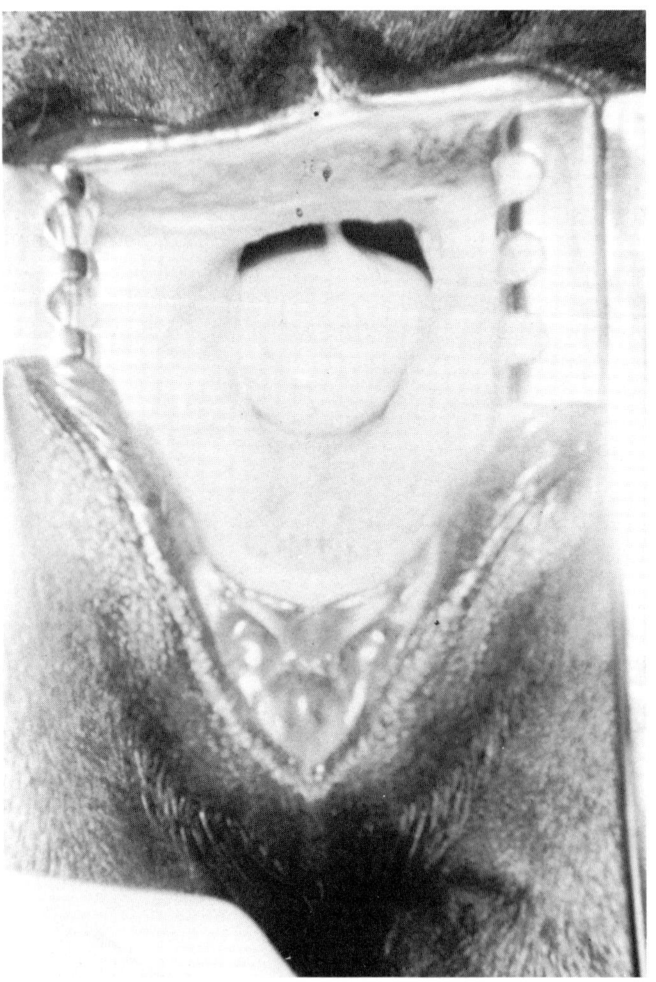

FIG. 47–5. A persistent hymen in a mare. The vulvar lips have been pulled to the side. This has a more bladder-like appearance than most persistent hymen and obstructs our view of the urethral orifice.

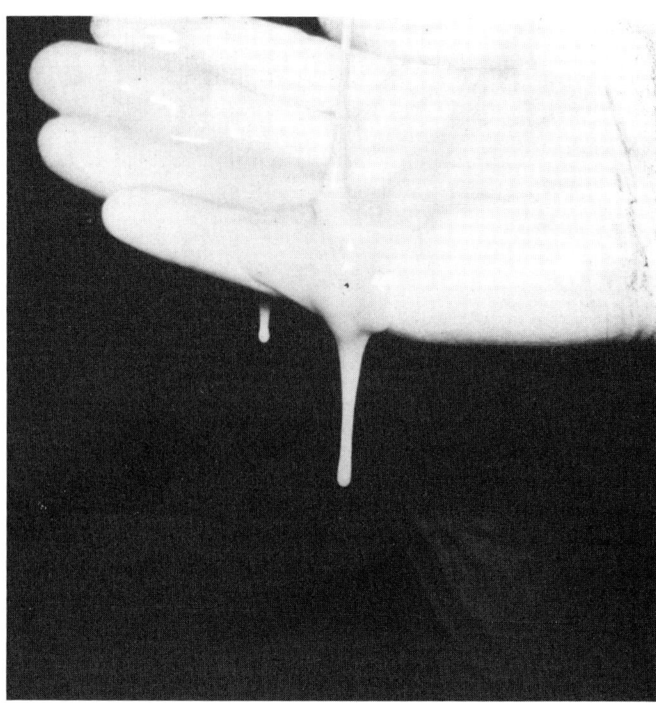

FIG. 47–6. Mucoid secretions that accumulated behind an intact persistent hymen.

A case of cervical hypoplasia was reported in a 2-yr-old Thoroughbred filly. The mare had persistent pneumovagina and a short cervix (1 to 1.5 cm), which was incompetent.[10] A pony mare with no cervix and no outlet from the uterus to the vagina has been described.[11]

A congenitally absent or short uterine body was reported in a 7-yr-old Quarter Horse mare with a history of repeated abortions. Abortion was attributed to insufficient placental surface leading to inadequate nutrition for the developing fetus.[12]

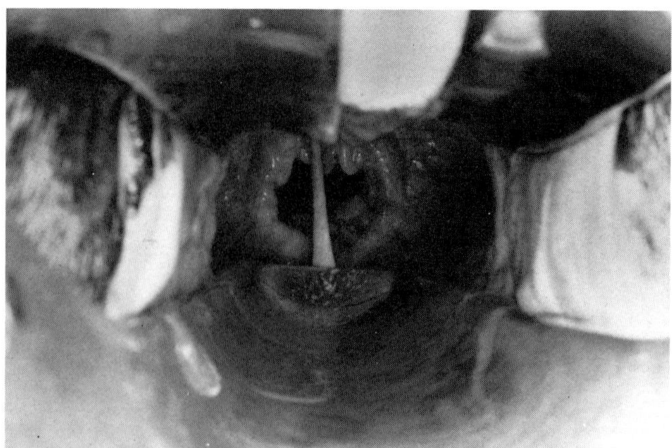

FIG. 47–7. Dorsoventral band in the anterior vagina across the external os of the cervix. These bands are considered to be remnants of the paramesonephric (müllerian) ducts.

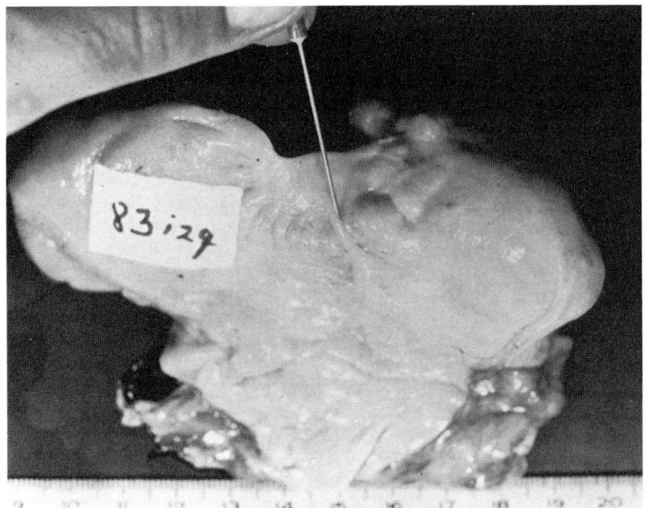

FIG. 47–8. A fibrous band between the ovary and uterus crossing the oviduct.

PERSISTENT HYMEN

Although not common, persistent hymen is certainly the most frequently observed developmental anomaly of the mare's tubular genital system[6] (Fig. 47–5). The hymen may be imperforate or be present in varying degrees because of failure of the caudal sections of the müllerian duct to fuse with the urogenital sinus. While the condition is not usually a threat to fertility, secretions may collect within the uterus with their outflow blocked by the imperforate hymen (Fig. 47–6). Chronic distension of the uterus or contamination of the secretions by bacteria may result in infertility.[13]

Failure of proper fusion of the müllerian ducts may result in a dorsoventral band in the anterior vagina across the external os of the cervix (Fig. 47–7). Easily snipped with scissors, the bands are no impediment to reproduction.

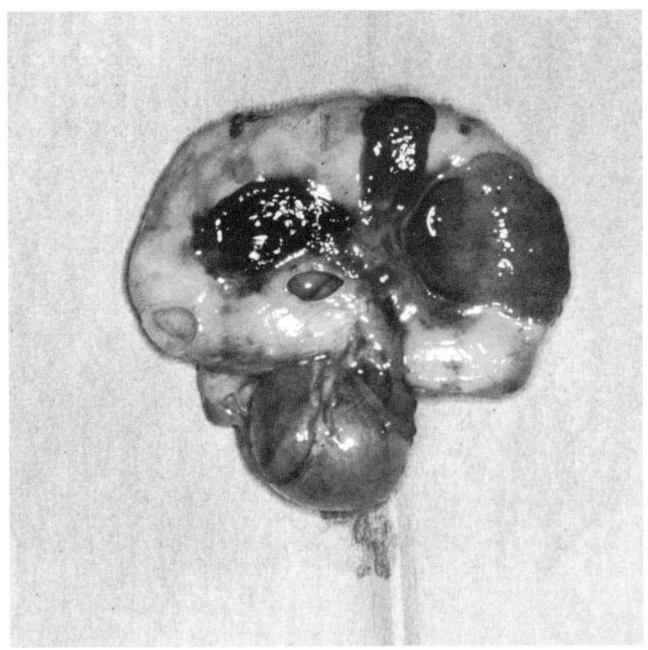

FIG. 47–10. A cyst in the region of the ovulation fossa. Cysts in this area are probably of paramesonephric (müllerian) origin.

FALLOPIAN TUBE (UTERINE TUBE)

Although adhesions of the infundibulum to the ovary, uterus, or mesovarial border of the broad ligament are common (Fig. 47–8), fallopian tube abnormalities of any consequence in the mare are rare.[6,13,14] A tubo-ovarian cyst has been described which contained 200 to 250 mL of clear fluid. The ovarian end of the uterine tube was attached to the ovary, forming a cyst. Whether the structure was congenital or the result of inflammation was unknown.[15]

Hydrosalpinx, distension of the uterine tube with fluid, is usually secondary to external pressure from adhesions obstructing the lumen.[6,13] I had one case of a

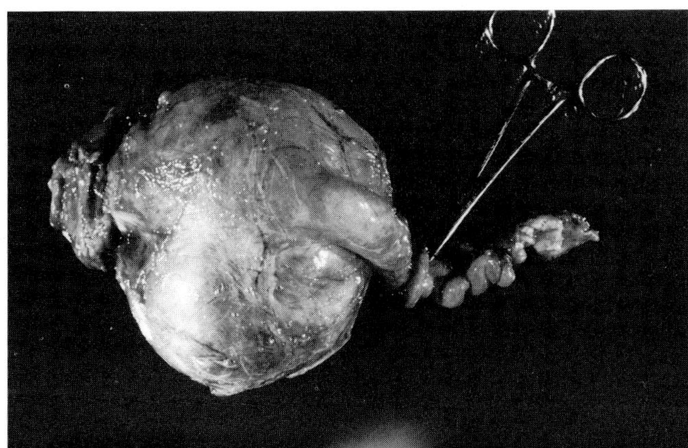

FIG. 47–9. A rare case of cystic hydrosalpinx. The uterine tube that continues from the cystic area is at the tip of the forceps.

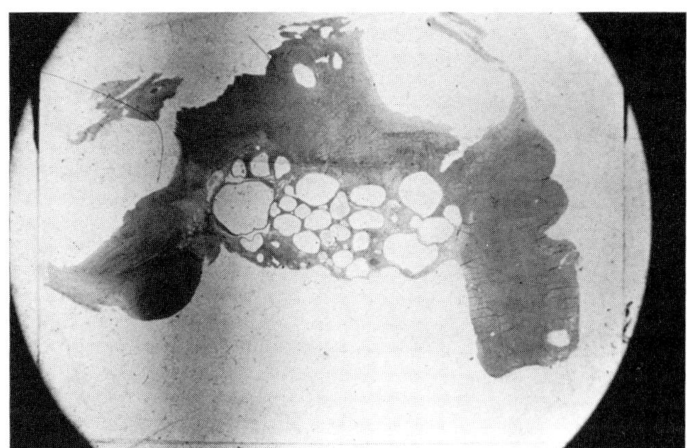

FIG. 47–11. Inclusion cysts within the ovarian tissue around the ovulation fossa. Formed in older mares, they may obstruct release of the ova.

cystic hydrosalpinx, which was probably a developmental anomaly (Fig. 47–9).

Cysts of various sizes are quite common in the region of the ovulation fossa around the ovary (Fig. 47–10), along the fimbria and mesovarium.[15–17] Cysts in the region of the ovulation fossa are of paramesonephric (müllerian) origin whereas the parovarian cysts are considered to be of mesonephric (wolffian) origin.[6,16,17] The cysts are of no clinical significance concerning reproductive performances. Inclusion cysts ("fossa cysts") are found within the ovarian tissue around the ovulation fossa and arise from the surface epithelium. These cysts become numerous in some older mares and may obstruct release of the egg from the ovulation fossa or render the ovary nonfunctional.[6,17] (Fig. 47–11).

Genital tracts were collected from 2297 mares at slaughter over a period of 3 yr. No congenital abnormalities of the reproductive tract were found in this study.[15]

Endometrial cysts are frequently found in the uterus of the mare (Fig. 47–12). Developing as cystic distension of uterine glands they may enlarge to extend beyond the surface of the endometrium as a fluid-filled sac[18] (Fig. 47–13). Lymphatic lacunae are cysts appearing as single or multisacular fluid-filled structures within the endometrium[18] (Fig. 47–14). They occur in older mares and have an uncertain pathogenesis. These endometrial cysts and lymphatic lacunae are not congenital. They can be confused with early stages of pregnancy both on palpation and ultrasonography of the uterus per rectum.

OVARY

As noted in Chapter 30, gonadal hypoplasia is most often associated with the following chromosomal abnormalities: 63,X; 64,XY; 63,X/64XX; 63X/64XY; 64,XX del Xp; 65XXX. The uteri and cervices of these mares are small and flaccid on rectal palpation, and an open cervix is found on speculum examination[19] (Fig. 47–15). The ovaries are small, smooth, and firm (Fig. 47–16), with follicles occasionally noted in the 63,X/64XX and the 64,XX del Xp. All mares with small ovaries are not chromosomally abnormal. Normal mares with small ovaries and in winter anestrus may also have little, if any, follicular activity.

Teratomas also are rarely seen in the mare (Fig. 47–17). I have observed teratomas containing cystic areas with hair or combinations of cysts with hair and firm areas of bone and/or cartilage. A teratoma in an 8-yr-old Arabian mare consisted of mineralyzed dental tissue, which resembled well-differentiated teeth with recognizable pulp cavities. The ovarian teratoma

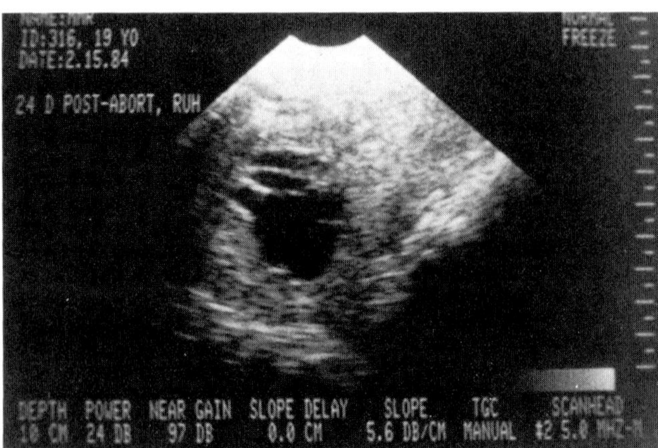

FIG. 47–12. Ultrasonic image of endometrial cysts.

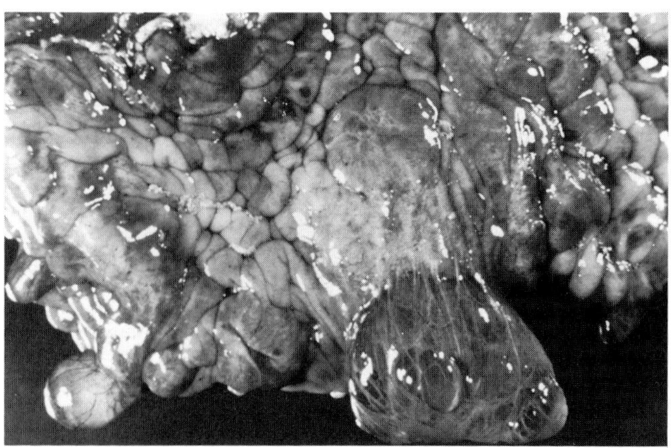

FIG. 47–13. Gross view of endometrial cysts extending beyond the surface of the endometrium.

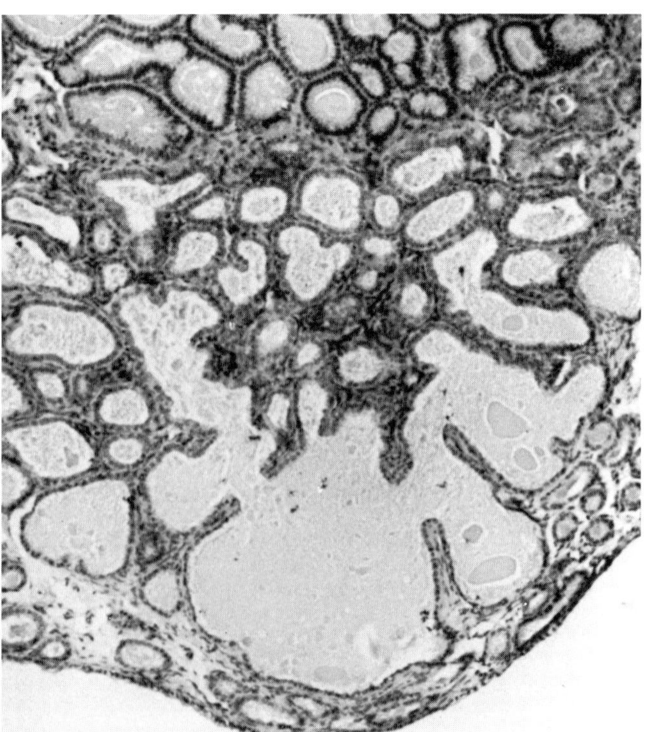

FIG. 47–14. Endometrium of a mare showing a developing lymphatic lacuna.

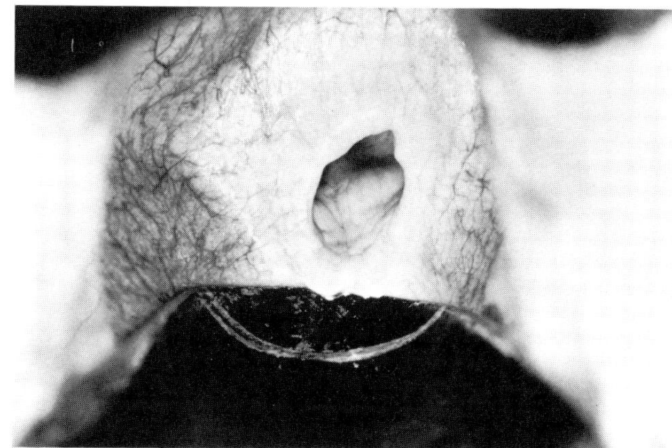

FIG. 47-15. An open cervix as often observed on speculum examination of the vagina of a mare with gonadal dysgenesis and a 63,X karyotype.

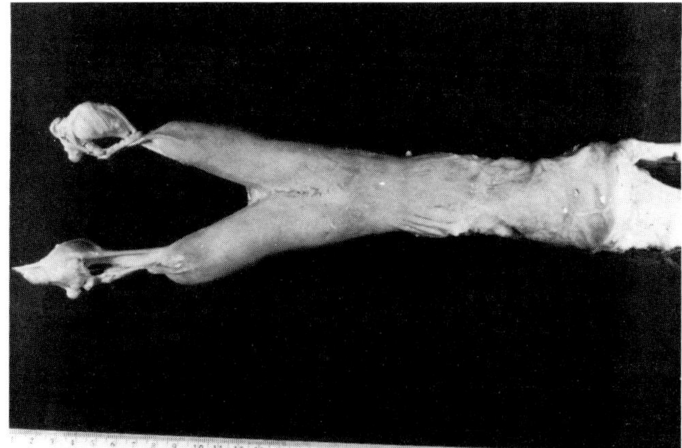

FIG. 47–16. Ventral view of the reproductive tract of a 63,X mare illustrating the small, smooth, and inactive ovaries.

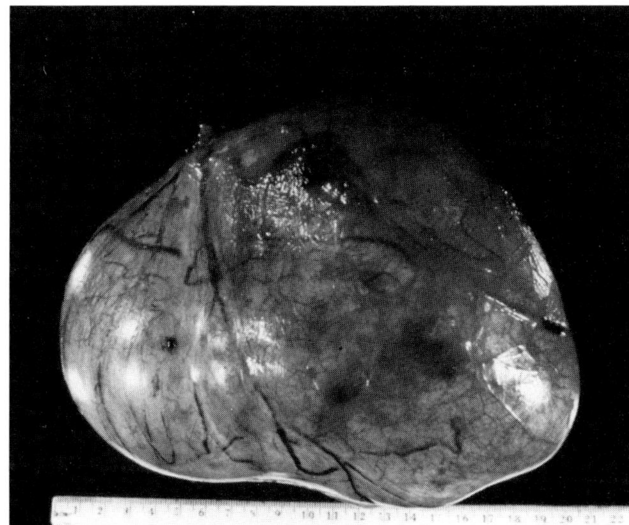

FIG. 47–17. A large teratoma removed from a maiden mare. On cross section this teratoma was made up of cartilage and a large cavity filled with hair.

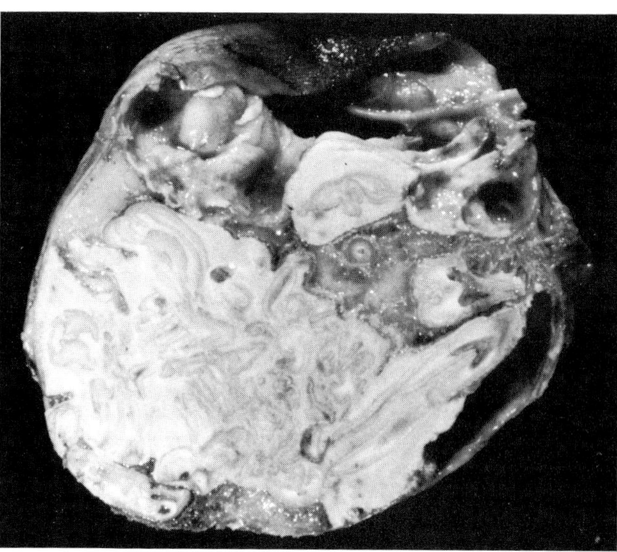

FIG. 47–18. Cross section of a large (2.3 kg) teratoma consisting of mineralized dental tissue.

weighed 2.34 kg and measured 14 × 11.5 cm. It did not affect the mare's estrous cycles or fertility (Fig. 47–18).

REFERENCES

1. Robboy, S.J., Lombardo, J.M., and Welch, W.R.: Disorders of abnormal sexual development. *In* Pathology of the Female Genital Tract. 3rd ed. Edited by R.J. Kurman. New York, Springer-Verlag, 1987, pp. 15–33.
2. Griffin, J.E., and Wilson, J.D.: The syndromes of androgen resistance. N. Engl. J. Med., *302:*198–209, 1980.
3. Ferm, V.H.: Developmental malformations as manifestations of reproductive failure. *In* Comparative Aspects of Reproductive Failure. Edited by K. Benirschke. New York, Springer-Verlag, 1966, pp. 246–255.
4. Meyers-Wallen, V.N., and Patterson, D.F.: Disorders of sexual development in the dog. *In* Current Therapy in Theriogenology 2. Edited by D.A. Morrow. Philadelphia, W.B. Saunders, 1986, pp. 567–574.
5. Shoemaker, C.F., Squires, E.L., and Shideler, R.K.: Safety of altrenogest in pregnant mares and on health and development of offspring. J. Equine Vet. Sci., *9:*69–72, 1989.
6. McEntee, K.: Reproductive Pathology of Domestic Animals. San Diego, Academic Press, 1990.
7. Volkmann, D.H., and Gilbert, R.O.: Uterus bicollis in a Clydesdale mare. Equine Vet. J., *21:*71, 1989.
8. Blue, M.G.: A uterocervical anomaly (uterus bicorpor bicollis) in a mare, and the manual disruption of early bilateral pregnancies. N.Z. Vet. J., *33:*17–19, 1985.
9. Macrae, D.R.: Double os uteri in a mare. Vet. Rec., *15:*1100, 1935.
10. Blanchard, T.L., et al.: Congenitally incompetent cervix in a mare. J. Am. Vet. Med. Assoc., *181:*266, 1982.
11. Schlotthauer, C.F., and Zollman, P.E.: The occurrence of so-called "white heifer disease" in a Shetland Pony mare. J. Am. Vet. Med. Assoc., *129:*309–310, 1956.
12. Meyers, P.J., and Varner, D.D.: Habitual abortion associ-

ated with a congenitally absent or short uterine body in a mare. J. Am. Vet. Med. Assoc. In press.

13. Jubb, K.V.F., and Kennedy, P.C.: Pathology of Domestic Animals. Vol. 1. 2nd ed. New York, Academic Press, 1970.
14. Henry, M., and Vandeplassche, M.: Pathology of the oviduct in mares. Vlaams Diergeneeskundig Tijdschr., *50:*301–325, 1981.
15. Blue, M.G.: A tubo-ovarian cyst, para ovarian cysts and lesions of the oviduct in the mare. N.Z. Vet. J., *33:*8–10, 1985.
16. Osborne, V.E.: Photographic display of various anomaloxis and aberrant fluid-filled sacs which may confuse diagnostic procedures and the accuracy of ultrasonic echography in the mare. J. Reprod. Fertil. Suppl., *35:*665, 1987.
17. Oshea, J.D.: A histological study of non-follicular cysts in the ovulation fossa region of the equine ovary. J. Mophol., *124:*313–320, 1968.
18. Kenney, R.M., and Ganjam, V.K.: Selected pathological changes of the mare uterus and ovary. J. Reprod. Fertil. Suppl., *23:*335–339, 1975.
19. Hughes, J.P., and Trommershausen-Smith, A.: Infertility in the horse associated with chromosomal abnormalities. Aust. Vet. J., *53:*253–257, 1977.

SECTION E

REPRODUCTIVE SURGERY OF THE MARE

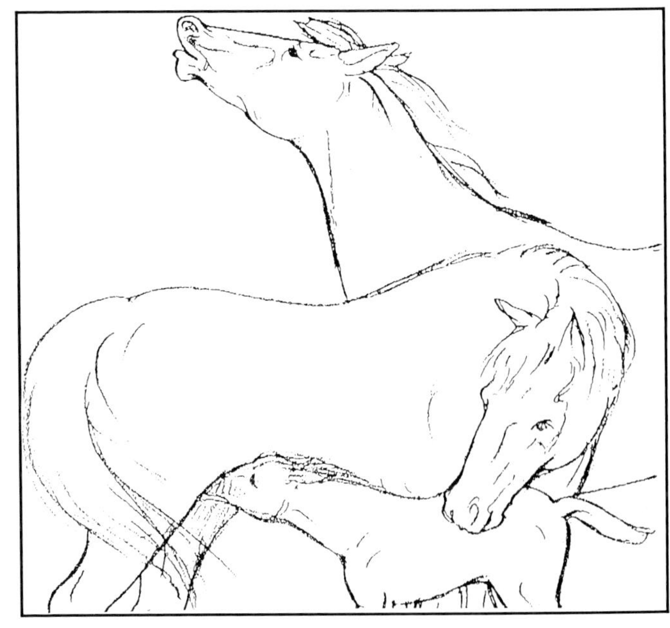

CHAPTER 48

SURGERY OF THE PERINEUM IN THE MARE

G.W. Trotter

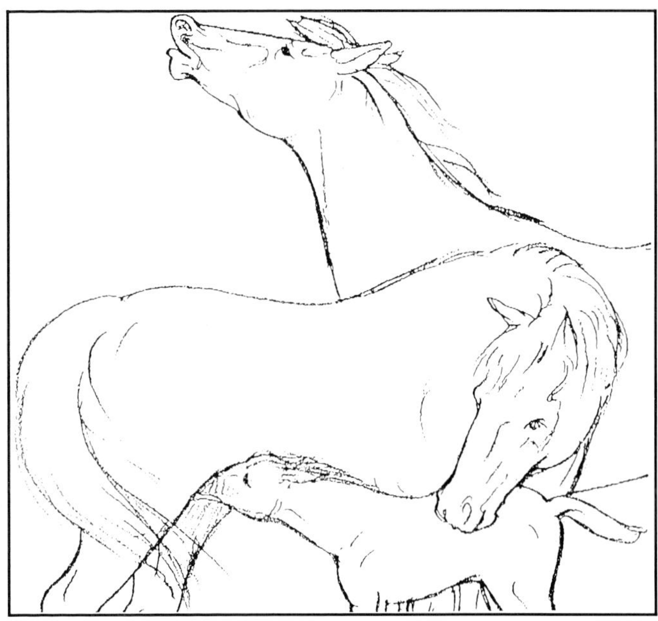

Perineal surgery in the mare is usually performed to correct inherent perineal conformation abnormalities or damage from breeding or foaling trauma. A common sequel to perineal trauma is disruption of protective barriers that prevent contamination of the cranial reproductive tract.[1–3] The constrictor vulvae muscles form the first barrier; the vestibular sphincter, the second; and the cervix, the third. When any of these protective barriers is rendered incompetent, contamination of the cranial reproductive tract can occur. Aspiration of air into the cranial vagina occurs initially (pneumovagina), but particulate matter and/or urine gain access to the vagina in more severely or chronically affected cases.

Many of the anatomic conditions that predispose to pneumovagina can also predispose to urovagina or urine pooling.[4] This should be considered when both evaluating and planning treatment for mares having poor reproductive performance. A combination of medical and surgical treatments may be necessary in a given mare to resolve reproductive problems. For a more complete discussion of perineal conformation, see Chapter 2.

PREOPERATIVE CONSIDERATIONS

Rectal palpation and ultrasonography of the uterus and a speculum examination of the vagina and vestibule should be done on any mare that has had a foaling injury. In addition, mares that have poor perineal conformation and unsatisfactory reproductive performance should be carefully evaluated (see Chapters 22 to 29 for detailed discussion on evaluation). If exudate is present at the cervix or in the vagina, a culture should be taken for bacterial isolation and sensitivity. An ancillary aid that should often be included is uterine biopsy. Although many mares with perineal lacerations and gross fecal contamination of the vagina will conceive after surgery, a uterine biopsy is justified to eliminate a mare from having surgery that has no chance of conception.[4] In mares for which pneumovagina is suspected, but cannot be confirmed on physical examination, ultrasonography can sometimes detect air in the uterus.[5] Other factors to consider before surgery for many conditions affecting the perineum include the age of the mare, her previous breeding history, whether artificial insemination is available or breeding must be by natural cover, potential heritability of the problem being treated, and whether surgery will offer only a short-term solution.[4]

SEDATION AND ANESTHESIA FOR PERINEAL SURGERY

Most surgical procedures involving the perineum, vestibule, or vagina are performed with the mare standing using local infiltration or epidural anesthesia. Appropriate restraint is essential. Xylazine in combination with butorphanol is an effective combination for standing perineal surgery.[6] In a clinical trial, detomidine alone was shown to provide excellent sedation and analgesia for completion of numerous reproductive surgical procedures on mares.[7] Both 20 μg/kg and 40 μg/kg dosages proved to be effective, with the only side effects being sweating, cutaneous hypersensitivity, and piloerection. It is recommended that local anesthetics be used in conjunction with detomidine. Other combinations of ataractic and analgesic drugs can also be used.

Local anesthetic infiltration is satisfactory for completion of a Caslick vulvoplasty. For other more invasive procedures, infiltration of local anesthetic into the perineal body may provide sufficient anesthesia to complete surgery. However epidural anesthesia provides the most complete perineal anesthesia per volume of anesthetic injected. A 2% lidocaine or mepivacaine solution is injected at the first intercoccygeal space at a dose of 1 mL/100 lb body weight, to a maximum of 7 to 8 mL total volume for most mares.[2] A 3.8-cm, 18-gauge needle is sufficient for most mares. The needle is directed at right angles to the skin, preferably through a small skin bleb of local anesthetic. Once the skin is penetrated, filling the hub of the 18-gauge needle with local anesthetic and watching for it to be drawn through the hub into the epidural space can assist with correct placement. Caudal analgesia of 90 to 150 min can be obtained using this technique.[8]

The use of xylazine as an epidural anesthetic has also been reported.[8,9] Xylazine reportedly gives profound analgesia without the side effect of ataxia that is sometimes seen with local anesthetics. In one study, xylazine was given at a dose of 0.17 to 0.22 mg/kg, diluted with saline to a volume of 10 mL, with analgesia persisting for 3.5 h.[9] The onset of analgesia is more rapid with local anesthetics than with xylazine (15 vs. 30 min), but the duration of action of xylazine is longer.[9] A perineal sweat dermatome also appears approximately 30 min after epidural administration of xylazine and reportedly corresponds both temporally and topographically with the area of regional analgesia.[9]

CONDITIONS REQUIRING SURGERY

PNEUMOVAGINA

Pneumovagina is well recognized as a cause of, or contributor to, reproductive inefficiency or failure in mares. Some mares are affected with both pneumovagina and urovagina.[1,3,10–12] Aspiration of air into the vagina can result from faulty perineal conformation, previous injury to perineal tissues, or poor body condition.[13] Older multiparous mares are more commonly affected with pneumovagina, but young mares with inverted or poorly formed labia can also develop pneumovagina. Pneumovagina can lead to vaginitis, cervicitis, and eventually metritis.

In some mares, pneumovagina may only occur during estrus when perineal tissues are more edematous and relaxed. Failure to conceive with a positive uterine culture may be the only suggestive sign of pneumovagina in other mares.[5] Occasionally a small volume of foamy-appearing exudate may accumulate on the cranial floor of the vagina, or air may be seen on ultrasonographic examination of the uterus.[5] A Caslick Index has been described for helping determine which mares may benefit from a Caslick vulvoplasty, but its use has not gained common acceptance.[10]

All contributory factors to pneumovagina must be effectively managed for the condition to be corrected. The mare in poor body condition must be examined and treated for causes of that problem, including a dental examination, and determination of her nutritional status and parasite control history. Some mares with pneumovagina may also suffer from urovagina, and more than one surgical procedure may be necessary.

Caslick Vulvoplasty

The vulvoplasty procedure was first described by Caslick in 1937.[1] Caslick noted that many mares that had repeated manual entry for uterine irrigation for metritis had their metritis temporarily worsen. Dramatic clinical improvement was seen when uterine irrigation was discontinued and the dorsal aspects of the vulvar labia were temporarily closed.[1]

A Caslick vulvoplasty is done in the standing mare and using local infiltration anesthesia of the margins of the vulvar labia. The procedure is completed in a stocks or with the surgeon protected by some other means from a kicking injury. The vulvar margins are distended with local anesthetic and an 8- to 10-mm strip of vulvar mucosa is removed from the level of the mucocutaneous margin craniad (Fig. 48–1A and B). Care should be taken that perineal skin is not removed as excessive fibrosis will develop and complicate the successful completion of subsequent vulvoplasties.[13] The strip of mucosa is removed from the level of the dorsal commissure to a point just below the level of the ischial arch. Alternatively, a scalpel blade may be used to incise distended labial margins until the desired tissue gap forms. Clo-

FIG. 48–1. *A*, Local anesthetic is injected along the mucocutaneous junction from just below the level of the ischium to the dorsal commissure. By using a 6.3-cm, 22-gauge needle, only one needle entry point needs to be made. *B*, A strip of mucosa is removed so the resulting exposed submucosal tissue gap is 8 to 10 mm wide. The mucosa should be removed from the mucocutaneous junction craniad. *C*, Sutures may be placed in an interrupted or a continuous fashion. Suture spacing should be such that fistula formation is discouraged. *D*, A "breeder's stitch" is often used to reinforce the primary suture line at the time of breeding.

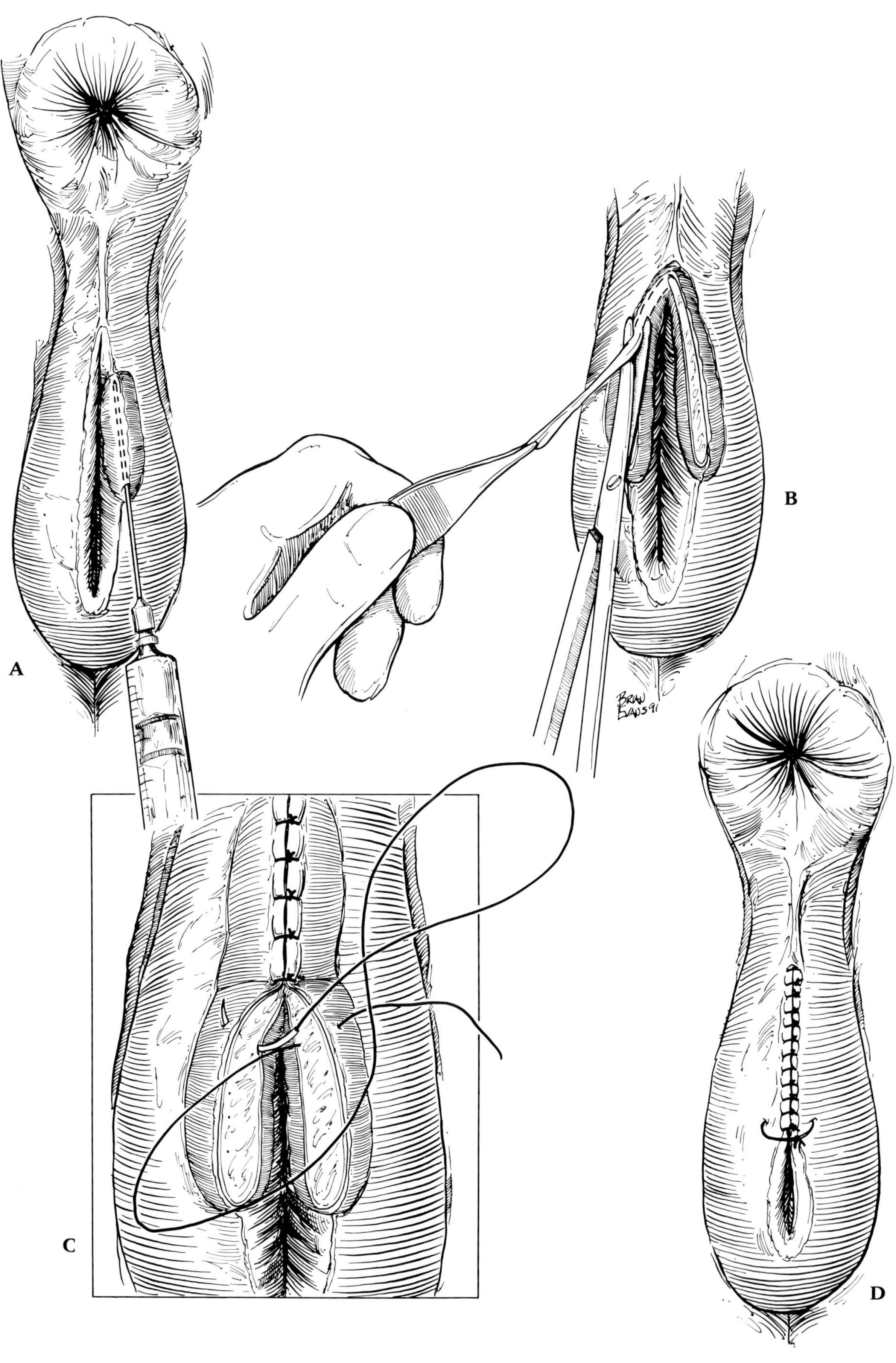
A
B
C
D
BRIAN EVANS 91

sure of the vulvar cleft is usually completed using #00 to #0 suture material in a continuous suture pattern. Suture placement should result in broad tissue apposition at the denuded tissue surfaces (Fig. 48–1C). Synthetic absorbable suture material is preferred by some, but polymerized caprolactam (Vetafil) is also used extensively[10,14,15] (K. Shiner, R. Magnuson, and B. David, personal communications). Some clinicians prefer to close the vulvar cleft until the remaining opening will just admit a tube speculum. (K. Shiner, personal communication). Sutures are often removed 10 to 12 days after closure, to minimize accumulation of feces and other debris along the suture line.[2,13] Examination for presence of fistula(s) should be done at suture removal.

Excessive closure of the vulvar cleft can contribute to forward splashback of urine and subsequent urovagina.[4,16] Positive uterine cultures were found in 5 of 18 mares that were considered to have excessive closure of the vulvar cleft. This forward reflux of urine could carry vulvar and vestibular contaminants into the vagina. Although the ventral limit of the closure will vary between mares, excessive closure is probably present if a tube speculum cannot be readily passed.[16]

A "breeder's stitch" is often placed at the ventral limits of the repair to protect the vulvoplasty at subsequent breeding[13,16] (Fig. 48–1D). This is usually a single large-diameter suture or umbilical tape, which is normally left in place until the mare is confirmed pregnant. Suture placement and the material used must be designed to protect the stallion's penis during coitus. This suture is usually placed just proximal to the ventral limit of the Caslick vulvoplasty. The suture loop is left sufficiently loose to allow for some local tissue expansion and to facilitate opening the vulvar cleft at breeding. (R. Magnuson and B. David, personal communications). Most mares can be naturally covered by manually elevating and opening the vulvar cleft and guiding the stallion's penis. The use of a breeding roll is recommended (see Chapter 85).

An episiotomy will be required before foaling and in some cases before breeding if the remaining vulvar cleft is too small for intromission. Closure of a vulvoplasty should also be delayed 2 to 3 days after foaling if significant vulvar edema is present. Closure is also delayed postfoaling if uterine irrigation is considered necessary.

Episioplasty

If both vulvar and vestibular barriers are ineffective, more extensive surgery will be required. If on minimal parting of vulvar labia a prominent inrush of air is heard, the vestibular sphincter is likely dysfunctional.[2] In mares that have had extensive or repeated second-degree perineal lacerations, or in multiparous mares that have suffered repeated stretching of the vulva and vestibule, an episioplasty may be necessary. Although the Caslick vulvoplasty is a form of episioplasty, the term "episioplasty" is more commonly used to describe this more extensive surgical procedure that has alternately been called a deep Caslick procedure, the Gadd technique, or perineal body reconstruction.[11,13] Episioplasty is meant to restore some degree of function to the perineal body.

Surgery is best completed with the mare standing and using epidural anesthesia. Perineal body infiltration with local anesthetic will also allow completion of the surgery. An incision is made along the mucocutaneous junction from the dorsal commissure of the vulva to end distally in a similar location to the distal extent of a Caslick vulvoplasty. The labia are retracted using stay sutures or towel clamps to expose the roof of the vestibule. A right-angled, triangular-shaped piece of mucosa is then removed from the dorsum of the vestibule. The base of each triangle is the cutaneous perineum, with the side of each triangle being the dorsal midline. The dorsal midline incision is extended from the cutaneous perineum to approximately the level of the vaginovestibular junction at the level of the external urethral orifice.[11,17] The cranial extent of the incision is also based somewhat on the degree of damage that the perineal body has incurred. The hypotenuse of each triangle is the line that connects the ventral limit of the base with the cranial limit of the side of the triangle (Fig. 48–2A). The mucosa is then excised to expose the submucosa (Fig. 48–2B). Vestibular mucosa is then apposed on midline using #00 absorbable suture material in a continuous pattern that inverts the mucosa into the vestibule (Fig 48–2C). Submucosal tissues are then apposed using #0 or #1 absorbable suture material in an interrupted pattern (Fig. 48–2D). It is important that the dorsal commissure of the vulva be retracted dorsad and caudad during closure so that the vulva assumes a more vertical orientation when closure is completed (Fig. 48–2E).

Breeding should not be attempted for 4 to 6 weeks after surgery. Because of the nature of the surgery, the dimensions of the vestibule are reduced and some mares will require an episiotomy at the time of foaling.

A similar, but much more extensive technique, has also been described for the correction of atonic vagina.[13] A triangular-shaped piece of mucosa is removed from the level of the cutaneous perineum to the level of the cervix. Submucosal tissues are subsequently apposed in an attempt to restore some tone to the flaccid vagina. This technique has not shown sufficient benefit over the previously described episioplasty for it to achieve popularity.

Perineal Body Transection

Perineal body transection has been described as a successful technique for correction of both pneumovagina and urovagina.[12] The procedure is recommended for some mares that have a sunken anus and forward sloping of the vagina and when success with other procedures is deemed unlikely[12,18] (Fig. 48–3). A detailed description of this procedure is presented in Chapter 49.

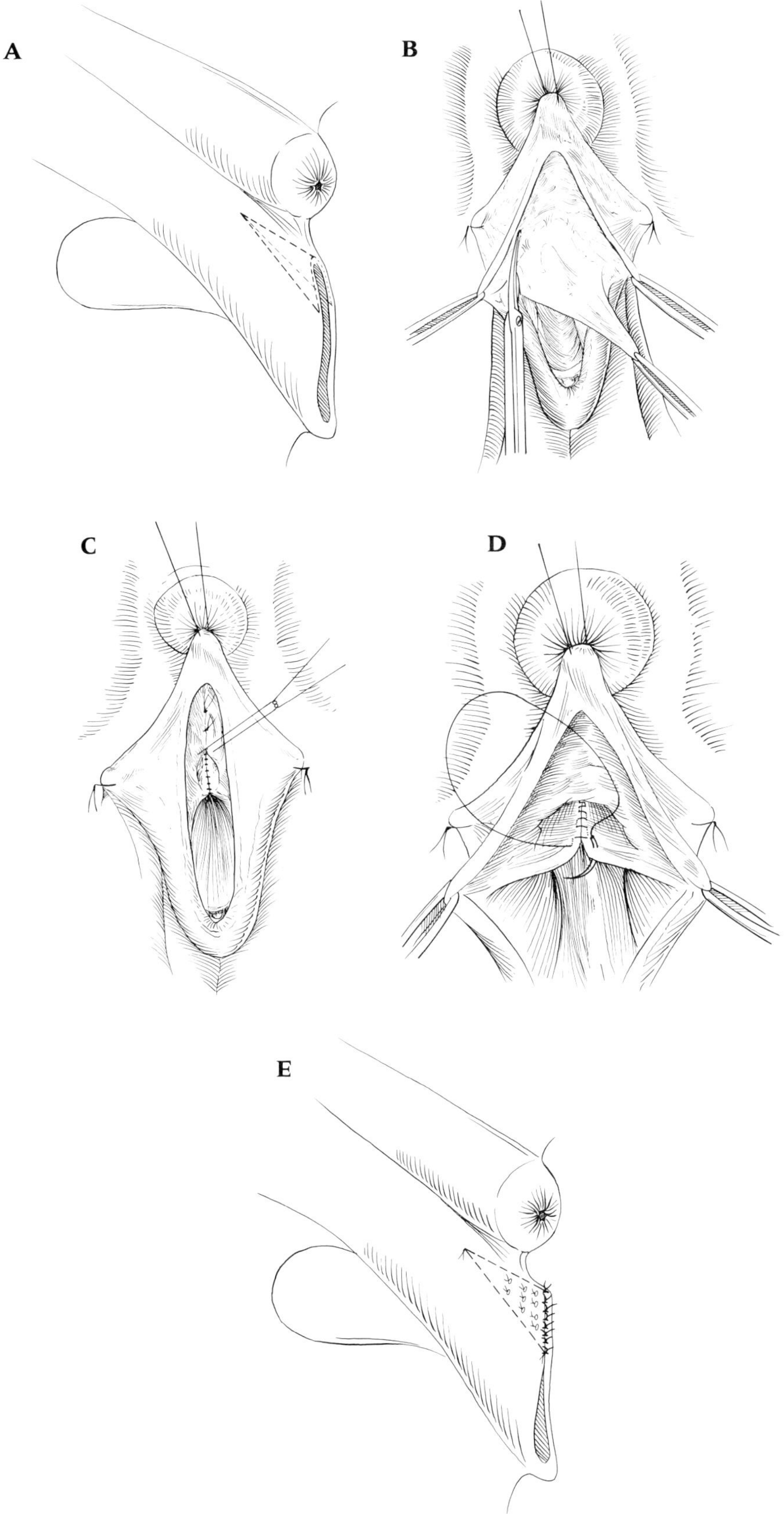

FIG. 48–2. *A,* The triangular area of mucosa to be removed in an episioplasty is outlined. *B,* After being dissected free from the submucosa, the mucosa is excised. *C,* The initial suture line is a horizontal mattress pattern that inverts mucosa into the vestibule. *D,* Submucosal tissues are apposed using interrupted sutures. The dorsal commissure should be retracted dorsad and caudad and be maintained in this position during closure. *E,* At the completion of surgery, the vulva should assume a more vertical orientation.

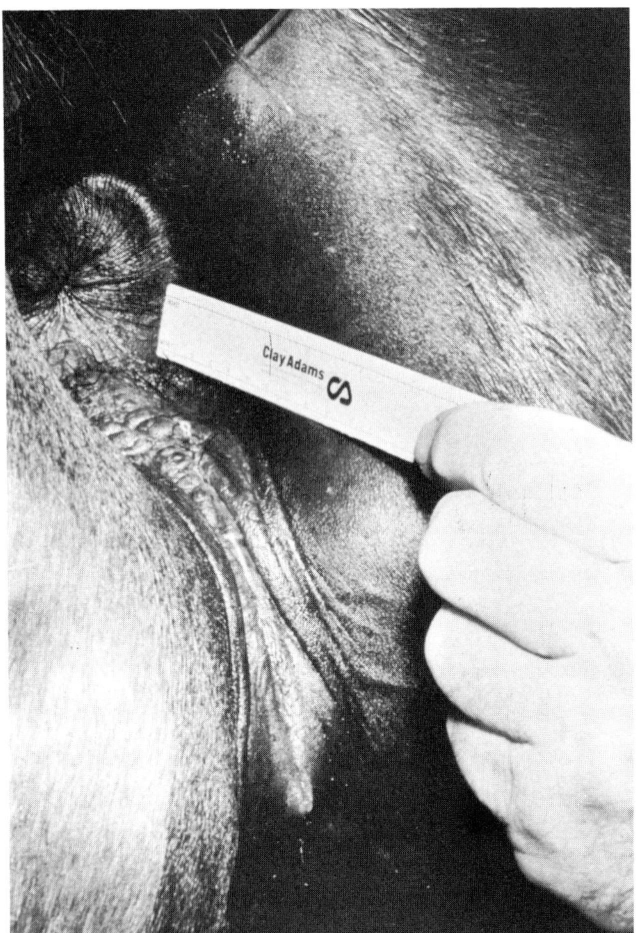

FIG. 48–3. A mare with the perineal conformation shown here would benefit from perineal body transection.

PERINEAL LACERATIONS

Most perineal injuries occur at the time of foaling, either as a result of an oversize or malpositioned fetus or because of excessive manipulation during assisted delivery. Although minor injuries or lacerations to the perineum do not require surgery, others will affect reproductive performance and require surgical correction.[17,19,20]

Damage from the majority of foaling injuries is restricted to the vulva and vestibule.[19] Lacerations that occur at parturition have been classified based on their extent into first-, second-, and third-degree lacerations.[13,19,20] First-degree lacerations involve only mucosa of the vestibule and skin of the dorsal commissure of the vulva. Second-degree lacerations involve both mucosa and submucosa of the dorsal vestibule, skin of the dorsal vulva, and some of the musculature of the perineal body, in particular the constrictor vulvae muscle. Third-degree lacerations extend from the vestibule through all muscles of the perineal body, enter the rectum, and also disrupt the anal sphincter.

Some minor first-degree lacerations require no treatment and will heal completely if left alone. Others may be able to be repaired at the time of occurrence, either with definitive repair of the laceration or by completing a Caslick vulvoplasty. Some second-degree lacerations also require no specific surgical treatment. However, if much of the perineal body is involved, the result of healing by second intention is a sunken dorsal aspect of the vulva with subsequent pneumovagina and aspiration of particulate material. Immediate reapposition of traumatized tissues can be done in selected cases where the degree of trauma is relatively minor. In most cases, a delay in surgery until local tissue edema and inflammation has subsided will be necessary. Episioplasty may then be needed.

Third-degree injuries usually occur in primiparous mares, and often those with an excitable temperament.[20] Presumably the foal's foot or nose catches on the dorsal vulvovaginal fold, and the expulsive effort forces the foot or nose through the perineal body into the rectum. If the appendage is withdrawn or replaced, the result is a rectovestibular fistula. If another expulsive effort is given, the appendage may be forced out through the anal sphincter completely dividing the perineal body. Some third-degree lacerations occur on midline and others tear the perineal body near its junction with the lateral aspect of the perineum (Fig. 48–4). Although tearing into the vagina can occur, tears of this extent are uncommon.

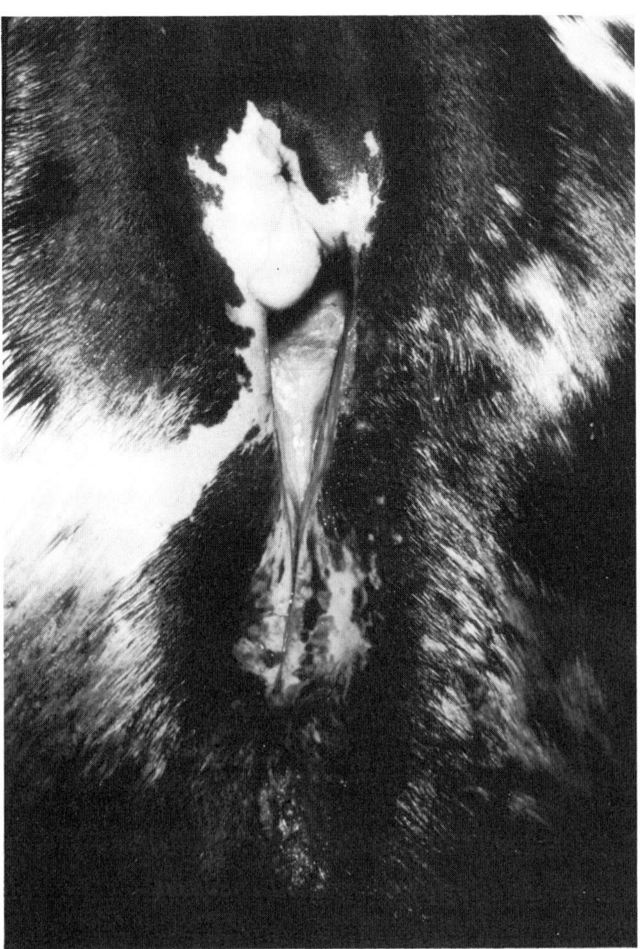

FIG. 48–4. The third-degree perineal laceration shown here was to the right of midline; much of the perineal body had undergone necrosis and sloughing.

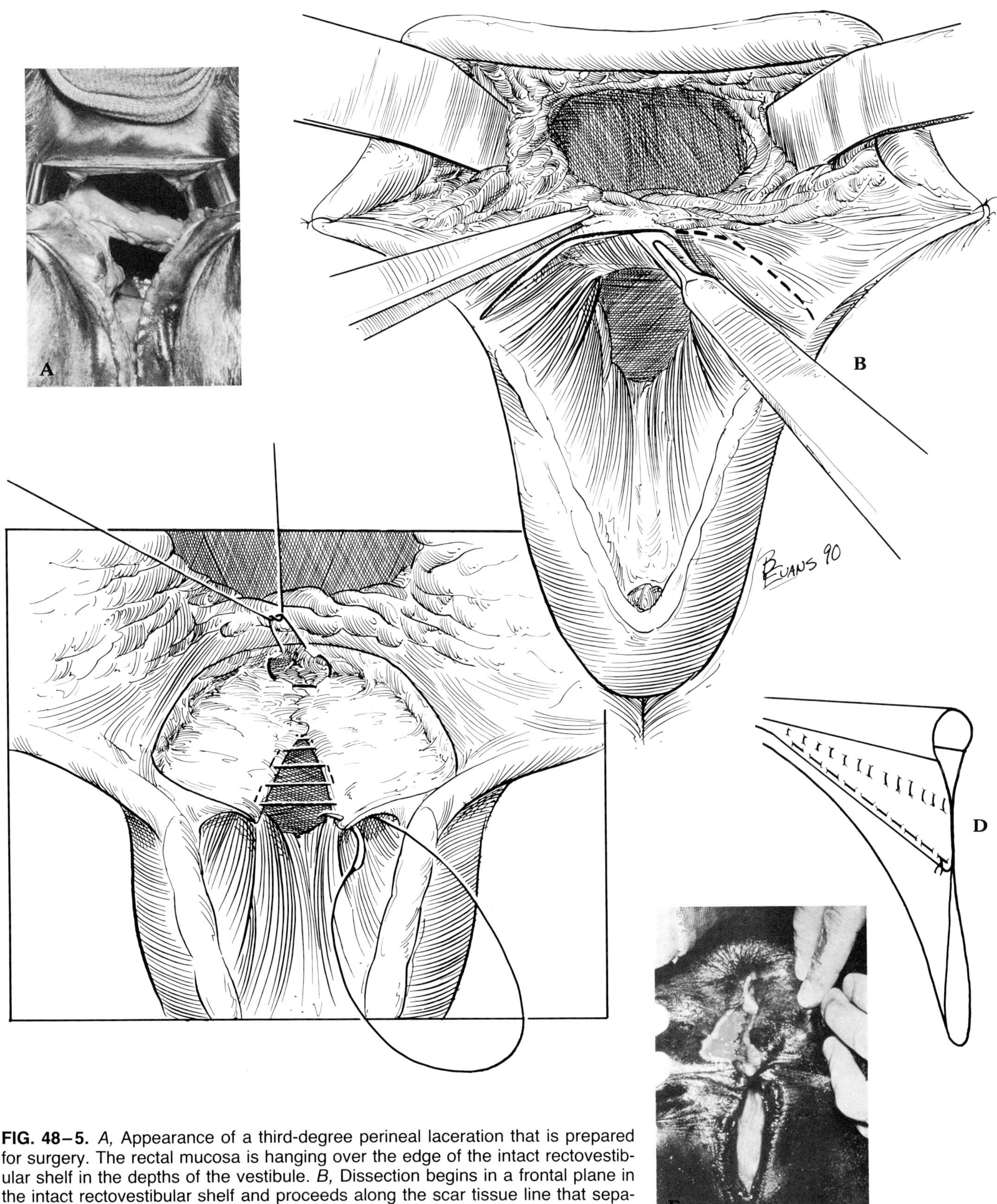

FIG. 48–5. *A,* Appearance of a third-degree perineal laceration that is prepared for surgery. The rectal mucosa is hanging over the edge of the intact rectovestibular shelf in the depths of the vestibule. *B,* Dissection begins in a frontal plane in the intact rectovestibular shelf and proceeds along the scar tissue line that separates rectum from vestibule. *C,* The initial suture line is a continuous horizontal mattress pattern that inverts vestibular mucosa into the vestibule. Submucosal tissues are apposed using large absorbable suture material placed in an interrupted fashion. *D,* Schematic representation of a completed first-stage repair, with the dorsal aspect of the perineal body left open. *E,* A completed first-stage repair.

Immediate repair of third-degree lacerations is rarely indicated. Degree of tissue trauma is usually such that total failure of an early repair will take place as local tissue edema and necrosis develop during the first few days after the injury and the repair.[17,19,20] Local tissue debridement will be necessary in some cases, and systemic antibacterial therapy for 5 to 7 days after the injury is recommended. The mare's tetanus prophylaxis status should also be current. Definitive surgical repair should be delayed for at least 3 weeks after injury. If a live foal was born, the surgery can usually be delayed until the foal is weaned. This avoids having the foal in a hospital environment and helps to prevent problems with the foal from the dietary changes the mare will be undergoing in the perioperative period. It necessarily delays rebreeding until the subsequent breeding season.

Preoperative planning includes evaluation of a uterine biopsy, and alteration of the mare's diet to ensure soft feces in the perioperative period. The mare's diet should be changed sufficiently prior to the planned surgery date so that feces are soft but not fluid-like in consistency. Numerous dietary regimens have been proposed to achieve soft feces, including numerous laxative agents that are administered by stomach tubes, the use of pelleted feeds or alfalfa, grazing at pasture, and the use of bran.[13,17,19,20] Geographic location and personal preference eventually dictate the method that is chosen. Although a definite advantage to using perioperative antibacterial therapy has not been proven, most recommend that they be used.[19,20] Perioperative anti-inflammatory therapy may also help minimize swelling and tenesmus that occasionally complicates the postoperative period.

Numerous surgical techniques or variations on techniques have been described.[13,17,19–23] The goal of all surgical procedures is re-establishment of a shelf between the rectum and vestibule and restoration of a functional perineal body. Broad tissue apposition under minimal tension must be established at surgery. The two most common procedures used are the two-stage repair described by Aanes[20] and the single-stage repair using a modification of the original Goetze method.[21,24]

Surgery is usually done with the mare standing and using epidural anesthesia. The tail should be elevated and tied overhead to provide some stability to the mare if mild ataxia develops from the epidural anesthetic. The perineum is prepared for aseptic surgery, and the vagina, vestibule, and rectum are irrigated using an antibacterial solution and cotton pledgets. All fluid should be removed before starting surgery. A cotton tampon placed in the rectum may prevent contamination of the surgical site during surgery. Special operating room arrangements can also be made so that surgery can be completed with the mare under general anesthesia and in sternal recumbency.[25] Adequate precautions must be taken so that inadvertent myositis is avoided from improper positioning and padding. Because of soft tissue impingement into the vestibule, surgery in lateral or dorsal recumbency is usually impossible.

A two-stage repair was developed so that obstipation that sometimes complicates the early postoperative period could be avoided.[20] The first stage of the repair involves reconstruction of a rectovestibular shelf without closure of most of the perineal body. The second stage of the repair is done 3 to 4 weeks later and involves closure of the remainder of the perineal body. Dissection begins cranially in a frontal plane at the level of the existing rectovestibular shelf (Fig. 48–5A and B). Dissection is continued laterad and caudad along the scar tissue line that separates the rectum from the vestibule. The dissection is continued caudad to the level of the cutaneous perineum. Lateral dissection proceeds into the submucosal tissues to a sufficient depth so that the vestibular tissue flaps that are created can be brought to midline under the minimal tension.

The initial suture line apposes the vestibular mucosa on midline. A continuous horizontal mattress pattern using #00 absorbable suture material is used to invert the vestibular mucosa into the vestibule (Fig. 48–5C). This pattern is temporarily interrupted midway along the repair to allow sufficient access for suture placement in the cranially located submucosal tissues. The initial submucosal sutures at the cranial limits of the dissection are placed in purse-string fashion. These sutures close the dead space under the intact rectovestibular shelf that lies craniad to the original defect. Where excessive tissue loss or inelastic cicatrix results in undue tension as these sutures are tightened, a transversely oriented tissue ridge forms in the rectal submucosa.[20] Subsequent obstipation and tenesmus may result in failure of the repair. A modification of the original repair has recently been described to manage this complication. A loosely placed purse-string suture is placed in a transverse plane and tightened until the transverse ridge just begins to form. Sagittally oriented interrupted sutures are then placed within the boundaries of the purse-string suture to appose rectal and vestibular submucosal tissues.[20] The remainder of the submucosal tissues caudal to the pre-existing rectovestibular shelf are then apposed using #2 synthetic absorbable suture material placed in a simple interrupted fashion (Fig. 48–5C). This suture line is continued to the level of the cutaneous perineum, with the majority of the dorsal perineal body being left open (Fig. 48–5D and E).

The second-stage repair is delayed for 3 to 4 weeks. The epithelium is removed from the surface of the remaining open perineal body, and submucosal tissues are apposed on midline using #0 or #1 absorbable suture material (Fig. 48–6A and B). Epithelial tissues within the rectum are apposed using #00 nonabsorbable suture material in a continuous pattern, and surgery is completed with a Caslick vulvoplasty. (Fig. 48–6C and D).

A rectal pullback technique has been described, which is a modification of the two-stage technique but which is completed in one stage.[19] The dissection is as previously described, with the exception that the intact rectal mucosa at the cranial aspect of the dissection is undermined craniad until the mucosa can be drawn caudad as close to the level of the anal sphincter as possible. As each of the subsequent purse-string or simple interrupted submucosal sutures is placed, rectal mucosa

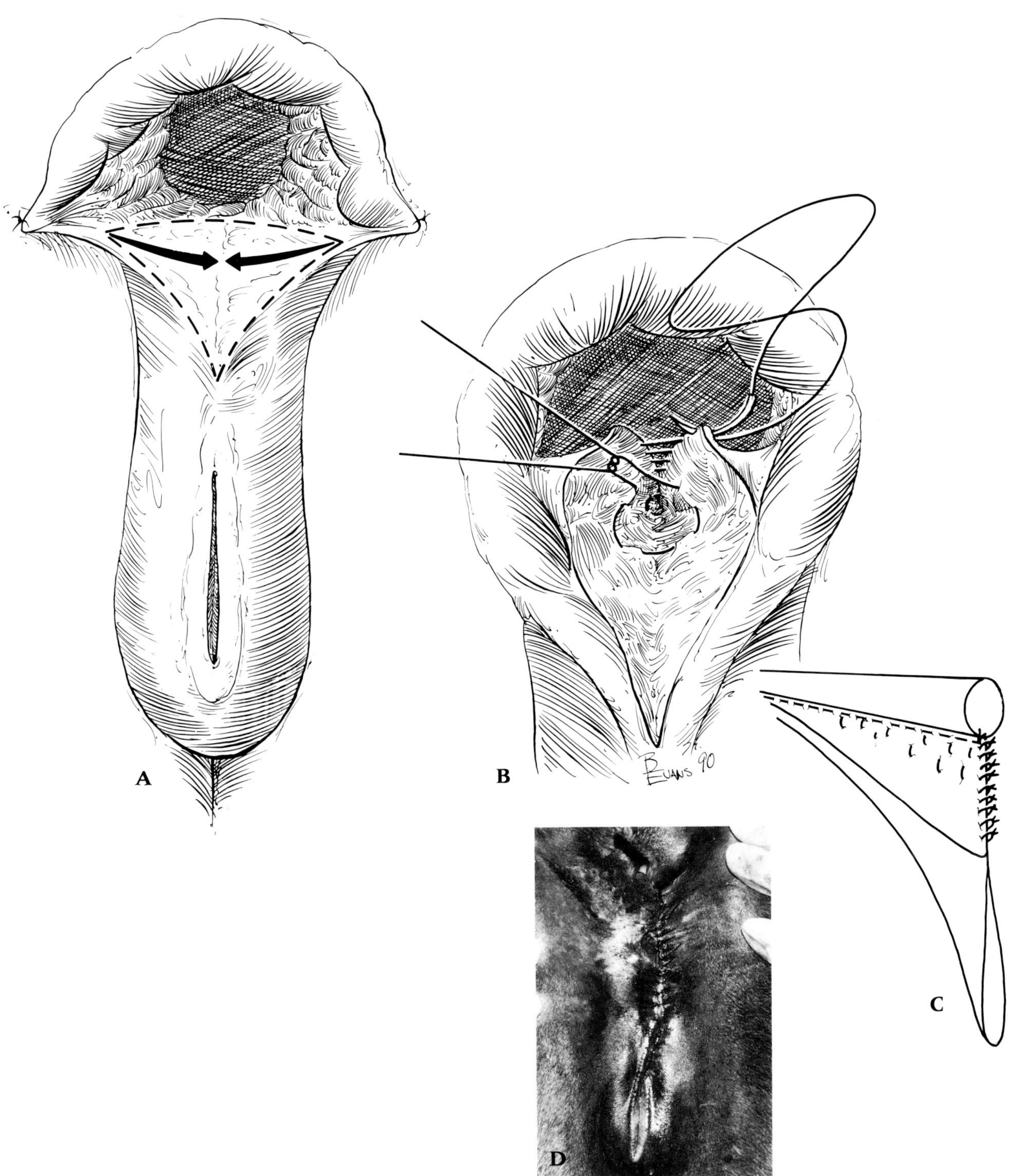

FIG. 48–6. Second-stage repair of a third-degree perineal laceration. *A,* The triangular area is outlined from which epithelium is removed from the open portion of the perineal body. *B,* Closure consists of buried absorbable sutures to close the perineal body; a continuous pattern is placed in the epithelial tissues within the rectum. *C,* Schematic representation of a completed second-stage repair. *D,* A completed second-stage repair.

is drawn caudad and a suture bite is taken in the rectal submucosa. This fixes the rectal mucosa in its retracted state. The retracted rectal mucosa thereby protects the underlying sutures from fecal contamination. When the level of the perineal body is reached, closure proceeds as described under episioplasty.

When the Goetze modification of the single-stage repair is used, two tissue flaps are created with the rectal flap being made thicker than the vestibular flap.[24] Apposition of the tissue flaps from each side is done using a six-bite suture pattern, and the suture knots are hand tied in the vestibule. Large-diameter nonabsorbable suture material is used, with consecutive tissue bites being taken in the left vestibular tissue flap well back from the incised margin, the left rectal submucosa to emerge near the rectal mucosa, the right rectal submucosa, deep in the right vestibular flap, the right vestibular mucosa, and the left vestibular mucosa (Fig. 48–7). When tightened, these sutures should appose rectal mucosa and evert vestibular mucosa into the vestibule. The suture ends in the vestibule are left long to facilitate removal in 12 to 14 days. This pattern is continued to within 4 to 6 cm of the cutaneous perineum. Dissection is then completed to expose the remainder of the perineal body. A combination of the six-bite pattern and simple interrupted sutures is then used to appose the tissues of the perineal body, and a Caslick vulvoplasty is completed.

For either surgical procedure, natural cover is not recommended for 2 to 4 months after surgery is completed, although artificial insemination may be considered in 3 to 6 weeks.[19,20] The conception rate after surgery has been reported to be as high as 75%, and retearing is a low-incidence complication.[20,23] Other complications that may occur include fistula formation, urine pooling, complete dehiscence of the repair, obstipation, and tenesmus. Eversion of the urinary bladder has also been reported in association with third-degree perineal lacerations.[26] If obstipation does occur, enemas administered carefully by dose syringe can relieve the obstipation with salvage of the repair in some cases (Fig. 48–8).

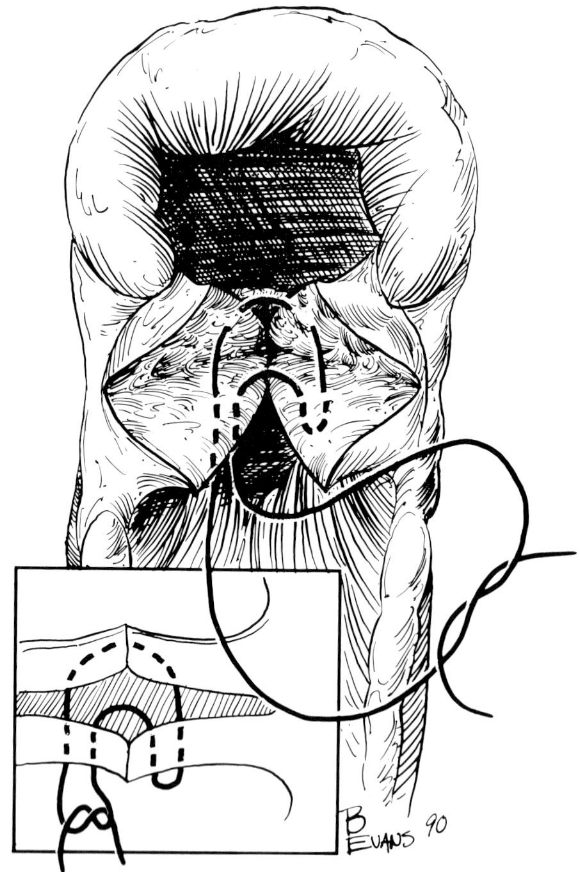

FIG. 48–7. Schematic representation of the six-bite suture pattern used in the single-stage repair for third-degree perineal lacerations.

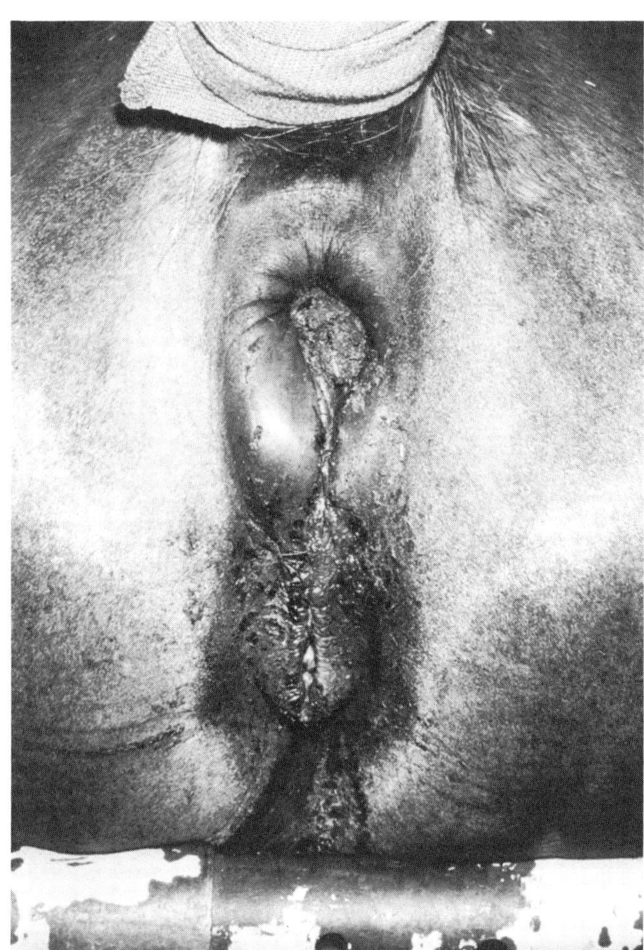

FIG. 48–8. Obstipation and swelling can complicate the early postoperative period leading to failure of the repair. Frequent enemas administered by dose syringe can relieve obstipation without failure of the repair in some cases.

RECTOVESTIBULAR FISTULA

A rectovestibular fistula is usually a result of a foaling injury, although they may also result from a breeding injury or sadism.[20] The fistula may occur relatively close to the cutaneous perineum or be more deeply located in the vestibule. Some small fistulas may close completely by second intention wound healing. Surgical repair of larger fistulas should again be delayed for 3 to 4 weeks until inflammation is minimal and epithelialization is complete. If the fistula is caudally located, converting the fistula to a third-degree perineal laceration is recommended. For a more deeply located fistula, a perineal body transection approach should be used. A transversely oriented incision is made through the perineal body and is continued craniad to end 3 to 4 cm cranial to the fistula.[19,20] Closure of the rectal portion of the fistula is completed using #1 or #2 absorbable suture material placed in Lembert fashion and in a transverse plane to coincide with the lines of stress within the rectum.[19] These sutures invert rectal mucosa into the rectum and should not penetrate the rectal mucosa. The vestibular portion of the fistula is then closed using the same suture material and pattern, but the suture line is placed in a sagittal plane. The space between the rectum and the vestibule is then closed using interrupted sutures of absorbable suture material.

An alternate technique involves general anesthesia with the mare placed in dorsal recumbency.[27] The fistula is approached through the vulva and vestibule and is converted into rectal and vestibular layers using a combination of sharp and blunt dissection. The repair is then completed as previously described.

REFERENCES

1. Caslick, E.A.: The vulva and the vulvo-vaginal orifice and its relation to genital health of the Thoroughbred mare. Cornell Vet., *27:*178–187, 1937.
2. Trotter, G.W., and McKinnon, A.O.: Surgery for abnormal vulvar and perineal conformation in the mare. Vet. Clin. North. Am., *4:*389–405, 1988.
3. Ansari, M.M.: The Caslick operation in mares. Compend. Contin. Educ. Vet. Practicing Vet., *5:*S107–S111, 1983.
4. Easley, K.J., Osborne, J., and Thorpe, P.E.: Surgery for conditions causing decreased fertility in mares: case selection: Vet. Clin. North Am., *4:*381–388, 1988.
5. McKinnon, A.O., et al.: Diagnostic ultrasonography of uterine pathology in the mare. Proc. Am. Assoc. Equine Pract., 605–622, 1987.
6. Tranquilli, W.: Injectable regimens for standing restraint and anesthesia. Compend. Contin. Educ. Practicing Vet., *121:*1283–1285, 1989.
7. McKinnon, A.O., Carnevale, E.M., Squires, E.L., and Jochle, W.: Clinical evaluation of detomidine hydrochloride for equine reproductive surgery. Proc. Am. Assoc. Equine Pract., 563–568, 1988.
8. Leblanc, P.H., et. al.: Epidural injection of xylazine for perineal analgesia in horses. J. Am. Vet. Med. Assoc., *193:*1405–1408, 1988.
9. Leblanc, P.H., and Caron, J.P.: Clinical use of epidural xylazine in the horse. Equine Vet. J., *22:*180–181, 1990.
10. Pascoe, R.R.: Observations on the length and angle of declination of the vulva and its relation to fertility in the mare. J. Reprod. Fertil. Suppl., *27:*299–305, 1979.
11. Gadd, J.D.: The relationship of bacterial cultures, microscopic smear examination and medical treatment to surgical correction of barren mares. Proc. Am. Assoc. Equine Pract., 362–368, 1975.
12. Pouret, E.J.M.: Surgical technique for the correction of pneumo- and urovagina. Equine Vet. J., *14:*249–250, 1982.
13. Vaughan, J.T.: The female genital system. *In* Textbook of Large Animal Surgery. 2nd ed. Edited by F.W. Oehme. Baltimore, Williams & Wilkins, 1988, pp. 559–584.
14. Belling, T.H.: Surgery of the vulva: modification of the traditional Caslick operation. Vet. Med., *78:*870–878, 1983.
15. Shires, G.M., and Kaneps, A.J.: A practical and simple surgical technique for repair of urine pooling in the mare. Proc. Am. Assoc. Equine Pract., 51–56, 1986.
16. Witherspoon, D.M.: Some reflections concerning Caslick's surgery, ultrasonography and the treatment of uterine cysts. Equine Pract., *11:*12–15, 1989.
17. Vaughan, J.T.: Equine urogenital system. *In* The Practice of Large Animal Surgery. Edited by P.B. Jennings, Philadelphia, W.B. Saunders, 1984, pp. 1122–1150.
18. Ricketts, S.W.: Perineal conformation abnormalities. *In* Current Therapy in Equine Medicine. 2nd ed. Edited by N.E. Robinson. Philadelphia, W.B. Saunders, 1987, pp. 518–520.
19. Embertson, R.H.: Perineal lacerations. *In* Current Practice of Equine Surgery. Edited by N.A. White and J.N. Moore. Philadelphia, J.B. Lippincott, 1990, pp. 669–704.
20. Aanes, W.A.: Surgical management of foaling injuries. Vet. Clin. North Am., *4:*417–438, 1988.
21. Straub, O.C., and Fowler, M.E.: Repair of perineal lacerations in the mare and cow. J. Am. Vet. Med. Assoc., *138:*659–664, 1961.
22. Stickle, R.L., Fessler, J.F., and Adams, S.B.: A single-stage technique for repair of rectovestibular lacerations in the mare. Vet. Surg., *8:*25–27, 1979.
23. Colbern, G.T., Aanes, W.A., and Stashak, T.S.: Surgical management of perineal lacerations and rectovestibular fistulae in the mare: A retrospective study of 47 cases. J. Am. Vet. Med. Assoc., *186:*265–269, 1985.
24. Vaughan, J.T.: Equine urogenital systems. *In* Current Therapy in Theriogenology 2. Edited by D.A. Morrow. Philadelphia, W.B. Saunders, 1986, pp. 756–775.
25. Robertson, J.T.: Cervical lacerations. *In* Current Practice of Equine Surgery. Edited by N.A. White and J.N. Moore. Philadelphia, J.B. Lippincott, 1990, pp. 696–699.
26. Haynes, P.F., and McClure, J.R.: Eversion of the urinary bladder: A sequel to third-degree perineal laceration in the mare. Vet. Surg., *9:*66–71, 1980.
27. Hilbert, B.J.: Surgical repair of recto-vaginal fistulas in mares. Aust. Vet. J., *57:*85–87, 1981.

CHAPTER 49

CORRECTION OF VESICOVAGINAL REFLUX

J. EASLEY

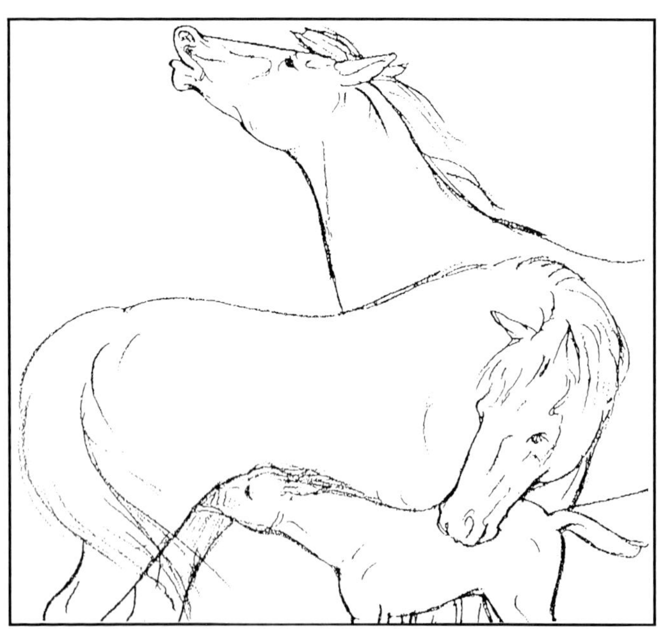

Vesicovaginal reflux (VVR), also known as urovagina and urine pooling, is the retention of incompletely voided urine in the cranial vaginal fornix.[1,2]

The caudal end of the reproductive tract is the vulva, which passes through the vestibule and opens into the vagina (see Chapters 1 and 2). The vagina extends craniodorsad. The urinary bladder lies just beneath the cranial vagina and cervix. Ventral to the cervix lies the vaginal fornix, the deepest and most cranial portion of the vaginal vault.

Ideally, urine is evacuated from the bladder into the vulvar vestibule and out the open vulvar labia, or lips. However, if the normal slope of the vulva is altered (approximately 10° from horizontal) or the genitourinary tract slopes cranioventrad, a splashback of urine can occur, whereby some urine refluxes back toward the cervix and uterus instead of out of the vulva. This condition can lead to accumulation of a variable amount of urine in the vaginal fornix.

Uterine secretions or urine accumulation in the vaginal fornix lead to and/or intensify vaginitis and cervicitis. During estrus, when the cervix relaxes and opens, urine may flow back into the uterus and cause endometritis. Chronic irritation from urine changes the pH of the vagina and affects sperm viability, which in turn compromises the mare's chances of becoming pregnant.[3,4]

Reduced conception rate is only one danger associated with vesicovaginal reflux. Allowed to persist, endometritis can lead to periglandular fibrosis, as well as premature regression of the corpus luteum, causing a deficiency of progesterone and early embryonic loss.

Factors responsible for VVR are many and varied and relate to the mare's conformation, age, and reproductive history. This chapter discusses diagnosis and treatment of VVR and establishment of a reproductive prognosis for the mare afflicted with this condition.

Infertility in the mare associated with VVR must be managed as a complex problem. Complete reproductive evaluation of the mare is necessary to establish the cause of VVR and for proper therapy to be recommended. Determining a prognosis for the mare's future breeding soundness is important to the horse owner and breeding manager. To achieve this, the clinician must remember that vesicovaginal reflux is almost always associated with other reproductive problems and successful treatment requires the condition be viewed in the context of the mare's overall reproductive health.

ETIOLOGY

A primary predisposing factor to urine pooling is pneumovagina, or the aspiration of air into the vaginal canal. The vulva is the first barrier protecting the reproductive tract from contamination by air or debris. If vulvar labia do not function properly, air may be drawn into the reproductive tract, inflating the vaginal vault and/or uterus, relaxing the reproductive tract and providing a potential space for urine to enter through an open second barrier, the vestibular sphincter. The problem occasionally can be corrected with a Caslick operation[5,6] (see Chapter 48).

The second and most effective barrier to ascending bacterial contamination is the vulvovaginal fold or vestibular sphincter, which in the normal mare is located cranially and dorsally to the urethral orifice, the structure which allows urine to enter the vulva during urination. The vulvovaginal fold consists of a transverse fold or remnant of the hymen and the pelvic floor ventrally, the caudal constrictor muscles laterally, and the perineal body dorsally[7] (see Chapter 1). When the vulvovaginal fold does not function properly or when its location is altered in relation to the urethral orifice VVR may occur.

In aged mares, where repeated foalings or second-degree perineal lacerations have disrupted the constrictor muscles of the vulva and vestibule, advanced cases of pneumovagina are often seen. Repair may be effected by an episioplasty.[8,9]

Speculum examination, vaginal examination, and breeding can break the vulvar barrier to air and cause a transient pneumovagina that can lead to a one-time, temporary vesicovaginal reflux. This condition can be alleviated by inserting an arm (in a lubricated glove) into the mare's rectum and applying ventral and caudal pressure on the reproductive tract to evacuate the air.

Another predisposing factor in VVR is an excessive Caslick operation or episioplasty that has extended too far ventrad and prevents passage of the proper outflow of urine from the vulvar area.

Many factors can change the effectiveness of the vulvovaginal fold. The most common scenario is found in multiparous mares with poor reproductive tract tone or damage to the vulval suspensory ligament, anal retractor muscle, and vulvar constrictor muscles. These individuals often suffer from splanchnoptosis or visceroptosis, a relaxation and falling of the pelvic and abdominal organs.[10] The pelvic viscera, vulva, and vagina are displaced in such a way that the reproductive tract then descends craniad and ventrad. The urethral orifice is then cranially displaced over the crest of the ischium, or pelvic floor, and a variable amount of urine flows into the vaginal fornix. This problem may be corrected surgically with a perineal body transection (perineoplasty).

Another frequent cause of VVR is the hormonal environment of the reproductive tract. Depending on stage of estrus and concentrations of estrogen and progesterone, the reproductive tract may be predisposed to urine pooling. Estrogens stimulate and maintain the tissues of the tubular reproductive tract by increasing vascularity and uterine secretions, therefore increasing the area's defense against mechanical insult and infection.[3] A side effect, however, is a mild edema of the tubular tract, vagina, and uterus, resulting from intracellular absorption of water. The pelvic structures and vulva then relax as the general perineal area enlarges, and cranial displacement of the reproductive tract follows, leading to vesicovaginal reflux. A progesterone-influenced vaginal canal is more susceptible to infection but maintains better tone and is somewhat less affected by urine pooling. Hormonal influences can lead to inconsistent clinical signs, depending on stage of the estrous cycle of the mare when examined. This phenomenon is extremely important when assessing mares which may be pooling urine.

Thin physical condition may also precipitate VVR, because malnutrition can cause poor tone of the reproductive tract and loss of pelvic fat, which leads to a sunken perineum and its attendant adverse effects.

Any substantial retention of uterine contents can predispose a mare to VVR, because added weight of the secretions may cause cranioventral displacement of the reproductive tract. Factors responsible for this retention include failure of the uterus to contract because of chronic irritation, endometritis, uterine enlargement caused by an insufficiency of blood or lymph resulting from the effects of age, multiparity, and cervical injury. Pyometra, or accumulation of exudate in the uterus, has also been reported in conjunction with urine pooling.[11]

Injury to the urethra secondary to foaling or a misplaced infusion pipette (or any other instrument used to examine or treat the vaginal area) can lead to vesicovaginal reflux. Injuries to the urethra allow urine to be sprayed out of the vaginal cavity through a fistula cranial to the normal transverse fold. Injury or scarring of the transverse fold of the urethra may lead to an incomplete vulvovaginal fold, which can in turn precipitate urine pooling.

A further condition which can lead to VVR is an ectopic ureter, or displacement of the tube that conveys urine from the kidney to the bladder. An ectopic ureter may empty urine into any area along the reproductive tract. Although the diagnosis of ectopic ureter is usually made in younger fillies, the occasional female may not suffer from perineal urine scald and will, therefore, escape early detection of the condition; these fillies can be candidates for VVR at a later age. Cystitis and/or urolithiasis can lead to incomplete voiding or dribbling of urine, which can allow urine to accumulate stagnantly in the vaginal vault or reflux back into the vaginal fornix.[12]

DIAGNOSIS

The diagnosis of VVR is based on demonstration of urine in the cranial portion of the reproductive tract. Usually, a speculum examination yields a visual observation of accumulation of urine in the vaginal fornix.

Differential diagnoses of urine pooling would be uterine infection with accumulation of exudate in the vaginal fornix; mucometra (mucus in the uterus); or other uterine discharge resulting from uterine infection, cysts, or tumors. Special laboratory techniques can ensure accuracy of a diagnosis. Most notable is an examination of pH of fluid found in the fornix; horse urine is slightly alkaline, whereas purulent exudate is usually more acidic. Cytologic evaluation of the fluid can reveal bacteria and white blood cells (WBC) or calcium carbonate crystals, the most prominent type of crystal found in horse urine.[13] Tests for creatinine and urea nitrogen can be valuable, because creatine levels in accumulated urine will be at least two or three times blood creatinine concentration.

When diagnosis of VVR has been made and the cause identified, a treatment regimen can be initiated. A complete reproductive examination should be performed at this time to provide a basis for comparison after treatment is completed. A thorough reproductive workup should include assessment of ovarian function and serum hormone analysis, as well as a complete examination of the uterus (to rule out functional disturbances and the presence of periglandular fibrosis), including uterine culture, cytology of uterine contents, and an endometrial biopsy. Hysteroscopy, or endoscopic inspection of the uterus, may be useful in evaluating the nature of the fluid and the lining of the uterus as well as in checking for structures within the uterine lumen (cysts, exudate, tumors, and foreign bodies). Ultrasonographic evaluation of the reproductive tract can add information regarding texture and thickness of the uterus and presence and nature of fluid content within the tubular organs. In general, many infections and uterine inflammatory changes will be reversed or more easily treated after VVR has been successfully treated.

TREATMENT

The highest priority goal of treatment must be to correct the specific cause of vesicovaginal reflux. The source and severity of the affliction will dictate the sophistication of treatment necessary to restore a healthy reproductive tract.

If urine pooling results from unfortunate conformation as a result of poor physical condition, the problem often can be alleviated by sexual rest and weight gain. Transient VVR sometimes found in postpartum mares will also frequently resolve after the uterus returns to its normal size. Oxytocin and prostaglandin have been used during estrus to improve uterine tone. Preovulation and postovulation uterine lavages with complete removal of all fluid from the uterus have been beneficial in improving uterine tone and removing toxic substances from the uterine cavity.

Another relatively elementary solution is available for some mares in the early stages of vesicovaginal reflux. Occasionally, evacuation of urine from the vaginal fornix before breeding will enable the mare to conceive. Addition of semen extender at the time of breeding also has been found to dilute the toxic effects of urine to spermatozoa and is, therefore, recommended.

In cases where injury to the transverse fold or vulvovaginal fold is present, surgery is required.[14] A Caslick procedure, perineal body reconstruction, and variations of these techniques are usually effective for a mare with poor perineal conformation, a sunken anus, or dorsally displaced vulva which has precipitated pneumovagina. Where urine pooling is present because of conformation or multiparity and splanchnoptosis, a vaginoplasty or perineoplasty is recommended. A urethral extension technique (urethroplasty) is usually required to correct more severe cases.

Surgical correction of VVR discussed herein addresses modified vaginoplasty, perineoplasty, and a modified urethral extension procedure which has recorded clinical success.[15–17]

CAUDAL RELOCATION OF THE TRANSVERSE FOLD

The aim of this technique is to promote proper evacuation of urine by relocating the transverse fold in a more caudal position. Originally referred to as a vaginoplasty, this surgical manipulation more correctly occurs in the vestibule.[17] The technique is appropriate for mares with mild conformational faults or transient VVR primarily caused by hormone-induced relaxation of the reproductive tract or secondary to foaling.

Caudal relocation of the transverse fold is routinely performed on the standing mare, using local infiltration anesthesia. No special surgical instruments are required; however, a set of long-handled instruments is helpful. Postoperative management is minimal.

The technique will not be satisfactory in all cases to prevent urine pooling. Caudal relocation of the transverse fold should not be performed on mares with severe vaginal slope, because it can lead to complications if a urethral extension procedure is required later.

Surgical Preparation

The surgery is performed on the standing, restrained mare. Tranquilization with xylazine hydrochloride and butorphanol tartrate or the use of a lip twitch is recommended.

The rectum is manually cleaned of fecal matter, the tail is wrapped and tied away from the surgical field, and the perineal area scrubbed with povidone-iodine soap. The vestibule and vagina are flushed with a 2% dilute providone-iodine solution in saline.

If a Caslick operation has been performed, a local anesthetic should be administered to the vulvar labia and the suture opened; if a Caslick procedure is anticipated after the operation, the area around the vulvar lips can be infiltrated with 2% mepivacaine hydrochloride before surgery.

Retraction sutures are set on either side of the vulvar lips and either held in place by an assistant or sutured to the buttocks, to allow adequate exposure to the vulvar area.

Surgical Procedure

The transverse fold looks like a flap of wrinkled tissue and runs horizontally across the vaginal floor, obscuring the urethral orifice. The transverse fold is grasped just left of center with a thumb forceps, and from just left of center, the tissue should be infiltrated with a 2% mepivacaine hydrochloride and include 5 to 7 cm of the vestibular wall. Local anesthesia is identically administered in the opposite side. Alternatively, an epidural anesthetic may be administered.

The transverse fold just left of center should be grasped with thumb forceps and retracted caudad 3 to 5 cm, preparatory to making an incision in the vestibular wall. To ascertain the line of the proposed attachment and incision, the transverse fold is positioned along the ventrolateral wall of the vestibule. Using a #10 scalpel blade, the incision is made from the point where the forceps are attached, extending to the junction of the transverse fold with the wall of the vestibule, then caudad 3 to 5 cm along the vestibular wall (Fig. 49–1A). The procedure is repeated on the right side.

The transverse fold is then grasped in the middle and retracted caudad. The incision along the left transverse fold is sutured to the incision on the lateral wall of the vestibule, beginning on the caudal end, in two everting layers. A minimal amount of tension must be exerted on the tissue when it is sutured into its new position (Fig. 49–1B).

The new urethral orifice should be approximately 2 to 2.5 cm from the floor of the vestibule, allowing sufficient size for normal urine flow while not protruding up into the vestibule so high as to risk tearing the orifice during copulation or vaginal examination. Finally, the vulvar labia are closed with a Caslick operation.

Postoperative Management

Postoperative management is basically threefold: tetanus prophylaxis, a course of antibiotics, and anti-inflammatory drugs are initiated preoperatively and continued postoperatively as needed; the vaginal area is not examined or manipulated for 2 weeks; and the mare is sexually rested for 30 to 60 days, during which time any uterine infection or disease may be treated.

PERINEAL BODY TRANSECTION (PERINEOPLASTY)

Mares with severely deformed perineal conformation (sunken anus and tilted vulva that have been pulled dorsad and craniad) because of hereditary predisposition, repeated foaling, or thinning of the perineal body present a special surgical problem. These mares suffer from pneumovagina and VVR that often requires such

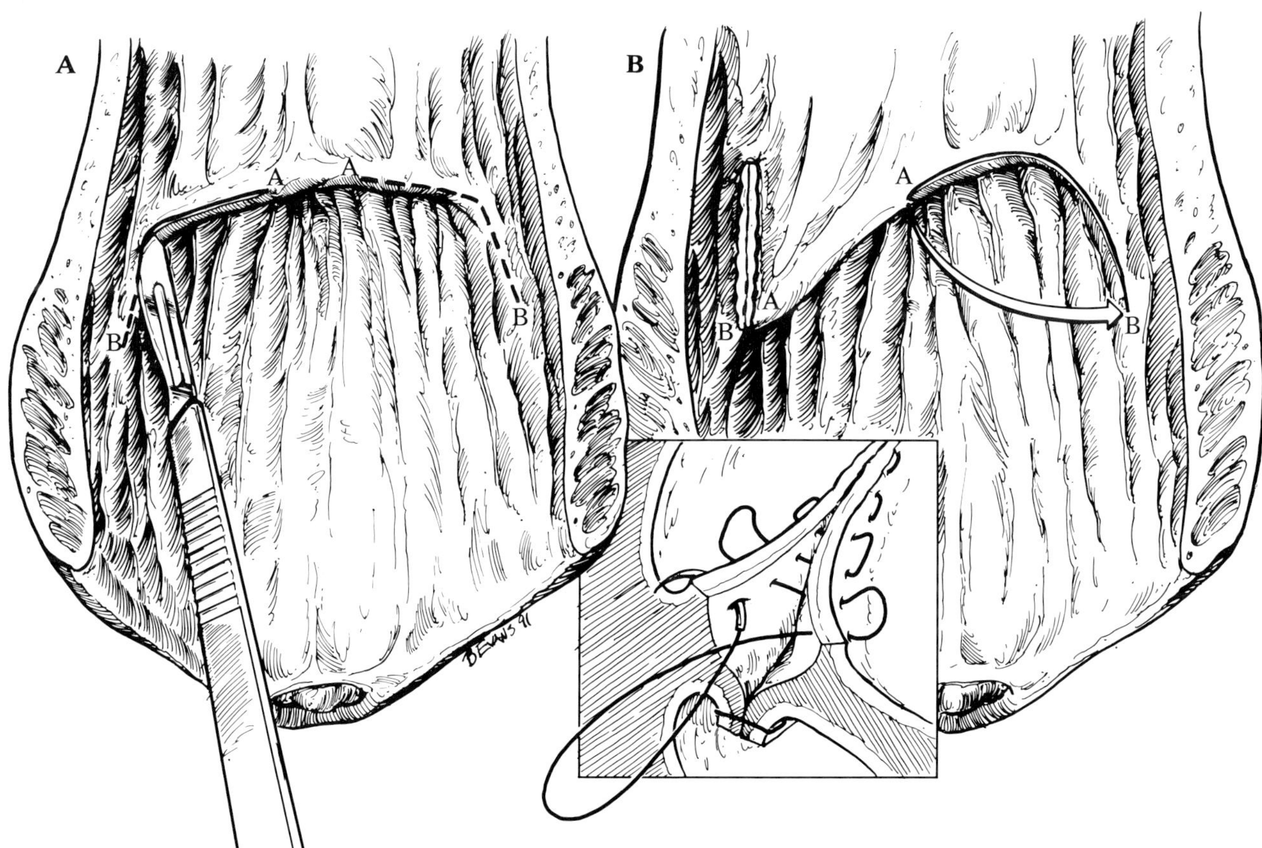

FIG. 49–1. *A*, Vaginoplasty technique to correct vesicovaginal reflux. The transverse fold is grasped (A) and retracted caudad and laterad (3 to 5 cm) to a desired point (B). An incision is then made on each side of the transverse fold and vestibular wall from points A to B. *B*, The transverse fold is retracted from points A to B and the cut edges closed in two layers of everting sutures. This brings points A and B into apposition. (Courtesy of Brian Evans and Dr. G.W. Trotter, Colorado State University.)

extensive episioplasty that the resulting vulvar opening is not of sufficient size to allow the mare to be bred. In correcting this condition, positive results have been achieved by using a modification of the technique described by Pouret and later modified by Trotter and McKinnon.[2,9]

The surgical procedure is designed to restore normal anatomic relationships of the caudal vagina, vestibule, and vulvar lips by separating muscular and ligamentous attachments of the caudal vagina from the pull of the dorsally displaced rectum.

Surgical Preparation

Before surgery, the mare should be placed on a diet that will encourage loose, moist manure. The surgical procedure should be performed while the mare is sedated and standing, restrained in the stocks. Epidural anesthesia can be used or the procedure may be carried out with local infiltration anesthesia; a combination of epidural and local infiltration anesthesia in the perineal body with lidocaine and 1:100 epinephrine is recommended. The local infiltration anesthesia helps separate the tissue plane between the rectum and the dorsal vaginal wall and aids in dissection. The tail should be wrapped, rectum evacuated of fecal matter, and perineal region prepared in the usual manner.

Surgical Procedure

A slightly curved 10 to 15-cm horizontal skin incision is made midway between the ventral border of the anus and the dorsal commissure of the vulva. The incision should be made 2 to 3 cm beyond the lateral borders of the perineum, with the curve following the line of the dorsal commissure of the vulva. Towel clamps or traction sutures can be placed on the dorsal and ventral edges of the wound to aid in the dissection.

A curved pair of long Nelson or Metzenbaum scissors with the blades pointed downward are then used to dissect through the muscles of the perineal body (Fig. 49–2A) Digital palpation, as well as applying traction on the wound edges while one hand palpates within the vestibule, is helpful in ascertaining the exact plane of dissection. The dissection should be carried out in a plane which leaves the predominant amount of tissue to be left with the rectum. Penetration of the rectum and vestibule should be avoided, because this could lead to fistula formation.

Dissection continues craniad for a variable distance (8 to 20 cm) until the vulva is vertically oriented without using traction (Fig. 49–2B). The dorsal and lateral edges of the vulva are secured to the skin of the perineum with stay sutures to avoid their being pulled dorsad as the wound contracts (Fig. 49–2C). The perineal plane of dissection is left open to heal by second intention, and the wound is packed with a roll of povidone-iodine–soaked gauze.

The packing is sutured in place and changed every 3 to 4 days, until the wound has closed. When the wound has granulated and epithelialized, the stay sutures should be removed. The open wound usually heals within 2 to 3 weeks. After the procedure, the mare may have a noticeable shelf between the dorsal commissure of the vulva and the anus where fecal balls may periodically rest. After the tissues have healed, the reproductive tract should be evaluated. Breeding can be resumed at that time.

URETHRAL EXTENSION (URETHROPLASTY)

Urethroplasty provides caudal extension of the urethra and is required in mares with VVR caused by a severe cranioventral slope (> 20°) to the vaginal vault. It is indicated when the transverse fold is displaced craniad and should be used if any question about the success of a vaginoplasty to correct vesicovaginal reflux exists.

Two techniques have been described: The first is the urethral extension delineated by Brown et al.[18] The procedure is no longer used by some clinicians because of problems of fistula formation and urinary obstruction leading to cystitis and nephritis.[12] The second technique, a urethroplasty described by McKinnon and Belden,[16] has the advantage of providing a wide, long, and strong tunnel for evacuation of urine. The technique requires special surgical instrumentation and expertise, and in my experience, provides the most reliable method of correcting VVR with the fewest postoperative complications.[16,19]

Surgical Preparation

The mare is sedated while standing and epidural anesthesia is induced using 2% lidocaine hydrochloride or xylazine.[20] If the mare has had a previous epidural, results may be unsatisfactory. Therefore, local infiltration of the perineal body and vaginal walls with a 2% mepavicaine hydrochloride may be necessary. The tail is wrapped and tied out of the field. Fecal material in the rectum is manually evacuated. The perineal area is scrubbed with povidone-iodine soap and the vaginal vault is lavaged with a dilute 2% povidone-iodine solution in saline and the fluid suctioned out of the surgical field.

The following special surgical instrumentation is recommended: (1) a head light or flexible light source; (2) a #3 long knife handle and #12 blade; (3) 28-cm (11-in.) curved Nelson or Metzenbaum scissors; (4) 23-cm (10-in.) tissue forceps with 2 × 3 teeth; (5) 25-cm (10-in.) needle holders; and (6) a self-retaining Glasser or Aanes (Scanlan Surgical Instruments, Englewood, CO) retractor. Hemorrhage can be controlled by ligation but is best dealt with by electrocautery or CO_2 laser dissection. Electrocautery requires the mare be in insulated stocks to prevent electrical shock or skin burn.

Surgical Procedure

Self-retaining retractors are placed in the vaginal vault to gain exposure of the surgical site. The central caudal border of the transverse fold is grasped with Allis tissue

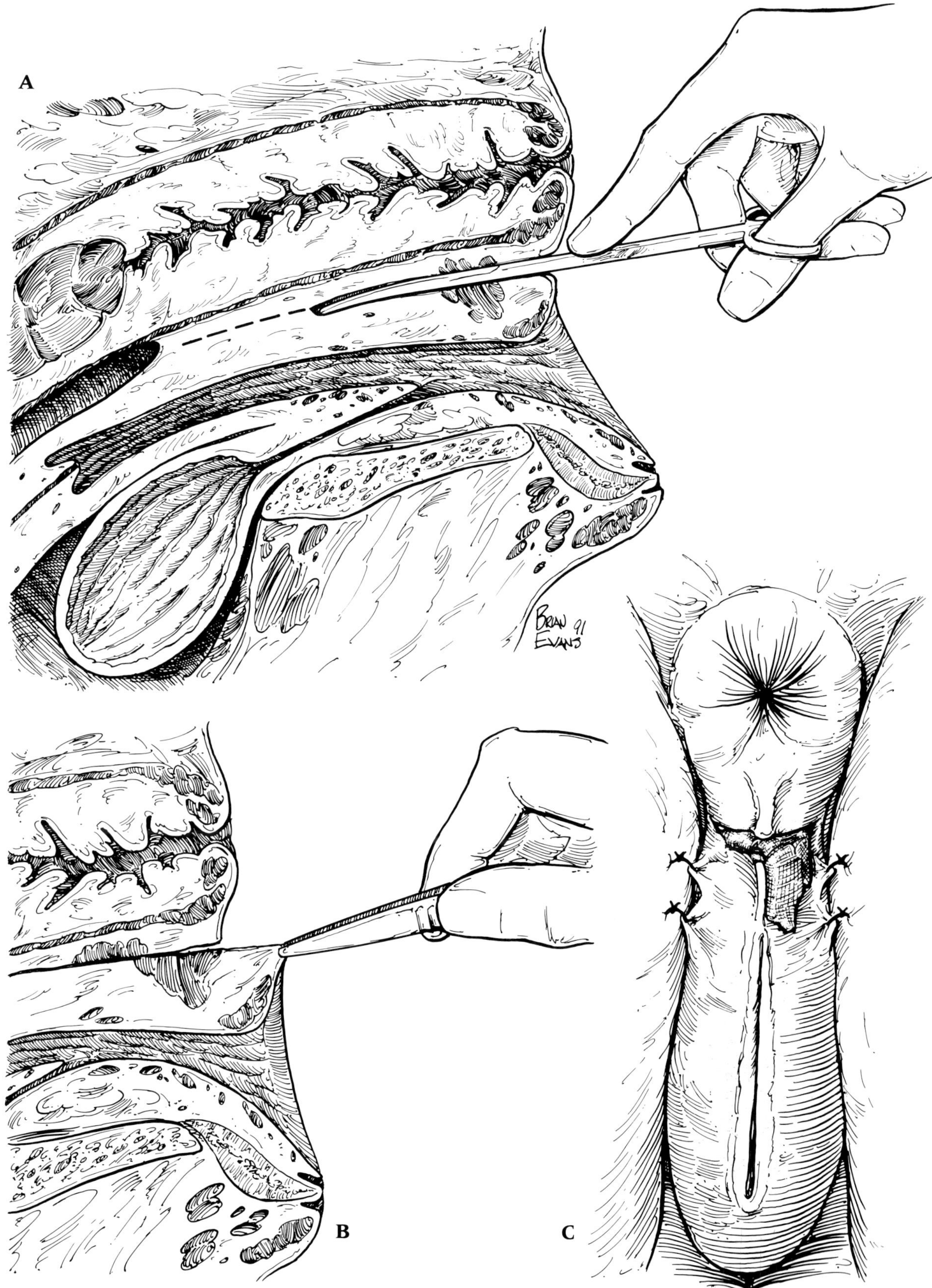

FIG. 49–2. *A,* The perineoplasty technique is performed by dissecting between the rectum and vagina to a depth of 8 to 20 cm separating these structures. *B,* The vaginal tissue is retracted caudad, bringing the vulva into a more vertical position. *C,* The vulvar tissue is secured with sutures to the skin lateral to the perineum. The perineal plane of dissection is packed with povidone-iodine–soaked roll gauze and allowed to heal by second intention. (Courtesy of Brian Evans and Dr. G.W. Trotter, Colorado State University.)

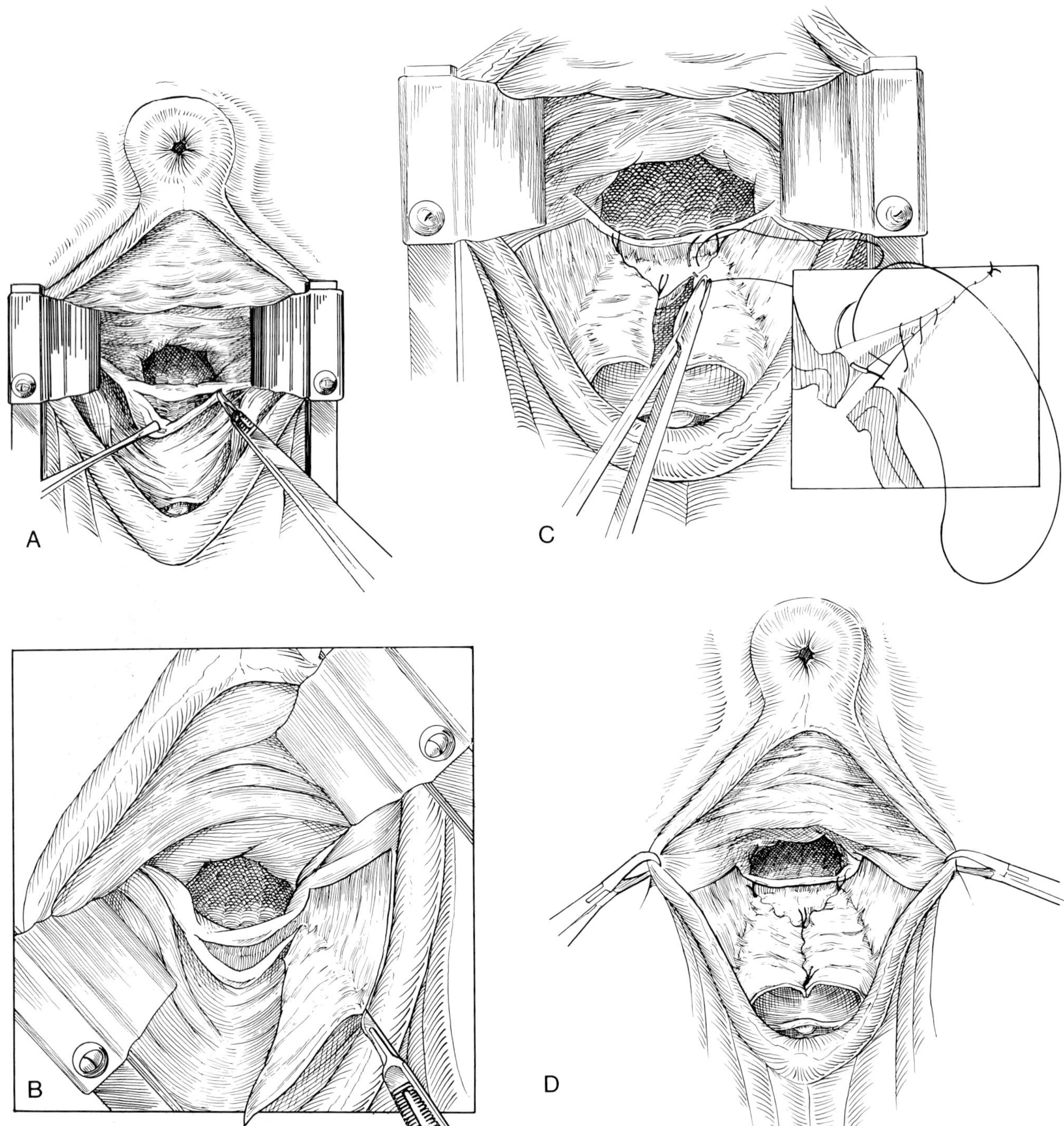

FIG. 49–3. *A,* To begin the urethral extension procedure, the vaginal vault has been exposed using self-retaining retractors. The transverse fold and right vestibular mucosa have been incised and a submucosal flap raised. *B,* The incision is extended laterad, curved slightly dorsad on the vestibular wall, and carried caudad to the labia at a point approximately half the distance between the vestibular floor and roof. *C,* The reflected submucosal flaps are apposed on their raw surfaces by sutures inverting the mucosa into the urethral tunnel. *D,* The finished urethral extension is in the shape of a *Y* with the base at the caudal end of the tunnel. (Adapted from McKinnon, A.O., and Beldon, J.O.: A urethral extension technique to correct urine pooling (vesicovaginal reflux) in mares. J. Am. Vet. Med. Assoc., *192:*647–650, 1988. *In* Trotter, G.W.: Surgical diseases of the caudal reproductive tract. *In* Equine Surgery. Edited by J.A. Auer. Philadelphia, W.B. Saunders. In press.)

forceps and retracted caudad. A horizontal incision with a #12 Bard-Parker blade across the dorsal edge of the transverse fold, 2 to 4 cm cranial to its caudal border, taking care to incise only through the dorsal mucosa and into the submucosa (Fig. 49–3A). The incision is then carried laterad and curved slightly dorsad upon the vestibular wall. The incision is extended caudad to the labia at a level of about half the distance between the vestibular floor and roof (Fig. 49–3B).

The caudal cut edge from the transverse fold incision and the ventral cut edge of the vestibular incision are dissected to free and raise a mucosal-submucosal flap. This continuous flap is reflected caudad and mediad, resulting in a Y-shaped configuration; the mucous membranes of the free-tissue flaps are ventral, and the raw submucosal edges, dorsal. The dissection is continued until the new caudal edge of the transverse fold flap can be reflected about 3 to 6 cm caudad and laterally cut edges of the vestibular portion of the flap can be apposed on the midline without tension (Fig. 49–3B).

An inverting suture pattern of #2-0 adsorbable suture is used to appose the submucosal tissue layer, beginning at the cranial end of one side of the union of the transverse fold and vestibular wall flaps and progressing caudad to the midline. A second suture is begun at the opposite cranial end and brought to meet the first suture on the midline (Fig. 49–3C). The inverting submucosal pattern is then continued caudad to the labia. The result is a strong, wide, extended tunnel from the urethral orifice (under the transverse fold) to the caudal vestibule. It is critical that the apposed submucosal edges be inverted with the raw edges in apposition and under minimal tension (Fig. 49–3D).

The denuded tissue created dorsally by the extensive dissection to create the tissue flaps is allowed to heal by granulation and epithelialization. If necessary a Caslick operation or perineoplasty can be performed at this time or delayed for 2 to 3 weeks.

Postoperative Management

Tetanus prophylaxis, a course of antibiotics and nonsteroidal anti-inflammatory drugs are initiated. To allow appropriate healing, the reproductive tract should not be examined for 2 to 4 weeks postoperatively.

The dissection must be carried out high enough on the vestibular walls to allow a 2- to 4-cm diameter urethral tunnel. A small tunnel can lead to urinary retention and predispose to cystitis or even nephritis. Several cases of such conditions have been seen following urethral tunnel procedures, using another urethral extension technique.[12] Fistula formation can occur, but in every case I have seen, it has been associated with previous unsuccessful urethral extension surgery and altered anatomy with scar tissue present at the surgical site. Early postoperative manipulation of the tissue with the hand or vaginal speculum can also lead to fistula formation. The urethral tunnel established with this technique occupies the ventral 2 to 3 cm of the vestibule. This is not a concern in a natural breeding situation, but precautions should be taken during vaginal examination to prevent iatrogenic injuries to the tunnel roof. Fistula formation at the surgical site does not always result in recurrence of urine pooling. The mare should, therefore, be examined several times for urovagina before recommending repair of the fistula.

Fistulas that result in VVR must be surgically repaired. Small holes can be repaired by careful dissection of the mucosal edge of the fistula to create dorsal and ventral tissue flaps. These mucosal flaps are closed in an everting pattern with #3-0 absorbable suture material. To repair a large defect in the urethral tunnel, the roof of the extended urethra is incised to the fistula and the mucosal edge is separated into dorsal and ventral layers. The layers are then closed separately everting the mucosal edges, following the basic principles of urogenital surgery.[21]

REFERENCES

1. Engle, M.J.: Urine pooling in the mare. Iowa State Vet., *1*:5–8, 1980.
2. Pouret, E.J.M.: Surgical techniques for correction of pneumo- and urovagina. Equine Vet. J., *14*:249–250, 1982.
3. Asbury, A.C.: Infections and immunologic considerations in mare infertility. Compend. Contin. Educ. Practicing Vet., *9*:585–592, 1987.
4. Pickett, B.W., et al.: Management of the stallion for maximum reproductive efficiency. Animal Reproduction Lab, General Series, No. 1005. Fort Collins, Colorado State University, 1981.
5. Ansari, M.M.: The Caslick's operation in mares. Compend. Contin. Educ. Practicing Vet., *5*:S107–S111, 1983.
6. Caslick, E.A.: The vulva and the vulvo-vaginal orifice and its relationship to genital health of the Thoroughbred mare. Cornell Vet., *27*:178–187, 1937.
7. Hinrichs, K., et al.: Clinical significance of aerobic bacterial flora of the uterus, vagina, vestibule and clitoral fossa of clinically normal mares. J. Am. Vet. Med. Assoc., *193*:72–78, 1988.
8. McIlwraith, C.W., and Turner, A.S.: Equine surgery advanced techniques. Philadelphia, Lea & Febiger, 1986, pp. 163–166.
9. Trotter, G.W., and McKinnon, A.O.: Surgery for abnormal vulvar and perineal conformation in the mare. Vet. Clin. North Am. Equine Pract., *4*:389–405, 1988.
10. Vaughan, J.T.: The practice of large animal surgery, edited by P.B. Jennings. Philadelphia, W.B. Saunders, 1984, pp. 1122–1140.
11. Pugh, E.G., and Caudle, A.B.: Equine pyometra: A case report. J. Equine Vet. Sci., *7*:92–93, 1987.
12. Ehnen, S.J., Divers, T.J., Gillette, D., and Reef, V.B.: Obstructive nephrolithiasis and ureterolithiasis associated with chronic renal failure in horses:. Eight cases (1981–1987). J. Am. Vet. Med. Assoc., *197*:249–253, 1990.
13. Slusher, S.H., Freeman, K.P., and Roszel, J.F.: Infertility diagnosis in mares using endometrial biopsy, culture and aspirate cytology. Proc. Am. Assoc. Equine Pract., 165–170, 1986.
14. Shires, G.M., and Kaneps, A.J.: A practical and simple

surgical technique for repair of urine pooling in the mare. Proc. Am. Assoc. Equine. Pract., 51–56, 1986.

15. Bowman, T.R.: A surgical solution to urine pooling. Mod. Horse Breeding, *3:*14–17, 1986.
16. McKinnon, A.O., and Belden, J.O.: A urethral extension technique to correct urine pooling (vesicovaginal reflux) in mares. J. Am. Vet. Med. Assoc., *192:*647–650, 1988.
17. Monin, T.: Vaginoplasty: A surgical treatment for urine pooling in the mare. Proc. Am. Assoc. Equine Pract., 99–192, 1972.
18. Brown, M.P., Colahan, P.T., and Hawkins, D.L.: Urethral extension for treatment of urine pooling in mares. J. Am. Vet. Med. Assoc., *173*:1005–1007, 1978.
19. Easley, K.J.: Diagnosis and treatment of vesicovaginal reflux in the mare. Vet. Clin. North Am. Equine Pract., *4:*407–416, 1988.
20. LeBlanc, P.H., et al.: Epidural injection of xylazine for perineal analgesia in horses. J. Am. Vet. Med. Assoc., *193:*1405–1408, 1988.
21. Embertson, R.M.: Urovagina. *In* Current Practice in Equine Surgery. Edited N.A. White, and J.N. Moore. Philadelphia, J.B. Lippincott, 1990, pp. 693–696.

CHAPTER 50

CESAREAN SECTION

T.S. Stashak
M. Vandeplassche

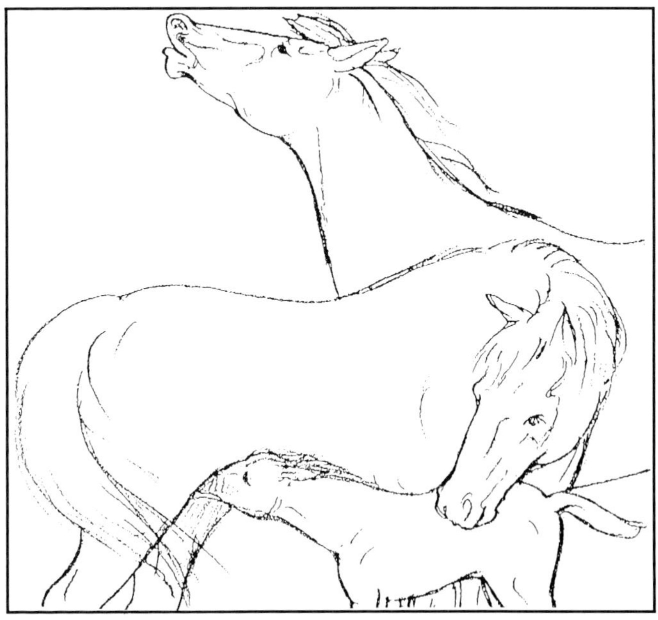

Cesarean section is indicated when vaginal delivery cannot be achieved in a dystocia[1–8] and may be required in certain cases of uterine tears (rupture)[9] and uterine torsion.[10] Reasons for elective cesarean section are the production of gnotobiotic foals[11] and the recognition of an undersize pelvic diameter before parturition.[12]

Malpositions (particularly transverse presentations) and fetal deformities (ankylosed joints, fetal monsters, and hydrocephalus) are the most common causes of dystocia requiring cesarean delivery.[1,6,7,12,13] Incidence of fetal deformities in a series of 601 severe dystocias was 30 to 35%[13] and in another series of 17 cases of cesarean delivery it was 37%.[12] Occasionally, an undersize (juvenile) pelvis or a pelvic mass that reduces its diameter or vaginal scarring may be the cause of dystocia. If these later conditions are recognized, elective cesarean section should be considered. Although in experienced hands most dystocias are managed by reposition, partial fetotomy of the dead foal, and traction, the decision for cesarean delivery should not be considered a last resort. Delay in decision for surgery usually results in more trauma to the mare and a greater chance of losing the mare and foal.[4]

Uterine tears may be caused by dystocia, uterine torsion and overzealous manipulation of the fetus in an attempt to deliver it.[9] When a uterine tear is diagnosed before the foal is delivered, cesarean section is indicated to reduce the chances of enlarging the tear, which would result in greater contamination of the abdominal cavity, and to prevent herniation of the abdominal viscera.[9] Once a cesarean delivery is completed and the uterine incision is closed, the tear is sutured.

Uterine torsion in the last trimester of pregnancy is often best managed by standing flank laparotomy and detorsion of the gravid uterus or by rolling the mare while under anesthesia[10,14] (see Chapters 53 and 68). However, if the mare is full-term, the uterus has ruptured, or the torsion cannot be corrected, a cesarean delivery is recommended. If the uterus can be untwisted easily, it is followed by delivery or cesarean section. If the detorsion is difficult, cesarean section precedes the untwisting of the torsion.[10] In the case of a uterine tear, it may be sutured after the hysterotomy incision is closed,[15] except when the tear is close to the cervix. In the latter case, the tear should be sutured first, because it may not be approachable after the uterus begins to contract.

SURGICAL PREPARATION AND ANESTHESIA

Administration of intravenous balanced electrolyte fluids and parenteral antibiotics should commence before surgery. Ideally, sufficient fluids are given to stabilize the patient physiologically before induction of anesthesia. The nonsteroidal anti-inflammatory agent flunixin meglumine (0.44 mg/kg body weight) can be administered intravenously if endotoxic shock is a concern.

Selection of an anesthetic regimen may vary whether

the foal is alive or dead. If the foal is dead, anesthesia is by personal choice, yet it is advisable to select an anesthetic agent that does not increase uterine bleeding. If the foal is alive, several anesthetic options may be considered to reduce pharmacologic fetal depression as well as reduce uterine bleeding. Although epidural anesthesia combined with chloral hydrate and guaifenesin and a low oblique flank celiotomy have been used successfully in Europe,[6] gas anesthesia, dorsal recumbency and ventral midline celiotomy are preferred in North America.[3,4,7,8,12]

Premedication with a low dose of acepromazine is acceptable followed by induction with guaifenesin and ketamine or guaifenesin and thiamylal sodium. Bolus administration of a thiobarbiturate is discouraged. Methohexital sodium was shown to be superior to thiopental sodium as an induction agent for obtaining live gnotobiotic foals by cesarean delivery.[11] Although halothane and oxygen have been used for maintenance of anesthesia and live foals have been obtained, this combination increases uterine incisional bleeding.[11] Methoxyflurane or isoflurane and oxygen are preferred because they are short acting and do not encourage uterine bleeding.

SURGERY

Once the patient is recumbent, aseptic preparation for surgery should progress rapidly. Two celiotomy approaches are used most commonly for cesarean delivery: the low oblique flank (Marcenac) and the ventral midline.[12] The Marcenac celiotomy is popular in Europe.[6] The left flank is preferred because the cecum is in the right flank region. The skin incision begins just caudal to the midcostal region and extends caudoventrad to just below the fold of the flank. The abdominal fascia (superficial and deep) is incised in a similar fashion and deepened to expose the muscular fibers of the external abdominal oblique. The muscular fibers of the external abdominal oblique are separated by blunt finger dissection in the same plane as the more superficial incision. Once the external abdominal oblique muscle fibers are retracted, the aponeurosis of the internal abdominal oblique muscle is exposed, and it is incised at right angles to the separated external abdominal oblique muscle fibers. Underlying the retracted internal abdominal oblique aponeurosis is the transversely oriented transverse abdominal oblique muscle. This muscle is separated in the direction of its fibers so as to bisect the right angles of the abdominal oblique muscles. The upper edge of the rectus abdominal muscle is encountered at the lower end of the incision and must be retracted ventrad. The retroperitoneal fat of the fascia transversalis and peritoneum are incised in the same plane as the skin incision. The incision is then retracted sufficiently to allow elevation of a gravid horn of the uterus into the incision.[6,7] Although the low oblique flank has been used successfully in a large series of cases, incision infection and partial wound dehiscence are complications.[6,11] In addition, this approach limits the access to the abdominal cavity compared with that of the ventral midline.

The caudoventral midline celiotomy is most popular in North America because abdominal entry is rapid, no muscles are encountered, bleeding is minimal, and the incision can be lengthened quickly if needed. The skin incision is begun just cranial to the mammary glands and extends craniad on the ventral midline for 30 to 40 cm. The subcutaneous tissue is incised sharply in a similar fashion to expose the narrow, slightly elevated fibrous linea alba. The linea is incised over its center along its length to expose the retroperitoneal fat of the fascia transversalis. The fat is separated by finger dissection and the peritoneum is opened by finger puncture followed by blunt separation longitudinally to correspond to the length of the skin incision. The initial concerns about postoperative incisional dehiscence with this approach have been unfounded.

In either celiotomy approach, the incision must be long enough to allow the surgeon's hands and arms to enter the abdominal cavity to palpate, manipulate, and elevate the gravid uterus. Uterine displacements are preferably corrected before the gravid horn is elevated. However if the correction of the displacement is difficult or the uterus appears edematous and friable, the cesarean delivery and suture closure of the hysterot-

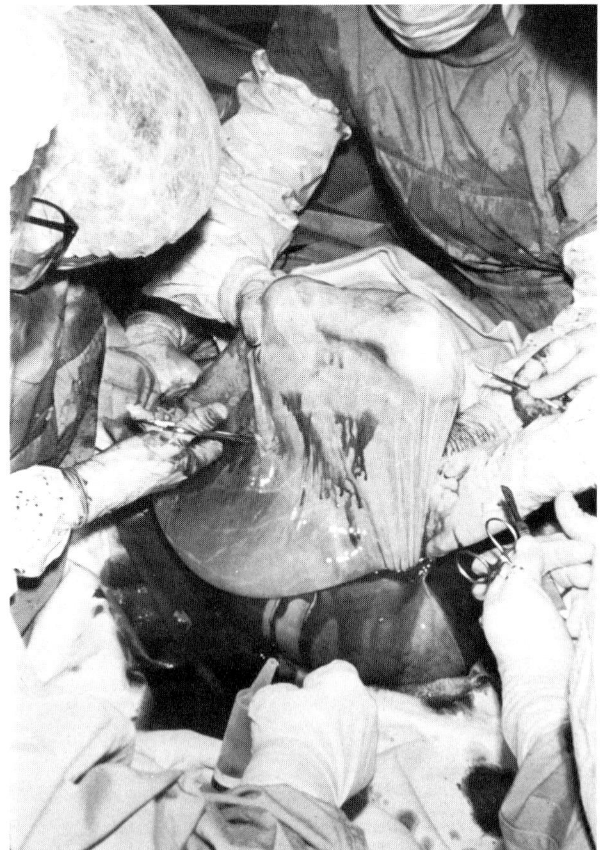

FIG. 50–1. The uterus has been incised with a scalpel and the amnion is being opened with scissors. Note the fetal limbs are visible through the amnionic membrane.

omy incision should precede correction of the displacement.[9,10,14] Once the gravid horn containing the limbs is elevated, the uterus is isolated from the abdominal incision and the abdominal cavity with laparotomy drapes. Rubberized laparotomy drapes that are impervious to fluid penetration are preferred. This is done because in all cases the uterine fluid should be considered contaminated. At this point the gravid exteriorized uterine horn can be stabilized by grasping a fetal limb(s) through the uterine wall. The uterine incision is made over the greater curvature of the gravid horn and it should be long enough to allow delivery of the fetus without risk of tearing the uterus. The incision, however, should not be extended to the uterine tip where the oviduct enters. Generally, with posterior presentation a longer hysterotomy incision will be needed, because the fetus's head and limbs are in one uterine horn. In contrast, an anterior presentation where only the feet and hind limbs are in the uterine horn, a smaller incision can be made.[7] The uterine incision is made with a scalpel. The placenta and amnion may be incised with the scalpel or scissors (Fig. 50–1). Considerable hemorrhage will be encountered from large vessels within the myometrium and subendometrial regions. Once the uterus is open, sterile obstetrical chains are placed around the limbs and the fetus is extracted by simultaneous lifting by the surgeon and pulling by an assistant (Fig. 50–2).

If the fetus is alive and apparently normal, it is laid down beside the mare until pulsations of the umbilical artery are decreased and breathing begins (Fig. 50–3). In most cases, this will occur within 5 min.[7] While in this position, nasopharyngeal and oral mucous are removed by wiping and suction. Bottled oxygen, intubation, and positive pressure ventilation may be needed (Fig. 50–4). Once arterial pulsations decrease and respiration begins, the umbilical cord may be broken or severed at the slight constriction a few centimeters from the cutaneous navel. This should be done without pulling excessively on the site of attachment to the foal, because it may predispose to an umbilical hernia.[7] Alternatively, the umbilicus may be crushed with a forcep some 5 cm from its cutaneous attachment, after which it is separated sharply. If bleeding persists in the uterine side, a ligature may be placed. An assistant should be available to attend to the foal's needs at this time. If the fetus is dead, it should be removed as quickly as possible and ligature of the umbilical vessels or clamping is acceptable if bleeding persists.

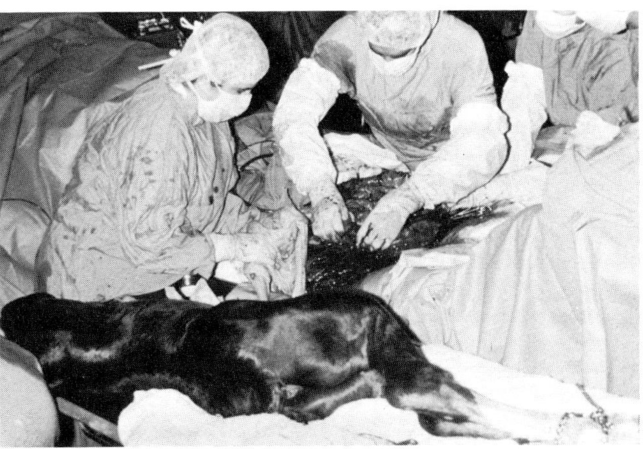

FIG. 50–3. The foal is laid down on a separate table beside the mare. Note the umbilical cord is still intact. The foal's head and neck (lower left) are off the end of the table where an assistant is cleaning the mucus out of its mouth.

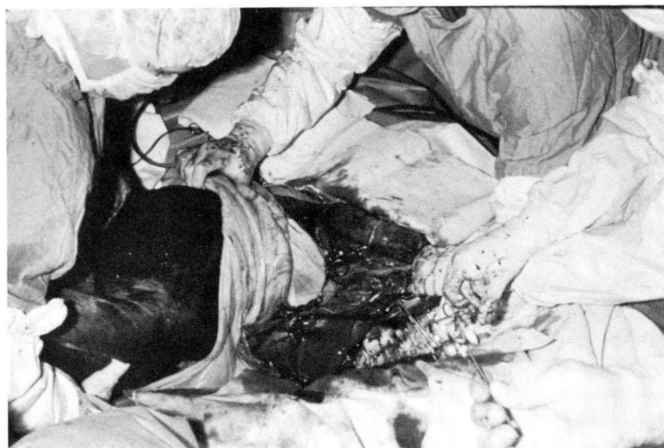

FIG. 50–2. Sterile obstetric chains have been applied to the fetus's hind limbs (not visible) and the surgeon is lifting the fetus while an assistant (not visible) is applying traction with the obstetric chains. The assistant surgeon (top right) is holding the uterus so it will not be pulled off the surgical field.

Once the fetus is delivered, the fluid remaining within the uterus is aspirated to reduce the chances of spillage and further contamination of the surgery site. Loosely adhered placentas are removed. This reduces the amount of postoperative care required to manage a retained placenta. If the placenta is adhered, it is separated manually from the endometrium for 5 to 10 cm around the circumference of the uterine incision. This is done so the placenta will not be included in the continuous through-and-through hemostatic suture pattern that will be applied to the edge of the uterine incision. The cavity of the uterus may be flushed with sterile physiologic saline solution, after which the fluid is aspirated, which is done to reduce the bacterial concentration. The addition of dilute antiseptic (i.e., 0.1% or 0.2% povidone-iodine solution) or an antimicrobial is by personal preference. However, remember that a greater concentration of povidone-iodine can inhibit white blood cell function and irritate the endometrial lining, which makes the uterus more susceptible to infection. Additions of some antimicrobials, particularly the sulfonamides, also act like higher concentrations of povidone-iodine and, therefore, should not be used.[16]

Closure of the uterus must take into account adequate hemostasis and the fact that the surgical field is contaminated. Although large subendometrial vessels can be ligated individually, this is usually not sufficient to control the mural hemorrhage that will continue to bleed into the uterine cavity following inverting suture

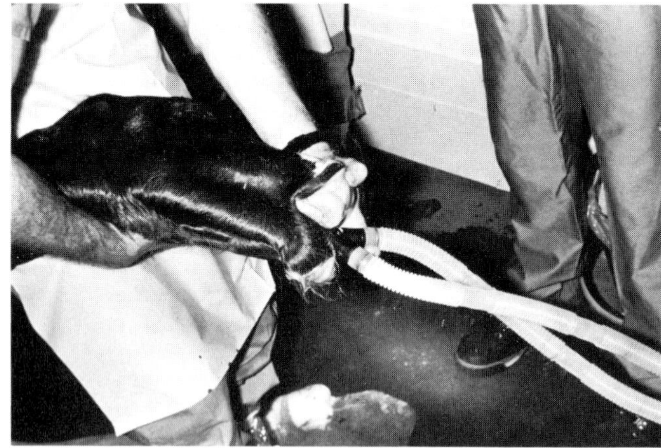

FIG. 50–4. Foal is still on the separate table. Because this foal was having difficulty breathing, an endotracheal tube was passed and oxygen delivered with positive pressure ventilation.

closure. Continued bleeding has been recognized as a significant cause of death in mares after cesarean section.[6] To prevent this, a continuous interlocking or simple continuous suture of #0 or #1 surgical gut is placed through all layers of the uterus (excluding the placenta) and around the entire circumference of the incision (Fig. 50–5).[4,6,12] The continuous suture must be placed tightly enough to effect good hemostasis. Following this, the cut margin of the uterus is cleansed with dilute antiseptic sterile physiologic saline solution after which the uterus is closed with a two-layer inverting pattern. Either continuous Cushing (the first author's preference) or a continuous Lembert suture of #0 surgical gut or #0 synthetic absorbable may be used. If the uterus is edematous or friable, surgical gut is recommended, because there is less tendency for this suture material to cut through the weakened wall of the uterus. In any case, the continuous suture should be pulled tightly enough so the sutures are buried and not exposed to the peritoneal cavity (Fig. 50–6). Cleansing the incision line with dilute antiseptic sterile physiologic saline solution after the first layer of closure is recommended to reduce bacterial contamination. After the uterus is closed with a second inverting suture layer, the blood clots on the outer surface of the uterus are removed by gentle wiping with dilute antiseptic sterile physiologic saline solution. The surgeon's gloves should be rinsed, after which the rubber drapes are removed and the rest of the uterus is examined for tears.

If a tear is found, it is sutured in a similar fashion as just described. In some cases, however, the continuous suture to stop myometrial bleeding may not be needed because hemorrhage may have ceased.[9] However, if any question exists, a continuous encircling suture is recommended. If the uterus was torn, the abdomen should be lavaged copiously with warm sterile physiologic saline solution to reduce the peritoneal contamination.[9] Before closure, a fenestrated tube drain (Ortho Tubing #621326, Biomet Friesen, Lakewood, CO) may be placed to remove the contaminated peritoneal fluid from the abdominal cavity in the postoperative period. The drain should be flushed with full-strength sterile heparin before placement in the abdomen to prevent fibrin clots from occluding the fenestrated openings. The drain is placed with the aid of a sharp trocar, which penetrates the abdominal wall in a dependent location adjacent to the celiotomy incision. The fenestrated portion of the drain remains in the abdominal cavity while the nonfenestrated portion exits through the abdominal wall to the exterior. The drain is sutured to the skin to fix it in place. Generally, the drain is removed within 12 h after recovery.

Before closing the celiotomy incision, the wound's edges should be cleansed with a dilute antiseptic sterile physiologic saline solution to ensure that all blood clots are removed. If the uterus was not ruptured, gowns, gloves, and instruments are changed for sterile ones and a new wound drape applied. Plastic drapes or soft rubberized drapes are preferred. Closure can commence without suturing the peritoneum. If a uterine rupture was found, the peritoneum may be sutured to create a barrier to contaminated abdominal contents. Simple continuous sutures of #2-0 synthetic absorbable suture is recommended for peritoneal closure, because less chances of visceral adhesion to the ventral midline exist. In this case the incision is lavaged after the peritoneum is closed and the surgical attire is changed, including drapes, after which the celiotomy incision is closed.

Closure of the low oblique flank incision is accomplished with interrupted or continuous sutures of #0 or #1 synthetic absorbable suture. Each layer is sutured independently and the skin can be apposed with surgical staples or nonabsorbable sutures. The placement of a drain between muscle layers is recommended and in all cases a stent bandage over the skin incision should be employed.

Closure of the ventral midline can be accomplished

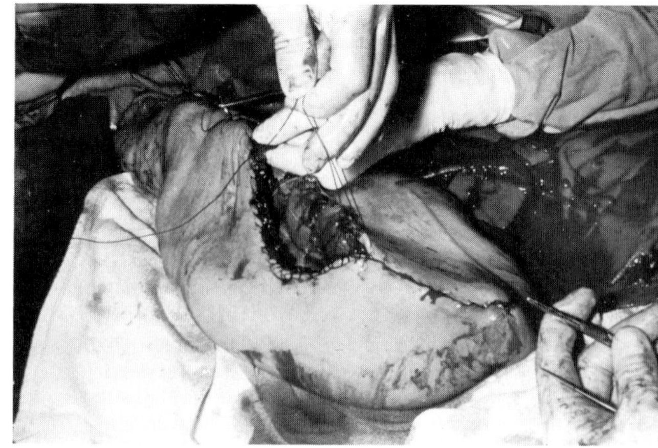

FIG. 50–5. The uterine incision is being sutured. *Center left,* The simple continuous hemostatic suture encircling the cut edge of the uterus is seen. *Lower right,* The first continuous Cushing suture pattern is being applied to close the uterine incision.

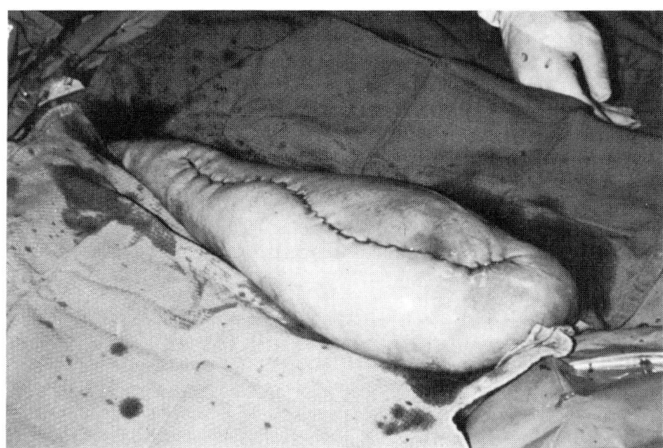

FIG. 50–6. Closure of the hysterotomy incision is complete. Note the suture and knots are buried. In addition, the uterus has been wiped clean and it is ready for replacement in the abdominal cavity.

with either doubled #2-0 synthetic absorbable suture in a continuous suture pattern or with a single strand of a like material placed in a simple interrupted or cruciate mattress pattern. The subcutaneous tissues are apposed with simple continuous #2-0 synthetic absorbable suture and the skin is apposed with surgical skin staples or continuous horizontal mattress of #2-0 monofilament nylon. The application of a stent bandage sutured over the celiotomy incision is recommended.

Upon completion of the abdominal closure, oxytocin (20 IU administered IV) may be given to aid in the expulsion of the remaining placenta and uterine fluid.[16] It also encourages involution of the uterus.

POSTOPERATIVE CARE AND COMPLICATIONS

Fluid therapy is continued until the patient is stable. Antibiotics are continued until the placenta has passed and the uterine lochia (fluid) appears clear after the lavage and siphonage. If the placenta was removed at surgery, the antibiotics are continued until the uterine fluids appear clear and nonodorus. Generally this is within 4 to 5 days. Oxytocin is administered to accelerate uterine contraction and detachment of the uterine membranes. A low dose of nonsteroidal anti-inflammatory drugs may be administered to reduce postoperative colic pain caused by uterine contractions.[17] Flunixin meglumine should be used if septicemia or toxemia are a problem. Tetanus prophylaxis is considered.

A major complication in the past was hemorrhagic shock from uterine bleeding and death within 24 to 48 h. With the advent of the continuous hemostatic suture placed in the uterine incisional margins, this problem has largely been obviated, however, anemia may be seen after cesarean section in the postoperative period.[12] Retained placenta is a common problem.[18] Retention of fetal membranes is observed in about 4% of mares following natural birth, and it occurs in about 30% of mares following cesarean section if the foal is dead and in about 50% following cesarean section if the foal is alive. Delayed involution of the uterus is common but variable. A combination of retained fetal membranes and delayed uterine involution predisposes to a polybacterial endometritis. With the added weight in the uterus it sinks farther into the abdomen, pulling the cervix and vagina cranioventrad. With this, urometria, which can seriously damage the endometrium, may be observed. The intravenous administration of oxytocin (20 IU) at the end of surgery may alleviate some of these complications.

If the fetal membranes are retained in the postoperative period, administration of 30 to 50 IU of oxytocin in 1 L of balanced electrolyte solution intravenously as a slow drip over a 1-h period is usually followed by passage of the placenta in about 80% of the cases.[1,18] Accumulation of uterine exudate may be removed by daily intrauterine lavage with sterile physiologic saline solution and siphonage. The procedure usually stimulates uterine contraction and some straining. Walking the mare for 5 to 10 min. after this is done appears to help with further evacuation of uterine fluid and seems to reduce the amount of straining when the mare is placed in the stall. Continued administration of nonsteroidal anti-inflammatory drugs is recommended to reduce straining after intrauterine lavage and the straining associated with retained placenta that may lead to uterine prolapse. Intrauterine flushes are continued until the placenta has passed and the uterine siphonage fluid appears clear and nonodorous. Antibiotics are continued as well. If there is any question remaining whether the fetal membranes were passed, antibiotics are continued through the next heat cycle.

Intrauterine scar tissue and parametrial scar tissue formation from the uterine incision have been associated with reduced fertility and particularly the latter with abortions of 7 to 10 months' gestation. Intrauterine scar reduces uterine milk and normal surface area for the maternal placenta to attach. The scar can be reduced somewhat by making the hysterotomy incision long enough so it does not tear during delivery of the foal, which may result in a uterine wall hematoma and vascular thrombosis. In addition, incorporation of excessive amounts of tissue in the continuous hemostatic suture is discouraged because ischemic necrosis of the uterine wall may develop, resulting in excessive uterine scar.

Parametrial adhesions may develop between the uterine incision, the abdominal wall, and the visceral peritoneum. Rectal examination on days 5 and 10 after surgery is done to identify soft fibrinous adhesions. If present, they can be broken down by gently separating them with the hand per rectum. In an attempt to avoid parametrial adhesions, the primary author no longer uses surgical gut, which is highly reactive when buried in tissue, for closure of the uterine incision. Braided synthetic absorbable suture is preferred. However, if the uterus is edematous and friable, surgical gut is still recommended. Lavage after the first inverting suture closure decreases the bacterial contamination and the potential for bacterial injury and inflammation that may follow. Tying the knots so they are buried and pulling the continuous inverting suture tight enough so the suture is not exposed is also important, because exposed suture material can result in adhesions. Finally, wiping the closed uterus with a mild antiseptic solution will remove blood clots and bacterial contaminants, which are implicated in adhesions.

Septic peritonitis as a complication after cesarean section can largely be avoided by extra-abdominal uterine incision, draping to create a barrier to the abdominal cavity and cleaning the outer surface of the uterus after it is closed. Septic peritonitis after a uterine tear can be reduced by proper suturing of the tear, cleansing the uterus and copious lavage of the abdominal cavity followed by suction. The placement of an intra-abdominal drain will also allow draining of the remaining contaminated abdominal fluid. The administration of continued antibiotics is without question.

Laminitis can often be avoided by careful attention to uterine treatment to prevent metritis and the administration of nonsteroidal anti-inflammatory drugs. Feeding laxative feed in the first week after cesarean section may reduce incidence of colic caused by intestinal displacements.

PROGNOSIS AND FERTILITY

An 80 to 90% survival rate can be expected in mares that have undergone cesarean section.[12,19,20] Foals survival rates after cesarean delivery range from 10[12] to 30%.[19] In the case series for which a 10% foal survival was observed, 33% of the foals were delivered alive but fetal deformity was a common reason for euthanasia.[12] In another case series for which eight elective cesarean sections were performed, all the mares survived and seven of eight foals were discharged from the hospital.[20]

Fertility after cesarean section appears to be reduced substantially.[2,5,12] However, conception rates after elective cesarean section appear to be higher than those observed after emergency cesarean section.[11] In Vandeplassche's cases (Table 50–1), that 58% (28/48) of the served mares became pregnant suggests that conception rates were almost normal. However, several of these mares needed services in 2 consecutive years to become pregnant, indicating an overall reduced fertility. Although overall reduced fertility is expected, some mares showed almost normal fertility after cesarean section. This was the case with 6 mares producing 18 pregnancies with one mare aborting.

Foaling rates in normal mares in North America range from 50 to 60%, and under intensive reproductive management, foaling rates may exceed 70%.[21] This is in contrast to a 36% collective foaling rate observed in 16 mares that were bred a total of 25 seasons after cesarean section.[12] However, a collective foaling rate of 50% was achieved in this same group of mares during the breeding seasons subsequent to the year of the operation. This suggests that a year should pass following cesarean section before the mare is rebred. This concept of delayed rebreeding has been advocated by Vandeplassche (Table 50–1) for whom 6 of 40 gestations ended in abortion, indicating a trend toward abortion, particularly in the first year after the mare undergoes operation. The trauma associated with attempted vaginal delivery and surgery, the delay in uterine involution, and the increased incidence of retained placenta are believed to be reasons for increased abortion.

TABLE 50–1. REPRODUCTIVE HISTORY OF 82 MARES AFTER CESAREAN SECTION

MARE CLASSIFICATION	NUMBER	PERCENT
Mares not bred after cesarean section	34	41.5
Mares bred	48	58.5
Mares not pregnant	20	41.7
Mares pregnant	28	58.3
Mares bred more than one season	28	58.3
Mares that produced only one foal	22	78.6
Mares that produced a foal more than one season: three mares produced two foals each; one, three; one, four; and one, five	6	21.4
Outcome in mares after cesarean section		
Normal foal at term	33	82.5
Interrupted gestation	7	17.5
Embryonic death	1	2.5
Abortion at 7 months	2	5.0
Abortion at 9 months	2	5.0
Abortion at 10 months	2	5.0

REFERENCES

1. Arthur, G.H.: The cesarean operation in the mare. *In* Veterinary Reproduction and Obstetrics. 3rd ed. Baltimore, Williams & Wilkins, 1975, pp. 325–329.
2. Colahan, T.T.: Female urogenital surgery. *In* Equine Medicine and Surgery. 3rd ed. Edited by R.A. Mansmann, and E.S. McAllister. Santa Barbara, CA, American Veterinary Publications, 1982, pp. 1373–1375.
3. Sloan, D.E.: Ovariectomy, ovariohysterectomy and cesarean section in mares. Vet. Clin. North Am. Large Anim. Pract., *4:*451–459, 1988.
4. Turner, A.S., and McIlwraith, C.W.: Cesarean section in the mare. *In* Techniques in Large Animal Surgery. 2nd ed. Philadelphia, Lea & Febiger, 1989, pp. 200–203.
5. Vandeplassche, M.M.: Cesarean section in horses. Vet. Ann., *14:*73–78, 1973.
6. Vandeplassche, M., Bouters, R., Spincemaille, J., and Bonte, P.: Cesarean section in the mare. Proc. Am. Assoc. Equine Pract., 75–79, 1977.
7. Vaughan, J.T.: Equine urogenital system. *In* The Practice of Large Animal Surgery. Edited by P.B. Jennings, Jr., Philadelphia, W.B. Saunders, 1984, pp. 1145–1147.
8. Walker, D.F., and Vaughan, J.T.: Bovine and Equine Urogenital Surgery. Philadelphia, Lea & Febiger, 1980.
9. Fisher, A.T., and Phillips, T.N.: Surgical repair of a rup-

tured uterus in five mares. Equine Vet. J., *18:*153–155, 1986.

10. Pascoe, J.R., Meagher, D.M., and Wheat, J.D.: Surgical management of uterine torsion in the mare: A review of 26 cases. J. Am. Vet. Med. Assoc., *179:*351–354, 1981.

11. Edwards, G.B., Allen W.E., and Newcombe, J.R.: Elective cesarean section in the mare for production of gnotobiotic foals. Equine Vet. J., *6:*122–126, 1974.

12. Juzwiak, J.J., Sloan, D.E., Santschi, E.M., and Mole, H.D.: Cesarean section in 19 mares: Results and postoperative fertility. Vet. Surg., *19*:50–52, 1990.

13. Vandeplassche, M.M.: The pathogenesis of dystocia and fetal malformation in the horse. J. Reprod. Fertil. Suppl., *35*:547–552, 1987.

14. Wheat, J.D., and Meagher, D.M.: Uterine torsion and rupture in mares. J. Am. Vet. Med. Assoc., *160:*881–884, 1972.

15. Hill, D.R.: Cesarean section and correction of uterine torsion in a mare. Vet. Med. Small Anim. Clin., *72:*1753–1758, 1977.

16. Vandeplassche, M.M.: Stimulation and inhibition of phagocytosis in domestic animals. Proceedings of the Tenth International Conference on Animal Reproduction and Artificial Insemination, 1984, p. 478.

17. Asbury, A.C.: The pregnant mare. *In* Equine Medicine and Surgery. 3rd ed. Edited by R.A. Mansmann, and G.S. McAllister. Santa Barbara, American Veterinary Publishing, 1982, pp. 1356–1361.

18. Vandeplassche, M.M., Spincemaille, J., and Bouters, R.: Etiology, pathogenesis and treatment of retained placenta in the mare. Equine Vet. J., *3:*144–147, 1971.

19. Vandeplassche, M.M.: Obstetrician's view of the physiology of equine parturition and dystocia. Equine Vet. J., *12:*45–48, 1980.

20. Watkins, J.P., et al.: Elective cesarean section in mares. J. Am. Vet. Med. Assoc., *197:*1639–1645, 1990.

21. Ginther, O.J.: Reproductive Biology of the Mare—Basic and Applied Aspects. Cross Plains, WI, published by the author, 1979.

CHAPTER 51

CERVICAL LACERATION(S)

W.A. Aanes

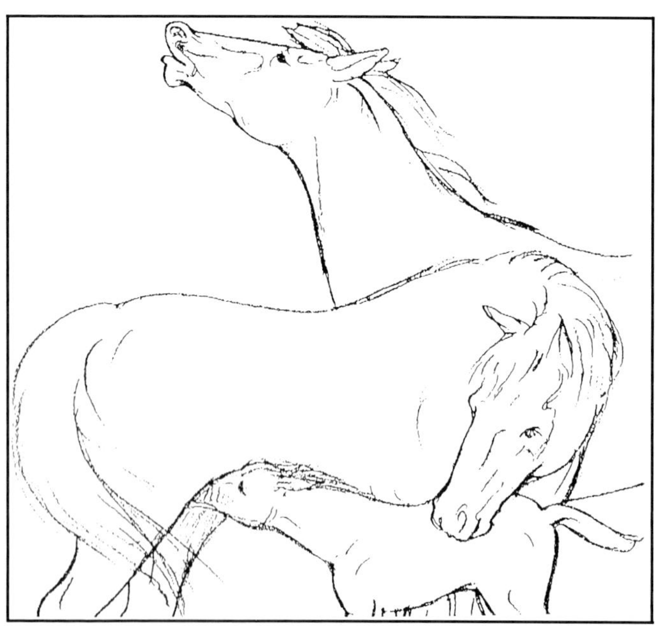

Injuries to the mare's cervix are usually associated with parturition (Fig. 51–1) Most cervical lacerations result from dystocia or induced parturition with dystocia, but they can occur in some apparently normal births. Severe bruising with hematoma formation and tearing of the fibromuscular layer of the cervix may cause incompetence without laceration of the mucosal layers of the cervix. Laceration of the cervix has been observed following copulation.[1] Congenital failure of proper cervical closure has also been reported.[2]

Diagnosis of cervical laceration(s) can be difficult. If the mare is in estrus or near estrus when examined, cervical folds may be so edematous that they cover the laceration and the cervix will appear normal (relaxed) in preparation for breeding. This should be considered in postpartum examinations, because lacerations can be easily missed. If on examination during estrus cervical incompetence is suspected, a second examination should be conducted during diestrus when the cervical folds are not conjested. During diestrus, the open incompetent cervix and cervical scars are identified more easily. To diagnose a cervical defect accurately, manual palpation of the entire cervix is essential. This is accomplished by inserting the thumb or index finger in the os of the cervix and palpating the entire circumference. A sterile sleeve should be used during this examination. Manual palpation of the cervix allows defects to be detected in the fibromuscular layer that are covered with intact mucous membrane and cannot be noticed by visual inspection.

Cervical lacerations may be diagnosed immediately after the injury, but cervical relaxation may obscure injuries. In many cases they are found during breeding soundness examinations performed at a later date, either because of failure to conceive or following return to estrus after early abortion. If the injury is detected at foaling, complete healing should occur (approximately 30 days) before surgical repair is attempted.

SURGERY

A technique for repair of cervical lacerations and incompetent cervix was described by Evans et al. in 1979.[3] In 1984, Brown et al. described the repair of the lacerated cervix using a similar but slightly modified technique.[4] In both techniques the defect was closed using three layers of suture. The internal layer was a continuous horizontal mattress pattern that everted the internal layer of mucosa into the cervical lumen, the second was a continuous layer that apposed the fibromuscular layer, and the third layer was a continuous horizontal mattress pattern that everted the external mucosal layer of the cervix.

When repairing lacerations of the cervix, limited access, visibility, and depth of the surgical field make instrument manipulation and suture placement difficult. The vagina of the mare is deep and cervical retraction is restricted. In previous descriptions of the repair, two- and three-bladed vaginal specula were used in conjunction with Knowles uterine forceps and/or tension su-

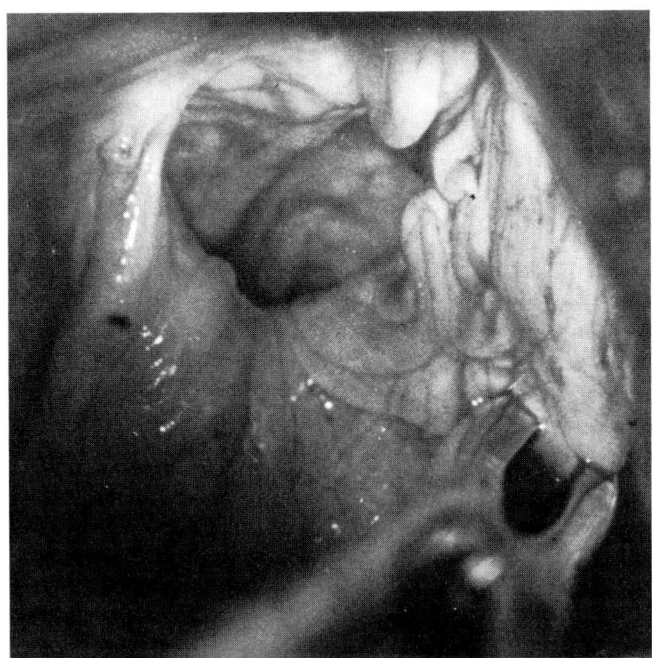

FIG. 51–1. Laceration of a mare's cervix at the 10 o'clock position. This laceration extended to the cranial os where the endometrium is visible.

tures placed on each side of the cervical defect to retract the cervix during surgery.[3,4] Long-handled scissors (36 cm or 14 in.) were used to debride up to 1.25 cm of mucosa from each side of the laceration to expose the fibromuscular layer. The layers were sutured with #1 catgut.[3] or #2-0 Vicryl,[4] using needle holders that had been lengthened by welding extensions onto the handles of heavy-duty needle holders. The surgery was performed with the mares standing in stocks. Epidural anesthesia was administered. Some mares were given 100 to 200 mg xylazine before and during surgery. Surgery can be performed with the mare, under a general anesthetic, suspended from the side of the operating table by the tail and a chest girth. The belly girth cannot be used because it forces abdominal contents against the vagina, distorting the normal anterior vagina.[3]

To accomplish successful repair of cervical injuries in the mare, special instrumentation is important in the performance and accuracy of the surgical technique. A set of instruments—40 to 50 cm or 16 to 20 in. length—composed of needle holders, thumb forceps, scissors, scalpel handle, and Knowles uterine forceps greatly facilitate a successful repair (Fig. 51–2).

In addition, adequate cervical exposure requires further special instrumentation. Suitable retraction of the vulva, vagina, and cervix is accomplished by using a modified Finochietto-type retractor with 28 cm (11-in.) removable blades (Scanlon Surgical Instruments, Inc., Englewood, CO) (Fig. 51–3). A fiberoptic light source and delivery system ensure adequate visualization. The fiberoptic light bundle is attached to the axial surface of one of the retractor blades to deliver light directly on the cervix during the surgical procedure (Fig. 51–4).

Mares are restrained in stocks, epidural anesthesia with sedation or a sedative/analgesic combination of xylazine and butorphanol, or detomidine hydrocloride is administered before surgery. General anesthesia may be necessary to operate on intractable mares. Infiltration of 30 to 60 mL of local anesthetic dorsal to the cervix facilitates retraction of the cervix. (A.O. McKinnon, personal communication).

After placing the mare in the stocks, feces are removed from the rectum, the bladder is emptied, and the tail is wrapped and tied in a dorsal position. The perineal area is prepared for aseptic surgery. Dilute iodophor solution is used to cleanse the vaginal canal and cervix. The retractor with the fiberoptic light cord attached is placed in the vagina and opened as wide as permitted by the conformation of the mare without applying excessive pressure on the vestibule and vagina. The laceration is identified and the caudal edge of the cervix grasped with Knowles uterine forceps on each side of the laceration. The cervix is retracted caudad as far as possible without excessive tension. The cicatrix at the junction of the external and internal layers of the cervical mucosa is identified, and an incision is made along the scar, extending from the caudal edge of the posterior os to the cranial end of the defect (Fig. 51–5A). The incision is extended 1 to 2 cm beyond the cranial end of the defect to ensure separation of intact internal and external layers of mucous membrane from the fibromuscular layer. The incision is continued from the cranial end of the laceration along the scar to the external os on the opposite side of the laceration. The incision separating the internal and external cervical mucous membranes is extended into the fibromuscular layer. Initially, the suture pattern used was a three-layer closure as described by others. Subsequently, a two-layer closure has been used with good success. The internal layer of suture is started at least 1 cm cranial to the separation of internal and external layers of the cervical laceration and is a continuous pattern placed through the internal mucous membrane into the fibro-

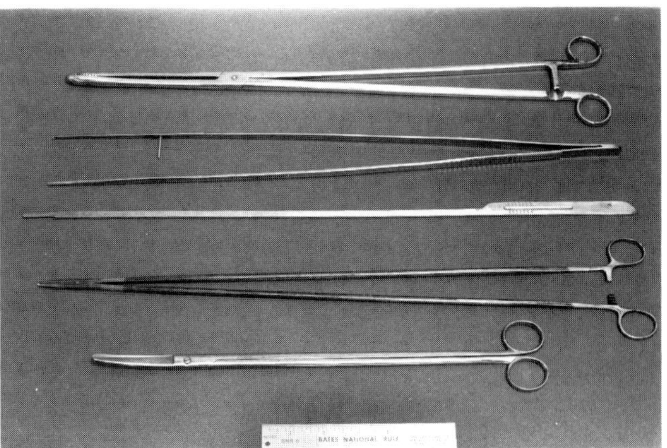

FIG. 51–2. Special 40- to 50-cm instruments used in repairing cervical laceration(s). From top to bottom: Knowles forceps, thumb forceps with pin guide, scalpel handle, needle holders, and curved scissors.

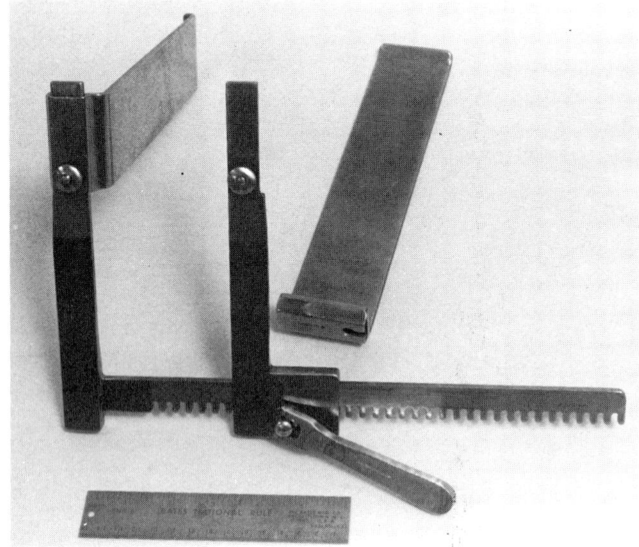

FIG. 51–3. The modified Finochietto-type retractor with 28-cm (11-in.) detachable blades used for surgery on the cervix.

muscular layer of the cervix (Fig. 51–5B). The suture pattern is continued to the external os where it is tied. Absorbable suture material in (# 0) with a swaged-on cutting needle is preferred. When placing the suture, the cervical lumen must be intermittently checked to ensure that it is not accidentally occluded by the suture. A second continuous layer of suture is placed in the external mucous membrane and the fibromuscular layer of the cervix (Fig. 51–5C). When this layer is completed, the patency of the cervical lumen should be reconfirmed before releasing the cervix (Fig. 51–5D).

Aftercare includes antibacterial treatment for several days. Phenylbutazone for 2 or 3 days helps reduce the discomfort associated with the procedure. The mare should not be examined for at least 2 weeks postoperatively, and the cervix should not be palpated until completely healed.

Brown et al. reported that five of eight mares bred after cervical laceration repair had conceived at the time of publication.[4] The experience at Colorado State University's Veterinary Teaching Hospital is in agreement, with a favorable prognosis for rebreeding. Mares bred by natural service may be partially protected by using a breeding roll at service. Some mares will reinjure the cervix at subsequent foalings. Careful postparturient examination is recommended on these mares, and if necessary, further surgical repair can be done.

Some mares with badly damaged cervices will conceive and may deliver live foals, but most will abort. Minor lacerations of the external os do not require repair. Lacerations extending into the fibromuscular layer of the cervix usually heal with a defect that results in incompetence. Tears extending from the external to the internal os of the cervix require surgical repair. Mares with a thin or badly damaged cervix with multiple tears that abort in early pregnancy may be candidates for cervical cerclage. Cervical incompetence without laceration of the mucosal layers may be repaired by excising the mucosal layers over the defect in the fibromuscular layer, excising scar tissue from the fibromuscular layer, and suturing as described for laceration of the cervix.

CERVICAL CERCLAGE

Cervical incompetence is a major problem in human obstetric practice. In dealing with the problem, numerous surgical, mechanical, and medical techniques have been tried. The number in use indicates none is ideal.[5] Several surgical techniques using cervical cerclage in the human have been described.[6–8] The success of these procedures was measured by increased percentage of live deliveries after cerclage, as compared with previous pregnancies in the same individuals.

Cervical cerclage has also been described for treating cervical incompetence in the mare.[3] The procedure has been used on mares with a history of abortion occurring 60 days to 5 months after conception. Mares found to have a flimsy cervix in early pregnancy tend to abort,

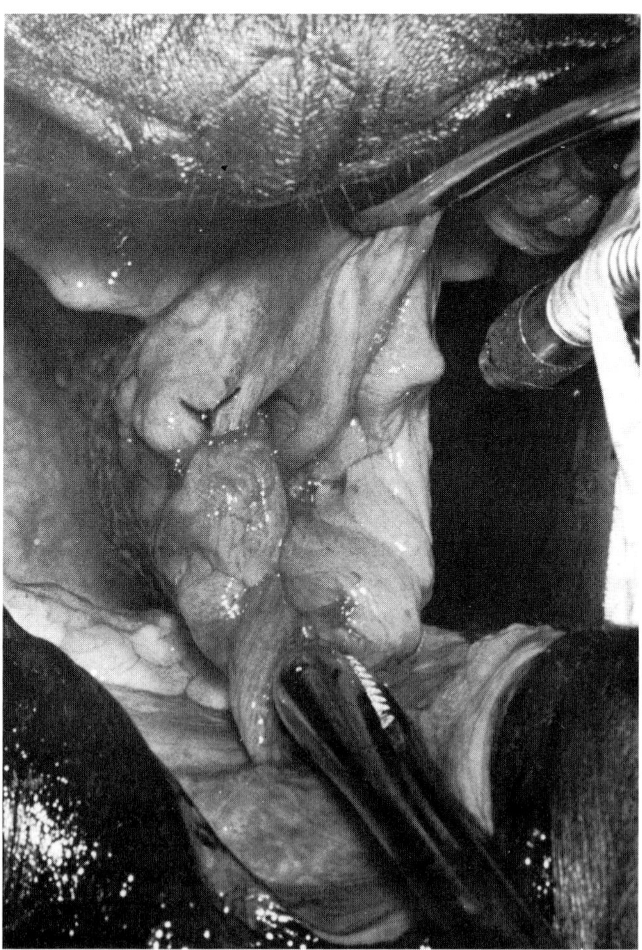

FIG. 51–4. The mare's cervix in Figure 51–1 after the first layer of suture was tied. Knowles uterine forceps are retracting the cervix. The fiberoptics light cable can be seen attached to the modified Finochietto-type retractor.

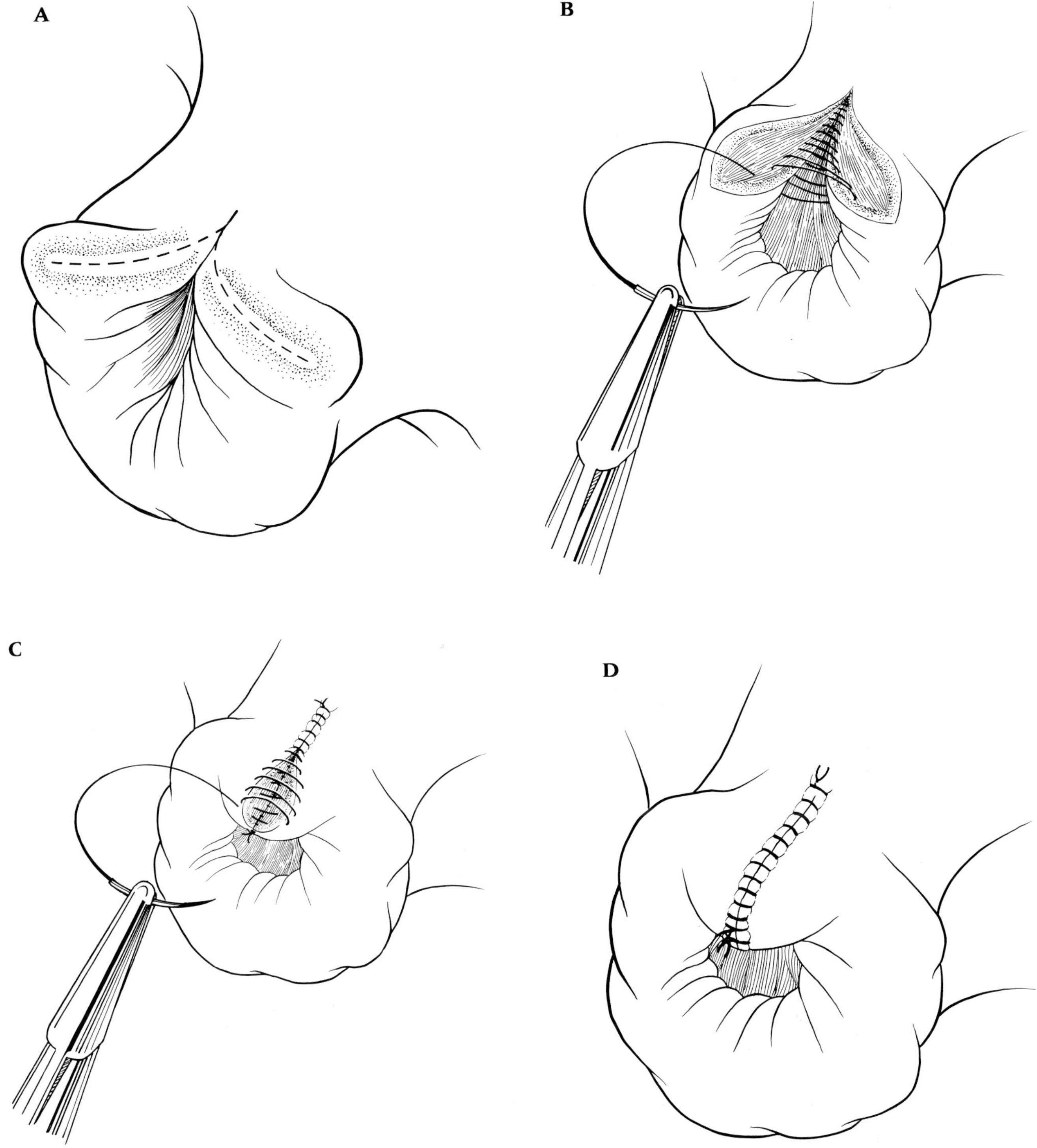

FIG. 51–5. *A,* Mare's cervix lacerated at the 12 o'clock position. The broken line represents the healed junction of the internal and external cervical mucous membranes. An incision is made along this line and extended into the fibromuscular layer. At the cranial end of the healed laceration, the incision is extended 1 to 2 cm beyond the original laceration to separate the intact internal and external mucosa and expose the fibromuscular layer. *B,* A continuous pattern of absorbable suture is placed through the internal cervical mucous membrane and inner portion of the fibromuscular layer. To reduce the risk of fistula formation, the suture pattern is started in the intact internal mucosa of the cervix cranial to the laceration. *C,* A second continuous absorbable suture is placed in the external mucous membrane and fibromuscular layer of the cervix. *D,* Completed suture patterns are tied at the external os. The cervical canal should be checked to be sure it is patent before releasing the cervix.

and mares with badly scarred cervices that are not amenable to repair of individual lacerations may benefit from this technique. A nonabsorbable suture (5-mm ribbon of Mersilene or two strands of #2 Mersilene) is used to support the incompetent cervix. The cervix is retracted using two tension sutures. Two small incisions are made through the vaginal mucosa of the cervix, one dorsal and one ventral, close to the cranial os of the cervix. With the surgeon's thumb or index finger of one hand in the cervical os to identify and stabilize the cervix, the nonabsorbable suture (treated with triple antibiotic ointment) is passed through the ventral mucosal incision, guided by the surgeon's other hand. The suture is passed through the fibromuscular layer of the cervix and out the dorsal mucosal incision. The other end of the suture is also passed through the ventral mucosal incision, through the contralateral side of the fibromuscular layer, and out the dorsal mucosal incision. Care must be exercised to be sure the nonabsorbable suture has not entered the cervical os during placement. After tightening and securely tying (with surgeons' and several overhand knots) the cerclage suture, the cervical canal should be checked for patency. If the canal is inadequately closed the suture should be replaced, with the ends of the suture exiting from the fibromuscular layer lateral to the dorsal mucosal incision, thereby placing more tension on the cervical tissues when the suture is tied. The mucosal incisions are closed with #2-0 chromic catgut to bury the nonabsorbable suture.

In a modification of this technique (Fig. 51–6A), the cervical mucosal incisions are no longer used when placing the nonabsorbable suture (#2 monofilament nylon) around the cranial cervical os (L.H. Evans, personal communication) (Fig. 51–6A). The suture enters the cervix on the ventral surface (6 o'clock position), is passed through the fibromuscular layer, and exits through the vaginal cervical mucosa lateral to the dorsal midline of the cervix (1 o'clock position). The same procedure is used to place the opposite end of the suture through the contralateral side of the cervix, exiting lateral to the dorsal midline of the cervix (11 o'clock position). This procedure ensures that when the suture is tightly tied (with surgeons' and several overhand ties), the cervical os will be closed (Fig. 51–6B). The ends of the suture are not buried under the mucosa. A liberal coating of antibiotic ointment is applied over the exposed section of the suture to reduce the risk of infection.

The recommended time of cerclage insertion was within 2 days after breeding and ovulation. Because mares with cervical incompetence usually have a history of uterine infection (poor defense mechanism), suturing within 2 days after breeding can result in return to estrus with an exudative endometritis. Antibiotic infusion for 2 days postbreeding and suturing with a modified pattern and minor cervical manipulation, only after early confirmation of pregnancy (via ultrasonography) is recommended (A.O. McKinnon, personal communication). The nonabsorbable suture must be removed a few days before foaling. No reports of the success of this procedure on incompetent cervix were found in the veterinary literature. The clinical impres-

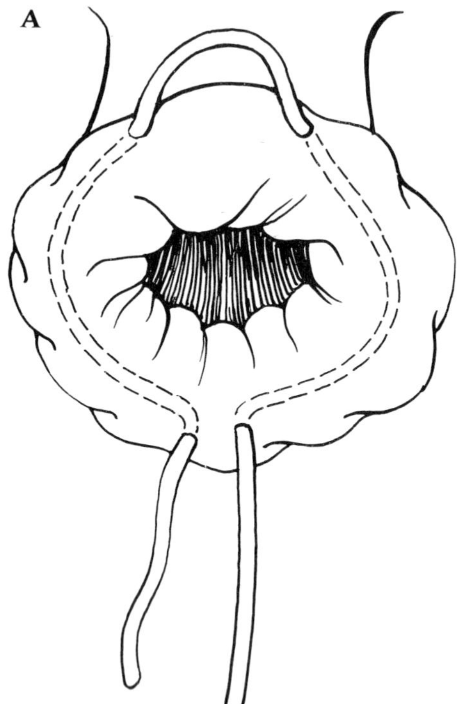

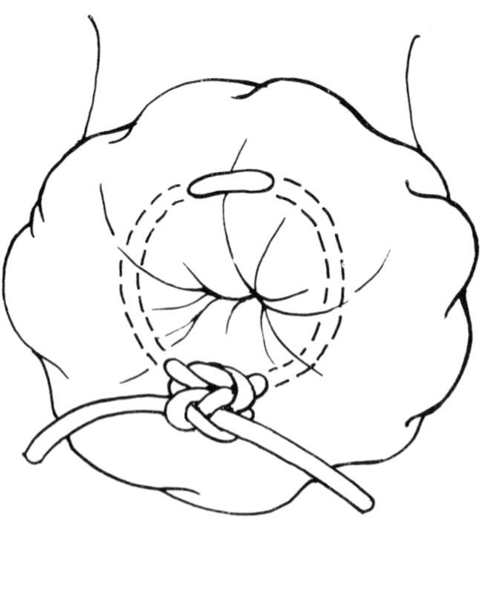

FIG. 51–6. *A*, Placement of the suture in the modified technique of cervical cerclage using doubled #2 monofilament nylon. *B*, The closed cervix after completion of surgery. A surgeon's knot and several overhand ties should be used.

sion is that abortion may be avoided in approximately 50% of the mares for which cerclage is used as a method of treatment for accurately diagnosed cervical incompetence (L.H. Evans, personal communication).

REFERENCES

1. Aanes, W.A.: Surgical management of foaling injuries. Vet. Clin. North Am. Equine Pract. Urogenital Surg., *4*:417–438, 1988.
2. Blanchard, T.L., et al.: Congenitally incompetent cervix in a mare. J. Am. Vet. Med. Assoc., *181*:266, 1982.
3. Evans, L.H., Tate, L.P., Jr., Cooper, W.L., and Robertson, J.T.: Surgical repair of cervical lacerations and the incompetent cervix. Proc. Am. Assoc. Equine Pract., 483–486, 1979.
4. Brown, J.S., Varner, D.D., Hinrichs, K., and Kenney, R.M.: Surgical repair of the lacerated cervix in the mare. Theriogenology, *22*:351–359, 1984.
5. Shortle, B., and Jewelewicz, R.: Cervical incompetence. Fertil. Steril., *52*:181–188, 1989.
6. Shirodkar, V.N.: A new method of operative treatment for habitual abortion in the second trimester of pregnancy. Antiseptic, *52*:299–300, 1955.
7. McDonald, I.A.: Suture of the cervix for inevitable miscarriage. Br. J. Obstet. Gynecol., *64*:346–350, 1957.
8. Novy, M.J.: Transabdominal cervicoisthmic cerclage for the management of repetitive abortion and premature delivery. Am. J. Obstet. Gynecol., *143*:44–54, 1982.

CHAPTER 52

OVARIECTOMY

G. T. Colbern

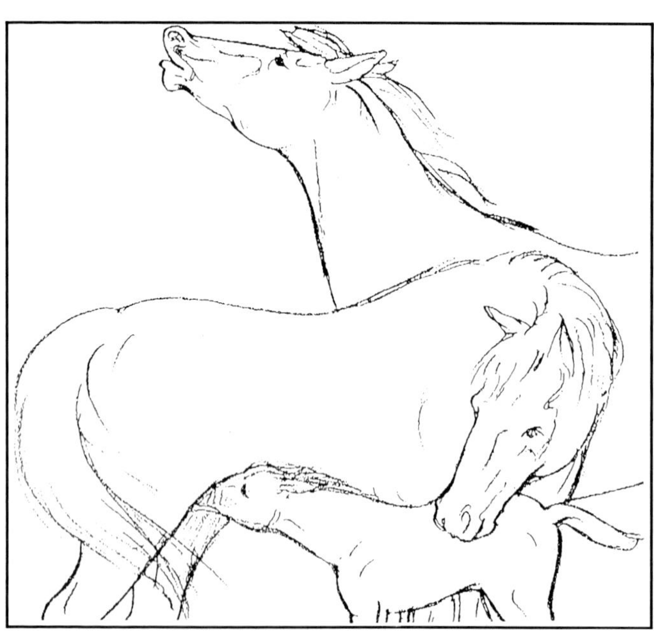

Classic indications for ovariectomy in mares are behavioral problems and ovarian tumors.[1–7] Estrous behavior can be objectionable in performance mares, especially if exhibited for extended time periods. Ovariectomy can alleviate this behavior in some cases. Ovarian tumors are relatively common in mares, especially granulosa-theca cell tumors (see Chapter 45). Progressive increase in size, hormone production, and infertility necessitate removal.[1] Removal of the affected ovary can permit normal reproductive potential by the contralateral ovary. Other ovarian tumors (teratoma, cystadenoma, adenocarcinoma, dysgerminoma, arrhenoblastoma, and ovarian lymphosarcoma) occur at much less common frequency and are handled similarly to granulosa/theca cell tumors.[7] Ovarian abscess or hematoma and ovarian cysts have also been reported as indications for ovariectomy.[7]

Economic value of performance or working mares can be enhanced by ovariectomy, because objectionable or cyclic reproductive behavior is eliminated. Ovariectomized mares have been found to be excellent embryo transfer recipients,[8–10] thus reducing the necessary number of recipient mares per donor. Ovariectomy can be valuable for biomedical research which requires elimination of ovarian hormones to evaluate other reproductive hormonal or biologic processes.[10]

Ovariectomy was first described prior to the twentieth century. Use of an écraseur, or crusher, to remove tumors was first described by Chassaignac as cited in Fleming's *Textbook of Operative Veterinary Surgery.*[11] In 1884, Fleming described several modifications of the instrument designed to crush vessels and induce hemostasis while removing vascular tissues.[11] In 1903, Williams described ovariectomy by colpotomy in the standing mare with maximal physical restraint.[6] With the advent of newer pharmaceutical agents and anesthetic techniques, both standing and recumbent ovariectomy techniques have become more acceptable.[3,5,12–15] Three abdominal approaches are currently used for ovariectomy: colpotomy (vaginal), flank grid celiotomy, and ventral midline celiotomy.[15] Selection of which abdominal approach depends on the specific indication for ovariectomy, economics, facilities available, and surgeon's preference.

OVARIECTOMY BY COLPOTOMY

Vaginal approach to the abdomen for ovariectomy has the advantage of requiring minimal equipment and trained personnel thus limiting cost. It also results in the most cosmetic postoperative appearance and least recuperative time for ovariectomy. Limitations for this technique are size of ovary to be removed (maximum ovarian diameter for this technique is approximately 10 cm), vaginal size, and palpation skills of the surgeon. Uterine or vaginal inflammation and infection, especially with purulent exudate, also preclude use of this technique.

PRESURGICAL PREPARATION

Feed but not water is withheld for 36 to 48 h before surgery. Withholding feed for only 24 h may make abdominal manipulation difficult. Procaine penicillin G (20,000 IU/kg) and tetanus toxoid are administered intramuscularly before surgical preparation. For surgery, the mare is placed in a stocks and restrained by cross-tie. The tail is bandaged and tied firmly over a beam above the stocks. This prevents the mare from squatting during surgery. The rectum is manually evacuated and the size and location of each ovary and the bladder is determined. The perineum and surrounding skin are scrubbed with antiseptic soap, such as povidone-iodine (Betadine Surgical Scrub). If necessary, bladder catheterization to remove urine is performed with care to prevent introduction of air into the bladder. The vagina is distended and lavaged with 1 L warm sterile saline and drained. The perineum is scrubbed again and sprayed with antiseptic solution (Betadine Solution). Use of alcohol or astringents should be avoided to prevent inflammation of the perineal tissues.

Standing chemical restraint and analgesia is administered during the scrub procedure. The combination of acetylpromazine, xylazine and butorphanol, or detomidine is recommended.[16–18] Epidural anesthesia can be performed but is not required with this analgesic regimen. After tranquilization, the tail rope can be tightened to prevent the mare from slumping during the surgical procedure. Normal surgical gowning and full-length rubber or plastic rectal sleeves are recommended. Gowning permits use of both hands without contamination during the surgical procedure.

An écraseur and guarded scalpel blade are the only instruments required. The author prefers the Hauptner écraseur with a ratchet-tightening mechanism. The vaginal incision is made with a sharp, curved bistoury, guarded scalpel, or sharp/sharp scissors. A sterile muslin or gauze pack should be available for application of lidocaine to the mesovarium. If gauze sponges are used, they should be sutured together before sterilization to prevent loss of sponges in the abdomen.

SURGERY

An assistant should be present at the mare's head to monitor heart rate and response to the procedure. A twitch can be applied to the patient's upper lip if necessary. The bistoury, guarded in the surgeon's hand, is passed to the cranial vagina. The blade is advanced approximately 2 cm past the surgeon's thumb and forefinger and grasped firmly. The incision is made in the right cranioventral quadrant of the vaginal cavity. A ventral midline incision is avoided because of proximity to the bladder and urethra. The oblique ventral incision avoids the rectum and facilitates orientation within the abdomen.

The incision is made at least 4 cm from the os cervix to avoid tearing the musculature of the cervix during digital enlargement of the incision. This is especially important when preparing embryo transfer recipients. The bistoury, blade directed ventrad, is thrust firmly into the tissue to the limits allowed by the thumb and forefinger. The blade is then rotated 180° and advanced craniad (1 to 2 cm) until the forefinger can pass into the vaginal incision. The incision is made through all vaginal tissue layers and the peritoneum. If the peritoneum is not penetrated, the surgeon's forefinger is thrust through the tissue into the peritoneal cavity. The incision is digitally enlarged to allow the surgeon's hand to enter the peritoneal cavity. The incision normally enters the peritoneal cavity in the vesicogenital peritoneal reflection, but occasionally will enter the rectogenital peritoneal reflection. The abdomen is thoroughly explored with special attention to location of the uterus and ovaries.

The muslin or gauze sponge pack is soaked in 30 mL sterile lidocaine solution. The pack is passed into the peritoneal cavity and applied to the mesovarium. Firm pressure is applied for a minimum of 30 s. The pack is removed, more lidocaine is applied, and the process is repeated with the contralateral mesovarium.

The écraseur is adjusted so that the chain is just long enough to allow passage of the ovary through the loop. The chain is looped over the surgeon's thumb and forefinger and passed into the peritoneal cavity. The ovary is located by tracing the uterine horn forward to the oviduct and ovary. This procedure prevents grasping the ovary through the mesocolon and removing a section of mesocolon. The ovary is grasped by thumb and forefinger and drawn through the loop of the écraseur. The écraseur is tightened by sliding the metal shaft forward until the loop fits snugly around the mesovarium. The area is carefully palpated to be sure that no intestine or other tissues are incorporated. The ovary is grasped and held while the surgeon slowly closes the écraseur loop using the ratchet mechanism. When the loop is completely closed, the ovary is drawn back into the vaginal cavity and removed. Connective tissue attachments frequently must be gently torn to remove the ovary. The ratchet is slowly released. The chain is advanced into the écraseur to form a loop of suitable size for the contralateral ovary. Écrasement of this ovary can be performed through the same incision with the same or opposite surgeon's hand, according to the surgeon's preference.

After completion of the procedure, each mesovarium is gently palpated for pulsations indicating hemorrhage. If pulsations are detected, the écraseur should be applied to the mesovarium again and held in place for several minutes. Both ovaries should be examined to ensure that all ovarian tissue has been removed. Closure or treatment of the vaginal incision is not attempted.

POSTSURGICAL CARE AND POTENTIAL COMPLICATIONS

Procaine penicillin G therapy is continued once daily (20,000 IU/kg IM) for 5 days postsurgery. The mare can be returned to a nonbedded or shavings-bedded stall after tranquilization has sufficiently resolved. Water can be made available immediately, but feed should be withheld for an additional 2 to 4 h. Immediately after surgery, some mares may exhibit abdominal discomfort and assume sternal recumbency. Postsurgical nonsteroidal anti-inflammatory therapy appears to alleviate this discomfort partially. Intravenous phenylbutazone (4 mg/kg) is given as needed for pain or straining. Flunixin meglumine (Banamine) (1 mg/kg) should be used for severe pain or signs of endotoxemia. At 7 days postsurgery, vaginal examination to determine the degree of healing of the vaginal wall can be performed. If the incision is sealed, the mare can be returned to pasture or light exercise at this time. Full exercise should not be resumed until 3 weeks postsurgery.

Delayed healing or abscess/hematoma formation in the vaginal incision are encountered but require minimal intervention and usually are not associated with clinical signs.[19] Adhesions of abdominal organs to the vaginal incision site are possible and may result in subsequent colic. Tearing of the musculature of the cervix can occur when the initial vaginal incision is made too close to the os cervix. This would result in an incompetent cervix, which could be important if the mare were to be used for reproductive purposes such as embryo transfer.[19] Peritonitis is a potential complication but appears to be less likely than with other abdominal approaches.[19] Good surgical technique and minimal operative time minimize peritoneal inflammation with this technique.[19]

Fatal complications have been reported. Surgical errors—penetration of the rectum, bladder, or great vessels in the pelvic region or removal of a section of intestine—are possible.[4,6] Ventrolateral vaginal incision, adequate fasting, maximal vaginal distension, and thorough intraoperative palpation of abdominal contents minimize these risks.[6,12] Hemorrhage from the mesovarium can occur with improper crushing. This can be prevented by ensuring that the écraseur chain is flat and straight before introduction of the ovary and by crushing the mesovarium slowly over a period of several minutes.[5,6] Palpation of the mesovarium at the completion of surgery might indicate hemorrhage and allow crushing again. Evisceration through the vaginal incision has been reported but is quite rare.[19]

OVARIECTOMY BY FLANK GRID CELIOTOMY

Flank grid approach to the abdomen for ovariectomy allows improved exposure of the mesovarium but it is still limited and only one ovary is accessible. If the contralateral ovary must be removed, the technique is similar to ovariectomy by colpotomy. Maximal ovarian diameter to be removed by this technique is much larger than by colpotomy but is still limited by size of the paralumbar fossa (25 cm). Surgical equipment, facilities, and trained personnel required for this technique are moderate, thus reducing the cost compared, with ventral midline celiotomy. This surgical approach allows for the least cosmetic result at completion of ovariectomy and a moderate recuperative time.

PRESURGICAL PREPARATION

Preparation for flank ovariectomy is similar to colpotomy ovariectomy. Feed is withheld for similar duration and antibiotic and tetanus prophylaxis are similar. The procedure can be performed in either standing or recumbent position. For the standing procedure, the mare is restrained in a stocks and the tail is bandaged and tied as for colpotomy. Standing chemical restraint and analgesia with a combination of acetylpromazine, xylazine and butorphanol, or detomidine is recommended. For the recumbent procedure, intravenous induction, endotracheal intubation, and inhalant general anesthesia are recommended. The paralumbar fossa, on the side of the affected ovary, is clipped in a wide area and the region of incision is shaved. The surgical site is prepared aseptically. For the standing procedure, local analgesia is administered by line block or inverted "L" block. The surgical site is given final preparation and draped with surgical linen.

A standard surgical instrument pack is minimal instrumentation. An écraseur is necessary if the contralateral ovary is to be removed. Sterile lidocaine should be available for application to the ovarian pedicle. Sterile rubber or plastic sleeves are required for abdominal manipulation. Synthetic absorbable suture (#0, 00, and 2) and nonabsorbable suture (#1) or staples are required. A suction drain can be used to prevent seroma formation in the incision.

SURGERY

The skin incision is made midway between the tuber coxae and last rib. Size of the incision will depend on ovarian diameter, from 15 cm for a normal to slightly enlarged ovary to 30 cm for a moderate tumor. The incision should be in the dorsal paralumbar fossa, beginning at the longissimus dorsi muscle,[20] regardless of incision length. The incision is continued through the subcutaneous tissue and hemorrhage is controlled.

Technique for penetration of the abdominal musculature depends on ovarian size. For a normal-size ovary and minimal necessary exposure, a true grid technique is used and each muscle layer is divided along the direction of the muscle fibers. For an enlarged ovary, a modified grid technique is used. A vertical incision is made through the fascia and muscle fibers of the external abdominal oblique muscle with internal abdominal oblique and transverse abdominus muscles divided along the direction of their fibers. Blunt dissection is used to incise internal abdominal oblique and transverse abdominus muscles and peritoneum to avoid penetration of viscera.

Thorough abdominal palpation is performed after entering the peritoneum. If the contralateral ovary is to be removed, it is removed first by the technique described in the previous section. If not greatly enlarged, the ipsilateral ovary can also be removed by this technique. If necessary, the ipsilateral ovary is identified and exteriorized. Lidocaine is applied to the mesovarium, by injection or topical application, before proceeding. Transfixion ligation of the mesovarium is performed using overlapping interrupted sutures of #2 synthetic absorbable suture.[21] All portions of mesovarium should be ligated. During ligation of the mesovarium, tension must be placed on the ovary for proper placement of ligatures. Tension should be released before tying each ligature to allow complete hemostasis.[21] Failure to release tension on the ovary before ligature may result in slippage and postoperative hemorrhage. Once ligation is complete, the ovary is removed and the mesovarium is examined carefully for hemorrhage. Areas with hemorrhage should be further ligated. The mesovarium can be oversewn with #00 synthetic absorbable suture to decrease adhesion formation.

The flank incision is closed in five layers.[20] Peritoneum and transverse abdominus muscle and internal abdominal oblique muscle are closed in two layers with simple interrupted sutures of #0 synthetic absorbable suture. A suction drain can be placed between the internal and external abdominal oblique muscles to prevent seroma formation and incisional complications. External abdominal oblique muscle is closed with simple interrupted sutures of #2 synthetic absorbable suture. Fascia of external abdominal oblique muscle is carefully apposed. Subcutis is closed in a simple continuous pattern of #0 synthetic absorbable suture. Skin is closed in simple interrupted sutures of #1 nonabsorbable suture or surgical staples.

POSTSURGICAL CARE AND POTENTIAL COMPLICATIONS

Procaine penicillin G therapy is continued once daily (20,000 IU/kg IM) for 5 days postsurgery. Flunixin meglumine (Banamine) (1 mg/kg) can be used for discomfort or signs of endotoxemia. Additional supportive care (intravenous fluids) should be administered as indicated by clinical signs. If a suction drain is used, it is taped to the patient's back and emptied frequently. The drain is removed when aspirated fluid content decreases (2 to 3 days). Skin sutures or staples are removed after 12 to 14 days. Following suture removal, the mare can be returned to pasture or light exercise. Full exercise should not be resumed until 6 weeks postsurgery.

Delayed healing or abscess formation in the incision occurs with relative frequency and can be difficult to manage and requires long-term care. Hematoma or adhesions of the mesovarium may result in clinical signs of colic. Use of anti-inflammatory medications in the immediate postoperative period may minimize colic at this time. Peritonitis can affect recovery. Good surgical technique and minimal operative time will minimize this complication.

Fatal complications have been reported. Flank incision dehiscence may result in evisceration. Good postoperative incision care should minimize this complication. Hemorrhage from the mesovarium can occur as a result of improper ecrasement or slippage of ligatures. Mesovarium should be palpated at completion of procedure to detect hemorrhage. Prolonged hemorrhage may require subsequent surgical intervention. Severe peritonitis and endotoxemia should not be encountered with good surgical technique.

OVARIECTOMY BY VENTRAL MIDLINE CELIOTOMY

Ventral midline abdominal approach for ovariectomy has the advantage of maximal exposure of the ovary and mesovarium during removal and ability to remove extremely large ovarian tumors. If ovarian size cannot be determined by rectal palpation, ventral midline approach is recommended.[21,22] Both ovaries can be accessed via the same abdominal incision. Surgical and anesthetic equipment, facilities, and trained personnel required for this technique are extensive, resulting in high surgical costs. Ventral midline incision allows cosmetic results if incisional complications are not encountered.

PRESURGICAL PREPARATION

Preparation for ventral midline ovariectomy is similar to colpotomy ovariectomy. Feed is withheld for 36 to 48 h but water is continued. Hydration should be well monitored for effects on anesthetic procedure. Oral fluids can be administered by stomach tube 2 to 4 h preoperatively to minimize hydration problems. Antibiotic and tetanus prophylaxis are administered before surgery. Flunixin meglumine (Banamine) is recommended preoperative to minimize postoperative problems.

Intravenous anesthetic induction, endotracheal intubation, and inhalant anesthetic maintenance are used. Intravenous fluids should be administered intraoperatively. The mare is placed in dorsal recumbency. A hydraulic surgery table that allows slight lowering of the mare's head can help during surgical manipulation of a large ovary. Anesthetic complications can occur in this position and should be monitored. The ventral abdomen, from mammary glands to xyphoid, is clipped, shaved, and aseptically prepared for surgery.

A standard laparotomy instrument pack is minimal instrumentation. Sterile lidocaine should be available for application to the mesovarium. Sterile rubber or plastic sleeves are required for abdominal exploration and manipulation. Synthetic absorbable suture (#0, 00, and 2) and nonabsorbable suture (#2) are required. Staples can be used in the skin but can be difficult to remove. Stapling equipment can also be used for mesovarium ligation.

SURGERY

The skin incision is made on ventral midline just cranial to the mammary glands. Incision length is variable and depends on size of the ovary to be removed. The incision is continued sharply through linea alba and bluntly through subcutaneous fat and peritoneum. Subcutaneous fat can be extensive in this region. Thorough abdominal exploration should be performed before exteriorization of the affected ovary. A large ovary may be difficult to exteriorize because of the short, broad attachment of mesovarium. Manual retraction and pressure on the body wall should allow adequate exteriorization. A very large ovary may require repositioning during ligation for adequate exposure. Use of Balfour or Finochietto retractors on the body wall may be helpful with small ovaries but may inhibit exteriorization of large ovaries.[21]

Before beginning ligation, lidocaine should be applied to the mesovarium. Lidocaine can be injected into the region or applied topically with gauze as in the previous procedures. Mesovarium is then relaxed for several minutes before beginning ligation. This procedure minimizes the drop in blood pressure associated with ligation and removal of the ovary.[21,23]

As described in the previous section, transfixion ligation of the mesovarium is performed using overlapping interrupted sutures of #2 synthetic absorbable suture.[21] All portions of mesovarium should be ligated. During ligation, tension must be placed on the ovary for proper placement of ligatures. Tension should be released before tying each ligature to allow complete hemostasis.[21] Failure to release tension on the ovary before ligature may result in slippage and postoperative hemorrhage. Extremely large ovaries may require partial ligation and severing, followed by repositioning the ovary to allow exposure of the entire mesovarium for ligation. The blood supply to a large pathologic ovary can be quite extensive and require significant ligation. Fibrosis around blood vessels may make ligation difficult.[21] Once the ovary is removed, the mesovarium should be carefully examined for hemorrhage. Areas of hemorrhage should be ligated again. The stump can be oversewn with #00 synthetic absorbable suture to reduce adhesion formation.

As an alternative to manual ligation, surgical stapling equipment can be used. The TA 90 surgical stapling device (United States Surgical Corporation) with the 3.5-mm loading base has been used successfully.[21]

Peritoneum can be closed with a simple continuous pattern using #0 synthetic absorbable suture. The linea alba is closed with simple interrupted or continuous sutures of #2 synthetic absorbable suture. Subcutaneous tissue is carefully closed over linea alba sutures with simple continuous sutures of #0 synthetic absorbable suture. All sutures in the linea alba should be buried by this layer to prevent ascending infection. The skin is closed with simple interrupted or continuous Ford interlocking sutures with nonabsorbable suture. Skin staples can be used but may be difficult to remove.

POSTSURGICAL CARE AND POTENTIAL COMPLICATIONS

Procaine penicillin G therapy is continued once daily (20,000 IU/kg IM) for 5 days postsurgery. Flunixin meglumine (Banamine) (1 mg/kg IV) should be administered daily for 3 days postsurgery to minimize abdominal discomfort. Additional supportive care (intravenous fluids) should be administered as indicated by clinical signs. Skin sutures or staples are removed at 12 to 14 days. Following suture removal, the mare should be confined to a small area for 2 to 4 additional weeks. Pasture or light exercise can be resumed at this time. Full exercise should not be resumed until 8 to 12 weeks postsurgery.

Complications with this technique are similar to those described for flank ovariectomy. Delayed healing or abscess or hematoma formation in the incision occur with less frequency but can be difficult to manage. Hematoma or adhesions of the mesovarium and peritonitis can also cause postoperative complications. Good surgical technique and minimal operative time will minimize these complications.

Fatal complications have also been reported. Ventral midline incision dehiscence, resulting in evisceration, can occur with incision complications. Postoperative incision care is imperative. Severe hemorrhage from the mesovarium can occur if ligatures slip and require further surgical intervention. Larger ovarian tumors are more difficult to remove and maintain adequate hemostasis and will have more frequent complications. Anesthetic complications can be severe with this procedure because of the marked decrease in blood pressure during ligation and removal of the ovary. Nerve paralysis (femoral, peroneal, or radial), general rhabdomyolysis or postoperative shock have all been reported.[23]

CONCLUSIONS

Ovariectomy is a valuable technique for several conditions of mares in equine practice. The technique used to perform the procedure depends on several considerations. The specific indication for surgery (ovarian size) may preclude use of colpotomy or flank celiotomy. Economic and cosmetic considerations may be more important for performance mares where behavior is a problem or for mares for research or embryo transfer purposes. Available facilities, equipment, and expertise of the practitioner are also considerations.

Client communications are important before performing this procedure. When a single tumorous ovary is removed, normal reproductive capacity is recovered in approximately 60 to 75% of mares over a period of 2 to 16 months.[1,23] When the procedure is used to control undesirable estrous behavior, success may be slightly lower. The submissive nature of estrous behavior causes the behavioral patterns to be repeated in certain situations. These patterns may be learned behavior and may not be controlled hormonally and may be continued after ovariectomy. The cosmetic defect caused by flank celiotomy can be quite distressing to some owners and should be stressed before selecting this technique. With appropriate client education, these techniques can be quite successful in many practices.

REFERENCES

1. Bosu, W.T.K., Van Camp, S.C., Miller, R.B., and Owen, R. ap R.: Ovarian disorders: Clinical and morphologic observations in 30 mares. Can. Vet. J., *23:*6–14, 1982.
2. Cox, J.E.: Surgery of the Reproductive Tract in Large Animals. Liverpool, Liverpool University Press, 1982.
3. Guard, W.F.: Surgical Principles and Techniques. Ann Arbor, Edwards Brothers, 1953.
4. Nickels, F.A.: Complications of urogenital surgery. Proc. Am. Assoc. Equine Pract., 261–265, 1978.
5. Scott, E.A., and Kunze, D.J.: Ovariectomy in the mare: Presurgical, surgical, and postsurgical considerations. J. Equine Med. Surg., *1:*5–12, 1977.
6. Wiliams, W.L.: Surgical and Obstetrical Operations. Ithaca, W.L. Williams, 1903.
7. Pugh, D.G., Bowen, J.M., and Gaughan, E.M.: Equine ovarian tumors. Compend. Contin. Educ. Practicing Vet., *7:*S710–S716, 1985.
8. Hinrichs, K., Sertich, P.L., Cummings, M.R., and Kenney, R.M.: Pregnancy in ovariectomised mares achieved by embryo transfer: A preliminary study. Equine Vet. J. Suppl., *3:*74–75, 1985.
9. Hinrich K., Sertich, P.L., and Kenney, R.M.: Use of altrenogest to prepare ovariectomized mares as embryo transfer recipients. Theriogenology, *26:*455–460, 1986.
10. McKinnon, A.O., Squires, E.L., Carnevale, E.M., and Hermenet, M.J.: Ovarectomized steroid-treated mares as embryo transfer recipients and as a model to study the role of progestins in pregnancy maintenance. Theriogenology, *29:*1055–1063, 1988.
11. Fleming, G. A Textbook of Operative Veterinary Surgery. New York, William R. Jenkins, 1884.
12. Berge, E., and Westheus, M.: Veterinary Operative Surgery. Baltimore, Williams & Wilkins, 1966.
13. Frank, E.R.: Veterinary Surgery. 6th ed. Minneapolis, Burgess Publishing, 1959.
14. Kersjes A.W., Nemeth, F., and Rutgers, L.F.E.: Atlas of Large Animal Surgery. Baltimore, Williams & Wilkins, 1985.
15. Vaughan, J.T.: Operative surgery of the cranial tract. *In* Practice of Large Animal Surgery. Edited by P.B. Jennings, Jr. Philadelphia, W.B. Saunders, 1984, pp. 1140–1143.
16. Taylor, P.M.: Chemical restraint of the standing horse. Equine Vet. J., *17:*269–273, 1985.
17. Muir, W.W., and Robertson, J.T.: Visceral analgesia: Effects of xylazine, butorphanol, meperidine and pentazocine in horses. Am. J. Vet. Res., *46:*2081–2084, 1985.
18. McKinnon, A.O., Carnevale, E.M., Squires, E.L., and Jochle, W.: Clinical evaluation of detomidine hydrochloride for equine reproductive surgery. Proc. Am. Assoc. Equine Pract., 563–568, 1988.
19. Colbern, G.T., and Reagan, W.J.: Ovariectomy by colpotomy in mares. Compend. Contin. Educ. Practicing Vet., *9:*1035–1041, 1987.
20. Turner, A.S., and McIlwraith, C.W.: Standing flank laparotomy. *In* Techniques in Large Animal Surgery. 2nd ed. Philadelphia, Lea & Febiger, 1989, pp. 248–253.
21. McIlwraith, C.W., and Turner, A.S.: Ovariectomy (tumor removal). *In* Equine Surgery Advanced Techniques. Philadelphia, Lea & Febiger, 1987, pp. 346–351.
22. Turner, A.S., and McIlwraith, C.W.: Ventral Midline Laparotomy and Abdominal Exploration. *In* Techniques in Large Animal Surgery. 2nd ed. Philadelphia, Lea & Febiger, 1989, pp. 240–247.
23. Meagher, D.M., et al.: Granulosa cell tumors of mares—A review of 78 cases. Proc. Am. Assoc. Equine Pract., 133–138, 1977.

CHAPTER 53

UTERINE TORSION

J.R. Vasey

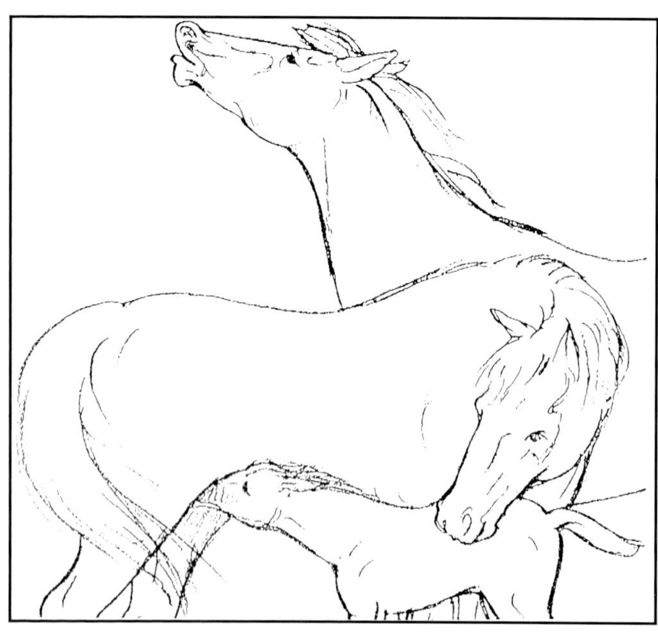

Uterine torsion is an infrequent but serious complication of pregnancy in mares. Initiating factors which cause uterine torsion are unclear. Fetal activity alone or in combination with the mare rolling may result in uterine torsion. The end result is a torsion of the uterine horns and body through 180 to 540° in either a clockwise or counterclockwise direction as viewed from the rear. The broad ligament, or mesometrium, which suspends the uterus has an extensive base in the sublumbar region, which limits incidence of uterine torsion in the mare compared with the cow. No breed or age predilection has been demonstrated in the horse.

In a review of 26 cases, torsion occurred at a mean of 9.6 months of gestation, with a range of 8 months to term.[1] In a survey of 42 cases in Belgium, about 50% of the uterine torsions were diagnosed during parturition, but this only accounted for 5 to 10% of the total number of dystocias.[2] In these later cases which occur near term, the fetus can assume an abnormal position which may contribute to the uterine torsion and thus the cause of dystocia.

DIAGNOSIS

A diagnosis of uterine torsion should always be considered in mares which exhibit mild signs of colic during the last trimester of gestation. Usually the mild, intermittent signs of colic respond only temporarily to analgesics. Signs of colic associated with uterine torsion include depression, periodic pawing, looking at the flank, kicking at the abdomen and rolling. Rectal temperature and heart and respiratory rates are within normal limits or only slightly elevated. Abdominal auscultation will reveal normal or reduced gastrointestinal sounds. Severity of pain is related to degree of torsion and/or concurrent involvement of the gastrointestinal tract. Dystocia may be the presenting sign if torsion of the uterus occurs near term (see Chapter 68). Usual abdominal contractions of foaling are absent as the torsion prevents the fetus from being delivered into the pelvic canal.

A definitive diagnosis is based on careful rectal examination. In late pregnancy, the broad ligaments are pulled tightly downward in front of the brim of the pelvis by the gravid uterus. Torsion of the uterus causes asymmetry of these ligaments. In the case of a counterclockwise torsion the left uterine ligament, which originates from the left sublumbar region, is strongly stretched and runs immediately downward under the uterine body. The right uterine ligament runs from its origin in the right sublumbar region to the left of the abdomen and then under the uterine body. When the torsion is clockwise and exceeds 180°, the right ligament is the more tense and runs immediately under the right side of the uterus; the left ligament is less tense and runs to the right, over the uterine body, and then under the uterus. Occasionally position and orientation of the rectum may be useful in establishing direction of uterine torsion. In a review of the literature, the authors concluded that the likelihood of rotation in either direction was equal.[1] Palpation of the body of the uterus may indicate it has become involved in the torsion, in which case the fetus cannot be readily palpated because of cranial displacement in the abdomen. Severity of the torsion is indicated by the amount of tension on the ligaments. Some constriction of the small colon may exist, depending on stage of gestation and degree and site of the torsion, which will restrict exploration of the abdomen. Tympany of small or large colon may also make rectal evaluation difficult. Evacuation of the rectum may be necessary to palpate the uterus and make a diagnosis of uterine torsion. All palpable organs within the abdominal cavity should be examined to rule out a concurrent or associated gastrointestinal condition. Any tense band in a pregnant mare needs to be carefully examined to distinguish between the taenia coli and the broad ligaments of the uterus.

The uterine wall should be carefully palpated to assess degree of congestion, necrosis, or possible rupture. Rupture of the uterus is not an uncommon sequela to prolonged uterine torsion, and position and extent will influence surgical access and resultant prognosis.

Abdominal paracentesis is indicated in mares with colic, particularly if rectal examination does not confirm a diagnosis of uterine torsion or a concurrent gastrointestinal lesion is suspected. Peritoneal fluid may be difficult to obtain from a mare in late pregnancy because the uterus occupies a large amount of the ventral abdomen.[3] Peritoneal fluid characteristics from mares prepartum and postpartum do not vary significantly from normal peritoneal fluid (D. Trout, personal communication).

All pregnant mares with undiagnosed colic should have a visual and manual examination of the vagina performed. However, only rarely will the cervix or vagina be involved in cases of uterine torsion, thus relying on vaginal examination alone for diagnosis of uterine torsion in the mare is unsatisfactory.

TREATMENT

NONSURGICAL CORRECTION

Manual Rotation Through the Cervix

When uterine torsion has been diagnosed at term, an attempt should be made to correct the torsion manually per vagina. Successful delivery depends on passage through the cervical canal of the clinician's well-lubricated hand and arm. This will usually only be possible if the torsion is less than 270°. If the fetal membranes are intact, they should be ruptured to release fluids and reduce the size and weight of the uterus and its contents.[4] It is essential that the mare remain standing throughout the procedure. Hence sedatives should be avoided but epidural anesthesia may help eliminate abdominal straining. Elevation of the mare's hindquarters on an inclined plane will provide more room in the posterior part of the abdominal cavity, as the large and small bowel will move forward. The clinician's hand and arm should be inserted as deeply as possible into the uterus and a substantial part of the fetus (upper forearm or body) should be grasped. The fetus and uterus are then rocked back and forth through small arcs (25 to 30 cm) until with an extra effort in a semicircular motion, opposite to the direction of the torsion, detorsion is accomplished. A second effort may be necessary for complete detorsion. Complete detorsion is recognized by normal dorsopubic delivery of the fetus, lack of twisting of the cervix or uterine body, and normal position of the uterine ligaments detected by rectal palpation. Following correction of the torsion the mare should spontaneously commence second-stage labor, although this may be delayed because vascular congestion and edema diminish uterine contractility. If the mare does not spontaneously deliver the foal following full dilation of the cervix, either the mare can be induced to foal with 40 to 60 IU of oxytocin or the foal can be delivered with manual assistance. Over 80% of the uterine torsions seen at parturition can be corrected by the described technique.[2]

Mares in advanced pregnancy with a partial uterine torsion in which the cervix is sufficiently dilated to deliver the foal need to be carefully evaluated.[5] Traction applied to the foal in this case may cause uterine rupture, resulting in fatal hemorrhage and peritonitis. Before attempting delivery, a rectal examination should establish if a uterine torsion exists and then appropriate corrective procedures need to be performed. Some uterine torsions of less than 180° may become corrected spontaneously.

Rolling

Rolling the anesthetized mare can be used to correct uterine torsion during the last trimester of pregnancy but should not be used near term because of the increased risk of uterine rupture.[6] The mare is anaesthetized and placed in lateral recumbency on the side toward which the torsion is directed. The mare is then turned quickly in the direction of the twist, with the objective of turning the body around the uterine axis. For example, if a clockwise torsion to the right is diagnosed the mare is positioned in right lateral recumbency and the mare rotated in a clockwise direction. This technique depends on inertia of the gravid uterus maintaining a constant fetal position while the maternal position changes. Occasionally rolling needs to be repeated or the mare rocked back and forth while positioned in dorsal recumbency to help correct the uterine torsion.[7]

A modification of this technique involves the use of a plank of wood to help stabilize the fetus while the mare is rotated[6,8] (Fig. 53–1). A person kneels on a board (2 to 3 m long and 20 to 30 cm wide) that has one end across the recumbent mare's upper paralumbar region and the other end on the floor near the mare's feet. The mare is then rolled as described above although more slowly to reduce risk of uterine rupture. In cases where the fetus is ballotable through the abdominal wall, the plank is repositioned during the rolling procedure as

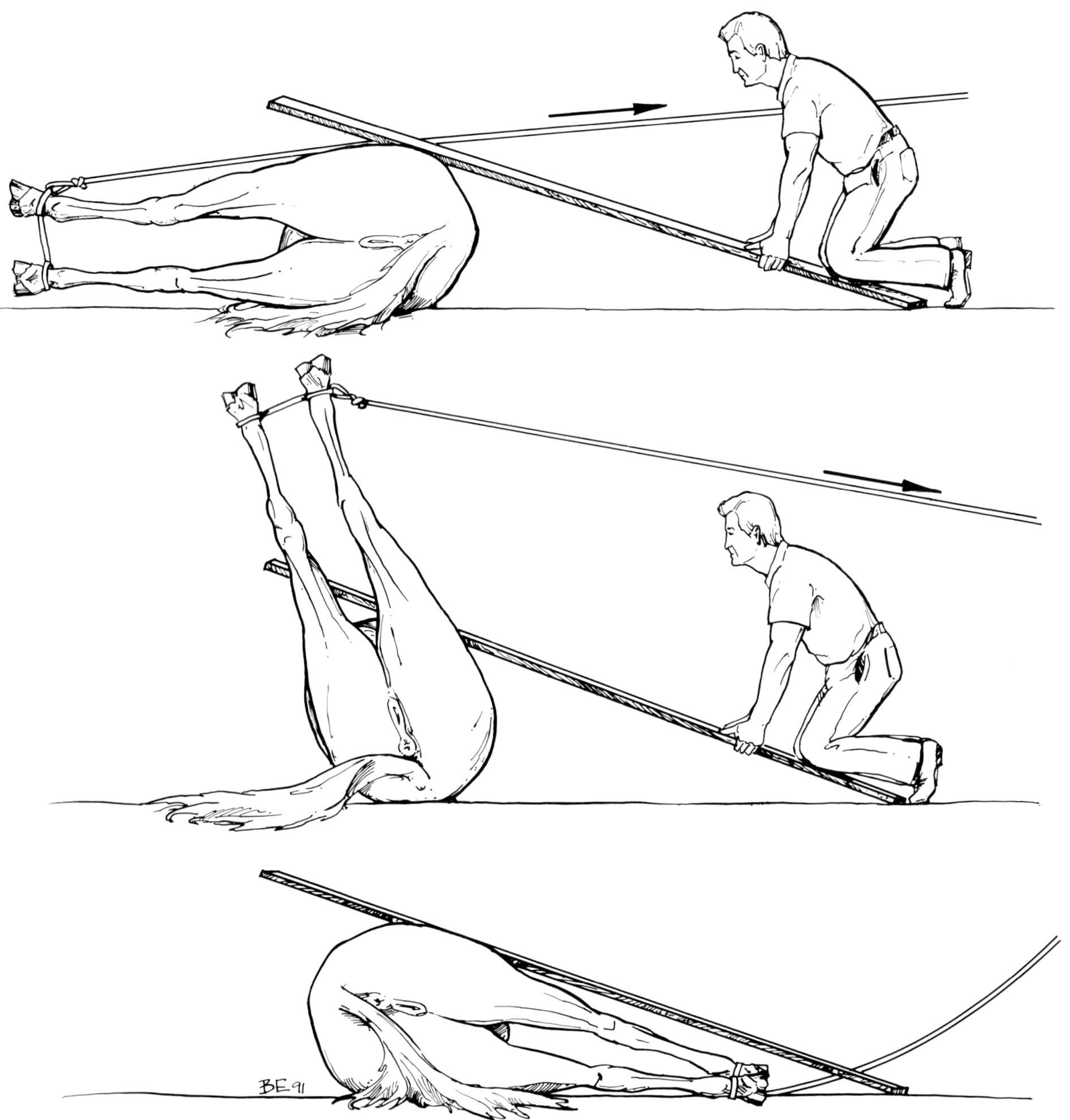

FIG. 53–1. Technique for nonsurgical correction of a uterine torsion. The mare is placed in lateral recumbency, the side the uterus has turned toward is down. In this case, the mare has a clockwise uterine torsion. The mare is slowly rolled over to the opposite side while a board and weight are used to keep the uterus from rotating with the mare. (Adapted from Bowen, J.M., Gaboury, C., and Bousquet, D.: Non-surgical correction of a uterine torsion in the mare. Vet. Rec., *99:*495–496, 1976.)

necessary to maintain maximal leverage on the fetus. To achieve correction, this procedure may need to be repeated up to five times.[6] Progress is assessed by rectal palpation, but that may be difficult on recumbent mares. Early reports using this nonsurgical method were associated with a high mortality rate of both mare and foal,[2] possibly because of separation of the allantochorion from the endometrium with subsequent abortion, premature birth, death of the fetus, or uterine rupture.[6] However more recent reports have given much better results,[6,7] possibly because of (1) an improved rolling technique, (2) the patient selection of nonparturient mares, and (3) the lack of interference with the cervix during corrective procedures.

SURGICAL CORRECTION

Standing Flank Laparotomy

In tractable mares, without evidence of uterine rupture, uterine torsion is best corrected by standing flank laparotomy. The flank incision is made on the side toward which the torsion is rotated. For example, in the case of a clockwise or right torsion, the incision is made in the right flank. It is easier to detorse the uterus by lifting and then repelling than by pulling, which may predispose rupture of the uterine wall.[1] If the direction of the torsion is not clear, then the incision should be made in the left flank to avoid the cecum.

The mare is placed in stocks and sedated only enough to ensure that she remain standing during the procedure. The appropriate paralumbar fossa is clipped and prepared for aseptic surgery. Skin and abdominal muscles are desensitized by local infiltration with 2% lidocaine in a vertical line. A modified grid approach is used incising the skin, cutaneous muscle, and external abdominal oblique muscle in a vertical direction and dividing the internal abdominal oblique and transverse abdominal muscles in the direction of their fibers. The peritoneum is punctured and then dilated to provide sufficient room for introduction of the surgeon's arm. Direction of the uterine torsion is confirmed by palpating the direction of displacement of the broad ligaments of the uterus and palpating the dorsal surface of the uterine body forward from the cervix. If the uterus is rotated toward the surgeon, the surgeon's arm is passed deeply along the body wall under the uterus and a prominant part of the foal is grasped through the uterine wall. Gentle rocking movements toward the surgeon followed by repulsion of the dorsal surface of the uterus will correct the torsion. In cases of prolonged, severe (greater than 240°) torsion in which the uterine wall is edematous and friable because of venous congestion, detorsion needs to be performed carefully to prevent uterine rupture. In these cases, lengthening the incision and inserting both arms to lift and repell the uterus concurrently may be helpful. Occasionally, dual flank incisions with two surgeons may be necessary to correct a difficult uterine torsion in mares in advanced pregnancy. Correction of the uterine torsion is confirmed by palpation of the broad ligaments and the dorsal surface of the uterus beginning at the cervix. Fetal viability is assessed by stimulating the foal to move by pinching an extremity. If the foal is definitely dead or the cervical mucus has been lost, the foal is removed by hysterotomy. Hysterotomy is performed under general anesthesia either through the flank approach, in which case exposure is improved by incising the internal abdominal oblique muscle ventral to the grid incision, or through a ventral midline incision. The abdomen is explored to rule out any concurrent gastrointestinal cause of colic. Closure is accomplished by suturing each muscle layer separately with #2 polyglactin 910 (Vicryl; Ethicon, Inc.), and the skin, with a nonabsorbable suture.

Ventral Midline Laparotomy

Following induction of general anesthesia, the mare is positioned in dorsal recumbency and a 25-cm-long ventral midline incision is made immediately cranial to the umbilicus. This approach allows better access to the abdomen and enables both arms to be inserted through the incision to correct the torsion. If a hysterotomy (see Chapter 50) is indicated, it can be performed and then the torsion more easily corrected. Advantages of the ventral midline approach include easier correction of uterine torsion in advanced pregnancy and better access. The midline makes it easier to (1) perform a hysterotomy if indicated, (2) repair uterine wall ruptures, (3) treat concomitant gastrointestinal problems, and (4) visualize the uterine wall viability. The disadvantages include (1) the stress of general anesthesia on the mare and foal, (2) the surgical facilities that are necessary, and (3) the severe strain on the ventral incision if the mare goes into labor soon after surgery.

Before surgery, the mare is given broad spectrum antibiotics and a nonsteroidal anti-inflammatory drug, such as flumixin meglumine (0.5 to 1.1 mg/kg IV), to counteract the risk of endotoxemia associated with abdominal surgery. Following surgery, antibiotics, intravenous fluids, and nonsteroidal anti-inflammatory drugs are given as necessary, and the mare is confined to a stall for 3 to 4 weeks. The mare should be observed for any signs of abortion such as loss of the cervical mucus plug, udder development, vulval discharge, or early signs of parturition.

PROGNOSIS

Survey results for survival of mares with uterine torsion treated surgically are 73%,[1] and nonsurgically from poor[2] to 85%.[6] In one survey of the fetuses determined to be alive at surgery, 20 of 26 foals were alive at the time of correction, but only 14 (70%) were born alive, i.e., 54% of the total were born alive.[1] Complications associated with correction of uterine torsion include (1) premature placental separation with subsequent fetal death and abortion, (2) uterine wall necrosis and rupture, (3) peritonitis, (4) partial or complete dehiscence of the incision, (5) endotoxic shock, and (6) recurrence of the torsion during the same pregnancy. In cases of uterine rupture in which the fetal fluids are fresh, prognosis for the mare is generally good, but when fetal fluids have become contaminated the prognosis is poor.

Nonsurgical or surgical correction of uterine torsion does not adversely affect mares' subsequent reproductive performance unless either uterine rupture has occurred or a cesarean section was performed.[1] Advanced pregnancy, extensive torsion, and delay in diagnosis and treatment of the condition significantly decrease prognoses of mares with uterine torsion.

The optimum treatment for a mare with uterine torsion will depend on (1) economics, (2) facilities available, (3) stage of pregnancy, (4) duration of clinical signs, and (5) whether signs of abortion or parturition are present. A quiet, valuable mare, 6 weeks or more from term, with a diagnosed uterine torsion would be best treated using a standing flank laparotomy. When facilities or economics preclude surgery, then rolling such a mare is indicated. For a mare at term, when the cervix has dilated, manual correction should be attempted through the cervix. If this is unsuccessful a ventral midline approach is indicated.

REFERENCES

1. Pascoe, J.R., Meagher, D.M., and Wheat, J.D.: Surgical management of uterine torsion in the mare: A review of 26 cases. J. Am. Vet. Med. Assoc., *179:*351–354, 1981.
2. Vandeplassche, M., Spincemaille, J., Bouters, R., and Bonte, P.: Some aspects of equine obstetrics. Equine Vet. J., *4:*105–113, 1972.
3. Pascoe, J.R., and Pascoe, R.R.: Displacement, malpositions and miscellaneous injuries. Vet. Clin. North Am., Equine Pract., *4*:439–450, 1988.
4. Freeman, D.E.: Uterine torsion. *In* Current Practice of Equine Surgery. Edited by N.A. White and J.N. Moore. Philadelphia, J.B. Lippincott, 1990, pp. 716–719.
5. Vaughan, J.T.: Surgery of the equine reproductive system. *In* Current Therapy in Theriogenology. Edited by D.A. Morrow. Philadelphia, W.B. Saunders, 1980, pp. 820–821.
6. Wichtel, J.J., Reinertson, E.L., and Clark, T.L.: Nonsurgical treatment of uterine torsion in seven mares. J. Am. Vet. Med. Assoc., *193:*337–338, 1988.
7. Guthrie, R.G.: Rolling for correction of uterine torsion in a mare. J. Am. Vet. Med. Assoc., *181:*66–67, 1982.
8. Bowen, J.M., Gaboury, C., and Bousquet, D.: Non-surgical correction of a uterine torsion in the mare. Vet. Rec., *99:*495–496, 1976.

CHAPTER 54

MAMMARY GLAND SURGERY

J. Easley

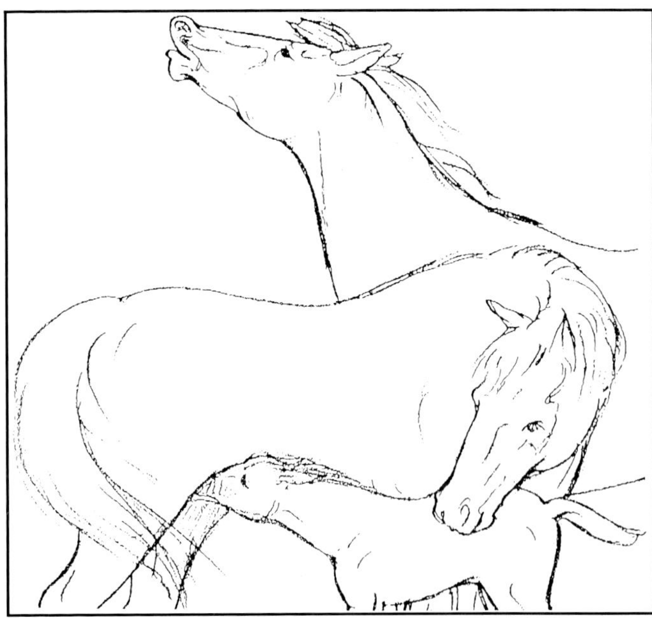

The udder of the mare is located ventrally on the abdomen between the two hind legs. This position affords it protection from traumatic injury and damaging effects of the sun. The mammary gland undergoes various changes associated with the stage of production. Dry mares possess an udder which is small, not well vascularized, and inconspicuous whereas lactating mares have an udder that appears more prominent both in size and vascularity.

Surgery of the mammary gland may be necessary in certain cases of chronic recurrent mastitis, tumors, and traumatic lacerations. Mastitis is usually seen in lactating mares and most often occurs following weaning.[1] Both clinical and subclinical mastitis are seen in the mare. Clinically, the mare's udder appears distended, warm, red, firm, and painful. Subclinically, the udder appears normal, but further examination of udder secretions reveal a high somatic cell count and abnormal cell structure.[2,3] Therefore, careful examination and palpation of the mammary gland and cytologic evaluation of mammary gland secretions are recommended as part of a reproductive examination of the mare and of those suspected of clinical mastitis.

Several different causes have been identified for clinical mastitis in mares. The most common bacteria isolated are those of the streptococcal and gram-negative species. In a recent study, these isolates were found to be most sensitive to antimicrobial combination of trimethoprim and sulfonamide.[2] These or other antibiotics are administered systemically or by intramammary infusion. Adjuncts to antibiotic therapy are administration of nonsteroidal anti-inflammatory drugs, frequent milkings, hot packing, and/or hydrotherapy. Sequelae to mastitis includes scar tissue and granuloma formation, which may lead to recurrent bouts of mastitis. This can further result in decreased milk production, decreased milk protein and calcium, and alterations of foal growth and development.[1] Staphylococcal bacteria have been documented to cause recurrent granulomatous mastitis (botryomycosis).[4] This disease is not responsive to medical therapy and may necessitate surgical removal of the affected udder.

Mammary neoplasia in mares is rare. Schmahl reported incidences between 0.11 and 1.99% in a European slaughter house study.[5] The tumors reported to affect the mammary gland are adenocarcinoma, melanoma, mastocytoma, and lymphosarcoma.[5–9] These tumors appear as multifocal cutaneous nodules or superficial ulcerations visible on the surface of the udder. The mammary gland does not necessarily appear enlarged but may have palpable nodules in the deeper mammary tissues. Lesions may present themselves in a nodular or ulcerative form and drip serosanguinous fluid. Such lesions can be misdiagnosed as habronemiasis or sarcoid neoplasia.[7] Therefore, accurate diagnoses require deep biopsy for adequate histopathologic evaluation. Early diagnosis is important because of the aggressive metastatic nature of mammary adenocarcinoma, which is the most commonly reported mammary tumor. These tumors have been known to metastasize through lymphatic and hematogenous routes.[7,8] Rectal palpation, abdominocentesis, and thoracocentesis may be valuable aids in determining whether metastasis has occurred. The treatment of choice with such lesions includes removal of the affected mammary gland as well as the regional lymph nodes. Nonmalignant tumors of the mammary gland may be dealt with via excision of the mass or cryotherapy.

Superficial melanomas with their typical dark pigmented surface are best left undisturbed unless they can be excised in their entirety. Inspection of the other hairless areas of the mare including, but not limited to, the vulva, perineum, and base of the tail may reveal other melanomas especially in older gray mares. These tumors are usually slow to metastasize to internal organs if simply left alone.

Other rarely malignant mammary growths, mastocytoma, equine sarcoid, or habronemiasis should be managed by total excision of the lesion. If the margins appear clear, the skin edges can be closed by first intention, taking the same precautions associated with laceration repair described in the next paragraph. If the growth cannot be removed totally, then it may be managed by local cryotherapy. Liquid nitrogen is used either by direct contact or by a brass cryoprobe to lower the temperature of the entire lesion rapidly to $-20°$ C with a slow thaw and refreeze technique.[10] The necrotic area that forms will slough. The eschar should be left dry and allowed to dislodge on its own. Systemic antibiotics and nonsteroidal anti-inflammatory drugs may be indicated during the postoperative period, but the defect left from this procedure usually heals within 6 weeks leaving a superficial nonpigmented scar.

Trauma, such as puncture wounds or lacerations to the mammary gland may necessitate surgery. Superficial laceration to the teat or udder are amenable to surgical repair. This can be done standing under sedation with local infiltration of anesthetic or under a short-acting general anesthetic. The wound edges are trimmed if jagged or devitalized tags of tissue are present. Deep wounds should be evaluated to determine whether lactiferous ducts or teat canals are involved. If so, these should be sutured with fine #2-0 to #4-0 absorbable suture, bringing the deep layers into apposition. Lacerations which do not involve the milk canals should be closed with skin sutures, avoiding burying the suture if possible. Tissue adhesive may also be used and has been shown to cause less tissue reaction and decreased healing time.[11]

MAMMARY GLAND AMPUTATION

Mammary gland amputation may be indicated in cases of mammary tumors or chronic recurrent mastitis that is nonresponsive to medical therapy. Amputation may be of one or both udders as the clinical diagnosis dictates. Surgery of the mammary gland is most successful when performed on nonlactating mares. This ensures minimal hemorrhage into the surgical field.

SURGICAL TECHNIQUE

Before surgery the mare should receive appropriate antibiotics and nonsteroidal anti-inflammatory drugs. The mare is anesthetized and placed in dorsal recumbency with the hind limbs in a relaxed abducted position. The surgical field, including the udder and peripheral abdominal and inguinal areas, is clipped and scrubbed, and the fluids are drained from the inguinal folds. Special consideration should be taken to remove all debris from the fold between the two halves of the udder. The surgical area is draped in normal fashion. An elliptical skin incision is made extending from the anterior to the posterior edge of the udder, centered over the teat. Using sharp scissor dissection, the skin flap is elevated from the deeper mammary tissue. This is continued with blunt finger dissection beginning on the caudal aspect of the mammary gland. This blunt dissection is continued both mediad and laterad in an anterior direction. Medially the gland is separated from the prominent median raphe, which separates the two halves of the udder. Laterally the gland is separated from the skin and body wall. When dissection is nearly complete, the gland is elevated from the body wall to expose vessels within the inguinal region. The external pudendal artery must be carefully exposed and double ligated close to the body wall before it branches into the cranial and caudal mammary artery. Other vessels encountered in this area are the obturator vein caudally and branches of the internal pudendal and contralateral external pudendal veins. This dissection may be carried out with the aid of electrocautery to minimize bleeding. The mammary gland is completely separated from the anterior body wall, taking care to identify and ligate the caudal superficial epigastric vein which enters the cranial most aspect of the udder.

After all mammary tissues have been dissected and removed, the superficial inguinal lymph nodes at the base of the udder should be examined and biopsied for histopathologic exam if indicated. A drain tube or gauze roll (soaked in povidone-iodine solution) is inserted into the vacated cavity. The gauze or drain should exit the most cranioventral aspect of the skin at least 2.5 cm away from the incision. This will allow easy retrieval postoperatively. The wound is closed in routine fashion, making every attempt to reduce dead space.

During recovery, the mare is placed in lateral recumbency with the affected area down, to reduce stress on the suture site. After recovery, the drain and incision area should be monitored. Normally, transudate should exit the drainage site for up to 10 days. As much as 50 mL of serosanguinous fluid exiting the drain is not abnormal. If more than this is detected or if the fluid becomes purulent, then the drain is acting as an infective wick and should be removed. If all progresses normally, the drain is removed in 10 to 14 days. The incision site is monitored carefully as this area is prone to infection. Its pendulous nature makes the mammary area susceptible to fluid accumulation and exuberant granulation tissue proliferation. This accumulation may delay first-intention healing for up to 3 to 4 weeks. This is especially true with bilateral mastectomy. If first-intention healing fails, then this area must be treated as an open wound with lavage and/or hydrotherapy to encourage second-intention healing. If histopathologic study reveals malignancy disease of the regional lymph nodes, radiation therapy may be indicated postoperatively.

REFERENCES

1. Rossdale, P.D., and Ricketts, S.W.: Equine Stud Farm Medicine. 2nd ed. London, Baillieri Tindall, 1980.
2. McCue, P.M., and Wilson, W.D.: A review of 28 cases of equine mastitis. Equine Vet. J., *21:*351–353, 1989.
3. Freeman, K.P., Roszel, J.F., Slusher, S.H., and Young, D.: Cytologic features of equine mammary fluids: Normal and abnormal. Compend. Contin. Educ. Practicing Vet., *10:*1090–1099, 1988.
4. Smith, H.A., Jones, J.C., and Hunt, R.D.: Veterinary Pathology. 4th ed. Philadelphia, Lea & Febiger, 1972.
5. Schmahl, V.W.: Solides Karzinom der mamma bei einen pferd. Ber. Munch. Tierarztl. Wochenschr., *85:*141–141, 1972.
6. Jubb, K.V.F., and Kennedy, P.C.: Pathology of domestic animals. 2nd ed. New York, Academic Press, 1970.
7. Foreman, J.H., Weidner, J.P., Parry, B.W., and Hargis, A.: Pleural effusion secondary to thoracic metastatic mammary adenocarcinoma in a mare. J. Am. Vet. Med. Assoc., *197:*1193–1195, 1990.
8. Surmont, J.: L epitheliome mammaire de la jument et ses metastases plumonires. Bull. Assoc. Frac. Etude. Can., *15:*98–101, 1926.
9. Acland, H.M., and Gillette, D.M.: Mammary carcinoma in a mare. Vet. Pathol., *19:*93–95, 1982.
10. Fritz, P.B., and Barber, S.M.: Prospective analysis of cryosurgery as the sole treatment of equine sarcoids. Vet. Clin. North Am. Small Anim. Pract., *10:*847–859, 1980.
11. Makady, F.M., Whitmore, H.L., Nelson, D.R., and Simon, J.: Effect of tissue adhesives and suture patterns on experimentally induced teat lacerations in lactating dairy cattle. J. Am. Vet. Med. Assoc., *198:*1932–1934, 1991.

CHAPTER 55

MANAGEMENT OF RECTAL TEARS

M.S. Spensley
M.D. Markel

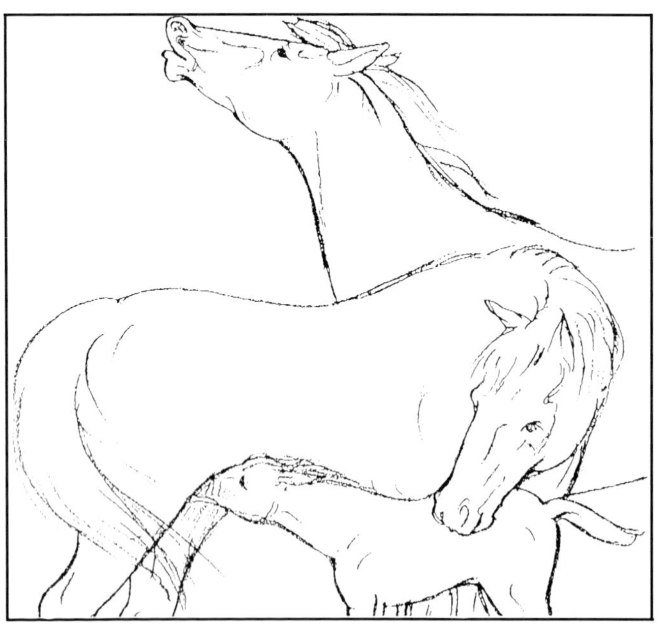

Since late in the nineteenth century, practitioners have recognized the potential for the occurrence of rectal tears and its associated complications.[1] At present, iatrogenic rectal tears and their complications represent one of the most frequent reasons for malpractice suits brought against the equine practitioner, with the incidence of claims increasing. Between 1976 and 1988, rectal tears accounted for 8% (181 of 2229) of the total resolved liability claims against equine practitioners (J.R. Dinsmore, personal communication). When a rectal tear is suspected, a definitive protocol needs to be followed to determine if a tear has occurred, to evaluate it in terms of possible treatment, and to protect it from further damage and contamination. It is imperative that immediate action be initiated after a rectal tear is diagnosed.

Previous reports indicated a high mortality rate in horses which sustained rectal tears[2–4] (J.R. Dinsmore, personal communication). Although the overall survival rate of horses with rectal tears in one retrospective study was 36%,[2] another survey indicated that only about 20% of horses with the more severe grade 3 or 4 tears survived.[3] Such reports suggest a need for early recognition of rectal tears and the development of better surgical techniques, which may result in improved survival rates. It should be emphasized that not all rectal tears are amenable to or require surgical repair; alternatives include conservative medical management and euthanasia.

The rectum extends from the terminal small colon, at about the pelvic inlet, to the anus, and is approximately 25 to 30 cm in length.[5] It is divided anatomically into a cranial, or peritoneal, portion and a caudal, or retroperitoneal, segment. The former is suspended by mesorectum; the latter is attached to surrounding pelvic structures by connective tissue and muscular bands.

Of particular importance is the short distance, approximately 15 to 20 cm in an adult light breed horse, between the peritoneal reflexion and the anus.[2] Most rectal tears occur at about the depth of, or cranial to, the pelvic inlet; that is, greater than 25 to 30 cm cranial to the anus. These are important relationships to remember when evaluating a rectal tear to determine if it extends into the retroperitoneal space or peritoneal cavity. In addition, most tears occur between the 10 and 2 o'clock positions in the dorsal rectal wall and most tears are longitudinally oriented. While rectal tears occur in horses of all ages, the injury happens most often in young horses, 1 to 5 yr of age.[2]

CAUSES

Rectal tears are usually iatrogenic, occurring during examination by palpatation per rectum[2–4,6–13] (J.R. Dinsmore, personal communication). Although palpation may be the ultimate determinant in the development of a rectal tear, spontaneous tears have been reported, indicating that ischemic vascular disease which causes devitalization of rectal tissue may predispose to rupture[2–14] (J.R. Dinsmore, personal communication). However, this group represents a minority of cases.

Other less common causes include the misdirected stallion penis, parturition/dystocia, and accidents associated with attempts to utilize enemas or forceps in removing meconium from foals.[2–11] There were 181 resolved rectal tear liability claims against equine practitioners between 1976 and 1988; of these, 33 (18.2%) involved colts, stallions, and geldings that sustained rectal tears during prepurchase, presurgical, and colic examinations; during cryptorchidectomy; or associated with exertional rhabdomyolysis. Regarding breed predisposition, Arabians have been incriminated as the breed in which the injury occurs most frequently. However, of the 181 resolved rectal tear suits between 1976 and 1988, 66 (36%) occurred in Quarter Horses, and 48 (27%) occurred in Arabians (J.R. Dinsmore, personal communication). It should be emphasized that experienced as well as inexperienced practitioners have had rectal tears occur while they were examining a horse. Therefore, experience is no guarantee that a serious rectal tear will be avoided during their career. Patient inexperience and refractoriness may represent significant predisposing factors for consideration. The inexperienced filly or mare, unaccustomed to procedures associated with examination per rectum, may be nervous. She may refuse to stand still, object to having her tail wrapped, and refuse to allow rectal introduction of the palpator's coned fingers. Nervousness may give way to fractiousness. Accordingly, prudent use of physical and chemical restraint techniques should be considered; however, selected procedures should be employed before the situation deteriorates to unmanageable extremes. Especially pertinent to inexperienced fillies and mares destined to be bred would be time spent familiarizing them with breeding farm procedures. Routine precautions should include wrapping the tail to prevent introduction of tail hair through the anus, liberal use of lubricant on the palpator's sleeved arm and hand, rectal introduction of the coned fingers, and gentle removal of feces to facilitate examination. Manipulations during examination by palpation must be performed gently. Palpation must cease immediately when the mare strains, the rectal wall becomes taut or a peristaltic contraction occurs.

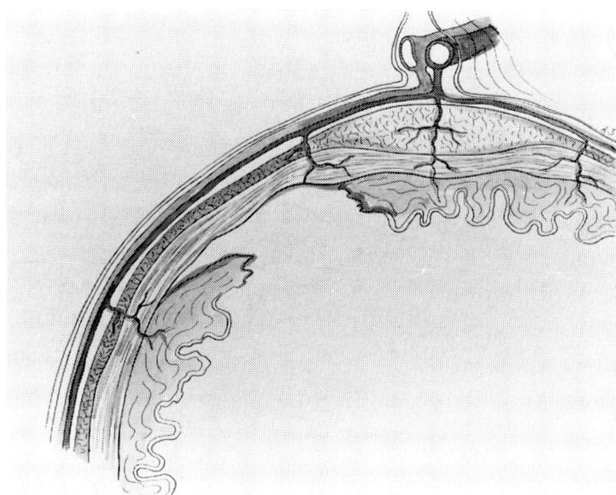

FIG. 55–1. Grade 1 tears involve only the mucosa or the mucosa and submucosa. (From Rick, M.C.: Management of rectal injuries. Vet. Clin. North Am., *5*:407–428, 1989.)

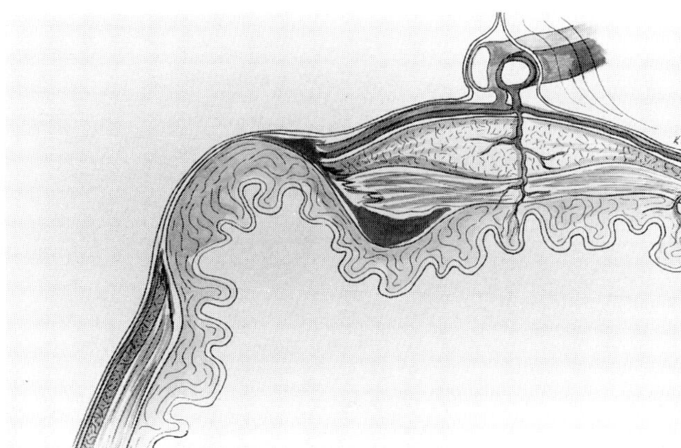

FIG. 55–2. In grade 2 tears, a separation defect persists in the muscularis, and a mucosa-submucosa hernia may be formed. (From Rick, M.C.: Management of rectal injuries. Vet. Clin. North Am., *5*:407–428, 1989.)

CLASSIFICATION

Rectal tears are classified as grades 1 through 4, according to the number of tissue layers perforated.[6] Grade 1 tears involve only the mucosa or mucosa and submucosa (Fig. 55–1). In grade 2 tears, only the muscularis is torn and a mucosal-submucosal hernia may develop. Grade 2 rectal tears usually represent only a theoretic event. However, such a pre-existing condition has been recognized and may contribute to some iatrogenic rectal tears. Histologic examination of sections taken from healing tear areas suggest that unless primary closure is achieved, a separation defect persists in the muscularis and a mucosal-submucosa hernia may be formed (Fig. 55–2). Grade 3 tears perforate the mucosa, submucosa, and muscularis, leaving only serosa or mesentery as the barrier to either the peritoneal cavity or retroperitoneal space (Fig. 55–3). All layers are perforated in grade 4 tears, and communication between the rectal lumen and the retroperitoneal space or peritoneal cavity exists (Fig. 55–4). Factors which determine the seriousness of a rectal tear and how it is managed include size, distance from the anus into the rectum and position on the rectal wall, layers which have been perforated, and time interval between occurrence and initiation of treatment. Rectal tears and their repair often become complicated because of tenesmus and fecal contamination. Consequences can be septicemic shock, dissecting cellulitis, abscessation, fistula formation, and severe peritonitis.

CLINICAL SIGNS/DIAGNOSIS

Presence of any amount of blood on the examination sleeve or on feces, no matter how small, should be considered significant evidence of rectal mucosal damage

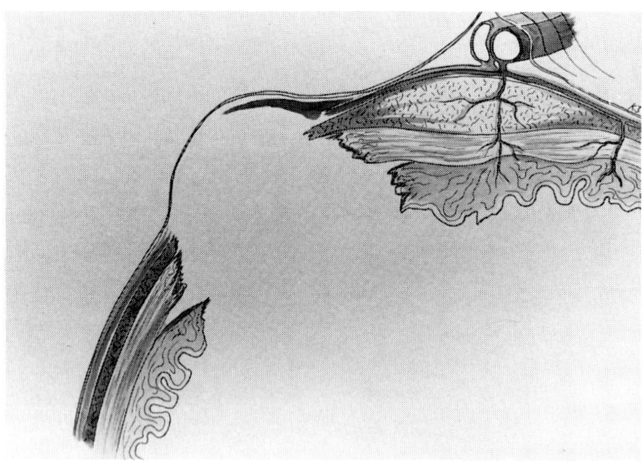

FIG. 55–3. Grade 3 tears perforate the mucosa, submucosa, and muscularis, leaving only serosa or mesentery as the barrier to either the peritoneal cavity or the retroperitoneal space. (From Rick, M.C.: Management of rectal injuries. Vet. Clin. North Am., *5*:407–428, 1989.)

and warrant, at least, that precautions be taken. Traces of blood-tinged fluid or small blood clots on the palpator's hand are not infrequently observed; this may occur particularly during serial palpations at the height of the breeding season or following palpation by multiple examiners or prolonged examination. Such observations are most likely associated with mucosal irritation without perforation. Persistent or increasing amounts of blood, and all cases of serious hemorrhage, must be investigated as potential tears by re-examination to confirm presence or absence of significant mucosal damage. Horses that have sustained a rectal tear during examination by palpation per rectum may manifest a spectrum of signs. These signs range from sudden relaxation of the rectum, with the presence of fresh blood on the examination sleeve, to no manifestation of rectal injury having occurred and the horse developing signs of acute abdominal disease soon after completion of the examination. Horses which have sustained grade 3 or 4 rectal tears, and even those with large grade 1 tears, may manifest anxiety or depression, anorexia, sweating, fever, and increased pulse and respiratory rates by virtue of peritonitis and septicemia soon after injury. In addition, variable signs of colic (including anorexia, scant diarrhea, splinted abdomen, and ileus) may be present.

A suspected rectal tear must be evaluated in a manner that will reveal the severity of injury without causing further damage. The horse should be sedated and peristalsis stopped to facilitate careful evacuation of the rectum. Following speculum examination of the injury, the examiner's hand is advanced into the rectum in 5 to 10 cm increments to remove feces, palpate the tear, and evaluate surrounding tissues. While some clinicians use a rectal sleeve or a latex glove, others prefer a non-gloved hand to digitally evaluate the tear. Xylazine (0.3 mg/kg IV) combined with butorphanol tartrate (0.1 mg/kg IV) has afforded sufficient sedation to allow thorough evacuation of feces and evaluation of many patients with rectal tears.[12] When necessary, caudal epidural anesthesia, lidocaine enema, or propantheline bromide has been employed to facilitate digital rectal evacuation, examination, and visual examination through a glass or disposable vaginal speculum.[10–13] While propantheline bromide (0.014 to 0.07 mg/kg IV) can be used to reduce peristalsis and relax the small colon and rectum, its use has been associated with abdominal discomfort. The administration of atropine (0.044 mg/kg IM or subcutaneously) has been found to be a reliable and safe means of depressing intestinal motility.[12]

The baseline values for temperature, pulse and respiratory rates, abdominal paracentesis, and hematologic parameters must be determined as soon as possible after a tear is suspected. Hematologic abnormalities frequently occur as clinical signs of peritonitis develop.[15] Initial peripheral neutrophil and plasma protein values may decrease because of effusion of white blood cells and exudation of protein into the peritoneal cavity. Accordingly, severity and progression of peritonitis can be monitored by serial abdominocenteses.

MEDICAL MANAGEMENT

The importance of communicating clearly to the owner or agent the nature of the injury and its potential seriousness, in event of a confirmed tear, cannot be overemphasized. Once the owner or agent has been informed of the situation, an appropriate therapeutic plan must be initiated. The patient's vital signs, hydration status, character of feces, tenesmus, and signs of colic must be intensively monitored. Colic and tenesmus are indicative of inflammation of tissues adjacent to the tear and of peritonitis. Tenesmus also enhances the likelihood of dissection of the tear between planes of rectal tissue. Once caudal epidural anesthesia and appropriate parasympatholytic drug therapy have been adminis-

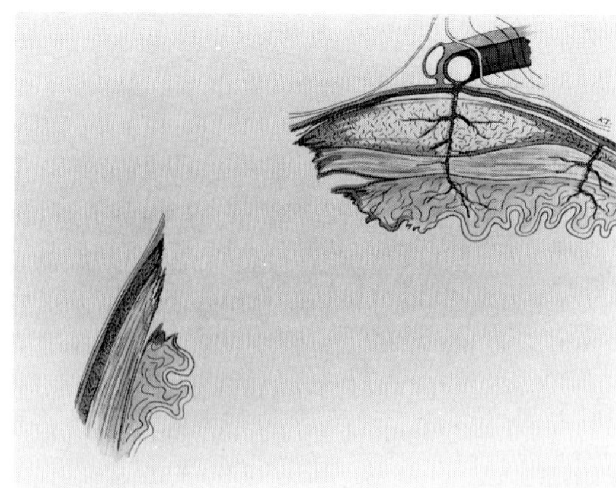

FIG. 55–4. All layers are perforated in grade 4 tears, and communication between the rectal lumen and the retroperitoneal space or the peritoneal cavity exists. (From Rick, M.C.: Management of rectal injuries. Vet. Clin. North Am., *5*:407–428, 1989.)

tered, the small colon or rectum cranial to the tear and the tear itself should be gently packed with gauze or cotton soaked in an organic iodine solution. Such packing may help prevent further fecal contamination and dissecting cellulitis between tissue layers involved in the rectal tear. In several horses with grade 3 rectal tears we have observed enlarging of the tear, marked inflammation, and distortion of the tissues incorporating the tear and/or development of a large subserosal pocket. A vicious circle ensues: fecal contamination of the tear leads to inflammation and straining; causing the tear to enlarge; causing more contamination, inflammation, and straining; and so on. Tetanus prophylaxis and broad-spectrum antibiotic therapy should be administered. The more severe grade 3 and 4 rectal tear patients are administered sodium or potassium penicillin G, an aminoglycoside, and metronidazole. Grade 1 tears, often presenting as mucosal flaps, are administered trimethoprim-sulfadiazine intravenously initially, followed by oral administration for several days. In the more severe grade 3 and 4 cases, nonsteroidal anti-inflammatory drugs and fluid therapy are begun immediately. Peritoneal lavage may be used in cases of severe peritonitis. Fluids are administered to rehydrate and/or maintain patient hydration and keep the feces soft. Fecal softeners (such as 5% dioctyl sodium sulfosuccinate or magnesium hydroxide) and an emollient (such as mineral oil) are administered. When indicated, the horse is referred to a surgical facility.

SURGICAL MANAGEMENT

Not all rectal tears require or are amenable to surgical repair. Unless the horse with a grade 4 tear is presented for surgery immediately on recognition of the tear and the tear is small, the prognosis for recovery is grave. Septicemia, peritonitis, and shock develop rapidly after peritoneal contamination. These patients and their owners are often better served by euthanasia than by unrealistic heroic attempts at surgical repair.

GRADE 1 TEARS

While most Grade 1 rectal tears can be successfully managed medically by administration of systemic antibiotics and fecal softeners/laxatives, large grade 1 tears should be repaired, usually by direct suturing techniques in the standing horse. If available, an expandable rectal speculum can be used to better visualize the tear (Fig. 55–5).[13] Alternately, a Caslick mare speculum and retractors have been used; however, mucosal folds tend to compromise visualization of and accessibility to the tear, and many such attempts have failed.[6]

Treatment may require administration of intravenous fluids if bowel stasis and dehydration occur. Unless deterioration of signs warrants further exploration, horses with grade 1 tears should not be palpated for at least 30 days after injury.[12]

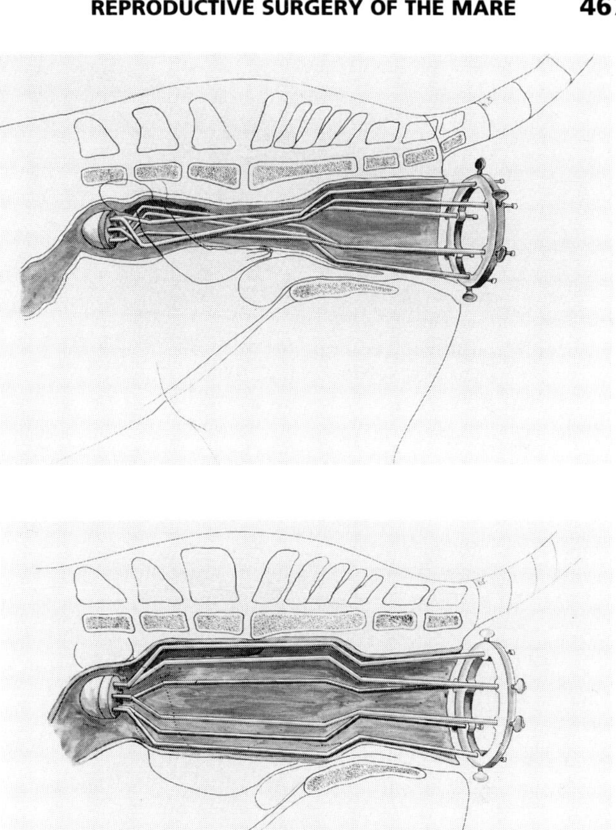

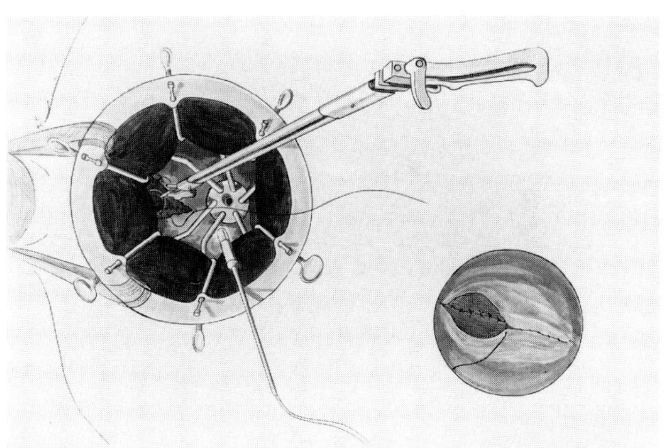

FIG. 55–5. Use of an expandable rectal speculum to visualize a rectal tear. *A*, The speculum is inserted into the rectum in its closed configuration. *B*, The expanded rectal speculum creates a cage through which rectal tears can be repaired. *C*, The expandable rectal speculum can be used to enhance visualization of rectal tears. Long-handled pistol-grip instruments facilitate surgical repair of tears. (From Rick, M.C.: Management of rectal injuries. Vet. Clin. North Am., *5*:407–428, 1989.)

GRADE 2 TEARS

As previously discussed, grade 2 tears are more a theoretical concern than a practical one. If a horse presents signs of colic or straining to defecate and palpation reveals a rectal diverticulum, the rectum should be carefully evacuated and evaluated. Ablation of the diverticulum is rarely, if ever, required because these horses usually respond to measures designed to maintain soft feces.

GRADE 3 AND 4 TEARS

Grade 3 tears almost always require surgical repair unless so much time has elapsed between occurrence of the tear and presentation of the horse that surgery will not benefit the animal. What period of time actually constitutes the "golden period" during which surgical repair is most readily accomplished is extremely variable between cases. Aggressive medical management as described in the previous section should be immediately instituted.

Horses with grade 4 tears, if immediately diagnosed and surgically treated, may survive. In general, though, widespread, massive fecal contamination, resulting in severe peritonitis has already occurred by the time the surgeon is able to repair the tear, giving horses with grade 4 tears a grave prognosis for survival.

Currently, surgical management of rectal tears is attempted by one of several possible approaches: (1) suture repair via celiotomy; (2) suture repair utilizing partial prolapse of the rectum; (3) temporary diverting colostomy, including "end-on" colostomy and loop colostomy; (4) suture repair via rectum; and (5) rectal liner.

Suture Repair via Celiotomy

Direct repair of rectal tears through a ventral midline celiotomy may be used but is rarely performed.[10] To be useful, the tear must be far enough cranial to allow exteriorization, or at least visualization, of the affected colon/rectum. Rectal tears are usually dorsal in the mesocolon and, combined with their tendency to be fairly far caudal, are often difficult or impossible to suture via this approach.

Suture Repair Utilizing Partial Prolapse of the Rectum

Rectal tears in the caudal two-thirds of the rectum can sometimes be repaired by partially prolapsing the rectum.[6] The technique works best in thin, older horses which tend to have more movable rectums. In young horses with a lot of pelvic fat, the rectum tends to be relatively immobile and partial prolapse of the rectum may not be feasible.

One or two Caslick speculums are used to dilate the rectum.[16] Stay sutures are placed cranial to the tear and used for traction when inverting the rectum. The tear is then sutured with a single continuous layer of #0 or #1 absorbable suture material such as polydiaxanone (PDS II). This technique works best if the rectum can be exteriorized to a sufficient extent as to allow direct visualization of the entire tear.

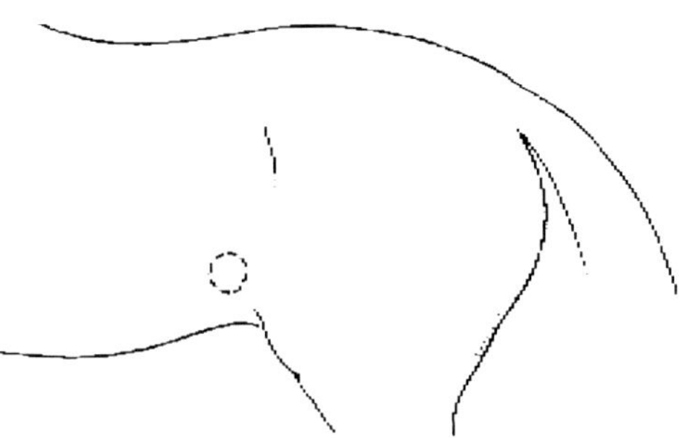

FIG. 55–6. The lower left flank is the optimum site for placement of the stoma for the end-on colostomy. (From Rick, M.C.: Management of rectal injuries. Vet. Clin. North Am., *5*:407–428, 1989.)

Temporary Diverting Colostomy

A temporary diverting colostomy, whether it be "end-on" or loop, has the advantage of diverting most or all of the feces away from the tear.[6,7,10,12,16–19] Both techniques usually require general anesthesia, because the majority of horses resent manipulation of the colon or rectum within an inflamed peritoneal cavity. If cost or medical condition of the horse precludes general anesthesia, these techniques may be performed, with difficulty, in the standing animal.

"End-on" Colostomy. An end-on colostomy can be performed through one or two incisions.[7,12,16–19] If there is minimal or no evidence of peritonitis and the surgeon believes the tear is incomplete, the entire procedure may be performed through a lower flank incision, which is used as the exit site for the small colon (Fig. 55–6). More often, a routine paralumbar flank incision is made through which the abdomen is explored. The lower flank incision is then used for the colostomy.

The section of small colon to be incorporated in the colostomy is located several feet cranial to the rectal tear. This allows for easier access to the small colon during the colostomy and, more important, will allow for the difficult reanastomosis which will follow. The caudal stump is flushed free of fecal material and is then closed in a double-row inverting pattern. The cranial segment is then oversewn or clamped, brought through the lower flank incision, and attached to the stomal site with a multiple-layered closure. After surgery, patients are placed on green pasture or given soaked alfalfa pellets with frequent administration of mineral oil. It is imperative that strict attention to diet is followed after surgery to avoid impaction at the surgical site.

Loop Colostomy. The loop colostomy is simpler to perform and only partially bypasses the distal segment of the small colon and the rectum. This may aid in prevention of distal segment atrophy, but also may pose a risk of further fecal contamination or trauma to the rectal tear. The approach utilizes a left paralumbar flank incision through which the colon loop is exteriorized.

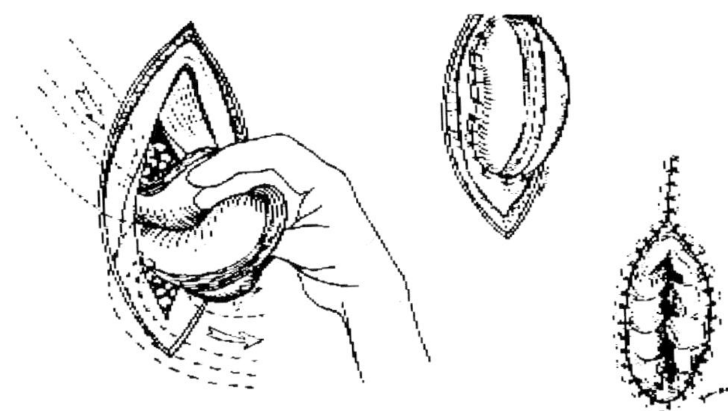

FIG. 55–7. The loop of colon is sutured to the external abdominal oblique muscle and fascia, and following incision through the antimesenteric band into the lumen of the colon, the mucosal lining is sutured to skin. (From Rick, M.C.: Management of rectal injuries. Vet. Clin. North Am., *5*:407–428, 1989.)

The colon is then placed so that the cranial segment is attached at the dorsal aspect of the incision.[10,11] An 8-cm loop of colon is sutured to the external abdominal oblique muscle and fascia and, following incision through the antimesenteric band into the colon's lumen, the mucosal lining is sutured to skin (Fig. 55–7).

Reanastomosis. The specifics of reanastomosis are beyond the scope of this chapter. Suffice it to say that reanastomosis, particularly of an end-on colostomy, is difficult. Unequal colon diameters, adhesions, and infection are just a few problems the surgeon faces. End-on colostomies are usually reanastomosed via a ventral midline approach, whereas loop colostomies are usually closed via the flank.

Suture Repair via Rectum

One-handed suture repair via rectum is often a time-consuming, tedious affair with variable results.[6,16] The horse is sedated and administered caudal epidural anesthesia. Repair is attempted with a large, curved, swaged-on needle with absorbable suture. The suture line is best started at the cranial aspect of the tear and completed in a continuous fashion. Frequently, the technique causes excessive trauma resulting in either further enlargement of the tear or inadequate closure. Adjacent folds of rectal mucosa may inadvertently be incorporated into the suture line making determination of complete closure difficult.

An expandable rectal speculum (see Fig. 55–5) has been used in standing or recumbent anesthetized horses to repair tears through the rectum.[13] This device is inserted in a closed position and, after expansion of the six-angled rods, allows excellent visualization of the tear. With specially designed long forceps and needle holders, the tear may be sutured under direct visualization as long as the tear is not close to or cranial to the rectal-colonic junction. Tears cranial to this site are difficult to access with this instrument.

Rectal Liner

Rectal liners recently have been described for the treatment of grade 3 and 4 rectal tears.[20] Through a ventral midline celiotomy, a distal segment of colon is exteriorized. The large colon is evacuated to minimize further fecal passage by the tear site. An assistant passes a plastic rectal ring and sleeve through the anus and small colon cranial to the tear. The surgeon then anchors the plastic ring to the wall of the small colon with retention sutures and oversews these sutures to infold the wall. It has been recommended that this technique be combined with partial or complete closure of the tear to minimize the lesion size and decrease the likelihood of a permanent fistula or ostomy formation. This device allows fecal material to pass the tear without further contaminating it.

POSTOPERATIVE MANAGEMENT

Horses with rectal tears, as outlined in the "medical management" section of this chapter, require aggressive and intense postoperative care. Broad-spectrum antimicrobial therapy; management of diet to maintain soft feces; treatment of ileus secondary to peritonitis; administration of heparin to minimize adhesions; anti-inflammatory/analgesic therapy to minimize peritonitis, adhesions, and signs of colic; and peritoneal lavage to lessen infection or inflammatory exudate from the abdomen are a few of the standard after-surgery treatments.

REFERENCES

1. Williams, W.: The Principles and Practice of Veterinary Medicine. New York, Wm. Wood and Co., 1883.
2. Arnold, J.S., Meagher, D.M., and Lohse, C.L.: Rectal tears in horses. J. Equine Med. Surg., *2*:55–61, 1978.
3. Fielden, E.D.: Rectal tears in horses. Paper presented at the Conference of Equine Practitioners, Auckland, New Zealand, February, 1982.
4. Stauffer, V.D.: Equine rectal tears—A malpractice problem (insurance note). J. Am. Vet. Med. Assoc., *178*:798–799, 1981.
5. Sisson, S., and Grossman, J.D.: Digestive system. *In* The Anatomy of Domestic Animals. 5th ed. Edited by R. Getty. Philadelphia, W.B. Saunders, 1975, pp. 454–497.
6. Arnold, J.S., and Meagher, D.M.: Management of rectal tears in the horse. J. Equine Med. Surg. *2*:64–71, 1978.
7. Azzie, M.A.J.: Temporary colostomy in the management of rectal tears in the horse. J. S. Afr. Vet. Assoc., *46*:121–122, 1975.
8. Lusk, N.D.: Clinical aspects of court trials. Proc. Am. Assoc. Equine Pract., 11–13, 1977.
9. Speirs, V.C., Christie, B.A., and Van Veenendaal, J.C.: The management of rectal tears in horses. Aust. Vet. J., *56*:313–317, 1980.
10. Brown, M.P.: Conditions of the rectum. *In* Equine Gas-

trointestinal Surgery: The Veterinary Clinics of North America: Large Animal Practice. Edited by C.W. McIlwraith. Philadelphia, W.B. Saunders, 1982, pp. 185–196.

11. Shires, G.M.H.: Rectal tears. *In* Current Therapy in Equine Medicine. 2nd ed. Edited by N.E. Robinson. Philadelphia, W.B. Saunders, 1987, pp. 75–79.

12. Rick, M.C.: Management of Rectal Tears. *In* Advances in Equine Abdominal Surgery: Veterinary Clinics of North America: Equine Practice. Edited by M.D. Markel and J.R. Snyder. Philadelphia, W.B. Saunders, 1989, pp. 407–423.

13. Spensley, M.S., Meagher, D.M., and Hughes, J.P.: Instrumentation to facilitate surgical repair of rectal tears in the horse: A preliminary report. Proc. Am. Assoc. Equine Pract., 553–563, 1985.

14. Slone, D.E., Homburg, J.M., Jagar, J.E., and Powers, R.D.: Noniatrogenic rectal tears in three horses. J. Am. Vet. Med. Assoc., *180:*750–751, 1982.

15. Markel, M.D.: Prevention and management of peritonitis in horses. *In* Management of Colic: The Veterinary Clinics of North America: Equine Practice. Edited by S.M. Stover. Philadelphia, W.B. Saunders, 1988, pp. 145–156.

16. Meagher, D.M.: Rectal surgery. *In* Current Practice of Equine Surgery. Edited by N.A. White and J.N. Moore. Philadelphia, J.B. Lippincott, 1990, pp. 357–365.

17. Herthel, D.J.: Colostomy in the mare. Proc. Am. Assoc. Equine Pract., 187–191, 1974.

18. McIlwraith, C.W., and Turner, A.S.: Temporary diverting colostomy for management of rectal tears. *In* Equine Surgery: Advanced Techniques. Philadelphia, Lea & Febiger, 1987, pp. 326–332.

19. Stashak, T.S., and Knight, A.P.: Temporary diverting colostomy for management of small colon tears in the horse: A case report. J. Equine Med. Surg., *2:*196–200, 1978.

20. Taylor, T.S., Watkins, J.P., and Schumacher, J.: Temporary indwelling rectal liner for use in horses with rectal tears. J. Am. Vet. Med. Assoc., *191:*677–680, 1987.

SECTION F

PREGNANCY, PARTURITION, AND THE PUERPERAL PERIOD

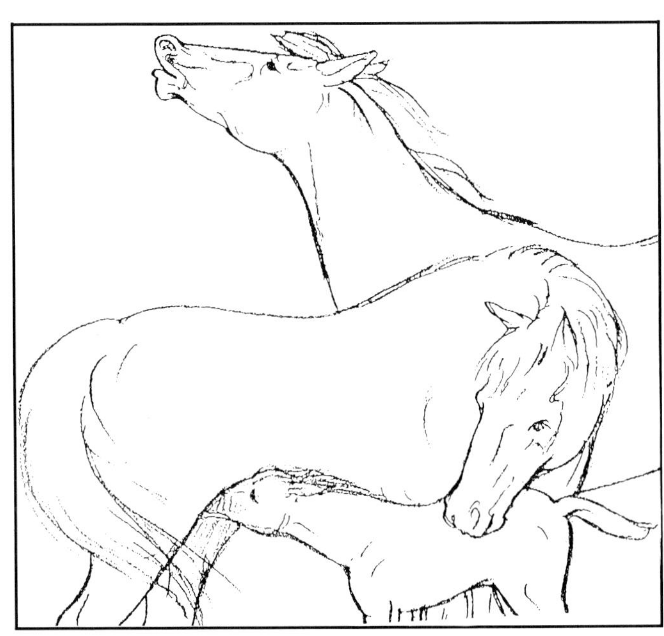

CHAPTER 56

FERTILIZATION, EARLY DEVELOPMENT, AND THE ESTABLISHMENT OF THE PLACENTA

P.F. Flood

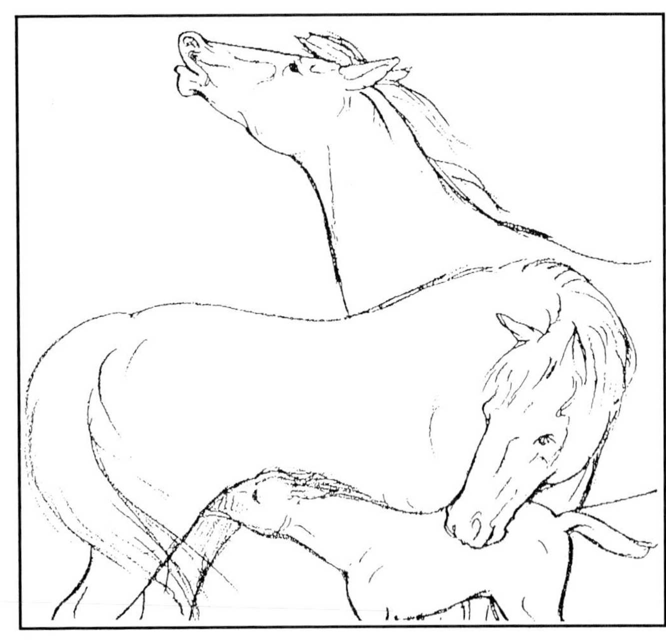

The purpose of this chapter is to describe the changes occurring between ovulation and the stage at which the placenta is fully established, though not perhaps mature—a time roughly at the end of the first third of pregnancy, when the entire uterine lining is involved in placenta formation and the microcotyledons are clearly recognizable. The chronology of these events is summarized in Table 56–1.[1-20]

THE CONCEPTUS BEFORE ATTACHMENT

The life of the unattached equine embryo can be divided into tubal and uterine phases. The tubal phase lasts 5 or 6 days, ending when the late morula or early blastocyst passes through the uterotubal junction. The uterine phase continues until the trophoblast and the uterine epithelium begin to adhere to one another around day 40. Thus the period when the conceptus lies within the uterus but is without firm attachment is extraordinarily protracted in the mare, exceeding that in any species yet described, with the exception of those showing an embryonic diapause.

EVENTS OCCURRING IN THE UTERINE TUBES

The uterine tubes of mares have attracted much attention since it was found that they usually contained several eggs, often in various stages of degeneration, regardless of the reproductive condition of the animal[20] (Fig. 56–1). This was perhaps the first intimation that the transport of mammalian eggs through the uterine tubes might be influenced by the eggs[1] viability and development: they were not mere passengers on a escalator.

Entry of the Egg into the Uterine Tube

Entry of the egg into the uterine tube of the mare has been little studied, but it is apparently an efficient process. The fact that the ovarian bursa is small and does not envelope the ovary is probably unimportant, because ovulation is restricted to the ovulation fossa and one of the frond-like extensions of the infundibular margin (one of the fimbriae) is always attached close to the point of ovulation. The equine oocyte with its "large sticky" cumulus[1] is therefore unlikely to avoid the sweeping action of the cilia lining the infundibulum. However, little of the follicular fluid seems to enter the uterine tube, because about four-fifths of it is extruded during the first 100 s of the ovulatory process and yet no large fluid accumulations can be seen in the uterine tube by echography.[21]

Some confusion still surrounds the exact state of the oocyte at the time of ovulation. Completion of the first meiotic division with extrusion of the first polar body possibly occurs close to the time of ovulation, because oocytes with a polar body have been recovered from gonadotrophin-stimulated large follicles,[1,22] and ova lacking a polar body have been reported in the uterine

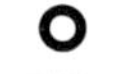
-position of ova

-tubal musculature and mesosalpinx

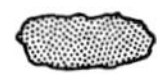
-"gelatinous" material

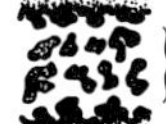
-tubal lumen

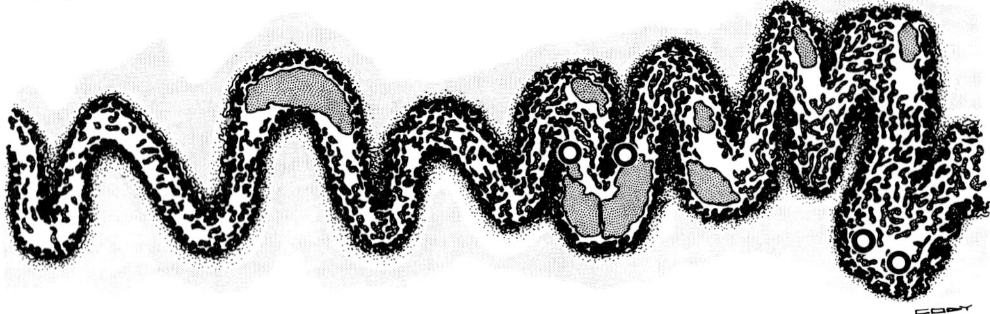

FIG. 56–1. A composite diagram made from several histologic sections of the middle third of an equine oviduct. The ampulla is to the right and the isthmus to the left. The fine stippling indicates related areas of the mesosalpinx. The coarse stippling with a heavy outline indicates gelatinous masses lying in the lumen. The positions but not the sizes of the retained eggs are shown by the black circles. (From Flood, P.F., Jong, A., and Betteridge, K.J.: The location of eggs retained in the oviducts of mares. J. Reprod. Fertil., *57:*291–294, 1979.)

tubes.[1,23] Nonetheless after reviewing the earlier literature and their own data, King et al. concluded that in the horse, as in most other mammals, the ovulating oocyte is normally in metaphase of the second meiotic division.[24]

Fertilization

Fertilization occurs in the ampulla of the uterine tubes. Its timing is such that embryos have developed to the two-cell stage by about 24 h after ovulation if ovulation is preceded by insemination; then capacitated spermatozoa are presumed to be present in the ampulla when the egg arrives there.[1,2] If, on the other hand, ovulation is succeeded by mating, events are delayed because of the time required for spermatozoal migration and capacitation; then the ova are still in the pronuclear stage 17 to 21 h postcoitum.[25] Under the later conditions, two activated ova were recovered 10 and 14 h postcoitum, and both were in telophase of the second meiotic division; the fertilizing sperm heads were found in slight protrusions of the cell surface and although their nuclei had expanded, no nuclear envelope was present. The pronuclei, when formed, are eccentric rather than central in position within the egg, and each pronuclear envelope is ruffled on the side that faces the other pronucleus.[25]

Following activation of the egg by the fertilizing spermatozoon, the cortical granules are reduced in number or disappear,[25,26] and the inner part of the zona seems to be rendered resistant to further sperm penetration. This is indicated by the frequency with which trapped spermatozoa are found in the outer half of the zona and the relative rarity of supernumerary spermatozoa within the perivitelline space.[2,3,25]

Cleavage

After reaching the two-cell stage about 24 h after ovulation, division of the blastomeres continues in a regular manner so that there are four to six cells at 48 h and eight to ten cells at 72 h.[1–3,27] During early cleavage, normal equine embryos have quite large amounts of cellular debris in the perivitelline space,[1–3,26] and they are often ellipsoidal in shape.[3,23] By 4 or 5 days after ovulation a morula is formed which rapidly undergoes compaction.[3]

Tubal Transport

Several eggs, in various stages of degeneration can usually be found in the oviducts of either cyclic, pregnant, or anestrous mares.[20,28–32] Furthermore, van Niekerk and Gernike's contention that the eggs accumulate from successive normal ovulations, and that only the fertilized eggs are reliably transported into the uterus,[20] is now widely accepted. It is supported by the finding of spermatozoa in the zonae of degenerate eggs recovered from the uterine tubes of mares 30 and 58 days after isolated matings[33] and by the remarkable correspondence between the known ovulatory history of pony mares and the number of eggs that can be flushed from their oviducts.[34] An alternative hypothesis, that the eggs are derived from the rupture of small "extra" follicles situated near the ovulation fossa, has also been advanced.[31]

TABLE 56–1. A CHRONOLOGY OF EVENTS DURING EARLY PREGNANCY IN THE MARE

EVENT	TIME AFTER OVULATION	SOURCE
Two-cell stage reached	24 h	1, 2
Morula formed	4–5 days	3
Blastocyst formed	5–6 days	4–8
Embryo enters uterus	5–6 days	4–8
Zona shed	7 days	3, 9
Blood islands form	14 days	10
Fixation	15–16 days (variable)	11, 12
Active vitelline circulation present	22 days	10
Amnion completed	21 days	13
Allantoic bud formed	21 days	10, 14
Capsule ruptures	22 days (limited data)	13
Allantochorion established	25 days	10
Chorionic girdle cells migrate	36 days	13, 15
Placentation involves the uterine body	56 days	16, 17
Primary chorionic villi well established	61 days	18
Uterus is fully occupied	77 days	16, 17
Microcotyledons are clearly defined	100 days	18
Endometrial cups regress	120 days (variable)	19

Fertilized eggs can pass unfertilized eggs lodged in the uterine tubes[34] but the mechanism remains mysterious. The number of old eggs in the tubes seems to be slightly reduced by mating,[28] but the effect is not confined to the side on which ovulation has occurred. Transport of the fertilized egg is not attributable to the presence of the corpus luteum in the ipsilateral ovary, but development beyond the first two or three cleavage divisions is required.[27,35]

Although it is tempting to hypothesize that differential egg transport in the mare is caused by changes in surface characteristics of the egg, transmission electron microscopy has failed to reveal any clear differences in the surface of the zonae pellucidae of fertilized and unfertilized eggs of a similar age. Nonetheless, after prolonged retention in the tubes, the zona acquires a smooth external surface[36] and a more homogeneous internal structure.[35]

The site of retention of unfertilized eggs is the middle third of the uterine tube,[28,30] and histologic examination of this region showed degenerate eggs lying free in the lumen without any special relationship with the endosalpinx (Fig. 56–1).[37] Often this part of the tubal lumen also contains irregular masses of collagenous material[30,37] that may contain proliferating cells akin to fibroblasts[37] or even, in one case examined 5.5 days after mating, compressed degenerating spermatozoa (Flood and Betteridge, personal observations). Such an accumulation of detritus suggests a general tendency for this part of the equine tube to retain materials that enter it. Even so, the isthmus of the tube does sometimes permit the passage of inert materials, because both degenerate eggs and irregular masses have been recovered from the uterus.[38,39]

The problem of differential tubal transport in the mare has recently been reanalyzed by Hunter, who proposed that unfertilized eggs become misshapen during their relatively long "normal" sojourn in the uterine tube and that this deformation may account for their retention.[40] While it is true that many retained eggs are grossly distorted, the critical evidence that unfertilized eggs are already misshapen by 5 days after ovulation is apparently still lacking. On occasion, as indicated above, old distorted eggs can enter the uterus.[38,39]

The possibility remains that the developing horse egg is master of its own fate and that its endocrine or metabolic products cause local changes in the tubal cilia or musculature that facilitate its progress toward the uterus. Similarly, changes in its charge, elasticity, or adhesiveness may exist that have a similar effect. In other species, fertilized and unfertilized eggs also behave differently in the uterine tubes. In the long-tongued bat, unfertilized ova degenerate without ever reaching the uterus but in this animal the fertilized embryo does not enter the uterus directly either: it implants at the uterotubal junction.[41] Fertilized eggs progress more rapidly through the uterine tubes of hamsters than do unfertilized ones,[42] and in rats, advanced embryos pass through the oviduct more rapidly than those that are less mature.[43]

Contraction of the mare's myosalpinx can be elicited by exogenous prostaglandin $F_2\alpha$, epinephrine, norepinephrine, or oxytocin,[44] and passage of a cannula through the cervix on day 3 or 4 seems to hasten transport of the fertile egg in some mares leading to the egg's arrival in the uterus on day 5.[45,46] Though, in these circumstances, it seemed likely that more rapid egg transport was associated with prostaglandin release, attempts to mimic the effect with exogenous prostaglandin were unsuccessful.[47] One product of the early embryo that might influence tubal transport is platelet-activating factor,[48] but more recent evidence implicates prostaglandin E_2 (PGE_2) in the mare. Infusion of PGE_2 into the uterine tube hastens egg transport, PGE_2 is produced by the egg at the appropriate time, and the uterine tube possesses PGE_2 receptors.[49,50]

Egg Coverings in Tubal Stages

At the time of ovulation the oocyte is enclosed by a bilaminar[51] or perhaps trilaminar[25] zona pellucida, which usually has a further gelatinous layer, or gel coat, on its outer surface. The gel coat is soon lost, particularly if the egg is fertilized, but may be replaced by a thin, smooth, outer layer late in the tubal period of development.[9,23,36]

THE UNATTACHED CONCEPTUS IN THE UTERUS

Embryo Coverings

Embryos recovered from the uterus on day 6 are either at the morula or early blastocyst stage and are surrounded by the zona pellucida with, perhaps, its additional smooth outer coat.[4–8] Such embryos soon embark on a period of rapid growth when the relative daily rate of increase in volume will be greater than at any other stage[3] (Figs. 56–2 and 56–3). From the beginning of blastocyst formation, this expansion is accompanied by the deposition of a novel, rather irregular, electron-dense layer on the inside of the zona pellucida.[9] During the first 48 h of intrauterine life, the new layer becomes thicker and more organized, and the attenuated zona is shed leaving the embryo encased only in the new covering, the capsule.[9] Though the capsule was clearly described in the nineteenth century,[52] it was later either ignored or misidentified.[53] Its serendipitous rediscovery[16] in the early 1970s rekindled interest, and by 1989, just 100 years after the original description, sufficient data had been accumulated to warrant an erudite and detailed review.[51]

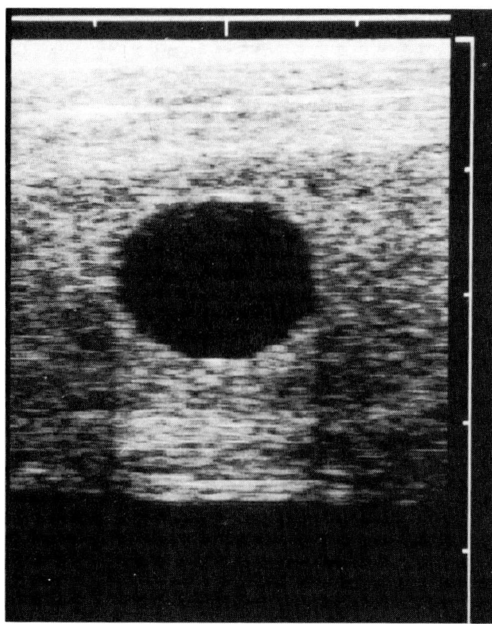

FIG. 56–3. A 13-mm diameter embryo in the uterus of a mare that had ovulated 14 days before examination. (Aloka DS-210 instrument with a 7.5-MHz intrarectal transducer.)

When fully developed, the equine embryonic capsule is about 4 μm thick and forms a spherical, resilient, glistening envelope around the cellular components of the embryo (Fig. 56–4). It is permeable to proteins with a molecular weight of 200,000 but hampers the diffusion of ferritin (450,000).[54] The capsule matrix is composed of a glycoprotein that can be readily distinguished from that of the zona pellucida by both its physicochemical and immunologic properties.[55] It does not appear to contain collagen and is remarkably resistant to a number of solubilizing agents and some proteases.[56] The origin of the capsular material is still obscure, but its quantity alone makes it seem most unlikely that it is entirely synthesized by the conceptus. An endometrial precursor is more probably precipitated by a trophoblastic enzyme or binding agent. This view is supported by two further observations: capsules do not form around equine demiembryos that have been deprived of their original coverings when they develop in vitro, although they do form in vivo,[5] and anticapsule antibodies no longer bind to the capsular matrix after they have been absorbed with uterine secretions.[55]

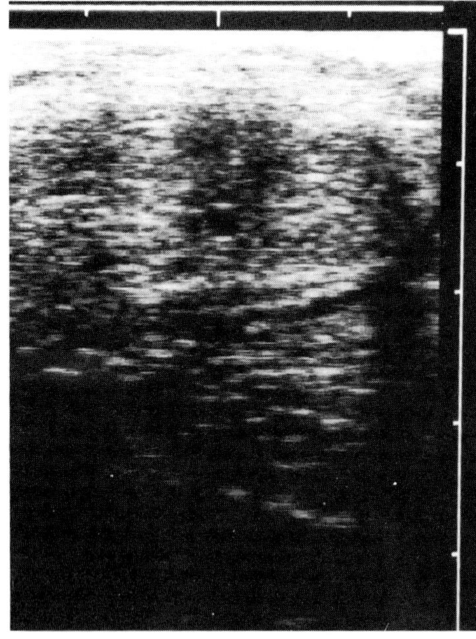

FIG. 56–2. A 2-mm diameter embryo in the uterus of a mare that had had twin ovulations 8 and 9 days before examination. (Aloka DS-210 instrument with a 7.5-MHz intrarectal transducer.)

The function of the capsule has not been demonstrated experimentally, but it probably provides the embryo with mechanical protection and support during the period of intrauterine migration; it may also give protection against intrauterine micro-organisms, because additional capsular material is deposited in response to a microbial threat.[57] The two common mammalian species known to have a capsule (or tertiary embryonic membrane) are the horse and the rabbit. Both have a postpartum estrus, and hence in both there is a possibility that the embryo will arrive in a poorly involuted and contaminated uterus. Perhaps the capsule also protects against potentially hostile maternal leucocytes and antibodies. It is interesting that loss of the capsule roughly coincides with completion of the amnion, an event occurring at about day 20.[13] Thus the embryo proper (as opposed to the embryonic membranes) is never exposed to the uterine lumen.

Unfortunately, information on the time of rupture of the capsule is somewhat sketchy and depends on only a few observations. Enders and Liu and I noted that two embryos examined on day 20 were still encapsulated

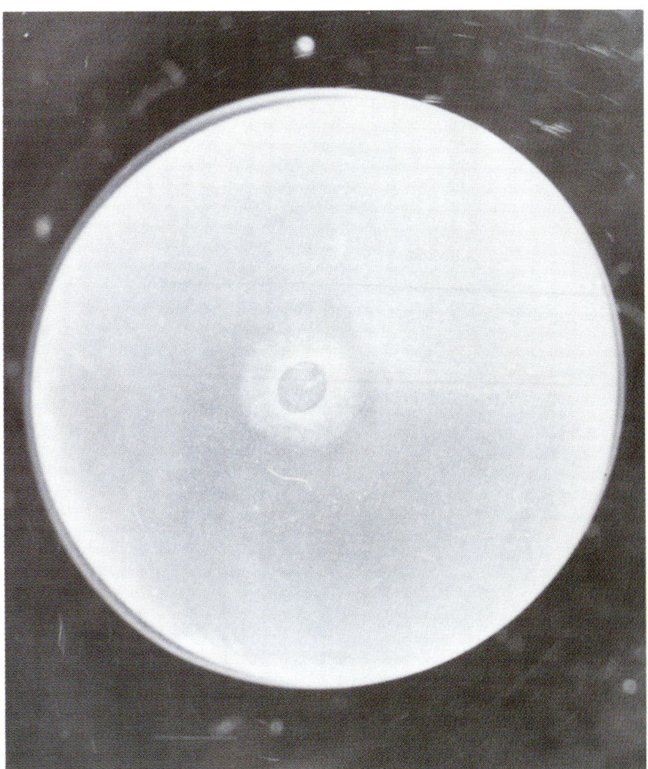

FIG. 56–4. A day-13 embryo that is 16 mm in diameter. The capsule is clearly visible where it is separated from the trophoblast by a fluid-filled space. The embryonic disc is central in position and roughly elliptical in shape with axes of 1.24 and 1.6 mm. About half of the long axis of the embryonic disc is occupied by the primitive streak. The halo surrounding the disc is created by the developing extraembryonic mesoderm.

(Fig. 56–5), but the capsule had been largely displaced from an adjacent pair of twin embryos on day 22.[13] The shed (or, because it is elastic, recoiled) capsular material disappears from the uterus rather slowly and fragments of it can be found in uterine flushings as late as day 28[58] and can be detected histologically until day 36.[13] In one case, the capsule was found intact a week after the death of an embryo at about day 13 of development.[59]

Migration

There is a strong tendency for horse embryos to attach in alternate uterine horns in successive breeding seasons,[60,61] but no correlation between the side of ovulation and the side of final attachment has been found.[62] This implies a remarkable degree of embryonic mobility, which has now been amply confirmed by transrectal echography.[11,63] The horse conceptus wanders throughout the uterus from at least the time it can first be detected by echography until day 15. Movement is maximal between days 11 and 14. On one occasion, an embryo was observed to pass from the caudal part of the left horn to its tip, back to the body, to the tip of the right horn, and back to the caudal part of the right horn during a single 2-h observation period.[11,63]

The function of these peregrinations would seem to be related to maternal recognition of pregnancy because an embryo that is denied access to the entire endometrium is likely to perish because of luteal insufficiency.[64] The migration of the horse conceptus, therefore, seems to have an analogous function to formation of the filamentous blastocyst in artiodactyls: it ensures that all parts of the endometrium receive the maternal recognition signal.

Pharmacologic inhibition of uterine contraction impairs embryonic mobility indicating that the myometrium is primarily responsible. However, artificial embryos do not move as much as authentic ones, suggesting the latter may stimulate the myometrium.[11] One embryonic product that might be expected to be involved is estradiol but exogenous estradiol failed to influence migration,[65] perhaps because local application is required or because stimulation was already maximal.

Fixation

The conceptus has normally become "fixed" or ceased to migrate by day 15 in ponies or day 16 in horses and adopts a position in the bend in the uterus at the caudal end of either the right or left horn.[11,12] Here it lies at the antimesometrial side of the uterine lumen and occupies an ellipsoidal nidation chamber with a craniocaudally directed long-axis.[13]

The reason the embryo always comes to rest at the caudal end of one of the horns is not clear. The endo-

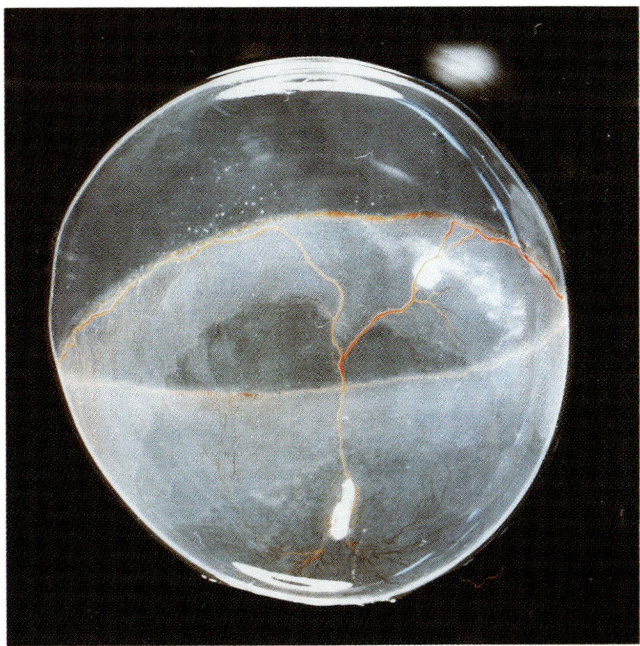

FIG. 56–5. A day-20 embryo measuring 66 by 58 mm. Careful inspection reveals the capsule is still present. The yolk sac vessels are well developed and the sinus terminalis is clearly visible. The sinus terminalis marks the boundary of a cloudy band that extends from the sinus toward the embryonic pole. The caudal end of the embryo shows some expansion, which may be caused by the allantoic primordium.

metrium at the fixation point is not obviously different from that elsewhere. However, the uterus does receive a large branch of the uterine artery at this point,[13] it is a point at which the uterus bends, and it would be the most ventral part of the organ if the uterus could hang freely without interference from the other viscera. Perhaps the bend and the ventral location progressively impede motion as the embryo enlarges. The increase in myometrial tone during pregnancy would seem to favor fixation, and perhaps local differences in tone also occur.[11,13] Steroid hormones may play a role in fixation, which does not seem to occur in the absence of progesterone. Whether this is a direct effect or a reflection of impending embryonic death is not clear.[66] Exogenous estradiol, on the other hand, may advance the time of fixation somewhat.[65]

Orientation

In most mammals, the conceptus becomes orientated in a consistent fashion in relation to the mesometrium: the mare is no exception and both ultrasonographic and conventional anatomic studies show that the embryonic disc is found on the antimesometrial side.[11,13] The time at which the embryo achieves its definitive orientation is not known but it probably occurs shortly after fixation.[11] An embryo examined on day 18 was apparently already orientated.[13] How orientation occurs is a matter of speculation; perhaps the embryonic pole is less flexible than the remainder of the blastocyst and the asymmetry of the uterine lumen is such that this part of the embryo comes to lie antimesometrially where the curvature is least acute.[11]

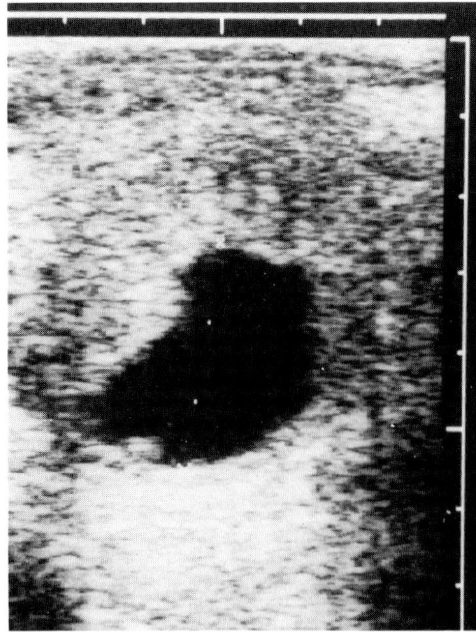

FIG. 56–6. A 29-mm diameter conceptus in the uterus of a mare that was last mated 23 days before examination. The embryo proper is visible in the bottom left of the conceptus. The regular outline of the conceptus has been lost perhaps, in part, because of rupture of the capsule. (Aloka DS-210 instrument with a 5-MHz intrarectal transducer.)

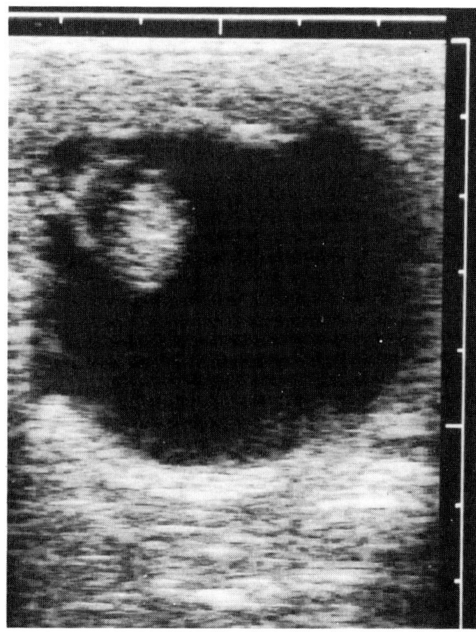

FIG. 56–7. A day 38-conceptus. The development of the allantois has pushed the embryo proper toward the mesometrial side of the uterus but the development of the umbilical cord is just beginning to allow it to move in an antimesometrial direction once again. (Aloka DS-210 instrument with a 5-MHz intrarectal transducer.)

The consistency of the initial orientation of the embryo ensures that when the major fluid-filled cavities of the conceptus—the yolk sac, amnion, and allantois—are formed, they too have a consistent relationship with the uterus. Because the embryonic disc is antimesometrial, it follows that the yolk sac is mesometrial and the amnion antimesometrial. For the same reason, the embryo proper (within the amnion) is first detected by ultrasonography in an antimesometrial position (Fig. 56–6). When, during the fourth week of pregnancy, the allantois begins to grow rapidly, it is obliged to occupy the antimesometrial side of the uterine lumen because the mesometrial angle is already filled by the yolk sac. As allantoic fluid accumulates, it moves the embryo mesometrially and it comes to lie close to the attachment of the broad ligament (Fig. 56–7). It is only with the eventual obliteration of the yolk sac and the formation of the umbilical cord that the fetus—as it may now be called—will descend once more. Detailed reviews of these events have been provided by Ginther[11,67] and van Niekerk and Allen.[10]

DIRECT CELLULAR INTERACTIONS BETWEEN THE TROPHOBLAST AND THE ENDOMETRIUM

Direct cellular interactions between the conceptus and the endometrium are obviously impossible before the retraction of the capsule. Shortly after this event at least two types of trophoblast become recognizable: the transparent placental trophoblast covering the majority of the conceptus and the specialized milky colored band that encircles the vitelline pole of the conceptus (Fig. 56–8). The latter is known as the chorionic girdle,[68] and it consists of invasive cells.[15]

FORMATION OF THE ENDOMETRIAL CUPS

The endometrial cups are distinctive, irregular, pallid plaques, usually about 2 cm across, that form a discontinuous ring centered on a point at the mesometrial side of the uterus at the caudal end of one horn. Because of the original orientation of the conceptus and the relationship of the chorionic girdle to the allantoic stalk, the umbilical cord always arises from the middle of the ring of cups.[67] The cups consist of colonies of trophoblast cells (Fig. 56–9) derived from the chorionic girdle and produce equine chorionic gonadotropin.[69]

The Chorionic Girdle

The chorionic girdle becomes visible to the unaided eye during week 4 of gestation and reaches maturity by day 35.[15] At this time it is a belt 6 to 8 mm wide that surrounds the conceptus at the level of the boundary between the areas of chorion supplied by the allantoic and vitelline circulations. Its translucent appearance contrasts sharply with the transparency of the remainder of the chorion. It consists of a stratified columnar epithelium with numerous mitoses.[13]

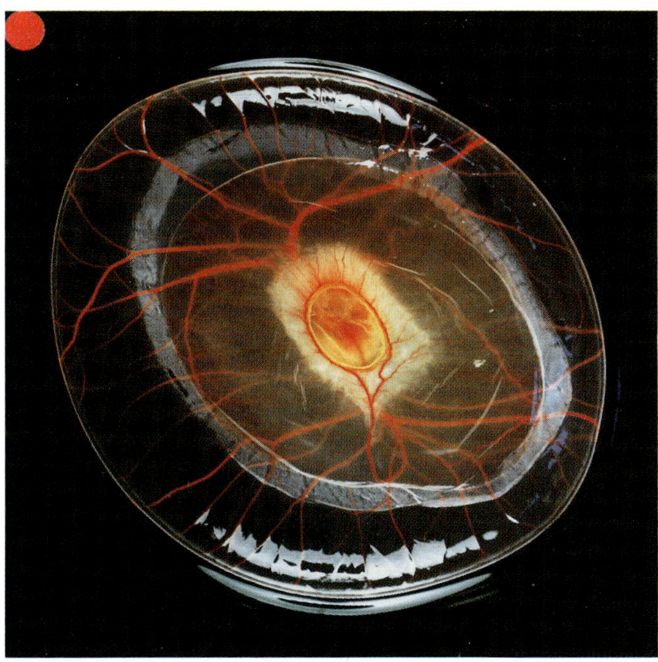

FIG. 56–8. A day-34 conceptus seen from the mesometrial pole. It was about 80 mm in diameter when lying on a flat surface but it probably had a slightly smaller diameter in utero where it adopted a more perfect sphere. The sinus terminalis is still visible as a loop surrounding an oval area of bilaminar omphalopleure at the center. Outside the sinus terminalis is a cream-colored zone that is probably associated with the trilaminar omphalopleure. The entire yolk sac is encircled by the pale chorionic girdle that lies about midway between the embryonic pole and the equator of the conceptus.

Invasion

By day 36 or 37, many of the trophoblast cells of the girdle, which are binucleate at this stage (F.B.P. Wooding, personal communication), have emigrated from the chorion, penetrated and then destroyed the adjacent uterine epithlium, and established themselves in the endometrial stroma.[15] Yet this would seem to be an imperfect process, because only irregular patches of the girdle cells cross to the maternal side;[13] perhaps these are the patches in particularly close contact with the endometrial folds and perhaps the irregularity of the migration process accounts for the irregular appearance of the cups themselves. Those girdle cells that fail to reach the endometrial stroma die and are replaced by a simple epithelial layer.[13]

The Established Endometrial Cups

The established trophoblast cells of the endometrial cups are epithelioid and very large (Fig. 56–9). They occupy much of the endometrial stroma, but they do not greatly damage the uterine glands. Dilated glands are often found, however, suggesting that their ducts are occluded to some degree. Almost as soon as the trophoblast cells enter the uterine connective tissue, the colonies they form are surrounded by a wall of lymphocytes. It also happens that the equine endometrium, including the region of the endometrial cups, is unusually well supplied with lymphatic vessels when compared with other species. It is not clear that these phenomena are connected, but it is likely that the vessels provide an important link in the efferent immune pathways that lead to the immunologic recognition of the trophoblast cells (see below).[13]

The Fate of the Cup Tissue

The endometrial cups persist for a variable period, but they have usually disappeared completely by day 130.[19] The mechanism of their demise has been the subject of much interest. Shortly after invasion of the uterus by the girdle cells, paternally directed cytotoxic antibodies appear in the maternal blood. No such antibodies are present in males, in maiden mares, or in pregnant females of other species.[70] Sixty to eighty days later, endometrial cups are invaded by leukocytes, although before this time most white cells are detained at the periphery of the colony of trophoblast cells. The cups then become necrotic and are sloughed from the endometrial surface. In some cases the sloughed debris forms the core of the allantoic pouches that frequently project into the allantoic cavity.[19]

The leukocytic response to the invading trophoblast is more severe and sloughing is hastened in mares mated

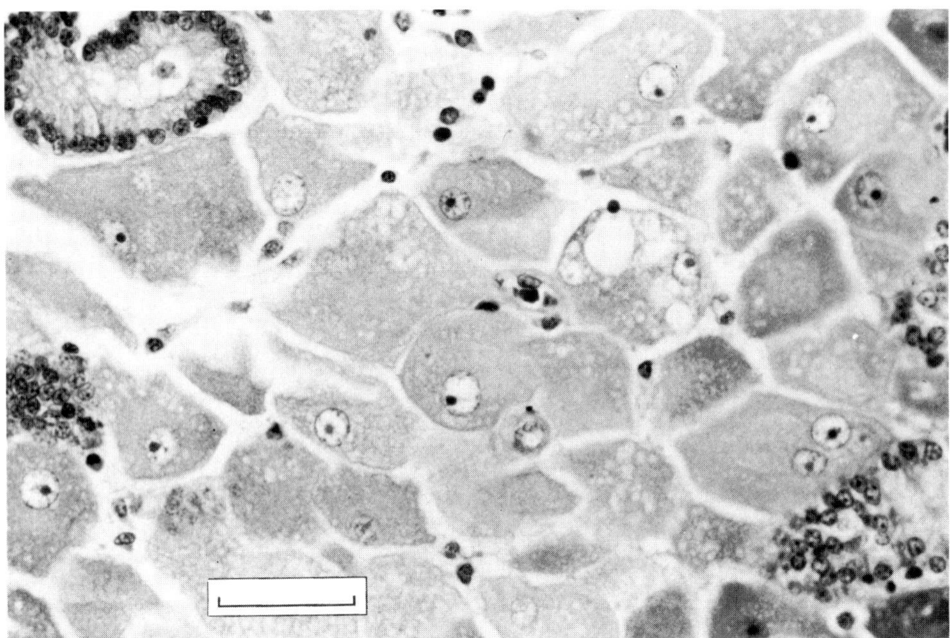

FIG. 56–9. Endometrial cup cells during month 4 of pregnancy. The center of the field shows several large epithelioid cells that are of trophoblastic origin. Occasional lymphocytes are visible between the trophoblast cells. Parts of several uterine glands are present around the edges. Stained with hematoxylin and eosin. Scale bar = 50 μm.

to donkeys,[70] but the endometrial cups apparently survive much longer than normal in mares carrying foals sired by their own cotwin.[71] The death of the cup cells therefore appear to have an immunologic component, and they are the only known placental tissue destroyed in this way. Meanwhile the placental trophoblast (to be discussed next) is entirely unaffected. The factors controlling the timing of cup cell rejection remain unexplained; certainly, a simple skin allograft would be rejected much more quickly. The cup cells probably produce steroids which might confer some protection,[72,73] and although the young, invading endometrial cup cells are unusually rich in major histocompatibility complex antigens, these antigens seem to be lost with time, which might also help to prolong the life of the cells.

FORMATION OF THE PLACENTA

Two critical features of any placenta are its vascular supply and the histologic relationship between the maternal and fetal tissues. In the horse, both present unusual and interesting features.

The Embryonic Blood Supply to the Placenta

The equine yolk sac circulation is remarkably well developed when compared with other ungulates. It first appears as a few islands of erythropoietic tissue in the extraembryonic mesoderm on day 14 and an active vitelline circulation is present on day 22 and possibly before[10] (Fig. 56–6). During week 4 of embryonic life, the yolk sac circulation remains predominant, but thereafter it is overwhelmed by the burgeoning allantois. Nonetheless it continues to appear active and retains a small area of contact with the endometrium until day 60 at least.[67] The equine yolk sac has been shown to have a steroidogenic function,[73] as well as the expected hemopoietic, absorptive, and excretory roles. Between days 25 and 32 the trophoblast overlying the yolk sac placenta becomes columnar especially in the region of the sinus terminalis (Figs. 56–5 and 56–8) forming the sinus terminalis complex.[13]

The allantois is not discernible until day 20 or 21[10,14] but then grows quickly to provide the dominant blood supply to the chorion 10 days later (Fig. 56–10). The fused allantois and chorion (the allantochorion) then attaches to the endometrium to form the definitive placenta.

Expansion of the Conceptus

The equine conceptus is more or less globular until the end of week 5 and is roughly ellipsoidal for some time thereafter.[10,16,67,74] Thus colonization of the uterus beyond the nidation chamber is relatively slow; however, the body of the uterus is occupied by fetal membranes on day 56, and the entire endometrial surface is involved in placenta formation by day 77.[16,17] Once a new area of the endometrium is invaded, it seems that placental development progresses fairly rapidly because the entire external surface of the allantochorion appears equally developed.

One unusual feature of the fetal membranes of the horse is the complete separation of the allantochorion and amnion by the expanding allantoic cavity. As a

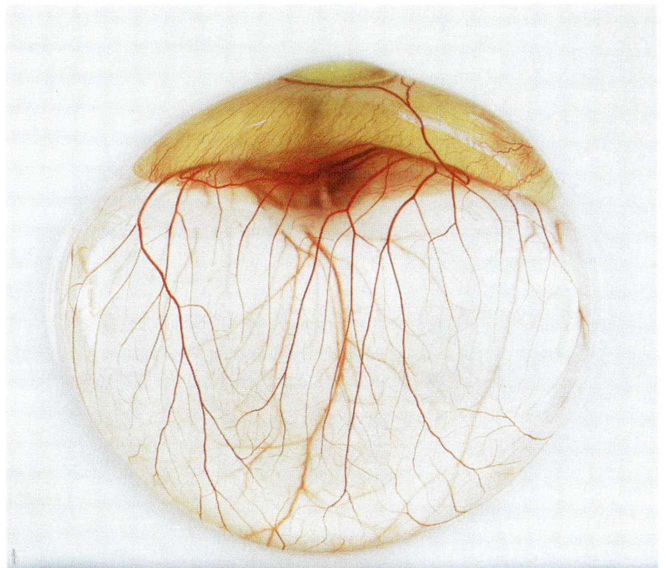

FIG. 56–10. The same conceptus as that shown in Figure 56–8. Lateral view. The mesometrial side is at the top. The sinus terminalis and the other delicate yolk sac vessels can be seen at the mesometrial pole which is readily recognizable by the yellowish yolk sac fluid. The more open allantoic vascular network is visible over the remainder of the surface. The chorionic girdle is just discernible immediately below the junction of the yolk sac and allantois. The embryo proper can be seen lying between the yolk sac and the allantoic cavity. Its outlines are indistinct, but the left forelimb bud can be seen clearly projecting toward the camera.

consequence, the umbilical cord is distinctly divided into allantoic and amniotic parts.

Villi and Microcotyledons

At first glance, the exterior of the established equine allantochorion appears to be remarkably uniform, with the exception of those areas that lie adjacent to the cervix and the endometrial cups, and do not take part in normal placental exchange, remaining pale and poorly vascularized. Yet on close examination the exposed chorionic surface is seen to be divided into thousands of polygonal areas 1 or 2 mm across. These are the microcotyledons. Each consists of a short thick central stem with secondary and even tertiary branches. In the intact placenta, they lie in complementary and equally elaborate invaginations of the endometrium. The endometrial glands, which are simple tubes, are numerous and open between the microcotyledons.

Formation of the Microcotyledons

From day 25 onward, the endometrial capillaries are dilated around the nidation chamber and the trophoblast and the uterine epithelium are closely aligned.[13] Even so there is no obvious attachment between the embryonic and maternal epithelia as late as day 35 but by day 40 the "conceptus pours hesitantly from the incised uterus."[67]

The primary villi that ultimately form the microcotyledons have been reported in a rudimentary form by day 40 in fresh specimens,[72] though their presence could not be confirmed in a day-42 perfusion-fixed preparation.[13] While there may be some variation in the time of appearance of the first villi, they are clearly present by day 61.[18] By this stage too, the fetal and maternal epithelia are attached to one another by a dense interlocking carpet of microvilli.[18] By day 100 the primary villi have developed branches, and later, the fusion of adjacent groups of villi leads to the formation of the definitive globular microcotyledons characteristic of the latter half of pregnancy.[18]

Maturation of the Interhemal Membrane

The interhemal membrane is the membrane separating the maternal and fetal circulations. Initially it is composed of the classic six cell layers and the basement membranes associated with them. These are the maternal and fetal endothelia, maternal and fetal connective tissue, uterine epithelium, trophoblast, and a total of four basement membranes (Fig. 56–11). This kind of structure was once viewed as a primitive arrangement and was assumed to have limited efficiency. This view seems intuitively unreasonable considering the vigor of the new-born foal and is belied by physiologic[75] and anatomic data.[76]

Detailed examination reveals that the equine placenta is exquisitely organized to promote efficient exchange of gases and electrolytes between maternal and fetal circulations. The thickness of the interhemal membrane is progressively reduced beginning as early as the eighth week of gestation.[13] This is achieved by the formation of ever-deepening grooves in the inner surface of the trophoblast for accommodation of the fetal capillaries and progressive thinning of the uterine epithelium; a process accompanied by almost complete elimination of fetal connective tissue. Eventually the distance between the two circulations is reduced to about one-third of the original.[77]

The arrangement of blood vessels within the placenta also enhances exchange. The oxygen-rich uterine arteries enter the placenta close to its fetal aspect and the uterine veins leave from the maternal side,[78] allowing the capillaries entering the umbilical veins to equilibrate with the most highly oxygenated maternal blood before leaving the microcotyledon. Thus, the oxygen tension in the umbilical vein can exceed that in the uterine vein under experimental conditions.[75]

The Arcade System and Histotrophic Nutrition

While the microcotyledons are apparently specialized for rapid interchange of small molecules, the areas between the microcotyledons are involved in histotrophic nutrition of the fetus. Here the trophoblast and the uterine epithelium are separated by the secretion of the endometrial glands, and the trophoblast has a tall columnar structure that is obviously absorptive.[79] The space receiving the secretion (Fig. 56–12) forms a continuous

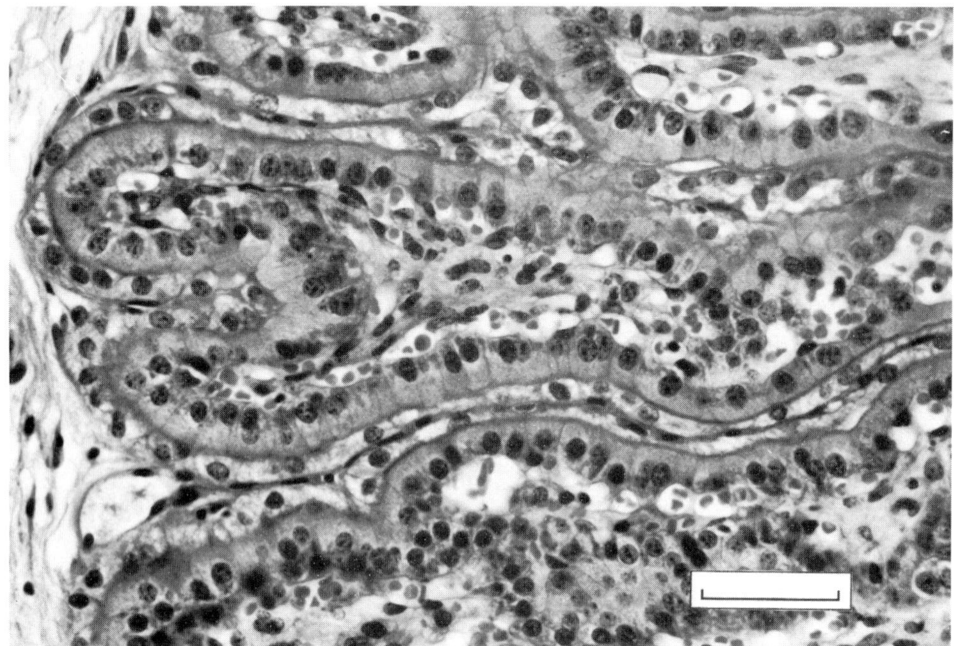

FIG. 56–11. Part of a microcotyledon of a mare destroyed on day 122 of pregnancy. The maternal side of the placenta is toward the left and the fetal side toward the right. Most of the field is occupied by a single trophoblastic villus and parts of neighboring villi. The central villus is delimited by a layer of columnar trophoblast which is directly apposed to the cuboidal maternal epithelium. On the fetal side there are numerous subepithelial capillaries that are just beginning to indent the basal surface of the trophoblast. The maternal capillaries are mainly empty and are less easy to identify. Fixed in Helly's fluid and stained with hematoxylin and eosin. Scale bar = 50 μm.

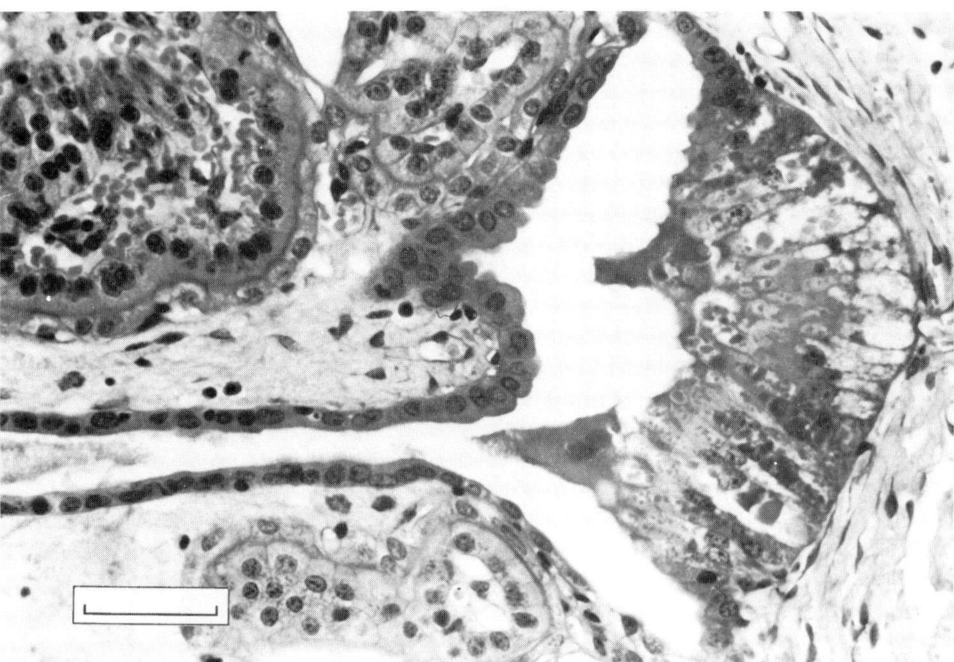

FIG. 56–12. Part of the histotrophic arcade system of a mare destroyed on day 122 of pregnancy. The maternal side of the placenta is toward the left and the fetal side toward the right. The duct of an endometrial gland can be seen entering from the left and opening into the arcade cavity close to the mouth of a neighboring, tangentially sectioned gland (above it in this illustration). The glandular and uterine epithelia are roughly cuboidal, but the histotrophic trophoblast has an exceptionally high columnar form with numerous cytoplasmic inclusions. The large empty cavity of the arcade is an artifact caused by tissue shrinkage. Part of an adjacent microcotyledon can be seen in the upper left. Fixed in Helly's fluid and stained with hematoxylin and eosin. Scale bar = 50 μm.

meshwork of channels that surround the microcotyledons and extends throughout the placenta. These structures, which are homologous with the areolae of other species,[80] are referred to as arcades.[65] The uterine glands themselves are normally found in groups of four and they are active throughout pregnancy.[79]

ACKNOWLEDGMENTS

I would like to dedicate this chapter to the late Arthur Marrable who taught embryology to so many at the University of Bristol and elsewhere. Arthur was the first to show me a real equine embryo and I shall always be in his debt. It is with no little poignancy now that I recall my feeling of astonishment when Arthur and I first examined, under a phase-contrast microscope, the structure that has come to be known as the capsule. Out of natural reticence Arthur avoided giving the extraordinary object a name but referred to the embryo as being "encapsulated." That which encapsulates soon becomes a "capsule."

I am most grateful to Drs. B.D. Murphy and R.A. Pierson for their most helpful criticism of the manuscript and to Dr. R.J. Bell for making the sonograms.

REFERENCES

1. Webel, S.K., Franklin, V., Harland, B., and Dzuik, P.J.: Fertility, ovulation and maturation of eggs of mares injected with hCG. J. Reprod. Fertil., *51:*337–341, 1977.
2. Bezard, J., Magistrini, M., Duchamp, G., and Palmer, E.: Chronology of equine fertilisation and embryonic development in vivo and in vitro. Equine Vet. J. Suppl., *8:* 105–110, 1989.
3. Betteridge, K.J., et al.: Development of horse embryos up to twenty-two days after ovulation: Observations on fresh specimens. J. Anat., *135:*191–209, 1982.
4. Oguri, N., and Tsutsumi, Y.: Non-surgical egg transfer in mares, J. Reprod. Fertil., *41:*313–320, 1974.
5. McKinnon, A.O., et al.: Bisection of equine embryos. Equine Vet. J. Suppl., *8:*129–133, 1989.
6. Skidmore, J., Boyle, M.S., Cran, D., and Allen, W.R.: Micromanipulation of equine embryos to produce monozygotic twins. Equine Vet. J. Suppl., *8:*126–128, 1989.
7. Müller, Z., and Cikryt, P.: A simple method for bisecting horse embryos. Equine Vet. J. Suppl., *8:*123–125, 1989.
8. Weimer, K.E., Casey, P.L., Mitchell, P.S., and Godke, R.A.: Pregnancies following 24-hour co-culture of equine embryos on foetal bovine uterine monolayer cells. Equine Vet. J. Suppl., Dtsch. *8:*117–122, 1989.
9. Flood, P.F., Betteridge, K.J., and Diocee, M.S.: Transmission electron microscopy of horse embryos 3–16 days after ovulation. J. Reprod. Fertil., *32:*319–327, 1982.
10. Van Niekerk, C.H., and Allen, W.R.: Early embryonic development in the horse. J. Reprod. Fertil. Suppl., *23:*495–498, 1975.
11. Ginther, O.J.: Ultrasonic Imaging and Reproductive Events in the Mare. Cross Plains, WI, Equiservices, 1986.
12. Ginther, O.J.: Fixation and orientation of the early equine conceptus. Theriogenology, *19:*613–623, 1983.
13. Enders, A.C., and Liu, I.K.M.: Lodgement of the equine blastocyst in the uterus from fixation through endometrial cup formation. J. Reprod. Fertil. Suppl., *44:*427–438, 1991.
14. Bergin, W.C., Gier, H.T., Frey, R.A., and Marion, G.B.: Developmental horizons and measurements useful for age determination of equine embryos and fetuses. Proc. Am. Assoc Equine Pract., 179–196, 1967.
15. Allen, W.R., Hamilton, D.W., and Moor, R.M.: Origin of the equine endometrial cups. 2. Invasion of the endometrium by trophoblast. Anat. Rec., *177:*485–502, 1973.
16. Marrable, A.W., and Flood, P.F.: Embryological studies on the Dartmoor pony during the first third of gestation. J. Reprod. Fertil. Suppl., *23:*499–502, 1975.
17. Douglas, R.H., and Ginther, O.J.: Development of the equine fetus and placenta. J. Reprod. Fertil. Suppl., *23:*503–505, 1975.
18. Samuel, C.A., Allen, W.R., and Steven, D.H.: Studies on the equine placenta I. Development of microcotyledons. J. Reprod. Fertil., *41:*441–445, 1974.
19. Clegg, M.T., Boda, J.M., and Cole, H.H.: The endometrial cups and allantochorionic pouches in the mare with emphasis on the source of equine gonadotropin. Endocrinology, *54:*448–463, 1954.
20. Van Niekerk, C.H., and Gerneke, W.H.: Persistence and parthenogenetic cleavage of tubal ova in the mare. Onderstepoort J. Vet. Res., *31:*195–232, 1966.
21. Townson, D.H., and Ginther, O.J.: Ultrasonic characterization of follicular evacuation during ovulation and fate of the discharged follicular fluid in mares. Anim. Reprod. Sci., *20:*131–141, 1989.
22. Palmer, E., et al.: Non-surgical recovery of follicular fluid and oocytes of mares. J. Reprod. Fertil. Suppl., *35:*689–690, 1987.
23. Hamilton, W.J., and Day, F.T.: Cleavage stages of the ova of the horse with notes on ovulation. J. Anat., *79:*127–129, 1945.
24. King, W.A., et al.: The meiotic stage of preovulatory oocytes in mares. Genome, *29:*679–682, 1987.
25. Enders A.C., et al.: The ovulated ovum of the horse: cytology of nonfertilized ova to pronuclear stage ova. Biol. Reprod., *37:*453–466, 1987.
26. Betteridge, K.J., Flood, P.F., and Mitchell, D.: Possible role of the embryo in control of oviductal transport in mares. *In* Ovum Transport and Fertility Regulation. Edited by M.K.J. Harper, et al. Copenhagen, Scriptor, 1976, pp. 381–389.
27. Peyrot, L.M., et al.: Autotransfer of day 4 embryos from oviduct to oviduct versus oviduct to uterus in the mare. Theriogenology, *28:*699–708, 1987.
28. Steffenhagen, W.P., Pineda, M.H., and Ginther, O.J.: Retention of unfertilized ova in the uterine tubes of mares. Am. J. Vet. Res., *33:*2391–2398, 1972.
29. Betteridge, K.J., and Mitchell, D.: Retention of ova by the fallopian tube in mares. J. Reprod. Fertil., *31:*515, 1972.
30. Oguri, N., and Tsutsumi, Y.: Studies on the lodging of equine unfertilized ova in fallopian tubes. Research Bulletin of the Livestock Farm, Hokkaido University, No. 6, *6:*32–43, 1972.
31. David, J.S.E.: A survey of eggs in the oviducts of mares. J. Reprod. Fertil. Suppl., *23:*513–517, 1975.
32. Onuma, H., and Ohnami, Y.: Retention of tubal eggs in mares. J. Reprod. Fertil. Suppl., *23:*507–511, 1975.
33. Betteridge, K.J., and Mitchell, D.: Direct evidence of retention of unfertilized ova in the oviduct of the mare. J. Reprod. Fertil., *39:*145–148, 1974.
34. Betteridge, K.J., and Mitchell, D.: A surgical technique applied to the study of tubal eggs in the mare. J. Reprod. Fertil. Suppl., *23:*519–524, 1975.

35. Betteridge, K.J., Eaglesome, M.D., and Flood, P.F.: Embryo transport through the mares oviduct depends upon cleavage but is independent of the ipsilateral corpus luteum. J. Reprod. Fertil. Suppl., *27:*387–394, 1979.
36. Betteridge, K.J., and Guillomot, M.: Scanning electron microscopy of the preattachment horse embryo. J. Reprod. Fertil. Suppl., *32:*623, 1982.
37. Flood, P.F., Jong, A., and Betteridge, K.J.: The location of retained eggs in the uterine tubes of mares. J. Reprod. Fertil., *57:*291–294, 1979.
38. Wilson, J.M., Kreider, J.L., and Potter, G.D.: Nonsurgical recovery of degenerative ova from the uterus of mares. Theriogenology, *23:*236, 1985.
39. Oguri, N., and Tsutsumi, Y.: Nonsurgical transfer of equine embryos. *In* In vitro fertilization and embryo transfer. Edited by E.S.E. Hafez and K. Semm. Lancaster, MTP Press, 1982, pp. 287–295.
40. Hunter, R.H.F.: Differential transport of fertilised and unfertilised eggs in equine fallopian tubes: A straightforward explanation. Vet. Rec. *125:*304, 1989.
41. Rasweiler, J.J. IV: Differential transport of embryos and degenerating ova by the oviducts of the long-tongued bat, Glossophaga soricina. J. Reprod. Fertil., *55:*329–334, 1979.
42. Ortiz, M.E., Bedregal, P., Carvajal, M.I., and Croxatto, H.B.: Fertilized and unfertilized ova are transported at different rates by the hamster oviduct. Biol. Reprod., *34:*777–781, 1986.
43. Ortiz, M.E., Llados, C., and Croxatto, H.B.: Embryos of different ages transferred to the rat oviduct enter the uterus at different times. Biol. Reprod., *41:*381–384, 1989.
44. Flood, P.F., and Porter, D.G.: A method for monitoring contractile activity of the myosalpinx in mares in vivo. Proceedings of the Society for the Study of Fertility. Winter meeting, Cambridge, 1980, abstract 11.
45. Oguri, N., and Tsutsumi, Y.: Non-surgical recovery of equine eggs, and an attempt at non-surgical egg transfer in horses. J. Reprod. Fertil., *31:*187–195, 1972.
46. Geary, R.T., Weber, J.A., and Woods, G.L.: Hastened transport of equine embryos through the oviduct of the mare. Theriogenology, *31:*973–978, 1989.
47. Hinrichs, K., and Riera, F.L.: Effect of administration of $PGF_2\alpha$ on embryo recovery from the uterus on day 5 after ovulation in mares. Am. J. Vet. Res., *51:*451–453, 1990.
48. Harper, M.J.K.: Platelet-activating factor: A paracrine factor in preimplantation stages of reproduction? Biol. Reprod., *40:*907–913, 1989.
49. Weber J.A., Freeman D.A., Vanderwall D.K., and Woods G.L.: Prostaglandin E_2 secretion by oviductal transport-stage equine embryos. Biol. Reprod., *45:*540–543, 1991.
50. Weber J.A., Freeman D.A., Vanderwall D.K., and Woods G.L.: Prostaglandin E_2 hastens oviductal transport of equine embryos. Biol. Reprod., *45:*544–546, 1991.
51. Betteridge, K.J.: The structure and function of the equine capsule in relation to embryo manipulation and transfer. Equine Vet. J. Suppl., *8:*92–100, 1989.
52. Bonnet, R.: Die Eihäute des Pferdes. Verh. Anat. Ges., *3:*17–38, 1889.
53. Zietzschmann, O., and Krölling, O.: Lehrbuch der Entwicklungsgeschichte der Haustiere, Paul Parey, Berlin, 1955.
54. Guillomot, M., and Betteridge, K.J.: Permeability of the capsule of the equine embryo. Proceedings of the Society for the Study of Fertility. Winter meeting, Cambridge, 1984, abstract 58.
55. Bousquet, D., Guillomot, M., and Betteridge, K.J., Equine zona pellucida and capsule: Some physicochemical and antigenic properties. Gamete Res., *16:*121, 1987.
56. Oriol, J.G., Beresford, B., Sharom, F.J., and Betteridge, K.J.: Biochemical composition of the equine capsule: a preliminary report. J. Reprod. Fertil. Suppl., *44:*639–641, 1991.
57. Schlafer, D.H., Dougherty, E.P., and Woods, G.L.: Light and ultrastructural studies of morphological alterations in embryos collected from maiden and barren mares. J. Reprod. Fertil. Suppl., *35:*695, 1987.
58. Denker, H.W., Betteridge, K.J., and Sirois, J.: Shedding of the 'capsule' and proteinase activity in the horse embryo. J. Reprod. Fertil. Suppl., *35:*703, 1987.
59. Hinrichs, K., and Watson, E.D.: Clinical report: Recovery of a degenerating 14-day embryo in the uterine flush of a mare seven days after ovulation. Theriogenology, *30:*349–353, 1988.
60. Allen, W.E., and Newcombe, J.R.: Relationship between early pregnancy site in consecutive gestations in mares. Equine Vet. J., *13:*51–52, 1981.
61. Pascoe, R.R.: Transuterine migration of the fetus in the mare between day 42 and parturition. J. Reprod. Fertil. Suppl., *32:*441–446, 1982.
62. Butterfield, R.M., and Matthews, R.G.: Ovulation and the movement of the conceptus in the first 35 days of pregnancy in Thoroughbred mares. J. Reprod. Fertil. Suppl., *27:*447–452, 1979.
63. Ginther, O.J.: Mobility of the early equine conceptus. Theriogenology, *19:*608–611, 1983.
64. McDowell, K.J., et al.: Restricted conceptus mobility results in failure of pregnancy maintenance in mares. Biol. Reprod., *39:*340–348, 1988.
65. Bessant, C., Cross, D.T., and Ginther, O.J.: Effect of exogenous estradiol on mobility and fixation of the early equine conceptus. Anim. Reprod. Sci., *16:*159–167, 1988.
66. Kastelic, J.P., Adams, G.P., and Ginther, O.J.: Role of progesterone in mobility, fixation, orientation, and survival of the equine embryonic vesicle. Theriogenology, *27:*655–663, 1987.
67. Ginther, O.J.: Reproductive Biology of the Mare: Basic and Applied Aspects. Equiservices, Cross Plains, WI, 1979.
68. Ewart, J.C.: A critical period in the development of the horse. London, Adam & Charles Black, 1897.
69. Murphy, B.D., and Martinuk, S.D.: Equine chorionic gonadotrophin. Endocr. Rev., *12:*27–44, 1991.
70. Antczak, D.F., and Allen, W.R.: Maternal immunological recognition of pregnancy in equids. J. Reprod. Fertil. Suppl., *37:*69–78, 1989.
71. Spincemaille, J., Bouters, R., Vanderplassche, M., and Bonte, P.: Some aspects of endometrial cup formation and PMSG production. J. Reprod. Fertil. Suppl., *23:*415–418, 1975.
72. Flood, P.F., and Marrable, A.W.: A histochemical study of steroid metabolism in the equine fetus and placenta. J. Reprod. Fertil. Suppl., *23:*569–573, 1975.
73. Heap, R.B., Hamon, M., and Allen, W.R.: Studies on oestrogen synthesis by preimplantation equine conceptuses. J. Reprod. Fertil. Suppl., *32:*343–352, 1982.
74. van Niekerk, C.H.: The early diagnosis of pregnancy, the development of the foetal membranes and nidation in the mare. J. S. Afr. Vet. Med. Assoc., *36:*483–488, 1965.
75. Comline, R.S., and Silver, M.: PO_2, PCO_2 and pH levels in the umbilical and uterine blood of the mare and ewe. J. Physiol. (Lond.), *208:*587–608, 1970.
76. Steven, D.H.: Placentation in the mare. J. Reprod. Fertil. Suppl., *31:*41–55, 1982.

77. Samuel, C.A., Allen, W.R., and Steven, D.H.: Studies on the equine placenta II. Ultrastructure of the placental barrier. J. Reprod. Fertil., *48:*257–264, 1976.

78. Steven, D.H., and Samuel, C.A.: Anatomy of the placental barrier in the mare. J. Reprod. Fertil., *23:*579–582, 1975.

79. Samuel, C.A., Allen, W.R., and Steven, D.H.: Studies on the equine placenta III. Ultrastructure of the uterine glands and the overlying trophoblast. J. Reprod. Fertil., *51:*433–437, 1977.

80. Flood, P.F.: The development of the conceptus and its relationship to the uterus. *In* Reproduction in Domestic Animals. Edited by P.T. Cupps. New York, Academic Press, 1991, pp. 315–360.

CHAPTER 57

MATERNAL RECOGNITION OF PREGNANCY

D.C. Sharp

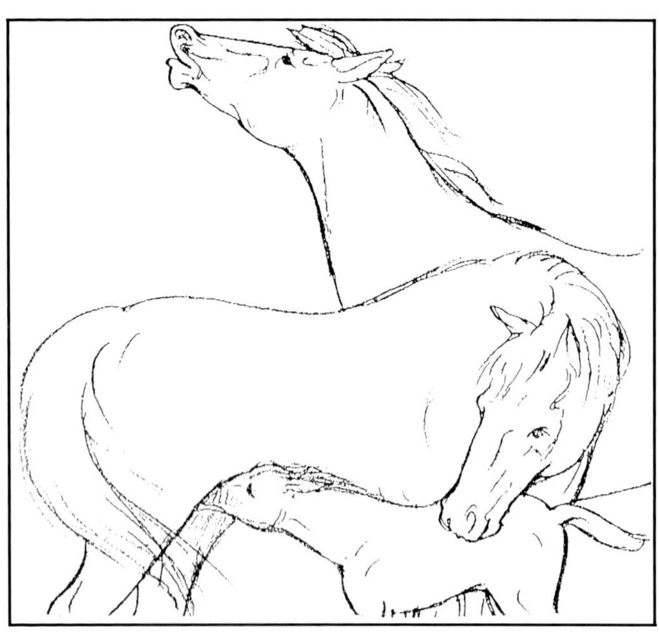

REGULATION OF THE ESTROUS CYCLE AND MECHANISMS OF CORPUS LUTEUM REGRESSION

As the name implies, the estrous cycle is a repetitive phenomenon that provides multiple opportunities for breeding, thus ensuring a reasonable chance of propagating the species. In order for the cycle to function well, mechanisms must exist which stimulate, or permit, smooth transition from one phase of the cycle to the next. The regression of the corpus luteum (CL) culminates the diestrous phase of the estrous cycle, permitting the renewed onset of estrous activity (see Chapter 18 for a detailed discussion of luteolysis). Mechanisms regulating regression of the CL must be averted at the time of maternal recognition of pregnancy. Thus, for the purpose of this discussion, the phrase "maternal recognition of pregnancy" will pertain to the events and/or mechanisms that prevent CL regression. An early form of pregnancy recognition takes place in the oviduct, which permits selective transport of 16-cell embryos or older but does not permit transport of unfertilized ova.[1,2] However, the successful "recognition" and transport of fertilized ova through the oviducts is no guarantee of successful accomplishment of the critical step of providing continuing luteal support for pregnancy establishment. As a consequence of CL maintenance, many other events of critical importance to the establishment of pregnancy may follow. Such events, while important to a successful pregnancy, are secondary to the task of maintaining CL function.

The uterus is necessary for regression of the CL in most mammalian species; the human is a notable exception. Loeb first hysterectomized guinea pigs and noted that the life span of the CL was extended far beyond normal.[3] Ginther and First reported the effects of complete and partial hysterectomy in pony mares, stating that complete hysterectomy resulted in maintenance of the CL in all mares, hemihysterectomy (one uterine horn and approximately one half of the uterine body removed) resulted in maintenance of the CL in about half of the mares, and the side of ablation relative to the side of the CL was not important.[4] Clinical observations of mares with extreme cases of pyometra with extensive damage to the endometrium have also revealed extended CL life span. Thus, the uterus, and more specifically the endometrial lining, plays an important role in the normal regression of the CL and, therefore, must somehow be involved in the mechanisms of maternal recognition of pregnancy.

REGULATION OF PROSTAGLANDIN $F_2\alpha$ SYNTHESIS

Douglas and Ginther measured prostaglandin $F_2\alpha$ ($PGF_2\alpha$) in the uterine veins of anesthetized pony mares and reported a significant increase in uterine venous $PGF_2\alpha$ on day 14 after ovulation.[5] Zavy et al. measured $PGF_2\alpha$ in the uterine lumen of cycling pony and horse mares and also reported a significant increase in uterine luminal $PGF_2\alpha$ on day 14.[6,7] These experimental approaches were necessary because $PGF_2\alpha$ has a short half-life in the periphery, and $PGF_2\alpha$ concentrations could not be detected in the peripheral circulation. Later studies using an assay system for 13,14-dihydro-15-keto metabolite (PGFM), which has a considerably longer half-life than $PGF_2\alpha$ and can be detected in the peripheral circulation, demonstrated a prominent rise in circulating PGFM concentrations beginning about day 14 after ovulation in horse mares.[8]

In attempts to determine the tissue source, as well as the potential steroid regulation of $PGF_2\alpha$ synthesis and secretion by the uterus, researchers incubated endometrial tissue harvested from cycling pony mares throughout the estrous cycle.[9] They reported that the $PGF_2\alpha$ content of endometrium increased on day 14 after ovulation, and more important, the in vitro production of $PGF_2\alpha$ increased markedly on day 14 after ovulation. Furthermore, using endometria collected from ovariectomized steroid-treated mares they showed that prior exposure of the endometrium to progesterone was essential for in vitro $PGF_2\alpha$ production and that estrogen treatment added to the incubations significantly enhanced the in vitro production of $PGF_2\alpha$.[9] In a later study, researchers from the same laboratory reported a small, but highly significant, increase in uterine luminal estrone and estradiol that coincided temporally with the increase in luminal $PGF_2\alpha$.[7] The source of the luminal estrogen is not known, but the temporal association with $PGF_2\alpha$ secretion is provocative, and a causal relationship can be reasonably suspected.

These studies, when taken together, indicate two key points: (1) the endometrium is clearly the tissue source of the $PGF_2\alpha$ secreted at the end of the luteal phase and (2) the timing of $PGF_2\alpha$ secretion is remarkably consistent, regardless of the laboratory or method used to quantify it. These points suggest that the timing of $PGF_2\alpha$ secretion, and thus, the regression of the CL, is a well-regulated phenomenon.

The events which lead up to and result in the release of PGF are not yet completely understood, but enough is known to permit some careful speculation. That progesterone is required for $PGF_2\alpha$ secretion is evident from the studies of Zavy et al.[6,7] and Vernon et al.,[9] who examined $PGF_2\alpha$ in uterine luminal washings, or in vitro endometrial incubations from mares with no circulating progesterone (i.e., estrous, ovariectomized, or anestrus). In all the above cases, little or no detectable $PGF_2\alpha$ was found. In intact, cycling mares, little increase in luminal or in vitro production of $PGF_2\alpha$ occurred until after day 12.[6,7,9] Because little $PGF_2\alpha$ secretion was observed until after about day 12 after ovulation the question of $PGF_2\alpha$ secretion regulation is raised. Is there a threshold of time of exposure to progesterone (i.e., $>$ 12 days) required for $PGF_2\alpha$ secretion or is some further signal required after exposure to progesterone? A reasonable guess is that some minimum exposure to progesterone is necessary, the duration of which is unknown at this time; however, the stimulus for synthesis and/or secretion may be independent of the progesterone priming and may even be derived from a set of seemingly dissociated events elsewhere in the reproductive axis. In this regard, the results of Vernon et al.,[9] which showed that in vitro administration of estrogen to endometria previously exposed (in vivo) to progesterone for 2 weeks resulted in a large increase in vitro $PGF_2\alpha$ production, agreed with the report of Zavy et al.[7] that a small, but highly significant, increase in both estradiol and estrone occurs in uterine luminal washings of cycling mares at about the time of $PGF_2\alpha$ increase. Therefore, the elevated uterine luminal estrogens could be involved in the stimulation of $PGF_2\alpha$ synthesis and/or secretion. However, the source of estrogens contributing to this temporally coincident rise remains to be determined.

MAINTENANCE OF THE CL

It is obvious that the death of the CL is likely an active event. In the absence of the uterus, the life span of the CL is quite long, suggesting that without uterine $PGF_2\alpha$ the CL is maintained for considerably longer periods than experienced in a normal estrous cycle. My colleagues and I monitored mares that had been hysterectomized 1 yr before the experiment. Interestingly, these mares displayed typical anestrous characteristics (i.e., small, atrophic ovaries with no discernible follicular development) and then underwent an apparently normal vernal transition, developing a series of anovulatory follicles, the course of which could not be distinguished from uterine-intact mares. At the first ovulation of the year (at the normally expected date), resulting CL were marked by administration of India ink, and half of the mares ($n = 6$) were ovariectomized 90 days later to identify whether the original CL were still existent. All mares had healthy appearing, marked CL at 90 days. The second group of mares ($n=6$) was ovariectomized at 180 days after ovulation, and four of six were observed to have marked CL still evident. Thus, these data indicate that the CL are capable of surviving a long time in the absence of uterine factors.

Unique among the farm species, the mare undergoes occasional periods of prolonged CL maintenance.[10] These periods (called prolonged luteal phase, prolonged diestrus, and pseudopregnancy) are clinically important because they can easily be mistaken for pregnancy unless careful attention to pregnancy diagnosis is taken. Furthermore, if undetected, these prolonged periods of inappropriate luteal activity can waste a lot of time in a breeding program. Although the advent of ultrasonography has done much to alleviate this diagnostic problem, many veterinarians and breeders do not have access to such equipment, and the problem of prolonged luteal phase remains. The frequency with which this occurs apparently varies, with reports of 5 to 7% to nearly 20% of mares in a given herd experiencing at least one bout of inappropriate CL maintenance during the breeding season.[11]

The reasons for prolonged luteal structures may vary, ranging from known to presumed failure of PGF secretion.[12] As mentioned previously, destruction of a major portion of the endometrial lining of the uterus, as with pyometra may lead to chronically prolonged corpora, similar to hysterectomy. Another possible mechanism involves formation of additional, or accessory, luteal structures during diestrus. As demonstrated by Vernon et al. newly formed corpora lutea do not have $PGF_2\alpha$ receptors by day 4 after ovulation and thus are not affected by $PGF_2\alpha$ secretion.[13] Therefore, if a luteal structure should form about day 10 or so after ovulation, it would be "immune" to the normally timed secretion of $PGF_2\alpha$ on or about day 14.[14] The result would be that the ovulatory CL would indeed be expected to regress, but the newly formed luteal structure would not, leading to prolonged luteal phase.

THE PRESENCE OF A CONCEPTUS

With the above as background for the events leading to CL regression, and the occasional aberrant maintenance of CL, the presence of a conceptus in a potential pregnancy is now considered. Zavy et al. reported that unlike cycling mares, no increase in uterine luminal $PGF_2\alpha$ around day 14 in pregnant mares was observed.[7] Likewise, Kindahl et al. reported failure to detect any increase in peripherally circulating $PGF_2\alpha$ metabolite in pregnant mares compared with nonpregnant mares,[8] and Douglas and Ginther reported that uterine venous samples had had significantly lower $PGF_2\alpha$ concentrations on day 14 in pregnant mares than in cycling mares.[5] Finally, Berglund et al. reported that endometria harvested from pregnant mares on day 14 and coincubated with conceptus tissue produced significantly less $PGF_2\alpha$ than did endometria alone.[15]

That the conceptus must be present for maternal recognition of pregnancy to occur is evident from a number of studies. However, one of the most compelling demonstrations is that it is possible to transfer a conceptus from one mare to an unbred mare, with pregnancy occurring in the unbred mare. Although the concept of embryo transfer is not new, it is relatively new to the horse industry. Walter Heape was the first to report transfer of rabbit embryos from one doe to another in 1891.[16] From this publication, it was 85 yr until embryo transfer was reported in mares by Allen and Rowson.[17]

Much has been said about a critical period during which the conceptus must be present for successful maternal recognition of pregnancy to occur. However, the phrase "critical period" implies a beginning and an end to the process, and current knowledge of conceptus-maternal interactions from the time of fertilization to the last stages of maternal pregnancy recognition is sparse. Clearly, there is a critical deadline by which the conceptus must act or suffer the consequences of CL regression and loss of vital uterine secretions, but relatively little is known about the early events which might be critical to the establishment of pregnancy. In practice, embryo transfers which are performed around day 6 to 8 after ovulation, result in successful pregnancies, but the success rate declines with age of the conceptus transferred. It is not clear whether the reduced success rate reflects (1) more difficult technical logistics of collecting and transferring a larger conceptus; (2) simple demographic emphasis, because relatively few researchers have even tried to transfer later stage conceptuses, or (3) a real physiologic phenomenon in which conceptus and/or maternal uterus have had insufficient time to interact in a vital way. The answer to this question will be an important part of the continuing quest for an understanding of the mechanisms of maternal pregnancy recognition.

The opposite experiment has also been done. That is, removal of the conceptus from bred mares at various intervals after ovulation to study the effects of conceptus removal on CL function has also shown that CL function may be maintained if the conceptus is removed after about day 16, but not if the conceptus is removed sometime before day 14 to 16.[18]

INHIBITION OF $PGF_2\alpha$ SECRETION

One of the critical requirements for maternal recognition of pregnancy is that the CL be maintained for continued progesterone secretion. The conceptus could conceivably accomplish that goal through one of several ways: (1) preventing the secretion of prostaglandin $F_2\alpha$ (i.e., a luteostatic effect), (2) altering the distribution of $PGF_2\alpha$ so that it does not reach the CL in appropriate form (also a luteostatic effect), or (3) secreting a substance that counteracts the effects of $PGF_2\alpha$ at the level of the CL (a luteotropic or antiluteolytic effect). Of these possible actions, the available evidence in mares best supports the first. Zavy et al. reported that $PGF_2\alpha$ concentrations in uterine flushings reached maximal on or about day 14 in nonbred mares but that $PGF_2\alpha$ concentration did not increase at all in uterine flushings recovered from pregnant mares.[7] Also, $PGF_2\alpha$ in uterine veins of pregnant mares was significantly lower on day 14 of pregnancy than on day 14 of the estrous cycle.[5] Finally, Kindahl et al. demonstrated that the major metabolite of $PGF_2\alpha$—PGFM, which can be measured in peripheral plasma—was essentially undetectable in the peripheral plasma of pregnant mares compared with nonpregnant mares around days 14 to 16.[8] These studies all suggested that in the presence of a conceptus, uterine production of $PGF_2\alpha$ is reduced or blocked altogether. This was further demonstrated by evidence that coincubation of conceptus tissue and endometrial explants resulted in significantly less $PGF_2\alpha$ production in vitro compared with $PGF_2\alpha$ production from endometrial explants alone.[15]

The possibility that a conceptus factor or factors inhibit $PGF_2\alpha$ production by endometrial tissue is intriguing and clearly needs further work. Coincubating endometrial explant tissue with conceptus membranes contained within small bags of dialysis tubing suggested that conceptus $PGF_2\alpha$-inhibitory factors may be relatively low molecular weight.[19] That is, $PGF_2\alpha$ production was inhibited by endometrial explants when conceptus membranes were contained within dialysis bags with molecular exclusion limits of 12,000 to 14,000, 6,000 to 8,000 and 3,500 but not 1,000. Thus, the failure of conceptus factors to interact with endometrial tissue at the molecular exclusion limit of 1,000 suggests that the conceptus factor is larger than most common ions, steroids, or even other prostaglandins. The $PGF_2\alpha$-inhibiting interaction of conceptus membranes contained within dialysis bags of larger molecular exclusion limits suggests that the factor(s) may be at least smaller than 6,000. This observation does not support the idea that equine maternal recognition of pregnancy is similar to other domestic species. In cattle and sheep, a group of proteins called trophoblastic proteins is synthesized and secreted from conceptus membranes at the time of maternal recognition of pregnancy.[20] These proteins are acidic with molecular weights of about 17,000 (sheep) to 21,000 (cattle). Assessment of conceptus-produced proteins from equine embryos did not reveal similar proteins.[21] Furthermore, studies in the author's laboratory have indicated that antibodies to ovine trophoblast protein (oTP1) do not cross-react with equine conceptus proteins. Therefore, little evidence exists for the argument that equine embryos accomplish the task of pregnancy recognition in a manner similar to that of cattle and sheep. In pigs, the conceptus factor which appears to be a major part of the recognition signal is estrogen. Estrogen from the pig conceptus alters the manner of $PGF_2\alpha$ secretion in pregnant gilts compared with nonpregnant gilts.[22] That is, in nonpregnant gilts, $PGF_2\alpha$ is secreted by uterine endometrium about day 15 into the myometrial side of the endometrium, where it gains access to the vascular tree and is carried to the CL. On the other hand, in pregnant gilts at day 15, $PGF_2\alpha$ is secreted primarily toward the luminal side of the endometrium where it is sequestered, preventing CL regression.[22] Evidence in support of this theory has come from a variety of experiments, but the most compelling have involved use of a two-chambered perfusion device.[23] With this device, endometrial tissue can be placed at the opening between the two chambers such that the secretion of $PGF_2\alpha$ toward myometrial and luminal sides can be studied. When such studies were conducted using endometrium from nonpregnant gilts, the majority of $PGF_2\alpha$ secreted was toward the myometrial side, whereas when endometrium from pregnant gilts was used, the majority of $PGF_2\alpha$ secreted was toward the luminal side.[24] A similar mechanism is not at work in the horse. In one study, uterine luminal $PGF_2\alpha$ concentrations were lower in pregnant mares compared with nonpregnant mares, suggesting a blockade of $PGF_2\alpha$ secretion, not a redirection of secretion as has been demonstrated in pigs.[7] Likewise, when equine endometrial tissue was studied with the LaCroix chambers, no sidedness to secretion of $PGF_2\alpha$ in either the nonpregnant or pregnant state was evident.[25]

ESTROGEN SECRETION

Because the equine conceptus produces prodigious amounts of estrogen,[26,27] as does the porcine conceptus,[28] comparison with the mechanism of maternal recognition of pregnancy in gilts had been natural. However, the comparison does not stand up to investigative scrutiny. As mentioned above, no sidedness to $PGF_2\alpha$ secretion in the mare exists and uterine luminal $PGF_2\alpha$ is decreased at the time of maternal recognition of pregnancy, not increased as it is in gilts.[29] Furthermore, no shift in secretion of $PGF_2\alpha$ toward luminal or myometrial side of the endometrium in mares has been demonstrated. Rather, the secretion of $PGF_2\alpha$ appears to be equally distributed toward both sides, regardless of pregnancy status.[25] Finally, the idea that estrogen is the conceptus' signal for maternal recognition of pregnancy in mares persists partially because of reports in the literature that estrogen administration leads to retained CL function.

Administration of estrogen—diethylstilbestrol, estradiol (5 mg/day, days 7 to 18), or estrone (100 mg/day, days 7 to 18)—to nonbred mares resulted in prolonged interovulatory interval.[30,31] Similarly, prolonged interovulatory intervals following administration of 0.1, 1.0, or 10.0 mg estradiol daily from the day of ovulation until the next ovulation has been reported.[32] These latter workers reported that CL of estrogen-treated mares underwent regression at the normally expected time (about days 14 to 16), as assessed by monitoring peripherally circulating progesterone, and concluded that the prolonged interovulatory interval was the result of suppressed follicular development, not failure of CL regression. Early investigators monitored primarily interovulatory interval, a potentially misleading end point in this case.[30,31] Nishikawa removed the ovaries of three estrogen-treated mares at various intervals after the primary ovulation and reported that they contained CL, but because the primary corpora were not marked, whether they were the primary CL or not is impossible to state. In contrast to these studies in which estrogen treatment was relatively prolonged, administration of estrogen over as short a period as 3 days (11 to 13) in gilts leads to prolonged luteal function.[20] Therefore, the assumption that estrogen is the embryonic signal for maternal recognition of pregnancy in mares as it appears to be in pigs is not in line with existing knowledge. However, that is not to say that embryonic estrogens are unimportant in the establishment of pregnancy in horses. In fact quite the opposite is likely true. Estradiol and estrone concentrations within the uterine lumen were markedly elevated in pregnant mares from days 10 to 20.[7] Similarly, uterine content of uteroferrin as well as other uterine-specific proteins have been shown to increase markedly during this same time.[7] The temporal association between elevated uterine estrogens and uterine specific proteins was found to be likely causal.[33] McDowell et al. reported that administration of progesterone to ovariectomized mares resulted in uteroferrin concentrations similar to those observed in uterine flushings of nonpregnant mares during the peak of the luteal phase but that the combined administration of progesterone and estradiol resulted in uteroferrin concentrations that were significantly elevated over progesterone treatment alone.[33] Thus at least certain uterine-specific proteins, thought to be important to the establishment of pregnancy, are enhanced by the actions of estrogen in concert with progesterone. It may be premature to state that elevated estrogens are necessary for successful pregnancy establishment and conceptus development, but it seems a plausible hypothesis at present. If so, pregnancy establishment in the mare presents the interesting situation in which conceptus factors provide some signal which ensures continued progesterone secretion (i.e., luteostasis) which drives the secretion of uterine secretions (histotrophe) thought to be essential in conceptus development. The secretion of these uterine factors then, could be further amplified by estrogens from the conceptus.

OVINE TROPHOBLASTIC PROTEIN 1

In sheep, a protein produced by the conceptus has been identified and appears to be a primary candidate for the role of conceptus signal for maternal recognition of pregnancy. This acidic protein, with a molecular weight of about 17,000 is called (ovine trophoblastic protein 1 (oTP1)[34] and was recently found to have a high homology with interferon-α and is relatively active in common antiviral assay systems.[35] Whether the antiviral activity is an essential part of the conceptus signal for maternal recognition of pregnancy (i.e., CL maintenance) or whether it serves an ancillary role by helping create a suitable uterine environment is unknown at present. However, as with many new findings, the existence of this interesting protein in sheep and cattle has prompted the question of its existence in horses. In that regard, equine uterine flushings, media from conceptus incubations, and yolk sac fluid have all been tested for antiviral assay systems similar to those in which oTP1 is highly active, and essentially no activity was found.[19] Furthermore, researchers failed to detect mRNA for interferon-α in equine conceptus membranes, utilizing Northern blot techniques.[36] Studies of equine conceptus secreted proteins did not reveal any proteins of molecular weight comparable to oTP1 during the time of maternal recognition of pregnancy.[21] In addition, antibodies raised against oTP1 do not cross-react with conceptus-conditioned media or with uterine flushings collected from pregnant mares.[19] Therefore, little evidence exists to suggest that an interferon-like protein which could participate in the maternal recognition of pregnancy is produced by the early equine conceptus.

CONCEPTUS MOBILITY

Early studies on the production of PGF from uterine endometrium in vitro indicated a paradoxical situation in that $PGF_2\alpha$ was produced by endometrium obtained from pregnant mares, yet uterine luminal $PGF_2\alpha$ concentrations were reduced in pregnancy.[6,9] This paradox was resolved, as mentioned, when it was shown that coincubations of endometrium from pregnant mares with conceptus membranes reduced the $PGF_2\alpha$ produced.[11,15,37] These observations led to the realization, however, that the inhibitory effects of conceptus products on endometrial $PGF_2\alpha$ production were likely short lived or transient. When Ginther published the interesting observation, determined with ultrasonography, that equine conceptuses are highly mobile from the time of first detection with ultrasound (day 10) until days 16 to 18, when they became trapped or lodged at the junction of the uterine horn and body,[38] the extensive mobility seems likely to be an important mechanism to ensure $PGF_2\alpha$ inhibition throughout the uterine horn. To test this hypothesis, conceptus mobility was restricted by ligating uterine horns at various locations and the events of maternal pregnancy recognition were studied.[39] Results of those studies revealed that pregnancy recognition was indeed jeopardized when conceptus mobility was restricted and that a crude relationship between amount of uterine luminal surface to which the conceptus had access and the success of pregnancy recognition existed.[39] That is, when conceptuses had access to most of the uterus (tip of uterine horn contralateral to side of ovulation ligated, i.e., surgical control) all mares recognized pregnancy as determined by CL maintenance (monitored via ultrasound observation and elevated progesterone concentrations), failure to display estrus, continued conceptus viability (monitored with ultrasound observation), and positive tests for equine chorionic gonadotropin (eCG) at day 40. When only about 50% of the uterus was accessible to conceptuses' migration (i.e., uterine horn contralateral to side of ovulation ligated at bifurcation), 50% of mares were unable to recognize pregnancy as determined by loss of the CL, return to estrus, and eventual loss of conceptus integrity. When conceptus mobility was severely restricted (i.e., uterine horn ipsilateral to side of ovulation ligated at bifurcation) only about 12% of mares were able to recognize pregnancy. Furthermore, in a second study, an additional group of mares was studied, with uteri ligated so as to restrict conceptus mobility maximally, but the synthetic progestin allyltrenbolone (Regumate, Hoescht-Roussel) was administered to provide a source of progestin. In this latter group, four of five mares maintained viable conceptuses, with a positive eCG test at day 40, indicating that the major cause of conceptus loss in the groups with maximal conceptus restriction was the loss of progestin. Thus conceptus mobility throughout the uterus clearly plays an important role in the blockade of $PGF_2\alpha$ at the time of maternal recognition of pregnancy. The extensive mobility may also permit conceptuses access to uterine histotrophe throughout the uterus. Conceptuses of the other domestic species undergo extensive elongation during the time of maternal recognition of pregnancy, which enables maximum exposure to endometrium. Mobility of the spherical equine conceptus may serve a similar purpose.

UTERINE PROTEINS

One of the consequences of progesterone production by the CL, is the secretion of uterine proteins. Researchers demonstrated that the pattern—and, more importantly, the quantity—of uterine proteins was altered (increased) with advancing days after ovulation and CL formation.[26,40] Similarly, others demonstrated that total uterine protein and uteroferrin increased with time of

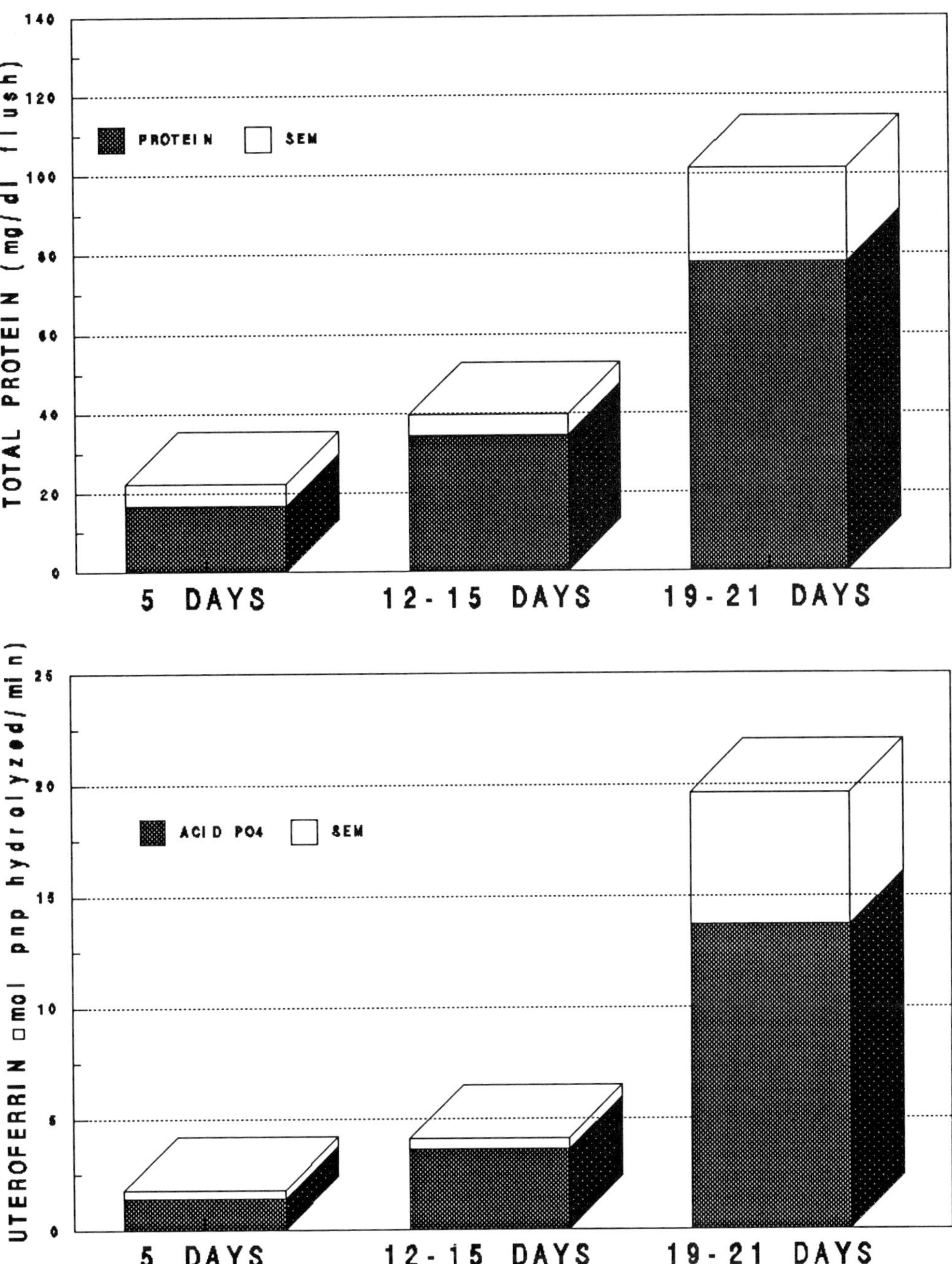

FIG. 57–1. Protein recovered in uterine flushings of ovariectomized mares treated with progesterone for 5, 12 to 15, or 19 to 21 days. *A,* Total protein, mg/dL flush recovered. *B,* Uteroferrin, estimated as acid phosphatase activity; µmol paranitrophenol hydrolyzed/min. (From Hinrichs, K., Kenney, R.M., and Sharp, D.C.: Differences in protein content of uterine fluid related to duration of progesterone treatment in ovariectomized mares used as embryo transfer recipients. Equine Vet. J. Suppl., *8:*49–55, 1989.

progesterone administration in ovariectomized mares[41] (Fig. 57–1).

UTEROFERRIN

Included in the milieu of proteins in uterine secretions is a relatively low molecular weight, basic glycoprotein called uteroferrin which has been identified in uterine flushings of pigs, horses, and late-pregnant cows and sheep. Uteroferrin is progesterone dependent, and does not appear in the uterine flushings of ovariectomized or estrogen-administered animals. A threshold amount of progesterone required for uteroferrin, as well as total protein, secretion seems to exist. Administration of increasing concentrations of progesterone to ovariectomized mares resulted in increased uteroferrin and total protein when 50 mg of progesterone were administered daily compared with vehicle controls. Administration of larger doses of progesterone (i.e., 200 or 400 mg daily) however, did not significantly increase the amount of total protein or uteroferrin recovered.[33] Others have reported that expression of the gene for porcine uteroferrin is differentially regulated by estrogen and progesterone.[42,43] Specifically, progesterone increased the steady-state levels of endometrial mRNA for uteroferrin, whereas estrogen diminished the steady-state levels of uteroferrin mRNA. Administration of estrogen to diestrous gilts results in a marked decrease in uterine luminal uteroferrin.[44] In contrast, others reported that uteroferrin continued to increase at the time of maternal recognition of pregnancy in mares.[40,44,45] The latter workers further demonstrated that uteroferrin concentrations were increased markedly in progesterone plus estrogen administered ovariectomized mares.[44,45] Thus, it seems that this uterine-specific protein which has so much in common in mares and gilts, may have some differences in regulation of the gene for expression of the protein.

The promoter region of the porcine gene for uteroferrin (a 2kb genomic fragment corresponding to −2005 to +48 nucleotides) requires an interaction between estrogen and prolactin in order for progesterone to be effective in eliciting promoter activity.[42] Thus, regulation of the gene for porcine uteroferrin is more complex than previously expected, and regulation of the gene for equine uteroferrin may also be as complex, although not necessarily identical. Studies are currently under way to examine the promoter region of the equine uteroferrin gene to see if similar hormonal requirements exist. Regardless, the observation that estrogen greatly enhances production of equine uteroferrin may be of some practical importance, because equine conceptuses produce prodigious amounts of estrogen during the time of maternal recognition of pregnancy. In a remarkably efficient and conservative design, the equine conceptus probably relies on maternal progesterone as the major gene regulatory agent, then simply increases or amplifies the production of uteroferrin through its secretion of estrogen. This is only speculation until more is known about the promoter region of the equine uteroferrin gene, but such speculation does not seem incautious at present.

PROGESTERONE

It has been shown that the conceptus requires progesterone or, more accurately, the uterine secretions which are stimulated by progesterone. Removal of the CL, either surgically or by administration of $PGF_2\alpha$ results in loss of the conceptus within 5 to 7 days. Similarly, when the maternal recognition of pregnancy was averted by restricting conceptus mobility, conceptuses were evident within the uterus by ultrasonography 2 to 3 days after mares returned to estrus (5 to 7 days after the progesterone decline associated with luteolysis).[39] Examination of conceptuses with ultrasonography did not reveal signs of gradual deterioration, although the health of the tissues themselves cannot be determined via ultrasonography. In some cases, when a distinct fluid-filled vesicle was no longer evident with ultrasonographic examination, conceptus membranes were recovered when the uterine lumen was flushed with saline. Occasionally, the ultrasonographic examination indicated small, nondiscrete nonechogenic areas, suggestive of fluid pools. Whether they represent the yolk sac fluid which had dispersed after rupture of the conceptus membranes is conjecture, but seems likely. This was especially true in ligated uterine horns where, ostensibly, fluid from ruptured conceptuses would not have been able to exit via the cervix.[39] What is interesting about these observations is not necessarily that the conceptus was eventually lost, but that conceptuses persisted for such a long time (5 to 7 days) after progesterone withdrawal. Zavy et al. reported that total uterine protein declined rapidly in uterine flushings (48 h) after CL regression, indicating that progesterone withdrawal was associated with a rapid decline in histotrophe;[26] however, in the report of McDowell, et al., conceptuses appeared to remain intact up to 7 days after luteolysis, suggesting the existence of energy and/or nutrient storage.[39] The yolk sac fluid, of course, is the likely candidate for that role. Of further interest, I have shown that administration of progesterone or the synthetic progestin Allyl trenbolone after loss of the corpus luteum can "rescue" the conceptus. In experiments to test this possibility, pregnant mares were administered a luteolytic dose of $PGF_2\alpha$ on day 14, then Regumate was administered 2, 3, or 4 days after (days 16, 17, and 18, respectively). The appearance as well as the diameter of the conceptus were monitored daily via ultrasound. Of interest, all conceptuses appeared to increase diametrically in a similar manner, even in experimental groups in which the conceptus was eventually lost. Of the three groups previously described, conceptuses were lost from only the 4-day group. That is, progestin administration at 2 or 3 days after a luteolytic dose of $PGF_2\alpha$ was sufficient to prevent loss of the conceptus, whereas all of the conceptuses were lost when progestin treatment was delayed until 4 days after initiation of luteolysis. These data suggest that the conceptus may contain enough nutrient store not only to maintain viability but to continue spherical expansion, although caution is necessary with the latter point, because spherical expansion may not necessarily indicate viability. It could also reflect inappropriate transport systems in the face of metabolic disturbances before death. However, the clear viability of conceptuses "rescued" with progestin as long as 3 days after initiation of luteolysis indicates that conceptuses remained viable at least that long. These studies raise the intriguing question of progesterone regulation of protein secretion. In the normal course of luteal formation and histotrophe secretion, total protein, generally, and uteroferrin, specifically, appear to require some length of time to be expressed.[7,41,46,47] The concentration of these proteins increases gradually in uterine flushings with advancing luteal phase, or progesterone administration. The time lag in the induction of uteroferrin mRNA levels by progesterone may reflect the requirement of endometrial cells to undergo a progesterone-mediated differentiation.[48] Does this gradual increase in concentration represent increasing recruitment of secretory cells or are essentially all glandular epithelial cells involved and production increased? The answer is unknown but presumably may have bearing on the important question of why some mares conceive readily, yet cannot carry a foal beyond 2 to 3 months. Such mares may simply be unable to provide an adequate uterine environment to support a developing fetus because of extensive periglandular fibrotic inclusions. Thus, the question of uterine secretion production may be an important one. Furthermore, what happens to the uterine histotrophe after administration of a luteolytic dose of prostaglandin (PGF), followed by progestin treatment some time later? The gene regulating transcription of certain uterine proteins, such as uteroferrin, may not be turned off immediately, but translation of the protein is halted so that it is soon lost from the uterine environment. Expression of the gene, however, can be initiated readily by treatment with progestin. By 4 days after initiation of luteolysis the gene may be completely switched off so that stimulation of transcription requires too much time to produce enough uterine histotrophe for conceptus survival. These thoughts are only speculative, of course, but seem worthy of verification or rejection by appropriate research techniques.

PRACTICAL CONSIDERATIONS

At first glance, understanding the mechanisms of maternal pregnancy recognition may seem a bit esoteric and of little use in the field but, as with all fresh knowledge, that simply reflects the incompleteness of understanding. Once a thorough understanding of the maternal recognition of pregnancy is available, many applications may suggest themselves. As already pointed out, the time of maternal pregnancy recognition is a time associated with extremely high conceptus mortality, the causes of which are not known, but may have some basis in inappropriate pregnancy recognition signals. Similarly, failure of luteal regression, leading to prolonged luteal phase, or pseudopregnancy (pseudopsyecis), occurs often enough to present a serious management problem, even if a simple, effective treatment exists. The difficulty with prolonged luteal phase is not the treatment, because many researchers have demonstrated that a single administration of $PGF_2\alpha$ is sufficient to cause luteal regression and return to estrus, but the burden is one of diagnosis, because mares with this problem often had been bred and whether the diagnosis of prolonged luteal phase is accurate or whether the mare is simply pregnant must be ascertained.

Once an understanding of the mechanisms of maternal pregnancy recognition has been obtained, new and more sophisticated diagnostic tests may be developed based on the same signal that the mare uses to recognize pregnancy. Furthermore, quantitative assessment of conceptus and/or maternal factors may help in monitoring the quality of the uterine environment. In addition, certain sire and dam characteristics may be reflected in conceptus-secreted products which could be used early in pregnancy to predict some aspects of conceptus development. For instance, sheep conceptuses secrete a protein, called oTP1, which likely serves as the conceptus signal for maternal pregnancy recognition in this species. Some component of the genetic ability of the conceptus to secrete oTP1 is derived from the sire, suggesting that sire selection for successful maternal pregnancy recognition might be a possibility. It is known, for example, that the sire exerts a marked effect on chorionic gonadotropin production in mares, with dramatic differences between stallions and jacks. Differences have also been observed within sire lines within a breed as well. Such genetic influences are thought not to be expressed until the time of endometrial cup formation in mares, but other conceptus-secreted products may also reflect sire inheritance, and these factors may serve similarly useful diagnostic or predictive purposes at the time of maternal recognition of pregnancy. Finally, once having understood the mechanisms of pregnancy recognition, it may be possible to develop clinical treatments that favor successful establishment of pregnancy.

REFERENCES

1. Van Niekerk, C.H., and Gernecke, W.H.: Persistence and parthenogenic cleavage of tubal ova in the mare. Onderstepoort J. Vet. Res., *31:*195–232, 1966.
2. Betteridge, K.J., Eaglesome, M.C., and Flood, P.F.: Embryo transport through the mare's oviduct depends upon cleavage and is independent of the ipsilateral corpus luteum. J. Reprod. Fertil. Suppl., *27:*387–394, 1979.
3. Loeb, L.: The effect of extirpation of the uterus on the life and function of the corpus luteum of the guinea pig. Proc. Soc. Exp. Biol. Med., *20:*441–443, 1923.
4. Ginther, O.J., and First, N.L.: Maintenance of the corpus luteum in hysterectomized mares. Am. J. Vet. Res., *32:*1687–1691, 1971.
5. Douglas, R.H., and Ginther, O.J.: Concentration of prostaglandins F in uterine venous plasma of anesthetized mares during the estrous cycle and early pregnancy. Prostaglandins, *11:*251–260, 1976.
6. Zavy, M.T., et al.: Uterine luminal prostaglandin F in cycling mares. Prostaglandins, *16:*643–648, 1978.
7. Zavy, M.T., Vernon M.W., Sharp, D.C., and Bazer, F.W.: Endocrine aspects of early pregnancy in pony mares: A comparison of uterine luminal and peripheral plasma levels of steroids during the estrous cycle and early pregnancy. Endocrinology, *115:*214–219, 1984.
8. Kindahl, H., Knudsen, O., Madej, A., and Edqvist, L.-E.: Progesterone, prostaglandin $F_2\alpha$, PMSG, and oestrone sulphate during early pregnancy in the mare. J. Reprod. Fertil. Suppl., *32:*353–359, 1982.
9. Vernon, M.W., Zavy, M.T., Asquith, R.L., and Sharp, D.C.: Prostaglandin $F_2\alpha$ in the equine endometrium: Steroid modulation and production capacities during the estrous cycle and early pregnancy. Biol. Reprod., *25:*581–589, 1981.

10. Hughes, J.P., Stabenfeldt, G.H., and Evans, J.W.: Clinical and endocrine aspects of the estrous cycle of the mare. Proc. Am. Assoc. Equine Pract., 119–148, 1972.
11. Sharp, D.C.: Factors associated with the maternal recognition of pregnancy in mares. *In* Veterinary Clinics of North America: Large Animal Practice. Edited by J.P. Hughes. Philadelphia, W.B. Saunders, 1980, pp. 277–289.
12. Neely, D.P., et al.: Prostaglandin release patterns in the mare: Physiological, pathophysiological, and therapeutic responses. J. Reprod. Fertil. Suppl., *27:*181–189, 1979.
13. Vernon, M.W., et al.: Specific PGF2 binding by the corpus luteum of the pregnant and nonpregnant mare. J. Reprod. Fertil. Suppl., *27:*421–429, 1979.
14. Townson, D.H., Pierson, R.A., and Ginther, O.J.: Characterization of plasma progesterone concentrations for two distinct luteal morphologies. Theriogenology, *32:*197–204, 1989.
15. Berglund, L.A., Sharp, D.C., Vernon, M.W., and Thatcher, W.W.: Effect of pregnancy status and collection technique on prostaglandin F in the uterine lumen of pony mares. J. Reprod. Fertil. Suppl., *32:*335–341, 1982.
16. Heape, W.: Preliminary note on the transplantation and growth of mammalian ova within a uterine foster mother. Proc. R. Soc. Lond., *48:*457–459, 1891.
17. Allen, W.R., and Rowson, L.E.A.: Surgical and nonsurgical egg transfer in horses. J. Reprod. Fertil. Suppl., *23:*525–530, 1975.
18. Hershman, E., and Douglas, R.D.: The critical period for the maternal recognition of pregnancy in pony mares. J. Reprod. Fertil. Suppl., *27:*395–401, 1979.
19. Sharp, D.C., McDowell, K.J., Weithenauer, J., and Thatcher, W.W.: The continuum of events leading to maternal recognition of pregnancy in mares. J. Reprod. Fertil. Suppl., *37:*101–107, 1989.
20. Bazer, F.W., et al.: Comparative aspects of maternal recognition of pregnancy between sheep and pigs. J. Reprod. Fertil. Suppl., *37:*85–89, 1989.
21. McDowell, K.J., Sharp, D.C., Fazleabas, A., and Roberts, R.M.: Two-dimensional gel electrophoresis of proteins synthesized and released by conceptuses and endometria from pony mares. J. Reprod. Fertil., *89:*107–115, 1990.
22. Bazer, F.W., and Thatcher, W.W.: Theory of maternal recognition of pregnancy in swine based on estrogen-controlled endocrine versus exocrine secretion of prostaglandin $F_2\alpha$ by the uterine endometrium. Prostaglandins, *14:*397–402, 1977.
23. LaCroix, M.C., and Kann, G.: Discriminating analysis of in vitro prostaglandin release by myometrial and luminal sides of the ewe endometrium. Prostaglandins, *25:*853–869, 1983.
24. Gross, T.S., et al.: Prostaglandin secretion by perifused porcine endometrium: Further evidence for an endocrine versus exocrine secretion of prostaglandins. Prostaglandins, *35:*327–341, 1988.
25. Franklin, K.J., Gross, T.S., Dubois, D.H., and Sharp, D.C.: In vitro prostaglandin secretion from luminal and myometrial sides of endometrium from cyclic and pregnant mares at day 14 post-estrus. Biol. Reprod. Suppl. 1, *40:*114, 1989.
26. Zavy, M.T., et al.: An investigation of the uterine luminal environment of nonpregnant and pregnant pony mares. J. Reprod. Fertil. Suppl., *27:*403–411, 1979.
27. Heap, R.B., Hamon, M., and Allen, W.R.: Studies on estrogen synthesis by the preimplantation equine conceptus. J. Reprod. Fertil. Suppl., *32:*343–352, 1982.
28. Perry, J.S., Heap, R.B., and Amoroso, E.C.: Steroid hormone production by pig blastocysts. Nature, *245:*45–47, 1973.
29. Frank, M., Bazer, F.W., Thatcher, W.W., and Wilcox, C.J.: A study of prostaglandin $F_2\alpha$ as the luteolysin in swine: IV. An explanation for the luteotrophic effect of estradiol. Prostaglandins, *15:*151–160, 1978.
30. Nishikawa, Y.: Studies on Reproduction in Horses. Tokyo, Japan Racing Association, 1959.
31. Berg, S.L., and Ginther, O.J.: Effect of estrogens on uterine tone and life span of the corpus luteum in mares. J. Anim. Sci., *47:*203–208, 1978.
32. Woodley, S.L., Burns, P.J., Douglas, R.H., and Oxender, W.D.: Prolonged interovulatory interval after estradiol treatment in mares. J. Reprod. Fertil. Suppl., *27:*205–209, 1979.
33. McDowell, K.J., Sharp, D.C., and Grubaugh, W.R.: Comparison of progesterone versus progesterone and estrogen on total and specific uterine proteins in pony mares. J. Reprod. Fertil. Suppl., *35:*335–342, 1987.
34. Godkin, J.D., et al.: Synthesis and release of polypeptides by pig conceptuses during the period of blastocyst elongation and attachment. Biol. Reprod., *27:*977–987, 1982.
35. Imakawa, K., et al.: Interferon-like sequence of ovine trophoblast protein secreted by embryonic trophectoderm. Nature, *330:*377–379, 1987.
36. Baker, C.B., Adams, M.H., and McDowell, K.J.: Lack of expression of alpha or omega interferons by the horse conceptus. J. Reprod. Fertil. Suppl., *44:*439–443, 1991
37. Sharp, D.C., et al.: The role of prostaglandins in the maternal recognition of pregnancy in mares. Anim. Reprod. Sci., *7:*269–282, 1984.
38. Ginther, O.J.: Mobility of the early equine conceptus. Theriogenology, *19:*603–661, 1983.
39. McDowell, K.J., et al.: Restricted conceptus mobility results in failure of pregnancy maintenance in mares. Biol. Reprod., *39:*340–348, 1988.
40. Zavy, M.T., et al.: Uterine protein secretions of the mare during the oestrous cycle and pregnancy. Identification of stage specific and hormonally induced polypetides using two-dimensional gel electrophoresis. J. Reprod. Fertil., *64:*199–207, 1982.
41. Hinrichs, K., Kenney, R.M., and Sharp, D.C.: Differences in protein content of uterine fluid related to duration of progesterone treatment in ovariectomized mares used as embryo transfer recipients. Equine Vet. J. Suppl., *8:*49–55, 1989.
42. Fliss, A.E., et al.: Regulation of the uteroferrin gene promoter in endometrial cells: Interactions between estrogen, progesterone and prolactin. Endocrinology, in press.
43. Simmen, R.C.M., Simmen, F.A., and Bazer, F.W.: Regulation of uterine secretory proteins: Evidence for differential induction of porcine uteroferrin and antileukoproteinase gene expression. Biol. Reprod., *44:*191–200, 1991.
44. Bazer, F.W., et al.: Role of conceptus secretory products in establishment of pregnancy. J. Reprod. Fertil., *76:*841–850, 1986.
45. McDowell, K.J., et al.: Characterization of an equine uteroferrin-like protein in the mare. J. Reprod. Fertil. Suppl., *32:*329–334, 1982.
46. Zavy, M.T., Bazer, F.W., Sharp, D.C., and Wilcox, C.J.: Uterine luminal proteins in the cycling mare. Biol. Reprod., *20:*689–698, 1979.
47. Roberts, R.M., and Bazer, F.W.: The properties, hormonal control and synthesis of uteroferrin, the purple protein of the pig uterus. *In* Steroid-induced Proteins. Edited by M. Beat. Amsterdam, Elsevier-North Holland, 1980, pp. 133–149.
48. Knight, J.W., Bazer, F.W., and Wallace, H.D.: Hormonal regulation of porcine uterine protein secretions. J. Anim. Sci., *36:*546–555, 1973.

CHAPTER 58

ENDOCRINOLOGY OF PREGNANCY

E.L. Squires

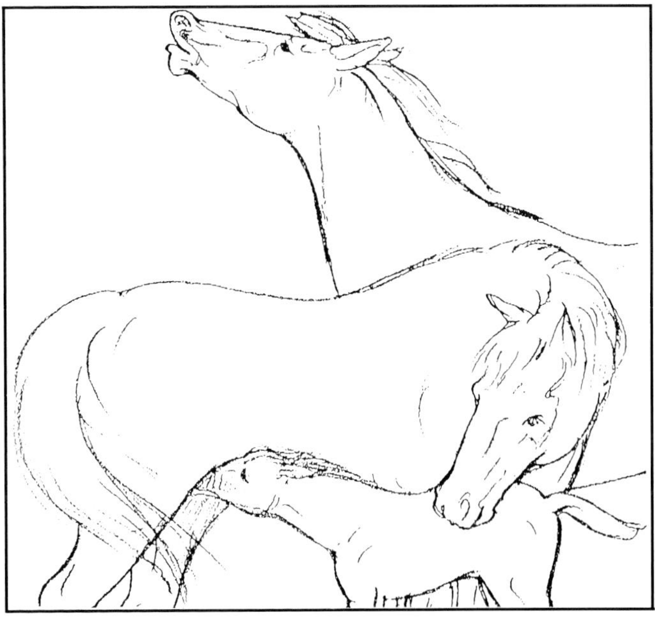

EVENTS DURING THE FIRST TRIMESTER

Continued high levels of progesterone are essential for pregnancy maintenance in mares. The mechanism used to ensure elevated concentrations of progesterone in the mare is unique. Initially the primary corpus luteum (1°CL), which forms at time of conception, is the sole source of progesterone. Secretion from the 1°CL results in an increase in progesterone from day 0 to day 8, then a gradual decrease until day 28 to day 30.[1–3] Apparently the 1°CL undergoes partial regression during this time of decreasing concentrations of progesterone. Concentrations of progesterone then increase dramatically between days 30 and 40.[1,3,4] The rise in secretion of progesterone is coincident with formation of endometrial cups and secretion of equine chorionic gonadotropins (eCG)[5–7] (see Chapter 9 for details). Squires and Ginther suggested that increased secretion of progesterone by the 1°CL may be from eCG stimulation.[3] Supporting evidence for the luteotropic role of eCG was the demonstration of increased secretion of progesterone from slices of 1°CL and the secondary corpus luteum (2°CL) incubated with eCG.[8] Progesterone concentrations peak at days 60 to 90 and plateau until days 120 to 150[1,3] (Fig. 58–1). Peak concentrations of progesterone are 10 to 20 ng/mL during days 60 to 90 of gestation. Elevated levels of progesterone at this time have been attributed to 2°CL formation. Formation of 2°CL during gestation is a unique feature of the mare. Numerous studies have attempted to determine the stimulus for follicular development in pregnant mares with subsequent 2°CL formation. In a series of studies, follicular and luteal changes in pregnant mares were characterized.[3,9,10] Number of large follicles (> 20 mm) and diameter of the largest follicle increased from days 20 to 60 of gestation. The diameter of largest follicle was significantly greater at day 60 than at any other day (Fig. 58–2). The decrease in number of large follicles after day 50 was attributed to formation of 2°CL. Allen examined per rectum the ovaries of 20 pregnant mares for the first 4 months of gestation.[11] Serial blood samples from 16 of the mares were assayed for eCG concentrations. A marked seasonal difference was noted for ovarian activity but not eCG concentrations. Those mares that conceived in April to July had greater ovarian and follicular sizes than mares that conceived between July and February. Because eCG is secreted during the time of greatest follicular activity, initially eCG was thought to be responsible for follicular activity in pregnant mares. However, growth of ovarian follicles during early pregnancy occurs before the earliest detectable appearance of eCG.[5] In addition, horse mares carrying donkey conceptuses have a complete absence of eCG and no 2°CL are present.[12] Therefore, other factors must be responsible for follicular growth in pregnant mares. Several authors have suggested that follicle-stimulating hormone (FSH), not eCG, is responsible for follicular activity in early pregnancy.[13,14] Surges in FSH were reported to occur at 10- to 11-day intervals during early pregnancy.[14]

Because follicular activity up to day 68 was similar in

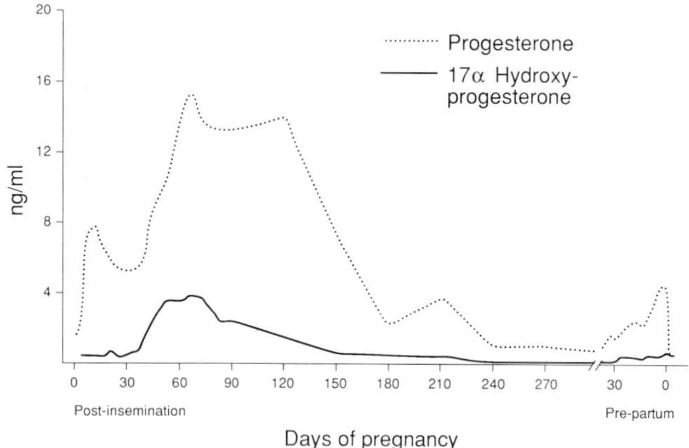

FIG. 58–1. Concentrations of progesterone (dotted line) and 17α-hydroxyprogesterone (solid line) during pregnancy in mares. (From Holtan, D.W., Nett, T.M., and Estergreen, V.L.: Plasma progestagens in pregnant mares. J. Reprod. Fertil. Suppl., *23:*419–424, 1975.)

hysterectomized and pregnant mares,[10] FSH would appear to be the major stimulus for follicular development during early pregnancy. The amount of follicular activity during early pregnancy is extremely variable among mares, with some mares having ovaries that contain several follicles larger than 30 mm and ovaries measuring more than 80 to 100 mm in length. Detailed studies in which concentrations of FSH were correlated with follicular activity have not been conducted. Regardless of the exact stimulus, once large follicles are formed, eCG induces maturation and ovulation or luteinization of follicles.

SECONDARY CORPORA LUTEA

Secondary corpora lutea first appear at approximately day 40 of pregnancy and the number of 2°CL increases up to approximately day 140. All 2°CL regress at days 180 to 200.[9,11,13] The number of 2°CL formed during pregnancy varies tremendously among mares, with some mares having no 2°CL and others forming 30 to 40 2°CL. The mean number of 2°CL reported in one study of pony mares was 2.8 at 70 days and 10.2 at 140 days.[9] It is still unclear as to what percentage of the 2°CL result from ovulations compared with luteinized anovulatory follicles. Squires et al. demonstrated that many of the 2°CL had nearly identical physical characteristics to the 1°CL (Fig. 58–3).[9] Those 2°CL that were mushroom shaped with a tract toward the ovulation fossa were considered to be formed from ovulatory follicles. Further evidence for occurrence of ovulation during pregnancy includes corpora hemorrhagica with ovulatory papillae, recently ovulated ova recovered from oviduct of mares necropsied, and a developmental change from a corpus hemorrhagicum to corpus luteum. Ginther reported that formation of 2°CL from ovulatory follicles is much more likely during days 40 to 70 than after day 70.[15] Secondary corpora lutea that are more rounded with a central cavity, filled with lymph-like fluid or plasma, are likely formed from unruptured, luteinized follicles. Regardless of the type of 2°CL, these structures secrete progesterone and are a supplementary source of progesterone in the pregnant mare. Contrary to earlier reports, the 1°CL does not regress after the first month of gestation but remains functional along with 2°CL until days 180 to 200. Apparently regression of all CL occurs once the luteotropic stimulus of eCG is no longer available. Concentrations of eCG are nearly nondetectable by day 120.[5]

EQUINE CHORIONIC GONADOTROPIN

Presence of eCG in the blood of pregnant mares was first reported in the 1930s and 1940s.[16] Since then, formation of endometrial cup and control of eCG secretion has been the subject of extensive investigation.[6–8,11,12,17] These investigators demonstrated that the trophoblastic cells of the chorionic girdle invade the uterine epithelium to form endometrial cups.[7] Endometrial cups become grossly visible as pale, swollen areas in uterine folds beginning at 38 to 40 days, with mature cups present on days 50 to 60 (Fig. 58–4). The mare eventually mounts an immune response, and the cups are sloughed from the uterine wall between 70 to 100 days. The cups are arranged in a semicircle in the horn of pregnancy with two sets present in mares with twins.

Equine chorionic gonadotropin is first detectable on days 37 to 42, with levels increasing rapidly to peak values at 55 to 65 days.[5] Thereafter concentrations decline slowly to nondetectable levels by days 120 to 150 (Fig. 58–5). Factors reported to influence eCG secretion from endometrial cups include size, parity, breed of mare, and number and genotype of fetuses.[5,17] Urwin and Allen examined the concentrations of FSH, luteinizing hormone (LH), eCG, and progesterone in mares and donkeys carrying normal intraspecies and mares carrying donkey conceptuses and donkeys carrying

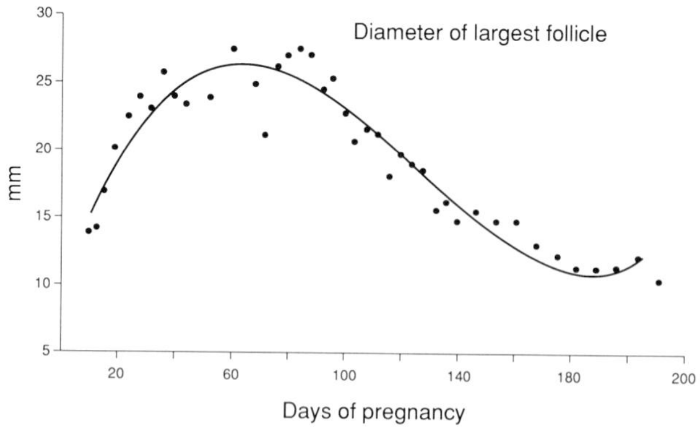

FIG. 58–2. Diameter of largest follicle in pregnant mares. (From Squires, E.L., Douglas, R.H., Steffenhagen, W.P., and Ginther, O.J.: Ovarian changes during the estrous cycle and pregnancy in mares. J. Anim. Sci., *38:*330–338, 1974.)

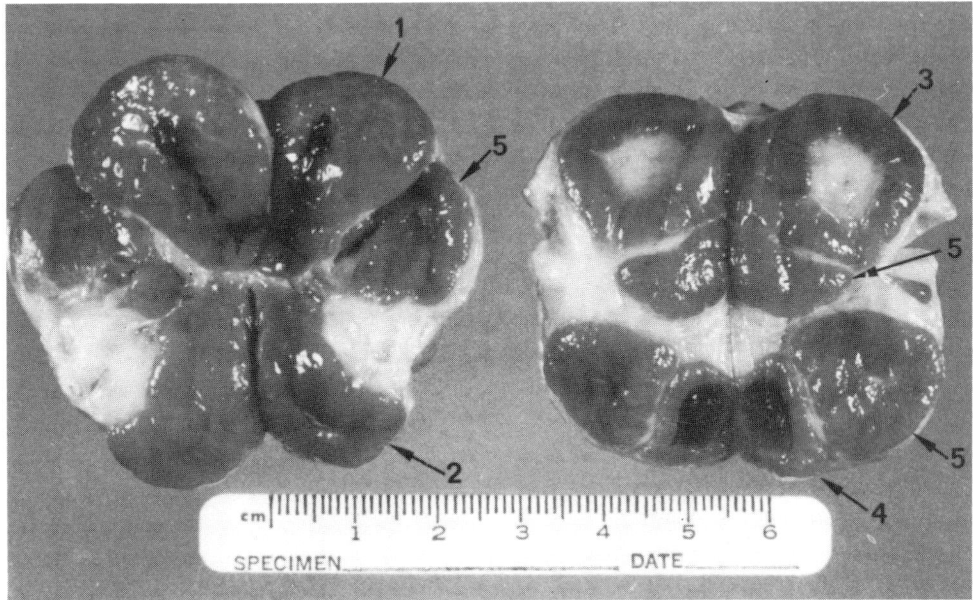

FIG. 58–3. Ovaries taken from a pregnant mare at day 100 of gestation, containing 1°CL with ink mark (1); a 2°CL, which is indistinguishable from 1°CL (2); 2°CL with spherical shape and central cavity (3); 2°CL with central cavity; secondary clot (4); and 2°CL that do not have noticeable central cavities (5). (From Squires, E.L., Douglas, R.H., Steffenhagen, W.P., and Ginther, O.J.: Ovarian changes during the estrous cycle and pregnancy in mares. J. Anim. Sci., *38:*330–338, 1974.)

horse conceptuses. These extraspecies pregnancies were prepared by embryo transfer. In horses carrying donkey conceptuses, a complete absence of eCG production was noted and seven of eight mares examined had no secondary rise in progesterone at the expected time.

The 1°CL and all 2°CL apparently regress at approximately days 180 to 200 of gestation. Although it has been suggested that CL regression occurs as a result of the disappearance of the luteotropin eCG, it seems unlikely because eCG levels are extremely depressed by day 120. Further studies are needed to determine the cause of CL regression during pregnancy.

SOURCES OF PROGESTERONE DURING LAST TRIMESTER

The importance of the ovary for pregnancy maintenance was determined in a series of studies in which the ovary was removed at various stages of pregnancy.[18] A total of 50 mares was bilaterally ovariectomized at selected days between 25 and 210 days of gestation over 3 separate years. After ovariectomy, the uterus was palpated daily for 4 days, on alternate days for the next 8 days, and once weekly thereafter. Abortion or resorption of the conceptus occurred in all 14 mares ovariectomized before day 50 of gestation. In contrast, 11 of 20 mares ovariectomized between 50 and 70 days maintained pregnancy, and pregnancy was not interrupted in any of 12 mares ovariectomized on day 140 or 210. Concentrations of progestagens dropped dramatically within 1 to 2 days of ovariectomy on days 25, 35, 45, 55, and 70. The results indicate that the primary (only) source of progesterone during early pregnancy is corpora lutea on the ovaries. The exact time when the placenta becomes a major source of progesterone has not been determined. However, progesterone concentrations in the uterine vein were significantly higher than those in jugular vein plasma at days 80 and 100, indicating a nonovarian source may be important in maintaining pregnancy after this time.[3]

Regression of all CLs (1° and 2°), around day 180, results in decreased concentrations of progesterone (Fig. 58–1). Holtan et al. reported a peak in progesterone at about day 64, and thereafter concentrations gradually decreased and reached a nadir between 240 and 300 days.[1] During the last 30 days of gestation, progesterone gradually increased to a peak 5 days before parturition. Another study reported the appearance of three unknown compounds between days 30 and 60.[19] Concentrations of these compounds increased gradually to day 300 (Fig. 58–6), but were not present during the postpartum period or during the estrous cycle. These compounds detected during pregnancy were later identified as 5α-pregnan-3,20-dione (DHP); 3β-hydroxy-5α-pregnan-20-one (3β-oL); and 20α-hydroxy-5α-pregnan-3-one (20α-oL).[19,20] In a subsequent study, the source of 5α-pregnanes during gestation in the mare was examined.[2] That study demonstrated that DHP was produced by the placenta and a maternal source, 20α-oL was primarily of maternal origin, and 3β-oL was formed primarily by the fetus. Because of the cross-

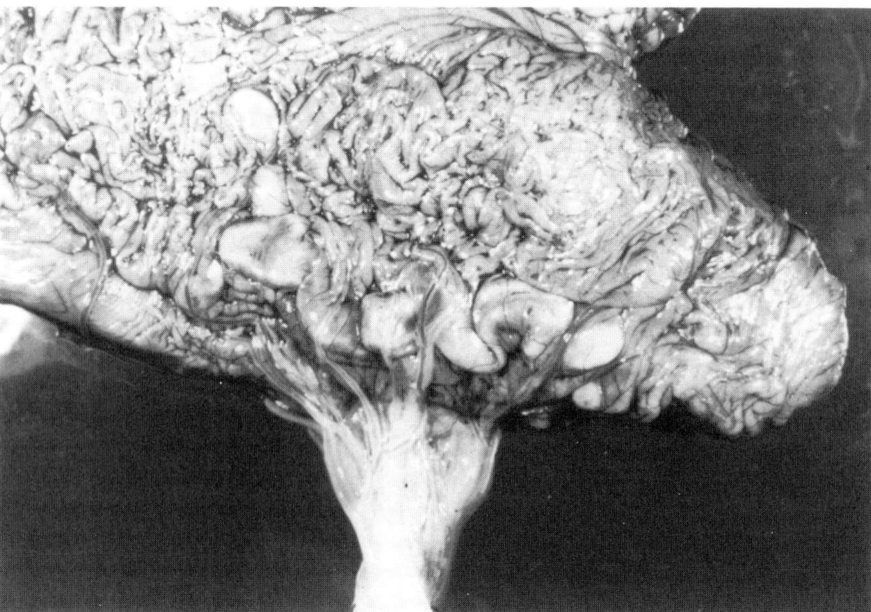

FIG. 58–4. Endometrial cups attached to the uterine lining.

reactivity of these compounds with progesterone, reported concentrations of progesterone during late pregnancy using conventional immunoassay techniques are questionable. This may explain the discrepancy in concentrations of progesterone reported in late pregnancy. Recently, gas chromatography mass spectrometry was used to quantify plasma progestagens during late pregnancy. Predominant steroids in plasma near term were 20α-hydroxy-5α-pregnan-3-one and 5α-pregnane-3β-20α-diol. These pregnanes were first detectable between 30 and 60 days of gestation and increased gradually until a more rapid increase 30 days prepartum. The exact function of these 5α-pregnanes apparently has not been determined.

ESTROGENS

Estrogenic compounds are contained in urine from mares during late pregnancy.[16,21] Eight estrogens have been isolated from urine; the most prominent are estrone, equilin, and equilenin. Equilin is only slightly less active biologically than estrone but more active than equilenin. Cox described a chemical method for assay of these estrogens in peripheral plasma.[22] Using gas-liquid chromatography, he reported a dramatic rise in concentrations of estrone during the fourth month of gestation. This high concentration was maintained for 4 to 5 months. During that same time, concentrations of equilin increased gradually, and a plateau was maintained from 180 days onward until a decline in the last month of pregnancy. In a similar study, concentrations of estrogens, LH, eCG, and prolactin were determined in peripheral circulation of mares throughout gestation.[23] Blood samples were collected from the jugular vein at 4-day intervals from mating until day 90 of gestation, monthly intervals until day 300, and thereafter at 4-day intervals until parturition. Samples were extracted and underwent chromatography such that estrone, equilin, and equilenin (E_1) eluted simultaneously and estradiol (E_2) eluted separately. Concentrations of E_1 and E_2 remained at basal levels until day 90. Concentrations of E_1 and E_2 increased steadily from days 90 to 210 (E_1) or 240 (E_2) of gestation. Thereafter, levels of E_1 and E_2 declined gradually until parturition (Fig. 58–7).

Although no significant changes in estrogen concentrations were reported by Nett et al.,[23] other researchers reported total (conjugated plus unconjugated) concentrations of estrogens during early gestation remained

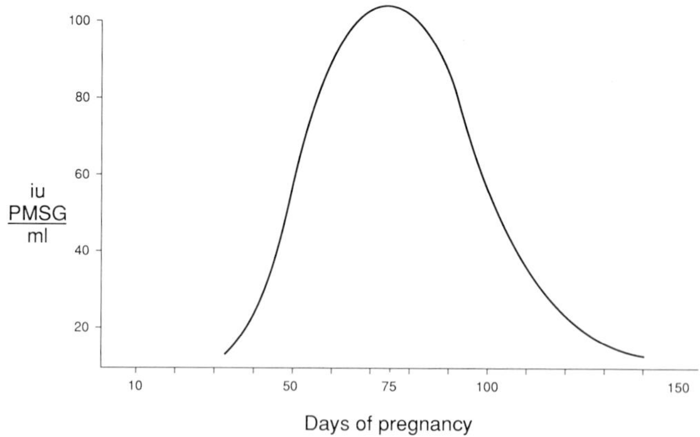

FIG. 58–5. Concentrations of equine chorionic gonadotropin. Peak concentrations at 55 to 65 days. (From Allen, W.R.: The immunological measurement of pregnant mare serum gonadotropin. J. Endocrinol., *43*:593–598, 1969.)

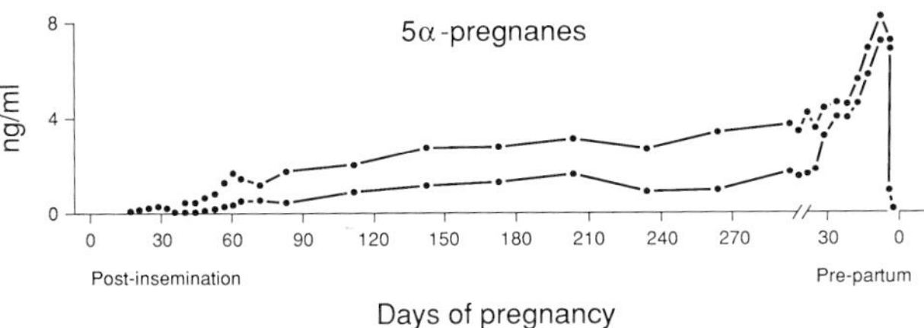

FIG. 58–6. Concentrations of two unidentified 5α-pregnanes during pregnancy in mares. The dots indicate more frequent sampling. (From Holtan, D.W., Nett, T.M., and Estergreen, V.L.: Plasma progestagens in pregnant mares. J. Reprod. Fertil. Suppl., *23*:419–424, 1975.)

similar to concentrations in diestrus until day 30, but rose significantly by day 45, were constant until day 64, and then increased sharply by day 90.[24–27] At exactly the same time estrogens rose around day 35, plasma progestagen levels increased. Interestingly, this is the same time eCG is first detected in mare's blood. Because concentrations of conjugated estrogens in mare plasma are 100 times higher than those of unconjugated estrogens, it is not surprising that Nett et al. failed to show any significant increase in estrogen secretion around day 37 when measuring unconjugated estrogens by radioimmunoassay.[23] Palmer and Joussett demonstrated that this rise in total estrogens during early pregnancy was of ovarian source because levels were depressed after ovariectomy.[28] The increase after day 60 was considered to be of fetoplacental origin, since levels at this time were not suppressed after ovariectomy. Raeside et al. stated that the large amount of estrogens in late pregnancy are formed by fetal gonads.[29] Urinary estrogens decreased markedly after fetal gonadectomy.

Measurement of estrone sulfate has been suggested as

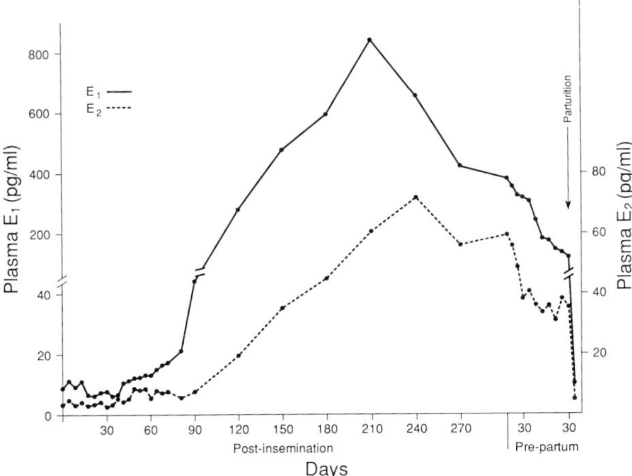

FIG. 58–7. Concentrations of estrone, equilin, equilenin (E_1) (solid line) and estradiol (E_2) (broken line) in pregnant mares throughout gestation. (From Nett, T.M., Holtan, D.W., and Estergreen, V.L.: Oestrogens, L.H., PMSG and prolactin in serum of pregnant mares. J. Reprod. Fertil. Suppl., *23*:457–462, 1975.)

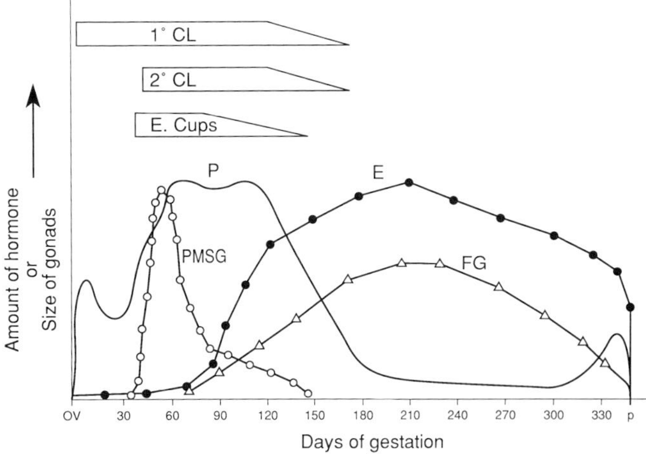

FIG. 58–8. Summary of hormonal events during gestation of mares. 1°CL, primary corpus luteum; 2°CL, secondary corpus luteum; E. cups, endometrial cups; P, progesterone; E, estrogens; PMSG, pregnant mares serum gonadotropin; FG, fetal gonads; OV, ovulation; and p, parturition.

an index for fetal viability.[24,27,30] Darenius et al. demonstrated that mares with fetal resorption had lower levels of eCG and slightly lower concentrations of estrone sulfate than those with normal fetal development.[26] Kindahl et al. stated that massive increase in estrone sulfate between days 75 and 100 is likely to occur only in mares with normal fetal development.[27] Recently, an enzyme immunoassay has been developed for measurement of plasma and fecal concentrations of estrogen conjugates.[30] Changes in estrogen conjugate were similar to those reported previously. Concentrations increased sharply beginning about day 35 of gestation, peaked at days 40 to 42, declined slightly through day 50 and increased rapidly after day 70. Stabenfeldt et al. suggested that the secretion before day 70 was of ovarian source and in response to eCG.[30] Workers in the same laboratory conducted a study to identify the ovarian compartment responsible for the estrogen rise between days 35 and 40 of pregnancy.[25] A total of 30 mares was divided into three groups: group 1 consisted of controls, group 2 was treated with Altrenogest from days 16 to 80, and group 3 was treated with a luteolytic dose of prostaglandin $F_2\alpha$ ($PGF_2\alpha$) on day 16 followed by Altrenogest treatment. Blood and urine were collected every second day from days 16 to 80. In group 3, 6 mares did not have an active CL from day 16 until after day 60, whereas the remaining 4 mares developed a new CL on days 32, 40, 43, and 49 of pregnancy, respectively. Mean concentrations of conjugated estrogens were not different between groups 1 and 2, and an increase in estrogens occurred between days 35 and 40. In contrast, mares in group 3 without an active CL had low levels of estrogen during the time of the expected rise. Thus increase in estrogen secretion observed between days 35 and 50 of pregnancy does not occur in the absence of a functional CL. Equine chorionic gonadotropin from the endometrial cups apparently stimulates luteal steroidogenesis, resulting in increased estrogen synthesis and secretion.

Figure 58-8 is a summary of hormonal events during pregnancy in the mare.

REFERENCES

1. Holtan, D.W., Nett, T.M., and Estergreen, V.L.: Plasma progestagens in pregnant mares. J. Reprod. Fertil. Suppl., *23*:419–424, 1975.
2. Moss, G.E., Estergreen, V.L., Becker, S.R., and Grant, B.D.: The source of the 5α-pregnanes that occur during gestation in mares. J. Reprod. Fertil. Suppl., *27*:511–519, 1979.
3. Squires, E.L., and Ginther, O.J.: Collection technique and progesterone concentration of ovarian and uterine venous blood in mares. J. Anim. Sci., *40*:275–281, 1975.
4. Kooistra, L., and Ginther, O.J.: Termination of pseudopregnancy by administration of prostaglandin $F_2\alpha$ and termination of early pregnancy by administration of prostaglandin $F_2\alpha$ or colchicine or by removal of embryo in mares. Am. J. Vet. Res., *37*:35–39, 1976.
5. Allen, W.R.: The immunological measurement of pregnant mare serum gonadotropin. J. Endocrinol., *43*:593–598, 1969.
6. Allen, W.R., and Moor, R.M.: The origin of the equine endometrial cups. I. Production of PMSG by fetal trophoblast cells. J. Reprod. Fertil., *29*:313–316, 1972.
7. Allen, W.R., Hamilton, D.W., and Moor, R.M.: The origin of equine endometrial cups. II. Invasion of the endometrium by trophoblast. Anat. Rec., *177*:485–501, 1973.
8. Squires, E.L., Stevens, W.B., Pickett, B.W., and Nett, T.M.: Role of pregnant mare serum gonadotropin in luteal function of pregnant mares. Am. J. Vet. Res., *40*:889–891, 1979.
9. Squires, E.L., Douglas, R.H., Steffenhagen, W.P., and Ginther, O.J.: Ovarian changes during the estrous cycle and pregnancy in mares. J. Anim. Sci., *38*:330–338, 1974.
10. Squires, E.L., Garcia, M.C., and Ginther, O.J.: Effects of pregnancy and hysterectomy on the ovaries of pony mares. J. Anim. Sci., *38*:823–830, 1974.
11. Allen, W.E.: Ovarian changes during early pregnancy in pony mares in relation to PMSG production. J. Reprod. Fertil. Suppl., *23*:425–428, 1975.
12. Urwin, V.E., and Allen, W.R.: Pituitary and chorionic gonadotrophic control of ovarian function during early pregnancy in equids. J. Reprod. Fertil. Suppl., *32*:371–381, 1982.
13. Allen, W.E.: Ovarian changes during gestation in pony mares. Equine Vet. J., *6*:135–138, 1974.
14. Irvine, C.H.G., and Evans, M.J.: The role of follicle stimulating hormone in early pregnancy in the mare. Proceedings of the International Congress on Animal Reproduction and Artificial Insemination, 1976, pp. 372–374.
15. Ginther, O.J.: Reproductive Biology of the Mare: Basic and Applied Aspects. Equiservices, Cross Plaines, WI, 1979.
16. Cole, H.H., and Saunders, F.J.: The concentration of gonad-stimulating hormone in blood serum and of oestrin in the urine throughout pregnancy in the mare. Endocrinology, *19*:199–208, 1935.
17. Allen, W.R.: Factors influencing pregnant mare serum gonadotropin production. Nature, *223*:64–66, 1969.
18. Holtan, D.W., Squires, E.L., Lapin, D.R., and Ginther, O.J.: Effect of ovariectomy on pregnancy in mares. J. Reprod. Fertil. Suppl., *27*:457–463, 1979.
19. Holtan, D.W., Ginther, O.J., and Estergreen, V.L.: 5α-pregnanes in pregnant mares. J. Anim. Sci., *41*:359, 1975.
20. Atkins, D.T., Sorensen, A.M., Jr., and Fleeger, J.L.: 5α-dihydroprogesterone in the pregnant mare. J. Anim. Sci., *39*:196–206, 1974.
21. Savard, K.: The estrogens of the pregnant mare. Endocrinology, *68*:411–416, 1961.
22. Cox, J.E.: Oestrone and equilin in the plasma of the pregnant mare. J. Reprod. Fertil. Suppl., *23*:463–468, 1975.
23. Nett, T.M., Holtan, D.W., and Estergreen, V.L.: Oestrogens, LH, PMSG and prolactin in serum of pregnant mares. J. Reprod. Fertil. Suppl., *23*:457–462, 1975.
24. Bosu, W.T.K., Turner, L., and Franks, T.: Estrone sulphate and progesterone concentrations in the peripheral blood of pregnant mares: Clinical implications. Proceedings of the International Congress on Animal Reproduction and Artificial Insemination, 1984, p. 78.
25. Daels, P.F., et al.: The corpus luteum: source of oestrogen during early pregnancy in the mare. J. Reprod. Fertil. Suppl., *44*:501–508, 1991.
26. Darenius, K., et al.: PMSG, progesterone and oestrone sulphate during normal pregnancy and early fetal death. J. Reprod. Fertil. Suppl., *32*:625–626, 1982.
27. Kindahl, H., Knudson, O., Madej, A., and Edqvist, L.E.: Progesterone prostaglandin $F_2\alpha$, PMSG and oestrone sulphate during early pregnancy in the mare. J. Reprod. Fertil. Suppl., *32*:353–359, 1982.
28. Palmer, E., and Joussett, B.: Urinary estrogens and plasma progesterone levels in nonpregnant mares. J. Reprod. Fertil. Suppl., *23*:213–221, 1975.
29. Raeside, J.I., Liptrap, R.M., and Milne, F.J.: Relationship of fetal gonads to urinary estrogen excretion by the pregnant mare. Am. J. Vet. Res., *34*:843–845, 1973.
30. Stabenfeldt, G.H., et al.: An oestrogen conjugate enzyme immunoassay for monitoring pregnancy in the mare: limitation of the assay between Days 40 and 70 of gestation. J. Reprod. Fertil. Suppl., *44*:37–43, 1991.

CHAPTER 59

DIAGNOSIS OF PREGNANCY

A.O. McKinnon

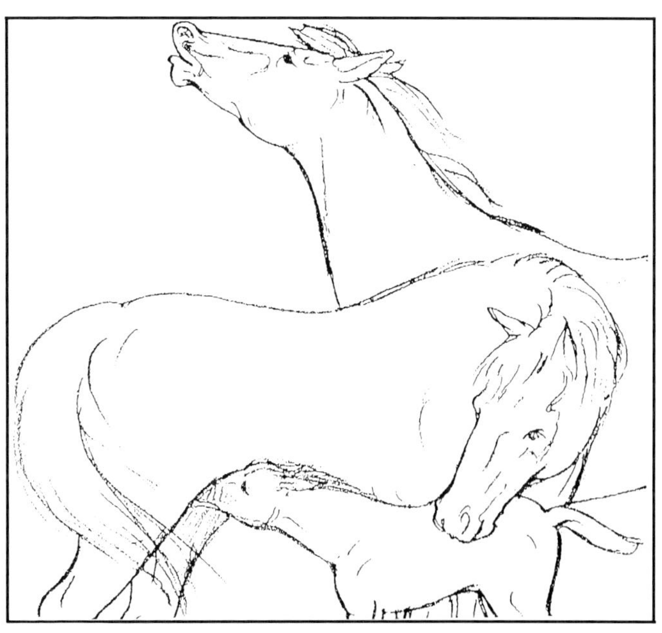

In mares, maternal recognition of pregnancy associated with production of an immunosuppressive agent, a pregnancy-specific protein called early pregnancy factor (EPF), may be as early as 48 h after conception.[1] Early pregnancy factor has been detected in mice, sheep, humans,[2] and mares,[1] and, in the future, may aid in detection of pregnancy and early embryonic death (EED). The second time for maternal recognition of pregnancy probably arises on or before day 5 or 6 after ovulation as fertilized ova are transported from the oviduct through the uterotubule junction into the uterus by 5 or 6 days after ovulation,[3] but unfertilized oocytes generally are retained in the oviducts.[4,5] The third time for maternal recognition (or reinforcement) of pregnancy occurs between 12 and 16 days. During this time, the conceptus is extremely mobile and probably secretes an antiluteolytic substance or prevents release of prostaglandin $F_2\alpha$ ($PGF_2\alpha$), thus maintaining the corpus luteum and preventing the mare from returning to estrus.[6–8]

Considerable pressure is put on the veterinarian to diagnose pregnancy as early as possible. However, because of the prevalence of EED attributable to uterine infection, hormonal imbalances, pathologic changes in uterine glands, endocrinologic imbalances, genetic abnormalities, and currently unrecognized factors, periodic examinations are necessary to monitor pregnancy. Accurate foaling rates can only be approximated when final pregnancy rates are determined after at least 50 days of fetal age. All methods of pregnancy diagnosis have limitations: (1) some laboratory tests for pregnancy may remain positive after EED has occurred, (2) ultrasonographic identification of a uterine cyst may be confused with an early embryonic vesicle; (3) unilateral twin pregnancies (fixed together) may not be detected utilizing rectal palpation, and (4) most methods of pregnancy diagnosis will fail to detect impending embryonic death.

PALPATION PER RECTUM

When mares that have been bred fail to return to estrus by 16 to 19 days after the last visible signs of estrus, pregnancy must be suspected. However, not all mares may be pregnant,[9] because of EED, prolonged maintenance of the corpus luteum (CL),[10] silent estrus, and occasionally, lactational anestrus after "foal heat."

Pregnancy of 15 to 18 days duration is recognized by determination of good to excellent uterine and cervical tone.[11] An embryonic vesicle at day 15 is approximately 15 to 20 mm in diameter and is not palpable per rectum. Uterine tone, particularly of the horns, is generally more pronounced, compared with that during diestrus or during prolonged maintenance of the CL. Progesterone-treated, ovariectomized, recipient mares pregnant from embryo transfer developed much more pronounced uterine tone at approximately 16 to 18 days of pregnancy (confirmed by ultrasonography) than did those progesterone-treated ovariectomized mares that were diagnosed as nonpregnant at the same interval after embryo transfer.[12] Thus, a fetal-maternal hormonal interaction probably is responsible for the increase in uterine tone.

With care and experience, palpation of the embryonic vesicle is possible by day 20 (Fig. 59–1A). The embryonic vesicle bulges ventrad in the uterus and most commonly will be located at one of the junctions between the uterine body and horn (corpus cornual junction). The technique for vesicle location is to palpate the ventral aspect of the uterus with the fingers bent over the cranial uterine margin and to reach under the uterine horns and body. The embryonic vesicle at day 20 is approximately 30 to 40 mm in diameter. Careful palpation should reveal a slight decrease in the tone of the uterine wall over the area of the vesicular bulge when compared with the remainder of the uterine horn. The fetus/embryo cannot be palpated at this stage because it is extremely small (1 to 2 mm). An early pregnancy can be confused with a large uterine cyst; however, with a cyst, the tone of the reproductive tract is usually not as firm.

Palpation per rectum is the most economical pregnancy-detection method when conducted after 30 days. The accuracy of rectal palpation for early determination of pregnancy depends largely on the skill of the examiner. By day 30 (Fig. 59–1B), the fetal-fluid bulge is 40 to 50 mm in diameter and more recognizable as a discreet fluid swelling at the corpus cornual junction. Uterine and cervical tone are excellent, but decreased tone associated with the vesicular bulge is more obvious. The slight enlargement of the previously gravid horn may, in instances of mares bred back at foal heat, result in improper diagnosis because of incomplete involution, which may resemble a fetal bulge. A distinct impression of fluid within the bulge is possible after 30 days and should permit detection of pregnancy rather easily. Veterinarians in equine reproductive practice must develop skills necessary to diagnose pregnancy at this stage. Elective abortion of twins before formation of the endometrial cups at approximately day 35 may be important, because abortion after this event occasionally results in failure of the mare to return to estrus for rebreeding during the current breeding season.

At day 40 (Fig. 59–1C), the fetal-fluid bulge is approximately 65 mm in diameter, and decreased tone at the site of the bulge associated with fetal growth is obvious. Tone of the pregnant uterine horn is slightly less than that observed previously, but cervical tone remains excellent. By day 50, the size of the fluid-filled vesicle is at least 8 cm in diameter and has extended from the

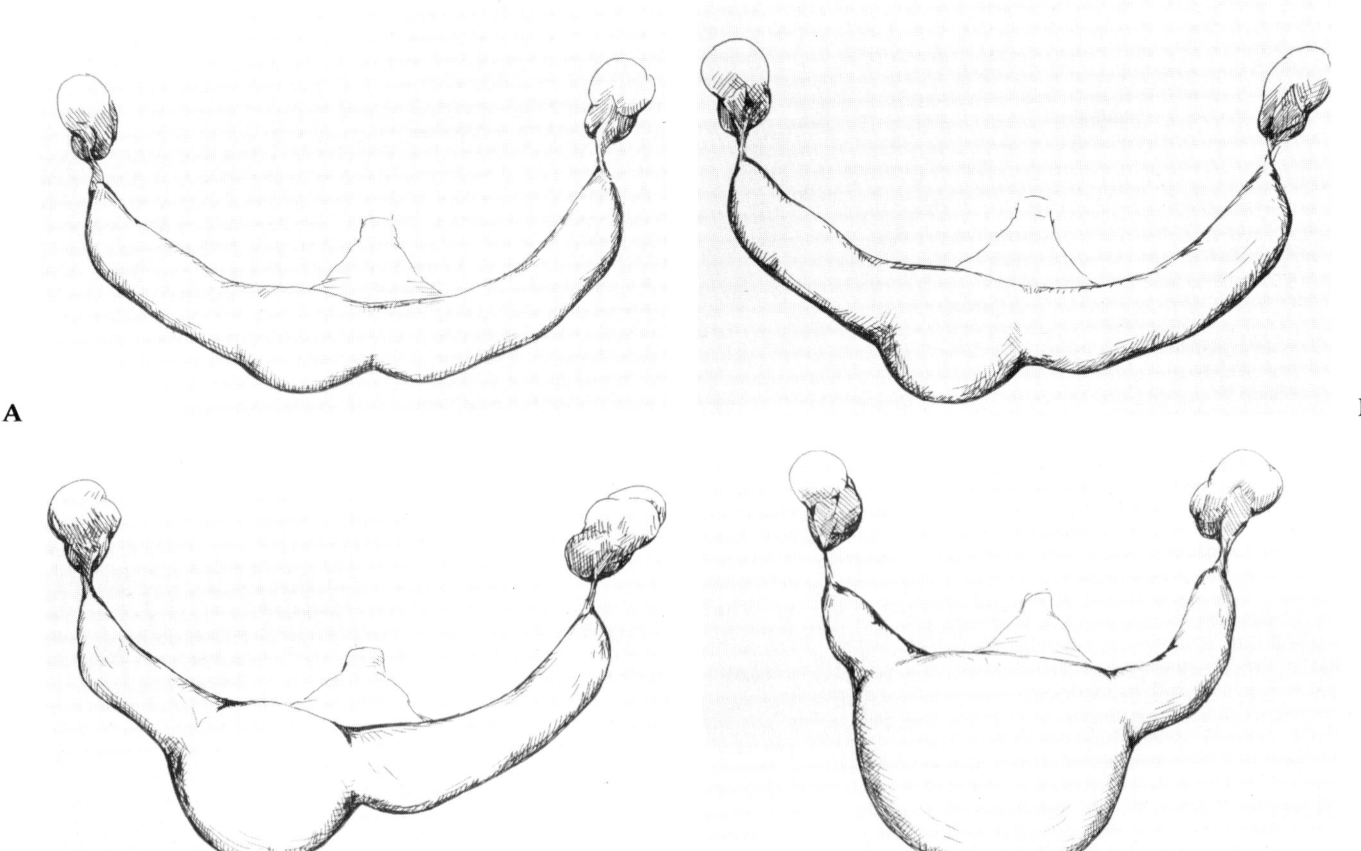

FIG. 59–1. Gross characteristics of the reproductive tract from a mare. *A*, 20 days pregnant; *B*, 30 days pregnant; *C*, 40 days pregnant, and *D*, 60 days pregnant.

corpus cornual junction into the uterine body. By day 60 (Fig. 59–1D), the tips of the uterine horn and cervix still have good tone. The bulge, which has extended into the uterine body, measures between 10 and 13 cm in diameter, and loss of tone to the bulge is more obvious. The uterus has begun a forward, downward descent into the abdomen, pulling the ovaries down and closer together. The bladder may then be mistaken for the fetal-fluid vesicle. By careful palpation, exploring the total reproductive tract continuously from one ovary to the other, the entire uterus can be examined, and pregnancy can be diagnosed.

Between days 60 and 100, the uterus increases in size and is drawn farther into the abdomen by the weight of the fetus. The ovaries are closer together and descend slightly more ventrad. At this stage, palpation, or ballottement, of the fetus is difficult. A mare with pyometra that has a fluid-filled uterus may be mistakenly diagnosed as pregnant, but lack of uterine tone, decreased elasticity of the uterus, and "sluggish, doughy feeling" to the uterine fluid and wall aid in distinguishing pyometra from pregnancy.

After approximately 3 to 4 months of gestation, the fetus can be palpated readily. However, on occasion, careful and repeated ballottement may be necessary to palpate the fetus. When the fetus can be palpated, or identified by ballottment, an approximate age determination can be made by comparison of the size of a fetal part such as head, trunk, or limbs with previously recorded age determinants.[13]

VAGINAL EXAMINATION

Pregnancy detection by speculum or manual examination of the vagina and cervix has been advocated.[14] Certain changes are suggestive of early pregnancy; however, none are totally diagnostic. A typical cervix in early pregnancy is elongated, tubular, and firm and can be ascertained by vaginal or rectal palpation of a mare that is 17 to 20 days pregnant. Cervical tone and consistency are generally more exaggerated in pregnant mares than in diestrous mares.

Frequently, pregnancy results in an increased "stickiness" of vaginal secretions. By 30 days of pregnancy, vaginal speculum examination reveals a pale cervix, comparable with that of a mare in anestrus. However, the cervix is obviously tight and frequently pulled to one side. Manual vaginal examination for detection of pregnancy may be performed late in gestation, particularly in mares that do not permit rectal palpation.[15] The aim of the examination is to detect fetal extremities. However, vaginal examination is recommended only as an adjunct to other methods of pregnancy diagnosis.

INDIRECT PREGNANCY TESTS

Many occasions exist when a blood or urine sample may be used to diagnose pregnancy. Generally, such tests are used to support diagnosis of pregnancy or when results of rectal palpation are inconclusive. Other reasons and situations for using laboratory methods for pregnancy detection are: (1) inadequate examination facilities; (2) vicious or nondomestic equids; (3) miniature horses or ponies; (4) horses that have had previous rectal tears; (5) to confirm early embryonic death; and (6) inexperienced veterinarians.

The interaction between maternal ovaries, fetal gonads, fetal-placental unit, and maternal pituitary gonadotropic hormones results in certain characteristic endocrinologic patterns during pregnancy (Fig. 59–2). Knowledge of these hormonal changes permits more accurate application and evaluation of laboratory tests. Laboratory tests are biologic, immunologic, or chemical, and most rely on detection of the hormones progesterone, equine chorionic gonadotropin (eCG) (pregnant mares serum gonadotropin, PMSG), or estrogens.

PROGESTERONE DETERMINATION

Progesterone is produced by the CL and is essential for maintenance of pregnancy. The CL forms from luteinization of granulosa cells and theca interna cells from the wall of an ovulated follicle.[16] The primary CL is formed from the follicle that released the oocyte that resulted in pregnancy. After fertilization and recognition of pregnancy, the primary CL is maintained beyond day 15 until at least days 140 through 180 and probably longer.[17] Progesterone concentrations peak at approximately day 20, then decline slightly until days 40 through 45 at which time secondary CL formation occurs, resulting in an increase until days 80 to 90 of pregnancy (Fig. 59–2). Secondary CL may form from follicles that are stimulated by 10-day cyclic pulses of follicle-stimulating hormone (FSH)[18] and either ovulation and/or luteinization[17] may be initiated by eCG.[19]

Ovariectomy commonly will result in abortion before day 60, but not after day 80.[20,21] Pregnancy is maintained by progestagens (progesterone-like compounds) produced by the placenta beginning around days 60 through 90, with increasing concentrations until parturition (Fig. 59–2).[22,23]

When used to assess ovarian activity in mares, measurement of plasma progesterone concentration is more reliable than observation of estrous behavior patterns.[24] Progesterone concentrations between 4 and 9 ng/mL are found 5 to 10 days after ovulation.[22,25] If pregnancy ensues, higher concentrations are observed during days 16 through 20, compared with mares destined to return to estrus. In one study, measurement of plasma progesterone concentration in nonpregnant and pregnant mares at days 13 through 17 and 18 through 22 postovulation was 3.08 and 0.77 ng/mL in nonpregnant and 7.72 and 6.34 ng/mL in pregnant mares, respectively.[26] Regardless, some pregnant mares will have low progesterone measurements and some diestrous mares (with a retained CL) will have high progesterone measurements similar to those in pregnant mares.[18,27]

There are numerous progestagens.[28] If the assay for progesterone is not highly specific,[22,23] many other

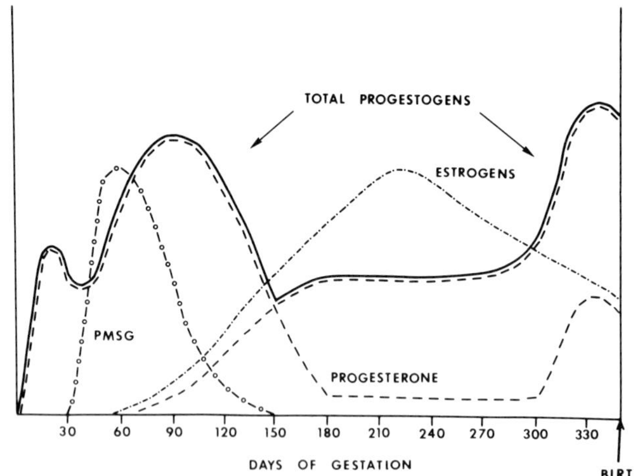

FIG. 59–2. Endocrinology of pregnancy.

progestagens, including progesterone metabolites, will be measured in the serum and milk, particularly after days 60 to 90 of gestation when progestagens from the fetal-placental unit are produced. In general, the radioimmunoassay (RIA) and enzyme-linked immunosorbent assay (ELISA) tests are highly specific for progesterone, whereas competitive protein-binding assay will detect progestagens as well.

EQUINE CHORIONIC GONADOTROPIN DETERMINATION

Equine chorionic gonadotropin is produced by fetal trophoblast cells that invade the maternal endometrium on days 35 through 38.[19] These cells form endometrial cups that are white, raised plaques that increase in size until day 60 of gestation.[29] A maternal immunologic rejection against the endometrial cups results in a decrease in their size beginning around day 70 and continuing through day 120 when they are no longer functional. Plasma concentrations of eCG parallel the growth and regression of endometrial cups and are first detected from days 35 through 40, peak between days 60 and 65, and decrease to low or nondetectable values between 120 and 150 days of gestation (Fig. 59–2). The exact function of eCG is undetermined. Current popular theory is that eCG is responsible for a luteinizing hormone-like activity that causes ovulation and/or luteinization of follicles, resulting in formation of secondary CL.[19] Serum analysis for eCG should be performed between days 40 and 110 of gestation.

When abortion occurs after day 35, endometrial cups may persist for a short time, which means that (1) eCG is still detectable and may be responsible for a false-positive pregnancy diagnosis and (2) these mares commonly fail to return to estrus. In addition, when mares are carrying a mule fetus, the immunologic rejection of the endometrial cups occurs much earlier and extremely low or nondetectable concentrations of eCG exist despite the persistence of pregnancy.[30]

Biologic tests rely on the effects of eCG obtained from mare serum on the reproductive tract of laboratory animals, e.g., stimulation of rabbit ovaries (Friedman test),[31] rat uterus,[32] mouse uterus,[33] and production of spermatozoa from male toads.[34] A practical, inexpensive bioassay involves the injection of 0.5 to 1 mL of mare serum subcutaneously into immature, 21-day-old female mice. Saline-injected mice serve as controls. The presence of eCG will cause enlargement and congestion of the mouse uterus compared with controls when examined at 72 h.[15] The sensitivity of the biologic assays is, in general, good. However, little diagnostic application exists for these assays, because of expense and time involved, ethical considerations, and excellent immunologic testing methods now available.

Immunologic methods of pregnancy diagnosis generally rely on an antigen-antibody reaction. The antibody is produced by hyperimmunization of another animal such as a rabbit, with eCG as the antigen.[35] Some reported immunologic assay systems are the mare immunologic pregnancy (MIP) test,[36–40] RIA,[41,42] direct latex agglutination (DLA),[43] and ELISA.[44–46] In addition, a radioreceptor assay has been described.[47]

Serum from pregnant mares (diagnosed by ultrasonography) has been used to compare the efficacy of the MIP test (Diamond Laboratories, Des Moines, IA), DLA assay (Rapitex, Institut Behring, Behringwerke, Morhing, Germany), and ELISA (D-TEC-MP ELISA test, Pitman-Moore Co., Washington Crossing, NJ).[48] The MIP test, or hemagglutination inhibition (HI) test, is based on the principle of inhibition of agglutination of sensitized red blood cells. If eCG is present in sufficient concentration in the serum, it competitively binds to the eCG antibody, thus preventing agglutination of the red blood cells. For the DLA test, if eCG is present in the serum, agglutination of polystyrene particles occurs within 2 min.[43,49] ELISA requires a specific antibody for eCG be adhered to a solid phase such as a microplate. If eCG is present in the mare's serum, it serves as an antigen and binds to the plate containing the antibody. An enzyme reaction and color change are used to quantitate the amount of eCG. None of the 7 samples from pregnant mares obtained on day 35 resulted in positive reactions with the HI or DLA assay, but 3 of 7 (43%) were diagnosed positive, using ELISA (Table 59–1).[48] On day 40, a greater ($p < 0.01$) number of mares was detected pregnant with the ELISA (16/16, 100%) compared with the HI (5/16, 31%) or DLA assay (6/16, 37%). Between days 45 and 100, no differences in efficacy among the 3 tests were found. At 50 days and later, efficacy of the 3 tests ranged from 90 to 100%. Sera collected from 10 nonpregnant mares were used as control samples. None of these samples resulted in positive reaction. The authors concluded that all 3 tests were simple, quick, methods that could be used for detection of pregnancy in mares.[48] Although the DLA assay was the easiest to conduct, all 3 assay procedures could be performed in <2 h, and the ELISA, because of increased sensitivity could be used to detect pregnancy slightly earlier than the other 2 methods.

ESTROGEN DETERMINATION

A minor maternal (ovarian) production of estrogen occurs between days 35 and 60 but appears to have little diagnostic significance. A major increase in plasma estrogen concentration occurs after day 60.[29,50] This increase originates from the fetal-placental unit and thus is not affected by ovariectomy. Concentrations of estrogen in urine and serum peak at about day 210 of gestation[42] (Fig. 59–2) and are thought to come from fetal gonads, which are enlarged at this time. If fetal gonads are removed, plasma estrogen concentrations drop immediately to low levels.[51]

In general, estrogen detection in serum or urine has only limited value for pregnancy diagnosis because it becomes reliable only relatively late in pregnancy. Earlier it was not recommended to test for estrogens before 150 days of pregnancy, but measurement of estrone sulfate (conjugated) for diagnosis of pregnancy and evidence of a viable conceptus is now advocated after day 60 of pregnancy.[52–54] Fetal death results in an immediate decrease in estrone sulfate concentration.[53] If a mare in the second or third trimester of pregnancy begins to lactate, measurement of estrone sulfate may provide an index of fetal viability. This may be particularly useful when other tests of fetal viability such as ultrasonography or electrocardiographic monitoring are not available.

Biologic, chemical, and immunologic tests are available for estrogen determination. Biologic tests such as increased nipple length in guinea pigs, or induction of vaginal cytologic findings typical of estrus in immature or ovariectomized mice are seldom used. They have been replaced by chemical tests, largely because of cost and time.

Chemical tests for urinary estrogen rely on color changes and fluorescence in the presence of warm, concentrated sulfuric acid. The tests of Cuboni,[55] Kober,[56] and Lunaas[57] have been compared,[58] and for field use the Cuboni method was best, being easy to interpret and simple to perform. The Kober method was too cumbersome, and the Lunaas method unreliable.

Radioimmunoassay can be used for determination of plasma total estrogen (conjugated plus unconjugated) concentration[50] or urinary estrone conjugates.[52] The method described for plasma analysis[50] requires enzymatic hydrolysis and extraction and may not reveal all estrone conjugates because the concentration of estrone sulfate is 1000 times higher in the urine.[52] Direct conjugated estrogen measurement on serum or milk has been described,[54,59] and differentiation between pregnancy and estrus was possible after approximately 50 days. In mares, an enzymatic determination of unconjugated estrogens in the feces for pregnancy diagnosis has been described.[60] Pregnancy was confirmed after 120 days of gestation, and because this technique may be totally noninvasive to the mare, some benefits to the equine reproductive industry may be realized.

TABLE 59–1. EFFICACY OF IMMUNOLOGICAL TESTS FOR EARLY PREGNANCY DETECTION IN MARES*

	STAGE OF GESTATION (DAYS)							
	35	40	45	50	70	80	90	100
Test	Percent Positive Diagnosis							
MIP†	0	31[a]‡	60	91	89	96	100	100
DLA§	0	37[a]	80	89	91	92	100	100
ELISA	43	100[b]	100	100	100	100	100	100
Total Number of mares	7	16	7	46	35	26	16	3

*Mares were confirmed pregnant with ultrasonography before immunologic testing.

†MIP = Mare immunological pregnancy test (also known as hemagglutination inhibition).

‡Means within column with different superscripts differ ($p < 0.01$).

§DLA = direct latex agglutination test.

(Adapted from Squires, E.L., Voss, J.L., and Villahoz, M.D.: Immunological methods for pregnancy detection in mares. Proc. Am. Assoc. Equine Pract., 45–51, 1983.)

ULTRASONOGRAPHY

The efficacy of ultrasonography for detection of pregnancy has been well documented.[61–69] A more detailed review of ultrasonography, including pregnancy diagnosis, is presented in Chapter 31. In addition to detection of pregnancy, twins, and EED, ultrasonography of the uterus can be used to monitor pathologic uterine changes, such as fluid accumulation.[65,70,71] Furthermore, uterine size can be measured and assessment of postpartum uterine involution can be used to manipulate breeding strategies.[70] Stage of estrus, status of preovulatory follicles, confirmation of ovulation, in vivo morphologic characteristics of the CL, and ovarian irregularities and pathologic features can also be evaluated with ultrasonography.[72]

For diagnosis of pregnancy at 11 to 12 days, accurate ovulation dates, careful examination and a 5- or 7.5-MHz transducer are needed.[63] However, because of embryonic loss in early pregnancy, the discontinuation of teasing mares after initial pregnancy examination is inappropriate. From a practical standpoint, the first examination could be postponed until approximately 18 to 20 days, thus eliminating scanning of mares that are destined to return to estrus. However, a major exception would be scanning of breeds that have a history of twinning or multiple ovulation (Thoroughbreds). These mares should be scanned between days 12 to 15 after ovulation to manage manual embryonic reduction most effectively. The frequency of subsequent scans will depend on such factors as availability of the mare, presence of twins, size and quality of the vesicle, and economics.

Regardless of side of entry into the uterus, the early equine conceptus is highly mobile and moves between the two uterine horns and uterine body.[73] Mobility begins to decrease by day 15, and after day 17, transuterine migration no longer can be detected (stage of fixation).[74] The yolk sac vesicle is spherical before day 16 but subsequently becomes quite irregular. Growth of the vesicle reaches a plateau between days 17 through 24, and then resumes at a slightly slower rate.[63]

When performing ultrasonography on mares that have been pregnant for 11 to 12 days, the transducer should be moved slowly so the image or tissue slice examined by the beam, which is only 2 to 3 mm wide, does not pass over the vesicle too rapidly. A systematic technique should be developed to avoid omitting or scanning too rapidly a portion of the reproductive tract. The most common mistakes associated with early pregnancy diagnosis are failure to detect a vesicle and inability to differentiate the vesicle from a uterine cyst. Inexperienced examiners often fail to detect small vesicles located in the caudal uterine body. Operator experience and quality of equipment are helpful in distinguishing a pregnancy from a cyst. In addition, accurate determination of vesicle location and subsequent reexamination before the end of the mobility phase are often rewarding.

The fetus within the vesicle is first detected ultrasonographically from days 20 through 23 and is commonly observed on the ventral aspect of the vesicle. The heartbeat has been reported to be detected around day 24,[61] although in our experience with more recent equipment the heartbeat should be observed as soon as the fetus is visible. An important aspect of embryologic development is the growth of the allantois, recognizable on day 24, and concurrent with its expansion, the contraction of the yolk sac. The interplay of growth between these two fluid-filled structures results in the fetus moving from the ventral (day 22) to the dorsal (day 40) aspects of the vesicle. By day 40, the yolk sac has degenerated, and the umbilical cord elongates from the dorsal pole, allowing the fetus to gravitate back to the ventral floor, where it is seen in dorsal recumbency from day 50 onward (see Chapter 31). The optimum time for determination of fetal sex would appear to be between days 59 and 78.[75] However, similar to some other aspects of reproductive ultrasonography, this technique is limited by quality of equipment and operator experience.

The apposition of the yolk sac and allantois result in an ultrasonographically visible line, normally orientated horizontally. On occasion, this junction can be observed in a vertical configuration, but apparently this has no deleterious effect on pregnancy. Vesicle walls of twin embryos when in contact, generally appear as an ultrasonographically visible, vertically orientated line (see Chapter 31). Knowledge of approximate gestational duration and growth characteristics of the conceptus helps the clinician decide between an abnormally oriented singleton and twins with apposition of both yolk sacs.

It is apparent from the preceding discussion that accurate aging of the young fetus is possible by ultrasonographic examination to assess development. The recognition of normal development and a heartbeat is critical to the diagnosis of pregnancy. Absence of a heartbeat can be observed in an otherwise normally developing fetus. In these cases, manual examination invariably suggests a normally developing pregnancy. However, deterioration of the conceptus and loss of uterine tone occur later.[76] Absence of heartbeat should be confirmed by a subsequent examination at least 24 h apart before diagnosis of EED is followed by $PGF_2\alpha$ administration. Because of these occurrences, we believe that the practice of early pregnancy diagnosis with ultrasonography and a final manual examination at approximately 45 days is obsolete and in many cases a disservice to the client. The client deserves to make a decision in regard to economics and practicality only after having limitations of each diagnostic procedure thoroughly explained.

REFERENCES

1. Gidley-Baird, A.A., and O'Neil, C.: Early pregnancy detection in the mare. Equine Vet. Data, *3:*42, 1982.
2. Rolfe, B.E.: Detection of fetal wastage. Fertil. Steril., *37:*655–660, 1982.
3. Oguri, N., and Tsutsumi, Y.: Non-surgical egg transfer in mares. J. Reprod. Fertil., *41:*313–320, 1974.
4. Betteridge, K.J., and Mitchell, D.: Direct evidence of retention of unfertilized ova in the oviduct of the mare. J. Reprod. Fertil., *39:*145–148, 1974.
5. Van Niekerk , C.H., and Gerneke, W.H.: Persistence and parthenogenetic cleavage of tubal ova in the mare. Onderstepoort J. Vet. Res., *33:*195–232, 1966.
6. Hershman, L., and Douglas, R.H.: The critical period for the maternal recognition of pregnancy in pony mares. J. Reprod. Fertil. Suppl., *27:*395–401, 1979.
7. McDowell, K.J., Sharp, D.C., Peck, L.S., and Cheves, L.L.: Effect of restricted conceptus mobility on maternal recognition of pregnancy in mares. Equine Vet. J. Suppl., *3:*23–24, 1985.
8. Sharp, D.C., and McDowell, K.J.: Critical events surrounding the maternal recognition of pregnancy in mares. Equine Vet. J. Suppl., *3:*19–22, 1985.
9. Lensch, J.: The early clinical diagnosis of pregnancy in mares. Proc. Am. Assoc. Equine Pract., 197–200, 1967.
10. Stabenfeldt, G.H., et al.: Spontaneous prolongation of luteal activity in the mare. Equine Vet. J., *6:*158–163, 1974.
11. Van Niekerk, C.H.: Early clinical diagnosis of pregnancy in mares. J. S. Afr. Vet. Med. Assoc., *36:*53–58, 1965.
12. McKinnon, A.O., Squires, E.L., Carnevale, E.M., and Hermenet, M.J.: Ovariectomized steroid-treated mares as embryo transfer recipients and as a model to study the role of progestins in pregnancy maintenance. Theriogenology, *29:*1055–1064, 1988.
13. Bergin, W.C., Gier, H.T., Frey, R.A., and Marion, G.B.: Developmental horizons and measurements useful for age determination of equine embryos and fetuses. Proc. Am. Assoc. Equine Pract., 179–196, 1967.
14. Roberts, S.J.: Gestation and pregnancy diagnosis in the mare. *In* Current Therapy in Theriogenology. Edited by D.A. Morrow. Philadelphia, W.B. Saunders, 1980, pp. 736–746.
15. Asbury, A.C.: The reproductive system. *In* Equine Medicine and Surgery. Vol. 2. 3rd ed. Edited by R.A. Mansmann, E.S McAllister, and P.W. Pratt. Santa Barbara, CA, American Veterinary Publications, 1982, pp. 1305–1367.
16. Ginther, O.J.: Reproductive Biology of the Mare: Basic and Applied Aspects. Equiservices, Cross Plaines, WI, 1979.
17. Squires, E.L., and Ginther, O.J.: Follicular and luteal de-

velopment in pregnant mares. J. Reprod. Fertil. Suppl., *23:*429–433, 1975.
18. Evans, M.J., and Irvine, C.H.G.: Serum concentrations of FSH, LH and progesterone during the oestrous cycle and early pregnancy in the mare. J. Reprod. Fertil. Suppl., *23:*193–200, 1975.
19. Allen, W.R.: Hormonal control of early pregnancy in the mare. Vet. Clin. North Am. Large Anim. Pract. Equine Reprod., *2:*291–302, 1980.
20. Holtan, D.W., Squires, E.L., Lapin, D.R., and Ginther, O.J.: Effect of ovariectomy on pregnancy in mares. J. Reprod. Fertil. Suppl., *27:*457–463, 1979.
21. Shideler, R.K., Squires, E.L., Voss, J.L., and Eikenberry, D.J.: Exogenous progestin therapy for maintenance of pregnancy in ovariectomized mares. Proc. Am. Assoc. Equine Pract., 211–220, 1981.
22. Ganjam, V.K., and Kenney, R.M.: Peripheral blood plasma levels and some unique metabolic aspects of progesterone in pregnant and non-pregnant mares. Proc. Am. Assoc. Equine Pract., 263–276, 1975.
23. Holtan, D.W., Nett, T.M., and Estergreen, V.L.: Plasma progestins in pregnant, postpartum and cyclic mares. J. Anim. Sci., *40:*251–260, 1975.
24. Hunt, B., Lein, D.H., and Foote, R.H.: Monitoring of plasma and milk progesterone for evaluation of postpartum estrous cycles and early pregnancy in mares. J. Am. Vet. Med. Assoc., *172:*1298–1302, 1978.
25. Hughes, J.P., Stabenfeldt, G.H., and Evans, J.W.: Clinical and endocrine aspects of the estrous cycle of the mare. Proc. Am. Assoc. Equine Pract., 119–151, 1972.
26. Sato, K.: Relationship between progesterone and oestrogens in serum for early pregnancy diagnosis in mares. Zuchthygiene, *12:*165–171, 1977.
27. Darenius, K., et al.: PMSG, progesterone and oestrone sulphate during normal pregnancy and early fetal death. J. Reprod. Fertil. Suppl., *32:*625–626, 1982.
28. Neeley, D.P.: Equine gestation. *In* Equine Reproduction. Edited by D.P. Neeley, I.K.M. Liu, and R.B. Hillman, Princeton Junction, NJ, Veterinary Learning Systems, 1983, pp. 57–70.
29. Cole, H.H., and Saunders, F.J.: The concentration of gonad-stimulating hormone in blood serum and of oestrin in the urine throughout pregnancy in the mare. Endocrinology, *19:*199–208, 1935.
30. Taylor, T.S., and Honey, P.G.: Use of immunological pregnancy testing in mares carrying mule fetuses. Equine Pract., *2:*25–28, 1980.
31. Barben, E.E.: A practical laboratory test for diagnosing pregnancy in the mare. Vet. Med., *64:*231–233, 1969.
32. Cole, H.H., and Hart, G.H.: The potency of blood serum of mares in progressive stages of pregnancy in effecting the sexual maturity of the immature rat. Am. J. Physiol., *93:*57–68, 1930.
33. McCaughey, W.J., Hanna, J., and O'Brien, J.J.: A comparison of three laboratory tests for pregnancy diagnosis in the mare. Equine Vet. J., *5:*94–95, 1973.
34. Berry, R.O., and Spalding, J.F.: The pregnancy test for mares using the male toad (Bufo). J. Anim. Sci., *11:*788–789, 1952.
35. Wide, M., and Wide, L.: Diagnosis of pregnancy in mares by an immunological method. Nature, *198:*1017–1018, 1963.
36. Allen, W.R.: A quantitative immunological assay for pregnant mare serum gonadotropin. J. Endocrinol., *43:*581–591, 1969.
37. Chak, R.M., and Bruss, M.: The MIP test for diagnosis of pregnancy in mares. Proc. Am. Assoc. Equine Pract., 53–55, 1968.
38. Jeffcott, L.B., Atherton, J.G., and Mingay, J.: Equine pregnancy diagnosis. A comparison of two methods for the detection of gonadotrophin in serum. Vet. Rec., *84:*80–82, 1969.
39. Mitchell, D.: Early fetal death in serum gonadotrophin test for pregnancy in the mare. Proc. Am. Assoc. Equine Pract., 55–65, 1970.
40. Parker, W.G., Sullivan, J.J., and Larson, L.L.: Comparison of the methods of rectal palpation and haemagglutination-inhibition assay for diagnosis of pregnancy in mares. J. Reprod. Fertil. Suppl., *23:*489–493, 1975.
41. Menzer, C., and Schams, D.: Radioimmunoassay for PMSG and its application to in-vivo studies. J. Repro. Fertil., *55:*339–345, 1979.
42. Nett, T.M., Holtan, D.W., and Estergreen, V.L.: Oestrogens, LH, PMSG and prolactin in serum of pregnant mares. J. Reprod. Fertil. Suppl., *23:*457–462, 1975.
43. De Coster, R., Cambiaso, C.L., and Masson, P.L.: Immunological diagnosis of pregnancy in the mare by agglutination of latex particles. Theriogenology, *13:*433–436, 1980.
44. Aloisi, G., Schmied, L., and Villahoz, M.D.: New method for detection of pregnancy in the mare. Proc. Sem. Mil. Vet., Buenes Aires, 7, 1981.
45. Aloisi, G., Schmied, L., and Villahoz, M.D.: Nuevo methodo de Deteccion de la prenez en la yegua. Rev. Mil. Ved., *140:*197, 1982.
46. Mia, A.S., Tierney, M., and Rohovsky, M.W.: A rapid micro ELISA test for detection of equine pregnancy. Proceedings of the Conference on Research Workers in Animal Diseases. Chicago, 1981, p. 18.
47. Fay, J.E., and Douglas, R.H.: The use of radioreceptor assay for the detection of pregnancy in the mare. Theriogenology, *18:*431–444, 1982.
48. Squires, E.L., Voss, J.L., and Villahoz, M.D.: Immunological methods for pregnancy detection in mares. Proc. Am. Assoc. Equine Pract., 45–51, 1983.
49. Frank, W.: Eine neue Methode der hormonal-immunologischen Trachtigkeits-diagnose bei der Stute mit Hilfe eines Latex-Testes, Prakt. Tierarzt., *63:*233–241, 1982.
50. Terqui, M., and Palmer, E.: Oestrogen pattern during early pregnancy in the mare. J. Reprod. Fertil. Suppl., *27:*441–446, 1979.
51. Raeside, J.I., Liptrap, R.M., and Milne, F.J.: Relationship of fetal gonads to urinary estrogen excretion by the pregnant mare. Am. J. Vet. Res., *34:*843–845, 1973.
52. Evans, K.L., et al.: Pregnancy diagnosis in the domestic horse through direct urinary estrone conjugate analysis. Theriogenology, *22:*615–620, 1984.
53. Jeffcott, L.B., et al.: Changes in maternal hormone concentrations associated with induction of fetal death at day 45 of gestation in mares. J. Reprod. Fertil. Suppl., *35:*461–467, 1987.
54. Sist, M.D., Williams, J.F., and Geary, A.M.: Pregnancy diagnosis in the mare by immunoassay of estrone sulfate in serum and milk. J. Equine Vet. Sci., *7:*20–23, 1987.
55. Cuboni, E.: A rapid pregnancy diagnoses test for mares. Clin. Vet. (Milano), *57:*85–93, 1934.
56. Kober, S.: Eine kolorimetrische bestimmung des bruns thromons (menformon). Biochem. Z., *239:*209, 1931.
57. Lunaas, T.: A rapid method for the quantitative estimation of urinary oestrogens in the pregnant mare. Acta Chem. Scand., *16:*2064–2065, 1962.
58. Cox, J.E., and Galina, C.S.: A comparison of the chemical

tests for oestrogens used in equine pregnancy diagnoses. Vet. Rec., *86:*97–100, 1970.

59. Hyland, J.H., Wright, P.J., and Manning, S.J.: An investigation of the use of plasma oestrone sulphate concentrations for the diagnosis of pregnancy in mares. Aust. Vet. J., *61:*123, 1984.
60. Bamberg, E., et al.: Enzymatic determination of unconjugated oestrogens in faeces for pregnancy diagnosis in mares. Equine Vet. J., *16:*537–539, 1984.
61. Allen, W.E., and Goddard, P.J.: Serial investigations of early pregnancy in pony mares using real time ultrasound scanning. Equine Vet. J., *16:*509–514, 1984.
62. Chevalier, F.E., and Palmer, E.: Ultrasonic echography in the mare. J. Reprod. Fertil. Suppl., *32:*423–430, 1982.
63. Ginther, O.J.: Ultrasonic evaluation of the reproductive tract of the mare: The single embryo. J. Equine Vet. Sci., *4:*75–81, 1984.
64. Pipers, F.S., et al.: Ultrasonography as an adjunct to pregnancy assessments in the mare. J. Am. Vet. Med. Assoc., *184:*328–334, 1984.
65. McKinnon, A.O., Squires, E.L., and Voss, J.L.: Ultrasound evaluation of the mare's reproductive tract: Part II. Compend. Contin. Educ. Practicing Vet., *9:*472–482, 1987.
66. Simpson, D.J., et al.: Use of ultrasound echography for early diagnosis of single and twin pregnancy in the mare. J. Reprod. Fertil. Suppl., *32:*431–439, 1982.
67. Torbeck, R.L., and Rantanen, N.W.: Early pregnancy detection in the mare with ultrasonography. J. Equine Vet. Sci., *2:*204–207, 1982.
68. Villahoz, M.D., Iuliano, M.F., and Squires, E.L.: The use of real-time ultrasound for pregnancy detection in embryo transfer mares. Theriogenology, *19:*149, 1983.
69. Villahoz, M.D., Squires, E.L., Voss, J.L., and Shideler, R.K.: Some observations on early embryonic death in mares. Theriogenology, *23:*915–924, 1985.
70. McKinnon, A.O., et al.: Ultrasonographic studies on the reproductive tract of postpartum mares: Effect of involution and uterine fluid on pregnancy rates in mares with normal and delayed first postpartum ovulatory cycles. J. Am. Vet. Med. Assoc., *192:*350–353, 1988.
71. McKinnon, A.O., et al.: Diagnostic ultrasonography of uterine pathology in the mare. Proc. Am. Assoc. Equine Pract., 605–622, 1987.
72. McKinnon, A.O., Squires, E.L., and Voss, J.L.: Ultrasound evaluation of the mare's reproductive tract. Part I. Compend. Contin. Educ. Practicing Vet., *9:*336–345, 1987.
73. Ginther, O.J.: Mobility of the early equine conceptus. Theriogenology, *19:*603–611, 1983.
74. Ginther, O.J.: Fixation and orientation of the early equine conceptus. Theriogenology, *19:*613–623, 1983.
75. Curran, S., and Ginther, O.J.: Ultrasonic diagnosis of equine fetal sex by location of the genital tubercle. J. Equine Vet. Sci., 9:77–83, 1989.
76. McKinnon, A.O., Squires, E.L., Pickett, B.W.: Equine reproductive ultrasonography. Colorado State University Animal Reproduction Bulletin No. 04. Fort Collins, 1988.

CHAPTER 60

THE PLACENTA

A.C. Asbury
M.M. LeBlanc

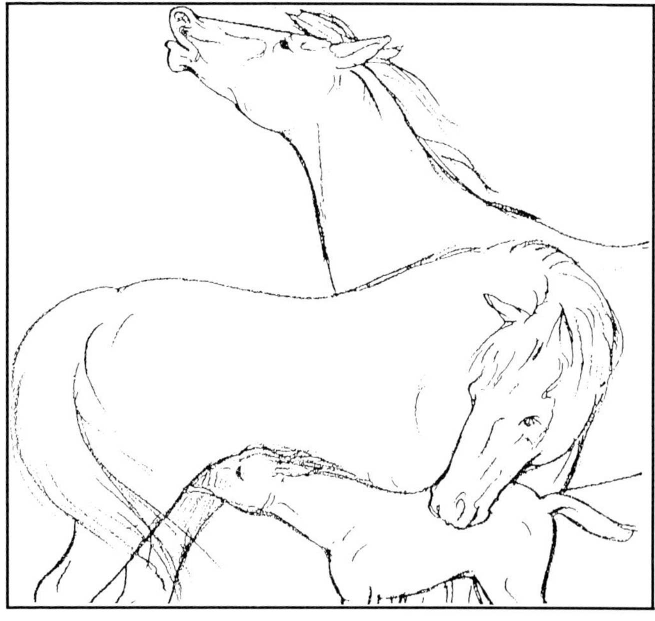

The equine placenta, a unique integration of fetal membranes with endometrium, provides useful information on the condition of the both the mare and foal to the clinician who makes the effort to examine it. Careful inspection of the membranes, particularly the chorionic surface of the allantochorion, reveals much about the apposing endometrium. In some cases, more can be learned about the cause of abortion from examining the membranes rather than the fetus. Clues to the future fertility of the mare and to potential septic conditions of the neonate are available by careful placental evaluation.

In short, familiarity with the normal and abnormal aspects of placentation may greatly improve the diagnosis, prognosis, and therapy of problems of perinatal diseases of horses. Knowledge of the structure, function, and abnormalities of the placenta is necessary to achieve these objectives.

ANATOMY OF THE PLACENTA AND FETAL MEMBRANES

The placenta, as described in this section, includes not only those portions of the fetal membranes that appose and fuse with the endometrium to achieve physiologic exchange but also the fetal membranes in their entirety. The entire complex of fetus, membranes, and maternal components function as a unit, and should be considered as such.

GROSS ANATOMY

Development of the equine placenta is essentially complete by day 150 of gestation. The embryologic aspects of this development have been presented in Chapter 56. By the latter half of gestation, other than some refinements and growth, the membranes are in their mature form.[1] Only membranes in their final configuration will be considered here.

The mature fetal membranes, which have previously been described,[2,3] are presented below and the relationships between them are illustrated in Figure 60–1. The membranes can be divided into three groups. First is the allantochorion, which is formed by fusion of the chorion to the allantois. The chorion apposes the endometrium throughout the uterus, with a small area at the internal os of the cervix (cervical star) excluded. Microcotyledons form over the entire area of interaction with the endometrium (diffuse placentation). The chorionic components of the microcotyledons are villous, and the endometrial side is made up of crypts corresponding to the villi. When the chorionic surface is separated from the endometrial surface, the chorionic villi appear as reddened, velvety tissue. The allantoic side of the membrane is smooth and bluish in color and the fetal blood vessels are prominent on its surface. Major and minor branches of the umbilical arteries and veins are the vessels noted. The allantoic space is that which is bounded entirely by allantois.

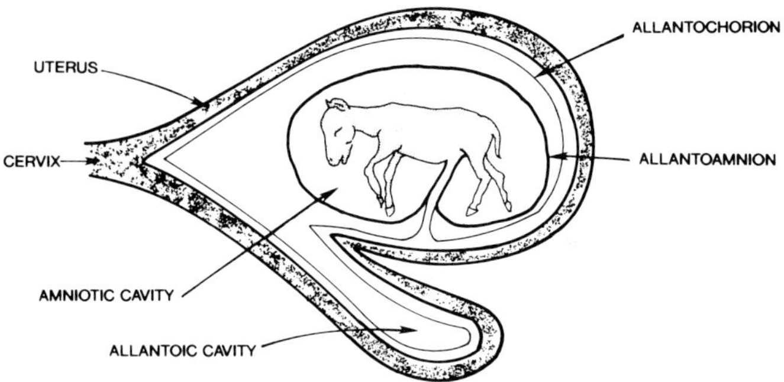

FIG. 60–1. Diagram of the mature fetal membranes, showing the relationships of the membranes to one another, and to the fetus.

Second is the allantoamnion, which is formed by the fusion of amnion to allantois. The resulting membrane is smooth and whitish in color and blood vessels are evident between the two layers of the membrane. The allantoamnion completely envelops the fetus, which has no attachment to the membrane except at the umbilicus. Small white plaques may appear over any portion of the amniotic side of the allantoamnion. These plaques consist of layers of ectodermal cells with or without a core of connective tissue.[4] The amniotic space is that which is bounded entirely by the amnion.[2] The allantoamnion attaches to the chorioallantois only at the base of the umbilical stalk, allowing great freedom of movement of the fetus within the uterus.

Third, the umbilical cord is made up of an amniotic portion and an allantoic portion, as it passes through the appropriate spaces. This structure contains two umbilical arteries and one umbilical vein, which provide the interchange of blood between the fetal and placental circulations. The cord also contains the urachus, a connection between the fetal bladder and the allantoic space. The equine umbilical cord is 50 to 100 cm long, enabling free rotation of the fetus on its long axis as well as great mobility.[2]

MICROSCOPIC ANATOMY

The equine placenta is characterized as epitheliochorial. This designates the layers separating the maternal from the fetal blood as two layers each of endothelium, connective tissue, and epithelium. These layers comprise the interhemal membrane, which in the term placenta becomes quite thin, because of the indentation of the chorionic epithelium by fetal capillaries and progressive thinning of the connective tissue.[5] Detailed histologic descriptions of the fetal and maternal apposition occurring in the microcotyledons have been presented in Chapter 56 and are illustrated in Figures 56–11 and 56–12.

An artist's rendition of the relationship between the maternal and fetal components of mature microcotyledons is depicted in Figure 60–2. The complex interdigitation between the chorionic epithelium and the endometrial epithelium is clear in this drawing. The relationship between uterine and umbilical circulation is also well represented. Maternal circulation to the microcotyledon is in the form of long, straight branches of the uterine artery that break over the rim on the microcotyledon and give rise to a dense vascular network in walls of the maternal crypts, then drain to a single uterine vein. The chorionic villi in apposition are fed and drained by branches of the umbilical arteries and veins, respectively. Maternal and fetal capillaries carry blood moving in opposite directions.[6]

The allantoamnion is made up of ectodermal tissue (amnion) and endodermal tissue (allantois) fused together around two layers of intervening connective tissue. In the mature membrane the endodermal and ectodermal layers undergo marked hyperplasia and thickening.[4]

FUNCTIONS OF THE PLACENTA

The equine placenta acts as an organ of respiratory and nutrient exchange between dam and fetus. It functions in hormone synthesis and metabolism, provides a depository for fetal wastes, and acts as a mechanical protectant for the fetus.

NUTRIENT AND GAS EXCHANGE

Molecular and gaseous exchange occurs throughout the placenta by a variety of processes. For example, gases and small molecules rapidly diffuse across the highly vascularized microcotyledons.[7] Large water-soluble molecules originating from uterine gland secretions, on the other hand, are pinocytosed by chorionic epithelium overlying uterine glands.[5]

The placenta permits the transport of sugars, amino acids, vitamins, and minerals to the fetus as substrates for fetal growth.[6] It also serves as a storage organ for glycogen and certain other substances such as iron. Glucose is the major metabolic fuel of the equine fetus and is transferred across the placenta by means of an active transport system.[8]

Because of the epitheliolchorial nature of the equine placenta, large molecules including proteins and immunoglobulins do not pass from dam to fetus, except when the placenta is compromised. In cases of severe placentitis, IgG, whole cells, and plasma proteins may leak through pores in the placental membrane. Anesthetics and drugs will rapidly diffuse across the placental barrier. In other species, certain drugs have been shown to effect the fetus adversely. Little is known about the effects of drugs on the well-being of the equine fetus.

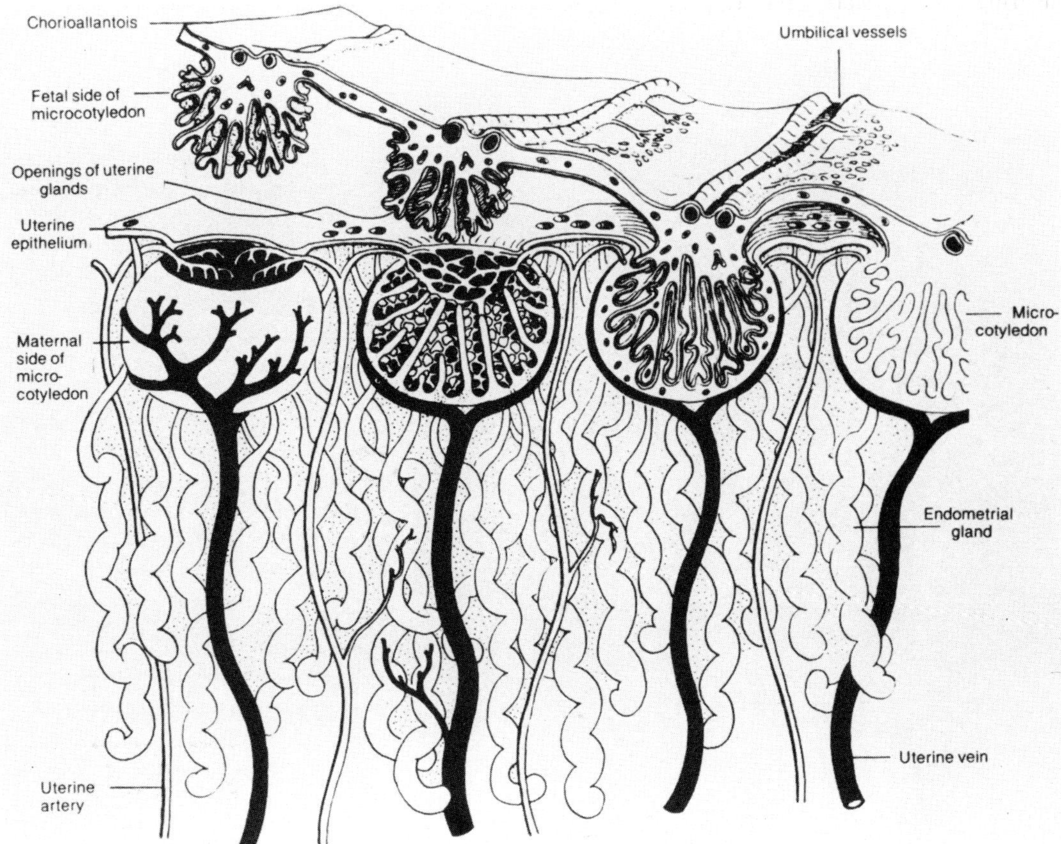

FIG. 60–2. Drawing of a portion of the mature equine placenta, showing the relationship between maternal and fetal sides of microcotyledons. (From Steven, D.H., and Samuel, C.A.: Anatomy of the placental barrier in the mare. J. Reprod. Fertil. Suppl., *23*:579–582, 1975.)

ENDOCRINE FUNCTION

The placenta is a transient endocrine organ like the corpus luteum (CL), which secretes both tropic and steroid hormones into the fetal and the maternal circulations. The term fetoplacental unit is used when discussing hormone production by the placenta or fetus because, by itself, each unit lacks specific enzymes essential for steroidogenesis. Integration of the steroidogenic functions of both the fetus and placenta, however, results in production of steroid hormones.[6]

Progesterone is necessary for pregnancy maintenance in the mare. Until day 80 of gestation, the CL is the primary source of progesterone. At this time, the fetoplacental unit begins to contribute to the pool of circulating maternal progestins by producing 5α-pregnanes. Plasma progesterone begins to decline by day 120 and only small amounts of progesterone are measurable in plasma by day 150. Presumably pregnancy is then maintained by placental progestin production.[9] Disagreement exists, however, on what is considered to be the normal concentration of plasma progesterone between day 120 and parturition. Daily progesterone values of 1 to 8 ng/mL have been reported as normal.[9,10] The discrepancy between reports can be attributed to cross-reaction of progesterone antiserum used in radioimmunoassays (RIA) with other progestins. Because of this cross-reactivity, interpretation of progesterone values obtained by RIA after 80 days of gestation must be made with caution. A low plasma progesterone value may be the result of a RIA that is extremely progesterone specific.

Measurement of plasma progesterone during mid- to late gestation may not directly reflect the fetoplacental environment. The predominant steroids in maternal plasma near term are not the same as those in the umbilical vein or artery (Table 60–1).[11] Fetal pregnenolone is converted to progesterone in the placenta, fetal adrenals and endometrium. Further 3β- and 20β-hydroxylation of progesterone occurs in the fetus and endometrium. In contrast, the 20α-hydroxylation compounds predominate on the maternal side and are not found in the fetoplacental unit. However, maternal progestins decrease in mares with severe colic and will drop to < 1 ng/mL in mares that abort.[12,13]

TABLE 60–1. PROGESTIN CONCENTRATIONS IN MATERNAL AND UMBILICAL BLOOD

LOCATION	PROGESTIN	CONCENTRATION (NG/ML)
Maternal plasma	20α-hydroxy-5-pregnane-3-one	400–2100
	5α-pregnane-3β,20α-diol (5α-DHP)	100–350
Umbilical vein	5α-DHP	220
	progesterone	5–20
Umbilical artery	pregnenolone	420
	5-pregnene-3β, 20β-diol	165
	5α-pregnane-3β, 20β-diol	105

(From Holtan, D.W., et al.: Plasma progestagens in the mare, fetus and newborn foal. J. Reprod. Fertil., *44*:517–528, 1991.

FUNCTION OF FETAL FLUIDS

The amniotic and allantoic fluids perform several functions vital to the fetus. Amniotic fluid protects the fetus from external shock, prevents adhesions between fetal skin and amniotic membranes, and assists in dilating the cervix and lubricating the birth canal during birth.[6] It is composed of fetal urine, secretions from the respiratory tract and buccal cavity, and fluid from the dam's circulation. As pregnancy progresses, the concentration of fetal urine in the amniotic space decreases and secretions from the respiratory tract increase, changing the consistency of the amniotic fluid from watery to mucoid. Amniotic fluid volume is low for the first 3 months of gestation then increases rapidly to equal the volume of allantoic fluid at midpregnancy. The amniotic fluid serves as a conduit for water exchange from dam to fetus and back to the dam. The fetus is also capable of removing water by either swallowing or by drawing amniotic fluid into its lungs during respiratory movements.

Allantoic fluid is composed of hypotonic urine and fetal excretory products that are not readily transferred back to the dam. Allantoic fluid also maintains the osmotic pressure of the fetal plasma and prevents fluid loss to maternal circulation. At parturition, the volume of amniotic fluid and allantoic fluid has been reported to be 3 to 5 and 8 to 15 L, respectively.[14] The hippomane—a smooth, discoid, rubber-like, dark brown calculus, consisting of concentric layers of cellular debris—floats within the allantoic fluid. Both fluid compartments contain high concentrations of fructose, various metabolic constituents, electrolytes, enzymes, hormones, and cells. Their functions have not been studied in the mare.

AMNIOCENTESIS

Amniocentesis is a procedure commonly performed in pregnant women to determine fetal karyotype and to assess fetal pulmonary and kidney maturation. In humans, fetal pulmonary maturity can be predicted accurately by determining the percentage of phosphatidylglycerol and the lecithin to spingomyelin ratio (L:S) from amniotic fluid phospholipids (surfactant). Evidence exists to suggest that fetal cortisol production is also associated with fetal lung maturation and that fetal creatinine excretion parallels kidney maturation and function.[15,16] Ultrasound-guided amniocentesis can be performed successfully in the late gestational mare.[17] In the mare, however, the percent of phosphatidylglycerol, L:S, and creatinine concentration in amniotic fluid do not differ in samples collected from mares between 290 days of gestation and parturition. Amniotic cortisol concentrations in these mares increased only at foaling.[18] At present, amniocenteses do not appear to be useful in determining fetal maturation.

PERIPARTURIENT DYNAMICS OF THE PLACENTA

Interaction between the uterus and placenta occurs before, during, and after parturition. Final maturation of the placental junction and the first steps involved in microcotyledon separation precede the onset of labor. During labor, respiratory exchange must continue until the foal is able to breathe. Once delivery is complete, the membranes normally release and are delivered in a set pattern. Variations from normal may be cause for concern.

MATURATION AND PLACENTAL RELEASE

Complex interactions of endocrine and physical events are involved in the final maturation of both the fetus and placenta before the onset of parturition. While the exact sequences and relationships are not well worked out, the steroid hormones and possibly corticoids are clearly involved in these processes early on.[19] Prostaglandins and finally oxytocin come into play as stimulants of myometrial contraction.[20] Maturation of the fetus and the placental attachments appears to be related to mammary development and the change in mammary secretions.[21] Early placental separation is often accompanied by premature lactation.[3]

Actual separation of the chorionic and endometrial elements of the placenta cannot be completed until the fetus is capable of its own oxygenation. That fact would argue for a major role of uterine contractions in third-stage labor to be the factor in final separation. It is interesting that electromyographic (EMG) activity of the uterus decreases dramatically in the last 2 to 4 h preceding delivery but abruptly increases when the allantochorion ruptures.[22] The interdigitating elements of the microcotyledon are likely squeezed apart by uterine contraction. Any swelling at those junctions, such as that caused by inflammatory edema, could cause a delay in the normal separation and, if widespread, cause placental retention.

MECHANICS OF NORMAL MEMBRANE DELIVERY

The first component of the fetal membranes to be delivered during normal parturition is the allantoamnion. This passage is accommodated by the rupture of the allantochorion at the cervical star, enabling the fetus to enter and pass through the birth canal, with the amnion intact around it.

The length of the umbilicus is such that the entire fetus can be delivered with the chorionic attachment still in contact with the endometrium. However, the amount of gaseous and nutrient exchange is probably minimal at this point. Blood flows from the placenta to the fetus after delivery via the umbilical vein for a few minutes after delivery, but it is probably not highly oxygenated.

Primary passage of the allantoamnion and umbilicus through the birth canal with the fetus causes tension on the allantoic side of the allantochorion, at its attachment to the umbilicus. Continuation of this tension as the third stage of labor commences causes the allantochorion to be delivered inverted, with the allantoic side outermost. This is the normal presentation of the allantochorion.

One variation in the normal process of placental mechanics at delivery is premature placental separation. This situation, which can jeopardize oxygenation of the foal, occurs when the allantochorion fails to rupture at the cervical star.[23] As a result, the mare attempts to deliver the entire fetoplacental unit with the chorion intact. When chorionic membrane, identified by its villous surface, is presented at the vulva, rapid intervention is indicated. The chorion must be cut or torn to allow delivery of the fetus in its amniotic membrane. The foal should be managed as if it were hypoxic, because the degree of chorionic separation is difficult to assess.

Delivery without allantochorion rupture may involve pathologic changes of the membrane at the cervical star, with resulting thickening of the tissue, or primary chorionic separation from the endometrium could be a factor. In the latter situation, the observation of hemorrhage, originating cranial to the cervix during the last few days of pregnancy, may provide a warning of the impending problem.

Another mechanical problem associated with delivery is compression of the umbilicus between the fetus and the maternal pelvis, inducing hypoxia. This situation is only of concern in posterior presentations and calls for immediate extra assistance in extraction of the foal, when the delivery is slowed by the size of the fetal thorax or shoulders.

SIGNIFICANCE OF PLACENTAL EXAMINATION

Placental examination and attention to any abnormalities indicated in that process are essential parts of the management of every foaling, whether normal or abnormal.

EXAMINATION OF THE PLACENTA

Systematic examination of the placenta will provide a wealth of information on the status of uterine health, the process of parturition, the completeness of the membranes delivered and on pathologic processes that may be of importance in management of the case. A practical and orderly examination process has been suggested, and is widely used.[24]

Assuming that the placenta has been delivered in the normal state (allantochorion inverted and allantoamnion evident), the intact membranes should be spread out on a clean flat surface. After identifying the cervical star and both horns, the allantochorion is arranged in a rough F configuration, as shown in Figure 60–3. The cervical star is at the bottom, with the membranes that occupied the uterine body forming the vertical part of the F. The wider and thicker membrane from the pregnant horn forms the upper arm of the F and the nonpregnant component the lower arm.

Consistent arrangement of the membranes in this manner leads to a repeatable and systematic examination. When the allantoic side of the membrane is outermost, it is easier to detect a missing piece of membrane by lining up the pattern of the blood vessels on the allantoic surface. Assurance that the entire placenta has been delivered is an important fact in managing the postpartum mare. Inspection of the allantoamnion and umbilicus is easiest when the membranes are arranged in the inverted position.

The allantochorion should then be reoriented to expose the chorionic surface. Arrangement of the tissues as described previously is helpful in correlating any observed changes with the corresponding part of the uterus (Fig. 60–4). The chorionic surface of a freshly delivered placenta provides unique insight into the condition of the entire endometrium. The major abnormalities encountered are described briefly in the next sections of this chapter.

Historically, total weight of fresh fetal membranes has been suggested as a guide to the health of the fetoplacental unit. Gross changes in total weight may be caused by inflammatory processes and particularly edema. Weights in the range of 6 to 7 kg for light breed horses have been proposed as normal. In our experience, a wide range of weight may result from fetal size, maternal age and size, and other nonspecific factors. Weighing the placenta should never become a substitute for a careful examination of the membranes.

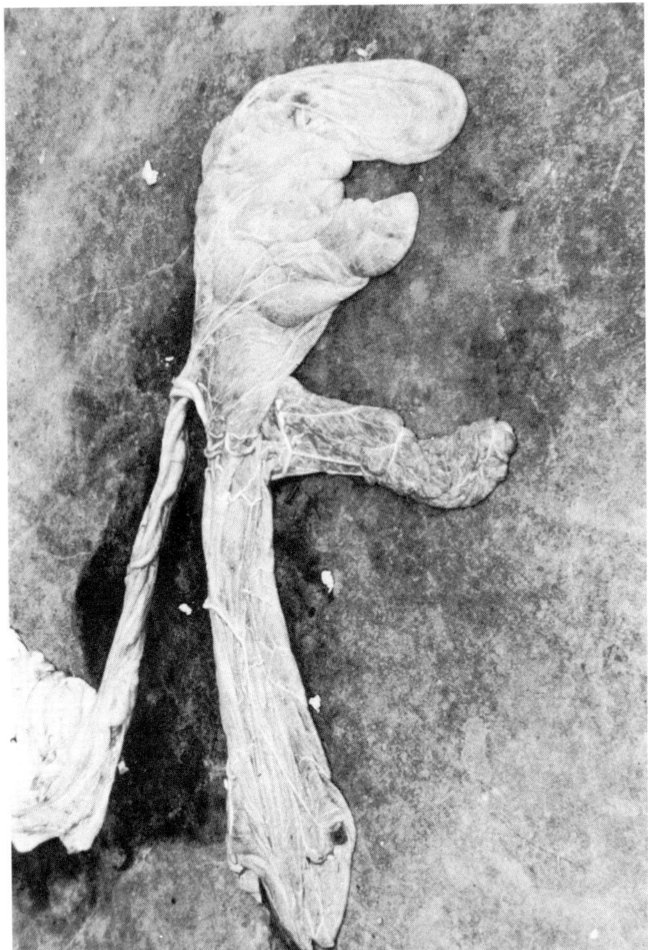

FIG. 60–3. Fetal membranes in the usual configuration when delivered, arranged for inspection. The allantochorion is inverted. The umbilical cord, connected to the allantoamnion is to the lower left.

PLACENTAL ABNORMALITIES

Changes evident from the gross inspection of the fetal membranes as described may provide information of importance to the health of the mare and foal and to the condition of the reproductive tract. Also, in cases of abortion, inspection of the fetal membranes is an essential part of the diagnostic procedure.[25] Gross abnormalities may also suggest further diagnostic work, such as culture or histopathologic examination, whether a live foal exists or not. Following is a list of major abnormalities seen, with brief comment on the significance of each.

Allantochorion

Areas Devoid of Chorionic Villi. Chorionic villi form only when chorionic membrane and healthy endometrium are placed in apposition. Therefore, areas devoid of villi are normal where the membrane meets the cervix (cervical star) or the endometrial cups or where the chorion is folded on itself. The latter situation results in long thin lines that are bare. Large areas where villi are absent or hypoplastic occur in twin pregnancy and in mares with significant degenerative change in the endometrium. Twin pregnancy invariably results in one chorion abutting the other, with no villous development. Even when a normal-size fetus is produced and its twin is small and inconsequential, the bare area should be evident somewhere on the chorionic surface of the membrane. Large areas of hypoplastic villi in singleton pregnancies are characteristic of older mares with degenerative endometrial changes. The resulting deficit of functional chorion usually produces a small, malnourished foal, often carried to abnormally long gestational ages. Mares tend to repeat this production pattern, because the endometrial changes are usually irreversible.

Inflammatory Changes of the Allantochorion. Chorionitis caused by bacterial or fungal agents is manifested as proliferative and exudative changes on either the chorionic surface or the entire thickness of the al-

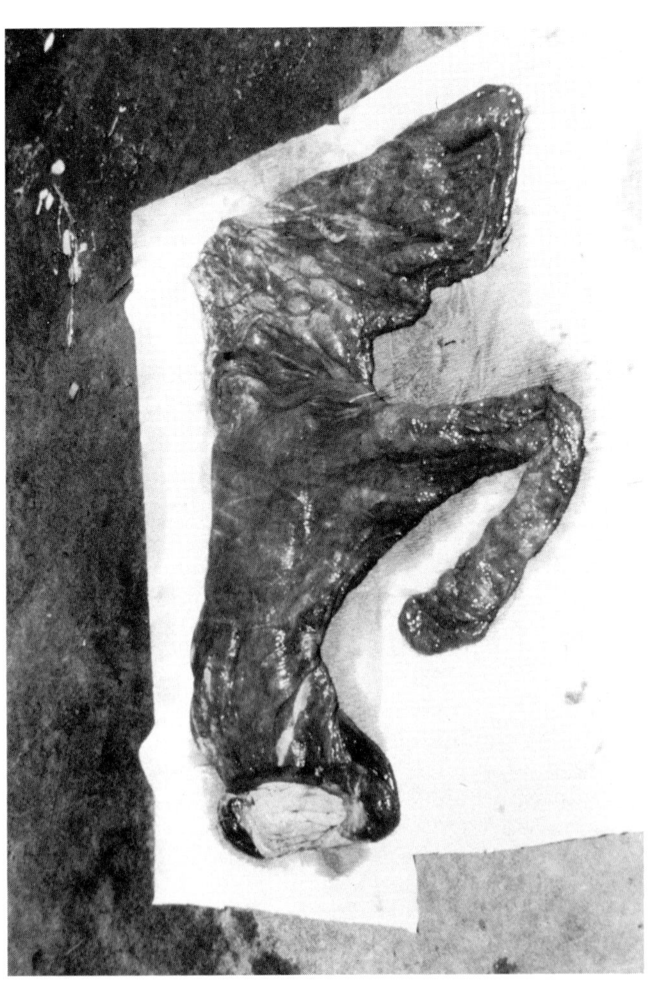

FIG. 60–4. Fetal membranes after orientation to expose the chorionic surface, arranged for inspection.

lantochorion. Large areas of the allantochorion may show edema with local areas of thickening as the result of the proliferative process. Typically, the lesions are focused in the area of the cervical star, suggesting that these infections are likely secondary to transcervical invasion.[23,26] Exudates are not characteristic enough to separate bacterial from fungal disease. The typical exudate is thick, mucoid, and adherent to the surface of the membrane. Culture and staining are necessary to identify the cause.

When placentitis lesions are discovered following delivery of a live foal, a high index of suspicion of a septicemic foal should exist and appropriate diagnostic and therapeutic actions should be taken. Initiation of treatment based on inspection of the placenta could be a significant step in saving the neonate.

Chronic placentitis may interfere with the transport of nutrients across the placenta, thus compromising growth and development of the fetus. Oxygenation of the fetus could also possibly be interfered with by the abnormal placenta, resulting in retardation of intrauterine growth, as has been reported in human fetuses.[27]

Allantoamnion

Inflammatory Changes of the Allantoamnion. Primary inflammation of the allantoamnion is rarely seen. Extension of allantochorionic lesions are more likely to be found on the allantoamnion. Their significance is questionable.

The Umbilical Cord

Major pathologic changes in the umbilical cord are usually associated with fetal death and abortion. Among the common abnormalities are increased cord length, which can cause strangulation of the fetus, and umbilical torsion, which may disrupt umbilical circulation or urachal flow.[28] In the live-born foal, evidence of the existence of these abnormalities may be noted in some minor degree. The presence of edema and excessive rotation of the cord are signs that some level of torsion had been present before delivery. If urachal obstruction occurred without killing the fetus, necrosis of the urachus, with subsequent leaking of urine, is a possibility in otherwise normal foals.[28]

REFERENCES

1. Samuel, C.A., Allen, W.R., and Steven, D.H.: Studies on the equine placenta. I. The development of the microcotyledons. J. Reprod. Fertil., *41:*441–445, 1974.
2. Roberts, S.J.: Veterinary Obstetrics and Genital Diseases. 2nd ed. Ithaca, NY, published by the author, 1971.
3. Asbury, A.C.: The pregnant mare. *In* Equine Medicine and Surgery. 3rd ed. Edited by R.A. Mansmann and E.S. McAllister. Santa Barbara, CA American Veterinary Publications, 1982, pp. 1343–1363.
4. Ginther, O.J.: Reproductive Biology of the Mare: Basic and Applied Aspects. Equiservices, Cross Plains, WI, 1979.
5. Samuel, C.A., Allen, W.R., and Steven, D.H.: Studies on the equine placenta. II. Ultrastructure of the placental barrier. J. Reprod. Fertil., *48:*257–264, 1976.
6. Jainudeen, M.R., and Hafez, E.S.E.: Gestation, prenatal physiology and parturition. *In* Reproduction in Farm Animals. 4th ed. Edited by E.S.E. Hafez. Philadelphia, Lea & Febiger, 1980, pp. 247–283.
7. Steven, D.H.: Placentation in the mare. J. Reprod. Fertil. Suppl., *31:*41–55, 1982.
8. Comline, R.S., and Silver, M.: Recent observations on the undisturbed foetus in utero and its delivery. *In* Recent Advances in Physiology. edited by R.J. Linden. London, Churchill Livingstone, 1974. pp. 406–454.
9. Holtan, D.W., Nett T.M., and Estergreen, V.L.: Plasma progestins in pregnant, postpartum and cycling mares. J. Anim. Sci., *40:*251–260, 1975.
10. Squires, E.L., Wentworth, B.C., and Ginther, O.J.: Progesterone concentration in blood of mares during the estrous cycle, pregnancy and after hysterectomy. J. Anim. Sci., *39:*759–767, 1974.
11. Holtan, D.W., et al.: Plasma progestagens in the mare, fetus and newborn foal. J. Reprod. Fertil. Suppl., *44:*517–528, 1991.
12. Santschi, E.M., LeBlanc, M.M., and Weston, P.G.: Progestin, oestrone sulphate and cortisol concentrations in pregnant mares during medical and surgical disease. J. Reprod. Fertil. Suppl., *44:*627–634, 1991.
13. Hamon, M., et al.: Production of 5α-dihydroprogesterone during late pregnancy in the mare. J. Reprod. Fertil. Suppl., *44:*529–535, 1991.
14. Arthur, G.H.: Veterinary Reproduction and Obstetrics. 4th ed., London, Bailliere Tindall, 1975, pp. 41–42.
15. Stahlman, M.T.: Acute respiratory disorders in the newborn. *In* Neonatology-Pathophysiology and Management of the Newborn. 3rd ed. Edited by G.B. Avery. Philadelphia, J.B. Lippincott, 1987, pp. 420–421.
16. McCarthy, T., and Saunders, P.: The origin and circulation of the amniotic fluid. *In* Amniotic Fluid-Research and Clinical Application. 2nd ed. Edited by B.V.I. Fairweather and T.K.A.B. Eskes. Oxford, Exerpta Medical, 1988, pp. 6–8.
17. Carleton, C.L., Schmidt, A.R., and Williams, M.A.: Amniocentiesis in the late gestational mare. Proceedings of the Second International Conference on Veterinary Perinatology. Cambridge, 1990, p. 37.
18. Williams, M.A., et al.: Amniotic fluid analysis for evaluation of equine foetal development. Proceedings of the Second International Conference on Veterinary Perinatology. Cambridge, 1990. p. 38.
19. Alm, C.C., Sullivan, J.J., and First, N.L.: The effect of a corticosteroid (dexamethasone), progesterone, oestrogen and prostaglandin $F_2\alpha$ on gestation length in normal and ovariectomized mares. J. Reprod. Fertil. Suppl., *23:*637–640, 1975.
20. Barnes, R.J., et al.: Foetal and maternal plasma concentrations of 13,14-dihydro-15-oxo-prostaglandin F in the mare during late pregnancy and at parturition. J. Endocrinol., *78:*201–215, 1978.
21. Jeffcott, L.B.: Observations on parturition in crossbred pony mares. Equine Vet. J., *4:*i–v, 1972.

22. Haluska, G.J., Lowe, J.E., and Currie, W.B.: Electromyographic properties of the myometrium correlated with the endocrinology of the pre-partum and post-partum periods and parturition in pony mares. J. Reprod. Fertil. Suppl., *35:*553–564, 1987.

23. Prickett, M.E.: Abortion and placental lesions in the mare. J. Am. Vet. Med. Assoc., *157:*1465–1470, 1970.

24. Whitwell, K.E., and Jeffcott, L.B.: Morphological studies on the fetal membranes of the normal singleton foal at term. Res. Vet. Sci., *19:*44–55, 1975.

25. Acland, H.M.: Abortion in mares: Diagnosis and prevention. Compend. Contin. Educ. Practicing Vet., *9:*318–324, 1987.

26. Platt, H.: Infection of the horse fetus, J. Reprod. Fertil. Suppl., *23:*605–610, 1975.

27. Koterba, A.M.: Effects of acute and chronic fetal hypoxia on the newborn. Proc. Soc. Theriogenol., 311–315, 1988.

28. Whitwell, K.E.: Morphology and pathology of the equine umbilical cord. J. Reprod. Fertil. Suppl., *23:*599–603, 1975.

CHAPTER 61

EMBRYONIC DEATH IN MARES*

B.A. Ball

*Portions of this chapter have been adapted from Ball, B.A.: Embryonic loss in mares: Incidence, possible causes, and diagnostic considerations. Vet. Clin. North Am. Equine Pract. *4*:263–290, 1988.

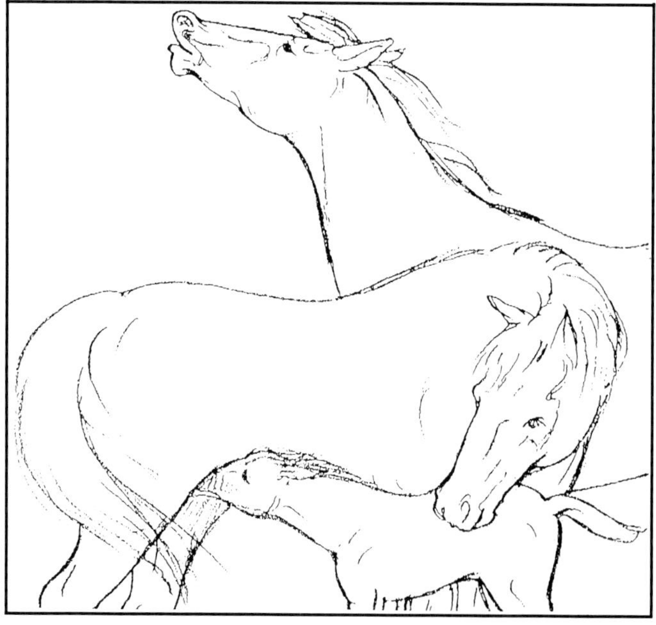

Research over the past 10 yr has demonstrated that early embryonic death is a major factor in subfertility and reduced reproductive efficiency in mares. The importance of embryonic death in mares has been demonstrated in clinical and research trials as well as in routine breeding management. Although understanding of embryonic death in mares has improved, understanding of its causes remains limited. Much of our knowledge comes from extrapolation of information from other species and from clinical anecdotal information. Because early pregnancy in the mare presents certain physiologic differences from other species, this extrapolation of information on embryonic death to the mare may be inappropriate in some cases.

FERTILIZATION RATES IN MARES

Information about the fertilization rate in mares is required to determine the magnitude of embryonic death that occurs before the earliest time of pregnancy detection. The fertilization rate is over 90% in fertile mares, comparable with other domestic species.[1,2] In subfertile mares, fertilization rates are also quite high with rates of 81 and 92% reported.[1,2] Fertilization failure, therefore, constitutes a relatively small portion of fertility losses when breeding management and stallion fertility are optimal, and embryonic death constitutes a major portion of reproductive inefficiency in mares.

INCIDENCE OF EMBRYONIC DEATH

Incidence of embryonic death in mares can be divided into losses before pregnancy detection (days 10 to 14) and losses confirmed by ultrasonography or palpation per rectum after pregnancy detection (days 14 to 40). Incidence of embryonic death between fertilization and day 14 was 9% for young fertile mares and 62 to 73% for aged subfertile mares.[1,2] A significant proportion of embryonic deaths in subfertile mares appears to occur by the time the embryo reaches the uterus at day 5 or 6, because embryo transfer studies show that recovery of embryos from the uterus of subfertile mares is reduced as early as days 6 to 8.

Estimates on the detected incidence of embryonic death vary, depending on method of pregnancy determination, interval of detection, and group of animals under study. Most investigators have detected an embryonic death rate between 5 and 24% in fertile mares (Tables 61–1 and 61–2). In subfertile mares, the detected embryonic death rate is even higher during this interval.[11] The combined incidences of embryonic death from fertilization through approximately day 40 appear to be near 20% in fertile mares and greater than 70% in subfertile mares. These estimates are combined across several studies but represent our best estimate of embryonic death in these two groups of mares (Fig. 61–1).

The period of greatest embryonic death in subfertile mares is clearly the interval before early pregnancy de-

TABLE 61–1. A REVIEW OF STUDIES ON PREGNANCY LOSS IN MARES DETECTED BY PALPATION PER RECTUM OR REAL TIME, TRANSRECTAL ULTRASONOGRAPHY

Type of Study Reference Number	Breed*	Day of Detection: First	Day of Detection: Last	Number of Losses/ Number of Pregnancies	Percent
Rectal Palpation					
3	TB	20–40	30–50	294/1,921	15
4	SB TB	20–24	40–50	27/386	7
5	Draft	21–35	70+	34/213	16
6	TB	18–30	90	932/11,098	8
7	—	18–28	43–49	84/767	11
Ultrasonography					
8	Trotter, Draft, Pony	23±6	43±10	69/1,295	5
9	TB	20	45	16/326	5
10†	Pony	11	40	37/154	24
	Horse	11	40	5/27	19
11†	—	15	50	61/354	17
12‡	SB, TB	14	48	42/404	10
13‡	SB, TB	14	48	60/559	11
14	TB	18	42	26/437	6

*TB, Thoroughbred; SB, Standardbred.
†Study included experimental animals.
‡Only singleton pregnancies included.
(From Ball, B.A.: Embryonic loss in mares. Vet. Clin. North Am. Equine Pract., *4*:263–290, 1988.)

tection with ultrasonography (days 10 to 14). Losses during this interval in subfertile mares occur before maternal recognition of pregnancy and appear to occur near the time the embryo enters the uterus. Embryonic death in fertile mares also occurs more often in the early period but without the dramatically high incidence reported in subfertile mares.

FACTORS CONSIDERED IN EMBRYONIC DEATH

Many factors serve as potential causes of embryonic death in mares. This chapter discusses maternal, external, and embryonic factors. Maternal factors include endocrine factors, oviduct, uterus, maternal age, and lactation/foal heat breeding. External factors include stress, seasonal factors, sire effects, and iatrogenic factors. Embryonic factors include genetic defects and immunogenetic factors. Several of the categories potentially overlap, and a single factor is frequently difficult to isolate.

MATERNAL FACTORS

Endocrine Factors

Progesterone is critical for continued maintenance of pregnancy in mares. During the embryonic period, the source of progesterone remains from the primary corpus luteum (CL) formed at the initial ovulation. Maintenance of the cyclic CL in pregnant mares depends on the ability of the conceptus to block endometrial production of prostaglandin $F_2\alpha$ in a process termed "maternal recognition of pregnancy."[16] After day 30, progesterone production by the primary CL is apparently stimulated by the production of equine chorionic gonadotropin (eCG) from the endometrial cups.[17]

Reduced progesterone concentrations leading to embryonic death can probably arise through at least three mechanisms, including failure of maternal recognition

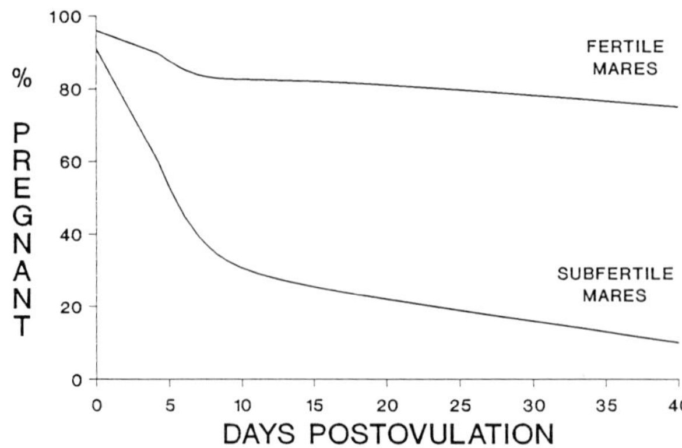

FIG. 61–1. Pregnancy rate for fertile and subfertile mares through day 40 postovulation. Data are combined across several studies and represent an estimate of embryonic loss during this interval.

TABLE 61–2. PERCENTAGES OF EMBRYONIC DEATH OCCURRING IN MARES DURING SPECIFIC INTERVALS OF GESTATION AS DETECTED BY ULTRASONOGRAPHY IN VARIOUS STUDIES

Reference Number	INTERVAL (DAYS) 11–15	15–20	20–25	25–30	30–35	35–40
10						
Ponies	18.2[a]*	3.3[b]	2.6[b]	0.0[b]	1.1[b]	1.1[b]
Horses	0.0	3.7	3.8	4.0	4.2	4.3
11	—	4.7[c]	2.5[d]	1.6[d]	5.8[c]	1.4[d]

Reference Number	INTERVAL (DAYS) 14–28	28–42	42–56
15	5.7[a]	2.2[b]	2.5[b]
13	5.2[c]	3.6	2.3[d]

*Loss rates within studies were different: a, b, $p < 0.01$; c, d, $p < 0.05$.
(From Ball, B.A.: Embryonic loss in mares. Vet. Clin. North Am. Equine Pract., *4*:263–290, 1988.)

of pregnancy, primary luteal insufficiency, and uterine-induced luteolysis caused by endometrial irritation.[18]

Maternal recognition of pregnancy relies on the ability of the equine conceptus to block luteolysis. This ability appears transient and must be accomplished before the proposed "critical deadline" for pregnancy recognition.[16] If development of the conceptus is retarded, then luteolysis occurs and the mare returns to estrus. These small-for-date conceptuses have a higher rate of embryonic death than normal conceptuses.[8,10,19] The reduced embryonic survival might be a result of asynchronous development of the conceptus and the maternal endometrium.

Embryo transfer studies also confirm the need for synchrony of the conceptus and the maternal endometrium.[20] However, requirements for synchrony between the embryo and uterus appear considerably broader in the mare than in other domestic animals.[21] The requirement for synchrony may be related to a time-dependent production of uterine proteins.[22] Secretion of certain uterine proteins in progesterone-treated ovariectomized mares is time dependent and relies on exposure of the endometrium to a brief period of estrogen followed by progesterone.[23]

Mobility of the equine conceptus appears to be a unique aspect of pregnancy recognition in the mare. Restricted mobility of the conceptus will result in embryonic death because of failure of pregnancy recognition.[24] Experimental restriction of the conceptus to one uterine horn resulted in a return to estrus and failure of maternal recognition of pregnancy, whereas pregnancy continued with exogenous progesterone therapy.[24] Although spontaneous clinical cases of impaired mobility of the conceptus have not been reported, such defects might result in failure of maternal recognition of pregnancy because of failure of the conceptus to interact with the maternal endometrium to block luteolysis. Certain pharmacologic agents, such as Clenbuterol, that impair uterine contractility[25] might result in embryonic death secondary to failure of mobility of the conceptus during the time of pregnancy recognition.

Luteal insufficiency has been proposed as an important factor in early embryonic death in a number of species. However, a primary luteal defect is difficult to establish. Both uterine-induced luteolysis and failure of maternal recognition of pregnancy can result in reduced progesterone because of prostaglandin $F_2\alpha$ release from the endometrium. Failure of pregnancy recognition might be expected to result in lower progesterone concentrations as early as day 11,[26,27] whereas uterine-induced luteolysis might lower progesterone concentrations after day 4 or 5.[17] A significantly higher progesterone concentration in pregnant versus nonpregnant mares has been found as early as day 11[28] or day 12.[29] Other studies, however, have failed to demonstrate a difference in progesterone concentrations until the time of luteolysis.[14] My own results indicated that serum progesterone concentrations through day 28 were significantly greater for aged, subfertile mares ($n = 8$) that established pregnancy with normal embryos, than for young, fertile mares ($n = 10$) that established pregnancy. Although these findings have several different interpretations, it is possible that aged, subfertile mares require higher progesterone concentrations for establishment and/or maintenance of pregnancy. To conclusively demonstrate a primary luteal defect, uterine-induced luteolysis secondary to endometritis or failure of pregnancy recognition must be excluded. This will require measurement of prostaglandin $F_2\alpha$ or its metabolite (PGFM) to exclude luteolysis.[30]

Embryonic deaths in mares have been associated with uterine-induced luteolysis. Adams et al. demonstrated uterine-induced luteolysis as a cause of reduced progesterone concentration and embryonic death in mares with ultrasonographic evidence of endometritis.[19] Intrauterine inoculation of yeast in pregnant mares resulted in endometritis, luteolysis, and embryonic death.[31] In these mares, embryonic death was coincident with a decline in serum progesterone; however, the effects of inflammation and the pathogen must also be considered as possible causes of embryonic death.[31]

Daels et al. have demonstrated embryonic death in mares through day 55 of gestation caused by endotoxin-mediated prostaglandin $F_2\alpha$ release.[32,33] Because endotoxemia is a potential complication of several disease conditions, luteolysis and embryonic death may be an important complication in these diseases. Although flunixin meglumine effectively blocks the release of prostaglandin $F_2\alpha$ as a result of endotoxemia, flunixin must be administered before the onset of endotoxemia to be effective. Therefore, administration of supplemental progesterone appears to be a better alternative to prevent embryonic death secondary to suspected endotoxemia. Administration of the synthetic progestin altrenogest (44 mg) within 12 h after endotoxemia effectively prevented embryonic death, and the clinician may have up to 48 h after endotoxemia to assess viability of the conceptus and begin progestin therapy.[33]

Progesterone appears to be the only ovarian substance required for pregnancy maintenance. Administration of progesterone allows establishment of pregnancy in ovariectomized, embryo-recipient mares at a rate comparable with intact mares.[34] Exogenous progesterone therapy in intact mares resulted in a significant increase in diameter of the early conceptus and an increase in yolk sac proteins.[35,36] Therefore, supplemental progesterone can influence uterine secretion and conceptus growth in the mare.

Estrogen

The equine conceptus produces detectable levels of estrogens in vitro as early as days 6 to 12 after ovulation.[37–39] Estrogen production by the conceptus has been postulated to be important in maternal recognition of pregnancy.[39,40] Estrogen also appears to be associated with increased uterine tone noted between days 16 and 20 of pregnancy.[41] Later in gestation, between days 35 and 40, a rise in plasma levels of conjugated estrogens[42,43] occurs that has been used to assess fetal viability.[44] Fetal death also resulted in a rapid decline in plasma estrone sulfate.[44,45] Similar declines in plasma estrone sulfate have been reported in pregnant mares that underwent spontaneous early fetal losses.[46,47]

Oviductal Environment

Oviductal function is important in many early events associated with embryonic development and has some features that are unique in the mare. The equine embryo remains in the oviduct longer and reaches a more advanced stage of development within the oviduct than in other domestic animals. Oviduct transport time is 5.5 days, and the embryo reaching the uterus at this time is a morula or early blastocyst.[48,49] Therefore, a substantial portion of early embryonic development, including blastulation, occurs in the oviductal environment.

Timing of oviductal transport appears critical to allow restoration of a favorable uterine environment after mating or insemination. If oviductal transport is significantly accelerated, the uterine environment may be unsuitable for embryonic survival. However, embryo transfer studies have demonstrated that the uterine environment is capable of supporting embryonic development as soon as day 4 after ovulation.[2] Likewise, if oviductal transport is significantly delayed, embryonic development might be impaired as shown for tubal-locked embryos in pigs.[50]

Another unique aspect of oviductal function in mares is differential transport of embryos versus unfertilized oocytes. This mechanism allows differential transport of fertilized oocytes but not unfertilized oocytes. Considerable latitude seems to exist in the mechanism as indicated by the ability of day-6 embryos to undergo oviductal transit after transfer into the oviduct at day 4 after ovulation.[51] Two recent reports demonstrate that the early embryo initiates oviductal transit by secretion of prostaglandin E_2.[52,53] Failure of the embryo to secrete adequate PGE_2 might result in failure of oviductal transit and loss of the conceptus, a possibility that requires further consideration.

Because of the importance of oviductal environment on early embryonic development, lesions of the oviduct may play a critical role in embryonic death. Oviductal lesions appear to increase with mare age and a positive correlation between endometritis and salpingitis is found in mares at slaughter.[54,55] The relationship between oviductal lesions and embryonic death has not been examined directly; however, a lower incidence of oviductal lesions occurred in pregnant versus nonpregnant mares at slaughter.[54]

Uterine Environment

The uterine environment is critical for continued support and development of the equine conceptus after day 6. Because microcotyledonary formation of the placenta occurs after day 40, nourishment of the developing equine conceptus relies heavily on secretion of histotroph (uterine milk) and its absorption across the choriovitelline (yolk sac) placenta or developing allantochorion. Production of uterine milk by the endometrial glands—which is stimulated by progesterone—is, therefore, critical for the entire embryonic period.

Stage-specific secretion of uterine proteins has been demonstrated for the mare with significant increases in protein content under the influence of progesterone.[23,56] These proteins include uteroferrin, an iron-containing acid phosphatase that is believed to be important in iron transport to the developing conceptus. Although endometrial proteins were influenced by progesterone, pregnant and diestrous mares had similar proteins at days 12 to 18.[56]

Clinically, the role of abnormal uterine environment in embryonic death has received considerable attention. These uterine abnormalities include endometritis and periglandular fibrosis. A relationship exists between severity of periglandular fibrosis and subsequent foaling rates (Table 61–3), and Kenney first proposed that periglandular fibrosis was a common cause of embryonic and early fetal death between days 40 and 90.[57]

The effect of periglandular fibrosis on fertility is complicated because severity of periglandular fibrosis increases with mare age.[61,62] Uterine environment of subfertile mares with periglandular fibrosis was comparable with that of fertile mares without fibrosis in ability to support normal embryos through day 28.[63] It appeared that embryonic defects or oviductal abnormalities may be more important in the high incidence of embryonic death noted in subfertile mares before day 14. However, the uterine environment of subfertile mares may be important in embryonic or early fetal death as metabolic demands of the conceptus increase beyond day 28.

As discussed earlier, endometritis could result in embryonic death because of luteolysis or because of the effect of inflammation or pathogens directly on the conceptus. Aged, subfertile mares may be more susceptible to endometritis after mating or insemination.[30,64] Failure to eliminate bacterial contaminants from the uterus may result in endometritis that persists into the luteal phase with subsequent embryonic death.

TABLE 61–3. ENDOMETRIAL BIOPSY GRADE AND FOALING RATES AS REPORTED IN SEVERAL STUDIES

		NUMBER OF MARES		
Reference Number	Biopsy Grade*	Bred	Foaling	Percent
57	I	60	41	68
	II	113	58	51
	III	71	8	11
58	I	42	31	74
	II	28	12	43
	III	16	3	19
59	I	36	28	78
	II	29	16	55
	III	14	5	36
60	I	198	121	61
	II	87	42	48
	III	37	13	36
61†	A	57	47	82
	B	209	155	74
	C	129	59	46
	D	8	0	0

*Biopsy grades as described by Kenney.[57]

†Biopsy grades similar to those of Kenney,[57] but with an additional category (D) for mares with severe, obliterating fibrosis.

(From Ball, B.A.: Embryonic loss in mares. Vet. Clin. North Am. Equine Pract., *4*:263–290, 1988.)

Maternal Age

Because mares are more likely to be maintained in a breeding herd until a relatively late age, the problem of declining fertility with maternal age is probably more pronounced in the mare than in other domestic animals. A reduced fertility occurs with increased age in the mare characterized by a decline in fertility after middle to late teens and a concomitant increase in embryonic death (Table 61–4). Luteal insufficiency has been proposed as a factor in aged, subfertile mares;[29] however, aged mares had significantly higher progesterone during diestrus than did young mares.[68] Embryonic defects appear to be a major factor in early embryonic death in these mares (see section on embryonic defects). Likewise, abnormal uterine environment, such as persistent endometritis, may increase embryonic death in aged mares.

Lactation and Postpartum Breeding

Several studies indicated that fertility in mares bred at the first postpartum estrus (foal heat) is reduced compared with that of mares bred at later postpartum estrous periods. Much of the reduced fertility in mares mated at foal heat appears to be related to embryonic death. Higher embryonic death rates have been reported in mares bred on foal heat in some studies but not in others (Table 61–5). Abnormalities of the uterine environment, such as delayed uterine involution or persistent endometritis, appear to be the major contributing factors responsible for embryonic death in mares mated at foal heat. Villahoz reported a higher incidence of embryonic death in mares mated at foal heat that had ultrasonographic or cytologic evidence of endometritis.[70] He suggested that uterine lavage in postpartum mares might improve uterine environment and reduce incidence of embryonic death.

Side of fixation of the conceptus in postpartum mares may also influence embryonic death. The equine conceptus becomes fixed more often in the previously nongravid uterine horn in mares mated at foal heat.[71] One report suggested a higher incidence of embryonic and early fetal death in mares in which pregnancy was established in the previously gravid uterine horn (C.H. Marlow and R.O. Gilber, personal communication). The reason for increased incidence of embryonic death in conceptuses fixed in the previously gravid horn is unknown, although differences in degree of histologic involution between previously gravid and nongravid horns might account for higher embryonic death when fixation occurred in the previously gravid horn.

In addition to foal heat matings, some investigators have reported a higher incidence of embryonic death in lactating than in nonlactating (maiden and barren) mares. Other investigators, however, have not been able to confirm this observation (Table 61–6). Differences between these studies may be the result of different management factors such as nutrition, which can influence the fertility of lactating mares.[72]

TABLE 61–4. MATERNAL AGE AND INCIDENCE OF PREGNANCY LOSS IN MARES AS REPORTED IN SEVERAL STUDIES

STUDY	AGE GROUPS (YR)	NUMBER OF PREGNANCIES	NUMBER OF PREGNANCY LOSSES	PREGNANCY LOSSES (%)
3*	3–6	675	102	15
	7–9	637	123	19
	10–12	507	109	22
	13–16	471	101	21
	>16	170	39	23
65†	2–4	177	4	2
	5–7	362	17	5
	8–10	220	12	5
	11–13	142	6	4
	14–16	67	9	12
	>16	42	6	13
66†	3–6	173	12	7
	7–10	205	23	11
	11–14	103	11	11
	15–18	52	8	15
	>18	14	4	29
67‡	<10	107	6	6
	10–15	37	2	5
	>15	21	5	24
13**	2–5	153	18	12
	6–9	177	24	14
	10–13	130	12	9
	14–17	34	8	24
	18–21	12	4	33

*Pregnancy losses from day 20 through term.
†Pregnancy losses from day 42 through term.
‡Embryonic deaths between days 17 and 40.
**Embryonic deaths between days 14 and 56.
(From Ball, B.A.: Embryonic loss in mares. Vet. Clin. North Am. Equine Pract., *4*:263–290, 1988.)

EXTERNAL FACTORS

Stress

Stress has been proposed as an important factor in embryonic death in mares.[73–75] Osborne examined mares at slaughter and proposed that a high rate of early fetal loss might be associated with handling or transporting mares.[74] However, Baucus et al. found no increase in embryonic death rates for small groups of mares that were transported for 9 h compared with mares that were not transported.[76] Transport did elicit changes in serum cortisol and progesterone concentrations indicative of stress.[76] Mitchell and Allen reported a 46% (44 of 95) incidence of embryonic and early fetal loss in mares first bred as yearlings (12 to 14 months) and proposed that many of the observed losses could have been caused by physical or nutritional stresses.[73] Van Niekerk reported a sharp decline in total peripheral progestogen concentrations in mares that experienced stress related to pain, infectious disease, or weaning after 100 days of gestation and proposed the decline in progestogen concentrations was the result of corticosteroid release.[75] The role of maternal stress and its possible relationship to progesterone levels and embryonic death in mares requires further study.

A relationship may also exist between level of nutrition (primarily protein or energy) and embryonic death in mares. Van Niekerk reported that mares on poor-quality pasture had more embryonic deaths between days 25 to 31 than did mares that received a supplement or better-quality grazing.[77] He also proposed this was a critical period during which mares that received poor nutrition were susceptible to embryonic death. Unfortunately, changes in body weight or condition of mares in this study were not reported, and other factors such as season or climate may have been important.

Influence of nutrition and body condition on reproductive performance of mares from 90 days prefoaling, through breeding, and to 90 days postfoaling was examined.[72] Lower day-30 pregnancy rates (4 of 8 vs. 8 of 8) and more pregnancy losses between days 30 and 90 (3 of 4 vs. 0 of 8) resulted when mares were fed a ration which resulted in loss of body condition during prepartum and postpartum intervals. In a related study, restricted energy intake resulted in a decrease in mare weight (0.76 kg/day) and in more pregnancy losses by

TABLE 61–5. A REVIEW OF DETECTED PREGNANCY LOSSES IN FOALING MARES THAT CONCEIVED AT FIRST, SECOND, OR LATER POSTPARTUM ESTROUS PERIODS

	NUMBER OF LOSSES/NUMBER OF PREGNANCIES (PERCENT)		
Reference Number	First Estrus	Second Estrus	Later Estrus
66*†	30/143 (21.0)	17/112 (15.2)	8/127 (6.3)
6*‡	150/716 (21.0)	141/1037 (15.2)	98/914 (6.3)
69†§	16/126 (12.7)		32/280 (11.4)
7‡	24/275 (8.7)	13/110 (11.8)	9/176 (5.1)
13†‖	18/157 (11)		24/203 (12)

*Difference ($p < 0.01$) in proportions between groups.
†Later estrus included mares bred on second estrus.
‡Detected pregnancy losses before days 70 to 90.
§Detected pregnancy losses between days 35 to 42 and term.
‖Embryonic deaths detected by ultrasonography between days 14 and 48.
(From Ball, B.A.: Embryonic loss in mares. Vet. Clin. North Am. Equine Pract., *4*:263–290, 1988.)

90 days than in control mares.[78] Mares on the restricted energy diet had higher progesterone and lower cortisol concentrations than control mares.[78] These studies indicate that the level of nutrition as it relates to body condition has a significant effect on embryonic and early fetal death in mares. Conversely, overfeeding did not adversely affect fertility in postpartum mares.[79]

Season and Environmental Temperature

Mares are seasonal breeders,[17] and seasonal influences probably affect embryonic death. Scherbarth found a higher incidence (7.7%) of embryonic and early fetal loss in Hanoverian mares in the early (March to May) breeding season than (2.7%) in the later breeding season (June).[7] Moberg also reported an apparently higher incidence of embryonic deaths in mares bred early in the breeding season.[5,80] Woods et al., however, found no significant difference in mean date of conception between mares that maintained pregnancy and mares that underwent embryonic death.[15] Swerczek proposed that mares bred early in the year (February and March) were more susceptible to early fetal losses (60 to 100 days of gestation) because of bacterial placentitis sec-

TABLE 61–6. REVIEW OF PREGNANCY LOSSES IN LACTATING AND NONLACTATING MARES

		MARE CLASSIFICATION*	
Reference Number	Interval of Loss (Days)	Lactating	Nonlactating†
3	20–150 d	186/1382 (13.5%)	160/1180 (13.6%)
6†‡	before 90	389/2667 (14.6%)	146/2564 (5.7%)
7	18–70	46/561 (8.2%)	34/175 (7.2%)
12§	14–48	30/259 (11.6%)	14/144 (10.4%)
13**	14–48	52/385 (13.5%)	28/215 (13.0%)

*Expressed as number of losses divided by number of pregnancies (percent).
†Includes mares classified as barren and maiden.
‡Difference ($p < 0.01$) in proportions between groups.
**Pregnancy detection by ultrasonography.
(From Ball, B.A.: Embryonic loss in mares. Vet. Clin. North Am. Equine Pract., *4*:263–290, 1988.)

ondary to cervical relaxation.[81] He also proposed that nutritional effects (such as lush pasture) or seasonal effects resulted in cervical dilation. Possible seasonal effects on embryonic death in mares require further investigation.

Unfortunately, no reports were found on the effect of environmental temperature on embryonic death in mares. In cattle, both rectal and uterine temperatures near the time of insemination appear related to pregnancy rates, and heat stress resulted in embryonic death before day 16.[82,83] Heifers exposed to elevated temperatures beginning at 30 h postestrus had more abnormal or degenerate day-7 embryos when compared with control heifers.[84] The potential role of heat stress on embryonic death in mares needs further study.

Sire Factors in Embryonic Death

Limited information is available regarding influence of stallion on embryonic death. Differences between fertility of stallions could be related to differences in fertilization rates or subsequent embryonic death rates; however, the relative magnitude of these factors is unknown. Some authors have reported high embryonic or early fetal death rates for particular stallions.[66,85] In laboratory rodents, females mated to subfertile males had a higher incidence of embryonic death as well as fertilization failure,[86] but little evidence is available to assess the incidence of embryonic death in mares mated to subfertile stallions. Transmission of specific venereal pathogens such as Klebsiella sp., Pseudomonas sp., Taylorella equigenitalum, equine viral arteritis, or nonspecific bacterial contaminants could also account for some sire-related embryonic deaths.[64,87–90]

The effect of mating practices on embryonic death should also be considered. The long duration of estrus, longevity of stallion sperm, and maintenance of sexual receptivity after ovulation make gamete aging a distinct possibility. In swine, aging of the ovum after ovulation can significantly increase incidence of polyspermia and subsequent embryonic death.[91] A recent study in mares indicated that mating postovulation resulted in a higher embryonic death rate particularly in mares inseminated 12 h or later after ovulation.[92] Timing of insemination or mating is therefore an important consideration in routine reproductive management of mares.

Iatrogenic Factors in Embryonic Death

Palpation per rectum was proposed as a factor in embryonic death when more losses were determined when pregnancy was first detected at days 20 to 30 than in a second year when pregnancy was first detected after day 42.[74] In another study, pregnancy losses were similar between years in which pregnancy was first detected by palpation per rectum at days 20 to 30 or after day 42.[4] An increased incidence of detected embryonic deaths might be expected with earlier pregnancy detection because this would include a time with a higher incidence of pregnancy losses (see section on fertilization and embryonic death rates). Voss et al. reported a significant decline in detected, first-cycle pregnancy rates in mares that were palpated daily during estrus compared with mares that were not palpated; however, palpation per rectum on a daily basis during the first 50 days of gestation did not appear to affect pregnancy loss rates.[93]

Safety of ultrasonography for early pregnancy detection in mares has not been critically tested.[94] Ginther suggested that frequent, repeated ultrasound examinations of the early pregnant uterus resulted in no apparent increase in embryonic deaths.[94] McKinnon et al. examined mares at 5-day intervals between days 15 and 50 via palpation per rectum or by palpation per rectum and ultrasonography and found no significant differences in pregnancy rates between techniques.[95] Vogelsang et al. also found no adverse effects of frequent ultrasound examinations on fertility or embryonic death.[96] Potential effects of both palpation per rectum and ultrasonography on embryonic death in mares require further controlled study.

Several exogenous hormones have been associated with embryonic death in mares. Squires et al. identified a tendency for an increased embryonic death rate in young mares that had previously received anabolic steroids.[97] Allen found that administration of three doses of 2000 IU of human chorionic gonadotropin (hCG) to pregnant pony mares between days 24 and 38 resulted in embryonic death, but administration of similar doses of hCG after day 39 did not result in pregnancy loss.[98] Embryonic death induced with hCG was apparently caused by reduced progesterone levels after administration of hCG, and exogenous progesterone was effective in preventing embryonic death.[99] The administration of $PGF_2\alpha$, or its analogues, has been shown to induce embryonic death between days 12 and 35.[100–104] Administration of prostaglandin to pregnant mares after day 35 resulted in early fetal losses but apparently required repeated administration to induce pregnancy loss effectively.[17,103,104]

EMBRYONIC FACTORS

Primary embryonic abnormalities are also important considerations in embryonic death in mares. Recovery of embryos from the uterus of subfertile mares is reduced (Table 61–7). Embryos recovered from subfertile mares were smaller and had more morphologic defects than embryos from fertile mares.[109,110] Because these embryos had been exposed to the uterine environment, uterine or oviductal abnormalities as well as primary embryonic defects must be considered as possible causes of these defects.

Observations on the transfer of day-7 or -8 embryos from subfertile mares appear to indicate a reduced viability after transfer to the uterus of normal recipient mares.[111] Embryos collected at day 4 from the oviduct of aged, subfertile donor mares had a significantly lower survival rate after transfer to normal recipient mares than embryos from young, fertile mares.[2] Defects in embryos from subfertile mares were present before ex-

TABLE 61–7. PERCENTAGE OF EMBRYOS RECOVERED FROM FERTILE AND SUBFERTILE MARES AT DAYS 7 TO 10 AS REPORTED IN SEVERAL STUDIES

REFERENCE NUMBER	FERTILE MARES*	SUBFERTILE MARES
105	56/100 (56%)	12/35 (34%)
106	128/160 (80%)	10/36 (28%)
107	29/49 (59%)	5/34 (15%)
15	29/42 (69%)	17/42 (40%)
108	334/442 (76%)	24/109 (40%)

*Difference between groups at $p < 0.05$ (*) or $p < 0.01$ (**).

(From Ball, B.A.: Embryonic loss in mares. Vet. Clin. North Am. Equine Pract., *4*:263–290, 1988.)

posure to uterine environment. Therefore, oviductal environment or primary embryonic defects must be considered in the high embryonic death rate observed in aged, subfertile mares.

Chromosomal and Genetic Abnormalities

Karyotypic abnormalities have been described in mares and stallions and have been proposed as a cause of embryonic death in mares.[112–116] Blue examined 22 embryos collected surgically from mares at days 28 to 64 but found no karyotypic abnormalities.[112] Romagnano et al. described a technique for chromosomal preparation from equine embryos, but did not report any detectable karyotypic abnormalities in 92 equine embryos examined between days 6 and 28 after ovulation.[117,118]

Bishop proposed that a considerable part of embryonic death was caused by genetically defective embryos that probably arise de novo within each parent generation and that this embryonic death should be regarded as a normal elimination of defective genotypes.[119] In support of Bishop's hypothesis, studies of human pregnancy loss indicated that 50 to 60% of spontaneous first trimester abortions have detectable chromosomal abnormalities. However, perhaps one should not extrapolate these results to domestic animals, because the incidence of identifiable chromosomal abnormalities in embryos of domestic animals is much lower (< 10%) than that reported in human pregnancy losses.[120–123] However, incidence of chromosomal abnormalities may vary with the population of embryos under study. In cattle, embryos with morphologic defects had a higher incidence of detectable chromosomal abnormalities,[124] and research is needed to determine whether the higher incidence of morphologic abnormalities in embryos from subfertile mares is also associated with more chromosomal defects. Furthermore, an apparently low incidence of karyotypic abnormalities does not eliminate possible influence of as yet unrecognized genetic defects in equine embryos.

Although heritable defects have been described, most numeric chromosome disorders are thought to arise as a result of errors in gametogenesis, fertilization, or early embryo cleavage.[119,125,126] Gamete aging and abnormalities of spermatozoal transport might be related to numeric chromosome abnormalities, but considerable research is required to investigate these possible factors in embryonic death.

Immunogenetic Factors

Immunogenetic aspects of pregnancy in equids are unique among domestic animals because of the pronounced maternal immune response to fetal major histocompatibility antigens associated with chorionic girdle cells.[127] This response is reflected in a marked cellular immune response to the endometrial cups as well as presence of serum antibody against paternal lymphocytes as early as days 45 to 70.[128] Failure of endometrial cup formation and equine chorionic girdle formation in interspecific transfer of donkey conceptuses to horse recipients resulted in a high incidence of fetal death between days 80 and 90.[127] Abnormalities in this immunologic response have been proposed as a factor in some spontaneous early fetal deaths.[127]

Immunogenetic regulation during the embryonic period is not as well described as that during the early fetal period. Antigens specific to equine trophoblast have been identified as early as day 12 after ovulation.[129] However, because the equine conceptus is surrounded by an acellular capsule until approximately day 21, any immunologic reaction to the conceptus would likely occur after this period.[127,129] The capsule would probably mask antigens expressed by the early conceptus as well as prevent maternal antibodies from reaching the conceptus.[127]

Antibodies to equine zona pellucida have been identified in infertile mares,[130] and immunization of mares with heterologous porcine zona pellucida has been used as a method of contraception.[131] The method of action of antizona antibodies, however, appears to be directed against spermatozoal binding at fertilization rather than embryonic survival.[131]

DIAGNOSTIC CONSIDERATIONS IN EMBRYONIC DEATH

ULTRASONOGRAPHIC CHARACTERISTICS OF SPONTANEOUS AND INDUCED EMBRYONIC DEATHS

The ultrasonographic morphologic features of spontaneous and induced embryonic deaths have been described.[8,19,94,101] Possible indications of impending embryonic death included (1) presence of intraluminal uterine fluid, (2) irregular shape of the embryonic vesicle, (3) prolonged mobility of the vesicle, (4) undersize vesicle, (5) loss of embryonic heartbeat, (6) dislodgment of the vesicle with loss of fluid, and (7) edema of the endometrial folds.[10,31,94,101] Many spontaneous embryonic deaths detected between days 11 and 20 were not preceded by ultrasonographically detectable changes in the embryonic vesicle or in the mare's uterus.[10,94,101] In 3 of 28 losses, small collections of free fluid were observed in the mare's uterine lumen.[10] Irregular vesicles were noted in a few cases before embryonic death between days 11 to 20; however, changes from early spherical shape of the vesicle were normally observed by days 17 to 19.[94] The embryonic vesicle is mobile within the uterus from time of first detection until days 15 to 16 when it becomes fixed at the base of one uterine horn.[132,133] Failure of fixation as indicated by prolonged mobility of the embryonic vesicle beyond day 17 has been observed in a few cases of spontaneous embryonic death.[10] A higher proportion of embryonic vesicles that were later lost were detected in the uterine body between days 11 and 14 than were embryonic vesicles that were maintained (30 of 50 vs. 70 of 189, respectively). Whether this difference in location of the embryonic vesicles was related to embryonic mobility was unclear.[92]

Undersize embryonic vesicles have been reported as a possible indicator of impending loss.[8,19,94] A total of 78% (96 of 144) of undersize vesicles (more than 1 standard deviation below the mean diameter of embryos of the same age),[8] and 62% (21 of 34) of the undersize vesicles (more than 2 standard deviations below the mean diameter) were lost by day 25.[10] In a study in which embryonic deaths were apparently related to uterine inflammation, the mean diameter of embryonic vesicles that were lost was significantly less by day 13 than that of embryonic vesicles that survived.[19] Many undersize vesicles that were subsequently lost continued to grow at an approximately normal rate until the loss was detected.[10,94] In contrast to undersize vesicles, oversize embryonic vesicles were not associated with an increased embryo death.[8,10]

Studies on ultrasonographic structure of induced embryonic deaths have provided a more consistent description of changes associated with embryonic death. Embryos were lost an average of 6.8 days after administration of 5 mg $PGF_2\alpha$ to pregnant mares at day 12.[101] In these mares, the embryonic vesicle was mobile beyond day 17 (failure of fixation), uterine tone decreased, and the yolk sac membrane separated from the endometrium.[101] All four mares given $PGF_2\alpha$ at day 12 had a patent cervix on the day of loss detection; however, it was unknown whether the embryonic vesicle was discharged through the cervix.[101]

Mean interval to complete loss of the conceptus after $PGF_2\alpha$ at day 30 was 8.5 days.[101] Within 1 to 3 days after $PGF_2\alpha$, the vesicle was dislodged from the base of either uterine horn and often moved into the uterine body[101] possibly caused by a loss of uterine tone as progesterone levels declined.[94] After administration of $PGF_2\alpha$ at day 30, a prominent edema of the endometrial folds was noted before embryonic death.[101] Loss of the conceptus following $PGF_2\alpha$ at day 30 was also characterized by a gradual decrease in fluid volume with a closed cervix and expulsion of the conceptus debris through the cervix when the mare returned to estrus.[94] In another study, fetal death was induced by administration of a hypertonic saline solution into the fetal sac of 10 mares at day 45. In this study, the fetal heartbeat was lost within 3 h and dissociation of the conceptus within the uterus within 2 to 3 days after administration.[45]

ENDOCRINOLOGY

Serum or plasma progesterone concentrations have been suggested as a method to predict impending embryonic death.[29,34,134,135] Practical use of this method requires knowledge of the considerable variation in blood progesterone concentrations during pregnancy and among animals.[136,137] Detection of progesterone concentrations under 4 ng/mL over 2 consecutive days has been suggested as a possible indicator of impending embryonic death with a significantly higher rate of embryonic death in mares with progesterone concentration under 2 ng/mL.[134] Research in ovariectomized, progesterone-treated, embryo-recipient mares indicated that progesterone concentrations above 2.5 ng/mL were adequate to maintain pregnancy in the absence of an endogenous source.[33] Effective use of blood progesterone concentrations requires rapid reporting of test results or the use of a synthetic progestin, such as altrenogest, which does not cross-react with radioimmunoassays for progesterone. Identification of a low progesterone concentration does not, however, indicate whether the cause is related to inappropriate luteolysis, luteal insufficiency, or failure of maternal recognition of pregnancy as discussed earlier.

Although estrone sulfate can be used to assess fetal viability after day 44,[44] no other readily available endocrinologic assays exist to assess the well-being of the equine conceptus during the embryonic period. Reports of use of an assay for early pregnancy factor (EPF) indicate that it may be possible to use a blood-based assay to assess pregnancy status of mares as early as day 7; however, the rosette-inhibition assay used to detect EPF is difficult to perform and is not widely available.[138,139]

PREVENTION, MANAGEMENT, AND THERAPY OF EMBRYONIC DEATHS

Because of the multifactorial nature of embryonic death in mares, no single therapeutic or management scheme is likely to be effective. Understanding of the processes associated with embryonic death in mares also limits our ability to effectively and rationally deal with mares with impending or repeated embryonic death.

Because of the importance of progesterone for pregnancy maintenance in mares, much attention has been placed on the use of exogenous progesterone as a method to prevent or treat impending embryonic death. Considerable controversy exists regarding merits of exogenous progesterone therapy as well as dosages and duration of therapy. Many dosages do not effectively elevate or maintain serum progesterone concentrations. Research in pregnant, ovariectomized mares indicated that 1000 mg repositol progesterone every 4 days or 22 to 44 mg altrenogest daily were adequate to maintain pregnancy.[134] Daily administration of 300 mg progesterone in oil or 22 mg altrenogest has been used to maintain pregnancy in ovariectomized recipient mares, although levels of 200 mg progesterone and 11 mg altrenogest appeared adequate for pregnancy maintenance in these mares as well.[34,140] Altrenogest does not appear to suppress endogenous progesterone secretion and provides a convenient method of oral supplementation of progesterone.[141] Clitoral enlargement has been reported in fillies born to dams treated with altrenogest, but no other adverse effects of prenatal altrenogest therapy on reproductive function were noted.[142]

Administration of exogenous luteinizing hormone (LH) in the form of human chorionic gonadotropin (hCG) (1000 IU on days 3, 4, and 5 postestrus) resulted in a significantly increased serum progesterone concentration in pregnant mares through day 30.[143] No clinical reports of attempts to stimulate endogenous progesterone secretion with luteotrophic hormones were found; however, this approach merits further research to determine if administration of hCG in the early luteal phase might be a method to enhance luteal function and progesterone secretion.

Duration of progestin therapy has also been debated. Most benefits of exogenous progesterone therapy are probably realized during the first 3 to 4 months of pregnancy. Placental production of progesterone is adequate to maintain pregnancy after days 50 to 70,[144] and concentrations of serum progesterone begin to decline after day 120.[17] In early pregnancy, high doses of exogenous progesterone can increase growth rate of the conceptus (as determined by diameter of the embryonic vesicle) and increase the amount of protein in yolk sac fluid.[35,145] This benefit is likely a result of increased secretion of histotroph stimulated by progesterone. The benefits realized from exogenous progesterone administration will likely occur during the first 90 to 120 days of gestation.

Nonsteroidal anti-inflammatory drugs, such as flunixin meglumine, have been used to block prostaglandin $F_2\alpha$ mediated luteolysis and subsequent embryonic death in mares that received endotoxin experimentally.[33] Long-term therapy with flunixin meglumine (1.1 mg/kg daily from days 10 to 60) has also been used to prevent luteolysis in a mare with repeated embryonic death, which was apparently related to chronic uterine inflammation.[30] However, safety of chronic flunixin meglumine therapy during early pregnancy in the mare has not been extensively tested. Long-term progestin therapy may be effective in preventing embryonic death secondary to reduced endogenous progesterone concentrations.

REFERENCES

1. Ball, B.A., Little, T.V., Hillman, R.B., and Woods, G.L.: Pregnancy rates at days 2 and 14 and estimated embryonic loss rates prior to day 14 in normal and subfertile mares. Theriogenology, *26*:611–619, 1986.
2. Ball, B.A., Little, T.V., Weber, J.A., and Woods, G.L.: Viability of day-4 embryos from young, normal mares and aged, subfertile mares after transfer to normal recipient mares. J. Reprod. Fertil., *85*:187–194, 1989.
3. Bain, A.M.: Foetal losses during pregnancy in Thoroughbred mares: a record of 2562 pregnancies. N. Z. Vet. J., *17*:155–158, 1969.
4. Irwin, C.F.P.: Early pregnancy testing and its relationship to abortion. J. Reprod. Fertil. Suppl., *23*:485–489, 1975.
5. Moberg, R.: The occurrence of early embryonic death in the mare in relation to natural service and artificial insemination with fresh or deep-frozen semen. J. Reprod. Fertil. Suppl., *23*:537–539, 1975.
6. Merkt, H., and Gunzel, A.: A survey of early pregnancy losses in West German Thoroughbred mares. Equine Vet. J., *11*:256–258, 1979.
7. Scherbarth, R.: On the occurrence of embryonic resorption by mares in the Hanoverian warm blood breed. DTW Dtsch. Tierarztl. Wochenschr, *87*:189–191, 1980.
8. Chevalier, F., and Palmer, E.: Ultrasonic echography in the mare. J. Reprod. Fertil. Suppl., *32*:423–430, 1982.
9. Simpson, D.J., et al.: Use of ultrasound echography for early diagnosis of single and twin pregnancy in the mare. J. Reprod. Fertil. Suppl., *32*:431–439, 1982.
10. Ginther, O.J., Bergfelt, D.R., Leith, G.S., and Scraba, S.T.: Embryonic loss in mares: Incidence and ultrasonic morphology. Theriogenology, *24*:73–86, 1985.
11. Villahoz, M.D., Squires, E.L., Voss, J.L., and Shideler, R.K.: Some observations on early embryonic death in mares. Theriogenology, *23*:915–923, 1985.
12. Woods, G.L., et al.: A field study on early pregnancy loss in Standardbred and Thoroughbred mares. J. Equine Vet. Sci., *5*:264–267, 1985.
13. Woods, G.L., et al.: Early pregnancy loss in broodmares. J. Reprod. Fertil. Suppl., *35*:455–459, 1987.
14. Forde, D., et al.: Reproductive wastage in the mare and its relationship to progesterone in early pregnancy. J. Reprod. Fertil. Suppl., *35*:493–495, 1987.
15. Woods, G.L., Baker, C.B., Hillman, R.B., and Schlafer, D.H.: Recent studies relating to early embryonic death in the mare. Equine Vet. J. Suppl., *3*:104–107, 1985.
16. Sharp, D.C., McDowell, K.J., Weithenauer, J., and Thatcher, W.W.: The continuum of events leading to maternal recognition of pregnancy in mares. J. Reprod. Fertil. Suppl., *37*:101–107, 1989.
17. Ginther, O.J.: Reproductive Biology of the Mare: Basic and Applied Aspects. Cross Plaines, WI, Equiservices, 1979.
18. Ginther, O.J.: Embryonic loss in mares: Incidence, time of occurrence, and hormonal involvement. Theriogenology, *23*:77–89, 1985.
19. Adams, G.P., Kastelic, J.P., Bergfelt, D.R., and Ginther, O.J.: Effect of uterine inflammation and ultrasonically-detected uterine pathology on fertility in the mare. J. Reprod. Fertil. Suppl., *35*:445–454, 1987.
20. Iuliano, M.F., Squires, E.L., and Cook, V.M.: Effect of

age of equine embryos and method of transfer on pregnancy rate. J. Anim. Sci., *60:*258–263, 1985.

21. Pope, W.F.: Uterine asynchrony: A cause of embryonic loss. Biol. Reprod., *39:*999–1003, 1988.
22. McDowell, K.J.: Establishment of pregnancy in mares: Interrelationships among uterine proteins, prostaglandin F2 alpha, and conceptus secretory proteins. Ann Arbor, University Microfilms, Inc., 1986.
23. Hinrichs, K., Kenney, R.M., and Sharp, D.C.: Differences in protein content of uterine fluid related to duration of progesterone treatment in ovariectomised mares used as embryo recipients. Equine Vet. J. Suppl., *8:*49–55, 1989.
24. McDowell, K.J., et al.: Restricted conceptus mobility results in failure of pregnancy maintenance in mares. Biol. Reprod., *39:*340–348, 1988.
25. Leith, G.S., and Ginther, O.J.: Mobility of the conceptus and uterine contractions in the mare. Theriogenology, *24:*701–711, 1985.
26. Betteridge, K.J., Renard, A., and Goff, A.K.: Uterine prostaglandin release relative to embryo collection, transfer procedures and maintenance of the corpus luteum. Equine Vet. J. Suppl., *3:*25–33, 1985.
27. Goff, A.K., Pontbriand, D., and Sirois, J.: Oxytocin stimulation of plasma 15-keto-13,14-dihydro prostaglandin $F_2\alpha$ release during the oestrous cycle and early pregnancy in the mare. J. Reprod. Fertil. Suppl., *35:*253–260, 1987.
28. Ginther, O.J., et al.: Embryonic loss in mares: Pregnancy rate, length of interovulatory intervals, and progesterone concentrations associated with loss during days 11 to 15. Theriogenology, *24:*409–417, 1985.
29. Douglas, R.H., Burns, P.J., and Hershman, L.: Physiological and commercial parameters for producing progeny from subfertile mares by embryo transfer. Equine Vet. J. Suppl., *3:*111–114, 1985.
30. Darenius, K., Fredriksson, G., and Kindahl, H.: Allyl trenbolone and flunixin meglumine treatment of mares with repeated embryonic loss. Equine Vet. J., Suppl., *8:*35–39, 1989.
31. Ball, B.A., et al.: Embryonic loss in pony mares induced by intrauterine inoculation of Candida parapsilosis. Theriogenology, *29:*835–848, 1988.
32. Daels, P., et al.: Effect of Salmonella typhimurium endotoxin on prostaglandin release and early fetal death in the mare. J. Reprod. Fertil. Suppl., *35:*485–492, 1987.
33. Daels, P.F., Stabenfeldt, G.H., Kindahl, H., and Hughes, J.P.: Prostaglandin release and luteolysis associated with physiological and pathological conditions of the reproductive cycle of the mare: A review. Equine Vet. J. Suppl., *8:*29–34, 1989.
34. McKinnon, A.O., Squires, E.L., Carnevale, E.M., and Hermenet, M.J.: Ovariectomized steroid-treated mares as embryo transfer recipients and as a model to study the role of progestins in pregnancy maintenance. Theriogenology, *29:*1055–1063, 1988.
35. Weithenauer, J., McDowell, K.J., Davis, S.D., and Rothman, T.K.: Effect of exogenous progesterone and estrogen on early embryonic growth in pony mares. Biol. Reprod. Suppl. 1, *34,* 102, 1986.
36. Weithenauer, J., Sharp, D.C., and Sheerin, P.C.: Use of vitellocentesis to investigate the effects of steroids on nutrients within the yolk-sac of day 18 pregnant mares. Equine Vet. J. Suppl., *8:*25–28, 1989.
37. Flood, P.F., Betteridge, K.J., and Irvine, D.S.: Oestrogens and androgens in blastocoelic fluid and cultures of cells from equine conceptuses of 10–22 days gestation. J. Reprod. Fertil. Suppl., *27:*413–420, 1979.
38. Heap, R.B., Hamon, M., and Allen, W.R.: Studies on oestrogen synthesis by the preimplantation equine conceptus. J. Reprod. Fertil. Suppl., *32:*343–352, 1982.
39. Marsan, C., Goff, A.K., Sirois, J., and Betteridge, K.J.: Steroid secretion by different cell types of the horse conceptus. J. Reprod. Fertil. Suppl., *35:*363–369, 1987.
40. Zavy, M.T., et al.: An investigation of the uterine luminal environment of nonpregnant and pregnant pony mares. J. Reprod. Fertil. Suppl., *27:*403–411, 1979.
41. Hayes, K.E.N., and Ginther, O.J.: Role of progesterone and estrogen in development of uterine tone in mares. Theriogenology, *25:*581–590, 1986.
42. Kindall, H., Knudsen, O., Madej, A., and Edqvist, L.E.: Progesterone, prostaglandin $F_2\alpha$, PMSG and oestrone sulphate during early pregnancy in the mare. J. Reprod. Fertil. Suppl., *32:*353–354, 1982.
43. Terqui, M., and Palmer, E.: Oestrogen pattern during early pregnancy in the mare. J. Reprod. Fertil. Suppl., *27:*441–446, 1979.
44. Kasman, L.H., et al.: Estrone sulfate concentrations as an indicator of fetal demise in horses. Am. J. Vet. Res., *49:*184–187, 1988.
45. Jeffcott, L.B., et al.: Changes in maternal hormone concentrations associated with induction of fetal death at day 45 of gestation in mares. J. Reprod. Fertil. Suppl., *35:*461–467, 1987.
46. Bosu, W.T.K., Turner, L., and Franks, T.: Estrone sulphate and progesterone concentrations in the peripheral blood of pregnant mares: Clinical implications. Proceedings of the International Congress on Animal Reproduction and Artificial Insemination, 1984, p. 78.
47. Darenius, K., Kindahl, H., and Madej, A.: Clinical and endocrine aspects of early fetal death in the mare. J. Reprod. Fertil. Suppl., *35:*497–498, 1987.
48. Betteridge, K.J., et al.: Development of horse embryos up to twenty-two days after ovulation: Observation on fresh specimens. J. Anat., *135:*191–209, 1982.
49. Betteridge, K.J., Eaglesome, M.D., and Flood, P.F.: Embryo transport through the mare's oviduct depends on cleavage and is independent of the ipsilateral corpus luteum. J. Reprod. Fertil. Suppl., *27:*387–394, 1979.
50. Murray, F.A., et al.: Developmental failure of swine embryos restricted to the oviductal environment. J. Reprod. Fertil. *24:*445–448, 1971.
51. Freeman, D.A., Weber, J.A., and Woods, G.L.: Transport of equine uterine embryos and rabbit embryos through the oviduct of the mare. Equine Vet. J. Suppl., *8:*86, 1989.
52. Weber, J.A., Freeman, D.A., Vanderwall, D.K., and Woods, G.L.: Prostaglandin E2 hastens oviductal transport of equine embryos. Biol. Reprod., *45:*1–3, 1991.
53. Weber, J.A., Freeman, D.A., Vanderwall, D.K., and Woods, G.L.: Prostaglandin E2 secretion by oviductal transport-stage equine embryos. Biol. Reprod., *45:*8–11, 1991.
54. Saltiel, A., Paramo, R., Murcia, C., and Tolosa, J.: Pathologic findings in the oviducts of mares. Am. J. Vet. Res., *47:*594–597, 1986.
55. Henry, M., and Vandeplassche, M.: Pathology of the oviduct in mares. Vlaams Diergeneesk Tijdschr., *50:*301–325, 1981.
56. McDowell, K.J., Sharp, D.C., Fazleabas, A.T., and Roberts, R.M.: Two-dimensional polyacrylamide gel electrophoresis of proteins synthesized and released by concep-

tuses and endometria from pony mares. J. Reprod. Fertil., *89:*107–115, 1990.

57. Kenney, R.M.: Cyclic and pathologic changes of the mare endometrium as detected by biopsy, with a note on early embryonic death. J. Am. Vet. Med. Assoc., *172:*241–262, 1978.

58. Shideler, R.K., et al.: Endometrial biopsy in the mare. Am. Assoc. Equine Pract., 97–103, 1977.

59. De la Concha-Bermejillo, A., and Kennedy, P.C.: Prognostic value of endometrial biopsy in the mare: A retrospective analysis. J. Am. Vet. Med. Assoc., *181:*680–681, 1982.

60. Shideler, R.K., McChesney, A.E., Voss, J.L., and Squires, E.L.: Relationship of endometrial biopsy and other management factors on the fertility of broodmares. Equine Vet. Sci., *2:*5–10, 1982.

61. Doig, P.A., McKnight, J.D., and Miller, R.B.: The use of endometrial biopsy in the infertile mare. Can. Vet. J., *22:*72–76, 1981.

62. Leishman, D., Miller, R.B., and Doig, P.A.: A quantitative study of the histologic morphology of the endometrium of normal and barren mares. Can. J. Comp. Med., *46:*17–20, 1982.

63. Ball, B.A., Hillman, R.B., and Woods, G.L.: Survival of equine embryos transferred to normal and subfertile mares. Theriogenology, *28:*167–174, 1987.

64. Hughes, J.P., and Loy, R.G.: The relation of infection to infertility in the mare and stallion. Equine Vet. J., *7:*155–159, 1975.

65. Badi, A.M., O'Byrne, T.M., and Cunningham, E.P.: An analysis of reproductive performance in Thoroughbred mares. Ir. Vet. J., *35:*1–12, 1981.

66. Platt, H.: Aetiological aspects of abortion in the Thoroughbred mare. J. Comp. Pathol., *83:*199–205, 1973.

67. La Cour, A., and Sprinkle, T.A.: Relationship of endometrial cytology and fertility in the broodmare. Equine Pract., *7:*27–36, 1985.

68. Fonda, E.S., Hackett, G.E., Burrill, M.J., and Cogger, E.A.: A comparison of LH and progesterone secretion in young and aged mares. J. Anim. Sci. Suppl. 1, *65:*429, 1988.

69. Loy, R.G.: Characteristics of postpartum reproduction in mares. Vet. Clin. North Am. Large Anim. Pract., *2:*345–359, 1980.

70. Villahoz, M.D.: Increased pregnancy rates in postpartum mares and early embryonic death. Proc. Soc. Theriogenol., 210–221, 1989.

71. Allen, W.E., and Newcombe, J.R.: Relationship between early pregnancy site in consecutive gestations in mares. Equine Vet. J., *13:*51–52, 1981.

72. Henneke, D.R., Potter, G.D., and Kreider, J.L.: Body condition during pregnancy and lactation and reproductive efficiency of mares. Theriogenology, *21:*897–909, 1984.

73. Mitchell, D., and Allen, W.R.: Observations on reproductive performance in the yearling mare. J. Reprod. Fertil. Suppl., *23:*531–536, 1975.

74. Osborne, V.E.: Factors influencing foaling percentages in Australian mares. J. Reprod. Fertil. Suppl., *23:*477–483, 1975.

75. Van Niekerk, C.H., and Morgenthal, J.C.: Fetal loss and the effect of stress on plasma progestogen levels in pregnant Thoroughbred mares. J. Reprod. Fertil. Suppl., *32:*453–457, 1982.

76. Baucus, K.L., et al.: Effects of transportation on early embryonic death in mares. J. Anim. Sci., *68:*345–351, 1990.

77. Van Niekerk, C.H.: Early embryonic resorption in mares. J. S. Afr. Vet. Med. Assoc., *36:*61–69, 1965.

78. Potter, J.T., et al.: Embryo survival during early gestation in energy deprived mares. J. Reprod. Fertil. Suppl., *35:*715–716, 1987.

79. Kubiak, J.R., et al.: Postpartum reproductive performance in the multiparous mare fed to obesity. Theriogenology, *32:*27–36, 1989.

80. Moberg, R.: Investigations concerning the occurrence of early embryonic death in the mare. Proceedings of the Sixth International Congress on Animal Reproduction and Artificial Insemination, 1968, pp. 1585–1587.

81. Swerczek, T.W.: Early fetal death and infectious placental disease in the mare. Proc. Am. Assoc. Equine Pract., 173–179, 1980.

82. Thatcher, W.W., and Collier, R.J.: Effects of climate on bovine reproduction. *In* Current Therapy in Theriogenology. 2nd ed. Edited by D.A. Morrow. Philadelphia, W.B. Saunders, 1986, pp. 301–309.

83. Tucker, H.A.: Seasonality in cattle. Theriogenology, *17:*53–59, 1982.

84. Drost, M., Thatcher, W.W., and Putney, J.D.: Effects of heat stress on fertility in dairy cattle. Proc. Soc. Theriogenol., 207–215, 1986.

85. Britton, J.W.: Clinical studies on early equine abortion. Cornell Vet., *37:*1–14, 1947.

86. Setchell, B.P., et al.: Is embryonic mortality increased in normal female rats mated to subfertile males?. J. Reprod. Fertil., *82:*575–579, 1988.

87. Ley, W.B.: Influence of the sire on early embryonic loss in domestic large animals. Compend. Contin. Educ. Practicing Vet., *7:*S277–S294, 1985.

88. Hughes, J.P., Asbury, A.C., Loy, R.G., and Burd, H.E.: The occurrence of Pseudomonas in the genital tract of stallions and its effects on fertility. Cornell Vet., *57:*53–69, 1967.

89. Timoney, P.J., McAdle, J.F., and O'Reilly, P.J.: Experimental reproduction of contagious equine metritis in pony mares. Vet. Rec., *102:*63, 1978.

90. Timoney, P.J., and McCullom, W.H.: The epidemology of equine viral arteritis. Proc. Am. Assoc. Equine Pract., 545–551, 1985.

91. Hunter, R.H.F.: Fertilization in the pig and horse. *In* A Comparative Overview of Mammalian Fertilization. Edited by B. Dunbar and M. O'Rand. New York, Plenum Press. In press.

92. Woods, J.A., Bergfelt, D.R., and Ginther, O.J.: Effects of time of insemination relative to ovulation on pregnancy rate and embryonic loss rate in mares. Equine Vet. J., *22:*410–415, 1990.

93. Voss, J.L., Pickett, B.W., Back, D.G., and Burwash, L.D.: Effect of rectal palpation on pregnancy rate of nonlactating, normally cycling mares. J. Anim. Sci., *41:*829–834, 1975.

94. Ginther, O.J.: Ultrasonic Imaging and Reproductive Events in the Mare. Cross Plaines, WI, Equiservices, 1986.

95. McKinnon, A.O., Squires, E.L., and Voss, J.L.: Ultrasonic evaluation of the mare's reproductive tract—Part II. Compend. Contin. Educ. Practicing Vet., *9:*472–482, 1987.

96. Vogelsang, M.M., Vogelsang, S.G., Lindsey, B.R., and Massey, J.M.: Reproductive performance in mares subjected to examination by diagnostic ultrasound. Theriogenology, *32:*95–103, 1989.

97. Squires, E.L., Voss, J.L., Maher, J.M., and Shideler, R.K.: Fertility of young mares after long-term anabolic steroid treatment. J. Am. Vet. Med. Assoc., *186:*583–586, 1985.

98. Allen, W.E.: Pregnancy failure induced by human chorionic gonadotrophin in pony mares. Vet. Rec., *96:*88–90, 1975.

99. Allen, W.E.: The effect of human chorionic gonadotropin and exogenous progesterone on luteal function during early pregnancy in pony mares. Anim. Reprod. Sci., *6:*223–228, 1983.

100. Allen, W.E.: Effect of prostaglandin analogue on progesterone-treated mares during early pregnancy. Equine Vet. J., *9:*92–95, 1977.

101. Ginther, O.J.: Embryonic loss in mares: Nature of loss after experimental induction by ovariectomy or prostaglandin $F_2\alpha$. Theriogenology, *24:*87–98, 1985.

102. Kooistra, L.H., and Ginther, O.J.: Termination of pseudopregnancy by administration of prostaglandin $F_2\alpha$ and termination of early pregnancy by administration of prostaglandin $F_2\alpha$ or colchicine or by removal of embryo in mares. Am. J. Vet. Res., *37:*35–39, 1976.

103. Squires, E.L., Hillman, R.B., Pickett, B.W., and Nett, T.M.: Induction of abortion in mares with Equimate: effect on secretion of progesterone, PMSG and reproductive performance. J. Anim. Sci., *50:*490–495, 1980.

104. Baucus, K.L., Squires, E.L., Morris, R., and McKinnon, A.O.: The effect of stage of gestation and frequency of prostaglandin injection on induction of abortion in mares. Proc. Equine Nutr. Physiol. Symp., *10:*255–258, 1987.

105. Douglas, R.H.: Some aspects of equine embryo transfer. J. Reprod. Fertil. Suppl., *32:*405–408, 1982.

106. Squires, E.L., Imel, K.J., Iuliano, M.F., and Shideler, R.K.: Factors affecting reproductive efficiency in an equine embryo transfer programme. J. Reprod. Fertil. Suppl., *32:*409–414, 1982.

107. Pascoe, D.R., Liu, I.K.M., Spensley, M.S., and Hughes, J.P.: Effect of endometrial pathology on the success of non-surgical embryo transfer. Equine Vet. J. Suppl., *3:*108–110, 1985.

108. Squires, E.L., Garcia, R.H., and Ginther, O.J.: Factors affecting success of equine embryo transfer. Equine Vet. J. Suppl., *3:*92–95, 1985.

109. Woods, G.L., Hillman, R.B., and Schlafer, D.H.: Recovery and evaluation of embryos from normal and infertile mares. Cornell Vet., *76:*386–394, 1986.

110. Schlafer, D.H., Dougherty, E., and Woods, G.L.: Light and ultrastructural studies of morphological alterations in embryos collected from maiden and barren mares. J. Reprod. Fertil. Suppl., *35:*695, 1987.

111. Vogelsang, S.G., and Vogelsang, M.M.: Influence of donor parity and age on the success of commercial equine embryo transfer. Equine Vet. J. Suppl., *8:*71–72, 1989.

112. Blue, M.G.: A cytogenetical study of prenatal loss in the mare. Theriogenology, *15:*295–309, 1981.

113. Dewes, H.F.: Thoroughbred breeding in New Zealand. Proc. Am. Assoc. Equine Pract., 39–48, 1973.

114. Halnan, C.R.E.: Sex chromosome mosaicism and infertility in mares. Vet. Rec., *116:*542–543, 1985.

115. McFeely, R.A.: A review of cytogenetics in equine reproduction. J. Reprod. Fertil. Suppl., *23:*371–374, 1975.

116. Trommershausen-Smith, A., Hughes, J.P., and Neely, D.P.: Cytogenetic and clinical findings in mares with gonadal dysgenesis. J. Reprod. Fertil. Suppl., *27:*271–276, 1979.

117. Romagnano, A., King, W.A., Richer, C.L., and Perrone, M.A.: A direct technique for the preparation of chromosomes from early equine embryos. Can. J. Genet. Cytol., *27:*365–369, 1985.

118. Romagnano, A., Richer, C.L., King, W.A., and Betteridge, K.J.: Analysis of X-chromosome inactivation in horse embryos. J. Reprod. Fertil. Suppl., *35:*353–361, 1987.

119. Bishop, M.W.H.: Paternal contribution to embryonic death. J. Reprod. Fertil., *7:*383–396, 1964.

120. Berepubo, N.A., and Long, S.E.: A study of the relationship between chromosome anomalies and reproductive wastage. Theriogenology, *20:*177–190, 1983.

121. Bolet, G.: Timing and extent of embryonic mortality in pigs, sheep and goats: genetic variability. *In* Embryonic Mortality in Farm Animals. Edited by J.M. Sreenan and M.G. Diskin. Dordrecht, M. Nijhoff, 1986, pp. 12–15.

122. Long, S.E., and Williams, C.: Frequency of chromosomal abnormalities in early embryos of the domestic sheep (Ovis aries). J. Reprod. Fertil., *58:*197–201, 1980.

123. Wilmut, I., Sales, D.I., and Ashworth, C.J.: Maternal and embryonic factors associated with prenatal loss in animals. J. Reprod. Fertil., *76:*851–864, 1986.

124. Salisbury, G.W., and Hart, R.G.: Gamete aging and its consequences. Biol. Reprod. Suppl., *2:*1–13, 1970.

125. King, W.A.: Intrinsic embryonic factors that may affect survival after transfer. Theriogenology, *23:*161–174, 1985.

126. Short, R.V.: Maternal Recognition of Pregnancy. Amsterdam, Excerpta Medica, 1979.

127. Antczak, D.F., and Allen, W.R.: Maternal immunologic recognition of pregnancy in equids. J. Reprod. Fertil. Suppl., *37:*69–78, 1989.

128. Antczak, D.F., Miller, J., and Remick, L.H.: Lymphocyte antigens of the horse II. Antibodies to ELA antigens produced during equine pregnancy. J. Reprod. Immunol., *6:*283–297, 1984.

129. Oriol, J.G., Poleman, J.C., and Antczak, D.F.: A monoclonal antibody specific for equine trophoblast. Equine Vet. J. Suppl., *8:*14–18, 1989.

130. Shivers, C.A., and Liu, I.K.M.: Inhibition of sperm binding to porcine ova by antibodies to equine zonae pellucidae. J. Reprod. Fertil. Suppl., *32:*315–318, 1982.

131. Liu, I.K.M., Bernoco, M., and Feldman, M.: Contraception in mares heteroimmunized with pig zonae pellucidae. J. Reprod. Fertil., *85:*19–29, 1989.

132. Ginther, O.J.: Mobility of the early equine conceptus. Theriogenology, *19:*603–611, 1983.

133. Leith, G.S., and Ginther, O.J.: Characterization of intrauterine mobility of the early equine conceptus. Theriogenology, *22:*401–408, 1984.

134. Shideler, R.K., et al.: Progestogen therapy of ovariectomized pregnant mares. J. Reprod. Fertil. Suppl., *32:*459–464, 1982.

135. Douglas, R.H.: Reproduction laboratory in Kentucky. J. Equine Vet. Sci., *4:*69–72, 1984.

136. Allen, W.R.: Is your progesterone therapy really necessary? Equine Vet. J., *16:*496–498, 1984.

137. Stabenfeldt, G.H., and Hughes, J.P.: Clinical aspects of reproductive endocrinology in the horse. Compend. Contin. Educ. Practicing Vet., *9:*677–686, 1987.

138. Gidley-Baird, A.A., and O'Neil, C.: Early pregnancy detection in the mare. Equine Vet. Data, *3:*42, 1982.

139. Branco, M.D.L., Kuchembuck, M.R.G., Papa, F.O., and Campos Filho, E.P.: Detection of early pregnancy in

mares by the Rosette inhibition test and measurement of serum progesterone. Equine Vet. J. Suppl., *8:*19–20, 1989.

140. Hinrichs, K., Sertich, P.L., Palmer, E., and Kenney, R.M.: Establishment and maintenance of pregnancy after embryo transfer in ovariectomized mares treated with progesterone. J. Reprod. Fertil., *80:*395–401, 1987.

141. Jackson, S.A., Squires, E.L., and Nett, T.M.: The effect of exogenous progesterone on endogenous progesterone secretion in pregnant mares. Theriogenology, *25:*275–279, 1986.

142. Naden, J., Squires, E.L., and Nett, T.M.: Effect of maternal treatment on age at puberty, hormone concentrations, pituitary response to exogenous GnRH, oestrous cycle characteristics and fertility of fillies. J. Reprod. Fertil., *88:*185–195, 1990.

143. Kelly, C.M., Hoyer, P.B., and Wise, M.E.: In-vitro and in-vivo responsiveness of the corpus luteum of the mare to gonadotrophin stimulation. J. Reprod. Fertil., *84:*593–600, 1988.

144. Holtan, D.W., Squires, E.L., Lapin, D.R., and Ginther, O.J.: Effect of ovariectomy on pregnancy in mares. J. Reprod. Fertil. Suppl., *27:*457–463, 1979.

145. Weithenauer, J., Sharp, D.C., and Sherrin, P.C.: The effects of steroids on nutrients in yolk sac fluid of day 18 pony conceptuses. Equine Vet. J. Suppl., *8:*25–28, 1989.

CHAPTER 62

MANAGEMENT OF TWIN EMBRYOS AND TWIN FETUSES IN THE MARE

G.L. Woods
A.L. Hallowell

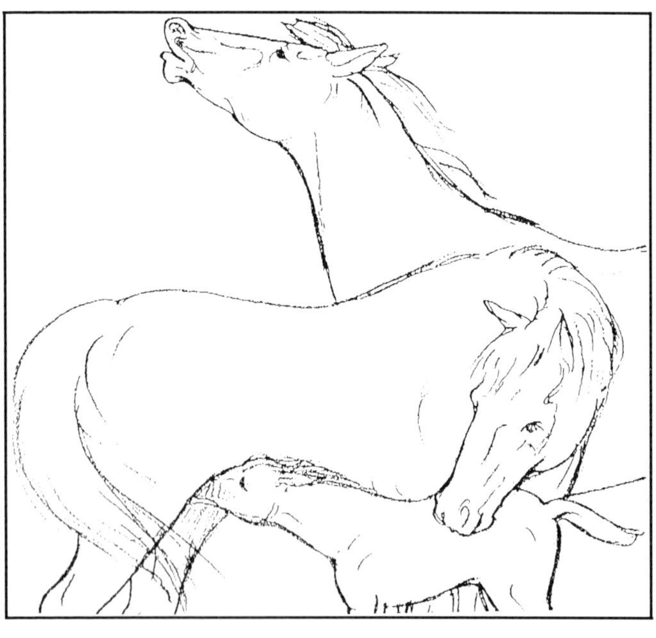

PHYSIOLOGY OF TWINS

ORIGIN OF TWINS

Equine twins originate from multiple ovulations as controlled ultrasonographic studies have documented a 93% correlation between the number of ovulations and the number of embryos[1] and because aborted or born equine twins are dizygotic.[2] Twin fetuses are dizygotic because they can be of opposite sex and have different markings as well as separate chorions and amnions.[2] Only one set of equine twins has been documented to have originated from a single ovulation.[3] In this case, the single ovarian follicle either ovulated two ova or the follicle ovulated one ovum, which became fertilized and subsequently split into two embryos.

Incidence of multiple ovulations is influenced by breed, age, and foaling status of the mare.[4] Draft and Thoroughbred mares, which are the largest horses, have the greatest incidence of multiple ovulations; Quarter Horse and Arabian mares, which are intermediate in size, have an intermediate incidence of multiple ovulations; and pony mares, which are smallest in size, have the lowest incidence of multiple ovulations. Older mares (6 to 10 yr old) have more multiple ovulations than do younger mares (2 to 5 yr old). Mares within 80 days following parturition have approximately twice the incidence of multiple ovulations as do other mares. In addition, multiple ovulations are repeatable within mares. Mares which have had multiple ovulations are twice as likely to have multiple ovulations on subsequent cycles. Ova from multiple ovulations are as fertile as ova from single ovulations; therefore, mares with multiple ovulations have a high incidence of twin embryos and a high overall pregnancy rate.[4]

Effect of Endometrial Cups

Endometrial cups, which are established by days 36 to 40 postovulation and maintained until approximately day 120 postovulation, are believed to prevent a mare from being rebred, even in the absence of a conceptus.[5] Therefore, if a mare is induced to abort after the endometrial cups are established, little opportunity exists for it to be rebred during that same breeding season. Many mares have secondary ovulations of pregnancy at 40 to 70 days of gestation.[5] Research should be conducted to determine whether ova from these secondary ovulations of pregnancy are fertile and if the uterus of an aborted mare with endometrial cups would maintain a pregnancy from one of these secondary ovulations.

REDUCTION OF ADJACENT TWIN EMBRYOS

The equine conceptus is classified as an embryo until day 40 postovulation and as a fetus after day 40 postovulation.[5] Embryos move throughout the mare's uterus from day 9 until day 16 postovulation.[4] Cessation of mobility, which is termed embryo fixation, occurs at the junction of one of the mare's uterine horns and the uterine body.[4] Twin embryos of dissimilar size and age (note that embryo size is correlated to embryo age) fix more frequently in the same uterine horn (unilateral fixation).[6] Twin embryos of similar size and age fix with equal frequency in the same uterine horn as in separate uterine horns (bilateral fixation).[6]

If twin embryos undergo unilateral fixation, their membranes, which serve as a nutrient exchange between the embryo and the mare's endometrium, will develop a nonfunctional membrane-to-membrane contact. This embryonic membrane-to-membrane contact usually results in the death of only one embryo by day 40, and the viability of the surviving embryo is apparently not diminished.[6] In contrast, if twin embryos undergo bilateral fixation, their membranes will not initially be in contact, and both embryos will usually survive beyond day 40. As the surviving bilaterally fixed twin fetuses develop, their membranes expand into the mare's uterine body where fetal membrane-to-membrane contact is eventually established. Fetal membrane-to-membrane contact, unlike embryo membrane-to-membrane contact, appears to result in gradual fetal weakening and the eventual abortion or birth of weak or dead twins.[2] The nonproductive membrane-to-membrane contact of the conceptuses has been hypothesized to be the underlying cause of the desirable selective death of only one twin embryo or the undesirable nonselective weakening or death of both twin fetuses.

MANAGEMENT OF TWINS

A program to minimize the number of twins should be cost effective. It should not decrease the mare's overall pregnancy rate; it should, during the same season, enable the rebreeding of mares which lose their pregnancies; and it should prevent the abortion or birth of weak or dead twin foals.

We recommend that

1. All mares be bred, whether they have single or multiple preovulatory follicles.
2. All breeds or types of mares which have a high incidence of multiple ovulations be examined for twins, whether single or multiple ovulations were detected.
3. Mares which have twin embryos be treated to prevent twin fetuses.

BREED ALL MARES

Mares with multiple preovulatory follicles should be bred, because mares with multiple ovulations have high pregnancy rates.[4] Programs to eliminate twins by restricting the breeding of mares with multiple preovulatory follicles are believed to have been unsuccessful because the incidence of twins was not decreased and the overall pregnancy rate may have been decreased.[4]

EXAMINE ALL BREEDS OR TYPES OF MARES THAT HAVE A HIGH INCIDENCE OF MULTIPLE OVULATIONS

Twins originate from multiple ovulations; therefore, to complete examinations for twins on mares which have a low incidence of multiple ovulations (e.g., pony mares) is not cost effective. In contrast, Thoroughbred or draft mares, which have a high incidence of multiple ovulations, should routinely be examined for twins. Under field conditions, in which ovulations were detected by rectal palpation, the majority of twin fetuses occurred in mares in which only one ovulation had been detected;[4,7] therefore, regardless of the number of ovulations detected, all mares which have a high incidence of multiple ovulations should be examined for twins. Misdiagnosis of multiple ovulations likely occurred under field conditions because (1) double ovarian follicles ovulated adjacently from the same ovary and they were detected as one ovulation or (2) a first ovulation was diagnosed, ovulation detection was discontinued, and a second ovulation subsequently occurred.

We recommend that the first routine examination for twins be at 14 days postovulation. This examination would then be at a time when the embryo is still mobile. The examination should be thorough and systematic. It should be completed by an operator who understands the developmental ultrasonographic structure of the equine embryo. A high-quality ultrasonographic machine with a 5 MHz linear array transducer is preferred to identify twin embryos.[4] Furthermore, the number of ovulations can be estimated by ultrasonographically scanning and counting corpora lutea on the mare's ovaries.[4]

Inexperience of the operator, improper ultrasonographic instruments, adjacent twin embryos, fractious or improperly restrained mares, rapid examinations, and endometrial cysts are possible reasons why twin embryos are misdiagnosed. Operators today, in contrast with those who first examined mares' reproductive tracts with ultrasonography, have the advantage of studying an excellent textbook which accurately describes the ultrasonographic structure of the equine embryo.[4] Knowledge of the expected size and structure of the equine embryo is essential for accurately interpreting ultrasonographic findings.

Adjacent twin embryos may be difficult to differentiate as two separate embryos. Their combined diameter will be larger than the expected diameter of a similarly aged single embryo; they may have a dorsoventral line, which represents their adjacent membranes; and there may be a cleavage between the two embryonic vesicles.[8] If adjacent twin embryos are suspected, reexamination of the mare for twins is recommended by day 29 postovulation. In the case of misdiagnosis, consolation can be found in the fact that many adjacent twin embryos reduce to one surviving embryo by day 40 postovulation. Fortunately, nonadjacent twin embryos, which usually do not reduce to one surviving embryo by day 40 postovulation, are easier to diagnose than are adjacent twins.

Uterine cysts, which occur primarily in aged mares, are another cause of misdiagnosis of twin embryos.[9,10] These cysts are fluid filled as are embryonic vesicles. Cysts can also be the same size and shape as embryonic vesicles. Careful recording of the location, size, and shape of uterine cysts at the beginning of the breeding season or shortly following ovulation will help on subsequent examinations to differentiate between uterine cysts and embryonic vesicles.[4] If multiple, fluid-filled structures are detected, we recommend that the size, shape, and location of the structures be recorded and the mare be re-examined 3 to 4 days later. If the structures do not change in size or shape and they do not develop an embryo proper with a heartbeat, they are likely to be uterine cysts. The embryo proper and heartbeat are accurately identified by day 28. We recommend the routine video recording of all ultrasonographic examinations, because it provides a simple and economical permanent record.

TREATMENT OF MARES WITH TWINS

Mares should routinely be examined three times for twins. First, before the expected detection of embryos for the identification and mapping of uterine cysts; second, at day 14 postovulation; and third, by day 29.

OBSERVATIONS AND RECOMMENDATIONS FOR THE DAY-14 PREGNANCY EXAMINATION

1. A. *Observation.* One detected embryo.
   B. *Recommendations.* Re-examine the mare for twins by day 29.

2. A. *Observation.* Two nonadjacent embryos.
   B. *Recommendations.* Crush the smallest conceptus by either compressing it ventrocaudad against the pelvis or crushing it between one's fingers and thumb.[4] (Note: One must be certain that one of the fluid-filled structures is not a uterine cyst.) Antiprostaglandins and progesterone therapy are not recommended in conjunction with the crushing technique because their use has not increased the success of the procedure.[11]

3. A. *Observation.* Two adjacent embryos.
   B. *Recommendations.* Attempt to manually separate the twins using an ultrasonographic probe (see chapter 31). If the embryos are post fixation (age greater than day 16) and vesicle separation is not possible, re-examine the mare for twins by day 29.

OBSERVATIONS AND RECOMMENDATIONS FOR THE DAY-29 PREGNANCY EXAMINATION

1. A. *Observation.* Two nonadjacent embryos.
   B. *Recommendations.* Crush one embryo. The success rate for crushing day-29 embryos is believed to be less than the success rate for crushing day-19 to -21 embryos.[11,12]

2. A. *Observation.* Adjacent twin embryos.
   B. *Recommendations.*
      i. If there is sufficient time remaining in the breeding season to recycle and rebreed the mare, one may consider aborting the mare with prostaglandin $F_2\alpha$ and subsequently rebreeding her.
      ii. If insufficient time remains in the breeding season to recycle and rebreed the mare, allow the pregnancy to advance with the hope that only one embryo will survive.

Mares with twin fetuses > 40 days postovulation are difficult to manage, because their endometrial cups have become established,[5] they have a low probability of spontaneously reducing to one fetus,[6] and the success rate of manually killing only one fetus is much lower than the success rate of manually killing only one embryo.[12] If the mare aborts the fetuses after the endometrial cups are established, she will probably not recycle for rebreeding until after day 120 when endometrial cups will have regressed.[5] Incidence of spontaneous reduction of one fetus is low for twin fetuses which were either adjacent as embryos and failed to reduce or which were nonadjacent as embryos and first established membrane-to-membrane contact as fetuses.[6] Killing one fetus by manual crushing usually results in the death of both fetuses.[12]

When considering the possible options for treating twin pregnancies, the clinician must consider the effect late-term twins will have on the mare's chances of becoming pregnant during the subsequent breeding season. Because the number of available days in a breeding season is limited, how many days of the subsequent season will be lost because of a full-term pregnancy must be considered. For example, if the expected parturition is to be in late May, the opportunity for that mare to again become pregnant during that season are low; therefore, to abort the mare early and have a better opportunity for a pregnancy during the next season may be economically prudent. Also, fertility of the mare may be decreased following abortion or birth of twins.[7]

One plausible approach to managing twin fetuses is to monitor the pregnancy by transrectal or transabdominal ultrasonography until approximately midpregnancy with the hope that only one fetus will spontaneously die. Accuracy of monitoring the fetuses by transrectal ultrasonography decreases as the size of the fetus increases.[4] A 3.5 MHz instead of a 5.0 MHz transducer might be beneficial, because the lower the frequency of the transducer, the greater its penetration.[4] Electrocardiography has also been used to detect twin fetuses accurately.[13]

If both fetuses survive to midpregnancy, the clinician might consider aborting the mare with prostaglandin $F_2\alpha$ and beginning the subsequent breeding season with a nonpregnant mare. An alternative treatment for midgestation twin fetuses is to ultrasonographically guide a needle into the heart of one fetus and inject potassium chloride solution.[14] If both fetuses fail to survive this procedure, the mare would begin the subsequent breeding season as a nonpregnant mare.

Additional research is required to understand fetal twins and the effect of twin abortions or births on the mare's subsequent fertility. Just as the recently acquired knowledge of twin embryo interactions now enables logical management of twin embryos, additional knowledge of twin fetuses may enable the logical management of twin fetuses.

REFERENCES

1. Ginther, O.J.: Relationships among number of days between multiple ovulations, number of embryos, and type of fixation in mares. J. Equine Vet. Sci., *7:*82–88, 1987.
2. Jeffcott, L.B., and Whitwell, K.E.: Twinning as a cause of fetal and neonatal loss in the Thoroughbred mare. J. Comp. Pathol., *83:*91–106, 1973.
3. Rooney, J.R.: Autopsy of the Horse. Baltimore, Williams & Wilkins, 1970.
4. Ginther, O.J.: Ultrasonic Imaging and Reproductive Events in the Mare. Cross Plaines, WI, Equiservices, 1986.
5. Ginther, O.J.: Reproductive Biology of the Mare: Basic and Applied Aspects. Cross Plaines, WI, Equiservices, 1979.
6. Ginther, O.J.: The nature of embryo reduction in mares with twin conceptuses: Deprivation hypothesis. Am. J. Vet. Res., *50:*45–53, 1989.
7. Pascoe, R.R.: Methods for the treatments of twin pregnancy in the mare. Equine Vet. J., *15:*40–42, 1983.
8. Simpson, R.E., et al.: Use of ultrasound echography for early diagnosis of single and twin pregnancy in the mare. J. Reprod. Fertil. Suppl., *32:*431–439, 1982.
9. Ginther, O.J.: The twinning problem: From breeding to day 16. Proc. Am. Assoc. Equine Pract., 11–26, 1983.
10. Zent, W.W.: Use of ultrasound in broodmare practice. Proc. Am. Assoc. Equine Pract., 53–57, 1983.
11. Pascoe, D.R., et al.: Management of twin pregnancy by manual embryonic reduction and comparison of two techniques and three hormonal therapies. J. Reprod. Fertil. Suppl., *35:*701–702, 1987.
12. Roberts, C.J.: Termination of twin gestation by blastocyst crush in the mare. Equine Vet. J., *15:*40–42, 1983.
13. Parkes, R.D., and Colles, C.M.: Fetal electrocardiography in the mare as a practical aid to diagnosing singleton and twin pregnancy. Vet. Rec., *100:*25–26, 1977.
14. Rantanen, N.W., and Kencaid, B.: Ultrasound guided fetal cardiac puncture: A method of twin reduction in the mare. Proc. Am. Assoc. Equine Pract., 173–179, 1989.

CHAPTER 63

INTERSPECIES AND EXTRASPECIES EQUINE PREGNANCIES

W.R. Allen, J.H. Kydd, D.F. Antczak

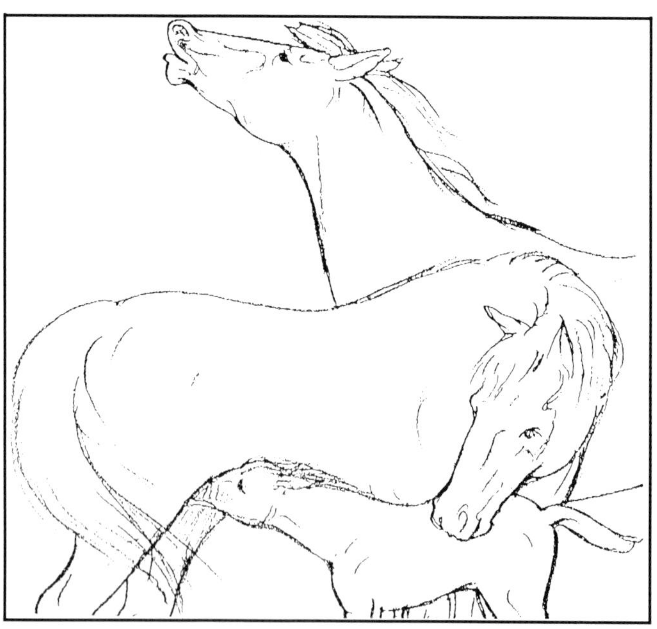

The genus Equus is unusual, but not unique, within the mammalian kingdom for the ability of its phenotypically and karyotypically diverse member species to interbreed freely to produce live, though infertile, offspring. Species range from the ancient horse of Mongolia (Equus przewalskii) with the highest diploid chromosome number of 66, through the many breeds and types of domestic horse (E. caballus, $2n = 64$), to the European ass or domestic donkey (E. asinus, $2n = 62$), to the many African and Asiatic species of wild ass (e.g., E. hemionus, $2n = 54$), to the Grévy's Zebra of Somalia and northern Kenya (E. grevyi, $2n = 46$), the many subspecies of common zebra in Central and East Africa (E. burchelli, $2n = 44$), and the now rare mountain zebra of southwest Africa (E. zebra, $2n = 32$). Cataloged evidence concerning the range of hybrid foals born during the past 100 yr makes it safe to assume that an adult cycling female from any of the species inseminated with fertile semen from a male of another species will conceive and give birth to a viable hybrid foal.[1–4]

The mule ($2n = 63$), the result of the mating of a horse mare (E. caballus) to a domestic jack donkey (E. asinus), and the reciprocal cross, the hinny ($2n = 63$), are by far the most common equine hybrids, simply because their parents are the only two species of equids to have been domesticated in significant numbers. The mule was man's first and only commercially viable interspecific hybrid,[5] and many millions of them have been produced since long before Christ to the present day, for the perfect blend of the physical and mental attributes of the two parental species. But, in addition to its physical prowess, the mule has intrigued and puzzled biologists and geneticists since the time of Aristotle.

As described so eloquently by Short,[5] "the clear and equal mixture in the mule of the phenotypic characteristics of both parents ran counter to Aristotle's 'seed and soil' view of reproduction in which the male provided the essential 'seed' for the new offspring while the female played an entirely passive role by supplying merely the 'soil' in which the male seed would grow." Much later, as Short quoted, "the Danish anatomist Stensen (1638–1686) and the Dutch biologist De Graaf (1641–1673) used the mule as an example in their proposals that the females of all mammalian species also contribute 'seed' toward the generation of new individuals. Stensen noted the presence of follicles in the ovaries of one of two female mules he was able to dissect, just as he had seen these fluid-filled 'eggs' in the ovaries of women, cattle, sheep, hares, and many other species."[5] And, as quoted by Jocelyn and Setchell,[6] De Graaf noted, "If a mare receives the semen of an ass, the fetus has the features not of the father alone, but those of both parents mixed together. . . . Mothers, therefore, as well as fathers have child-producing semen."

In more recent times the infertility of mules and hinnies has similarly aroused the interest of geneticists. Wodsedalek was first to conclude that spermatozoa are not produced in the testes of male mules because of an incompatability between the paternal and maternal sets of chromosomes leading to a block in meiosis.[7] More than 50 yr later, Taylor and Short demonstrated that the same chromosomal incompatibility leads to partial meiotic arrest in female mules and hinnies, which results in a severely depleted stock of oocytes at birth in these hybrids.[8]

Thus equine hybrids, especially the mule, have proved to be of scientific interest as well as commercial value for many centuries past. But perhaps of equal and more modern scientific interest are the immunologic and developmental questions posed by the discovery that at least the horse, donkey, and mule within the equine family will accept, carry to term, give birth to and rear successfully true xenogeneic extraspecific foals following the use of the technique of between-species embryo transfer.[9]

In this chapter we attempt to review some of the more puzzling immunologic and endocrinologic aspects of the establishment of pregnancy and the survival of the xenogeneic fetus in mares and other equids when they are carrying hybrid interspecific and transferred extraspecific foals.

INTERSPECIES PREGNANCIES

THE MULE AND HINNY

There seems little doubt that the interspecies mating of the jack donkey and the horse mare is just as fertile, in terms of conception rates, as the straightforward intraspecies mating between either of the parental species. Many millions of mules have been produced during the centuries in the Asian and Indian subcontinents, in Southern Europe and North Africa and, in more recent times, in North and South America. These pregnancies have been established both by natural mating and by artificial insemination, and although strict comparisons of conception rates achieved per insemination or per estrous cycle have not been reported in the scientific literature, it is a situation for which common knowledge and practical horsemanship dictates that the interspecies mating for mule production is of normal fertility.

This high fertility of the mating to produce the mule is certainly not matched when attempting to produce the reciprocal hybrid, the hinny, by mating jenny donkeys to horse stallions.[10,11] Once again, the situation does not appear to have been researched thoroughly or recorded in any detail in the literature. However, few confirmed hinnies exist in countries like Spain, Portugal, Greece, and India where enormous numbers of mules are still produced and used routinely by small holders and peasant farmers. Enquiry of such farmers always yields the same response, namely, "the horse stallion is much less aroused by the estrous display of the jenny donkey than vice versa and hence he is less than keen to mate with her. But even if mating is achieved, only rarely does conception occur."

This relative infertility of the hinny mating is also the experience of the authors. During a 7-yr period in two laboratories (Cambridge, UK, and Cornell University), a total of 159 attempts were made in successive breeding seasons to establish hinny pregnancies in 51 jenny donkeys. These jennies appeared to be of normal fertility and were cycling normally and ovulating regularly. A total of 6 pony and horse stallions, all of proven high fertility, were used with a mixture of natural matings and artificial insemination on alternate days during estrus. In 125 instances, the mated/inseminated jenny donkey was left untouched in the hope of establishing a normal ongoing hinny pregnancy; this occurred in 18 cases to give a conception rate of only 14.4%. In the other 34 instances, the uterus of the donkey was flushed nonsurgically on day 7 or 8 after ovulation (n = 29) or the ipsilateral oviduct was flushed on day 2 or 3 (n = 5) as described previously[12] in an attempt to recover a hinny embryo for transfer to another recipient animal; this was successful in 5 cases to give an embryo recovery rate of only 14.7%; much lower than the recovery rates of 60 to 70% obtained when flushing mares or jenny donkeys following normal intraspecific matings or inseminations[12] (Table 63–1).

This striking disparity in fertilization and/or pregnancy rates when carrying out reciprocal hybrid matings has parallels in other species. In sheep-goat crosses, for example, Hancock and his colleagues reported high fertilization rates when inseminating female goats with ram semen, but many fewer conceptions (± 10%) when reciprocally inseminating ewes with goat semen.[13–15] Similarly, hybrid matings between the hare (Lepus americanus) and the rabbit (Oryctolagus cuniculus) produce high rates of fertilization when rabbits are inseminated with hare semen whereas <10% of hare oocytes are fer-

TABLE 63–1. CONCEPTION RATES ACHIEVED IN 51 JENNY DONKEYS MATED TO HORSE STALLIONS OR INSEMINATED WITH FRESH STALLION SEMEN IN REPEATED ESTROUS CYCLES

	NUMBER OF MATED/INSEMINATED ESTROUS CYCLES	NUMBER OF CONFIRMED HINNY PREGNANCIES	NUMBER OF HINNY EMBRYOS RECOVERED AT DAYS 3 TO 8 AFTER OVULATION	CONCEPTION RATE (%)
	125	18	—	14.4
	34	—	5	14.7
Totals	159	23		14.5

tilized by rabbit semen.[16] The mechanisms responsible for these large differences in fertilization rates in interspecies matings have yet to be determined, although the phenomenon of gene imprinting could possibly play a role.[17]

OTHER EQUINE HYBRIDS

As mentioned previously, to create viable hybrid offspring from the crossing of any two of the considerable array of equine species seems likely. Hybrids that have been produced have been well cataloged,[3,18] and they include such unlikely combinations as the progeny of the domestic donkey (Equus asinus) mated to (1) the Somali, African, and Asiatic wild asses; (2) Przewalski's and domestic horses; and (3) Burchell's, Grévy's, and mountain zebras (Fig. 63–1). Similarly, a wide range of hybrids has been produced by mating domestic horses (E. caballus) to all the main zebra species, including Burchell's, Chapman's, Grant's, Hartmann's, and Grévy's (Fig. 63–2), and to a wide range of the wild asses, including Abyssinian, Asiatic, Tibetan, Indian, and Persian subspecies. In all these cases of successful birth, the female of the partnership was the horse, in a similar manner to the production of mules. In any instances in which reciprocal crosses were attempted by mating a male domestic horse to a female wild ass or zebra, conceptions failed to occur.[3] This seems to mimic the previously described situation of a greatly reduced conception rate when attempting to produce hinnies compared with mules. To speculate that fertilization may occur readily in any cross where the sire has a lower diploid chromosome complement than the dam is tempting (e.g., a domestic horse mare [E. caballus, $2n = 64$] mated to a domestic jack donkey [E. asinus, $2n = 62$] or to a male Grant's Zebra [E. burchelli, $2n = 44$]. Conversely, conception rate is greatly reduced in any combination in which the sire has a higher diploid number of chromosomes than the dam (e.g., E. caballus ♂ × E. asinus ♀ or E. zebra ♀ × E. asinus ♂).

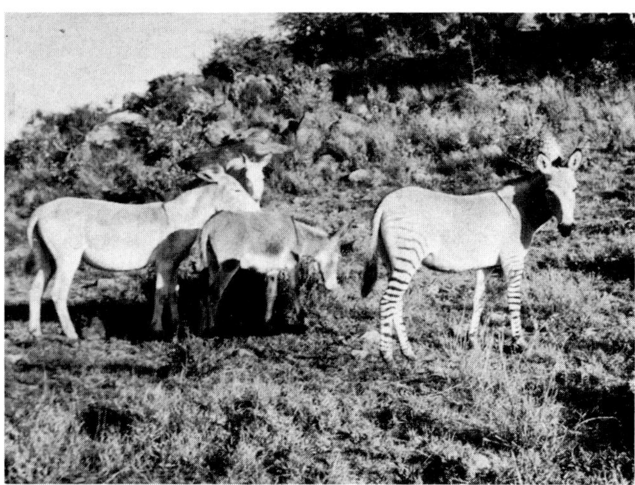

FIG. 63–1. F1-interspecies hybrid "zebronkey," which resulted from the mating of a male Burchell's zebra (Equus burchelli böhmii, $2n = 44$) to a European jenny donkey (E. asinus, $2n = 62$). (From King, J.M.: Comparative aspects of reproduction in Equidae. Ph.D. thesis. University of Cambridge, 1965.)

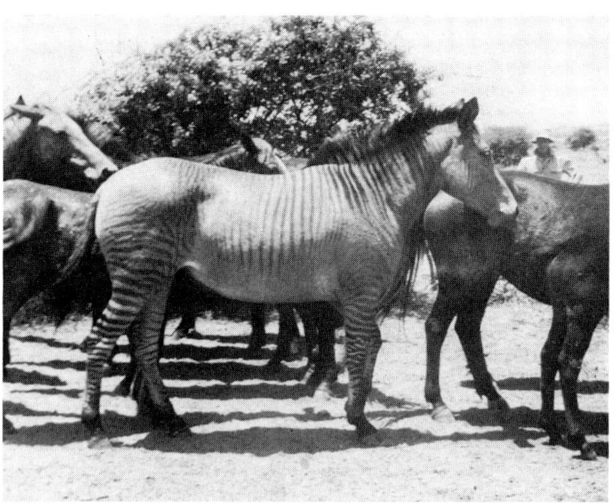

FIG. 63–2. F1-interspecies hybrid "zebrorse" that was produced by the mating of a male Grévy's Zebra (Equus grevyi, $2n = 46$) to a domestic horse mare (E. caballus, $2n = 64$). (From King, J.M.: Comparative aspects of reproduction in Equidae. Ph.D. thesis. University of Cambridge, 1965.)

FERTILITY OF EQUINE HYBRIDS

The infertility of mules has perplexed and fascinated horse breeders and scientists through the ages. Wodsedalek was first to provide the real explanation of the situation when, after studying the testes of three male mules histologically, he concluded that spermatozoa could not be produced because of the incompatibility between the paternal (donkey) and maternal (horse) sets of chromosomes resulting in a block in meiosis.[7] This breakdown of spermatogenesis at the pachytene stage of meiotic prophase was confirmed in male mules and hinnies,[19] and the same sort of chromosomal incompatibility, causing partial meiotic arrest in oogenesis during fetal life, was described in female mules and hinnies.[8]

A number of isolated and unverified reports of individual fertile female mules were made during the early part of the twentieth century.[3,20] The most notable of which was an animal named "Old Bec" that was owned by Texas A&M College in the 1920s. She had all the morphologic characteristics of a mule and was reported to have given birth to two foals in her lifetime. One of these, sired by a jack donkey, was a female, was typically mule-like in appearance, and was infertile. The other, a colt sired by a horse, was completely horse-like in appearance and was apparently fully fertile; he sired many male and female foals that were all horse-like in appearance and were fertile.[21] However, some years later another allegedly fertile female mule was karyotyped and it was discovered to be a normal donkey.[22]

This revelation, and the finding of few spermatozoa in the centrifuged ejaculates of male mules and hinnies,[19] led Short to declare firmly that all mules and hinnies, without exception, should be considered infertile unless conclusive proof to the contrary was provided.[5] Curiously, such proof was soon forthcoming, and during the past 10 yr, no fewer than three female mules, one in China,[23,24] one in Nebraska,[25] and one in Brazil (M. Henry, personal communication) have all been karyotyped as mules and have all been shown conclusively to have produced one or more foals.

Similarly, a female hinny in China has been karyotyped correctly as a hybrid and has produced a donkey-like foal after having been mated to a jack donkey.[26] Chandley discussed at some length the mechanisms which might function to enable these odd female mules and hinnies to be fertile.[27] She favored Michie's[28] earlier hypothesis of "affinity," whereby chromosomally balanced haploid gametes might occasionally be produced by the movement of centromeres of similar ancestry to opposite poles at anaphase I of meiosis. This could leave the whole set of female parental chromosomes remaining in the oocyte with subsequent elimination to the polar body of the paternal set. Elimination of the donkey paternal set of chromosomes from the mule oocyte would leave only the maternal horse set remaining so that another mule would be produced if the animal was mated to a jack donkey, whereas a pure horse would result if the mating were to a horse stallion. This is exactly what appears to have happened in the case of "Old Bec's" mule and horse foals in the 1920s, the mule foal from the mule in Nebraska in 1985, and the three progeny produced by the fertile female mule in Brazil. However, when the offspring of the fertile mule and the hinny in China were investigated by Chandley and her colleagues,[23,24,26] they showed a mixture of horse and donkey chromosomes and, therefore, demonstrated random inheritence of both paternal and maternal chromosomes in the oocyte that was fertilized.

Not all the possible equine hybrids seem to be as infertile as the mule and hinny. Both the male and female offspring ($2n$ = 65) of the cross between Przewalski's Horse (Equus przewalski $2n$ = 66) and the domestic horse (E. caballus, $2n$ = 64) are fully fertile[29–31] (Fig. 63-3). Furthermore, Gray lists a number of examples where hybrids between the domestic donkey (E. asinus, $2n$ = 62) and both Burchell's Zebra (E. burchelli, $2n$ = 44) and Chapman's Zebra (E. burchelli antiquorum, $2n$ = 44) were reported to be fertile,[3] although none of these cases were verified. On the other hand, examples of hybrids between the domestic donkey and other members of the wild ass family, including the Persian Wild Ass (E. hemionus onager) and the Somali Wild Ass (E. asinus africanus) have been reported as being sterile, as have hybrids between the various species of zebra and the domestic horse.

EXTRASPECIES PREGNANCIES

The use of between-species embryo transfer to establish xenogeneic equine pregnancies has highlighted some unexpected and intriguing interacting influences of fetal genotype and maternal uterine environment on placental development and implantation. Horse embryos were first successfully transferred to donkey recipients and, vice versa, donkey embryos were transferred to horses in our laboratories in 1979, and further transfers of more exotic equine embryos to domestic horses or donkeys have been undertaken in collaboration with other laboratories since then. In all instances, the techniques used for synchronizing and diagnosing ovulation in donor and recipient animals, and the methods employed for the nonsurgical recovery of embryos from donors and their surgical transfer to recipients, were similar.

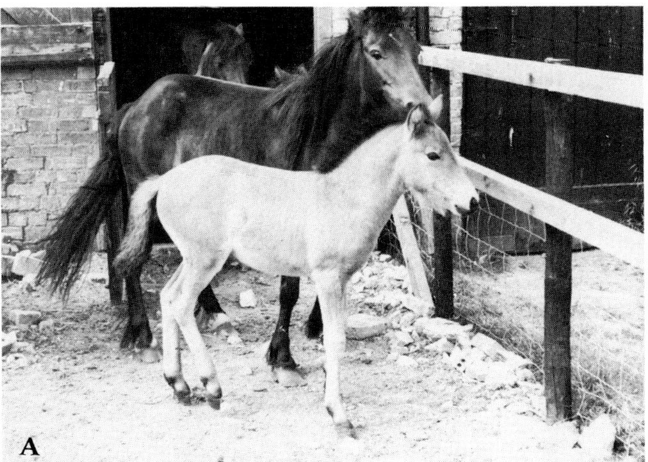

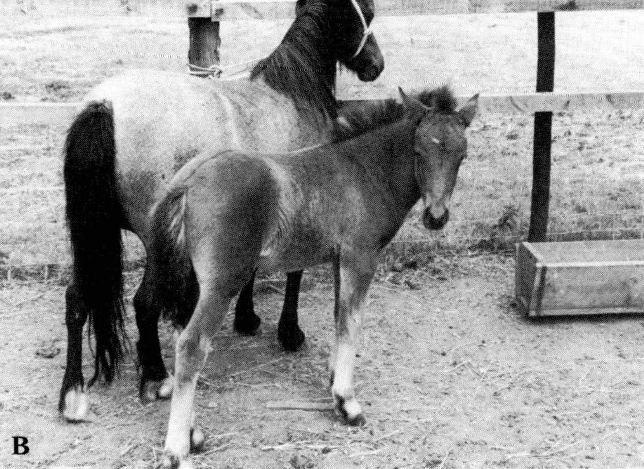

FIG. 63–3. F2-interspecies foals produced by mating a male Przewalski's Horse × domestic horse F1 hybrid to two domestic horse mares. *A*, The F2-filly foal had a karyotype of $2n$ = 65 and was similar to Przewalski's horse in appearance, whereas the F2-colt foal *(B)* had a karyotype of $2n$ = 64 and, apart from a prominent dorsal stripe, was indistinguishable from a normal horse foal.

EMBRYO RECOVERY AND TRANSFER

The stages of the estrous cycles of the donor and recipient animals, and the occurrence of ovulation in both groups, were determined by measuring progesterone concentrations in samples of peripheral plasma recovered daily during estrus and for 2 to 3 days after the end of estrous signs. Only rarely were the ovaries of either the donor or the recipient animals palpated or scanned per rectum, both as a major saving of animal handling time and because of the impossibility of undertaking such manipulative procedures when using wild zoo species as donors. Initially, progesterone concentrations were measured by radioimmunoassay,[32] but in the latter part of the study, the amplified enzyme-linked immunoassay (AELIA) developed for use in bovine milk[33] and subsequently adapted for equine serum[34] was used. Day 0 was taken as the last day on which plasma progesterone concentrations were < 1 ng/mL.

For embryo recovery, a 20- or 24-French gauge flexible two-way polythene catheter (Franklin Medical, Middlesex, UK) was passed through the diestrous cervix into the lumen of the uterine body. The cuff was inflated with 40 mL of air to seal the internal os of the cervix and the uterus was then filled to distension with flushing medium [Dulbecco's phosphate-buffered saline (DPBS) containing 1% w:v bovine serum albumin (BSA)[12]]. The medium was recovered from the uterus under gravity flow, with the operator's arm within the rectum to massage the uterus and so aid in recovering the maximum amount of medium. The flushing process was repeated three times with each donor.

On some occasions the cylinders of medium were left to stand on the laboratory bench (22° to 25° C) for 10 to 20 min to allow the embryo to sink to the bottom before sucking off the bulk of medium using a vacuum pump. At other times the medium was passed through an embryo filter with a pore size of 75 μm (Immuno Systems, Inc., Madison, WI). The small volume of residual medium in each method was then searched with the aid of a binocular dissecting microscope. When located, the embryo was washed four times by passing it through drops of transfer medium (DPBS containing 20% w:v BSA). It was then held in a larger volume of transfer medium at 37° C until transferred to the selected recipient.

Almost all the transfers were carried out surgically via midventral laparotomy performed under general anaesthesia. The anterior third of one of the uterine horns was exposed and the embryo injected into the uterine lumen using a flame-polished Pasteur pipette passed through a small hole made in the uterine wall with a blunted 18-gauge needle.[12] A few embryos were transferred nonsurgically via the cervix using a sterile bovine insemination catheter.

The great majority of embryos were recovered on days 7 or 8 after ovulation and were, therefore, at the early blastocyst or expanded blastocyst stages when transferred. Similarly, most of the recipients had ovulated synchronously with, or 1 to 2 days *after,* the donor. On a few occasions recipients were used that had ovulated 1 day before, or 3 days after, the donor. Although some pregnancies were achieved at these levels of asynchrony, the success rate was lower than that obtained when working within the donor/recipient synchrony range of 0 to −2 days.[12]

Pregnancy in the recipients was diagnosed by a combination of palpation and real-time ultrasound scanning of the uterus per rectum,[35] commencing 8 to 10 days after transfer and with repeat examinations at intervals of 10 to 14 days until around day 100 of gestation. Jugular vein blood samples were recovered three times a week throughout gestation from all pregnant recipients to monitor routinely profiles of equine chorionic gonadotropin (eCG),[36] progesterone[32,34] and, occasionally, the onset, specificity, and titer of maternal antibodies to paternal lymphocyte alloantigens.[37] Most pregnancies were left untouched to proceed to term or to abort spontaneously, whichever was destined to be the outcome. In other pregnancies, especially in horse mares carrying donkey fetuses and vice versa in jenny donkeys carrying horse fetuses, the conceptus was electively removed from the uterus via midline hysterotomy under general anesthesia for gross and histologic examinations of many parameters, including fetal growth; endometrial cup development and/or degeneration, and the rate of growth, degree of interdigitation, and general histologic appearance of the noninvasive allantochorion-endometrium interface.[9]

HORSE-IN-DONKEY PREGNANCY

Six extraspecies horse-in-donkey pregnancies were created over a 3-yr period. These arose from nine transfers (67%) of single horse embryos recovered on days 7 or 8 after ovulation; the nine embryos were obtained from 13 recovery attempts (77%). On one occasion the horse embryo was transferred to a jenny donkey that had been mated to a jack donkey in the previous estrus. This animal successfully implanted the two conceptuses—her own intraspecific donkey embryo conceived normally and the extraspecific horse conceptus transferred to her subsequently.

Of these six horse-in-donkey pregnancies, two were allowed to continue uninterrupted to term and the jennies gave birth to healthy horse foals on, respectively, days 336 and 363 of gestation.[9] Both foals were slightly smaller at birth than expected (Fig. 63-4), probably because of the restrictive effects of the physically smaller uteri of the donkey surrogate mothers, compared with the uterine and general body size and "roominess" of the true genetic horse mothers. Nevertheless, both foals were robust and they stood and sucked unaided. Two other singleton horse-in-donkey conceptuses were removed by surgical hysterotomy on days 59 and 62 and the donkey carrying the intraspecific donkey and extraspecific horse twin conceptuses was killed on day 63 for recovery of the gravid uterus. In all three of these recipient donkeys, a horseshoe or semicircle of large endometrial cups was associated with the horse conceptus. These cups were relatively broad and they

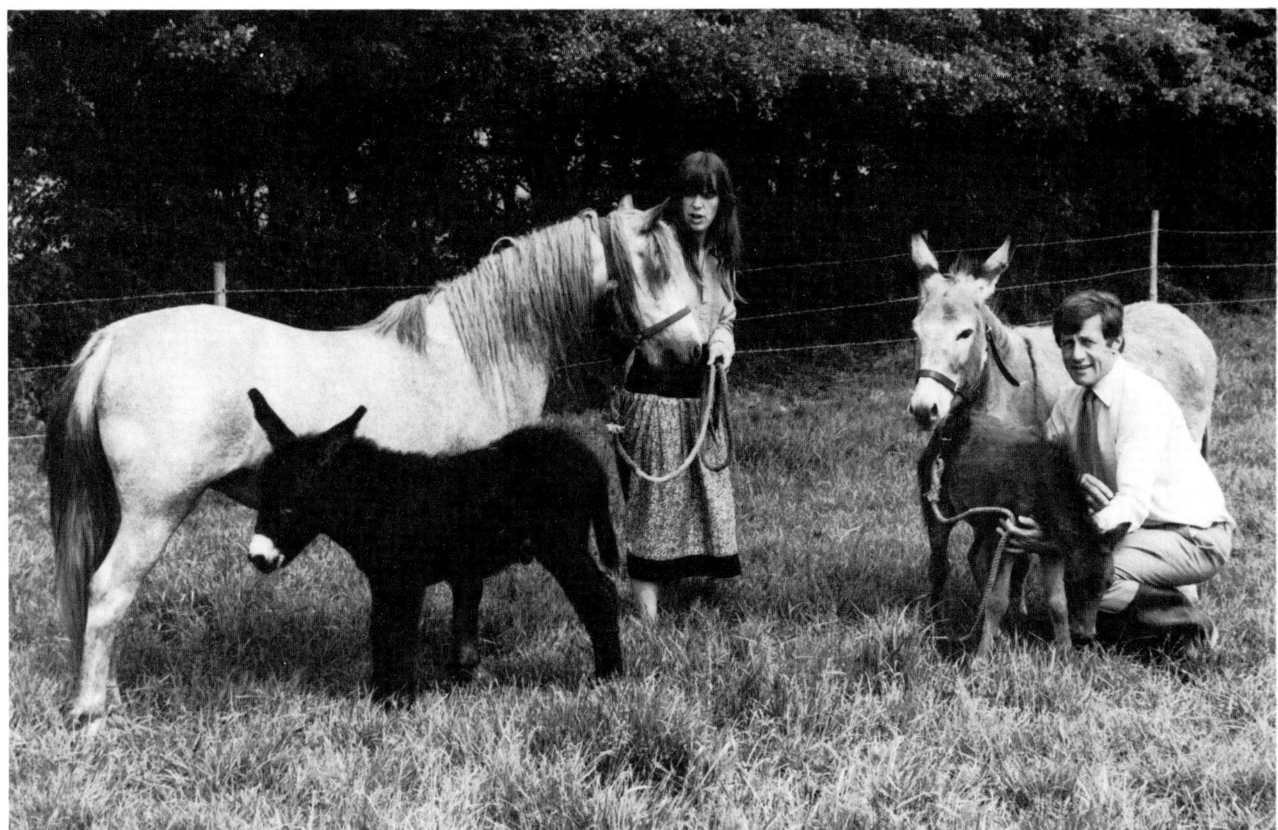

FIG. 63–4. Donkey and horse extraspecific foals with their horse and donkey surrogate mothers. Note how big and robust the donkey foal is compared with the horse foal, which developed in the smaller uterus of its donkey surrogate mother.

protruded prominently from the luminal surface of the endometrium, just as in donkeys carrying interspecific hinny conceptuses.[10] In the donkey carrying the twins, however, the endometrial cups associated with the intraspecies donkey conceptus were, typically, much narrower and generally smaller than those associated with the horse conceptus (Fig. 63-5). This striking difference in the size and general development of the endometrial cups between the horse and donkey conceptuses in the same animal reflected the pronounced influence of fetal genotype on the development of the placental progenitor of the cups, the chorionic girdle[9,11] (see Chapter 9).

In another parallel to hinny pregnancy, the ovaries of the recipient donkeys carrying horse fetuses were greatly enlarged because of the development of multiple secondary corpora lutea and luteinized follicles[10] (Fig. 63-5). This, in turn, led to extremely high concentrations of progesterone in maternal peripheral plasma[38] (Fig. 63–6) and was almost certainly the result of the higher ratio of follicle-stimulating hormone–like to luteinizing hormone–like biologic activities in eCG, causing hyperstimulation of the surrogate donkey ovaries (see Fig. 63–5), as described previously in donkeys carrying interspecies hinny conceptuses.[39]

Histologic examination of the placental interface in these three donkeys carrying extraspecific horse conceptuses revealed that implantation and placentation

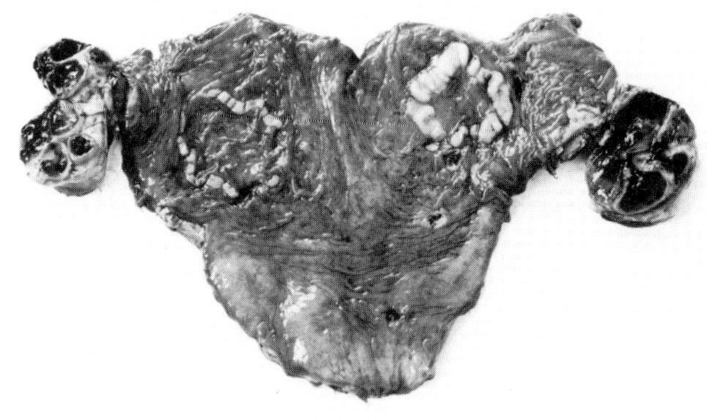

FIG. 63–5. Opened uterus of a jenny donkey carrying its own intraspecific donkey fetus and a transferred extraspecific horse fetus, at day 63 of gestation. The conceptuses have been removed to show the small narrow donkey endometrial cups in the left uterine horn and the circle of much larger and more active horse endometrial cups in the right horn. Note the secondary corpora lutea and luteinized follicles in the hyperstimulated maternal ovaries.

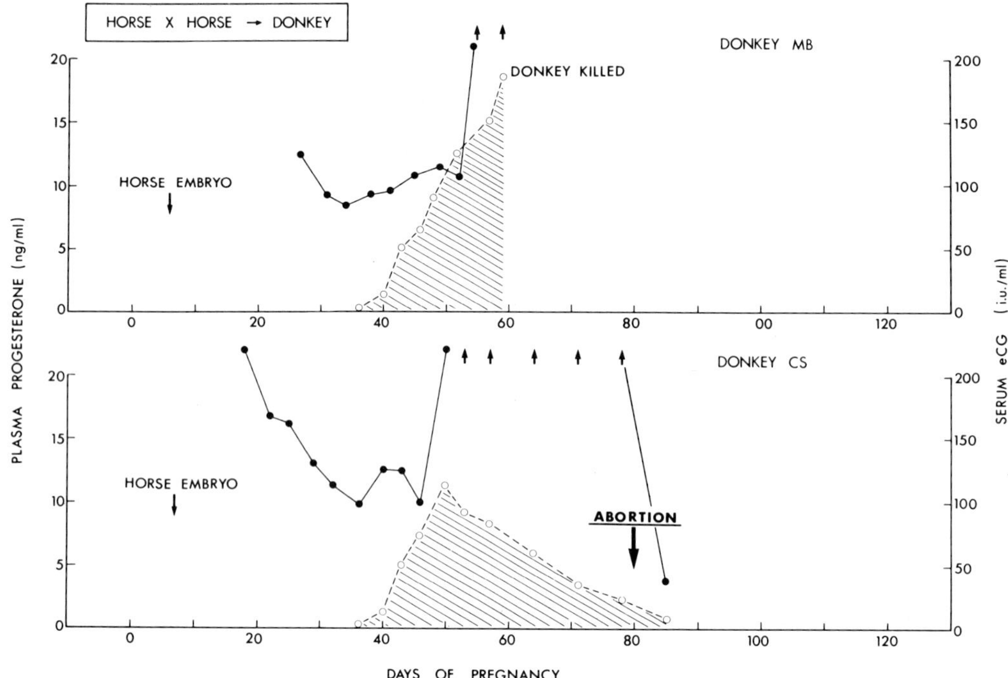

FIG. 63–6. Peripheral plasma progesterone (solid circles) and serum eCG (open circles) concentrations measured during early pregnancy in two surrogate jenny donkeys carrying transferred extraspecies horse conceptuses. Note the high plasma progesterone concentrations in both animals. The donkey in the top graph was killed on day 59, whereas the donkey in the lower graph aborted spontaneously on day 80 when serum eCG concentrations had fallen rapidly and prematurely to < 5 IU/mL.

were proceeding normally. The horse allantochorion was well interdigitated with the donkey endometrium and a firm microvillous attachment existed between the trophoblast and the endometrial epithelium. No sign of any leukocyte aggregations were evident at this junction. The horse endometrial cups were large and the majority of the binculeate eCG-secreting cup cells appeared viable and active. Large numbers of lymphocytes were aggregated around each cup, and in a manner similar to interspecies hinny pregnancy but in contrast to the situation in interspecies mule pregnancy, the accumulated cells remained clustered in the surrounding endometrial stroma, with little invasion and destruction of the cup tissue itself.

Thus it was apparent that endometrial cups had developed as expected and implantation and placentation were occurring normally in these three recipient donkeys, as clearly it had done in the two which carried their foals to term. However, the remaining donkey carrying a horse conceptus aborted spontaneously on day 80, following an atypical steep decline in maternal serum eCG concentrations from day 64 onward (Fig. 63-

TABLE 63–2. RECOVERY AND TRANSFER OF HORSE (E. CABALLUS) AND DONKEY (E. ASINUS) EMBRYOS TO F1 HYBRID CYCLING AND ANESTROUS PROGESTAGEN-TREATED FEMALE MULES

TYPE OF TRANSFER	NUMBER OF EMBRYOS TRANSFERRED	NUMBER OF RECIPIENTS PREGNANT (%)	OUTCOME OF PREGNANCIES
Horse to cycling mule	5	3(60)	2 foaled (days 344 and 366) 1 removed (day 73)
Donkey to cycling mule	3	1(33)	Foaled (day 357)
Horse to anestrous mule	4	1(25)	Resorbed (day 55)
Donkey to anestrous mule	1	0	

(Data from Antczak, D.F., Davies, C.J., Kydd, J., and Allen, W.R.: Immunological aspects of pregnancy in mules. Equine Vet. J., *3(Suppl.)*:68–72, 1985; and Shaw, E., and Haupt, K.A.: Pre- and post partum behaviour in mules impregnated by embryo transfer. Equine Vet. J., *3(Suppl.)*:73, 1985.)

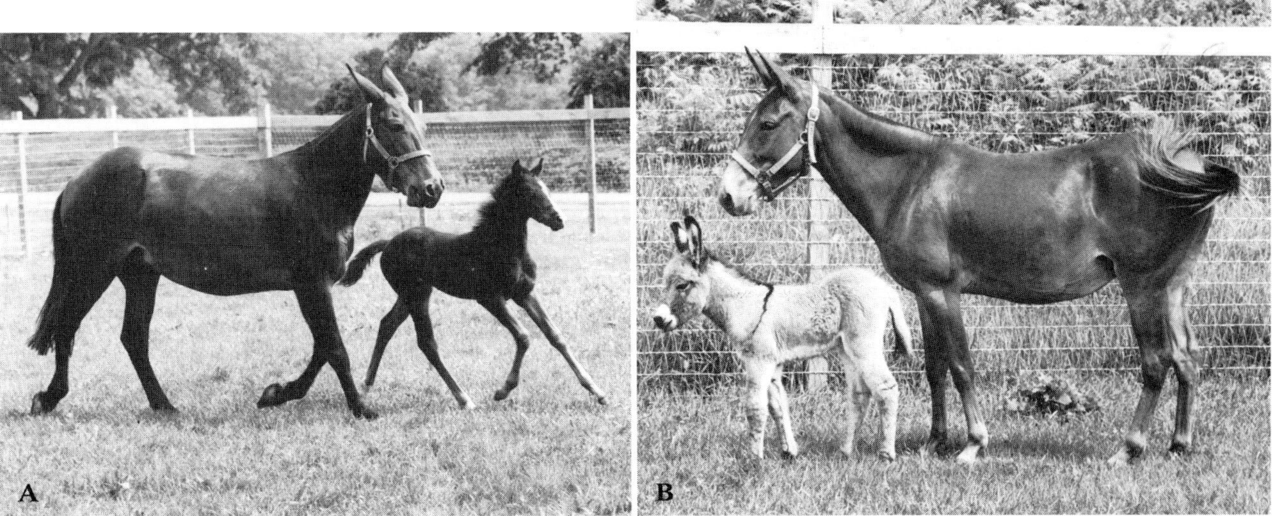

FIG. 63–7. Surrogate F1 mule mothers with their horse *(A)* and donkey *(B)* foals following embryo transfer. Note the vitality and forward development of both foals following their gestation in the uteri of the large recipient mules.

6). An endometrial biopsy recovered nonsurgically on the day after abortion showed an intense inflammatory reaction of neutrophils and lymphocytes.

EMBRYO TRANSFER IN MULES

To compare the humoral and cell-mediated maternal immune responses of the F1 interspecies mule to antigens expressed by the fetuses of its component parental species, five horse and six donkey embryos were transferred surgically to cycling female mules. Four other horse embryos and a donkey embryo were transferred to noncycling mules with streak gonads; these animals were given a daily oral dose of 27.5 mg of the synthetic progestagen Altrenogest (Regumate, Hoechst Animal Health, Milton Keynes, UK), beginning 5 days before transfer, to simulate diestrus. The results of this experiment were described previously.[40,41]

One donkey and three horse pregnancies became established in the cycling recipient mules, and one horse pregnancy got underway in a progestagen-treated anestrous mule (Table 63–2). One donkey and two of the horse foals were carried safely to term and were born healthy and robust between days 344 and 366 (Fig. 63–7); all three of the mule surrogate mothers lactated normally and showed strong maternal behavior toward their foals.[42] One horse-in-mule conceptus was removed by surgical hysterotomy at day 73 for gross and histologic examinations of the endometrial cups and noninvasive placenta. In the progestagen-treated acyclic pregnant mule recipient, the fetus died spontaneously around day 55, and the resorbing conceptus was expelled a few days later. This animal was also subjected to hysterotomy on day 84 to recover persisting endometrial cup tissues for histologic evaluation.

Both the amounts of eCG secreted and the duration of eCG secretion differed markedly between the two pregnancy genotypes in these hybrid surrogate mothers. For example, peak serum eCG concentrations in the four mules carrying horse fetuses ranged from 38 to 352 IU/mL, and eCG remained detectable until days 92 to 119 of gestation (Fig. 63–8). Thus the profiles were essentially similar to those found in mares carrying normal intraspecies horse pregnancies.[43] In the mule carrying the donkey fetus, on the other hand, serum eCG concentrations peaked at only 10 IU/mL, and the hormone had become undetectable by as early as day 84 of gestation[41] (see Fig. 63–7). Thus, in this animal the se-

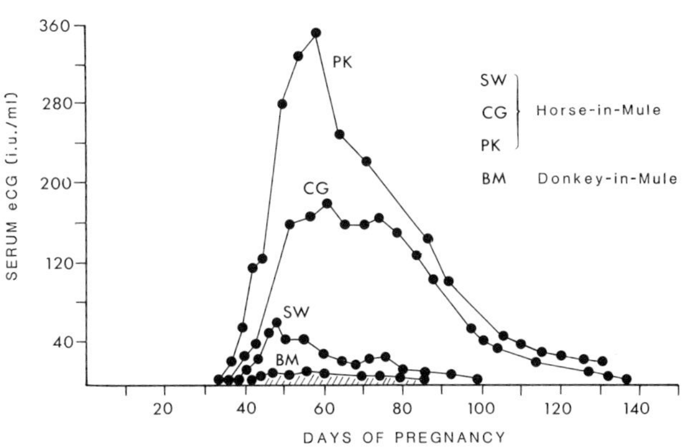

FIG. 63–8. Serum eCG profiles measured between 40 and 140 days of gestation in four pregnant female mules, three of which were carrying a horse conceptus and the other a donkey conceptus following embryo transfer. (From Antczak, D.F., Davies, C.J., Kydd, J., and Allen, W.R.: Immunological aspects of pregnancy in mules. Equine Vet. J., *3(Suppl.)*:68–72, 1985.)

cretion pattern was much more like that described in mares carrying interspecies mule fetuses.[44]

Striking differences existed also in the gross and histologic appearances of the endometrial cups recovered from two of the mules carrying horse fetuses. In the animal that underwent hysterotomy at day 73 while still pregnant, the cups were already cheesy and yellowish in appearance as a result of a significant degree of cell degeneration and a copious amount of eCG-rich exocrine secretion accumulated on their luminal surfaces. Histologically, most of the cup tissue was already necrotic and had become mixed with the liberated gland secretions to give the honey-colored pabulum trapped between the luminal surface of the cup and the overlying allantochorion. An extremely dense band of maternal lymphocytes and other leukocytes surrounded the cup, completely separating it from the adjacent maternal tissues (Fig. 63–9A). In marked contrast, the endometrial cups recovered on day 84 from the allyl trenbolone–treated mule that had undergone spontaneous fetal death some 30 days previously were pale, convex rather than saucer-shaped in outline, and still clearly viable and active. Histologically, the endometrium of this acyclic animal was immature and prepubertal in general appearance, with few endometrial glands that were straight and nonbranched. The persisting endometrial cups were composed, typically, of the mass of large, binucleated eCG-secreting endometrial cup cells of fetal origin. However, as a consequence of the loose and immature architecture of the endometrial stroma, the cup cells were much less densely packed together than normal, so the cup as a whole had an edematous appearance (Fig. 63–9B). But most striking of all, few lymphocytes had accumulated in the stroma around the cup, thereby giving a picture more like the histologic appearance of the endometrial cups in intraspecies donkey pregnancy,[9,10] in complete contrast to the dense aggregation of lymphocytes around the

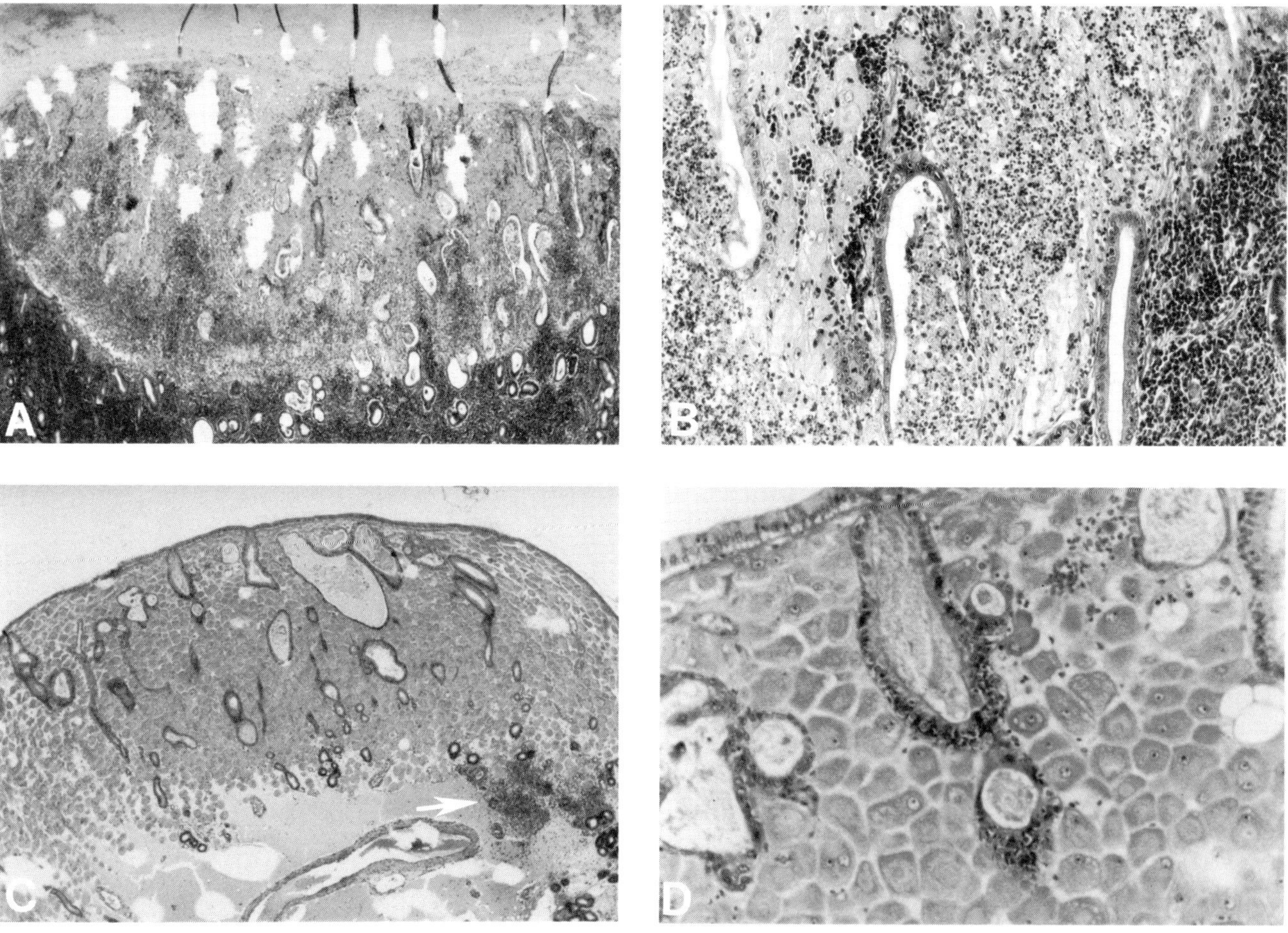

FIG. 63–9. Histologic sections of endometrial cups recovered from a female mule carrying a viable transferred horse fetus at day 73 of gestation (*A*, × 10; *B*, × 50) and from a noncycling progestagen-treated female mule that had aborted a transferred horse fetus 30 days previously at day 54 of gestation (*C*, × 10; *D*, × 50). Note the pronounced contrast between these two animals in the viability of the fetal cup cells and in the intensity of the maternal leukocyte accumulation around the cups. Only a small patch of lymphocytes was observed around the cups from the mule that aborted its conceptus (arrow in *C*). Sections were fixed in Bouin's solution and stained with hematoxylin and eosin.

cups in the other mule still carrying a viable horse fetus at day 73.

This big difference in the intensity of the leukocyte accumulations around the endometrial cups in the two horse-in-mule pregnancies was almost certainly caused by the absence of the fetus and noninvasive placenta from the second animal. A similar marked decline in the intensity of maternal leukocyte response to the endometrial cups, and consequently a longer persistence of viable cups in the endometrium, has been observed on a number of occasions in mares that have spontaneously aborted their normal, intraspecies horse conceptus soon after development of the endometrial cups at day 40. The equally large differences in eCG production and endometrial cup life span between the horse-in-mule and the donkey-in-mule pregnancies further highlighted the profound and interactive influences of fetal genotype and maternal uterine environment on the development and invasiveness of the chorionic girdle and on the expression of, and maternal cell-mediated responses to, fetal antigens on these specialized trophoblast cells.

EMBRYO TRANSFER IN EXOTIC EQUIDS

Over a 2-yr period attempts were made at the Zoological Society of London to recover embryos nonsurgically from two Przewalski's Horse mares (Equus przewalskii, $2n = 66$) and two Grant's Zebra mares (E. burchelli, $2n = 44$) for transfer to domestic Pony mares (E. caballus, $2n = 64$) and jenny donkeys (E. asinus, $2n = 62$).[45,46]

Estrus in the donor animals was induced by an IM injection, given between days 6 and 14 of diestrus, of 250 μg of the prostaglandin analogue cloprostenol (Estrumate, Coopers Animal Health, Berkhamstead, UK), which was delivered by a compressed air dart from a blowgun. The treated animals were placed in a pen with the appropriate male for 1 h each day and observed for signs of estrus and successful mating. Ovulation was assumed to have occurred during the 24-h period before the cessation of estrous behavior and embryo recovery attempts were carried out between 6 and 10 days later, mostly on days 7 or 8.[45] Briefly, the zebra or Przewalski's Horse donor mare was tranquilized by an IM injection of 1.1 to 2.9 mg etorphine-hydrochloride and 4 to 12 mg acepromazine maleate (0.9 to 1.2 mL Large Animal Imobilon, C-Vet Ltd., Suffolk, UK). The sedated animal was then blindfolded and restrained standing or in sternal recumbancy. A flexible 24-French gauge Gibbon balloon-flushing catheter was passed through the cervix and the uterus was then irrigated three times, each with 700 to 1000 mL of flushing medium, as described previously. When located, the embryo was transferred to 5 mL of fresh transfer medium in a sterile plastic tube. This was placed in a shirt breast pocket and driven 72 miles by car to Cambridge (1.5 to 2 h transit time) for surgical or nonsurgical transfer to the selected, synchronized recipient pony mare or jenny donkey.[45]

The embryo recovery and pregnancy rates achieved in these experiments are summarized in Table 63–3. Eleven Przewalski's Horse embryos were obtained from 18 recovery attempts performed on the two donor mares (61%). Of these embryos, 9 were transferred surgically and 2 were transferred nonsurgically to recipient pony mares. This resulted in seven pregnancies initially (64%), as diagnosed by ultrasonographic scanning of the uterus between days 15 and 18 after ovulation.[36] However, an embryo did not appear after day 21 in 2 of these conceptuses, which then diminished steadily in size and finally disappeared during the next 12 days. A third conceptus was aborted spontaneously between days 85 and 101. The other four pregnancies proceeded to term and three live and healthy foals were born (Fig. 63–10). The fourth mare foaled unobserved in the pad-

TABLE 63–3. RECOVERY AND TRANSFER OF PRZEWALSKI'S HORSE (E. PRZEWALSKII) AND GRANT'S ZEBRA (E. BURCHELLI) EMBRYOS TO DOMESTIC HORSE (E. CABALLUS) AND DONKEY (E. ASINUS) RECIPIENTS

TYPE OF TRANSFER	EMBRYO RECOVERY ATTEMPTS	NUMBER OF EMBRYOS RECOVERED (%)	NUMBER OF EMBRYOS TRANSFERRED/ NUMBER OF RECIPIENTS PREGNANT (%)	OUTCOME OF PREGNANCIES
Przewalski's horse to horse	18	11 (61)	11/7 (64)	2 resorbed (days 20 to 40) 1 resorbed (days 85 to 101) 1 stillborn at term 3 live foals
Zebra to horse	25	14 (56)	5/3 (60)	1 resorbed (days 59 to 64) 1 stillborn (day 350) 1 live foal
Zebra to donkey			8/2 (25)	1 resorbed (days 53 to 64) 1 aborted (day 292)

(Data from Kydd, J., et al.: Transfer of exotic equine embryos to domestic horses and donkeys. Equine Vet. J., *3(Suppl.)*:80–84, 1985; and Summers, P.M., et al.: Successful transfer of the embryos of Przewalski's horse (Equus przewalskii) and Grant's zebra (E. burchelli) to domestic mares (E. caballus). J. Reprod. Fertil., *80*:13–20, 1987.)

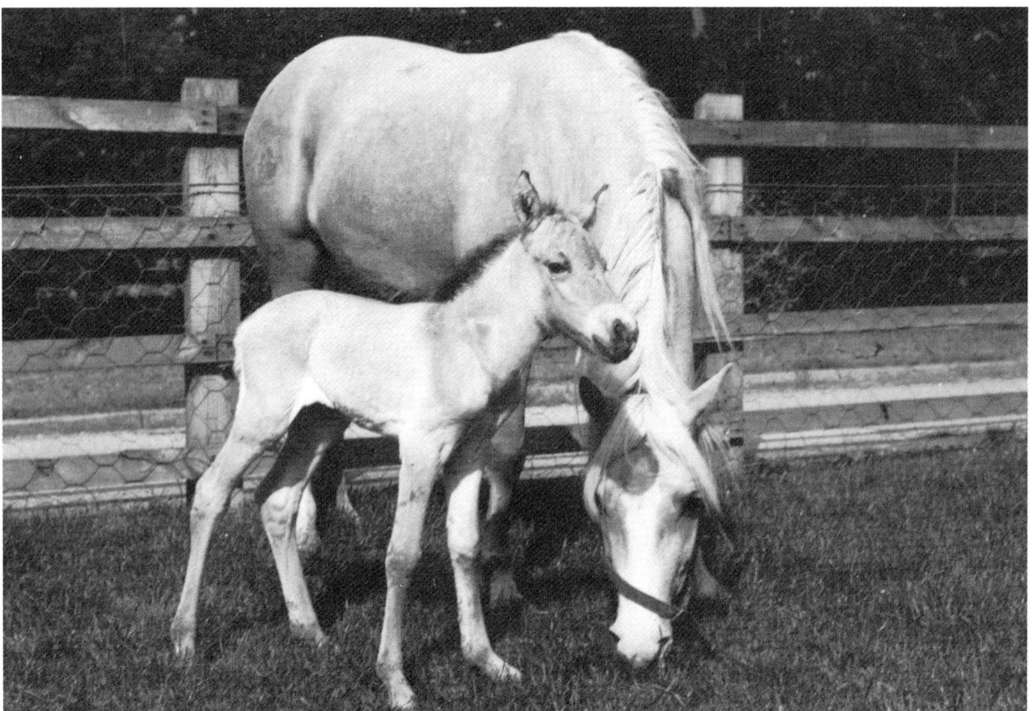

FIG. 63–10. Surrogate domestic horse mare (E. caballus, $2n = 64$) with her newborn Przewalski's Horse foal ($2n = 66$), resulting from embryo transfer on day 7 after ovulation. (From Kydd, J., et al.: Transfer of exotic equine embryos to domestic horses and donkeys. Equine Vet. J., *3(Suppl.)*:80–84, 1985.)

dock, and her foal was unfortunately suffocated by the amnion.

Fourteen zebra embryos were obtained from a total of 25 embryo recovery attempts (56%) performed on the 2 donor zebra. Of these, 5 embryos were transferred surgically to recipient pony mares, which resulted in three established pregnancies (60%). However, 1 fetus died and the conceptus was resorbed between days 59 and 66 and a second foal was stillborn by cesarean section performed on day 350. This mare had shown increasingly severe polyarthritis during the previous 3 weeks. The condition was considered likely to be the manifestation of some form of immunologically based pregnancy toxemia, because the joint swelling and soreness disappeared completely within a few hours after removing the conceptus. The third foal was born alive and robust at day 367, and it was reared successfully by its surrogate horse mother (Fig. 63–11A). Of the original zebra embryos, 7 were transferred surgically to synchronized recipient jenny donkeys to yield only 2 pregnancies. One of these was resorbed between days 53 and 64, whereas the other foal was born prematurely at day 292 and lived for only 3 h before succumbing to respiratory incompetence (Fig. 63–11B). This surrogate donkey mother also showed clinical signs of severe polyarthritis for 5 days before the premature birth (Table 63–3).

Thus, from the total of seven Przewalski's Horse and five Grant's Zebra pregnancies established initially in the recipient mares and jenny donkeys, only three Przewalski's Horse and one zebra foal were born alive. The two Przewalski's Horse conceptuses that were resorbed before day 40 were most likely to have failed as a result of lethal damage to the inner cell mass (ICM) sustained during the recovery, transport, and transfer procedures which then lead to the development of anembryonic trophoblast vesicles.[47] The one Przewalski's Horse and two Grant's Zebra conceptuses that failed between days 53 and 101 may not have implanted properly for reasons that are not understood. One possibility, however, is that the xenogeneic conceptus may have elicited a generalized cell-mediated rejection response from the maternal immune system. The donkey and the horse recipients that aborted well-developed zebra foals near term both showed clinical signs of severe noninfective polyarthritis before the abortion. Both these surrogate mothers also exhibited high concentrations of antigen-antibody complexes in their peripheral blood at this time. For these reasons, and because the changes resolved rapidly after expulsion of the pregnancy from the uterus, the problem was thought likely to reflect a sort of pregnancy toxemia, resulting from maternal immunologic recognition of, and response to, zebra-specific antigens expressed at the fetomaternal interface.[46] However, these untoward signs were not exhibited by the other pony mare that gave birth to the live zebra foal, nor by an aged Quarter Horse mare in Kentucky that also carried an extraspecific zebra foal to term after nonsurgical transfer.[48]

In endocrinologic terms, the Przewalski's Horse-in-

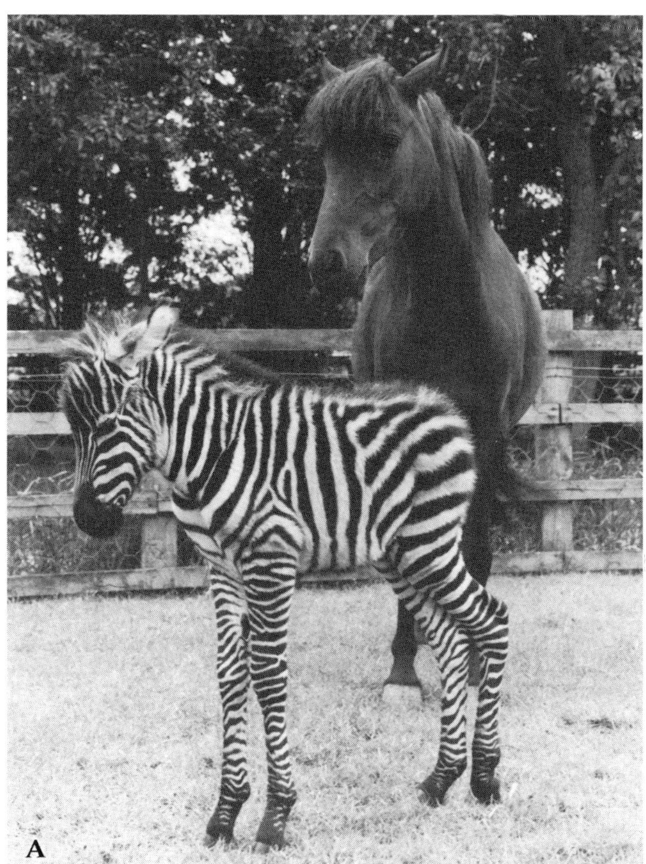

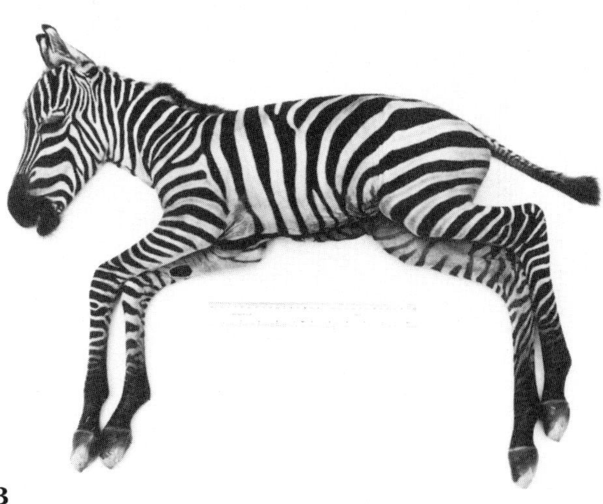

FIG. 63–11. *A,* A 3-day-old Grant's Zebra foal (Equus burchelli, $2n = 44$) with its surrogate domestic horse mother (E. caballus, $2n = 64$). *B,* A well-formed Grant's Zebra fetus aborted by its surrogate jenny donkey mother (E. asinus, $2n = 62$) on day 292 of gestation.

horse pregnancies were characterized by serum eCG profiles that were essentially similar to those measured in normal, intraspecies horse-in-horse pregnancies.[43,46] Considerable variation existed, however, among the four animals involved, both in the peak concentrations (5 to 135 IU/mL) and in the stage of gestation when eCG disappeared from the blood (55 to 95 days). In contrast, minimal amounts of eCG (0.5 to 1.5 IU/mL) were detected for only a few days of gestation between days 40 and 56 in the three mares carrying zebra conceptuses, whereas the peak concentrations were higher (7 to 22 IU/mL) and eCG secretion was more prolonged (days 39 to 83) in both the donkeys carrying zebra fetuses.[46] These big differences in serum eCG concentrations between the different pregnancy genotypes probably reflected differences in the breadth and overall development of the progenitor chorionic girdle. Similarly, the equally large variation in the duration of eCG secretion no doubt mirrored differences in the surrogate maternal cell-mediated responses to xenogeneic fetal antigens expressed at the fetomaternal interface. Certainly, the most striking examples of both these aspects were seen in the three mares carrying zebra conceptuses. The low concentrations of eCG indicated a greatly reduced development of the zebra chorionic girdle in the horse uterus compared with the degree of development in the zebra uterus, as evidenced by the much higher concentrations of eCG measured in the blood of the two donor Grant's Zebra mares when carrying their own interspecies zebra conceptuses at the conclusion of the embryo-transfer experiment.[46] Similarly, the brief period when eCG was present in maternal blood indicated an even more rapid cell-mediated destruction of the small zebra-in-horse endometrial cups that occurs in mares carrying interspecies mule conceptuses.[9,10]

THE DONKEY-IN-HORSE MODEL OF PREGNANCY FAILURE

The one example of equine extraspecific pregnancy that seems to differ markedly from the other types examined to date is that created when a donkey embryo (Equus asinus, $2n = 62$) is transferred to the uterus of a horse recipient (E. caballus, $2n = 64$). In this situation, the donkey chorionic girdle develops as an extremely narrow and scanty band of trophoblast tissue compared with its counterpart in intraspecies horse pregnancy, and it fails completely to invade the surrogate horse endometrium at days 36 to 38 to form endometrial cups. This results in total absence of eCG in maternal blood at any time during gestation.[9] Nevertheless, the donkey fetus and its membranes continue to grow and develop until around days 60 to 65, but in most cases without the normal interdigitation of allantochorionic villi with crypts in the endometrium that commences around day 42 in conventional intraspecies equine pregnancy.[9,49]

In around 70% of donkey-in-horse pregnancies, im-

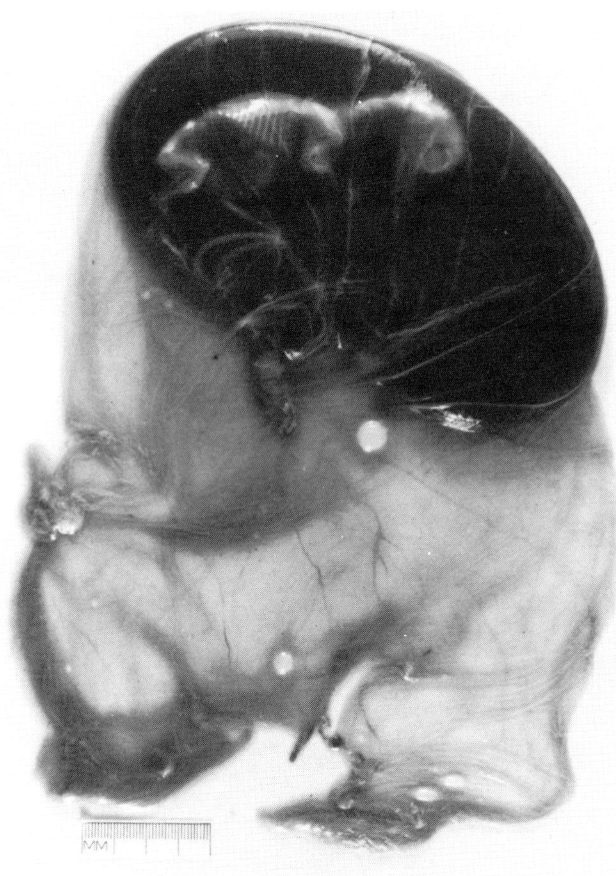

FIG. 63–12. A degenerating donkey conceptus (Equus asinus, $2n = 62$) aborted by its surrogate horse mother (E. caballus, $2n = 64$) at day 83 of gestation. Note the pale and bloodless allantochorion and the cachectic fetus within the heavily blood-stained amniotic fluid.

plantation does not occur at all, with the result that the fetus becomes increasingly starved and stressed until it finally dies and is aborted between days 80 and 100 (Fig. 63–12). Furthermore, this process of fetal degeneration is accompanied by a generalized infiltration of lymphocytes and other leukocytes into the area of endometrium that is in contact with the poorly attached donkey trophoblast; this response has the appearance of a cell-mediated rejection reaction, mounted in this case in response to maternal recognition of xenogeneic donkey antigens at the poorly developed placental interface (Fig. 63–13). In the other 30% of donkey-in-horse pregnancies, however, the rate of attachment and interdigitation of the allantochorion and endometrium is somewhat slower than it is in either intraspecies horse or donkey pregnancy. It eventually occurs, and these "successful implanters" seem to develop relatively normally until at or near term, at which time a second clear division occurs. In about half the cases, a live and particularly large and robust donkey foal is born, having clearly benefited in utero from the larger area of placental exchange in the bigger uterus of the recipient mare (see Fig. 63–7).

But in the other half, the donkey foal is either aborted during the last 4 to 8 weeks of pregnancy or is born live but weak, dysmature, and nutrionally deprived at or near term. This latter group show a placenta that is much smaller and lighter than normal because of the combination of fewer and less well developed microcotyledons per area of tissue. This, in turn, is clearly related to the slower rate of differentiation and interdigitation of the allantochorion much earlier in pregnancy. Thus, a complete gradation appears to exist within this one type of extraspecific donkey-in-horse pregnancy in terms of implantation, placentation, and fetal survival. This ranges from apparently normal

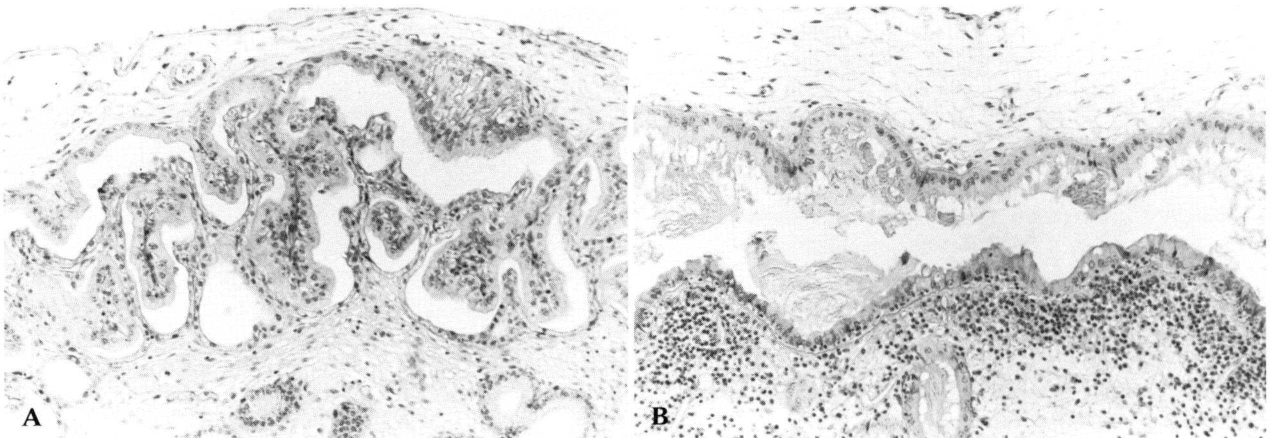

FIG. 63–13. Histologic sections of the allantochorion-endometrium interface in *(A)* a mare carrying a viable intraspecies horse conceptus at day 60 of gestation and *(B)* a mare carrying a transferred extraspecies donkey conceptus at day 71. The typical, branched chorionic villi interdigitating with endometrial crypts of the implanting horse-in-horse pregnancy are absent in the failing donkey-in-horse pregnancy. Instead, appreciable quantities of exocrine secretion tend to separate the trophoblast from the endometrial epithelium while large numbers of lymphocytes and other leukocytes accumulate in the endometrial stroma (× 100).

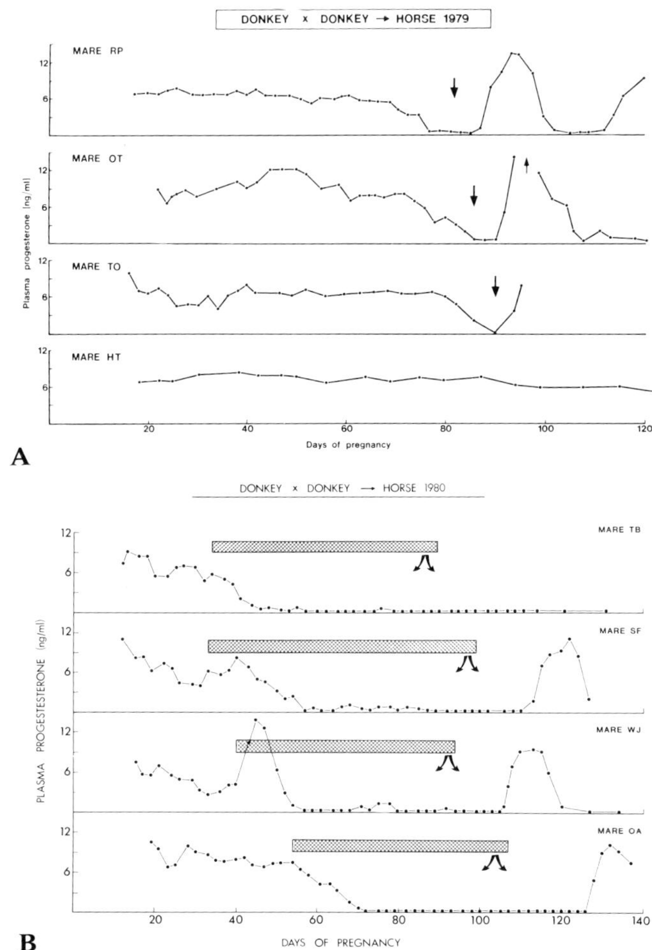

FIG. 63–14. Peripheral plasma progesterone concentrations measured in mares carrying transferred extraspecies donkey conceptuses that were *(A)* not given any exogenous hormonal therapy and *(B)* given 30 mg allyl trenbolone daily from around day 35 of gestation onward (hatched horizontal bar). The vertical arrows in *A* show the days on which three of the untreated mares aborted their degenerating conceptus. The curved arrows in *B* indicate the period of gestation when the fetus died and resorption of the conceptus began in all four of the allyl trenbolone–treated mares. Note the premature decline in endogenous plasma progesterone concentrations in the treated group of animals. (From Allen, W.R.: Immunological aspects of the endometrial cup reaction and the effect of xenogeneic extraspecies pregnancy in horses and donkey. J. Reprod. Fertil. Suppl., *31*:57–94, 1982.)

in those few mares that give birth to big and robust donkey foals to another small "just made it" group that give birth to small but dysmature foals at or beyond term to another small "almost made it" group that abort severely undernourished foals within a few weeks before term to the majority of "didn't have a chance" animals that undergo the now well-characterized pattern of failed implantation and inadequate placentation leading to fetal starvation, death, and abortion before day 100.

During the past decade we have carried out a variety of experiments aimed at elucidating the underlying causes of the high rate of pregnancy failure in the donkey-in-horse model, which differs so strikingly from its counterparts among the range of equine extraspecies pregnancies. Initially, hormonal deficiency seemed likely to play an important part in the syndrome, because the failure of endometrial cup development meant that (1) eCG was completely absent from maternal blood during the first half of pregnancy, (2) the normal rises in plasma progesterone concentrations after day 40[50] did not occur in most animals because of an absence of secondary luteal development,[9] and (3) the normal sharp rise in plasma conjugated estrogen concentrations between days 36 and 40 resulting from eCG stimulation of the maternal ovaries[51,52] also failed to occur.[53] Moreover, plasma progesterone concentrations declined steadily over a 15- to 20-day period in mares destined to abort their donkey conceptuses during the first 100 days of pregnancy, and the levels reached baseline coincidentally with expulsion of the degenerating fetus and membranes (Fig. 63–14A).

However, supplementation of four mares carrying donkey conceptuses with high daily doses of the orally active synthetic progestagen allyl trenbolone (Regumate, Hoechst Animal Health, Milton Keynes, UK) failed to prevent fetal death during the characteristic period in all four animals. Furthermore, the exogenous progestagen hastened the demise of the primary corpus luteum in the treated mares, as evidenced by a more rapid decline of plasma progesterone concentrations to basal values compared with the situation in the untreated mares (Fig. 63–14B). Similarly, fetal death and abortion occurred during the characteristic period (days 83 to 105) in 6 of 7 mares carrying donkey conceptuses that were given high doses (20,000 to 300,000 IU) of partially purified eCG on one or more occasions be-

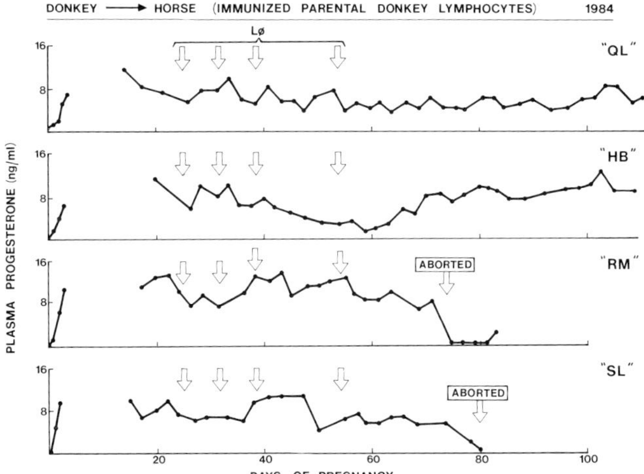

FIG. 63–15. Peripheral plasma progesterone concentrations measured in four mares carrying transferred extraspecies donkey conceptuses that were each immunized four times between days 28 and 52 of gestation with washed parental donkey lymphocytes. In the two mares that aborted (arrows), plasma progesterone concentrations were equal to or higher than those in the two mares that remained pregnant.

TABLE 63–4. THE EXTRASPECIES DONKEY-IN-HORSE PREGNANCY MODEL OF PREGNANCY FAILURE: ENDOCRINOLOGIC TREATMENTS

TREATMENT	NUMBER OF MARES	NUMBER ABORTED BEFORE DAY 120	FETAL SURVIVAL (%)
None (control)	12	11	8
Progestagen (allyl trenbolone from day 36)	4	4	0
Equine chorionic gonadotropin (20,000 to 300,000 IU repeatedly from day 38)	7	6	14

tween days 38 and 60 of gestation and which showed measurable eCG concentrations in their serum after this exogenous treatment (Table 63–4).

Two types of immunologic therapy have been applied to the model, and both seem to have increased the rate of fetal survival and the chance of successful pregnancy in treated animals.[54] The first of these was a type of passive immunization whereby six mares carrying donkey fetuses were given repeated intravenous infusions, every 5 days between days 40 and 80 of gestation, of large volumes (0.75 to 1.2 L) of serum recovered from mares carrying normal intraspecific horse conceptuses at equivalent stages of gestation. Three of these mares (50%) then carried their donkey foals to term whereas both of the control mares infused with nonpregnant mares' serum aborted at the usual time (Table 63–5).

The second type of immunologic treatment involved active immunization, following reports in the literature concerning the successful treatment of women with histories of repeated spontaneous abortion by immunization with paternal or third-party lymphocytes.[55] Nine mares carrying donkey pregnancies were immunized, on four occasions between days 28 and 52 after ovulation, with approximately 200×10^6 mixed washed peripheral blood lymphocytes recovered either from the donkey sire and dam of the particular donkey embryo being carried or from a panel of four unrelated male and female donkeys. Six of the nine lymphocyte-treated mares remained pregnant to > 150 days of gestation to give an overall improved fetal survival rate of 67%[54] (Table 63–5). None of the immunized mares showed any detectable eCG in their blood at any stage, and as judged by the relatively flat peripheral plasma progesterone profiles exhibited between days 40 and 100, none of them had any secondary luteal development. Nevertheless, on the basis of plasma progesterone assays and other clinical parameters, it was impossible to predict prospectively, or to determine retrospectively, why the three mares still aborted their donkey conceptuses despite having been immunized (Fig. 63–15).

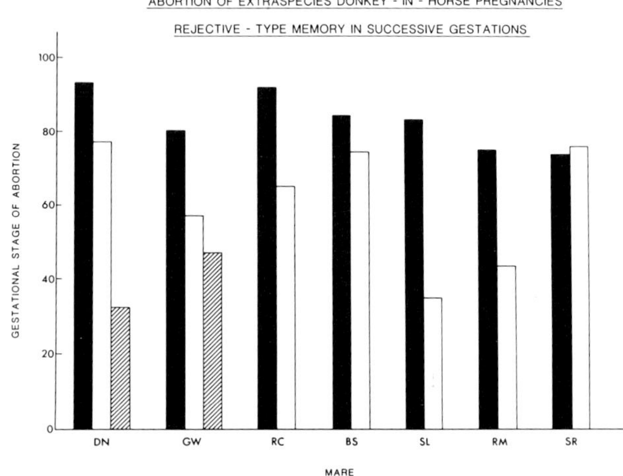

FIG. 63–16. The successively earlier stages of gestation when abortion occurred in seven pony mares carrying their first (filled bar), second (open bar), and third (hatched bar) successive transferred donkey-in-horse pregnancies.

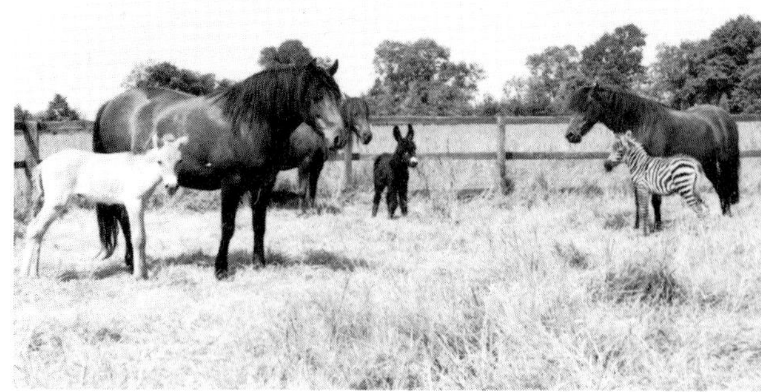

FIG. 63–17. Genetic drift in the equine nursery. Surrogate domestic horse (Equus caballus, $2n = 64$) mothers with their transferred extraspecific foals; a Przewalski's Horse (E. przewalskii, $2n = 66$), a domestic donkey (E. asinus, $2n = 62$) and a Grant's Zebra (E. burchelli, $2n = 44$).

TABLE 63–5. THE EXTRASPECIES DONKEY-IN-HORSE PREGNANCY MODEL OF PREGNANCY FAILURE: IMMUNOLOGIC TREATMENTS GIVEN

TREATMENT	NUMBER OF MARES	NUMBER ABORTED BEFORE DAY 120	FETAL SURVIVAL (%)
None (control)	24	19	21
Infusions of pregnant mares serum	6	3	50
Immunized with donkey lymphocytes	9	3	67

These striking and inexplicable differences in the responses of individual mares carrying donkey conceptuses to immunologic and other forms of treatment attempted so far leave a question as to whether the whole phenomenon of early pregnancy failure in this model is mediated immunologically or whether it has a genetic basis. Unfortunately, the difficulty and cost of establishing such xenogeneic pregnancies makes it virtually impossible to carry out controlled experiments with sufficient numbers of replicates to provide statistically valid results and comparisons. Nevertheless, one striking observation that has emerged from the results of the experiments undertaken so far points strongly to the involvement of both genetic and immunologic factors in the process. Namely, the high correlation that exists between the outcome of successive pregnancies in individual mares to which donkey conceptuses were transferred in successive breeding seasons. For example, of 10 mares that carried their first donkey pregnancies to term, no fewer than 9 carried a second donkey conceptus successfully; 2 of these same mares were given a third successive donkey pregnancy and these were also carried successfully without any form of exogenous therapy.[54] Conversely, all of 7 mares that aborted their first donkey pregnancies aborted second donkey conceptuses in the following breeding season; six of these seven second abortions occurred significantly earlier in gestation and both of the third successive abortions occurred even earlier (Fig. 63–16). This positive correlation between the outcome of the first and subsequent donkey pregnancies points strongly toward a genetic basis for the phenomenon (Fig. 63–17). On the other hand, the pronounced decrease in the interval from embryo transfer to abortion in second and later donkey-in-horse pregnancies is reminiscent of immunologic memory, one of the hallmarks of the immune system.

In summary, strong suggestive evidence exists that the characteristic degeneration leading to death and expulsion of the fetus and membranes which occurs between days 80 and 100 of gestation in around 70% of the extraspecific donkey-in-horse pregnancies involves a vigorous maternal cell-mediated rejection response to the mare's recognition of foreign fetal antigens. Enormous numbers of lymphocytes accumulate in the endometrium in contact with the degenerating allantochorion (see Fig. 63–13B), and these have been observed tracking through the endometrial epithelium, apparently en route to attack the xenogeneic trophoblast cells.[9,54] Furthermore, the severe hemolysis of the fetal red blood cells that occurs before the death of the donkey fetus is also a characteristic feature of another murine model of early pregnancy failure, namely, that which occurs when rare Mus caroli (mouse) embryos are transferred to the uteri of the common laboratory mouse (M. musculis).[56] But whether these immunologic changes are actually the cause of fetal death leading to abortion, or whether they occur merely as a consequence of developmental placental failure enabling maternal recognition of fetal antigens that would otherwise remain masked, is far from clear.

REFERENCES

1. Tegetmeier, W.B., and Sutherland, C.L.: Horses, Asses, Zebras, Mules and Mule Breeding. London, Horace Cox, 1895.
2. Ewart, J.C.: On zebra-ass hybrids; with observations on the relationships of the zebras. Veterinarian, *71:*185–202, 1898.
3. Gray, A.P.: Mammalian Hybrids. Slough, UK, Commonwealth Agricultural Bureaux, 1971.
4. Short, R.V.: The evolution of the horse. J. Reprod. Fertil. Suppl., *23:*1–6, 1975.
5. Short, R.V.: The contribution of the mule to scientific thought. J. Reprod. Fertil. Suppl., *23:*359–364, 1975.
6. Jocelyn, H.D., and Setchell, B.P. (trans.): Regnier de Graaf on the human reproductive organs. J. Reprod. Fertil. Suppl., *17,* 1972.
7. Wodsedalek, J.E.: Causes of sterility in the mule. Biol. Bull. Mar. Biol. Lab. Woods Hole, *30:*1–56, 1916.
8. Taylor, M.J., and Short, R.V.: Development of the germ cells in the ovary of the mule and hinny. J. Reprod. Fertil., *32:*441–445, 1973.
9. Allen, W.R.: Immunological aspects of the equine endometrial cup reaction and the effect of xenogeneic extraspecies pregnancy in horses and donkey. J. Reprod. Fertil. Suppl., *31:*57–94, 1982.
10. Allen, W.R.: The influence of fetal genotype upon endometrial cup development and PMSG and progestagen production in equids. J. Reprod. Fertil. Suppl., *23:*405–413, 1975.
11. Allen, W.R.: Maternal recognition of pregnancy and im-

munological implications of trophoblast-endometrium interactions in equids. *In* Maternal Recognition of Pregnancy. CIBA Foundation Symposium No. 64. Amsterdam, Excerpta Medica, 1979, pp. 323–352.

12. Allen, W.R.: Embryo transfer in the horse. *In* Mammalian Egg Transfer. Edited by C.E. Adams. Boca Raton, CRC Press, 1982, pp. 126–154.
13. Hancock, J.L.: Animal hybrids: Causes of death before birth. New Scient., *35:*504, 1967.
14. Hancock, J.L., and McGovern, P.T.: The transport of sheep and goat spermatozoa in the ewe. J. Reprod. Fertil., *15:*283–287, 1964.
15. Hancock, J.L., McGovern, P.T., and Stamp, J.T.: Failure of gestation of goat × sheep hybrids in goats and sheep. J. Reprod. Fertil. Suppl., *3:*29–36, 1968.
16. Chang, M.C., Marston, J.H., and Hunt, D.M.: Reciprocal fertilization between the domesticated rabbit and the snowshoe hare with special reference to insemination of rabbits with an equal number of hare and rabbit spermatozoa. J. Exp. Zool., *155:*437–445, 1964.
17. Barton, S.C., Surani, M.A.H., and Norris, M.L.: Role of paternal and maternal genomes in mouse development. Nature, *311:*374–376, 1984.
18. King, J.M.: Comparative aspects of reproduction in Equidae. Ph.D. thesis. University of Cambridge, 1965.
19. Chandley, A.C., et al.: Meiosis in interspecific equine hybrids. I. The male mule (Equus asinus × E. caballus) and hinny (E. caballus × E. asinus). Cytogenet. Cell. Genet., *13:*330–341, 1974.
20. Bielanski, W.: Observations on ovulation processes in she-mules. Bull. Acad. Pol. Sci. *3:*243–247, 1955.
21. Anderson, W.S.: Fertile mare mules. J. Hered., *30:*549–551, 1939.
22. Benirschke, K., Low, R.J., Sullivan, M.M., and Carter, R.M.: Chromosome study of an alleged fertile mare mule. J. Hered., *55:*31–38, 1964.
23. Rong, R., Cai, H., and Wei, J.: Fertile mule in China and her unusual foal. J. R. Soc. Med., *78:*821–825, 1985.
24. Chandley, A.C., and Clarke, C.A.: Cum mula peperit. J. R. Soc. Med., *78:*800–801, 1985.
25. Ryder, D.A., Chemmick, L.G., Bowling, A.T., and Benirschke, K.: Male mule qualifies as the offspring of a female mule and jack donkey. J. Hered. *76:*379–381, 1985.
26. Rong, R., et al.: A fertile mule and hinny in China. Cytogenet. Cell Genet., *47:*134–139, 1988.
27. Chandley, A.C.: Fertile mules. J. R. Soc. Med., *81:*2, 1988.
28. Michie, D.: Affinity: a new genetic phenomenon in the house mouse, evidence from distant crosses. Nature, *171:*26–27 1953.
29. Koulischer L., and Frechkof, S.: Chromosome complement: A fertile hybrid between Equus przewalskii and Equus caballus. Science, *151:*93–95, 1966.
30. Short, R.V., Chandley, A.C., Jones, R.C., and Allen, W.R.: Meiosis in interspecific equine hybrids. II. The Przewalski horse/domestic horse hybrid (Equus przewalskii × E. caballus). Cytogenet. Cell. Genet., *13:*465–478, 1974.
31. Chandley, A.C., Short, R.V., and Allen, W.R.: Cytogenetic studies of three equine hybrids. J. Reprod. Fertil. Suppl., *23:*365–370, 1975.
32. Newcomb, R., Booth, W.D., and Rowson, L.E.A.: The effect of oxytocin treatment on the levels of prostaglandin F in the blood of heifers. J. Reprod. Fertil., *49:*17–24, 1977.
33. Stanley, C., et al.: Use of a new and rapid milk progesterone assay to monitor reproductive activity in the cow. Vet. Rec., *118:*664–667, 1986.
34. Allen, W.R., and Sanderson, M.W.: The value of a rapid progesterone assay (AELIA) in equine stud veterinary medicine and management. *In* Bain-Fallon Memorial Lectures. Sydney, Australian Equine Veterinarian Association, 1987, pp. 75–82.
35. Simpson, D.J., et al.: Use of ultrasound echography for early diagnosis of single and twin-pregnancy in the mare. J. Reprod. Fertil. Suppl., *32:*431–439, 1982.
36. Allen, W.R.: A quantitative immunological assay for pregnant mare serum gonadotrophin. J. Endocrinol., *43:*581–591, 1969.
37. Kydd, J., Miller, J., Antczak, D.F., and Allen, W.R.: Maternal anti-fetal cytotoxic antibody responses of equids during pregnancy. J. Reprod. Fertil. Suppl., *32:*361–369, 1982.
38. Sheldrick, E.L., Wright, P.J., Allen, W.R., and Heap, R.B.: Metabolic clearance rate, production rate and source of progesterone in donkeys with fetuses of different genotypes. J. Reprod. Fertil., *51:*473–476, 1977.
39. Stewart, F., Allen, W.R., and Moor, R.M.: Influence of foetal genotype on the follicle-stimulating hormone luteinizing hormone ratio of pregnant mare serum gonadotrophin. J. Endocrinol., *73:*419–425, 1977.
40. Davies, C.J., Antczak, D.F., and Allen, W.R.: Reproduction in mules: Embryo transfer using sterile recipients. Equine Vet. J. *3(Suppl.):* 63–67, 1985.
41. Antczak, D.F., Davies, C.J., Kydd, J., and Allen, W.R.: Immunological aspects of pregnancy in mules. Equine Vet. J., *3(Suppl.):*68–72, 1985.
42. Shaw, E., and Haupt, K.A.: Pre- and post partum behaviour in mules impregnated by embryo transfer. Equine Vet. J., *3(Suppl.):*73, 1985.
43. Allen, W.R.: The immunological measurement of pregnant mare serum gonadotrophin. J. Endocrinol., *43:*593–598, 1969.
44. Allen, W.R.: Factors influencing pregnant mare serum gonadotrophin production. Nature, *223:*64–66, 1969.
45. Kydd, J., et al.: Transfer of exotic equine embryos to domestic horses and donkeys. Equine Vet. J., *3(Suppl.):*80–84, 1985.
46. Summers, P.M., et al.: Successful transfer of the embryos of Przewalski's horse (Equus przewalskii) and Grant's zebra (E. burchelli) to domestic mares (E. caballus). J. Reprod. Fertil., *80:*13–20, 1987.
47. Skidmore, J., Boyle, M.S., Cran, D., and Allen, W.R.: Micro-manipulation of equine embryos to produce monozygotic twins. Equine Vet. J., *8(Suppl.):*126–128, 1989.
48. Bennett, S.D., and Foster, W.R.: Successful transfer of a zebra embryo to a domestic horse. Equine Vet. J., *3(Suppl.):*78–79, 1985.
49. Samuel, C.A., Allen, W.R., and Steven, D.H.: Ultrastructural development of the equine placenta. J. Reprod. Fertil. Suppl., *23:*575–578, 1975.
50. Squires, E.L., and Ginther, O.J.: Follicular and luteal development in pregnant mares. J. Reprod. Fertil. Suppl., *23:*429–433, 1975.
51. Terqui, M., and Palmer, E.: Oestrogen pattern during early pregnancy in the mare. J. Reprod. Fertil. Suppl., *27:*441–446, 1979.
52. Kindahl, H., Knudsen, O., Madej, A., and Edqvist, L.E.: Progesterone, prostaglandin $F_2\alpha$, PMSG and oestrone sulphate during early pregnancy in the mare. J. Reprod. Fertil. Suppl., *32:*353–359, 1982.
53. Urwin, V.E., and Allen, W.R.: Pituitary and chorionic gonadotrophin control of ovarian function during early

pregnancy in equids. J. Reprod. Fertil. Suppl., *32:*371–382, 1982.

54. Allen, W.R., Kydd, J.H., Boyle, M.S., and Antczak, D.F.: Extra-specific donkey-in-horse pregnancy as a model of early fetal death. J. Reprod. Fertil. Suppl., *35:*197–209, 1987.

55. Mowbray, J.F., et al.: Controlled trial of treatment of recurrent spontaneous abortion by immunisation with paternal cells. Lancet, *1:*941–943, 1985.

56. Croy, A.B.: Use of experimental embryo transfer to study the role of the immune system in embryonic death. Equine Vet. J., *3(Suppl.):*49–52, 1985.

CHAPTER 64

ABORTION IN MARES

H.M. Acland

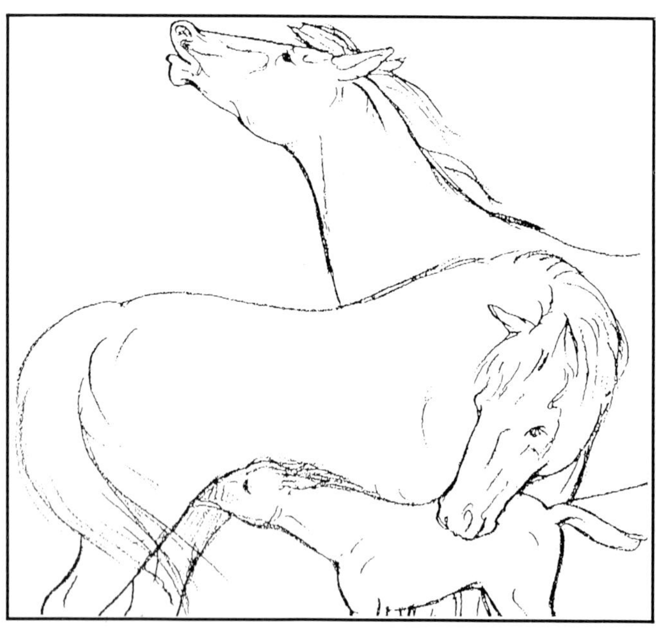

Abortion continues to be a problem in equine reproduction. The subject has been well reviewed,[1–9] yet after abortions as a result of twinning and equine herpesvirus type 1 infection are accounted for, diagnosticians are all too often ignorant of the cause. In a study of Thoroughbreds, an overall abortion rate of 19% was found, with a rate of 9.3% occurring after 60 days gestation.[10]

Normal gestation length in the Thoroughbred mare is approximately 340 days. Strictly, abortion means the termination of pregnancy before 300 days, and stillbirth refers to fetal loss after 300 days gestation, at which time a foal born alive may be capable of survival. In this chapter, both are considered abortion.

Most equine abortions are sporadic, although in some years, the incidence of abortion has been high because of an epizootic of equine herpesvirus type 1 infection. The placenta is frequently delivered with the fetus. The premature onset of lactation may be a sign of impending abortion. Most aborted fetuses are freshly dead, however mummification is not uncommon in one of a set of twins.

METHOD OF INVESTIGATION

Important facts to be sought in the history are gestational age of the fetus, vaccination history of the mare, illnesses experienced by the mare or other members of the group, and past reproductive performance of the mare. The likelihood of reaching an etiologic diagnosis for abortion is always greater if both the fetus and placenta are examined. The fetus and placenta should be sent to a diagnostic laboratory, to take advantage of the specialty training of the personnel and the environment better suited to aseptic collection of specimens for microbiologic examination. Because of the constraints of time, money, and availability of services, the practitioner is often obliged to perform a field necropsy. A suggested kit is given in Table 64–1 and the range of specimens to collect is shown in Table 64–2.

EXAMINATION OF THE FETUS

The aborted fetus is examined externally and internally for gross abnormalities, and specimens are collected for microscopic and microbiologic evaluation. Contamination of specimens for bacteriology, mycology, and virology is avoided by harvesting relevant tissues as they are exposed and before they are handled.

The general nutritional condition of the fetus is noted first. Crown-rump length and the presence or absence of hair on the mane, muzzle, eyelids, and coronary bands are recorded for later reference to a chart that allows the estimation of fetal age.[7,11] The limbs are then reflected and the abdomen is opened. Two pieces of liver (up to 50 g each) are collected aseptically, one for bacteriologic examination and one for virus isolation. The organs are examined for any abnormal location, size, color, or consistency. Any edema at the root of the

TABLE 64–1. CONTENTS OF KIT FOR COLLECTION OF LABORATORY SPECIMENS FROM ABORTED FETUSES

ITEM	PURPOSE
Steel rule	Measurement of crown-rump length and measurement of umbilical cord length
Knife and steel	Necropsy
4 sets sterile forceps and scissors	Collecting specimens for microbiology
String	Tying off the fetal stomach for culture of contents
8 sterile containers packed in ice	Holding and transporting specimens for bacterial and fungal culture and for virology
Fixative, at least 100 mL	Histopathology

greater mesentery is noted. The stomach is tied off so that its contents are retained for bacterial culture. Small pieces (1 × 2 × 2 cm) of a range of tissues (liver, lymph node, adrenal, and spleen) are placed in 10% buffered formalin or Bouin's fluid for histology. Next, the diaphragm is cut away from the ribs and the amount of fluid in the thorax noted. Immediately and aseptically, samples of lung are collected for bacteriology and virology, and a sample of thymus is collected for virology. Lung and thymus specimens are taken for histology. If fluorescent antibody staining is available for diagnosis of equine herpesvirus type 1 infection, a range of unfixed tissues (lung, thymus, lymph node, spleen, and adrenal) should be taken and held chilled or frozen. The heart is then examined externally and internally, followed by the other structures of the thorax, and the neck and head. A check is made for fractured ribs, hemarthrosis of the shoulder, and subcutaneous edema of the head.

EXAMINATION OF THE PLACENTA

The normal equine placenta is described and discussed in Chapter 60. Postfoaling or postabortion examination of the placenta should be a standard practice. Valuable clues to the cause of abortion are often found in the placenta. Unless the examination is methodical, some of these clues could be easily missed. Visualizing all surfaces—chorion, allantois, amnion, and cord—is an essential part of a thorough examination of the placenta.[12] Note whether the placenta has everted and the foal exited through the cervical star area (as in most normal deliveries) or whether the chorion side is presented outward and the membranes have been ruptured at a place corresponding to a location in the uterine body unrelated to the cervix. Put the free end of the cord in a tube and milk several milliliters of blood into the tube. Turn the chorionic side out and examine for nonvillous areas or areas discolored from the normal pink-brown or thickened areas. Take pieces of allantochorion from near the cervical star and elsewhere as well as pieces of allantoamnion for bacterial and fungal cultures and for histology.

CAUSES OF EQUINE ABORTION

GENERAL COMMENTS

Discrepancies between the actual and expected fetal crown-rump length and hair development for gestational age[11] indicate an error in the records or fetal growth retardation. Often the latter can be linked with an inflammatory or noninflammatory placental lesion. The lesion causes a chronic placental insufficiency.

Fetuses can have a set of nonspecific gross lesions associated with death in the preparturient, parturient, or even the immediate postparturient period. A convenient diagnostic term of "neonatal asphyxia" has been ap-

TABLE 64–2. SPECIMENS TO COLLECT FROM ABORTED FETUSES FOR LABORATORY EXAMINATION

	PURPOSE			
	Virus Isolation			
Specimen	EHV 1	EVA	Bacterial/Fungal Culture	Histology
Placenta		x	x	x
Spleen	x	x		x
Liver	x		x	x
Lymph nodes	x	x		x
Adrenal	x			x
Kidney			x	x
Stomach contents			x	
Lung	x		x	x
Thymus	x	x		x
Heart				x

plied.[13] The lesions include petechial and ecchymotic hemorrhages on the parietal and visceral pleura, tracheal, and bronchial mucosa, and the epicardium and endocardium. Yellow edematous fluid may be present in the root of the great mesentery. Causes of neonatal asphyxia can be placental disease, premature placental separation, congenital cardiac abnormalities, fetal infections, and dystocia. In the latter condition, broken ribs and hemarthrosis of the shoulder are often present as well.

Microscopically, a common finding in the pulmonary alveoli of aborted fetuses or dead neonates is clusters of epithelial squames from fetal skin, some with yellow granules of meconium. Multishaped eosinophilic bodies in fetal alveoli have been identified as congealed amnionic fluid.[14] These materials apparently enter the lung as a result of fetal respiratory movements in utero. Sometimes a mild inflammatory response occurs. The amount of amnionic debris in the lungs of fetuses and foals varies greatly; large amounts may be an indication of fetal distress.

The causes of equine abortion can broadly be divided into infectious, noninfectious, and unknown. Most reports categorize about 40% of abortions as of unknown cause,[1,7,13,15] although one large survey has only 12.6% undetermined.[16] For those of known cause, the split between infectious and noninfectious varies widely; infections are found to be responsible for between 16.2% and 47.5% of abortions.

NONINFECTIOUS ABORTION

Twinning

Sophisticated management of the mare and the widespread use of ultrasonography should dramatically reduce the prevalence of twinning, but historically twins have been the single most important cause of abortion

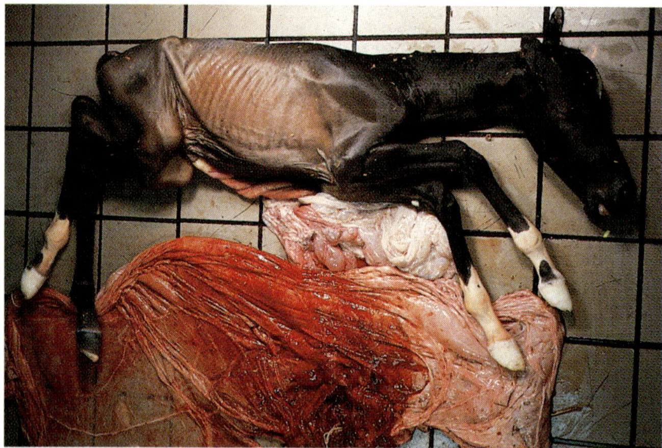

FIG. 64–1. Aborted twin fetus. The left two thirds of the chorion has normal villi, while the right one third has no villi. Note the thin condition of the fetus. (From Acland, H.M.: Abortion in mares: diagnosis and prevention. Compend. Contin. Educ. Practicing Vet., *9*:318–326, 1987.)

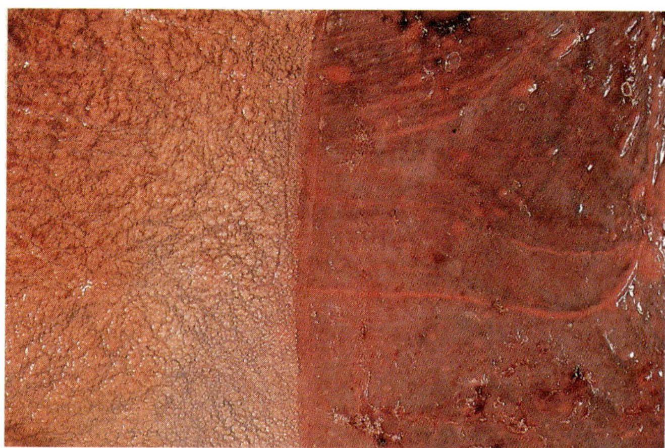

FIG. 64–2. Chorion of an aborted twin fetus. In this close-up view, the normal part of the chorion (on the left) is sharply demarcated from the part of the chorion that was in contact with the chorion of the twin and has no villi. (From Acland, H.M.: Abortion in mares: diagnosis and prevention. Compend. Contin. Educ. Practicing Vet., *9*:318–326, 1987.)

in Thoroughbreds. Twins are dizygotic. Briefly, three main distributions of twins exist in the uterus. The most common pattern (about 80%) has the larger twin occupying all of one horn and most of the body, leaving the smaller twin only a small portion of the body and the other horn. These pregnancies frequently end in abortion or stillbirth of one or both twins, many at 8 to 9 months' gestation. The other two patterns are seen with about equal frequency. In one, the villous surface area is more or less equally divided, so that each fetus occupies one horn and part of the body; both twins are usually born alive, but many are destroyed because of weakness, poor conformation, or small size. In the third type, much greater disparity exists, with the smaller twin occupying only a part of one horn and dying early and becoming mummified, while the larger twin is usually born alive with a fair chance of survival.[17] Twinning is discussed in detail in Chapter 62.

Although the diagnosis is obvious when twins are aborted, they should be submitted to a diagnostic laboratory for the purpose of ruling out concurrent infectious disease. When only one twin is found, it is still possible to make the diagnosis of twin pregnancy by the appearance of the placenta. The key finding is a large smooth area of chorion (Figs. 64–1 and 64–2). The contact area between the chorions of the two twins is smooth because villi do not develop where the chorion does not make contact with endometrium. Villi (2 to 5 mm long) are densely packed all over the outer surface of the chorion of the normal singleton foal, except for five areas where no contact with endometrium exists—cervical star, the openings of the two uterine tubes, the endometrial cups, and where the chorion is folded on itself over the large allantoic blood vessels.[12]

Abortion of twins can occur at any stage of pregnancy. Fetal death is attributed chiefly to placental insufficiency. The combined functional surface area of the chorions of both twins is only slightly larger than that for a single normal foal. The fetuses are thin, with prominent ribs and often exhibit growth retardation. Aborted twin fetuses often appear to have died at different times. In one study, in 59% of twin pregnancies the smaller twin died first, while in 20% of pregnancies the larger twin died first.[17] It is difficult to explain why a lack of consistency in the order of death of dissimilar size twins occurs and why some die early in the pregnancy before the uterine wall has reached its maximum capacity to enlarge.[6]

Abnormalities of the Placenta

Umbilical Cord. The length of the cord in 95% of normal Thoroughbreds is less than 84 cm.[18] Excessive length or shortness of the cord may interfere with survival. Increased length has been associated with excessive torsion and allantochorionic necrosis at the cervical pole. In many cases of abortion of undiagnosed cause between 7 and 10 months, the cords are over 80 cm long. On the other hand, abnormal shortness of the umbilical cord has been shown to cause stillbirth owing to premature intrapartum rupture of the cord and fetal asphyxia.[6]

Torsion of the umbilical cord is often considered to be the cause of fetal death. Normally, much twisting of the cord occurs. Only when localized swelling and discoloration accompanying the twisting are present should the diagnosis of death caused by vascular obstruction be made. Fluid-filled sacs in the amnionic part of the cord are likely to be local distentions of the urachus. They are not incompatible with survival and occur with lesser degrees of torsion, as the urachus is much more compressible than the umbilical blood vessels.

Allantochorion. ***Premature Placental Separation.*** Premature placental separation may cause the death of full-term fetuses as a result of anoxia. In the more common type, the allantochorion bulges out of the vulva with the cervical star intact. An incomplete or complete tear occurs in the middle of the body of the allantochorion.[4,13,19] The fetus may be delivered through the tear. In another type of premature placental separation, the allantochorion detaches from the endometrium of the horns some time before the start of labor.[13] If such a placenta is examined soon after delivery, the detached areas can be distinguished because they are dry and brown. The causes of premature placental separation are unknown.

Body Pregnancy. Examination of the expelled placenta shows the proportion of the membranes corresponding to the two uterine horns to be small, suggesting the fetus largely occupied the uterine body, rather than the body and a horn. Growth of the fetus is retarded. Presumably, abortion occurs when the nutritional demands of the fetus can no longer be met. Body pregnancy is rare.[6,13]

Villous Atrophy or Hypoplasia. Although little opportunity for verification has been found, the chorionic surface seems to give a mirror-image impression of the endometrial surface with which it was in contact. Areas with no villi or with small villi should reflect areas with no or small endometrial glands, most likely because of scarring. Examination of one mare slaughtered after parturition has provided confirmation of the observation of the relationship of abnormal areas of chorion to areas of endometrial fibrosis and atrophy.[6] Additional less-direct or exact evidence includes the frequent association between extensive endometrial scarring in uterine biopsy specimens and a history of abortion in that individual in previous years.[20,21]

Developmental Anomalies

Many developmental anomalies have been reported in aborted fetuses,[1,6] and a detailed discussion appears in Chapter 71. Some may be incompatible with fetal life, others may be incidental to the cause of abortion. Autolysis hinders the cytogenetic study of aborted embryos and fetuses.[22] Many chromosomal defects likely cause embryonic death rather than abortion (see Chapter 30).

INFECTIOUS ABORTION

The main agents of infectious abortion are viruses, bacteria, and fungi, although mycoplasmas and protozoa also cause abortion.

Viruses

Equine Herpesvirus Type 1. Equine herpesvirus type 1 (EHV 1) is the single most important infectious cause of equine abortion. This virus is capable of causing respiratory, nervous, or fetal/perinatal disease.[23] Analysis of restriction fragments of viral DNA has shown respiratory and aborted fetal isolates of the virus to be distinctly different.[24,25] Considerable differences in biologic behavior exist and less than 20% homology is found between subtype 1 (the type associated with abortions and neurologic disease and a small proportion of respiratory tract infections) and subtype 2 (the type associated with the large proportion of respiratory tract infections).[26] A molecular epizootiologic study on viruses isolated between 1960 and 1982 in Kentucky showed that within subtype 1 relatively little genetic heterogeneity was found compared with the large number of cocirculating genetically distinct strains found for other herpesviruses.[27] However, in 1982, the situation changed; the predominant electrophoretotype of subtype 1 was displaced by a previously uncommon one.[28]

After respiratory infection with subtype 1, the virus infects vascular endothelium and blood leukocytes. A cell-associated viremia occurs and is possible even in mares with high levels of neutralizing antibody, showing that the transport mechanism is immunologically privileged. Transplacental migration of a virus-carrying cell is probably an accident and explains the great variability in time between infection and abortion, such as 14 to 120 days in one experiment.[29] The first event in the process of abortion appears to be a rapid separation of the placenta from the endometrium, with the fetus dying of suffocation; near-term fetuses may be born alive. Abortion occurs between 7 months gestation and term, with no maternal illness at the time.

The placenta may be normal or edematous. It may cover the fetus at the time of abortion or be shed later. Some or all of the following gross lesions may be seen in the fetus: subcutaneous edema, jaundice, increased fluid in the abdominal and thoracic cavities, and enlarged liver with a few 1-mm yellow-white areas (Fig. 64–3). Histologically, the characteristic lesion is small areas of necrosis with minimal inflammation and few to many large intranuclear eosinophilic inclusion bodies (Fig. 64–4). Fixation with formalin is adequate, but the inclusion bodies are more obvious if the tissues have been fixed in Bouin's fluid. Lymphoid tissues are the most commonly affected, including lymph nodes, spleen, thymus, and Peyer's patches. Mild multifocal necrotizing inflammation is often seen in the liver and adrenal cortex. In the lung, a hyperplastic necrotizing bronchiolitis is found. It is prudent to process a wide range of tissues for histopathology, because the microscopic lesions in an individual foal may involve most or only a few of the target tissues. No specific microscopic lesions are present in the placenta.

When the effectiveness of various commonly available diagnostic methods is compared, fluorescent antibody staining of fetal tissues is found to be the best method, followed closely by virus isolation, and then by the observation of viral inclusion bodies in liver, lung, and thymus.[30] Fetal serology has aided in the diagnosis of EHV 1 infection and is useful for those cases in which histologic lesions are not apparent and attempted virus isolation is unsuccessful.[31] Fetal response is likely to vary with antigen, but equine fetuses were found to be capable of producing antibody to the antigens of coliphage T2 at 200 days gestation.[32] Hybridization of cloned fragments of subtype 1 viral DNA to EHV 1 in tissues of aborted fetuses has been confirmed as specific, but it is less sensitive as a diagnostic method than classic techniques. The dot blot, however, has potential as a rapid diagnostic test.[33]

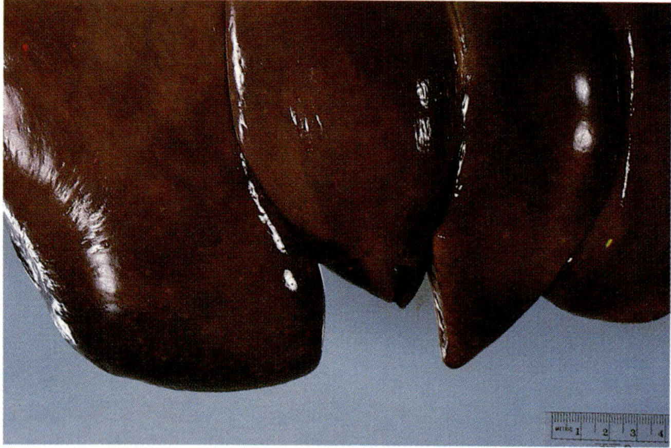

FIG. 64–3. Fetal liver with numerous 1-mm yellow-white areas of necrotizing hepatitis caused by EHV 1 infection. In most cases, the foci are much more difficult to observe. (From Acland, H.M.: Abortion in mares: diagnosis and prevention. Compend. Contin. Educ. Practicing Vet., *9*:318–326, 1987.)

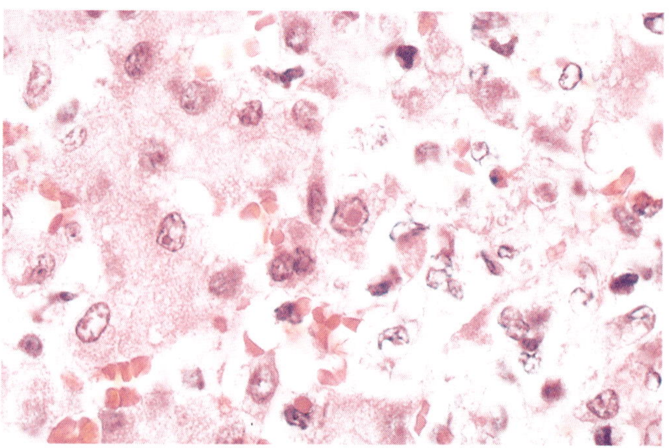

FIG. 64–4. Fetal liver with a large intranuclear eosinophilic inclusion body typical of EHV 1 infection. (From Acland, H.M.: Abortion in mares: diagnosis and prevention. Compend. Contin. Educ. Practicing Vet., *9*:318–326, 1987.)

Equine Viral Arteritis (EVA). In 1953, equine viral arteritis virus was recognized as a cause of illness and abortion in mares.[34] Inapparent to moderate clinical disease (fever, leukopenia, lacrimation, conjunctivitis, and nasal discharge) and generalized vascular necrosis were recorded in adult horses, with abortion occurring within a few days of the onset of clinical illness. Virus could be recovered from aborted fetuses, but vascular lesions were not observed. Experimental infection of mares produced acute multifocal myometritis, without arteritis in the uterus.[35] This work suggested that fetal death occurs because of anoxia secondary to compression of myometrial vessels by edema, with the additional effect of decreased progesterone production by the injured placenta.

Between 1953 and 1984 few reports were made of EVA outbreaks. In the 1984 outbreak in Kentucky, no unequivocally confirmed field occurrences of abortion were noted.[36] However, 10 of 14 mares aborted in a group involved in an investigation of the 1984 virus. Abortions occurred on postexposure days 23 to 57, and from 6 to 29 days after the onset of fever. The mares were infected by viral transmission either sexually or by contact. Two historically common features of the disease—edema in infected mares and autolytic changes in aborted fetuses—were not observed. No lesions were found in placentas or fetuses, apart from moderate arteritis in the myocardium of two fetuses.[37] In additional outbreaks of EVA confirmed since 1984, abortion did occur, although at a low incidence.[38]

Bacteria

A large number of bacterial species are capable of causing abortion in the mare.[7] Bacteria may be in the uterus at the time of conception, or ascend through the cervix in early pregnancy, or (uncommonly in the mare) arrive hematogenously. Ascending infections in late pregnancy are thought to be rare.

The responsible organisms are mostly residents of the posterior genital tract. Relaxation of the cervix at the time of secondary ovulations or vaginitis secondary to pneumovagina may precede the entry of organisms. Streptococcus sp. are the bacteria most frequently recovered from aborted fetuses. Other commonly encountered organisms are Escherichia coli, Pseudomonas, Klebsiella, and Staphylococcus sp. Taylorella equigenitalis, the cause of contagious equine metritis, a true venereal disease of the equine species, has been recovered from a few fetuses.[39] Placental and fetal lesions produced by the various bacterial species are not distinguishable from one another.

The ascending route, via the cervix, is the most common manner of infection, judging by the frequency with which inflammation of the allantochorion is most severe opposite the cervix. There the placenta is edematous and the chorionic surface is brown with a small amount of fibrinonecrotic exudate (Figs. 64–5 and 64–6). Fluid in the allantoic cavity may be cloudy, and the allantoamnion may become thick and opaque. Infection spreads to the fetus, and organisms can be recovered from many organs and consistently from the stomach.[40] Fetal gross lesions are nonspecific and may be no more than enlarged liver and increased fluid in body cavities. Abortion is caused by either fetal death from septicemia or by expansion of the area of chorionitis to the extent that placental insufficiency occurs.[6] Placental and fetal disease can be so low grade that the fetus is born alive, but ill.

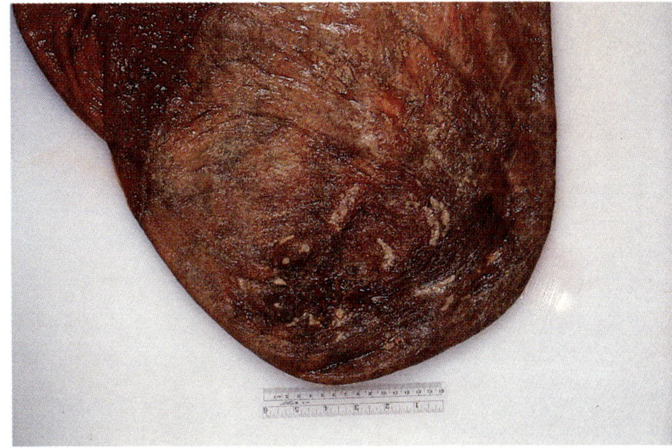

FIG. 64–6. Cervical star area of allantochorion from Figure 64–5. The membrane is brown and edematous and a small amount of fibrinonecrotic debris exists. (From Acland, H.M.: Abortion in mares: diagnosis and prevention. Compend. Contin. Educ. Practicing Vet., *9*:318–326, 1987.)

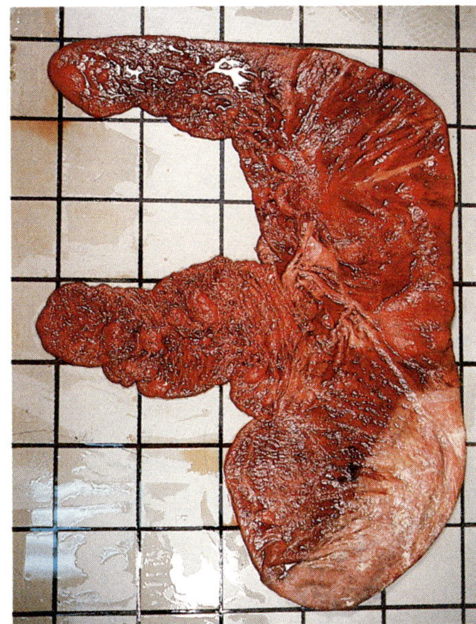

FIG. 64–5. Allantochorion of a fetus aborted following bacterial infection. Infection started opposite the cervix (at the bottom of the picture) and extended ventrad into the uterine body to produce the light brown discoloration of the chorion. (From Acland, H.M.: Abortion in mares: diagnosis and prevention. Compend. Contin. Educ. Practicing Vet., *9*: 318–326, 1987.)

Fungi

The pathogenesis of fungal disease, with inflammation of the chorion starting at the cervical pole, and the gross appearance of the placenta and fetus are similar to those in bacterial abortions. Microscopically, fungal hyphae are plentiful. Aspergillus is the most frequently encountered fungus.[41] It generally does not affect the amnion, whereas mucoraceous fungal infections sometimes cause amnionitis and fetal pulmonary granulomas.[40] Occasionally, fetal mycotic dermatitis occurs (Fig. 64–7). A feature of the normal placenta is small (1 to 2 mm) yellow nodules of hyperkeratosis on the amnionic (fetal) side of the allantoamnion near the cord and overlying major vessels and on the cord. The nodules should not be mistaken for fungal plaques.

PREVENTION OF ABORTION

Selection Against Mares Likely to Abort

The extensiveness and severity of endometrial periglandular fibrosis seen on uterine biopsy can be used to predict the incapability of a mare's uterus to carry a foal to term. Mares with widespread fibrosis commonly become detectably pregnant but lose the fetus before 90 days of pregnancy.[21]

Medical and Surgical Treatment of Abortion-Prone Mares

Progesterone, orally or parenterally, is administered in an attempt to prevent abortion. Once the placenta has

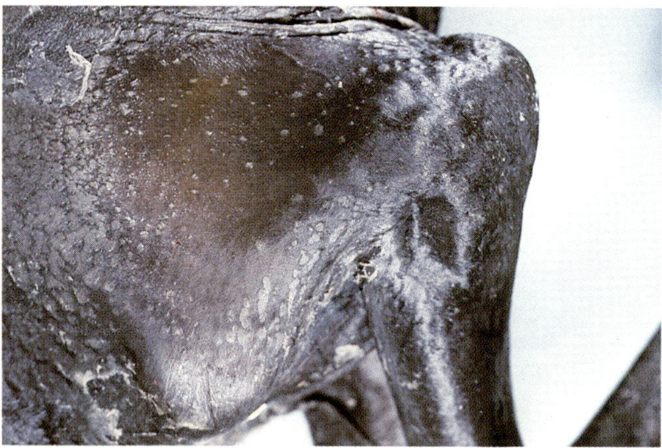

FIG. 64–7. Thorax of an aborted foal. Gray plaques of mycotic dermatitis are present, a rare occurrence in abortion caused by fungal infection. (From Acland, H.M.: Abortion in mares: diagnosis and prevention. Compend. Contin. Educ. Practicing Vet., *9*:318–326, 1987.)

taken over progesterone production from the ovary (around day 70 of gestation) exogenous supplementation is unlikely to be necessary.[8] Whether luteal inadequacy or poor placental progesterone production occurs is controversial.

Twin Abortion

The prevention and management of twin conceptions are considered in Chapter 62.

Bacterial and Fungal Abortion

Hygiene at breeding and parturtion are important to prevent entry of organisms into the uterus. Resolution of a postabortion endometritis should be achieved before rebreeding. A postbreeding Caslick procedure may help reduce vaginal contamination.

Equine Herpesvirus Type 1 Abortion

The respiratory tract is the portal of entry for all forms of EHV 1 infection—respiratory, abortigenic, and neurologic. Respiratory symptoms may be severe—as they often are in young horses—or mild—as they can be in horses of all ages. Clinical signs of respiratory disease caused by subtype 1 or subtype 2 of EHV 1 are indistinguishable from one another. Almost all subtype 2 infections are restricted to the respiratory tract and its lymph nodes, whereas subtype 1 infections involve the respiratory tract, vascular endothelium, and circulating blood leukocytes, which may transfer the virus to the uterus or central nervous system (CNS). The majority of epizootics of upper respiratory tract disease in young horses are caused by subtype 2, and therefore, pose little threat to pregnant mares. The few epizootics of respiratory disease caused by subtype 1 constitute emergencies that warrant the separation of affected animals from pregnant mares.[26] Using subtype specific monoclonal antibodies, enzyme immunofiltration and indirect immunofluorescence, EHV 1 can be subtyped within 3 h after virus isolation.[42]

Abortions that occur without an episode of respiratory disease in the preceding months are difficult to explain. Possibly, earlier respiratory disease did occur, but was subclinical or so mild that it escaped notice. Or possibly, activation of a latent infection occurred. In other species, herpesviruses are well known for setting up latent or persistent infection, yet little information exists on latent EHV 1 infection. Some evidence has been found that the phenomenon occurs in the horse. Reactivated subtype 1 virus has been recovered after immunosuppression by administration of corticosteroids.[43] Cells of the lymphoid system are likely to be the site of latency, rather than nerve ganglia as in herpesvirus infections in most other species.

Naturally acquired immunity after EHV 1 infection is short lived. It lasts only a few weeks or months, and then reinfection is possible. With repeated challenge, horses eventually develop resistance to diseases caused by EHV 1. Even though clinical signs may not recur on re-exposure, infection exists, along with the production and shedding of virus, and, in the case of subtype 1, leukocyte-associated viremia and the possibility of abortion.

In experimental infections, and probably in natural infections as well, initially little cross-protection between the two subtypes exists. After several spaced infections, some cross-protection develops.

Vaccination of horses is approached on the strategy of mimicking natural infection. A horse has numerous exposures over a lifetime, with brief protection after each. Immunity is gained as the result of repeated exposures.

A killed virus vaccine and an attenuated live virus vaccine are commercially available in the United States. The killed virus vaccine is marketed for the prevention of abortion in mares, and the manufacturer advises that it be given each year at 5, 7, and 9 months gestation. The live subtype 1 vaccine is currently labeled only for the prevention of the respiratory form of the disease but is being used to prevent abortion, by inoculating pregnant mares every 2 or 3 months throughout gestation.[2] Reports on the value of vaccination are conflicting. For instance, in one documented vaccination program, frequent booster doses of the killed vaccine was thought to keep abortion rates at a minimum level,[44] whereas in a trial in which pregnant mares were challenged with subtype 1 virus, the killed vaccine did not protect against abortion.[45] In Kentucky, in the first 4 yr after the use of the killed vaccine, the incidence of abortion caused by EHV 1 in vaccinated mares was 1.7/1000 compared with 2.9/1000 for the entire population.[26]

Management practices play a role in the reduction of disease caused by EHV 1. Stress should be avoided, by such means as dividing mares into foaling groups and dividing mares and foals into weaning groups. Newly arrived animals should never be mixed with pregnant mares on a farm.[16] The environment should be regarded as contaminated for 3 weeks after an infected animal has been present. On farms with multiple abortions, a common thread of overcrowding, frequent traffic in horses, and unsystematic vaccination records is seen.[27]

Equine Viral Arteritis Abortion

A mean of 30 to 35% of naturally infected stallions become persistently infected with the equine viral arteritis (EVA) virus and constantly shed the virus in their semen. Those carrier stallions probably play a major role in the perpetuation of the virus from year to year. Control of the disease revolves around the strategic vaccination of seronegative stallions, the treatment of carrier stallions by physical isolation, breeding only with immune mares, and isolation of the mares for 3 weeks.[38]

REFERENCES

1. Platt, H.: Aetiological Aspects of abortion in the Thoroughbred mare. J. Comp. Pathol., *83:*199–205, 1973.
2. Neely, D.P., Liu, I.K.M., and Hillman, R.B.: Equine Reproduction. Veterinary Learning Systems, 1983.
3. Mahaffey, L.W.: Abortion in mares. Vet. Rec., *82:* 681–687, 1968.
4. Prickett, M.E.: Abortion and placental lesions in the mare. J. Am. Vet. Med. Assoc., *157:*1465–1470, 1970.
5. Rossdale, P.D., and Ricketts, S.W.: Equine abortion. Vet. Ann., *16:*133–141, 1976.
6. Whitwell, K.E.: Investigations into fetal and neonatal losses in the horse. Vet. Clin. North Am. Large Anim. Pract. Equine Reprod., *2:*213–331, 1980.
7. Roberts, S.J.: Veterinary Obstetrics and Genital Diseases (Theriogenology). 3rd ed. Woodstock, VT, published by the author, 1986.
8. Hyland, J., and Jeffcott, L.B.: Abortion. *In* Current Therapy in Equine Medicine 2. Edited by N.E. Robinson. Philadelphia, W.B. Saunders, 1987, pp. 520–525.
9. Asbury, A.C.: Abortion in mares. *In* The Mare and Foal: Proceedings of the Ninth Bain-Fallon Memorial Lectures. Edited by P. Huntington and N.S.W. Artarmon. Syndney, Australian Equine Veterinary Association, 1987, pp. 117–120.
10. Bain A.M.: Foetal losses during pregnancy in the Thoroughbred mare: A record of 2,562 pregnancies. N. Z. Vet. J., *17:*155–158, 1969.
11. Bergin, W.C., Gier, H.T., Frey, R.A., and Marion G.B.: Developmental horizons and measurements useful for age determination of equine embryos and fetuses. Proc. Am. Assoc. Equine Pract., 179–196, 1967.
12. Whitwell, K.E., and Jeffcott, L.B.: Morphological studies on the fetal membranes of the normal singleton foal at term. Res. Vet. Sci., *19:*44–55, 1975.
13. Rooney, J.R.: Autopsy of the Horse. Baltimore, Williams & Wilkins, 1970.
14. Simpson, C.F., and Buergelt, C.D.: Congealed amnionic fluid in the alveoli of lungs of aborted foals. Equine Vet. J., *13:*109–111, 1981.
15. Dimock, W.W., Edwards, R.P., and Bruner, D.W.: Infections observed in equine fetuses and foals. Cornell Vet., *37:*89–99, 1974.
16. Bryans, J.T.: Application of management procedures and prophylactic immunization to the control of equine rhinopneumonitis. Proc. Am. Assoc. Equine Pract., 259–272, 1980.
17. Jeffcott, L.B., and Whitwell, K.E.: Twinning as a cause of foetal and neonatal loss in the Thoroughbred mare. J. Comp. Pathol., *83:*91–106, 1973.
18. Whitwell, K.E.: Morphology and pathology of the equine umbilical cord. J. Reprod. Fertil. Suppl., *23:*599–603, 1975.
19. Franco, O.J.: Gross lesions as an aid in the diagnosis of equine abortions. Proc. Am. Assoc. Equine Pract., 257–261, 1976.
20. Doig, P.A., McKnight, J.D., and Miller, R.B.: The use of endometrial biopsy in the infertile mare. Can. Vet. J., *22:*72–76, 1981.
21. Kenney, R.M.: Cyclic and pathologic changes of the mare endometrium as detected by biopsy, with a note on early embryonic death. J. Am. Vet. Med. Assoc., *172:*241–262, 1978.
22. Blue, M.D.: A cytogenetical study of prenatal loss in the mare. Theriogenology, *15:*295–305, 1981.
23. Campbell, T.M., and Studdert, M.J.: Equine Herpesvirus type 1 (EHV1). Vet. Bull., *53:*135–146, 1983.
24. Studdert, M.J., Simpson, T., and Roizman B.: Differentiation of respiratory and abortigenic isolates of equine herpesvirus 1 by restriction endonucleases. Science, *214:*562–564, 1981.
25. Turtinen, L.W., Allen, G.P., Darlington, R.W., and Bryans, J.T.: Serologic and molecular comparisons of several equine herpesvirus type 1 strains. Am. J. Vet. Res., *42:*2099–2104, 1981.
26. Allen, G.P., and Bryans, J.T.: Molecular epizootiology, pathogenesis, and prophylaxis of equine herpesvirus-1 infections. Prog. Vet. Microbiol. Immunol. *2:*78–144, 1986.
27. Allen, G.P., et al.: Molecular epizootiologic studies of equine herpesvirus-1 infections by restriction endonuclease fingerprinting of viral DNA. Am. J. Vet. Res., *44:*263–271, 1983.
28. Allen, G.P., Yeargan, M.R., Turtinen, L.W., and Bryans, J.T.: A new field strain of equine abortion virus (equine herpesvirus-1) among Kentucky horses. Am. J. Vet. Res., *46:*138–140, 1985.
29. Doll, E.R., and Bryans, J.T.: Incubation periods for abortion in equine viral rhinopneumonitis. J. Am. Vet. Med. Assoc., *141:*351–354, 1962.
30. Whitwell, K.E.: An assessment of the criteria used to diagnose virus abortion: A review of 100 cases. J. Reprod. Fertil. Suppl., *32:*632–633, 1982.
31. Crandell, R.A., and Angulo, A.B.: Equine herpesvirus-1 antibodies in stillborn foals and weak neonates. Vet. Med., *80:*73–75, 1985.
32. Martin, B.R., and Larson, K.A.: Immune response of equine fetus to coliphage T2. Am. J. Vet. Res., *34:*1363–1364, 1973.
33. Morris, C.M., and Field, H.J.: Application of cloned fragments of equine herpesvirus type-1 DNA for detection of virus-specific DNA in equine tissues. Equine Vet. J., *20:*335–340, 1988.
34. Doll, E.R., Bryans, J.T., McCollum, W.H., and Crowe M.E.W.: Isolation of a filterable agent causing arteritis of horses and abortion by mares. Its differentiation from the equine abortion (influenza) virus. Cornell Vet., *47:*3–41, 1975.
35. Coignoul, F.L., and Cheville, N.F.: Pathology of maternal genital tract, placenta, and fetus in equine viral arteritis. Vet. Pathol., *21:*333–340, 1984.
36. Timoney, P.J., and McCollum, W.H.: The epidemiology of equine viral arteritis. Proc. Am. Assoc. Equine Pract., 545–551, 1986.
37. Cole, J.R., et al.: Transmissibility and abortigenic effect of equine viral arteritis in mares. J. Am. Vet. Med. Assoc., *189:*769–771, 1986.

38. Timoney, P.J., and McCollum, W.H.: Equine viral arteritis. Can. Vet. J., *28:*693–695, 1987.

39. Nakashiro, H., et al.: Isolation of Haemophilus equigenitalis form an aborted equine fetus. Natl. Inst. Anim. Health Q. Jpn., *21:*184–185, 1981.

40. Platt, H.: Infection of the horse fetus. J. Reprod. Fertil. Suppl., *23:*605–610, 1975.

41. Mahaffey, L.W., and Adam, N.M.: Abortions associated with mycotic lesions of the placenta in mares. J. Am. Vet. Med. Assoc., *144:*24–32, 1964.

42. Yeargan, M.R., Allen, G.P., and Bryans, J.T.: Rapid subtyping of equine herpesvirus 1 with monoclonal antibodies. J. Clin. Microbiol., *21:*694–697, 1985.

43. Edington, N., Bridges, C.G., and Huckle, A.: Experimental reactivation of equid herpesvirus 1(EHV 1) following the administration of corticosteroids. Equine Vet. J., *17:*369–372, 1985.

44. Burki, F.: Equine rhinopneumonitis—An unsettled problem. J. Equine Vet. Sci., *8:*65–69, 1988.

45. Burrows, R., Goodridge, D., and Denyer, M.S.: Trials of an inactivated equid herpesvirus 1 vaccine: Challenge with a subtype 1 virus. Vet. Rec., *114:*369–374, 1984.

CHAPTER 65

INDUCTION OF ABORTION DURING EARLY TO MID GESTATION

E.L. Squires
W.T.K. Bosu

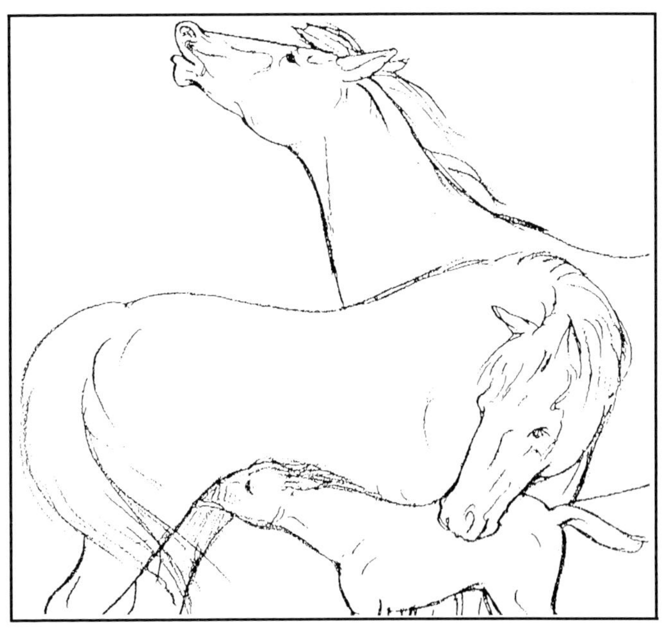

Veterinarians and/or breeders are often requested to induce abortion in mares during the first trimester of gestation. Abortion is generally performed on mares that are mismated, purchased as open mares and later found to be in foal, involved in a change of ownership or function, or used for teaching and research purposes. In addition, twin pregnancies that are diagnosed after day 35 are generally aborted. This chapter reviews induction of abortion during early and midpregnancy.

Continual secretion of progesterone from corpora lutea (CL) on the ovary is paramount for maintenance of pregnancy.[1] Thus lowering progesterone levels is one sure way of inducing abortion. Ovariectomy has been used as a research tool to determine at what stage of pregnancy ovaries of the pregnant mare are no longer required for pregnancy maintenance.[2] A total of 50 mares were bilaterally ovariectomized at selected days between 25 and 210 days of gestation. Abortion or resorption of the conceptus occurred in all 14 mares ovariectomized before day 50 of gestation. Of 20 mares ovariectomized between 50 and 70 days, 11 maintained pregnancy, and pregnancy was not interrupted in any of 12 mares ovariectomized on day 140 or 210. Shideler et al. ovariectomized mares on days 34 or 35 of gestation and gave various regimens of exogenous progestagens.[3] However, the control group received no progesterone; all 8 control mares aborted in a mean of 4.5 days. In a subsequent study pregnancies were established in ovariectomized–progestin-treated mares by way of embryo transfer.[4] The dose of progesterone was slowly decreased from day 35 to day 50. Pregnancy losses occurred once concentrations of progesterone decreased below 2.5 ng/mL of blood. Ovariectomy, however, would not be a practical way of inducing abortion; thus, the most common means of decreasing concentrations of progesterone in early gestation and inducing abortion is the administration of prostaglandins $F_2\alpha$ or a $PGF_2\alpha$ analogue.

INDUCTION OF ABORTION WITH PROSTAGLANDINS

No reliable method of preventing pregnancy is available for use within the first 5 days after ovulation. The developing CL is refractory to lysis by prostaglandins for approximately 5 days after ovulation.[5] Uterine lavage during the first 5 days after ovulation is also ineffective in interrupting pregnancy because the embryo is still in the oviduct.[6] However, between day 5 and before formation of endometrial cups and secretion of equine chorionic gonadotropin (eCG) at days 38 to 40,[7] a single injection of $PGF_2\alpha$ or $PGF_2\alpha$ analogue has been shown to efectively induce abortion.[8–10] Treatment of pregnant mares with a single injection of 1.25 mg $PGF_2\alpha$ on day 32 resulted in termination of pregnancy in each of four mares.[8] In another study, a $PGF_2\alpha$ analogue (Equimate) was given to eight pregnant mares on day 35 of gestation.[9] About 3 to 4 days after a single injection, seven of eight mares aborted. Prostaglandins and an analogue of $PGF_2\alpha$ (Luprostiol) were both highly effective (15 of

16 and 17 of 17) in inducing abortion in mares at 30 to 35 days of gestation.[10] In a group of mares at 26 to 31 days of gestation, 5 mg prostaglandin given on two consecutive days caused abortion and estrus 3 to 5 days after abortion.[11] Abortion of twin pregnancies before day 35 with a single injection of $PGF_2\alpha$ has also been reported.[12] Thus, if a mare is mismated, the simplest procedure is to administer a single injection of $PGF_2\alpha$ after the CL is fully formed, at least 5 days after ovulation.

Because twinning is one of the leading causes of spontaneous abortion, the veterinarian is faced with how to selectively eliminate one conceptus without affecting the viability of the second conceptus. One common method for elimination of twin conceptuses is "crushing" the fetoplacental unit. Studies have shown that crushing of one twin between 16 to 22 days results in one viable conceptus in 95% of the cases.[13] However, if crushing a twin is delayed until more than 30 days, the success of eliminating only one conceptus is 50% or less.

Even though reduction of twins to a singleton by manual crushing is less successful after day 30, an attempt at crushing may still be made, and in those cases where twin reductions are not successful, $PGF_2\alpha$ can be given to induce abortion. Unfortunately, a single injection of $PGF_2\alpha$ will result in loss of both conceptuses and thus cannot be used to selectively eliminate only one twin.

If an equine conceptus is crushed or removed by physical means after the signal for maternal recognition of pregnancy,[14] the CL will often be retained for 10 to 90 days causing a delay in return to estrus. Uterine and cervical tone in mares with retained CL are similar to that of pregnancy. Suggested treatment consists of a single injection of $PGF_2\alpha$ or $PGF_2\alpha$ analogue. A normal luteolytic dose should cause the onset of estrus in 4 to 5 days after treatment.[15] Fertility during the estrus after abortion of mares between days 5 to 35 of gestation is similar to that of untreated, normally cycling mares.

Multiple injections of $PGF_2\alpha$ or $PGF_2\alpha$ analogues are usually required to abort a mare once the endometrial cups have formed. Endometrial cups are formed between days 38 to 40 and eCG is secreted until days 110 to 120.[16] Douglas et al. evaluated various $PGF_2\alpha$ treatments for inducing abortion in pony mares at 40 to 150 days of gestation.[17] A single injection of 0, 1.25, or 2.50 mg $PGF_2\alpha$ terminated pregnancy in 0 of 7, 3 of 7, and 4 of 8 mares, respectively. Incidence of abortion was not related to stage of gestation. Twice daily injections (12-h intervals) of 2.50 mg $PGF_2\alpha$ resulted in 13 of 13 mares aborting after an average of 3.7 injections. Mean interval from first injection to abortion was 39 h. Mares that were 80 to 90 days pregnant tended to have a shorter interval from abortion to estrus and ovulation compared with those beyond 160 days of gestation. The effectiveness of Equimate for induction of abortion in light horse mares when given before and after the appearance of eCG was examined.[9] A total of 32 mares was assigned to one of four treatments: (1) injected with 250 μg of Equimate on day 70 and again on day 77 if abortion had not occurred, (2) injected with 250 μg Equimate on day 70 and every 24 h or (3) every 12 h until abortion occurred, and (4) injected with 250 μg Equimate once only on day 35 of gestation. Mares were observed four times daily for incidence of abortion and side effects. Estrous behavior and follicular activity were monitored after abortion. A single injection of Equimate terminated pregnancy in all but 1 mare injected on day 35, but none of the mares given an injection on days 70 and 77 aborted. In contrast, multiple injections of Equimate beginning on day 70 terminated pregnancy in all mares. Fewer injections to abortion were required for mares given daily treatments (3.6) than those treated twice daily (7.4). Concentrations of progesterone decreased in all mares injected with $PGF_2\alpha$ analogue, but concentrations were greater ($p < 0.05$) for mares injected once on day 70 than for those in the other three groups. Thus multiple injections of $PGF_2\alpha$ analogue will cause CL regression. However, Equimate did not affect secretion of eCG in the day-70 groups.

Rothwell et al. reported no effect of daily injections of $PGF_2\alpha$ on function of endometrial cups and secretion of eCG.[18] Because of continued high levels of eCG after abortion, estrus and ovulation are delayed. It remains unclear as to how eCG can be stimulatory to the ovary during pregnancy and subsequently inhibit follicular development after abortion. The interval from abortion to first day of estrus and ovulation was less for mares injected with Equimate once on day 35 than for those injected either daily or twice daily beginning on day 70. None of the estrous periods immediately after abortion were anovulatory for mares treated on day 35, whereas 6 of 8 mares in each of the day-70 groups exhibited at least one anovulatory estrus before estrus accompanied by ovulation. Intervals to estrus and ovulation after abortion at day 70 were approximately 40 and 50 days, respectively.[9] Thus follicular development appears to be suppressed until endometrial cups are sloughed from the uterus at days 110 to 120 of gestation and eCG levels are low. Therefore, if mares abort late in the breeding season and are ≥ 35 days of gestation, rebreeding in the same season may be difficult. Currently no treatment for hastening disappearance of endometrial cups is available.

Two subsequent studies were conducted to evaluate the effect of stage of gestation and frequency of injection on induction of abortion with $PGF_2\alpha$ or $PGF_2\alpha$ analogue.[10] In the first study, mares were assigned to 1 of 3 groups: (1) control, 1 mL propylene glycol (vehicle) IM; (2) 7.5 mg Luprostiol, IM; and (3) 7.5 mg $PGF_2\alpha$ IM. Mares were treated on days 30 to 35 and pregnancy was monitored daily with ultrasonography for 2 weeks or until fetal expulsion/resorption. Within 4 to 5 days of injection, 4 of 15, 17 of 17, and 15 of 16 mares aborted, respectively. Mares in the second study were given a single injection or 3 daily injections of Luprostiol beginning on day 50 of gestation. The number of mares aborting was similar for each group—7 of 10 and 10 of 10, respectively. Based on several studies, the response to a single injection of Luprostiol appeared to be more variable if given after day 35 of gestation (Table 65–1).

Induction of abortion with prostaglandins after eCG has not been adequately studied. In one study, mares were given 2.5 mg $PGF_2\alpha$ at 12-h intervals during days 160 to 180 (n = 3) and > 300 days (n = 7).[17] All mares aborted after three to four injections, and the interval from first injection to abortion averaged 41 and 33 h, respectively. No significant differences were found in the mean number of injections given before abortion occurred or the mean interval from injection to abortion among three stages of gestation (80 to 90, 160 to 180, or > 300 days). However, the interval from abortion to estrus and ovulation did appear to be shorter for mares that were 80 to 90 days pregnant than for those 160 to 180 or > 300 days pregnant. In a clinical trial, mares on day 100 to 245 of gestation were treated daily with $PGF_2\alpha$ (1 mg/45 kg) until abortion occurred. The percentages of mares aborting during weeks 1, 2, 3, and 4 of treatment were 75%, 12%, 4%, and 8%, respectively.[19]

OTHER METHODS OF ABORTION

During the period when endometrial cups are functional (days 40 to 120), pregnancy may also be terminated by intrauterine infusion of large volumes of saline (1 to 2 L). However, we prefer to administer three to four daily injections of prostaglandins, and then if mares do not abort, the cervix is penetrated and saline infused. If abortion has not occurred within 24 h of uterine infusion, the infusion process is repeated. It is recommended that, if the cervix is penetrated for infusion of saline, antibiotics should be added to the flushing medium or the uterus irrigated with a saline-iodine solution. Pretreatment with 10 mg estradiol, 24 h before flushing, may facilitate and hasten abortion by causing cervical relaxation.[15] Even though infusion of saline can be used to induce abortion, eCG production and function of the endometrial cups remain unaltered. Thus, the time to estrus and ovulation after abortion is delayed and similar to that of $PGF_2\alpha$-induced abortions. Lofstedt reported that flushing the uterus for induction of abortion before day 80 results in fluid separating the microvilli from the endometrium, whereas after day 80, the allantochorion is ruptured and the fetus is gently removed by traction.[15] The placenta will usually be readily expelled because placental attachment is not well developed. If the allantochorion is merely ruptured and the fetus is not withdrawn, abortion usually occurs in 2 to 7 days.[15] A variation of intra-allantoic infusions for termination of pregnancy during midgestation involves single infusions of dexamethasone solution. Infusion of 15 mL of an aqueous solution containing 30 mg dexamethasone terminated pregnancy in four mares that were at days 167 to 174. Paccamonti stated that uterine infusions terminated pregnancies either directly through embryotoxic effects or indirectly by stimulating release of prostaglandins.[20]

Other methods for induction of abortion, that have limited applicability, include injection of colchicine[8] or potassium chloride[21] into the conceptus. A needle is guided, using ultrasonography, into the heart. Repeated injections of human chorionic gonadotropin (hCG)[22] or estrogens have also been shown to cause abortion.[15]

TABLE 65–1. RESPONSE OF MARES TO $PGF_2\alpha$ OR $PGF_2\alpha$ ANALOGUE FOR INDUCTION OF ABORTION

REFERENCE NUMBER	INJECTION TREATMENT	DAY OF PREGNANCY	NUMBER OF MARES		INTERVAL (DAYS)	
			Treated	Aborted	Abortion	Estrus
8	Single 1.25 mg $PGF_2\alpha$	32	4	7	2–5	—
9	Single 250 μg Equimate	35	8	7	3.7	11.2
10	Single 7.5 mg Luprostiol	30–35	17	17	4.2	—
10	Single 7.5 mg $PGF_2\alpha$	30–35	15	16	4.7	—
17	Single 1.25 or 2.5 mg $PGF_2\alpha$	40–60	6	4	10	—
10	Single 7.5 mg Luprostiol	50	10	7	2.6	—
10	3 consecutive days 7.5 mg Luprostiol	50	10	10	2.4	—
9	Single 250 μg Equimate	70	8	0	—	—
9	250 μg Equimate every 24 h	70	8	8	3.6	45
9	250 μg Equimate every 12 h	70	8	8	7.4	36
17	Single 1.25 mg $PGF_2\alpha$	70–90	4	2	14	—
17	Single 2.5 mg $PGF_2\alpha$	100–150	5	1	3	—
17	2.5 mg $PGF_2\alpha$ every 12 h	80–90	2	2	2.3	2
17	2.5 mg $PGF_2\alpha$ every 12 h	160–180	3	3	1.7	25
		> 300	7	7	4.2	—

Three injections of 2000 IU hCG on alternate days beginning before day 39 resulted in four of four abortions, whereas treatment started on days 40 to 97 had no effect on pregnancy. The mechanism of hCG-induced abortion is unknown, but eCG may have a protective effect such that repeated injections of hCG will not result in abortion once eCG is secreted. Further studies are needed to determine the efficacy of other hormones for induction of abortion besides $PGF_2\alpha$. Although estrogens have been suggested as a method of inducing abortion in early gestation, documented controlled studies are lacking.

REFERENCES

1. Squires, E.L., Douglas, R.H., Steffenhagen, W.P., and Ginther, O.J.: Ovarian changes during the estrous cycle and pregnancy in mares. J. Anim. Sci., *38:*330–338, 1974.
2. Holtan, D.W., Squires, E.L., Lapin, D.R., and Ginther, O.J.: Effect of ovariectomy on pregnancy in mares. J. Reprod. Fertil. Suppl., *27:*456–463, 1979.
3. Shideler, R.K., et al.: Progestagen therapy of ovariectomized pregnant mares. J. Reprod. Fertil. Suppl., *32:*459–464, 1982.
4. McKinnon, A.O., Squires, E.L., Carnevale, E.M., and Hermenet, M.J.: Ovariectomized steroid-treated mares as embryo transfer recipients and as model to study the role of progestins in pregnancy maintenance. Theriogenology, *29:*1055–1063, 1988.
5. Douglas, R.H., and Ginther, O.J.: Effect of prostaglandin $F_2\alpha$ in ewes and pony mares. J. Anim. Sci., *37:*308–312, 1973.
6. Squires, E.L., Cook, V.M., and Voss, J.L.: Collection and transfer of equine embryos. Colorado State University, Animal Reproduction Laboratory Bulletin No. 01. 1985, pp. 12–15.
7. Allen, W.R.: The immunological measurement of pregnant mare serum gonadotropin. J. Endocrinol., *43:*593–598, 1969.
8. Kooistra, L., and Ginther, O.J.: Termination of pseudopregnancy by administration of $PGF_2\alpha$ and termination of early pregnancy by administration of $PGF_2\alpha$ or colchicine or by removal of embryo in mare. Am. J. Vet. Res., *37:*35–39, 1976.
9. Squires, E.L., Hillman, R.B., Pickett, B.W., and Nett, T.M.: Induction of abortion in mares with Equimate: Effect on secretion of progesterone, PMSG and reproductive performance. J. Anim. Sci., *50:*490–495, 1980.
10. Baucus, K.L., Squires, E.L., Morris, R., McKinnon, A.O.: The effect of stage of gestation and frequency of prostaglandin injection on induction of abortion in mares. Proc. Equine Nutr. Phys. Soc., 255–258, 1987.
11. Penzhorn, B.L., Bertschinger, H.J., and Coubrough, R.I.: Reconception of mares following termination of pregnancy with prostaglandin $F_2\alpha$ before and after day 35 of pregnancy. Equine Vet. J., *18:*215–217, 1986.
12. Squires, E.L., and McKinnon, A.O.: Management of twins and early embryonic death. Proc. N. Z. Vet. Assoc. Contin. Educ. Short Course, 36–53, 1987.
13. Pascoe, D.R., et al.: Comparison of two techniques and three hormone therapies for management of twin conceptuses by manual embryonic reduction. J. Reprod. Fertil. Suppl., *35:*701–702, 1975.
14. Hershman, L., and Douglas, R.H.: The critical period for maternal recognition of pregnancy in pony mares. J. Reprod. Fertil. Suppl., *27:*395–401, 1979.
15. Lofstedt, R.M.: Termination of unwanted pregnancy in the mare. *In* Current Therapy in Theriogenology. 2nd ed. Edited by D.A. Morrow. Philadelphia, W.B. Saunders, 1986, pp. 715–718.
16. Allen, W.R., and Moor, R.M.: The origin of the equine endometrial cups. I. Production of PMSG by fetal trophoblast cells. J. Reprod. Fertil., *29:*313–316, 1972.
17. Douglas, R.H., Squires, E.L., and Ginther, O.J.: Induction of abortion in mares with prostaglandin $F_2\alpha$. J. Anim. Sci., *39:*404–407, 1974.
18. Rothwell, A.C., Asbury, A.C., Hansen, P.J., and Archbald, L.F.: Reproductive function of mares given PGF-2α daily from Day 42 of pregnancy. J. Reprod. Fertil. Suppl., *35:*507–508, 1987.
19. Ginther, O.J.: Reproductive Biology of the Mare: Basic and Applied Aspects. Cross Plaines, WI, Equiservices, 1979.
20. Paccamonti, D.L.: Elective termination of pregnancy in mares. J. Am. Vet. Med. Assoc., *198:*683–689, 1991.
21. Rantanen, N.W., and Kincaid, B.: Ultrasound guided fetal cardiac puncture: A method of twin reduction in the mare. Proc. Am. Assoc. Equine Pract., 173–180, 1988.
22. Allen, W.E.: Pregnancy failure induced by human chorionic gonadotropin in pony mares. Vet. Rec., *96:*88–90, 1975.

CHAPTER 66

PARTURITION

C.E. Card
R.B. Hillman

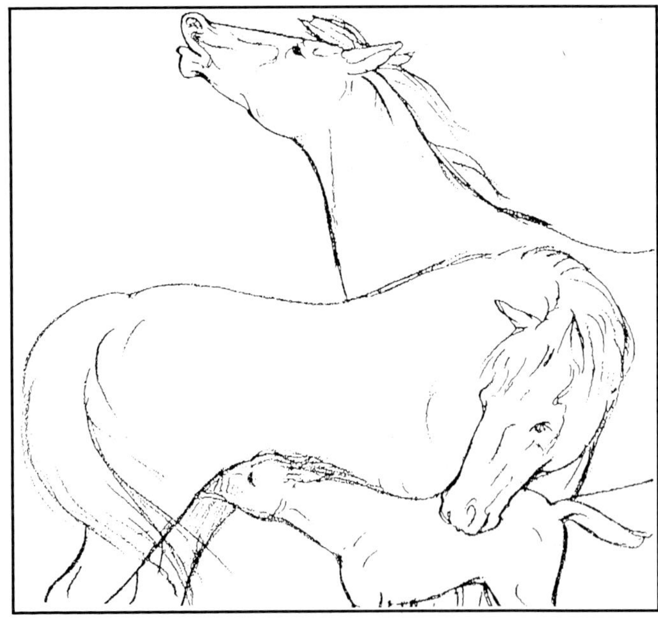

Parturition is a unique physiologic process that terminates pregnancy and begins the extrauterine existence of the foal. Relatively little is known about preparation of the fetus for independent life, the process of preparation of the mare for labor, the hormonal interplay between mother and fetus, and changes in the uterus which ready and finally activate the myometrium to initiate labor.

PREPARATION OF FETUS FOR INDEPENDENT LIFE: PHYSIOLOGIC PREPARATION OF THE EQUINE FETUS

Survival of the neonate is related to terminal developmental events in utero. In preparation for birth, the fetal musculoskeletal, cardiovascular, nervous, respiratory, digestive, and endocrine systems mature. Regular fetal motion is necessary for normal musculoskeletal development and prepares the fetus to attain actively the correct posture and position during labor. The regulation of fetal cardiovascular function is complex and involves the autonomic nervous system. This is evident in late gestation when the fetal heart rate accelerates in response to exercise. At birth, the fetal pattern of circulation changes and the neonatal pattern begins. The respiratory and digestive systems become activated. Prepartum hormonal signals, such as increased cortisol secretion are probably involved in the final stages of lung and intestinal maturation.

Clinical evaluation of the health and preparedness of the fetus for birth is difficult. However, ultrasonographically the fetal heart may be seen and this provides useful information about normal fetal cardiac function.

Prepartum, the normal mean fetal heart rate is around 76 ± 18 beats per minute. Fetal activity is reflected in heart rate accelerations from 25 to 40 beats per minute and 23 to 36 s in duration. Fetal heart rate accelerations are frequent (10 accelerations in a 10-min period).[1] Fetuses with heart rates or patterns markedly divergent from this may be compromised. Fetal activity is greatest at 5 to 72 h before parturition. In Stage I and Stage II of delivery the fetal heart rate (54 to 60 beats per min) is similar to the fetal heart rate (62 beats per min) the day before delivery.[2] During oxytocin-induced parturition in mares, vigorous labor is associated with increases in fetal heart rate.[1] Presumably, intense uterine contractions may be related to the increase in fetal heart rate. The heart rate of the normal newborn rises rapidly to >100 beats per minute.

Ultrasonographically, prepartum changes are evident in fetal fluids. Echogenic particles increase in density and number in most mares 10 days before delivery, but aging changes are not detectable in the placenta before delivery as reported in other species.[1]

In summary, antepartum periods of fetal rest and activity are normal, and fetal activity produces fetal heart rate accelerations. During spontaneous labor and delivery, mean fetal heart rate is unchanged. A possible causal relationship exists between myometrial contractions and fetal heart rate. A prepartum increase in echogenic particulate density and number is normal.

Hematologic assessment of the foal is performed as a diagnostic aid when prematurity is suspected. Recent hematologic studies performed on fetuses and the newborn have revealed indexes for assessing fetal maturation.[3,4] The red blood cell (RBC) count, packed cell volume (PCV), hemoglobin content (HBG), and erythrocyte size (MCV) at birth are indicative of fetal maturity. The normal term values are RBC count, 11.9 ± 0.3 ($\times 10^{12}$/L); PCV, 0.42 ± 0.0 (L/L); HBG, 14.2 ± 0.2 (g/dL); MCV, 35.0 ± 1.0 (fL).[3] The white blood cell (WBC) count and the neutrophil to lymphocyte ratio also give an indication of the foal's readiness for birth and can be used as a diagnostic aid to predict its chance of survival. The normal WBC count is 7.8 ± 0.3 ($\times 10^9$/L). The neutrophil to lymphocyte ratio of healthy spontaneously delivered foals is >2.5 at birth and will continue to rise for up to 24 h. The increase is primarily the result of a neutrophilia[3] and may be related to adrenal cortical activity. A neutrophil to lymphocyte ratio of <1 indicates immaturity and a grave prognosis for foal survival. Fetal RBC are smaller and have a higher oxygen carrying capacity than foal RBC. Transition to the neonatal red cell begins before delivery.[3]

PREPARATION OF THE MARE FOR LABOR

PHYSIOLOGIC ADAPTATIONS BEFORE PARTURITION

The most reliable indicators of approaching delivery are changes in mammary size and secretion.[5,6] Udder growth begins around 1 month before parturition, with the major increase in size occurring during the last 2 weeks.[5] The changes in the volume of mammary secretion and the character of the secretion occur gradually. Twice a day observation and palpation of the udder will reveal mammary engorgement 24 to 48 h before foaling.[7] Distention of the teats with colostrum usually occurs 24 to 48 h before foaling.[7] Waxing is observed in many mares within 24 h of foaling, but may occur 1 to 2 weeks before parturition or not at all.[5,8,9] Mares may leak milk a week or more before foaling,[5] and colostrum may need to be harvested and kept frozen if this leakage is excessive. The parity of the mare will influence the size of the udder and the amount of secretion present; maiden mares may foal with minimal mammary changes.[7]

Prefoaling mammary secretions may be used to help predict the time of foaling.[8,10–14] Mammary secretion changes are variable but typically change from a honey-like clear fluid to a gray, or straw-colored thin, milk-like fluid near parturition and finally to a thick, white milk (colostrum).[8] Changes occur in the concentrations of ions in the mammary secretion as foaling approaches. A variety of commercial kits are available which detect changes in the calcium and/or magnesium ions in the secretion.[11,14–16] Magnesium ion concentrations begin increasing (12 days prepartum) in milk first with calcium ion concentrations rising steeply over the last 3 to 4 days before parturition.[8] Calcium ion concentrations in a large proportion of mares spontaneously foaling typically exceed 10 mmol/L.

Studies comparing commercially available test kits found these tests easy to perform and adaptable for on-the-farm use.[10,14] Test results varied both within and between mares, as well as between tests. Approximately 10% of mares did not foal for 2 or 3 days after the readiness point was achieved with several mares maintaining a maximum score for 5 to 16 days.[10,14] Some mares (6 to 27%) never reached a readiness score before foaling.[10,14] The authors concluded that these kits are most useful in determining when mares do not need to be attended overnight, rather than predicting the exact day of foaling. The total calcium ion concentration in mammary secretions is useful in predicting foal survival before induction and, therefore, may be useful as a clinical aid in differentiating mares that have short gestational durations from mares in premature labor.[11,12]

Late in pregnancy, the sacrosciatic ligaments relax, and obvious sinking alongside the tail head and palpable softening may be noted.[5,6] Visible relaxation was observed in only 12 of 22 foaling mares over 3 days before delivery, indicating the necessity of palpating these ligaments to detect the softening.[9] These changes may be more obvious in older mares. The elongation, swelling, and relaxation of the vulva are subtle in the mare; the most obvious changes occur a few hours before birth.[5,17] A slight amount of blood-tinged mucus may be seen in some mares associated with cervical dilation, but it is uncommon.[5]

A circadian variation in core body temperature has been reported in spontaneously foaling mares.[9] Peak temperatures are recorded in the evening (3:00 to 11:00 p.m.); the lowest temperatures are recorded in the morning (7:00 a.m.). Some authors report a significant decline in mares' evening temperatures as indicative of imminent parturition,[9,18] whereas other authors failed to detect significant temperature changes before foaling.[19] Foaling mares spend significantly more time lying down and walking on the evening of parturition.[18]

GESTATIONAL DURATION

The duration of normal pregnancy is variable but averages 335 to 342 days.[7] Extremes of gestation ranging from 305 days to more than 400 days have been reported with normal foals being born.[20–22] Mares foaling in winter or early spring have gestational durations that are around 10 days longer than summer-foaling mares.[23] Increasing the photoperiod of pregnant mares to 16 h of daylight beginning on December 1 shortened gestation by 10 days.[24] Although no direct information exists on pregnant mares, melatonin may be involved in translating photoperiod information to the mare which then physiologically alters the duration of pregnancy.[25] Some degree of circadian perception occurs in mares, as more than 70% of mares foal between 10:00 p.m. and

2:00 a.m.[9,26,27] Male foals may have gestational durations 2 to 3 days longer than female foals.[5,28]

HORMONAL INTERPLAY BETWEEN MOTHER AND FETUS

PROGESTERONE

Extensive studies using gas chromatography/mass spectrometry have been performed to quantify plasma progestagens near parturition in maternal peripheral blood, uterine blood, fetal umbilical blood, and neonatal peripheral blood.[29] The predominant steroids in the maternal peripheral blood near parturition are 20α-hydroxy-5α-pregnen-3-one (400 to 2100 ng/mL), and 5α-pregnane-3β,20α-diol (100 to 350 ng/mL). These show a rapid rise in the last 30 days of pregnancy, peak 2 to 3 days before delivery and decrease prepartum. Maternal peripheral progesterone concentrations are typically undetectable or low (0.5 to 1.0 ng/mL) during mid- and late pregnancy. Uterine venous blood contains concentrations of these steroids similar to that in the peripheral blood; however, uterine arterial blood concentrations of these steroids are about 50% lower.[29]

Fetal arterial blood contains pregnenolone (420 ng/mL) at 250 to 300 days of pregnancy, along with 5-pregnane-3β,20β-diol (165 ng/mL), 5α-pregnane-3β,20β-diol (105 ng/mL) and 3β-hydroxy-5α-pregnen-20-one (85 ng/mL). The 5α-pregnene-3,20-dione concentrations are around 30 ng/mL in late pregnancy. The fetal umbilical venous blood has high levels of 5α-dihydroxyprogesterone (5α-DHP) and measurable levels of progesterone (5 to 20 ng/mL). Pregnenolone is, therefore, probably converted into progesterone and 5α-DHP by the placenta with continued hydroxylation into 3β and 20β metabolites.[29,30]

The major source of progesterone in late pregnancy in the mare is the placenta with some of this progesterone likely converted to 5α-DHP locally. The fetal plasma does not contain 20α-hydroxylated metabolites, and these may reflect maternal endometrial metabolism and not involve the fetoplacental unit.[30]

ESTROGENS

The horse has a true fetoplacental unit for estrogen production and synthesizes phenolic estradiol and estrone, as well as B ring saturated equilin and equilenin compounds prepartum.[31] Higher peak estrogen concentrations are present in pony mares associated with long days than in horse mares.[32,33] Relatively stable plasma concentrations of estradiol-17β are found before parturition, concurrent with declining concentrations of progestagens detected during the last 24 h preceding parturition.[29,33] These hormonal changes alter the ratio of estrogen to progestagens, which provides a stimulus for the evolution of labor though a series of changes in receptor numbers and myometrial gap-junction formation.

RELAXIN

Relaxin is a polypeptide hormone secreted primarily by the placenta in the horse.[34] Prepartum plasma relaxin concentrations in intensively sampled mares range between 4 to 7 ng/mL, with peak concentrations reached during the second stage of labor at 11 ng/mL.[34] This relaxin surge is temporally related to increased oxytocin secretion, which also occurs during the second stage of labor.[33,35] Researchers do not know whether oxytocin exerts its effect on relaxin directly or indirectly through alterations in blood flow or uterine contractions.[34]

The tissue content of relaxin in term-delivered placentas is low, which suggests that the placenta does not store large amounts of relaxin. Maternal concentrations of relaxin decline after delivery of the placenta and are undetectable in normal mares by 36 h, indicating relaxin has a relatively long half-life.[34] Possible roles for relaxin include changes in connective tissue allowing relaxation of ligaments of the birth canal and the cervix before parturition.[36] The absence of a large prepartum surge of relaxin may explain the subtle nature of these changes in the mare.

LUTEINIZING HORMONE AND FOLLICLE-STIMULATING HORMONE

Plasma concentrations of luteinizing hormone (LH) and follicle-stimulating hormone (FSH) in mares prepartum are low, and LH and FSH pulses are synchronous.[37,38] The basal levels of LH and FSH are unaffected by ovariectomy prepartum, indicating that a conceptus product (such as placental progestagens and estrogens) modulates gonadotropin secretion. An increase in LH and FSH pulse frequency occurs, but pulse amplitude decreases, and mean FSH concentrations are elevated on the day of foaling.[39] This pattern of release is consistent with one hypothalamic-releasing hormone for LH and follicle-stimulating hormone.[39]

PROSTAGLANDIN

A gradual increase in prostaglandin metabolite (PGFM) is noted in pony mares carrying catheterized fetuses in the last few months of gestation.[40] Significant increases in PGFM occur during the last 2 weeks before parturition.[41,42] High plasma PGFM concentrations are measured a few hours prepartum, with peak levels reached before delivery in spontaneously foaling mares.[41] Fetal PGFM levels are higher than maternal levels.[43] Allen and Pashen[44] proposed that the fetoplacental unit is the primary site of prostaglandin production and the maternal uterine tissues are primarily responsible for metabolism of the prostaglandins. Mares carrying gonadectomized fetuses have low circulating concentrations of PGFM and estrogen. Parturition in these mares resulted in fetal malposition and ineffective abdominal straining.[44] The terminal rise in maternal PGFM may relate to gradual maturational changes in the fetus which alter the synthesis of the hormone. High concentrations of estrogen and prostaglandin are important for normal parturition. Prostaglandin F (PGF) and oxytocin are suggested to be acute regulators of myometrial activity.[40,41]

OXYTOCIN

No information is available on oxytocin binding in the pregnant mare uterus, but oxytocin has been shown to bind to the myometrium of the cyclic mare.[45] During the estrous cycle, oxytocin has been reported to be secreted in a pulsatile fashion. Rising maternal plasma oxytocin concentrations are detected before presentation of the chorioallantois, suggesting that oxytocin may be the initiator of Stage II labor and that mares may have a means of controlling the delivery-triggering release of oxytocin.[33]

PROLACTIN

Early studies of plasma prolactin concentrations in mares using heterologous radioimmunoassays report no clear rise in prolactin prepartum, but later studies report dramatic elevations in prolactin in the last week of pregnancy.[46–48] The rise in prolactin suggests that as in other species it is involved in the onset of lactogenesis. The origin of the signals which result in rising prolactin levels is unknown.

INSULIN

Marked changes in carbohydrate metabolism and pancreatic β cell function occur during late pregnancy in mares.[49] These metabolic adjustments include a lower insulin concentration in late (>270 days) pregnant mares versus early pregnant mares, a tendency toward lower maternal glucose concentrations in the fed state, a reduction in the effectiveness of insulin, and hypoglycemia during fasting. The reduction in the effectiveness of insulin and lower insulin concentrations after 270 days of gestation conserve glucose for the fetus. A relationship between hypoglycemia and increases in uterine prostaglandin production appears to exist.[40,49,50]

Insulin is detected in fetal plasma in late gestation. During late gestation insulin secretion is affected by fetal infusion of glucose, arginine, and endogenous variations in glucose. A significant positive correlation exists between the plasma concentrations of insulin and glucose. The maturity of the foal also influences the β cell responsiveness and insulin levels in the immediate postnatal period.[51]

CATECHOLAMINES

At birth, active adrenal glands are essential for survival. Adrenal medullary activity is reflected in peripheral plasma concentrations of epinephrine and norepinephrine. The foal is delivered extremely rapidly, hence intrapartum oxygenation, metabolic status, and catecholamine concentrations may be unaffected resulting in normal values being attained immediately postpartum.[52]

ENDORPHINS

Opioid peptides are believed to be related to stress and secretion of these peptides is believed to be an adaptive function to ease stress of delivery.[53] Spontaneously delivered foals had higher umbilical blood levels of β-endorphin (717 ± 116 pg/mL arterial, 609 ± 84 pg/mL venous) than maternal venous blood (337 ± 126 pg/mL).

CORTISOL

The weight of the fetal adrenal gland increases near term and the increase in weight has been reported to be largely an increase in the growth of the zona fasciculata.[54,55] Survival of the newborn has been shown to be related to the maturity of its adrenal glands.[56]

Evidence of a prepartum surge in fetal plasma cortisol remains equivocal because of the paucity of information from chronically catheterized fetuses delivered at term.[57,58] High prolonged doses of glucocorticoid (Dexamethasone) will induce parturition.[59] Substantial umbilical arteriovenous differences are detected at birth, indicating enhanced adrenal activity before birth.[60,61]

In ruminants, activation of the fetal hypothalamus-hypophyseal-adrenal axis is responsible for fetal cortisol secretion which decreases maternal progesterone concentrations and increases maternal estradiol-17β.[62]

Reports have been made of gradual increases in fetal cortisol during late pregnancy but not of a distinct prepartum rise.[57,58,60] Recently devised techniques have been used to maintain catheterized placental vessels, and Figure 66–1 shows the daily changes in fetal cortisol concentrations prepartum in a spontaneously foaling (342 days) Standardbred mare. These preliminary data suggest that cortisol may play a greater role in parturition than previously recognized and warrants further study.

CHANGES IN THE UTERUS

ACTIVATION OF THE MYOMETRIUM

Myometrial activation is a key event in initiating labor.[63] Haluska et al.[64] proposed that the myometrium responds to changes in estradiol, progesterone, or the estradiol to progestagen ratio and that relaxin is a key hormonal substance in maintaining uterine quiescence in late pregnancy. Increased myometrial activity has been reported in the last week of pregnancy, which further increased during the last 4 h before delivery.[64] In pony mares, a decrease in electromyography (EMG) activity was reported 2 to 4 h before delivery, with a rapid

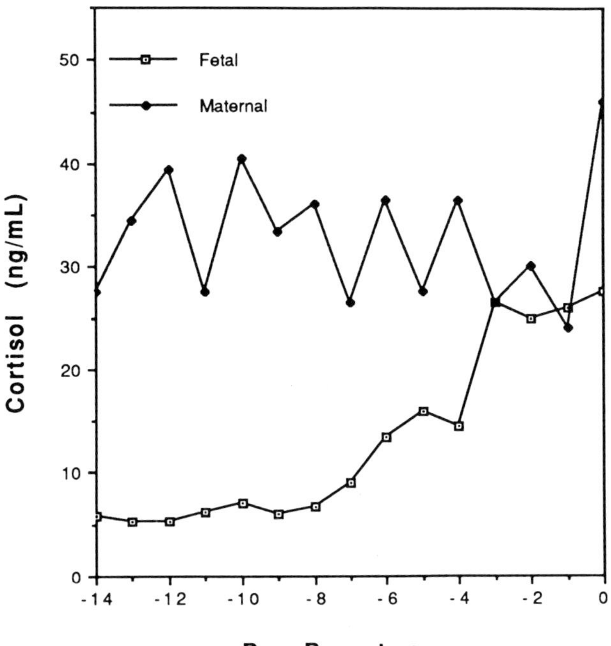

FIG. 66–1. Fetal and maternal cortisol concentrations in a spontaneously foaling Standardbred mare at 342 days of pregnancy.

increase at rupture of the chorioallantois. At delivery, EMG activity was characterized by 10 to 13 rapid bursts of activity. After delivery of the fetus, the uterus becomes more quiescent until Stage III labor. A decrease in maternal progesterone during the 24 h before delivery is thought to be the key to activating the myometrium, and the final activity is probably the result of the effects of oxytocin and prostaglandin $F_2\alpha$ overcoming the inhibitory effects of relaxin.[64] In other species, relaxin decreases myosin light chain kinase activity of the myometrium and elevates myometrial intracellular cyclic adenosine monophosphate (cAMP), which causes sequestration of calcium. Calcium is necessary for myometrial contractions.

STAGES OF PARTURITION

The onset of parturition in the mare is preceded by the physical changes which develop in response to the previously discussed hormonal changes occurring at the termination of gestation. Filling of the udder accompanied by distention of the teats with colostrum, "waxing" of the teats, relaxation of the sacrosciatic ligaments and vulva, and softening of the cervix herald the onset of impending parturition.

Foaling is a continuous process which has been divided into three stages for descriptive purposes.[65] Before the onset of parturition, the fetus is normally resting in a dorsopubic position with the front legs flexed at the carpus and the head resting between the knees. The start of Stage I is difficult to ascertain as no overt signs signal the increase in myometrial activity which begins hours before delivery and marks the onset of parturition.[64] Although no visible signs of straining occur during Stage I, patchy sweating is often noted behind the elbows, in the flanks, and along the neck as early as 4 h before birth of the foal.

Other signs that may be noted during Stage I include increased restlessness with the mare pacing the stall, lying down and getting up frequently, switching her tail, stretching as if to urinate, and looking at her flanks. Frequent passage of small amounts of feces and yawning are also seen. The increased myometrial activity occurring during Stage I stimulates the fetus to reposition itself to a dorsosacral position with its front legs and head extended. The cervix dilates in response to myometrial contractions and the pressure of the fluid-distended chorioallantoic membrane pushing against it. As the fetus passes through the cervix into the birth canal, the chorioallantoic membrane ruptures marking the end of Stage I. If the mare is disturbed or becomes excited, Stage I signs can occasionally be interrupted and foaling may be delayed for several hours or even days.[7] Should the red, velvet-like chorioallantoic membrane with its cervical star appear intact at the lips of the vulva, it should be broken immediately, because this indicates premature placental separation which, if allowed to continue, will result in a severely hypoxic foal.

Stage II labor begins with the rupture of the chorioallantoic membrane and the passage of allantoic fluid from the vulva ("breaking water"). As the fetus enters the birth canal it stretches the soft tissue of the pelvic cavity initiating powerful contractions of the abdominal muscles and diaphragm together with a closing of the glottis (Ferguson's reflex).[65] With the appearance of the transparent, bluish white amnion at the lips of the vulva, the mare assumes lateral recumbency and forceful contractions begin in groups of three or four followed by rest periods of 2 to 3 min. Most mares get up and change position during Stage II labor. During a normal delivery, the foal usually presents with one foreleg preceding the other by 10 to 15 cm. The most forceful contractions occur when the head and then the shoulders pass through the pelvis. When the foal's hips clear the vagina, straining stops and Stage II ends. Although Stage II labor can be completed in less than 10 min, it usually averages about 20 min and may rarely proceed for up to 60 min.[7,65] Following delivery of the foal, the mare usually lies quietly for 10 to 15 min, often resting with the foal's rear legs still within the vagina. Although some clinicians recommend that care be taken to ensure the umbilical cord is not broken for several minutes following delivery to allow completion of blood flow from the placenta to the foal's circulatory system,[66] some research has demonstrated that separation of the cord immediately after birth had no harmful effect on the foal.[67]

Stage III of parturition involves passage of the placental membranes. Although visible straining stops with delivery of the foal, myometrial contractions continue. With the birth of the foal, the vessels in the fetal placenta collapse and the villi become shrunken and begin to separate from the uterus.[65] The apex of the chorioallantoic sac becomes inverted and, as the sac is "rolled" down the uterine horn, the fetal villi are freed from the maternal crypts.[7] Because of this inversion, the placenta is normally expelled with the allantoic surface outermost. The mare frequently shows mild signs of colic during passage of the placental membranes; this can include uneasiness, pawing, lying down, and rolling. If the mare becomes unduly distressed, walking her until the placenta is passed usually avoids complications. The placenta is normally passed within 0.5 to 3 h after delivery of the foal and Stage III of parturition is complete.

REFERENCES

1. Adams-Brendenmuehl, C., and Pipers, F.S.: Antepartum evaluations of the equine fetus. J. Reprod. Fertil. Suppl., *35*:565–573, 1987.
2. Too, K., Kanagawa, H., and Kawata, K.: Fetal and maternal electrocardiograms during parturition in the mare. Jpn. J. Vet. Res., *15*:5–13, 1967.
3. Jeffcott, L.B., Rossdale, P.D., and Leadon, D.P.: Haematological changes in the neonatal period of normal and induced premature foals. J. Reprod. Fertil. Suppl., *32*: 537–544, 1982.
4. Rossdale, P.D., Ousey, J.C., Silver, M., and Fowden, A.: Studies on equine prematurity 6: Guidelines for assessment of foal maturity. Equine Vet. J., *16*:300–302, 1984.
5. Evans, J.W., and Torbeck, R.L. (eds.): Breeding Management and Foal Development. Tyler, TX, Equine Research, 1982.
6. Arthur, G.H.: Veterinary Reproduction and Obstetrics. 4th ed. London, Bailliere Tindall, 1975.
7. Rossdale, P.D., and Ricketts, S.W.: Equine Stud Farm Medicine. 2nd ed. Philadelphia, Lea & Febiger, 1980.
8. Peaker, M., Rossdale, P.D., Forsyth, I.A., and Falk, M.: Changes in mammary development and the composition of secretion during late pregnancy in the mare. J. Reprod. Fertil. Suppl., *27*:555–561, 1979.
9. Haluska, G.J., and Wilkins, K.: Predictive utility of prepartum temperature changes in the mare. Equine Vet. J., *21*:116–118, 1989.
10. Ley, W.B., et al.: Daytime foaling management of the mare. 2. Induction of parturition. J. Equine Vet. Sci., *9*:95–99, 1989.
11. Ley, W.B., et al.: Daytime management of the mare. 1. Prefoaling mammary secretions testing. J. Equine Vet. Sci., *9*:88–93, 1989.
12. Ousey, J.C., Dudan, F., and Rossdale, P.D.: Preliminary studies of mammary secretions in the mare to assess foetal readiness for birth. Equine Vet. J., *16*:259–263, 1984.
13. Leadon, D.P., Jeffcott, L.B., and Rossdale, P.D.: Mammary secretions in normal spontaneous and induced premature parturition in the mare. Equine Vet. J., *16*:256–259, 1984.
14. Ousey, J.C., Delclaux, M., and Rossdale, P.D.: Evaluation of three strip tests for measuring electrolytes in mare's prepartum mammary secretions and for predicting parturition. Equine Vet. J., *21*:196–200, 1989.
15. Cash, R.S.G., Ousey, J.C., and Rossdale, P.D.: Rapid strip test method to assist management of foaling mares. Equine Vet. J., *17*:61–62, 1985.
16. Brooke, D.: Evaluation of a new test kit for estimating the foaling time in the mare. Equine Pract., *9*:34–36, 1987.
17. Neely, D.P., Liu, I.K.M., and Hillman, R.B.: Equine Reproduction. Princeton Junction, NJ, Veterinary Learning Systems, 1983.
18. Shaw, E.B., Houpt, K.A., and Holmes, D.F.: Body temperature and behaviour of mares during the last two weeks of pregnancy. Equine Vet. J., *20*:199–202, 1988.
19. Ammons, S.F., Threlfall, W.R., and Kline, R.C.: Equine body temperature and progesterone fluctuations during estrus and near parturition. Theriogenology, *31*: 1007–1019, 1989.
20. Hintz, H.F., Hintz, R.L., Lein, D.H., and Van Vleck, L.D.: Length of gestation periods in Thoroughbred mares. J. Equine Med. Surg., *3*:289–292, 1979.
21. Law, J.: Diseases of the generative organs. *In* Diseases of the Horse. Edited by A.D. Melvin. Washington, D.C., U.S. Government Printing Office, 1911, pp. 142–189.
22. Vandeplassche, M.M.: Delayed embryonic development and prolonged pregnancy in mares. *In* Current Therapy in Theriogenology. 2nd ed. Edited by D. Morrow. Toronto, W.B. Saunders, 1986, pp. 685–692.
23. Howell, C.E., and Rollins, W.C.: Environmental sources of variation in the gestation length of the horse. J. Anim. Sci., *10*:789–796, 1951.
24. Hodge, S.L., et al.: Influence of photoperiod on the pregnant and postpartum mare. Am. J. Vet. Res., *43*: 1752–1755, 1982.
25. Sharp, D.C.: Transition into the breeding season: Clues to the mechanisms of seasonality. Equine Vet. J., *20*: 159–161, 1988.
26. Rossdale, P.D., and Short, R.V.: The time of foaling in Thoroughbred mares. J. Reprod. Fertil., *13*:341–343, 1969.
27. Bain, A.M., and Howey, W.P.: Observations on the time of foaling in Thoroughbred mares in Australia. J. Reprod. Fertil. Suppl., *23*:545–546, 1975.
28. Roipha, R.T., et al.: The duration of pregnancy in Thoroughbred mares. Vet. Rec., *84*:552–555, 1969.
29. Holtan, D.W., et al.: Plasma progestagens in the mare, fetus and newborn foal. J. Reprod. Fertil. Suppl., *44*:517–528, 1991.
30. Hamon, M., et al.: Production of 5α-dihydroprogesterone during late pregnancy in the mare. J. Reprod. Fertil. Suppl., *44*:529–535, 1991.
31. Pashen, R.L.: Maternal and foetal endocrinology during late pregnancy and parturition in the mare. Equine Vet. J., *16*:233–238, 1984.
32. Nett, T.M., Holtan, D.W., and Estergreen, V.L.: Plasma estrogens in pregnant and postpartum mares. J. Anim. Sci., *37*:962–970, 1973.
33. Haluska, G.J., and Currie, W.B.: Variation in plasma concentrations of oestradiol-17β and their relationship to those of progesterone, 13,14-dihydro-15-ketoprostaglandin $F_2\alpha$ and oxytocin across pregnancy and at parturition in pony mares. J. Reprod. Fertil., *84*:635–646, 1988.
34. Stewart, D.R., Stabenfeldt, G.H., and Hughes, J.P.: Relaxin activity in foaling mares. J. Reprod. Fertil. Suppl., *32*:603–609, 1982.
35. Ginther, O.J.: Reproductive Biology of the Mare: Basic and Applied Aspects. Cross Plaines, WI, Equiservices, 1979.
36. Bryant-Greenwood, G.D.: Relaxin a new hormone. Endocr. Rev. *3*:62–90, 1982.
37. Nett, T.M., Shoemaker, C.F., and Squires, E.L.: Changes in serum concentrations of luteinizing hormone and follicle-stimulating hormone following injection of gonadotropin-

releasing hormone during pregnancy and after parturition in mares. J. Anim. Sci., *67:*1330–1333, 1989.

38. Turner, D.D., et al.: FSH and LH concentrations in peri-parturient mares. J. Reprod. Fertil. Suppl., *27:*547–553, 1979.
39. Hines, K.K., Fitzgerald, B.P., and Loy, R.G.: Effect of pulsatile gonadotrophin release on mean serum LH and FSH in peri-parturient mares. J. Reprod. Fertil. Suppl., *35:*635–640, 1987.
40. Barnes, R.J., et al.: Foetal and maternal plasma concentrations of 13,14-dihydro-15-oxo-prostaglandin F in the mare during late pregnancy and at parturition. J. Endocrinol., *78:*201–215, 1978.
41. Stewart, D.R., Kindahl, H., Stabenfeldt, G.H., and Hughes, J.P.: Concentrations of 15-keto-13,14-dihydro-prostaglandin $F_2\alpha$ in the mare during spontaneous and oxytocin induced foaling. Equine Vet. J., *16:*270–274, 1984.
42. Haluska, G.J.: Electromyographic analysis of the myometrium of the mare correlated with the endocrinology of pregnancy, parturition and the postpartum period. Ph.D. thesis. Cornell University, 1985.
43. Silver, M., et al.: Prostaglandins in maternal and fetal plasma and in allantoic fluid during the second half of gestation in the mare. J. Reprod. Fertil. Suppl., *27:*531–539, 1979.
44. Allen, W.R., and Pashen, R.L.: The role of prostaglandins during parturition in the mare. Acta Vet. Scand., *77:*279–298, 1981.
45. Stull, C.L., and Evans, J.W.: Oxytocin binding in the uterus of the cycling mare. Equine Vet. Sci., *6:*114–119, 1986.
46. Forsyth, I.A., Rossdale, P.D., and Thomas, C.R.: Studies on milk composition and lactogenic hormones in the mare. J. Reprod. Fertil. Suppl., *23:*631–635, 1975.
47. Nett, T.M., Holtan, D.W., and Estergreen, V.C.: Oestrogens, LH, PMSG, and prolactin in serum of pregnant mares. J. Reprod. Fertil. Suppl., *23:*457–462, 1975.
48. Worthy, K., et al.: Plasma prolactin concentrations and cyclic activity in pony mares during parturition and early lactation. J. Reprod. Fertil., *77:*569–574, 1986.
49. Fowden, A.L., Comline, R.S., and Silver, M.: Insulin secretion and carbohydrate metabolism during pregnancy in the mare. Equine Vet. J., *16:*239–246, 1984.
50. Silver, M., and Fowden, A.L.: Uterine prostaglandin F metabolite production in relation to glucose availability in late pregnancy and a possible influence of diet on time of delivery in the mare. J. Reprod. Fertil. Suppl., *32:*511–519, 1982.
51. Fowden, A.L., et al.: Studies on equine prematurity 3: Insulin secretion in the foal during the perinatal period. Equine Vet. J., *16:*286–291, 1984.
52. Rose, R.J., Rossdale, P.D., and Ledon, D.P.: Blood gas and acid-base status in spontaneously delivered, term-induced and induced premature foals. J. Reprod. Fertil. Suppl., *32:*521–528, 1982.
53. Dudan, F.E., et al.: Circulating immunoreactive beta endorphin concentrations in the perinatal foal. Equine Vet. J. Suppl., *5:*46–49, 1988.
54. Comline, R.S., and Silver, M.: Catecholamine secretion by the adrenal medulla of the foetal and new-born foal. J. Physiol., *216:*659–682, 1971.
55. Webb, P.D., and Steven, D.H.: Development of the adrenal cortex in the fetal foal: An ultrastructural study. J. Dev. Physiol., *3:*59–73, 1981.
56. Webb, P.D., Leadon, D.P., Rossdale, P.D., and Jeffcott, L.B.: Studies on equine prematurity 5: Histology of the adrenal cortex of the premature newborn foal. Equine Vet. J., *16:*297–299, 1984.
57. Nathanielsz, P.W., Rossdale, P.D., Silver, M., and Comline, R.S.: Studies on fetal, neonatal, and maternal cortisol metabolism in the mare. J. Reprod. Fertil. Suppl., *23:*625–630, 1975.
58. Rossdale, P.D., et al.: Plasma cortisol in the foal during the late fetal and early neonatal period. Res. Vet. Sci., *15:*395–397, 1973.
59. Alm, C.C., Sullivan, J.J., and First, N.L.: Induction of premature parturition by parenteral administration of dexamethasone in the mare. J. Am. Vet. Med. Assoc., *165:*721–722, 1975.
60. Silver, M.S., et al.: Studies on equine prematurity 2: Post natal adrenocortical activity in relation to plasma adrenocorticotrophic hormone and catecholamine concentrations in term and premature foals. Equine Vet. J., *16:*278–286, 1984.
61. Hillman, R.B., and Gangam, V.K.: Hormonal changes in the mare and foal associated with oxytocin induction of parturition. J. Reprod. Fertil. Suppl., *27:*541–546, 1979.
62. Challis, J.R.G., and Olson, D.M.: Parturition. *In* The Physiology of Reproduction. Edited by S.E. Knobil, et al. New York, Raven Press, 1988, pp. 61–129.
63. Haluska, G.J., Lowe, J.E., and Currie, W.B.: Electromyographic properties of the myometrium of the pony mare during pregnancy. J. Reprod. Fertil., *81:*471–478, 1987.
64. Haluska, G.J., Lowe, J.E., and Currie, W.B.: Electromyographic properties of the myometrium correlated with the endocrinology of the pre-partum and post-partum periods and parturition in pony mares. J. Reprod. Fertil. Suppl., *35:*553–564, 1987.
65. Roberts, S.J.: Veterinary Obstetrics and Genital Diseases (Theriogenology). 3rd ed. Woodstock, VT, published by the author, 1986.
66. Rossdale, P.D.: Clinical studies on the newborn Thoroughbred foal. 1. Perinatal behavior. Br. Vet. J. *123:*470–481, 1967.
67. Doran, R.T., Threlfall, W.R., and Kline, R.: Umbilical blood flow and the effects of premature severence in the neonatal horse. Proc. Soc. Theriogenol., 175–178, 1985.

CHAPTER 67

INDUCTION OF PARTURITION

M.M. LeBlanc

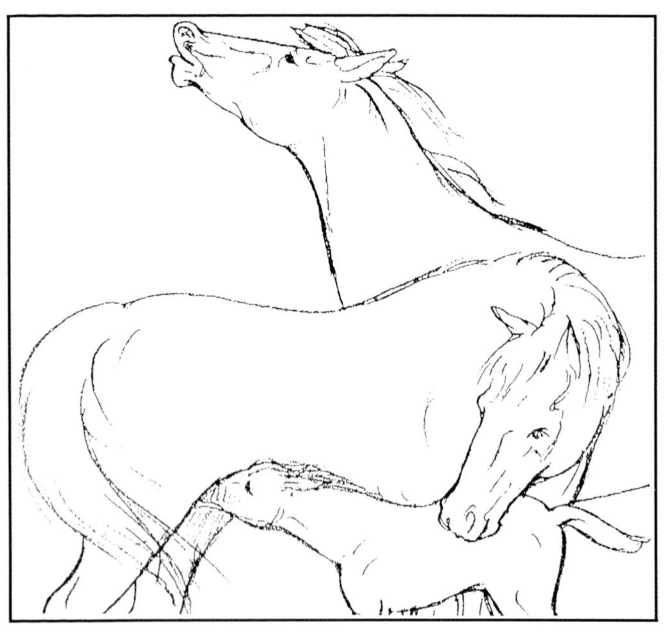

Induction of parturition in the mare permits professional assistance at foaling. Because the majority of mares foal at night or in the early morning hours, efforts to ensure a safe, attended delivery of the foal are labor intensive and costly. Inducing parturition is, therefore, frequently performed for the convenience of farm managers, farm personnel, and veterinarians. Clients may place considerable pressure on a veterinarian to induce a mare, particularly if the client is a nervous owner of a single mare that has a gestational length greater than 335 days. Mares must be carefully selected, however, because fetal maturity is difficult to ensure. If mares are induced too early, a dysmature or premature foal may be delivered. The potential problems associated with the induction procedure need to be explained carefully to the mare owner.

INDICATIONS

Indications for induction of parturition include a history of premature placental separation, delayed parturition attributable to uterine atony (usually seen in older, multiparous mares), delivery of a foal with neonatal isoerythrolysis, rectovaginal fistula, and physical damage, especially in mares with reduced pelvic canal size. Other indications include preparturient colic, excessive ventral edema., impending rupture of the prepubic tendon, and imminent death of the mare. Mares may also be induced for teaching purposes, and research investigations and to be used as nurse mares.[1–3]

DETERMINATION OF FETAL MATURITY

Fetal maturity is a prerequisite for induction. In women and domestic species other than the horse, gestational age is related to fetal maturation, and parturition can be induced safely in the last 5 to 10% of gestation. In the horse, fetal maturation cannot be predicted by gestational age because of extreme variability in duration of normal gestation (320 to 365 days) and the apparent narrow window of neonatal viability in the species.[4]

Clinical signs of impending parturition (e.g., udder enlargement with the presence of colostrum, relaxation of perineal region, and cervical relaxation[1–3]) are not always reliable for predicting fetal maturation or time of foaling.[1] Colostrum may be present in the udder for days or only for hours. The cervix may remain firmly closed and covered with tacky mucus until the end of first stage of labor or it may be open sufficiently to admit the entire hand several weeks before calculated term. Because of this variability, induction of parturition can be a precarious procedure if not adequately timed.

Electrolyte changes in prepartum mammary secretions of the mare have been shown to be associated with fetal maturity.[5,6] As the mare approaches parturition, total calcium concentrations in the mammary secretions rise (Fig. 67–1). Concentrations > 40 mg/dL are usually associated with a mature fetus, whereas val-

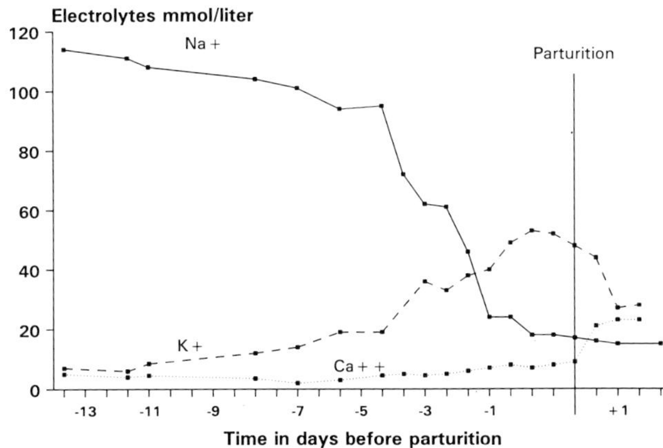

FIG. 67–1. Electrolyte changes in prepartum mammary secretions. Calcium concentrations are expressed in mEq/L. (Adapted from Ousey, J.C., Dudan, F.E., and Rossdale, P.D.: Preliminary studies of mammary secretions in the mare to assess foetal readiness for birth. Equine Vet. J., *16*:259–263, 1984.)

ues of 12 mg/dL are indicative of fetal immaturity and hence poor neonatal viability.[5] In conjunction with the rise in calcium concentration, an inversion of sodium and potassium concentrations in the mammary secretions occurs (Fig. 67–1). Sodium concentrations are significantly greater than those of potassium until close to term, at which time sodium concentrations fall dramatically and potassium concentrations rise above those of sodium. Mature foals have been delivered safely if parturition is induced after calcium concentrations in mammary secretions rise above 40 mg/dL and after the inversion of sodium and potassium concentrations.

A scoring system using the values of those three electrolytes has also been developed to enable successful induction of parturition and to predict the time of foaling (Table 67–1). The clinician gives 5, 10, or 15 points to each of the three electrolyte values; the maximum score possible is 45 points on the day of foaling and the minimum score possible is zero.[5] An ionic score of 35 points or more suggests that a mare is within 24 h of foaling. When mares in this category were induced, mature, term foals were delivered, whereas mares induced with ionic scores between 20 and 30 points delivered premature, weak foals.

TABLE 67–1. SCORING SYSTEM FOR PREPARTUM COLOSTRAL ELECTROLYTE CONCENTRATIONS*

CALCIUM (MG/DL)	SODIUM (MEQ/L)	POTASSIUM (MEQ/L)	POINTS FOR EACH ELECTROLYTE
≥40	≤30	≥35	15
≥28	≤50	≥30	10
≥20	≤80	≥20	5

*A total score of ≥35 suggests safe induction is possible.

(Adapted from Ousey, J.C., Dudan, F., and Rossdale, P.D.: Preliminary studies of mammary secretions in the mare to assess foetal readiness for birth. Equine Vet. J., *16*:259–263, 1984.)

Electrolytes in mammary secretions can be measured by automated chemistry techniques or by rapid strip test methods.[7–10] The strip tests quantitate calcium concentrations within a sample. There are five rapid test kits available: kit 1 is the Predict-a-Foal Test (Animal Healthcare Products, Chino, CA);[8] kit 2 is a strip test kit developed by Cash et al. (Newmarket, UK);[7] and kit 3 (Sofchek Test Strips, Environmental Test Systems, Elkhart, IN), kit 4 (Titrets Calcium Hardness Test Kits, Chemetrics, Inc., Calverton, VA), and kit 5 (Merchoquant No. 10017; Darmstadt, West Germany) are commercial water hardness test strips.[9,10]

The first two kits measure calcium and magnesium and consist of test strips with either four (kit 1) or five (kit 2) reaction zones per strip. The greater the number of zones showing a color change, the greater the concentrations of calcium and/or magnesium. Parturition can be safely induced after day 330 of gestation, when at least four color bar changes occur in the Predict-a-Foal Test[8] or when three of four color bar changes occur in the test developed by Cash et al. The other test strips are used in the water-quality industry and measure calcium (kits 4 and 5) or water hardness (kit 3). These strips consist of a single reaction zone which changes, depending on the concentration of calcium in the test solution, from white to light yellow, orange, or red. Samples of mammary secretions are diluted in a 1:6 ratio with double distilled water for the Sofchek and Titrets strips and 1:4 for the Merchoquant No. 10017 strip. Parturition can be safely induced when ≥250 ppm water hardness is found with the Sofchek test, ≥250 ppm calcium carbonate content is found with the Titrets Test, and ≥12 mmol/L calcium is found with the Marchoquant No. 10017 test. All methods accurately measure calcium and/or magnesium. These test kits are not particularly accurate in predicting time of parturition. Maximum calcium scores frequently occur on more occasions before the day of birth than on parturition.[10] These kits may be more helpful in indicating when it is not necessary to attend a mare at night.[9]

METHODS OF INDUCTION

Methods of elective induction of parturition in the mare include oxytocin and prostaglandins. Oxytocin is the most frequently used.[11,12] Various techniques, including intravenous or intramuscular administration and high (40 to 120 IU) or low (2.5 to 10 IU) doses of oxytocin have been advocated. Low doses given intravenously are preferred over high doses given intramuscularly.[12] Lower doses of oxytocin (<20 IU) are associated with lesser degrees of discomfort in the mare and shorter delivery times than are higher doses (>40 IU). Higher doses (40 to 120 IU) appear to be unnecessary and may be potentially dangerous to the foal.[13] After intravenous administration of oxytocin, foaling ordinarily begins within 15 to 30 min and is completed within 1 h. Intravenous oxytocin can be administered as multiple small injections of 2.5 to 10 IU diluted in 30 to 60 mL of isotonic saline, repeated every 20 min or as a single 20 IU bolus. Before administration, an in-dwelling catheter should be placed in the jugular vein of the mare, her perineum should be thoroughly washed, and a wrap should be placed around her tail.

Mares should be induced in a quiet, clean, dry area, preferably removed from other farm activities. Resuscitation equipment and a small surgical pack should be available for possible complications. Following oxytocin administration, mares will become restless and colicky, swish their tails, and frequently get up and down and stretch. Sweat will appear over their shoulders, on their necks, behind their elbows, and in their flanks within 20 min. Rupture of the chorioallantoic membrane and strong abdominal straining usually occur within 20 to 30 min.

If strong abdominal contractions are present but the chorioallantoic membrane does not rupture or signs of immediate parturition are not present within 20 min of oxytocin administration, a manual vaginal examination using a sterile glove should be performed. I perform a vaginal manual examination on all mares 20 min after the first injection of oxytocin to determine progress of delivery of the foal. Premature separation of the placental membranes occurs commonly, and if present, the chorioallantois should be incised with scissors or knife and the foal immediately delivered. Premature placental separation is diagnosed by vaginal palpation of a thick membrane lying freely within the uterine lumen or by the appearance of a large red sac at the lips of the vulva.

The majority of mares will foal within 60 min of administration of oxytocin. If the placenta is not passed within 3 h of delivery of the foal, treatment for retained placenta should be instituted. Oxytocin will stimulate parturition in the late-term pregnant mare after 300 days of gestation.[14] The ability of oxytocin to override the physiologic events responsible for normal parturition, without regard for fetal maturation in utero, makes this hormone clinically dangerous when used without supportive evidence to indicate the foal's and the mare's readiness for birth. Therefore, mares must be carefully evaluated before its use if a mature, viable, foal is to be delivered.

In the late 1970s and early 1980s the use of a synthetic prostaglandin analogue (fluprostenol, 250 to 1000 g IM) was advocated for induction of parturition, because it did not initiate parturition in mares unless the fetus was ready for birth.[15–18] In those studies, prostaglandin appeared to be a somewhat capricious inducing agent, resulting in the induction of labor some 1 to 6 h after administration. Serious complications including cervical rupture and poor fetal viability were reported.

Recently, Ley et al. have shown that mares may be induced with either prostalene (4 mg subcutaneously) or fenprostalene (two 0.5 mg doses at 2-h intervals subcutaneously).[19] Mares were induced when electrolyte concentrations in mammary secretions, as measured by commercial test kits, indicated the foal's readiness for birth. All 17 mares receiving fenprostalene delivered viable foals at a mean of 3.9 h from initial injection; 75% of the 16 mares receiving prostalene for induction delivered viable foals at a mean of 3.7 h from injection time. Mares that failed to respond produced viable foals spontaneously 30 to 56 h later. The number of foaling complications in the induced group did not differ from the number of complications in the spontaneously foaling group.

COMPLICATIONS

Adverse effects associated with induction include delivery of premature or dysmature foals, decreased passive transfer of immunoglobulins, hyperstimulation of the myometrium, myometrial spasm, premature placental separation, malpresentation, and prolonged placental retention.[3,11,20]

In my experience, mares undergoing severe stress such as anterior enteritis, colic and acute laminitis and mares that are receiving high doses of nonsteroidal anti-inflammatory drugs may not respond even to high doses of oxytocin. These mares frequently experience premature placental separation without proper positioning of the foal. Dystocia results and the foals must be delivered per vagina with the mares under general anesthesia. In cases such as these, proper facilities must be available to accommodate serious complications.

REFERENCES

1. Purvis, A.D.: Elective induction of labor and parturition in the mare. Proc. Am. Assoc. Equine Pract., 113–118, 1972.
2. Hillman, R.B., and Lesser, S.A.: Induction of parturition. Vet. Clin. North Am. Large Anim. Pract., *2:*333–344, 1980.
3. Hillman, R.B.: Induction of parturition in mares. J. Reprod. Fertil. Suppl., *23:*641–644, 1975.
4. Silver, M., and Fowden, A.L.: Induction of labour in domestic animals: Endocrine changes and neonatal viability. *In* The Endocrine Control of the Fetus. Edited by W. Kunzel and A. Jensen, Berlin, Springer-Verlag, 1988, pp. 403–411.
5. Ousey, J.C., Dudan, F., and Rossdale, P.D.: Preliminary studies of mammary secretions in the mare to assess foetal readiness for birth. Equine Vet. J., *16:*259–263, 1984.
6. Leadon, D.P., Jeffcott, L.B., and Rossdale, P.D.: Mammary secretions in normal spontaneous and induced premature parturition in the mare. Equine Vet. J., *16:*256–259, 1984.
7. Cash, R.S.G., Ousey, J.C., and Rossdale, P.D.: Rapid strip test method to assist management of foaling mares. Equine Vet. J., *17:*61–62, 1985.
8. Brook, D.: Evaluation of a new test kit for estimating the foaling time in the mare. Equine Pract., *9:*34–36, 1987.
9. Ley, W.B., et al.: Daytime management of the mare. 1: Prefoaling mammary secretions testing. J. Equine Vet. Sci., *9:*88–94, 1989.
10. Ousey, J.C., Delclaux, M., and Rossdale, P.D.: Evaluation of three strip tests for measuring electrolytes in mares' pre-partum mammary secretions and for predicting parturition. Equine Vet. J., *21:*196–200, 1989.

11. Jeffcott, L.B., and Rossdale, P.D.: A critical review of current methods for induction of parturition in the mare. Equine Vet. J., *9:*208–215, 1977.
12. Pashen, R.L.: Oxytocin—The induction agent of choice in the mare? J. Reprod. Fertil. Suppl., *32:*645, 1982.
13. Pashen, R.L.: Low doses of oxytocin can induce foaling at term. Equine Vet. J., *12:*85–87, 1980.
14. Leadon, D.P., et al.: A comparison of agents for inducing parturition in mares in the pre-viable and premature periods of gestation. J. Reprod. Fertil. Suppl., *32:*597–602, 1982.
15. Ousey, J.C., Dudan, F.E., Rossdale, P.D., and Silver, M.: Effects of fluprostenol administration in mares during late pregnancy. Equine Vet. J., *16:*264–269, 1984.
16. Rossdale, P.D., Pashen, R.L., and Jeffcott, L.B.: The use of synthetic prostaglandin analogue (fluprostenol) to induce foaling. J. Reprod. Fertil. Suppl., *27:*521–529, 1979.
17. Rossdale, P.D.: Foaling induced by a synthetic prostaglandin analogue (fluprostenol). Vet. Rec., *99:*26–28, 1976.
18. Rose, R.J.: Experiences with fluprostenol as an induction agent in Thoroughbred mares. J. Reprod. Fertil. Suppl., *32:*645, 1982.
19. Ley, W.B., et al.: Daytime foaling management of the mare. 2: Induction of parturition. J. Equine Vet. Sci., *9:*95–99, 1989.
20. Townsend, H.G.G., Tabel, H., and Bristol, F.M.: Induction of parturition in mares. Effect on passive transfer of immunity to foals. J. Am. Vet. Med. Assoc., *182:*255–257, 1983.

CHAPTER 68

DYSTOCIA

M. Vandeplassche

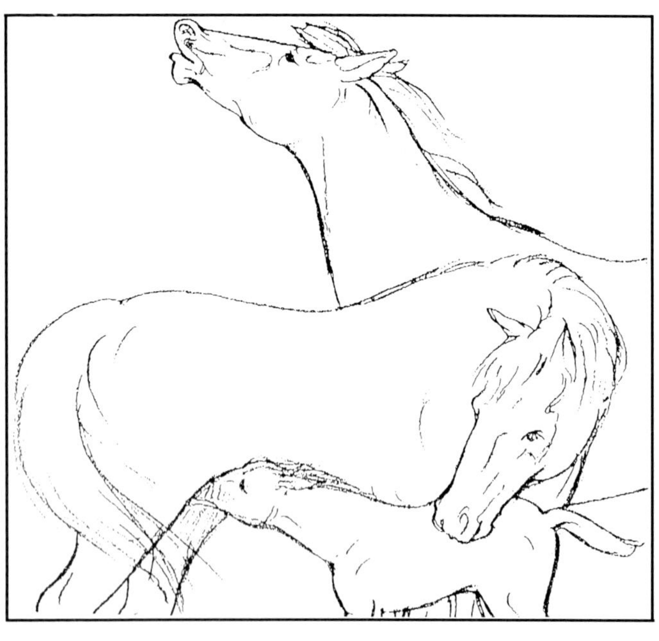

Dystocia in mares is a serious problem that can cause life-threatening risks for both dam and fetus, if proper obstetric assistance is not given immediately. Incidence of dystocia varies with different breeds. Difficult foaling occurs in about 4% of Thoroughbred and Trotter births. In Belgian Draft Horses, the incidence is about 10%, primarily caused by a fetal muscular hypertrophy comparable with double muscling in some cattle breeds. This results in a more difficult passage of the increased fetal diameter through the bony birth canal. In Shetland Ponies, the incidence of dystocia is approximately 8% and is mainly caused by an oversize skull approaching hydrocephaly in some cases. Incidence of dystocia is also markedly higher in young primiparous than older multiparous mares, which can be explained by an increased disproportion between fetal cross diameter and the pelvic passage. However, dystocia is most often caused by abnormal presentation, position, or posture with long fetal extremities predisposing the mare to problems in delivery.[1]

Personal observations over a period of 45 yr concern a total of about 1000 cases of dystocia of which accurate detailed notes could be gathered for 601 mares. About 60% of them were Belgian Draft mares, 15% Trotters and Thoroughbreds, 15% Saddle Horses, and 10% pony and Haflinger mares.

The objective of a veterinary clinician is to save, whenever possible, the life of both dam and fetus. To accomplish this, a mare in dystocia must be considered as a double patient, i.e., the dam and fetus. A thorough history along with a general and genital examination are paramount to arrive at a correct diagnosis and planned treatment. The treatment approach to any dystocia is selected from four different obstetric methods: reposition, traction, fetotomy, and cesarean section. In selecting a treatment plan, priority should be first to the dam, then the fetus, economic interests of the owner, and last and least the interests of the veterinarian. Equine dystocia should always be considered as cases of emergency. The fetus is particularly at risk for hypoxemia from exhaustion of the dam, progressing involution, detachment of the placenta, and damage to the respiratory center. Postpartum care should also be planned at the same time a treatment for dystocia is developed. For the well-being of the dam the clinician must consider and prepare for puerperal and parturient problems and for a living foal (artificial respiration, supply of oxygen, stimulation of the cardiovascular system, etc.).

A skilled clinician needs first-quality instruments to correct difficult dystocia. Some heroic instruments of the past belong in a museum. Remarkable improvement in instrumentation has occurred, which has greatly reduced the unnecessary fight between mare and clinician. A Thygesen's wire saw fetotome and accessories are a must for the veterinarian wishing to do a fetotomy.

Drugs which can be useful in treating dystocia cases include tranquilizers (be cautious if the fetus is alive), anesthetics, antibiotics, spasmolytics, oxygen, oxytocin, prostaglandins, analeptics such as doxapram, glucocorticosteriods, and lubricants (e.g., carboxymethylcellulose, mineral oil, petroleum jelly).

The clinician should select an area with sufficient space for working on a standing or recumbent mare, enabling hygienic manipulations with minimal contamination and trauma to the genital tissues.[2–4] The clinician must also be aware of personal danger (kicking, sudden going down of the mare, etc.); the use of a nose twitch as well as a rope side line to secure the hindlegs are indicated.[5]

After correction of dystocia, the clinician must remember that the normal uterine defense includes bacterial phagocytosis by neutrophils and macrophages. This important defense mechanism can be destroyed by antiseptics and some irritating antibiotics[2,4] (Fig. 68–1).

POSITION OF FETUS

Any fetal displacement which causes a substantial increase of the cross diameter of the fetus hinders normal birth. Fetal disposition involves presentation (anterior, posterior, and transverse), position (dorsal, lateral, and ventral), and posture (head, neck, and limbs in anterior, posterior, and transverse presentation). Previously, only a limited number of dystocia cases were reported for which reliable data were available on the incidence of various maldisposition causes of dystocia. Presented in Table 68–1 are data from 601 mares with dystocia for which the maldisposition was recorded.

From these data note that posterior and transverse presentations greatly increased the percentage of dystocia cases. Vandeplassche and Lauwers showed that the incidence (< 2%) of posterior presentation is the result of a strongly preferential final rotation of the fetus at about 7 to 8 months of gestation.[6] No explanation for the cause and low incidence of transverse presentations is known. Some simple maldispositions are corrected by veterinarians in practice, and these cases are often not recorded. Therefore, the incidence of fetal maldisposition presented to a referral clinic does not fully correspond with what occurs in practice. Nevertheless, the comparative figures are so unexpectedly different, that maldisposition must be a common cause of dystocia.

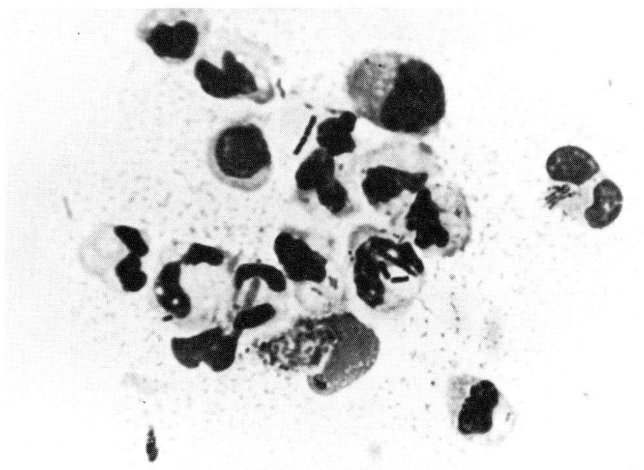

FIG. 68–1. Gram-stained smear of uterine exudate from postpartum mare. Phagocytosis and advanced digestion of bacteria by neutrophils and free bacteria are evident. This natural defense mechanism can be altered by harsh chemicals and chemotherapeutic agents.

TABLE 68–1. A COMPARATIVE STUDY OF FETAL PRESENTATION IN A POPULATION OF APPROXIMATELY 170,000 FOALING MARES COMPARED WITH 601 MARES WITH DYSTOCIA; BOTH SPREAD OVER A PERIOD OF 40 YR

	NORMAL POPULATION OF 170,000 FOALING MARES	MARES WITH DYSTOCIA* (N = 601)
Anterior presentation	168,130 (98.9%)	408 (68%)
Posterior presentation	1,700 (1.0%)	95 (16%)
Transverse presentation	170 (0.1%)	98 (16%)

*Treated in clinic.

The causes of dystocia in 408 mares delivered with the fetus in anterior presentation are shown in Table 68–2, and the methods of correction for those with reflected head are summarized in Table 68–3.

ANTERIOR PRESENTATION

Reflected Head and Neck

A reflected head and neck (Fig. 68–2) was diagnosed in 58% (237/408) of dystocias with the fetus in anterior presentation and in 39% (237/601) of all dystocia in mares brought to our clinic. Methods of correction included reposition, fetotomy, and cesarean section. Reposition should be attempted first in all cases in which the fetus is alive. Success depends on a favorable ratio of fetal size to space in the uterus and pelvic inlet, degree of uterine tonicity, arm length of the clinician, his or her skill and the existence of torticollis and face scoliosis.[7]

When treating a dystocia, the hindquarters of the mare should be elevated when possible. Furthermore, maldisposition is more easily corrected under epidural anesthesia and with copious application of the fetus and genital tract with a nonirritating lubricant. Petroleum jelly is preferred in our clinic. The clinician should first

TABLE 68–2. CAUSES OF DYSTOCIA IN 408 MARES IN WHICH THE FETUS WAS IN AN ANTERIOR PRESENTATION

CAUSES	NUMBER	PERCENT
Reflected head and eventually limbs	237/408	58
Abnormal posture, malformed front limbs, ventral position, oversize fetus, hydrocephalus, etc.	171/408	42

TABLE 68–3. METHOD OF DELIVERY IN 237 CASES OF DYSTOCIA WITH FETUS IN ANTERIOR PRESENTATION AND REFLECTED HEAD

METHOD	NUMBER	PERCENT
Reposition	64/237	27
Fetotomy	154/237	65
Cesarean section	19/237	8

identify a reference point on the fetal head such as an ear, one or both orbits, or the mouth. In some cases, eyehooks can be fixed in the lacrimal canals to maintain the reference of the fetal head. No serious damage is caused to the eyes with this procedure. Before pulling on the head, maximal repulsion of the fetal trunk deeply into the uterus is absolutely necessary to provide sufficient free room for stretching the head and neck into the birth canal.

When reposition is unsuccessful, cesarean section is indicated for a living fetus. However, the clinician must take into consideration the rather frequent presence of a wryneck deformation, which may recover in an otherwise vital foal[7] (Fig. 68–3). When the fetus is dead, partial fetotomy is the method of choice for correction. If a wire saw leader can be passed through the split of the concave side of the bent neck, a simple longitudinal section can be made by applying the head of the fetotome halfway on the convex side of the neck. Usually the amputated head of the fetus can be removed before extraction of the remaining fetus. When removal of the amputated head turns out to be difficult, the clinician

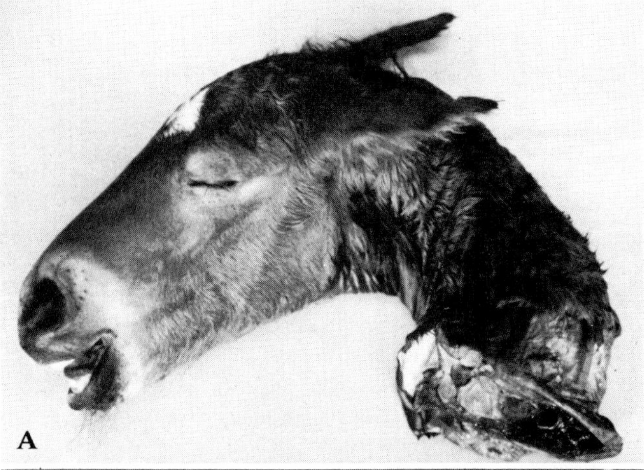

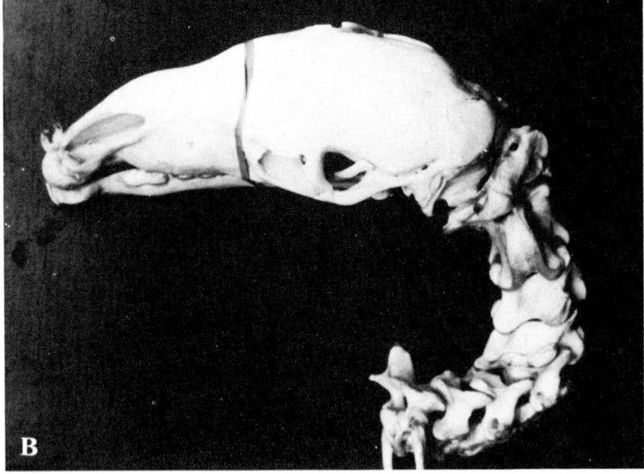

FIG. 68–2. *A*, Foal from a partial bicornual gestation, delivered by cesarean section. Note scoliotic head and wryneck. *B*, Partial skeleton of same foal. Note malformed vertebrae, particularly C4, C5, and C6.

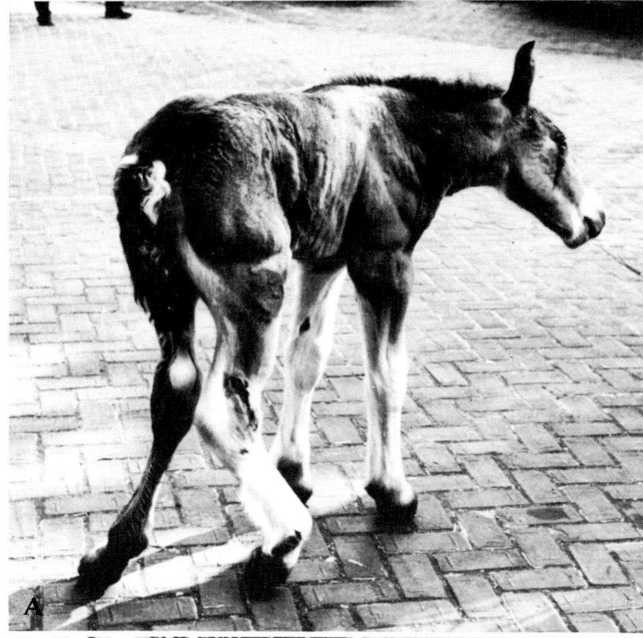

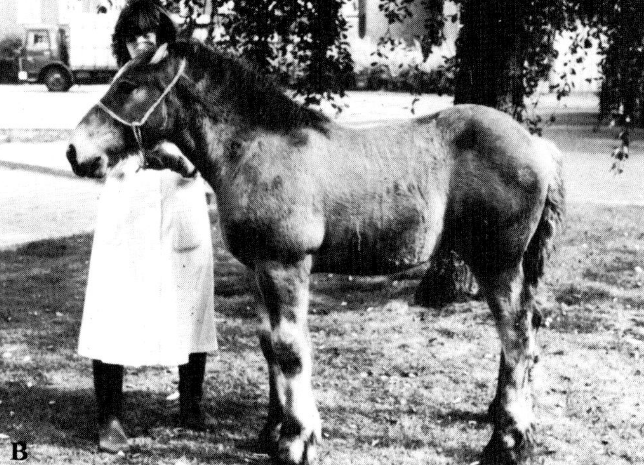

FIG. 68–3. *A*, Foal delivered by cesarean section from an incomplete bicornual gestation. Although foal was alive, reposition was impossible because the foal was oversize and grossly malformed (scoliosis of the head, torticollis, and malformed hindlegs). *B*, Same foal almost fully recovered at age of 3 months. (From Vandeplassche, M.: Embryotomy and cesarotomy. *In* Textbook of Large Animal Surgery. 2nd ed. Edited by F.W. Oehme. Baltimore, Williams & Wilkins, 1982, pp. 598–622.)

may find it preferable to push it deeper into the uterus, and to extract first the fetus and then the head.

In exceptional cases, the head can be reflected so far backward and the neck bent so intensely, that the clinician cannot get a wire saw leader around the neck. If the fetus is dead, the simplest way of delivery is to amputate the easiest-to-reach forelimb by an oblique section in which the head of the fetotome is fixed on the top of the scapula while the wire saw loop runs in the axilla. After removal of one forelimb, the thoracic girdle is markedly diminished, so that the fetal body penetrates sufficiently deeper into the cranial pelvic ring to get the wire saw leader around the neck for amputation. Two fetotomy cuts can be performed in half an hour or less.

Incomplete Extension of the Elbows

Incomplete extension of the elbows is uncommon in most horse breeds, but does occur in strongly muscled draft horses. Diagnosis can be made by inspection, because the hooves lie at the same level as the fetal muzzle. Reposition can easily be performed on the standing mare, by retropulsion of the head and the body of the fetus after epidural anesthesia and lubrication of the genital tract. Extension of the limbs, one by one, is usually followed by a normal birth.

Carpal Flexion Posture

Carpal flexion can be unilateral or bilateral. By itself such posture does not provoke a severe dystocia, if it is not accompanied by flexion of the elbow and of the scapulohumeral joint. Correction of the flexed carpal joint is usually easy if the basic conditions for reposition have been fulfilled (epidural anesthesia, copious lubrication, elevating hindquarters of mare, etc.). Retropulsion of the fetus and manipulations of fetal parts are always easier if the clinician can create free space in the uterine body. If the fetus is dead or extension of the carpal joint is difficult or impossible as in case of ankylosis, a cross-sectional fetotomy cut through the middle of the carpal joint is the most desirable method of correction. After removal of the amputated metacarpus, the fetus should be retropulsed to facilitate extension of the elbow and shoulder. Normal expulsion of the fetus follows, assisted by traction when necessary.

Shoulder Flexion Posture

Retention of one or of both forelimbs will cause dystocia. When the size of the fetus and favorable uterine space is available, a postural correction in two phases should be attempted. First, the shoulder flexion is reduced to a carpal flexion and, second, the carpal flexion is extended. The clinician should remember that such a reposition, usually of both limbs, can be difficult and time consuming, reducing the chances of a live foal. In most cases, cesarean section is indicated.

When the fetus is dead, amputation of a forelimb can be considered. If a wire saw leader can be passed through the axilla, the head of the fetotome is then fixed on the upper line of the scapula, which results in a longitudinal section that amputates a complete forelimb. After removal of that limb, a substantial increase of uterine space is obtained, sufficient for manual extension of the second limb and a normal birth.

Foot-Nape Posture

An upward displacement—usually of both forelegs, which lie in the vagina above the extended head—hinders spontaneous expulsion of the fetus. This condition can represent a serious danger for rupture of the roof of the vagina and sometimes perforation of the rectum as a consequence of strong abdominal straining. To correct this dystocia, the fetus must be repulsed backward and downward into the uterus. In some instances, the limbs must be removed from perforations in the dorsal vagina. Correction is best accompanied with the mare standing, utilizing epidural anesthesia and after injection of 100 to 200 mg of a tocolytic drug such as isoxsuprine lactate (Duphospasmin-Duphar, B.V., Weesp, Holland). Once free space has been obtained cranial to the pelvic inlet, both forelimbs can be brought under the head. After extension of the forelimbs, head, and neck, the foal can be delivered with adapted traction. In most cases, ruptures of the vagina and rectum are retroperitoneal, so little direct risk of peritonitis exists. Depending on the place and size of ruptures, surgical correction can be attempted immediately after delivery or several weeks later when inflammation has totally subsided.

POSTERIOR PRESENTATION

Abnormal Position

In 95 mares delivering foals in posterior presentation, 47 (50%) also were in lateral or ventral position, compared with only 13% (52/408) for fetuses presented in anterior presentation. A logical explanation for such a remarkable difference is difficult. However, no doubt exists that lateral and especially ventral fetal positions provoke severe dystocia. The reason is that the fetus, by being out of its normal position, loses the advantage of pelvic space because its convex rigid backbone misses the excavated roof of the pelvic canal and becomes blocked by the bony pelvic brim or shaft of the ilium. Manual correction toward a dorsal position can be done on the standing or recumbent mare, but optimal preparations are necessary for sufficient obstetric room combined with profuse lubrication. A substantial amount of manual correction can be obtained from well-adapted traction on both limbs crossed in such a way that a mechanical torsion effect is produced. In a living fetus, this is more easily achieved with a "position reflex" of the fetus. Correction of a ventral position can be quite difficult. Correction depends on the size of the fetus, the free obstetric space, a well-relaxed uterus, and the strength of the clinician.

TABLE 68–4. POSTURE OF 95 EQUINE FETUSES PRESENTED IN POSTERIOR PRESENTATION

POSTURE	NUMBER	PERCENT
Extended hindlimbs	24/95	25
Hip flexion (94% bilateral)	47/95	50
Hock flexion (90% bilateral)	24/95	25

Hip Flexion and Hock Flexion Postures

Of 95 dystocias in mares with posterior presentation, 94% of those with hip flexures and 90% with hock flexures were bilateral (Table 68–4). When the fetus is alive, the clinician should attempt to correct the posture manually. However, be aware that only exceptionally will a living foal be born from such a dystocia. Consequently, reposition should only be attempted when a favorable relationship exists between fetal size and free uterine space. A hip flexion must first be changed to a hock flexion, which then must be extended. Correction of a hock flexion is particularly dangerous because of the possibility of perforation of the roof of the uterine body by the hock joint. Cesarean section or fetotomy seem to be preferable, even when the fetus is already dead.

For a dead fetus in the hock flexion posture, an embryotomy cut just below the hock joints, can be performed easily and with little danger. After removal of the amputated metatarsi, the fetal body is repulsed into the uterus, to facilitate extension of the thighs and delivery is usually normal.

In evaluating data from 95 mares in dystocia caused by posterior presentation (Table 68-5), 46% of the deliveries were made by fetotomy, needing an average of 2.8 sections. That can be explained, at least partly, by the fact that about half of the 95 deliveries occurred in a period (from 1940 to 1970) when cesarean section was not yet fully accepted by most horse breeders. No doubt a much higher percentage of those mares should have had cesarean sections.

TRANSVERSE PRESENTATION

For a transverse presentation to occur, the fetus normally develops in one horn and uterine body and expands from the early pregnant horn into the opposite horn. Because of the crosslike structure of the equine uterus, with both horns transversely directed on the uterine body, the result is a bicornual gestation with the body containing the whole or partial fetus (Fig. 68–4).

From a large number of observations made on pregnant uteri at slaughter and on the structure of afterbirths, the fetus in transverse presentation appears to be tightly packed in both horns, and this is frequently aggravated by an oversize fetus developed from an extra large placenta. These two factors can lead to malformation of the forelimbs and head and neck (wryneck).[7,8] The observations indicated that a transverse presentation will almost never develop or disappear at parturition (Table 68–6). Therefore, complete and incomplete transverse presentations at term originate from bicornual gestations. Ventrotransverse presentations are the rule and dorsotransverse presentations are exceptional.

TABLE 68–5. METHOD OF CORRECTION AND DELIVERY IN 95 MARES WITH DYSTOCIA IN WHICH THE FETUS WAS PRESENTED IN POSTERIOR PRESENTATION

METHOD	NUMBER	PERCENT	SURVIVAL RATE	PERCENT
Reposition	20	21	4	20
Fetotomy	44	46	0	0
Cesarean	12	13	7	58
Traction	19	20	6	32

Fetuses in transverse presentation at birth totally prevent spontaneous parturition. Labor only increases the blockage of the fetus in both horns, and reflexive abdominal straining is usually absent. The diagnosis is easy to make. In cases of complete bicornual pregnancy, the hand and fingertips of the clinician can hardly touch the fetus. In cases of partial bicornual gestation, only one or more limbs can be palpated deeply in the birth tract. However, the fetal trunk, head, and neck remain out of reach.

When the fetus is alive, delivery method of choice is cesarean section. Reposition can be considered, when all obstetric circumstances are extremely favorable. However, the procedure will often take too much time and the fetus will likely die before delivery. In case of incomplete bicornual gestation, with a dead fetus, an experienced clinician can perform a partial fetotomy followed by reposition to a longitudinal fetal presentation and normal delivery.

Presented in Table 68–7 are the methods of handling 98 mares in dystocia with foals in transverse presentation. The data represent mares seen between 1940 and 1970, a period in which cesarean section was not yet considered a fully justified delivery method for mares. Note that 47% of the deliveries made by fetotomy needed an average of 3.3 sections (Fig. 68–5). This is explained by the exceptionally well trained clinicians experienced in fetotomy. Most, if not all, of the fetoto-

TABLE 68–6. TRANSVERSE PRESENTATION (PARTIAL OR COMPLETE BICORNUAL GESTATION) IN 98 MARES AT SLAUGHTER

CORNUAL GESTATION	NUMBER	PERCENT
Complete	47	48
Partial	51	52

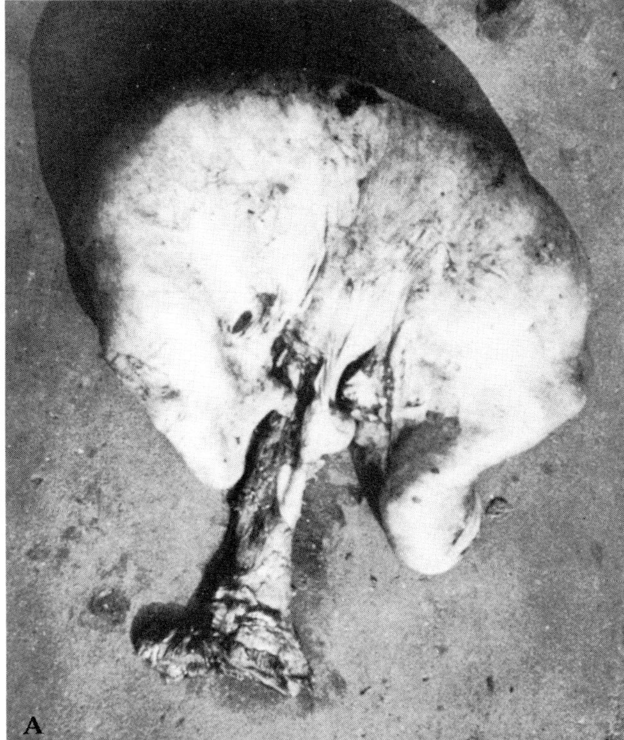

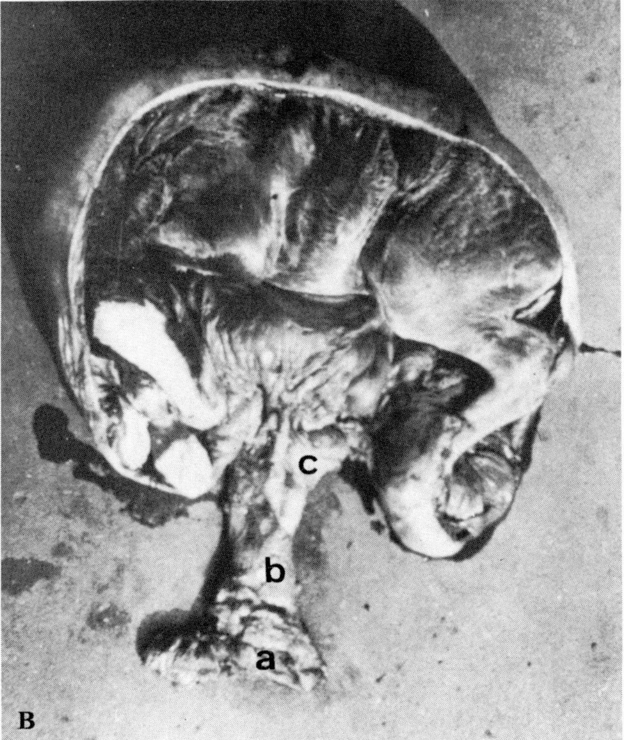

FIG. 68–4. *A,* A complete bicornual pregnancy. Intact uterus was removed at necropsy. Note contracted tips of uterine horns and small uterine body. *B,* Uterus has been opened to view the transverse presentation of fetus. a, the vulva; b, the vagina; c, the cervix. (From Vandeplassche, M.: Embryotomy and cesarotomy. *In* Textbook of Large Animal Surgery. 2nd ed. Edited by F.W. Oehme. Baltimore, Williams & Wilkins, 1982, pp. 598–622.)

TABLE 68–7. TREATMENT METHOD OF 98 MARES IN DYSTOCIA WITH FETUSES IN TRANSVERSE PRESENTATION (BICORNUAL GESTATION)

METHOD	NUMBER	PERCENT
Cesarean	46	47
Fetotomy (mean of 3.3 cuts)	47	47
Reposition	5	6

mies for fetuses in transverse presentation requiring more than two sections should actually be replaced by cesarean section.

UTERINE TORSION

About 50% of uterine torsions in mares occur during parturition. The remaining cases of uterine torsion occur before parturition from 7.5 months of gestation until term.[1,9,10] Methods of correcting uterine torsion that do not occur at parturition are discussed in detail in Chapter 53. In addition to the twisted uterus, the position of the fetus is disturbed and can vary from ventral to dorsal and again ventral, depending on the degree of torsion. The torsion is undoubtedly the main cause of the dystocia; however, the abnormal fetal position is also a contributing factor.

A history of slow signs of labor and colic often suggest uterine torsion.[11] Confirmation is usually easy by

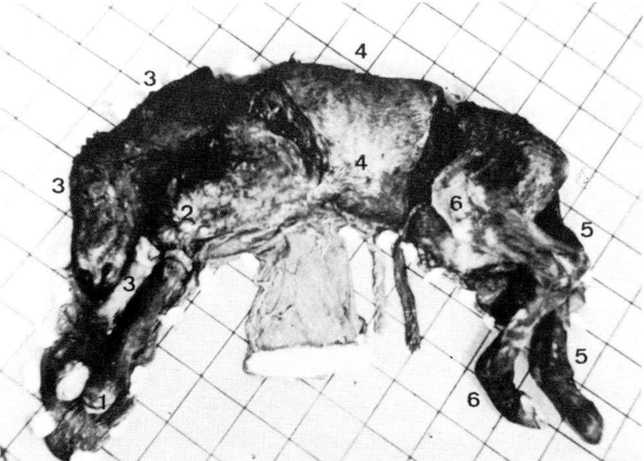

FIG. 68–5. Total fetotomy in which a foal was sectioned into six fetal pieces (labeled 1 through 6). The sections have been replaced in their original position of the ventral transverse presentation (total bicornual pregnancy). Two clinicians needed 2 h to complete this extremely difficult embryotomy. A cesarean section would be a better treatment approach. (From Vandeplassche, M.: Embryotomy and cesarotomy. *In* Textbook of Large Animal Surgery. 2nd ed. Edited by F.W. Oehme. Baltimore, Williams & Wilkins, 1982, pp. 598–622.)

vaginal and rectal palpation. At vaginal palpation, clear torsion folds of the vaginal wall are uncommon but are more pronounced in the cervix of some mares. A diagnosis of torsion is best established by rectal palpation. Characteristically, the fetus that is repulsed deeply into the lumen of the uterus cannot be reached because of the twisted walls of the uterine body and by the crossed broad ligaments of the uterus. These ligaments provide a good estimation of degree of torsion and a conformation of the direction of torsion. In case of a left (counterclockwise) torsion, the left uterine ligament (starting from the lumbar region) is strongly stretched and runs immediately downward under the uterine body. The right ligament runs directly from the lumbar region to the left and farther under the uterine body. When the torsion is clockwise and exceeds 180°, the right ligament is under strong tension and runs immediately under the right side of the uterus; the left ligament is more flabby and runs to the right side and under the uterus.

Successful detorsion depends mainly on whether the hand and arm of the clinician can pass through the cervical canal.[12,13] Entry may at first seem impossible; however, with adequate lubrication of the torsion folds and gentle persistence, the hand can usually be inserted through the cervix far enough to fix the head or hindquarters of the fetus. To do detorsion, an epidural helps eliminate abdominal straining and the hindquarters of the mare should be elevated by 15 to 20 cm. This will provide more room in the posterior part of the abdominal cavity, because the large and small bowel will move forward and the pregnant uterus can be detorsed with minimal resistance from friction on adjacent structures. The clinician inserts the hand and arm as deeply as possible into the uterus and under a substantial part of the fetus (do not grasp the feet). The uterus and fetus are then rocked back and forth until with an extra effort and in a semicircular movement—opposite to the direction of the torsion—the uterus and fetus are rotated over a sort of dead point, thus correcting the torsion. A second similar detorsion technique may be necessary for a complete detorsion. Complete detorsion is almost always characterized by a projection and rupture of the allantochorion, dorsal position of the fetus, and a normal position of the uterine ligaments on rectal palpation. After detorsion, the clinician should determine if the fetus is alive or dead. Delivery of the foal after detorsion usually requires some time as vascular congestion and edema diminish uterine contractions. The birth canal from the cervix to the vulva may need massage to help relaxation and full dilation.

More than 80% of the uterine torsions seen at parturition can be corrected by the above technique. Unsuccessful cases are often complicated by an oversize dead fetus, a rupture of the uterus, or large accumulation of fetal fluids. Correction by rolling the mare or use of a plank,[14] are controversial and generally disappointing when hand passage of the cervix is impossible.

When the hand of the operator cannot pass through the cervix, a standing laparotomy can be performed to correct the torsion (see Chapter 53). If the torsion cannot be corrected by laparotomy, the incision can be extended and a cesarean performed (see Chapter 50).

TRACTION

More than 90% of foalings are spontaneous, because uterine contractions and expulsive efforts of the mare are sufficient to accomplish the first and second stages of parturition. However, natural events can fail in the first stage of labor from uterine inertia or perhaps be insufficient in the second stage of labor because of an unfavorable relationship between the cross diameter of the fetus (the thoracic and pelvic girdle) and the space in the pelvic canal.

Traction can be used to assist a protracted birth, prevent needless exhaustion of the dam, and improve the chances for survival of the fetus. Traction remains an important benefit for delivery in mares, on the condition that it is applied "lege artis." The basic rules to assist parturition with traction in cases of dystocia are summarized in Table 68–8.

When dystocia is caused by uterine inertia (relapses may occur in consecutive years in the same mare), the defective labor should be supported by an injection of oxytocin, eventually combined with an intravenous infusion of calcium gluconate. Obstetric manipulations and traction also stimulate the release of endogenous oxytocin. Traction is preferentially made by two or exceptionally three medium- to above-average-strength individuals, which means a traction force of no more than 250 to 300 kg is applied. When lay help is not available, a fetal extractor equipped with a force-control system can be used by an experienced veterinarian. Excessive traction signifies a serious risk for the dam (contusions and lacerations of the uterus and birth canal and traumatic lesions of the obturator nerves and more particularly the gluteal nerves, which may cause paralysis of the hindlimbs often followed by muscular atrophy) and for the fetus (damage of vertebrae, ribs, and limbs and sometimes rupture of the liver).

The most important indications for obstetric traction in mares are insufficient uterine contractions, oversize fetus, and/or a narrow pelvis (mainly in primiparous mares). Occasionally traction on a fetus in anterior presentation succeeds in passage to its thoracic girdle, but

TABLE 68–8. RULES TO BE RESPECTED WHEN TRACTION IS USED IN EQUINE OBSTETRICS

1. Traction is first of all a diagnostic method to be stopped before it becomes dangerous.
2. The birth tract should be fully relaxed and lubricated.
3. Traction is to support maximal natural expulsive forces.
4. Traction should be minimal to help, not to replace, the natural expulsive forces of dam.
5. Never use "forced extraction."
6. Synchronize traction with abdominal straining.

the pelvic ring becomes blocked in the pelvis of the dam (hip lock). When the fetus is still alive, a slight retropulsion enables a copious smearing of the hindquarters with lubricant. After repulsion and lubrication, rotation of the fetus to the right and to the left, and traction together with abdominal straining of the dam usually frees the fetus. Once the fetus is dead, fetotomy is indicated. A transverse section in the lumbar region followed by a longitudinal section of the hindquarters in two halves will allow removal of the fetus.

A special case report of dystocia should be mentioned. A heavy Belgian Draft mare (950 kg after delivery) for which excessive traction was used (six men) delivered a live foal weighing 136 kg. The foal died 10 min later; the dam was fully intact. No doubt such mares are an absolute indication for cesarean section. However, the clinician and client are frequently too anxious to deliver the fetus and excessive traction is applied before this is recognized.

Some authors suggest an episiotomy in cases of difficult parturition. The real resistance for fetal expulsion rarely originates from a narrow vulva; lubrication and massage of the vestibulum and the vulva and a little patience have always been effective in our hands. We consider an episiotomy contraindicated for dystocia in mares.

FETOTOMY (EMBRYOTOMY)

All fetotomy operations are understood to be percutaneous, using a Thygesen-fetotomy set and accessories (Fig. 68–6). Other embryotomy instruments are much more limited in their use and are a risk of trauma to the dam. The objective of a fetotomy is to save the mare's life and her subsequent fertility, occasionally sacrificing a living fetus, especially if the owner is unwilling to select cesarean section.

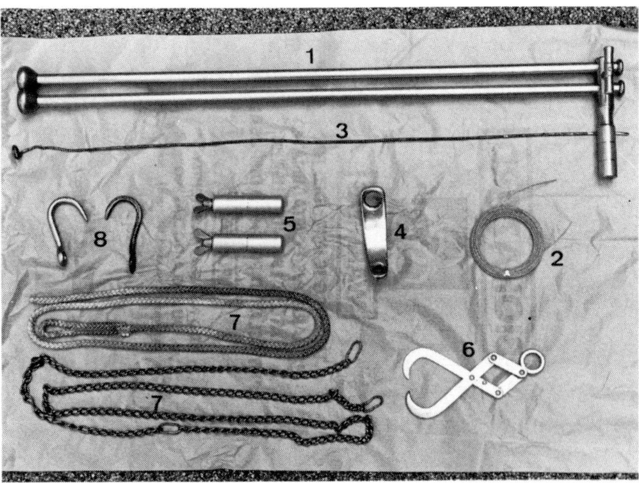

FIG. 68–6. Thygesen's fetotome and accessories. 1, Thygesen's fetotome, (85 cm); 2, wire saw, Liess model; 3, wire saw sounding line; 4, wire saw leader; 5, handgrips for wire saw; 6, double-jointed hook of Krey-Shöttler; 7, obstetric snare and chain; 8, eyehooks.

MATERIALS AND METHODS

About 500 fetotomies have been performed at our obstetric or ambulatory clinic of which 80% were partial and 20% total. About 60% of the patients were of the Belgian Draft Horse breed. Almost all partial fetotomies were made with the mare standing, whereas total fetotomies, as a rule, were made on mares in lateral recumbency. The policies listed in Table 68–9 were applied to all fetotomy procedures.

A clinician has several options to avoid breaking one of the "ten commandments of fetotomy" (Table 68-9).

1. Elevation of the hindquarters of the mare (about 20 cm) will provide additional free abdominal space to

TABLE 68–9. THE TEN COMMANDMENTS FOR FETOTOMY IN THE MARE

1. A well-immobilized dam (standing or in lateral recumbency) with elevated hindquarters.
2. Abolish or diminish abdominal straining by epidural anesthesia.
3. Prevent spasmodic uterine ring formations with a uterine relaxant.
4. Copious use of a nonirritating lubricant.
5. For most transverse and oblique cuts, first introduce, before the wire saw loop is brought forward, the head of the fetotome to its final desired location in the dorsal half of the genital tract. The head of the fetotome is in the hollow of the hand and permanent finger contact with the fetus is essential.
6. For some longitudinal sections, start by introducing the wire saw leader around the neck or a limb, then thread the wire saw through the second tube of the fetotome and adapt the fetotome to the fetal part for section.
7. A solid fixation of the head of the fetotome in longitudinal and lateral locations is necessary.
8. Prevent breaking of the wire saw by palpating after each section for any broken wire. Any break in one of the 27 strands of the wire can mean a serious risk for the wire to break during the next cut.
9. Prevent all needless entering and internal maneuvres in the genital tract. This will minimize trauma of the uterus and birth canal and reduce contamination.
10. An experienced, skillful clinician is essential for good results.

repel the fetus away from the birth canal into the uterus, which facilitates obstetric manipulations and reduces trauma to sensitive genital tissues.
2. Epidural anesthesia is valuable in substantially reducing the expulsive efforts of the dam. It is more effective in the standing than recumbent mare. The injection site is between the first and second coccygeal vertebra and 7 to 10 mL of 2% lidocaine is usually injected. To prevent excessive repulsive efforts in mares in lateral recumbency, a general anesthetic may be necessary. Good results can be obtained with glyceryl guaiacolate, 30 to 50 g in a 10% solution given intravenously or other short-acting anesthetic agents.
3. In case of a contracted uterus, particularly when spasmodic ring formations are present, an injection of a tocolytic drug may relax the uterus and reduce the trauma to the reproductive tract.
4. Putting and keeping the head of the fetotome in its definite place must be done by the clinician; an assistant is responsible for sawing.
5. Fetotomy requires much more training and experience to reach a level of proficiency than cesarean section.

INDICATIONS AND METHODS OF FETOTOMY

Most of the indications and results of fetotomy have been described under the headings of reposition and traction and in Tables 68–2, 68–3, 68–5, and 68–7. In the mare and cow only partial fetotomy is easily performed. The drawbacks of a total embryotomy are related to time, trauma, and danger to the life and future fertility of the dam. Cesarean section is usually preferable to total fetotomy. However, some special indications for fetotomy do exist.

Hydrocephalus

Hydrocephalus is not unusual in the mare, particularly in Ponies, and cause such a substantial increase of the cross diameter of the head, that eutocia becomes impossible. Hydrocephalus is when the bones of the skull have enlarged because of increased intracranial pressure, resulting in a hard, bony deformity that almost doubles the size of the head. Hydrocephalus is usually easily differentiated from encephalocele in which excessive accumulation of liquid in the lateral ventricles has forced a soft sac through a split in the skull. Some fetuses with encephalocoele will be born normally. The diagnosis is easy for fetuses in anterior presentation. In rare cases of posterior presentation, hydrocephalus should be suspected when fetal expulsion is stopped after normal passage of the hindquarters and trunk.

Delivery is usually simple in cases of encephalocoele. A perforating incision results in the evacuation of fluid, reducing head size to normal. For a hydrocephalic fetus, a wire saw loop is placed behind the ears of the fetus and the head of the fetotome is fixed in the mouth. A longitudinal section will remove the dorsal half of the fetal head.

A Double-Headed Fetus

A double-headed fetus causes impossible delivery. To amputate one head, the wire saw loop is passed around the throat area and the head of the fetotome is placed to the caudodorsal part of the fetal head. The resulting cut will produce a slightly obliqual-transverse section, amputating one of the two fetal heads. Normal expulsion of the fetus can follow.

Other Fetal Malformations

For a small, dead fetus, fetotomy can be indicated when not more than two embryotomy cuts are required. For large fetuses with severe malformations, cesarean section is preferable.

THE OBSTETRIC RESULTS OF FETOTOMY

Results obtained with fetotomy are presented in Tables 68–5 and 68–10. The results are less favorable because total fetotomies have been included. Although 90% of the mares undergoing fetotomy recovered, note that even with partial fetotomy some contusion and superficial lesions occur in the genital tract. This may cause local inflammation, scar tissue formation, and subsequent adhesions. After fetotomy, involution is often prolonged but varies from mare to mare. An increased incidence of retained placenta compared with normal parturition[3,15] and an increase in puerperal endometritis[16,17] occur. Because of the increased risks of retained placenta and endometritis, especially in cases of atonic uterus, administration of systemic antibiotics is indicated.[1] If uterine involution is delayed and oxytocin is ineffective in reducing its size, infusion of the uterus for a few days

TABLE 68–10. OUTCOME OF 202 FETOTOMIES IN MARES (69 WERE TOTAL AND 133 PARTIAL FETOTOMIES)

CAUSE OF DYSTOCIA	NUMBER OF MARES	NUMBER OF RECOVERED
Reflected head and neck (some ankylotic)	102	98
Partial transverse presentation; fetus dead	37	30
Breech presentation with deformity or ankylosis of hindlegs; fetus dead	25	21
Deformity, ankylosis, or reflexion of forelegs	19	17
Oversize, dead fetus	12	9
Hydrocephalus or double head	7	7
Total	202	182 (90%)

after fetotomy with chemotherapeutic agents is indicated.

Fertility is lowered in cases of dystocia corrected by fetotomy. Future breeding soundness may be improved by giving a season's rest after fetotomy. However, a mare with an incomplete transverse presentation of the fetus in its first pregnancy was delivered by a relatively difficult (three sections) fetotomy. The mare recovered quite well and became pregnant from a breeding 52 days postpartum. At foaling, a circular ring of hard fibrous tissue, over a length of about 10 cm, was noted, leaving an opening of only 4 cm in diameter near the hymen. A normal foal was delivered by cesarean section. With some assistance, the placenta passed through the narrow scar tissue ring.

REFERENCES

1. Roberts, S.J.: Veterinary Obstetrics and Genital Diseases (Theriogenology). 3rd ed. Woodstock, VT, published by the author, 1986.
2. Vandeplassche, M., and Bouters, R.: Phagocytosis in the blood and uterine exudate of mares, cows and sows. Proceedings of the International Symposium of the World Association of Veterinary Laboratory Diagnosticians. Vol. 1. 1983, pp. 83–89.
3. Vandeplassche, M., et al.: Observations on involution and puerperal endometritis in mares. Irish Vet. J., *37:* 126–132, 1983.
4. Vandeplassche, M.: Stimulation and inhibition of phagocytosis in domestic animals. Proceedings of the International Congress on Animal Reproduction and Artificial Insemination, 1984, pp. 475–477.
5. Vandeplassche, M.: Obstetrician's view of the physiology of equine parturition and dystocia. Equine Vet. J., *12:*45–49, 1980.
6. Vandeplassche, M., and Lauwers, H.: The twisted umbilical cord: An expression of kinesis of the equine fetus. Anim. Reprod. Sci., *10:*163–175, 1986.
7. Vandeplassche, M., et al.: Aetiology and pathogenesis of congenital torticollis and head scoliosis in the equine fetus. Equine Vet. J., *16:*419–424, 1984.
8. Vandeplassche, M.: The pathogenesis of dystocia and fetal malformation in the horse. J. Reprod. Fertil. Suppl., *35:*547–552, 1987.
9. Pascoe, J.R., Meagher, D.M., and Wheat, J.D.: Surgical management of uterine torsion in the mare: A review of 26 cases. J. Am. Vet Med. Assoc., *179:*351–354, 1981.
10. Wichtel, J.J., Reinertson, E.L., and Clark, T.L.: Nonsurgical treatment of uterine torsion in seven mares. J. Am. Vet. Med. Assoc., *193:*337–338, 1988.
11. Wheat, J.D., and Meager, D.M.: Uterine torsion and rupture in mares. J. Am. Vet. Med. Assoc., *160:*881–884, 1972.
12. Vandeplassche, M., Paredis, F., and Bouters, R.: Flanksnede bij de rechstaande of neerliggende merrie voor het ontdraaien van torsio uteri. Vlaams Diergeneeskd. Tijdschr., *30:*1–2, 1961.
13. Spincemaille, J., Vandeplassche, M., and Bouters, R.: Optreden en behandeling van torsio uteri bij de merrie. Vlaams Diergeneeskd. Tijdschr., *39:*653–662, 1970.
14. Bowen, J.M., Gaboury, C., and Bousquet, D.: Non-surgical correction of a uterine torsion in a mare. Vet. Rec., *99:*495–496, 1976.
15. Vandeplassche, M., Spincemaille, J., and Bouters, R.: Aetiology, pathogenesis and treatment of retained placenta in the mare. Equine Vet. J., *3:*144–147, 1971.
16. Vandeplassche, M.: Immunité et métrite. Recl. Med. Vet., *163:*127–133, 1987.
17. Vandeplassche, M.: L'endométrite puerpérale chez la jument. Pratique Vet. Equine, *21:*1013, 1989.

CHAPTER 69

LACTATION

P.M. McCue

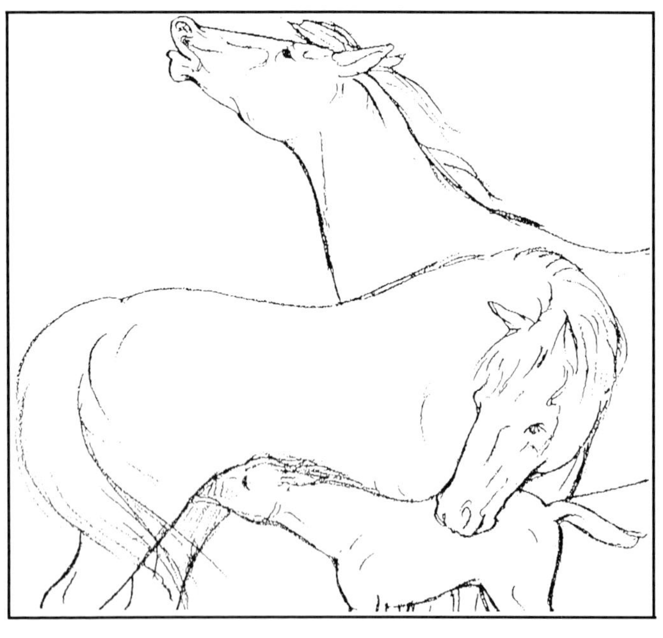

The mammary gland plays a key role in allowing the fetus to survive outside the uterus. It is responsible for providing the neonate with immunoglobulins critical to survival and supplies nutrition to the foal during the first few months of life. This chapter reviews the anatomy of the equine mammary gland and function of lactation; describes the primary components of colostrum, milk, and milk replacers; and discusses alterations of lactation, lactation-associated diseases, and selected diseases of the mammary gland.

ANATOMY OF THE MAMMARY GLAND

The mammary gland of the mare consists of paired mammae, separated by a fascial septum, each with a glandular body and teat.[1] The glandular portion of each half is divided by fibroelastic capsules into two, or occasionally three, lobes.

Milk is secreted by specialized epithelial cells into the lumen of alveoli and small ducts. Myoepithelial cells surround the alveoli and are important in the ejection of milk following a sucking stimulus.[2] Milk passes through progressively larger lactiferous ducts and then into the teat cistern before exiting at the teat orifice. Each of the mare's teats serves a cranial and caudal lobe of mammary tissue and has two corresponding teat orifices. See Chapter 1 for greater detail of anatomy of the mammary gland.

PHYSIOLOGY OF LACTATION

Development of the mammary gland and onset of lactation are complex processes under control of the hypothalamic-pituitary axis, ovaries, and placenta. Mammary growth and galactopoiesis are influenced by ovarian and adrenal steroids, prolactin, oxytocin, growth hormone, insulin, thyroid hormones, and other factors. Estrogen induces development of the mammary ducts. Progesterone stimulates lobuloalveolar growth, while at the same time inhibiting lactogenesis.[2] The trigger that initiates lactogenesis is thought to be the decline in progesterone and increase in prolactin that occurs late in gestation.[2]

Plasma prolactin concentration in the mare increases during the last week of gestation and remains elevated during early lactation before declining to baseline by 1 to 2 months postpartum.[3] Production of prolactin by lactotrophs in the anterior pituitary is regulated by hypothalamic secretion of a prolactin-inhibiting factor, thought to be dopamine. The presence of a placental lactogen as exists in primates, rodents, and ruminants has not been demonstrated in the mare.[4]

Oxytocin is synthesized in the supraoptic and paraventricular nuclei of the hypothalamus. Nursing by the foal stimulates the release of oxytocin from the neurohypophysis.[5] Oxytocin release induces contraction of myoepithelial cells surrounding the alveoli, causing expulsion of milk from the alveoli and small ducts into the larger lactiferous ducts and teat cisterns. Milk ejec-

TABLE 69–1. IMMUNOGLOBULIN CONTENT (MEAN ± SEM) OF COLOSTRUM AND SERUM OF STANDARDBRED MARES COLLECTED WITHIN 6 TO 12 H AFTER FOALING

IMMUNOGLOBULIN CLASS	COLOSTRUM (MG/DL)	SERUM (MG/DL)
IgG	8911.9 ± 1047.0	2463.9 ± 225.9
IgM	122.9 ± 12.9	136.4 ± 36.8
IgA	957.0 ± 183.8	305.2 ± 40.1

(Adapted from Kohn, C.W., et al.: Colestral and serum IgG, IgA, and IgM concentrations in Standardbred mares and their foals at parturition. J. Am. Vet. Med. Assoc., *195*:64–68, 1989.)

tion in the mare can also occur in the absence of tactile stimulation or a measurable oxytocin release.[6]

COMPONENTS OF COLOSTRUM AND MILK

The epitheliochorial placenta of the mare prevents transfer of maternal antibodies to the fetus in utero. The foal depends entirely on passive transfer of antibodies in colostrum for protection against infection during the early neonatal period (see Chapter 111). The mammary gland selectively concentrates immunoglobulins from the blood of the mare during the last 2 weeks of pregnancy.[7] After ingestion of colostrum, specialized enterocytes in the small intestine absorb the immunoglobulins by pinocytosis and transfer them to the systemic circulation of the foal. Absorptive capacity of the intestine is greatest during the first few hours after birth. Within 24 h after birth, the specialized enterocytes are replaced by cells incapable of transferring immunoglobulins.

Equine colostrum contains high concentrations of IgG, which decline rapidly during the first 24 h after foaling,[7–11] whereas the concentration of IgM and IgA in equine colostrum is relatively low (Table 69–1).[8] Premature lactation can significantly decrease the amount of immunoglobulins available to the neonate and may result in failure of passive transfer. The concentration of colostral immunoglobulins can be quantitated using radial immunodiffusion or estimated by measurement of specific gravity using a commercial colostrometer.[12]

Concentrations of total solids, protein, and amount of gross energy decrease abruptly during the first 12 h following foaling and continue to decline slowly throughout lactation[13,14] (Table 69–2). Conversely, lactose concentrations tend to rise slowly throughout lactation.[14] The mare has milk that is low in total solids, fat, and protein but high in lactose, which is somewhat rare in mammals.[15,16]

Mineral composition of mare's milk also varies with stage of lactation. Concentrations of total solids, ash, calcium, phosphorus, magnesium, copper, and zinc all decrease as lactation progresses[17–19] (Table 69–3). Composition of milk from nondomestic equids is similar to that of the domestic horse.[16] Mineral and electrolyte concentrations in prepartum mammary secretions can be used as an indicator of impending parturition and to evaluate fetal readiness for birth.[20–22] Concentrations of calcium and potassium increase while concentration of sodium decreases progressively in mammary secretions as parturition draws near. An increase in calcium concentration is the most reliable indicator of impending parturition.[20–22] Commercial kits are available to estimate calcium concentrations in prepartum mammary secretions and therefore predict the interval to spontaneous parturition (Predict-a-Foal, Animal Healthcare Products, Vernon, CA).

Lactation in the mare peaks at 1 to 2 months postpartum. Average daily milk production in Quarter horse mares ranges from 11.8 kg on day 30 of lactation to 9.8 kg on day 150 of lactation.[13] Daily milk production in the mare is equivalent to 2.1 to 3.4% of body weight.[13,23]

TABLE 69–2. COMPOSITION OF EQUINE MILK

WEEKS OF LACTATION	ENERGY (KCAL/100 G)	PROTEIN (%)	FAT (%)	LACTOSE (%)	TOTAL SOLIDS (%)
1–4	58	2.7	1.8	6.2	10.7
5–8	53	2.2	1.7	6.4	10.5
9–21	50	1.8	1.4	6.5	10.0

(Adapted from National Research Council: Nutrient Requirements of Horses. 5th ed. Washington, D.C., National Academy Press, 1989.)

TABLE 69–3. MINERAL CONSTITUENTS OF EQUINE MILK

Weeks of Lactation	CONCENTRATION (UG/G OF FLUID MILK)						
	Ca	P	Mg	K	Na	Cu	Zn
1–4	1200	725	90	700	225	0.45	2.5
5–8	1000	600	60	500	190	0.26	2.0
9–21	800	500	45	400	150	0.20	1.8

(Adapted from National Research Council: Nutritional Requirements of Horses. 5th ed. Washington, D.C., National Academy Press, 1989.)

MILK REPLACERS

It may become necessary to provide a foal with an alternative source of milk because of death or injury to the dam, rejection of the foal by the mare or inadequate lactation. Orphaned neonates must first be provided an adequate quantity of colostrum with a high immunoglobulin content. Foals should receive 250 mL of colostrum every hour for the first 6 h of life.[24] This may be accomplished via a bottle or passage of a small nasogastric tube. Once the foal has been given colostrum, the optimal approach would be to foster the foal onto a nurse mare if one is available.[25,26] Alternatively, orphaned foals have been fostered successfully onto cows or goats.[26]

If the foal cannot be fostered onto a nurse mare, it can be hand reared on a milk substitute such as fortified cow's milk or a commercial milk replacer (Table 69–4). Cow's milk (whole) has almost twice the fat content and only two-thirds the sugar content of mare's milk. Low-fat cow's milk (2% milk fat) can be used as a substitute for mare's milk if 20 g dextrose are added per liter. Fortified cow's milk should be fed to a total volume of 10% of the foal's body weight at 1 day of age.[25] The amount fed should be gradually increased to 25% of body weight per day from day 10 until weaning.

Many mare's milk replacer powders are commercially available (Table 69–5). Milk replacers should contain about 15% fat and 22% crude protein and have a fiber content of less than 0.5%. Manufacturers of milk replacers often recommend feeding a solution more concentrated than normal mare's milk. However, Naylor and Bell recommend that foals be fed a more dilute (12.5%) solution when using commercial milk replacers to avoid potential problems with constipation and dehydration.[24] Therefore, a greater volume of diluted milk replacer solution should be fed to provide the recommended total dry matter intake.

Foals can be artificially reared using a bottle, or they can be taught to drink from a bucket. Foals nurse from their dam more frequently during the first week of life than at any other age.[27] Consequently, recommended frequency of feeding orphan foals gradually decreases from every 1 to 2 h during the first few days after birth to every 4 to 6 h after 2 weeks of age.[24] Overall weight gains in foals reared on an artificial diet have been reported to be similar to gains in foals allowed to nurse from their dams.[28,29]

DIETARY REQUIREMENTS FOR LACTATION

Foaling mares should be fed good-quality roughage of at least 1 to 2% of body weight of dry matter per day. Supplementation with concentrates should be based on quality of the roughage, environmental conditions, nutritional status of the mare, and stage of lactation. Nutrient requirements of mares during early lactation are substantially greater than those of the pregnant or open mare.

Energy requirements during early and late lactation are 1.7 and 1.5 times, respectively, greater than neces-

TABLE 69–4. COMPARISON OF THE COMPOSITION OF MARE'S MILK WITH VARIOUS SUBSTITUTES

ITEM	MARE'S MILK	MILK REPLACER*	COW'S MILK	GOAT'S MILK
Fat, % of dry matter (DM)	15	14.4	29	34
Protein, % of DM	22.8	20.2	27	25
Sugar, % of DM	58.8	52.6	38	31
Fiber, % of DM	0	0.2	0	0
Total solids	11.6	20	12.3	13.2

*Foal-Lac, Borden, Inc., Hampshire, IL.

(Adapted from Naylor, J.M., and Bell, R.: Raising the orphan foal. Vet. Clin. North Am. Equine Pract., *1*:169–178, 1985.)

TABLE 69–5. COMMERCIAL MILK REPLACERS FOR ARTIFICIAL REARING OF FOALS

NAME	MANUFACTURER
Foal-Lac	Borden, Inc., Hampshire, Il.
Foal-Mate	Manna Pro, Los Angeles, CA
Nutrequin	Vetrepharm, Inc., London, Ont.
Wet Nurse	Prairie Microtech, Inc., Regina, Sask.

sary for maintenance in an open mare.[30] The National Research Council indicated that the percentage of dietary protein, calcium, and phosphorus during early lactation are approximately 1.7, 2.2, and 2.0 times that required for maintenance.[30] A 450-kg mare in early lactation, for example, would require a diet that contained 25.6 Mcal digestible energy, 12% protein, 0.47% calcium, and 0.30% phosphorus. Those requirements could be provided by feeding a ration of 6 kg of alfalfa hay and 4.1 kg of grain per day.

All horses should have free access to a clean water supply and a salt-mineral supplement. Water requirements of a lactating mare may be 50 to 70% above that required for a nonpregnant mare.[30] See Chapter 75 for additional information on nutritional requirements of pregnant mares.

WEANING

Foals are commonly weaned at 4 to 6 months of age. Weaning of individual foals may be accomplished by removing the dam from the box stall of the foal to another area of the farm, which is out of visual and auditory contact with the foal. After a few days in the stall, the foal may be placed into a small paddock with other weanlings. Alternatively, groups of foals housed with their dams in large paddocks may be weaned together by removing one or two mares every other day over a period of 1 to 2 weeks. An old gentle mare may be left with the weaned foals to have a quieting effect.[26]

Alveolar cells continue to secrete milk as long as milk is removed regularly from the mammary gland. After nursing ceases, mammary glands may become mildly distended with milk. Accumulation of milk initiates involutional changes in the mammary gland, resulting in decreased milk synthesis and glandular regression. Glandular distension will gradually subside without treatment. Mastitis occasionally occurs in the mare after abrupt weaning of the foal. Therefore, the mammary gland should be routinely monitored for development of mastitis for several weeks after weaning.

ECLAMPSIA

Lactation tetany, or eclampsia, is an uncommon disease that may occur in lactating mares in the early postpartum period or after weaning.[31,32] Mares producing large quantities of milk that are subjected to hard physical work or prolonged transport are most commonly affected. The syndrome is characterized by low serum calcium levels (4 to 6 mg/dL) and occasionally low magnesium levels. Severity of clinical signs—which may include a stiff gait, tachypnea, synchronous diaphragmatic flutter, and muscle tremors—is related to the degree of hypocalcemia. Without treatment, tetanic convulsions begin within 24 h and death occurs within 48 h. Treatment with a 20% calcium gluconate solution (250 to 500 mL per 450 kg, diluted 1:4 in saline or dextrose) results in a rapid recovery. Calcium solutions should be administered slowly intravenously while monitoring cardiovascular function. Retreatment may be required in some cases.

AGALACTIA

Agalactia is the failure of the mammary gland to secrete colostrum or milk following parturition. The clinical consequences of agalactia or hypogalactia in the periparturient mare are failure of passive transfer of immunoglobulins and inadequate milk supply to the neonate.

The factor most often incriminated in the pathogenesis of agalactia in mares in the United States is ingestion of fescue grass infected with the ergot alkaloid producing fungus Acremonium coenophialum.[33–35] In Brazil, ergot-alkaloid–induced agalactia has been reported to follow ingestion of oats infected with the fungus Claviceps purpurea.[36]

Pregnant mares maintained on pastures contaminated with a fungus-producing ergot alkaloid may exhibit a lack of udder development and agalactia, thickened fetal membranes that may be retained following parturition, prolonged gestation, abortion, uterine rupture, dystocia, and rebreeding problems.[35,36]

Agalactic mares often have serum prolactin concentrations that are lower than concentrations in normal lactating mares.[35,37] Ergot alkaloids depress prolactin secretion by their action as dopamine agonists and serotonin antagonists.[38] Administration of thyrotropin-releasing hormone (TRH) has been shown to stimulate prolactin secretion in the mare.[37,39,40] Other agents that cause an increase in prolactin by blocking the inhibitory action of dopamine include reserpine, phenothiazine tranquilizers, butyrophenones, metoclopramide, and sulpiride.[33,40–42]

Treatment of mares with fescue-induced agalactia is based on stimulation of pituitary prolactin synthesis. Induction of galactopoiesis in agalactic mares has been reported after administration of TRH,[39] reserpine,[33] and perphenazine[34] (Table 69–6).

Management recommendations for the prevention of fescue-associated reproductive problems include overseeding fescue pastures with legumes, removal of pregnant mares from fescue pastures 3 months before foaling, or supplementation with a nonfescue hay, such as alfalfa.[33,35]

Causes of lactation failure in the mare other than ergot alkaloid ingestion are not well documented. Factors

TABLE 69–6. MEDICATIONS USED TO STIMULATE LACTOGENESIS IN AGALACTIC MARES

DRUG	DOSE	ROUTE	REFERENCE
TRH	2.0 mg	SQ, bid	39
Reserpine	0.5–2.0 mg	IM q 48 h	33
Perphenazine	0.3–0.5 mg/kg	PO, bid	34

that may lead to hypogalactia include inadequate nutrition, selenium deficiency, and stress.[33] Further research is necessary to define the pathophysiologic conditions of lactation failure and to determine effective treatment regimens.

GALACTORRHEA

PREMATURE LACTATION

Pregnant mares may exhibit mammary development and begin lactation weeks or months before the expected foaling date. The causes of premature udder development and lactation in pregnant mares include impending abortion, in utero death of one twin fetus, placental separation, and bacterial or fungal placentitis.[7,43,44] Occasionally a pregnant mare will, for unknown reasons, show mammary enlargement during mid- to late gestation, which subsequently spontaneously regresses.

Premature lactation is one of the most important causes of failure of passive transfer caused by the loss of colostrum.[7] Lactation that occurs even a few hours before foaling may significantly reduce the quantity of immunoglobulins available to the neonate. Immunoglobulin content of presuckle colostrum of mares that have run milk before foaling should be evaluated by estimation of colostral specific gravity. Foals born to mares that lactated significantly before foaling should be supplemented with stored colostrum and their plasma immunoglobulin content subsequently assessed.

No specific treatment for premature lactation exists, because it is usually a symptom of another underlying disease. The efficacy of progestagen therapy for mares that have premature udder enlargement and lactation during midgestation is not known.

INAPPROPRIATE LACTATION

Neonates occasionally exhibit precocious mammary development with associated secretory activity, referred to as "witch's milk." This phenomenon, which has been observed in most domestic large animal species, has been attributed to elevations of lactogenic hormones of maternal origin in fetal circulation.[45] The incidence of galactorrhea in human infants has been reported to be approximately 6%.[46]

Transient glandular development and lactation are also occasionally observed in weanling foals, yearlings, and adult mares with no previous history of pregnancy or lactation. Causes of galactorrhea in these animals are not well defined. In humans, the most common cause of inappropriate lactation is an elevation in plasma prolactin concentration.[47] Treatment of choice for galactorrhea secondary to hyperprolactinemia in women has been bromocriptine or other dopamine agonists.[48] Bromocriptine is a semisynthetic ergot alkaloid which, like dopamine, directly inhibits prolactin secretion from pituitary lactotrophs, resulting in a decrease in lactogenesis. Bromocriptine mesylate (CB-154) administered at a dose of 10 mg has been reported to suppress prolactin concentrations when administered when basal levels of serum prolactin are at their seasonal high.[49] However, the dosage, efficacy, and safety of bromocriptine administration to horses as a treatment for inappropriate lactation has not been reported.

MASTITIS

Incidence of mastitis, or inflammation of the mammary gland, is much lower in mares than in dairy cattle. Clinical signs associated with mastitis include a warm, swollen, and painful udder; ventral edema; and fever.[50] Occasionally, systemic signs of illness, such as depression and anorexia or a mild degree of lameness in the hindlimb adjacent to the affected mammary gland will be exhibited. Mastitis usually occurs in adult horses, but has been reported in a 15-week-old filly.[51] A seasonal predilection for mastitis has been reported, with most mares affected during the summer.[50] Mastitis occurs most commonly during lactation or within 8 weeks after weaning a foal.[50,52,53] However, mastitis can occur in mares that have never been pregnant or have not lactated in over a year.[50,54–57]

Diagnosis of mastitis is usually made on the basis of clinical signs. Cytologic evaluation and culture of milk or mammary exudate may be used to confirm presence of mastitis. Cytologic evaluation of milk samples from mares with clinical and subclinical mastitis often show large numbers of neutrophils.[50,58] The most common bacterial organism obtained from aerobic culture of aseptically collected samples is Streptococcus zooepidemicus[50,53,56,59] (Table 69–7).

A combination of frequent milking, hotpacks or hydrotherapy, systemic antibiotics (i.e., trimethoprim-sulfamethoxazole), and possibly infusion of an intramammary antibiotic preparation is recommended for the treatment of equine mastitis. Nonsteroidal anti-inflammatory drugs such as flunixin meglumine or phenylbutazone may be indicated to relieve patient discomfort, decrease inflammation and stabilize an elevated body temperature. Clinical signs are usually abated within 2 to 3 days after medical treatment and the udder is almost normal within 1 week.

TABLE 69–7. ORGANISMS CULTURED FROM MILK OR MAMMARY EXUDATE OF MARES WITH CLINICAL MASTITIS

ORGANISM	NUMBER OF ISOLATES	PERCENT OF ALL ISOLATES
Streptococcus zooepidemicus	7	36.8
S. viridans	1	5.3
S. agalactiae	1	5.3
Staphylococcus sp.	2	10.5
Actinobacillus suis sp.	2	10.5
Pasteurella ureae	1	5.3
Enterobacter aerogenes	1	5.3
Klebsiella pneumoniae	2	10.5
Escherichia coli	1	5.3
Pseudomonas aeroginosa	1	5.3

(From McCue, P.M., and Wilson, W.D.: Equine mastitis—A review of 28 cases. Equine Vet. J., *21*:351–353, 1989.)

MISCELLANEOUS CAUSES OF MAMMARY GLAND ENLARGEMENT

UDDER EDEMA

Accumulations of ventral edema during the last weeks of gestation and the periparturient period may result in mammary gland enlargement. Affected mares may exhibit mild discomfort, a reluctance to move and may refuse to allow their foal to nurse.[60] Physiologic udder edema is most common in primiparous mares. Treatment, which is usually not necessary, consists of light controlled exercise, hydrotherapy, and possibly diuretics.

ABSCESSATION OF THE MAMMARY GLAND

Abscessation of the mammary gland or adjacent lymph nodes in California is most commonly associated with Corynebacterium pseudotuberculosis infections. Other bacteria cultured from mammary abscesses include Streptococcus zooepidemicus, S. equi, Staphylococcus sp., Peptostreptococcus anaerobius and Actinomyces naeslundii. Clinical signs include a unilaterally swollen, painful mammary gland, ventral edema, and often lameness. Abscessation is usually not associated with lactation. Treatment includes the establishment of ventral drainage, lavage, hotpacks or hydrotherapy, and occasionally antimicrobial agents and nonsteroidal anti-inflammatory drugs.

TUMORS OF THE MAMMARY GLAND

Tumors of the equine mammary gland are rare,[61] especially compared with the incidence in certain other domestic animals such as the bitch.[62] Recent reports of mammary carcinomas in three horses involved extensive metastases that spread by lymphatic channels and/or hematogenous routes.[63–65] Acland and Gillette reported a mammary carcinoma with metastases limited to the regional lymph nodes.[61] A total of 45 cases of mammary tumors were found during examinations of approximately 20,000 mares in a Paris abattoir.[66]

REFERENCES

1. Getty, R.: Sisson and Grossman's The Anatomy of the Domestic Animals. Philadelphia, W.B. Saunders, 1975, pp. 296–297.
2. Mepham, T.B.: Physiology of Lactation. Milton Keynes, Open University Press, 1987, pp. 109–127.
3. Worthy, K., et al.: Plasma prolactin concentrations and cyclic activity in pony mares during parturition and early lactation. J. Reprod. Fertil., *77*:569–574, 1986.
4. Forsyth, I.A., Rossdale, P.D., and Thomas C.R.: Studies on milk composition and lactogenic hormones in the mare. J. Reprod. Fertil. Suppl., *23*:631–635, 1975.
5. Sharma, O.P.: Release of oxytocin elicited by suckling stimulus in mares. J. Reprod. Fertil., *37*:421–423, 1974.
6. Ellendorff, F., and Schams, D.: Characteristics of milk ejection, associated intramammary pressure changes and oxytocin release in the mare. J. Endocrinol., *119*:219–227, 1988.
7. Jeffcott, L.B.: Passive transfer of immunity to foals. *In* Current Therapy in Equine Medicine. 2nd ed. Edited by N.E. Robinson. Philadelphia, W.B. Saunders, 1987, pp. 210–215.
8. Kohn, C.W., et al.: Colostral and serum IgG, IgA, and IgM concentrations in Standardbred mares and their foals at parturition. J. Am. Vet. Med. Assoc., *195*:64–68, 1989.
9. Lavoie, J.P., Spensley, M.S., Smith, B.P., and Mihalyi, J.: Colostral volume and immunoglobulin G and M determinations in mares. Am. J. Vet. Res., *50*:466–470, 1989.
10. Pearson, R.C., et al.: Times of appearance and disappearance of colostral IgG in the mare. Am. J. Vet. Res., *45*:186–190, 1984.
11. Rouse, B.T., and Ingram D.G.: The total protein and immunoglobulin profile of equine colostrum and milk. Immunology, *19*:901–907, 1970.
12. LeBlanc, M.M., McLaurin, B.I., and Boswell, R.: Relationships among serum immunoglobulin concentration in foals, colostral specific gravity, and colostral immunoglobulin concentration. J. Am. Vet. Med. Assoc., *189*:57–60, 1986.
13. Gibbs, P.G., Potter, G.D., Blake, R.W., and McMullan, W.C.: Milk production of Quarter Horse mares during 150 days of lactation. J. Anim. Sci., *54*:496–499, 1982.
14. Ullrey, D.E., Struthers, R.D., Hendricks, D.G., and Brent, B.E.: Composition of mare's milk. J. Anim. Sci., *25*:217–222, 1966.
15. Lukas, V.K., Albert, W.W., Owens, F.N., and Peters, A.: Lactation of Shetland mares. J. Anim. Sci., *34*:350, 1972.
16. Oftedal, O.T., and Jenness, R.: Interspecies variation in milk composition among horses, zebras and asses (Perissodactyla: Equidae). J. Dairy Res., *55*:57–66, 1988.
17. Linton, R.G.: The composition of mare's milk. II. The

variation in composition during lactation. J. Dairy Res., *8:*143–172, 1937.
18. Schryver, H.F., et al.: A comparison of the mineral composition of milk of domestic and captive wild equids (Equus Przewalski, E. zebra, E. burchelli, E. caballus, E. assinus). Comp. Biochem. Physiol., *85A:*233–235, 1986.
19. Schryver, H.F., et al.: Lactation in the horse: The mineral composition of mare milk. J. Nutr., *116:*2142–2147, 1986.
20. Peaker, M., Rossdale, P.D., Forsythe, I.A. and Falk, M.: Changes in mammary development and the composition of secretion during late pregnancy in the mare. J. Reprod. Fertil. Suppl., *27:*555–561, 1979.
21. Leadon, D.P., Jeffcott, L.B., and Rossdale, P.D.: Mammary secretions in normal spontaneous and induced premature parturition in the mare. Equine Vet. J., *16:*256–259, 1984.
22. Ousey, J.C., Dudan, F., and Rossdale, P.D.: Preliminary studies of mammary secretions in the mare to assess foetal readiness for birth. Equine Vet. J., *16:*259–263, 1984.
23. Oftedal, O.T., Hintz, H.F., and Schryver, H.F.: Lactation in the horse: milk composition and intake by foals. J. Nutr., *113:*2096–2106, 1983.
24. Naylor, J.M., and Bell, R.J.: Feeding the sick or orphaned foal. *In* Current Therapy in Equine Medicine. 2nd ed. Edited by N.E. Robinson. Philadelphia, W.B. Saunders, 1987, pp. 205–209.
25. Naylor, J.M., and Bell, R.: Raising the orphan foal. Vet. Clin. North Am. Equine Pract., *1:*169–178, 1985.
26. Rossdale, P.D., and Ricketts, S.W.: Equine and Stud Farm Medicine. 2nd ed. Philadelphia, Lea & Febiger, 1980.
27. Carson, K., and Wood-Gush, D.G.M.: Behaviour of Thoroughbred foals during nursing. Equine Vet. J., *15:* 257–262, 1983.
28. King, S.S., and Nequin, L.G.: An artificial rearing method to produce optimum growth in orphaned foals. J. Equine Vet. Sci., *9:*319–322, 1989.
29. Knight, D.A., and Tyznik, W.J.: The effect of artificial rearing on the growth of foals. J. Anim. Sci., *60:*1–5, 1985.
30. National Research Council: Nutrient Requirements of Horses. 5th ed. Washington, D.C., National Academy Press, 1989.
31. Blood, D.C., Radostits, O.M., and Henderson, J.A.: Veterinary Medicine. 6th ed. London, Bailliere Tindall, 1983.
32. Hintz, H.F.: Eclampsia. *In* Current Therapy in Equine Medicine. Edited by N.E. Robinson. Philadelphia, W.B. Saunders, 1983, p. 111.
33. Cowles, R.R.: Lactation failure in the mare. Proc. Soc. Theriogenol., 222–233, 1983.
34. Green, E.M., and Loch, W.E.: Fescue-induced agalactia in mares: management and treatment. Proc. Am. Coll. Vet. Intern. Med. Forum, 551–553, 1990.
35. Henton, J.E., Lothrop, C.D., Dean, D., and Waldrop, V.: Agalactia in the mare: A review and some new insights. Proc. Soc. Theriogenol., 203–221, 1983.
36. Riet-Correa, F., et al.: Agalactica, reproductive problems and neonatal mortality in horses associated with the ingestion of Claviceps purpurea. Aust. Vet. J., *65:*192–193, 1988.
37. Lothrop, C.D., Henton, J.E., Cole, B.B., and Nolan, H.L.: Prolactin response to thyrotrophin-releasing hormone stimulation in normal and agalactic mares. J. Reprod. Fertil. Suppl., *35:*277–280, 1987.
38. Floss, H.G., Cassady, J.M., and Robbers, J.E.: Influence of ergot alkaloids on pituitary prolactin and prolactin-dependent processes. J. Pharm. Sci., *62:*699–715, 1973.
39. Caudle, A.B., et al.: Effects of thyrotropin releasing hormone in agalactic mares. Proc. Soc. Theriogenol., 235, 1984.
40. Johnson, A.L. and Becker, S.E.: Effects of physiologic and pharmacologic agents on serum prolactin concentrations in the nonpregnant mare. J. Anim. Sci., *65:*1292–1297, 1987.
41. Brander, G.C., Pugh, D.M., and Bywater, R.J.: Veterinary Applied Pharmacology & Therapeutics. 4th ed. London, Bailliere Tindall, 1982.
42. Loch, W., Worthy, K., and Ireland, F.: The effect of phenothiazine on plasma prolactin levels in non-pregnant mares. Equine Vet. J., *22:*30–32, 1990.
43. Shideler, R.K.: Prenatal lactaton associated with twin pregnancy in the mare: a case report. J. Equine Vet. Sci., *7:*383–385, 1987.
44. Whitwell, K.E.: Fetal membrane abnormalities. *In* Current Therapy in Equine Medicine. 2nd ed. Edited by N.E. Robinson. Philadelphia, W.B. Saunders, 1987, pp. 528–531.
45. Roberts, S.J.: Veterinary Obstetrics and Genital Diseases (Theriogenology). 3rd ed. Woodstock, VT, published by the author, 1986.
46. Madlon-Kay, D.J.: Witch's milk. Am. J. Dis. Child., *140:*252–253, 1986.
47. Schindler, A.M.: Galactorrhea in a young teenage girl. Hosp. Pract., *23:*21–28, 1988.
48. Ho, K.Y., and Thorner, M.O.: Therapeutic applications of bromocryptine in endocrine and neurologic diseases. Drug, *36:*67–82, 1988.
49. Johnson, A.J., and Becker, S.E.: Effects of physiologic and pharmacologic agents on serum prolactin concentrations in the nonpregnant mare. J. Anim. Sci., *65:* 1292–1297, 1987.
50. McCue, P.M., and Wilson, W.D.: Equine mastitis—A review of 28 cases. Equine Vet. J., *21:*351–353, 1989.
51. Pugh, D.G., Magnusson, R.A., Modransky, P.D., and Darnton, K.R.: A case of mastitis in a young filly. J. Equine. Vet. Sci., *5:*132–134, 1985.
52. Addo, P.B., Wilcox, G.E., and Taussig, R.: Mastitis in a mare caused by C. ovis. Vet. Rec., *95:*193, 1974.
53. Al-Graibawi, M.A.A., Sharma, V.K., and Ali, S.I.: Mastitis in a mare. Vet. Rec., *115:*383, 1984.
54. O'Reilly, L.M.: The isolation of Bazeley and Battle's type 5 Streptococcus from a case of equine mastitis. Irish Vet. J., *19:*198–202, 1965.
55. Prentice, M.W.M.: Mastitis in the mare. Vet. Rec., *94:*380, 1974.
56. Welsh, R.D.: The significance of Streptococcus zooepidemicus in the horse. Equine Pract., *6:*6–16, 1984.
57. Roberts, M.C.: Pseudomonas aeruginosa mastitis in a dry non-pregnant pony mare. Equine Vet. J., *18:*146–147, 1986.
58. Freeman, K.P., Roszel, J.F., Slusher, S.H., and Young, D.: Cytologic features of equine mammary fluids: Normal and abnormal. Compend. Contin. Educ. Practicing Vet., *10:*1090–1099, 1988.
59. Strong, M.G.: Mastitis in the mare. Vet. Rec., *94:*526, 1974.
60. Spensley, M.S.: Alterations in lactation, *In* Large Animal Internal Medicine. Edited by B.P. Smith. St. Louis, C.V. Mosby, 1990, pp. 258–262.
61. Acland, H.M., and Gillette, D.M.: Mammary carcinoma in a mare. Vet. Pathol., *19:*93–95, 1982.

62. Moulton, J.E.: Tumors in Domestic Animals. Berkeley, University of California Press, 1961.

63. Munson, L.: Carcinoma of the mammary gland in a mare. J. Am. Vet. Med. Assoc., *191:*71–72, 1987.

64. Schmahl, V.W.: Solides karzinom der mamma bei einem pferd. Berl. Munch. Tierarztl. Wochenschr., *85:*141–142, 1972.

65. Foreman, J.H., Weidner, J.P., Parry, B.W. and Hargis, A.: Pleural effusion secondary to thoracic metastatic mammary adenocarcinoma in a mare. J. Am. Vet. Med. Assoc., *197:*1193–1195, 1990.

66. Martel, H.: Cancer in horses. Am. Vet. Rev., *44:*299–300, 1913–14.

CHAPTER 70

MISCELLANEOUS DISEASES OF PREGNANCY AND PARTURITION

R.M Lofstedt

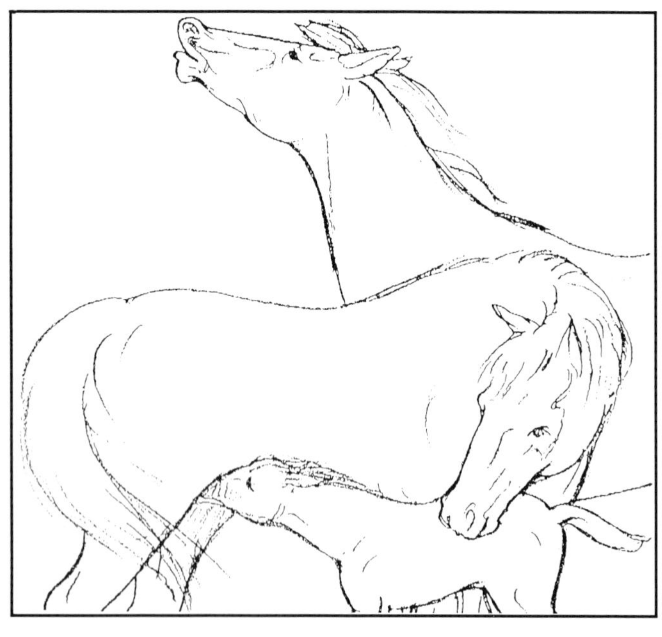

FETAL MALFORMATION CAUSED BY TRANSVERSE AND POSTERIOR PRESENTATION

The position of the fetus within the uterus appears to affect the incidence of fetal malformation in horses. In 601 cases of dystocia,[1] fetal anomalies were found to be disproportionally common when the fetus developed in posterior or transverse presentation. When the general incidence of posterior presentation was considered, the proportion of fetal malformation was almost 20 times higher than expected. In transverse presentations it was about 200 times higher than expected. These findings led to the suggestion that malformations occurred because the forequarters of the fetus became wedged within the narrow apex of the uterine horn in both presentations.[1] This constraint on fetal development may be particularly severe when the foal is transverse and the broad uterine body is unavailable to accommodate the fetus.

When live birth via caesarian section is possible, many foals with severe malformations (scoliosis, torticollis, and limb deformities) may recover spontaneously.[1] Therefore, decisions for euthanasia should be delayed in such cases.

UTERINE TORSION

Uterine torsion during advanced pregnancy is an important cause of uterine rupture and an occasional cause of serious hemorrhage; therefore, it is introduced briefly in this chapter. Uterine torsion is covered in detail in Chapters 53 and 68.

Mares with uterine torsion and impending rupture are seldom presented with acute abdominal pain, although this can occur when a loop of bowel has been strangulated by the twisted uterus. When the uterus becomes friable because of vascular strangulation, it can rupture spontaneously or during an attempt at correcting the torsion. Although uterine rupture can result in exsanguination and death, in my experience and that of others the fetus may come to lie in the abdomen while the mare appears to be in little or no distress. In such cases, laparotomy, fetal delivery, and hysteropexy should be performed immediately.[2–7]

HYDROPS OF THE FETAL MEMBRANES

Excess fluid can accumulate in the amnion (hydramnion, hydramnios, or hydrops amnion)[8,9] as well as the allantois (hydrallantois or hydrops allantois)[8,10–13] in mares. Hydrops allantois is more commonly reported, but both conditions are rare. The presence of hydrops amnion has been substantiated by drainage of fluid from a fetal sac that was specifically identified as the amnion by its palpable characteristics (well-developed blood vessels that diminish in size toward term).[8] Amnionic fluid can also be identified by its high sodium content (> 100 mmol/L).[8] In another case, the affected amnion was seen during postmortem examination.[9] A specific diagnosis of hydrops allantois can be made by drainage of large volumes of fluid after penetrating the chorioallantois.[10-13]

Normal volumes of allantoic fluid in mares vary from 8 to 18 L at term.[7] Comparative volumes of amnionic fluid vary from 3 to 7 L. Also, the normal weight of the placenta varies between 2.2 and 6.4 kg in various breeds.[10,14] Therefore, hydrops (of either or both fetal membranes) is likely if a mare experiences a total weight loss of more than the weight of the foal + 18 kg + 7 kg + 6.4 kg, or the weight of the foal + 31.4 kg during foaling.

The incidence of hydrops amnion is too low to develop general characteristics, but cases appear to be similar to those of hydrops allantois.[8-10] Mares of any age or breed appear to be susceptible to hydrops allantois. They are usually presented after 7 months of gestation with a history of rapid abdominal enlargement over the previous 10 to 14 days. They may have abdominal discomfort and labored breathing because of pressure on the diaphragm. In some cases, fluid accumulation in the uterus may be so dramatic that the mares walk with difficulty. They may even become recumbent. Severe ventral edema, abdominal pain, rupture of the abdominal muscles,[15] inguinal hernias, and uterine rupture[10,12] can also occur. The clinician usually finds it difficult or impossible to palpate a fetus, probably because the weight of the uterus makes it so dependent. Distension of the uterus may also restrict palpation of the fetus.

If spontaneous abortion is not in progress,[10] treatment should be directed at aborting the pregnancy. Abortion is usually induced by gradual cervical dilation (over 15 to 20 min), drainage of fetal fluid and forced extraction of the fetus. Forced extraction is typical because of uterine inertia. In most cases of hydrops, induction of abortion with oxytocin is not effective,[10,16] but if gestation is almost complete, oxytocin may be useful.[13] Because of a sudden loss of pressure on the abdominal vessels, a tendency for blood to pool in the abdomen is found, and severe shock and death can ensue. Therefore, fluid should be drained gradually from the uterus and intravenous fluid administered concomitantly to maintain blood pressure. When the acute phase has passed, oral electrolyte mixtures can be given to save on the cost of treatment.

In some cases of hydrops, the chorioallantois may be difficult to rupture by digital pressure because it can be thickened and edematous. In this instance, the chorioallantois should be drawn into the cranial vagina where it can be punctured more easily.[10] Upon rupture of the chorioallantios, the normally expected rush of fetal fluid may be absent,[8,10] probably because of extreme uterine atony.

Fetuses associated with hydrops allantois have been delivered alive. Some were normal, but too premature to survive, whereas others had abnormalities including severe ventral herniation,[8] growth retardation, wryneck, abnormal presentation (see the section on fetal malformation earlier in this chapter) limb ankylosis and deformity,[15] brachygnathia inferior, hydrocephalus, multiple mesotheliomas,[10] scoliosis, and hydrancephaly.[11] Hydrops allantois[12] and hydrops amnion[8-10] have both occurred in polytocous pregnancies, but neither condition is typically associated with twins or triplets.

Despite uterine inertia caused by hydrops, uterine involution appears to be almost normal once the fluid has been removed.[10] Presence of uterine fluid should be monitored by transrectal ultrasonography and drainage should be repeated as necessary.

Information on the fertility of mares that have been treated for either form of hydrops is lacking, but in two cases of hydrops allantois, the mares conceived after treatment and one of them delivered a normal foal.[10,13]

In most cases the origin of hydrops remains unknown; several causes may exist. One case of hydrops amnion was probably caused by blood vascular embarrassment, which was secondary to torsion of the amnion and umbilicus.[9] Hydrops allantois has been related to placentitis,[13,15] and a heritable cause is also possible.[11] A heritable cause is particularly likely because normal pregnancies occasionally follow hydroptic pregnancies.[10] For this reason, affected mares should probably be bred to different stallions if rebreeding is considered.

RUPTURE OF THE UTERUS BEFORE TERM

Uterine rupture usually occurs during the peripartum period as a result of mutation and fetotomy[7,17] or possibly because of violent intrapartum movement.[18,19] These problems are discussed in other chapters. However, in cases of uterine torsion and hydrops, the uterus can rupture before term.[2,9]

When the uterus ruptures before term, the mare may not show pain beyond that which is consistent with uterine torsion. In fact, if the fetus escapes into the abdomen and hemorrhage is not severe, uterine involution may occur and the entire episode may pass unnoticed by the owner. In one such case, the rupture was not detected during subsequent rectal palpation and the mare was diagnosed as nonpregnant (T.L. Clark, personal communication). Subsequent insemination caused peritonitis and death of the mare. During the postmortem examination, a near-term fetus was discovered in the peritoneal cavity (Fig. 70-1). In most cases of uterine rupture, severe hemorrhage appears to be unusual, despite the excellent blood supply to the uterus.[2,9] However, the possibility for exsanguination does exist.[7]

Diagnosis of uterine rupture may be facilitated by palpation of the uterus per rectum, by fetal examination, abdominal centesis (large volumes of clear fluid at multiple sites), and a history of moderate to severe abdominal pain during the last trimester of pregnancy. When the uterus is still twisted or distended with excessive fetal fluid, these features can be appreciable by rectal palpation. However, once the uterus has ruptured and its contents have escaped, the uterine wall may feel thickened and corrugated, because the uterus contracts and begins to involute almost immediately. If the fetus

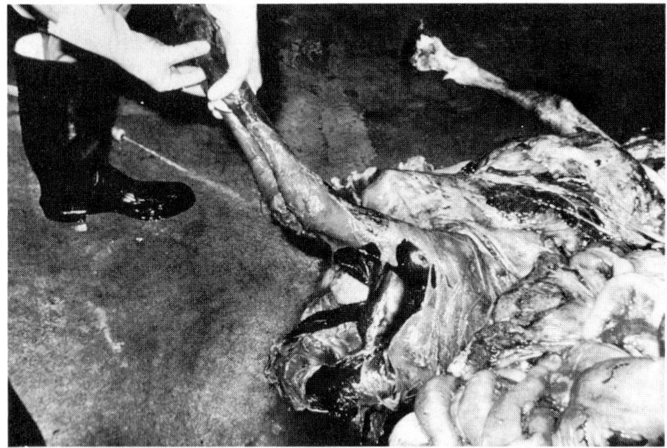

FIG. 70–1. Uterine rupture in a mare. The foal is being extracted from the abdominal cavity after death of the mare caused by peritonitis following artificial insemination. (Courtesy T.L. Clark, Iowa State University.)

is lying in the ventral abdomen, the operator will be struck by the absence of a fetus that is normally palpable per rectum. If the site of rupture is within reach, it may be palpable, but in most cases this is impossible, especially when the uterus has begun to contract and the wound margins are approaching apposition. The site of rupture may be equally difficult to demonstrate by transrectal ultrasonography. However, by transabdominal ultrasonography, the fetus may be seen on the floor of the abdomen.[9] Fetal ultrasonography[9] and electrocardiography[20] may add to the diagnosis because absence of a heartbeat is consistent with most cases of antepartum uterine rupture.[2] A definitive diagnosis is made via laparotomy.

Uterine rupture is usually repaired through a ventral midline incision,[2] but repair via uterine prolapse has also been described.[21] However, the latter approach was used at term when a fetus had already been delivered. Nevertheless, an adaption of the latter technique could be considered for field use if it were possible to extract the fetus per vagina.

FETAL MUMMIFICATION AND MACERATION

Mummification of one member of a set of twins happens occasionally during normal gestation and has no apparent significance in terms of the reproductive capacity of the mare. The mummified fetus may advance into the third trimester before dying but more commonly, it is small and dies during embryonal development. Therefore, when the fetal membranes are examined at foaling, the mummified cotwin is barely recognizable as an embryo. The reason for the death of an early embryo is obscure but when both concepti survive into the fetal stage, the death of one fetus probably occurs because the endometrial area is insufficient to maintain twin concepti. The death of the fetus is followed by its mummification.

Mummification and maceration of a single fetus is rare in horses. Some cases may arise when fetal problems prevent foaling[22] and others may occur when uterine torsion causes fetal death and then resolves spontaneously. Infectious or genetic causes of mummification and maceration condition are unknown in horses. Clinicians generally assume that an equine mummy can only exist when a cotwin is present to produce progestagens for the maintenance of pregnancy.[7] However, I and others have encountered singleton pregnancies either undergoing mummification or in a state of complete mummification (Fig. 70–2) or maceration (Fig. 70–3) (J.P. Hughes, personal communication; T.L. Clark, personal communication).[22]

Mares undergoing mummification may show signs of mammary enlargement and lactation such as those that are harbingers of abortion, but premonitory signs may be slight and can go unnoticed by the owner.[22] As a result, mummies are usually detected after mares have passed their expected foaling dates. A palpable absence of fetal fluid exists and the uterus is contracted around the fetus. If the fetus has been dead for some time and has become dehydrated, the angularity of the skeleton will be obvious. A highly echogenic mass can be seen during transrectal ultrasonography. If the cervix is open, the fetus and placenta may become infected and can undergo maceration. In those mares, a vulvar discharge may be seen. In cases of fetal mummification and maceration seen by me and others, little or no systemic involvement occurred, which is remarkable when related to the systemic condition of mares with retained placenta and severe metritis. However, it is consistent with the absence of systemic signs seen in cases of pyometra[23] and most likely demonstrates an intact endometrium. Whether mares with macerated or mummified fetuses are consistently anestrous, as is the case in cattle, is not known. Affected mares may experience variable cyclicity like those with pyometra.[23]

The mummified or macerated fetus can be removed by dilating the cervix over a period of 15 to 20 min.

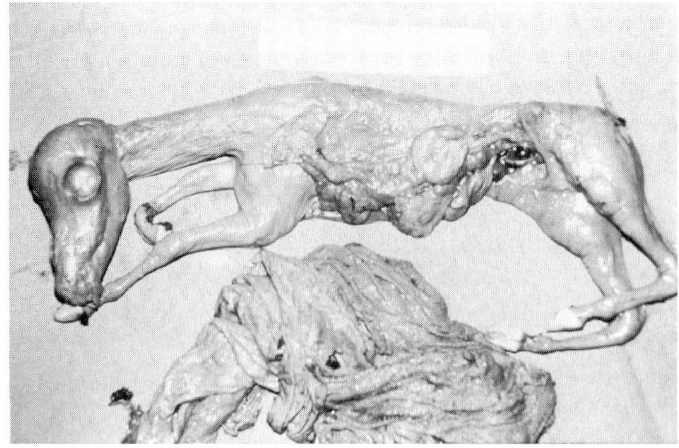

FIG. 70–2. A mummified equine fetus unaccompanied by a living cotwin. The fetus appeared to have died at approximately 5 months of gestation and was discovered when the mare passed her foaling date. (Courtesy T.L. Clark, Iowa State University.)

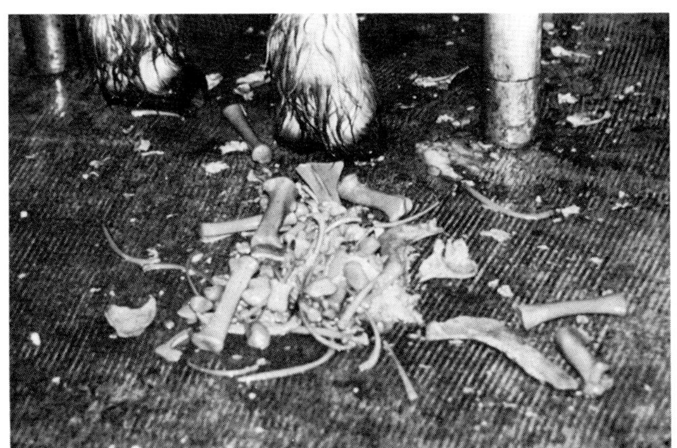

FIG. 70–3. The bones of a macerated equine fetus withdrawn from a mare that was systemically normal but had a history of a vulvar discharge.

When the cervix has been sufficiently dilated, the uterine contents are extracted. Pretreatment with 10 to 15 mg estradiol cypionate 24 h before attempting extraction may facilitate cervical dilation, but it does not have proven value and is not essential. After the mummified or macerated fetal parts have been removed, the uterus should be flushed with saline and antibiotics. Further use of antibiotics should be based on culture and sensitivity results. If the fetus is large and difficult to remove without causing uterine damage, it should be carefully removed by caesarian section.[22] The reproductive potential of mares treated for fetal mummification and maceration is unknown, but is probably compromised.

VENTRAL RUPTURES: RUPTURE OF THE PREPUBIC TENDON AND THE ABDOMINAL MUSCLES

Ventral herniation and rupture of the prepubic tendon are often discussed under separate headings. However, in this chapter ventral herniation of the abdominal wall (rupture of the oblique and transverse abdominis muscles), rupture of the prepubic tendon, and rupture of the rectus abdominis muscle will be discussed under the collective heading of ventral ruptures. In pregnant mares, these conditions can occur together,[15] can appear to have the same predisposing causes, can have similar or identical clinical presentations, and are frequently difficult or impossible to distinguish from one another in the living mare. In some cases, postmortem examination may be the only method by which to make a definitive diagnosis.

Rupture of the ventral abdominal musculature and the prepubic tendon occur in mares of all breeds during late gestation but draft mares may be predisposed to these problems.[7,15,24] Among 11 cases reviewed, the average age of mares was 11 y, suggesting that the conditions are more common in older mares.[7,15,24,25] A reference to idleness also conveys the impression that a lack of muscle tone predisposes a mare to ventral ruptures.[7] Extraordinary uterine weight as a result of twins or hydrops of fetal membranes are additional predisposing causes.[7,15] However, in most cases there is no obvious predisposing cause for musculotendinous failure.

Mares with ruptured ventral abdominal structures are typically close to foaling and are presented with abdominal pain and reluctance to walk. The abdominal pain can be confused with the pain of colic but can usually be differentiated from colic pain by discomfort shown when the caudal abdomen is palpated. The abdomen is usually dependent (Fig. 70–4) or may bulge ventrolaterad, but complete eventration is rare. Affected mares invariably show a thick plaque of ventral edema as well. This is far more obvious than the mild ventral edema that is commonly seen in normal mares at the end of pregnancy and does not disappear with exercise. The origin of this severe edema is not certain, but it probably arises because of uterine pressure on the caudal epigastric and caudal superficial epigastric veins (and possibly their cranial counterparts as well). The ventral abdomen is drained by these vessels. Edema may also be caused by trauma to the abdominal muscles.

If the prepubic tendon or rectus abdominis muscle ruptures completely and transversely, abdominal tension on the pecten of the pelvis is lost, causing a characteristic elevation of the ischial tuberosities.[7] The same phenomenon causes the udder to move craniad (Fig. 70–5). Sometimes edema around the mammary gland may cause the teats to become indistinct and the neonate may have difficulty suckling. In addition, tension on the mammary gland can cause rupture of its blood vessels, resulting in blood in the milk.

If a mare with a ventral abdominal defect has a gestation length of greater than 330 days, foaling should be induced,[26] because rupture of uterine blood vessels can occur[7] and abdominal discomfort and weakness can progress to a point at which the mare is no longer ambulatory. Although spontaneous foaling is possible,[24] traction is usually required because the mare is not able to exert an abdominal press. Passive immunity in the

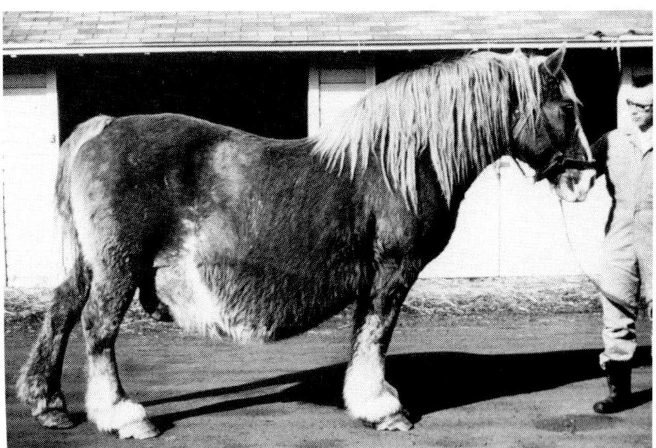

FIG. 70–4. A pregnant Suffolk-type Draft mare with rupture of either the prepubic tendon or rectus abdominis muscles. (Courtesy T.L. Clark, Iowa State University.)

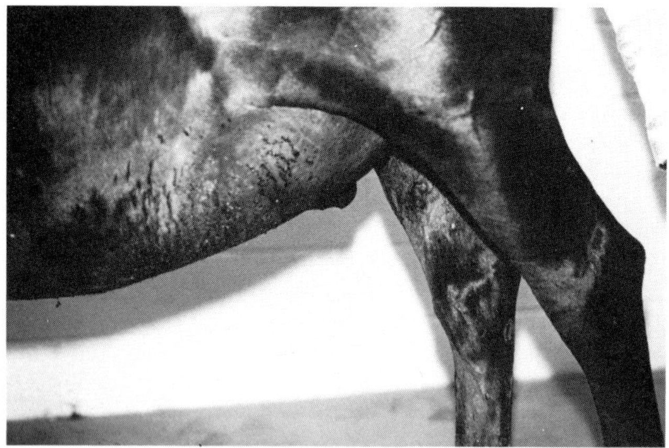

FIG. 70–5. A pregnant Standardbred mare with rupture of either the prepubic tendon or rectus abdominis muscles. Note how the mammary gland is drawn craniad and the teats are almost obliterated by edema.

foal should also be monitored, because it may be incomplete when foaling is induced.[27] If pregnancy is not sufficiently advanced, abdominal support (in the form of a special abdominal bandage or wrapping with wide adhesive tape) should be supplied until induction of parturition is feasible. In addition, a laxative diet should be fed to decrease tenesmus during defecation.

Immediately after the transverse and oblique abdominal muscles have ruptured[15] the site of rupture may not be distinct, but as edema resolves after foaling, the hernia can be delineated (Fig. 70–6). Repair of ventral abdominal defects after foaling has been described and appears to be highly effective.[25] However, the postoperative reproductive capacity of these mares has not been reported. I suggest that repair should only be contemplated if a chance exists that the inciting cause of the rupture will not recur, e.g., if the rupture was caused by hydrops allantois (see section on hydrops of the fetal membranes in this chapter) or external trauma. In most other cases, clinicians find little point in repairing structures that failed under the stress of normal pregnancy. If surgery is not performed, partial reduction of ventral ruptures can occur and the defect may become invisible after several weeks. If additional pregnancies are required and breed regulations allow it, embryo transfer should be considered. A few mares have delivered foals from subsequent pregnancies without complication but such cases require constant supervision and may have sudden remission.

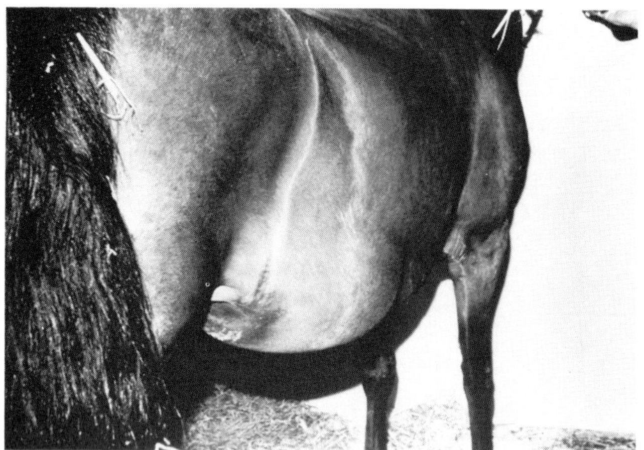

FIG. 70–6. A Standardbred mare with rupture of the right ventrolateral abdominal muscles 2 days after foaling. Because of extensive prepartum edema, the margins of the hernia only became evident after foaling, when some of the edema had resolved.

PROLONGED GESTATION

Prolonged gestation caused by abnormalities of the hypothalamic-hypophyseal-adrenal axis is well known in ruminants,[7] but does not seem to occur in horses. Gestation usually lasts for 310 to 374 days,[28] but normal pregnancies can be as long as 399 days.[29] Foals born from such pregnancies are not usually oversize as in cattle and do not predispose the mare to dystocia.[29] Little is known of this syndrome, but prolonged gestation has been attributed to delayed embryonic development, especially during the first 2 months of gestation.[29]

The duration of gestation is partly controlled by nutrition and the genotype of the foal,[28,30] but mares themselves may also control the duration of gestation. Based on the finding that average gestational durations were longer for mares bred earlier in the season, Ginther suggested that mares may be able to make limited adjustments to gestation so that their foals are born with an optimal chance for survival.[30] The physiologic control of this phenomenon is unknown, but it may be related to photoperiod. Although the capacity to prolong gestation (embryonal diapause or delayed embryonic development) may be unique to the horse among domestic animals, it is well known in other mammals.[31]

Many clients become concerned when their mares have not foaled by 11.5 months of gestation and begin to exert pressure on the veterinarian to induce foaling. If fetal movement is palpable, but no mammary development has occurred, the clinician should not yield to this pressure,[27] even if the duration of gestation is longer than 1 yr. Instead, the owner should be reassured that this is probably a normal phenomenon and that waiting should result in a normal foal, with adequate colostrum and normal passive immunity.

HEMORRHAGE ASSOCIATED WITH PREGNANCY AND PARTURITION

HEMORRHAGE FROM THE UTERUS DURING PREGNANCY AND FOALING

Fatal extrauterine hemorrhage can occur during pregnancy when major uterine vessels rupture. This may be caused by uterine torsion, uterine rupture, or trauma experienced during violent exercise or transport.[7] However, most cases of hemorrhage occur at foaling. Rupture can involve the uterine (middle uterine) arteries, utero-ovarian arteries, or external iliac arteries.[32] Severe intrauterine hemorrhage can also be seen when foaling trauma exists or when retained placentas are forcibly removed.

Older mares are especially predisposed to rupture of major vessels during pregnancy. In three studies that incorporated a total of 30 mares, the average age of 25 mares that died from hemorrhage was 18.5 yr.[32–34] The youngest mare was 12 yr old. A subgroup of 5 mares that only had hematomas of the broad ligament appeared to be slightly younger, with a mean age of about 12 yr.[34] Therefore, rupture of major vessels is associated with aging. In one study, a possible causal link was also established between serum copper concentrations, aging, and vascular degeneration.[33] The researchers showed that aged mares had significantly lower serum copper concentrations than young mares. Serum copper was also lower ($p < 0.05$) in mares that suffered fatal vascular ruptures than in unaffected mares. Mares that were able to recover after experiencing hemorrhage, had intermediate serum copper concentrations. The data on aging correlate well with degenerative changes and aneurisms described in other mares with ruptured uterine arteries.[32] Aging and repeated pregnancies also cause increased pressure within arteries as a result of dilation of the vessels (Laplace's law). Together with excessive tension on the arteries, these factors contribute to rupture.

The birth of a foal can exert pressure on the external iliac arteries and can also cause vascular rupture. In the iliac arteries, pressure from the fetus may cause local vascular hypoxia, damage to the arterial walls, and subsequent rupture.[32] This theory is tenable, because no direct tension on these arteries exists during pregnancy and no aneurisms have been seen in the iliac arteries during postmortem examinations.[32]

Of some interest was the finding that the majority of ruptured uterine blood vessels occurred on the right-hand side. This was associated with the presence of the caecum in the right flank, causing displacement of the uterus to the left with increased tension on the right uterine artery.[34] When ruptured uterine and external iliac arteries were examined by culture and biopsy, no infectious organisms or parasites were observed. In ruptured ovarian and uterine vessels, varying degrees of degeneration of the vessel walls occurred. By contrast, damage to the iliac arteries appeared to be more acute and was characterized by damage to the intima, with subsequent thrombus formation and eventual division of blood through the damaged vessel wall.[32]

When a vessel ruptures, hemorrhage may be contained within the mesometrium, but in some cases, arteries rupture directly into the abdomen. Sometimes bleeding can dissect the mesometrium until it ruptures and acute exsanguination may then occur.[32] The mare may die even if hemorrhage is contained within the mesometrium.

When a large artery ruptures during foaling, it may not be noticed immediately, because the discomfort of normal parturition and placental expulsion may mask the hemorrhage. However, classic signs of vascular rupture will soon be recognized.[17] These signs include colic, sweating, rapid pulse, anemia, and death. In some cases, death may occur within 30 min after foaling, but when delayed rupture of a hematoma occurs, death may occur after several weeks.[34] Palpation of a hematoma is often possible and usually causes discomfort, but in some cases, the hematoma cannot be felt per rectum and is only discovered when surgery is performed to investigate the cause of abdominal pain. In some mares, palpable masses may remain in the mesometrium for a long time after the event.[35]

When severe intrauterine hemorrhage occurs, e.g., when a placenta has been removed forcibly, a form of tamponade occurs and hemorrhage is not usually fatal. In such cases, broad-spectrum antibiotic coverage should be supplied and the clotted blood should be left in the uterus so that it is expelled as part of the lochia. Occasionally, these mares return to normal reproductive function.

Treatment of severe hemorrhage from ruptured arteries can be surgical or nonsurgical, but a high death rate can be expected in both cases. Little success may be found with blood transfusion,[36] but it is an attractive alternative to laparotomy because surgical risk is significant. Transfusion should begin as soon as possible after foaling, and plasma expansion therapy should be used as well. When the packed-cell volume is less than 20%, and blood is required for transfusion, the approximate amount of blood required (in liters) can be calculated by multiplying 8% of the body weight of the mare by the *missing fraction* of the normal packed-cell volume (PCV). For example, for a mare weighing 450 kg, the volume of whole blood required is $0.08 \times 450 \times 0.55$ (if the PCV measures 18%, i.e., if the PCV is 55% lower than normal) = 19.8 L. Up to 8 L blood can be removed from a healthy horse without adverse effect, and although this is not sufficient to raise the PCV of the affected mare to a normal level, it will raise it to above critical levels. Blood can be collected in a 4% solution of sodium citrate. A total of 1 L blood can be administered every 10 min,[37] but when exsanguination is occurring, the rate of administration can be faster. If the mare survives, blood typing should be done to assess the possibility of neonatal isoerythrolysis in future pregnancies. Movement of the mare should be restricted to decrease the possibility of dislodging blood clots and reinitiating bleeding.

As a result of the peracute nature of many cases of uterine hemorrhage and the difficulty of surgical intervention, the precise site of hemorrhage is usually unknown. Although the administration of oxytocin will have no value when the external iliac or major uterine arteries have ruptured, it may decrease hemorrhage when it is myometrial in origin or if bleeding is occurring into the uterine lumen. Therefore, doses of 40 to 60 IU q 30 min should be used in all cases of peripartum hemorrhage. Because of the severe discomfort associated with mesometrial hemorrhage, analgesics such as flunixin meglumine (1.0 mg/kg) and butorphanol tartrate (0.01 mg/kg) may be used as well.

HEMORRHAGE CAUSED BY VAGINAL AND VESTIBULAR TRAUMA DURING FOALING

Occasionally blood vessels in the vagina and vestibulum are damaged during foaling. Fortunately, most of these cases are not serious and require no treatment, except the administration of tetanus antitoxin and toxoid. Even when third-degree lacerations of the perineum exist, hemorrhage is seldom life threatening. If the hemorrhage is profuse and the damaged vessels cannot be ligated, a large tampon made of rolled cotton and umbilical tape may be used as a pressure bandage. It should be covered with petroleum jelly and an oily antibiotic preparation, such as a mastitis preparation.

When there are large hematomas in the vagina (Fig. 70–7), they may cause some difficulty in defecation. In such cases, the mare should be given a laxative diet until the hematoma becomes reduced in size. Hematomas can also be drained when the damaged blood vessel has been given time to heal.

HEMORRHAGE FROM THE EXTERNAL GENITALIA DURING PREGNANCY

Although the placenta is well vascularized, placental detachment, placentitis, and impending abortion are not usually associated with hemorrhage from the cervix. Therefore, owners can be assured that blood seen at the vulvar lips is usually unimportant and most likely originates from vaginal varicosities or vulvar trauma. An examination with a vaginal speculum will confirm this diagnosis. Blood can also originate from the urinary tract because of cystitis or urolithiasis; therefore, exclusion of urinary tract disease is also important.

In older mares, varicose veins occasionally develop in the vagina during pregnancy and in estrus. The reason for their presence is obscure because no effect of gravity on vaginal veins exists. Weakening of the veins with age, increased blood flow to the genitalia under the influence of estrogens, and retrograde pressure because of abdominal filling during advanced pregnancy may all be contributing causes. Occasionally these veins may rupture and are a source of hemorrhage from the vulva. Hemorrhage is seldom severe, but it can provoke suspicions of impending abortion.

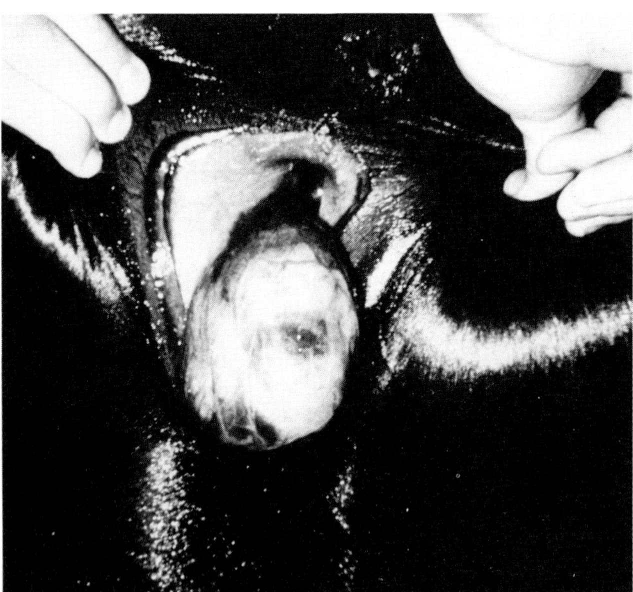

FIG. 70–7. A vaginal hematoma caused by foaling trauma. (Courtesy T.L. Clark, Iowa State University.)

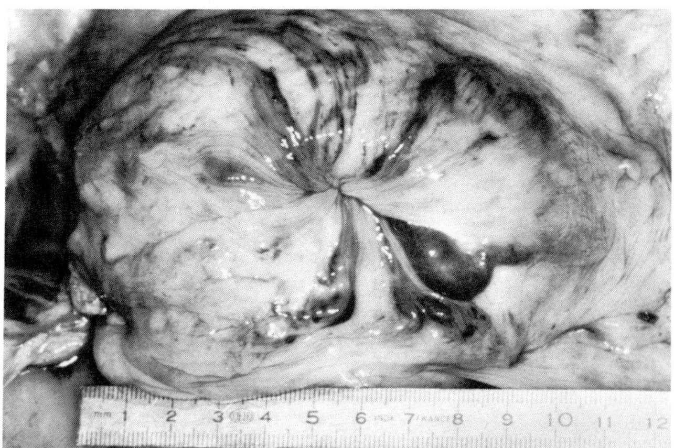

FIG. 70–8. A vaginal varicose vein in an aged mare. The vagina of this postmortem specimen has been everted to demonstrate the affected vessels.

Vaginal varicose veins can be up to 4 or 5 mm in diameter (Fig. 70–8) and are usually most obvious in the dorsal vaginal wall, just cranial to the urethral opening. These vessels can be ligated if hemorrhage is significant or persistent, but treatment is usually not required because the varicosities often shrink when pregnancy ends.

REFERENCES

1. Vandeplassche, M.M.: The pathogenesis of dystocia and fetal malformation in the horse. J. Reprod. Fertil. Suppl., *35:*547–552, 1987.
2. Pascoe, J.R., Meagher, D.M., and Wheat, J.D.: Surgical management of uterine torsion in the mare: A review of 26 cases. J. Am. Vet. Med. Assoc., *179:*351–354, 1981.
3. Wichtel, J.J., Reinertson, E.L., and Clark, T.L.: Nonsurgical treatment of uterine torsion in seven mares. J. Am. Vet. Med. Assoc., *193:*337–338, 1988.
4. Jones, R.D.: Diagnosis of uterine torsion in the mare and correction by standing flank laparotomy. Can. Vet. J., *17:*111–113, 1976.
5. Maxwell, J.A.L.: The correction of uterine torsion in a mare by caesarian section. Australian Vet. J., *55:*33–34, 1979.
6. Wheat, J.D., and Meager, D.M.: Uterine torsion and rupture in mares. J. Am. Vet. Med. Assoc., *160:*881–884, 1972.
7. Roberts, S.J.: Veterinary Obstetrics and Genital Diseases (Theriogenology). 3rd ed. Woodstock, VT, published by the author, 1986.

8. Allen, W.E.: Two cases of abnormal equine pregnancy associated with excess foetal fluid. Equine Vet. J., *18:*220–222, 1986.
9. Honnas, C.H., et al.: Hydramnios causing uterine rupture in a mare. J. Am. Vet. Med. Assoc., *193:*332–336, 1988.
10. Vandeplassche, M., et al.: Dropsy of the fetal sacs in mares: Induced and spontaneous abortion. Vet. Rec., *99:*67–69, 1976.
11. Waelchli, R.O., and Ehrensperger, F.: Two related cases of cerebellar abnormality in equine fetuses associated with hydrops of fetal membranes. Vet. Rec., *123:*513–514, 1988.
12. Blanchard, T.L., et al.: Hydrallantois in two mares. Equine Vet. Sci., *7:*222–225, 1987.
13. Koterba, A.M., Haibel, G.K., and Grimmet, J.B.: Respiratory distress in a premature foal secondary to hydrops allantois and placentitis. Compend. Contin. Educ. Practicing Vet., *5:*S121–S125, 1983.
14. Jennings, W.: Some common problems in horse breeding. Cornell Vet., *31:*197–216, 1941.
15. Hanson, R.R., and Todhunter, R.J.: Herniation of the abdominal wall in pregnant mares. J. Am. Vet. Med. Assoc., *189:*790–793, 1986.
16. Lofstedt, R.: Termination of unwanted pregnancy. *In* Current Therapy in Theriogenology. 2nd ed. Edited by D.A. Morrow. Philadelphia, W.B. Saunders, 1986, pp. 715–718.
17. Walker, D.F., and Vaughan, J.T.: Bovine and equine urogenital surgery. Philadelphia, Lea and Febiger, 1980
18. Patel, J., and Lofstedt., R.M.: Uterine rupture in a mare. J. Am. Vet. Med. Assoc., *189:*806–807, 1986.
19. Brooks, D.E., McCoy, D.J., and Martin, G.S.: Uterine rupture as a postpartum complication in two mares. J. Am. Vet. Med. Assoc., *187:*1377–1379, 1985.
20. Buss, D.D., Asbury, A.C., and Chevalier, L.: Limitations of equine fetal electrocardiography. J. Am. Vet. Med. Assoc., *177:*174–176, 1980.
21. Fischer, A.T., and Phillips, T.N.: Surgical repair of a ruptured uterus in five mares. Equine Vet. J., *18:*153–155, 1986.
22. Gilbert, R.O., et al.: Intrauterine death and onset of mummification of a single equine foetus. Equine Vet. J., *21:*301–302, 1989.
23. Hughes, J.P., et al.: Pyometra in the mare. J. Reprod. Fertil. Suppl., *27:*321–329, 1979.
24. Jackson, P.G.G.: Rupture of the prepubic tendon in a Shire mare. Vet. Rec., *111:*38, 1982.
25. Tulleners, E.P., and Fretz, P.B.: Prosthetic repair of large abdominal wall defects in horses and food animals. J. Am. Vet. Med. Assoc., *182:*258–262, 1983.
26. Carleton, C.L., and Threlfall, W.R.: Induction of parturition in the mare. *In* Current Therapy in Theriogenology. 2nd ed. Edited by D.A. Morrow. Philadelphia, W.B. Saunders, 1986, pp. 689–692.
27. Townsend, H.G.G., Tabel, H., and Bristol, F.M.: Induction of parturition in mares: Effect of passive transfer of immunity to foals. J. Am. Vet. Med. Assoc., *182:*255–257, 1983.
28. Rossdale, P.D., and Ricketts, S.W.: The practice of equine stud medicine. Baltimore, Williams and Wilkins, 1974.
29. Vandeplassche, M.: Obstetrician's view of the physiology of equine parturition and dystocia. Equine Vet. J., *12:*45–49, 1980.
30. Ginther, O.J.: Reproductive Biology of the Mare—Basic and Applied Aspects. Cross Plains, WI, published by the author, 1979.
31. Rowlands, I.W., and Weir, B.J.: Mammals: Non-primate eutherians. *In* Marshall's Physiology of Reproduction. Vol. 1. 4th ed. Edited by G.E. Lamming. Edinburgh, Churchill Livingstone, 1984, pp. 455–658.
32. Rooney, J.R.: Internal hemorrhage related to gestation in the mare. Cornell Vet., *54:*11–17, 1964.
33. Stowe, H.D.: Effects of age and impending parturition upon serum copper of Thoroughbred mares. J. Nutr., *95:*179–183, 1968.
34. Pascoe, R.R.: Rupture of the utero-ovarian or middle uterine artery in the mare at or near parturition. Vet. Rec., *104:*77, 1979.
35. Wenzel, J.G.W., Caudle, A.B., and White, N.A.: Treating for uterine intramural hematoma in a horse. Vet. Med., *80:*66–69, 1985.
36. Asbury, A.C.: The reproductive system. *In* Equine Medicine and Surgery. 3rd ed. Edited by R.A. Mannsman and E.S. McAllister. Santa Barbara, CA, American Veterinary Publications, 1982, pp. 1305–1367.
37. Becht, J.L., and Gordon, B.J.: Blood and plasma therapy. *In* Current Therapy in Equine Medicine. 2nd ed. Edited by N.E. Robinson. Philadelphia, W.B. Saunders, 1987, pp. 317–322.

CHAPTER 71

CONGENITAL DEFECTS IN FOALS

H.W. Leipold
S.M. Dennis

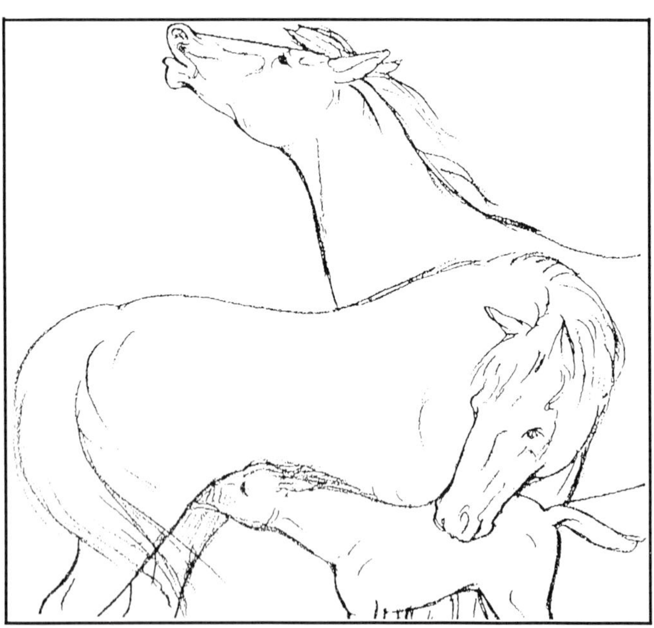

A wide spectrum of defects has been recorded in newborn foals, mostly from single case reports. Although defects are usually obvious at birth, diagnosis depends on the nature of such defects. Many defective foals are unnoticed and unrecorded and only a fraction comes to the attention of investigators interested in studying such defects. Presented in this chapter is a review of congenital defects in foals.

NATURE AND EFFECT AND CAUSES

Congenital defects are abnormalities of structure, function, and formation present at birth. Thus a defective neonate is an adapted survivor from a destructive event in the sequence of embryologic and fetal developmental processes. That disruptive event may lead to embryonic mortality, fetal death, abortion, stillbirth, or a defective neonate. Susceptibility to various teratogenic or genetic factors varies with the developmental stage and decreases with fetal development.

Congenital defects may involve a structure, several structures, a single function, or a syndrome combining various structures or functions. Differences occur among animals regarding which parts of the body are involved. In the horse, musculoskeletal and urogenital systems seem to be affected most commonly. Effects of congenital defects are many and diverse. They lower economic value of the mare and stallion involved and that of other relatives. Furthermore, embryonic death, fetal loss, and neonatal mortality lessen genetic gain, and control measures in breeding programs may require costly changes. In addition, congenital defects may cause a considerable emotional stress in people involved with the well-being of their horses.

FREQUENCY

The frequency of congenital defects in horses varies among breeds and geographical areas. The absolute frequency is difficult to obtain because many defects are identified only at necropsy and others are not reported. Incidence of congenital defects has been estimated as 3 to 4% of all foals born.[1] However, risk of foals being affected with congenital defects has been estimated to be intermediate between the low risk in cats and high risk in pigs.[2] Platt estimated that 3.5% of all live foals are affected with deformities.[3] The figures of Crowe and Swerczek are similar.[4] Among a total of 137,717 cases in clinics of veterinary colleges in the United States and Canada, 6,455 patients with congenital defects were reported; 17.5% were horses.[2] The most common equine congenital defects were cryptorchidism, contracted tendons, and dislocation of patella.[2]

CAUSES

Many reported defects in horses have no established cause. A total of 608 foals afflicted with congenital defects was examined between 1970 and 1982 in Kentucky. The breeds represented were 545 Thoroughbred, 53 Standardbreds, 4 Quarter Horses, 5 American Saddle Horses, and 1 mixed-ancestry foal. The most commonly diagnosed defect was tendon contracture in 202 cases (33.2%), followed by multiple defects (5.3%), microphthalmia (4.6%), craniofacial defects (3.5%), umbilical defect (3.5%), and hydrocephalus (3.0%); the remainder were less frequently diagnosed defects.[4] A recent review identified about 100 different congenital defects in horses.[5] Environmental factors have been incriminated only in a few. In contrast with other domestic animals, prenatal viral infections have not been identified as causes of defects in foals.

Poisoning by plants such as Astragalus mollisimus has resulted in abortions and congenital defects such as limb defects.[6] Arthrogryposis in foals has been linked to pregnant mares eating Sorghum vulgare during pregnancy.[7] The use of cambendazole for parasite control in pregnant Shetland Pony mares was incriminated in 3 deformed foals among 83 births.[8] Congenital defects observed were twisting of limbs below the tarsus in the first foal; multiple defects such as a short lower jaw, large eyes, deformed legs, and a constriction in the aorta in the second foal; and only deformed hind legs in the third foal.[8]

A total of 14 foals were reported with congenital musculoskeletal abnormalities; 10 had low total serum concentrations of triiodothyronine (T_3) and/or thyroxine (T_4) suggestive of hypothyroidism and 6 foals had histologic lesions of thyroid hyperplasia. Musculoskeletal lesions encountered were forelimb contracture, ruptured common digital extension tendon, short face, skeletal hypoplasia, and combinations of these defects.[9]

The cause of a congenital syndrome, consisting of torticollis, scoliosis of the head, and frequently malformation of one or more limbs, was linked to intrauterine fetal positioning. Deformed foals were more frequently in caudal and, in particular, transverse presentation.[10]

GENETIC FACTORS

Hereditary defects are pathologic or pathophysiologic results of mutant genes or chromosomal aberrations. Cytogenetic studies in horses have not attained the diagnostic significance they have in man. Chromosomal aberrations have been described in the horse and have been summarized[5,11] (see Chapter 30).

No recent guidelines for studying genetic diseases and defects in horses exist. Diagnosis of genetic defects is based on the rule that defects run in families. That requires collecting information on the family and establishing and enumerating normal and abnormal offspring. Statistical methods are applied to the data to analyze intragenerational and intergenerational transmission patterns and to determine if data are compatible with simple or more complex transmission patterns.

SPECIFIC DEFECTS

The following sections review congenital defects usually diagnosed in neonatal foals. The defects are discussed by the principal body system involved. The list is not complete, but the review gives an insight into congenital defects in foals. Further discussion of congenital defects and diseases in foals may be found in other reviews.[4,5,11]

SKELETAL DEFECTS

Skeletal defects may be single and involve a specific body region (such as facial, cranial, axial, or appendicular) or may involve the entire skeletal system.

Regional Skeletal Defects

A variety of regional skeletal defects has been described in foals. Cleft palate occurs and varies in degree ranging from fissure of both soft and hard palates to a cleft in the soft palate only. Foals affected with cleft palate do poorly, and food, milk, or water may discharge from one or both nostrils. The cause is not established. Secondary inhalation pneumonia is common.[4,12–15] Defects of lips have not been described in horses. Disparity of length of upper and lower jaw are important in the foal. Short upper jaw (brachygnathia superior) appears to be less common than brachygnathia (shorter than normal mandible) (Fig. 71–1). Brachygnathia has frequently been repaired, a practice that should be discouraged, because the defect is suspected to be genetically transmitted as a simple autosomal recessive.

In one study, 8.8% of foals had craniofacial defects, with 1.8% having wryface.[4] The cause of the defect is unknown. Another study described a syndrome of wryhead, scoliosis of the neck, and limb malformation in various Belgian breeds. The mares were presented to a veterinary clinic because of severe dystocia. No genetic factor could account for the defect, and investigators

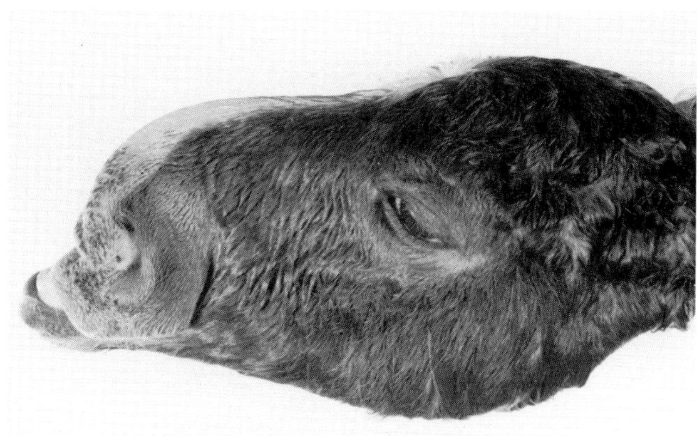

FIG. 71–1. Quarter Horse filly with a facial defect. Note shortened twisted upper jaw.

postulated that intrauterine space limits resulted in this syndrome.[10]

Vertebral Column

Defects of the vertebral column occur as single regional malformations or in association with defects of the limbs, such as arthrogryposis. Atlanto-occipital fusion in Arabian horses may be recognized at birth or later in life because of resulting spinal cord damage. It is characterized by fusion of the atlas to the occiput and the dens of the axis is hypoplastic. The problem appears to be of genetic cause.[16] Recently, a variant of this defect was reported. In addition to occipito-atlanto-axial malformation, the atlas was duplicated. The foal was unable to rise after birth and had signs of spastic tetraparesis from spinal cord compression.[17]

Other defects include kyphosis (dorsal deviation), lordosis (ventral deviation), scoliosis (lateral deviation), torticollis (twisted neck), and various combinations (Fig. 71–2). Aborted, newborn, and older contracted foals have bilateral contractures of the legs and may have a combination of twisted head, twisted neck, and scoliosis. Associated defects may include defects of the ventral abdominal wall and diaphragm and also hypoplasia and malformations of joint surfaces. The intrauterine position of the fetus and space limitations have been postulated as causative factors.[10] Lordosis (swayback) of unknown cause was ascribed to faulty alignment of intervertebral joints probably because of hypoplasia of joint surfaces.[5]

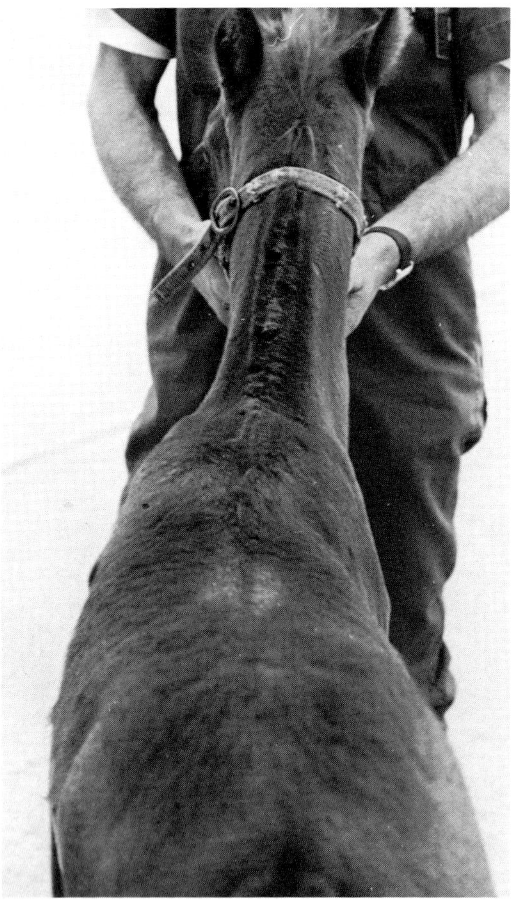

FIG. 71–2. Scoliosis in the thoracic area of 3-month-old Arabian female foal.

Appendicular Skeleton

Polydactylism, defined as duplication of all or part of a digit, has been seen most commonly on the left front leg. Location of the supernumerary digit was usually medial. Occasionally, other developmental defects may have been present. Various breeds were involved, and the defect has been attributed to a dominant gene with incomplete penetrance.[18] However, confirmation of genetic transmission is lacking.

Lack of development of front legs has been referred to as amelia anterior; no associated defects were found. Foals of both sexes were involved. Foals affected with anterior amelia are nonviable and must be euthanatized. The condition has been referred to as abrachia, amelia, and hemimelia, and part or total absence of one or both forelimbs occurs.[19] Unilateral agenesis of the radius was described in one foal.[20]

Unilateral or bilateral phalangeal hypoplasia occurred sporadically in various breeds of horses and may come to the attention of the owner or veterinarian because of lameness and discrepancy in hoof growth (Fig. 71–3). Radiographs disclosed hypoplasia of the third phalanx and partially or completely absent navicular bone.[21–23] In one case, clenbuterol administered to the pregnant mare was discussed as a possible cause of this defect.[23]

Several congenital defects involving size and position of the patella have been described. Agenesis of the patella is rare.[24] Patellar ectopia is characterized by bilateral posterior and lateral dislocation of patellas to the lateral epicondyles. Foals have a squatting stance. No primary abnormality is known that causes this defect, e.g., the femoral condyles and femoropatellar ligaments are normal.[25,26] Genetic causes have not been demonstrated, whereas lateral luxation of the patella is considered to be the result of homozygosity of a simple autosomal recessive gene.[27] Foals affected with lateral luxation of the patella exhibit a squatting stance with hips, stifles, and hocks in extreme flexion. The condition may be unilateral or bilateral, and the lateral ridge of the femoral trochlea is hypoplastic.[28]

Unilateral or bilateral upward fixation of the patella caught on the medial femoral trochlea and resulting in extension of one or both hind legs is a fairly common defect. It is thought to be hereditary. Horses predisposed to upward patella fixation have a straighter hind leg conformation.[29]

Contracted foals have been described in aborted fetuses and neonatal and yearling foals. The syndrome consists of asymmetric skull development, torticollis, scoliosis of thoracolumbar area, bilateral flexion contracture of distal limbs more commonly involving front limbs, and defects of the ventral abdominal wall. The

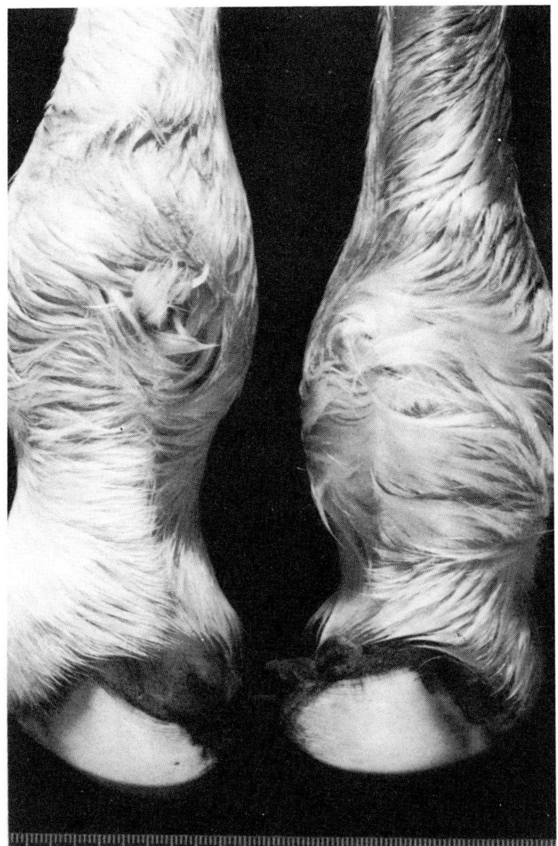

FIG. 71–3. Volar view of both hind feet of a Quarter Horse filly with phalangeal hypoplasia.

syndrome varies from mild, reversible, and flexion contractures to severe lesions of skull and vertebral column combined with joint contractures.[30–32]

No significant gross or microscopic changes were observed in brain, spinal cord, peripheral nerves, tendons, ligaments, and muscles. Intervertebral and costovertebral joint surfaces were smaller on the convex side of the lesion. Furthermore, hypoplasia and malformation of the shafts of metacarpal III and metatarsal III or both were found. Aberrations observed in 3-month-old, contracted fetuses suggested either defective mesenchymal or cartilaginous models.[30] In one study, contracted foal was the most commonly diagnosed congenital defect.[4] Bilateral contracture of both hind and front legs was seen, ranging from mild to severe. In addition, scoliosis and/or torticollis were encountered, ranging from mild to severe. The third component was curvature of the head.[10] The cause of this syndrome has been ascribed to intrauterine positioning.[10]

Generalized bone defects in the horse seemed to be limited to multiple exostoses characterized by numerous bony protuberances located most commonly on ribs close to costochondral junctions. Long bones and pelvic bone may also be involved. Exostoses develop from cartilage and are remodeled to bone, and growth ceases with closure of the epiphyseal plates. The trait has been confirmed to be dominant.[33,34]

JOINTS

Joint defects may be generalized or restricted to a single joint. However, little information is available in horses. Only hip dysplasia has been reported, involving one or both acetabulums that were shallow and the femoral head flattened. Subluxation may result, and degenerative joint disease follows. The cause is unknown.[35,36]

MUSCULAR SYSTEM

Arthrogryposis

Arthrogryposis is defined as permanent joint contracture at birth and may be neurogenic, myogenic or caused by lesions in joint surfaces. It may involve front or hind legs and may have associated defects such as cleft palate, brachygnathia superior, and torticollis (Fig. 71–4). A newborn Thoroughbred foal had arthrogryposis of the left hind leg.[37] The number of large motor neurons of the ventral horn was reduced involving the left side of the spinal cord from L3 to S4. Hypoplasia of nerves, muscles, and bone was also seen in the affected left hindleg.[37] In Norwegian Fjord Horses, the syndrome of bimelic posterior arthrogryposis associated with cleft palate, brachygnathia superior, and polydactylism of the hind leg was lethal and considered to be genetically transmitted.[38]

Tendons

Weak flexor tendons may be self-correcting or need supportive treatment or surgery. The condition is characterized by bilateral overextension of phalangeal joints. Prematurity or dysmaturity has been postulated as the causal factor.[39,40]

Contracted digital flexor tendons is fairly common, and various causes such as genetic factors, positioning

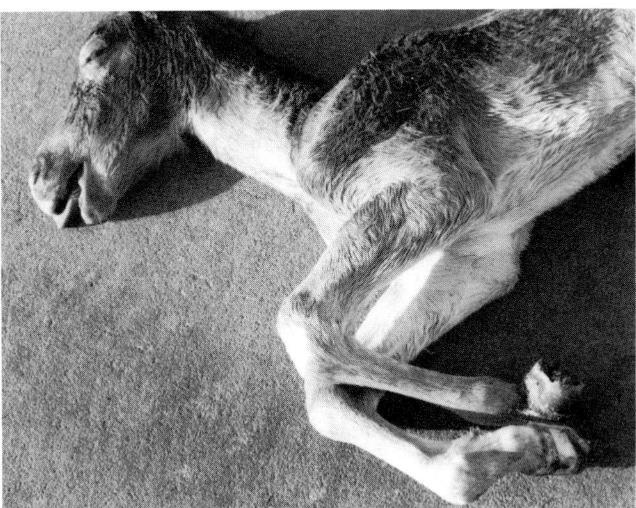

FIG. 71–4. Arthrogryposis involving both front legs in a neonatal male grade Quarter Horse.

in utero, or nutritional deficiency have been postulated[8] (see Chapter 116).

Myotonia

Myotonia is an uncommon disease of presumably familial origin in horses. The gait is stiff, and upon palpation, the muscles of the hind legs give an impression of knotting.[41,42]

CENTRAL NERVOUS SYSTEM

Congenital defects of brain and spinal cord are common in foals and may involve the central nervous system only or may be combined with skeletal lesions. These defects are best classified by combining anatomical and functional factors: cerebral defects and malformations involving only or mainly the cerebrum, defects involving only or mainly the cerebellum and brain stem, and spinal cord defects.[43–45] Equine central nervous system defects were common in one study and ranged from cyclopia to hydrocephalus.[4] Unfortunately, etiologic studies of the defects in horses appear to be rare. Frequency of these defects is not a fixed proportion of all foal births but varies by genetic and environmental factors. Neurologic abnormalities are common in the newborn foal and may be the result of sepsis, electrolyte disturbances, hypoglycemia, hypoxic or ischemic injuries, and congenital defects.[46] Morphologic information obtained by computed tomography (CT) scanning will greatly improve the diagnosis and prognosis of neonatal neurologic disorders.[43]

Cerebral Defects

Agenesis of the Corpus Callosum. Agenesis of the corpus callosum is commonly associated with other defects such as hydranencephaly, agenesis of the septum pellucidum, internal hydrocephalus, porencephaly or microencephaly, or Dandy-Walker syndrome.[43]

Anencephaly. Anencephaly is a combination of nonclosure of the anterior portion of the neural tube and failure of cranial development, but eyes, base of cranium, and cerebellum usually are present. The pituitary may be present or defective, leading to prolonged gestation in cattle. No reports are available for foals.

Hydranencephaly. The complete or almost complete absence of cerebral hemispheres is called hydranencephaly. The cranium has normal conformation, and the resulting space is filled with cerebrospinal fluid surrounded by a thin membranous cerebral tissue. The defect is uncommon in horses, and its cause is unknown. It may be associated with hydrops allantois.[44]

Internal Hydrocephalus. Excessive fluid accumulating in the cranial cavity within the ventricular system (internal hydrocephalus) may cause dystocia, because of the large size of the head. Hydrocephalus is a commonly reported defect of unknown origin in horses.[46]

Meningocele and Meningoencephalocele. Meningocele and meningocephalocele are protrusions of meninges and brain tissue through a cranial cleft (cranioschisis), forming a large liquid-filled sac. These defects are rare in foals.[4]

Microencephaly, or Microcephaly. An abnormally small but grossly normal brain, called microencephaly, has been described in foals.[45]

Defects of the Cerebellum and Brain Stem

Dandy-Walker Syndrome. Dandy-Walker syndrome consists of hydrocephalus, aplasia, or hypoplasia of cerebellar vermis and cystic enlargement of the fourth ventricle covered by a markedly thinned medullary velum. The syndrome has associated tela chorioidea, and an inner ependymal layer representing the roof of the expanded fourth ventricle is found.[43] It is rare in foals.[43]

Cerebellar Hypoplasia. The clinical signs present at birth for cerebellar hypoplasia are recumbency with extended limbs, intermittent opisthotonos, and ataxia. Whereas earlier investigators invariably incriminated hereditary causes in cerebellar disease in calves, researchers have documented that intrauterine fetal infection with bovine virus diarrhea virus causes cerebellar hypoplasia.[45] No prenatal viral infection is reported to be teratogenic in foals.

Cerebellar Disease in Arabian Horses. Signs of cerebellar disease are present at birth or appear at 3 to 6 months of age and are characterized by intention tremor (Fig. 71–5). Histologic lesions include degeneration of Purkinje cells and mineralized neurons in the thalamus.[47]

Spinal Cord

Spina bifida, defective closure of the dorsal vertebral laminae, has been described in foals. Other rare spinal cord defects reported are atlanto-occipital fusion and spinal dysraphism.[46,48]

OCULAR DEFECTS

A variety of ocular defects has been described in foals, either single or multiple defects or associated with defects of other organs (Fig. 71–6). Unilateral or bilateral smallness of the eye globe (microphthalmia) is seen in all breeds.[4] It is usually associated with other ocular defects such as cataracts. Complete mature cataracts may be genetic and occasionally are associated with microphthalmia. They are considered to be the most common cause of blindness in young horses and usually in-

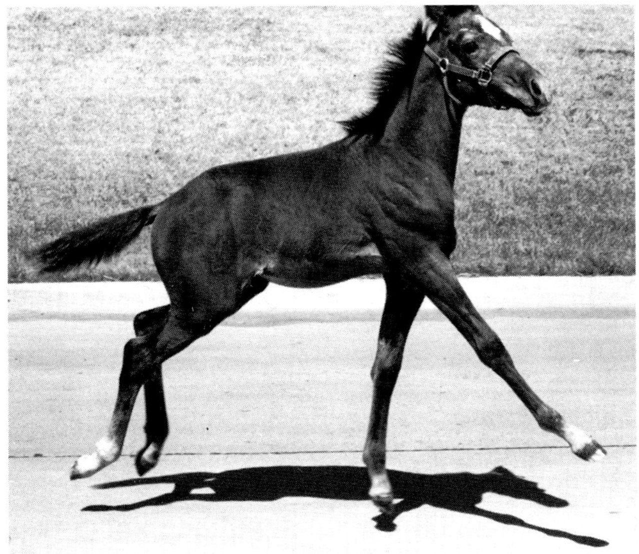

FIG. 71–5. A 3-month-old Arabian colt with cerebellar disease.

SKIN

Congenital defects involving skin and andexa, with a few exceptions, are rare in horses and may be localized or generalized. Lethal white (ileocolonic aganglionosis) in Paint Horses is described with the digestive system defects. "Albinism" in horses characterized by white coat color, pink skin, and almost complete lack of pigment in the iris is caused by an autosomal dominant gene *(W)*, which is lethal in the homozygous condition *(WW)* (Fig. 71–7). Matings between white horses *(Ww)* and white horses *(Ww)* have a 25% probability of producing nonviable embryos *(WW)*.[56,57]

Epitheliogenesis imperfecta has been reported in most species including the horse and is characterized at birth by lack of development of the epithelium in patches, usually just above carpal and tarsal area. The tongue may have similar lesions, and one or more hooves may be partially or completely missing. The disease is fatal. The defect is most likely transmitted as a simple autosomal recessive trait.[58–60]

Curly coat was reported in Percherons and was con-

volve bilateral opacity of the entire lens.[49] Nuclear cataract is opacity of the center of the lens.[29] The cause is unknown, as is the origin of Y-shaped cataracts. Both conditions are present at birth.[29,50] Opacity of the posterior capsule of the lens combined with persistence of the hyaloid artery is not common and is of unknown cause.[29] Bilateral absence of iris, referred to as aniridia, has been reported most commonly in the Belgian breed. It is considered to be a genetic defect most probably transmitted as a simple autosomal recessive. Cataracts develop within a few months after birth.[51,52] Bilateral subluxation of the lens may also lead to cataracts.[53] Abnormal color of the iris consisting of white, brown, and blue parts is most commonly seen in white, spotted, and chestnut horses as well as Palominos. No defects are associated with the condition.[53]

Bilateral optic nerve hypoplasia may occur in eyeballs that are grossly normal or affected with microphthalmia, cataracts, or retinal detachment. It is an uncommon defect and characterized by blindness; the cause is not known.[53,54] Entropion, inversion of the eyelid, and ectropion, eversion of the eyelid, are of unknown origin in horses. They are not common and may be corrected surgically.[53] Retinal detachment, encountered most commonly in Standardbreds and Thoroughbreds, is usually bilateral and complete and results in blindness. Histologic examination of such retinas disclosed dysplasia.[55] Retinal detachment has been described in a foal that also had microphthalmia and unilateral cataract.[55] Microcornea, defined as a small cornea, is usually seen in eyes affected with microphthalmia.[53] Centrally located melanosis of the cornea is a rare defect of unknown cause.[53] Corneal opacities in thin linear arrangements and bands are seen rarely in foals and are attributed to a thin and abnormal Descemet's membrane.[53]

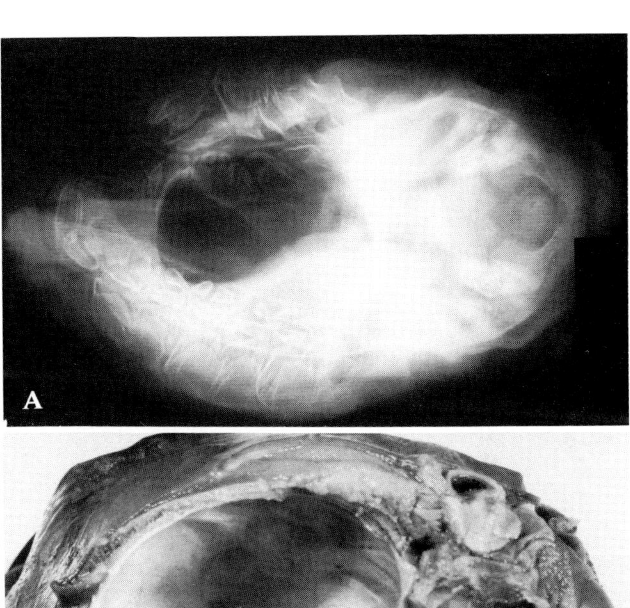

FIG. 71–6. *A*, Radiograph of a 7-month-old aborted female fetus with facial deformity and orbital meningocele. *B*, Associated defects were anophthalmia on the left side and cleft palate.

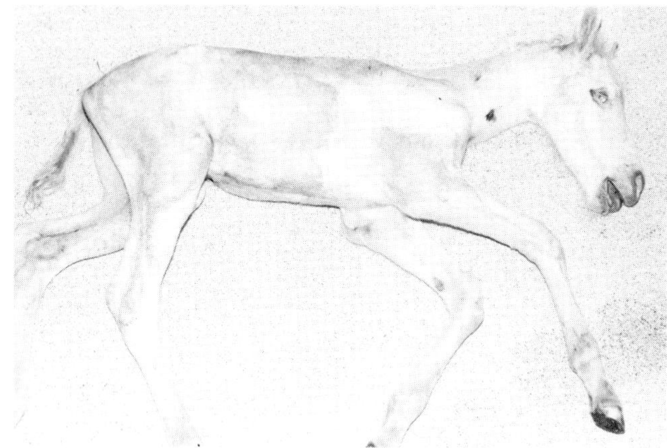

FIG. 71–7. White foal lethal in a Paint Horse. Note white coat and blue eyes.

sidered to be caused by homozygosity of a simple autosomal recessive trait. The trait did not affect the health and well-being of the foals.[61]

Melanomas may be present in a foal at birth.[62,63] Papillomatosis, possibly caused by infection in utero, may also be seen at birth.[64,65] Dentigerous cysts are abnormalities of the first branchial arch and contain tooth remnants. They are located in the skin at the base of the ear.[66]

Hereditary junctional mechanobullous disease has been described in Belgian foals. The foals were 6 and 12 days old and had multiple epidermal defects and separation of the hooves from the coronet bands.[67–69] Ultrastructural studies confirmed light microscopic changes, indicating that separation occurred through the lamina lucida of the basement membrane.[68]

Inherited connective tissue disease, characterized by hyperextensible fragile skin, occurs in horses later in life.[70]

CARDIOVASCULAR SYSTEM

Congenital heart and vascular defects may come to the attention of owners and veterinarians at birth, or affected horses may do poorly or have impaired usefulness. Most reports are case reports and do not contain data about frequency of these defects. In addition, nothing is known about their cause.

Interventricular septal defect is the most common heart defect in young horses.[4] They are poor doers and may have intolerance to exercise. The defect is around 2.5 cm in diameter and located in the upper part of the membranous septum.[71,72] Tetralogy and pentalogy of Fallot are rare defects in horses and, in addition to an interventricular defect, are associated with pulmonic stenosis, dextroposition of aorta, and right ventricular hypertrophy.[73,74] The pentalogy of Fallot also has a patent ductus arteriosus. Multiple heart defects in foals ranging in age from 2 h to 3 weeks were characterized by high ventricular septal defects, stenosis of pulmonary artery, and persistence of common truncus arteriosus.[75] Neonatal death has been attributed to persistence of the foramen ovale.[76] Various defects of the large vessels such as patent ductus arteriosus have occurred in foals.[75] Persistence of the right aortic arch and dextroposition of aorta are also rare defects in horses.[77,78] In summary, all these cases require careful clinical examination and confirmation at necropsy, if indicated.

BLOOD

Hemophilia A (factor VIII deficiency) is the most commonly reported genetic coagulation defect in domestic animals. It is the only one reported in horses and is a sex-linked recessive trait. The disease is characterized by hematomas, especially around joints and body prominences in young foals.[79–83]

DIGESTIVE SYSTEM

Ileocolonic aganglionosis has been reported in white foals of the Paint Horse breed, resulting from mating overo to overo.[84–87] Affected foals have blue irises and white bodies (Fig. 71–7). They are normal at birth but develop colic within 5 to 24 h. The defect is genetic, but its transmission pattern needs to be elucidated. The defect is characterized by a small narrow segment of large intestine. Histologically, the myenteric and submucosal neuronal plexuses are not developed in the large intestine and part of the small intestine.[85–87]

Atresia coli has also been encountered in foals. The cause was not determined.[5] Atresia ani, nonpatency of the anus, has been reported in foals. It may be associated with rectourethral or rectovaginal fistula, depending on sex and/or absence of coccygeal vertebrae.[88–90]

LARGE BODY CAVITIES

Umbilical hernia is common in foals and usually is discernible from birth to 7 days of age. Studies of its frequency are lacking. The genetic transmission has not been clarified.[29,91–93]

Inguinal hernia, characterized by protrusion of loops of intestines through the inguinal canal, is not a common problem.[90,91] It occurs among animals in veterinary hospitals as 1.13 cases/1000 admissions and appears to be inherited.[92]

Closure defects of the ventral abdominal wall are rare, and schistosoma reflexum and schistocele have been reported infrequently; all are of unknown origin.[94–96]

URINARY SYSTEM

Bladder defect is characterized by a defect or tear in the dorsal or ventral surface of the urinary bladder near the urachus (see Chapter 114). The defect may be developmental or traumatic, because of rupture of a filled bladder during parturition. It has been reported rather frequently. It is characterized by frequent straining with little urine being voided and urine accumulating within the abdominal cavity.[97]

A pervious urachus is common in foals and is characterized by urine dripping from the umbilical area. This is particularly seen during micturition. The cause is twisting of the umbilical cord.[98]

Ectopic ureters are bilateral or unilateral and are characterized by urinary incontinence. Hydronephrosis may be induced by the defect.[99,100]

Unilateral kidney agenesis has occurred in horses in Switzerland; the cause was unknown.[101]

Small thin-walled cysts of approximately 1.5 cm in diameter replaced cortex and medulla of polycystic kidneys and were grossly enlarged up to 12 kg. The condition appears to be rare in frequency and of unknown cause.[102] Bilateral renal hypoplasia in four young horses was characterized by stunted growth, weight loss, anorexia, and depression. Two of the horses had been poor doers since birth. The cause was not determined.[103] Another foal was described as being affected with bilateral renal hypoplasia and dysplasia associated with dysgenesis of the ureters, atresia ani, and bilateral cryptorchidism.[104] Recently, a neonatal foal was described as being affected with bilateral renal dysplasia and nephron hypoplasia.[105]

METABOLIC AND ENDOCRINE DEFECTS

Overfeeding of iodine (83 mg/day) to pregnant mares may have led to birth of weak foals, which may die shortly after birth. The affected foals had goiter.[106] Dietary imbalance was also suspected in retarded bone development and contracture of tendons. Incoordination and poor reflexes, low body temperature, and goiter were present.[106]

Episodic weakness, muscular tremors, and collapse lasting minutes to hours associated with intermittent serum hyperkalemia have been reported in young Quarter Horses.[107,108] It appears to be inherited. Simple autosomal recessive inheritance was described in a family of Quarter Horses in Canada, whereas one study presented data compatible with dominant transmission.[109,110]

REFERENCES

1. Rossdale, P.D.: Modern concepts of neonatal diseases in foals. Equine Vet. J., *4:*117–128, 1972.
2. Priester, W.A., Glass, M.D., and Waggoner, N.S.: Congenital defects in domesticated animals: General considerations. Am. J. Vet. Res., *31:*1871–1879, 1970.
3. Platt, H.: Etiologic aspects of perinatal mortality in the Thoroughbred. Equine Vet. J., *5:*116–120, 1973.
4. Crowe, M.W., and Swerczek, T.W.: Equine congenital defects. Am. J. Vet. Res., *46:*353–358, 1985.
5. Leipold, H.W., Saperstein, G., and Woollen, N.: Congenital defects in foals. *In* Large Animal Internal Medicine. Edited by B.P. Smith. St. Louis, C.V. Mosby, 1990, pp. 1567–1597.
6. McIlwraith, C.W., and James, L.F.: Limb deformities in foals associated with ingestion of locoweed by mares. J. Am. Vet. Med. Assoc., *181:*255–258, 1982.
7. Prichard, J.T., and Voss, J.L.: Fetal ankylosis in horses associated with hybrid sudan pasture. J. Am. Vet. Med. Assoc., *150:*871–873, 1967.
8. Drudge, J.H., Lyons, E., Swerczek, E.T., and Tolliver, S.C.: Cambendazole for strongyle control in a Pony band: Selection of a drug-resistant population of small strongyles and teratologic implications. Am. J. Vet. Res., *44:*110–114, 1983.
9. McLaughlin, B.G., Doige, C.E., and McLaughlin, P.S.: Thyroid hormone levels in foals with congenital musculoskeletal lesions. Can. Vet. J., *27:*264–267, 1986.
10. Vandeplassche, M., et al.: Aetiology and pathogenesis of congenital torticollis and head scoliosis in the equine fetus. Equine Vet. J., *16:*419–424, 1984.
11. Willer, S., Willer, H., and Wiesner, E.: Chromosomenaberrationen beim Pferd. Mh. Vet. Med., *36:*386–394, 1981.
12. Batstone, J.H.F.: Cleft palate in a horse. Br. J. Plast. Surg., *19:*327–331, 1966.
13. Jones, R.S., et al.: Surgical repair of cleft palate in the horse. Equine Vet. J., *7:*86–90, 1975.
14. Kendrick, J.W.: Cleft palate in a horse. Cornell Vet., *40:*188–189, 1950.
15. Stickle, R.L., Goble, D.O., and Braden, T.D.: Surgical repair of cleft soft palate in a foal. Vet. Med., *68:*159–162, 1973.
16. Mayhew, I.G., Watson, A.S., and Heissan, J.A.: Congenital occipito-atlanto-axial malformations in the horse. Equine Vet. J., *10:*103–113, 1978.
17. DeLahunta, A., Hatfield, C., and Dietz, A.: Occipitoatlantoaxial malformation with duplication of the atlas and axis in a half Arabian foal. Cornell Vet., *79:*185–193, 1989.
18. Frew, D.G., and Wright, I.M.: Supernumerary digits in the horse. Equine Pract., *12:*21–26, 1990.
19. DeBowes, R.M., and Leipold, H.W.: Anterior amelia. Equine Vet. J., *4:*133–135, 1984.
20. McFarland, L.Z., and Denis, E.: Unilateral agenesis (phocomelia) in a foal. Anat. Rec., *109:*236–240, 1961.
21. Bertone, A.L., and Aanes, W.A.: Congenital phalangeal hypoplasia in equidae. J. Am. Vet. Med. Assoc., *185:*554–556, 1984.
22. Modransky, P., Thatcher, C.D., and Welker, F.M.: Unilateral phalangeal dysgenesis and navivicular bone agenesis in a foal. Equine Vet. J., *19:*347–349, 1987.
23. Smith, D.R.K., Leach, D.H., and Bell, R.I.: Phalangeal and navicular bone hypoplasia and hoof malformation in the hind limbs of a foal. Can. Vet. J., *27:*28–34, 1986.
24. Kostyra, J.: Congenital absence of patella in a foal. Vet. Med., *19:*95–97, 1963.
25. Finocchio, E.J., and Guffy, M.M.: Congenital patellar ectopia in a foal. J. Am. Vet. Med. Assoc., *156:*222–223, 1970.
26. Van Pelt, R.W., Keahey, K.K., and Dalley, J.B.: Congenital bilateral patellar ectopia in a foal. Vet. Med., *66:*445–447, 1971.
27. Hermans, W.A., et al.: Investigation into the hereditary of congenital lateral patellar (sub)luxation in the Shetland Pony. Vet. Q., *9:*1–8, 1987.
28. Rooney, J.R., Rake, C.W., and Harmany, K.J.: Congenital lateral luxation of the patella in the horse. Cornell Vet., *61:*670–673, 1971.

29. Catcott, E.J., and Smithcors, J.F.: Equine Medicine and Surgery. 2nd ed. Wheaton, American Veterinary Publisher, 1972, pp. 365–366.
30. Rooney, J.R.: Contracted foals. Cornell Vet., *56:*172–187, 1966.
31. Finocchio, E.J.: A cause of contracted foal syndrome. Vet. Med., *68:*1254–1255, 1973.
32. Boyd, J.S.: Congenital deformities in two Clydesdale foals. Equine Vet. J., *8:*161–164, 1976.
33. Gardner, E.J., Shupe, J.L., Leone, N.C., and Olson, A.E.: Hereditary multiple exostosis. J. Hered., *66:*318–322, 1975.
34. Li, K.K.J. et al.: DNA polymorphism analysis of hereditary multiple exostoses in horses. Am. J. Vet. Res., *50:*978–983, 1989.
35. Jogi, P., and Norberg, I.: Malformation of the hip joint in a Standardbred horse. Vet. Rec., *74:*421–422, 1962.
36. Manning, J.P.: Hip dysplasia-osteoarthritis. Mod. Vet. Pract., *44:*44–45, 1963.
37. Mayhew, I.G.: Neuromuscular arthrogryposis multiplex congenita in a Thoroughbred foal. Vet. Pathol., *21:*187–192, 1984.
38. Nes, N., Lomo, O.M., and Bjerkas, I.: Hereditary lethal arthrogryposis (muscle contracture) in horses. Nord. Vet. Med., *31:*425–430, 1982.
39. Adams, O.R.: Lameness in Horses. 3rd ed. Philadelphia, Lea & Febiger, 1974, pp. 344–345.
40. Fackelman, G.E., and Lodins, L.: Surgical correction of the digital hyperextension deformity in foals. Vet. Med., *67:*1116–1123, 1972.
41. Jamison, J.M., Baird, J.D., and Smith-Maxie, L.L.: A congenital form of myotonia with dystrophic changes in a Quarterhorse. Equine Vet. J., *19:*353–358, 1987.
42. McKerrell, R.E.: Myotonia in man and animals. Confusing comparisons. Equine Vet. J., *19:*266–267, 1987.
43. Cudd, T.A., Mayhew, I.G., and Cottrill, C.M.: Agenesis of the corpus callosum with cerebellar vermian hypoplasia in a foal resembling the Dandy-Walker syndrome: Pre-mortem diagnosis by clinical evaluation and CT scanning. Equine Vet. J., *21:*378–381, 1989.
44. Waelchli, R.O., and Ehrensberger, F.: Two related cases of cerebellar abnormality in equine fetuses associated with hydrops of fetal membranes. Vet. Rec., *123:* 513–514, 1988.
45. Leipold, H.W., and Troyer, D.L.: Congenital neurological abnormalities. Proc. Am. Coll. Vet. Int. Med., *8:*611–615, 1990.
46. Adams, R., and Mayhew, I.G.: Neurologic disease. Vet. Clin. North Am., *1:*209–234, 1985.
47. Turner-Beatty, M., et al.: Cerebellar disease in Arabian horses. Proc. Am. Assoc. Equine Pract., 241–255, 1986.
48. Cho, D.Y., and Leipold, H.W.: Myelodysplasia in a foal. Equine Vet. J., *9:*195–197, 1977.
49. Gelatt, K.N., Myers, V.S., and McClure, J.R.: Aspiration of congenital and soft cataracts in foals and young horses. J. Am. Vet. Med. Assoc., *165:*611–616, 1974.
50. Walde, I.: Some observations on congenital cataracts in the horse. Equine Vet. J. Suppl., *2:*27–36, 1983.
51. Erickson, K.: Hereditary aniridia with secondary cataract in horses. Nord. Vet. Med., *7:*773–793, 1955.
52. Joyce, J.R.: Aniridia in a Quarterhorse. Equine Vet. J. Suppl., *2:*21–22, 1983.
53. Latimer, C.A. and Wyman, M.: Neonatal ophthalmology. Vet. Clin. North Am., *1:*235–260, 1985.
54. Gelatt, K.M., Leipold, H.W., and Coffman, J.R.: Bilateral optic nerve hypoplasia in a colt. J. Am. Vet. Med. Assoc., *155:*627–631, 1969.
55. Rebhun, W.C.: Equine retinal lesions and retinal detachments. Equine Vet. J. Suppl., *2:*86–90, 1983.
56. Pulos, W.L., and Hutt, F.G.: Lethal dominant white in horses. J. Hered., *60:*59–63, 1969.
57. Salisbury, G.W., and Britton, J.W.: The inheritance of equine coat color. J. Hered., *32:*255–260, 1941.
58. Berthelsen, H., and Ericksson, K.: Epitheliogenesis imperfecta neonatorum in a foal, possibly of a hereditary nature. J. Comp. Pathol., *48:*285–287, 1935.
59. Butz, M., and Meyer, H.: Epitheliogenesis imperfecta in foals. DTW Dtsch. Tierarztl. Wochenschr., *64:*555–559, 1957.
60. Crowell, W.A., Stephenson, C., and Gosser, H.S.: Epitheliogenesis in a foal. J. Am. Vet. Med. Assoc., *168:*56–58, 1976.
61. Blakeslee, L.H., Hudson, R.S., and Hunt, H.R.: Curly coat in horses. J. Hered., *34:*115–118, 1943.
62. Hamilton, D.P., and Byerly, C.S.: Congenital malignant melanoma in a foal. J. Am. Vet. Med. Assoc., *164:*1040–1041, 1974.
63. Cox, J.M., DeBowes, R.M., and Leipold, H.W.: Congenital malignant melanoma in two foals. J. Am. Vet. Med. Assoc., *194:*944–947, 1989.
64. Schueler, R.L.: Congenital equine papillomatosis. J. Am. Vet. Med. Assoc., *162:*640, 1973.
65. Njoku, C.O., and Burwash, W.A.: Congenital cutaneous papillomas in a foal. Cornell Vet., *62:*54–57, 1972.
66. Markus, G.: Die Angeborene Ohrfistel beim Pferd. DTW Dtsche. Tierarztl. Wochenschr., *81:*505–506, 1976.
67. Kohn, C.W., et al.: Mechanobullous disease in two Belgian foals. Equine Vet. J., *21:*297–307, 1989.
68. Johnson, G.C., et al.: Ultrastructure of junctional epidermolysis bullosa in two Belgian foals. J. Comp. Pathol., *98:*329–336, 1981.
69. Frame, S.R., et al.: Hereditary junctional mechanobullous disease in a foal. J. Am. Vet. Med. Assoc., *193:*1420–1424, 1988.
70. Hardy, M.H., et al.: An inherited connective tissue disease in the horse. Lab. Invest., *59:*253–262, 1988.
71. Reef, V.B.: Cardiovascular disease in the equine neonate. Vet. Clin. North Am., *1:*117–129, 1985.
72. Reef, V.B.: Problems in Equine Medicine. Philadelphia, Lea & Febiger, 1989, pp. 122–137.
73. Greene, H.J., Wray, D.D., and Greenway, J.A.: Two equine congenital cardiac anomalies. Irish Vet. J., *29:*115–117, 1975.
74. Prickett, M.E., Reeves, J.T., and Zent, W.W.: Tetralogy of Fallot in a Thoroughbred mare. J. Am. Vet. Med. Assoc., *162:*552–555, 1973.
75. Rooney, J.R., and Franks, W.C.: Congenital cardiac anomalies in horses. Pathol. Vet., *1:*454–464, 1964.
76. Wilson, A.P.: Persistent foramen ovale in a foal. Vet. Med., *38:*491–492, 1943.
77. Bartels, J.E., and Vaughan, J.T.: Persistent right aortic arch in the horse. J. Am. Vet. Med. Assoc., *154:*406–409, 1969.
78. Vitums, A., et al.: Transposition of the aorta and atresia of the pulmonary trunk in a horse. Cornell Vet., *63:*41–57, 1973.
79. Archer, R.K.: True haemophilia (haemophilia A) in horses. Vet. Rec., *73:*338–340, 1961.
80. Archer, R.K., and Allan, B.V.: True haemophilia in horses. Vet. Rec., *91:*655–656, 1972.
81. Henninger, R.W.: Hemophilia A in two related Quarterhorse colts. J. Am. Vet. Med. Assoc., *193:*91–94, 1988.
82. Hutchins, D.R., Lepherd, E.E., and Crook, I.G.: A case of equine haemophilia. Aust. Vet. J., *43:*83–87, 1967.

83. Sanger, V.L., Mairs, R.E., and Trapp, A.L.: Hemophilia in a foal. J. Am. Vet. Med. Assoc., *144:*259–264, 1964.
84. Trommershausen, A.: Lethal white foals in mating overo spotted horses. Theriogenology *8:*303–309, 1977.
85. Schneider, J.E., and Leipold, H.W.: Recessive lethal white in two foals. J. Equine Med. Surg., *2:*479–482, 1978.
86. Hultgren, B.D.: Ileocolonic aganglionosis in white progeny of overo spotted horses. J. Am. Vet. Med. Assoc., *180:*289–292, 1982.
87. Vonderfecht, S.L., Trommershausen-Bowling, B.A., and Cohen, M.: Congenital intestinal aganglionosis in white foals. Vet. Pathol., *20:*65–70, 1983.
88. Gideon, L.: Anal agenesis with rectourethral fistula in a colt. Vet. Med., *72:*238–240, 1977.
89. Kingston, R.S., and Park, R.D.: Atresia ani with urogenital tract anomalies in foals. Equine Pract., *4:*32–34, 1982.
90. Robertson, J.T., and Embertson, R.M.: Surgical management of congenital and perinatal abnormalities of the urogenital tract. Vet. Clin. North Am., *4:*359–379, 1988.
91. Spurlock, G.M., and Robertson, J.T.: Congenital hernias associated with a rent in the common vaginal tunic in five foals. J. Am. Vet. Med. Assoc., *193:*1087–1088, 1988.
92. Hayes, H.M., Jr.: Congenital umbilical and inguinal hernias in cattle, horses, swine, dogs and cats: Risk by breed and sex among hospital patients. Am. J. Vet. Res., *35:*839–842, 1974.
93. Hance, R.S., DeBowes, R.M., Clem, M.F., and Welch, R.D.: Umbilical, inguinal, and ventral hernias in horses. Compend. Contin. Educ. Practicing Vet., *12:*862–871, 1990.
94. Addo, P.B., Cook, J.E., and Dennis, S.M.: Schistocelia in a twin foal. Equine Vet. J., *16:*69–71, 1984.
95. Allen, W.E.: Two cases of abnormal equine pregnancy associated with excess fetal fluid. Equine Vet. J., *18:*220–222, 1986.
96. Irwin, M.R., and Pulley, L.T.: Schistosomus reflexus in an equine fetus. Vet. Med., *70:*44–45, 1975.
97. Richardson, D.W.: Urogenital problems in the neonatal foal. Vet. Clin. North Am., *1:*179–188, 1985.
98. Turner, T.A., Fessler, J.F., and Ewert, K.M.: Patent urachus in foals. Equine Pract., *4:*24–31, 1982.
99. Houlton, J.E.F., et al.: Urinary incontinence in a Shire foal due to ureteral ectopia. Equine Vet. J., *19:*244–247, 1987.
100. Sullins, K.E., et al.: Ectopic ureter managed by unilateral nehprectomy in two female horses. Equine Vet. J., *20:*463–466, 1988.
101. Hofliger, H.: Zur Kenntnis der Kongenitalen Unilateralen Nierenagenesis bei Haustieren. Schweiz. Arch. Tierheilkd., *113:*330–337, 1971.
102. Ramsey, G., et al.: Polycystic kidneys in an adult horse. Equine Vet. J., *19:*243–244, 1987.
103. Andrews, F.M., et al.: Bilateral renal hypoplasia in four young horses. J. Am. Vet. Med. Assoc., *189:*210–212, 1986.
104. Brown, C.M., et al.: Bilateral renal dysplasia and hypoplasia with an imperforate anus. Vet. Rec., *122:*91–92, 1988.
105. Zicker, S.C., et al.: Bilateral renal dysplasia with nephron hypoplasia in a foal. J. Am. Vet. Med. Assoc., *196:*2001–2005, 1990.
106. Irvine, C.H.G.: Hypothyroidism in foals. Equine Vet. J., *16:*306–312, 1984.
107. Cox, J.H.: An episodic weakness in four horses associated with intermittent serum hyperkalemia and the similarity of the disease to hyperkalemic periodic paralysis in man. Proc. Am. Assoc. Equine Pract., 383–392, 1985.
108. Spier S.J., et al.: Hyperkalemic periodic paralysis in horses. J. Am. Vet. Med. Assoc., *197:*1009–1017, 1990.
109. Steiss, J.E., and Naylor, J.M.: Episodic muscle tremors in a Quarterhorse: Resemblance to hyperkalemic periodic paralysis. Can. Vet. J., *27:*332–335, 1986.
110. Naylor, J.M., et al.: Hyperkalemic periodic paresis may be inherited as an autosomal dominant with incomplete penetrance. J. Vet. Intern. Med., *3:*115, 1989.

CHAPTER 72

RETAINED PLACENTA

W.R. Threlfall

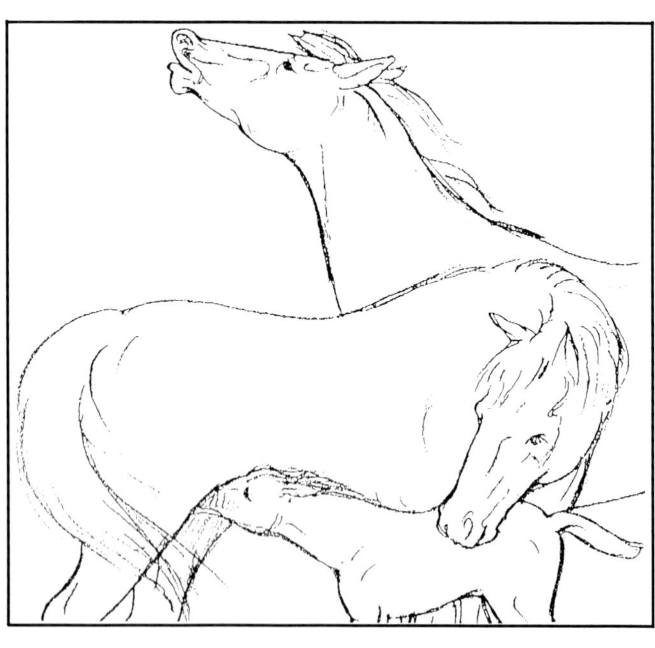

Retained placenta, also referred to as retained afterbirth and fetal membranes, has a variable definition in the literature. All authors consider retained placenta to be failure of passage of part or all of the allantochorionic membrane with or without the amnionic membrane within a specific period of time. This length of time postpartum, however, varies and has included 30 min,[1] 1 h,[2] 1.5 h,[1] 2 h,[3] 3 h,[4] and 6 to 12 h.[5] Retained placenta is reported to be the most common postpartum problem in the mare.[6]

Incidence of this condition is difficult to assess because of lack of a specific postpartum time interval in the definition, but has, however, been reported to be between 2 and 10.5% of foalings.[7] Authors report a higher incidence in draft mares,[8,9] and after dystocia,[7] prolonged gestation,[10] hydrops,[11] and cesarean.[7] Although retained placentas have been reported to occur at a higher incidence in association with abortion, stillbirth, and twinning in lightweight horses, one report indicated no increase with these conditions if they occurred without dystocia.[12] Furthermore, the reported occurrence of retained placenta did not differ between the birth of a weak or diseased foal and that of a healthy foal. Sex of foal did not influence incidence of retained placenta. Age of mare may be related to incidence of retained placenta on some farms; the reason for this farm effect has not been reported. Mares older than 15 yr may have a significantly higher incidence of retained placenta than younger mares. Time of year appeared to influence incidence of retained placenta only on certain farms; when a difference existed a higher incidence occurred after March 31. Mares that were barren or maiden or had foaled the previous year had no difference in retained placental incidence after foaling. No difference in placental passage in mares artificially bred at foal heat versus mares artificially bred at other heats was reported. Mares bred naturally versus by artificial insemination at these heats reportedly experience an increased incidence of retained placentas at foal heat breeding.[13]

In uncomplicated placental retention cases, pregnancy rates after first breeding, at the end of the breeding season, at midgestation, and at term may[6,14] or may not[12] be affected by foal heat breeding. Mares that have had retained placentas before demonstrated a three times greater probability of having retained placenta after foaling than mares without this history.[12] A possible reason for this increase is that formation of pathologic adherences between the endometrium and chorion during the first retention of the placenta may recur at subsequent pregnancies. Mares that develop uterine or systemic infections before or during pregnancy have an increased occurrence of retained placentas. Any debilitating condition such as senility, excessive fatigue, poor condition, or poor environment may increase incidence of retained placenta and puerperal infections. Retained placenta occurrence is reportedly 28% after fetotomy and averages 50% following cesarean, with the percentage occurring with a live fetus at the beginning of surgery twice that with a dead fetus.[15]

In the mare, normal separation of trophoblastic cells

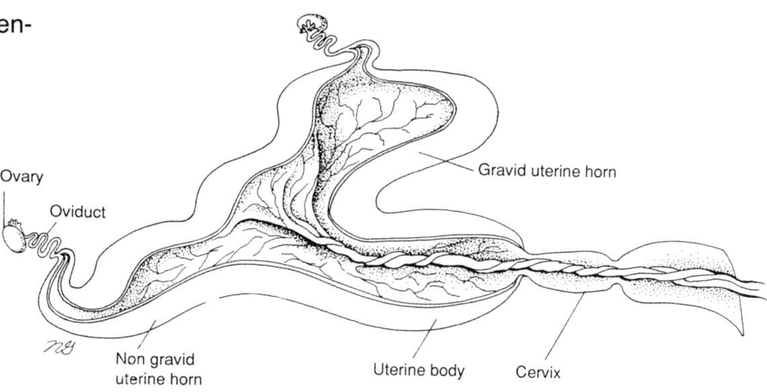

FIG. 72–1. Postpartum uterus with placenta attached to endometrial surface.

from the uterine epithelium and expulsion of placenta through the cervix and vagina occur in the third stage of labor[6] (Fig. 72–1). Rupture of the umbilical cord is assumed to cause collapse of fetal placental vessels and shrinkage of chorionic villi[1] (Fig. 72–2). Postpartum uterine contractions reduce uterine size and probably the amount of blood circulating within the endometrium; maternal crypts relax. Uterine contractions, originating at the apices of the horns and progressing toward the cervix, evert the apical pole of the allantochorion, squeezing the base of endometrial crypts and dilating them. Moving toward the cervix, the everted allantochorion pulls the chorionic villi from endometrial crypts (Fig. 72–3). Presence of the allantochorion at the cervix stimulates oxytocin release and additional uterine contractions, which are accompanied by further abdominal expulsive efforts. Portions of freed placenta pass through the vagina and vulva adding weight of the placenta to the expulsive efforts of the abdomen and uterus. Oxytocin seems to play a role in postpartum uterine contractions, because an increased concentration is found in the blood during the third stage of labor.[17]

CAUSES

The cause for retained placentas is unclear. Attachment of the microcotyledons (microvilli) are tightly adhered by the seventh month of gestation.[7] This attachment makes complete separation difficult to impossible unless the microvilli are released. Either the gravid horn or the nongravid horn allantochorion of a retained placenta is attached to the endometrium, thus preventing expulsion.[18,19] Another report stated that neither horn is attached but actually the area between the two horns remains attached.[20] The generalized opinion today is that areas of allantochorion near the tip of the nonpregnant horn have failed to separate. Clinical and pathologic observations suggest mechanical interference and hormonal imbalance as possible causes. Allantochorion thickness, length of villi, and degree of attachment of the placenta increase from gravid to nongravid horn. An explanation for these characteristics includes the presence of more developed microvilli in uterine horns than in the body plus microvilli are more branched and larger in the nonpregnant horn.[15] Furthermore, folding of the placenta and endometrium within the nongravid horn is more pronounced.[21] Last, uterine involution occurs at a slower rate in the nongravid than gravid horn. These events, working in combination or alone, help explain slower release of the placenta from the nongravid horn. Placental edema is reported to be partially responsible for retention.[22] Presence of edema and increased weight supposedly led to weighing of placentas. The placenta should reportedly weigh 6.4 kg. However, the weights of 200 normal Thoroughbred placentas ranged from 4 to 8 kg. Furthermore, edema is apparently more prevalent in the gravid than nongravid horn.

Blood-borne or ascending infection after cervical re-

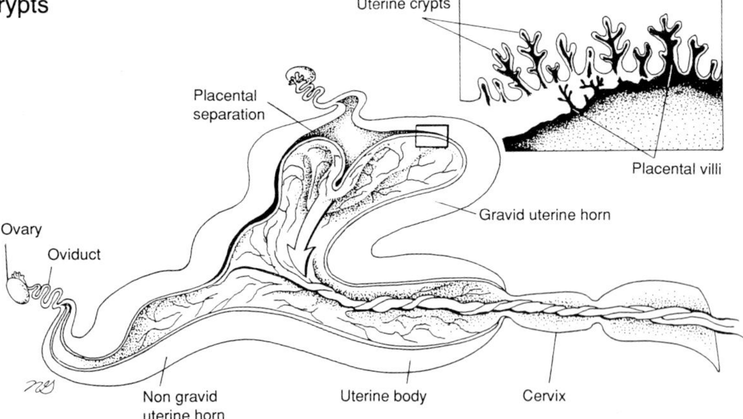

FIG. 72–2. Separation of microvilli from endometrial crypts beginning within gravid horn.

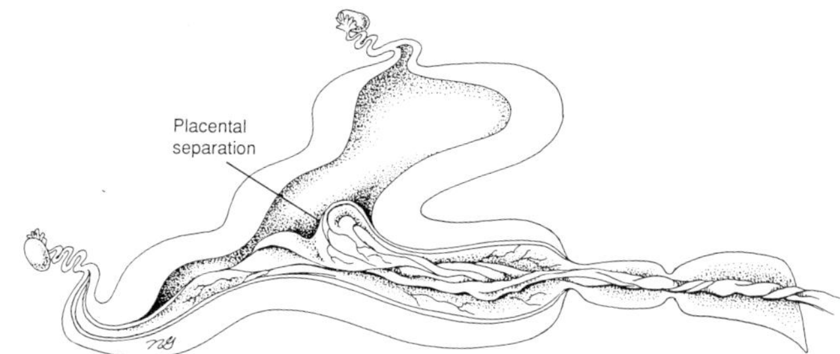

FIG. 72–3. Continued separation with eversion of placenta.

laxation and endometritis during pregnancy could induce inflammatory choriouterine adherences and delay separation of the placenta.[1] This type of lesion, along with placentome sclerosis, has also been observed in the cow with retained placenta and after experimental infections with Brucella abortus and Aspergillus spp. Roberts has suggested that contaminated air entering the uterus at time of parturition could carry in bacteria that could reduce speed of placental passage.[1] That the contaminating bacteria could have such an effect within 30 to 60 min is difficult to imagine. Bacteria more likely enter at the time of breeding or foaling, because of poor hygiene, and could have an effect on the next parturition. Mares that have uterine infections before breeding, that become infected at breeding, or that are bred to an infected stallion may have retarded placental separation at the following parturition.[1]

Infection as a cause of retained placenta may not be as important as was once thought, because infections between endometrium and placenta are usually present near the internal os and surrounding area.[1] These infections have not lead to placental retention and do not account for the last attachment freed being located near the tip of the uterine horn.

Many authors believe that retained placentas are primarily the result of uterine inertia and hormonal imbalance because mares affected with retained placentas do not exhibit the mild signs of colic associated with postpartum uterine contractions.[23] This hormonal imbalance could result in abnormal myometrial activity, not necessarily decreased movement or contractions. Excellent results obtained with treatment of retained placenta with oxytocin suggest a possible deficiency or lack of this hormone in the circulation.[7,24] One report on a limited number of pony mares revealed that oxytocin increased in the serum during the second and third stages of a normal labor.[17] Furthermore, when oxytocin was used to induce parturition, increasing doses shortened time to the second and third stages of labor.[25]

Although some authors believe uterine inertia can cause retained placenta in the cow, it probably is not a cause in the mare because, reportedly, uterine tone frequently increases after dystocia with placental retention.[7] Uterine inertia can be caused by low blood calcium, overstretching of the myometrium as in hydrops allantois, twinning and oversize fetus, myometrial degeneration resulting from bacterial infection, and myometrial exhaustion after dystocia in poorly conditioned animals.[1] Uterine inertia was also incriminated in premature delivery when the normal sequence of hormonal changes had not occurred. Low concentrations of circulating cortisol at calving have been associated with retained placenta, which has not been reported in the mare. Decrease in plasma progesterone before calving was slower in cows that retained the placenta. High blood concentrations of progesterone at calving interfered with uterine contractions and with detachment and expulsion of the placenta. A report on one mare with a retained placenta indicated serum progesterone remained elevated at prepartum concentrations instead of decreasing as occurred in all mares that passed the placenta within 30 min.[26] Another report indicated that relaxin activity remained elevated in a mare with a retained placenta, possibly because the presence of the placenta within the uterus acted as a source of relaxin.[27] The role of prostaglandins (PG) in passage of the placenta remains unknown. A report on retained placentas in cows indicated that $PGF_2\alpha$ decreased and PGE_2 increased in association with retained placenta.[28]

SIGNS

The most obvious sign of a mare with a retained placenta is the appearance of that tissue protruding from the vulva. It may be from slightly visible to dragging the ground. A retained placenta present with no placenta visible is usually caused by a portion of the placenta remaining attached to the endometrium rather than the entire placenta being present within the uterus, although the latter is possible.

Mares that normally pass the placenta during stage three of parturition show slight to mild colic because of uterine contractions.[1] Mares with retained placentas infrequently demonstrate this activity, and when present it is diminished. A retained placenta protruding from the vulva and touching the hocks should be tied up away from the hocks below the vulva[29] (Fig. 72–4). This procedure will reduce the probability that the mare will kick at the placenta and in doing so possibly injure the foal.[1] The mare will also be less likely to step on the

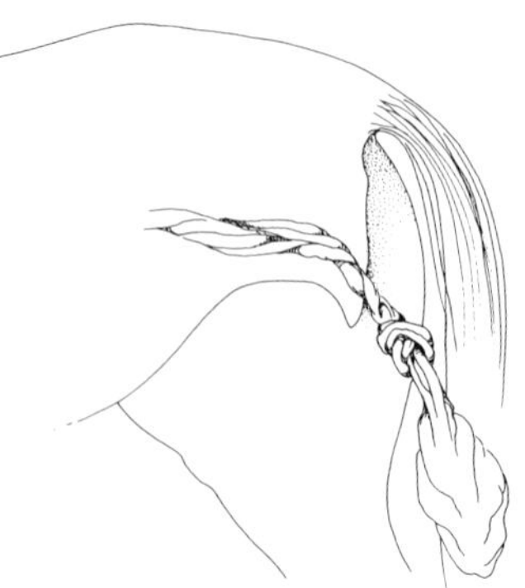

FIG. 72–4. Placenta tied in knot to avoid hocks.

placenta, causing it to tear or causing the tip of the uterine horn to invaginate within itself or to evert through the vulva.

COMPLICATIONS OF RETAINED PLACENTA

Sequellae of retained placenta in the mare may vary from none to metritis, laminitis, septicemia, or death.[30] Acute metritis and laminitis, as described in heavy breeds, are not as commonly seen in Thoroughbreds and other light breeds. Older literature suggests the longer the placenta is present the greater the risk of uterine infection and greater delay in uterine involution.[31] A major concern regarding a retained placenta to most veterinarians and horse owners is that the mare may develop laminitis.[32] Laminitis has been reported to be more common in draft horses, and it occurs especially with a profuse uterine discharge. The suggested mechanism of action was that delayed uterine involution resulted in autolysis of the placenta within the uterus. This condition provided the environment in which bacteria could rapidly multiply, resulting in local inflammation and absorption of uterine contents that created a septicemia or toxemia.

Although Streptococcus zooepidemicus is the predominant infective organism within the uterus at time of a retained placenta,[1] other gram-negative bacteria capable of endotoxin and histamine production may be more important. Furthermore, laminitis has been attributed to degenerative changes in connective tissue within the foot and not to the typical toxic capillary injury and edema.[33]

A study of 356 retained placentas in Standardbreds treated without manual removal reported no cases of laminitis, toxemia, septicemia, or acute metritis.[12] Postparturient laminitis is considered the result of a systemic acute metritis with[34] or without[35] a retained placenta. Most veterinarians would agree that this metritis creates an abnormal condition within the uterus and consider it to be septicemic or toxemic, because it involves sensitive laminae of the hoof and possibly body temperature, disposition, and appetite. Occurrence of postpartum laminitis in association with a retained placenta is often the result of either retention of many microvilli in large areas when they are broken free from their attachments to the remainder of the placenta, which can occur during manual removal, or separation of the apex of the placenta in the nongravid horn from the remainder of the placenta.[1] These placental remnants serve as a focus of infection, and the uterus fills with fluid. The importance of placental examination following passage becomes obvious. Laminitis is caused by the effects of septic uterine contents and possibly by the release of histamines. The actual mechanism producing laminitis is not certain. Two suggested possibilities involve a vasoactive component and a coagulation component.[36] The vasoactive component may be related to hormones or toxins acting on digital vessels or shunts, thus altering blood circulation through the foot. Hood et al. suggested that peripheral blood circulation increases immediately postpartum because of decreased uterine size and this blood is involved in the vasoactive component.[37] The coagulation component is related to intravascular coagulation,[38] alterations in the intrinsic coagulation system, platelet numbers, and fibrinogen degradation products;[37] incidence of laminitis can be reduced with heparin administration.[38]

The laminitis observed is similar to that of gastrointestinal origin in that in 2 to 4 days the animal exhibits a foundered gait with the hind limbs placed well forward under the body to reduce some of the weight from the front legs. The hooves are warmer than normal to the touch and the digital artery pulse is increased. The animal may spend the majority of its time lying down or may refuse to lie down. Milk production decreases rapidly, and the foal becomes hungry and looks for food.

THERAPY CONSIDERATIONS

Some authors recommend treating any animal with a retained placenta to prevent laminitis. Recommended treatments have consisted of cold water or ice to hooves, suitable supportive footing and uterine and systemic antibiotic therapy to prevent septic metritis. Antihistamines,[39] phenylbutazone,[22] nonsteroidal anti-inflammatory drugs,[22] and tranquilizers have also been included in recommended therapy. Antihistamines, however, reportedly neither prevent nor cure laminitis after a retained placenta.[7] In addition, the quantity of roughage being fed should be reduced and grains possibly eliminated from the diet.[1] Although many clinicians recommend flushing the uterus of a mare that has septic or toxic metritis or manually removing the placenta, I am opposed to both practices. The less conservative treatments described in the literature rely on manual removal of the placenta and flushing the uterus in an attempt to reduce uterine debris. The disadvantage of this technique is that the treatment itself will increase absorption of septic or toxic material during removal and flushing and the mare's condition will deteriorate before she can improve. This action may result in more damage to the feet or in death. Excellent results have been obtained with conservative therapy involving systemic therapy and supportive care plus antibiotic therapy of the uterus the first or possibly first 2 days. The conservative approach is based on helping the mare establish the normal uterine barrier, which develops by approximately day 3 postpartum. This assistance is accomplished primarily by systemic antibiotics, anti-inflammatory drugs such as butezolidin or flunixin meglumine, and systemic fluids if necessary. This approach will result in improvement of the mare's condition within 24 to 48 h. Once this improvement has occurred, more localized treatment of the uterus can begin. Frequent temperature and complete blood count monitoring in mares treated in this manner will demonstrate slight subclinical relapses in progress after every uterine manipulation for 2 to 3 days. However, this result is more desirable than the less conservative therapies.

TREATMENTS

Treatments for retained placenta vary with each possessing advantages and disadvantages. The most conservative treatment in my opinion is the use of oxytocin. Several descriptive doses and routes of administration are available in the literature. Oxytocin can be administered in slow IV drip form by placing 30 to 60 units of oxytocin in 1 to 2 L of saline and administering it over an hour[7] or 80 to 100 units in 500 cc of saline and administering it over a 30-min period.[22] Oxytocin can also be administered in a bolus form (IV or IM);[2,32] doses range from 20 to 120 units. Doses can be repeated at 1.5- to 2-h intervals until passage of the placenta or 7 h postpartum. Disadvantage of the bolus form of administration include intense and only spasmodic contractions when "large" doses are administered and were believed to be of no value.[7] Furthermore, colic appeared to be more of a problem with bolus administration;[24] cramping may have been related to dosage. I have not encountered excessive colic with 20 units of oxytocin administered IM every 1 to 2 h. Furthermore, colicky signs, if they occur, can be eliminated with sedation or analgesics.[39] The dose of oxytocin can be increased with additional time postpartum without colicky signs.[25]

Antibiotics have been used in the therapy of retained placentas by most clinicians. One author suggested oxytetracycline hydrochloride in capsule form as the antibiotic of choice.[40] In my experience, use of powdered antibiotics (or antibiotics in capsule or tablet form) is considered undesirable because the antibiotic is unable to make contact with much of the endometrial surface. Other antibiotics used in the treatment of retained placentas have included sulfanilamide,[39] penicillin,[39] polymyxin, amikacin, ticarcillin,[22] and others. Administration of antibiotics intrauterine has been recommended to commence at 8 h following delivery. Antibiotics are thought to be an important part of retained placenta treatment because of their ability to control numbers of contaminating bacteria that enter the uterus at parturition or during attempts to manually remove the placenta. The placental attachment should be examined each time before treatment. Mares treated intrauterinely with antibacterial agents for placental retention reportedly have a significantly higher pregnancy rate after the breeding season than mares that had no intrauterine therapy for retained placenta.[12] However, because of a higher pregnancy loss, both groups had the same foaling percentage the following year. In a study of intrauterine combined with systemic antibiotic therapy versus only oxytocin therapy, 5 h following treatment 55% of the intrauterine-treated mares had not passed the placenta compared with 19% of those treated with oxytocin.[12]

Manual removal was the first reported treatment for retained placentas.[7] The literature describes five methods for manual removal of a placenta. The first consists simply of grasping the protruding free portion of the placenta and applying traction. This method does not require entry into the uterus if the placenta is exposed. Another method involves placing of the hand between the chorion and the endometrium to separate them. A third method also involves placing the hand between the chorion and the endometrium; however, the allantochorionic membrane is massaged free from the endometrium.[29] A fourth method involves grasping the allantochorionic membrane and twisting it into a tight cord.[1,39] The chorion is separated from the endometrium. The last method utilizes a wooden ring placed between the chorion and the endometrium such that the chorion separates as the ring is advanced. The time between parturition and recommended manual removal varies from immediately to 24 hs. Early removal could avoid a delay causing retarded uterine involution and a predisposition to uterine infection. However, in the same article the researcher reported that manual removal will delay uterine involution. Several visits to the mare at 4- to 12-h intervals may be necessary to remove a placenta manually without injury to the mare.[29] Arthur et al. suggest not working longer than 10 min on the placenta's removal at each visit.[39]

Although reported by many authors as the treatment of choice, manual removal of a placenta has many undesirable complications occurring after treatment. The first complication of manual removal of the placenta is severe hemorrhage.[7] The mare may lose large amounts of blood into the uterus, and blood serves as an excellent environment for bacterial growth. Furthermore, pulmonary emboli have been reported following this procedure, apparently the result of dislodgement of naturally occurring emboli from the uterine vein.[7]

Invagination or intussusception of the uterine horn attached to the placenta can occur at the time of manual removal. Another reproductive complication is a delay in uterine involution.[7] One study reported a "vastly" increased amount of fluid accumulated within the uterus after manual removal of the placenta.[39] The reason given for this increase was that during manual removal only central branches of the chorionic villi were removed and all microvilli were broken off and retained within the endometrium. In addition, rupture of endometrial and subendometrial capillaries may occur, adding to the fluid within the lumen of the uterus. Microvilli will need to be released and then flushed by natural uterine secretions from their crypts. These microvilli were related to increased occurrence of tissue debris, endometritis, laminitis, uterine spasm, and delayed involution.[39] One report acknowledged that manual removal should be discouraged because of the induced trauma, hemorrhage, and infection.[40] However, the treatment was recommended after other methods had failed.

Held suggested that manual removal of the placenta can result in permanent endometrial damage.[22] I have observed that damage has occurred in some mares 3 to 14 yr of age which had normal fertility until manual removal of a placenta. Following manual removal, I have found a decrease in fertility, and endometrial biopsies revealed classifications of categories IIB and III based on presence of scar tissue. The cervix also remains open longer when the placenta is manually removed.[7] Arthur et al. suggested that manual removal of the placenta has been continued from a time when draft horses predominated and retained placentas were more of a problem.[39]

Antiseptics placed into the uterus have been suggested as another method of therapy. Betadine in 5 to 8 gal of warm water has been placed into the uterus and inside the placenta.[2] Another method describes the placement of 10 to 12 L of povidine-iodine into the allantochorionic space followed by closure of the hole in this membrane (Fig. 72–5A), trapping the fluid within the allantoic cavity[30] (Fig. 72–5B). This procedure aids expulsion by stretching the uterus and causing endogenous oxytocin release and separation of microvilli from their attachments. The placenta should be passed within 30 min. The exact effect of this procedure on microvilli separation has not been reported. One disadvantage of antiseptic use was that it could depress phagocytosis. The importance of this effect is unknown.[6]

Flushing and siphoning[39] of fluid from the uterus have been reportedly successful in treatment of retained placentas.[29] Roberts stated that douching the uterus is of questionable value.[1] Infusing the uterus with 42° C water has been used with apparently beneficial results.[14] Flushing the uterus with large volumes of saline containing antibiotics reportedly prevented or cured laminitis.[2] Much diversity in regard to uterine therapy and its importance obviously exists.

Tetanus protection in the form of antitoxin,[39] or preferably toxoid, is recommended. Placement of Caslick sutures or clips in the dorsal vulva after foaling have been recommended to reduce uterine contamination.[1]

The importance of intrauterine therapy or need to remove the placenta rapidly is not established. Systemic oxytocin treatment for uncomplicated retained placenta apparently is superior to all others in the nondraft breed. A report on a heavy hunter mare that was treated solely with systemic antibiotics after a cesarean passed the placenta 5 days following parturition with no adverse side effects.[41] The animal was not treated intrauterinely because of its disposition. A second mare was first examined 5 days following foaling.[42] She had passed the placenta that day and had received no prior treatment. The mare's temperature was normal, there was no laminitis, and she was eating and drinking. The only reason the owners realized a problem existed was the passage of the foul-smelling placenta. I have treated one mare following an abortion at 9 months with intrauterine oxytetracycline for 3 days and then 2% Lugol's solution every other day until placental passage. She received phenylbutazone for the first 4 days. The placenta was passed 13 days following the abortion. The uterus was cultured at 34 days and contained no bacteria. She was bred at approximately 60 days postabortion and conceived, maintaining the pregnancy and delivering a healthy foal. This case is the longest I have had a mare retain a placenta. Adequate examination and treatment of the mare with a retained placenta must be provided. The clinician must realize manual removal of the placenta is not the treatment of choice.

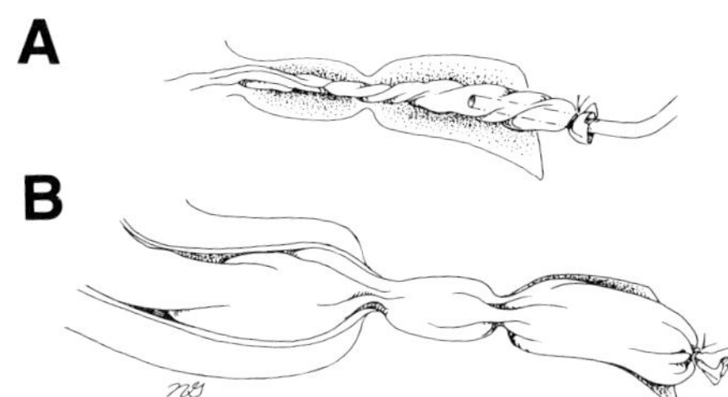

FIG. 72–5. *A*, Placement of fluid inside choriallantoic membrane. Tube is inserted into placenta for placement of fluid and a suture is made to aid in fluid retention. *B*, Fluid-filled placenta to aid in expulsion.

SUBSEQUENT EXAMINATION

Subsequent followup examination of mares with retained placentas should be mandatory regardless of treatment. The uterus must be determined to be normal whether or not the mare is to be bred again that year. Rectogenital examination, uterine culture, endometrial biopsy and ultrasonographic examination are recommended techniques that can be employed in this evaluation. Endometrial cytology and endoscopic examination can also be used. My recommendation is to wait approximately 25 days following placental passage before breeding. However, late in the breeding season mares have conceived and maintained pregnancies when bred at 10 to 20 days postpartum. The latter is recommended only at the end of the breeding season when no other option is available. The placenta when passed should be examined for completeness and obvious abnormalities. This is often difficult because of deterioration of tissue.

INFLUENCE OF RETAINED PLACENTA ON FUTURE REPRODUCTION

No difference in pregnancy rates after first breeding, pregnancy rates after the breeding season, pregnancy loss rates, and foaling rates between normal foaling mares and mares with retained placentas has been reported.[12] This lack of a difference was evident regardless of the duration of time the placenta was retained. No manual removal was used in this study.

SUMMARY OF TREATMENT

A three-paragraph correspondence by Kelly in 1944 probably described treatment of the retained placenta as well as anyone.[43] Placentas which cannot be removed "easily" should not be removed; give "appropriate" medication and wait. Recommendations regarding retained placentas include initiation of therapy at 3 h postpartum. This therapy is accomplished most conveniently by dispensing oxytocin to the owner with written instructions for administration of 20 units of oxytocin IM every 1 to 2 h to mares not passing the placenta within 3 h of parturition. This action permits commencement of treatment in the middle of the night that otherwise may not occur. The low dose administered IM has not been associated with severe colicky signs but has been observed at the time of cesarean operations to cause muscular contractions of the uterus. An examination of the mare within 12 to 18 h of foaling is imperative to distinguish an uncomplicated retained placenta from one that could be more severe. This examination consists of rectogenital palpation and is performed regardless of placental passage. Decreased uterine tone is an excellent indicator of potential complications. No vaginal examination is performed or treatment administered if the placenta has passed and the uterus has good to excellent tone at the time of the examination. If the placenta is present and the uterus has good to excellent tone, the uterus is infused with 5 to 8 g oxytetracycline in 500 mL of saline. I am uncertain whether this is necessary. If the uterine tone is diminished the volume of infusion is increased. In lightweight breeds, no other treatment is given. In draft breeds or in any mare following a severe dystocia, animals are administered systemic penicillin with or without gentomycin and flunixin meglamine. Mares that have experienced severe dystocias appear to be at most risk for developing complications from retained placenta or to the dystocia itself. Systemic treatment is continued for 3 to 7 days depending on the animal's condition. Uterine infusions are switched from oxytetracycline to 2% Lugol's solution on days 2 to 4 to enhance the contractibility of the uterus. The volume of Lugol's solution is determined by the size of the uterus and may vary from 500 cc to 6 L. The important factor to remember regarding Lugol's administration is not to overfill the uterus. I have used 2 to 10% Lugol's solutions to treat uterine infections and inflammation as well as retained placentas without any adverse effects on the endometrium as determined by endometrial biopsy and endoscopy. Lugol's solution, however, placed into the vagina will cause straining and the development of fibrous connective tissue bands across the vaginal lumen.

Mares with a history of retained placenta should be treated with oxytocin immediately after foaling and treated again as described previously. Mares over 15 yr old may be candidates for postpartum treatment with oxytocin, and although the author does not routinely do this, it is a consideration and is used selectively. Intrauterine medication may prove to be unnecessary or detrimental in uncomplicated cases of retained placentas. Although a concern, the importance of laminitis and the effect of retained placenta on future reproduction in lighter breeds does not appear to be a major problem if treatment is initiated early.

REFERENCES

1. Roberts, S.J.: Veterinary Obstetrics and Genital Diseases. 3rd ed. Woodstock, VT, published by the author, 1986.
2. White, T.E.: Retained placenta. Mod. Vet. Pract., *61:*87–88, 1980.
3. Shipley, W.D., and Bergen, W.C.: Care of the foaling mare and foal. Vet. Med., *64:*63–70, 1969.
4. Sager, F.C.: Examination and care of the genital tract of the brood mare. J. Am. Vet. Med. Assoc., *115:*450–455, 1949.
5. Wright, J.G.: Parturition in the mare. J. Comp. Pathol., *53:*212–219, 1943.
6. Asbury, A.C.: Management of the foaling mare. Proc. Am. Assoc. Equine Pract., 487–490, 1972.
7. Vandeplassche, M., Spincemaille, J., and Bouters, R.: Aetiology, pathogenesis and treatment of retained placenta in the mare. Equine Vet. J., *3:*144–147, 1971.
8. Jennings, W.E.: Some common problems in horse breeding. Cornell Vet., *31:*197–215, 1941.
9. Williams, W.L.: The Diseases of the Genital Organs of Domestic Animals. 3rd ed., Ithaca, NY, published by the author, 1943.
10. Blanchard, T.L., et al.: Sequelae to percutaneous fetotomy in the mare. J. Am. Vet. Med. Assoc., *182:*1127, 1983.
11. Vandeplassche, M., Bouters, R., Spincemaille, J., and Bonte, P.: Dropsy of the fetal sacs in mares: Induced and spontaneous abortion. Vet. Rec., *99:*67–69, 1976.
12. Provencher, R., Threlfall, W.R., Murdick, P.W., and Wearly, W.K.: Retained fetal membranes in the mare: A retrospective study. Can Vet. J., *29:*903–910, 1988.
13. Jennings, W.E.: Twelve years of horse breeding in the army. J. Am. Vet. Med. Assoc., *116:*11–16, 1950.
14. Sager, F.C.: Management and medical treatment of uterine disease. J. Am. Vet. Med. Assoc., *153:* 1567–1569, 1968.
15. Vandeplassche, M, Spincemaille, J., Bouters, R., and Bonte, P.: Some aspects of equine obstetrics. Equine Vet. J., *4:*105–109, 1972.
16. Steven, D.H., Jeffcott, L.B., and Mallon, K.A.: Ultrastructural studies of the equine uterus and placenta following parturition. J. Reprod. Fertil. Suppl., *27:*579–586, 1979.
17. Allen, W.E., Chard, T., and Forsling, M.L.: Peripheral plasma levels of oxytocin and vasopressin in the mare during parturition. J. Endocrinol., *57:*175–176, 1973.
18. Van der Kaay, F.C.: Cursus Nota's. Faculteit Diergeneeskunde, Utrecht, 1945.
19. Alhnelt, E.: Tiergeburtshilte 2e Aufl. Berlin, P. Pary, 1960.
20. Derivauz, J.: Obstetrique Veterinaire. Paris, Vigot Freres, 1957.
21. Arthur, G.H.: Wright's Veterinary Obstetrics. 3rd ed. Baltimore, Williams & Wilkins 1964.
22. Held, J.P.: Retained placenta. *In* Current Therapy in Equine Medicine, 2nd ed. Edited by N. Edward Robinson. Philadelphia, W.B. Saunders, 1987, pp. 547–550.
23. Berthelon, M., and Tournut, J.: Retention of the placenta in domestic animals. Rev. Med. Vet., *104:*529–538, 1953.
24. Cox, J.E.: Excessive retainment of the placenta in a mare. Vet. Rec., *89:*252–253, 1971.
25. Hillman, R.B.: Induction of parturition in mares. J. Reprod. Fertil. Suppl., *23:*641–644, 1975.
26. Seamans, K.W., Harms, P.G., Atkins, D.T., and Fleeger,

J.L.: Serum levels of progesterone, 5 alpha-dihydroprogesterone and hydroxy-5 alpha prenanones in the prepartum and postpartum equine. Steroids, *33:*55–63, 1979.

27. Stewart, D.R., Stabenfeldt, G.H., and Hughes, J.P.: Relaxin activity in foaling mares. J. Reprod. Fertil. Suppl., *32:*603–609, 1982.
28. Horta, A.E.M., Chassagne, M., and Brochart, M.: Prostaglandin F_2alpha and prostacyclin imbalance in cows with placental retention. Ann. Res. Vet., *17:*395–400, 1986.
29. Allen, W.E.: Fertility and Obstetrics in the Horse. Boston, Blackwell Scientific, 1988.
30. Burns, S.J., Judge, N.G., Martin, J.E., and Adams, L.G.: Management of retained placenta in mares. Proc. Am. Assoc. Equine Pract., 381–390, 1977.
31. Rossdale, P.D., and Ricketts, S.W.: Equine Stud Farm Medicine. 2nd ed. Philadelphia, Lea & Febiger, 1980.
32. Hafez, E.S.E.: Reproduction in Farm Animals. 5th ed. Philadelphia, Lea & Febiger, 1987.
33. Obel, N.: Contribution to our knowledge of the aetiology and pathogenesis of the foaling laminitis. Scand. Vet. Tidsskr., *33:*41–46, 1943.
34. Adams, O.R.: Lameness in Horses. 3rd ed. Philadelphia, Lea & Febiger, 1974.
35. Threlfall, W.R., and Carleton, C.L.: Treatment of uterine infections in the mare. *In* Current Therapy in Theriogenology. 2nd ed. Edited by D.A. Morrow. Philadelphia, W.B. Saunders, 1986, pp. 730–737.
36. Hood, D.M. and Stephens, K.A.: Physiology of equine laminitis. Compend. Contin. Educ. Practicing Vet., *3:*454–460, 1981.
37. Hood, D.M., et al.: Update on laminitis: Physiopathology and treatment. Paper presented at the Annual Meeting of the American Veterinarian Medical Association, Washington, D.C., July 20–24, 1980.
38. Hood, D.M., et al.: Equine laminitis III: Coagulation dysfunction in the developmental and acute disease. J. Equine Med. Surg., *3:*355–361, 1979.
39. Arthur, G.H., Noakes, D.E., and Pearson, H.: Veterinary Reproduction and Obstetrics. 5th ed. London, Bailliere Tindall, 1982.
40. Neely, D.P., Liu, I.K.M., and Hillman, R.B.: Equine Reproduction. Nutley, NJ, Veterinary Learning Systems, 1983.
41. Mason, T.A.: Retention of the placenta in the mare. Vet. Rec., *89:*546, 1971.
42. Alexander, R.W.: Excessive retainment of the placenta in the mare. Vet. Rec., *89:*175–176, 1971.
43. Kelly, E.V.: Retained placenta in the mare. Vet. Rec., *56:*296, 1944.

CHAPTER 73

UTERINE INVOLUTION AND POSTPARTUM BREEDING

T.L. Blanchard
D.D. Varner

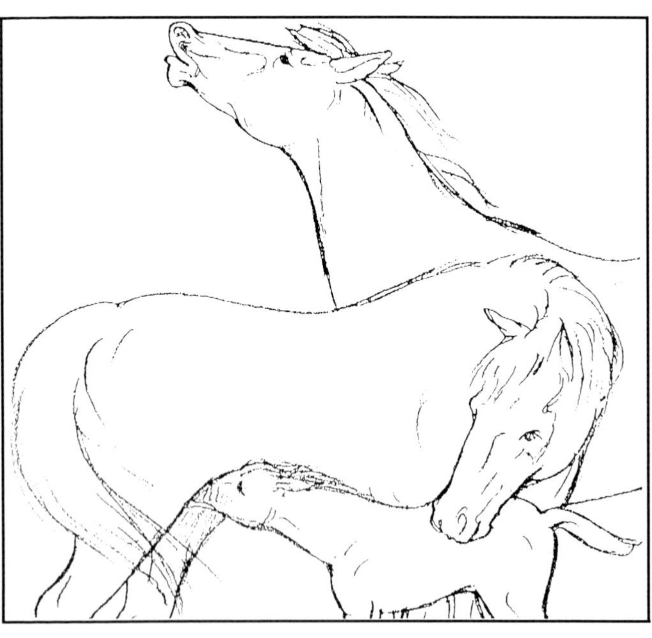

The relatively long gestational period of the mare (average of 340 days) permits, on average, only 25 days from parturition to conception if foals are to be produced at yearly intervals. Adaptation has resulted in a rate of uterine involution and return to ovarian cyclicity that is more rapid and dynamic in the equine than in other domestic large animal species. Rapid uterine involution and the relatively short interval from parturition to onset of a fertile estrus often result in the establishment of pregnancy quite early in the postpartum period (e.g., within 1 to 2 weeks following parturition).

PHYSIOLOGIC CHANGES OF UTERINE INVOLUTION

Hormonal changes that occur in late gestation to prepare the uterus for the strong contractions necessary for delivery of the fetus are thought also to contribute to expulsion of the placenta and uterine involution. Plasma progesterone concentration drops in late pregnancy and remains low from parturition until the first postpartum ovulation. Plasma estrogen concentration is low immediately following parturition but begins to rise within a few days because of follicular recruitment and maturation, which initiates the first postpartum estrus.[1,2] Progesterone blocks myometrial contractions,[3] while estrogens enhance myometrial activity, perhaps by increasing populations of oxytocin and prostaglandin receptors in the myometrium.[4] Prostaglandin $F_2\alpha$ and oxytocin contribute to increased uterine contractility and are elevated during the first few days postpartum in normally foaling mares.[5,6] The function of those hormones in stimulating uterine contractions and involution during the postpartum period is incompletely understood. However, they are likely to play an instrumental role.

Uterine contractility plays an important part in rapidly reducing the size of the postparturient uterus to its pregravid state. Following delivery of the fetus, myometrial contractions decrease temporarily but then resume to aid in placental expulsion.[7] Uterine contractions are orderly, commencing at the apices of the uterine horns as peristaltic waves, which progress toward the cervix.[8] This abrupt increase in uterine activity probably results from removal of the myometrial inhibitors, progestins and relaxin, which are contained in the placenta. Long bursts of electromyographic (EMG) activity (which is correlated with uterine contractility) are replaced gradually over the first few days postpartum with a more continuous, low-level, and erratic electrical activity.[7]

Concurrent with this decrease in uterine size, a significant amount of lochial fluid is discharged from the uterine lumen.[8] This normal uterine discharge progressively decreases through the first postpartum ovulation,[9] and ultrasonographically detected fluid in the uterine lumen gradually decreases; no fluid should be detectable by day 15 postpartum.[10] The histologic character of the endometrium correspondingly reverts to a condition more conducive to embryonic support.[8] Uterine horns return to pregravid size by day 32 postpartum, whereas involution of the endometrium occurs more rapidly. Overlying luminal epithelium is intact by days 4 to 7 postpartum,[11,12] and resorption of microcaruncles is essentially complete by day 7 postpartum. Endometrial gland dilation is absent by day 4 postpartum and glandular activity increases, as indicated by taller epithelial cells with increased mitotic activity, to day 12 postpartum.[12] The endometrium usually has a normal pregravid histologic appearance by day 14 postpartum.[11]

CHARACTERISTICS OF FIRST POSTPARTUM ESTRUS

The mare is unique among domestic animals in that the first postpartum estrus is ovulatory. This estrus, commonly referred to as foal heat, is characterized by normal follicular development and ovulation within the first 20 days postpartum.[13] The onset of the foal heat occurs within 5 to 12 days after parturition in > 90% of mares.[14] In a study involving 470 mares, 43% had ovulated by day 9, 93% by day 15, and 97% by day 20 after parturition.[13] The average interval to first ovulation was 10.2 ± 2.4 days. Although season does not affect interval from parturition to onset of foal heat, it does affect both duration of the first postpartum estrus and interval from parturition to ovulation;[13,14] both decrease as day length increases. Loy found that only 33% of mares foaling in January to February ovulated before day 10 postpartum, whereas 83% of mares foaling in May ovulated before day 10 postpartum.[13] Mares foaling late in the season (May) were more likely to have double ovulations during foal heat than mares foaling earlier in the year (January to March).[13] An additional noteworthy seasonal effect is that mares bred early in the breeding season have a gestational period approximately 10 days longer than mares bred late in the breeding season.[14]

Pregnancy rates achieved by breeding during foal heat are generally reported to be 10 to 20% lower than those obtained by first breeding at subsequent estrous periods;[13–15] however, management practices are likely to affect the potential difference in pregnancy rates achieved by breeding on the first, or a later, postpartum estrous period. While controversy still exists regarding whether a greater incidence of pregnancy loss occurs in mares conceiving during foal heat breedings,[14] when management differences and variation over years are taken into account, the rate of pregnancy loss is probably not significantly different from that occurring in mares bred first during later estrous periods.[13]

MANAGEMENT CONSIDERATIONS FOR BREEDING ON THE FIRST POSTPARTUM ESTRUS

The major constraints to maximize the number of foals produced per dam lifetime are the long gestational period in the mare and the restricted operational breeding season which is often imposed. Because the birth date of foals is universally January 1 for the majority of breed registrations in the Northern Hemisphere, and horses are generally required to compete in performance at a very early age (i.e., 1 to 2 yr), great pressure exists to produce foals with birth dates early in the year. As a result, "late-foaling" mares are not rebred until the following season. Failure to produce foals on a yearly basis culminates in irretrievable economic loss, because of expenses for feed and housing, transportation, animal care, and perhaps nonproductive breeding fees. While more estrous periods are required to produce foals from mares bred during the foal-heat compared with mares first bred during later postpartum estrous periods (2.3 estrous periods/live foal vs. 1.9 estrous periods/live foal), failure to establish pregnancy by breeding on the foal heat results in an 18-day drift toward a later conception and a corresponding delay in the foaling date the following year. Cumulative season pregnancy and foaling rates are similar between mares bred on the foal heat and mares first bred on later postpartum estrous periods.[13] The time-saving advantage is, therefore, the primary impetus for breeding mares during their foal heat.

The decreased pregnancy rate associated with foal heat breedings has been suggested to be caused by the failure of the uterus, particularly the endometrium, to be completely involuted and, therefore, ready to support a developing embryo.[8,14] In support of this hypothesis, the pregnancy rate from foal heat breedings is higher in mares that ovulate after 10 days postpartum compared with those that ovulate before this time.[13] Because a 5-day interval following ovulation is required before the embryo enters the uterus,[14] ovulation after day 10 postpartum ensures that the histioarchitecture of the endometrium has returned to normal before embryo entry. Attempts to improve pregnancy rates from breeding in the early postpartum period have been centered around either attempting to enhance the rate of uterine involution or delaying breeding until involution is complete. Presence of fluid in the uterine lumen during the first postpartum ovulatory period has been correlated with decreased pregnancy rates.[10] Removal of uterine fluid containing bacteria, blood, and cellular debris by uterine lavage with 8 to 20 L of various solutions has been advocated as a method of increasing pregnancy rate on foal heat breedings,[16,17] but critical investigations have not found lavage to enhance either uterine involution[18,19] or pregnancy rates achieved by breeding on the first postpartum estrus[20] in normally foaling mares.

The administration of ecbolic agents (e.g., oxytocin and prostaglandin) has been advocated as a method to enhance uterine involution. Administration of oxytocin, prostaglandins, and prostaglandin analogues to nonpregnant, fully involuted mares stimulates uterine contractions.[21,22] Although administration of oxytocin or a prostaglandin analogue twice daily to a limited number of mares for the first 10 days postpartum did not enhance uterine involution,[23] administration of a prostaglandin analogue twice daily for 9 to 10 days postpartum has been reported to improve pregnancy rates from foal heat breedings.[22] Further investigation of methods to enhance uterine involution is warranted before sound recommendations can be made regarding their effectiveness.

Basically, two methods are currently employed to delay breeding in the postpartum period until normal pregnancy rates can be achieved: (1) to shorten the interval to the second postpartum estrus and (2) to delay the onset of the foal heat. Administration of prostaglandin 6 to 7 days after the first postpartum ovulation will hasten onset of the second postpartum estrus, which normally occurs approximately 30 days postpartum.[24] While this management technique is expected to increase pregnancy rate at the first breeding postpartum, such is not always the case.[25] In addition, when compared with breeding during the foal heat, the parturition to breeding interval will be delayed approximately 2 weeks (i.e., approximately 1 week is saved compared with waiting and breeding on the second postpartum estrus). The authors believe the best method for using this technique is to monitor postpartient mares closely for ovulation and breed on the foal heat if they do not ovulate before day 10 postpartum and little or no fluid remains in the uterus. Normal pregnancy rates can be expected in these mares, even though they are bred on foal heat. If ovulation is anticipated to occur before day 10 postpartum, or if significant fluid accumulation is present in the uterus, instead of breeding during the foal heat the mare can be injected with prostaglandin 1 week later and bred on the induced estrus.

Pregnancy rates achieved by breeding on the foal heat appear to be higher in mares in which estrus is delayed by hormonal therapy.[10,26,27] Altrenogest is given daily for 8 days,[10] but prostaglandin should be administered on the last day of treatment, because progesterone therapy alone may not prevent ovulation from occurring even though estrus is suppressed.[28–30] Daily treatment with a combination of progesterone and estradiol-17β for 5 days will delay onset of the first postpartum estrus and ovulation.[30] Treatment should commence as soon as practical on the day of foaling. Delaying the first postpartum ovulation with hormonal therapy until after day 10 postpartum allows more complete uterine involution to occur, as evidenced by greater proliferation of endometrial glands and increased endometrial gland density and ciliation of luminal epithelial cells.[28,29,31] The uterine environment and endometrial secretions necessary for conceptus development may thus be more favorable when the foal heat is delayed.[32,33] Whether the endometrial changes that occur are the result of the longer interval from parturition to onset of estrus and ovulation or to stimulatory effects of exogenously administered steroids has not been determined.[31] The major objection to the use of steroid therapy for several consecutive days, beginning at the time of foaling, is that the treatment delays the onset of the first postpartum estrus sufficiently so that foaling intervals are not significantly reduced. If treatment of postparturient mares for 2 or 3 days after foaling would only delay ovulation until just after day 10 postpartum, steroid treatment might offer the best method for increasing pregnancy rate without significantly extending the parturition to breeding interval in early postparturient mares. Preliminary trials using 150 mg progesterone and 10 mg estradiol-17β for the first 2 days postpartum have been encouraging in that respect. (F.M. Bristol, personal communication; H. Brady-Blue et al., personal communication).

REFERENCES

1. Hillman, R.B. and Loy, R.G.: Estrogen secretion in mares in relation to various reproductive states. Proc. Am. Assoc. Equine Pract., 111–119, 1969.
2. Nett, T.M., Holtan, D.W., and Estergreen, V.L.: Plasma estrogens in pregnant and postpartum mares. J. Anim. Sci., *37:*962–970, 1973.
3. McDonald, L.W.: Veterinary Endocrinology and Reproduction. 3rd ed. Philadelphia, Lea & Febiger, 1980.
4. Windmoller, R., Lye, S.J., and Challis, J.R.G.: Estradiol modulation of ovine uterine activity. Can. J. Physiol. Pharmacol., *61:*722–728, 1983.
5. Vandeplassche, M., et al.: Observations on involution and puerperal endometritis in mares. Ir. Vet. J., *37:*126–132, 1983.
6. Stewart, D.R., et al.: Concentrations of 15-keto-13,14-dihydro-prostaglandin $F_2\alpha$ in the mare during spontaneous and oxytocin induced foaling. Equine Vet. J., *16:*270–274, 1984.
7. Haluska, G.J., Lowe, J.E., and Currie, W.B.: Electromyographic properties of the myometrium correlated with the endocrinology of the pre-partum and post-partum periods and parturition in Pony mares. J. Reprod. Fertil. Suppl., *35:*553–564, 1987.
8. Roberts, S.J.: Veterinary Obstetrics and Genital Diseases (Theriogenology). 3rd ed. Woodstock, VT, published by the author, 1986.
9. Koskinen, E., and Katila, T.: Uterine involution, ovarian activity, and fertility in the postpartum mare. J. Reprod. Fertil. Suppl., *35:*733–734, 1987.
10. McKinnon, A.O., et al.: Ultrasonographic studies on the reproductive tract of mares after parturition: Effect of involution and uterine fluid on pregnancy rates in mares with normal and delayed first postpartum ovulatory cycles. J. Am. Vet. Med. Assoc., *192:*350–353, 1988.
11. Gygax, A.P., Ganjam, V.K., and Kenney, R.M.: Clinical, microbiological and histological changes associated with uterine involution in the mare. J. Reprod. Fertil. Suppl., *27:*571–578, 1979.
12. Bailey, J.V., and Bristol, F.M.: Uterine involution in the mare after induced parturition. Am. J. Vet. Res., *44:*793–798, 1983.
13. Loy, R.G.: Characteristics of postpartum reproduction in mares. Vet. Clin. N. Amer. Large Anim. Prac., *2:*345–358, 1980.
14. Ginther, O.J.: Reproductive Biology of the Mare: Basic and Applied Aspects. Cross Plaines, WI, Equiservices, 1979.
15. Lieux, P.: Comparative results of breeding on the first and second post-foaling heat periods. Proc. Am. Assoc. Equine Pract., 129–132, 1980.

16. Lenz, T.R.: One practitioner's approach to foal heat breeding. Proceedings of the Annual Meeting of the Society of Theriogenology. 1986, pp. 111–119.

17. Webb, G., Kreider, J., Potter, G. and Bowen, J.: Fertility and uterine histology of foaling mares infused with antibiotic, estradiol or hypertonic saline. Proceedings of the Equine Nurtritional and Physiology Symposium. 1983, pp. 301–307.

18. Shideler, R.K., McChesney, A.E., Squires, E.L., and Osborne, M.: Effect of uterine lavage on clinical and laboratory parameters in postpartum mares. Equine Pract., *9:*20–26, 1987.

19. Blanchard, T.L., et al.: Effects of postparturient uterine lavage on uterine involution in the mare. Theriogenology, *32:*527–536, 1989.

20. McCue, P.M., and Hughes, J.P.: The effect of postpartum uterine lavage on foal heat pregnancy rate. Theriogenology, *33:*1121–1129, 1990.

21. Goddard, P.J., and Allen, W.E.: Genital tract pressures in mares II. Changes induced by oxytocin and prostaglandin $F_2\alpha$. Theriogenology, *24:*35–44, 1985.

22. Ley, W.B., Purswell, B.J., and Bowen, J.M.: Prostaglandin $F_2\alpha$ as an uterine myometrial stimulant and effect on post-partum pregnancy rate in the mare. Proc. Soc. Theriogenol., 287–299, 1986.

23. Blanchard, T., et al.: Effects of myotonic agents on uterine involution in the mare. Theriogenology, *36:*559–572, 1991.

24. Kenney, R.M., Ganjam, V.K., and Bergman, R.V.: Non-infectious breeding problems in mares. Vet. Scope, *19:*16–24, 1975.

25. Burns, S.J., Irvine, C.H.G., and Amoss, M.S.: Fertility of prostaglandin-induced oestrus compared to normal post-partum oestrus. J. Reprod. Fertil. Suppl., *27:*245–250, 1979.

26. Bell, R.J., and Bristol, F.: Fertility and pregnancy loss after delay of foal oestrus with progesterone and oestradiol-17β. J. Reprod. Fertil. Suppl., *35:*667–668, 1987.

27. Loy, R.G., Evans, M.J., Pemstein, R., and Taylor, T.B.: Effects of injected ovarian steroids on reproductive patterns and performance in postpartum mares. J. Reprod. Fertil. Suppl., *32:*199–204, 1982.

28. Loy, R.G., Hughes, J.P., Richards, W.P.C., and Swan, S.M.: Effects of progesterone on reproductive function in mares after parturition. J. Reprod. Fertil. Suppl., *23:*291–295, 1975.

29. Pope, A.M., Campbell, D.L., and Davidson, J.P.: Endometrial histology of postpartum mares treated with progesterone and synthetic GnRH (ay-24,031). J. Reprod. Fertil. Suppl., *27:*587–591, 1979.

30. Bristol, F.M., Jacobs, K.A., and Pawlyshyn, V.: Synchronization of estrus in post-partum mares with progesterone and estradiol-17β. Theriogenology, *19:*779–785, 1983.

31. Sexton, P.E., and Bristol, F.M.: Uterine involution in mares treated with progesterone and estradiol-17β. J. Am. Vet. Med. Assoc., *186:*252–256, 1985.

32. Hafez, E.S.E., and Ludwig, H.: Scanning electron microscopy of the endometrium. *In* Biology of the Uterus. Edited by R.M. Wynn. New York, Plenum Press, 1977, pp. 309–336.

33. Allen, W.R., Hamilton, D.W., and Moore, R.M.: The origin of equine endometrial cupps. II. Invasion of the endometrium by trophoblasts. Anat. Rec., *177:*485–502, 1973.

CHAPTER 74

PARENTAGE TESTING

E. Bailey
E.G. Cothran
K.A. Graves

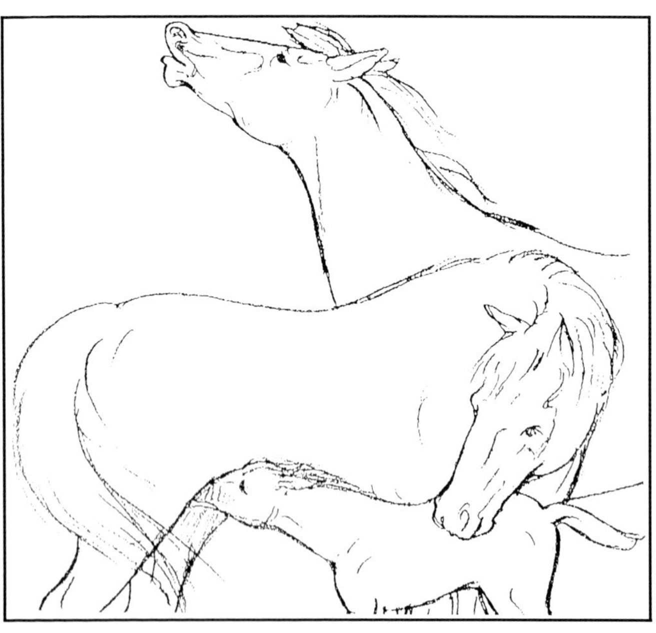

Genetic marker testing, commonly referred to as blood typing, is used for parentage verification and identification of horses. These tests were first developed in the 1950s and 1960s based on blood group tests and biochemical tests previously developed for humans, cattle, and other species.[1–7] Although genetic markers can be tested in other tissues, blood samples are easy to collect. Blood is also a diverse tissue that contains red blood cells; a variety of white blood cells, including lymphocytes, monocytes, and polymorphonuclear cells; and large molecules such as proteins, steroids, fats, and carbohydrates, which are secreted into the blood plasma by other tissues. At present, routine horse blood typing is based on tests of red blood cells and serum proteins.

Most horse blood typing laboratories belong to the International Society of Animal Genetics (ISAG), which conducts biennial comparison tests to standardize nomenclature and recognize new genetic systems in domestic animals. The tests considered by ISAG include blood group tests and biochemical marker tests.

BLOOD GROUP TESTS

The first blood typing tests were those for blood groups.[1,2,7–10] Blood group tests detect differences in red blood cell surface markers, called antigens. Tests used to detect these antigens are similar to those used to detect the ABO and Rh blood group antigens in humans, i.e., antibodies for these antigens are used to detect presence of the marker in agglutination or hemolytic tests. However, blood types of horses are different from those of humans and other species. Blood typing reagents specific to horses are used in horse blood typing tests. So far, no genetic or serologic homology has been found between human and equine blood groups. The equine blood group systems recognized by ISAG are listed in Table 74–1.

BIOCHEMICAL MARKERS

Serum is used to study proteins and enzymes which are secreted by other tissues and carried in blood. Red blood cells are lysed and intracellular enzymes tested for biochemical differences. The specific methods used to detect these proteins include starch-gel electrophoresis (STAGE), polyacrylamide electrophoresis (PAGE), 2-dimensional gel electrophoresis, and isoelectric focusing (IEF). The description of the methods can be found elsewhere.[3,5,6,11–14] The equine biochemical systems recognized by ISAG are listed in Table 74–2.

BASIS OF PARENTAGE ANALYSIS

No laboratory tests horses routinely for all 27 genetic systems listed in Tables 74–1 and 74–2. Testing would be too costly and some systems are not useful in some breeds. For example, Thoroughbred horses have rela-

TABLE 74–1. **EQUINE BLOOD GROUP SYSTEMS AND GENES FOUND IN EACH SYSTEM***

A Blood Group	C Blood Group	D Blood Group
adf	*a*	*ad*
adg	—	*adn*
a	K Blood Group	*bc*
b	*a*	*cgm*
c	—	*cgmp*
e	U Blood Group	*cfm*
bc	*a*	*cegimn*
be	—	*cefgm*
bce	P Blood Group	*cfgkm*
ce	*a*	*d*
cd	*ac*	*dn*
abdg	*acd*	*de*
—	*ad*	*deo*
O Blood Group	*b*	*dek*
abc	*bd*	*dfk*
ac	*d*	*dgh*
b	—	*dghp*
c		*dk*
—		—

*The lower case letters below each blood group system are names for the antigens known in that system and the combination of antigens are the known alleles.

tively little variation in the catalase system, and therefore, laboratories specializing in Thoroughbred testing do not use that system. Based on cost and effectiveness, most laboratories use between 12 and 17 systems routinely. At the University of Kentucky, routine blood typing tests include the A, C, D, K, P, Q, and U blood group systems as well as the albumin (Al), transferrin (Tf), A1b glycoprotein (Xk), protease inhibitor (Pi), serum carboxylesterase (Es), vitamin D binding protein (Gc), 6-phosphogluconate dehydrogenase (PGD), phosphoglucomutase (PGM), glucose phosphate isomerase (GPI), and α-hemoglobin (Hb) biochemical tests.

A blood type is the particular combination of genes expressed by a horse in all systems. The frequency of genes in the blood typing systems differ between breeds.[15,16] The most common blood types within each breed detected with the 17 systems listed above occur with the following frequencies: Thoroughbreds, 2.5 in 10,000; Standardbreds, 1.9 in 100,000; American Saddlebred horses, 1.7 in 1,000,000; and Quarter Horses, 6.6 in 10,000,000. Clearly, these figures demonstrate that even the most common blood type in each breed is not common. Herein lies the power of blood typing.

PARENTAGE ANALYSIS

Use of the markers in parentage depends on knowing the mode of inheritance of the genes. Each horse can possess up to two forms (alleles) of each gene, one inherited from the sire and one inherited from the dam. For example, albumin markers *A* and *B* are found in Thoroughbreds. (Albumin allele *I* is either absent or rare among Thoroughbred horses.) Based on these two alleles, a Thoroughbred horse may have the following albumin types: *AA, BB,* and *AB,* denoting inheritance of one albumin allele from the sire and one from the dam. Knowing this, albumin can be used for parentage analysis.

If a stallion has the albumin type *AA,* then he can only contribute the gene for *A* albumin to his offspring; all its offspring must have at least one copy of the *A* allele. He cannot have any offspring with type *BB.*

At the same time, the genes found in the offspring must be present in the parents. If a foal has albumin type *AB,* then at least one of its parents must possess each allele. The foal is excluded from parentage if both parents have the *AA* albumin type or both have the *BB* type.

In a similar fashion, parentage analysis is conducted for each system. When a genetic system with more alleles is used, such as Tf, Es, and Pi biochemical systems and the A, D, P, and Q blood groups, the number of possible types increases and the system becomes more powerful. Table 74–3 presents a sample parentage case. This case represents a situation in which a mare was bred to two stallions during a single estrous cycle. Either of the stallions could be the sire of the offspring. The analysis of the results is as follows:

1. *Albumin.* The offspring has only the allele for *Al-A.* Therefore, both parents must have at least one allele

TABLE 74–2. **EQUINE BIOCHEMICAL MARKER SYSTEMS AND GENES FOUND IN EACH SYSTEM***

Albumin (Al)	Glucosephosphate Isomerase (GPI)
A, B, I	*F, I, L, S*
Serum Carboxylesterase (Es)	Catalase (Cat)
F, G, I, L, M, O, R, S	*F, S*
Transferrin (Tf)	Carbonic Anhydrase (CA)
D, D2, E, F1, F2, F3, G,	*E, F, I, L, O, S*
H1, H2, J, M, O, R, X	Plasminogen (Plg)
Protease Inhibitor (Pi)	*1, 2*
E, F, G, H, I, J, K, L, L2, N,	NADH Diaphorase (DIA)
O, P, Q, R, S T, U, V, W, X, Z	*F, S*
A1B Glycoprotein (Xk)	Mannose Phosphate Isomerase (MPI)
F, K, S	*F, S*
Vitamin D Binding Protein (Gc)	Acid Phosphatase (AP)
F, S	*F, S*
6-Phosphogluconate Dehydrogenase (PGD)	
D, F, S	
α-Hemoglobin (Hb)	Malic Enzyme (ME)
A, AII, BI, BII	*F, S*
Phosphoglucomutase (PGM)	Haptoglobin (Hp)
F, V, S	*1, 2*
	Peptidase A (Pep)
	F, S

*The parentheses enclose the internationally (ISAG) recognized abbreviation of the marker system. The letters and/or numbers below the systems are the names of the alleles of that system.

TABLE 74–3. PARENTAGE ANALYSIS: DAM WAS BRED TO TWO STALLIONS DURING A SINGLE ESTROUS CYCLE*

	ALBUMIN	TRANSFERRIN	D BLOOD	ESTERASE	PI	K BLOOD
Stallion 1	*AB*	*F2O*	*ad, dfk*	*IS*	*LN*	*Ka*
Stallion 2	*AA*	*DO*	*de, dfk*	*FF*	*LS*	—
Dam	*AB*	*F2R*	*bc, dk*	*FS*	*LS*	—
Offspring	*AA*	*F2R*	*ad, bc*	*FI*	*LN*	*Ka*

*The dam, offspring, and two stallions are blood typed to determine which stallion is the sire. Stallion 2 is excluded as explained in the text.

for *Al-A*. The dam and both stallions have *Al-A*. Consequently, they all qualify as parents based on the albumin system.

2. *Transferrin*. The offspring has alleles for *F2* and *R*. The dam also has these transferrin alleles and may have contributed either one of them. Stallion 1 has *Tf-F2*, which it may have contributed to the offspring. Stallion 2 has neither *Tf-F2* nor *Tf-R*. Furthermore, the offspring does not have the *D* or *O* transferrin allele from stallion 2. Therefore, stallion 2 cannot be the sire of the offspring and is excluded.
3. *D blood group*. The offspring has blood group antigens *bc* and *ad*. Because the dam has the *bc* antigen and not the *ad* antigen, it must have contributed the allele for *bc* to the offspring. Therefore, the sire must have contributed the *ad* antigen. Stallion 1 has that antigen whereas stallion 2 does not have that antigen. Furthermore, the offspring does not have the *de* or *dfk* antigen from stallion 2. Consequently, stallion 2 is disqualified from parentage based on the D blood group system.
4. *Serum carboxylesterase*. The foal has *Es-F* and *Es-I*. The dam has the *F* esterase allele but not the *I* esterase allele. Because we know that the dam is correct, the sire must have contributed the allele for the *I* esterase. Stallion 1 has the *Es-I*, but stallion 2 does not. Therefore, stallion 2 is again disqualified from paternity.
5. *Protease inhibitor*. The offspring has Pi alleles for *L* and *N*. The dam has the *Pi-L* but not the *Pi-N*. Because we know that the foal is a product of this dam, then the *Pi-N* must have come from the sire. Stallion 1 has the *Pi-N* and stallion 2 does not. Therefore, stallion 2 cannot be the sire of the offspring.
6. *K blood group*. The foal has *Ka*, which is not present in the dam. Therefore, it must have come from the sire. Only stallion 1 has the *Ka* antigen, and consequently stallion 2 is disqualified from parentage.

The conclusion is that stallion 2 cannot be the sire of this foal. Because the only other stallion to which the mare was bred was stallion 1, and it was not disqualified, he must be the sire.

When a horse is excluded from parentage it is certain that the offspring is not a product of that mating. Exclusion in only a single one of the 17 systems is sufficient to warrant exclusion, thus constituting proof of nonpaternity. Paternity cases, as described above, will be solved 95 to 98% of the time based on the gene frequencies in different breeds and assuming random occurrence of the genetic markers in the two possible sires. If the two sires are related as father and son or as siblings, the probability of solution will decrease. A case where neither stallion can be excluded is given in Table 74–4. When cases are not solved by routine tests, further tests may be conducted including some of the additional systems from Table 74–2 or other systems such as lymphocyte typing.[17]

ROUTINE PARENTAGE SCREENING

In addition to solving specific parentage questions, breed registries use blood typing routinely to screen registered horses and detect instances of incorrectly assigned parentage. Although fraudulent representation is one possibility, other causes of incorrect parentage are found more commonly such as accidentally switching

TABLE 74–4. A SECOND PARENTAGE CASE*

	ALBUMIN	TRANSFERRIN	D BLOOD	ESTERASE	PI	K BLOOD
Stallion 1	*AB*	*F2O*	*ad, dkf*	*IS*	*LN*	*Ka*
Stallion 2	*AA*	*DF2*	*ad, de*	*FI*	*NS*	*Ka*
Dam	*AB*	*F2R*	*bc, dk*	*FS*	*LS*	—
Offspring	*AA*	*F2R*	*ad, bc*	*FI*	*LN*	*Ka*

*The same type of parentage analysis as was described for Table 74–3, except here neither stallion can be excluded, even though the two stallions have different alleles for each system.

foals in pasture or accidentally breeding mares to sexually precocious colts sharing a pasture. These accidents may be undetected until the horses are blood typed.

The power of routine blood typing to detect these errors depends on the circumstances. When both parents are incorrectly identified as in the case of foals becoming switched, the probability of detection is higher than when just the sire is incorrect. Nevertheless, for the following example we use the conservative estimates of 95 to 99% detection of parentage errors.

If errors of management led to misidentification of parentage at a rate of 1 in 100 registrations, a parentage verification program would reduce the error rate by detecting 95 to 99% of these errors, i.e., only 1 in 2,000 to 1 in 10,000 horses would have an incorrectly identified pedigree and not be detected by blood typing. In this way, routine parentage analysis can improve pedigree records within a breed.

PROOF OF PARENTAGE

For other questions, routine blood typing tests are less satisfactory. When a horse does not match its color description, i.e., the horse has white markings which are not on its papers, strong evidence is needed to counteract observations indicating that a switch has occurred. Parentage analysis can be done. However, as noted above, there will be a 1 to 5% chance that parentage will qualify even when the horse has been switched. In the face of strong evidence or suspicion that a switch has taken place 95 to 99% efficacy is not good enough.

For difficult parentage cases in people, researchers have adopted more powerful tests like lymphocyte typing and, more recently, DNA typing. In coupling with these tests a statistic called "proof of parentage" was developed.

Proof of parentage is actually a statistical statement that the likelihood of another set of parents producing an offspring with this genetic type approaches zero. Specifically, when an offspring has a blood type that is so unusual that the only reasonable conclusion is that it was derived from the stated parents, then parentage is considered to be proven, statistically.

For example, the albumin *I* allele is rare in Standardbred horses. If a Standardbred offspring had the albumin *II* type and both parents had albumin *I* genes, this would constitute a virtual proof of parentage because the likelihood of another randomly selected pair of parents being able to produce an individual with this albumin type would be 1 in 250,000. When genetic markers in other systems are considered, the likelihood that these were not the parents would easily exceed 1 in 1,000,000.

Unfortunately, all horses do not have rare blood typing genes detectable in current tests such that their parentage will be unique. Therefore, the next step in blood typing research is to identify even more powerful systems to determine parentage. It is readily apparent that the next generation of tests will be based on DNA testing.

ADVENT AND POTENTIAL USE OF DNA TESTS

Molecules of DNA are more complex than the proteins they encode, which are detected in blood typing tests. During the last 15 yr, several types of test have been developed for detecting genetic variation at the DNA level. These tests include the Southern blot using allele-specific probes, minisatellite probes, microsatellite testing oligonucleotide probes, and direct sequencing of genes. More genetic markers should be uncovered using these tests than can be identified with current tests. Tests based on DNA are also attractive because of the possibility to perform all testing using a single technique rather than mastering and maintaining current tests, which employ agglutination, hemolysis, STAGE, PAGE, IEF, and a variety of enzyme staining procedures.

Some tests for genetic variation at the DNA level have been reported for horses.[18–27] Nevertheless, additional research and development is needed for DNA-based marker testing in horses. At this writing, three major obstacles need to be overcome:

1. The cost of DNA based tests is currently high; however, the cost is dropping as technology evolves and the price of reagents decreases.
2. So far no satisfactory method exists for storing DNA "fingerprint" results; as a result, the sire, dam, and offspring must be retested each time a parentage question is investigated. This increases the number of tests required and adds a cost for long-term storage of DNA samples.
3. Researchers have not yet described as much genetic variation at the DNA level as is known based on current blood typing tests; the techniques exist and the potential is clear, but the work remains to be done.

These problems clearly will be resolved within the next 5 yr. As they become available, DNA-based tests will supplement current blood typing techniques to resolve those cases not solved by routine blood typing. Once these tests are as efficacious as blood typing and more cost effective, genetic marker testing in horses will be DNA based.

REFERENCES

1. Podliachouk, L.: Les Groupes sanguins des equides (cheval, mulet, ane). Ann. Inst. Pasteur, *95:*7–22, 1958.
2. Stormont, C., Suzuki, Y., and Rhode, E.A.: Serology of horse blood groups. Cornell Vet., *54:*439–452, 1964.
3. Braend, M., and Stormont, C.: Studies on hemoglobin and transferrin types of horses. Nord. Vet. Med., *16:*31–37, 1964.
4. Stormont, C., and Suzuki, Y.: Genetic systems of blood groups in horses. Genetics, *50:*915–929, 1964.
5. Stormont, C., and Suzuki, Y.: Genetic control of albumin phenotypes in horses. Proc. Soc. Exp. Biol. Med., *114:*673–675, 1963.

6. Gahne, B.: Studies on the inheritance of electrophoretic forms of transferrins, albumins, prealbumins and plasma esterases of horses. Genetics, *53:*681–694, 1966.
7. Stormont, C., and Y. Suzuki: Paternity tests in horses. Cornell Vet., *15:*365–377, 1965.
8. Sandberg, K.: Blood typing of horses: Current status and application to identification problems. Proceedings of the First World Congress on Genetic Applications of Livestock Production. Madrid, Garsi, 1974, pp. 253–265.
9. Suzuki, Y.: Studies on blood groups of horses. Mem. Tokyo Univ. Agric., *20:*1–50, 1978.
10. Bell, K.: The blood groups in domestic animals. *In* Red Blood Cells of Domestic Mammals. Edited by N.S. Agar and P.G. Board. Amsterdam, Elsevier Biomedical Press, 1983, pp. 133–169.
11. Braend, M.: Genetics of horse acidic prealbumins. Genetics, *65:*495–503, 1970.
12. Bengtsson, S., and Sandberg, K.: A method for simultaneous electrophoresis of four horse red cell enzyme systems. Anim. Blood Grp. Biochem. Genet., *4:*83–87, 1973.
13. Pollitt, C.C., and Bell, K.: Protease inhibitor system in horses: Classification and detection of a new allele. Anim. Blood Grp. Biochem. Genet., *11:*235–244, 1980.
14. Weitkamp, L.R., Costello-Leary, P., and Guttormsen, S.A.: Equine marker genes: Polymorphism for plasminogen. Anim. Blood Grp. Biochem. Genet., *14:*219–223, 1983.
15. Bowling, A.T., and Clark, R.S.: Blood group and protein polymorphism gene frequencies for seven breeds of horses in the United States. Anim. Blood Grp. Biochem. Genet., *16:*93–108, 1985.
16. Cothran, E.G., MacCluer, J.W., Weitkamp, L.R., and Bailey, E.: Genetic differentiation associated with gait within American Standardbred horses. Anim. Genet., *18:* 285–290, 1987.
17. Bailey, E.: Usefulness of lymphocyte typing to exclude incorrectly assigned paternity in horses. Am. J. Vet. Res., *45:*1979–1983, 1984.
18. Kay, P.H., Dawkins, R.L., Bowling, A.T., and Bernoco, D.: Heterogeneity and linkage of equine C4 and steroid 21-hydroxylase genes. J. Immunogenet., *14:*247–253, 1987.
19. Georges, M., et al.: DNA fingerprinting in domestic animals using four different minisatellite probes. Cytogenet. Cell Genet., *47:*127–131, 1988.
20. Bailey, E., Woodward, J.G., Albright, D.G., and Alexander, A.J.: RFLP marker genes for physiologically and serologically identified traits of the equine MHC. *In* The Molecular Biology of the Major Histocompatibility Complex of Domestic Animal Species. Edited by C.M. Warner, M.F., Rothschild, and S.J. Lamont. Iowa State University Press, Ames, 1988, pp. 135–153.
21. Li, J.K.K., et al.: DNA polymorphism analysis of hereditary multiple exostoses in horses. Am. J. Vet. Res., *50:*978–983, 1989.
22. Bailey, E., and Rossi, A.M.K.: Restriction fragment length polymorphisms of the immunoglobulin gamma chain constant region genes of the horse. Anim. Biotech., *1:*11–19, 1990.
23. Albright, D.L., Bailey, E., and Woodward, J.G.: Nucleotide sequence of a cDNA clone of the horse DRA gene. Immunogenetics, *34:*136–138, 1991.
24. Lear, T.L., and Bailey, E.: Southern blot studies of the MET locus in horses and cattle. Anim. Genet., *22:*307, 1991.
25. Bailey, E., Lear, T.L., and Cothran, E.G.: Association of MspI RFLPs with transferrin in horses. Anim. Genet., *22:*436, 1991.
26. Ellegren, H., Johansson, M., Sandberg, K., and Andersson, L.: Cloning of highly polymorphic microsatellites in the horse. Anim. Genet. In press.
27. Bernoco, D., and Byrns, G.R.: DNA fingerprint variation in horses. Anim. Biotech. In press.

CHAPTER 75

NUTRITION OF THE BROOD MARE

H.F. Hintz

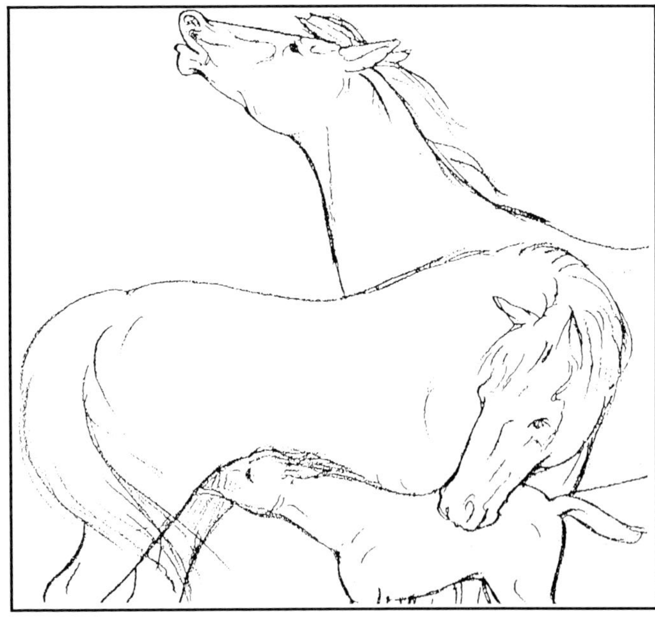

Many opinions exist as to the best way to feed the brood mare and as to the importance of nutrition. Some mares continue to produce in spite of apparently poor nutrition. Feral horses in the western United States do not get any grain or mineral supplements or even good-quality hay in the winter, but they continue to produce foals. Eberhardt et al. reported that the apparent rates of increase for two feral horse herds in Oregon could only be achieved if the survival rates were high and the rate of reproduction exceeded that normally expected from domestic horses.[1] Of course, the feral mares have the benefit of ready access to stallions, and they do not have their activity restricted by artificial birthdays. Garrot and Taylor reported that the foaling rates for feral mares of reproductive age ranged from 35 to 65% annually over a study of several years.[2] The Jockey Club reported that 56 and 59% of the Thoroughbred mares bred in 1988 and 1989, respectively, had live foals.[3] However, most equine nutritionists would probably agree with Donoghue et al. who stated that the cumulative nutritional demands on good brood mares are great.[4]

Unfortunately research on the requirements of brood mares is lacking for many nutrients. Few universities or experiment stations have adequate numbers of mares to study requirements, but the situation is improving. Studies from France and Germany have been particularly helpful for the estimation of nutrient requirements and for better understanding of brood mare nutrition. More universities in the United States are investigating the nutrition of the brood mare.

REQUIREMENTS

ENERGY

Energy is the nutritional factor that is usually of greatest concern in feeding of mares as in other horses and animals. In the past, obesity was commonly thought to be a significant cause of reduced fertility of mares. This concept may have arisen because many barren mares were fat. But Roberts pointed out that whether the mares were barren because they were fat or fat because they were barren was unclear.[5] Nevertheless the practice of flushing, that is, getting the mares into thin condition and then increasing the plane of nutrition was thought to be an excellent method of improving reproductive efficiency. However, university studies and observations made by farm managers have changed clinicians' ideas.[6,7] Mares that are in good or better condition are now considered to be more likely to conceive than mares that are thin.

An organized system for the visual appraisal of mares is useful. Systems such as those developed by Henneke et al.[8] and Carroll and Huntington[9] have been helpful. Based on field observations and university experiments, Hennecke et al. concluded that Quarter Horse mares at breeding time should have a minimum score of 5 and that 6 was probably better (based on a scale of 1 to 9).[6] Their studies also confirmed the earlier observation that thin mares fed an increased energy intake were more likely to get pregnant than thin mares fed to maintain weight. That is, flushing works. But they concluded that keeping mares in reasonable condition is more efficient than reducing and increasing weight.

Clinicians have wondered whether mares can get too fat. Kubiak et al.[10] and Goater et al.[11] found no adverse effects of obesity caused by overfeeding on incidence of foaling difficulties, foal size, or subsequent rebreeding efficiency. The obese mares in the study by Kubiak et al. had an average body score of 8.8 compared with 6.0 for control mares. However, Zimmerman and Greene reported obese mares were likely to have smaller foals and reduced rebreeding efficiency.[12] Overfeeding could also predispose the mares to metabolic conditions such as founder. Overfeeding mares, particularly of the pony breeds, could predispose to hyperlipemia.[13] Furthermore, feeding to obesity is a waste of money and feed.

Thus, although mares with body scores of 5 or above may have a higher reproductive efficiency than mares with a body score of 4 and lower, no justification exists for obesity. Harper suggested that because of many articles in lay horse publications concerning importance of body condition, more owners might tend to overfeed and incidence of obesity in brood mares could increase.[14]

Should the fat mare be put on a diet if the breeding season is near? Morris et al. studied fat mares fed either low- or high-energy diets.[15] Fat mares fed the high-energy diet had greater follicular activity and more mares ovulated than the fat mares fed low-energy diets. They concluded that fat mares entering the breeding season should not be fed a low-energy diet.

The role of exercise in breeding management of mares is poorly understood. Most farm managers do not exercise mares other than allowing time in paddocks. Some farm managers, particularly those in northern climates where outside exercise time may be limited in the winter, believe that treadmill exercise may be beneficial for mares. Improved muscle and uterine tone have been suggested. Other managers reported they did not observe any benefits from treadmill exercise and found the process to be labor consuming.

The National Research Council (NRC) suggested that digestible energy (DE) requirements for pregnant mares was the same as that for maintenance during the first 8 months of gestation.[16] Requirements for maintenance can be calculated by the formula DE (mcal/day) = 1.4 + 0.03 W where W is the weight of the horse in kilograms. Based on studies of fetal composition, the NRC estimated that the digestible energy requirements for months 9, 10, and 11 of gestation were 1.11, 1.13, and 1.20, respectively, times that of maintenance.[16] Birth weight of the foal was assumed to be 9 to 10% of the prepregnant weight of the mare. The council also suggested that the voluntary intake of hay may decrease during the last month of gestation presumably because of less-available abdominal space because of fetal development. Therefore, to provide adequate energy, some intake of grain may be needed. For example, the NRC suggested mares at maintenance may eat 1.5 to 2 kg of hay per 100 kg of body weight.[16] Mares in late gestation may eat 1 to 1.5 kg of hay and 0.5 to 1.0 kg of grain per 100 kg of body weight. But as with all classes of horses, the important aspect is body condition. If mares are too fat, decrease intake—if too thin, feed more.

Can other guidelines such as weight gains during gestation be used? The use of scales on farms is increasing; therefore, rules of thumb about weight gains might be useful. The NRC provides information about nutrient requirements but does not provide data about optimal weight gains of the mare for fetal development and for subsequent rebreeding.[16]

Assuming a foal weighs 9 to 10% of the mare's weight and that placenta and amniotic fluids could weigh as much as 20 kg, a 500-kg mare would seem to need to gain at least 65 kg during pregnancy unless body reserves were used.[5]

Bradley concluded that a 500-kg mare should gain 50 kg during the last 3 months of gestation.[17] Rich suggested that mares should gain 70 to 90 kg during the last third of gestation.[18] However, Banach and Evans reported that restriction of energy intake during the last 90 days of gestation such that mares lost 26 kg did not influence birth weight of foals.[19]

Jordan fed pony mares to maintain or lose 10 or 20% of the maintenance weight during gestation.[20] Treatment had no effect on foal birth weight or foal weight gains during the first 30 days of lactation. He concluded that initial condition had a significant influence on the amount of weight a mare could lose and still produce a viable foal.

Gallagher and McMeniman studied the weight gains of three pregnant mares and three nonpregnant mares grazing on pasture.[21] Pregnant mares gained an average of 40 kg during the last 90 days of gestation and nonpregnant mares gained 20 kg. All three pregnant mares had healthy foals and were in foal again within 32 days after foaling.

Kubiak et al. reported no differences in the birth weight of foals or incidence of foaling problems in mares fed to gain an average of 48 kg versus those fed to gain 123 kg during the last 45 to 75 days of pregnancy.[10] Mares in the first group had a prepartum body score of 5.9 compared with 8.8 for those in the latter group. On the other hand, Zimmerman and Greene reported that highly conditioned mares fed to gain 21 kg during the last 60 days of gestation had foals with a birth weight of 52 kg compared with 48 kg for foals from mares fed to gain 50 kg.[12] Thus they suggested obesity decreases birth weight. Reproductive efficiency was also decreased in the group that gained 50 kg.

Powell et al. studied mares that gained weight during the second third of gestation and plateaued during the last third.[22] Condition score, rump fat and thickness, and estimated body fat also increased during the second third of the gestation period. The latter criterion decreased during the last third even though body weight was maintained. Thus, they concluded that mobilization of body reserves occurred during the last third of gestation to support foal growth.

Kowalski et al. weighed 10 Thoroughbred mares (6

to 16 yr) every 14 days during the last 3 months of gestation.[23] Heights of the mares at the withers ranged from 151 to 165 cm. A total of 5 of the mares were bred to the same Dutch Warmblood stallion (650 kg) and 5 to 3 different Thoroughbred stallions (average weight, 555 kg). Of the mares bred to the Warmblood stallion, 3 were maiden mares. After foaling, the mares and foals were weighed every 7 days. The mares did not gain significant amounts of weight during the 3 months before foaling. No obvious differences between weight gains of mares bred to the Dutch Warmblood stallion and those bred to Thoroughbred stallions were noted. Weights of the mares also remained relatively constant during the month after foaling. The average weight just before foaling was 654 kg and the average weight after foaling was 573 kg. The average birth weight was 57 kg. Thus the foals weighed 8.7% of prefoaling and 9.9% of the postfoaling mare weight.

Two of the foals had lower birth weights than the others. This may have been because they were from maiden mares. The researchers could not compare effect of breed of sire on birth weight because three of the mares bred to the Dutch Warmblood stallion were maidens and none of the mares bred to the Thoroughbred stallions were maidens. However, a sire effect would not likely have been found in any case. Platt stated that paternal influence was much less than maternal influence on foal birth weight and early growth of the foal.[24]

The slope of weight gains against time was similar for all foals studied by Kowalski. The growth pattern observed by Kowalski et al.[23] was linear as was expected for horses.[25] Average daily gain for the first month was 1.55 kg per day, which was similar to the value of 1.5 kg per day previously reported for Thoroughbred foals.[24]

Neither the data of Powell et al.[22] nor the data of Kowalski et al.[23] can be used to answer the question of how much weight a mare should gain during the last third of gestation. However, both studies and those of Jordan[20] and Banach and Evans[19] demonstrated that mares can have foals of reasonable birth weight even though they do not gain any weight or even lose weight during the last 3 months of gestation. The important criteria are body condition and energy reserves of the mares. Further studies are needed to determine whether an optimal weight gain exists. Furthermore, studies with other species indicate carryover effects might be found. Therefore, the studies should be conducted over at least two gestational periods.

Other factors that may influence birth weight include age of the mare and time of year at birth. A study was conducted of weight gains of 1992 foals born over an 18-yr period.[25] Foals from dams under 7 yr of age and from dams over 11 yr of age were lighter at birth than foals from mares 7 to 11 yr of age. Foals born in April, May, and June were heavier than foals born in January, February, and March.

Nutrition of the lactating mare has been reviewed by the NRC,[16] Doreau et al.[26] and Donoghue et al.[4] The NRC concluded that mares of light breeds appear to produce amounts of milk equivalent to 3% of body weight per day during early lactation (1 to 12 weeks) and 2% of body weight during late lactation (13 to 24 weeks). Respective values for Pony mares were 4 and 3% of body weight. Researchers assumed that 792 kcal of DE were required to produce 1 kg of milk. Thus a 545-kg mare in early lactation would require 17.75 mcal of DE for maintenance and 12.95 for milk or a total of 30.7 mcal of DE. Expected intake according to the NRC would be 1 to 2 kg of forage and 1 to 2 kg of grain per 100 kg of body weight. An average intake of about 7 kg of hay and 6 kg of grain would provide 31 mcal, which would be equivalent to 2.4% of body weight.

Doreau et al. pointed out that energy requirements of lactating mares are generally calculated by a factorial method in which estimates of maintenance requirements, milk yield, energy value of milk, and efficiency of energy utilization are needed.[26] They reviewed the literature and found that values obtained for those parameters and basis for calculations vary from report to report. But now the good news. According to Doreau et al., little variation exists among the values recommended by the United States and several European groups. For example, the value for a 500-kg mare given by the NRC was 28.3 mcal of DE compared with 28.9 for Norway, 27.4 for Germany, and 30.3 for France.

Body condition at foaling will influence response of the mare to energy intake. Doreau et al. reported that mares fat at foaling but fed same energy intakes as mares thin at foaling gained 9 kg compared with 31 kg for the thin mares but foals of thin mares grew more slowly than foals of fat mares.[26] That is, thin mares provided with the same amount of energy as fat mares apparently diverted more energy to restore body reserves and less for milk than did fat mares.

Pagan et al. reported that mares could use body reserves to maintain milk production and foal growth; however, they suggested that it was an inefficient practice.[27] Doreau et al. concluded that lactating mares are often underfed and mares should be in good condition at the onset of lactation.[26]

The NRC suggested that mares during early lactation be fed diets containing about 50 parts hay and 50 parts grain to maintain a reasonable energy density in the diet.[16] A low DE concentration could limit energy intake. Doreau et al. reported that lactating mares could be fed diets containing 90 parts hay to 10 parts grain satisfactorily when the hay was of reasonable quality.[26] However, they concluded that poor-quality forages such as straw would limit performance and were unsuitable for lactating mares. Response of the lactating mare to increased energy intake could be quite variable because mares in the United States have not been selected for milk production and thus may not have genetic potential to respond.

Few studies have been conducted on the effect of diet of the mare on milk composition. Increasing energy intake by feeding more grain could increase milk yield but a decrease in milk energy concentration could occur.[26,28] Addition of 5% fat to the grain mixture increased fat content of mare's milk.[29] The NRC reviewed several reports on composition of mare's milk.[16] Milk collected during weeks 1 to 4 averaged 10.7% solids, 2.7% protein, 1.8% fat, and 6.2% lactose and contained 58 kcal per 100 g. Concentration of nutrients decreased throughout lactation. Milk collected during weeks 9 to 21 averaged 10.0% solids, 1.8% protein, 1.4% fat, and only 50 kcal per 100 gram.

PROTEIN

Protein requirements for mares at maintenance can be calculated according to the equation: 40 g of crude protein per mcal of DE.[16] Pregnant mares during late gestation need 44 g of crude protein per mcal of DE. The NRC calculated requirements for lactating mares assuming that milk contained 2.1% protein and the efficiency of conversion of crude protein into milk protein was 36%.[16] Therefore, when using conventional feedstuffs, mature horses at maintenance require 7 to 8% protein in the total ration (90% dry matter basis). Pregnant mares would require 9 to 10% and lactating mares would need 12% during early lactation and 10% during late lactation.

Obviously, no protein supplement would be needed for mares at maintenance fed conventional feedstuffs. Pregnant mares fed alfalfa hay would probably not need a protein supplement. That is, if the alfalfa contained 14% protein and was fed at a ratio 70 parts hay to 30 parts grain, no protein supplement would need to be added to the grain. If pregnant mares were fed grass hay containing 8% protein and a ratio of 70% hay and 30% grain were used, the grain mixture would need to contain about 14% protein to balance protein in the hay. Lactating mares fed alfalfa hay and grain in a 50:50 ratio would need a grain mixture containing at least 10% protein (assuming 14% protein in the alfalfa) to provide 12% in the total ration. If grass hay containing 8% protein were fed, the grain mixture would need 16% protein.

A deficiency of protein can cause a rough hair coat, decreased birth weight of foals, and slow growth rate of suckling foals because of reduced milk production.

MINERALS

The NRC reported that calcium (Ca) requirement for mature horses could be estimated by the equation Ca (g/day) = 0.04 × body weight (kg).[16] The requirements for pregnancy were based on studies of fetal composition. The NRC suggested that calcium uptake by the fetus corresponded to energy deposition. Therefore, the equation Ca (g/day) = 1.90 × mcal of DE was developed. For lactating mares in early lactation, the equation Ca (g/day) = maintenance Ca + [(0.03 body weight × 1.2)/0.5] and for late lactation the equation Ca (g/day) = maintenance Ca + [(0.02 body weight × 1.2/0.5)] can be used. Therefore, diets for mares at maintenance, pregnancy, and lactation should contain about 0.2, 0.4, and 0.5% calcium, respectively. Some controversy exists concerning the calcium requirement of mares. Krook and Maylin suggested the NRC value was excessive.[30] They theorized that high calcium intake would increase the amount of calcitonin produced and lead to development of osteochondrosis in the fetus. However, this theory has not been tested experimentally.

Free-choice feeding of mineral salts containing calcium can be used to increase calcium intake but mares do not have a "calcium sense." They will eat the mineral mixture to get salt. Thus, when possible, calcium should be added to the grain mixture if needed. If a legume hay is used, calcium supplements may not be necessary. If grass hay is used, the grain mixture should contain at least 0.6% calcium. Most commercial grain mixtures contain added calcium.

Phosphorus content of the ration should never greatly exceed that of calcium because phosphorus interferes with calcium absorption. The NRC suggests that diets for pregnant and lactating mares should contain at least 0.3% phosphorus.[16] The diet for maintenance should contain at least 0.15% phosphorus (90% dry matter basis).

Although clinicians generally agree that trace mineral deficiencies can cause reproductive problems, no evidence has been found that high levels of minerals increase fertility. Ley et al. compared reproductive performance of mares that had been barren for at least the previous 12 months and were fed at least the NRC levels with those given additional inorganic minerals (zinc, copper, and manganese) and chelated minerals.[31] No difference between the groups was found. However, the authors pointed out that to find a 10% difference in first-service conception rate, 115 mares per group may be necessary.

A great amount of interest has been shown in copper and zinc in recent years. The NRC suggested rations of mares should contain at least 10 mg copper and 40 mg zinc per kilogram of dry matter.[16] Knight et al. suggested that higher levels of copper and zinc may help prevent developmental orthopedic disease (DOD), particularly osteochondrosis.[32] They found fewer lesions in foals when the mares were fed 32 mg copper per kilogram of feed and foals were creep fed diets containing 55 mg copper compared with foals from mares fed 13 mg copper and given 15 mg copper in the creep feed. The NRC concluded that data were not sufficient to justify increasing estimates of copper and zinc requirements.[16] However, I believe copper and zinc status should be evaluated on farms which have DOD in foals.

Iodine deficiency in mares can result in weak, hairless, or dead foals or foals with goiter (enlarged thyroid). However, use of iodized or trace mineralized salt has effectively prevented the conditions. Requirement for the mare is estimated to be equivalent to 0.1 mg iodine per kilogram of diet or about 1 mg/day.[16] Feeding excessive amounts of iodine to the mare can cause problems and many clinical cases of iodism have been reported. Iodine readily passes the placenta and mammary gland. Pregnant mares fed more than 50 mg iodine daily are likely to have foals with goiter, retarded skeletal and muscular development, and weakened condition.[16] Sources of excessive iodine include overuse of supplements, particularly those containing seaweed or ethylenediamine hydroiodide. Mares with affected foals may appear normal. However, large doses such as 350 mg daily can cause goiter in the mare and abortion.[33]

Selenium has been written about extensively, and the dangers of selenium deficiency and selenium toxicity have been widely publicized. However, both situations continue to occur.[34,35] Feeding selenium-deficient diets to mares can result in foals with nutritional myopathy, causing weakness, impaired locomotion, difficulty in suckling and swallowing, respiratory distress, and impaired cardiac function. The NRC estimated that diets containing 0.1 mg selenium per kilogram would be adequate for mares.[16] However, my observation is that the NRC's concentration may not always support adequate blood concentrations. Selenium status should be evaluated by blood selenium or glutathione peroxidase levels on farms with low reproductive efficiency or weak foals. Selenium toxicity causes loss of hair from the mane and tail and sloughing of hoofs. The maximal tolerable level has been set at 2 mg per kilogram of diet.[16] Selenium toxicity has been reported in western states that have soils with a high selenium content and in horses given excessive amounts of supplements.

Vitamin nutrition of the brood mare has received little attention from scientists. Need for vitamin supplementation depends on the vitamin content of forage, because grains are usually lacking in vitamins. Because monitoring vitamin content of forage is expensive, most commercial grain mixtures are fortified with vitamins. In those cases, additional vitamin supplements are not usually needed.[36] Vitamin A and its precursor, carotene, have received the most attention. Vitamin A has many functions. Thus, a deficiency can lead to many signs such as reduced fertility, excessive lacrimation, spontaneous fractures, rough hair coat, elevated spinal fluid pressure, night blindness, convulsive seizures, and increased incidence of respiratory infections. The NRC recommended that mares be fed diets containing at least 3,000 IU but not more than 16,000 IU of vitamin A per kilogram of feed.[16] Bone fragility, rough hair coat, loss of hair, poor muscle tone, and depression have been observed in horses fed high intakes of the vitamin. Vitamin A activity in natural feedstuffs comes from carotene. Data on conversion of carotene to vitamin A by the horse are limited, but the NRC concluded that 1 mg of β-carotene ought to be considered equivalent to no more than 400 IU of vitamin A activity.[16] Toxicity of carotene is unknown, but apparently it is much less than that of vitamin A. According to the NRC, Kentucky bluegrass pasture may contain 480 mg carotene per kilogram of dry matter.[16] A 500-kg horse on pasture could eat 10 kg of dry matter daily and thus ingest 4,800 mg carotene. If 1 mg carotene provides 400 IU vitamin A activity, the horse would obtain 192,770 IU vitamin A per kilogram of feed, or 1,927,770 IU daily. However, although many horses graze such pasture, no reports of carotene toxicity in horses have been made. Thus carotene does not seem to be as toxic as vitamin A. Perhaps the decreased toxicity is because estimated efficiency of carotene conversion to vitamin A is incorrect or perhaps the estimate of maximum tolerable concentrations of vitamin A is too conservative.

Carotene is also of interest because of suggestions that carotene has specific functions beyond that of being a precursor to vitamin A. Carotene can serve as an antioxidant. Certain cancers are associated with low concentrations of plasma carotenoids. Interest in use of β-carotene to enhance fertility of mares was sparked by reports that β-carotene improved reproductive performance of cows even when plasma vitamin A concentrations were in the normal range.[37]

Ahlswede and Konermann reported that normal blood carotene concentrations in horses were much lower than that found in cattle, but horses on pasture had β-carotene plasma concentrations 8 to 13 times as high as horses kept in stables.[38] Therefore, the carotene plasma concentration of stabled horses could be increased by carotene supplementation. They also reported a tendency for carotene supplementation to improve ovarian activity.

Van der Holst reported that β-carotene supplementation improved conception rates in pony mares and that mares receiving β-carotene supplementation had stronger signs of estrus.[39] Early embryonic mortality tended to be reduced.

Ferrero and Cote reported that feeding 100 mg β-carotene per day seemed to enhance earlier and stronger heats and improve conception rates and maintenance of pregnancy.[40] However, other studies have found no benefit from β-carotene supplementation to horses. Eitzer and Rapp reported no benefit from the feeding of 400 mg β-carotene daily to mares normally fed a ration providing 70 to 80 mg β-carotene per day.[41] The supplement was fed from January 1 to April 5. Mares fed the control diet had β-carotene concentrations similar to those reported for stabled horses by Ahslwede and Konermann (about 10 micrograms per 100 mL plasma).[38] Carotene supplementation increased the plasma concentration to about 20 μg per 100 mL, but no differences in reproductive performance were noted. The NRC concluded that carotene supplements will not likely be beneficial if the mares are on pasture or fed forage containing high levels of carotene.[16]

Vitamin D is required for calcium utilization and bone formation. However, vitamin D deficiency has never been demonstrated in horses that are exposed to sunshine. Ultraviolet rays convert compounds formed by the animals into vitamin D. If mares are not exposed to sunshine, the diet should contain 600 IU vitamin D per kilogram of dry matter.[16] Excessive intakes of vitamin D cause soft tissue calcification. Several clinical cases of toxicity caused by overzealous use of supplements or mixing mistakes have been reported. The NRC suggested that the maximum tolerable dietary level of vitamin D_3 was 2200 IU per kilogram of feed.[16]

Vitamin E has received a great deal of attention in recent years. Recommended intake levels for many species has been increased. The NRC increased the recommended level from 15 IU per kilogram of feed in the 1978 publication to 50 IU per kilogram for maintenance and 80 IU per kilogram of feed for working, breeding, or growing animals.[16] Using the new values, brood mares should get about 800 to 1000 IU vitamin E daily compared with the old value of 150. The increase was based on several studies, including one which suggested the immune response was improved at the higher level. Vitamin E has several functions. It interacts with selenium in prevention of nutritional myopathy. Vitamin E deficiency has also been implicated in development of degenerative myelopathy. Six Przewalski Horses at the Bronx Zoo in New York were diagnosed with the condition.[42] Ataxia characterized by uncoordinated movement of the hindlimbs and an abnormally wide-based gait and stance was noted. Histologic lesions were found in neural processes. Low plasma concentrations of vitamin E and low concentrations of vitamin E in the feed led to the conclusion that a chronic vitamin E deficiency was present. Mayhew et al. suggested degenerative myelopathy might be caused by vitamin E deficiency in certain bloodlines of domestic horses.[43] That is, a vitamin E-genetic interaction existed. Some reports indicated that massive doses of vitamin E could be used to treat some cases of degenerative myelopathy in domestic horses.[44] Further studies are needed to evaluate effectiveness of high doses. Fortunately, no reports of vitamin E toxicity have been made for horses.

Biotin has often been advocated for treatment of horses with poor quality (shelly, flaky) hooves. Clinical reports indicated that such horses treated with 15 mg biotin showed improvement in hardness, integrity, and conformation of the hoof horn.[45] The NRC concluded insufficient evidence existed to establish a requirement for biotin.[16]

Requirements have not been established for vitamin C, niacin, pantothenic acid, pyridoxine, and vitamin B_{12}, but thiamin and riboflavin requirements were estimated to be 3 and 2 mg per kilogram of diet, respectively.[16]

In summary, vitamins are necessary for reproductive function. No doubt deficiency of vitamins can impair fertility. However, little evidence is found to suggest that megadoses of multivitamins will enhance reproduction. Addition of a vitamin supplement to a diet of mixed grain and mixed hay did not improve reproductive performance in a study with 54 mares.[36]

EXAMPLES OF REQUIREMENTS

In the past the 454-kg (1000-lb) mare was frequently used for examples. The 1000-lb weight was convenient to use and clinicians thought it was reasonably representative. But when clinicians started weighing Quarter Horse and Thoroughbred mares, they noted that 545 kg (1200 lb) was a more representative weight. Therefore, the values in Table 75–1 were calculated for a 545 kg mare based on the equations published by NRC.[16]

THE OLDER MARE

Are the requirements of the older mare different from those for the younger mare? Donoghue et al. suggested that part of the lower racing performance of progeny of mares over 10 yr of age when compared with progeny of mares 10 yr or younger might be caused by suboptimal nutrition.[4] Ralston et al. suggested that aged horses at maintenance had reduced apparent digestibility of protein and phosphorus.[46] Thus aged mares may be

TABLE 75–1. ESTIMATED DAILY REQUIREMENTS FOR A MARE WITH A MATURE WEIGHT OF 545 KG BASED ON EQUATIONS DEVELOPED BY THE NRC (1989)

		PREGNANCY (MONTHS)			LACTATION	
	Open	9	10	11	Early	Late
Energy (mcal)	17.8	19.8	20.1	21.4	30.7	26.4
Protein (g)	712	871	884	942	1555	1235
Calcium (g)	22	37	38	40	61	48
Phosphorus (g)	15	28	29	31	39	24
Copper (mg)	90	100	105	110	120	100
Zinc (mg)	360	400	420	440	480	400
Iodine (mg)	0.9	0.9	1.0	1.0	1.3	1.1
Selenium (mg)	0.9	0.9	1.0	1.0	1.3	1.1
Vitamin A (1000 IU)	16.5	33	33	33	33	33
Vitamin E (IU)	450	900	900	900	900	900
Hay (kg)*	9.4	7.5	7.5	7.5	7.0	7.5
Grain (kg)†	—	1.8	1.9	2.4	5.8	4.0

*Assuming 1.9 mcal of DE per kilogram, 90% dry matter (DM) basis.
†Assuming 3 mcal of DE per kilogram, 90% DM basis.

susceptible to nutrient deficiencies because of the cumulative demands of producing foals and because of decreased nutrient utilization. Donoghue et al. recommended that aged breeding stock should receive individual attention and any signs of poor status should prompt a thorough clinical examination.[4]

SOURCES OF NUTRIENTS

Any of the conventional feeds can be fed to brood mares. Use of oats may decline in the future because of reduced availability and economics. Amount of acreage planted in oats has been steadily decreasing and increased interest in oats as a human food has also influenced its price. The impact of the long-term effect the oat bran fad for humans will have on the supply of oats for horses remains to be seen. Corn and barley can be effectively used to replace oats when their nutritional characteristics are considered. Both contain less fiber and a higher concentration of digestible energy than that found in oats.

For many farms, managers note the practical and economical advantages of buying a commercial grain rather than mixing their own. Feed companies can use nutritious by-products and mix the micronutrients more precisely. Furthermore, companies will custom mix feed and formulate according to the forage used on the farm.

Considerable interest exists in the addition of fat to horse rations. Several advantages such as reduced dangers of founder, improved coat quality, and improved athletic performance have been suggested. Davison et al. fed mares a conventional pelleted concentrate or one with 5% added fat.[29] Mares fed added fat required less grain. No difference was noted in birth weights of foals from mares fed fat and control mares, but foals from mares fed fat gained 1.85 kg/day during the first week after foaling compared with 1.5 kg/day for foals from control mares.

Recently considerable interest has arisen in use of probiotics in horse rations. Live yeast cultures have been reported to improve fiber nitrogen and phosphorus utilization in horses by enhancing microbial hemicellulolytic and cellulolytic fermentation and decreasing endogenous fecal nitrogen. Glade reported a study in which five mares were given 10 g live yeast culture daily during late gestation and early lactation and five mares were controls.[47] The addition of yeast improved ration digestibility and increased energy and fat content of milk. Foals from yeast-fed mares were 21 kg heavier and 11.2 cm taller than foals from control mares at 8 weeks postfoaling.

Choice of hay depends on area. In the Northeast, grass or mixed grass-legume hays are most commonly fed, whereas in the West, legume or cereal hays are fed. The most important criterion is not which species of hay but rather what is the quality of hay and what is the cost of nutrients.

PROBLEM FEEDS

Feeds designed for other species containing additives such as ionophores or horse feed contaminated with ionophores have killed many horses. Monensin is the most common culprit but other ionophores such as salinomycin and lasalocid can also cause problems.[48] Feed refusal, colic, and profuse sweating are early signs. Muscle weakness will progress to recumbency. Death is a result of cardiac failure. Horses that survive may have a variety of cardiac arrhythmias.[48]

Blister beetle poisoning causes colic, fever, diarrhea, tachycardia, and death. Most of the reported cases have involved contaminated alfalfa from Southern and Southwestern states.[48]

Any moldy feeds should be avoided.[49] Mold-contaminated feeds have been reported to cause a wide range of problems in horses, including colic, feed refusal, brain damage, abortion, hemorrhage, increased respiratory problems, and death. Moldy corn disease (leukoencephalomalacia) is usually more common following periods of drought during the growth season and rain during the harvest season.

Fescue toxicity is probably the most widely publicized mold-related disease in horses. The toxicity is caused by an endophyte (Acremonium coenophialum). Signs in mares include decreased blood prolactin concentration and increased incidence of dystocia, prolonged gestation, weak or dead foals, agalactia, and thickened placenta. The prolonged gestation results in large foals, which can be a factor in an increased incidence of dystocia. Earle et al. reported four of seven mares grazing infested fescue died as a result of dystocia.[50] Problems can be prevented by planting endophyte-free seed or removing pregnant mares from pasture. Ireland et al. concluded that modifying hormone concentrations by use of dopamine receptor antagonist drugs could prevent adverse symptoms of fescue toxicosis.[51] Overseeding with legumes to dilute the endotoxin might also be helpful.

Legumes, particularly red clover, infested with the mold Rhizoctonia leguminicola causes the slobbering syndrome. O'Dell et al. reported several cases of profuse slobbering by horses fed infested red clover hay.[52] One mare became weak and aborted. Sudangrass or sorghum-sudangrass hybrids are not recommended for horse pastures. Mares may develop cystitis and have abortions and deformed foals.[53]

MANAGEMENT

The most important nutritional aspect of brood mare management is maintenance of proper body condition. Individual feeding of mares is one method of accomplishing this goal but can be labor consuming. Run-in sheds with partitions have been successfully used at Standardbred farms to regulate intake. If partitions are not used, the boss mare will usually eat more than her share of grain in a group-feeding situation. Holmes et

TABLE 75–2. ESTIMATES OF FEED NEEDED BY MARES WITH A MATURE WEIGHT OF 545 KG*

	HAY (POUNDS)	GRAIN (POUNDS)	HAY (FLAKES)	GRAIN (QUARTS)
Open	20	—	4	
Pregnant (month 9)	16	4	3+	3
Pregnant (month 10)	16	4	3+	3
Pregnant (month 11)	16	5	3+	4
Early lactation	15	12	3	9
Late lactation	16	8	3+	6

*As discussed in text, the volume of hay and grain needed depends on several factors; the weight of hay and grain needed depends on quality of feed and individuality of the horse.

al. concluded that head partitions on a trough facilitate feeding by subordinate horses in the presence of dominant pen-mates and thus provide a more equitable distribution of food resources.[54]

Horses should be fed by weight not volume. The density of grain varies greatly. For example, poor-quality, high-fiber oats may weigh less than 450 g per quart whereas high-quality oats may weigh more than 675 g per quart. Naked or hull-less oats can weigh even more. Shelled corn may weigh 800 g per quart and ground corn could weigh less.[55] Whole barley may weigh 675 g per quart whereas a quart of ground barley may weigh only 500 g.[55] Extruded feeds may weigh only half as much per unit of volume as do pelleted feeds.[56]

The weight of a bale of hay and thus the weight of a flake depends on many factors such as the condition of the hay, the type of hay, and the method of baling. Nevertheless, many horse owners feed by quarts or coffee cans and flakes. Therefore, owners may find it helpful to use average intakes expressed in terms of quarts and flakes as is shown in Table 75–2. The calculations assume that sweet feed weighs approximately 585 g per quart and that a string-tied bale of hay weighs 18 kg and flakes weigh 1.8 to 2.3 kg. But, of course, the most important factor is the body condition of the horse. Feed must be regulated to maintain the proper body condition.

REFERENCES

1. Eberhardt, L.L., et al.: Apparent rates of increase for two feral horse herds. J. Wildl. Manag., *46*:367–374, 1982.
2. Garrot, R.A., and Taylor, L.: Dynamics of a feral horse population in Montana. J. Wildl. Manag., *54*:603–612, 1990.
3. Bowen, E.L.: Breeding Records. Blood Horse, *114*:4341, 1990.
4. Donoghue, S., Meacham, T.N., and Kronfeld, D.S.: A conceptual approach to optimal nutrition of brood mares. Vet. Clin. North Am. Equine Pract., *6*:373–392, 1990.
5. Roberts, S.J.: Veterinary Obstetrics and Genital Diseases (Theriogenology). 3rd ed. Woodstock, VT, published by the author, 1986.
6. Henneke, D.R., et al.: Body condition during pregnancy and lactation and reproductive efficiency of mares. Theriogenology, *21*:987–909, 1984.
7. Kubiak, J.R., et al.: The influence of energy intake and percentage of body fat on the reproductive performance of non-pregnant mares. Theriogenology, *28*:587–598, 1987.
8. Henneke, E.R., et al.: Relationship between condition score, physical measurements and body fat percentages in mares. Equine Vet. J., *15*:371–372, 1983.
9. Carroll, C.L., and Huntington, P.J.: Body condition scoring and weight estimation of horses. Equine Vet. J., *20*:41–45, 1988.
10. Kubiak, J.R., et al.: Parturition in the multiparous mare fed to obesity. J. Equine Vet. Sci., *8*:135–140, 1988.
11. Goater, L.E., et al.: The effect of feeding excess energy to mares during late gestation. Proceedings of the Equine Nutrition and Physiology Symposium. Warrentown, 1981, pp. 111–116.
12. Zimmerman, R.A., and Greene, D.E.: Calorie allowance for gestating mares. J. Anim. Sci., *46* (Suppl. 1):326, 1978.
13. Jeffcott, L.B., and Field, J.R.: Current concepts of hyperlipaemia in horses. Vet. Rec., *116*:461–466, 1985.
14. Harper, F.:Feeding the Broodmare. Tennessee Horse Express. University of Tennessee Agricultural Extension Service, No. 9. Knoxville, TN, 1990, pp. 1–4.
15. Morris, R.P., et al.: Follicular activity in transitional mares as affected by body condition and dietary energy. Proceedings of the Equine Nutrition and Physiology Symposium. Fort Collins, CO, 1987, pp. 93–95.
16. National Research Council: Nutrient Requirements of Horses. Washington, DC, National Academy of Sciences, National Research Council, 1989.
17. Bradley, M.: Horses: A Practical and Scientific Approach. New York, McGraw-Hill, 1981.
18. Rich, G.: Feeding mares from maximum reproductive efficiency. Proceedings of the Colorado State Short Course on Equine Management. Fort Collins, CO, 1986, pp. 9–11.
19. Banach, M.A., and Evans, J.W.: Effects of inadequate energy during gestation and lactation on the estrous cycle and conception rates of mares and on their foal weights. Proceedings of the Equine Nutrition and Physiology Symposium. Warrentown, 1981, pp. 97–100.
20. Jordan, R.M.: Weight changes in pregnant pony mares. J. Anim. Sci. Suppl. 1, *55*:208, 1982.
21. Gallagher, J.R., and McMeniman, N.P.: The nutritional status of pregnant and non-pregnant mares grazing southeast Queensland pastures. Equine Vet. J., *20*:414–416, 1988.
22. Powell, D.M., Lawrence, L.M., Parrett, D., and DePietro, J.: Body composition in broodmares. Proceedings of the Equine Nutrition and Physiology Symposium. Stillwater, 1989, pp. 91–94.
23. Kowalski, J., Hintz, H.F., and Williams, J.: Weight gains in pregnant mares. Equine Pract., *12*:6–9, 1990.
24. Platt, H.: Growth of the equine foetus. Equine Vet. J., *16*:247–252, 1984.
25. Hintz, H.F., and Hintz, R.L.: Growth rate of Thoroughbreds. J. Anim. Sci., *48*:480–487, 1979.
26. Doreau, M., Martin-Rosset, W., and Boulot, S.: Energy requirements and the feeding of mares during lactation: A review. Livestock Prod. Sci., *20*:53–68, 1988.

27. Pagan, J., Hintz, H.F., and Rounsaville, T.R.: The digestible energy requirements of lactating pony mares. J. Anim. Sci., *58:*1382–1387, 1984.

28. Pagan, J., and Hintz, H.F.: Composition of milk from pony mares fed various levels of digestible energy. Cornell Vet., *76:*139–148, 1986.

29. Davison, K.E., et al.: Lactation and reproductive performance of mares fed added dietary fat during late gestation and early lactation. Proceedings of the Equine Nutrition and Physiology Symposium. Fort Collins, CO, 1987, pp. 87–92.

30. Krook, L., and Maylin, G.: Fractures in Thoroughbred race horses. Cornell Vet. Suppl. 2, *78:*1–33, 1988.

31. Ley, W.B., Thatcher, C.D., Swecker, W.S., and Lessard, P.N.: Chelated mineral supplementation in the barren mare: A preliminary trial. J. Equine Vet. Sci., *10:*176–181, 1990.

32. Knight, D.A., et al.: Copper supplementation and cartilage lesions in foals. Proc. Am. Assoc. Equine Pract., 191–194, 1987.

33. Silva, C.A.M., et al.: Jodvergiftung bei vollblutfohlen. Pferdeheilkunde, *3:*3–6, 1987.

34. Dill, S., and Rebhun, W.: White muscle disease in foals. Compend. Contin. Educ. Practicing Vet., *7:*S627–S631, 1985.

35. Traub-Dargatz, J.L., and Hamar, D.W.: Selenium toxicity in horses. Comp. Compend. Contin. Educ. Practicing Vet., *8:*771–776, 1986.

36. Voss, J., and Pickett, W.: Effect of a nutritional supplement on pregnancy rate in nonlactating mares. J. Am. Vet. Med. Assoc., *165:*702–703, 1974.

37. Lotthammer, J., et al.: Untersuchungen uber eine spezifische Vitamin A-unabhangige Wirkung des beta carotins auf die Fertilitat des Rindes. DTW Dtsch. Tierarztl. Wochenschr., *83:*353–357, 1976.

38. Ahlswede, L., and Konermann, H.: Erfahrungen mit der oralen und parenteralen applikation von beta-carotin beim pferd. Prakt. Tierarzt., *61:*47–51, 1980.

39. Van der Holst, M.: Experiences with oral administration of beta-carotene to pony mares in early spring. Proceedings of the Annual Meeting of the European Association of Animal Production. Paris, 1984, p. 6.

40. Ferraro, J., and Cote, J.F.: Broodmare management techniques improve conception rates. Standardbred, *12:* 56–58, 1984.

41. Eitzer, P., and Rapp, H.J.: Zur Oralen Anwendung von Synthetischen Beta-Carotin bei Zuchstuten. Prakt. Tierarzt., *66:*123, 1985.

42. Liu, S.K., Dolensek, E.P., Adams, C.R., and Tappe, J.P.: Myelopathy and vitamin E deficiency in six Mongolian wild horses. J. Am. Vet. Med. Assoc., *183:*1266, 1983.

43. Mayhew, I.G., et al.: Equine degenerative myeloencephalopathy: A vitamin E. deficiency that may be familial. J. Vet. Intern. Med., *1:*45–50, 1987.

44. Forfa, T.: Working on a wobblers cure. Equus, *120:*65–68, 1987.

45. Comben, N., Clark, R.J., and Sutherland, D.J.B.: Clinical observations on the response of equine hoof defects to dietary supplementation with biotin. Vet. Rec., *115:*642, 1984.

46. Ralston, S.L., et al.: Hematoligic, metabolic and digestive changes in aged horses. Proceedings of the Equine Nutrition and Physiology Symposium. Fort Collins, CO, 1987, pp. 545–549.

47. Glade, M.: Effect of Yea-Sace fed to lactating mares on feed digestibility, milk biological value and foal growth. Alltech Research and Technology Bulletin. 1989, p. 8.

48. Whitlock, R.H.: Feed additives and contaminants as a cause of equine disease. Vet. Clin. North Am. Equine Pract., *6:*467–478, 1990.

49. Hintz, H.F.: Molds, mycotoxins and mycotoxicosis. Vet. Clin. North Am. Equine Pract., *6:*419–432, 1990.

50. Earle, W.F., Cross, D.L., and Hudson, L.W.: Effect of energy supplementation on gravid mares grazing endophyte infected fescue. Proceedings of the Equine Nutrition and Physiology Symposium. Stillwater, 1989, p. 175–177.

51. Ireland, F.A., Loch, W.E., Anthony, R.V., and Worthy, K.: The use of bromocriptine and perpheazine in the study of fescue toxicosis in pregnant pony mares. Proceedings of the Equine Nutrition and Physiology Symposium. Stillwater, 1989, p. 202–204.

52. O'Dell, B.L., et al.: A study of the toxic principle in red clover. University of Missouri, Agricultural Experiment Station Research Bulletin No. 702. Columbia, MO, 1959, p. 1–12.

53. Morgan, S.E., Johnson, B., Brewer, B., and Walker, J.: Sorghum cystitis ataxic syndrome in horses. Vet. Hum. Toxicol., *32:*582, 1990.

54. Holmes, L.N., Song, G., and Price, E.O.: Head partitions facilitate feeding by subordinate horses in the presence of dominant pen-mates. Appl. Anim. Behav. Sci., *19:* 179–182, 1987.

55. Morrison, F.B.: Feeds and Feeding. 22nd ed. Ithaca, NY, Morrison, 1956.

56. Hintz, H.F., Scott, J.K., and Hernandez, T.M.: Extruded feeds for horses. Proceedings of the Cornell Nutrition Conference. 1986, pp. 81–85.

PART II

THE STALLION

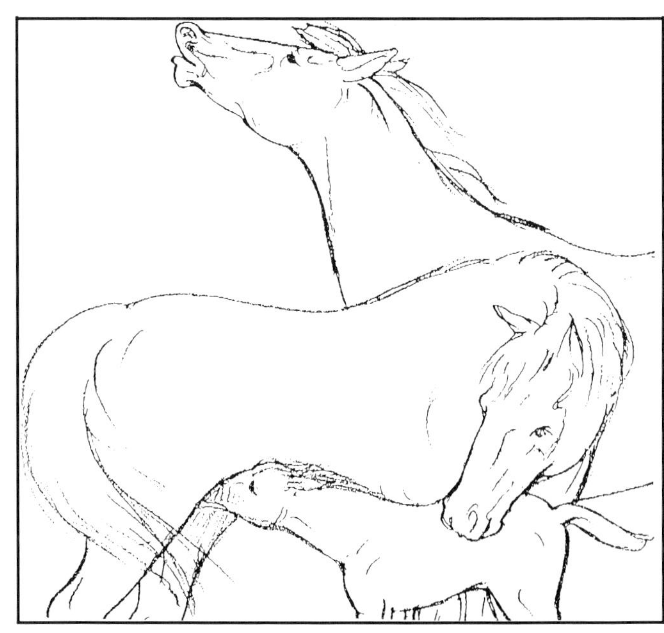

SECTION A

ANATOMY, PHYSIOLOGY, AND ENDOCRINOLOGY

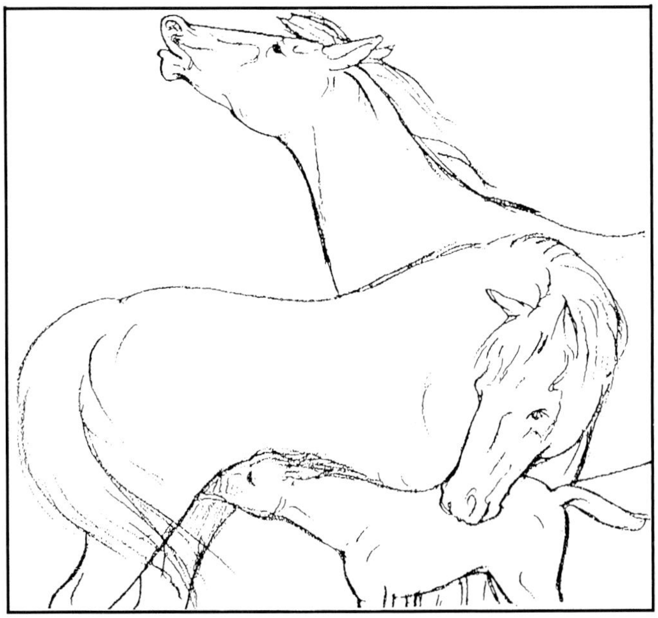

CHAPTER 76

FUNCTIONAL ANATOMY OF THE ADULT MALE

R.P. Amann

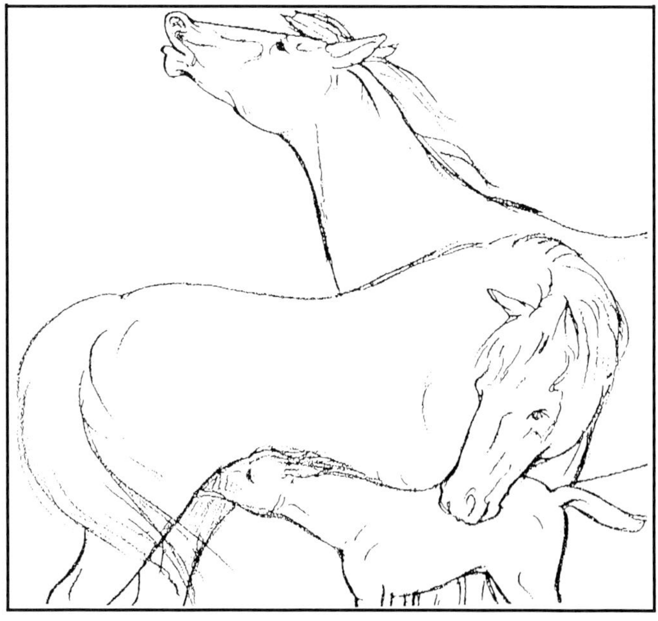

To evaluate properly a stallion suspected of having reproductive problems, the normal location, shape, and size of each organ must be known. The male reproductive organs consist of two testes, each suspended by a spermatic cord and external cremaster muscle; two epididymides; two deferent ducts each with an ampulla; paired vesicular glands; a prostate gland; paired bulbourethral glands; the penis; and the associated urethralis, ischiocavernosus, bulbospongiosus, and retractor penis muscles* (Fig. 76–1). The vesicular glands, prostate gland, and bulbourethral glands often are termed the accessory sex glands. The reproductive tract is supported within the pelvic cavity by the hammock-like genital fold and externally by the scrotum and prepuce.

SCROTUM

The scrotum is an outpouching of skin composed of two scrotal sacs, one for each testis, separated by the septum scroti. The sacs lie on either side of the penis (Fig. 76–2). If one testis is larger than the other, the scrotum may appear asymmetric or lopsided. The scrotum consists of four layers. The outermost layer is the skin, which contains an unusually large number of sweat glands. Underlying the skin and associated connective tissue is the tunica dartos. The tunica dartos is a layer of smooth muscle fibers intermingled with connective tissue, rather than a discrete muscle. This layer forms the outermost component of each scrotal sac and by raising or lowering the testis, the smooth muscle fibers aid in control of testicular temperature.

The third layer is loose connective tissue, or scrotal fascia, which allows the testis great mobility for vertical or horizontal movement within the scrotal sac. Normally, the loose connective tissue prevents 180° rotation of the testis within the scrotal sac, although in certain stallions such rotation does occur.[7–9] The impact of rotation of a testis on reproductive capacity is discussed in Chapter 82.

The innermost layer of the scrotum is the parietal vaginal tunic (some anatomists consider this covering as part of the testis). The parietal vaginal tunic (lamina parietalis of tunica vaginalis, also called the common vaginal tunic) is a membranous sac that extends from the abdominal cavity through the inguinal canal (cannalis inguinalis, an opening in the abdominal wall through which the spermatic cord passes) to the bottom of the scrotum. Part of this membrane covers the testis and epididymis and also contributes to the spermatic cord (funiculus spermaticus). The space within the vaginal cavity (cavum vaginale)—between the parietal vaginal tunic and visceral vaginal tunic (lamina visceralis of tunica vaginalis), which is the outermost covering around the testis and epididymis (Fig. 76–2)—contains a watery, serous fluid, which serves as a lubricant and facil-

*The general anatomic description is based on the authors' observations[1] and standard texts.[2–6] References for newer anatomic observations and for specific physiologic principles are supplied in the text.

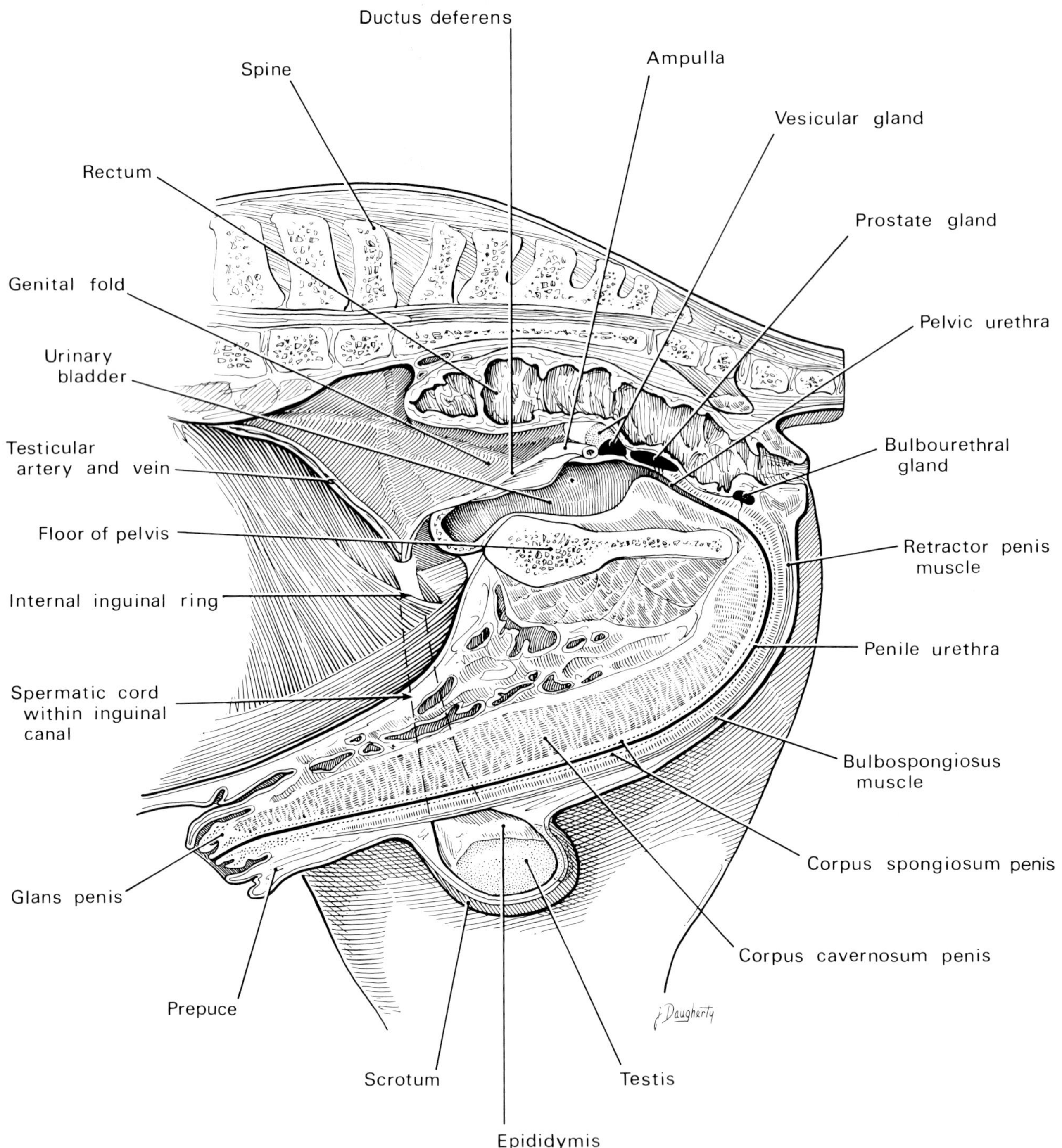

FIG. 76–1. Drawing of the reproductive tract of the stallion as seen in a left lateral dissection. (Modified from Pickett, B.W., et al.: Management of the Stallion for Maximum Reproductive Efficiency. II. Animal Reproduction Laboratory Bulletin No. 05. Fort Collins, Colorado State University, 1989.)

itates movement of the testis within the sac formed by the parietal vaginal tunic. In older stallions, adhesions sometimes develop between the parietal vaginal tunic and the visceral vaginal tunic, which covers the testis. Possibly, adhesions arise following slight hemorrhage from capillaries within the tunics, induced by slight trauma to the scrotum and testes as part of normal actions of a stallion. Such adhesions impede mobility of the testis and may reduce effectiveness of temperature-control mechanisms.

Descent of the testes into the scrotum[10] is described and diagramed in Chapter 77. The truly cryptorchid testis, one retained within the abdominal cavity, apparently occurs when the testis fails to enter the inguinal

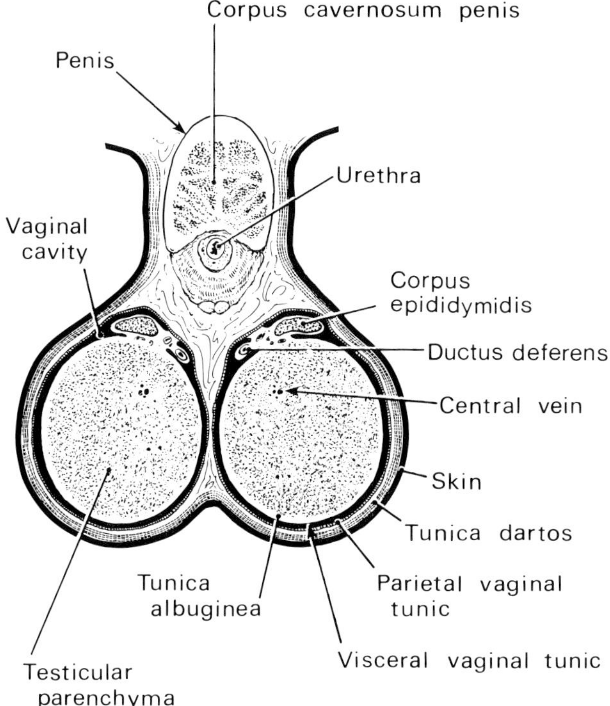

FIG. 76–2. Drawing of the penis, scrotum and testes of the stallion as seen in a vertical cross-section. (Modified from Pickett, B.W., et al.: Management of the Stallion for Maximum Reproductive Efficiency. II. Animal Reproduction Laboratory Bulletin No. 05. Fort Collins, Colorado State University, 1989.)

canal before closure of the internal inguinal ring (annulus inguinalis profundus) during the first 2 weeks after birth. The high incidence of failure of the left testis to descend[9] might result from the relatively slow rate of descent of the left epididymis and testis. Obviously, this could result in a higher incidence of retention of the left testis compared with the right.

Diagnosis of cryptorchidism should include careful external palpation of the scrotum and external inguinal ring, as well as palpation per rectum of the internal inguinal ring and pelvic area. Alternatively, cryptorchidism can be diagnosed by ultrasonography.[11] During the first several weeks after birth, the gubernaculum may be quite large and should not be confused with a testis. At birth, the weight of each testis is 5 to 20 g, and testicular size increases very little through 10 months of age. More rapid development of the testes generally starts around 12 to 18 months of age, but the age at which rapid growth of the testes commences varies considerably.

TESTIS

The testis is the male gonad and the site of production for both spermatozoa and the predominant male sex hormone, testosterone. The testes are ovoid, slightly compressed from side to side with their long axis almost horizontal (Fig. 76–1). When a testis is retracted, the long axis becomes more vertical, so the cauda epididymidis becomes ventrally rather than caudally located. Testes of postpubertal stallions range considerably in size. An average testis might measure 80 to 140 mm in length by 50 to 80 mm in width and weigh about 225 g. However, age and season greatly affect testis weight; no definitive data show that draft stallions have larger (or smaller) testes than light horse breeds, but for cattle, significant breed differences have been reported.[12]

If the testis is exposed, as during open castration, the thick tunica albuginea is seen (Fig. 76–2). Fused to the outer surface of this connective tissue capsule is the thin visceral vaginal tunic. Supporting strands of connective tissue extend from the tunica albuginea to divide the testis into lobules (lobuli testis).

The parenchyma, or noncapsular part of the testis, is lightly pigmented in a young postpubertal stallion, moderately pigmented in a 4- to 5-yr-old stallion, and darkly pigmented in an aged stallion.[13] The testicular parenchyma consists of seminiferous tubules (tubuli seminiferi) and interstitial tissue (Fig. 76–3). The seminiferous tubules (tubuli seminiferi contorti) (Fig. 76–4) are lined by a seminiferous epithelium (epithelium spermatogenicum) that consists of different types of germinal cells (cellulae spermatogenicae) (see Chapter 77) and the Sertoli cells (sustentacular cells).

The seminiferous tubule is limited by a lamina pro-

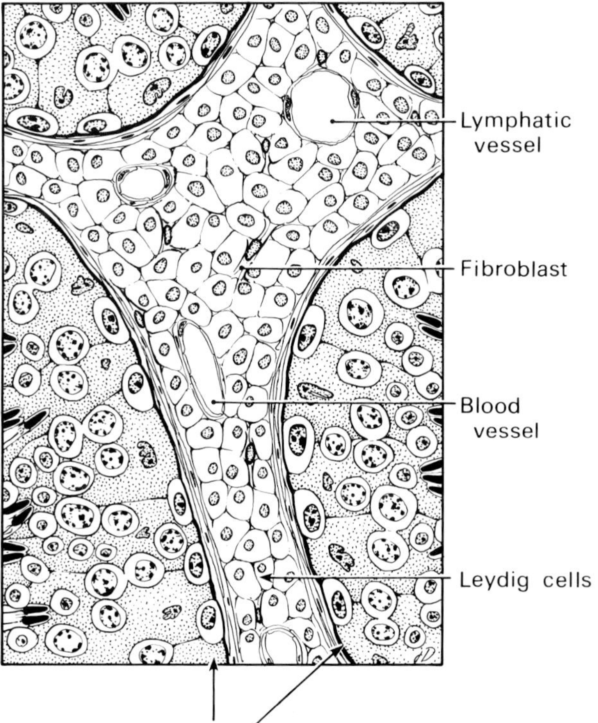

FIG. 76–3. Drawing of a stallion testis showing the relationship among the blood vessels, lymphatic vessels and Leydig cells of the interstitial tissue and seminiferous tubules. (From Pickett, B.W., et al.: Management of the Stallion for Maximum Reproductive Efficiency. II. Animal Reproduction Laboratory Bulletin No. 05. Fort Collins, Colorado State University, 1989.)

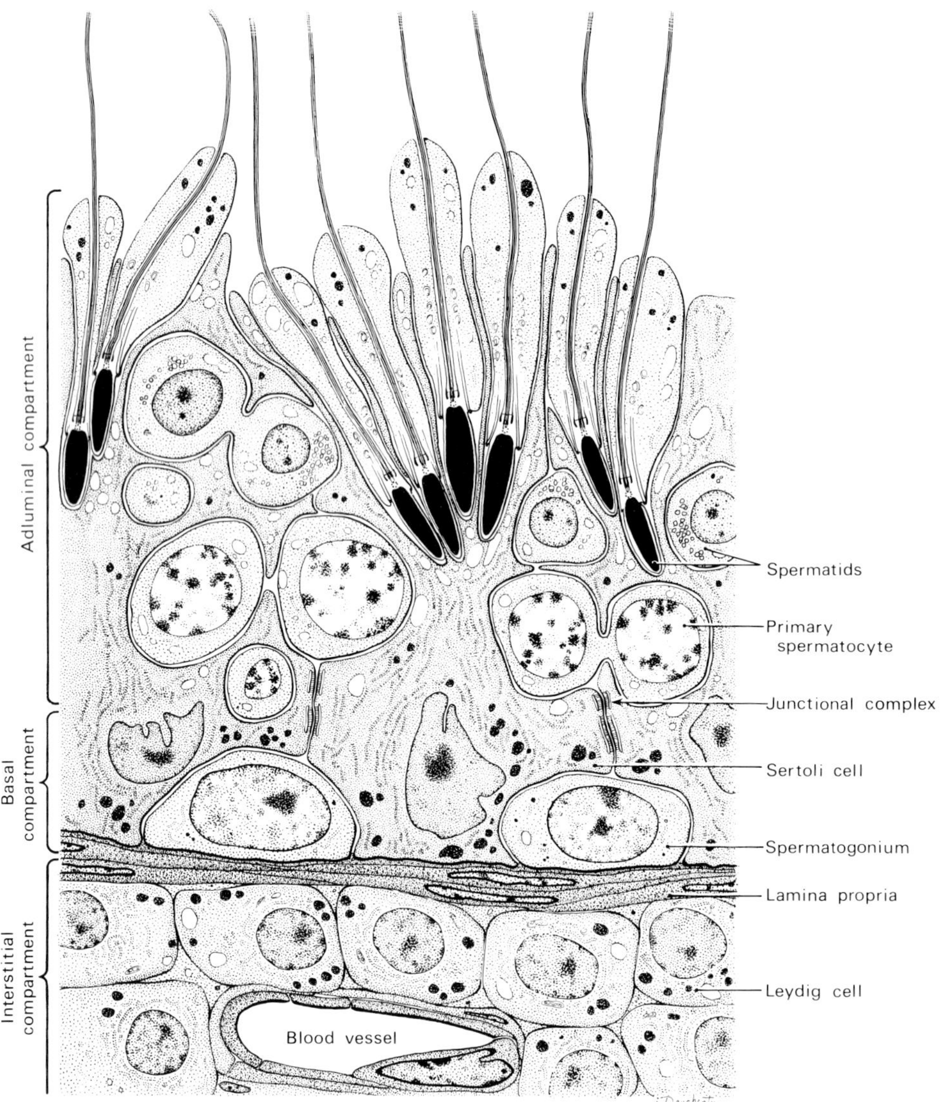

FIG. 76–4. Drawing of a section of a stallion seminiferous tubule showing the relationship of germinal cells and adjacent Sertoli cells in seminiferous epithelium. Spermatogonia, primary spermatocytes, secondary spermatocytes, and spherical spermatids all develop in the space between two or more Sertoli cells and are in contact with them. Primary spermatocytes are moved, by the Sertoli cells, from the basal compartment through the junctional complexes and into the adluminal compartment. During elongation of spermatids, they are repositioned by the Sertoli cells to become embedded within long pockets in cytoplasm of individual Sertoli cells. Note the intercellular bridges between adjacent germinal cells in the same cohort or generation. (From Pickett, B.W., et al.: Management of the Stallion for Maximum Reproductive Efficiency. II. Animal Reproduction Laboratory Bulletin No. 05. Fort Collins, Colorado State University, 1989.)

pria consisting of fibroblasts, myoid cells (specialized smooth muscle cells), and laminin. Rhythmic contractions of the myoid cells presumably help to move spermatozoa and fluids from the seminiferous tubules. The germinal cells are the most conspicuous feature of the seminiferous epithelium, but the Sertoli cells have a pivotal role in coordinating germinal cell differentiation and isolating most germinal cells from the host stallion's immune system. Junctional complexes between adjacent Sertoli cells (Fig. 76–4) form the major component of the blood-testis barrier and divide the seminiferous epithelium into two functional compartments, or regions: basal (peripheral) and adluminal (inner).

The blood-testis barrier isolates the more differentiated germinal cells from the immune system of the host stallion. Because the developing immune system is not exposed to differentiated spermatocytes or spermatids, it considers them to be foreign cells. Therefore, except for this isolation provided by the blood-testis barrier, germinal cells would be destroyed. Damage to the blood-testis barrier is rare in stallions, but can cause damage to the testis, reduce spermatozoal production, or induce sterility. Because Sertoli cells largely surround developing germinal cells, the immediate environment around all germinal cells, except spermatogonia, is controlled by Sertoli cells.[14–17] Sertoli cells produce several proteins needed to carry vitamin A, iron, and copper to developing germ cells and also a number of unique proteins involved in regulating formation of spermatozoa. Many compounds adversely affecting spermatogenesis probably act on Sertoli cells rather than directly on germinal cells. Furthermore, the general number of Sertoli cells per testis and maximum number of germinal cells per Sertoli cell are characteristics of a species,[18] but the number of Sertoli cells per testis is a trait with high heritability.[19] Any treatment that decreases the number of Sertoli cells formed before puberty or alters Sertoli cell function will probably adversely affect spermatozoal production.

The interstitial tissue (interstitium testis) includes blood vessels, lymphatic channels, nerves, connective tissue, and Leydig cells (endocrinocytus interstitialis). Leydig cells, which are responsible for production of steroid hormones including testosterone, are the major component of the interstitial tissue in adults.[13] As a stallion grows older, postpubertal Leydig cells are gradually replaced by adult Leydig cells, which contain abundant pigmented lipids and are interconnected by numerous interdigitations,[20] and they may produce more testosterone per cell than Leydig cells of younger stallions. The percentage composition of the testis, on a volume basis, changes with age. The ratio of Leydig cells to seminiferous tubules increases from 1:12 in stallions 2 to 3 yr old to 1:4 for those 13 to 20 yr old

TABLE 76–1. AGE-RELATED DIFFERENCES IN TESTICULAR COMPOSITION*

	AGE (YR)		
	2–3	4–5	13–20
Testicular weight (g)			
Parenchyma	105[a]	146[b]	184[c]
Tunica albuginea	12[a]	15[b]	29[c]
Parenchymal composition (%)			
Leydig cells	6[a]	12[b]	18[c]
Other interstitial tissue	22[a]	16[b]	10[c]
Seminiferous tubules	72	72	72
Seminiferous tubule			
Diameter (m)	212[a]	230[b]	242[b]
Length/testis (m)	2040[a]	2390[ab]	2790[b]
Daily spermatozoal production (10^9/testis)	1.3[a]	2.7[b]	3.2[b]

*Means in the same row with different superscripts differ ($p < 0.05$).

(Adapted from Johnson, L. and Neaves, W.B.: Age-related changes in Leydig cell population, seminiferous tubules, and sperm production in stallions. Biol. Reprod. *24*:703–712, 1981.)

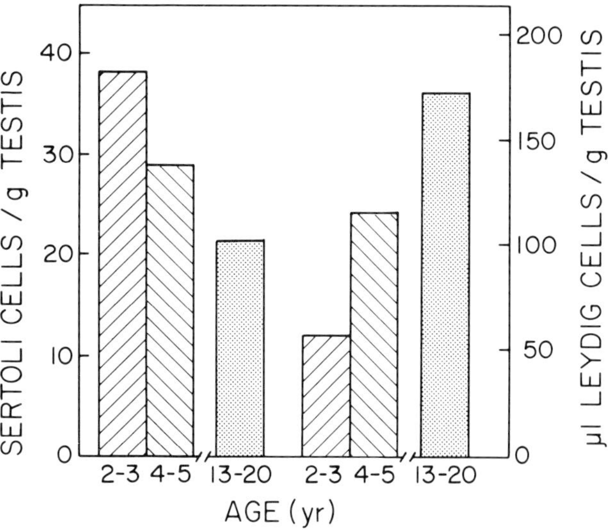

FIG. 76–5. Effect of age on number of Sertoli cells and volume of Leydig cells per gram of testicular parenchyma. Data for Sertoli cells are for testes collected in June and July and data for Leydig cells are for testes obtained between February and May. (From Pickett, B.W., et al.: Management of the Stallion for Maximum Reproductive Efficiency. II. Animal Reproduction Laboratory Bulletin No. 05. Fort Collins, Colorado State University, 1989.)

(Table 76–1). Although certain of the changes presented in Table 76–1 are a consequence of testicular growth, composition of the testis on a per gram basis also changes with age. This is especially evident for the number of Sertoli cells per gram of testicular parenchyma,[21] and the decline with advancing age (Fig. 76–5) may be partially responsible for the decline in daily spermatozoal production which occurs in some older stallions. Although percentage of the testis occupied by seminiferous tubules does not change with age (Table 76–1), total volume of Leydig cells per gram of testicular parenchyma increases more than threefold with age (Fig. 76–5). The total length of seminiferous tubules in the testis also increases by about one-third.[13]

A seminiferous tubule is arch shaped and consists of three zones. The major portion of a seminiferous tubule, the convoluted seminiferous tubule, is highly coiled and is the site of spermatozoal production. A convoluted seminiferous tubule is lined by a seminiferous epithelium, which contains Sertoli cells and several types of germinal cells.[1,2,13–15,17,21–27] Sertoli cells and spermatogonia line the basement membrane of the tubules, and Sertoli cells extend toward the lumen in a radial pattern (Fig. 76–4) to occupy 15 to 25% of the seminiferous epithelium in an adult stallion. Although it is conventionally accepted that Sertoli cells do not divide after puberty,[8,14,16,27] the results of recent research demonstrate that Sertoli cells in the stallion proliferate as the breeding season approaches.[21,24,28,29] The number of Sertoli cells in a testis is an important determinator of the number of spermatozoa that a testis can produce.[22]

Both ends of a convoluted seminiferous tubule continue as tapered transitional zones leading to the straight portions of the seminiferous tubule. Straight tubules (tubuli seminiferi recti) are the first component of the passageway through which spermatozoa pass from the seminiferous epithelium to the epididymis. Straight tubules converge in the cranial two-thirds of the testis[30] in an area termed the rete testis (Figs. 76–6 and 76–7). Tubules of the intratesticular rete testis penetrate the tunic albuginea and continue as an extratesticular rete.[30] Eventually, each rete tubule fuses with one of the 13 to 15 efferent ducts (ductuli efferentes testis) that lead to the epididymal duct (ductus epididymidis).[31]

Horses are seasonal breeders and characteristics of the testes (Table 76–2) change markedly throughout the year. However, unlike some seasonal breeders, stallions continue to produce spermatozoa throughout the year. Maximum testicular development and function occur in May, June, and July.[23,29,32–34] From September through February, the testes are regressed; they are probably minimal in size and function from November to January. At that time of year, the testes of typical stallions are 25% lighter; contain about 35% fewer Leydig cells and consequently less smooth endoplasmic reticulum (SER), the part of the cell involved in production of testosterone; contain 31% fewer Sertoli cells; and produce 40 to 50% fewer spermatozoa (Table 76–2). Concentrations in the blood of hormones involved in control of reproductive function also tend to be lower in the nonbreeding season.

SPERMATIC CORD

The spermatic cord extends from the abdominal inguinal ring to its attachment on the testis. It suspends the testis in the scrotum and acts as a passageway for the deferent duct (ductus deferens), nerves, and blood vessels associated with the testis (Fig. 76–8). The external cremaster muscle is conspicuous on the lateral aspect of the spermatic cord, although it is not part of the cord. This striated muscle helps to support the testis and aids in control of testicular temperature.

The spermatic cord includes the highly coiled testicular artery (Fig. 76–7). The veins draining the testis form

TABLE 76–2. EFFECT OF SEASON ON CHARACTERISTICS OF TESTES OF STALLIONS 4 TO 20 YR OLD*

	BREEDING	NONBREEDING	DIFFERENCE (%)†
Parenchyma weight, paired testes (g)	154	116	−25
Leydig cells			
(10^6/g testis)	22	20	−9
(10^9/2 testes)	7.26	4.70	−35
Leydig cell SER‡ (mL/2 testes)	34.0	22.2	−35
Testosterone			
(μg/g testis)	700	580	−17
(mg/2 testes)	224	154	−31
Sertoli cells			
(10^6/g testis)	24.2	23.6	−2
(10^9/2 testes)	3.69	2.54	−31
Elongated spermatids per Sertoli cell	9.36	7.54	−19
Daily spermatozoal production			
(10^6/g testis)	19.1	14.6	−23
(10^9/2 testes)	5.96	3.53	−41
Serum			
FSH§ (ng/mL)	108	81	−21
LH‖ (ng/mL)	36	22	−39
testosterone (ng/mL)	0.36	0.27	−25

*Not all data are for the same stallions. For most values $n \geq 48$.

†Not all differences between the breeding and nonbreeding seasons were statistically significant in the original studies. Because data were compiled across studies, statistical significance was not determined.

‡Smooth endoplastic reticulum.

§Follicle-stimulating hormone.

‖Luteinizing hormone.

(Based on Johnson, L., and Thompson, D.L., Jr.: Seasonal variation in the total volume of Leydig cells in stallions is explained by variation in cell number rather than cell size. Biol. Reprod., *35*:971–979, 1986; and Johnson, L. and Thompson, D.L., Jr.: Effect of seasonal changes in Leydig cells and intratesticular testosterone content in stallions. J. Reprod. Fertil., *81*:227–232, 1987. From Pickett, B.W., et al.: Management of the Stallion for Maximum Reproductive Efficiency. II. Animal Reproduction Laboratory Bulletin No. 05. Fort Collins, Colorado State University, 1989.

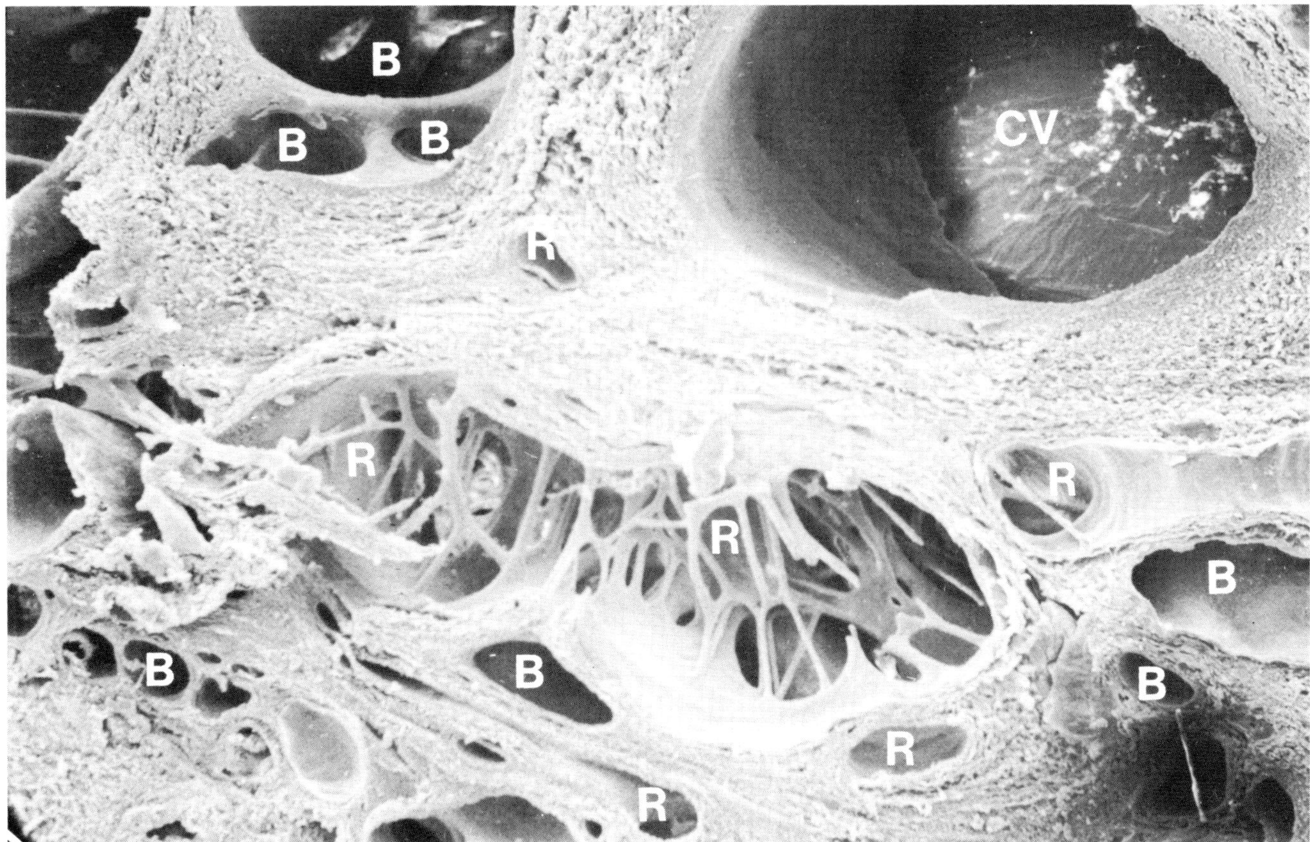

FIG. 76–6. A scanning electron micrograph (× 50) of the interconnecting tubules within the rete testis near the central vein (CV). Rete tubules (R) and smaller blood vessels (B) are comingled in that area. (From Amann, R.P., Johnson, L., and Pickett, B.W.: Connection between the seminiferous tubules and the efferent ducts in the stallion. Am. J. Vet. Res. *38:*1571–1579, 1977.)

an intimate network of small veins around the highly coiled artery.[35] This network of veins is called the pampiniform plexus and serves as a heat exchange system.

EXCURRENT DUCT SYSTEM

After penetrating the tunica albuginea, each rete tubule fuses with an efferent duct. These, in turn, lead to the epididymal duct (ductus epididymidis), which continues as the deferent duct, and terminates in the colliculus seminalis.

EPIDIDYMIS

The epididymis is divided anatomically into three parts: caput, corpus, and cauda. The caput curves around the testis and lateral aspect of the spermatic cord (Figs. 76–1 and 76–7) and continues as the corpus of the epididymis. The caput is rather flat, has a J shape and is closely attached to the testis. The corpus epididymidis is a cylindric structure loosely attached to the dorsal surface of the testis (Fig. 76–2). The cauda epididymidis is large, bulbous, and loosely attached to the caudal pole of the testis.

The proximal caput epididymidis actually contains the distal ends of 13 to 15 highly coiled efferent ducts that lead from the tubules of the extratesticular rete testis.[30,31] Within the caput epididymidis, efferent ducts fuse into a single duct termed the epididymal duct.[31] This single duct, possibly 45 m long, is folded in pleats and continues in a tortuous pattern (Fig. 76–7) through the caput, corpus, and cauda epididymidis and is continuous with the deferent duct. Based on cellular structure, six to eight regions can be distinguished in the stallion epididymis, and the function of each region is probably different.[36]

From a functional point of view (see Chapter 77), the epididymis has three segments.[37–40] Epithelia of the efferent ducts plus the initial segment of the caput (Figs. 76–9 and 76–10) are involved in resorption of most of the fluid and solutes entering from the testis and also secrete some compounds. The middle segment includes major portions of the caput and corpus epididymidis and is involved in spermatozoal maturation, a process that depends on specific secretions of the epithelium. The terminal segment is composed of the

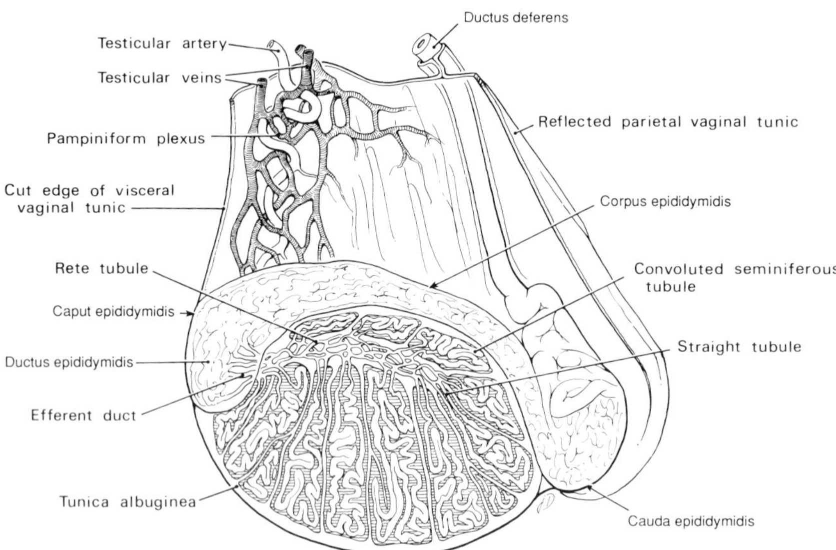

FIG. 76–7. Diagrammatic view showing the location of straight tubules and rete testis in the stallion testis. The straight tubules converge in a group of interconnecting rete tubules that penetrate the tunica albuginea and fuse with the efferent ducts. The efferent ducts merge in the epididymal duct. The testicular artery becomes highly coiled in the pampiniform plexus. After emerging from the pampiniform plexus, the testicular artery passes along the dorsal aspect of the testis to the caudal pole where it starts to branch to vascularize the parenchyma. Venous drainage of the parenchyma is via the central vein and superficial testicular veins. After leaving the testis, the veins form an anastomosing plexus of veins, termed the pampiniform plexus, which is in intimate contact with the testicular artery. About 7 to 10 cm above the testis, the veins converge into the testicular vein. (Modified from Pickett, B.W., et al.: Management of the Stallion for Maximum Reproductive Efficiency. II. Animal Reproduction Laboratory Bulletin No. 05. Fort Collins, Colorado State University, 1989.)

cauda epididymidis (Fig. 76–11) and proximal deferent duct and is involved in storage of fertile spermatozoa.

DEFERENT DUCT

The deferent duct (ductus deferens) is a continuation of the epididymal duct and extends from the cauda epididymidis through the spermatic cord to the pelvic urethra (Figs. 76–1 and 76–7). The deferent duct of the stallion has an extremely thick wall of smooth muscle. Thus the proximal deferent duct can be palpated readily through the scrotal skin.

As the deferent duct approaches the pelvic urethra, it widens into a structure termed the ampulla of the deferent duct (Figs. 76–1 and 76–12). The ampulla is about 18 mm in diameter compared with 4 to 5 mm for the deferent duct. The increased diameter in the ampullar region is primarily caused by a thickening of the wall associated with the presence of crypts and glands, although luminal diameter does increase slightly.

ACCESSORY SEX GLANDS

The accessory sex glands (glandulae genitales accessoriae) are sometimes considered to include the ampulla of the deferent duct, but herein are considered to include only the glandula vesicularis, prostata, and glandula bulbourethralis. Functions of these glands, and their contributions to semen are considered in Chapter 77.

The two vesicular glands (previously termed seminal vesicles) are elongated, hollow pouches about 15 to 20

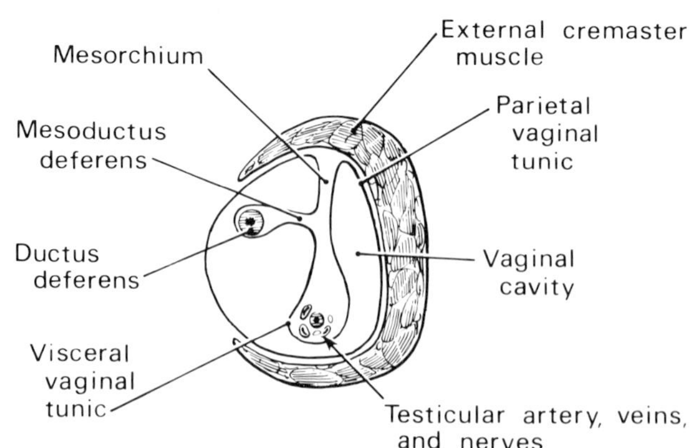

FIG. 76–8. Drawing showing a cross section through the right spermatic cord and external cremaster muscle above the pampiniform plexus. (From Pickett, B.W., et al.: Management of the Stallion for Maximum Reproductive Efficiency. II. Animal Reproduction Laboratory Bulletin No. 05. Fort Collins, Colorado State University, 1989.)

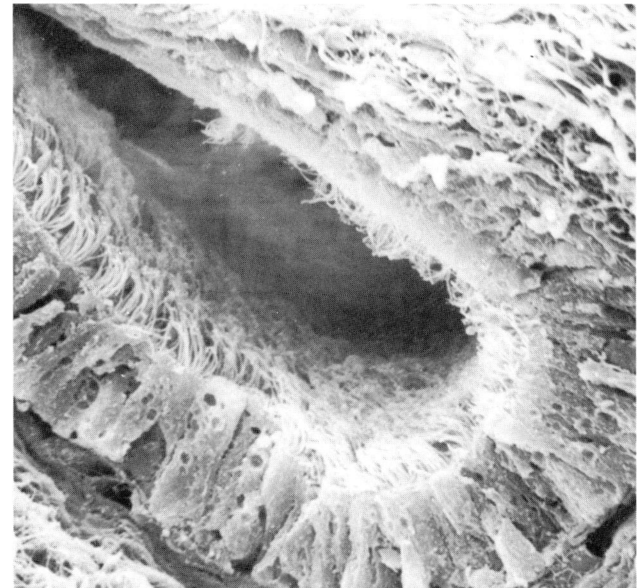

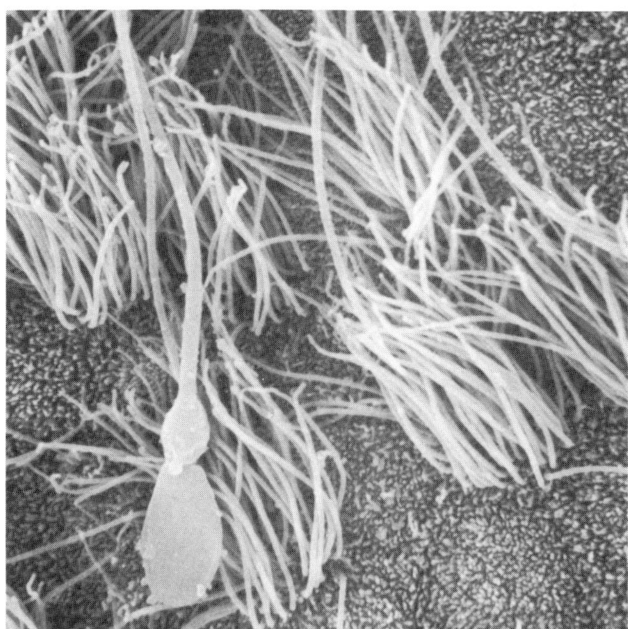

FIG. 76–9. *A,* Section through an efferent duct showing ciliated and nonciliated cells in this epithelium (× 725). *B,* The luminal surface of an efferent duct and a spermatozoon with a proximal cytoplasmic droplet (normal for a spermatozoon from this region) also are shown (× 3075). (From Johnson, L., Amann, R.P., and Pickett, B.W.: Scanning electron microscopy of the epithelium and spermatozoa in the equine excurrent duct system. Am. J. Vet. Res. *39:*1428–1434, 1978.)

cm long and 5 cm in diameter (Fig. 76–12). In spite of the common use of the term seminal vesicles to describe these glands, the vesicular glands do not serve as a storage organ for spermatozoa. The prostate gland is a single, firm, nodular gland (Fig. 76–12) with two narrow lobes (each 7 × 4 × 1 cm) connected by a thin transverse isthmus (about 3 cm long). The two bulbourethral glands (previously termed Cowper's glands) are positioned on either side of the pelvic urethra near the ischial arch (Figs. 76–1 and 76–12).

URETHRA

The urethra is a long mucous-secreting tube that extends from the bladder to the free end of the penis. The pelvic portion of the urethra is overlaid by a thick, striated muscle termed the urethralis muscle (Fig. 76–12), which contracts vigorously during ejaculation. The urethra terminates in a free extension called the urethral process (processus urethrae) (Fig. 76–13). The penile urethra is surrounded by the corpus spongiosum penis (Fig. 76–14), which is an area of cavernous, erectile tissue. The urethra serves as the joint excretory canal for urine and semen.

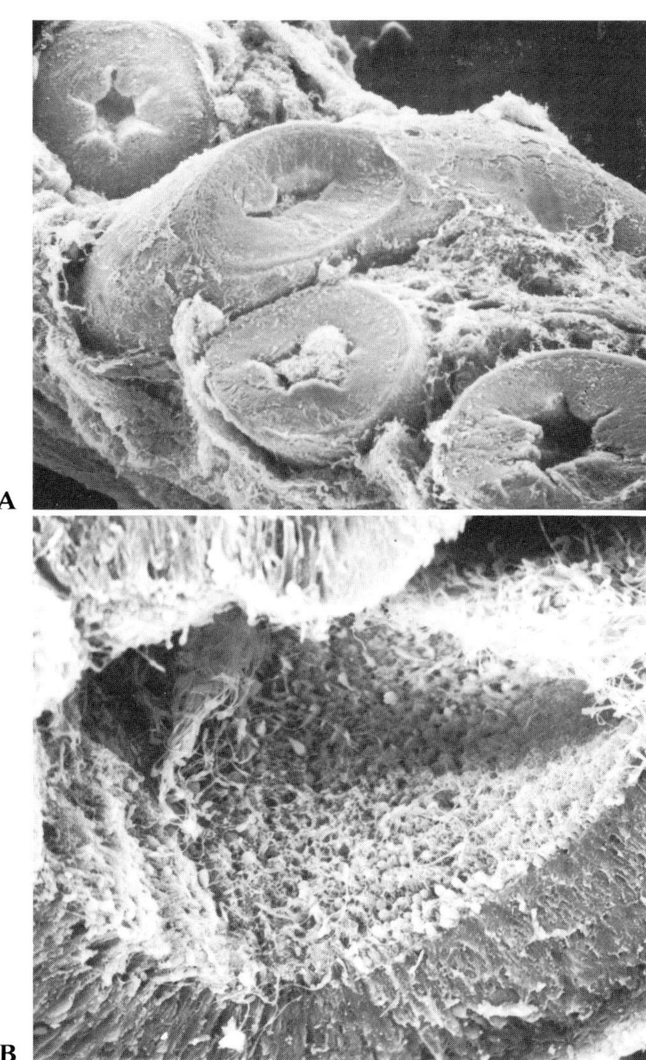

FIG. 76–10. Sections through the caput epididymidis showing *(A)* the epithelium and thin layer of smooth muscle (× 60) and *(B)* the surface of the epithelium and spermatozoa within the duct (× 300). (From Johnson, L., Amann, R.P., and Pickett, B.W.: Scanning electron microscopy of the epithelium and spermatozoa in the equine excurrent duct system. Am. J. Vet. Res. *39:*1428–1434, 1978.)

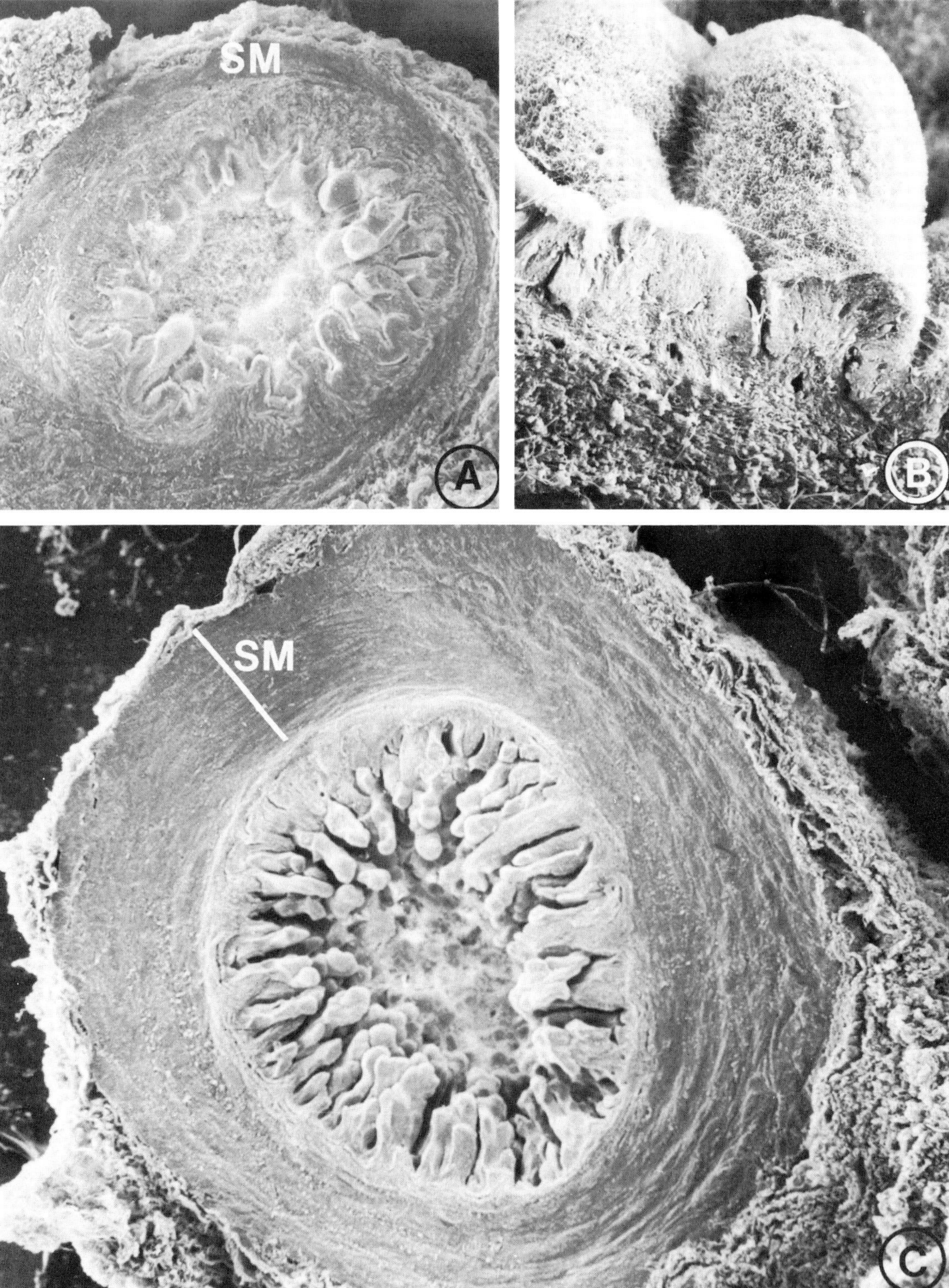

FIG. 76–11. Sections through the cauda epididymidis. *A,* In the proximal cauda, projections of epithelium radiate from the wall of the duct and the smooth muscle layer is of moderate thickness (× 53). *B,* Details of the projections and smooth muscle (SM) (× 225). *C,* In the distal cauda, projections are much longer and the smooth muscle layer is thick (× 35). (From Johnson, L., Amann, R.P., and Pickett, B.W.: Scanning electron microscopy of the epithelium and spermatozoa in the equine excurrent duct system. Am. J. Vet. Res. *39:*1428–1434, 1978.)

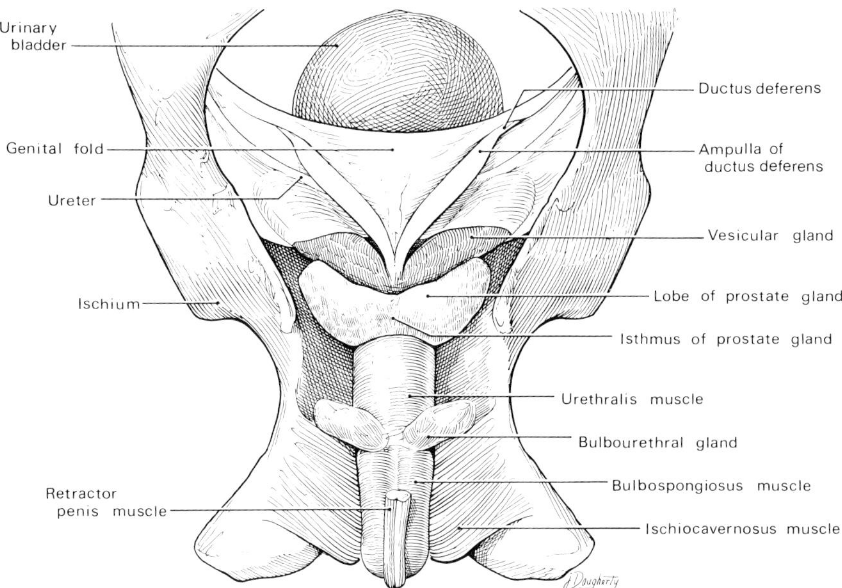

FIG. 76–12. Drawing showing a dorsal view of the pelvic portion of the reproductive tract. The connective tissue and fat have been dissected away to expose the genital fold that supports the pelvic portion of the tract. (From Pickett, B.W., et al.: Management of the Stallion for Maximum Reproductive Efficiency. II. Animal Reproduction Laboratory Bulletin No. 05. Fort Collins, Colorado State University, 1989.)

PENIS

The penis is the male organ of copulation and consists of three regions (Fig. 76–13): the root, which is the site of attachment to the skeletal system; the body or shaft, which is the main portion of the penis; and the glans penis, which is the enlarged, free end of the penis. The primary functional components of the penis are the corpus cavernosum penis; corpus spongiosum penis, which is continuous with the corona glandis of the glans penis; urethra; bulbospongiosus muscle; and associated blood vessels and nerves (Fig. 76–14). The stallion penis is a musculocavernosus type and undergoes considerable enlargement in length and diameter during erection, which is in contrast to the fibroelastic penis of the bull, which becomes straight and stiff during erection, but does not increase in size. The stallion penis contains a large amount of erectile tissue, some of which surrounds the urethra, but most of which is enclosed in a connective tissue capsule, the tunica albuginea (Fig. 76–14).

The root of the penis is tightly attached to the tuber ischii by the paired crua, overlain by the paired ischiocavernosus muscles and stabilized by two suspensory

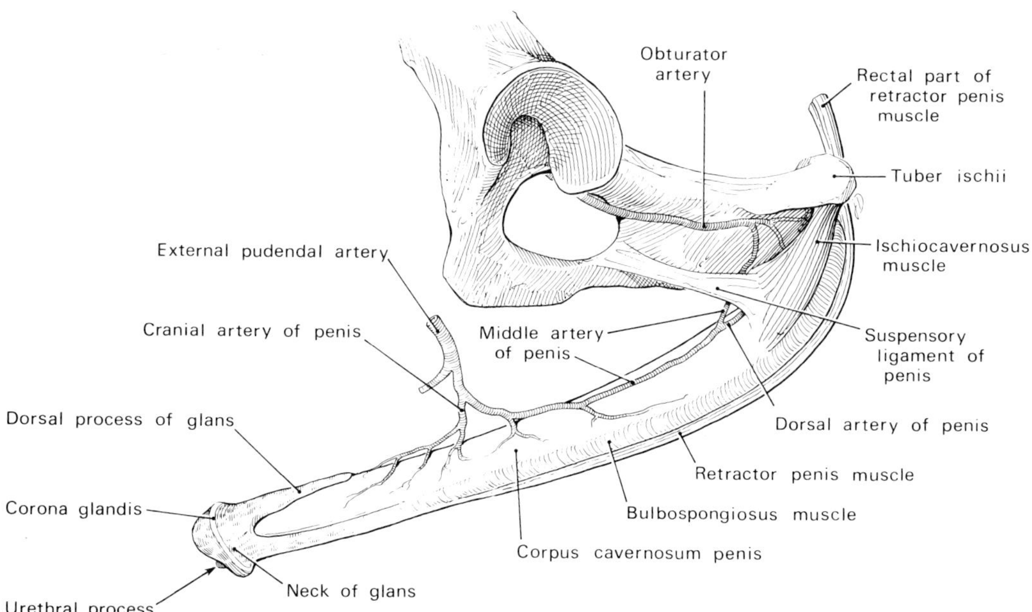

FIG. 76–13. Drawing showing a left lateral view of the penis and its attachment to the ischium. (From Pickett, B.W., et al.: Management of the Stallion for Maximum Reproductive Efficiency. II. Animal Reproduction Laboratory Bulletin No. 05. Fort Collins, Colorado State University, 1989.)

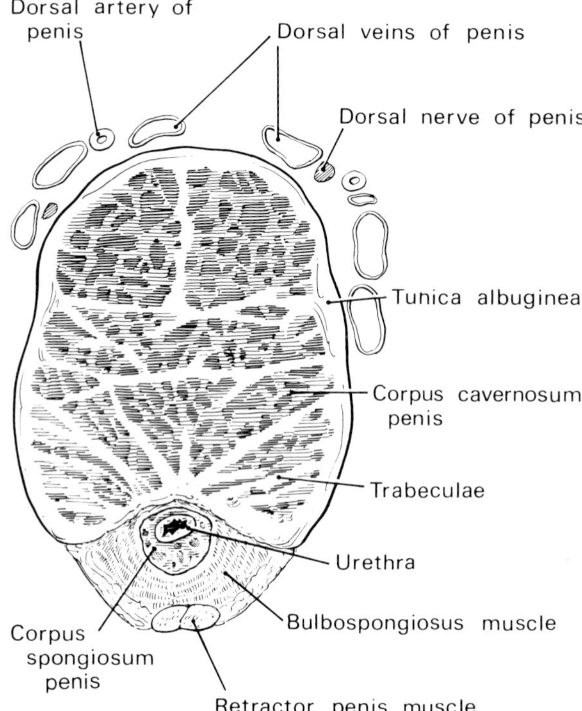

FIG. 76–14. Drawing showing a cross section through the body of the penis. (Adapted from Pickett, B.W., et al.: Management of the Stallion for Maximum Reproductive Efficiency. II. Animal Reproduction Laboratory Bulletin No. 05. Fort Collins, Colorado State University, 1989.)

ligaments (Fig. 76–13). When viewed in cross section (Fig. 76–14), the corpus cavernosum penis forms the major component of the body of the penis. The corpus cavernosum penis is spongy, erectile tissue, which is continuous with veins draining the penis. The corpus spongiosum penis is a small area of spongy, erectile tissue that immediately surrounds the urethra but is not enclosed by the tunica albuginea. The corpus spongiosum penis is continuous into the glans penis (Fig. 76–15), which is richly endowed with nerve endings. The corpus spongiosum penis and corona glandis become engorged with blood and erect during sexual excitement.

When not erect, the penis is about 50 cm long by 2.5 to 5.0 cm in diameter. About 15 to 20 cm are free in the prepuce (Fig. 76–15). Erection increases the length and diameter of the penis about 50%, whereas the glans penis increases 300 to 400% in diameter through engorgement.

HYPOTHALAMUS AND ADENOHYPOPHYSIS

The hypothalamus and adenohypophysis are described in Chapter 1. Their secretions are pivotal in the regulation of male reproductive function as considered in Chapters 77 and 89.

REFERENCES

1. Pickett, B.W., et al.: Management of the Stallion for Maximum Reproductive Efficiency. II. Animal Reproduction Laboratory Bulletin No. 05. Fort Collins, Colorado State University, 1989.
2. Banks, W.J.: Applied Veterinary Histology. 2nd ed. Baltimore, Williams & Wilkins, 1986.
3. Dyce, K.M., Sack, W.O., and Wensing, C.J.G.: Textbook of Veterinary Anatomy. Philadelphia, W.B. Saunders, 1987.
4. Krolling, O., and Grau, H.: Lehrbuch der Histologie und Vergleichenden Microskopischen Anatomie der Haustiere. Berlin, Paul Parey, 1960.

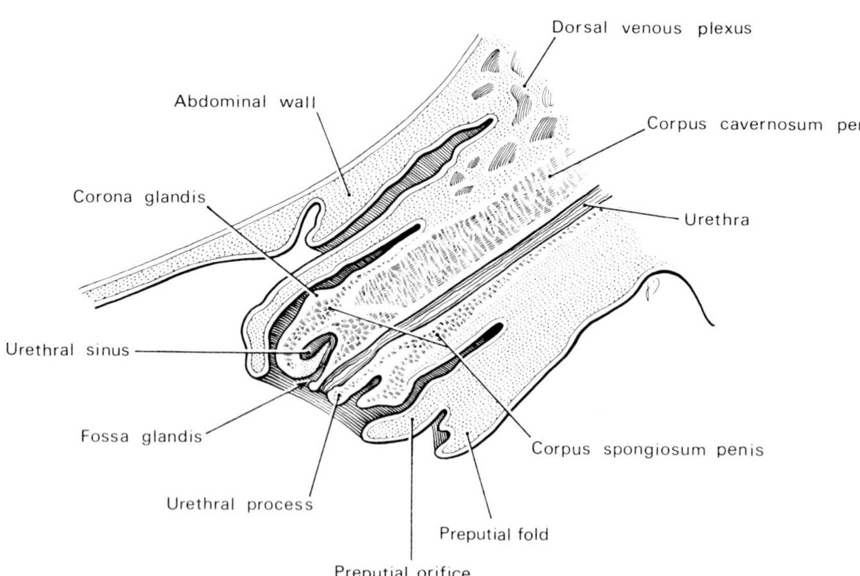

FIG. 76–15. Drawing showing a left lateral view of the glans penis and prepuce. (Adapted from Pickett, B.W., et al.: Management of the Stallion for Maximum Reproductive Efficiency. II. Animal Reproduction Laboratory Bulletin No. 05. Fort Collins, Colorado State University, 1989.)

5. Montane, M., Bourdelle, E., and Bressou, C.: Anatomie Regionale des Animaux Domestiques. I. Equides. 9th ed. Paris, J.B. Bailliere, 1949.
6. Nickel, R., Schummer, A., Seiferle, E., and Sack, W.O.: The Viscera of the Domestic Mammals. New York, Springer-Verlag, 1973.
7. Pickett, B.W., et al.: Seminal characteristics and total scrotal width (T.S.W.) of normal and abnormal stallions. Proc. Am. Assoc. Equine Pract., 487–518, 1988.
8. Setchell, B.P., and Brooks, D.E.: Anatomy, vasculature, innervation and fluids of the male reproductive tract. *In* The Physiology of Reproduction. Edited by E. Knobil and J. Neill. New York, Raven Press, 1988, pp. 753–836.
9. Stickle, R.L., and Fessler, J.F.: Retrospective study of 350 cases of equine cryptorchidism. S. Am. Vet. Med. Assoc., *172:*343–346, 1978.
10. Bergin, W.C., Gier, H.T., Marion, G.B., and Coffman, J.R.: A developmental concept of equine cryptorchism. Biol. Reprod., *3:*82–92, 1970.
11. Varner, D.D., Schumacher, J., Blanchard, T.L., and Johnson, L.: Diseases and Management of Breeding Stallions. Galeta, CA, American Veterinary Publications, 1991.
12. Lunstra, D.D., Ford, J.J., and Echternkamp, S.E.: Puberty in beef bulls: Hormone concentrations, growth, testicular development, sperm production and sexual aggressiveness in bulls of different breeds. J. Anim. Sci., *46:*1054–1062, 1978.
13. Johnson, L., and Neaves, W.B.: Age-related changes in the Leydig cell population, seminiferous tubules, and sperm production in stallions. Biol. Reprod., *24:*703–712, 1981.
14. De Kretser, D.M., and Kerr, J.B.: The cytology of the testis. *In* The Physiology of Reproduction. Edited by E. Knobil and J. Neill. New York, Raven Press, 1988, pp 837–932.
15. Fawcett, D.W.: Ultrastructure and function of the Sertoli cell. *In* Handbook of Physiology. Vol. 5. Edited by D.W. Hamilton and R.O. Greep. Washington, D.C., American Physiology Society, 1975, pp. 21–55.
16. Setchell, B.P.: The Mammalian Testis. Ithaca, NY, Cornell University Press, 1978.
17. Hochereau-de Reviers, M.-T., et al.: Spermatogenesis in mammals and birds. *In* Marshall's Physiology of Reproduction. Vol. 2. Reproduction in the Male. 4th ed. Edited by G.E. Lamming. London, Churchill Livingstone, 1990, pp. 106–182.
18. Lok, D., Weenk, D., and De Rooij, D.G.: Morphology, proliferation, and differentiation of undifferentiated spermatogonia in the Chinese hamster and the ram. Anat. Rec., *203:*83–99, 1982.
19. Hochereau-de Reviers, M.-T., Monet-Kuntz, C., and Courot, M.: Spermatogenesis and Sertoli cell numbers and function in rams and bulls. J. Reprod. Fertil. Suppl., *34:*101–114, 1987.
20. Almahbobi, G., Papadopoulos, V., Carreau, S., and Silberzahn, P.: Age-related morphological and functional changes in the Leydig cells of the horse. Biol. Reprod., *38:*653–665, 1988.
21. Johnson, L., and Thompson, D.L., Jr.: Age-related and seasonal variation in the Sertoli cell population, daily sperm production and serum concentrations of follicle-stimulating hormone, luteinizing hormone and testosterone in stallions. Biol. Reprod., *29:*777–789, 1983.
22. Berndtson, W.E., Igboeli, G., and Parker, W.G.: The numbers of Sertoli cells in mature Holstein bulls and their relationship to quantitative aspects of spermatogenesis. Biol. Reprod. *37:*60–67, 1987.
23. Berndtson, W.E., Squires, E.L., and Thompson, D.L., Jr.: Spermatogenesis, testicular composition and the concentration of testosterone in the equine testis as influenced by season. Theriogenology, *20:*449–457, 1983.
24. Johnson, L.: A new approach to quantification of Sertoli cells that avoids problems associated with the irregular nuclear surface. Anat. Rec., *214:*231–237, 1986.
25. Johnson, L., Amann, R.P., and Pickett, B.W.: Scanning electron and light microscopy of the equine seminiferous tubule. Fertil. Steril., *29:*208–215, 1978.
26. Swierstra, E.E., Gebauer, M.R., and Pickett, B.W.: Reproductive physiology of the stallion. I. Spermatogenesis and testis composition. J. Reprod. Fertil., *40:*113–123, 1974.
27. Fawcett, D.W.: Observations on the organization of the interstitial tissue of the testis and on the occluding cell junctions in the seminiferous epithelium. Adv. Biosci., *10:*83–99, 1973.
28. Johnson, L., and Nguyen, H.B.: Annual cycle of the Sertoli cell population in adult stallions. J. Reprod. Fertil., *76:*311–316, 1986.
29. Johnson, L., and Tatum, M.E.: Sequence of seasonal changes in numbers of Sertoli, Leydig, and germ cells in adult stallions. Proceedings of the Eleventh International Congress on Animal Reproduction and Artificial Insemination. Dublin, 1988, p. 373.
30. Amann, R.P., Johnson, L., and Pickett, B.W.: Connection between the seminiferous tubules and the efferent ducts in the stallion. Am. J. Vet. Res., *38:*1571–1579, 1977.
31. Hemeida, N.A., Sack, W.O., and McEntee, K.: Ductuli efferentes in the epididymis of boar, goat, ram, bull, and stallion. Am. J. Vet. Res., *39:*1892–1900, 1978.
32. Clay, C.M., Squires, E.L., Amann, R.P., and Pickett, B.W.: Influences of season and artificial photoperiod on stallions: Testicular size, seminal characteristics and sexual behavior. J. Anim. Sci., *64:*517–525, 1987.
33. Clay, C.M., Squires, E.L., Amann, R.P., and Nett, T.M.: Influences of season and artificial photoperiod on stallions: Luteinizing hormone, follicle stimulating hormone and testosterone. J. Anim. Sci., *66:*1246–1255, 1988.
34. Clay, C.M., Squires, E.L., Amann, R.P., and Nett, T.M.: Influences of season and artificial photoperiod on stallions: Pituitary and testicular responses to exogenous GnRH. J. Anim. Sci., *67:*763–770, 1988.
35. Ippensen, E., Klug-Simon, C., and Klug, E.: Der Verlauf der Blutgefasse vom Hoden des Pferdes im Hinblick auf eine Biopsiemoglichkeit. Zuchthygiene, *7:*35–45, 1972.
36. Nicander, L.: Studies on the regional histology and cytochemistry of the ductus epididymidis in stallions, rams and bulls. Acta Morphol. Neerl. Scand., *1:*337–362, 1958.
37. Amann, R.P.: Function of the epididymis in bulls and rams. J. Reprod. Fertil. Suppl., *34:*115–131, 1987.
38. Amann, R.P.: Maturation of spermatozoa. Proceedings of the Eleventh International Congress on Animal Reproduction and Artificial Insemination. Dublin, 1988, pp. 320–328.
39. Glover, T.D., and Nicander, L.: Some aspects of structure and function in the mammalian epididymis. J. Reprod. Fertil. Suppl., *13:*39–50, 1971.
40. Johnson, L., Amann, R.P., and Pickett, B.W.: Scanning electron microscopy of the epithelium and spermatozoa in the equine excurrent duct system. Am. J. Vet. Res., *39:*1428–1434, 1978.

CHAPTER 77

PHYSIOLOGY AND ENDOCRINOLOGY

R.P. Amann

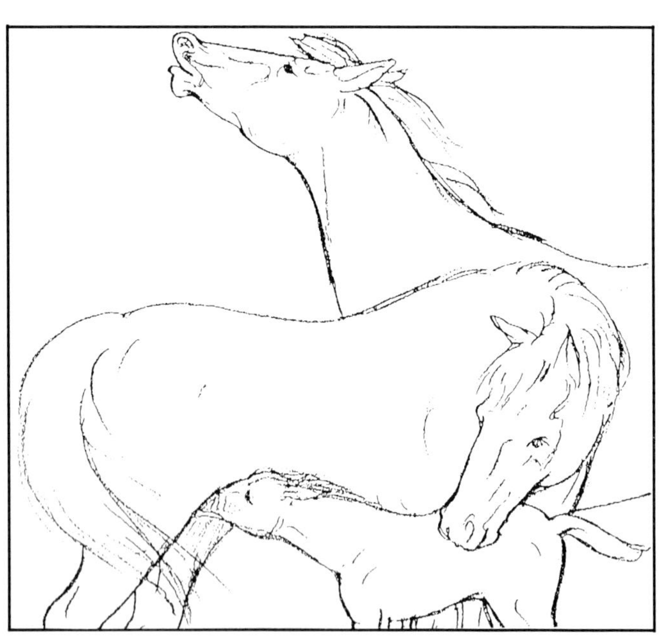

The production and ejaculation of normal spermatozoa in numbers adequate for conception is imperative for reproduction. Unfortunately, one or more of the reproductive organs may not function normally, and the probability of conception and development of a normal embryo is reduced. Development of a prognosis and effective treatment for such stallions, or effective management of a normal stallion, require an understanding of normal reproductive function. The testes have a pivotal dual role: (1) production of spermatozoa and (2) secretion of hormones essential for normal function of the epididymis and accessory sex glands as well as expression of sexual behavior. Consequently, knowledge of testicular function is crucial for people working with stallions, so they can avoid actions which interfere with normal testicular function or recognize possible origins of detected alterations in spermatozoal production. In addition, some knowledge of the role of the epididymis and accessory sex glands is desirable because their functions influence spermatozoal quality. Because of the predilection of horse owners and some veterinarians to administer hormones to normal stallions, endocrine regulation of reproductive function in adult stallions is considered in detail in this chapter to provide a basis for consideration of changes involved in puberty and to serve as a setting for Chapter 89. Finally, the process of ejaculation is briefly considered.

THE TESTES

The gross anatomy and microanatomy of the testis are considered in Chapter 76. To learn about testis function, examine Figures 76–3, 76–4, and 76–5 and read the associated text. These figures show how the testis is organized, and familiarity with the figures is assumed herein.

THERMOREGULATION OF TESTICULAR TEMPERATURE

The scrotum serves to cover and protect the testes (see Fig. 76–2), but its primary function is regulation of temperature in the testis and cauda epididymidis. This is accomplished by two basic mechanisms: vascular transfer of heat and changes in position relative to the abdominal wall. The first is a cooling mechanism whereas the latter can facilitate or minimize heat loss. A stallion's testes must be below body temperature (Fig. 77–1) for normal spermatogenesis.

Based on research with other species,[1–5] if intratesticular temperature is elevated to body temperature for a long interval, or to 40.5° C for as little as 2 h, certain germinal cells developing within seminiferous tubules will be affected and die. Especially sensitive to heat are certain pachytene primary spermatocytes, but B-spermatogonia and spherical spermatids can also be affected. Consequently, a transitory decrease in number of spermatozoa ejaculated would be expected starting

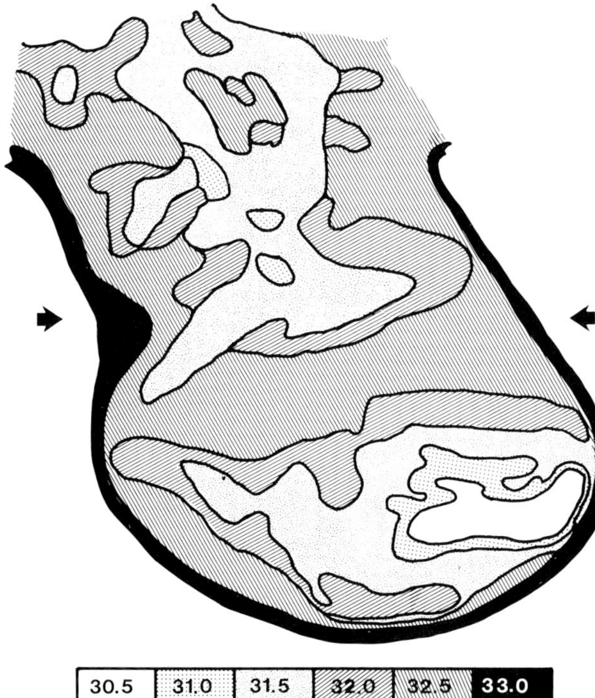

FIG. 77–1. Drawing showing temperatures at different points within the scrotum and adjacent tissue as measured by thermography. The globular left testis is the major tissue mass in the lower portion of the figure and the arrows designate the approximate level of the abdominal wall. The central core of cool tissue, leading from the testis, is the pampiniform plexus. Note that the area near the cauda epididymidis was the coolest tissue (white). The scale shows the temperature of designated areas. The recording was made when air temperature was 28.5° C. (From Pickett, B.W., et al.: Management of the Stallion for Maximum Reproductive Efficiency. II. Animal Reproduction Laboratory Bulletin No. 05. Fort Collins, Colorado State University, 1989.)

about 40 days later (Fig. 77–2). With an exposure of only a few hours, the maximum depression of number of spermatozoa ejaculated should occur at about 50 days and improvement should be detected within 2 weeks thereafter. However, it would take ≥ 70 days after cessation of elevated testicular temperature before seminal characteristics should approach normal. The influence of elevated temperature on spermatozoa within the epididymis has not been delineated for stallions. In other species, however, prolonged elevation of intrascrotal temperature affects the quality and functionality of spermatozoa within the epididymis,[4,6] although conflicting data exist.

A stallion might have normal fertility for 3 to 4 days after a severe traumatic injury to the testes, scrotal swelling or a marked increase in body temperature. However, the increased temperature within the cauda epididymidis, induced by such an event, might cause a decline in seminal quality as soon as 4 days later, as evidenced by spermatozoa with detached tails.[7] A severe decline in spermatozoal quantity and quality should be anticipated in 1 to 2 months (Fig. 77–2), because of impaired spermatogenesis resulting from the temporary rise in testicular temperature.

Thermal regulation of the testis and epididymis depends on the combined action of the scrotum, pampiniform plexus (see Fig. 76–7), tunica dartos muscle, and external cremaster muscle. Based on data for sheep (temperature values given are for rams), blood within surface veins of the testis is cooled through evaporation of moisture from the scrotal skin.[2,3] Thus, the temperature of testicular venous blood (33° C) is similar to that beneath the scrotal skin. The cooler venous blood enters the pampiniform plexus, which serves as a countercurrent heat exchange area and functions similarly to the radiator of an automobile. Heat is transferred from warm arterial blood (39° C) to cooler venous blood so that arterial blood leaving the pampiniform plexus (34° C) is cooler than that in the testicular artery just above the pampiniform plexus. Thus, arterial and capillary blood perfusing the testis is several degrees cooler than the blood in visceral organs, and tissue temperature remains low (34° C). The extent of cooling of arterial blood passing through the pampiniform plexus is governed by temperature of the venous blood.

Position of the testis relative to the abdominal wall is determined by two muscles. In cold weather, the tunica dartos muscle fibers, within the scrotal wall, contract to raise the testes close to the warm abdominal wall and heat loss is minimized by decreasing the area of the scrotal surface. In warm weather, the tunica dartos relaxes to make the scrotum more pendulous and maximize cooling of testicular venous blood by evaporation from scrotal skin. The external cremaster muscle can contract to raise the testis for a short interval.

SPERMATOGENESIS

Spermatogenesis is the sum of cell divisions and cellular changes that result in formation of spermatozoa from spermatogonia. A more complete definition is that sper-

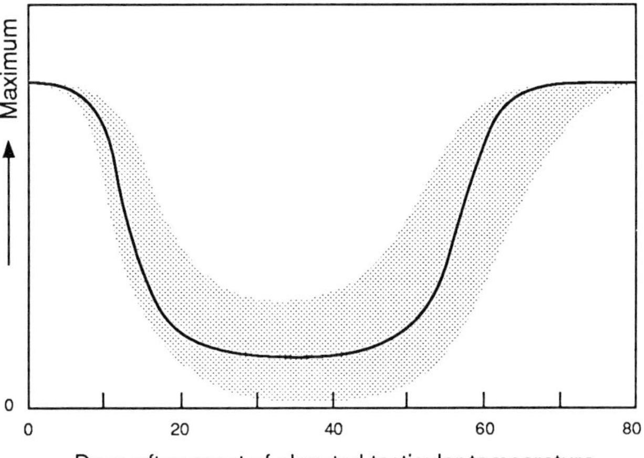

FIG. 77–2. The pattern of changes in spermatozoal output and morphology after 48 h of elevated testicular temperature (intrascrotal temperature averaged 37.3° C). Based on data for 12 stallions. (Data kindly provided by S.E. Heath.)

matogenesis is the lengthy, chronologic process whereby a few stem spermatogonia divide by mitosis to maintain their own number and to cyclically produce differentiated spermatogonia that divide by mitosis to produce primary spermatocytes that, in turn, undergo meiosis to produce spermatids which differentiate into spermatozoa. This chapter explains spermatogenesis using available data for stallions,[7-22] but some details of the process must be extrapolated from data for other species.[2,23-32]

Spermatozoa are produced within the seminiferous epithelium (epithelium spermatogenicum) of the convoluted seminiferous tubules (tubuli seminifer convolutus). The seminiferous epithelium of a mature stallion is composed of somatic cells, termed Sertoli cells (epitheliocytus sustentans), and different types of germinal cells (cellulae spermatogenicae), namely spermatogonia, primary spermatocytes, secondary spermatocytes, and spermatids (Fig. 77–3). In a cross section of a normal seminiferous tubule, four or five generations of developing germinal cells are arranged in well-defined cellular associations.[12,13,20,21] In the stallion, each succeeding layer or generation of germinal cells within a cellular association is 12.2 days more advanced toward spermatozoa.[23] The time required to produce a spermatozoon from a committed spermatogonium, or duration of spermatogenesis, is not influenced by season. The duration of spermatogenesis is about 57 days in stallions,[7,12,23,24] rather than 55 days as previously reported.[21] Consequently, the interval between an event detrimental to spermatogenesis and a decline in seminal quality might be as long as 2 months. An interval of at least 2 months may be required for restoration of normal spermatogenesis after damage from an increase in testicular temperature or administration of drugs such as steroids.

The duration of spermatogenesis (57 days) represents three phases: spermatocytogenesis (19.4 days), characterized by mitosis and differentiation of spermatogonia; meiosis (19.4 days), characterized by exchange of genetic material between homologous chromosomes in primary spermatocytes, followed by the two divisions of meiosis, producing haploid spermatids; and spermiogenesis (18.6 days), characterized by differentiation and specialization of function to result in fully differentiated spermatids, which are termed spermatozoa after release from the seminiferous epithelium.

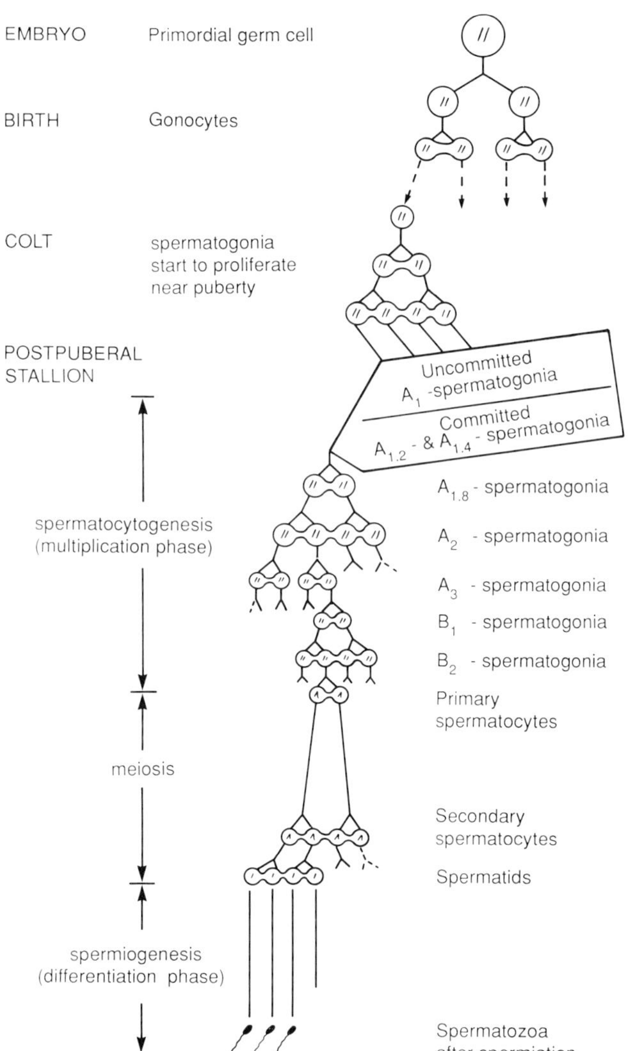

FIG. 77–3. The pattern of spermatogenesis in stallions during development of spermatogonia to form primary spermatocytes, secondary spermatocytes, spermatids, and spermatozoa. The horizontal connections between adjacent germ cells in a cohort depict intercellular bridges that connect germ cells. A cohort is a group of two or more germ cells that are the progeny of a less-developed type of germ cell. The vertical lines show the pattern of cell division and dashed lines designate that some potential germinal cells degenerate. The pattern of spermatogonial division and approximate life spans of the several types of spermatogonia are detailed in Figure 77–13. (From Pickett, B.W., et al.: Management of the Stallion for Maximum Reproductive Efficiency. II. Animal Reproduction Laboratory Bulletin No. 05. Fort Collins, Colorado State University, 1989.)

SERTOLI CELLS

As noted in Chapter 76, Sertoli cells rest on the lamina propria of the seminiferous tubule and their extensive cytoplasm extends around the germinal cells to the tubular lumen (see Fig. 76–4). All details of the role of Sertoli cells in spermatogenesis are unknown, but they play a pivotal role in the process. In addition, the more Sertoli cells a testis contains, the more spermatozoa that testis can produce.[12,16,17,22,26,30] The probable functions of Sertoli cells include (1) formation of the blood-testis barrier, (2) structural support for and nutrition of germinal cells, (3) movement of developing germinal cells within the seminiferous epithelium, (4) discharge of mature spermatids by a process termed spermiation, (5) phagocytosis of degenerating germinal cells and residual bodies of cytoplasm left behind as mature spermatids undergo spermiation, (6) secretion of fluids and proteins to bathe the developing germinal cells and convey spermatozoa through the seminiferous tubules to the rete testis, and (7) cell-to-cell communication with developing germinal cells, the underlying myoid cell layer (part of the lamina propria), and Leydig cells.

Junctional complexes between adjacent Sertoli cells form a blood-testis barrier functionally dividing the seminiferous epithelium into basal and adluminal compartments. Spermatocytogenesis occurs in the basal compartment, where spermatogonia and preleptotene primary spermatocytes are found. In the early leptotene phase of meiosis, primary spermatocytes migrate through the blood-testis barrier, by a process analogous to moving a ship through a pair of locks, into the adluminal compartment where meiosis continues and spermiogenesis occurs. Integrity of the blood-testis barrier is maintained by forming new junctional complexes below the leptotene primary spermatocytes before dissolution of junctional complexes above the cells.

The blood-testis barrier isolates spermatocytes and spermatids from the immune system of the host stallion. Because the developing immune system is not exposed to differentiated spermatocytes or spermatids, it considers them to be foreign cells and would react to antigens expressed on their surface. Therefore, except for this isolation provided by the blood-testis barrier, germinal cells would be destroyed and sterility would ensue. Damage to the blood-testis barrier can cause damage to the testis, reduce spermatozoal production, or induce sterility. Although rare in stallions, it is common in black mink.[33] The blood-testis barrier also restricts the flux of macromolecules and other components of interstitial fluid to spermatocytes and spermatids.

Sertoli cells provide structural support for developing germinal cells, as evident from their intimate contact, interdigitation of plasma membranes, and cellular specializations allowing communication. During spermiogenesis, spherical spermatids are moved, by actions of microtubular and microfibrillar components of Sertoli cells, toward the basal membrane and then back toward the luminal face; these changes occur concomitantly with changes in shape of spermatids, which are at least partially induced by Sertoli cells.

As spermiation approaches, mature spermatids are pushed out into the tubular lumen, but remain attached by a thin stalk (Fig. 77–4) to the major portion of the cytoplasm, contained in a residual body. The cytoplasmic residual body remains surrounded by Sertoli cells, and after rupture of the stalk, resulting in spermiation and discharge of spermatozoa, the residual bodies are phagocytized by Sertoli cells. Many germinal cells die during the process of spermatogenesis and these dead cells are rapidly phagocytized by Sertoli cells. Although degenerating cells can be seen within the seminiferous epithelium, because of their rapid phagocytosis by Sertoli cells, the number of degenerating cells seen does not accurately reflect the effect of cell death on the potential production of spermatozoa.

Sertoli cells secrete a number of products into the fluid surrounding the germinal cells and hence into the luminal fluid of the seminiferous tubule. Although certain of the products are unique and not produced elsewhere in the body, others are similar to secretions of

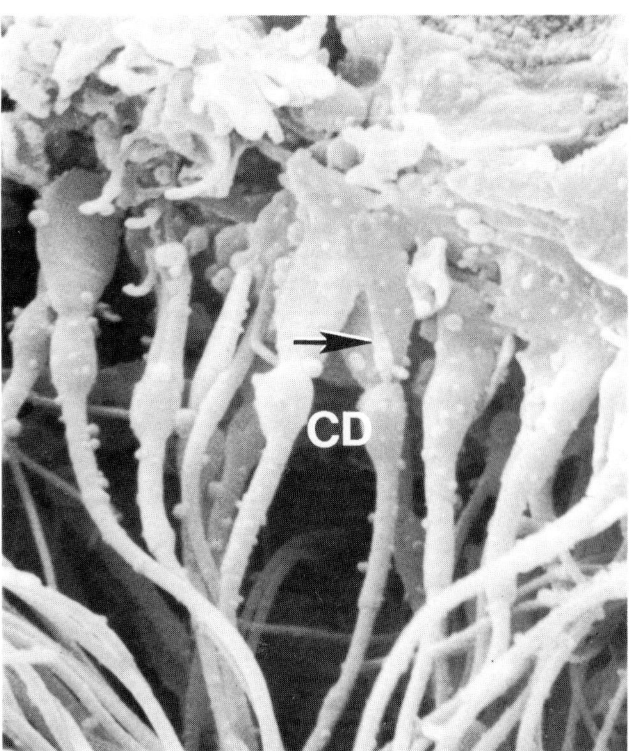

FIG. 77–4. A scanning electron micrograph (× 4500) of stallion spermatozoa just as they complete spermatogenesis and are about to be released from the seminiferous epithelium into the lumen of a convoluted seminiferous tubule. After their release by breakage of their cytoplasmic stalks (arrow), spermatozoa are washed into the straight seminiferous tubules by flowing fluid. Proximal cytoplasmic droplets (CD) are normal components of such spermatozoa. (From Johnson, L., Amann, R.P. and Pickett, B.W.: Scanning electron and light microscopy of the equine seminiferous tubule. Fertil. Steril., *29:*208–215, 1978.)

the epididymis or other organs. Lactate is secreted as an energy source for developing germinal cells. Published reviews provide an excellent overview of the biochemical nature of more complex secretions.[29,34,35] Some serve as transport molecules to move essential metals, vitamins, or hormones from Sertoli cells to developing germinal cells, whereas others may help in the regulation of epididymal function. Some secretions of Sertoli cells, such as the protein hormone inhibin, are secreted both from the luminal face of the seminiferous tubule to enter the epididymis in rete testis fluid and also from the basal aspect of Sertoli cells to pass into the interstitial fluid of the testis and ultimately enter by the lymphatic and venous drainage.

The function of Sertoli cells depends on two hormones: follicle-stimulating hormone (FSH) and testosterone. In addition, in the last several years it has become evident that Sertoli cells participate in two-way communication with both germinal cells and Leydig cells. For example, both Sertoli cells and Leydig cells apparently secrete or are responsive to a variety of regulatory factors such as β-endorphin, produced by Leydig cells apparently to cause cessation of mitosis of indifferent supporting cells before puberty.[36] Insulin-like growth factor (IGF), epidermal growth factor (EGF), and transforming growth factor-β (TGF-β) also may have a role in regulating testis function. Mitogenic polypeptides produced by Sertoli cells may stimulate or coordinate mitosis and meiosis of germinal cells.[36,37]

Many compounds adversely affecting spermatogenesis probably act on Sertoli cells rather than directly on germinal cells. Furthermore, the number of Sertoli cells per testis and the maximum number of germinal cells per Sertoli cell are characteristic of a species,[32] but the number of Sertoli cells per testis is a trait with high heritability.[26,30] In bulls, a direct relationship is found between the number of Sertoli cells in the testis and daily spermatozoal production by that testis. A treatment that decreases the number of Sertoli cells formed before puberty or that alters Sertoli cell function will probably adversely affect spermatozoal production.

SPERMATOGENESIS: A SPECIES COMPARISON

In the adult stallion, billions of spermatozoa are produced daily in the convoluted seminiferous tubules.[7–9,12,15–20,22,38–40] A comparison of productivity of the stallion testis with data for other species is presented in Table 77–1. Although the two testes of an adult stallion produce about 70,000 spermatozoa each second during the breeding season, production of each individual spermatozoon requires about 57 days. When spermatozoa are liberated from seminiferous epithelium (Fig. 77–4), fluid carries them from the convoluted seminiferous tubules into straight seminiferous tubules and the tubules of the rete testis where additional fluid may be added. The suspension of spermatozoa is moved rapidly through ductuli efferentes testis into the proximal epididymis.

THE CYCLE OF THE SEMINIFEROUS EPITHELIUM

From histologic examination of stallion testes, researchers have determined that adjacent cross sections through the seminiferous tubules are usually different. Detailed analyses have enabled recognition of eight different cellular associations, or stages, based on four or five specific types of germinal cells grouped together.[12,13,20,21] The exact number of cellular associations depends on the criteria used for identification of each grouping of germinal cells.[2,12,25,27–29,41–43] In each stage or cellular association, the four or five types of germinal cell are associated in a specific layered pattern (Figs. 77–5 and 76–4). Each layer is one generation of germinal cells, which is 12.2 days more developed than the layer below. The youngest generation is located along the wall or lamina propria of the seminiferous tubule. Older generations are found closer to the tubular lumen. In a normal testis, germinal cells are always found in these specific cellular associations or stages. The cells present in each cellular association can be determined by reading upward in a column (Fig. 77–5) from the lamina propria toward the tubular lumen (generations five to one). The width of each column in Figure 77–5 depicts the relative duration of each cellular association.

If a fixed point within a seminiferous tubule were viewed over time, germinal cells developing at that point would sequentially acquire the appearance of

TABLE 77–1. A COMPARISON BETWEEN SPERMATOGENESIS IN STALLIONS AND OTHER MAMMALS

		DAILY SPERM PRODUCTION			
	Paired Testes Weight (g)	Per Gram Parenchyma (10^6/g)	By Both Testes (10^9)	Duration of Cycle (days)*	Duration Spermatogenesis (days)†
Human	34	4.4	0.125	16.0	72
Bull					
Hereford	650	10	5.9	13.5	61
Dairy	725	12	7.5	13.5	61
Dog	34	12	0.37	13.6	61
Stallion‡	340	16	5.37	12.2	57
Ram, Ile de France	500	21	9.5	10.4	47
Boar	720	23	16.2	8.6	39
Rat, Wistar	3.7	24	0.086	13.3	60
Rabbit	6.4	25	0.160	10.7	48

*Duration of one cycle of the seminiferous epithelium.

†Duration of spermatogenesis, assuming that it requires 4.5 cycles of the seminiferous epithelium, except for stallions for which a value of 4.7 cycles was used.

‡Averaged across ages and seasons, see also Figures 77–12, 77–13, and 77–15.

(From Pickett, B.W., et al.: Management of the Stallion for Maximum Reproductive Efficiency. II. Animal Reproduction Laboratory Bulletin No. 05. Fort Collins, Colorado State University, 1989.)

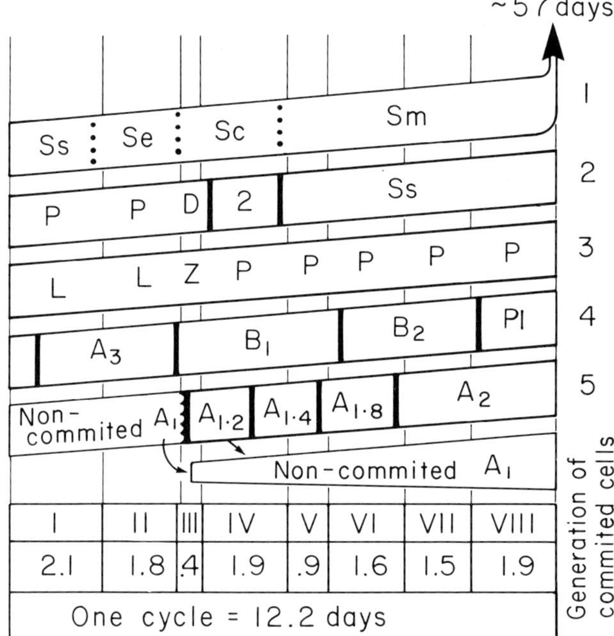

FIG. 77–5. The cycle of the seminiferous epithelium in the stallion. The lamina propria is at the bottom, and the lumen of the seminiferous tubule is at the top. Each of the five upper rows represents one generation of germinal cells that are increasingly (from bottom to top) more mature. The columns represent the eight cellular associations as explained in the text. Germinal cells present in each cellular association can be discerned by reading up in each column. The complete series of cellular associations is termed the cycle of the seminiferous epithelium. In the stallion, duration of 1 cycle of the seminiferous epithelium is 12.2 days. Duration of each cellular association is also shown. Spermatogenesis starts when a single A_1-spermatogonium divides to form a pair of A_1-spermatogonia (designated $A_{1\cdot2}$), this is the commitment of these germinal cells to divide further and differentiate into A_2-spermatogonia and ultimately give rise to spermatids and spermatozoa. Other germinal cells are designated: B_1-, B_1-spermatogonia; B_2-, B_2-spermatogonia; Pl, preleptotene; L, leptotene; Z, zygotene; P, pachytene; and D, diplotene primary spermatocyte; 2, secondary spermatocyte; and Ss, Se, Sc, and Sm, progressively more mature spermatids. Approximately 4.7 cycles of the seminiferous epithelium pass between division of a single A_1-spermatogonium into a pair of committed $A_{1\cdot2}$-spermatogonia and release of resulting spermatozoa from the seminiferous epithelium. Thus duration of spermatogenesis is 57 days in the stallion. (From Pickett, B.W., et al.: Management of the Stallion for Maximum Reproductive Efficiency. II. Animal Reproduction Laboratory Bulletin No. 05. Fort Collins, Colorado State University, 1989.)

each of the eight cellular associations (Figs. 77–6 to 77–9) characteristic of stallions.[7,12,13,20,21] This progression through the series of cellular associations occurs repeatedly in a predictable manner. The complete series of cellular associations (Fig. 77–5) is termed the cycle of the seminiferous epithelium. The interval required for one complete series of cellular associations to occur at one point within the tubule is termed the duration of the cycle of the seminiferous epithelium.

Swierstra et al. used 12 stallions to study spermatogenesis and was able to identify eight stages in the cycle of the seminiferous epithelium.[21] The cycle was divided into eight stages, based on the structure of the germinal cells and their relative position within the seminiferous epithelium (Figs. 77–6 to 77–8). A current interpretation of descriptions of each stage or cellular association follows.[12,20,21]

Stage I. From complete disappearance of mature spermatids lining the tubular lumen to onset of elongation of spermatid nuclei.

Stage II. From onset of elongation to end of elongation of spermatid nuclei.

Stage III. From end of elongation of spermatid nuclei to start of the first meiotic division.

Stage IV. From start of the first to end of the second meiotic division.

Stage V. From end of the second meiotic division to initial appearance of type B_2-spermatogonia.

Stage VI. From initial appearance of type B_2-spermatogonia to when all bundles of elongated spermatids begin to migrate toward the lumen of the seminiferous tubule.

Stage VII. From the time all bundles of elongated spermatids have begun to migrate toward the tubular lumen until they reach the lumen and B_2-spermatogonia are no longer present.

Stage VIII. From appearance of preleptotene primary spermatocytes and when elongated spermatids line the tubular lumen until complete disappearance of mature spermatids lining the tubular lumen.

The relative frequency of occurrence of the eight stages was expressed as a percentage of the total number of tubular cross sections evaluated for each testis (Table 77–2). Two generations of primary spermatocytes are found in stages I through III (Fig. 77–5), and thus about 35% of cross sections through seminiferous tubules should contain two generations of primary sper-

TABLE 77–2. RELATIVE FREQUENCY AND MEAN DURATION OF STAGES OF THE CYCLE OF THE SEMINIFEROUS EPITHELIUM*

STAGE	RELATIVE FREQUENCY (%)	DURATION (DAYS)
I	16.9	2.1
II	14.9	1.8
III	3.2	0.4
IV	15.8	1.9
V	7.4	0.9
VI	13.5	1.6
VII	12.6	1.5
VIII	15.7	1.9

*Mean for 18 stallions.

(Adapted from Swierstra, E.E., Gebauer, M.R., and Picket, B.W.: Reproductive physiology of the stallion. I. Spermatogenesis and testis composition. J. Reprod. Fertil., *40:*113–123, 1974.)

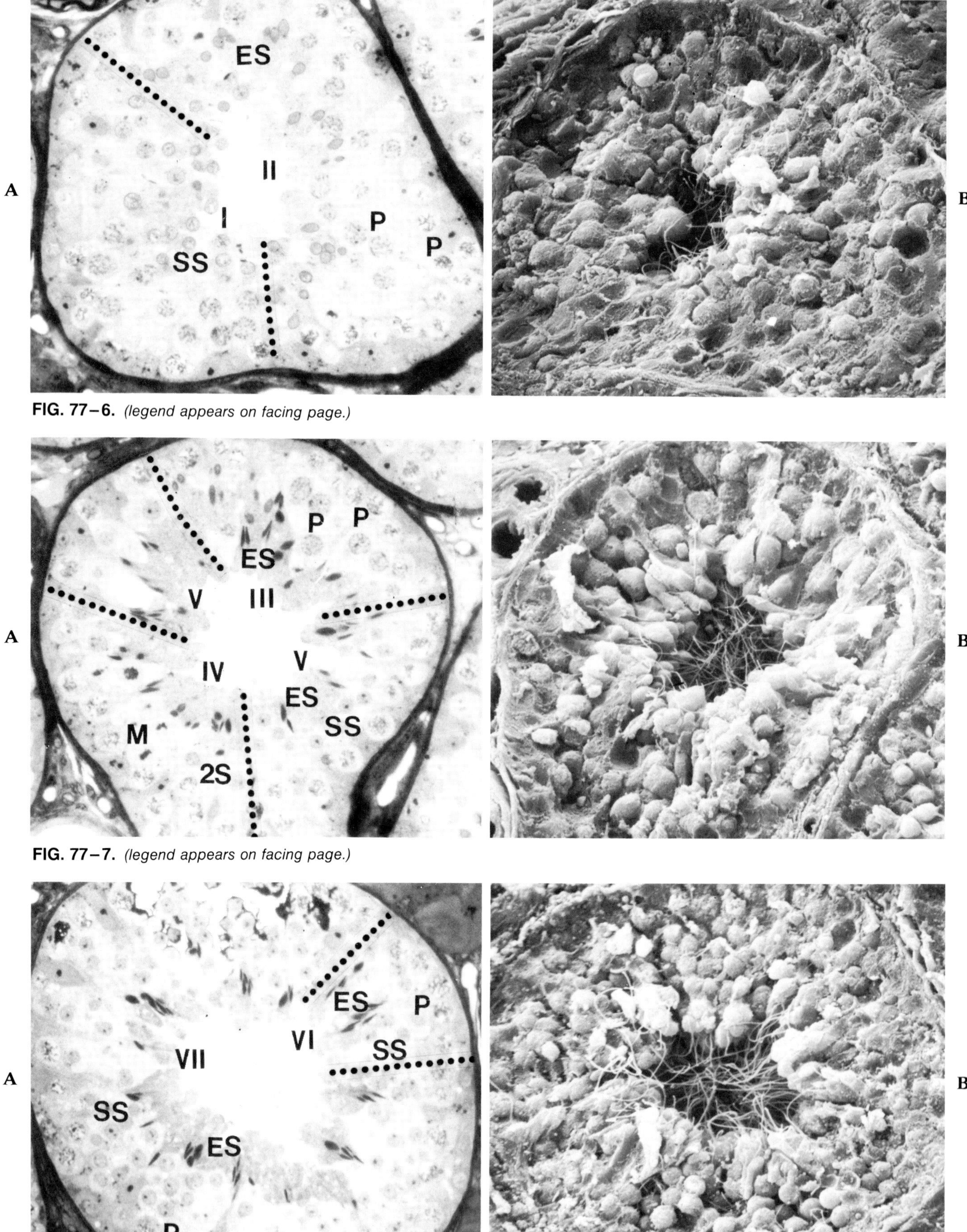

FIG. 77–6. *(legend appears on facing page.)*

FIG. 77–7. *(legend appears on facing page.)*

FIG. 77–8. *(legend appears on facing page.)*

FIG. 77–6. Photomicrograph *(A)* and scanning electron micrograph *(B)* of the same cross section of a seminiferous tubule showing stages I and II. Both cellular associations contain two generations of primary spermatocytes (P) and one generation of spermatids. The spermatids are spherical (SS) in stage I and elongating (ES) in stage II (× 510). (Modified from Johnson, L., Amann, R.P., and Pickett, B.W.: Scanning electron and light microscopy of the equine seminiferous tubules. Fertil. Steril., *29:*208–215, 1978.)

FIG. 77–7. Photomicrograph *(A)* and scanning electron micrograph *(B)* of the same cross section of a seminiferous tubule showing stages III, IV, and V. Stage III is characterized by two generations of primary spermatocytes (P) and deeply embedded bundles of elongated spermatid nuclei (ES). In stage IV, metaphase figures (M) and secondary spermatocytes (2S) are seen. Stage V contains newly formed spermatids with spherical nuclei (SS) and older spermatids with elongated nuclei (× 510). (Modified from Johnson, L., Amann, R.P., and Pickett, B.W.: Scanning electron and light microscopy of the equine seminiferous tubules. Fertil. Steril., *29:*208–215, 1978.)

FIG. 77–8. Photomicrograph *(A)* and scanning electron micrograph *(B)* of the same cross section of a seminiferous tubule showing stages VI and VII. Both stages are characterized by elongated spermatid nuclei (ES), spherical spermatid nuclei (SS) and one generation of primary spermatocytes (P). In stage VI, bundles of elongated spermatid nuclei are deeply embedded, while in stage VII the elongated spermatids have begun to migrate toward the lumen (× 510). (Modified from Johnson, L., Amann, R.P., and Pickett, B.W.: Scanning electron and light microscopy of the equine seminiferous tubules. Fertil. Steril., *29:*208–215, 1978.)

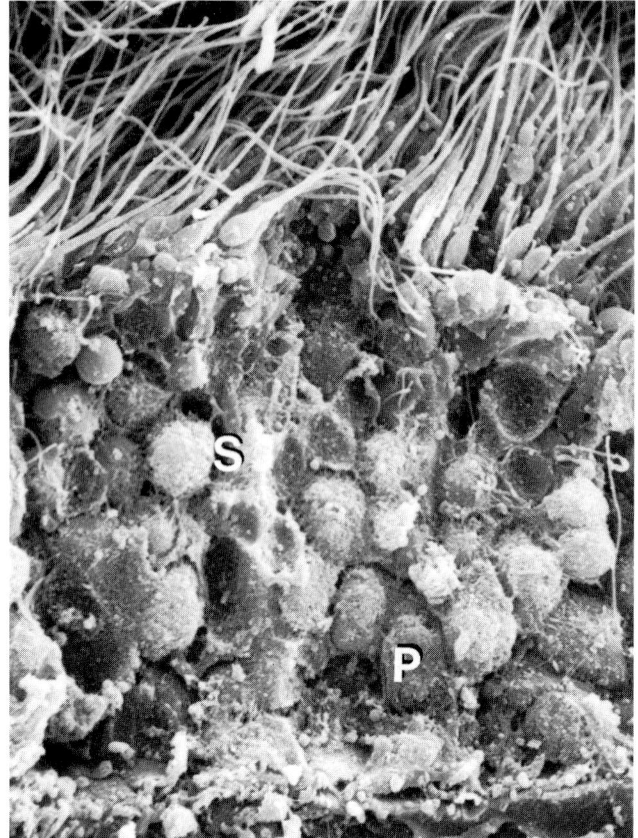

FIG. 77–9. Scanning electron micrograph of the seminiferous epithelium in late stage VIII, showing the entire length of the elongated spermatids extending into the tubule lumen. A Sertoli cell (S) and primary spermatocyte (P) are seen. The basement membrane is visible at the bottom of the picture (× 970). (From Johnson, L., Amann, R.P., and Pickett, B.W.: Scanning electron and light microscopy of the equine seminiferous tubules. Fertil. Steril., *29*:208–215, 1978.)

matocytes in a normal testis. Similarly, two generations of spermatids are found in stages V through VIII so that about 50% of cross sections in a normal testis should contain two generations of spermatids, and 16% should have spermatids lining the tubular lumen (stage VIII).

Although most cross sections through seminiferous tubules of a stallion testis contain a single cellular association, some cross sections contain two or three stages of cellular associations.[13,20] These cross sections presumably represent locations within a seminiferous tubule where different cellular associations adjoin.[23,29]

Knowledge of time required to produce a spermatozoon is essential for understanding the time course of events after drug injection or trauma to the testis. Swierstra et al. measured duration of the cycle of the seminiferous epithelium using six stallions. This was accomplished by injecting a radioisotope, [^{3}H]thymidine, into both testicular arteries of each stallion.[20,21] The compound [^{3}H]thymidine was taken up by germinal cells that were synthesizing DNA at the time of injection, and such cells or their progeny were identified on the basis of their radioactivity. The 12 testes from these stallions were removed 4.5 h to 35 days after injection of [^{3}H]thymidine. Radioactive germinal cells were detected by coating the histologic sections with a photographic emulsion. When the film was developed, black "grains" were evident over each radioactive germinal cell in a histologic section.

At 4.5 h after injection of [^{3}H]thymidine, young (leptotene) primary spermatocytes in stage I were the most mature radioactive germinal cells. For horses castrated at longer intervals after injection of the radioisotope, progressively more advanced germinal cells were labeled. By analyzing these data, Swierstra et al. concluded that duration of one cycle of seminiferous epithelium was 12.2 days.[20,21] Thus at any particular point within a seminiferous tubule the same cellular association or stage is repeated every 12.2 days. Cells in stage I, which were young (leptotene) primary spermatocytes in generation 3 (Fig. 77–5), will be old (pachytene) primary spermatocytes 12.2 days later (in generation 2) and spherical spermatids after another 12.2 days in generation 1 (Fig. 77–10). Using information on relative frequency for each stage and data for duration of the cycle of the seminiferous epithelium, absolute duration of each stage was calculated (Table 77–2). The life spans of primary spermatocytes, secondary spermatocytes, and spermatids are 18.7, 0.7, and 18.6 days, respectively.

DURATION OF SPERMATOGENESIS

At a given point within a seminiferous tubule, A_1-spermatogonia periodically produce committed $A_{1\text{-}2}$-spermatogonia (Figs. 77–3 and 77–5); this occurs only at an interval equal to the duration of one cycle of the seminiferous epithelium.[2,7,12,23,28,29,43] Similarly, at some point in the cycle, groups of mature spermatids, originating from spermatogonia committed to differentiate approximately 4.7 cycles earlier, are released from the seminiferous epithelium (Fig. 77–10). Thus, because of the division of A_1-spermatogonia every 12.2 days,[20] a new cohort (family or chain) of germinal cells begins to develop every 12.2 days, and all cells in this cohort develop synchronously (Fig. 77–10). Because total duration of spermatogenesis apparently is 4.7 cycles of the seminiferous epithelium (12.2 days), spermatogenesis requires about 57 days in the stallion. Because A_1-spermatogonia at different sites in the testis develop asynchronously, hundreds of spermatogonia committed to form spermatozoa are produced every second. Therefore, spermatozoa are released continuously from seminiferous tubules.

DAILY SPERMATOZOAL PRODUCTION

Daily spermatozoal production (DSP) is the number of spermatozoa produced per day by a testis or the two testes of a stallion.[23] Efficiency of spermatozoal production is the number of spermatozoa produced per gram of testicular parenchyma. During the breeding season, effi-

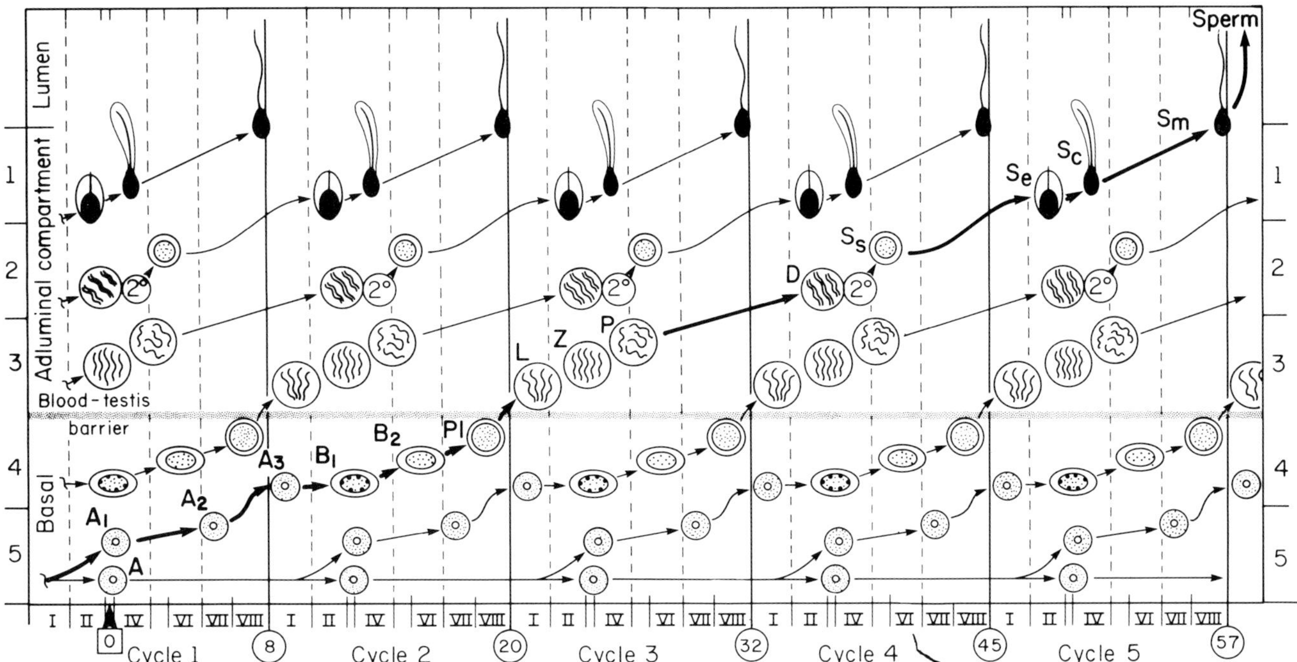

FIG. 77–10. Spermatogenesis in the stallion. Four or five generations (cohorts) of germinal cells develop simultaneously and synchronously at any point in a seminiferous tubule. Spermatogenesis is a continuous process and involves an infinite number of subtle changes at a given point in the tubule. These changes in cellular association have been classified as eight stages; some of them are depicted and demarcated by light vertical lines. The complete sequence of stages occurs at a given point in a tubule over an interval (12.2 days) termed the duration of the cycle of the seminiferous epithelium. Because development of generations is synchronized, the same stages recur every 12.2 days in stallions. The figure depicts (from left to right) changes over time, at a given point, in a seminiferous tubule during 57 days, or 4.7 cycles of the seminiferous epithelium, required for the complete process of spermatogenesis. Cellular associations are designated as stages I to VIII along the *x*-axis and their width is proportional to their duration. The four or five generations of germinal cells in any stage are designated along the *y*-axis, and designated: A_1-, A_2-, A_3-, B_1-, and B_2-spermatogonia; Pl, preleptotene; L, leptotene; Z, zygotene; P, pachytene; and D, diplotene primary spermatocyte; 2°, secondary spermatocyte; and Ss, Se, Sc, and Sm, progressively more mature spermatids. Development of one A_1-spermatogonium through spermatogenesis, to form a spermatozoon can be followed by the dark path. Near the beginning of the leptotene phase of development, new junctional complexes between adjacent Sertoli cells form below these germinal cells and the old junctions disappear. In this way, integrity of the blood-testis barrier (stippled band) is maintained. In stallions, one, but occasionally two or three, stages (usually sequential ones) are typically found in one cross section through a seminiferous tubule. Details of spermatogonial renewal have been simplified (see Fig. 77–14). (From Pickett, B.W., et al.: Management of the Stallion for Maximum Reproductive Efficiency. II. Animal Reproduction Laboratory Bulletin No. 05. Fort Collins, Colorado State University, 1989.)

ciency of spermatozoal production is reasonably similar for normal stallions, although testicular size may differ greatly among stallions.[8,9,11,12,16,17,22] Consequently, spermatozoal production can be estimated with fair accuracy by measuring testis size. Because testis size increases as a stallion grows from 2 or 3 yr old to a sexually mature stallion, DSP also increases[12,17] (Fig. 77–11). Daily sperm production also is affected by season (Chapter 78), as is especially evident for 6- to 20-yr-old stallions (Fig. 77–11). The magnitude of this decline during the nonbreeding season averages 50% in stallions 6 to 20 yr old (6.40 vs. 3.19 billion spermatozoa per day). Data for groups of similar adult stallions slaughtered in each month of the year are shown in Figure 77–12. Daily sperm production was low from September through February but increased by March.[12,16] Maximum DSP occurred in May and June, whereas values for July and August were markedly lower. However, DSP is not influenced by frequency of use for breeding.

Efficiency of spermatozoal production in a stallion during the breeding season averages 19 million spermatozoa per day per gram of testicular parenchyma,[8,9,11,12,15–17,26,40] and declines to about 15 million per day per gram in the nonbreeding season. It is evident (Fig. 77–11) that for stallions 6 to 12 and espe-

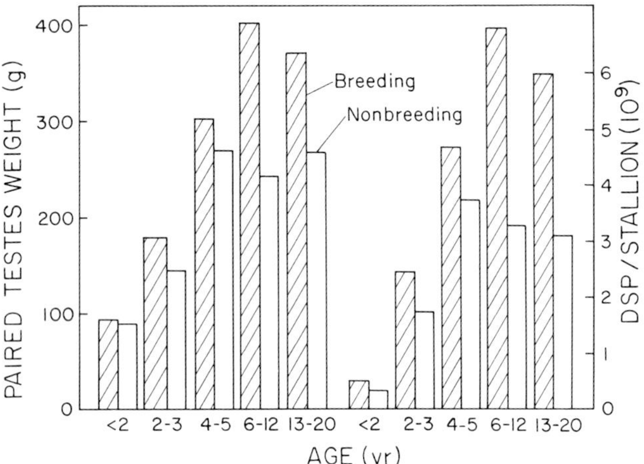

FIG. 77–11. Effects of age and season on testes weight and daily spermatozoal production (DSP) of stallions. Stallions were slaughtered during June and July (breeding season) and December and January (nonbreeding season). Means for 7 to 15 stallions in each group. For testicular weight or DSP, means (pooled across season) were significantly different for stallions < 2, 2 to 3, and 4 to 20 yr old. Effects of season also were significant as were interactions of age and season. (From Pickett, B.W., et al.: Management of the Stallion for Maximum Reproductive Efficiency. II. Animal Reproduction Laboratory Bulletin No. 05. Fort Collins, Colorado State University, 1989.)

cially 13 to 20 yr old, the decline in DSP during the nonbreeding season appears to be greater than that for testicular weight (49 vs. 29% for 13- to 20-yr-old stallions).[17] Differences in efficiency of spermatozoal production between breeding and nonbreeding season for stallions 2 to 3, 4 to 5, 6 to 12, and 13 to 20 yr old were −21%, −12%, −19%, and −34%, respectively.[17] Moreover, for stallions 13 to 20 yr old, the tunica albuginea represents a larger proportion of testicular weight than in stallions 4 to 8 or 2 to 3 yr old (14%, 9%, and 10%, respectively).[15] The efficiency of spermatozoal production in stallions is greater than in bulls, but less than in rams or boars (Table 77–1). However, because of difference in testicular size, DSP is similar for bulls and stallions.

GERMINAL CELL DEGENERATION AND RENEWAL OF SPERMATOGONIA

In stallions, spermatozoa are produced continuously after puberty. This is accomplished by continuous production of differentiated spermatogonia that produce primary spermatocytes, which ultimately give rise to spermatids (Figs. 77–3 and 77–10). At the same time, uncommitted spermatogonia must be replaced so that spermatogenesis will not stop because the seminiferous epithelium becomes depleted of spermatogonia.[2,8,12,25,27–29,31,43] Details of the process in stallions are now being unraveled[10–12,16] (L. Johnson, personal communication) (Fig. 77–13).

Present interpretations of data from ongoing research with stallions, based on personal communications with L. Johnson and published data,[18] and data for other species,[29,31] are as follows:

1. An isolated, uncommitted A_1-spermatogonium divides to form either two new uncommitted A_1-spermatogonia, which then are moved apart and serve as new "stem cells," or two cells that remain together joined by an intercellular bridge as a pair of A_1-spermatogonia (designated $A_{1\cdot2}$-spermatogonia in Fig. 77–13) that continue to divide by mitosis to form a chain of eight aligned A_1-spermatogonia (designated $A_{1\cdot8}$-spermatogonia).
2. Some of the A_1-spermatogonia degenerate, especially in the nonbreeding season, but in the breeding season most $A_{1\cdot8}$-spermatogonia divide to form A_2-spermatogonia that are termed "differentiated" cells because they are functionally different from A_1-spermatogonia.
3. A_2-spermatogonia divide by mitosis to form further differentiated A_3-spermatogonia, which in turn divide into morphologically different B_1-spermatogonia, although in the nonbreeding season some of A_3-spermatogonia degenerate.
4. B_1-spermatogonia divide by mitosis to form B_2-spermatogonia, which in turn divide into preleptotene primary spermatocytes, although in the breeding season some B_2-spermatogonia degenerate.
5. Soon after their formation, preleptotene primary spermatocytes enter the long prophase of the first division of meiosis, ultimately to give rise to secondary spermatocytes, then spermatids.

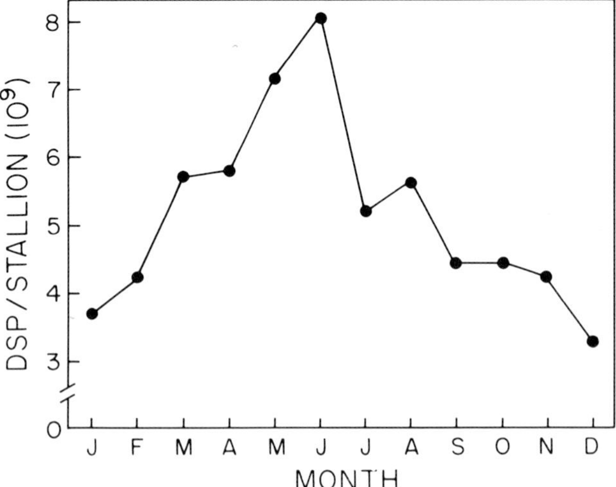

FIG. 77–12. Daily spermatozoal production (DSP) of stallions in each month of the year. Data for 13 to 17 stallions, 4 to 20 yr old, slaughtered in each month. Daily sperm production was estimated by morphometric analysis of spermatids with a spherical nucleus (similar to columns designated Ss in Fig. 77–10). (From Pickett, B.W., et al.: Management of the Stallion for Maximum Reproductive Efficiency. II. Animal Reproduction Laboratory Bulletin No. 05. Fort Collins, Colorado State University, 1989.)

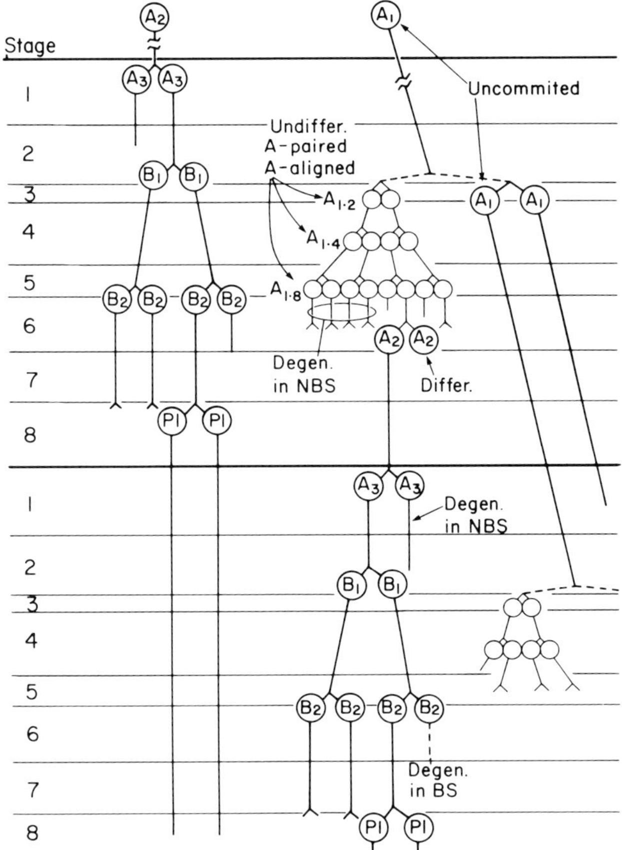

FIG. 77–13. A possible pattern for the process of spermatogonial renewal (formation of two new isolated and uncommitted A_1-spermatogonia) and commitment of A_1-spermatogonia toward differentiation by forming a pair of undifferentiated $A_{1\cdot 2}$-spermatogonia that divide to form a chain of committed, but undifferentiated, $A_{1\cdot 4}$- and then $A_{1\cdot 8}$-spermatogonia. Formation of a pair of committed $A_{1\cdot 2}$-spermatogonia is considered to be the onset of spermatogenesis (see Fig. 77–3). Commitment of another A_1-spermatogonium to form a pair of $A_{1\cdot 2}$-spermatogonia occurs only in stage III of the cycle of the seminiferous epithelium, once every 12.2 days at a given point in a seminiferous tubule. In theory, each differentiated A_2-spermatogonium could give rise to 64 spermatozoa. Much less than this number is produced because of degeneration of germinal cells. Although degeneration of potential spermatozoa can occur at any point in spermatogenesis, degeneration during the breeding season involves mostly B_2-spermatogonia, whereas in the nonbreeding season it involves $A_{1\cdot 8}$- and A_3-spermatogonia. Pl, Preleptotene; NBS; BS. (From Pickett, B.W., et al.: Management of the Stallion for Maximum Reproductive Efficiency. II. Animal Reproduction Laboratory Bulletin No. 05. Fort Collins, Colorado State University, 1989.)

Another population of A-spermatogonia, few in number, termed reserve spermatogonia, exist, but are not shown in Figure 77–13. Their life span is unknown, but is probably > 60 days. Normally, they do not participate in spermatogenesis but serve as a source of germinal cells to repopulate the testis in seasonal breeders in which the testes "shut down" completely except in the breeding season (such as mule deer) or after an event that causes loss of most or all of the regular germinal cells (exposure to a toxin).

Not all spermatozoa, which potentially should be produced by the seminiferous epithelium actually are formed and released from seminiferous epithelium (Figs. 77–11 and 77–13). Considerable degeneration of germinal cells occurs in normal stallions even during the breeding season. Because testicular weight decreases in the nonbreeding season (Fig. 77–11), researchers find it most informative to consider degeneration of germinal cells in terms of number of spermatozoa that theoretically should be produced per gram of testis. During the breeding season an excessive number of B_2-spermatogonia are produced and 32% of the potential number of "young" primary spermatocytes are not formed (Fig. 77–14). Presumably, this is because each Sertoli cell can accommodate only about 9 or 10 spermatids of a given generation and proportionately fewer primary spermatocytes (about 2.5 of a given generation).[10,17,22] Virtually all primary spermatocytes formed ultimately give rise to four spermatozoa.[11] However, during the nonbreeding season, 35% fewer A-spermatogonia per gram of testis are found and 40% fewer B_2-spermatogonia.[11,16,18] Nearly all B_2-spermatogonia give rise to two "young" primary spermatocytes, so that the number of these cells per gram of testis is not different in nonbreeding and breeding seasons (Fig. 77–14). However, in the nonbreeding season, about 23% of the potential number of spherical spermatids are not formed; germinal cells apparently degenerate during aberrant meiotic divisions or as newly formed spermatids. Presumably, the environment provided by Sertoli cells is deficient in some way, as evidenced by the reduced number of germinal cells per Sertoli cell.[11,12,30] As was true for the breeding season, in the nonbreeding season virtually all spherical spermatids that develop for 2 or 3 days are transformed into spermatozoa. The result is that in the nonbreeding season, only 75% as many spermatozoa are formed per gram of testis as in the breeding season. However, because of differences in testis weight, DSP per stallion is reduced by 20% for stallions 4 to 5 yr old and by 50% for stallions 6 to 20 yr old (Fig. 77–11). In addition to environmental factors such as day length or temperature, drugs or unknown factors can lead to increased degeneration of germ cells.[2,12,29,44,45]

LEYDIG CELLS

Within the interstitial tissue, Leydig cells (endocrinocytus interstitialis) are in close proximity to blood vessels and lymphatic channels, as well as the basal lamina of the seminiferous tubules. The primary role of Leydig cells is secretion of steroid hormones, which help to regulate function of the seminiferous epithelium, the hypothalamic-hypophyseal axis, and the accessory sex glands. Trivial names used for steroid hormones are testosterone (17β-hydroxy-androst-4-en-3-one), andro-

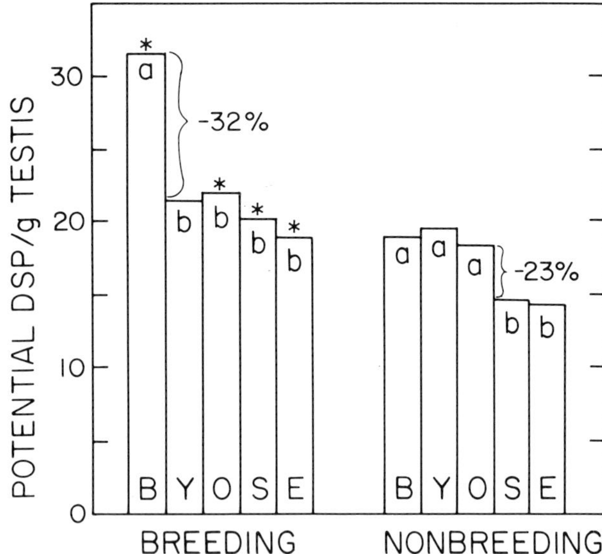

FIG. 77–14. Effects of season on degeneration of potential spermatozoa. Potential daily spermatozoal production (DSP) per gram of testicular parenchyma was calculated assuming all cells of a given type resulted in the theoretical number of spermatozoa without degeneration. Values for potential DSP/g testis were calculated from morphometric determinations of numbers of B_2-spermatogonia (B); preleptotene, leptotene, plus zygotene spermatocytes (Y); pachytene plus diplotene spermatocytes (O); spherical spermatids (S); and elongated spermatids (E) in testes of 28 stallions slaughtered in the breeding season (June and July) and 28 stallions slaughtered in the nonbreeding season (December and January). (From Pickett, B.W., et al.: Management of the Stallion for Maximum Reproductive Efficiency. II. Animal Reproduction Laboratory Bulletin No. 05. Fort Collins, Colorado State University, 1989.)

stenedione (3,17-diketoΔ^4-androstene), androstenediol (3β$_2$17β-dihydroxyΔ^5-androstene), dihydrotestosterone (17β-hydroxy-5α-androstan-3-one), 3α-androstanediol (5α-androstan-3α,17β-diol), 3β-androstanediol (5α-androstane-3β,17β-diol), progesterone (pregn-4-ene-3,20-dione), estrone [3β-hydroxyestra-1,3,5(10)-triene-17-one], and estradiol [estra-1,3,5(10)-triene-3β,17β-diol]. Because Leydig cells are the site of production for most of these hormones, interstitial fluid contains a much higher concentration of testosterone and other secretory products of Leydig cells than does peripheral blood (e.g., serum from blood drawn from the jugular vein). Concentration of testosterone averaged 416 ng/g and 640 ng/g parenchyma in two studies,[8,46] although these values might be artifactually high because of continued production of testosterone by the tissue after cessation of blood flow from the testis.

Leydig cells constantly secrete basal amounts of testosterone and several other hormones. However, periodically Leydig cells are stimulated to increase their production of testosterone. Thereafter, twofold to fourfold elevations of testosterone concentration, each lasting 2 to 4 h, are found in peripheral blood.[47] Three to eight episodic bursts of testosterone production occur each day in most, but not all, stallions. Consequently, if a single blood sample from a stallion is analyzed for concentration of testosterone, an unusually high value may be obtained that is not typical of peripheral concentrations in blood of that horse.

During episodic production of testosterone, concentrations of testosterone within the testis are probably elevated to >10 times basal concentration. Consequently, seminiferous tubules are continuously exposed to a high concentration of testosterone. This high concentration of testosterone around seminiferous tubules is probably essential for normal spermatogenesis, as has been shown with other species.[2,3,29,35,41,48] However, minimum concentration of testosterone necessary within the seminiferous epithelium for normal spermatogenesis in stallions is unknown. Researchers do not know whether normal intratesticular concentrations of testosterone could be maintained by injecting stallions with massive doses of testosterone. This is possible with rats[48] but not humans (E. Steinberger, personal communication).

The concentration of total 17β-hydroxy-androgen in blood leaving the testis through the testicular vein is about 45 times the concentration in blood taken concurrently from the jugular vein[49] (Table 77–3). During intervals when Leydig cells are under maximal stimulation of endogenous luteinizing hormone (LH), concentrations of testosterone in testicular vein blood can exceed 500 ng/mL, or approximately 100-fold typical concentrations of testosterone in jugular vein blood.[49,50]

In stallions, Leydig cells secrete greater amounts of estrogens than testosterone, although testosterone is the steroid of greatest physiologic importance. In addition to estrone and estradiol, the stallion testis also secretes estriol and two unusual compounds, equilin and equilenin[51–56] (Fig. 77–15). Although testicular vein blood contains extraordinarily high concentrations of free estrone and estradiol, most estrogen secreted by the stallion testis is conjugated with a sulfate (or glucuronide) side chain. This makes the compound more water soluble and restricts bioactivity. The biologic role of the conjugated estrogens produced by the equine testis remains obscure.

Enzymes involved in production of steroid hormones in Leydig cells are localized on the smooth endoplasmic reticulum and mitochondria.[57,58] No evidence exists to

TABLE 77–3. HORMONAL CONCENTRATIONS IN TESTICULAR VEIN AND JUGULAR VEIN BLOOD

	TESTIS VEIN	JUGULAR VEIN
17β-hydroxy-androgen (ng/mL)	61.5	1.3
Total nonconjugated estrogen (ng/mL)	25.4	0.058

(From Amann, R.P., and Ganjam, V.K.: Effects of hemicastration or hCG-treatment on steroids in testicular vein and jugular vein blood of stallions. J. Androl., *2*:132–139, 1981.)

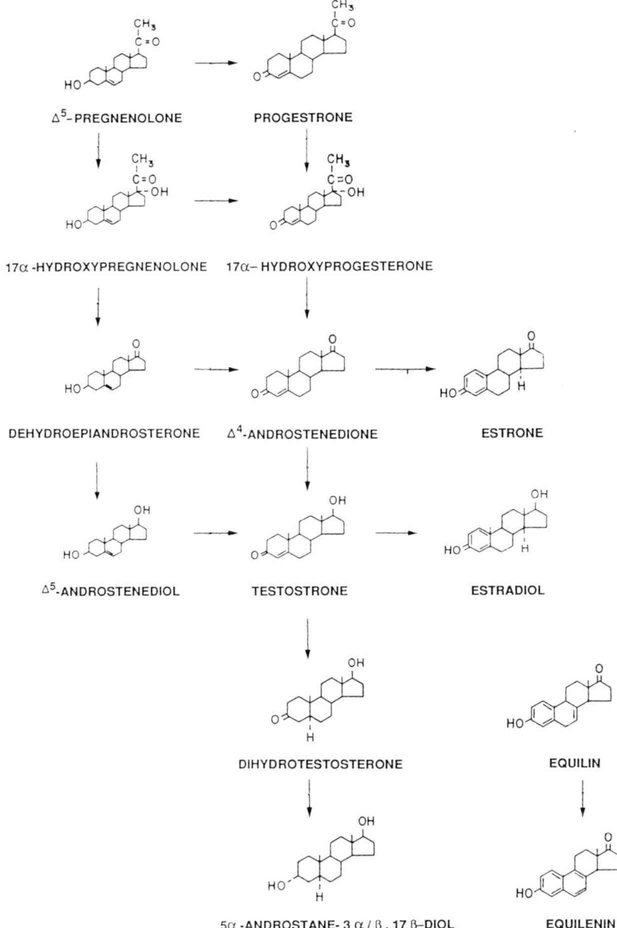

FIG. 77–15. The pathway for steroid biosynthesis in the stallion testis. Pregnenolone, formed from cholesterol, is converted by one of several possible pathways to androstenediol or androstenedione, which are the two immediate precursors of testosterone; the exact pathway is unknown for stallions. A portion of the androstenedione produced by Leydig cells is converted to estrone, rather than testosterone, and secreted as estrone sulfate. Testosterone in turn can be converted to dihydrotestosterone or 3α-androstanediol (androgens active in many tissues) or to estradiol (generally considered as a female sex hormone although it also may be important in the male) and secreted as estradiol sulfate. Note the structural similarity of many of these hormones. Synthetic compounds having a similar structure may affect a stallion by blocking or mimicking an action of a natural hormone. Two estrogens unique to horses, equilin and equilenin, also are depicted. (Modified from Pickett, B.W., et al.: Management of the Stallion for Maximum Reproductive Efficiency. II. Animal Reproduction Laboratory Bulletin No. 05. Fort Collins, Colorado State University, 1989.)

support the notion that other elements of interstitial tissue, or seminiferous tubules, produce steroid hormones. The first step in steroidogenesis is formation of cholesterol, either by de novo synthesis or breakdown from low-density lipoproteins of blood origin. Based on data for rodent and human testes,[59] researchers logically assume that in a stallion testis secreting testosterone at a minimal level most cholesterol is derived from intra-Leydig cell sources (cholesterol droplets). However, during stimulation by LH, or exogenous human chorionic gonadotropin (hCG), most of the cholesterol is probably derived from blood-borne low-density lipoprotein. The steroidogenic pathway begins with conversion of cholesterol to pregnenolone, which occurs within the mitochondria. Pregnenolone is transported to the smooth endoplasmic reticulum where other enzymes involved in the pathway (Fig. 77–15) are located. Detailed consideration of the enzymes and thermodynamics involved in steroidogenesis are outside the scope of this chapter, but excellent reviews are available.[57,58]

Figure 77–15 shows that two general pathways exist from pregnenolone to testosterone: (1) the so-called Δ^5 pathway through dehydroepiandrosterone and Δ^5-androstenediol and (2) the Δ^4 pathway via progesterone and Δ^4-androstenedione. Which pathway, or combination of pathways, predominates in equine Leydig cells is unknown. However, in rat Leydig cells the Δ^4 pathway predominates, whereas in rabbit Leydig cells the Δ^5 pathway is used almost exclusively.[60] Because steroidogenic enzymes are localized on the smooth endoplasmic reticulum, a direct and linear relationship exists between total surface area of smooth endoplasmic reticulum associated with Leydig cells of a testis and its ability to secrete testosterone. The relationship even holds true across species.[60]

Luteinizing hormone or hCG stimulates steroidogenesis by Leydig cells. This stimulatory effect probably is a consequence of LH stimulating transport of cholesterol from intracellular stores to the outer mitochondrial membrane, and also within the mitochondria, to provide cholesterol to the side-chain cleavage enzyme (a mitochondrial cytochrome P_{450} enzyme), which converts cholesterol to pregnenolone in a three-step sequence of reactions.[58] Thus conversion of cholesterol to pregnenolone is the rate-limiting step in production of testosterone. With gonadotropin stimulation, production of pregnenolone increases and this enables increased production of testosterone and estrogens.

Leydig cells contain specific receptors for LH integral to their plasma membrane. Binding of LH to the membrane receptor activates a guanosine triphosphate-(GTP-) binding protein which, in turn, stimulates adenylate cyclase and increases local concentration of cyclic adenosine monophosphate (cAMP).[58] Cyclic AMP, in turn, phosphorylates specific proteins by a post-translational modification; in this case a cholesterol-ester hydrolase becomes more active and releases increased amounts of free cholesterol for transport by microfilaments to mitochondria. Because the process does not involve synthesis of a new protein and enzymes involved in conversion of pregnenolone to testosterone are working far below their maximum capacity, Leydig cells rapidly increase production of testosterone in response to LH stimulation. Other proteins probably exist for which function is modified by LH stimulation to increase the transport flux of cholesterol to the inner mitochondrial membrane where the side-chain cleavage enzyme is located.

EPIDIDYMIS

Most aspects of epididymal function have not been studied in the stallion. However, from available data,[14,61] and those from other species,[62–69] the function of the excurrent duct can be deduced. After leaving the testis, spermatozoa enter the ductuli efferentes testis and then are transported, successively, through several zones of the epididymis. These include the initial segment of the epididymal duct (ductus epididymidis), two or three spermatozoal maturation zones in the caput and corpus epididymidis, and a zone where fertile spermatozoa are stored in the cauda epididymidis until ejaculated (Fig. 77–16). Most of the fluid, protein, and other material entering from the testis is resorbed in the ductuli efferentes and proximal caput epididymidis, to be replaced by secretions of the epididymal epithelium. However, spermatozoa are not normally removed in the epididymis. The composition of luminal fluid surrounding spermatozoa is different in successive functional zones and regional differences in mechanisms regulating epithelial function exist. Spermatozoa leaving the testis are infertile, whereas spermatozoa recovered from the cauda epididymidis are fertile.[62,63,65,66] The process by which spermatozoa develop capacity for fertilization is termed spermatozoal maturation, but this is only one aspect of a continuous spectrum of changes in these cells from when they are formed until they fertilize an egg[63] (see Fig. 80–1). Spermatozoal maturation depends on sequential exposure of spermatozoa to epididymal fluids of differing composition. Enzymes and other proteins in the fluid modify the plasma membrane and certain other components, of spermatozoa (Fig. 77–16). Availability of testosterone to the epithelium, especially in the caput and corpus epididymidis,[62,65,66] is essential for secretion of certain proteins by the epididymal epithelium, although other secretions are produced without androgenic stimulation.

Evidence for spermatozoal maturation includes acquisition of fertilizing capacity and progressive motility as well as changes in spermatozoal structure, characteristics of the plasma membrane of spermatozoa, and spermatozoal metabolism.[14,61,63,65–68] However, simple retention of spermatozoa within a given segment of the ductus epididymidis is insufficient to induce spermatozoal maturation.[65,66,68]

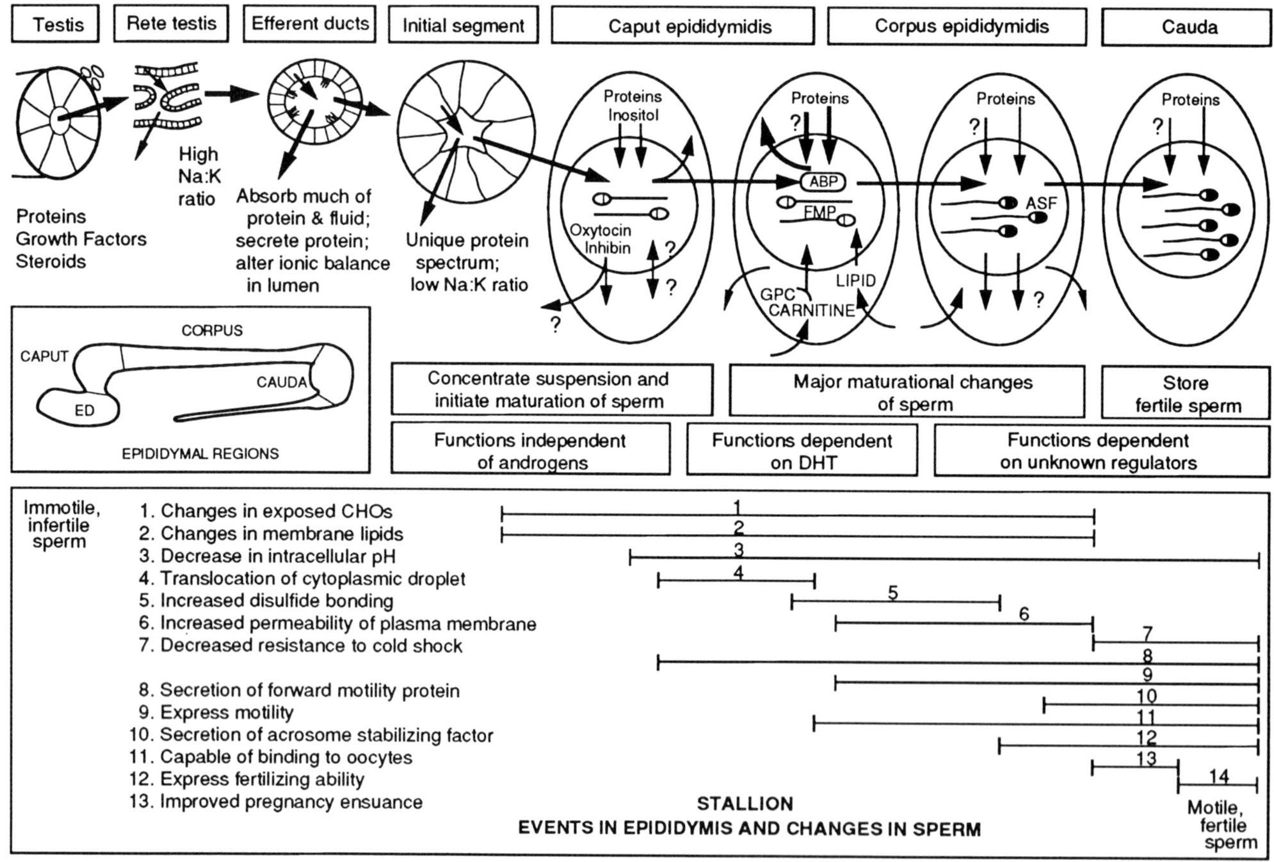

FIG. 77–16. A diagrammatic representation of the regional compartmentalization of epididymal function and changes in spermatozoa, associated with maturation, as they are transported through the epididymis. In the inset, the efferent ducts are designated as ED. Molecules present in the luminal fluid include: ABP, androgen binding protein; ASF, acrosome stabilizing factor; DHT, dihydrotestosterone; FMP, forward motility protein; and GPC, glycerylphosphorylcholine. Deduced from the literature, primarily for bulls, rams, and rats.

Equine spermatozoa from the caput or proximal corpus epididymidis are immotile when released into a physiologic salt solution (Table 77–4). However, the percentage of motile spermatozoa in samples removed from the cauda epididymidis and diluted in buffer is similar to that in ejaculates collected from the same stallions. Thus, as measured by progressive motility, maturation of stallion spermatozoa is completed before spermatozoa enter the cauda epididymidis.[14] As accessed by ability of their plasma membrane to exclude the pink dye eosin, spermatozoa from all regions of the epididymis are resistant to "cold shock," induced by rapid cooling to 0° C. Ejaculated spermatozoa, however, are altered by this treatment (Table 77–4). Based on these and other observations, Johnson et al. concluded that maturation of spermatozoa in the stallion was not completed until spermatozoa left the corpus epididymidis.[14] This is consistent with data for other species,[62,65–67] although changes in spermatozoa that result in a greater percentage of surviving embryos occur in the cauda epididymidis, at least in rams.[62] Available laboratory data and limited data on fertility of stallion spermatozoa from the cauda epididymidis lead to the conclusion that spermatozoa from the cauda epididymidis of a valuable stallion could be used to inseminate mares, if such spermatozoa were recovered within a few hours after death or castration.[70]

Although spermatozoa are found throughout the epididymis,[21,23,38,69,71] the cauda epididymidis and deferent duct (including the ampulla) are the major spermatozoal storage areas (Table 77–5). The two caudae epididymidum of a typical adult stallion (5 to 16 yr old) contain about 54 billion spermatozoa (Table 77–5), or 61% of the total number found within the excurrent duct system.[38] In stallions, the caudae epididymidum contain more spermatozoa than the caudae from a bull, but a much lower number than the caudae from a ram or boar. Sufficient numbers of spermatozoa are present within the caudae epididymidum in the horse for several ejaculates.[23,38] Testis size, daily spermatozoal production, and number of spermatozoa stored within the epididymis are influenced by age.

TABLE 77–4. CHANGE IN SPERMATOZOA DURING PASSAGE THROUGH THE EPIDIDYMIS

		UNSTAINED SPERMATOZOA (%)	
Spermatozoa from	Progressive Motility (%)	Not Cooled	Cooled to 0° C in ≤2 min
Central caput	0	96	96
Proximal corpus	0	97	95
Distal corpus	11*	93	93
Central cauda	56†	90	87
Ejaculated	64	68	27‡

*Spermatozoa from two of five stallions were progressively motile.

†The percentage of motile spermatozoa was similar ($p > 0.05$) to that in ejaculated semen.

‡The percentage of unstained spermatozoa was reduced ($p < 0.05$) by cold shock.

(Adapted from Johnson, L., Amann, R.P., and Pickett, B.W.: Scanning electron and light microscopy of the equine seminiferous tubule. Fertil. Steril., *29*:208–215 1978.)

TABLE 77–5. SPERMATOZOAL RESERVES IN THE ADULT STALLION*

SEGMENT OF EXCURRENT DUCT	SPERMATOZOA IN BOTH SIDES (10^9)	RELATIVE DISTRIBUTION (%)
Caput epididymidis	12	13
Corpus epididymidis	17	19
Cauda epididymidis	54	61
Deferent duct	4	2
Ampulla of deferent duct	2	2

*Data for stallions 5 to 16 yr old.

(Adapted from Amann, R.P., Thompson, D.L., Jr., Squires, E.L., and Pickett, B.W.: Effects of age and frequency of ejaculation on sperm production and extragonadal sperm reserves in stallions. J. Reprod. Fertil. Suppl., *27*:1–6, 1979.)

Spermatozoa do not swim through the epididymis and deferent duct. Movement of spermatozoa through the epididymal duct is primarily by continuous peristaltic contractions of smooth muscle in the wall of the duct within the caput and corpus epididymidis. In the cauda, the epididymal duct normally is inactive, except when smooth muscle is stimulated to contract. Consequently, time required for movement of spermatozoa through the caput and corpus epididymidis is not altered by ejaculation and averages about 4.1 days in stallions.[21,23,38,71]

Fertility of spermatozoa is usually not depressed in males ejaculating frequently, because rate of spermatozoal transport through the caput and corpus epididymidis is not influenced by ejaculation; decreased fertility could result if number of spermatozoa ejaculated were less than the number required for maximum reproductive efficiency. Extensive data for bulls ejaculating daily, or at a similar high frequency, show that spermatozoal fertility is equivalent, if not slightly superior, to that for bulls ejaculating once a week[72–74] (J.O. Almquist, personal communication). When seven successive ejaculates were collected from beef bulls and the spermatozoa was used to artificially inseminate cattle, fertility did not differ among the seven successive ejaculates.[75] Fertility of stallion spermatozoa used for artificial insemination should be similar whether stallions are collected daily, every other day, or every 4 days.

The interval that spermatozoa spend in the cauda epididymidis is influenced by ejaculation.[23,38] The number of spermatozoa in the cauda epididymidis is maximal in sexually rested stallions and is reduced in males ejaculating daily or every other day.[38] Because fewer spermatozoa are present in the cauda epididymidis of a stallion ejaculating regularly than in an inactive male, transit time for spermatozoa through the cauda epididymidis of a sexually active stallion is reduced by 2 or 3 days from the 10 days characteristic of a sexually rested stallion.[21,38,71] Although the time required for movement of spermatozoa through the caput and corpus epididymidis is reasonably similar among species,[23] the interval that spermatozoa spend in the cauda epididymidis differs greatly, and ranges from < 4 days in humans and some beef bulls to > 12 days in rams.

Spermatozoa are produced continuously, regardless of ejaculation frequency. Because spermatozoa enter the epididymis at a constant rate, they must also leave the excurrent duct system at a relatively constant rate, although this rate is altered by ejaculation. Based on research with several species,[76,77] all spermatozoa that enter the excurrent duct system of a stallion likely leave through the urethra. Resorption of spermatozoa probably does not occur within the excurrent duct system.[23,76,77] In bulls and rams, spermatozoa that are not ejaculated at copulation or voided by masturbation are eliminated periodically during urination.[77] Probably in a normal, sexually inactive stallion, spermatozoa intermittently pass from the deferent duct into the pelvic urethra (pars pelvina) and are voided during urination. The direct cause for or interval between such emissions is unknown. Certain stallions accumulate an abnormally large number of spermatozoa in the epididymis and perhaps to some extent in the deferent duct, including the ampulla. In such a horse, spontaneous emissions probably do not occur and spermatozoa accumulate in the epididymis until the limit of distensibility of the epididymal duct is reached. As a consequence of this accumulation, storage interval of spermatozoa in the cauda epididymidis of such a stallion is much longer than 7 to 10 days, and spermatozoa may undergo marked alterations. Much lower percentages of spermatozoa are structurally normal or motile in the first several ejaculates collected from a stallion accumulating spermatozoa than in a normal horse because of the prolonged storage interval.

ACCESSORY SEX GLANDS

Collectively, the prostate gland, bulbourethral glands, and vesicular glands are termed the accessory sex glands (glandulae genitales accessoriae) (see Figs. 76–1 and 76–12). These glands contribute most of the fluid to the ejaculate. Spermatozoa from the cauda epididymidis and deferent duct are immotile until mixed with accessory sex gland fluids at ejaculation (or mixed with a buffer by human intervention). Exact factors causing initiation of motility are unknown, but intracellular pH may be involved. Although certain proteins in accessory sex gland fluids are bound by spermatozoa, exposure to these fluids is not essential for normal fertility of the spermatozoa; cells from the cauda epididymidis are of normal fertility. Indeed, increasing evidence is accumulating that for some stallions a component of seminal plasma may be responsible for reduced survival of sperm during storage or low fertility.

Normal function of all accessory sex glands depends on availability of testosterone in peripheral blood.[78] The secretion of the prostate gland is thin and watery.[79] This secretion probably helps cleanse the urethra during ejaculation and also constitutes a major portion of seminal plasma, especially if a second ejaculation occurs 1 to 3 h after an earlier ejaculation. Depending on season and individual stallion, fluid secreted by the vesicular glands may (or may not) contribute a major portion of seminal plasma in an ejaculate. The gelatinous material often found in seminal plasma, especially in April to July is secreted by these glands.[79] This seasonal change in secretion of gel by the vesicular glands, as well as the stallion-to-stallion difference, may reflect differences in concentration of testosterone in blood. Two bulbourethral glands are positioned on either side of the pelvic urethra near the ischial arch. Their secretion contributes to the seminal plasma but probably only a minor portion in terms of volume.

ENDOCRINE HORMONES

Function of reproductive organs is controlled by the neuroendocrine system. The neuroendocrine system includes specialized groups of nerve cell bodies and endocrine tissues that secrete chemical messengers termed hormones (Chapter 3), which are carried through the blood from one organ to control the function of another organ. The autonomic nervous system has a role in controlling function of the reproductive organs; transport of spermatozoa from the testes through the epididymides and deferent ducts; and the processes of erection, emission, and ejaculation. However, maintenance of normal function of reproductive organs depends more on the neuroendocrine system.

HYPOTHALAMIC-HYPOPHYSEAL AXIS

The hypothalamus (see Fig. 1–1) is part of the diencephalon of the brain, but its exact boundaries have not been defined critically in the horse (Chapter 1). From work with other species, the hypothalamus seems to be involved in regulation of appetite and thirst, body temperature, vasomotor activity, emotion, use of body nutrient reserves, activity of the intestinal tract and bladder, states of sleep and wakefulness, sexual behavior, and release of tropic hormones. This latter role is essential for controlling reproductive function.

The hypophysis is connected to, and extends downward from, the hypothalamus. The adenohypophysis synthesizes and discharges a number of hormones that control reproductive processes in the stallion and mare.[80,81] The neurohypophysis, on the other hand, does not produce hormones but simply serves as a storage reservoir for hormones produced by neural tissue within the brain. The hypothalamus and adenohypophysis are linked by portal vessels, which extend from the hypothalamus through the infundibulum to the pars distalis. Within this portal system, blood normally flows directly from the hypothalamus to the pars distalis. The portal vessels are the only direct link between the hypothalamus and the adenohypophysis.

Under appropriate neural stimulation, the hypothalamus synthesizes and discharges a number of "releasing hormones." The releasing hormone directly involved in controlling reproductive function is gonadotropin-releasing hormone (GnRH) (Chapter 4). GnRH is discharged by the hypothalamus in short, pulsatile bursts. This fact, coupled with rapid removal of GnRH from the blood, results in a pulsatile stimulation of the gonadotropin-secreting cells in the adenohypophysis. A large number of compounds similar to GnRH, called structural analogues, have been synthesized and used in research to study and control reproductive function. Two types of analogues of GnRH are available: those that block the action of the natural hormone and those that are more effective in evoking a response than natural GnRH.

The adenohypophysis produces at least six tropic hormones, but only two or three have a direct role in male reproduction. The adenohypophysis produces LH and FSH in direct response to stimulation by GnRH. Luteinizing hormone and FSH (Chapter 5) are gonadotropic hormones because they act on the gonads (testes in males) and stimulate their function, including production of steroid hormones and spermatozoa. Although details of the secretory pattern of GnRH are not available for stallions, GnRH must be secreted in a pulsatile manner. Only pulsatile secretion of GnRH could account for secretion of LH as a series of distinct pulses.[82–85] However, in some stallions, pulsatile secretion of LH is not evident from analyses of jugular blood, especially during the breeding season.[47,85] Secretion of FSH also is pulsatile, although more short-term variability exists,[47,85] possibly reflecting intermittent discharges of small amounts of hormone. Pulsatile secretion of FSH is generally associated with an episode of LH secretion. Although several studies of concentrations of hormones in blood of stallions have been made,[17,44,47,56,78,82–91] concepts for endocrine control of reproductive function are based primarily on data from other species.[34,58,80,92,93] The concepts outlined herein are true regardless of season or age. However, great seasonal differences occur in secretory rates and concentrations of all hormones in blood.

TESTICULAR HORMONES

Steroid hormones produced by Leydig cells (Fig. 77–15) are the primary endocrine product of the testes. However, in the last decade the importance of other hormones secreted by the testes has become evident. Sertoli cells secrete inhibin and activin, a pair of related glycoprotein hormones, which share a common subunit.[94] As detailed in Chapter 12, the inhibin/activin family include three subunits: α, β_A and β_B. Inhibin is the combination α/β_A or α/β_B, and activin is the combinations β_A/β_B, β_A/β_A, or β_B/β_B. The relative amounts of different inhibins, or activins, secreted differ as a function of cell type (Sertoli cells of male or granulosa cells of female, species, and stage of development). Although stallion Sertoli cells secrete inhibin and activin, the exact molecular form(s) of each remains to be established.

Numerous reports have been made of secretion of GnRH-like peptides by the rat testis. This appears to be unique to rats, because attempts to detect secreted GnRH or responses of testicular tissue to applied GnRH in other species all have been unsuccessful. No such study with stallion tissue has been reported.

Based on data for rats and rams, Leydig cells likely secrete oxytocin into the interstitial fluid.[95,96] Apparently, oxytocin facilitates rhythmic contraction of seminiferous tubules to help evacuate sperm. Oxytocin seems to be transported by Sertoli cells into the luminal fluid or secreted by the rete testis, because in rams the rete testis fluid draining the testis contains about 550 pg/mL as compared with 124 pg/mL in serum from testicular venous blood.[96] Oxytocin may be important in facilitating contractions of the efferent ducts and proximal epididymal duct. Veeramachaneni and Amann speculated that a deficiency of testicular oxytocin in fluid entering the excurrent ducts or its uptake by the epithelium therein could be a cause of sperm stasis and formation of granulomatous lesions (common in cattle, sheep, and goats, but the frequency in horses is unknown).[97]

Research in the coming decade certainly will reveal an abundance of regulatory peptides, important for signaling between Leydig cells, Sertoli cells, and germinal cells. The testes may secrete unidentified hormones that act on other reproductive organs or the hypothalamic-hypophyseal axis. Certainly progesterone and conjugated estrogen may have some systemic role.

REGULATION OF HORMONE SECRETION

In the adult male, production of testosterone is controlled by episodic bursts of LH secretion, which periodically elevate the concentration of LH in blood reaching the testis far above the basal level. Consequently, basal

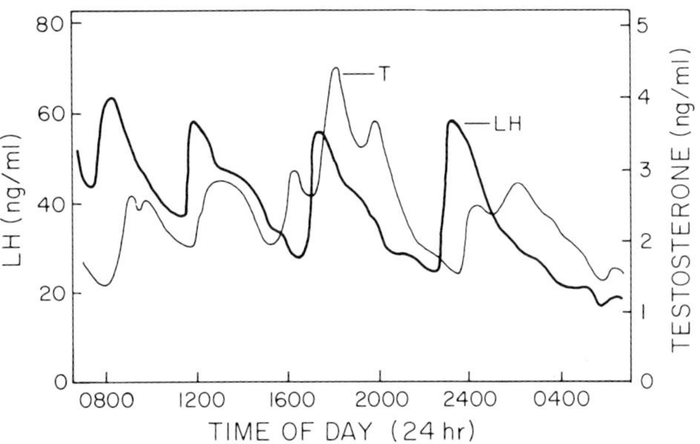

FIG. 77–17. Concentrations of LH and testosterone (T) in serum from jugular blood taken every 20 min from a stallion. Although pulsatile secretion of both LH and testosterone is not always as evident as in this example, pulsatile secretion of LH was evident for 96% of 231 such sequences of blood samples (72 samples/sequence) taken from 21 stallions in all seasons of the year. (From Pickett, B.W., et al.: Management of the Stallion for Maximum Reproductive Efficiency. II. Animal Reproduction Laboratory Bulletin No. 05. Fort Collins, Colorado State University, 1989.)

production of testosterone is augmented by episodic bursts of production of testosterone[49,54,82,85,87,90] (Fig. 77–17).

Testosterone produced by Leydig cells enters venous blood draining the testis, passes into the general circulation, and then moves to the hypothalamus and adenohypophysis (Fig. 77–18). In this manner, testosterone feeds back via a long loop and modulates discharge of GnRH and LH.[78,83] If the concentration of testosterone reaching the hypothalamus and adenohypophysis is relatively high, discharge of GnRH by the hypothalamus is suppressed and response of the adenohypophysis to available GnRH also is suppressed. This negative effect of gonadal steroids has been attributed to testosterone

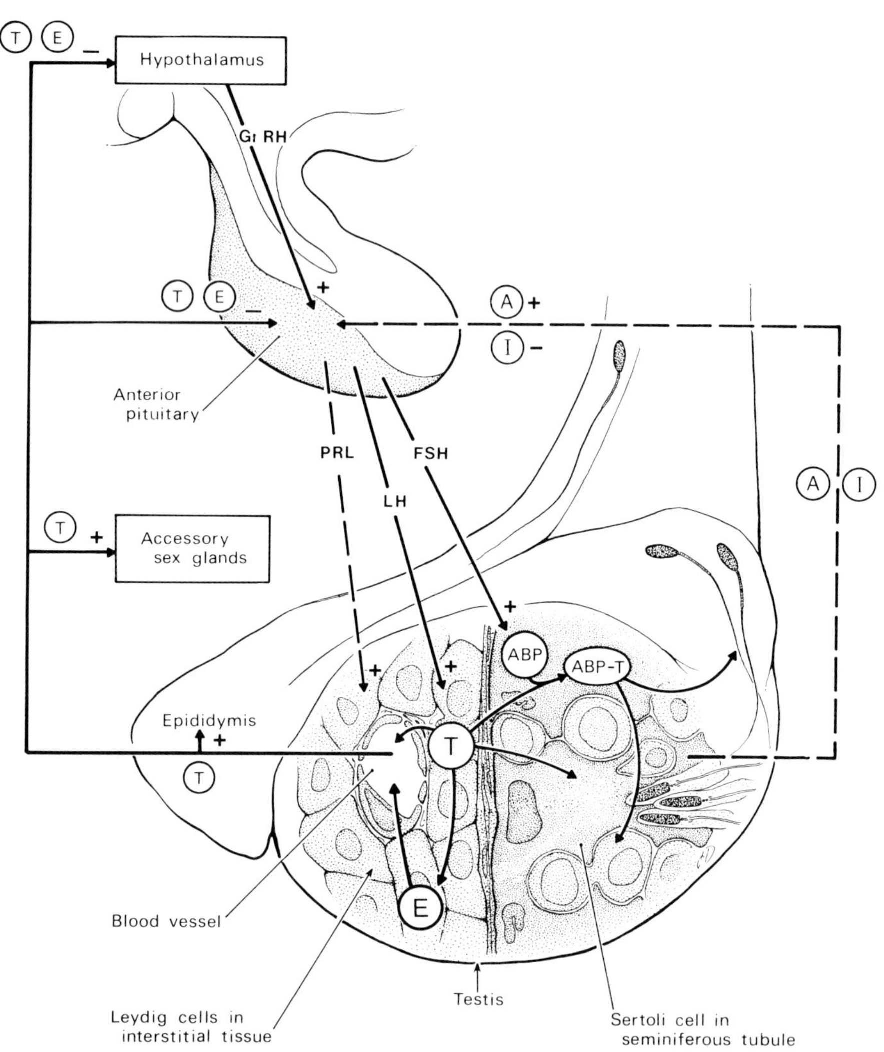

FIG. 77–18. Diagram showing interrelationship of hypophyseal hormones acting on Leydig cells and Sertoli cells of the seminiferous tubules and feedback control of gonadal hormones on the hypothalamus and adenohypophysis. An increased level of testosterone in peripheral blood, either as a result of increased production by the testes or after injection of hormone, feeds back on the hypothalamus and adenohypophysis to suppress discharge of GnRH and LH, respectively. Therefore, Leydig cells produce less testosterone and concentration of testosterone around the seminiferous tubules drops. Circulating FSH acts directly on Sertoli cells, which secrete two protein hormones: inhibin, which acts on the adenohypophysis to suppress selectively the amount of FSH secreted in response to GnRH, and activin, which stimulates FSH secretion. Adequate concentrations of testosterone and FSH must be present to stimulate Sertoli cells to produce an environment appropriate for normal spermatogenesis. A, activin; ABP, androgen-binding protein; E, estradiol or other estrogens; GnRH, gonadotropin-releasing hormone; I, inhibin; LH, luteinizing hormone; FSH, follicle-stimulating hormone; PRL, prolactin; T, testosterone. (Modified from Pickett, B.W., et al.: Management of the Stallion for Maximum Reproductive Efficiency. II. Animal Reproduction Laboratory Bulletin No. 05. Fort Collins, Colorado State University, 1989.)

per se, but it could result from a combined effect of testicular testosterone, estradiol, and possibly progesterone. Furthermore, testosterone might be converted to estradiol in the target cells of the hypothalamus or adenohypophysis. That negative effects of steroids are expressed on both the hypothalamus and adenohypophysis is likely, but unproven. In any case, because of this negative feedback, concentration of LH would be low in blood entering the testis so Leydig cells would be exposed to a low concentration of LH, and consequently, Leydig cells would only secrete testosterone at a basal rate. As concentration of testosterone in peripheral blood declines, the negative block is removed and episodic discharge of GnRH from the hypothalamus can occur. This is followed by a discharge of LH from the adenohypophysis, an elevated concentration of LH in blood flowing to the testis, and rapid stimulation of Leydig cells to produce and discharge testosterone (compare data for LH and testosterone in Fig. 77–17). Thus, Leydig cells, the hypothalamus, and the adenohypophysis are involved in a circular feedback loop that regulates concentrations of LH and testosterone in peripheral blood (Fig. 77–18).

Although secretion of FSH also is stimulated by GnRH, secretion of FSH and LH must be controlled by different mechanisms. Bursts of secretion of LH are sometimes not accompanied by a discharge of FSH and vice versa.[47,85] Furthermore, a differential effect of season on secretion of LH and FSH occurs. Synthesis and secretion of FSH may be much less dependent on GnRH than secretion of LH.[98] Based on research with nonequine species, FSH seems to act exclusively on Sertoli cells within the seminiferous tubules.[3,34] Among the products of Sertoli cells are several protein hormones, including closely related inhibin and activin (Chapter 12). Among other functions, these hormones act on the adenohypophysis to suppress (inhibin) or stimulate (activin) secretion of FSH, with little or no effect on secretion of LH. Thus, the inhibin/activin system and probably the ratio of testosterone to estradiol impinging on the adenohypophysis control the relative amounts of LH and FSH secreted in response to GnRH from the hypothalamus.

Although the stallion testis produces uniquely high concentrations of estrogens, researchers are not certain if estrogens are produced in Sertoli cells, Leydig cells, or some other component of the testis. Figure 77–18 incorporates the speculation that a portion of testosterone produced by Leydig cells is transformed within Leydig cells to estradiol or other estrogens. In any case, blood draining from the stallion testis contains high concentrations of estrogens, and high concentrations of estrogens in blood flowing to the hypothalamus and adenohypophysis may suppress discharge of GnRH or LH and FSH in a negative feedback loop.[78,98] Because of feedback loops involving the hypothalamus, adenohypophysis, and testis, injecting hormones will alter the delicate hormonal balance in a stallion and may profoundly disturb reproductive function. Sequelae of such manipulations, often with undesirable results, are detailed in Chapter 89.

HORMONAL CONTROL OF SPERMATOGENESIS

The hormonal requirements for normal spermatogenesis in a stallion are unknown. Based on research with rats, duration of the cycle of seminiferous epithelium and total duration of spermatogenesis are probably not modified by hormonal balance within the testis.[2,27,29,43] However, degree of germ cell degeneration is partially under hormonal control.[2,27,41,43,99] Seminiferous tubules are surrounded by Leydig cells producing testosterone, so the seminiferous epithelium is exposed to a higher concentration of testosterone than found in peripheral blood. This high level of testosterone is essential for normal spermatogenesis.[41,99] In rams, FSH is necessary for spermatogenesis[30,41,99] and LH may have a direct role in regulating division of spermatogonia in addition to its role at stimulating production of testosterone.[99] The role of FSH in bringing about normal development of spermatids apparently is mediated via Sertoli cells.[30] Definitive conclusions on hormonal control of spermatogenesis in stallions must await data obtained with stallions, because some differences among species exist.[99]

DESCENT OF THE TESTES

A description of the embryologic development of the equine reproductive system is beyond the scope of this chapter. However, understanding the process by which the testes normally descend from the abdominal cavity into the scrotum is essential. In the normal colt, both testes should descend into the scrotum between 30 days before and 10 days after birth.[100,101] Failure of normal testicular descent is common in horses[102] and is termed cryptorchidism.

By day 40 of gestation, the testis is suspended from the abdominal wall (Fig. 77–19) and the mesonephric duct, which later gives rise to the epididymis and ductus deferens, leads into the pelvic area.[100] A narrow evagination, termed the vaginal process (process vaginalis peritonei), starts to form about day 43 of gestation and progressively develops to form the inguinal canal (canalis inguinalis) (Fig. 77–19). Around day 150, the developing cauda epididymidis is drawn to or just within the internal inguinal ring (annulus inguinalis profundus) (Fig. 77–20), but the testis is large and cannot enter the inguinal canal.[100] Entrance of the testis into the inguinal canal typically begins between 270 and 300 days of gestation.[100] This occurs only after the vaginal process and internal inguinal ring have been stretched sufficiently by the enlarging cauda epididymidis (Fig. 77–21) to allow entrance of the testis that has diminished in size from 50 to 30 g. Pressure from fluid in the abdominal cavity, and possibly from the intestines, forces the testis down through the inguinal canal. This descent places the lamina visceralis or the tunica vaginalis—the outer covering of the testis—into apposition with the lamina parietalis of the tunica vaginalis—the former vaginal process—separated by the cavum vaginale (Fig. 77–21).

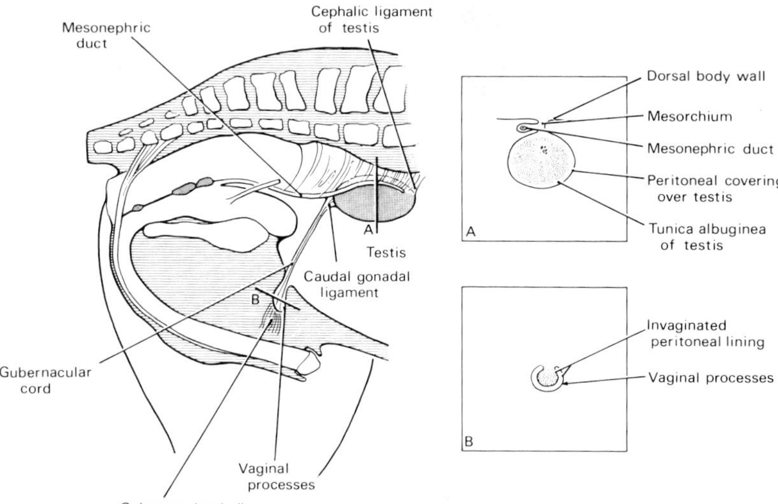

FIG. 77–19. Drawing of a horse fetus at 75 days of gestation. The testis is suspended within the abdominal cavity by a thin double-layered band of fused tissue termed the mesorchium. The caudal gonadal ligament, extending from the testis to its point of fusion with the mesonephric duct (future epididymis and ductus deferens), is continuous with the gubernacular cord that extends to the gubernacular bulb. The vaginal process (future lamina parietalis of the tunica vaginalis) encloses about one third of the gubernacular bulb. (Modified from Pickett, B.W., et al.: Management of the Stallion for Maximum Reproductive Efficiency. II. Animal Reproduction Laboratory Bulletin No. 05. Fort Collins, Colorado State University, 1989.)

Bergin et al. reported that the earliest complete descent of both testes was at 315 days of gestation, about 25 days before parturition.[100] In 32 fetuses between 9 months of gestation and birth, descent of the right testis was more advanced than the left in 78% of the fetuses, while the left testis was more advanced in only 3%. Of 12 fetuses collected at term, 42% had completely descended testes, 25% had both testes within the inguinal canals, 17% had one testis in the scrotum and one in the inguinal canal, and 17% had both testes within the abdominal cavity. A total of 5 of 9 colts less than 1 week old had complete bilateral descent of the testes into the scrotum.

As reviewed by Bergin et al., failure of the testes to descend has been attributed to abnormalities of the testis, development of adhesions between the testis and adjacent structures, or an abnormal outpouching of the vaginal process.[100] Bergin et al. discounted these factors as causes of cryptorchidism and suggested that the most obvious reasons for the testis to remain in the abdominal cavity included the following:

1. Insufficient abdominal pressure to properly expand the vaginal process.
2. Stretching of the gubernacular cord (chorda gubernaculi).
3. Insufficient growth of the gubernaculum and cauda epididymidis so that they are unable to expand the inguinal ring sufficiently to allow entrance of the testis.
4. Displacement of the testis to a position where intestinal pressure prevents tension from the gubernaculum, via the gubernacular cord, pulling the testis into the vaginal process.

PUBERTY

At birth, the testis contains few (if any) functional Leydig cells and only indifferent supporting cells and gonocytes (progenitors of Sertoli cells and spermatogonia). The stallion soon enters the infantile stage of its life. Based on data for other species, this infantile stage is characterized by a declining number of gonocytes, virtual absence of gonadotropin secretion by the adenohypophysis, and limited steroidogenesis (at least in terms of testosterone) by Leydig cells.[41,103–107] Spermatozoa are not produced. This infantile stage continues through ≥ 6 months in stallions, when changes are initiated which continue through a prepubertal stage and culminate in puberty. Timing of the prepubertal changes differs among stallions and might be influenced by breed and season of birth. Puberty (meaning "to beget") is the time when a stallion is first capable of successfully participating in reproduction. In literature on domestic animals, puberty is considered to be a definitive end point—being capable of reproduction—and, by definition, implies achievement of spermarche (production of first spermatozoa) and completion of prepubertal events. In literature pertaining to humans, however, the term puberty has no specific end point, but refers rather to the series of events termed the prepubertal stage herein. With some stallions, a few spermatozoa are available for ejaculation by 14 months of age. Follow-

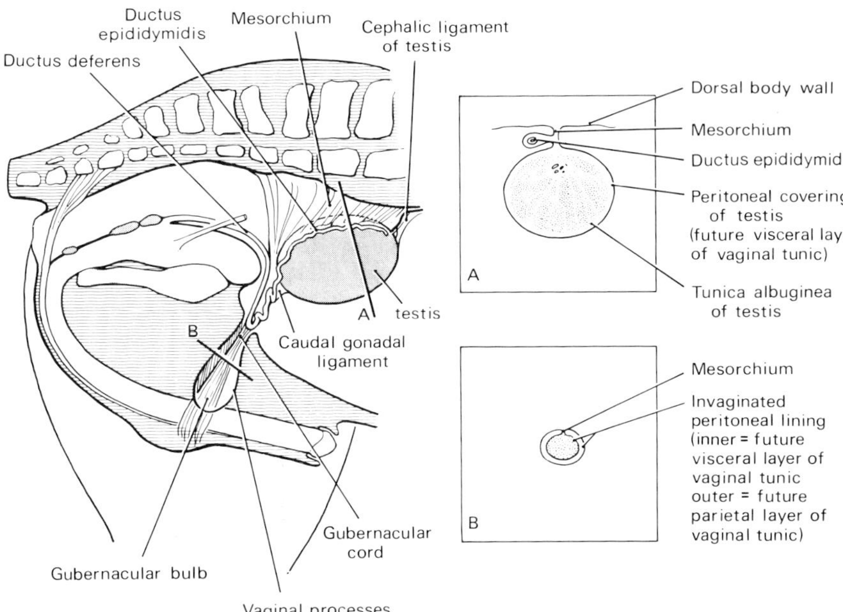

FIG. 77–20. Drawing of a horse fetus at 175 days of gestation. The vaginal process extends almost to the scrotum and has virtually enclosed the gubernacular bulb. The mesorchium is continuous from the gubernaculum and the vaginal process to the testis. The epididymis and ductus deferens have formed from the mesonephric duct and the future cauda epididymidis will form where the duct is sharply reflected. (Modified from Pickett, B.W., et al.: Management of the Stallion for Maximum Reproductive Efficiency. II. Animal Reproduction Laboratory Bulletin No. 05. Fort Collins, Colorado State University, 1989.)

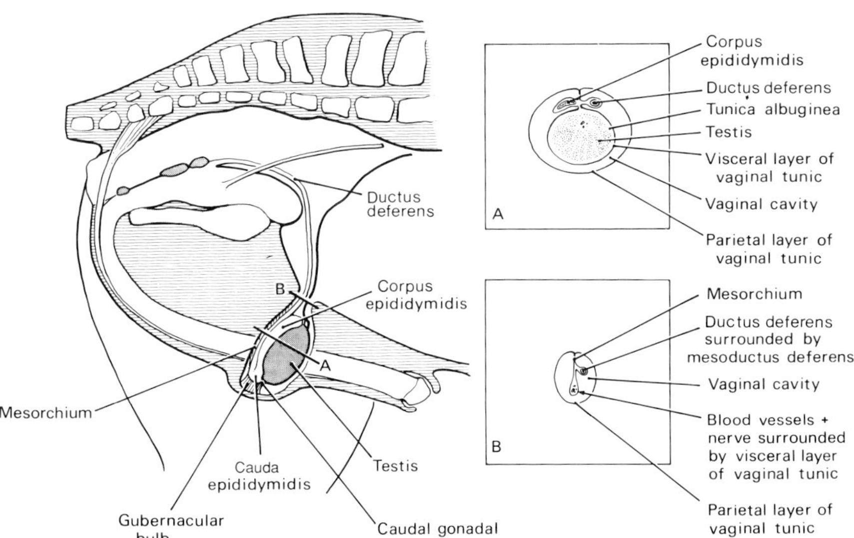

FIG. 77–21. Drawing of a horse fetus near term. The testis has passed through the inguinal canal, but is not fully within the scrotum. The gubernacular bulb, gubernacular cord, cauda epididymidis, and caudal gonadal ligament all have regressed. The testis now is connected by the mesorchium to the dorsal wall of the lamina parietalis of the tunica vaginalis (formally the vaginal process). The deferent duct, blood vessels and lymphatics are connected to the lamina parietalis of the tunica vaginalis by folds of the mesorchium. (Modified from Pickett, B.W., et al.: Management of the Stallion for Maximum Reproductive Efficiency. II. Animal Reproduction Laboratory Bulletin No. 05. Fort Collins, Colorado State University, 1989.)

ing puberty, development of reproductive capacity continues (postpubertal stage), and 2 to 4 yr after puberty, a stallion achieves sexual maturity (maximum reproductive capacity). Years later, reproductive senescence may occur. For most stallions, no change in DSP between 4 and 20 yr of age occurs.[22]

Little is known about testicular function or changes in the neuroendocrine system of stallions during the infantile stage of development or exactly when the prepubertal stage is initiated. Timing of specific events likely ranges considerably, especially comparing light horse and draft breeds. Starting at about 9 months, concentrations of FSH and especially LH in blood increase (Fig. 77–22) and around 12 months, the testes start to grow and develop rapidly.[88,108,109] Several months later, they gradually begin to produce spermatozoa.[88,110] Total scrotal width increases in a linear manner from 42 mm at 42 weeks to 85 mm at 96 weeks of age (about 1 mm/week), based on data for 15 colts born in July and early August.[88] Increased production of testosterone by Leydig cells after 80 weeks of age is evident from concentrations of testosterone in jugular vein blood (Fig. 77–22).[88] These prepubertal developments are culminated in puberty when a stallion produces spermatozoa and would be fertile if allowed to breed a mare.

For 15 colts born in July and early August, and carefully monitored for reproductive development, age at puberty averaged 83 weeks (puberty defined as first ejaculate containing 50 million spermatozoa of which ≥ 10% are motile).[88] A total of 11 of the 15 colts attained puberty by 90 weeks of age. After puberty, the quantity and quality of spermatozoa produced slowly increased (Table 77–6). At 2 yr of age, ejaculates contained 3.3 billion spermatozoa, although percentages of

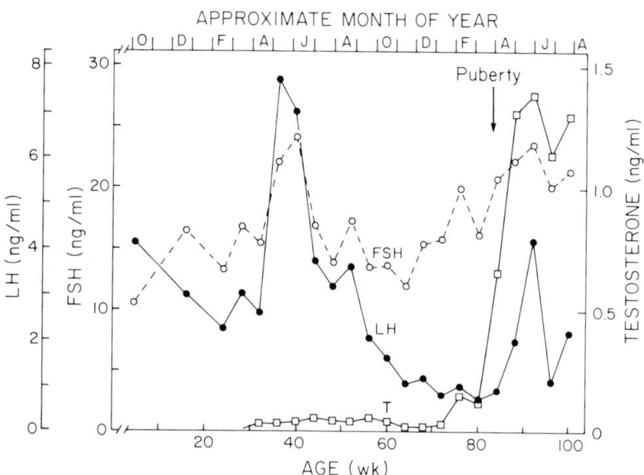

FIG. 77–22. Concentrations of LH, FSH, and testosterone in serum prepared from jugular blood. Age at puberty averaged 83 weeks, but ranged from 56 to 97 weeks (based on seminal characteristics). Based on data for eight colts born in July or early August. Blood samples were taken from each colt at 8, 16, and 24 weeks of age and every 4 weeks thereafter. (From Pickett, B.W., et al.: Management of the Stallion for Maximum Reproductive Efficiency. II. Animal Reproduction Laboratory Bulletin No. 05. Fort Collins, Colorado State University, 1989.)

TABLE 77–6. CHARACTERISTICS OF LIGHT HORSE STALLIONS AND THEIR SEMEN AT PUBERTY* AND 96 WEEKS OF AGE

CHARACTERISTIC	PUBERTY	96 WEEKS†
Total scrotal width (mm)	77	88
Gel-free seminal volume (mL)	12	21
Sperm concentration (10^6/mL)	99	162
Total sperm per ejaculate (10^9)	1.1	3.3
Motile spermatozoa (%)	26	26
Morphologically normal spermatozoa (%)	33	44

*Puberty was defined as the first ejaculate that contained 50 × 10^6 spermatozoa of which ≥ 10% were motile. Age at puberty averaged 83 weeks, but ranged from 56 to 97 weeks for the 15 colts.

†Seminal data are averages for nine ejaculates per colt, collected every third day.

(From Naden, J., Amann, R.P., and Squires, E.L.: Testicular growth, hormone concentrations, seminal characteristics and sexual behavior in stallions. J. Reprod. Fertil., *88*:167–176, 1990.)

motile and structurally normal spermatozoa still were low. With bulls, fertility of spermatozoa increases for about 6 months after puberty (J.O. Almquist, personal communication).

In the absence of complete information for stallions, changes in the hypothalamic-hypophyseal-testicular axis must be deduced based on information for bulls, rams, and other species.[92,93,103–107] Typically, little secretion of LH, FSH, or testosterone occurs in the infantile stage, but transition from the infantile to prepubertal stage is evidenced by a marked increase in frequency and amplitude of discharges of LH.[92,93,103,105] The relatively low secretion rate of LH in stallions before about 36 weeks of age (Fig. 77–22) probably reflects a low concentration of GnRH receptors in the adenohypophysis (based on data for bulls)[105] and little secretion of GnRH from the hypothalamus. In bulls, high secretion of LH, evidenced by frequent discharges of high amplitude, starts at 10 to 12 weeks of age and continues for about 6 weeks.[103] A similar event apparently occurs in stallions, as evidenced by the high concentrations of LH in jugular-vein blood between 36 and 45 weeks of age (Fig. 77–22). In stallions, however, the surge of LH secretion may reflect simply a change in amplitude of LH pulses rather than a combined effect of increased frequency of discharges of LH with each discharge containing more hormone; in adult stallions, the seasonal rise of serum concentration of LH was solely caused by an increase in LH pulse amplitude.[47,82,57] The stallion hypophysis has the capability to secrete considerably more LH at 32 weeks of age than actually is secreted,[89] although the amount of LH released after GnRH administration increased from 32 to 48 weeks of age.

For the eight stallions studied by Naden et al., Leydig cells were unresponsive to the increased LH-stimulation which occurred from 36 to 45 weeks of age because no change in testosterone concentration occurred in peripheral blood[88] (Fig. 77–22). This also is true for bulls, for which more extensive data are available.[92,93,103,105] Prolonged stimulation of Leydig cells by LH likely is necessary to complete their differentiation so that they can secrete testosterone. In stallions, an interval of almost 12 months is seen between initial increase of LH concentration in the blood and increase of testosterone concentration[88] (Fig. 77–22), whereas in bulls the interval is about 3 months.[103] Perhaps this difference is a consequence of the more pronounced seasonal effect on reproductive function in stallions than in bulls, coupled with the fact that in Naden's study Leydig cells were exposed to high concentrations of LH in May to July, and about 3 months later the effect of season may have suppressed secretion of testosterone that otherwise might have occurred.[88] In adult stallions, secretion of testosterone is reduced and blood concentrations are low during September through January.[88] With onset of the next breeding season, secretion of LH, FSH, and testosterone all increased in the young colts born in July and early August (Fig. 77–22).

What causes inactivity of the neuroendocrine system during the infantile stage? Extrapolating from data for bulls and rams,[99,103–105] I speculate that in stallions an estradiol-mediated block suppresses secretion of GnRH by the hypothalamus before about 16 weeks of age. Then pulsatile discharge of GnRH begins or increases, provided neurochemical stimuli are present. Concomitantly, an increased concentration of estradiol receptors in the adenohypophysis might allow initiation of positive feedback of estradiol on this organ, with a resultant increase in concentration of GnRH receptors in the adenohypophysis and increased responsiveness of the adenohypophysis to discharges of GnRH initiated concurrently. This course of events allows secretion of limited amounts of LH by 16 weeks of age (Fig. 77–22), although the gland is not operating at maximum capacity. Continued GnRH stimulation of the adenohypophysis presumably induces greatly increased synthesis of mRNA for the β-subunit of LH between 20 and 32 weeks of age, which, coupled with increased stimulation from GnRH, enables copious production of LH present at 32 to 45 weeks of age.

Naden et al. speculated that the testicular secretion involved in maturation of the hypothalamic-hypophyseal axis might be estradiol or androstenedione, rather than testosterone.[88] Secretion of a gonadal steroid, other than testosterone, which acts on the hypothalamic-hypophyseal axis, could be a cause of the seasonal suppression in LH secretion from 55 to 85 weeks of age in the colts studied[88] (Fig. 77–22). The interplay between hypophyseal stimulation of Leydig cells and the seminiferous epithelium and between Leydig cells and the seminiferous epithelium are unknown for stallions. For other species, however, indifferent supporting cells apparently must be exposed to FSH and receive androgenic stimulation to complete their differentiation into Sertoli cells capable of supporting spermatogenesis. Given the data depicted in Figure 77–22, sufficient androgenic stimulation appears to be provided by the intratesticular milieu at 70 to 75 weeks of age to enable onset of spermatogenesis and ejaculation of spermatozoa at 83 weeks of age (puberty), although secretion of testosterone continued to increase for at least several months after the initial rise around 72 weeks of age. Based on data for bulls and rats,[23,106,107] the efficiency of spermatozoal production in stallions likely increases rapidly through the interval from puberty to > 100 weeks of age, although no data exist for stallions.

EJACULATION

The process commonly considered to be ejaculation actually involves three sequential processes: erection, emission, and ejaculation. Erection is the lengthening and stiffening of the penis, resulting from engorgement with blood of the corpus cavernosum penis and, later, the corpus spongiosum penis. Emission is the movement and deposition of spermatozoa and fluid from the ductus deferens and cauda epididymidis, as well as fluids from the accessory sex glands, into the pelvic urethra (pars pelvina). Ejaculation is the actual expulsion of semen through the urethra.

Erection of the penis is initiated by sensory stimuli of the glans penis or psychic stimulation of the cerebral cortex. Erection is initiated during teasing because visual stimuli presented by location or teaser animal (or dummy) initiates responses in the cerebrum. Parasympathetic impulses pass from the second, third, and fourth sacral segments of the spinal cord, via splanchnic nerves, to the penis. This overrides sympathetic stimulus normally keeping the arterioles in the penis partly constricted and causes dilation of penile arterioles. More blood enters the corpus cavernosus penis and corpus spongiosum penis. Concurrently, extrinsic muscles of the penis (i.e., ischiocavernosus, bulbospongiosus, and urethralis) contract and compress the deep and dorsal veins of the penis against the ischial arch, impeding venous return from the cavernous bodies of the penis. Consequently, a shunting of blood to fill and distend the corpus cavernosum penis and corpus spongiosum penis occurs, and enlargement of the penis results. Cardiac output may also increase. The penis returns to its flaccid state when the arteries constrict to their normal state as a result of sympathetic impulses, and pressure on the veins is relieved by relaxation of the ischiocavernosus and bulbospongiosus muscles.

In the stallion, emission (caused by sympathetic impulses) and ejaculation (caused by parasympathetic stimulation) occur as a series of strong, pulsatile contractions of the urethralis and bulbospongiosus muscles so that several successive jets of semen are ejaculated.[111] The general sequence is probably that the prostate gland secretes a watery fluid into the pelvic urethra and some prostatic fluid is probably ejaculated as a prespermatozoal fraction. Next, emission and ejaculation of the spermatozoal-rich fraction occurs. This fraction consists of spermatozoa and epididymal secretions and probably prostatic fluids and watery bulbourethral gland fluid. Typically, three to six sequential discharges of sperm-rich fluid occur. Although not always present, the gel or postspermatozoal fraction is derived from the vesicular glands. The function of the gel is unknown, but it is not necessary for fertility. Some ejaculates, especially the second ejaculate in a 2-h period, contain little or no gel. Little is known about the secretions of the glands in the ampulla of the ductus deferens or urethra in terms of chemical composition or contribution to an ejaculate.

The characteristics of semen from a given stallion vary greatly as a function of season, age, testicular size (a highly heritable trait), interval of abstinence since the previous ejaculation(s), and the extent of sexual arousal or courtship before ejaculation. Composition of semen and details of spermatozoal structure and function are presented in the chapter on spermatozoal function (Chapter 80).

REFERENCES

1. Harrison, R.G.: Effect of temperature on the mammalian testis. *In* Handbook of Physiology. Vol. 5. Section 7. Edited by D.W. Hamilton and R.O. Greep. Washington, D.C., American Physiology Society, 1975, pp. 219–223.
2. Setchell, B.P.: The Mammalian Testis. Ithaca, Cornell University Press, 1978.
3. Setchell, B.P., and Brooks, D.E.: Anatomy, vasculature, innervation and fluids of the male reproductive tract. *In* The Physiology of Reproduction. Edited by E. Knobil and J. Neill. New York, Raven Press, 1988, pp. 753–836.
4. Waites, G.M.H.: Temperature and fertility in mammals. Proceedings of the Sixth International Congress on Animal Reproduction and Artificial Insemination. Vol. 1. Paris, 1968, pp. 235–256.
5. Waites, G.M.H., and Ortavant, R.: Effets precoces d'une breve elevation de la temperature testiculaire sur la spermatogenese du Belier. Ann. Biol. Anim. Biochim. Biophys., *8:*323–331, 1968.
6. Austin, J.W., Hupp, E.W., and Murphree, R.L.: Effect of scrotal insulation on semen of Hereford bulls. J. Anim. Sci., *20:*307–310, 1961.
7. Pickett, B.W., et al.: Management of the Stallion for Maximum Reproductive Efficiency. II. Animal Reproduction Laboratory Bulletin No. 05. Fort Collins, Colorado State University.
8. Berndtson, W.E., Squires, E.L., and Thompson, D.L., Jr.: Spermatogenesis, testicular composition and the concentration of testosterone in the equine testis as influenced by season. Theriogenology, *20:*449–457, 1983.
9. Johnson, L.: Increased daily sperm production in the breeding season of stallions is explained by an elevated population of spermatogonia. Biol. Reprod., *32:* 1181–1190, 1985.
10. Johnson, L.: A new approach to quantification of Sertoli cells that avoids problems associated with the irregular nuclear surface. Anat. Rec., *214:*231–237, 1986.
11. Johnson, L.: Effect of season on spermatocytogenesis in stallions. Proceedings of the Annual Meetings of the American Association of Veterinary Anatomists, New Orleans, 1987, p. 28.
12. Johnson, L.: Spermatogenesis. *In* Reproduction in Domestic Animals. 4th ed. Edited by P.T. Cupps. New York, Academic Press, 1990, pp. 173–219.
13. Johnson, L., Amann, R.P., and Pickett, B.W.: Scanning electron and light microscopy of the equine seminiferous tubule. Fertil. Steril., *29:*208–215, 1978.
14. Johnson, L., Amann, R.P., and Pickett, B.W.: Scanning electron microscopy of the epithelium and spermatozoa in the equine excurrent duct system. Am. J. Vet. Res., *39:*1428–1434, 1978.
15. Johnson, L., and Neaves, W.B.: Age-related changes in the Leydig cell population, seminiferous tubules, and sperm production in stallions. Biol. Reprod., *24:*703–712, 1981.
16. Johnson, L., and Tatum, M.E.: Sequence of seasonal changes in numbers of Sertoli, Leydig and germ cells in adult stallions. Proceedings of the Eleventh International Congress on Animal Reproduction and Artificial Insemination. Vol. 3. Dublin, 1988, pp. 373–374.
17. Johnson, L., and Thompson, D.L., Jr.: Age-related and seasonal variation in the Sertoli cell population, daily sperm production and serum concentrations of follicle-stimulating hormone, luteinizing hormone and testosterone in stallions. Biol. Reprod., *29:*777–789, 1983.
18. Johnson, L.: Seasonal differences in equine spermatocytogenesis. Biol. Reprod., *44:*284–291, 1991.
19. Johnson, L., Varner, D.D., and Thompson, D.L., Jr.: Effect of age and season on the establishment of spermatogenesis in the horse. J. Reprod. Fertil. Suppl., *44:*87–97, 1991.
20. Swierstra, E.E., Gebauer, M.R., and Pickett, B.W.: Reproductive physiology of the stallion. I. Spermatogenesis and testis composition. J. Reprod. Fertil., *40:*113–123, 1974.
21. Swierstra, E.E., Pickett, B.W., and Gebauer, M.R.: Spermatogenesis and duration of transit of spermatozoa through the excurrent ducts of stallions. J. Reprod. Fertil. Suppl., *23:*53–57, 1975.
22. Johnson, L., Varner, D.D., Tatum, M.E., and Scrutchfield, W.L.: Season but not age affects Sertoli cell number in adult stallions. Biol. Reprod., *45:*404–410, 1991.
23. Amann, R.P.: A critical review of methods for evaluation of spermatogenesis from seminal characteristics. J. Androl., *2:*37–58, 1981.
24. Amann, R.P., Johnson, L., Thompson, D.L., Jr., and Pickett, B.W.: Daily spermatozoal production, epididymal spermatozoal reserves and transit time of spermatozoa through the epididymis of the Rhesus monkey. Biol. Reprod., *15:*586–592, 1976.
25. Berndtson, W.E.: Methods for quantifying mammalian spermatogenesis: A review. J. Anim. Sci., *44:*818–833, 1977.
26. Berndtson, W.E., Igboeli, G., and Parker, W.G.: The numbers of Sertoli cells in mature Holstein bulls and their relationship to quantitative aspects of spermatogenesis. Biol. Reprod., *37:*60–67, 1987.
27. Clermont, Y.: Kinetics of spermatogenesis in mammals: Seminiferous epithelium cycle and spermatogonial renewal. Physiol. Rev., *52:*198–236, 1972.
28. Courot, M., Hochereau-de Reviers, M.-T., and Ortavant, R.: Spermatogenesis. *In* The Testis. Vol. 1. Edited by A.D. Johnson, W.R. Gomes, and N.L. VanDemark. New York, Academic Press, 1970, pp. 339–342.
29. de Kresta, D.M., and Kerr, J.B.: The cytology of the testis. *In* The Physiology of Reproduction. Edited by E. Knobil and J. Neill. New York, Raven Press, 1988, pp. 837–932.
30. Hochereau-de Reviers, M.-T., Monet-Kuntz, C., and Courot, M.: Spermatogenesis and Sertoli cell numbers

and function in rams and bulls. J. Reprod. Fertil. Suppl., *34:*101–114, 1987.

31. Lok, D., Weenk, D., and De Rooij, D.G.: Morphology, proliferation, and differentiation of undifferentiated spermatogonia in the Chinese hamster and the ram. Anat. Rec., *203:*83–99, 1982.
32. Russell, L.D., and Peterson, R.N.: Determination of the elongate spermatid-Sertoli cell ratio in various mammals. J. Reprod. Fertil., *70:*635–641, 1984.
33. Tung, K.S.K., Teuscher, C., and Meng, A.L.: Autoimmunity to spermatozoa and testis. Immunol. Rev., *55:*217–255, 1981.
34. Bardin, C.W., Chang, C.Y., Musto, N.A., and Gunsalus, G.L.: The Sertoli cell. *In* The Physiology of Reproduction. Edited by E. Knobil and E. Neill. New York, Raven Press, 1988, pp. 933–974.
35. Purvis, K., and Hansson, V.: Hormonal regulation of spermatogenesis. Int. J. Androl. Suppl., *3:*81–143, 1981.
36. Wright, W.W.: Intragonadal control of testis function. *In* Medically Assisted Contraception. Washington, D.C., National Academy Press. 1989, pp. 191–210.
37. Belvé, A.R.: The molecular biology of mammalian spermatogenesis. Oxf. Rev. Reprod. Biol. *1:*159–261, 1979.
38. Amann, R.P., Thompson, D.L., Jr., Squires, E.L., and Pickett, B.W.: Effects of age and frequency of ejaculation on sperm production and extragonadal sperm reserves in stallions. J. Reprod. Fertil. Suppl., *27:*1–6, 1979.
39. Berndtson, W.E., Hoyer, J.H., Squires, E.L., and Pickett, B.W.: Influence of exogenous testosterone on sperm production, seminal quality and libido of stallions. J. Reprod. Fertil. Suppl., *27:*19–23, 1979.
40. Gebauer, M.R., Pickett, B.W., and Swierstra, E.E.: Reproductive physiology of the stallion. II. Daily production and output of sperm. J. Anim. Sci., *39:*732–736, 1974.
41. Courot, M., et al.: Endocrinology of spermatogenesis in the hypophysectomized ram. J. Reprod. Fertil. Suppl., *26:*165–173, 1979.
42. Ellery, J.C.: Spermatogenesis, accessory sex gland histology and the effects of seasonal change in the stallion. Ph.D. thesis. St. Paul, University of Minnesota, 1971.
43. Steinberger, E., and Steinberger, A.: Spermatogenic function of the testis. *In* Handbook of Physiology. Vol. 5. Section 7. Edited by D.W. Hamilton and R.O. Greep. Washington, D.C., American Physiology Society, 1975, pp. 1–19.
44. Hoyer, J.: The effect of testosterone on reproductive function in stallions. M.S. thesis. Fort Collins, Colorado State University, 1978.
45. Squires, E.L., Todter, G.E., Berndtson, W.E., and Pickett, B.W.: Effect of anabolic steroids on reproductive function in young stallions. J. Anim. Sci., *54:*576–582, 1982.
46. Johnson, L., and Thompson, D.L., Jr.: Effect of seasonal changes in Leydig cell number on the volume of smooth endoplasmic reticulum in Leydig cells and intratesticular testosterone content in stallions. J. Reprod. Fertil., *81:*227–232, 1987.
47. Clay, C.M.: Influences of season and artificial photoperiod on reproduction in stallions. Ph.D. thesis. Fort Collins, Colorado State University, 1988.
48. Berndtson, W.E., Desjardins, C., and Ewing, L.L.: Inhibition and maintenance of spermatogenesis in rats implanted with polydimethylsiloxane capsules containing various androgens. J. Endocrinol., *62:*125–135, 1974.
49. Amann, R.P., and Ganjam, V.K.: Effects of hemicastration or hCG-treatment on steroids in testicular vein and jugular vein blood of stallions. J. Androl., *2:*132–139, 1981.
50. Seamans, M.C., et al.: Gonadotrophin and steroid concentrations in jugular and testicular venous plasma in stallions before and after GnRH injection. J. Reprod. Fertil. Suppl., *44:*57–67, 1991.
51. Silberzahn, P., et al.: Testosterone response to human chorionic gonadotropin injection in the stallion. Equine Vet. J., *20:*61–63, 1988.
52. Bedrak, E., and Samuels, L.T.: Steroid biosynthesis by the equine testis. Endocrinology, *85:*1186–1195, 1969.
53. Gaillard, J.-L., and Silberzahn, P.: Aromatization of 19-norandrogens by equine testicular microsomes. J. Biol. Chem., *262:*5717–5722, 1987.
54. Ganjam, V.K.: Episodic nature of the Δ^4-ene and Δ^5-ene steroidogenic pathways and their relationship to the adrenogonadal axis in stallions. J. Reprod. Fertil. Suppl., *27:*67–71, 1979.
55. Lindner, H.R.: Androgens and related compounds in the spermatic vein blood of domestic animals. IV. Testicular androgens in the ram, boar and stallion. J. Endocrinol., *23:*171–178, 1961.
56. Raeside, J.I.: Seasonal changes in the concentration of estrogens and testosterone in the plasma of the stallion. Anim. Reprod. Sci., *1:*205–212, 1979.
57. Ewing, L., and Brown, B.L.: Testicular steroidogenesis. *In* The Testis. Vol. 4. Edited by A.D. Johnson and W.R. Gomes. New York, Academic Press, 1977, pp. 239–287.
58. Hall, P.F.: Testicular steroid synthesis: Organization and regulation. *In* The Physiology of Reproduction. Edited by E. Knobil and J. Neill. New York, Raven Press, New York, 1988, pp. 975–998.
59. Zirkin, B.R., Samfulli, R., Awoniyi, C.A., and Ewing, E.L.: Maintenance of advanced spermatogenic cells in the adult rat testis: Quantitative relationship to testosterone concentrations within the testis. Endocrinology, *124:*3043–3049, 1989.
60. Zirkin, B.R., Ewing, L.L., Kormann, N., and Cochran, R.C.: Testosterone secretion by rat, rabbit, guinea-pig, dog, and hamster testes perfused in vitro: Correlation with Leydig cell ultrastructure. Endocrinology, *107:* 1867–1874, 1980.
61. Lopez, M.L., de Souza, W., and Bustos-Obregon, E.: Cytochemical analysis of the anionic sites on the membrane of the stallion spermatozoa during the epididymal transit. Gamete Res., *18:*319–332, 1987.
62. Amann, R.P.: Function of the epididymis in bulls and rams. J. Reprod. Fertil. Suppl., *34:*115–131, 1987.
63. Amann, R.P.: Maturation of spermatozoa. Proceedings of the International Congress of Animal Reproduction and Artificial Insemination. Vol. 5. Dublin, 1988, pp. 320–328.
64. Hamilton, D.W.: Structure and function of the epithelium lining the ductuli efferentes, ductus epididymidis, and ductus deferens in the rat. *In* Handbook of Physiology. Vol. 5. Section 7. Edited by D.W. Hamilton and R.O. Greep. Washington, D.C., American Physiology Society, 1975, pp. 259–301.
65. Orgebin-Crist, M.-C., Danzo, B.J., and Davies, J.: Endocrine control of the development and maintenance of sperm fertilizing ability in the epididymis. *In* Handbook of Physiology. Vol. 5. Section 7. Edited by D.W. Hamilton and R.O. Greep. Washington, D.C., American Physiology Society, 1975, pp. 319–338.
66. Robaire, B., and Hermo, L.: Efferent ducts, epididymis, and vas deferens: Structure, functions, and their regula-

tion. *In* The Physiology of Reproduction. Edited by E. Knobil and J. Neill. New York, Raven Press, 1988, pp. 999–1080.

67. Glover, T.D., and Nicander, L.: Some aspects of structure and function in the mammalian epididymis. J. Reprod. Fertil. Suppl., *13:*39–50, 1971.

68. Cooper, T.G.: The Epididymis, Sperm Maturation and Fertilization. Berlin, Springer-Verlag, 1986.

69. Nicander, L.: Studies on the regional histology and cytochemistry of the ductus epididymis in stallions, rams and bulls. Acta Morphol. Neerl. Scand., *1:*337–362, 1957.

70. Barker, C.A.V., and Gandier, J.C.C.: Pregnancy in a mare resulting from frozen epididymal spermatozoa. Can. J. Comp. Med. Vet. Sci., *21:*47–51, 1957.

71. Gebauer, M.R., Pickett, B.W., and Swierstra, E.E.: Reproductive physiology of the stallion. III. Extra-gonadal transit time and sperm reserves. J. Anim. Sci., *39:*737–742, 1974.

72. Almquist, J.O., Hale, E.B., and Amann, R.P.: Sperm production and fertility of dairy bulls at high collection frequencies with varying degrees of sexual preparation. J. Dairy Sci., *41:*733, 1958.

73. Hafs, H.D., Hoyt, R.S., and Bratton, R.W.: Libido, sperm characteristics, sperm output, and fertility of mature dairy bulls ejaculated daily or weekly for thirty-two weeks. J. Dairy Sci., *42:*626–636, 1959.

74. Martig, R.C., and Almquist, J.O.: Reproductive capacity of beef bulls. III. Postpuberal changes in fertility and sperm morphology at different ejaculation frequencies. J. Anim. Sci., *28:*375–378, 1969.

75. Martig, R.C., Almquist, J.O., and Foster, J.: Reproductive capacity of beef bulls. V. Fertility and freezability of successive ejaculates collected by different methods. J. Anim. Sci., *30:*60–62, 1978.

76. Amann, R.P., Kavanaugh, J.F., Griel, L.C., Jr., and Voglmayr, J.K.: Sperm production of Holstein bulls determined from testicular spermatid reserves, after cannulation of rete testis or vas deferens, and by daily ejaculation. J. Dairy Sci., *57:*93–99, 1974.

77. Lino, B.F., and Braden, A.W.H.: The output of spermatozoa in rams. I. Relationship with testicular output of spermatozoa and the effect of ejaculations. Aust. J. Biol. Sci., *25:*351–358, 1972.

78. Thompson, D.L., Jr., Pickett, B.W., Squires, E.L., and Nett, T.M.: Effect of testosterone and estradiol-17β alone and in combination on LH and FSH concentrations in blood serum and pituitary of geldings and in serum after administration of GnRH. Biol. Reprod., *21:*1231–1237, 1979.

79. Mann, T., and Lutwak-Mann, C.: Male Reproductive Function and Semen. Berlin, Springer-Verlag, 1981.

80. Cupps, P.T.: Reproduction in Domestic Animals. 4th ed. New York, Academic Press, 1991.

81. Waites, G.M.H., and Setchell, B.P.: Physiology of the testis. *In* Marshall's Physiology of Reproduction. 4th ed. Edited by G.E. Lamming. London, Churchill Livingstone, 1981, pp. 1–105.

82. Clay, C.M., Squires, E.L., Amann, R.P., and Nett, T.M.: Influences of season and artificial photoperiod on stallions: Luteinizing hormone, follicle stimulating hormone and testosterone. J. Anim. Sci., *66:*1246–1255, 1988.

83. Irvine, C.H.G., Alexander, S.L., and Turner, J.E.: Seasonal variation in the feedback of sex steroid hormones on serum LH concentrations in the male horse. J. Reprod. Fertil., *76:*221–230, 1986.

84. Thompson, D.L., Jr., Johnson, L., St. George, R.L., and Garza, F., Jr.: Concentrations of prolactin, luteinizing hormone and follicle stimulating hormone in pituitary and serum of horses: Effect of sex, season and reproductive state. J. Anim. Sci., *63:*854–860. 1986.

85. Thompson, D.L., Jr., St. George, R.L., Jones, L.S., and Garza, F., Jr.: Patterns of secretion of luteinizing hormone, follicle stimulating hormone and testosterone in stallions during the summer and winter. J. Anim. Sci., *60:*741–748, 1985.

86. Clay, C.M., Squires, E.L., Amann, R.P., and Nett, T.M.: Influences of season and artificial photoperiod on stallions: Pituitary and testicular responses to exogenous GnRH. J. Anim. Sci., *67:*763–770, 1988.

87. Irvine, C.H.G., Alexander, S.L., and Hughes, J.P.: Sexual behavior and serum concentrations of reproductive hormones in normal stallions. Theriogenology, *23:*607–617, 1985.

88. Naden, J., Amann, R.P., and Squires, E.L.: Testicular growth, hormone concentrations, seminal characteristics and sexual behavior in stallions. J. Reprod. Fertil., *88:*167–176, 1990.

89. Naden, J., Squires, E.L., Nett, T.M., and Amann, R.P.: Effect of maternal treatment with altrenogest on pituitary response to exogenous GnRH in pubertal stallions. J. Reprod. Fertil., *88:*177–183, 1990.

90. Squires, E.L., et al.: Effect of ejaculation on systemic levels of testosterone and LH in stallions. Proceedings of the Annual Meetings of the American Society of Animal Science. Madison, WI, 1977, p. 210.

91. Thompson, D.L., Jr., Pickett, B.W., and Nett, T.M.: Effect of season and artificial photoperiod on levels of estradiol-17β and estrone in blood serum of stallions. J. Anim. Sci., *47:*184–187, 1978.

92. Lacroix, A., Garnier, D.-H., and Pelletier, J.: Temporal fluctuations of plasma LH and testosterone in Charolais bull calves during the first year of life. Ann. Biol. Anim. Biochim. Biophys., *17:*1013–1019, 1977.

93. McCarthy, M.S., Convey, E.M., and Hafs, H.D.: Serum hormonal changes and testicular response to LH during puberty in bulls. Biol. Reprod., *20:*1221–1227, 1979.

94. Bardin, C.W.: Inhibin structure and function in the male. Ann. N. Y. Acad. Sci., *564:*102–123, 1989.

95. Pickering, B.T., et al.: Oxytocin in the testis: What, where and why? Ann. N. Y. Acad. Sci., *564:*198, 1989.

96. Knickerbocker, J.J., et al.: Evidence for the presence of oxytocin in the ovine epididymis. Biol. Reprod., *39:*391–397, 1988.

97. Veeramachaneni, D.N.R., and Amann, R.P.: Oxytocin in the ovine ductuli efferentes and caput epididymides: Immunolocalization and evidence for receptor-mediated endocytosis. Endocrinology, *126:*1156–1164, 1990.

98. Garcia, F., Jr., et al.: Active immunization of intact mares against gonadotropin releasing hormone: Differential effects on secretion of luteinizing hormone and follicle stimulating hormone. Biol. Reprod., *35:*347–352, 1986.

99. Courot, M.: The effects of gonadotrophins on testicular function (spermatogenesis). Proceedings of the International Congress on Animal Reproduction and Artificial Insemination. Vol. 5. Dublin, 1988, pp. 311–319.

100. Bergin, W.C., Gier, H.T., Marion, G.B., and Coffman, J.R.: A developmental concept of equine cryptorchism. Biol. Reprod., *3:*82–92, 1970.

101. Gier, H.T., and Marion, G.B.: Development of the mammalian testis. *In* The Testis. Vol. 1. Edited by A.D. Johnson, W.R. Gomes and N.L. VanDemark. New York, Academic Press, 1970, pp. 1–45.

102. Stickle, R.L., and Fessler, J.F.: Retrospective study of 350 cases of equine cryptorchidism. J. Am. Vet. Med. Assoc., *172:*343–346, 1978.
103. Amann, R.P.: Endocrine changes associated with the onset of spermatogenesis in Holstein bulls. J. Dairy Sci., *66:*2606–2622, 1983.
104. Amann, R.P., and Schanbacher, B.D.: Physiology of male reproduction. J. Anim. Sci., *57*(Suppl. 2):380–403, 1983.
105. Amann, R.P., Wise, M.E., Glass, J.D., and Nett, T.M.: Prepubertal changes in the hypothalamic-pituitary axis of Holstein bulls. Biol. Reprod., *34:*71–80, 1986.
106. Robb, G.W., Amann, R.P., and Killian, G.J.: Daily sperm production and epididymal sperm reserves of pubertal and adult rats. J. Reprod. Fertil., *54:*103–107, 1978.
107. Curtis, S.K., and Amann, R.P.: Testicular development and establishment of spermatogenesis in Holstein bulls. J. Anim. Sci., *53:*1645–1657, 1981.
108. Glassneck, H.W.: Histometrische Untersuchungen uber die Entwicklung des Pferdehodens zwischen 1. und 18. Lebensmonat. DMV dissertation. Tierarztliche Hochschule Hannover, 1978.
109. Nishikawa, Y.: Studies on Reproduction in Horses. Tokyo, Japan Racing Association, 1959.
110. Cornwell, J.C., Hauer, E.P., Spillman, T.E., and Vincent, C.K.: Puberty in the Quarter Horse colt. J. Anim. Sci., *36:*1215, 1973.
111. Tischner, M., Kosiniak, K., and Bielanski, W.: Analysis of the pattern of ejaculation in stallions. J. Reprod. Fertil., *41:*329–335, 1974.

SECTION B

BREEDING MANAGEMENT

CHAPTER 78

FACTORS AFFECTING SPERM PRODUCTION AND OUTPUT

B.W. Pickett

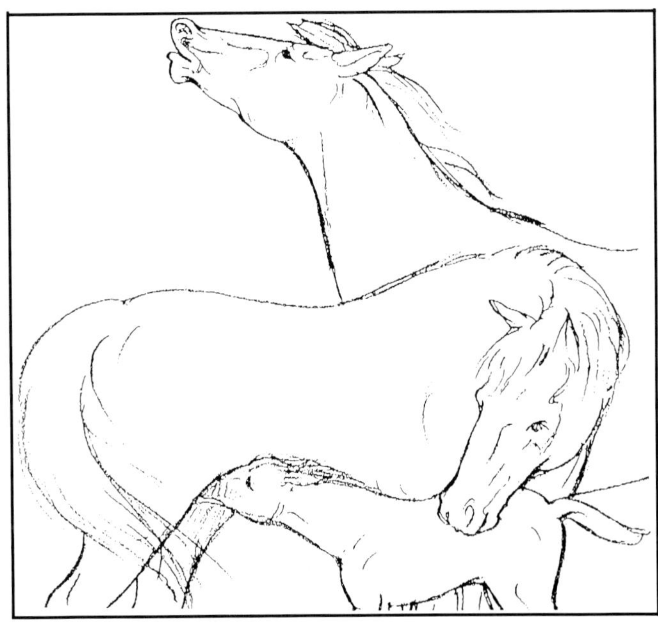

Principal factors determining sperm output are season, testicular size, age, and frequency of ejaculation. Although each factor will be discussed separately, they are so interrelated that the discussions will have some overlap. This should not be construed to mean these are the only factors that affect efficiency of sperm production; environmental factors, hormonal status, and drugs can also play important roles.

SEASON

Both the mare and stallion are seasonal breeders. Generally, changes in the stallion's seminal characteristics and sexual behavior, because of season, coincide with the natural breeding season of mares.[1-5] Estrus can be induced in anestrous mares by artificial lights.[2,6] From a practical standpoint, exposing dry mares to 16 h of light beginning about mid-December, stimulates them to establish a normal cycle earlier in the breeding season, resulting in earlier foals.[2,6] The effects of season on stallion seminal characteristics and sexual behavior have been reported.[7] However, effects of artificial light on reproductive function of the stallion have received far less attention.

SEASON AND SEMINAL CHARACTERISTICS

Studies were designed to determine effect of season on seminal characteristics so that a potential fertility evaluation could be conducted on a stallion any time of the year and the results related to the breeding season. Furthermore, stallion owners need this information to manage their stallion(s) for maximum reproductive efficiency.

First and second ejaculates of semen were collected with an artificial vagina (AV) from each of five aged Quarter Horse (QH) stallions each week from May of 1 yr through May of the next. The second ejaculate typically was collected 1 h after the first.

Presented in Figure 78–1 are monthly means of gel-free seminal volume. The average gel-free volume of first ejaculates was 58 mL, while that of second ejaculates was 50 mL. The volume of first ejaculates ranged from 45 mL in February to 81 mL in June. Second ejaculates varied from 42 mL in March to 63 mL in June. This was an increase of approximately 40% from the low months to the peak of the breeding season.

Total volume of first ejaculates averaged 66 mL. The range was from 45 mL in January to 104 mL in June. Second ejaculates averaged 52 mL, ranging from 42 mL in March to 68 mL in June (Fig. 78–2). Total seminal volume was greatly influenced by season, but most of the difference between first and second ejaculates was the result of the greater volume of gel in first ejaculates.

The mean number of spermatozoa per first ejaculate was 15 billion and ranged from 10 billion in January to 22 billion in July. Second ejaculates averaged 8 billion and ranged from 5 billion in December to 12 billion in

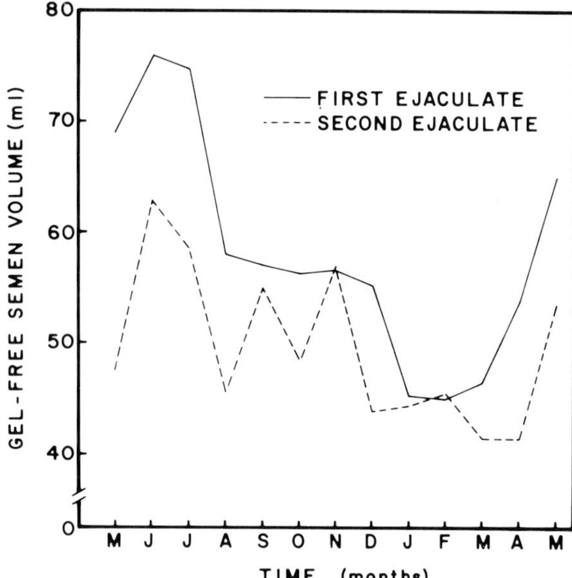

FIG. 78–1. Effect of season on gel-free seminal volume. Data for first ejaculates are represented by the solid line and second ejaculates, collected 1 h later, are represented by the dashed line. (Adapted from Pickett, B.W., et al.: Reproductive physiology of the stallion. VI. Seminal and behavioral characteristics. J. Anim. Sci., *43:*617–625, 1976.)

July (Fig. 78–3). Because the five stallions were collected each Tuesday, these sperm numbers represent several days' production. Sperm output during the lowest months was approximately 50% of the higher month's output (50 and 39% for first and second ejaculates, respectively). This dramatic seasonal decrease in sperm output reflected a decrease in spermatogenesis.

Remember that when the breeding season starts (February), stallion managers are working with a stallion that is producing only 50% of the spermatozoa he will produce in May. A stallion, whose mares are presented early in the breeding season, may have more difficulty settling them than when his mares are presented later in the season. If the stallion is normal the number of mares in an artificial insemination (AI) program and the frequency of ejaculation in natural service will be the principal factors determining fertility early in the season. The difference in sperm output between first and second ejaculates, collected approximately 1 h apart, was 54.7%. This relationship is important in the potential fertility evaluation of stallions and in determining the intervals at which a stallion may be used per day.

Because the data presented in Figure 78–3 are from stallions collected twice a week, the number of spermatozoa per first ejaculates does not represent what happens under practical conditions. Therefore, single ejaculates were collected daily for 10 weeks from two groups of mature stallions (Fig. 78–4). Group I consisted of four Quarter Horse (QH) stallions, and group II, of one Thoroughbred (TB) and six QH stallions. Seminal collections of group I stallions began April 27 and ended June 4. Because daily sperm output (DSO) may not have peaked on June 4, when the experiment had to be terminated, the study was repeated the following year. Seminal collections from stallions in group II were obtained daily from April 24 to July 2.[8]

Large numbers of spermatozoa were obtained during the first few days of daily collections. The number of spermatozoa collected per ejaculate stabilized by days 5 to 7 of the collections and for the following week varied between 2.6 and 3.6 billion.[8] The range in DSO averaged 3.2 to 6.6 billion (mean 4.8 billion) and 3.3 to 5.8 billion (mean 4.3 billion) during daily collections for 10 weeks from stallions in groups I and II, respectively. The first seven ejaculates averaged 5.3 billion spermatozoa per ejaculate in both studies. This difference of approximately 2 billion spermatozoa per ejaculate between the first and second weeks was because epididymal sperm reserves became depleted the second week. After a stallion has had several days of sexual rest, he can breed a larger number of mares per day for a few days until his sperm reserves are again depleted.[9] From these data, the researchers concluded that sperm output is seasonal.[8,10,11]

PHOTOPERIOD AND SEASON

It has been amply demonstrated that certain seminal and hormonal characteristics, and many aspects of sexual behavior, are affected by season. Because humans have imposed an artificial breeding period on domesticated horses, clinicians sometimes find it desirable to al-

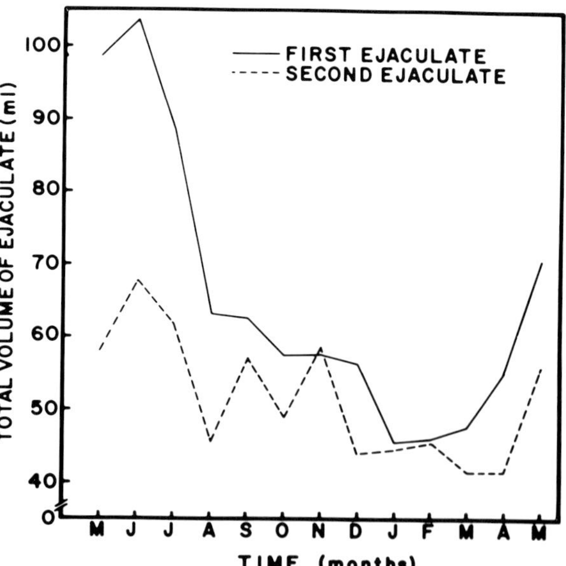

FIG. 78–2. Effect of season on total seminal volume by month. First ejaculate, solid line; second ejaculate, dashed line. (Adapted from Pickett, B.W., et al.: Reproductive physiology of the stallion. VI. Seminal and behavioral characteristics. J. Anim. Sci., *43:*617–625, 1976.)

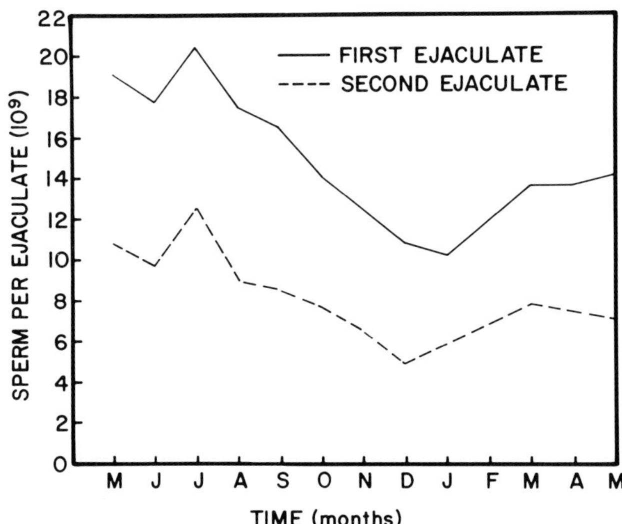

FIG. 78–3. Effect of season on mean number of spermatozoa per ejaculate (billions). First ejaculate, solid line; second ejaculate, dashed line. (Adapted from Pickett, B.W., et al.: Reproductive physiology of the stallion. VI. Seminal and behavioral characteristics. J. Anim. Sci., *43:*617–625, 1976.)

ter the stallion's reproductive capacity to coincide with these demands. Therefore, the following are some basic concepts of photoperiodism that have been developed for other animals. An understanding of the concept of refractoriness is central to understanding circannual or seasonal rhythms in photoperiodic (seasonal breeding) animals such as the horse (see Chapter 19). In general, the term "refractory" is used to describe a condition in which an animal is no longer sensitive or responsive to some prior stimulus that initiated a response. With seasonal breeders, this prior stimulus can be long days or short days. For example, suppose response to artificial light is controlled by an internal trigger-firing mechanism. Thus a long day acts to pull the trigger and fire the mechanism(s) that sets into motion events leading to heightened reproductive capacity. However, after a period of time these events will cease as the animal enters a period of reproductive quiescence. Until the trigger is reset, no amount of pulling, i.e., continued exposure to long days, will fire the mechanism(s) again. This is the condition of photorefractoriness and is why alternating periods of short and long days are essential. However, a further complication is that circannual rhythms in seasonal breeders are often endogenous, i.e., they are set internally. Therefore, the seasonal cycle will be expressed in the absence of changes in day length, but the changes in day length act to synchronize the cycle.

Photosensitive animals can be classified according to the concepts of refractoriness. Long-day breeders, such as the stallion, often are classified into two categories: scotorefractory and photorefractory. The term "scotorefractory" describes animals in which spontaneous gonadal recrudescence occurs when the animal is maintained continuously in inhibitory photoperiods. This means that short days followed by re-exposure to long days (stimulatory photoperiods) are required to abolish this refractory state. The term "photorefractory" describes animals in which spontaneous gonadal regression occurs as a result of continuous, prolonged exposure to stimulatory photoperiods. In this case, long days followed by re-exposure to short days are necessary to abolish this photorefractoriness and sensitize the animal so that exposure to long days will result in gonadal recrudescence.

With these concepts in mind, an experiment was conducted to determine: (1) if stallions maintained continuously in long days will become photorefractory and (2) if stallions maintained in long or short days will continue to exhibit a seasonal reproductive cycle.[12] A total of 21 stallions of light horse breeds, 4 to 15 yr old, was assigned to one of three treatments (7 per group): (1) controls, exposed to natural day length; (2) S-L, exposed to 8 h light and 16 h dark (8:16) for 20 weeks beginning July 16, 1982, then switched to 16:8 on December 2, 1982, and exposed to 16:8 until March 1984; (3) S-S, exposed to an 8:16 photoperiod from July 16, 1982, until March 1984 (Fig. 78–5). Before July 16, 1982, all stallions were housed in a nonlighted barn. On July 15, 1982, the 14 stallions in groups S-L and S-S were moved to a barn containing two separate lightproof areas in which photoperiod could be controlled independently. Each stall was illuminated by two 300-W incandescent bulbs. The 7 control stallions remained in the original barn and were exposed to natural day length. Temperature was not controlled, but it was measured and was similar for all three groups. Total scrotal width was measured every 4 weeks by two technicians three times each.

Semen was collected during 10 collection periods: June, September, and November 1982, February, April, June, August, October, and December 1983, and Febru-

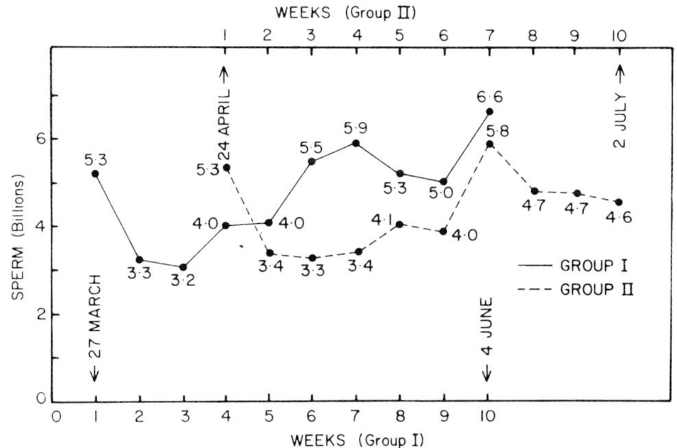

FIG. 78–4. Average daily sperm output from two groups of stallions over a 10-week period. Group I, solid line; group II, dashed line. (Adapted from Sullivan, J.J., and Pickett, B.W.: Influence of ejaculation frequency of stallions on characteristics of semen and output of spermatozoa. J. Reprod. Fertil. Suppl., *23:*29–34, 1975.)

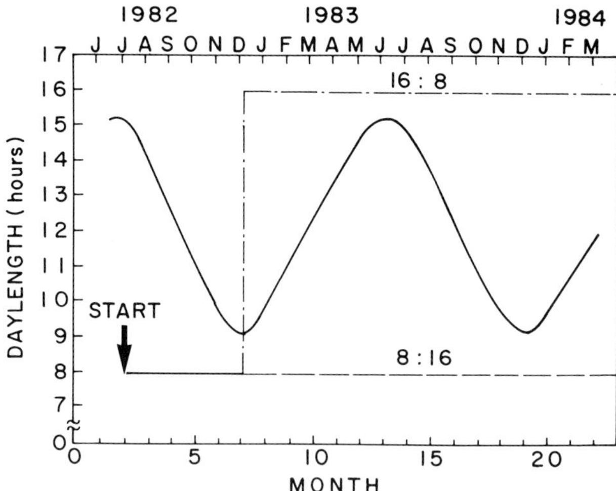

FIG. 78–5. Experimental design for study on effects of photoperiod on seminal and hormonal characteristics. Solid line indicates natural photoperiod, 16:8 indicates 16 h of light and 8 h of dark, 8:16 indicates 8 h of light and 16 h of dark. (From Clay, C.M., Squires, E.L., Amann, R.P., and Pickett, B.W.: Influences of season and artificial photoperiod on stallions: Testicular size, seminal characteristics and sexual behavior. J. Anim. Sci., *64:*517–525, 1987.)

ary 1984. For each period, seven ejaculates were collected to deplete extra-gonadal sperm reserves, then an additional nine ejaculates to assess daily sperm output. Each ejaculate was evaluated for gel volume, gel-free seminal volume, sperm concentration (millions) per milliliter of gel-free semen, sperm per ejaculate (billions), pH of gel-free semen, and percentage of progressively motile spermatozoa. On each of the last 9 collection days, sexual behavior of stallions was assessed by timing intervals: (1) to erection, (2) to first mount with an erection and intromission, and (3) from erection to ejaculation. The number of mounts per ejaculation was also recorded.

The exposure of S-L and S-S stallions to an 8:16 photoperiod in July did not hasten the normal seasonal regression of testicular size (Fig. 78–6). However, the S-L stallions responded to the stimulatory 16:8 photoperiod with an increase in total scrotal width so that by February they had significantly larger ($p < 0.05$) testes than either the control or S-S stallions. This trend continued through March. Thereafter, testicular size of S-L stallions regressed, which was presumably a consequence of photorefractoriness. A photorefractory state was also likely responsible for regression in testicular size exhibited by control stallions in mid- to late summer. The annual fluctuation of testicular size was similar in S-S and control stallions.

During June (pretreatment), sperm output averaged 6.4, 7.8, and 6.8 billion per day ($p > 0.05$) for control, S-L, and S-S stallions, respectively (Fig. 78–7). By September, sperm output was lower than in June for all groups, and means for all groups were similar (4.9 billion, 4.0 billion, and 4.1 billion; $p > 0.05$). As for testicular size, annual fluctuation in sperm output for S-S stallions was similar to that for controls. Within 2 months after switching S-L stallions to the 16:8 photoperiod, their sperm output (10.4 billion) was greater ($p < 0.05$) than that for controls (7.1 billion) and S-S stallions (6.0 billion). Thus, by exposing S-L stallions to short days then an increased day length, the researchers were able to hasten testicular recrudescence so that maximum sperm output occurred at least 2 months earlier than in control stallions. The increase in sperm output exhibited by S-L stallions occurred virtually coincident with an increase in testicular size. The continued exposure of S-L stallions to a 16:8 photoperiod did not prolong the cycle, and regression occurred, albeit somewhat earlier than in the other two groups. This observation supports the conclusion that induction of earlier sexual recrudescence in the stallion might result in an earlier regression.[13]

These data clearly demonstrate a stimulatory effect of increased day length, following 20 weeks of short days, on testicular size and daily sperm output of stallions. However, normal seasonal recrudescence, as exhibited by control stallions, did not appear to be initiated by long days. This is because recrudescence, leading to peak reproductive capacity in early summer or late spring, appeared to be initiated during the fall when day length was declining. In this experiment, the nadir in sperm output occurred in September to October and gradually increased until May or June.

Because testicular size and sperm output eventually decreased, stallions seemed to become photorefractory in a manner analogous to that described for birds.[14] Based on this observation, photostimulation at, or after, the summer solstice would not likely be effective in

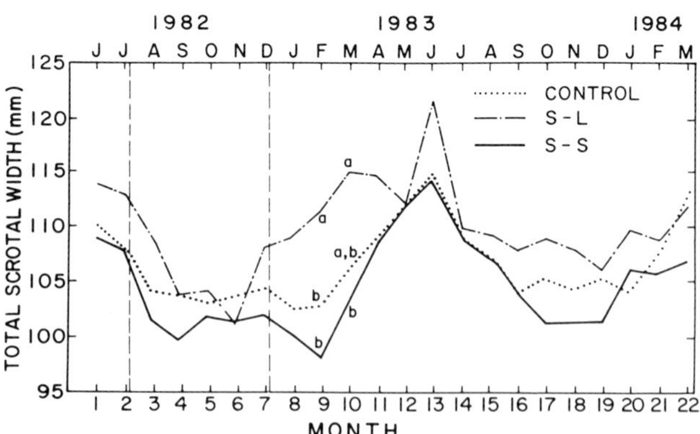

FIG. 78–6. Effect of photoperiod on total scrotal width of stallions exposed to natural day length (dotted line). S-L = 8 h of light and 18 h of dark from July 16, 1982, to December 2, 1982, then exposed to 16:8 until March 1984 (dashed and dotted line); S-S = exposed to an 8:16 photoperiod from July 16, 1982, until March 1984 (solid line). The points with different letters represent significant differences. (From Clay, C.M., Squires, E.L., Amann, R.P., and Pickett, B.W.: Influences of season and artificial photoperiod on stallions: Testicular size, seminal characteristics and sexual behavior. J. Anim. Sci., *64:*517–525, 1987.)

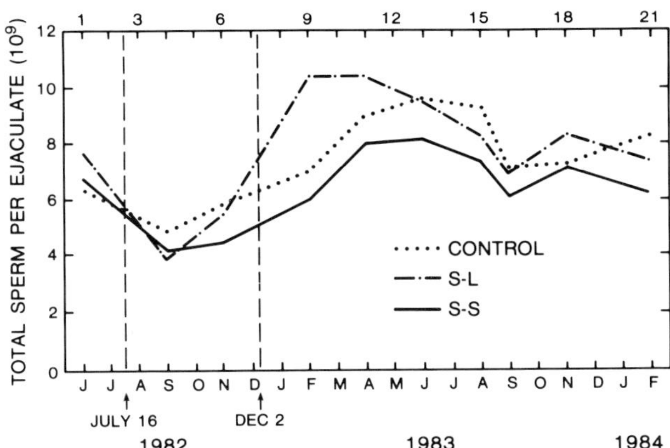

FIG. 78–7. Effect of photoperiod on sperm output. Control, dotted line; S-L, dashed and dotted line; S-S, solid line. (Adapted from Clay, C.M., Squires, E.L., Amann, R.P., and Pickett, B.W.: Influences of season and artificial photoperiod on stallions: Testicular size, seminal characteristics and sexual behavior. J. Anim. Sci., *64:*517–525, 1987.)

prolonging heightened reproductive function or delaying testicular regression. The normal, physiologic role of short days during the fall may not be to terminate the breeding season but rather to abolish a refractory condition and re-establish a mechanism whereby the stallion will again be sensitive to increasing day length or long days. Thus, termination of photorefractoriness allows subsequent photoinduction.

Gel-free seminal volume was lower ($p < 0.05$) for S-L and S-S stallions during November 1982 and February and June 1983 (Fig. 78–8) compared with controls. The reason for consistently lower seminal volumes in ejaculates of treated stallions is not known. The clinician should recognize, however, that other factors, such as sexual stimulation, may influence ejaculate volume. Furthermore, low seminal volume is not necessarily indicative of depressed or enhanced reproductive capacity, because during February, S-L stallions had a higher sperm output than control stallions yet mean gel-free seminal volume of ejaculates of S-L stallions was 36 mL compared with 50 mL for controls. Once again, this is evidence of the relative unimportance of seminal volume as an indicator of reproductive function. The percentage of progressively motile spermatozoa was not affected by treatment ($p > 0.05$) nor did it fluctuate with season (Fig. 78–9).

Although not significant, a trend toward a shorter time interval to erection for S-L stallions in March and May was noted (Fig. 78–10). A similar trend was noted for the mean time required to mount an estrous mare. Furthermore, total time to ejaculation was reduced ($p < 0.05$) for S-L stallions in both March and May compared with control or S-S stallions. When compared with control stallions, a reduction ($p < 0.05$) in number of mounts per ejaculation in March was observed (Fig. 78–10). Whether this reduction was actually caused by photostimulation is not clear, because this group was not different ($p > 0.05$) from S-S stallions, and in general, control stallions required more mounts to ejaculate than either S-S or S-L stallions. In any event, note that the improvement in libido, as assessed by a reduced time to ejaculation, was a result of photostimulation. The researchers concluded that stallions possess an endogenous circannual rhythm for which changes in day length act only as the primary synchronizer. Thus, in the absence of photoperiodic changes, the endogenous cycle still is manifested. Without annual synchronization by short days, this annual cycle would probably "free-run" eventually, resulting in a drift of the annual interval of maximum reproductive potential.[15]

Manipulation of photoperiod apparently could be used to increase reproductive capacity and sexual behavior of stallions early in the year. This would require exposure to a period of 8-h days before exposure to long days. In this experiment, a period of 20 weeks of 8-h days was used, although a shorter period may have been adequate.

Increasing day length can be used to maximize reproductive efficiency early in the breeding season (February to April). Exposure of stallions to 16 h of light and 8 h of dark starting in mid- to late December in northern latitudes and maintaining them on this photoperiod until natural day length approximates 16 h (early June) will provide maximum stimulation. For this procedure to be effective, the stallions must be allowed to be exposed to the decreasing day lengths of fall, because stallions, like most seasonal breeders, require alternating periods of long and short days for proper synchronization of circannual cycles. In addition, the farm managers must decide whether this schedule fits their particular breeding program. If the majority of mares are to be bred between February and June, then a lighting program may be suitable. If, however, mares are going to be bred in the late spring or early summer, a lighting program will be unsatisfactory and the stallions should

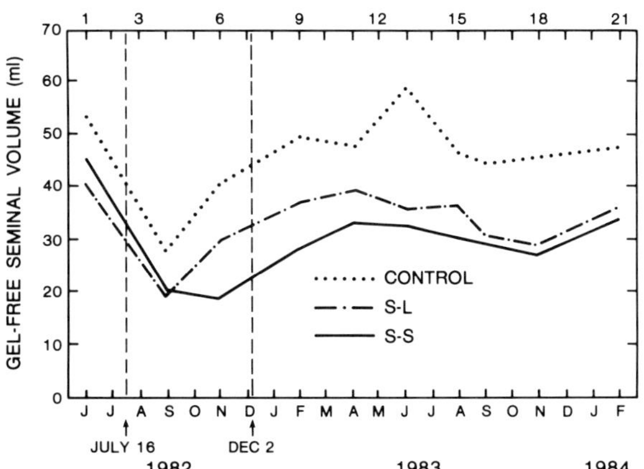

FIG. 78–8. Effect of photoperiod on gel-free seminal volume. Control, dotted line; S-L, dashed and dotted line; S-S, solid line. (Adapted from Clay, C.M., Squires, E.L., Amann, R.P., and Pickett, B.W.: Influences of season and artificial photoperiod on stallions: Testicular size, seminal characteristics and sexual behavior. J. Anim. Sci., *64:*517–525, 1987.)

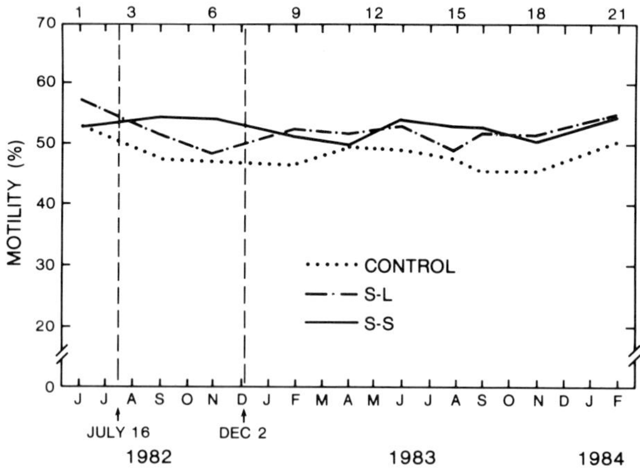

FIG. 78–9. Effect of photoperiod on stallion sperm motility. Control, dotted line; S-L, dashed and dotted line; S-S, solid line. (Adapted from Clay, C.M., Squires, E.L., Amann, R.P., and Pickett, B.W.: Influences of season and artificial photoperiod on stallions: Testicular size, seminal characteristics and sexual behavior. J. Anim. Sci., *64*:517–525, 1987.)

be allowed to cycle normally. Exposure of stallions to an artificial photoperiod in late winter and early spring will result in peaking of the breeding season earlier in the year.

TESTICULAR SIZE

Daily sperm production (DSP) is the number of spermatozoa produced per day by the testes. Daily sperm output (DSO) is the number of spermatozoa harvested per day, after extra-gonadal sperm reserves have been depleted, expressed on a per day basis. The efficiency of sperm production is the number of spermatozoa produced per day per gram of testicular tissue.[16]

The number of spermatozoa that an animal can produce depends largely on the amount of functional testicular tissue. Testicular size is an important factor in selecting and managing a stallion for maximum reproductive efficiency, assuming testicular consistency is satisfactory. Testicular measurements can be used to estimate sperm production and output, to identify individual stallions with a potentially high or low output, and perhaps to enable the prediction of how many mares can be bred under natural or AI management programs.

MEASURING THE TESTES

Testicular measurements are made from the left side of the horse with a pair of calipers (Fig. 78–11). Both testes are forced down into the scrotum with the left hand (Fig. 78–12). The calipers are positioned on the left and right sides of the scrotum so as to span the distance between the greatest curvatures of the left and right testes. The greatest curvature of the right testis is located with the little finger, and the greatest curvature of the left testis is determined visually (Fig. 78–13). The distance between the two points is total scrotal width (TSW). A certain amount of replication is obviously necessary to obtain an accurate estimate of testicular size. Therefore, to minimize error, at least three independent measurements should be taken by one individual, and these measurements should be averaged to obtain a value for TSW.

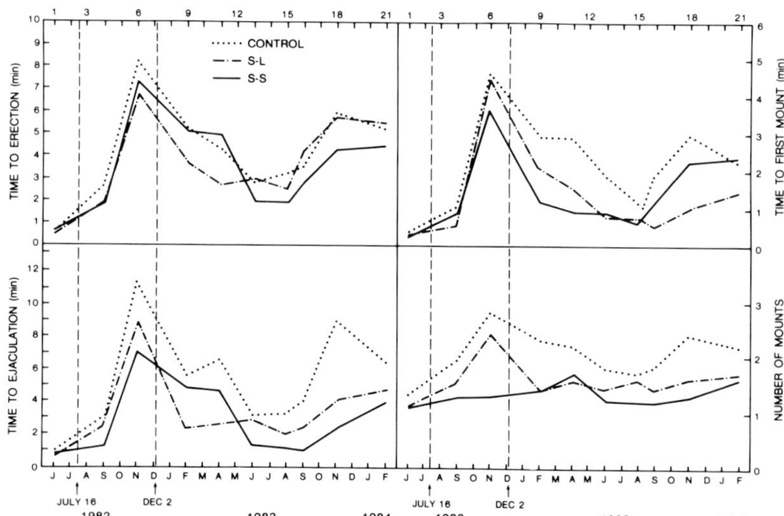

FIG. 78–10. Effect of photoperiod on sexual behavior of stallions. Control, dotted line; S-L, dashed and dotted line; S-S, solid line. (Adapted from Clay, C.M., Squires, E.L., Amann, R.P., and Pickett, B.W.: Influences of season and artificial photoperiod on stallions: Testicular size, seminal characteristics and sexual behavior. J. Anim. Sci., *64*:517–525, 1987.)

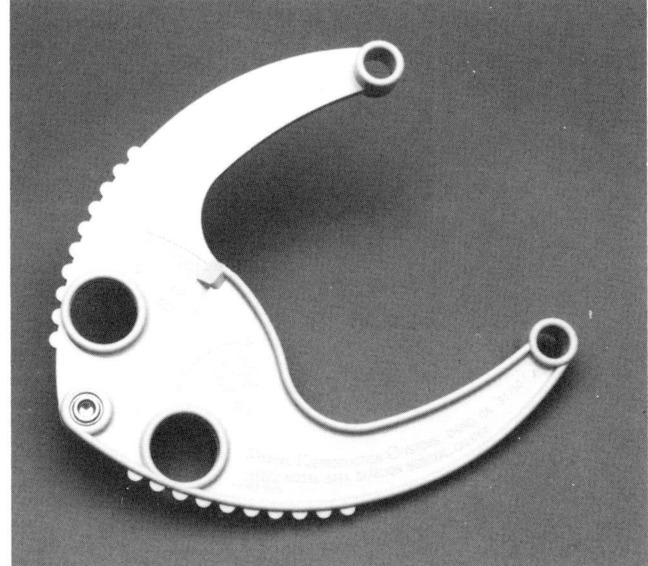

FIG. 78–11. Calipers used at our laboratory to measure total scrotal width to the nearest millimeter. (From Pickett, B.W., et al.: Management of the Stallion for Maximum Reproductive Efficiency. II. Animal Reproduction Laboratory Bulletin No. 05. Fort Collins, Colorado State University, 1989.)

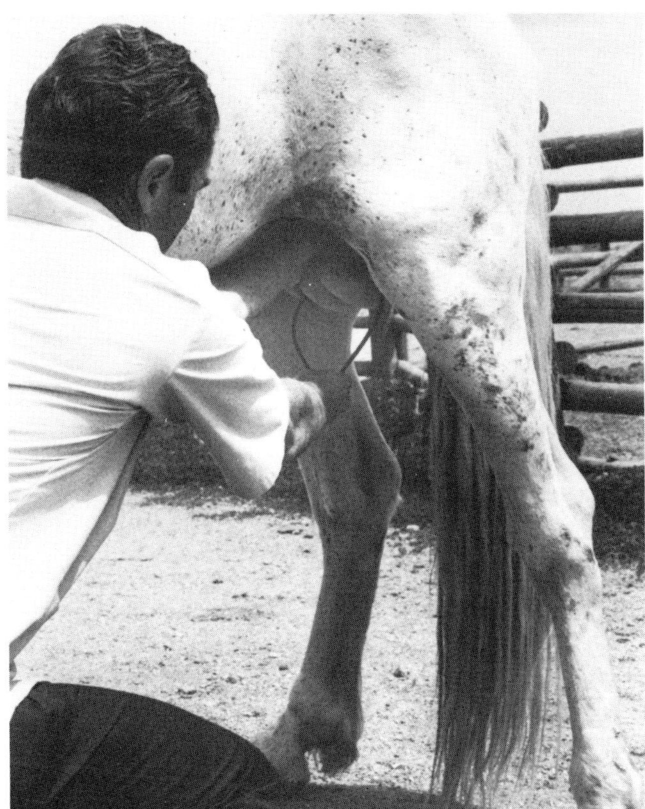

FIG. 78–12. Positioning the testes for measurement of total scrotal width. (From Pickett, B.W., et al.: Management of the Stallion for Maximum Reproductive Efficiency. II. Animal Reproduction Laboratory Bulletin No. 05. Fort Collins, Colorado State University, 1989.)

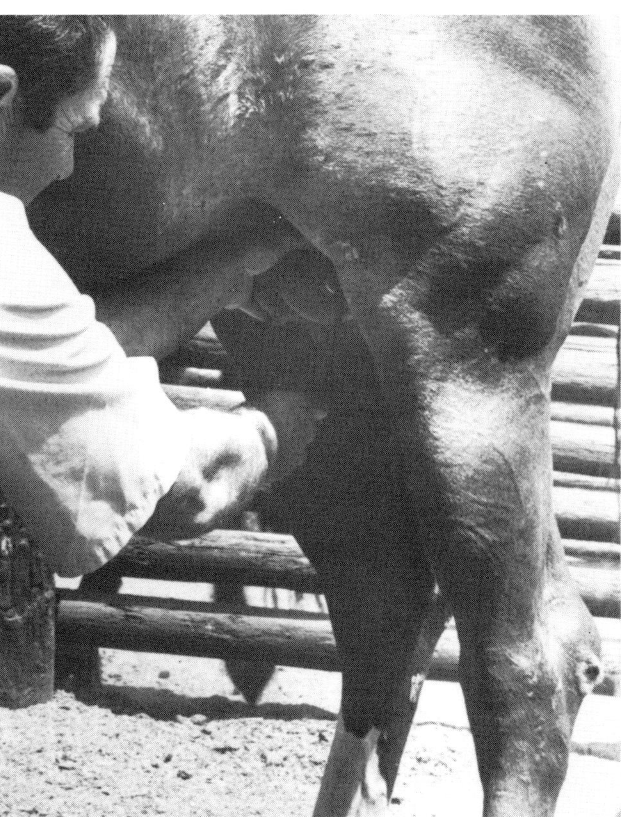

FIG. 78–13. Measuring total scrotal width of a stallion. (From Pickett, B.W., et al.: Management of the Stallion for Maximum Reproductive Efficiency. II. Animal Reproduction Laboratory Bulletin No. 05. Fort Collins, Colorado State University, 1989.)

REPRODUCTIVE CHARACTERISTICS RELATED TO TESTICULAR SIZE

Forty-three clinically normal stallions of light horse breeds, aged 2 to 16, were used in a study conducted at Colorado State University.[17] The TSW and the width and length of each testis were measured with calipers five times by each of two technicians on each of 6 days. Immediately after removal at castration, each testis was weighed; the tunica albuginea was removed, cleaned, and weighed; and the parenchyma weight was determined by difference. Daily sperm production was determined from analyses of testicular parenchyma.[18] Presented in Table 78–1 are average testicular measurements as well as means of other reproductive characteristics. Average TSW for all stallions, across age, was 102 mm.

The correlation coefficients among testicular measurements, parenchymal weight, DSP, and DSO (Table 78–1) are presented in Table 78–2. These values provide an estimate of the relationship between two variables. For example, the highest correlation coefficient was found between scrotal width and parenchymal weight ($r = 0.83$). This means that TSW accounted for 69% ($0.83 \times 0.83 \times 100$) of the variation in weight of

TABLE 78–1. REPRODUCTIVE CHARACTERISTICS OF STALLIONS*

CHARACTERISTICS	MEAN†
Measurement (mm)	
Total scrotal width	102±9.9
Left width	58±5.2
Right width	56±5.8
Left length	103±8.2
Right length	108±8.0
Parenchyma weight, paired (g)	328±104
Daily sperm	
Production (10^9)	4.55±1.46
Output (10^9)	3.35±1.41

*$n = 43$.

†Means are presented plus or minus standard deviation.

(Adapted from Thompson, D.L., Jr., Pickett, B.W., Squires, E.L., and Amann, R.P.: Testicular measurements and reproductive characteristics in stallions. J. Reprod. Fertil. Suppl., *27*:13–17, 1979.)

the testes. In addition, TSW accounted for approximately 55% of the variation in daily sperm production. Therefore, measurement of length and width of the individual testis contributed little additional information. Consequently, TSW is the only testicular measurement normally taken at our laboratory during a potential fertility examination.

The most useful application of measuring TSW is for predicting DSP in the intact animal. Because testicular size is highly heritable in other species,[19] stallions with a scrotal width of two standard deviations less than the mean value reported in Table 78–1 should not be used for breeding, if maximum reproductive capacity is a desirable characteristic to promote within a breed. Although TSW accounted for only 39% of the variation in DSO and it was not an accurate approach to estimate DSO (Table 78–2), in certain cases a general estimate of DSO may be useful. If semen is collected daily for 1 week or every other day for 2 weeks, DSO can be estimated to within ± 40%. The choice of technique to estimate DSO depends on the relative accuracy with which the estimate must be known and the amount of time and labor available for the estimate.

A small study was conducted to compare DSO of a stallion (Herb) with large testes (137 mm) and a stallion (BJ) with small testes (79 mm).[11] Semen was collected from each stallion at a frequency of six times per week for 1 month (Table 78–3). Sperm output for Herb was 20.7 billion per ejaculate for the first 6 days, while extragonadal reserves (EGR) were being depleted. During the following 3 weeks, weekly means were 12.9, 12.0, and 11.7 for a DSO of approximately 12 billion spermatozoa. Assuming that 500 million motile spermatozoa are needed per natural cover, how many mares could Herb breed? If 50% of the spermatozoa ejaculated were progressively motile—a conservative estimate—Herb was ejaculating sufficient spermatozoa to impregnate 12 mares per day in natural service. Obviously this is no problem with AI, but impossible under natural conditions, even if the covers were equally distributed (every 2 h) throughout the day. Therefore, in Herb's case, sex drive becomes the limiting factor in number of mares that can be bred in a natural breeding program. If 100 million motile spermatozoa were used in an AI program, Herb ejaculated sufficient spermatozoa to inseminate 60 mares per day, or approximately 120 on an every-other-day collection schedule.[20] On the other hand, BJ ejaculated 5.9 billion spermatozoa per ejaculate during week 1 of collection, which decreased to a DSO of 1.8 billion in week 4. His DSO was so low by week 4 that BJ could impregnate less than two mares per day naturally or with AI, using 500 million motile spermatozoa. When BJ was castrated and the testes were examined histologically, the testicular tissue was only 58% efficient, which was consistent with his low daily sperm output. Many stud managers believe that volume of ejaculate is important in fertility. However, little difference in volume ejaculated existed between Herb and BJ. Therefore, volume is not an important consideration in fertility of the stallion.[20]

Testicular size is highly heritable in bulls (65% or more). Therefore, if a stallion is presented to our laboratory with a TSW of 80 mm or less, he will not be approved as a sound breeder even though his seminal characteristics are normal, because the condition (hypoplasia) may be heritable and the stallion is a potentially poor producer of spermatozoa.

TESTICULAR CONSISTENCY

In addition to testicular size, consistency or tone of testicular tissue must be considered. Each testis is positioned between the thumb and fingers by pushing the opposite testis upward, and passing each testis through the thumb and fingers. Any abnormality of these structures should be recorded. If, upon palpation, the epididymis, particularly the tail, is found to be hard and small, some fibrosis probably has occurred, reducing the ca-

TABLE 78–2. CORRELATION COEFFICIENTS BETWEEN TESTICULAR MEASUREMENTS AND REPRODUCTIVE CHARACTERISTICS*

MEASUREMENT (MM)	PARENCHYMAL WEIGHT (G)	DSP (10^9)	DSO (10^9)
Total scrotal width	0.83†	0.75	0.55
Left width	0.82	0.68	0.50
Right width	0.82	0.76	0.61
Left length	0.57	0.52	0.34‡
Right length	0.61	0.59	0.50

*$n = 43$.

†r-value.

‡$p > 0.05$; all others significant, $p < 0.01$.

(Adapted from Thompson, D.L., Jr., Pickett, B.W., Squires, E.L., and Amann, R.P.: Testicular measurements and reproductive characteristics in stallions. J. Reprod. Fertil. Suppl., *27*:13–17, 1979.)

TABLE 78–3. SEMINAL VOLUME AND TOTAL SPERMATOZOA PER EJACULATION AT A FREQUENCY OF ONE COLLECTION PER DAY, 6 DAYS PER WEEK

	STALLION			
	Herb*		BJ†	
Weeks	Volume (mL)	Spermatozoa (10^9)	Volume (mL)	Spermatozoa (10^9)
1	85	20.7	76	5.9
2	74	12.9	72	3.7
3	90	12.0	63	2.6
4	75	11.7	56	1.8

*TSW = 137 mm.
†TSW = 79 mm.
(From Pickett, B.W., et al.: Management of the Stallion for Maximum Reproductive Efficiency. II. Animal Reproduction Laboratory Bulletin No. 05. Fort Collins, Colorado State University, 1989.)

pacity to store spermatozoa. Reduction of storage capacity results in breeding fewer mares per day.

Measuring TSW will provide a general estimate of a stallion's ability to produce and ejaculate spermatozoa. The time interval required for formation (57 days), transport (7 to 9 days), and ejaculation of spermatozoa totals about 65 days. Estimation of DSO via scrotal measurements will not provide information on motility or morphology of spermatozoa being produced.[21] Moreover, stallions can have testes of normal size and consistency and yet be azoospermic.[22] Thus, some type of seminal evaluation must be performed if fertility is to be predicted. Objective information obtained from testicular measurements can be used to identify horses with hypoplasia in contrast to those with a low efficiency of sperm production, but only if the low efficiency does not result in a reduction in testicular size or consistency.

Despite the variability associated with measuring TSW, it is a recommended part of a routine potential fertility evaluation. Good stallion management should include measurement of TSW at least once each month and results plotted for each stallion. By maintaining and using such a plot, the clinician may be able to predict potential problems and take steps to alter management before a serious reduction in fertility occurs. In addition to measuring TSW, each testis should be palpated for abnormalities and consistency. Clinicians cannot rely solely on seminal characteristics to predict testicular function.

AGE

Determining the number of mares that a given stallion can breed, either naturally and/or through AI, is important for appropriate stallion management. All too often, a young horse is overused and an older stallion is underused. Age of stallion is one of the more important factors affecting sperm production and output and the number of mares that can be bred.[17,23,24]

SPERM RESERVES

The number of spermatozoa ejaculated and quality of those spermatozoa determine relative fertility of an ejaculate. The number of spermatozoa available for ejaculation depends on reserves in the tails of the epididymides, deferent ducts, and ampullae.[17,23,25] Spermatozoa in the head and body of the epididymides are not available for ejaculation. The number available for ejaculation is profoundly influenced by interval since previous ejaculation(s), testicular size, and age. Stallions that have large sperm reserves in the tails of the epididymides can impregnate more mares in a shorter period of time than stallions with low reserves.

A study was conducted to determine effect of age and ejaculation frequency on epididymal sperm reserves.[23] In addition, the relationship between DSP and epididymal sperm reserves was investigated. Stallions of light horse breeds were sexually rested for at least 12 days, and then five ejaculates were collected at 1-h intervals or the stallions were ejaculated twice (1 h apart) every 4 days, once every 2 days, or once a day for at least 3 weeks. The total number of spermatozoa recovered in each ejaculate was calculated. The 54 stallions were unilaterally or bilaterally castrated 1 to 2 h, 24 h, or 12 days after the last ejaculation. Sperm reserves in 71 epididymides were determined. Daily sperm production was calculated by analyzing testicular tissue.[23]

Presented in Table 78–4 are sperm reserves of 16 sexually rested stallions. Sperm reserves of sexually rested stallions increased with advancing age. Although the increase was not significant for the head, approximately twice the number of spermatozoa was present in the body of the epididymis from 10- to 16-yr-old stal-

TABLE 78–4. EFFECT OF AGE ON SPERM RESERVES OF SEXUALLY RESTED STALLIONS*

	SPERMATOZOA PER SIDE (BILLIONS)			
Structure	2 to 4 Years (5)†	5 to 9 Years (5)	10 to 16 Years (6)	Percentage
Efferent ducts	0.3	0.1	0.1	0.6
Epididymis				
Head	4.0	5.0	6.4	14.3
Body	4.2	7.8	9.5	19.4
Tail	18.7	25.8	28.0	61.7
Proximal deferent duct	1.2	2.1	1.4	4.0
Total	28.5	40.8	45.4	

*$n = 16$.
†Numbers in parentheses represent the number of stallions in that age group.
(Adapted from Amann, R.P., Thompson, D.L., Jr., Squires, E.L., and Pickett, B.W.: Effect of age and frequency of ejaculation on sperm production and extragonadal sperm reserves in stallions. J. Reprod. Fertil. Suppl., *27*:1–6, 1979.)

TABLE 78–5. EFFECT OF AGE ON TESTICULAR SIZE (MM) IN STALLIONS

	AGE (YEARS)		
Measurements	2 to 3 (11)*	4 to 6 (14)	≥ 7 (18)
Scrotal width			
Mean	96†	100[b]	109[c]
67% of population	88–103	93–107	102–117
95% of population	81–111	85–115	95–124
Left width			
Mean	55[b]	57[b]	61[c]
67% of population	50–59	53–62	57–65
95% of population	45–63	49–66	52–70
Right width			
Mean	53[b]	55[b]	60[c]
67% of population	48–58	50–60	55–64
95% of population	43–62	45–65	50–69

*Numbers in parentheses represent the number of stallions in that age group.
†Means with different superscripts differ ($p < 0.05$).
(Adapted from Thompson, D.L., Jr., Pickett, B.W., Squires, E.L., and Amann, R.P.: Testicular measurements and reproductive characteristics in stallions. J. Reprod. Fertil. Suppl., *27*:13–17, 1979.)

lions (9.5 billion) than 2- to 4-yr-olds (4.2 billion). The total number of spermatozoa in sperm reserves of 2- to 4-, 5- to 9-, and 10- to 16-yr-old stallions was 29, 41, and 45 billion, respectively. Thus, older stallions have a much larger storage capacity for spermatozoa than 2- to 3-yr-old stallions. Regardless of age, the tail of the epididymis contained about 62% of the sperm reserves and served as the major site for sperm storage. Neither daily ejaculation nor a series of five ejaculations at hourly intervals reduced the number of spermatozoa within the head or body of the epididymis. Thus, sperm transit through these portions of the epididymides, which are presumed to be involved in sperm maturation, is not altered by frequency of ejaculation. However, ejaculation either 24 or 48 h before a seminal collection reduced the number of spermatozoa in the tail of the epididymis by 15 to 30%.

Contrary to popular belief, ejaculation frequency has little or no effect on fertility of the individual spermatozoon ejaculated during mating. A common belief presumes that if ejaculation occurs too frequently, the stallion will ejaculate immature spermatozoa. No scientific evidence supports that belief.

Testicular size, DSP, and EGR increased for several years after puberty. Based on these studies, the researchers concluded that DSP and EGR in a normal 3-yr-old stallion should be adequate to permit use once a day during the breeding season, provided testicular size is normal and sex drive is adequate. The reproductive capacity of older stallions should be adequate to permit use at least two or three times a day during spring and summer. For most mature, normal stallions, sex drive is the limiting factor in number of mares that can be bred per day by natural service.

TESTIS SIZE IN RELATION TO AGE

A series of studies were conducted to determine the relationship of age of stallion with testicular measurements.[17] A total of 48 stallions of light horse breeds, 2- to 16-yr of age, were used. Testicular measurements were made from the left side of the stallion on six separate days by each of two technicians. Age of stallions significantly affected testicular size (Table 78–5). The testes of stallions 7 yr or older were larger than those of younger horses. Average TSW for stallions 2 to 3, 4 to 6, and 7 yr old or older was 96, 100, and 109 mm, respectively. Ranges are presented that represent 67 and 95% of the population. Thus, in a given population of stallions, 66% should have a TSW within the first range of values. If 95% of the stallions are included, obviously the range is increased. These ranges should be considered when evaluating a stallion for breeding soundness.

The correlation coefficient between TSW and age was 0.64 ($p < 0.01$) (Fig. 78–14), which is another example of the interrelationships that affect sperm production and output. Approximately 40% of variation in testis size could be accounted for by age. Although scrotal width was correlated significantly with body weight, when body weight and age were considered together only age accounted for a significant amount of variation. Thus, for a given age, scrotal width was independent of body weight.

SUCCESSIVE EJACULATES

A study was conducted to determine seminal characteristics of five successive ejaculates and to determine the influence of age on characteristics of those ejaculates.[24] Two groups of clinically normal stallions of light horse breeds ranging in age from 2 to 16 yr were used. The effect of age on seminal characteristics is presented in

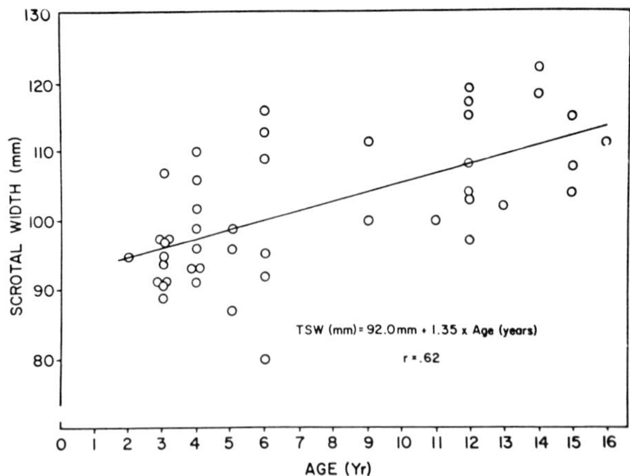

FIG. 78–14. Total scrotal width as a function of age. TSW (mm) = 92 mm + 1.35 × Age (yr); $r = 0.62$. (From Pickett, B.W., et al.: Management of the Stallion for Maximum Reproductive Efficiency. II. Animal Reproduction Laboratory Bulletin No. 05. Fort Collins, Colorado State University, 1989.)

TABLE 78–6. EFFECT OF AGE ON SEMINAL CHARACTERISTICS OF STALLIONS

Characteristics*	AGE (YEARS) 2 to 3 (7)†	4 to 6 (16)	9 to 16 (21)
Seminal volume (mL)			
Gel	2.1	5.1	13.3
Gel free	14.2	26.2	29.8
Total	16.2	31.4	43.2
Spermatozoa			
Concentration (10^6/mL)	120.4	160.9	161.3
Total (10^9)	1.8	3.6	4.5
Motility (%)	55.0	63.1	59.9
pH	7.68	7.64	7.59

*Means of five successive ejaculates.
†Numbers in parentheses represent the number of stallions in each age group.
(Adapted from Squires, E.L., Pickett, B.W., and Amann, R.P.: Effect of successive ejaculation on stallion seminal characteristics. J. Reprod. Fertil. Suppl., *27*:7–12, 1979.)

Table 78–6. Values for some characteristics declined markedly with successive ejaculates. Stallions in the 4- to 6- and 9- to 16-yr-old groups produced more gel-free semen and more total volume than 2- to 3-yr-old stallions. The amount of gel in ejaculates of older stallions (13 mL) appeared to be greater than that for young stallions (2 mL), although the difference was not significant. The number of spermatozoa per milliliter was similar for stallions in all three age groups (120 million, 161 million, and 161 million). Fewer spermatozoa were obtained in ejaculates from 2- to 3-yr-old stallions than from 9- to 16-yr-olds. Although the difference was not significant, twice the number of spermatozoa was obtained in the average ejaculate from 4- to 6-yr-old stallions (3.6 billion) than from 2- to 3-yr-old stallions (1.8 billion). Number of spermatozoa per ejaculate was similar for 4- to 6- and 9- to 16-yr-old stallions. This is additional proof that stallions do not become sexually mature until 6 yr of age or older and sperm output in normal older stallions remains relatively high.

Quality of spermatozoa was similar for all age groups as evidenced by means of 55%, 63%, and 60% motile spermatozoa for 2- to 3-, 4- to 6-, and 9- to 16-yr-olds, respectively. This was not surprising because the stallions had been evaluated before initiation of the experiment and were classified as normal. Many stallion managers erroneously believe that seminal quality of a young stallion is inferior to a more mature stallion.

The influence of age on number of spermatozoa in successive ejaculates was most evident in first ejaculates collected 1 h apart (Fig. 78–15). Major differences in sperm output were noted between 2- to 3-yr-old stallions and the other groups, but not between 4- to 6- and 9- to 16-yr-old stallions. Number of spermatozoa per ejaculate was less ($p < 0.05$) for 2- to 3-yr-old stallions than from 9- to 16-yr-olds in the first and second ejaculates but not in subsequent ejaculates. The first ejaculates from 4- to 6-yr-old stallions contained more ($p < 0.05$) spermatozoa than ejaculates from 2- to 3-yr-old stallions, but slightly less than from 9- to 16-yr-olds. Total number of spermatozoa per ejaculate decreased with each successive ejaculate for 2- to 3-yr-old stallions, but this decrease was not significant. Number of spermatozoa obtained in five ejaculates from 2- to 3-yr-olds (8.9 billion) was less ($p < 0.05$) than the 22.3 billion spermatozoa obtained from 9- to 16-yr-old stallions. Spermatozoa obtained in five ejaculates from 4- to 6-yr-old stallions was intermediate at 18.0 billion (Table 78–7).

By the fifth successive ejaculation, nearly half of the ejaculates from young stallions contained fewer than 200 million spermatozoa. Thus 2- to 3-yr-old stallions cannot be used with the same frequency as older stallions without lowering fertility. Because these stallions had at least 12 days of sexual rest, they probably could not be used daily in a natural service program. In contrast, all second ejaculates from 4- to 6- and 9- to 16-yr-old stallions contained more than 200 million spermatozoa. These aged stallions probably could be used several times per day and not alter fertility in a natural service program. The clinician cannot assume that the fifth ejaculate from all aged stallions would provide satisfactory fertility, even after 12 days' sexual rest, because of incomplete ejaculations. This is one of the advantages of an AI program, spermatozoa are counted in each ejaculate to ensure that minimal numbers of motile spermatozoa are available.

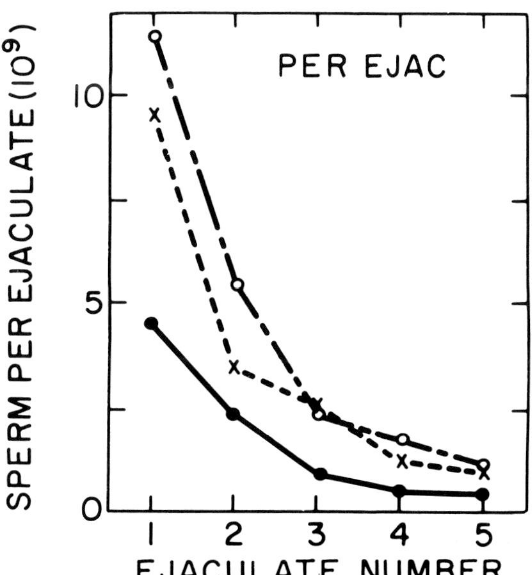

FIG. 78–15. Influence of age of stallion on sperm output in five successive ejaculates. 2- to 3-yr-olds, solid line; 4- to 6-yr-olds, dashed line; 9- to 16-yr-olds, short and long dashed line. (Adapted from Pickett, B.W., et al.: Management of the Stallion for Maximum Reproductive Efficiency. II. Animal Reproduction Laboratory Bulletin No. 05. Fort Collins, Colorado State University, 1989.)

TABLE 78–7. EFFECT OF AGE AND EJACULATE NUMBER ON TOTAL SPERM PER EJACULATE (BILLION)

	AGE (YEARS)		
Ejaculate	2 to 3 (7)*	4 to 6 (16)	9 to 16 (21)
1	4.5	9.5	11.4
2	2.4	3.5	5.5
3	0.9	2.6	2.4
4	0.6	1.3	1.8
5	0.5	1.1	1.2
Total	8.9	18.0	22.3

*Numbers in parentheses represent the number of stallions in that age group. (Adapted from Squires, E.L., Pickett, B.W., and Amann, R.P.: Effect of successive ejaculation on stallion seminal characteristics. J. Reprod. Fertil. Suppl., *27*:7–12, 1979.)

Based on data in Table 78–8, a normal, fertile, sexually rested, mature stallion could successfully impregnate five or more mares in one day by natural service. The willingness and ability of a normal aged stallion to mount and ejaculate may determine number of mares that can be bred on a given day. Stallions with a large reproductive capacity and excellent sex drive could have their breeding season shortened by synchronizing estrous cycles of mares, thus allowing a stallion to breed his mares in a shorter period. This may be extremely useful for a stallion with a heavy show or performance schedule.

These data can be used to manage stallions for maximum reproductive efficiency. All too often, economic pressure and popularity determine the size of a stallion's book, when it should be determined by reproductive capacity. The number of mares booked to some young stallions should be reduced, whereas in some cases, the number for older stallions could be increased without causing a decrease in fertility.

FREQUENCY OF EJACULATION

Frequency of ejaculation is one of the most important factors affecting sperm output. As frequency of ejaculation increases, number of spermatozoa per ejaculation decreases, providing frequency exceeds one ejaculate every other day.[9] If a stallion's sex drive is sufficiently high, fertility may decline because of overuse, i.e., ejaculation of insufficient spermatozoa, particularly early in the breeding season when sperm output may be only 50% as high as at the peak of the breeding season.[7,9] In fact, sex drive (libido) may be the limiting factor early in the breeding season when libido is normally low and toward the end of the season when the stallion is sexually satiated.

Two questions frequently asked are "How often can I use my stallion in a natural service program?" and "How many mares can I book to my stallion in an AI program?" To study the effects of frequency of ejaculation on some seminal and behavioral characteristics, nine QH and TB stallions were assigned randomly to three groups.[9] The groups were assigned to a seminal collection frequency of one time (1×), three times (3×), or six times (6×) per week for 4 weeks (one collection period). Stallions in the 1× group were collected once a week; 3× stallions, every other day; and 6× stallions, daily except Sunday. At the end of each collection period, stallions were sexually rested for 1 week, and groups were reassigned to a different collection period. This protocol was continued until each stallion had been collected at each frequency for 4 weeks.

Evaluation of the results of this experiment was limited to data obtained during the last 2 weeks of the collection period, after EGR had stabilized (Table 78–9). No differences ($p > 0.05$) occurred in gel volume, gel-free seminal volume, or total seminal volume per ejaculate as a result of frequency of ejaculation. Volume of gel for the 1×, 3×, and 6× frequencies averaged 18, 8, and 6 mL per ejaculate, respectively. Gel volume, gel-free seminal volume, and total volume per ejaculate were different ($p < 0.01$) among stallions. Although effect of frequency of ejaculation was not significant, the more frequently the animals were collected, the lower the gel volume.

A total of 47, 56, and 51 mL of gel-free semen was collected at frequencies of 1×, 3×, and 6×, respectively, but no differences in seminal volume caused by frequency of seminal collection were noted. Thus, a stallion can ejaculate large volumes of seminal plasma quite independently of concentration of spermatozoa. Obviously, sperm number is more important than volume for maximum fertility. Total volumes per collection were 65 mL for 1×, 54 mL for 3×, and 57 mL for 6×. The differences were primarily the result of volume of gel, not gel-free semen. Sperm concentration averaged 288 million, 248 million, and 142 million per milliliter, respectively, for 1×, 3×, and 6× treatments. In spite of two additional collections per week, the difference in spermatozoa per milliliter between 1× and 3× groups was only 40 million per milliliter. Although sperm concentration was similar when a stallion's semen was col-

TABLE 78–8. PERCENTAGE OF EJACULATES WITH 200 MILLION OR LESS SPERMATOZOA PER EJACULATE

	AGE (YEARS)		
Ejaculate	2 to 3 (7)*	4 to 6 (16)	9 to 16 (21)
1	0	0	0
2	29	0	0
3	14	6	5
4	14	12	0
5	43	6	10

*Numbers in parentheses represent the number of stallions in that age group. (From Pickett, B.W., et al.: Management of the Stallion for Maximum Reproductive Efficiency. II. Animal Reproduction Laboratory Bulletin No. 05. Fort Collins, Colorado State University, 1989.)

TABLE 78–9. EFFECT OF FREQUENCY OF EJACULATION ON MEAN STALLION SEMINAL CHARACTERISTICS OVER THE LAST 2 WEEKS OF A 4-WEEK COLLECTION PERIOD

	FREQUENCY OF EJACULATION PER WEEK		
Characteristic	1×	3×	6×
Volume/ejaculate (mL)			
Gel	18	8	6
Semen, gel-free	47	56	51
Total	65	64	57
Spermatozoa			
Concentration/mL (10^6)	288[a]*	248[a]	142[b]
Total/ejaculate (10^9)	11.4[a]	11.7[a]	5.9[b]
Total/week (10^9)	11.4[a]	35.2[a]	35.3[a]
Motility (%)	54	52	56
pH	7.56[c]	7.48[d]	7.58[c]
Sexual behavior			
Mounts/ejaculate	1.2	1.4	1.4
Reaction time (min)	1.75	1.93	2.10

*Row means with different superscripts are significantly different: a,b, $p < 0.01$; c,d, $p < 0.05$.

(Adapted from Pickett, B.W., Sullivan, J.J., and Seidel, G.E., Jr.: Reproductive physiology of the stallion. V. Effect of frequency of ejaculation on seminal characteristics and spermatozoal output. J. Anim. Sci., *40*:917–923, 1975.)

lected once per week or every other day, when he was collected 6× per week, the mean was only 50% of the number obtained at the 1× or 3× frequencies.

The stallions averaged 11.4 billion spermatozoa per ejaculate at 1× and 11.7 billion at 3×, but only 5.9 billion at 6× ($p < 0.05$). Thus, a stallion being used every other day ejaculates as many spermatozoa per cover as he would being used once or less per week. Total sperm output per week averaged 11.4 billion, 35.2 billion, and 35.3 billion at frequencies of 1×, 3×, and 6×, respectively. Thus, fewer spermatozoa were collected at the 1× frequency than 3× or 6×. When EGR became stable, sperm output per week was identical at the 3× and 6× frequencies. This indicates that increasing frequency of collection above once every other day will not result in more spermatozoa per week or per ejaculation. With an every-other-day seminal collection schedule, all spermatozoa that are available for ejaculation are being collected. Therefore, for maximum use of the stallion, with a minimum amount of labor, stallions should be collected every other day and all mares in standing heat for 2 days or longer should be inseminated.

Percentage of progressively motile spermatozoa averaged 54%, 52%, and 56%, respectively, for 1×, 3×, and 6× frequencies. Thus, these frequencies of ejaculation had no detrimental effect on sperm quality as measured by motility. Reaction time and number of mounts per ejaculation were not affected by these frequencies of ejaculation. Thus, sex drive of a well-adjusted stallion will remain as high on a daily collection schedule as on a schedule of once per week.

TWO VS. FOUR COLLECTIONS PER WEEK

In another experiment, eight mature stallions of the Arabian, Connemara, QH, and Welsh Pony breeds were randomly assigned to ejaculation frequencies of two times (2×) or four times (4×) per week for 4 weeks (one collection period).[9] For the lower frequency of ejaculation, one ejaculate was collected per day on Tuesday and Friday of each week, whereas for the higher frequency, two ejaculates were collected per day on Tuesday and Friday of each week. The study consisted of three 4-week collection periods. Thus, stallions in group I were collected at frequencies of 2×, 4×, and 2× per week for the three collection periods. At the same time, stallions in group II were collected 4×, 2×, and 4×.

Increasing ejaculation frequency from one to two ejaculates per day, twice a week, increased ($p < 0.01$) seminal volume obtained on 1 day. The volume of second ejaculates collected on the same day was lower ($p < 0.01$) than that of first ejaculates (58 vs. 49 mL) (Table 78–10).

More spermatozoa were collected in two ejaculates than in one, but mean concentration of spermatozoa in the two ejaculates collected on the same day was lower ($p < 0.05$) than that of a single ejaculate. This was primarily caused by the lower ($p < 0.01$) concentration of spermatozoa in the second ejaculate. As a result of

TABLE 78–10. EFFECT OF FREQUENCY OF EJACULATION ON STALLION SEMINAL CHARACTERISTICS

	FREQUENCY OF EJACULATION PER WEEK	
Characteristic*	2×	4×
Seminal volume (mL)		
Gel-free, 1st ejaculate	55	58
Gel-free, 2nd ejaculate	—	49
Total	55	107
Spermatozoa		
Concentration/mL, 1st ejaculate (10^6)	272	222
Concentration/ml, 2nd ejaculate (10^6)	—	145
Mean concentration/mL (10^6)	272	196
Total/1st ejaculate (10^9)	13.1	12.0
Total/2nd ejaculate (10^9)	—	5.5
Total/week (10^9)	26.2	35.1
Sperm motility (%)		
1st ejaculate	49	58
2nd ejaculate	—	61
Mean	49	59
Seminal pH		
1st ejaculate	7.65	7.59
2nd ejaculate	—	7.75
Mean	7.65	7.65

*Eight stallions collected from November 12 through February 21.

(Adapted from Pickett, B.W., Sullivan, J.J., and Seidel, G.E., Jr.: Reproductive physiology of the stallion. V. Effect of frequency of ejaculation on seminal characteristics and spermatozoal output. J. Anim. Sci., *40*:917–923, 1975.)

lower seminal volume and concentration of spermatozoa, number of spermatozoa in the second ejaculate was 45.8% less ($p < 0.01$) than in first ejaculates collected the same day. Nevertheless, sperm per week for the 4× frequency was 25.4% higher ($p < 0.01$) than at the 2× frequency. Percent motile spermatozoa in first and second ejaculates at the 4× frequency tended to be higher than at the 2× frequency (58 vs. 49%). Likewise, no difference ($p > 0.05$) occurred in percent motility between first and second ejaculates.

Sperm output for stallions on the 3× and 6× frequencies (Table 78–9) was the same as the 4× frequency. When two successive ejaculates were collected on the same day, number of spermatozoa in the second ejaculate decreased by approximately 50% (45.8%). This relationship between first and second ejaculates is extremely valuable in evaluation of stallions for breeding soundness.[7]

A practical ejaculation frequency for stallions in an AI program, in breeds where semen cannot be stored, would be one ejaculate on alternate days. Two ejaculates per week might provide maximal number of spermatozoa per ejaculate and be a practical ejaculation frequency, if semen were to be frozen and stored. Another advantage of these seminal collection frequencies, compared with daily collections, is that a smaller percentage of spermatozoa are lost in the collection equipment and gel;[26] this can be an important factor when a large number of mares are booked to a stallion.

ONE VS. TWO COLLECTIONS PER DAY

A total of 10 stallions of light horse breeds, between the ages of 3 and 23 yr, were subjected to two frequencies of ejaculation in a double switchback experiment.[27] Semen was collected from stallions either once (1×) or twice (2×) per day. Before beginning the experiment, all stallions were placed on a 1× ejaculation frequency for 8 days. After the 8-day stabilization period, 5 stallions (group 1) were placed on a 1× daily seminal collection schedule, while the other 5 stallions (group 2) were collected 2× per day. This schedule was maintained for 14 days. At the end of the collection period, group 1 stallions were switched to 2× and vice versa. During each collection period, the first 6 days were used as an additional stabilization period; data from the remaining 8 days were used to evaluate treatments. Second ejaculates from stallions on the 2× schedule were collected approximately 8 h after first ejaculates.

Total spermatozoa available for insemination was lower ($p < 0.001$) for the 2× frequency, because when semen was collected twice a day, more spermatozoa were lost in the collection equipment and gel. However, spermatozoa ejaculated were the same (7.5 billion vs. 7.4 billion) for the two frequencies of ejaculation, when ejaculations were corrected for sperm losses. Concentration of spermatozoa per milliliter of gel-free semen was lower ($p < 0.001$) for the 2× frequency (59 million vs.

TABLE 78–11. MEAN 8-DAY SPERM OUTPUT IN BILLIONS CORRECTED FOR SPERM LOSSES

GROUP	FREQUENCY OF EJACULATION		
	1×	2×	1×
1	56.7	55.2	53.9
	2×	1×	2×
2	63.3	63.4	64.5

(From Neil, J.R.: Ejaculation frequency, sperm loss in collection equipment and training stallions to a phantom. M.S. thesis. Fort Collins, Colorado State University, 1983.)

134.4 million) because of the higher ($p < 0.001$) gel-free seminal volume. Presented in Table 78–11 is sperm output for the two groups of stallions at the two frequencies of ejaculation. In spite of a concerted effort to divide the stallions into two equal groups with respect to sperm output, a difference of 7.4 billion spermatozoa in favor of group 2 was noted over the 8-day period.

The most important observation in this experiment was the almost identical (7.5 billion vs. 7.4 billion) sperm output within groups, regardless of frequency of ejaculation.[27] It must be concluded that increasing frequency of ejaculation from 1× to 2× per day did not result in an increase in sperm output. Thus, only so many spermatozoa are available per day and increasing frequency of breeding beyond once every other day will not increase daily sperm output. Therefore, for each mare to have an equal opportunity to become pregnant with natural service, the intervals between breedings must be long enough to ensure that each mare gets sufficient spermatozoa for maximum reproductive efficiency. As any good stallion manager knows, each stallion must be treated as an individual when determining number of breedings per day, week, month, and season.

DAILY COLLECTIONS

To answer the question "How often can I use my stallion?" 11 stallions, ranging in age from 3 to 13 yr old were collected daily during the breeding season.[10] Sperm output data for the first 14 days of collection are presented in Table 78–12. Based on number of spermatozoa collected per ejaculate, EGR had stabilized by days 5 to 7 of consecutive daily collections. Thus, mean DSO by week 2 of daily collections should represent the true DSO of a stallion for that particular time of the year.

The large number of spermatozoa collected during the first week of daily collections was attributed to accumulations in the EGR during the week of sexual rest. Thus, to obtain actual DSO for a particular time of year, semen must be collected from stallions daily for approximately 1 week before collecting sperm output data. Af-

TABLE 78–12. SPERMATOZOAL OUTPUT (BILLIONS) THE FIRST 14 DAYS OF DAILY COLLECTION*

DAY OF COLLECTION	SPERMATOZOA (BILLION)	CONFIDENCE INTERVAL (95%)
1	8.8	±3.6
2	6.9	±2.5
3	6.9	±2.1
4	4.4	±1.8
5	3.8	±1.6
6	3.9	±1.5
7	2.6	±1.4
8	4.1	±1.3
9	2.7	±1.2
10	3.4	±1.1
11	2.9	±1.1
12	3.0	±1.0
13	3.6	±1.0
14	3.5	±1.0

*Not corrected for spermatozoa lost in the collection equipment and gel.
(Adapted from Gebauer, M.R., Pickett, B.W., Voss, J.L., and Swierstra, E.E.: Reproductive physiology of the stallion: Daily sperm output and testicular measurements. J. Am. Vet. Med. Assoc., *165:*711–713, 1974.)

ter EGRs have been stabilized, accuracy of estimating actual DSO depends on number of consecutive days that ejaculates are collected. The number of spermatozoa obtained on day 7 of daily collections should approximate daily sperm output.

The number of mares that can be bred by natural service can only be rationally established by the individual(s) most familiar with that stallion, because in many cases sex drive is the limiting factor. For maximum reproductive efficiency the stallion must be managed to maintain maximum sex drive throughout the breeding season. His sex drive may change; thus, management must be realistic, intelligent, and observant.

REFERENCES

1. Ginther, O.J.: Occurrence of anestrus, estrus, diestrus, and ovulation over a 12-month period in mares. Am. J. Vet. Res., *35:*1173–1179, 1974.
2. Kooistra, L.H., and Ginther, O.J.: Effect of photoperiod on reproductive activity and hair in mares. Am. J. Vet. Res., *36:*1413–1419, 1975.
3. Nishikawa, Y.: Studies on Reproduction in Horses. Tokyo, Japan Racing Association, 1959.
4. Osborne, V.E.: An analysis of the pattern of ovulation as it occurs in the annual reproductive cycle of the mare in Australia. Aust. Vet. J., *42:*149–153, 1966.
5. Sharp, D.C. III, and Ginther, O.J.: Stimulation of follicular activity and estrous behavior in anestrous mares with light and temperature. J. Anim. Sci., *41:*1368–1372, 1975.
6. Burkhardt, J.: Transition from anoestrus in the mare and the effects of artificial lighting. J. Agr. Sci., *37:*64–68, 1947.
7. Pickett, B.W., et al.: Reproductive physiology of the stallion. VI. Seminal and behavioral characteristics. J. Anim. Sci., *43:*617–625, 1976.
8. Sullivan, J.J., and Pickett, B.W.: Influence of ejaculation frequency of stallions on characteristics of semen and output of spermatozoa. J. Reprod. Fertil. Suppl., *23:*29–34, 1975.
9. Pickett, B.W., Sullivan, J.J., and Seidel, G.E., Jr.: Reproductive physiology of the stallion. V. Effect of frequency of ejaculation on seminal characteristics and spermatozoal output. J. Anim. Sci., *40:*917–923, 1975.
10. Gebauer, M.R., Pickett, B.W., Voss, J.L., and Swierstra, E.E.: Reproductive physiology of the stallion: Daily sperm output and testicular measurements. J. Am. Vet. Med. Assoc., *165:*711–713, 1974.
11. Pickett, B.W., et al.: Management of the Stallion for Maximum Reproductive Efficiency. II. Animal Reproduction Laboratory Bulletin No. 05. Fort Collins, Colorado State University, 1989.
12. Clay, C.M., Squires, E.L., Amann, R.P., and Pickett, B.W.: Influences of season and artificial photoperiod on stallions: Testicular size, seminal characteristics and sexual behavior. J. Anim. Sci., *64:*517–525, 1987.
13. Burns, P.J., et al.: Effects of season, age and increased photoperiod on reproductive hormone concentrations and testicular diameters in Thoroughbred stallions. J. Equine Vet. Sci., *4:*202–208, 1984.
14. Follett, B.K.: Photoperiodism and seasonal breeding in birds and mammals. *In* Control of Ovulation. Edited by G.E. Lamming and D.B. Crighton. London, Butterworth, 1978, pp. 267–293.
15. Davis, E.E.: Endogenous cycles. *In* Testicular Development, Structure, and Function. Edited by A. Steinberger and E. Steinberger. New York, Raven Press, 1980, pp. 359–366.
16. Amann, R.P.: A critical review of methods for evaluation of spermatogenesis from seminal characteristics. J. Androl., *2:*37–58, 1981.
17. Thompson, D.L., Jr., Pickett, B.W., Squires, E.L., and Amann. R.P.: Testicular measurements and reproductive characteristics in stallions. J. Reprod. Fertil. Suppl., *27:*13–17, 1979.
18. Amann, R.P., Johnson, L., Thompson, D.L., Jr., and Pickett, B.W.: Daily spermatozoal production, epididymal spermatozoal reserves and transit time of spermatozoa through the epididymis of the Rhesus monkey. Biol. Reprod., *15:*586–592, 1976.
19. Coulter, G.H., Rounsaville, T.R., and Foote, R.H.: Heritability of testicular size and consistency in Holstein bulls. J. Anim. Sci., *43:*9–12, 1976.
20. Voss, J.L., and Pickett, B.W.: Reproductive Management of the Broodmare. Animal Reproduction Laboratory General Series Bulletin No. 961. Fort Collins, Colorado State University, 1976.
21. Voss, J.L., Pickett, B.W., and Squires, E.L.: Stallion spermatozoal morphology and motility and their relationship to fertility. J. Am. Vet. Med. Assoc., *178:*287–289, 1981.
22. Pickett, B.W., Voss, J.L., and Squires, E.L.: Impotence and abnormal sexual behavior in the stallion. Theriogenology, *8:*329–347, 1977.
23. Amann, R.P., Thompson, D.L., Jr., Squires, E.L., and Pickett, B.W.: Effect of age and frequency of ejaculation on sperm production and extragonadal sperm reserves in stallions. J. Reprod. Fertil. Suppl., *27:*1–6, 1979.

24. Squires, E.L., Pickett, B.W., and Amann, R.P.: Effect of successive ejaculation on stallion seminal characteristics. J. Reprod. Fertil. Suppl., *27*:7–12, 1979.
25. Gebauer, M.R., Pickett, B.W., and Swierstra, E.E.: Reproductive physiology of the stallion. III. Extra-gonadal transit time and sperm reserves. J. Anim. Sci., *39*:737–742, 1974.
26. Neil, J.R.: Ejaculation frequency, sperm loss in collection equipment and training stallions to a phantom. M.S. thesis. Fort Collins, Colorado State University, 1983.
27. Pickett, B.W., Neil, J.R., and Squires. E.L.: The effect of ejaculation frequency on stallion sperm output. Proceedings of the Ninth Equine Nutrition and Physiology Society Symposium, 1985, pp. 290–295.

CHAPTER 79

COLLECTION AND EVALUATION OF STALLION SEMEN FOR ARTIFICIAL INSEMINATION

B.W. Pickett

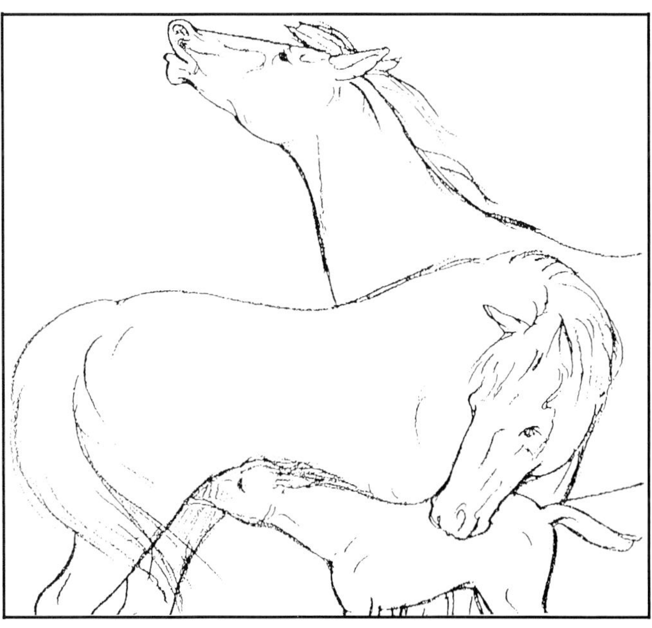

Because the stallion does not respond favorably to electroejaculation, an artificial vagina (AV) is essential to collect high-quality semen. Several models of AVs and their modifications have been described for collection of stallion semen. The Colorado Model AV has been used extensively in our laboratory since 1967.[1] An improved AV, the CSU Model, has been developed in cooperation with Animal Reproduction Systems (Chino, CA).[2] The CSU Model is a modification of the Missouri-USDA, Cambridge, and Colorado models (Fig. 79–1).

ASSEMBLY OF THE CSU MODEL AV

The casing of the CSU Model is plastic, and the posterior end, through which the stallion's penis enters, is fitted with a heavy rubber collar to prevent injury (Fig. 79–1). There are two rubber liners: one is the same width throughout its entire length and is called the inner liner, the other is tapered and is designated the combination liner and cone.

To assemble the AV, the inner liner is placed inside the casing with approximately equal lengths protruding at each end. The inner liner is then reflected over the rubber collar at the posterior end. Although the posterior end is flared by the rubber collar, at least one rubber band should be used to hold the liner in place to prevent leakage of water. Next, the inner liner is straightened and stretched the desired amount and reflected over the anterior end of the casing. This is the first point in assembling the AV at which it is possible to adjust the internal diameter and ultimately the internal pressure. Increasing the tautness, i.e., the amount the inner liner is stretched before it is reflected over the anterior end of the casing, reduces the amount of water that can be added and thus increases the internal diameter. Conversely, a loose inner liner will allow more water to be added, which decreases internal diameter and increases internal pressure. When the inner liner is in place, the inside should resemble a smooth tube with the rubber stretched equally all the way around the inside of the casing (Fig. 79–2).

Combination liners and cones are available in disposable plastic or reusable rubber. Convenience, cost, and the stallion's preference should be taken into account when making a selection. The rubber combination liner and cone is inserted through the AV casing and reflected over the posterior end of the casing and inner liner. It must be free of twists and wrinkles and reflected completely over the rubber collar to prevent slipping during collection. Stretching the rubber combination liner and cone over the posterior end of the AV is an art. The rubber is relatively thick and sufficiently smaller in diameter than the flared, posterior end of the AV that considerable stretching is necessary to reflect the rubber over the posterior end. Thus no rubber band is necessary. Unfortunately, if the stretching and reflecting is not done in one smooth movement, the rubber will most likely tear, especially if brute force is used.

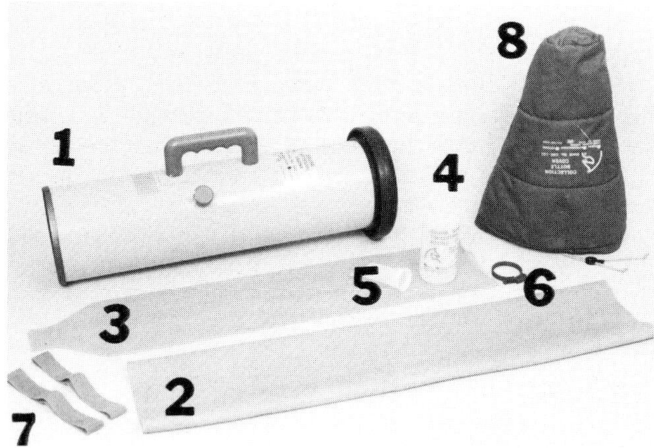

FIG. 79–1. Individual parts of the CSU Model AV. 1, casing; 2, inner liner; 3, combination liner and cone; 4, collection bottle; 5, filter assembly; 6, clamp; 7, rubber bands; 8, protector jacket. (From Pickett, B.W., Squires, E.L., and McKinnon, A.O.: Procedures for Collection, Evaluation and Utilization of Stallion Semen for Artificial Insemination. Animal Reproduction Laboratory Bulletin No. 03. Fort Collins, Colorado State University, 1987.)

This should be avoided because rubber liners are relatively expensive.

A disposable, plastic combination liner and cone is more likely to become twisted and wrinkled than rubber. Therefore, more precautions are necessary to position the plastic properly to avoid the considerable danger of puncturing the liner with the fingers when the AV is lubricated. Once the plastic liner is appropriately positioned, the flared end is reflected over the posterior end of the artificial vagina. Because the plastic has little or no stretch, a clamp must be used to hold the liner in place.

The AV is now ready to be filled with water at ~57° C (~135° F). During filling, the clinician is advised to pull on the tapered end of the liner to ensure that wrinkles and twists do not develop, particularly when a plastic liner is being used. Although disposable liners have the advantage of not having to be washed, some stallions object to them and are more difficult to collect, particularly in late fall and winter. We suggest that you try to collect your stallion a few times with the plastic liner. If the horse works well, continue to use them, otherwise use the rubber combination liner and cone. Every good equine seminal collector recognizes that many stallions have idiosyncracies. The better these are understood and compensated for, the more successful the seminal collection.

The second opportunity to adjust the internal pressure of the AV is when filling with water. A blunt object, *not the stem of the thermometer,* can be inserted through the valve, through which water is introduced, to stretch the rubber inner liner, thus allowing more water to be added. However, the clinician must be quick to remove the blunt object and replace the cap to prevent excess water from escaping once pressure is released.

After the AV is filled with water, a dial thermometer is placed inside to monitor temperature (Fig. 79–3). The temperature may continue to rise for 10 to 20 min while the temperature of the unit is stabilizing. If the AV is used before the temperature has risen to the maximum, it can become so hot that it injures the stallion and/or damages the spermatozoa. Many stallions have been burned by someone who has filled an AV and used it as soon as the thermometer registered the desired temperature. Only when the internal temperature has stabilized at ~44° to 50° C (~111° to 122° F) is the AV ready for lubrication.

Early or late in the breeding season, or any other time when the stallion becomes slow to mount and/or reluctant to ejaculate, internal temperature can be increased to ~52° to 54° C (~126° to 129° F) without damaging spermatozoa, provided that certain precautions are taken during collection.[3] Regardless of how accurate collectors think they may be in determining the internal temperature with their hands, a thermometer should *always* be used. Furthermore, at least once a month the accuracy of all laboratory thermometers, particularly dial thermometers, should be checked against boiling water (212° F = 100° C), and/or iced water (32° F = 0° C), or against a good-quality mercury thermometer. To aid in filling the AV with water at the appropriate temperature, a temperature-monitoring device can be installed in the plumbing system (Fig. 79–4). Such a device conserves time and water and heightens the awareness of laboratory personnel to the necessity of temperature control.

In summary, the sequence of events in preparing for seminal collection are as follows:

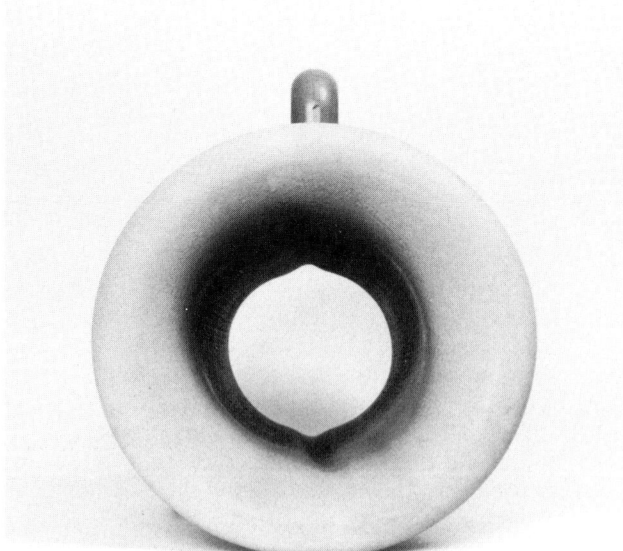

FIG. 79–2. Casing with inner liner appropriately positioned. (From Pickett, B.W., Squires, E.L., and McKinnon, A.O.: Procedures for Collection, Evaluation and Utilization of Stallion Semen for Artificial Insemination. Animal Reproduction Laboratory Bulletin No. 03. Fort Collins, Colorado State University, 1987.)

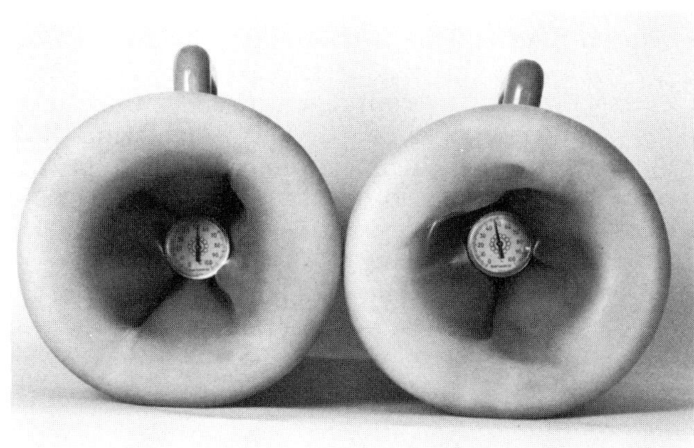

FIG. 79–3. Dial thermometers to monitor internal temperature within the artificial vagina. (From Pickett, B.W., Squires, E.L., and McKinnon, A.O.: Procedures for Collection, Evaluation and Utilization of Stallion Semen for Artificial Insemination. Animal Reproduction Laboratory Bulletin No. 03. Fort Collins, Colorado State University, 1987.)

1. Be sure all equipment to be used is at the appropriate temperature.
2. Turn on all equipment that will be needed, such as sperm counter, warming table, microscope, etc., well before semen is collected.
3. Remove the clean equipment, i.e., rubber material, AV casing, clamps, etc., from dust-free cabinets.
4. Assemble the AV correctly.
5. Place a dial thermometer in each AV after it has been filled with water to monitor temperature.
6. Allow the temperature of the AV to stabilize while the mare is being prepared for seminal collection.

PREPARATION OF THE MARE FOR SEMINAL COLLECTION

In spite of the fact that numerous stallions are injured by mares each year during attempts at seminal collection or during natural service, many breeding managers still do not believe it is necessary to hobble the mare. Their rationale appears to be to let the stallion learn a lesson. This "lesson" can result in serious physiologic and psychologic injury to the stallion, from which he may not fully recover. We have treated many cases of abnormal sexual behavior each year, of which many are the result of the stallion having been kicked during breeding or seminal collection.[4] In the event that the scrotum or penis is kicked, the stallion may become sterile or highly infertile (Chapter 96). A set of hobbles has been designed that has distinct advantages over most other designs. It effectively restrains the mare, fits snugly over the hocks without sliding down, allows the mare to move and be moved without removing the hobbles, causes minimal stress to the mare, and can be removed quickly in case of an emergency.

The teaser mare should be in good estrus and readily allow the stallion to mount.[5] The hobbles have a large leather strap that buckles around the mare's neck. This strap can be adjusted to fit mares of almost any size. A large leather strap also goes between the mare's front legs with a buckle that permits further adjustment. Fleece is sewn inside the leather straps that go around the hocks to keep the hobbles from sliding down. Attached to each end of a 2-cm-diameter nylon rope is a panic snap, which allows immediate release in awkward situations. The rope passes through a pulley, which also has a panic snap that attaches to a D-ring in the leather strap between the mare's front legs. The panic snaps at ends of the rope are attached to D-rings on the hock straps (Fig. 79–5).

The mare's tail should be completely enclosed or wrapped. This is easily done with a large athletic sock. The sock is turned wrong side out over one hand. The hair on the mare's tail is formed into a ball, and clasped through the sock. The opposite hand is used to pull the sock up over the mare's tail. The sock is then taped into place at the base of the tail. When a mare's tail is so wrapped, better sanitary control is permitted and the chance of injury to the stallion's penis from loose hair across the opening of the artificial vagina is minimized. On many farms, there is sufficient personnel in the breeding shed for one person to hold the mare's tail to the opposite side during seminal collection or natural service. In that case, the base of the mare's tail can be wrapped for 20 to 30 cm with gauze or some other disposable material.

When a stallion mounts a mare for seminal collection

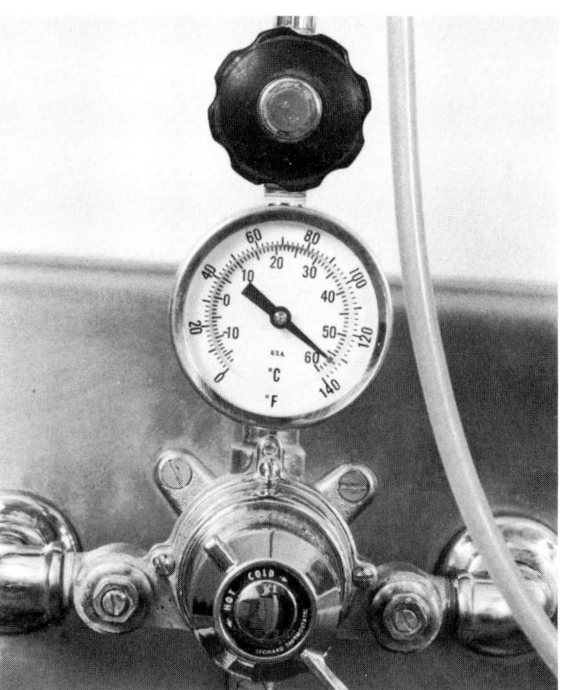

FIG. 79–4. Temperature-monitoring device in the plumbing system. (From Pickett, B.W., Squires, E.L., and McKinnon, A.O.: Procedures for Collection, Evaluation and Utilization of Stallion Semen for Artificial Insemination. Animal Reproduction Laboratory Bulletin No. 03. Fort Collins, Colorado State University, 1987.)

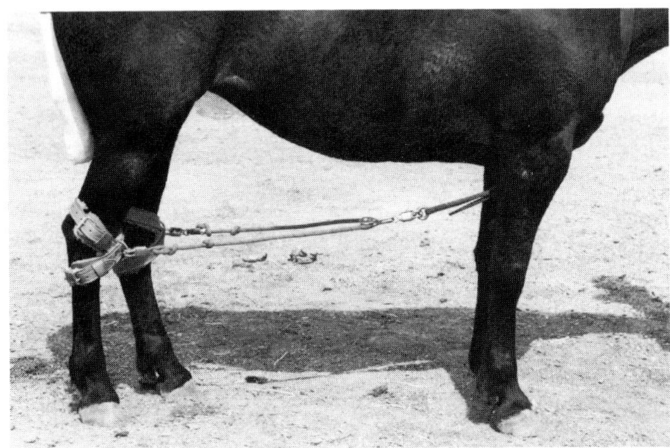

FIG. 79–5. Estrous mare appropriately hobbled for aid in seminal collection. (From Pickett, B.W., Squires, E.L., and McKinnon, A.O.: Procedures for Collection, Evaluation and Utilization of Stallion Semen for Artificial Insemination. Animal Reproduction Laboratory Bulletin No. 03. Fort Collins, Colorado State University, 1987.)

or natural service, a considerable amount of clear fluid is commonly emitted from the penis. Generally, the mare and stallion move quite a bit with the result that the fluid is spread over the mare's buttocks, flanks, tail, etc. This fluid may be nature's way of cleansing the stallion's reproductive tract before sexual contact. If so, this fluid could be heavily laden with bacteria.[6] Therefore, the mare must be washed between stallions, because the next stallion may touch the areas on the mare where this pre-ejaculatory fluid was sprayed and pick up whatever organisms were shed by the previous stallion. The mare's tail wrap should also be changed between stallions.

The mare should be washed with a tamed iodine solution wherever the stallion's penis is likely to come into contact with hair or skin. The individual doing the washing should wear disposable gloves (Fig. 79–6). Furthermore, when paper toweling or cotton pledgets are used to cleanse the mare, they should be discarded after use. Never put an item that has touched the mare back into the bucket, because this contaminates the washing fluid.

FINAL ASSEMBLY OF THE AV

When the mare has been prepared and the AV has reached proper, stable temperature, a collection bottle is removed from an incubator, which is maintained at body temperature ~38° C (~100° F), and fitted with a nylon filter[7] (Fig. 79–7). A lip on the plastic ring to which the nylon filter is attached prevents the filter assembly from falling into the collection bottle. The collection bottle, with filter assembly, is placed into the tapered end of the combination liner and cone and held in place with a clamp (Fig. 79–8). The protector jacket is then removed from a warming device, placed over the collection bottle and fastened to the AV casing. The device used to warm the inside of the protector jacket is composed of a rheostat and two light bulbs fitted with wire protectors to prevent direct contact with the lining of the protector jacket. The rheostat, similar to a dimmer switch, regulates amount of current flowing to the light bulbs and determines the inside temperature of the protector jacket. The light bulbs should be at 40° C (104° F). All areas of the AV, except around the anterior end, have more than one layer of material. Therefore, that is the area where most of the heat escapes. When the protector jacket is in place, heat that escapes is trapped by the protector jacket, thus the collection bottle remains at an acceptable temperature regardless of environmental temperature.

FIG. 79–6. Washing the tease mare before collecting another stallion. (From Pickett, B.W., Squires, E.L., and McKinnon, A.O.: Procedures for Collection, Evaluation and Utilization of Stallion Semen for Artificial Insemination. Animal Reproduction Laboratory Bulletin No. 03. Fort Collins, Colorado State University, 1987.)

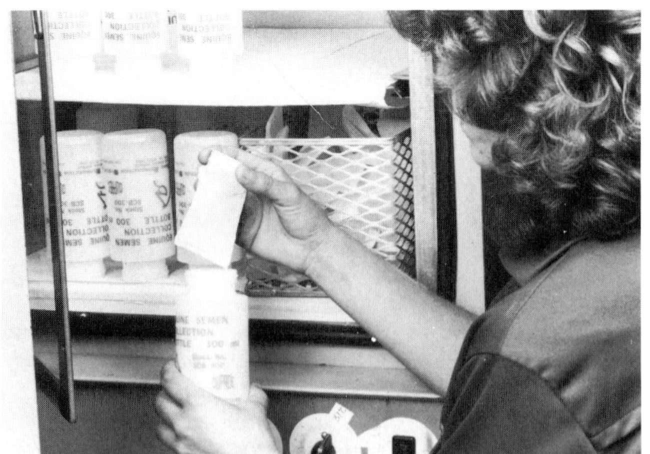

FIG. 79–7. Placing a nylon filter into the collection bottle. (From Pickett, B.W., Squires, E.L., and McKinnon, A.O.: Procedures for Collection, Evaluation and Utilization of Stallion Semen for Artificial Insemination. Animal Reproduction Laboratory Bulletin No. 03. Fort Collins, Colorado State University, 1987.)

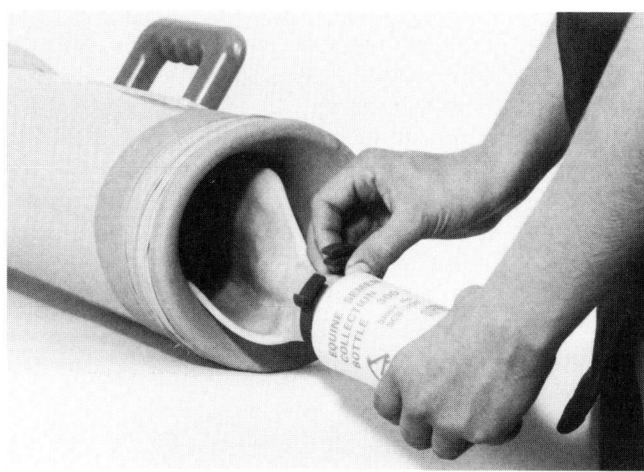

FIG. 79–8. Clamping the collection bottle into the combination liner and cone. (From Pickett, B.W., Squires, E.L., and McKinnon, A.O.: Procedures for Collection, Evaluation and Utilization of Stallion Semen for Artificial Insemination. Animal Reproduction Laboratory Bulletin No. 03. Fort Collins, Colorado State University, 1987.)

The next step is to lubricate the AV. Although there are numerous products on the market, we recommend K-Y lubricating jelly, because it has excellent lubricating properties and has proved not to be spermicidal when it was evaluated against other lubricants.[8] Place approximately 28 to 42 g of jelly into the palm of the right hand, which is covered by a shoulder-length plastic sleeve, and apply it inside the AV along two-thirds of its length. The largest quantity of lubricant should be placed in the first one-third of the AV. The hand is then pushed forward to the point at which the internal pressure of the AV holds the sleeve and allows the hand to be withdrawn, leaving the sleeve inside.

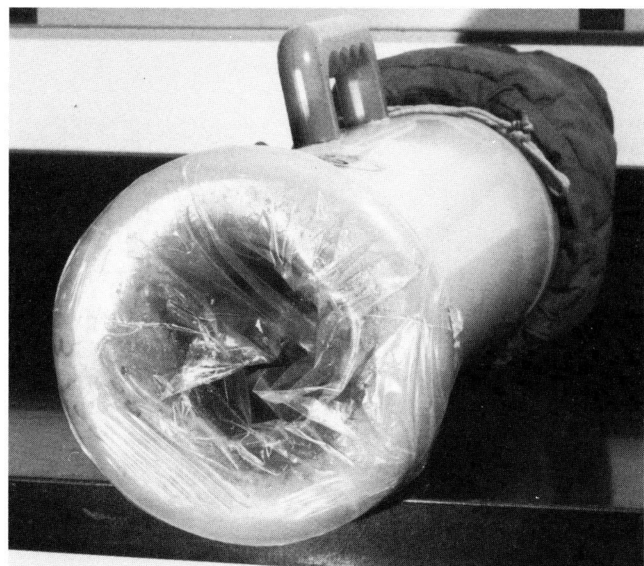

FIG. 79–9. Completely assembled AV with shoulder-length sleeve reflected over the posterior end. (From Pickett, B.W., Squires, E.L., and McKinnon, A.O.: Procedures for Collection, Evaluation and Utilization of Stallion Semen for Artificial Insemination. Animal Reproduction Laboratory Bulletin No. 03. Fort Collins, Colorado State University, 1987.)

If a twist or wrinkle is noted when the AV is being lubricated, it must be removed, although this is difficult. Occasionally, the problem can be corrected without starting over if someone pulls on the tapered end of the rubber combination liner and cone while another person pushes with the hand from inside the AV. A plastic liner is virtually impossible to straighten without removing water from the AV.

Once the liner is smooth, the outside, or shoulder portion, of the glove is reflected over the posterior end of the AV until time to collect the stallion. This prevents contamination and reduces heat loss (Fig. 79–9). We generally recommend that the AV lubricant be kept in an incubator. Warm lubricant can be used to adjust internal temperature of the AV by 2 to 6° C; it can be warmed more quickly by placing it into a bucket of hot water or it can be kept at room temperature or in cold water. For example, if the AV is slightly warmer than ideal, cold lubricant can be used to adjust the temperature and vice versa. This can prevent delays in synchronizing readiness of the AV with that of the stallion.

PREPARATION OF THE STALLION FOR SEMINAL COLLECTION

Ability to handle a stallion in a manner that will elicit maximal favorable sexual response with a minimum of difficulty is an art. In general, some basic rules exist, but each handler is different, as is each stallion. Therefore, what may work in one situation may not apply in another. The amount of restraint necessary for a stallion to react favorably and still ensure the safety of mare, handler, and collector should be applied. Some stallions respond to voice commands and need only a minimum of restraint to be under complete control. Others need a

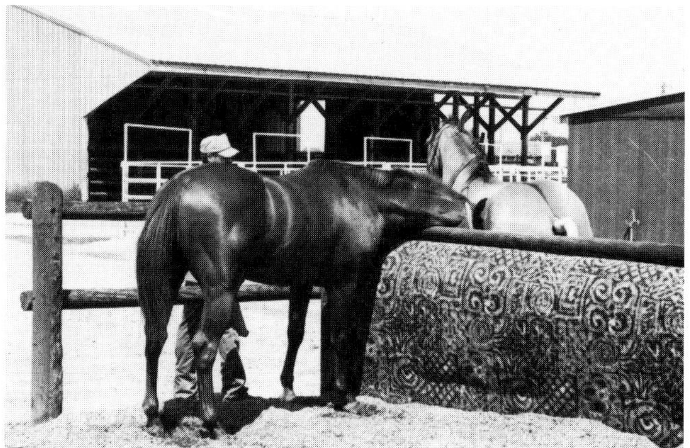

FIG. 79–10. Stallion teasing a mare over a padded barrier. (From Pickett, B.W., Squires, E.L., and McKinnon, A.O.: Procedures for Collection, Evaluation and Utilization of Stallion Semen for Artificial Insemination. Animal Reproduction Laboratory Bulletin No. 03. Fort Collins, Colorado State University, 1987.)

chain through the mouth or a severe bit, plus physical barriers. We strongly recommend that every farm have facilities that will permit a stallion to tease a mare safely (Fig. 79–10) so that he may become sexually stimulated while his penis is being washed. Furthermore, the washing procedure should constitute a sexually stimulating experience.

WASHING THE STALLION'S PENIS

In recent years, considerable controversy has existed about what type of soap and/or disinfectants should be used to wash and/or rinse a stallion's penis. Jones et al. have shown that once the breeding season is under way, no advantage was found to using anything other than warm water.[9] Therefore, warm water ~42° C (~108° F) is placed into a bucket protected with a plastic liner that is secured with a stout rubber band. Again, measure the temperature, *do not estimate.* A container for rinsing the stallion's penis is placed into the bucket. The stallion is then brought from his stall and presented to an estrous mare positioned behind a well-padded barrier (Fig. 79–10). The stallion should be allowed to tease the mare with as much freedom as possible without endangering himself, the mare, or the personnel. When an appropriate erection is attained, the handler puts some restraint on the stallion to permit quick, effective washing.

The individual who washes the stallion should wear plastic, disposable gloves. Washing is generally somewhat easier and quicker with most stallions, if someone holds the bucket while the stallion is being washed. The stallion's erect penis should be deflected, not grasped, and moistened with water and then massaged gently, but thoroughly. More water is added as necessary. The penis should be observed closely during the washing procedure for lesions, inflamed urethral orifice, etc. When it is suitably cleaned, the penis is thoroughly rinsed (Fig. 79–11); drying is not necessary. If the stallion's penis becomes contaminated after washing but before collection, it should be rinsed with warm water. In natural service, the stallion's penis should be washed with warm water before and after breeding, but most particularly after breeding (Chapter 85).

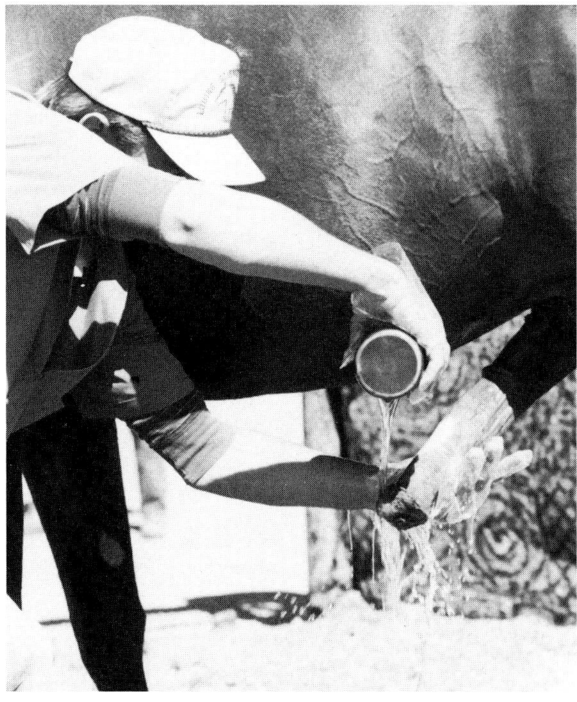

FIG. 79–11. Rinsing the stallion's penis. (From Pickett, B.W., Squires, E.L., and McKinnon, A.O.: Procedures for Collection, Evaluation and Utilization of Stallion Semen for Artificial Insemination. Animal Reproduction Laboratory Bulletin No. 03. Fort Collins, Colorado State University, 1987.)

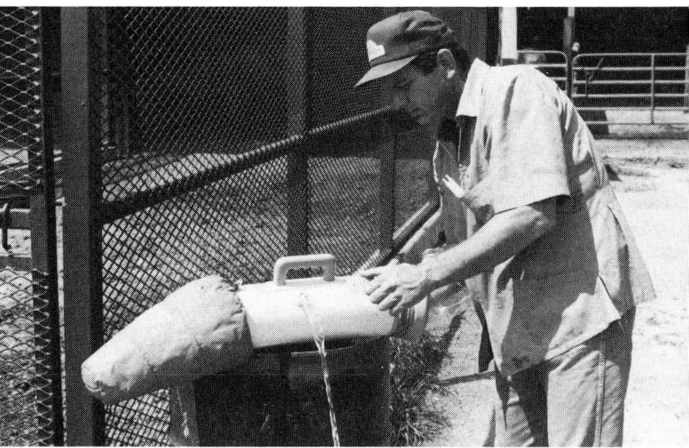

FIG. 79–12. Adjusting the internal pressure of the artificial vagina. (From Pickett, B.W., Squires, E.L., and McKinnon, A.O.: Procedures for Collection, Evaluation and Utilization of Stallion Semen for Artificial Insemination. Animal Reproduction Laboratory Bulletin No. 03. Fort Collins, Colorado State University, 1987.)

SEMINAL COLLECTION

While the stallion's penis is being washed, the mare is positioned and restrained with a twitch. Meanwhile, the collector observes the stallion and adjusts internal pressure of the AV (Fig. 79–12). When the washing procedure is completed, everything should be ready so that the stallion can be presented to the mare immediately. The mare should be positioned in a location that has good footing. Extreme caution should be taken to ensure that conditions are ideal before seminal collection is attempted. If conditions are not completely satisfactory, return the stallion to his stall and correct the deficiencies. Failure to follow this procedure is the most common cause of avoidable accidents during collection or breeding.

The collector should be positioned on the near side and slightly behind the stallion handler where he or she can observe the mare and the stallion (Fig. 79–13). The collector should direct mare and stallion handlers, just as the breeding shed manager does when natural ser-

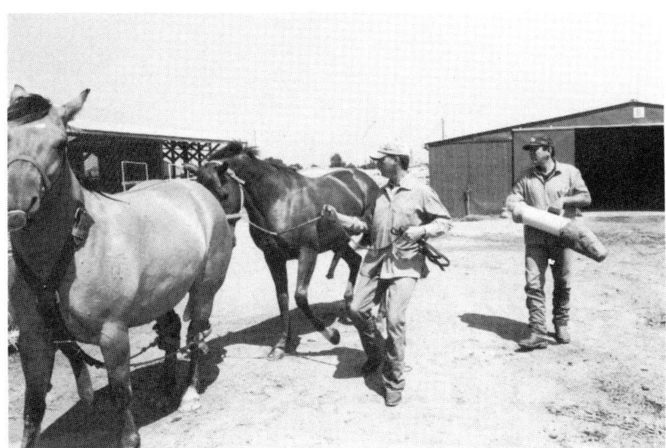

FIG. 79–13. Appropriate position for the mare, stallion, stallion handler, and collector. (From Pickett, B.W., Squires, E.L., and McKinnon, A.O.: Procedures for Collection, Evaluation and Utilization of Stallion Semen for Artificial Insemination. Animal Reproduction Laboratory Bulletin No. 03. Fort Collins, Colorado State University, 1987.)

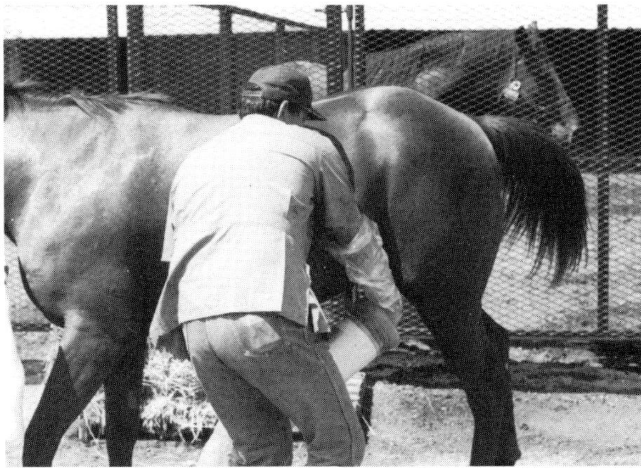

FIG. 79–15. Lowering the AV as the stallion completes ejaculation. (From Pickett, B.W., Squires, E.L., and McKinnon, A.O.: Procedures for Collection, Evaluation and Utilization of Stallion Semen for Artificial Insemination. Animal Reproduction Laboratory Bulletin No. 03. Fort Collins, Colorado State University, 1987.)

vice is being practiced. The stallion is allowed to approach the mare and mount immediately, if he has an erection. The handler should make sure that plenty of slack exists in the shank. The collector then steps forward and deflects the stallion's penis into the AV. The AV should be held at an angle that is comfortable for the stallion. As the stallion thrusts, the collector should manipulate the AV to provide maximal sexual stimulation. The left hand remains on the handle of the AV, while the right hand holds the AV from the bottom (Fig. 79–14). The weight of the AV is supported by pushing it against the mare with the ribs or hip.

Pushing the AV upward against the stallion's abdomen is usually more stimulating than pushing it down on the penis. When the stallion begins to ejaculate, spurts of semen (pulsations) through the urethra can be felt if the collector slides the hand on the AV to the bottom of the penis. These pulsations are usually associated with a pumping movement of the tail called flagging. After two or three pulsations, the anterior end of the AV should be lowered gradually. At this point the collector should grasp the stallion's penis and continue to lower the AV until it is almost vertical, as the stallion loses his erection (Fig. 79–15). If the AV is lowered too rapidly, the stallion will experience discomfort and that may interfere with ejaculation. Lowering the AV also permits more efficient separation of the sperm-rich fraction from the gel fraction as gel enters at the end of ejaculation. The collector examines the stallion's urethral orifice for presence of a white, frothy secretion, which is further evidence that ejaculation has occurred.

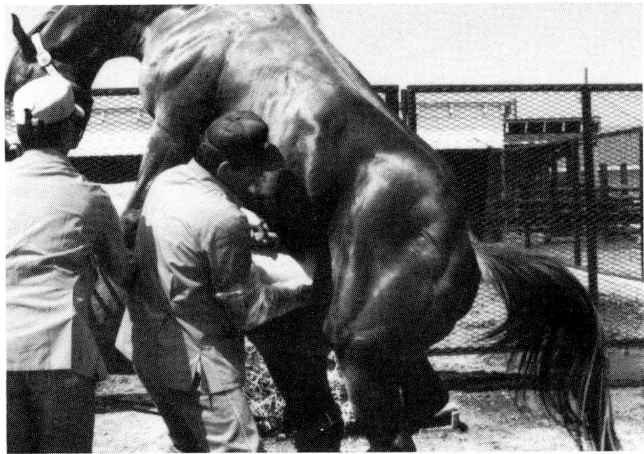

FIG. 79–14. Correct method of holding the AV while the stallion is thrusting. (Courtesy of Colorado State University.)

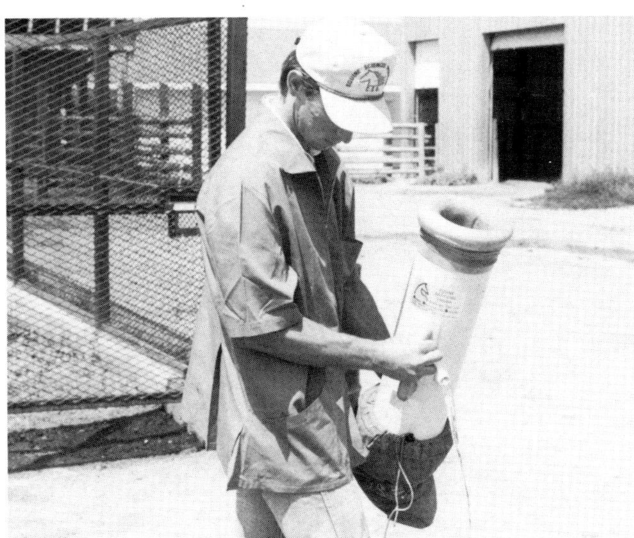

FIG. 79–16. Releasing water from the AV while it is in a vertical position. (From Pickett, B.W., Squires, E.L., and McKinnon, A.O.: Procedures for Collection, Evaluation and Utilization of Stallion Semen for Artificial Insemination. Animal Reproduction Laboratory Bulletin No. 03. Fort Collins, Colorado State University, 1987.)

If ejaculation occurred, the collector immediately steps away from the stallion, holding the AV in a vertical position, and removes the filler cap, to allow water to run out and reduce internal pressure (Fig. 79–16). This permits any semen that may have been ejaculated toward the posterior (open) end of the AV to drain into the collection bottle. The collection procedure should be such that semen was deposited into the tapered end of the combination liner and cone. The collector should proceed immediately to the laboratory with the AV and semen.

Immediately after the stallion dismounts, the mare handler should pull the mare to the left and forward. The stallion handler should back the stallion a few steps and also turn him to the left. This prevents the horses' buttocks from touching and minimizes risk of injury from kicking. However, the mare handler should not move the mare before the stallion's forefeet have touched the ground, lest they become tangled in the hobbles.

HANDLING AND EVALUATION OF SEMEN AFTER COLLECTION

After semen is collected, it should be taken immediately to the laboratory. The AV is placed on a countertop or in a rack designed to prevent it from rolling. The plunger in the slip lock is pulled so the drawstring holding the protector jacket onto the AV can be loosened. The protector jacket is removed, the AV tilted, and combination liner and cone stretched to ensure that all semen has drained into the collection bottle. The clamp is released, and the bottle is removed from the tapered end of the combination liner and cone. The filter is removed and discarded. Spillage can occur if the collection bottle is removed too quickly, because excessive gel or inversion of the filter may prevent drainage of semen into the bottle.

Spermatozoa, particularly from some stallions, are fragile. Therefore, the clinician must not expose the collection bottle to a cold countertop or anything that will rapidly alter the temperature of the semen. A warmed (~38° C, ~100° F) graduated cylinder is removed from the incubator and tilted to about a 30° angle so that semen can be poured slowly down the side. The objective is to get semen into a warmed graduated cylinder, for measurement, as soon as possible after collection. Once semen is in the graduated cylinder, it should be identified and placed in an incubator and the volume should be recorded.

The next step is to evaluate semen for percentage of progressively motile spermatozoa (motility). This should be done as accurately and quickly as possible. To obtain an accurate estimate of motility, the semen must be diluted or extended in an appropriate fluid, which will hereafter be designated as an "extender." Spermatozoa in raw semen tend to clump or agglutinate, making an accurate estimate of percentage of progressively motile spermatozoa in raw semen impossible.[10] The fluid we recommend to extend the semen is E-Z Mixin (Animal Reproduction Systems). The extender is prepared, and 4.75-mL aliquots are pipetted into 8-mL glass vials, which are then warmed to ~38° C (~100° F) before the addition of 0.25 mL semen. This dilution of 1:20 is sufficient to disperse spermatozoa and permit observation of an individual spermatozoon. If the semen is highly concentrated, a smaller volume may be added to the extender and vice versa.

Once semen is added to extender, the vial is inverted several times to ensure thorough mixing. The vial is placed on a warming table and allowed to sit for a moment before estimation. This waiting period is not necessary in most cases, but occasionally motility will improve if spermatozoa have an opportunity to acclimate to the extender. Presented in Figure 79–17 is a warming table maintained at ~38° C (~100° F). On the table are volumetric pipettes for measuring semen, pasteur pipettes for transferring semen, glass slides, and cover slips. Everything that comes into contact with the semen should be clean and maintained at body temperature. The extended semen should be kept on this table or in an incubator.

To prepare a sample for estimation of motility, place one drop of extended semen on each end of a clean glass slide. Cover each drop with a clean coverslip, taking care to avoid trapping air bubbles in the semen, then place the slide on a microscope stage. In the event that the microscope stage is not temperature controlled at ~38° C (~100° F), the slide should be placed in a stage incubator. The specimen must be kept warm during evaluation.

To estimate motility accurately, a phase-contrast microscope is essential (Fig. 79–18). This type of microscope permits clear resolution of materials of similar optical density. The specimen should be observed at 200 magnifications. The clinician should observe three to five fields per coverslip and be certain the fields are near the center. Estimates from each field should be aver-

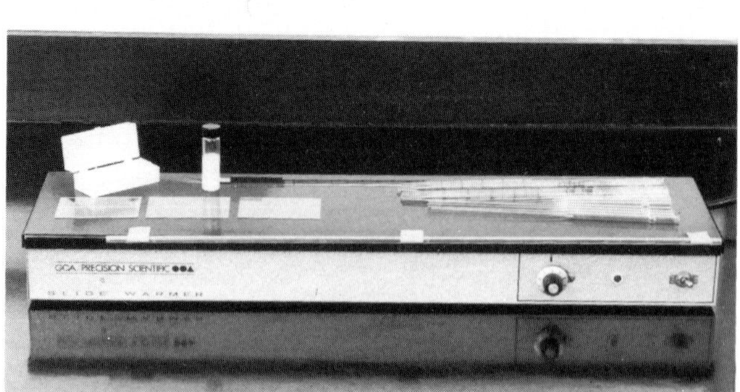

FIG. 79–17. Warming table for maintaining temperature of extended semen and glassware to be used in estimation of sperm motility. (From Pickett, B.W., Squires, E.L., and McKinnon, A.O.: Procedures for Collection, Evaluation and Utilization of Stallion Semen for Artificial Insemination. Animal Reproduction Laboratory Bulletin No. 03. Fort Collins, Colorado State University, 1987.)

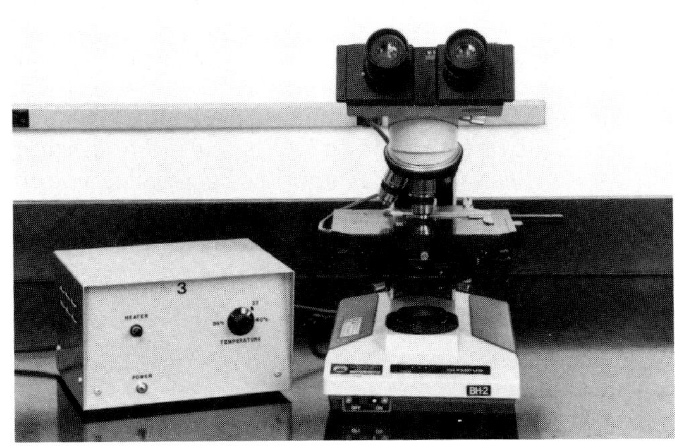

FIG. 79–18. Phase-contrast microscope and stage-temperature regulator. (From Pickett, B.W., Squires, E.L., and McKinnon, A.O.: Procedures for Collection, Evaluation and Utilization of Stallion Semen for Artificial Insemination. Animal Reproduction Laboratory Bulletin No. 03. Fort Collins, Colorado State University, 1987.)

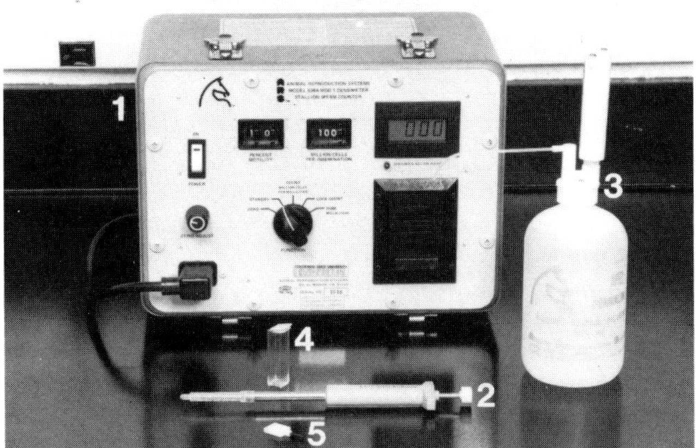

FIG. 79–19. Equipment for estimating number of spermatozoa per milliliter of gel-free semen; 1, densimeter; 2, semen pipettor; 3, formalin dispenser; 4, plastic cuvette with cap; 5, calibration device. (From Pickett, B.W., Squires, E.L., and McKinnon, A.O.: Procedures for Collection, Evaluation and Utilization of Stallion Semen for Artificial Insemination. Animal Reproduction Laboratory Bulletin No. 03. Fort Collins, Colorado State University, 1987.)

aged. If the difference between two estimates is greater than 10%, a new slide should be prepared. Accuracy is improved if two individuals make estimates. Also, the same sample can be estimated several times over an hour. In spite of bias caused by the original estimate, this procedure increases confidence.

Many spermatozoa that are moving may not be progressively motile. For a spermatozoon to be called progressively motile, it must move across the microscopic field reasonably rapidly and, with each back and forth lash of the tail, the head must rotate 360°. Spermatozoa with any other type of motility should be considered dead. This estimation of motility is greatly complicated when some spermatozoa are exhibiting normal motility and others are going in circles and not rotating, while others are lashing their tails with no forward movement or rotation. Because approximately 50% of all stallion spermatozoa have abaxial midpieces, they move in a circle if they do not rotate.

ESTIMATING THE NUMBER OF SPERMATOZOA

Once motility has been evaluated, which should not require more than 2 to 5 min, the number of spermatozoa per milliliter of semen must be estimated. In Figure 79–19 is the instrument and equipment for this purpose. The instrument must be turned on at least 10 min before use. A total of 3.42 mL formalin in 0.9% sodium chloride solution is placed into a cuvette with an automatic pipettor. The plastic cuvette is clear on two sides and ribbed on the other two. Care should be used to touch the cuvette only on ribbed sides. In the event that lint, dust, fingerprints, etc. need to be removed from the clear sides, it should be done with lint-free paper such as Kimwipe. The cuvette containing 3.42 mL formalin–sodium chloride solution is placed into the counting chamber of the densimeter with ribbed sides out. The counting chamber door is closed, the indicator knob is turned to zero, and the zero-adjust knob is rotated until 0.00 appears on the display panel.

The automatic semen pipettor must be calibrated before each use with the standard provided by the manufacturer. An aliquot of raw semen (0.18 mL) is drawn into the automatic semen pipettor, and excess semen is removed from the outside with a Kimwipe. Care must be exercised to avoid removing even the slightest amount of semen from inside the pipettor. Semen is then dispensed into the formalin–sodium chloride solution in the cuvette, without touching the tip of the pipettor into the solution. A plastic cap is fitted into the cuvette, and the semen and diluting fluid are slowly and thoroughly mixed by inverting the cuvette repeatedly. Before returning the cuvette to the counting

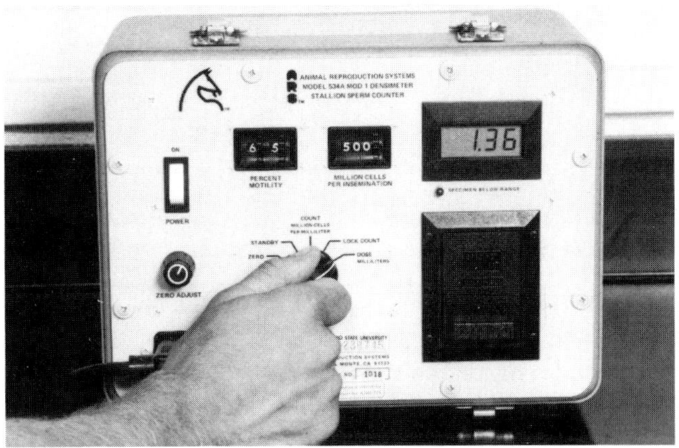

FIG. 79–20. Calculating the volume of gel-free semen necessary to provide 500 million motile spermatozoa (1.36 mL). (Courtesy of Colorado State University.)

chamber, be sure that semen is thoroughly mixed with diluting fluid; that there are no air bubbles adhering to the sides of the cuvette; and that any dirt, lint, fingerprints, etc. have been removed from the clear sides of the cuvette.

The cuvette is then placed into the densimeter in exactly the same position in which it was placed when the instrument was adjusted to 0.00. As soon as the cuvette is in place and the chamber door is closed, the knob is turned to *count.* A number will immediately appear on the display screen. However, it may change rapidly for 10 to 30 s, depending on number of spermatozoa in the sample. The counting process is based on an optical system that incorporates a beam of visible light, which is directed through the specimen and recorded on a photodetector. The signal from the photodetector is converted to an absorbance value, which is electronically programmed to convert the value to a measure of sperm density. Once the count on the display screen has stabilized, the knob should be turned to *lock count.* The number on the display screen represents the number of spermatozoa per milliliter of gel-free semen in millions.

After the count has been locked into the instrument, the percent motility that was estimated with the phase-contrast microscope is manually entered into the machine, in the case described here 65, along with the desired number of motile spermatozoa (500 million) per insemination dose. The knob is then turned to *dose milliliters,* and the volume of semen containing the desired number of progressively motile spermatozoa is displayed on the screen, which is 1.36 mL in Figure 79–20. The insemination volume should be 1.5 mL of gel-free semen.

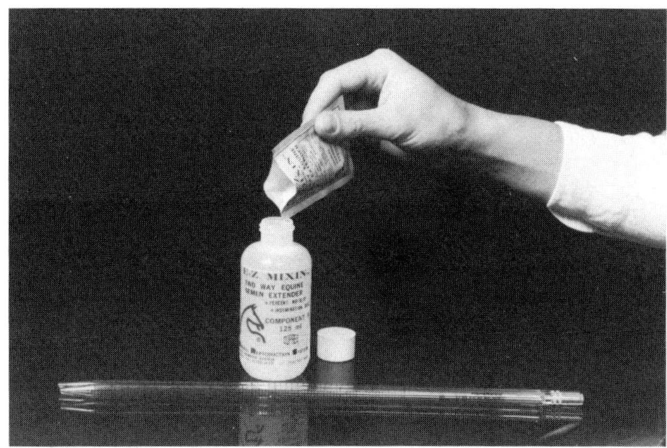

FIG. 79–21. Preparing the E-Z Mixin extender. (From Pickett, B.W., Squires, E.L., and McKinnon, A.O.: Procedures for Collection, Evaluation and Utilization of Stallion Semen for Artificial Insemination. Animal Reproduction Laboratory Bulletin No. 03. Fort Collins, Colorado State University, 1987.)

PREPARATION OF EXTENDER

A commercially prepared extender, E-Z Mixin, is used. The material is received in two components: component A is 125 mL of water in a plastic bottle and component B is a foil-lined packet containing the other ingredients. Component A may be warmed to 38° C (~100° F) and component B added or they can be mixed and then warmed. The dry ingredients should be kept in a cool, dry place, whereas the water can be stored at room temperature. The extender is prepared by placing the contents of component B into component A (Fig. 79–21). After addition of component B, the ingredients should be mixed thoroughly, but gently. The extender is then prepared, and providing it is at ~38° C (~100° F), it is ready to use.

REFERENCES

1. Pickett, B.W., and Back, D.G.: Procedures for Preparation, Collection, Evaluation, and Insemination of Stallion Semen. Animal Reproduction Laboratory General Series Bulletin No. 935. Fort Collins, Colorado State University, 1973.
2. Pickett, B.W., Squires, E.L., and McKinnon, A.O. Procedures for Collection, Evaluation and Utilization of Stallion Semen for Artificial Insemination. Animal Reproduction Laboratory Bulletin No. 03. Fort Collins, Colorado State University, 1987.
3. Hillman, R.B., Olar, T.T., Squires, E.L., and Pickett, B.W.: Temperature of the artificial vagina and its effect on seminal quality and behavioral characteristics of stallions. J. Am. Vet. Med. Assoc., *177:*720–722, 1980.
4. Pickett, B.W., Squires, E.L., and Voss, J.L.: Normal and Abnormal Sexual Behavior of the Equine Male. Animal Reproduction Laboratory General Series Bulletin No. 1004. Fort Collins, Colorado State University, 1981.
5. Voss, J.L., and Pickett, B.W.: Reproductive Management of the Broodmare. Animal Reproduction Laboratory General Series Bulletin No. 961. Fort Collins, Colorado State University, 1976.
6. Kenney, R.M., Bergman, R.V., Cooper, W.L., and Morse, G.W.: Minimal contamination techniques for breeding mares: Technique and preliminary findings. Proc. Am. Assoc. Equine Pract., 327–336, 1975.
7. Amann, R.P., Loomis, P.R., and Pickett, B.W.: Improved filter system for an equine artificial vagina. J. Equine Vet. Sci., *3:*120–125, 1983.
8. Froman, D.P., and Amann, R.P.: Inhibition of motility of bovine, canine and equine spermatozoa by artificial vagina lubricants. Theriogenology, *20:*357–361, 1983.
9. Jones, R.L., et al.: The effect of washing on the aerobic bacterial flora of the stallion's penis. Proc. Am. Assoc. Equine Pract., 9–16, 1984.
10. Pickett, B.W.: Collection and evaluation of stallion semen. Proceedings of the National Association of Animal Breeders Technical Conference on Artificial Insemination and Reproduction, 1968, pp. 80–87.

CHAPTER 80

SPERMATOZOAL FUNCTION

R.P. Amann
J.K. Graham

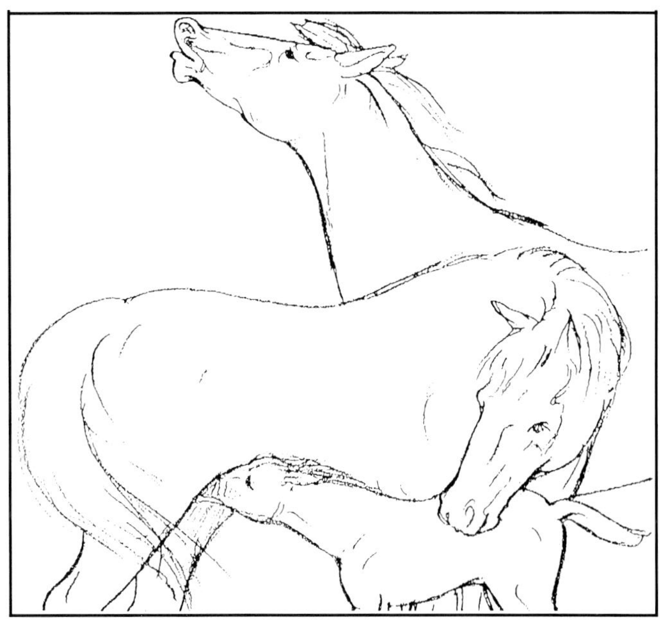

Spermatozoa are unique among cells produced by a stallion, not only by virtue of their haploid number of chromosomes but especially because of their highly specialized function and limited capacity for repair. Although spermatozoa are released from the seminiferous epithelium at the time of spermiation, designating the end of spermatogenesis, this represents but one point in a continuous process of cell modification (Chapter 77). The saga of the spermatid/spermatozoon is initiated with formation of spermatids, their development in the seminiferous epithelium during spermatogenesis, and their release as spermatozoa; continues with modifications, termed spermatozoal maturation, resulting from changes induced by components of luminal fluid within the epididymis; further continues with admixture of spermatozoa and seminal fluids at emission and ejaculation; progresses with exposure to the environment of the female reproductive tract and entrance into the microenvironment of the oocyte; and is culminated following penetration into the investments around the oocyte and ultimately the oocyte proper (Fig. 80–1).[1] Unfortunately, veterinarians and reproductive biologists tend to consider spermatozoa from the perspective of their own narrow interests, such as characteristics of ejaculated spermatozoa, preservation of ejaculated spermatozoa, or in vitro fertilization. This approach ignores the fact that an event modifying a spermatid/spermatozoon at any time during its normal 5-week life span can reduce the ability of that spermatozoon to fertilize an oocyte.

During spermatogenesis, organelles of the spermatid are modified in shape and function from those characteristic of a somatic cell into those appropriate for a cell designed to fertilize an oocyte.[2–5] Nuclear shape is modified from that of a sphere, and the chromatin is condensed and compacted to minimize its volume within the nucleus. A propulsion mechanism is provided as the axoneme, dense fibers, and the fibrous sheath; mitochondria are arrayed in close proximity to the proximal portion of the propulsion system to facilitate transport of adenosine triphosphate (ATP) from the mitochondria to the contracting elements of the axoneme; and a highly specialized structure, the acrosome, which contains hydrolytic enzymes, is placed over the rostral portion of the nucleus to facilitate penetration by the spermatozoon of the investments around the oocyte. Finally, the plasma membrane is anchored to underlying structures at several points over the tail of the spermatozoon but is relatively unattached to underlying structures in the head region. The major portion of the cytoplasm, including organelles characteristic of a somatic cell, is left behind as a residual body retained by the seminiferous epithelium at the time of spermiation. Consequently, although spermatozoa have the capacity for both aerobic and anaerobic metabolism of glucose, lactate, or pyruvate, and oxidation of certain amino acids and lipids, they lack the conventional machinery for biosynthesis and cell repair.

For a spermatozoon to fertilize an oocyte, it must develop and retain at least five general attributes:[6,7]

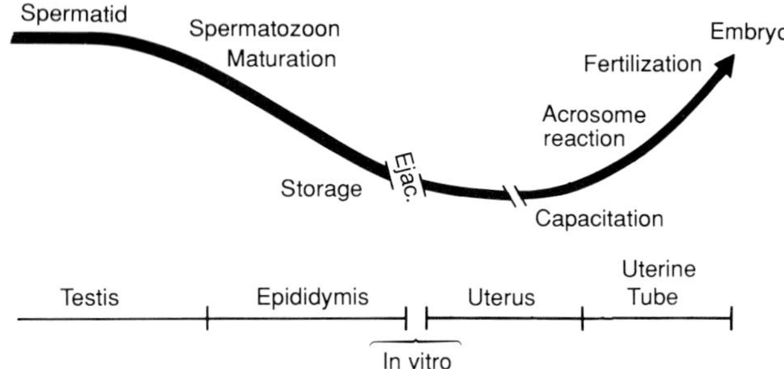

FIG. 80–1. The saga of the stallion spermatid/spermatozoon. An abnormal event, or human intervention, at any point on the lifeline can alter subsequent events. An alteration may be apparent immediately, but it often is not apparent until later in the life line or even by failure of a 4- or 8-cell embryo to develop into a foal. (Adapted from Amann, R.P.: Maturation of spermatozoa. Proceedings of the Eleventh International Congress on Animal Reproduction and Artificial Insemination. Dublin, 1988, pp. 320–328.)

1. Metabolism for production of energy.
2. Progressive motility.
3. Enzymes, located within the acrosome, that are essential for penetration of the spermatozoon through structures surrounding the oocyte.
4. Proper distributions of lipids in the plasma and acrosomal membranes to stabilize these structures until fertilization and ultimately allow membrane fusion at the proper time.
5. Proteins in the plasma membrane that are essential for survival of a spermatozoon within the female reproductive tract, by locally suppressing the immune system and also providing needed interactions with epithelial cells at selected sites and for attachment of the spermatozoon to the plasma membrane of the oocyte at the time of fertilization.

Although certain of these attributes are provided during spermatogenesis, their final development is not completed until maturation of spermatozoa within the epididymis and admixture of spermatozoa with seminal plasma[1,8] (Chapter 77). Although the exact nature and sequence of the multiple changes involved in developing a fertile spermatozoon are unknown for the stallion, researchers have no doubt that each of the attributes listed above is crucial for accomplishment of its task. Furthermore, although spermatozoa from the distal cauda epididymidis are equally as effective as ejaculated spermatozoa for fertilizing oocytes, with resulting embryos developing into newborns, seminal plasma alters spermatozoa in a manner presumed to be beneficial. Although seminal plasma probably is important in modifying spermatozoa,[9] as well as providing a large volume to facilitate their distribution within the uterus of a mare, it is not an ideal medium for storage of spermatozoa[10] and sometimes contains deleterious components.

Even what appear to be normal spermatozoa may not be competitive. Spermatozoa from some males are able to "beat out" spermatozoa from another male, or several males, when deposited simultaneously in the female reproductive tract by heterospermic insemination[11] or sequentially, as might happen in the wild when several males copulate with an estrous female. This probably is an evolutionary feature to help perpetuate a species.[12] Similarly, strains of mammals or poultry can be selected for fertility. A horse breeder who goes to extreme efforts to obtain progeny of a subfertile male by application of techniques of modern animal biotechnology is imprudent, because that might only perpetuate undesirable reproductive traits.

STRUCTURE OF EQUINE SPERMATOZOA

A spermatozoon usually is considered as having a head, neck, middle piece, principal piece, and end piece[2,13–17] (Fig. 80–2). Each of these five structural regions will be considered in detail, together with functions of the components of each region. However, from the perspective of storage of spermatozoa for use in artificial insemination, either at 5° C or especially −196° C, it is more relevant to consider spermatozoa as consisting of a highly condensed nucleus and microtubular, fibrous, and membranous structures, because of the differential response of these types of structural components to cold shock, reduced temperature, or cryopreservation.[18–20] Microtubular and fibrous structures are important for spermatozoal motility, because they constitute the doublets of the axoneme and the dense fibers and fibrous sheath of the middle piece and principal piece. However, membranous structures are more important from the perspective of cold shock. Cold shock is a type of damage which could be inadvertently caused during handling of spermatozoa associated with seminal collection or artificial insemination, even when semen is not intentionally cooled in preparation for storage.[20] Because of the importance of the changes in spermatozoa invoked by thermal stress, the topic is considered in detail in a following section.

PLASMA MEMBRANE

The plasma membrane encompasses the entire spermatozoon and is its outermost component. Although it is continuous over the surface of the spermatozoa except after the acrosome reaction, which is a prelude to fertilization, or with senescence and death, the nature and function of the plasma membrane differs regionally. Not all regional differences in function of the plasma membrane are known, but portions over the rostral and caudal surfaces of the head, middle piece, and principal piece have different roles in spermatozoal function and survival. Regardless of location in a spermatozoon, the plasma membrane consists of three zones: lipid bilayer, phospholipid-water interface, and glycocalyx (Fig. 80–3). In addition, proteins can be adsorbed to the surface of the membrane.

The lipid bilayer is composed of polar phospholipids

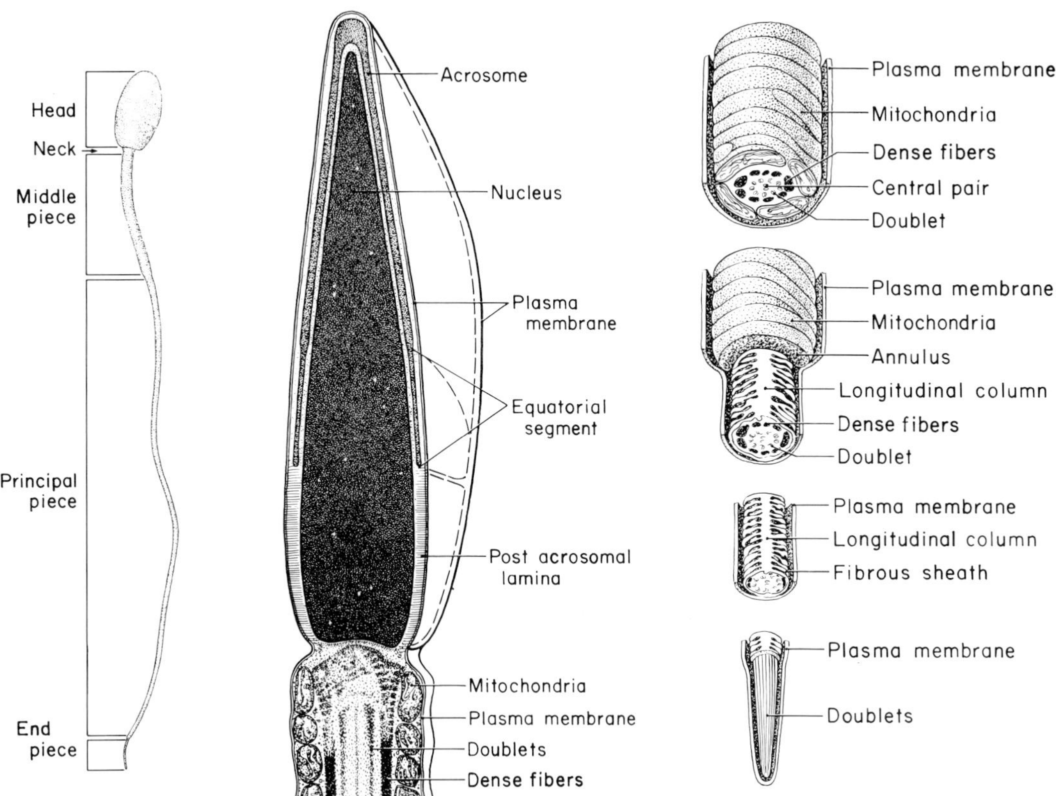

FIG. 80–2. Diagrams of a stallion spermatozoon. The entire spermatozoon is overlaid by the plasma membrane, which usually is in apposition with the underlying structures and is anchored to the caudal margin of the head, at the annulus, and along the longitudinal columns of the principal piece. The head includes the nucleus (containing the genetic information in highly condensed DNA), the bag-like acrosome (containing enzymes necessary for fertilization), a specialized portion of the acrosome termed the equatorial segment, and the postacrosomal lamina. The neck is the point of attachment of the tail to the head, by a ball-and-socket arrangement. The central pair and nine doublets of microtubules, which constitute the axoneme, are surrounded by nine dense fibers. All extend from the neck region, through the middle piece and principal piece, into the end piece where they terminate at slightly different sites. Because these dense fibers are tapered, the tail becomes progressively thinner. The doublets are the contractile elements which contract differentially to induce a sliding motion and flex the tail in a helical pattern. This propels the spermatozoon. Mitochondria are membranous structures where most of the energy necessary for spermatozoal motion is produced. The longitudinal columns and fibrous sheath of the principal piece and the dense fibers provide the rigidity necessary for normal motion of the tail. Dimensions of stallion spermatozoa are approximately as follows: head length, 7 μm; middle piece length, 10 μm; middle piece diameter, 0.9 μm; principal piece length, 40 μm; principal piece diameter, 0.6 to <0.5 μm; and end piece length, 4 μm. (Modified from Amann, R.P., and Pickett, B.W.: Principals of cryopreservation and a review of cryopreservation of stallion spermatozoa. J. Equine Vet. Sci., *7*:145–173, 1987.)

oriented with their hydrophobic fatty acyl chains directed internally and hydrophilic, charged polar headgroups directed externally toward the polar solvent, water[7,18,19] (Fig. 80–4). The predominant lipids are phospholipids and cholesterol. Proteins are intermingled with the lipids and represent about 50% of the weight of the membrane. Proteins within these lipids are considered either integral (essential for structure of the membrane) or peripheral (associated with the membrane, but easily removed). Some integral proteins serve as pores or channels through the membrane or are surface receptors for other molecules, whereas others are found between the two bilayers of the membrane. Many proteins on the external surface contain carbohydrate side chains, which tend to have a net negative charge and attract, and loosely bind, other proteins in the medium around the spermatozoon. Because of this adsorbed material, the outer aspect of the glycocalyx region of a spermatozoon can change, depending on its history and the medium it is in.

Only limited data exist on the composition of the plasma membranes of stallion spermatozoa.[21] The cholesterol to phospholipid ratio in the plasma membrane is 0.36, which is midway between values for boar and bull spermatozoa. As in spermatozoa from other domestic species, choline, ethanolamine, and sphingomyelin are the major phospholipid classes. In spermatozoa from common mammals, composition and localized distribution of phospholipids, and the nature of their fatty acyl side chains, differ within certain domains or regions of the plasma membrane. This probably also is true of stallion spermatozoa. Normally, different phos-

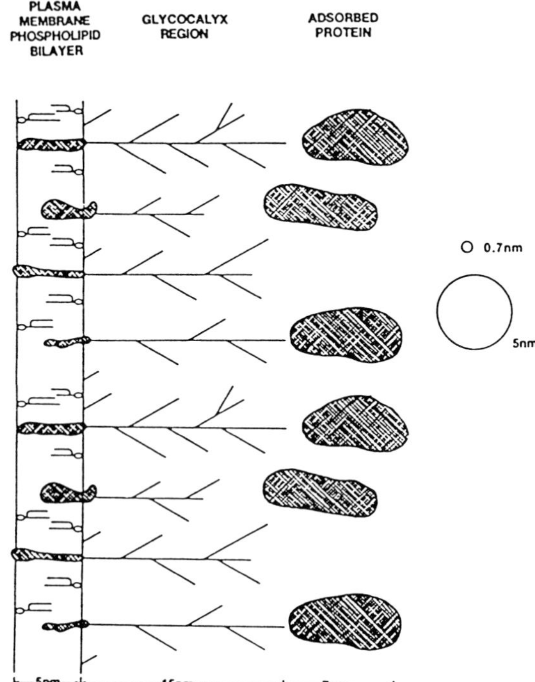

FIG. 80–3. Functional view of the plasma membrane of a spermatozoon, showing spatial relationships and distances. Both small (molecular weight 20,000) and large (molecular weight 60,000) solutes that might approach the membrane are depicted. Their approach to the lipid bilayer is influenced by the nature and amount of proteins adsorbed to the glycocalyx and the nature of the glycocalyx per se. (From Hammerstedt, R.H., Graham, J.K., and Nolan, J.P.: Cryopreservation of mammalian sperm: What we ask them to survive. J. Androl., *11*:73–88, 1990.)

pholipids are randomly arranged in a lamellar fashion and are free to move about laterad within one leaflet of the membrane bilayer.[7,18] This is because membranes are fluid at body temperature. Furthermore, the lipid molecules are in a liquid rather than a gel or crystalline state. The ratio of cholesterol to phospholipids with polyunsaturated acyl side chains, as well as the nature of the phospholipid, determines fluidity of the membrane. In general, the more cholesterol present, the less fluid or flexible is that portion of the membrane. Cholesterol aids in keeping the phospholipids in a random, lamellar arrangement.

Normally, an adequate amount of cholesterol and the random distribution of integral membrane proteins impose a lamellar configuration on phospholipids and a normal bilayer is maintained. Under certain conditions, however, the lipids may change into crystalline arrays (because of a phase transition) and the proteins become aggregated.[18] This induces instability in the membrane and the membrane may be damaged irreversibly. Cooling is one factor inducing such changes.

At least three areas of specialization of the plasma membrane serve to anchor it to underlying structures.[4,5] These are over the caudal ring of the head, the annulus, and the principal piece (Fig. 80–5). The plasma membrane overlaying the caudal ring, around the caudal end of the nucleus, is characterized by a striated band of intramembrane particles and fusion of the plasma membrane and the posterior ring. Over the annulus, the plasma membrane contains a densely packed band of particles which probably are involved in attachment of these structures. Finally, the principal piece has a longitudinal row of particles in or on the plasma membrane called the zipper. This is presumed to provide a firm attachment of the membrane and underlying structures in the principal piece. The plasma membrane overlaying the postacrosomal lamina may also be stabilized to underlying structures, because it is much less susceptible to vesiculation such as occurs during the acrosome reaction or senescent degeneration; alternatively it may have a unique lipid composition.

HEAD

The head of a spermatozoon includes the nucleus with its nuclear envelope, the acrosome, postacrosomal lamina, and the plasma membrane (Fig. 80–5). The shape

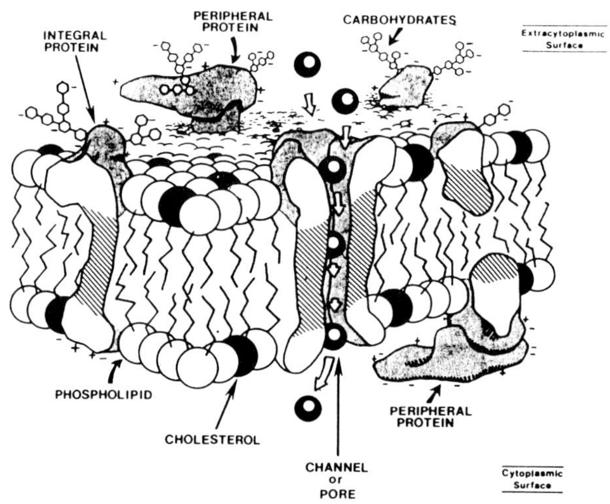

FIG. 80–4. A diagrammatic representation of the plasma membrane with the outer face up. This figure is an oversimplification, but it illustrates the complexity of membranes. Other membranes in a spermatozoon are similar in nature, but they may lack the extensive array of exposed carbohydrates constituting the glycocalyx. The membrane is composed of lipids (mainly phospholipids and cholesterol) and proteins (peripheral and integral). The structure of integral proteins allows formation of both hydrophilic (dark gray) and hydrophobic (striped) regions. The hydrophobic regions allow intercalation of proteins into the hydrophobic interior of the lipid bilayer. Carbohydrate groups (depicted on the upper surface) probably are found only on the extracellular side of plasma membranes. The channel, or pore, facilitates transport of small molecules through the membrane. The head groups of phospholipids are depicted as spheres, although in actuality they differ in size and shape, as does the nature of fatty acyl side chains. (From Zafian, P.T.: Plasma membrane alterations induced in bovine spermatozoa by cryopreservation. M.S. thesis. Colorado State University, 1984.)

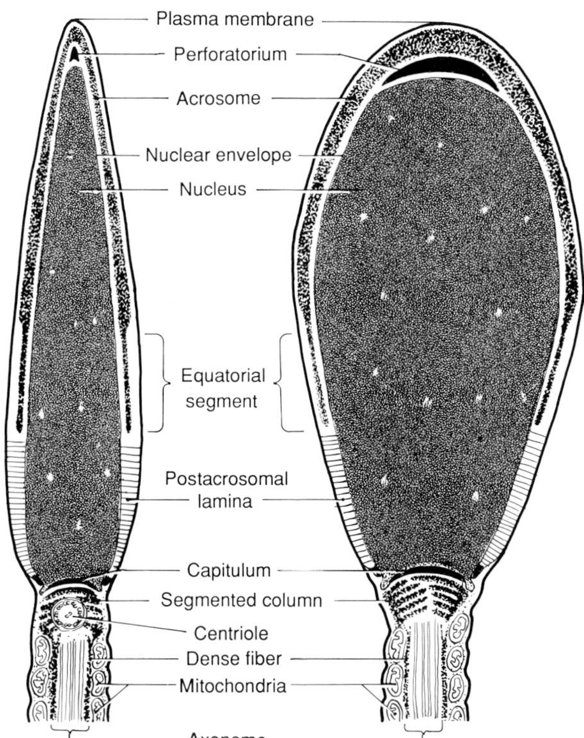

FIG. 80–5. Scale drawings of the head of a stallion spermatozoon. The head and neck are shown in longitudinal section and as viewed from the broad aspect. Major components include plasma membrane, acrosome, equatorial segment region of acrosome, postacrosomal lamina, and proximal centriole. Not shown is the close apposition of the plasma membrane and the underlying structures or its attachment to the underlying nuclear envelope at the caudal ring.

of the head is determined primarily by shape of its nucleus. For stallion spermatozoa, the head and nucleus are broad and relatively flat. The nucleus is gradually tapered from a narrow rostral end to a thicker caudal end, with maximum width of the broad aspect in the center (Fig. 80–5). The nucleus contains the highly condensed chromatin, DNA complexed with protamine, which typically is homogenous in appearance when viewed by an electron microscope. The nucleus is enclosed by the double-layered nuclear envelope, which contains few pores.

The rostral portion of the nucleus is overlain by the acrosome, which is a specialized vesicle formed from a double-layered membrane (Fig. 80–6). The acrosome in turn is overlain by the plasma membrane.[2,4,5,16,17,22] The acrosome contains glycolipids and enzymes, at least some of which are bound to the inner face of the inner acrosomal membrane rather than being contained in the contents (which appears amorphous under the electron microscope). Hyaluronidase, proacrosin/acrosin, and lipases are the primary enzymes. In stallion spermatozoa, the acrosome is slightly thickened but sharply tapered at the rostral end.[16,17] No conspicuous thickening is found on one side (apical segment or ridge) as is

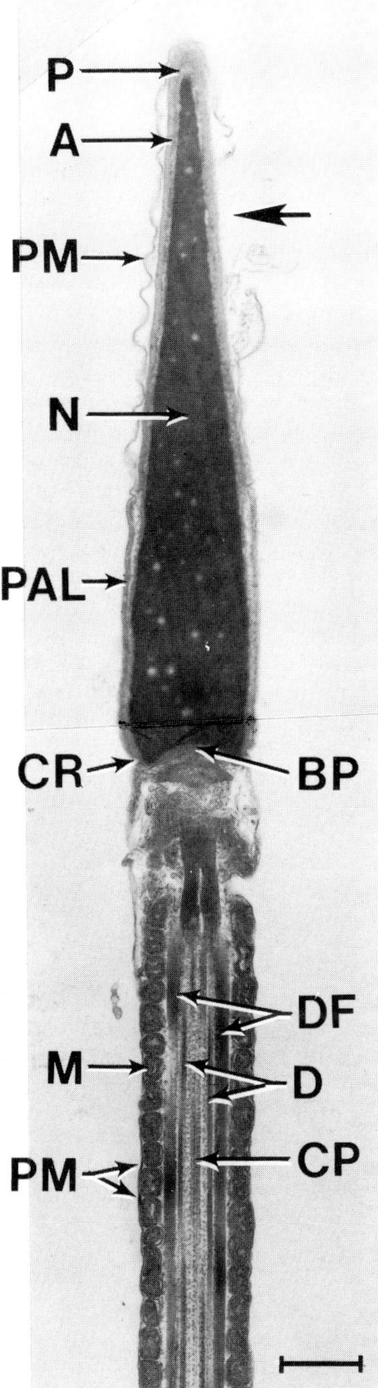

FIG. 80–6. The head, neck, and proximal middle piece of a stallion spermatozoon. In the head, perforatorium (P), acrosome (A), plasma membrane (PM), nucleus (N) with nuclear vacuoles, postacrosomal lamina (PAL), caudal ring (CR), and basal plate (BP) are evident. In the neck and middle piece, the mitochondria (M), plasma membrane (PM), two dense fibers (DF), two doublets (D), and the central pair (CP) are designated. A tear or vesiculation of the plasma membrane, evident on the right side (arrow), is a common artifact seen in transmission electron micrographs of spermatozoa. Bar is 0.5 μm; magnification ×23,000.

characteristic of bull, boar, and ram spermatozoa. Occasionally, evidence for a stabilizing structure, the perforatorium, can be seen under the rostral aspect of the acrosome. Caudad, the acrosome is thinner and this area is termed the equatorial segment. The outer acrosomal membrane rostral to the equatorial segment is uniquely fusogenic, and fuses with the plasma membrane during the acrosome reaction, which precedes fertilization (Chapter 56). The equatorial segment of the acrosome does not contain enzymes and is not involved in the acrosome reaction, but the plasma membrane in this area fuses with that of the oocyte.

The postacrosomal lamina covers the caudal portion of the nucleus, equatorial segment of the acrosome, and posterior ring (see Figs. 80–2 and 80–5). This ill-defined structure may have a secondary role in attachment of a spermatozoon to the plasma membrane of the oocyte at fertilization. The caudal ring is a point of fusion between the plasma membrane and the nuclear envelope, at the caudal end of the head.

The implantation fossa, at the base of the head, is a ball-and-socket articulation which serves to attach the neck (and the rest of the spermatozoon) to the head. The outer layer of the double-layered nuclear envelope lining the implantation fossa is thickened into a distinct basal plate. The basal plate provides the actual attachment with the neck. This attachment is fragile. In stallion spermatozoa, in contrast to those from other common mammals, the implantation fossa often is acentric in position, with respect to the breadth of the cell, and thus about 50% of stallion spermatozoa have an "abaxial tail"[23] (Fig. 80–7). In the rare cases when a spermatozoon actually has two tails, two implantation fossae exist.

NECK

The neck is the connection between the middle piece and the head (Fig. 80–8). It contains a complex structure termed the connecting piece, the proximal centriole, several small mitochondria, and redundant nuclear envelope.[2,4,5,17] The neck region is fragile, and the connecting piece contains several specialized elements, namely the segmented columns and capitulum. Malconnection of the head and neck may occur during spermatogenesis as a hereditary defect, or separation can be induced because of hereditary epididymal malfunction or other reasons.[13]

The nine segmented columns are formed from a series of about 15 overlapping plate-like structures, formed from a fibrous protein. Each segmented column is fused, in the neck region, to the rostral origin of one of the nine dense fibers (Fig. 80–8), which are components of the middle and principal pieces. The segmented columns are not continuous with the dense fibers. Two pairs of the nine segmented columns are fused together over most of their length to form two major segmented columns; the remaining five are termed minor segmented columns. The two major segmented columns differ in shape (Figs. 80–7 and 80–8). The primary one bends sharply and gives rise to the major portion of the capitulum, which is an enlarged head or ball which serves as the attachment with the basal plate of the head. The two stacks of plates in the other major segmented column are not fused together until they are rostral to the centriole, and then extend as a single fused stack of plates fused to the capitulum. Together, the two major segmented columns and capitulum form a continuous, elongated, articulation which has its long

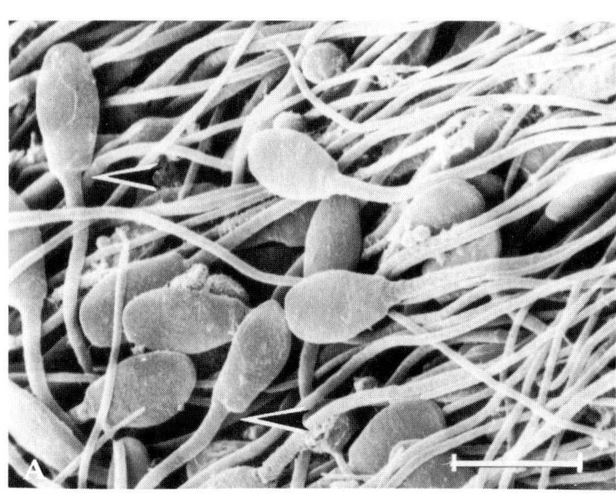

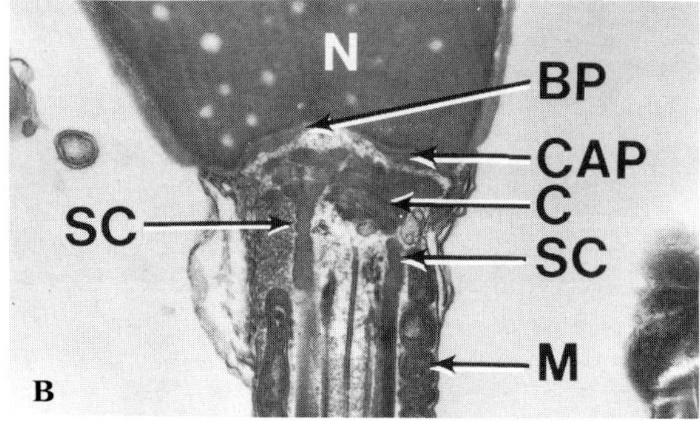

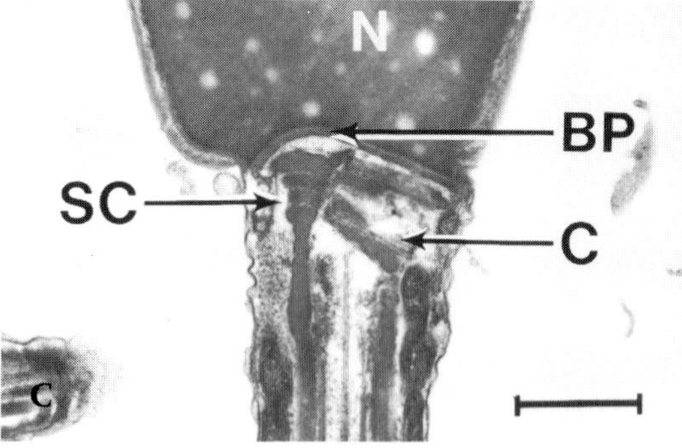

FIG. 80–7. *A,* Scanning electron microscopic view of spermatozoa with axial or abaxial (arrows) attachment of the tail. Bar is 5.0 μm, magnification ×34,000. The implantation fossa and neck region of spermatozoa with a central attachment *(B)* or an abaxial attachment *(C)* of the tail, as viewed by transmission electron microscopy. The nucleus (N), basal plate (BP), capitulum (CAP), centriole (C), segmented columns (SC), mitochondria (M), and dense fibers plus axoneme of the middle piece are evident. Bar is 0.5 μm; magnification ×26,600.

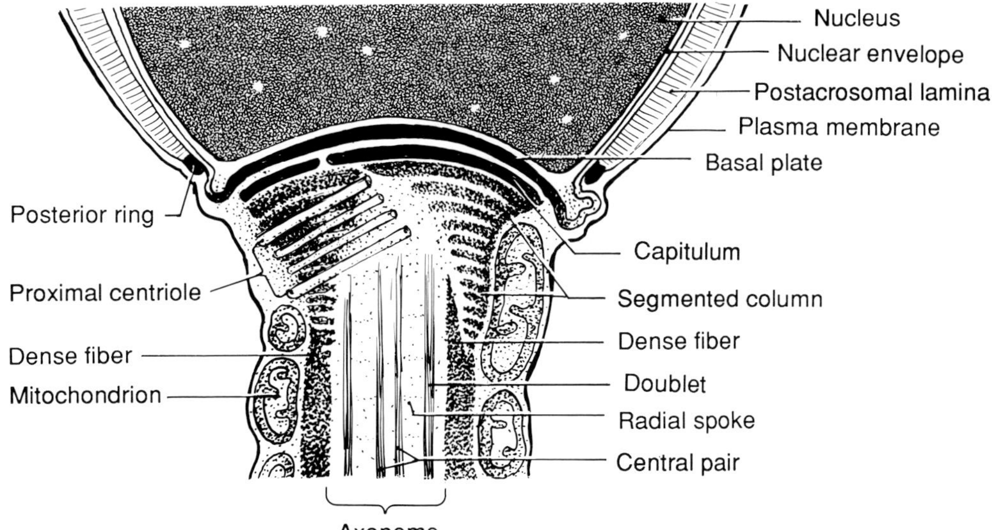

FIG. 80–8. Sketch of the neck region of a spermatozoon. The implantation fossa, at the base of the head, includes the basal plate which is attached to the capitulum, the most proximal structure of the principal piece. The capitulum consists of the cranial segments of the segmented columns which are coupled to the dense fibers. When the tail is detached from the head, usually it is because of separation of the basal plate and capitulum.

axis in the same plane as the broad axis of the spermatozoal head. Thus, the major segmented columns might be thought of as running up the "sides" of the neck. The five minor segmented columns bend over and merge with the capitulum on the dorsal and ventral aspects of the neck area.

The proximal centriole is located between the major segmented columns, within the anterior end of the connecting piece. This centriole has the characteristic nine-fibril structure and is positioned at a 45° to 60° angle to the tail axis. In stallion spermatozoa, the proximal centriole is relatively large in comparison with diameter of the neck, and typically one end is near the plasma membrane (see Fig. 80–7). The proximal centriole and connecting piece likely constitute the site where beat of the tail is initiated in mature spermatozoa. The distal centriole, seen in the neck region of a spermatid during development, disappears during formation of the connecting piece. A membranous outpocketing of redundant nuclear envelope lies lateral to the connecting piece. These loops or scrolls represent excess nuclear envelope remaining as the spermatid nucleus underwent condensation and a reduction in volume during spermiogenesis.

MIDDLE PIECE

The middle piece extends from the caudal end of the neck, distad through the annulus.[2,4,5,17] It is characterized by the presence of numerous mitochondria arranged circumferentially, end to end, in a continuous double spiral (Figs. 80–9 and 80–10). The terminations of two mitochondria in one winding of the coil are bordered by the middle of individual mitochondria in the turns above and below. A typical stallion spermatozoon has about 50 gyri, or helical turns, of mitochondria. Cristae are clearly visible by transmission electron microscopy within individual mitochondria. The mitochondria contain the enzymes and cofactors necessary for production of ATP (see next section). The exact mechanism by which energy stored in ATP is converted to contractile activity of the tail is unknown. The outer shell or membrane of a mitochondrion is rich in thiol bonds, and resistant to dissolution. Mitochondrial DNA is present, but its role in cellular function or reproduction is obscure.

Central to the gyri of mitochondria are the nine dense fibers. These have a tough, keratin-like fibrous structure. They extend from their origin in apposition to segmented columns, in the neck of the spermatozoon, through the length of the middle piece and most of the principal piece. They gradually taper away in the caudal principal piece and are not present in the end piece. Among the nine outer dense fibers (see Fig. 80–9), numbers 1, 5, and 6 are larger than the rest; number 9 is intermediate in size; and the rest are small. The dense fibers do not contract, but probably dampen the arc of flagellar beat by providing rigidity concurrently with flexibility.

A convention exists for numbering the dense fibers and doublets. A line tangential to the midpoints of the microtubules in the central pair divides the axoneme and dense fibers into halves (see Fig. 80–9). Four dense fibers or doublets are in either half, and one (pair) is bisected. The bisected dense fiber or doublet is called doublet 1, and doublet 2 is that on the side of doublet 1 to which its arms point. Dense fibers are numbered the same as the corresponding doublet.

The axoneme of a spermatozoon, central to the dense fibers, is identical in organization with the contractile

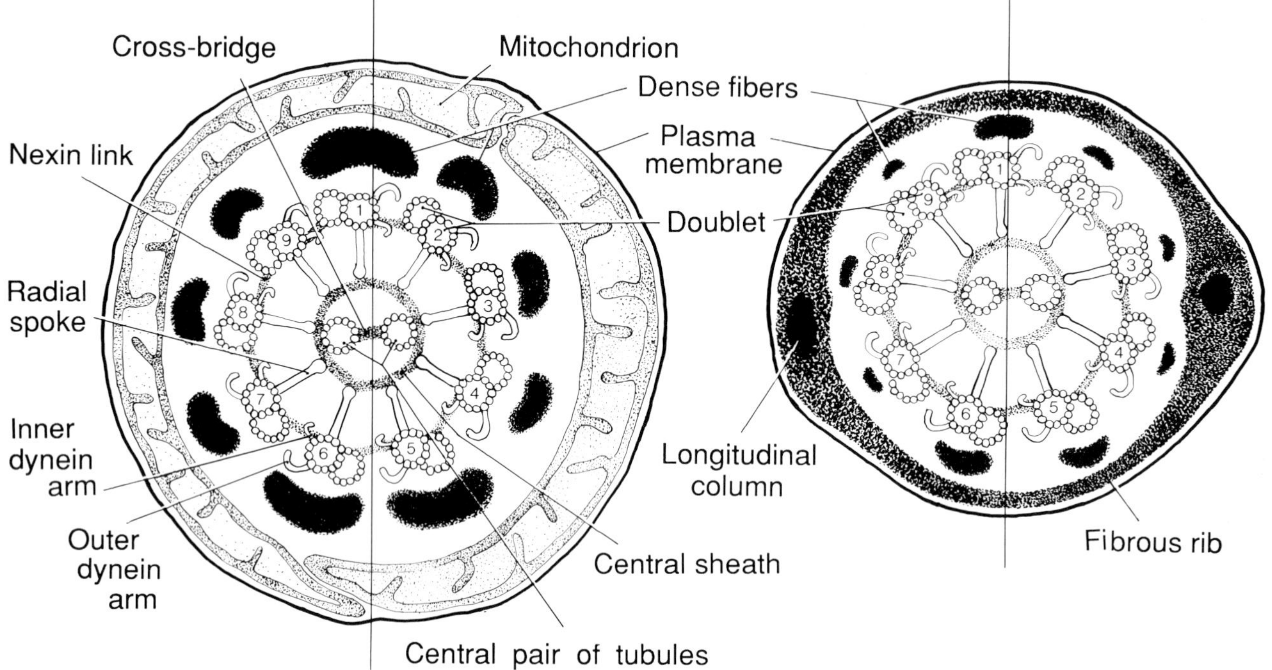

FIG. 80–9. Sketch of the middle piece (left) and principal piece (right) showing the plasma membrane, mitochondria or fibrous ribs, and nine dense fibers arranged around the axoneme, consisting of nine doublets and the central pair. Dense fibers and doublets are numbered as designated. Passing distally through the principal piece, the dense fibers become thinner and terminate; dense fibers 1, 5, and 6 are the longest.

structures of motile cilia of the trachea or certain microorganisms. The axoneme is the propulsive element of a spermatozoon, and the method by which spermatozoa move is considered in a subsequent section. The axoneme consists of a central pair of microtubules surrounded by a ring of nine doublets (Fig. 80–11). The role of the central pair is unclear. Each doublet is composed of a small cylindrical A microtubule, with an attached C-shaped B microtubule[5] (Figs. 80–9 and 80–11). The cylindrical A microtubule has two longitudinal rows of arms pointing toward the next doublet. Both microtubules of a doublet contain tubulin molecules arranged to form 13 protofilaments in the A microtubule and 9 or 10 in the B microtubule. The arms contain dynein, which is rich in ATPase and transduces chemical energy to mechanical motion. The entire doublet is about 70% tubulin and 15% dynein. The doublets are interconnected by nexin links, and a series of nine radial spokes extend from the central pair to the doublets (see Fig. 80–10). The nexin links probably are elastic and maintain symmetry while regulating displacement of the doublets during their sliding and contraction. The spokes probably provide structural support.

The annulus is an electron-dense structure which lies between the caudal-most gyrus of mitochondria and the rostral end of the fibrous sheath of the principal piece (see Fig. 80–10). Thus it demarcates the end of the middle piece. In cross section, the annulus appears as an isosceles triangle with its base against the mitochondria. The annulus is a point where the plasma membrane is firmly attached.

PRINCIPAL PIECE

The dense fibers and axoneme of the middle piece continue through the principal piece, although the dense fibers become narrower and terminate in the caudal principal piece.[2,4,5,17] First dense fibers 3 and 8 taper away, then dense fibers 4 and 7, then dense fiber 9, and finally dense fibers 1, 5, and 6.

The unique feature of the middle piece is the fibrous sheath with its fibrous ribs and longitudinal columns, both of proteinaceous material. In a sagittal section through the principal piece (see Figs. 80–9 and 80–10), the fibrous ribs are cut in cross section, and appear as dense strands, which pass halfway around the fibrous sheath, from one longitudinal column to the other. Sometimes the fibrous ribs branch. Longitudinal columns run the length of the principal piece, and overlay doublets 3, 4, and 8. Thus longitudinal columns are found on the dorsal and ventral aspects of the principal piece. Progressing caudad, the fibrous sheath lies closer to the axoneme, as the dense fibers taper away. The fibrous sheath probably provides the structural support plus flexibility essential for effective translation of sliding motion and contraction of the doublets into flagellar beats of defined flexure and amplitude.

END PIECE

The doublets and central pair of the axoneme continue intact about halfway through the end piece, and then taper out over a short distance of 1 to 2 μm. Thus the

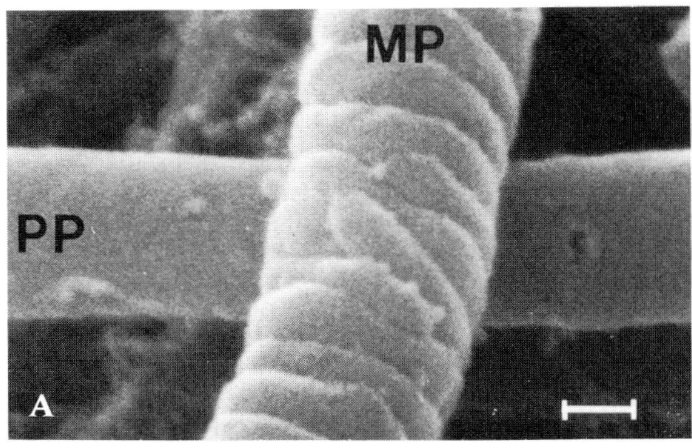

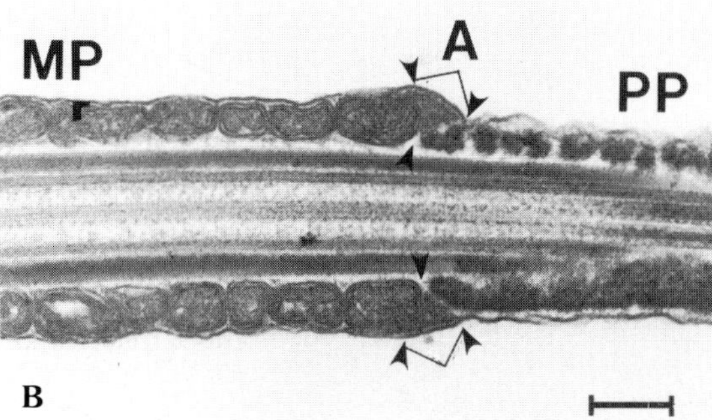

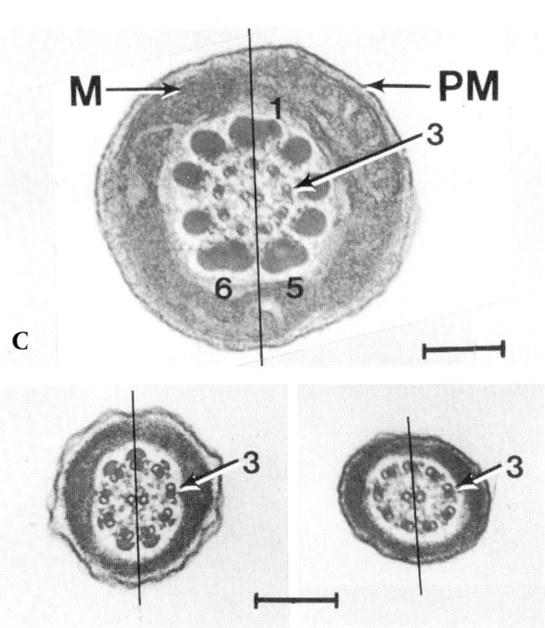

FIG. 80–10. *A*, Surface views by scanning electron microscopy of a middle piece (MP) and a principal piece (PP) of spermatozoa. Bar is 0.2 μm; magnification ×41,000. *B*, Longitudinal section through the middle piece and principal piece, showing the annulus (A). Bar is 0.2 μm; magnification ×45,000. *C*, Cross sections through the middle and principal piece. Compare with Figure 80–9. The vertical line bisects dense fiber 1 and the central pair and passes between dense fibers 5 and 6. Dense fibers 1, 5, and 6 and doublet 3 are designated. Bars are 0.2 μm, and magnifications are ×60,000.

9 + 2 pattern is lost in the caudal end of the end piece.

BIOCHEMISTRY AND METABOLISM OF SPERMATOZOA

SEMEN

The chemical compositions of stallion semen, seminal plasma, and spermatozoa have been tabulated.[24,25] Although there have been few comprehensive studies of either seminal plasma or spermatozoa, biochemical characteristics of stallion semen are similar to those for semen from other domestic mammals.[26] However, distinctive features are noted. Stallion semen contains considerable glucose and very little fructose, 0.82 and 0.02 mg/mL, respectively, unlike bull or ram semen in which fructose is the main glycolyzable sugar.[25] Stallion semen also contains a high concentration of sorbitol and a substantial amount of lactic acid.[26] The pH of normal stallion semen is 6.2 to 7.8, and the osmolality is between 300 and 334 mOsm/kg.[24,25] Differences in pH between first and second ejaculates (7.47 vs. 7.59) have been reported.[27] Season also affects seminal pH and osmolality (see Chapter 79).

Stallion semen contains glyceryl phosphoryl choline (GPC), ergothioneine, and citric acid which are produced by the epididymis, ampullary glands, and vesicular glands, respectively. Analysis of semen for these compounds can provide information concerning the secretory contribution by each of these glands to a given ejaculate.[24] When several ejaculates from a single stallion were analyzed, GPC, ergothioneine, and citric acid were present at 3.8, 0.8, and 2.6 mg/mL of semen.[24]

The sequence in which fluids from these glands are expelled during ejaculation has been determined by analyzing fractions collected at 5- to 10-s intervals during ejaculation.[24,26,28] Ejaculation begins with a presperm fraction, which is watery in appearance and contains no spermatozoa, GPC, ergothioneine, or citric acid. It prob-

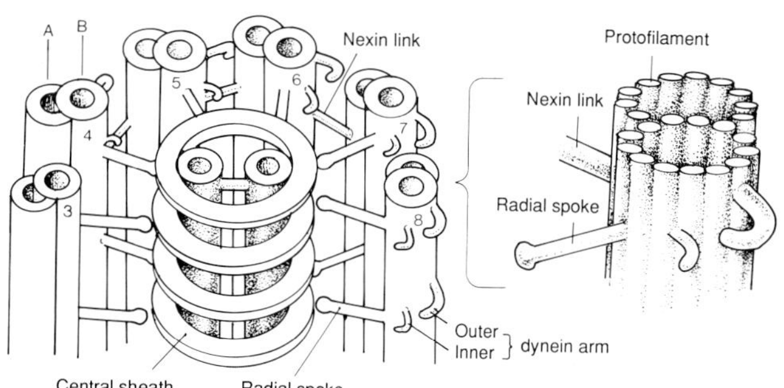

FIG. 80–11. Sketches of the axoneme showing the relationship between the A and B microtubules, dynein arms, nexin links, radial spokes, and central pair of microtubules. (Adapted from Satir, P.: How cilia move. Sci. Am., *231:*44–52, 1974; and Linck, R.W.: Advances in the ultrastructural analysis of the sperm flagellar axoneme. *In* The Spermatozoon. Edited by D.W. Fawcett and J.M. Bedford. Baltimore, Urban and Schwarzenberg, 1979, pp. 99–115.)

ably is from the bulbourethral glands and prostate gland. The second fraction is delivered a few seconds later. This fraction, which may encompass several jets of semen, has a milky appearance, is rich in spermatozoa, GPC, and ergothioneine but contains little citric acid or gel. This fraction, therefore, contains secretions from the epididymis (spermatozoa and GPC) and ampulla of the ductus deferens, but not the vesicular glands. The third fraction, contains few spermatozoa or ergothioneine, but large quantities of gel and citric acid. This fluid originates primarily from the vesicular glands and washes out the few spermatozoa remaining in the urethra. The final fraction, postcoital fluid which drips from the stallion's penis at dismount, has a watery appearance and contains few spermatozoa and little ergothioneine. It is not characteristic of the entire ejaculate.[24] Occasionally, infertility might result from defective function of the epididymis, ductus deferens, ampulla, or vesicular glands or from disturbances in sequence of the ejaculatory process (vesicular gland secretions discharged before or simultaneously with the sperm-rich fraction).[26]

COMPOSITION OF SPERMATOZOA

Only limited information exists on lipid composition of stallion spermatozoa.[21,29] Total lipid content of stallion spermatozoa is 14.2% (w:w), and the ratio of cholesterol to phospholipid is 0.23.[29] By comparison, cholesterol to phospholipid ratios are 0.22 for ejaculated bull spermatozoa[30] and 0.44 for ram cauda epididymal spermatozoa.[31] Parks et al. reported that the plasma and outer acrosomal membranes contain different lipid and protein compositions.[30] Presumably, regional differences in lipid composition give the different membrane compartments their specific functions (see previous section).

Analysis of the lipid composition of ram epididymal spermatozoa revealed that the major phospholipids were phosphatidylcholine (63%), phosphatidylethanolamine (15%), and lysophosphatidylcholine (10%); diphosphatidylglycerol, phosphatidylinositol, and phosphatidylserine were present in minor quantities (<10%).[30] The fatty acid docosahexanoic acid (22 carbons and 6 double bonds) is unique to spermatozoa and makes up about 50% of the total fatty acids in spermatozoa. Palmitic acid, a 16-carbon saturated fatty acid, makes up about 30% of the total spermatozoal fatty acids, while myristic acid (14 carbons, saturated) and stearic acid (18 carbons, saturated) each constitute about 10% of the total fatty acids in ram spermatozoa.[30]

Proteins constitute >50% of the total weight of spermatozoa.[24] Although many of these are histone proteins involved in DNA packaging,[24] others are involved as enzymes in the acrosome, receptors on the plasma membrane, elements of membrane function (ion and carbohydrate transport), and cytoskeletal structures (giving shape to head or providing filaments of the tail). Nothing is known about specific proteins in stallion spermatozoa, and a detailed discussion of these proteins would be beyond the scope of this book. Several surface proteins have been visualized in spermatozoa from other species using fluorescently labeled lectins[32,33] and antibodies.[34–36] The distribution patterns (quantity and location) of some of these proteins change during epididymal maturation and during capacitation. Immunosuppressive proteins in seminal plasma apparently bind to spermatozoa.[37] Other proteins originating from epididymal or seminal plasma are removed from spermatozoa during capacitation to facilitate membrane fusion and exposure of spermatozoa-oocyte receptors.[9,37] However, functions of most proteins on the plasma membrane remain unknown.

METABOLISM OF SPERMATOZOA

Spermatozoa are unique in that they lack the capability to divide and have only limited biosynthetic capacity.[38] Mature spermatozoa lack systems to repair cell damage or synthesize new enzymes. Therefore, most constituents necessary for spermatozoal function or metabolism are synthesized during spermatogenesis, and spermatozoa only perform maintenance functions and produce needed energy. Energy is used by spermatozoa to (1) initiate catabolic processes such as glycolysis, (2) maintain motility, and (3) maintain ion balance and miscellaneous cell functions.[38,39]

Spermatozoa rely primarily (about 90%) on extracellular substrates to meet their energy requirements. This energy is principally derived from carbohydrates (Fig. 80–12). Spermatozoa readily metabolize monosaccharides such as glucose and fructose but do not metabolize all sugars or more complex carbohydrates.[24,39] Stallion spermatozoa, however, possess limited capacity to use fructose when compared with spermatozoa from other species and cannot metabolize sorbitol, a major component of stallion seminal plasma.[24] Other exogenous substrates used by spermatozoa include lactic acid, glycerol, fatty acids, and amino acids.[24] Extensive use of exogenous glucose and fructose by ram[24] and bull[40] spermatozoa has been demonstrated. Ram spermatozoa in neat (undiluted) semen will metabolize all available monosaccharides in seminal plasma within 15 to 20 min at 37° C and stop swimming,[24] but this is not a problem with stallion spermatozoa.

Metabolizable sugars are transported across the plasma membrane by specific transport proteins, a process which has not been studied in stallion spermatozoa. In bull spermatozoa, however, the transport of glucose is the rate-limiting step in metabolism of exogenous sugars.[39] Glucose transport in spermatozoa is an ATP-dependent process which can be blocked by inhibitors such as cytochalasin B,[41] and is not coupled to Na^+ or K^+ transport[39] as is the case for many other cell types. At least in bull spermatozoa, the glucose transport protein has only limited capability to transport fructose.[39] A separate fructose transport protein may be

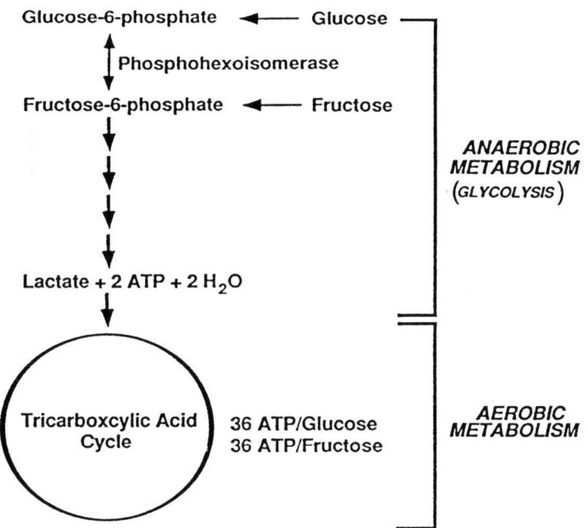

FIG. 80–12. Overview of carbohydrate metabolism in stallion spermatozoa. Not all metabolites are shown. Glucose is readily metabolized to fructose-6-phosphate and then to lactate and energy. Alternatively, fructose can enter the glycolytic pathway one reaction step below glucose. Both substrates yield identical end products and identical amounts of energy (2 ATP during anaerobic metabolism and 36 ATP during aerobic metabolism).

present in bull and ram spermatozoa, which enables them to readily metabolize fructose. A fructose transport protein may be absent in stallion spermatozoa, which would explain the limited capability of stallion spermatozoa to metabolize fructose.

Metabolism of endogenous compounds contributes about 10% of the cell's energy and ATP production in a physiologic state.[42] Spermatozoa can metabolize endogenous substrates, such as by oxidation of phospholipids in the mitochondria.[24,42] Spermatozoa have no glycogen stores and lack the enzymes necessary to use glycogen as an energy source.[38] In bull spermatozoa, ATP production from endogenous substrates remains constant regardless of the presence or absence of exogenous substrates or the temperature of the cell.[38] However, production of ATP from exogenous substrates, and hence total production of ATP, is temperature dependent.

Use of ATP also has been studied, but not for stallion spermatozoa. In bull spermatozoa, about 60% of ATP produced is used to maintain motility, but nearly 40% of ATP produced by spermatozoa is wasted by substrate cycling. Substrate cycling is the repeated phosphorylation and dephosphorylation of glycolytic intermediates,[43,44] so that no net production of ATP occurs. Spermatozoa are different from other cell types, in that they spend very little energy on transmembrane ion movement.[44] Only negligible amounts of ATP are used for maintenance of ion pumps and all other cell processes.

Several external ions affect spermatozoal motility and respiration. Compounds which stimulate spermatozoa include PO_4^- and $Na_2HCO_3^{--}$ and low concentrations of K^+ or Mg^{++}.[24,45–48] Ions which inhibit spermatozoal motility and metabolism include H^+, Mn^{++}, Ca^{++}, and high concentrations of Mg^{++}.[24]

Species differences exist in the capability of spermatozoa to use aerobic respiration. Bull and ram spermatozoa can use anaerobic respiration at a much higher rate than stallion spermatozoa, which rely heavily on aerobic metabolism.[24] Glycolytic breakdown of certain monosaccharides, especially glucose for stallion spermatozoa, provides the major source of ATP in spermatozoa. Human spermatozoa maintain a high rate of glycolysis even during aerobic respiration and maintain motility in the absence of oxygen and/or in the presence of mitochondrial inhibitors; thus, they have only a limited need for aerobic respiration.[49,50]

One consequence of aerobic metabolism is production of hydrogen peroxide in the mitochondria, which induces peroxidation of lipids in the plasma membrane.[51–55] Lipid peroxidation causes disfunction of certain metabolic enzymes; increases permeability of the plasma membrane;[53] and is deleterious to structural integrity, motility, and viability of spermatozoa.[51] Lipid peroxidation is depressed by seminal plasma and antioxidants such as butylated hydroxytoluene (BHT).[51,55]

When neat or extended semen remains undisturbed, aerobic metabolism exhausts the oxygen dissolved in the extender or seminal plasma and the spermatozoa are forced to rely on anaerobic metabolism. This occurs, for example, when semen is cooled slowly from body temperature to 5° C. After oxygen is depleted, spermatozoa use only glycolytic metabolic pathways and the end product is lactic acid.[24] Accumulation of lactic acid reduces the pH of the medium, which may cause a decrease in metabolism and ATP production with a resulting loss in spermatozoal motility. Rabbit spermatozoa rapidly die when exposed to a pH of less than 5.8.[24] Maintaining a proper intracellular pH for stallion spermatozoa (accomplished by maintaining the extracellular medium at a pH between 6.2 and 7.8) is an important factor in sustained spermatozoal motility and metabolism.

Maintenance of proper intracellular pH is complicated during storage of spermatozoa at low temperatures, because pH of the extender is affected by temperature, buffer(s) in the extender, buffer capacity, organic cosolvents used as cryoprotectants, and increased ionic strength of the medium during freezing when water leaves the solution by crystallizing into ice. Changes in pH caused by reduced temperature arise in part from changes in the pH scale, which is temperature dependent, and changes in the acid dissociation constant (pKa) of water and many biologic buffers; both are markedly affected by temperature. Taylor illustrated this pH dependence on temperature by the pH of water at 25° C (pH 7.0), 0° C (pH 7.47), and −35° C (pH 8.4).[56] Changes in pH induced by organic cosolvents are typified by addition of dimethyl sulfoxide to aqueous solutions, which can increase the pH by 0.1 to 0.2 pH units.[57] Increased ionic strength, incurred during freezing, lowers hydrogen activity coefficients and therefore alters pH.[58]

COMPARTMENTALIZATION OF SPERMATOZOAL FUNCTION

Spermatozoa contain only those cellular components necessary for them to traverse the female reproductive tract and fertilize an oocyte. Specialized compartments include the plasma membrane, nucleus, acrosome, neck, mitochondria, and axoneme. Each has a specific function and consists of several classes of molecules (i.e., lipids and proteins), which because of the molecules and/or their stoichiometry, make each compartment different from all others. Some compartment differences are easily recognizable. For example, the spermatozoal nucleus contains the DNA, the middle piece contains all mitochondria, and the axoneme contains primarily microtubules and contractile microfilaments. Other, more subtle, differences can also be detected within many compartments. Most intracellular compartments are bound by a membrane which has a distinct composition of lipids and proteins, different from all other compartmental membranes, which impart a designed characteristic to that compartment. Mixing of membrane proteins or lipids from one compartment to another rarely occurs. However, transfer of molecules between the acrosomal and plasma membranes does occur during the acrosome reaction when vesiculation of those membranes occurs.

Uniqueness of the lipid and protein constituents of each compartment membrane is obvious from several types of evidence. The plasma and acrosomal membranes contain different relative amounts of phospholipid and cholesterol. Molar cholesterol to phospholipid ratios of 0.38 for plasma membrane and 0.26 for acrosomal membrane are reported.[30] Differences exist in abundance and location of individual peripheral proteins as detected by antibodies.[34–36] Differences in carbohydrate residues on membrane proteins, detected using lectins, also exist.[33,59,60] These techniques reveal that although proteins are specific to certain membrane compartments, they can migrate to other membrane compartments. Differences in membrane potential, specific protein content, and macromolecular permeability between compartments have made it possible to analyze the integrity of each compartment in a spermatozoon. Specific fluorescent stains specific for DNA have been used to assess the status of this cell compartment.[61–64] Integrity of the plasma membrane covering the head can be assessed using specific stains,[13,65–67] whereas the integrity of the plasma membrane covering the tail can be assessed using a hypo-osmotic swelling assay[68] or column filtration using Sephadex or glass wool.[69,70]

The acrosome contains hydrolytic enzymes (including acrosin, acid phosphatases, β-glucuronidase, neuraminidase, N-acetylglucosaminidase, and hyaluronidase), at least some of which are required for fertilization.[5,71] The acrosome includes a large amount of carbohydrate which enables staining of the acrosome using the periodic acid-Schiff reaction.[72] The acrosome also can be visualized by other stains[73] and the acrosomal contents of spermatozoa from several species, including the stallion, specifically bind Pisum sativum agglutinin (PSA) lectin.[73–76] A specific monoclonal antibody to acrosomal protein(s) in stallion spermatozoa is available.[77] All of these probes can be used to assess acrosomal integrity in stallion spermatozoa with a reasonable degree of accuracy. Fluorescent probes also have been developed for assessment of mitochondrial function.[75,78,79]

The ability to use multiple assays for individual spermatozoal compartments illustrates the uniqueness of each compartment and the functional isolation of one compartment from all others. The underlying principle is that any spermatozoon capable of fertilizing an oocyte must have each of at least four attributes or functions operational at 100% of normal at the correct time, when it approaches the oocyte. The proportion of completely functional spermatozoa in a sample can be determined only by evaluating individual spermatozoa for each of a battery of important traits. Population averages are less sensitive; for a given characteristic, a value of 0.2 might result because 20% of all spermatozoa gave a 100% response (a potentially desirable situation) or because 100% of the cells gave a 20% response (a potentially undesirable situation). The percentage of motile cells is useful information because it distinguishes between these two cases. However, oxygen consumption or acrosin content of a spermatozoal population (rather than for individual cells) is less informative. Multiparameter tests of individual spermatozoa[75,78,80,81] circumvent this problem.

HOW SPERMATOZOA SWIM

MECHANICS OF DOUBLET SLIDING

Forward motion of a spermatozoon results from bending of the flagellum, a consequence of coordinated bending waves propagated from the neck. The bending movement probably results from the interplay of two systems: (1) a sliding filament system in the doublets, which generates the force for the bending wave, and (2) a control system, which coordinates the sliding and regulates flagella beat.[5,82–84] The ultimate pattern of bending of the flagellum results from active forces within the tail, working against constraints imposed by the nexin links, radial spokes, dense fibers, and fibrous sheath. The viscosity of the surrounding medium also alters beat frequency and bending pattern of the flagellum.[85]

Bending of the tail results from shear forces generated between neighboring doublets which cause one doublet to slide, temporarily, a short distance past the other.[5,82,83] Dynein arms are the pivotal component of this sliding system, and the vigor of sliding depends on ATP and a cyclic adenosine monophosphate (cAMP) dependent protein kinase. The sliding or shear force is not developed simultaneously over the entire length of a doublet, but probably is localized in a portion of a doublet(s). Doublets 1 to 4 alternate contractions with doublets 6 to 9, and the site of localized contractions may pass around the nine doublets in a circular manner.

How do the doublets slide to induce contraction? In the neutral or immotile state, dynein arms extending from microtubule A are long and associated with microtubule B of the adjacent doublet[5,82,83] (Fig. 80–13). Although the dynein arm is permanently attached to microtubule A, attachment with microtubule B is transitory and broken by availability of ATP. Thus local availability of ATP causes the dynein arm to detach from microtubule B and, concurrently, to shorten. This shortening is similar to ATP-driven contraction of a muscle fiber. The free arm then tilts at an angle of about 40°, elongates, and reattaches to microtubule B at a new site. Contraction and return of the attached arm to a 90° (horizontal) angle with the doublet creates a shear or sliding force sufficient to move the second doublet past the first doublet, toward the tip of the axoneme. By this slight movement of about 16 nm, the dynein arms attached to microtubule A "walk" along microtubule B of the neighboring doublet. The initial detachment and shortening of the dynein arm occur only with availability of ATP, tilting to a 40° angle and elongation of the detached dynein arm depend on hydrolysis of ATP to provide needed energy, and final shortening of the arm is independent of ATP because it is the "resting state" (Fig. 80–13). Although both the inner and outer dynein arms probably contribute an equivalent sliding force, contraction can occur in the absence of the outer dynein arms.

Sliding per se cannot create the bending motion of the flagellum. Presumably, bending is induced by anchorage of the doublets and dense fibers in the neck region and resistance offered along the entire length of the tail by the nexin links and other structures. Bends appear to form passively, some distance from the point of active formation and breaking of dynein attachments, as a consequence of resistance to displacement of the microtubules. As noted above, the doublets on one side of the axoneme contract more or less in synchrony. Thus a planar tail beat results from active shear forces

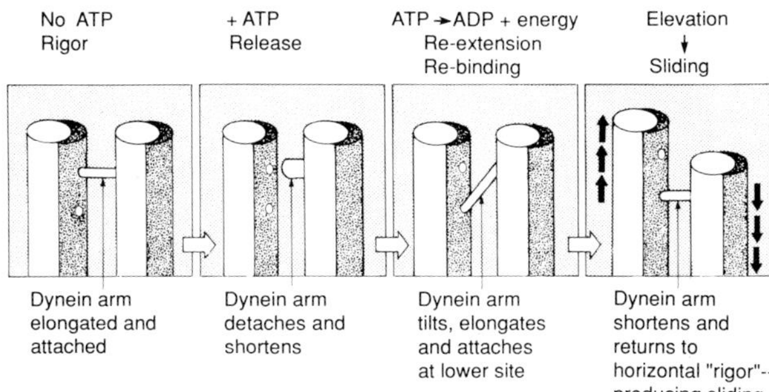

FIG. 80–13. Mechanism of doublet sliding within the axoneme resulting from detachment, shortening, elongation, and reattachment of the dynein arms in a localized region (only one is depicted), followed by return to the horizontal and rigor position. The return to horizontal slides one doublet relative to the other. (Adapted from Satir, P.: The generation of ciliary motion. J. Protozool., *31*:8–12, 1984.)

and sliding on one side of the axoneme, induced by the dynein arms, concurrent with passive sliding and relaxation on the opposite side. In the case of a helical tail beat, frequently evident as spermatozoa rotate or roll along their long axis, a slight twisting may be generated as the bending motion progresses along the principal piece, because of a staggered or rotational activation of dynein arms in doublets 1 through 9, rather than synchronous contractions of doublets 1 to 4 or 6 to 9. The control mechanism activating opposing groups of doublets to contract possibly is modulated by Ca^{++}, acting through calmodulin.

Initiation or maintenance of spermatozoal motility depends on maintenance of a necessary intracellular concentration of cAMP, synthesized from ATP by adenylate cyclase, and the calcium/calmodulin system is involved.[5,38,44] In addition, adenosine, bicarbonate, and the protein carboxymethylation enzyme system also are likely involved. The interactions of these regulatory systems are unclear for mammalian spermatozoa in general and have not been studied for stallion sperm.

THE PATTERN OF SPERMATOZOAL MOTION

To a casual observer viewing spermatozoa through a microscope, not all stallion spermatozoa swim in a similar manner. Detailed analysis of the motion characteristics of motile spermatozoa can be achieved by computer-assisted image analysis; comprehensive discussions of these instruments have been published.[86–90] Systems for computer-assisted analysis of spermatozoal motion are accurate if properly used.[87,91,92] Basically, the microscopic image of a sample of spermatozoa in an optically clear medium is detected by a video camera and sent, either directly or via a videotape interface, to a computer which captures information in 15 to 60 frames (typically 0.5 to 1.0 at 30 frames/s), locates each spermatozoon in each frame, and reconstructs their paths. The conventional terminology used to describe spermatozoal motion is summarized in Table 80–1 and Figure 80–14. Several instruments are available from commercial vendors. Although all use similar principles, actual algorithms and strategies for considering spermatozoa which collide or leave the field of view differ. Thus slightly different data will be obtained with each brand of instrument even if the same samples are analyzed. Also, values selected for user-defined settings can influence results. If properly used, these instruments can provide valuable objective data on spermatozoal motion, but data for other attributes also should be considered when predicting potential fertility of a stallion.

Although some spermatozoa are immotile, and may actually be dead, other spermatozoa pause momentarily and appear immotile only to resume swimming after a short interval. Watching motile spermatozoa, a researcher might note that they swim with different velocities, in a rather progressive manner with or without rotation along the long axis of the cell or sometimes swim in a curvilinear manner. This is evident in

TABLE 80–1. NOMENCLATURE USED TO DESCRIBE SPERMATOZOAL MOTION*

TERM	DESCRIPTION
Curvilinear velocity (VCL)	The centroid-to-centroid path, and velocity along that path
Average path velocity (VAP)	The smoothed centroid-to-centroid path, as calculated by one of several smoothing algorithms, and velocity along that path
Straight-line velocity (VSL)	The linear path between the first and last centroid in a sequence, and velocity along that path
Linearity (LIN)	VSL/VCL
Straightness (STR)	VSL/VAP
Wobble (WOB)	VAP/VCL
Motile spermatozoa (MOT)	Spermatozoa with a VAP or VCL > v μm/s
Progressively motile spermatozoa (PMOT)	Spermatozoa with a VAP or VCL > v μm/s and a LIN or STR >1
Circularly motile spermatozoa (CIR)	Spermatozoa with a VAP or VCL > v μm/s and radius of the average path < r μm
Lateral head displacement (LHD)	Mean distance of the centroids from the average path
Beat cross frequency (BCF)	The number of times the curvilinear path crosses the average path, expressed as intersections per second

*Distance is expressed as μm and velocity as μm/s. Note that VCL > VAP > VSL for any given spermatozoon (see Fig. 80–13). In determining if a spermatozoon is motile, a minimum cutoff value can be selected, but in some instruments it is for VCL and for other instruments it is for VAP. In most cases, an equine spermatozoon with VCL <15 or 20 μm/s or VAP <10 or 15 μm/s should be considered as immotile.

computer-based analysis of spermatozoal motion (Fig. 80–15). Other spermatozoa might actually be swimming backward, because of a 180° reflection of the tail near the juncture of the principal piece and middle piece. In addition, the pattern of flagellar beat and the nature of head motion can be influenced by the viscosity and chemical composition of the medium in which the spermatozoa are suspended, temperature, and depth of the preparation.[85,88,93]

Given the size of a stallion spermatozoon, the ampli-

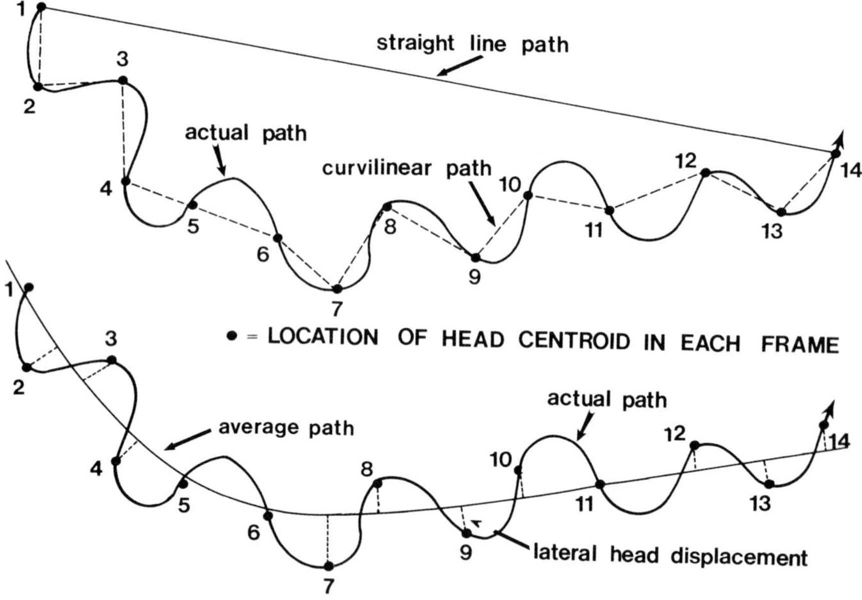

FIG. 80–14. Path of the centroid (midpoint) of a spermatozoal head and some parameters measured or typically reported. The curvilinear path joins the centroids, and the average path is calculated by a smoothing algorithm. The straight line path connects the first and last centroid. Lateral head displacement is the distance between a centroid and the average path, and beat cross frequency is the number of times the curvilinear path crosses the average path. (From Amann, R.P.: Relationship between computerized evaluations of spermatozoal motion and competitive fertility index. Proceedings of the National Association of Animal Breeders Technical Conference. Milwaukee, 1988, pp. 38–44.)

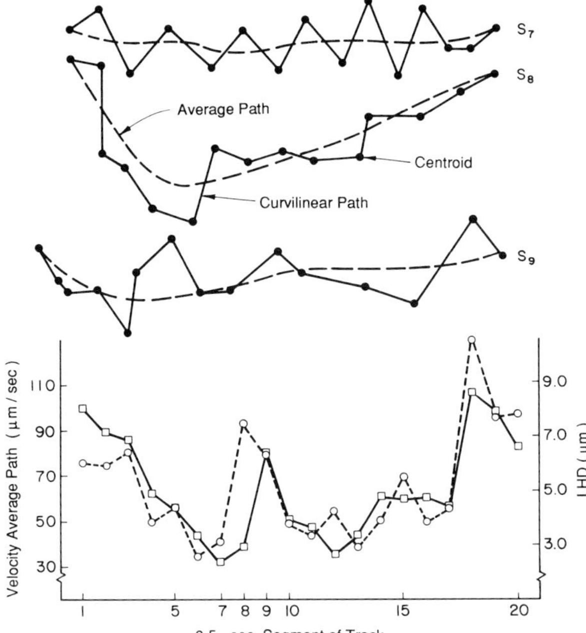

FIG. 80–15. Motion of a typical stallion spermatozoon over 10 s. The centroid location, curvilinear path, and average path during three 0.5-s segments (segments 7, 8, and 9) are shown in the upper portion of the figure. Mean path velocity (velocity over the average path, open squares) and lateral head displacement (LHD, open circles) are shown for all 20 segments in the lower portion. For all 20 segments, curvilinear velocity (centroid-to-centroid), path velocity, and LHD averaged 65 μm/s, 94 μm/s, and 5.1 μm/s. For segments 7, 8, and 9, values were 48, 81, and 102 μm/s for curvilinear velocity, 32, 39, and 81 μm/s for path velocity, and 3.1, 7.5, and 6.4 μm for LHD. Although curvilinear velocity was 68% greater during segment 8 than during segment 7, path velocity was only 22% greater; this was because LHD was large. (Modified from Amann, R.P.: Computerized evaluation of stallion spermatozoa. Proc. Am. Assoc. Equine Pract., 453–473, 1988.)

tude of flexations of the tail around the theoretical longitudinal axis of a swimming cell, and the wobble of the head as a spermatozoon rotates around its longitudinal axis, unfettered motion of a spermatozoon requires a sample depth of at least 50 μm and possibly 100 μm. Unfortunately, microscopic examination of spermatozoa in a preparation with a depth ≥50 μm is impossible with conventional instruments, because of the mutual exclusivity of the requirements for adequate magnification and retention of a motile cell within the depth of field of the microscope objective viewing the preparation.[93] Thus, to enable critical observation of spermatozoal motility, we must restrict the freedom of spermatozoal movement, in the belief that this does not negate validity of the observations. This assumption probably is correct if the depth of the preparation is ≥10 to 12 μm, but if depth of the preparation is ≤10 μm, spermatozoa find it increasingly difficult to move.[93,94] Erroneous conclusions are likely if depth of the preparation is <10 μm.

Preparations typically used by a theriogenologist are 15 to 30 μm in depth, assuming an appropriate-sized drop on a microscope slide is overlain with a cover glass. Restriction of the sample to a depth of 15 to 20 μm facilitates viewing and is obligatory with most computer-assisted systems for automated analysis of spermatozoal motion.[86,87] This can be achieved by placing 7 μL under an 18- × 18-mm cover glass,[95] 10 μL under a 22- × 22-mm cover glass, or use of special chambers (μ-Cell, Fertility Technologies, Inc., Natick, MA) made for computer-assisted analysis of spermatozoal motion. For visual observation, with continuous focusing on different levels in the preparation, volumes of 12 to 18 μL under a 22- × 22-mm cover glass are better.

The problem of sample thickness must be solved by compromise; use of a preparation ≥12 μm deep, but not so deep as to make use of the microscope difficult. Using an HTM-2000 motility analyzer (Hamilton-Thorne Research, Danvers, MA), with dark field illumination and infrared light, Amann et al. studied the motility of spermatozoa in a flat capillary tube 200 μm deep and in a preparation about 16 μm deep on a glass slide.[88] Semen was diluted to 25 × 10^6 spermatozoa/mL in an optically clear medium (10 g sucrose plus 3 g ovine serum albumin per 100 mL water). They found that sample thickness affected percentage of motile spermatozoa, straight-line velocity, lateral head displacement, and linearity (Table 80–2). In other words, spermatozoa swam differently in the 16-μm preparation than in the deep capillary tube, where proximity to a glass surface did not impede their motion. Surprisingly, a lower percentage of spermatozoa were motile in capillary tubes than on slides, but they had higher straight-line velocities and linearities.

The authors gave no explanation for the differences

TABLE 80–2. MOTION CHARACTERISTICS OF STALLION SPERMATOZOA ON A MICROSCOPIC SLIDE OR IN A CAPILLARY TUBE*

CHARACTERISTICS	SLIDE†	CAPILLARY†
Total motile spermatozoa (% ≥5 μm/s)	58	44[a]
Motile spermatozoa (% ≥20 μm/s)	55	42[a]
Progressively motile spermatozoa (%)‡	31	28
Average path velocity (μm/s)	91	98
Straightline velocity (μm/s)	46	57[b]
Lateral head displacement (μm)	13	11[a]
Linearity	0.51	0.56[b]

*Means for spermatozoa from 10 ejaculates extended in 10% (w:v) sucrose plus 3% (w:v) bovine serum albumin and evaluated 5 to 20 min and 95 to 110 min after collection, using five fields per evaluation; variance associated with time was not significant. Values designated by *a* or *b* differ ($p < 0.05$ or <0.01).

†The slide sample had a depth of about 16 μm and each field was scanned twice. The capillary had a depth of 200 μm and each field was scanned once.

‡Spermatozoa with a path velocity >5 μm/s and a straightness >0.5.

(Adapted from Amann, R.P.: Computerized evaluation of stallion spermatozoa. Proc. Am. Assoc. Equine Pract., 453–473, 1988.)

in velocity,[88] and none is evident for the difference in percentage of motile spermatozoa. However, a reasonable conclusion is that restrictions imposed by upper and lower surfaces of the 16-μm preparation precluded many spermatozoa from rotating smoothly about their long axis and caused them to thrash their heads and flagella more to complete each 180° rotation. If this assumption is correct, it could explain the increased lateral head displacement (a measure of how much the head is wobbling around the general path of movement) and decreased linearity and straight-line velocity (measures of how effectively a spermatozoon is moving from point A to point B in a linear manner). Changes detected probably should be interpreted as evidence that the 16-μm preparation somewhat restricts movement of a spermatozoon from point A to point B within such a preparation (Table 80–2). Nevertheless, the evaluation of percentage of motile spermatozoa was not compromised by use of preparations only 16 μm deep.

Effects of temperature on spermatozoal motion often are ignored by clinicians, because they are considered to be unimportant or because adequate temperature control of equipment used to prepare the slide, and of the slide during viewing, requires extra effort or expense. None of these reasons for inadequate control of temperature while viewing a sample of semen is justified and, depending on environmental conditions, can lead to erroneous results. Under most environmental conditions, failure to control temperature adequately while performing a seminal evaluation will provide incorrect information to the client; because the clinician should have known better, this is malpractice.

Effects of temperature on motion of stallion spermatozoa[88] when suspended in a 200-μm-deep flat capillary tube are summarized in Table 80–3. Temperature affected all parameters of spermatozoal motion ($p < 0.05$), although spermatozoa in some ejaculates were affected more than those in others; the ejaculate by temperature interaction was significant for percentage of motile spermatozoa, velocity parameters, and lateral head displacement. The important point is that at 22° C, essentially room temperature, the percentages of motile spermatozoa or progressively motile spermatozoa were significantly lower than at higher temperatures. Maximum percentage of motile spermatozoa was obtained only at 37° or 42° C.[86,88] Spermatozoa swam with greater velocity and linearity at higher temperatures, and more spermatozoa had a velocity of >60 μm/s for observations at 37° or 42° C than at cooler temperatures (Fig. 80–16). However, the effect of temperature on velocity characteristics is at least partially independent of its effect on percentage of motile spermatozoa.

What does this mean for a clinician? It is unlikely that a clinician will consider a spermatozoon with a linear velocity <20 μm/s as motile. Assuming this to be correct, and based on the data summarized in Table 80–3, Amann et al. calculated that for a sample in which 72% of spermatozoa were motile at 37° C, only 56% would be judged to be motile at 22° C.[86,88] Thus, failure to have a controlled temperature introduced a 22% reduction, or error, in the percentage of motile spermatozoa. A different human observer might require a spermatozoon to be moving at 30 or even 40 μm/s to be considered motile. In these cases, the errors would be 33 and 51%, respectively. However, if the observers requiring motile spermatozoa to be moving 30 or 40 μm/s had been evaluating samples at 37° C, the errors would have been only 4 and 14%, respectively. Thus, adequate temperature control at 37° C is essential to allow spermatozoa to swim with their potential charac-

TABLE 80–3. EFFECTS OF TEMPERATURE ON MOTION CHARACTERISTICS OF STALLION SPERMATOZOA*

CHARACTERISTIC	22° C	27° C	32° C	37° C	42° C
Total motile spermatozoa (% ≥5 μm/s)	53^a	66^b	66^b	68^b	66^b
Motile spermatozoa (% ≥20 μm/s)	49^a	63^b	64^b	67^b	63^b
Progressively motile spermatozoa (%)	33^a	46^b	53^c	58^d	56^{cd}
Curvilinear velocity (μm/s)	87^a	100^b	107^c	114^d	117^d
Average path velocity (μm/s)	51^a	57^b	62^c	69^d	75^e
Straight-line velocity (μm/s)	28^a	35^b	42^c	51^d	56^e
Linearity	34^a	36^b	42^c	47^d	50^e
Lateral head displacement (μm)	7.0^a	8.1^b	8.4^b	8.4^b	8.6^b

*Based on analyses of spermatozoa in each of five ejaculates; semen was diluted in an aqueous solution of 10% (w:v) sucrose and 3% (w:v) bovine serum albumin and held at about 30° C until analysis. All analyses using an HTM-2000 instrument were completed within 3 h of seminal collection, and each sample was evaluated in order of ascending temperature; time probably had a minimal effect in confounding effects of temperature. Means in a row with a different superscript differ ($p < 0.05$).

(Adapted from Amann, R.P.: Computerized evaluation of stallion spermatozoa. Proc. Am. Assoc. Equine Pract., 453–473, 1988.)

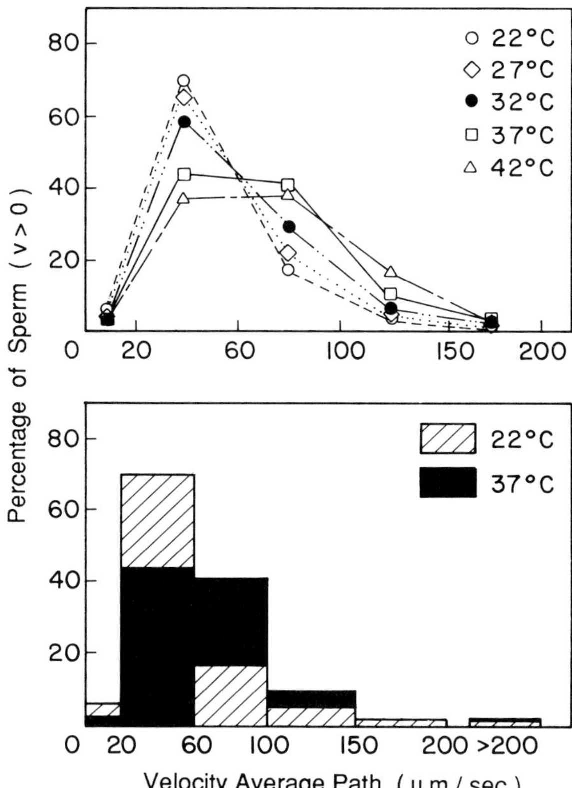

FIG. 80–16. Effect of temperature on average path velocity of stallion spermatozoa. Expressed as the percentage of distribution for about 800 spermatozoa with v >0 in each of five ejaculates, as determined using an HTM-2000 instrument. Although means for average path velocity differed ($p > 0.05$) at 22°, 27°, 32°, 27°, and 42° C, distributions at 22° and 27° C were similar, as were those at 37° and 42° C (upper; ignores values for v >200). The distribution was different ($p < 0.01$) at 22° and 37° C (lower). (Modified from Amann, R.P.: Computerized evaluation of stallion spermatozoa. Proc. Am. Assoc. Equine Pract., 453–473, 1988.)

teristics. More important, observation at 37° C is essential to minimize differences from sample to sample associated with velocity of spermatozoa within that sample or among observers. The take-home message is obvious: failure to evaluate samples at 37° C might preclude 30% of potentially motile spermatozoa from swimming with sufficient velocity to be considered motile by a human observer. Therefore, evaluations of seminal quality at room temperature often will lead to invalid estimates of spermatozoal quality.

No doubt the nature of the medium in which spermatozoa are suspended[10,85,93] and the physiologic status of the cells[92,96] influence how spermatozoa swim. However, the important question is not what are the motion characteristics of spermatozoa in vitro when in medium A or B or even how spermatozoa swim at sites U, I, or F within the female reproductive tract. The important questions are whether evaluations of spermatozoal motility, either subjectively by a human observer or by a computer-assisted system, accurately portray the quality of spermatozoa in a given sample and whether they indicate the potential for those cells to achieve fertilization.[6] The answer to both questions probably is a qualified yes,[6,70,86,87,89] but the important proviso is that spermatozoal motility is not the only attribute required for survival within the female reproductive tract or achievement of fertilization.

No data for motion characteristics of spermatozoa in vivo within the uterus or uterine tube exist, but spermatozoa do not necessarily swim in the same manner as they do in vitro. Indeed, based on studies focused on in vitro fertilization, clinicians have concluded that spermatozoa which have undergone the acrosome reaction, a prelude to fertilization, swim differently from spermatozoa which have not undergone this modification of the plasma membrane and underlying structures.[97]

As outlined previously in this chapter, a successful spermatozoon must have attributes in addition to those of "a good dancer" to fertilize an ovum. The successful spermatozoon must elude the natural defense mechanisms of the female, receive nurturing at receptive sites, retain the ability to respond to chemoattractants produced by oocytes (if they exist in mammals), and ultimately penetrate the investments of the oocyte. Motility certainly is a prerequisite for normal fertilization in terms of penetration through the zona pellucida and attachment to the plasma membrane of the oocyte. However, this does not mean that all spermatozoa which are motile when examined in vitro have the necessary attributes to fertilize an oocyte. Indeed, recent research strongly supports the conclusion that a subpopulation of motile spermatozoa, shortly after ejaculation or after preservation at 5° or −196° C, have altered plasma membranes which probably preclude their successful participation in fertilization.[70] Thus, not all motile spermatozoa are capable of fertilizing an ovum, although most motile spermatozoa likely have the potential to achieve this task.

RESPONSES OF SPERMATOZOA TO THERMAL STRESS

Cooling stallion spermatozoa to 5° C is necessary for storing spermatozoa to be used within a few days either at the location of collection or after shipment to another location or as a prerequisite for cryopreservation.[23] Cooling stallion spermatozoa, however, stresses the cell and can cause cellular injury.[20,22,98] Understanding the causes of cooling damage and how to minimize it is essential if spermatozoa stored at low temperatures are to retain maximal fertility.

Cellular injury can be caused directly by affecting cellular structures (such as by rupturing membranes) or indirectly by altering cellular functions (such as slowing down metabolic processes).[20] Rapid cooling of stallion spermatozoa from 20° C (room temperature) to 5° C induces partially irreversible damage characterized by an abnormal pattern of swimming, rapid loss of motility, damage to acrosomal and plasma membranes, reduced metabolism, and loss of intracellular components. Collectively, this damage is termed cold shock.[7,20,99] Stallion spermatozoa are susceptible to cold shock,[16] and cooling damages several spermatozoal membrane compartments (Table 80–4). Indirect cooling damage is more difficult to discern and may not be evident until sometime after the spermatozoa have reached 0° to 5° C.[7,99]

RESPONSES OF MEMBRANES TO COOLING

To understand how cooling and/or cold shock damages spermatozoa, the clinician must consider both spermatozoal structure (see Fig. 80–2) and function. The original concepts of the fluid-mosaic membrane model[100] provided a membrane model of proteins floating like icebergs in a sea of lipids composed primarily of phospholipids and cholesterol. The membrane consists of a bilayer having the hydrophilic portions of both lipids and proteins oriented externally and their hydrophobic portions oriented toward the bilayer center.[100–102] Modifications of this model include asymmetry of membrane lipids and proteins and complex interactions between lipids and proteins that regulate membrane receptors, ion pores or enzymes, and ultimately membrane function.[18,101,102] In addition, alternative forms of lipid aggregates exist within a membrane.[101–103] A minor lipid aggregate form, the hexagonal-II phase (Fig. 80–17), provides a point defect capable of inducing membrane fusion rather than maintaining a permeability barrier.[104] However, a similar aggregation to a hexagonal-II phase may be necessary for the acrosome reaction and fertilization. Under stress, such as induced by cooling, membranes may undergo rearrangement into the hexagonal-II phase, and the formed point defects then may induce excessive membrane permeability or even membrane disruption.[18]

Each spermatozoal membrane (e.g., plasma, acrosomal, and mitochondrial) is a unique aggregate of lipids and proteins arranged in a bilayer. The lipid and protein compositions of each membrane are unique, and little or no exchange of lipid or protein among them occurs. This compartmentalization arises during spermiogenesis and is maintained during epididymal modifications; it permits each membrane to maintain its unique function.[4,102,105] Few data are available on the lipid composition of membranes from stallion spermatozoa. However, cholesterol is the major sterol in stallion spermatozoa, and the cholesterol to phospholipid ratio for whole stallion spermatozoa is 0.36.[21] Glycolipids make up <10% of the polar lipids in stallion spermatozoa.[21]

More complete biochemical analyses are available for bull spermatozoa.[30] In addition to lipid analysis of whole spermatozoa, the isolation of membranes from individual compartments of bull spermatozoa revealed compositional differences. The plasma membrane of a bull spermatozoon has a higher cholesterol to phospholipid ratio (0.38) than the outer acrosomal membrane (0.26). Differences in amounts of individual phospholipid species also were detected between membrane compartments.[30]

TABLE 80–4. DAMAGE TO SPECIFIC MEMBRANE COMPARTMENTS OF STALLION SPERMATOZOA AFTER COLD SHOCK (%)

MEMBRANE COMPARTMENT STATUS	CONTROL 30° C	COLD SHOCKED* 0° TO 4° C
Intact plasma membrane; intact acrosome	81	36
Damaged plasma membrane; intact acrosome	9	23
Damaged plasma membrane; damaged acrosome	11	42

*Cells were cold shocked by immersion into water at 0° to 4° C.

(Data from Watson, P.F., Plummer, J.M., and Allen, W.E.: Quantitative assessment of membrane damage in cold-shocked spermatozoa of stallions. J. Reprod. Fertil. Suppl., *35*:651–653, 1987.)

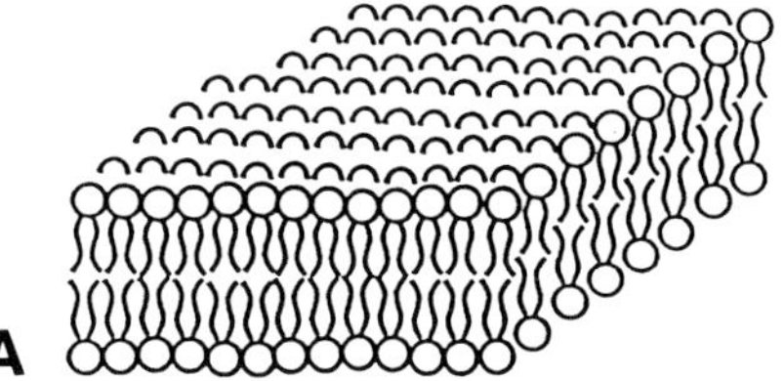

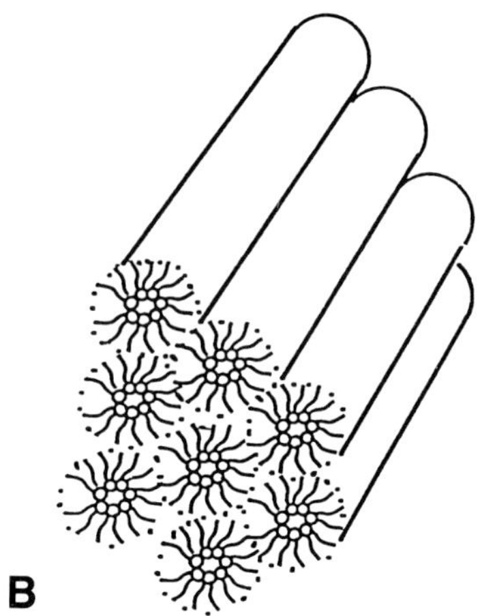

FIG. 80–17. Schematic representation of the two polymorphic phase forms for lipid in biologic membranes. Normally, the bilayer *(A)* has a planar configuration with phospholipid heads (spheres) oriented toward the bulk water and fatty acyl chains inward. The bilayer forms a continuous permeability barrier excluding polar molecules. *B*, The relatively rare hexagonal-II phase has a cylindric form with phospholipid head groups toward the center and hydrocarbon tails oriented outward. This structure weakens the permeability barrier but may play an important role during physiologic fusion of membranes. (Adapted from Hammerstedt, R.H., Graham, J.K., and Nolan, J.P.: Cryopreservation of mammalian sperm: What we ask them to survive. J. Androl., *11*:73–88, 1990.)

Lipid composition is important in membrane function, because each lipid species contributes its unique characteristics to the membrane. Lipids undergo a phase transition, from a fluid or liquid-crystalline state, in which the fatty acyl chains are relatively disordered, to the gel state, in which the fatty acyl chains are increasingly rigid and parallel to each other as temperature is reduced. Proper membrane function requires a fluid membrane. Each lipid species undergoes this phase transition at a temperature specific for that lipid. The phase transition temperature of a lipid is determined by the nature of the head group, length of fatty acyl chains (short chains have a lower transition temperature), and degree of unsaturation of fatty acyl chains (chains with more unsaturated bonds have lower transition temperatures). When the temperature of a membrane is decreased below the transition temperature of an individual lipid species, that lipid (but not other lipids) will undergo a phase transition and aggregate in microdomains of lipid gel in an otherwise liquid membrane. This has two effects. First, lipids which were randomly dispersed throughout the membrane interacting with specific lipid species and proteins aggregate into microdomains and no longer interact with their specific membrane partners. Second, borders between gel microdomains and fluid portions of the membrane create ion-permeable gaps which are unstable and can lead to membrane fusion or rupture.

Lipid asymmetry is an additional level of molecular complexity beyond the uniqueness of each membrane compartment. Membranes of cells consist of a stabile bilayer having the total phospholipid pool equally allocated to the inner and outer leaflets of the bilayer. Each phospholipid species, however, has a preference for one of these two leaflets. Phosphatidylcholine and sphingomyelin prefer the outward facing leaflet, whereas phosphatidylethanolamine, phosphatidylserine, and phosphatidylinositol prefer the inner, cytosolic leaflet. Membrane stressors (i.e., cooling) that alter orientations of lipids could affect membrane stability, particularly as each lipid species has an individual preference for the bilayer or hexagonal-II phase states when under stress.[106]

Lipid-protein interactions provide another level of membrane molecular complexity. Not all lipids in a membrane prefer the bilayer orientation. In a stable bilayer membrane, these lipid species, which tend to impede retention of a bilayer, are found in close association with integral membrane proteins.[106] These lipid-protein interactions mediate smooth melding of the protein into the bilayer, eliminating holes or pores where proteins contact the lipids of the bilayer, and may be requisite to proper function of the protein as an enzyme, receptor, or ion channel by inducing proper protein conformation.[102]

For each membrane compartment in a stallion spermatozoon, the proper lipid and protein constituents have evolved to permit proper function when the membrane is in the fluid state at 39° C. As spermatozoa are cooled, the bulk membrane undergoes a phase transition into the gel state. This occurs at 20.7° C for stallion spermatozoa.[21] In addition, individual lipid species undergo a phase transition and aggregate into microdomains, the proteins associated with these lipids may cease to function as designed because lipid-protein interactions are disrupted (Fig. 80–18). Upon rewarming, the nonbilayer-preferring lipids within any microdomain may not return to apposition with the proper protein but aggregate in a hexagonal-II phase.[106]

Aggregation of lipids into gel-phase microdomains forces membrane proteins of the glycocalyx to aggregate in the remaining fluid lipid domains.[101] Function of such glycocalyx components can be altered as stoichiometry of proteins in the membrane is altered. This can be caused by alterations in attachment of integral pro-

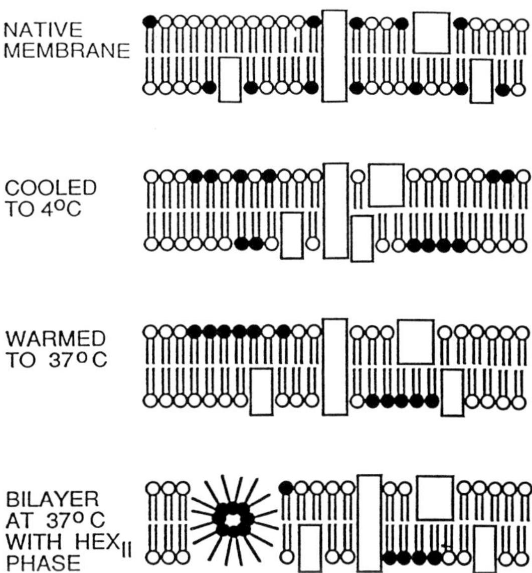

FIG. 80–18. Schematic representation of probable effects of cooling and rewarming on distribution of lipids around integral membrane proteins. The native membrane represents the spermatozoal plasma membrane at seminal collection; lipids tend to impede retention of bilayer associated with integral membrane proteins (blocks). Cooling to 4° C causes lipids tending to impede bilayer formation to undergo a phase transition and cluster together in the gel state; this forces membrane proteins to cluster together and associate with lipids tending to favor retention of the bilayer. However, clustering of membrane proteins alters membrane function. Rewarming to 37° C produces a membrane that has lipid-protein associations different from those of the native membrane, and lipid-lipid associations may form hexagonal-II configurations. A complete return to the native membrane configuration will occur only if lipid mobility is sufficient to allow all membrane components to find their "original" partners. (Adapted from Hammerstedt, R.H., Graham, J.K., and Nolan, J.P.: Cryopreservation of mammalian sperm: What we ask them to survive. J. Androl., *11*:73–88, 1990.)

teins with cytoskeletal assemblies or by protein coupling.[101,107]

RESPONSES OF PROTEINS TO COOLING

Intracellular proteins are affected by cooling. For example, as temperature is reduced, enzyme function is reduced. The relative rate of activity of adenylate cyclase was reduced by 90%, from 1630 pmol cAMP formed per minute per milligram protein when bull spermatozoa were cooled from 37° to 10° C.[108] Phosphodiesterase activity decreased similarly.[108]

Proteins involved in transport of substances across the membrane also have reduced activity at low temperature. Proteins which form the Na^+/K^+ and Ca^{++} pumps are decreased to 0.25% of their activity at 37° C when at ≤6° C. This decrease in pumping ability appears to be associated with the protein itself and not the surrounding lipids.[109] Glucose transport in the red blood cell is reduced at 0° C to <0.1% of its transport at 37° C.[109]

Reductions in both enzyme and transport activities can be caused by combination of (1) decreased kinetics of molecules at lower temperatures; (2) altered pH of aqueous portions of the cell and surrounding medium at low temperature, inducing a change in pK of the protein, its electrical charge, and its function;[109,110] (3) altered lipid-protein interactions, because of removal of preferred lipids (those tending to prefer the hexagonal-II phase) from the protein and reduced lateral movement of proteins in membranes in which lipids are in the gel phase;[101] and (4) irreversible denaturation of proteins.[107,110]

COOLING AND COLD SHOCK

With the preceding background on effects of cooling on cell components, one can begin to understand effects of cooling on spermatozoa. Rapid cooling of spermatozoa induces cold shock, but slow cooling does not entirely circumvent the problem.[20] Spermatozoa stored at 5° C undergo changes observed in cells undergoing senescence (see later), but at a reduced rate.[99]

Cooling appears to dissociate decreased fertility and decreased motility in contrast to senescence. Cooled ram spermatozoa maintain motility (upon warming), but have reduced fertility, whereas aged spermatozoa lose both attributes simultaneously.[99,107] This dissociation probably arises from differences in the composition of the membrane compartments. Cooling a membrane induces gel state microdomains with leaky borders. Normally, ions which leak into the cell (Na^+ and Ca^{++}) are pumped back out by ion transporters. However, at 5° C permeability of spermatozoal membranes to Ca^{++} is increased[107] and the effectiveness of the Ca^{++} transporter is decreased;[107,109] thus Ca^{++} accumulates in the cell. Probably the acrosomal membrane becomes more permeable to Ca^{++} at 5° C than mitochondrial membranes associated with motility, and the high Ca^{++} concentration in the acrosome induces a premature vesiculation of these membranes.[107] Differences in the biochemical composition of these membrane compartments (acrosome vs. mitochondria) may explain why fertility declines more rapidly than motility in cooled spermatozoa.

Cold-shocked spermatozoa exhibit acute and extensive damage. Changes in spermatozoal motion are easily recognized (Fig. 80–19). The percentage of motile cells is decreased[7,20,98,107] and motion characteristics of the motile spermatozoa are altered. In spermatozoa from many species, a nonreversible bending of the middle piece and coiling of the tail occurs which causes the tail to fold back on itself and the spermatozoa to swim backward.[20,107]

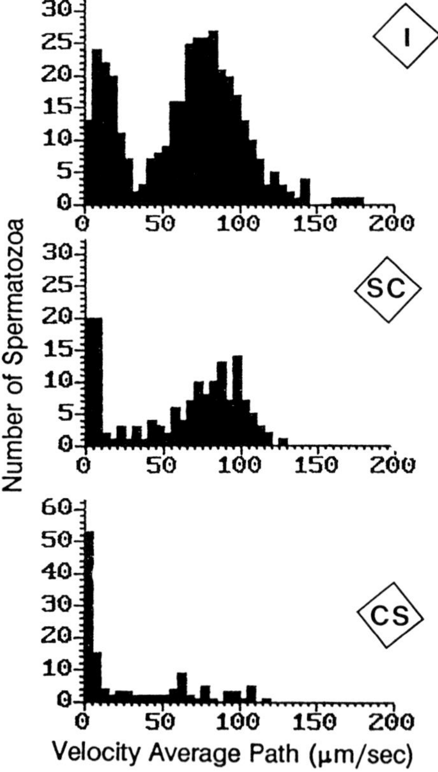

FIG. 80–19. Effects of slow cooling to 4° C and cold shock, by direct immersion of vial containing extended semen in 4° C water, on velocity of spermatozoa. Velocity for most spermatozoa in semen extended in E-Z Mixin shortly after ejaculation was >30 μm/s (I) and averaged 84 μm/s. After cooling extended semen slowly to 4° C, the velocity distribution for motile spermatozoa was not greatly altered (SC) and still averaged 84 μm/s; fewer spermatozoa were motile (73 vs. 84%, initially). For spermatozoa subjected to cold shock (CS), however, few spermatozoa had a velocity >30 μm/s. Means are for one ejaculate from each of three stallions. Semen are extended to 25 × 10^6/mL in E-Z Mixin. Samples were evaluated with a *Stromberg-Mika Cell Motion Analysis System* (SM-CMA, 4.3 Bad Fellienbach, Germany).

Investigations on metabolism of cold-shocked ram and bull spermatozoa revealed decreased anaerobic glycolysis[111] and respiration.[107,111] This was caused by losses of ATP, glycolytic enzymes, and cytochrome c as a result of membrane damage. However, uptake of a fluorescent dye, rhodamine 123, by mitochondria was evidence that the mitochondria still were functioning.[107]

Microscopic examinations of cold-shocked ram spermatozoa revealed increased permeability of the plasma membrane to vital stains, localized swellings of the flagellum, and damage to the acrosome (swollen, broken, or missing) in a high proportion of spermatozoa.[107] Electron microscopic evaluation revealed that the plasma membrane overlying the acrosome was particularly vulnerable to damage and damage was accompanied by loss of the acrosomal matrix.[107]

Stallion spermatozoa subjected to cold shock exhibit similar cellular damage as ram and bull spermatozoa.[112] Extensive disruption of the plasma membrane covering the head of stallion spermatozoa was noted. In contrast to ram spermatozoa, mitochondria in stallion spermatozoa also were damaged, indicating that cold stress directly affected the mitochondrial cristae.[112] Subtle mitochondrial damage probably is the cause of loss of motility, because little structural damage was observed in the spermatozoal middle piece or principal piece.

Although cooling spermatozoa to 4° or 5° C has some deleterious effects on spermatozoal function, when properly done it reduces metabolism and the rate of senescence so that a high proportion of spermatozoa are motile and fertilizing capacity is retained after 24 h at 5° to 8° C.[98,113–116]

MINIMIZING THERMAL STRESS

The maturity of spermatozoa affects their susceptibility to thermal stress. Epididymal spermatozoa are more resistant to cold shock than are ejaculated spermatozoa.[1] Although no data for stallion spermatozoa exist, incubation for ≥20 min in seminal plasma possibly will reduce sensitivity to cold. Indeed, boar spermatozoa are sensitive to cold shock immediately after ejaculation, but acquire resistance to cold-shock damage after incubation in seminal plasma.[117,118] A similar but less pronounced change is observed with ram spermatozoa.[107]

A variety of additives reduce cold-shock injury in spermatozoa.[99,107] Compounds such as ethylenediaminetetraacetic acid (EDTA), which bind Ca^{++} and Mg^{++}, are likely to reduce leakage of Ca^{++} into the cell. Most other protective compounds contain lipids or lipophilic molecules and likely affect the plasma membrane, although the exact mechanism by which they affect the cell is unknown.

Phillips and Lardy demonstrated that egg yolk protected bull spermatozoa from cold shock.[119] Egg yolk also protects ram spermatozoa[120] and stallion spermatozoa[121–123] but fails to protect boar spermatozoa from cold shock.[124] The protective action is provided by the low-density lipoproteins of the egg yolk,[125–129] especially phospholipids.[125,128,130–132] Phospholipids are believed to stabilize the membrane, but their mode of interaction is not understood. Lipid composition of the membrane apparently is not altered after addition of egg yolk,[125,130] and washing spermatozoa free of egg yolk removes its protective capabilities.[128,130,131]

Extenders containing skim milk or cream have been used for preservation of stallion spermatozoa.[23,98,113–115,133] Little research has been done investigating the mechanism of milk's protective action against cold-shock damage to spermatozoa. However, milk lipoproteins probably act similarly to egg yolk lipoproteins in protecting spermatozoal membranes. Milk proteins also may act by directly stabilizing protein elements in the spermatozoal membrane.[99]

Other additives, such as butylated hydroxytoluene (BHT)[134–137] and phosphatidylserine,[138,139] have been used with bull and boar spermatozoa. These compounds directly alter the composition of the plasma membrane and affect the membrane's fluidity and susceptibility to cold-shock damage.[99,134]

Whatever their mechanism for minimizing cold-shock injury to spermatozoa, these compounds permit the cooling of spermatozoa for storage as liquid semen or in conjunction with cryopreservation. Spermatozoa cooled to or stored at 5° C maintain fertilizing capacity, although cooled spermatozoa possess slightly altered function (motility and acrosomal integrity) upon rewarming and insemination.

To maximize retention of fertilizing capacity, stallion spermatozoa should be (1) mixed with at least three volumes of an appropriate extender, (2) cooled no faster than 0.05° C/min between 18° and 8° C,[107] and (3) incubated at low temperature (3° to 6° C) for as short an interval as possible and preferably <36 h.

CHANGES IN SPERMATOZOA OCCURRING BEFORE FERTILIZATION OR DURING AGING AND SENESCENCE

THE BIOCHEMISTRY OF CAPACITATION AND THE ACROSOME REACTION

Freshly ejaculated stallion spermatozoa, like spermatozoa from all mammals, are unable to fertilize oocytes without undergoing further modification (see Fig. 80–1). One major modification involves changes in the spermatozoal plasma membrane which facilitate fusion of the plasma membrane with the outer acrosomal membrane during the acrosome reaction. In addition, spermatozoal motion is modified and spermatozoa change from moving progressively forward to a nonprogressive motion in which a spermatozoon exhibits whiplash-like tail movements causing the head of the spermatozoon to move in a star-like or figure-eight pattern. This modified motility is referred to as hyperactivated motility or hyperactivation.[5,140] The processes which induce these spermatozoal modifications are referred to as spermatozoal capacitation. Some of these processes are enhanced by the female reproductive tract and its secretions, but most will proceed to some extent in vitro.

Spermatozoa undergo aging and senescence after ejaculation as well, which include spontaneous changes in the spermatozoal plasma membrane and metabolism that render spermatozoa infertile. These changes are similar to changes seen during spermatozoal capacitation.

The requirement for spermatozoal modification before fertilization first was observed in 1949 by Noyes, Finkle, and Rock, although never published,[141] and was reported by Austin[142] and Chang.[143] Austin coined the term *capacitation* to describe these changes.[144] Spermatozoal capacitation is defined as changes in a spermatozoon, particularly the plasma membrane, that allow the cell to undergo the acrosome reaction, which is a reaction to physiologic concentrations of free Ca^{++} which induces vesiculation of the plasma membrane and outer acrosomal membrane and is accompanied by an altered beat pattern of the flagellum resulting in hyperactivated motility.[4,5,145] These changes require 18 to 20 h for stallion spermatozoa in vitro.[146] However, the time required for capacitation to occur in utero is not known. Comprehensive studies of this process have been difficult because no obvious morphologic change occurs in spermatozoa during capacitation.[147]

Reviews of molecular mechanisms underlying capacitation and the acrosome reaction are available.[140,145,147–152] However, clinicians should be aware of the reversible changes in spermatozoal metabolism, cell surface components, and membrane alterations that occur during capacitation as a prelude to the acrosome reaction and hyperactivated motility.

After ejaculation, major changes occur in surface components of spermatozoa during capacitation. Although the female tract supplies spermatozoa with energy substrates, this environment is not necessarily optimal for spermatozoa. Therefore, spermatozoa acquire a glycoprotein coat during epididymal transit, secreted by epididymal epithelium, to which is added proteins from the seminal plasma upon ejaculation. These proteins help maintain membrane integrity during their sojourn in the female reproductive tract. One important part of capacitation is the gradual removal or alteration of the adsorbed protein coat to alter transmembrane ion flux, to expose spermatozoal membrane receptor sites, and to remove compounds covering the tail which may restrict flagellar hyperactive motion.[141] Similar changes occur over the caudal and rostral portion of the spermatozoal head, the middle piece, and principal piece. Changes in the plasma membrane over the head facilitate binding of the spermatozoon to the zona pellucida and occurrence of the acrosome reaction. Changes in the plasma membrane over the tail facilitate hyperactive motility, and those over the mitochondria facilitate increased energy output.[140]

In addition to changes in the glycoprotein coat covering the spermatozoal plasma membrane, the plasma membrane itself undergoes specific changes during spermatozoal capacitation. One major change is efflux of cholesterol from the plasma membrane.[150,153] Cholesterol is transferred nonspecifically to albumins in the female tract and is transferred to a high-density lipoprotein of follicular origin (apolipoprotein A-I) in the uterine tube by a specific transfer protein.[153] Cholesterol plays a significant role in stabilizing membranes. Thus, loss of cholesterol tends to destabilize the spermatozoal plasma membrane, particularly that portion over the acrosome, because this portion of the plasma membrane has a high concentration of phospholipids containing docoshexanoic acid, a fatty acid which enhances membrane fluidity. Destabilization of the membrane by removal of cholesterol permits reorganization of components in the bilayer, including redistribution of integral proteins. Clustering of these proteins facilitates receptor-ligand interactions, exposure of membrane-bound enzymes, and alters binding characteristics of surface receptors.[153] Destabilization affects the lipid portion of the membrane altering ion permeability, particularly Ca^{++}, and membrane fusogenic properties, both of which are important for the acrosome reaction.[140]

During capacitation, spermatozoal metabolism increases before onset of hyperactivated motion. Respiration of rabbit spermatozoa increases fourfold during that time and appears to be directly linked to an increase in intracellular cAMP.[148] Increased ATP production is required as spermatozoal velocity and the amplitude of flagellar movement increase during capacitation.[148]

Hyperactivated motility of spermatozoa at the site of fertilization may be necessary for spermatozoa to escape binding to epithelial cells of the uterine tube and to penetrate through the zona pellucida.[154] The time required to induce these changes, via capacitation, ensures induction of the acrosome reaction at the surface of the zona pellucida and not earlier during a spermatozoon's passage up the female tract. The acrosome reaction must occur in the vicinity of the egg, because fusion of the outer acrosomal membrane with the overlying plasma membrane releases the acrosomal enzymes needed for spermatozoal penetration through the zona pellucida;[140] premature loss of those enzymes would preclude fertilization. In addition, loss of the outer acrosomal/plasma membrane vesicles after the acrosome reaction exposes the inner acrosomal membrane, which contains receptors for sperm-egg binding.[140] Spermatozoa with an intact outer acrosomal membrane cannot bind to the egg plasma membrane and initiate fertilization.

THE BIOCHEMISTRY OF SPERMATOZOAL SENESCENCE INDUCED BY AGING

The natural saga for ejaculated stallion spermatozoa includes (1) deposition into the reproductive tract of the mare, (2) transport through the female tract (i.e., through cervical mucus, uterus, and uterine tube[155]), (3) capacitation, (4) exhibition of the acrosome reaction and hyperactived motility, (5) binding to and passing through the zona pellucida, (6) penetration of the plasma membrane of the oocyte, and (7) nuclear and chromosome decondensation and union of male and female pronuclei to produce a one-cell fertilized egg.[152,156] In horses, this sequence usually progresses normally if the stallion breeds the mare or artificial insemination occurs within 0 to 36 h before ovulation. If deposition of spermatozoa into the mare occurs 0 to 6 h after ovulation, fertility will not be greatly reduced, but deposition of semen in the mare 12 to ≥24 h after ovulation will result in reduced fertility and foaling rate (Chapter 83). The stallion, type of sperm (fresh cooled or frozen-thawed), and mare all probably affect the interval after ovulation when a successful insemination can occur.

If spermatozoa are deposited in the mare early or after spermatozoa have been stored in vitro (i.e., when spermatozoa are stored at 5° C or frozen-thawed), the timing of this sequence of events may be altered. Changes from this scenario arise because of spermatozoal aging. Although no research reports the effects of aging on stallion spermatozoa, stallion spermatozoa likely respond in a manner similar to spermatozoa from other species. Roche et al. demonstrated that when freshly collected rabbit spermatozoa were mixed in equal numbers with rabbit spermatozoa aged for 24 h at 5° C, the freshly collected spermatozoa were responsible for 95% of the resulting offspring.[157] Thus spermatozoal senescence can occur before insemination and during normal handling of spermatozoa between the time of semen collection and insemination. Aging also can occur in the female tract if spermatozoa are inseminated too early before ovulation and must reside in the female tract longer than is optimal.[158]

It is difficult to distinguish aging phenomenon from capacitation because some results of both processes are similar.[159] However, aging results in decreased fertilizing capacity, decreased spermatozoal motility, and increased embryonic mortality. Spermatozoal capacitation leads to a spermatozoon becoming competent to fertilize an egg.

Inseminating females with spermatozoa that had been stored for 1 to 5 days before insemination revealed gradually reduced pregnancy rates in mares, cattle, and rabbits (Table 80–5). However, fertility often is greater on day 2 than on day 1. Storage of spermatozoa for 4 to 5 days resulted in lower pregnancy rates.

Assessing spermatozoal fertility can be difficult because fertility and pregnancy rates are not the same because of embryonic loss. This discrepancy arises because defective as well as physiologically fit spermatozoa can initiate embryonic development.[164] Perhaps for this reason, fertility of semen stored for short periods of time resulted in higher fertilization rates than semen used immediately. An ejaculate may contain defective spermatozoa which can compete with normal spermatozoa immediately after ejaculation, but these spermatozoa may not survive storage and are unable to compete with normal spermatozoa when insemination occurs after 2 or 3 days of storage.[159,162]

The loss of fertility resulting from aged spermatozoa probably is caused by the inability of aged spermatozoa to initiate fertilization because of defective motility, capacitation, acrosome reaction, acrosomal enzymes, binding capability, or genomic abnormality. Rabbit or hamster spermatozoa aged in the uterus gave a decreased fertilization rate and development of resulting embryos was slower than normal. However, no increase in percentage of embryos with chromosomal abnormalities was noted.[163,165] Rabbit spermatozoa aged in vitro at 5° C for 5 h or 5 days resulted in kindling rates of 87 and 44% of ovulated oocytes, respectively.[165] Part of the decrease in live young was caused by abnormal embryonic development resulting from aged spermatozoa. Size of 6-day-old embryos was reduced for embryos resulting from spermatozoa aged 5 days (9 μL volume) compared with embryos resulting from fresh spermatozoa (26 μL volume). Embryonic death accounted for about one-third of the difference in kindling rate after insemination of aged rather than fresh spermatozoa. Maurer et al.[164] concluded that when aged spermatozoa fertilize an oocyte, embryonic development is delayed which, in some cases, results in embryonic death. However, most of these embryos result in live young. Mammalian (cow) and amphibian (frog) embryos resulting from aged spermatozoa lack several proteins found in normal embryos, probably because of defective genome translation, and this arrests embryonic development.[162,166] However, the major loss in offspring born, accounting for about two-thirds of the differences in kindling rates, was not attributed to increased embryonic mortality. Rather, reduced fertilization rate by aged spermatozoa was the major cause of

TABLE 80–5. EFFECT OF AGING OF SPERMATOZOA IN VITRO ON FERTILITY (%)*

	AGE OF SEMEN AT TIME OF INSEMINATION (DAYS)					
SPECIES	1	2	3	4	5	REFERENCE
Horse†	71	85	50	67	—	160
Cattle†	64	65	61	54	49	161
Cattle†	55	66	63	54	39	162
Rabbit‡	73	52	95	63	27	163

*Based on use of aliquots of the same semen sample each day.
†Fertility reported is 180-day nonreturn rate.
‡Fertility based on number of 6-day embryos and corpora lutea.

reduced kindling rate.[164] No critical study using aged stallion spermatozoa has been reported.

Use of transported semen is increasing and some reduction in fertility by aged spermatozoa might be expected. Therefore, age-related changes in spermatozoal function will be considered in detail. The physiochemical changes that occur during storage in vitro and in utero are largely irreversible.[167] Spermatozoal defects induced by aging can be classified as (1) nuclear instability, (2) membrane defects, (3) loss of intracellular components (enzymes, ions, metabolites, etc.), and (4) lipid peroxidation.

Nuclei of spermatozoa are altered during long incubation at 37° or 5° C.[159] The actual DNA content of the spermatozoon remains unchanged during storage,[159,167] but DNA-protein associations change.[167] Samples of bull semen in which a high proportion of the spermatozoa had altered DNA packaging had low fertility.[61,62] This also may be true for stallion spermatozoa,[168] but additional studies are necessary. Therefore, alterations in DNA-protein associations, induced by aging, are likely to affect fertility of spermatozoa adversely.

As spermatozoa age, plasma membrane defects arise. The acrosomal membrane swells, and all membranes become increasingly permeable.[159] Permeability changes can be detected with live-dead or differential stains.[73]

Increased membrane permeability results in an inability to maintain proper intracellular ionic concentrations, because Ca^{++} leaks into the cell faster than it can be pumped out. In addition, aged spermatozoa lose ATP and are incapable of resynthesizing it.[159] Acrosomal enzymes, glycolytic enzymes, and transaminase enzymes also are lost. The loss of glutamic-oxaloacetic transaminase (GOT) has been correlated with spermatozoal damage.[169–171]

Lipid peroxidation is detrimental to spermatozoa. Lipid peroxidation is the interaction of oxygen with unsaturated fatty acids to produce hydrogen peroxide. This reaction occurs in spermatozoa from all species examined,[54,172,173] with docoshexanoic acid, a primary fatty acid of spermatozoa, being especially vulnerable to peroxidation. The resulting lipid peroxides affect membranes, altering their permeability and inducing breakage.[172] Because docoshexanoic acid comprises up to 67% of the lipids in the acrosomal membranes,[172] acrosomal swelling and disintegration are commonly seen as a result of spermatozoal aging.[159]

The percentage of motile mouse spermatozoa decreases in a linear fashion as extent of peroxidation increases.[54] Lipid peroxidation is a major cause of the membrane defects seen in aged spermatozoa. Permeability of the plasma membrane increases, so that vital stains, such as eosin, enter the cell. Similarly, intracellular constituents, such as glycolytic enzymes, leak out.[172] Lipid peroxides also directly destroy and/or inactivate certain proteins and enzymes. Enzymes of the acrosome are susceptible to inactivation by lipid peroxidation.[172] Loss of enzymes through inactivation, as well as membrane leakage, radically alter spermatozoal metabolism, resulting in a rapid and irreversible loss of motility and fertilizing capacity.[54,172]

Seminal plasma contains several substances that help minimize lipid peroxidation. Naturally occurring antioxidants containing thiols, such as ergothioneine, glutathione, and cysteine, are effective in eliminating peroxides.[54] Stallion semen contains relatively high concentrations of ergothioneine (76 μg/mL semen) when compared with bull semen (trace amounts).[24] Bull spermatozoa receive protection from their seminal plasma, which contains proteins which virtually eliminate lipid peroxidation, but seminal plasma of the stallion, ram, and human lack such proteins.[172]

Lipid peroxidation also is affected by diluent and handling procedures. Diluents containing a high concentration of K^+ increase the rate of peroxidation,[54] while addition of egg yolk decreases peroxidation,[172] as do added antioxidants.[174] In addition, rapid cooling, cold shock, and centrifugation increase peroxidation rates, whereas slow cooling and passing carbon dioxide gas over semen reversibly arrests motility, metabolism, and peroxidation.[167]

In summary, in early stages of senescence, lipid peroxidation triggers degenerative changes in spermatozoal membranes. These lead to acrosomal swelling and increased permeability of the acrosomal and plasma membranes. Increased membrane permeability results in loss of essential substances (both ions and enzymes), decreased metabolism and motility, and decreased fertility. Inclusion of certain additives in a seminal extender and avoidance of deleterious handling procedures can minimize this damage to spermatozoa.

POTENTIAL FOR SEPARATING X- AND Y-CHROMOSOME–BEARING SPERMATOZOA

Interest in determining the sex of offspring was expressed as early as 460–370 B.C. but only recently has been achieved. Unfortunately, even methods proven effective with mammalian spermatozoa in controlled small-scale studies, and carefully documented in the literature,[175–178] are not appropriate for use in commercial artificial insemination, for which numerous doses of $>300 \times 10^6$ spermatozoa are needed.

Two basic approaches exist for altering sex ratio at birth by manipulating spermatozoa before artificial insemination.[179,180] The first is a physical separation to provide at least one population, if not two populations, enriched for either spermatozoa bearing an X chromosome or spermatozoa bearing a Y chromosome (hereafter termed X-spermatozoa and Y-spermatozoa). Obviously, enrichment to 80 to 85% for either type of spermatozoa would be of great economic importance, provided that fertility was not suppressed and that losses of spermatozoa in the separation procedure were minimal. This is the concept usually thought of for sexing sperm. However, a second and equally valid approach would be to selectively alter the function of either X-spermatozoa or Y-spermatozoa by a procedure that caused death of one type or enhanced the probability that spermatozoa of one type would fertilize the oocyte. With this strategy, a functional advantage is established, rather than a physical separation.

Less than 30 years ago the critical role of the Y chromosome in determining the sex of mammals was established. Based on data for several species of mammals, evidence shows that if the primitive gonads develop as fetal testes, during the second month of gestation for colts, the previously bipotential reproductive system will develop into one characteristic of a male; following birth and puberty, the testes will produce spermatozoa. This is because the fetal testes secrete hormones, including testosterone and müllerian-inhibiting substance.[181] In a normal fetus, the presence of a Y chromosome induces development of the gonads as testes. After a furious research effort during the past decade, researchers established that a single gene on the Y chromosome is responsible for determining how the primitive gonad develops. Based on data for mice and humans, the *Sry* gene is located on the Y chromosome; it encodes for a factor which is obligatory for making a male gonad.[182–185] This gene apparently is conserved across all common mammals and is expressed in somatic cells of the genital ridge only for a short interval just before overt testis differentiation. Animals with a Y chromosome lacking this gene develop as phenotypic females. Animals with two X chromosomes, one of which contains a translocated *Sry* gene, develop as sex-reversed phenotypic males rather than females. However, certain genes present on the X chromosome and autosomes, in addition to the *Sry* gene, are necessary for complete expression of maleness in the adult.

Occasionally, the *Sry* gene and other nearby genes are translocated from the Y chromosome to the X chromosome, as an aberration occurring in the primary spermatocyte that gave rise to the fertilizing spermatozoon. Such an XX embryo would develop as a male, because of presence of the translocated portion of the Y chromosome.[184] Nevertheless, in most cases an XX embryo will develop as a mare and an XY embryo will develop as a stallion.

X-spermatozoon contains more DNA than a Y-spermatozoon. For common domesticated mammals, this difference is about 3.5% of the total amount of DNA.[63] However, because of variations in components of spermatozoa other than DNA content, scientists have been unable to separate X-spermatozoa from Y-spermatozoa consistently by techniques relying on total mass, size, or sedimentation velocity.[179,180] A recent brief report, however, provided evidence that serial passage of bull spermatozoa through two 10-layer Percoll gradients gave a separation of X- and Y-spermatozoa.[186] Confirmation of this report is awaited.

With a technique termed flow sorting, scientists theoretically can distinguish an X-spermatozoon from a Y-spermatozoon on the basis of DNA content and collect spermatozoa of the desired type.[63,64,175,178] Until recently, the problem had been that the treatments imposed on spermatozoa to enable precise quantitation of their DNA content, and thus separation, killed the spermatozoa. This problem has been overcome by modifying the treatment imposed on the spermatozoa, so that viable spermatozoa emerge from the flow sorting instrument.[175–178] U.S. Department of Agriculture (USDA) scientists developing this procedure have applied for a patent, and the USDA has licensed the procedure. If a patent is granted, the exclusive license for use of this process will influence attempts to use the technology. In any case, access to an instrument costing at least $300,000 would be necessary.

Publications document birth of cattle, rabbits, and swine sired with spermatozoa isolated by flow sorting.[175,177,178] Although fertility rates were low, the sex ratios of animals born were skewed in the expected directions (Table 80–6). Improvements in both the efficacy of separation and fertility of spermatozoa subjected to this procedure are likely to occur in the coming years. Unfortunately, use of this procedure probably will be restricted to sorting spermatozoa in a few samples from truly superior sires, to enhance the probability of obtaining male or female offspring from such individuals. This technique is likely to be used with in vitro fertilization of oocytes obtained from very valuable females. Appropriate methods are in place for cattle and could be developed for horses, if the techniques were not precluded by breed registry associations. At least for

TABLE 80–6. SUCCESS IN PREDETERMINING SEX OF OFFSPRING BY ARTIFICIAL INSEMINATION OF FLOW-SORTED SPERMATOZOA

				SEX OF OFFSPRING			
Species	Type of Species Sperm	Number of Females	Fertility (%)	Male (No.)	Female (No.)	Correct Sex (%)	Reference
Cattle	X	75	15	3	8	73	175
	Y	75	27	12	8	60	
Rabbit	X	60	32	4	15	79	175
	Y	60	35	10	11	48	
Rabbit	X	14	21	1	15	94	177
	Y	16	31	17	4	81	
	X + Y	17	29	6	8	—	

cattle, sufficient spermatozoa can be obtained by flow sorting to enable success using conventional artificial insemination, although with low fertility.

Success with separating X-spermatozoa from Y-spermatozoa by flow sorting[175–178] or possibly Percoll gradients[186] has not eliminated the need for development of a technique for isolating large populations of cells highly enriched for either X-spermatozoa or Y-spermatozoa of normal fertility or for differentially blocking fertilizing capacity of one type of spermatozoa. No information exists to convince a knowledgeable individual that a given procedure works consistently with spermatozoa from stallions. To conveniently obtain numerous, large samples of sperm treated to predetermine sex of offspring remains an unsolved intellectual challenge. Availability of samples highly enriched for either X-spermatozoa or Y-spermatozoa with intact plasma membranes should facilitate development of large-scale methods. For example, several groups have attempted to detect proteins in the plasma membrane which are specific to either X-spermatozoa or Y-spermatozoa and use antibodies against sex-specific plasma membrane proteins to isolate, inactivate, or kill one type of spermatozoa.[187] Although this approach has not proven successful, access to populations of viable spermatozoa isolated by flow sorting should facilitate development of this approach, if sex-specific plasma membrane proteins actually exist.

Both the scientific literature and popular magazines are filled with articles and anecdotal data purporting to prove or disprove that a given method for treating semen alters sex ratio at birth. Virtually without exception, these reports should be given little credence. Reasons for discounting most literature on this popular topic have been discussed elsewhere.[177,178] Most publications purporting to prove or disprove that a given procedure results (or does not result) in an alteration of sex ratio of embryos or offspring are meaningless, because the authors have failed to consider limitations imposed by binomial variation (male vs. female). If the true sex ratio was 70:30 rather than 50:50, then 125 observations of embryos or offspring from treated spermatozoa and 125 observations for control spermatozoa would be needed to have a 95% chance of detecting a difference for that sample of processed semen. However, if the true sex ratio was 80:20, then only 50 observations would be needed. Most publications, however, contain far fewer than 100 observations on treated semen and 100 observations on contemporaneous control semen from the same males.

REFERENCES

1. Amann, R.P.: Maturation of spermatozoa. Proceedings of the Eleventh International Congress on Animal Reproduction and Artificial Insemination. Vol. 5. Dublin, 1988, pp. 320–328.
2. Johnson, L.: Spermatogenesis. *In* Reproduction in Domestic Animals. 4th ed. Edited by P.T. Cupps. New York, Academic Press, 1991, pp. 173–219.
3. Hochereau-de Reviers, M.-T., Courtens, J.L., Courot, M., and de Reviers, M.: Spermatogenesis in mammals and birds. *In* Marshall's Physiology of Reproduction. Vol. 2. 4th ed. Edited by G.E. Lamming. London, Churchill Livingstone, 1990, pp. 106–182.
4. Eddy, E.M.: The spermatozoon. *In* The Physiology of Reproduction. Edited by E. Knobil and J. Neill. New York, Raven Press, 1988, pp. 27–68.
5. Bedford, J.M., and Hoskins, D.D.: The mammalian spermatozoon: Morphology, biochemistry and physiology. *In* Marshall's Physiology of Reproduction. Vol. 2. Male Reproduction. Edited by G.E. Lamming. London, Churchill Livingstone, 1990, pp. 379–568.
6. Amann, R.P.: Can the fertility potential of a semen sample be predicted accurately? J. Androl., *10:*89–98, 1989.
7. Amann, R.P., and Pickett, B.W.: Principals of cryopreservation and a review of cryopreservation of stallion spermatozoa. J. Equine Vet. Sci., *7:*145–173, 1987.
8. Amann, R.P.: Function of the epididymis in bulls and rams. J. Reprod. Fertil. Suppl., *34:*115–131, 1987.
9. Metz, K.W., Berger, T., and Clegg, E.D.: Adsorption of seminal plasma proteins by boar spermatozoa. Theriogenology, *34:*691–700, 1990.
10. Jasko, D.J., Moran, D.M., Farlin, M.E., and Squires, E.L.: Effect of seminal plasma dilution or removal on spermatozoal motion characteristics of cooled stallion semen. Theriogenology, *35:*1059–1067, 1991.
11. Saacke, R.G., et al.: Semen quality and heterospermic insemination in cattle. Proceedings of the Ninth International Congress on Animal Reproduction and Artificial Insemination. Vol. 5. Madrid, 1980, pp. 75–78.
12. Small, M.F.: Sperm wars. Discover, 48–53, 1991.
13. Barth, A.D., and Oko, R.J.: Abnormal Morphology of Bovine Spermatozoa. Ames, Iowa State University Press, 1989.
14. Garner, D.L.: Artificial insemination. *In* Reproduction in Domestic Animals. 4th ed. Edited by P.T. Cupps. New York, Academic Press, 1991, pp. 251–278.
15. Setchell, B.P.: Male reproductive organs and semen. *In* Reproduction in Domestic Animals. 4th ed. Edited by P.T. Cupps. New York, Academic Press, 1991, pp. 221–249.
16. Johnson, L., Amann, R.P., and Pickett, B.W.: Maturation of equine epididymal spermatozoa. Am. J. Vet. Res., *41:*1190–1196, 1980.
17. Baumgartl, C.: Licht- und elektronenmikroskopische Untersuchungen über Veranderungen der Plasmamembran und Akrosomstruktur von Pferdespermien. DMV dissertation. Tierärztliche Hochschule Hannover, 1980.
18. Hammerstedt, R.H., Graham, J.K., and Nolan, J.P.: Cryopreservation of mammalian sperm: What we ask them to survive. J. Androl., *11:*73–88, 1990.
19. Hammerstedt, R.H., and Graham, J.K.: Cryopreservation of poultry sperm: The enigma of glycerol. Cryobiology, *29:*26–38, 1992.
20. Watson, P.F.: Artificial insemination and the preservation of semen. *In* Marshall's Physiology of Reproduction. Vol. 2. Male Reproduction. Edited by G.E. Lamming. London, Churchill Livingstone, 1990, pp. 747–869.
21. Parks, J.E., and Lynch, D.V.: Lipid composition and thermotropic phase behavior of boar, bull stallion and rooster sperm membranes. Cryobiology, in press.
22. Baumgartl, C., Bader, H., Drommer, W., and Lüning, I.: Ultrastructural alterations of stallion spermatozoa due to semen conservation. Proceedings of the Ninth Interna-

tional Congress on Animal Reproduction and Artificial Insemination. Vol. 5. Madrid, 1980, pp. 134–137.

23. Pickett, B.W., Squires, E.L., and McKinnon, A.O.: Procedures for Collection, Evaluation and Utilization of Stallion Semen for Artificial Insemination. Animal Reproduction Laboratory Bulletin No. 03. Fort Collins, Colorado State University, 1987.
24. Mann, T.: Metabolism of semen: Fructolysis, respiration and sperm energetics. *In* The Biochemistry of Semen and of the Male Reproductive Tract. Edited by T. Mann. New York, Barnes and Noble, 1964, pp. 265–307.
25. Polakoski, K.L., and Kopta, M.: Seminal plasma. *In* Biochemistry of Mammalian Reproduction. Edited by L.J.D. Zaneveld and R.T. Chatterton. New York, John Wiley & Sons, 1982, pp. 89–118.
26. Mann, T.: Biochemistry of stallion semen. J. Reprod. Fertil. Suppl., *23:*47–52, 1975.
27. Pickett, B.W., Faulkner, L.C., and Voss, J.L.: Effect of season on some characteristics of stallion semen. J. Reprod. Fertil. Suppl., *23:*25–28, 1975.
28. Tischner, M., Kosiniak, K., and Bielanski, W.: Analysis of the pattern of ejaculation in stallions. J. Reprod. Fertil., *41:*329–335, 1974.
29. Komarek, R.J., Pickett, B.W., Gibson, E.W., and Lanz, R.N.: Composition of lipids in stallion semen. J. Reprod. Fertil., *10:*337–342, 1965.
30. Parks, J.E., Arion, J.W., and Foote, R.H.: Lipids of plasma membrane and outer acrosomal membrane from bovine spermatozoa. Biol. Reprod., *37:*1249–1258, 1987.
31. Parks, J.E., and Hammerstedt, R.H.: Developmental changes occurring in the lipids of ram epididymal spermatozoa plasma membrane. Biol. Reprod., *32:*653–668, 1985.
32. Koehler, J.K.: Lectins as probes of the spermatozoon surface. Arch. Androl., *6:*197–217, 1981.
33. Magargee, S.F., Kunze, E., and Hammerstedt, R.H.: Changes in lectin-binding features of ram sperm surfaces associated with epididymal maturation and ejaculation. Biol. Reprod., *38:*667–685, 1988.
34. Eddy, E.M., et al.: Immunodissection of sperm surface modifications during epididymal maturation. Am. J. Anat., *174:*225–237, 1985.
35. Feuchter, F.A., Vernon, R.B., and Eddy, E.M.: Analysis of the sperm surface with monoclonal antibodies: Topographically restricted antigens appearing in the epididymis. Biol. Reprod., *24:*1099–1110, 1981.
36. Chakraborty, J., Constatinou, A., and McCorquodale, M.: Monoclonal antibodies to bull sperm surface antigens. Anim. Reprod. Sci., *9:*101–109, 1985.
37. Hunter, A.G., and Nornes, H.O.: Characterization and isolation of a sperm-coating antigen from rabbit seminal plasma with capacity to block fertilization. J. Reprod. Fertil., *20:*419–427, 1969.
38. Inskeep, P.B., and Hammerstedt, R.H.: Endogenous metabolism by sperm in response to altered cellular ATP requirements. J. Cell Physiol., *123:*180–190, 1985.
39. Hiipakka, R.A., and Hammerstedt, R.H.: 2-deoxyglucose transport and phosphorylation by bovine sperm. Biol. Reprod., *19:*368–379, 1978.
40. Flipse, R.J.: Metabolism of bovine semen. XI. Factors affecting the transport of fructose in bovine spermatozoa. J. Dairy Sci., *45:*917–920, 1962.
41. Peterson, R.N., Bundman, D., and Freund, M.: Binding of cytochalasin B to hexose transport sites in human spermatozoa and inhibition of binding by purines. Biol. Reprod., *17:*198–206, 1977.
42. Hammerstedt, R.H., and Lovrien, R.E.: Calorimetric techniques for metabolic studies of cells and organisms under normal conditions and stress. J. Exp. Zool., *228:*459–469, 1983.
43. Hammerstedt, R.H.: Use of sperm cells as a model for the study of metabolism. *In* Biochemistry of Metabolic Processes. Edited by D.L.F. Lennon, F.W. Stratman, and R.N. Zahlten. New York, Elsevier, 1983, pp. 29–38.
44. Hammerstedt, R.H., Volonte, C., and Racker, E.: Motility, heat, and lactate production in ejaculated bovine sperm. Arch. Biochem. Biophys., *266:*11–123, 1988.
45. Hoskins, D.D., Brandt, H., and Acott, T.S.: Initiation of sperm motility in the mammalian epididymis. Fed. Proc., *37:*2534–2542, 1978.
46. Vijayaraghavan, S., Critchlow, L.M., and Hoskins, D.D.: Evidence for a role for cellular alkalization in the cyclic adenosine 3′,5′-monophosphate-mediated initiation of motility in bovine caput spermatozoa. Biol. Reprod., *32:*489–500, 1985.
47. Wales, R.G., and Murdoch, R.N.: Factors influencing the response of ram spermatozoa to bicarbonate and carbon dioxide. Aust. J. Biol. Sci., *24:*345–354, 1971.
48. Peterson, R.N., and Freund, M.: Effects of [H+], [N+], [K+] and certain membrane-active drugs on glycolysis, motility, and ATP synthesis by human spermatozoa. Biol. Reprod., *8:*350–357, 1973.
49. Peterson, R.N.: The sperm tail and midpiece. *In* Biochemistry of Mammalian Reproduction. Edited by L.J.D. Zaneveld and R.T. Chatterton. New York, John Wiley & Sons, 1982, pp. 153–173.
50. Setchell, B.P.: Spermatogenesis and spermatozoa. *In* Reproduction in Mammals. I. Germ Cells and Fertilization. 2nd ed. Edited by C.R. Austin and R.V. Short. New York, Cambridge University Press, 1982, pp. 63–101.
51. Jones, R., Mann, T., and Sherins, R.: Peroxidative breakdown of phospholipids in human spermatozoa, spermicidal properties of fatty acid peroxides, and protective action of seminal plasma. Fertil. Steril., *31:*531–537, 1979.
52. Holland, M.K., and Storey, B.T.: Oxygen metabolism of mammalian spermatozoa. Generation of hydrogen peroxide by rabbit epididymal spermatozoa. Biochem. J., *198:*273–280, 1981.
53. Alvarez, J.G., and Storey, B.T.: Assessment of cell damage caused by spontaneous lipid peroxidation in rabbit spermatozoa. Biol. Reprod., *30:*323–331, 1984.
54. Alvarez, J.G., and Storey, B.T.: Lipid peroxidation and the reactions of superoxide and hydrogen peroxide in mouse spermatozoa. Biol. Reprod., *30:*833–841, 1984.
55. Aitken, R.J., and Clarkson, J.S.: Significance of reactive oxygen species and antioxidants in defining the efficacy of sperm preparation techniques. J. Androl., *9:*367–376, 1987.
56. Taylor, M.J.: The meaning of pH at low temperatures. Cryoletters, *2:*231–239, 1981.
57. Taylor, M.J.: Acid dissociation constants for some biological buffers in aqueous solutions containing dimethylsulfoxide at 25° C and −12° C. Cryoletters, *1:*449–460, 1980.
58. Taylor, M.J.: Physico-chemical principles in low temperature. *In* The Effects of Low Temperatures on Biological Systems. Edited by B.W.W. Grout and G.J. Morris. Baltimore, Edward Arnold, 1987, pp. 3–71.
59. Sinowatz, F., and Friess, A.E.: Localization of lectin receptors on bovine epididymal spermatozoa using a colloidal gold technique. Histochemistry, *79:*335–344, 1983.

60. Friess, A.E., and Sinowatz, F.: Con A- and WGA-binding sites on bovine spermatozoa: TEM of specimens in toto. Biol. Cell, *50:*279–284, 1984.
61. Evenson, D.P., Darzynkiewicz, Z., and Melamed, M.R.: Relation of mammalian sperm chromatin heterogeneity to fertility. Science, *210:*1131–1133, 1980.
62. Ballachey, B.E., Evenson, D.P., and Saacke, R.G.: The sperm chromatin structure assay relationship with alternate tests of semen quality and heterospermic performance of bulls. J. Androl., *9:*109–115, 1988.
63. Garner, D.L., et al.: Quantification of the X- and Y-chromosome-bearing spermatozoa of domestic animals by flow cytometry. Biol. Reprod., *28:*312–321, 1983.
64. Pinkel, D., et al.: Flow cytometric determination of the proportions of X- and Y-chromosome-bearing sperm in samples of purportedly separated bull sperm. J. Anim. Sci., *60:*1303–1307, 1985.
65. Mayer, D.T., Squires, C.D., Bogart, R., and Oloufa, M.M.: The technique for characterizing mammalian spermatozoa as dead or living by differential staining. J. Anim. Sci., *10:*226–235, 1951.
66. Swanson, E.W., and Bearden, H.J.: An eosin-nigrosin stain for differentiating live and dead bovine spermatozoa. J. Anim. Sci., *10:*981–987, 1951.
67. Hancock, J.L.: A staining method for the study of temperature shock in semen. Nature, *167:*323–324, 1951.
68. Jeyendran, R.S., et al.: Development of an assay to assess the functional integrity of the human sperm membrane and its relationship to other semen characteristics. J. Reprod. Fertil., *33:*113–118, 1984.
69. Graham, E.F., Schmehl, M.K.L., and Evensen, B.K.: An overview of column separation of spermatozoa. Proceedings of the Seventh National Association of Animal Breeders Technical Conference on Artificial Insemination and Reproduction. Milwaukee, 1978, pp. 69–73.
70. Samper, J.C., Hellander, J.C., and Crabo, B.G.: Relation between the fertility of fresh and frozen stallion semen and semen quality. J. Reprod. Fertil. Suppl., *44:*107–114, 1991.
71. Bhattacharyya, A.K., and Zaneveld, L.J.D.: The sperm head. *In* Biochemistry of Mammalian Reproduction. Edited by L.J.D. Zaneveld and R.T. Chatterton. New York, John Wiley & Sons, 1982, pp. 119–152.
72. Leblond, C.P., and Clermont, Y.: Definition of the stages of the cycle of the seminiferous epithelium in the rat. Ann. N.Y. Acad. Sci., *55:*548–573, 1952.
73. Cross, N.L., and Meizel, S.: Methods for evaluating the acrosomal status of mammalian sperm. Biol. Reprod., *41:*635–641, 1989.
74. Cross, N.L., and Overstreet, J.W.: Glycoconjugates of the human sperm surface: Distribution and alterations that accompany capacitation in vitro. Gamete Res., *16:*23–35, 1987.
75. Graham, J.K., Kunze, E., and Hammerstedt, R.H.: Analysis of sperm cell viability, acrosomal integrity, and mitochondrial function using flow cytometry. Biol. Reprod., *43:*55–64, 1990.
76. Farlin, M., Jasko, D.K., Graham, J.K., and Squires, E.L.: Assessment of Pisum sativum agglutinin in identifying acrosomal damage in stallion spermatozoa. Mol. Reprod., in press.
77. Blach, E.L., et al.: Use of a monoclonal antibody to evaluate integrity of the plasma membrane of stallion sperm. Gamete Res., *21:*233–241, 1988.
78. Evenson, D.P., Darzynkiewicz, Z., and Melamed, M.R.: Simultaneous measurement by flow cytometry of sperm cell viability and mitochondrial membrane potential related to cell motility. J. Histochem. Cytochem., *30:*279–280, 1982.
79. Auger, J., Ronot, X., and Dadoune, J.P.: Human sperm mitochondrial function related to motility: A flow image cytometric assessment. J. Androl., *10:*439–448, 1989.
80. Evenson, D.P., and Ballachey, B.E.: Flow cytometric evaluation of bull sperm chromatin structure, mitochondrial activity, viability and concentration. Proceedings of the Eleventh National Association of Animal Breeders Technical Conference on Artificial Insemination and Reproduction. Milwaukee, 1986, p. 109.
81. Didion, B.A., Dobrinsky, J.R., Giles, J.R., and Graves, C.N.: Staining procedure to detect viability and the true acrosome reaction in spermatozoa of various species. Gamete Res., *22:*51–57, 1989.
82. Satir, P.: How cilia move. Sci. Am., *231*(10):44–52, 1974.
83. Satir, P.: The generation of ciliary motion. J. Protozool., *31:*8–12, 1984.
84. Linck, R.W.: Advances in the ultrastructural analysis of the sperm flagellar axoneme. *In* The Spermatozoon. Edited by D.W. Fawcett and J.M. Bedford. Baltimore, Urban and Schwarzenberg, 1979, pp. 99–115.
85. Rikmenspoel, R.: Movements and active moments of bull sperm flagella as a function of temperature and viscosity. J. Exp. Biol., *108:*205–230, 1984.
86. Amann, R.P.: Computerized evaluation of stallion spermatozoa. Proc. Am. Assoc. Equine Pract., 453–473, 1988.
87. Budworth, P.R., Amann, R.P., and Chapman, P.L.: Relationships between computerized measurements of motion of frozen-thawed bull sperm and fertility. J. Androl., *9:*41–54.
88. Amann, R.P., Squires, E.L., and Pickett, B.W.: Effects of sample thickness and temperature on spermatozoal motion. Proceedings of the Eleventh International Congress on Animal Reproduction and Artificial Insemination. Vol. 3. Dublin, 1988, pp. 221a–221c.
89. Amann, R.P.: Relationship between computerized evaluations of spermatozoal motion and competitive fertility index. Proceedings of the Twelfth National Association of Animal Breeders Technical Conference on Animal Reproduction and Artificial Insemination. Milwaukee, 1988, pp. 38–44.
90. Boyers, S.P., Davis, R.O., and Katz, D.F.: Automated semen analysis. Curr. Probl. Obstet. Gynecol. Fertil., *12:*173–199, 1989.
91. Varner, D.D., Vaughan, S.D., and Johnson, L.: Use of a computerized system for evaluation of equine spermatozoal motility. Am. J. Vet. Res., *52:*224–230, 1991.
92. Jasko, D.K., Lein, D.H., and Foote, R.H.: The repeatability and effect of season on seminal characteristics and computer-aided sperm analysis in the stallion. Theriogenology, *35:*317–327, 1991.
93. Amann, R.P., and Hammerstedt, R.H.: Validation of a system for computerized measurements of spermatozoal velocity and percentage of motile sperm. Biol. Reprod., *23:*647–656, 1980.
94. Makler, A.: The thickness of microscopically examined seminal sample and its relationship to sperm motility estimation. Int. J. Androl., *1:*213–219, 1978.
95. Jasko, D.J., Lein, D.H., and Foote, R.H.: A comparison of two computer-automated semen analysis instruments for the evaluation of sperm motion characteristics in the stallion. J. Androl., *11:*453–459, 1990.
96. Blach, E.L., Amann, R.P., Bowen, R.A., and Frantz, D.: Changes in quality of stallion spermatozoa during cryo-

preservation: Plasma membrane integrity and motion characteristics. Theriogenology, *31*:283–298, 1989.

97. Robertson, L., Wolf, D.P., and Tash, J.S.: Temporal changes in motility parameters related to acrosomal status: Identification and characterization of populations of hyperactivated human sperm. Biol. Reprod., *39*:797–805, 1988.

98. Kayser, J.-P., et al.: Effects of linear cooling rate on motion characteristics of stallion spermatozoa. Theriogenology, in press.

99. Watson, P.F.: The effects of cold shock on sperm cell membranes. *In* Effects of Low Temperatures on Biological Membranes. Edited by G.J. Morris and A. Clarke. London, Academic Press, 1981, pp. 189–218.

100. Singer, S.J., and Nicholson, G.L.: The fluid mosaic model of the structure of cell membranes. Science, *175*:720–731, 1972.

101. Houslay, M.D., and Stanley, K.K. (eds.): Dynamics of Biological Membranes. New York, John Wiley & Sons, 1982.

102. Aloia, R.C., Curtin, C.C., and Gordon, L.M. (eds.): Lipid Domains and the Relationship to Membrane Function. New York, Liss, 1988.

103. Cullis, P.R., and Hope, M.J.: Physical properties and functional roles of lipids in membranes. *In* Biochemistry of Lipids and Membranes. Edited by D.E. Vance and J.E. Vance. Menlo Park, Benjamin/Cummings, 1985, pp. 25–72.

104. Ohki, S., et al. (eds.): Molecular Mechanisms of Membrane Fusion. New York, Plenum, 1988.

105. Hammerstedt, R.H., and Parks, J.E.: Changes in sperm surfaces associated with epididymal transit. J. Reprod. Fertil. Suppl., *34*:133–149, 1987.

106. Quinn, P.J.: Principles of membrane stability and phase behavior under extreme conditions. J. Bioenerg. Biomembr., *21*:3–19, 1989.

107. Watson, P.F., and Morris, G.J.: Cold shock injury in animal cells. *In* Temperature and Animal Cells. Edited by K. Bowler and B.J. Fuller. Cambridge, Company of Biologists Limited, 1987, pp. 311–340.

108. Hammerstedt, R.H., and Hay, S.R.: Effect of incubation temperature on motility and cAMP content of bovine sperm. Arch. Biochem. Biophys., *199*:427–437, 1980.

109. Ellory, J.C., and Hall, A.C.: Temperature effects on red cell membrane transport processes. *In* Temperature and Animal Cells. Edited by K. Bowler and B.J. Fuller. Cambridge, Company of Biologists Ltd., 1987, pp. 53–66.

110. Morris, G.J., and Clarke, A.: Cells at low temperatures. *In* The Effects of Low Temperatures on Biological Systems. Edited by B.W.W. Grout and G.J. Morris. London, Edward Arnold, 1986, pp. 72–119.

111. Morris, G.J.: Direct chilling injury. *In* The Effects of Low Temperatures on Biological Systems. Edited by B.W.W. Grout and G.J. Morris. London, Edward Arnold, 1986, pp. 120–146.

112. Watson, P.F., Plummer, J.M., and Allen, W.E.: Quantitative assessment of membrane damage in cold-shocked spermatozoa of stallions. J. Reprod. Fertil. Suppl., *35*:651–653, 1987.

113. Douglas-Hamilton, D.H., et al.: A field study of the fertility of transported equine semen. Theriogenology, *22*:291–303, 1984.

114. Province, C.A., Squires, E.L., Pickett, B.W., and Amann, R.P.: Cooling rates, storage temperatures and fertility of extended equine spermatozoa. Theriogenology, *23*: 925–933, 1985.

115. Francl, A.T., Amann, R.P., Squires, E.L., and Pickett, B.W. Motility and fertility of equine spermatozoa in a milk extender after 12 or 24 hours at 20° C. Theriogenology, *27*:517–525, 1987.

116. Varner, D.D., Blanchard, T.L., Meyers, P.J., and Meyers, S.A.: Fertilizing capacity of equine spermatozoa stored for 24 hours at 5° or 20° C. Theriogenology, *32*: 515–525, 1989.

117. Pursel, V.G., Johnson, L.A., and Schulman, L.L.: Effect of dilution, seminal plasma and incubation period on cold sock susceptibility of boar spermatozoa. J. Anim. Sci., *37*:528–531, 1973.

118. Berger, T., and Clegg, E.D.: Effect of male accessory gland secretions on sensitivity of porcine sperm acrosomes to cold shock, initiation of motility and loss of cytoplasmic droplets. J. Anim. Sci., *60*:1295–1302, 1985.

119. Phillips, P.H., and Lardy, H.A.: A yolk-buffer pablum for the preservation of bull sperm. J. Dairy Sci., *23*:399–404, 1940.

120. Blackshaw, A.W.: The prevention of temperature shock of bull and ram semen. Aust. J. Biol. Sci., *7*:573–582, 1954.

121. Nishikawa, Y., Waide, Y., and Shinomiya, S.: Studies on deep freezing of horse spermatozoa. Proceedings of the Sixth International Congress on Animal Reproduction and Artificial Insemination. Vol. 2. Paris, 1968, pp. 1589–1596.

122. Oshida, H., et al.: Fertility of frozen stallion semen and some factors affecting to it. Proceedings of the Sixth International Congress on Animal Reproduction and Artificial Insemination. Vol. 2. Paris, 1968, pp. 1597–1599.

123. Pickett, B.W., Burwash, L.D., Voss, J.L., and Back, D.G.: Effect of seminal extenders on equine fertility. J. Anim. Sci., *40*:1136–1143, 1975.

124. Pursel, V.G., Johnson, L.A., and Schulman, L.L.: Interactions of extender composition and incubation period on cold shock susceptibility of boar spermatozoa. J. Anim. Sci., *35*:580–584, 1972.

125. Kampschmidt, R.F., Mayer, D.T., and Herman, H.A.: Lipid and lipoprotein constituents of egg yolk in the resistance and storage of bull spermatozoa. J. Dairy Sci., *36*:733–742, 1953.

126. Masuda, H., and Nishikawa, Y.: Studies on the substances in egg yolk effective on viability and metabolism of spermatozoa. III. Substances in the non-dialyzable portion of egg yolk effective on the survival of spermatozoa of goats, bull and horses. Jpn. J. Zootech. Sci., *43*:355–359, 1972.

127. Pace, M.M., and Graham, E.F.: Components of egg yolk which protect bovine spermatozoa during freezing. J. Anim. Sci., *39*:1144–1149, 1974.

128. Watson, P.F.: The protection of ram and bull spermatozoa by the low density lipoprotein fraction of egg yolk during storage at 5° C and deep-freezing. J. Thermal Biol., *1*:137–141, 1976.

129. Foulkes, J.A.: The separation of lipoproteins from egg yolk and their effect on the motility and integrity of bovine spermatozoa. J. Reprod. Fertil., *49*:277–284, 1977.

130. Quinn, P.J., Chow, P.Y.W., and White, I.G.: Evidence that phospholipid protects spermatozoa from cold shock at the plasma membrane site. J. Reprod. Fertil., *60*:403–407, 1980.

131. Parks, J.E., Meacham, T.N., and Saacke, R.G.: Cholesterol and phospholipids of bovine spermatozoa. II. Effect of liposomes prepared from egg phosphatidylcholine and cholesterol on sperm cholesterol, phospholipids and via-

bility at 4° C and 37° C. Biol. Reprod., *24:*399–404, 1981.
132. Evans, R.W., and Setchell, B.P.: Association of exogenous phospholipids with spermatozoa. J. Reprod. Fertil., *53:*357–362, 1978.
133. Kenney, R.M., et al.: Minimal contamination techniques for breeding mares: Techniques and preliminary findings. Proc. Am. Assoc. Equine Pract., *21:*327–336, 1975.
134. Hammerstedt, R.H., et al.: Use of spin labels and electron spin resonance spectroscopy to characterize membranes of bovine sperm: Effect of butylated hydroxytoluene and cold shock. Biol. Reprod., *14:*381–397, 1976.
135. Pursel, V.G.: Effect of cold shock on boar sperm treated with butylated hydroxytoluene. Biol. Reprod., *21:* 319–324, 1979.
136. Watson, P.F., and Anderson, W.J.: Influence of butylated hydroxytoluene (BHT) on the viability of ram spermatozoa undergoing cold shock. J. Reprod. Fertil., *68:*229–235, 1983.
137. Graham, J.K., and Hammerstedt, R.H. Differential effects of butylated hydroxytoluene (BHT) analogs on bull sperm subjected to cold-induced membrane stress. Cryobiology, *29:*106–107, 1992.
138. Butler, W.J., and Roberts, T.K.: Effects of some phosphatidyl compounds on boar spermatozoa following cold shock or slow cooling. J. Reprod. Fertil., *43:* 183–187, 1975.
139. Graham, J.K., and Foote, R.H. Effect of several lipids, fatty acyl chain length, and degree of unsaturation on the motility of bull spermatozoa after cold shock and freezing. Cryobiology, *24:*42–52, 1987.
140. Yanagimachi, R.: Capacitation and the acrosome reaction. *In* Gamete Physiology. Edited by R.H. Asch, J.P. Balmaceda, and I. Johnston. Norwell, MA, Serono Symposia, 1990, pp. 31–42.
141. Noyes, W.R.: The fertilizing capacity of spermatozoa. West. J. Surg. Obstet. Gynecol., *61:*342–349, 1953.
142. Austin, C.R.: Observations on the penetration of the sperm into the mammalian egg. Aust. J. Sci. Res. Ser. B, *4:*581–596, 1951.
143. Chang, M.C.: Fertilizing capacity of spermatozoa deposited into the fallopian tubes. Nature, *168:*697–698, 1951.
144. Austin, C.R.: The "capacitation" of the mammalian sperm. Nature, *170:*326, 1952.
145. Bedford, J.M.: Significance of the need for sperm capacitation before fertilization in eutherian mammals. Biol. Reprod., *28:*108–120, 1983.
146. Brackett, B.G., Cofone, M.A., Boice, M.L., and Bousquet, D.: Use of zona-free hamster ova to assess sperm fertilizing ability of bull and stallion. Gamete Res., *5:*217–227, 1982.
147. Fraser, L.R.: Sperm capacitation and its modulation. *In* Fertilization in Mammals. Edited by B.D. Bavister, J. Cummins, and E.R.S. Roldan. Norwell, MA, Serono Symposia, 1990, pp. 141–154.
148. Rogers, B.J., and Brentwood, B.J.: Capacitation, acrosome reaction and fertilization. *In* Biochemistry of Mammalian Reproduction. Edited by L.J.D. Zaneveld and R.T. Chatterton. New York, John Wiley & Sons, 1982, pp. 203–230.
149. Clegg, E.D.: Mechanisms of mammalian sperm capacitation. *In* Mechanism and Control of Animal Fertilization. Edited by J.F. Hartmann. New York, Academic Press, 1983, pp. 177–212.
150. Langlais, J., and Roberts, K.D.: A molecular membrane model of sperm capacitation and the acrosome reaction of mammalian spermatozoa. Gamete Res., *12:*183–224, 1985.
151. Oliphant, G., Reynolds, A.B., and Thomas, T.S.: Sperm surface components involved in the control of the acrosome reaction. Am. J. Anat., *174:*269–283, 1985.
152. Yanagimachi, R.: Mechanisms of fertilization in mammals. *In* Fertilization and Embryonic Development in Vitro. Edited by L. Mastroianni and J.D. Biggers. New York, Plenum Press, 1981, pp. 81–182.
153. Parks, J.E., and Ehrenwald, E.: Cholesterol eflux from mammalian sperm and its potential role in capacitation. *In* Fertilization in Mammals. Edited by B.D. Bavister, J. Cummins, and E.R.S. Roldan. Norwell, MA, Serono Symposia, 1990, pp. 155–164.
154. Suarez, S.S., Drost, M., Redfern, K., and Gottlieb, W.: Sperm motility in the oviduct. *In* Fertilization in Mammals. Edited by B.D. Bavister, J. Cummins, and E.R.S. Roldan. Norwell, MA, Serono Symposia, 1990, pp. 111–124.
155. Overstreet, J.W., and VandeVoort, C.A.: Sperm transport in the female genital tract. *In* Gamete Physiology. Edited by R.H. Asch, J.P. Balmaceda, and I. Johnston. Norwell, MA, Serono Symposia, 1990, pp. 43–52.
156. Fraser, L.R., and Ahuja, K.K.: Metabolic and surface events in fertilization. Gamete Res., *20:*491–519, 1988.
157. Roche, J.F., Dziuk, P.J., and Lodge, J.R.: Competition between fresh and aged spermatozoa in fertilizing rabbit eggs. J. Reprod. Fertil., *16:*155–157, 1968.
158. Tesh, J.M.: Effects of ageing of rabbit spermatozoa in utero on fertilization and prenatal development. J. Reprod. Fertil., *20:*299–306, 1969.
159. Mann, T., and Lutwak-Mann, C.: Biochemical aspects of aging in spermatozoa in relation to motility and fertilizing ability. *In* Aging Gametes: Their Biology and Pathology. Edited by R.J. Blandau. New York, S. Karger, 1975, pp. 122–150.
160. Hughes, J.P., and Loy, R.G.: Artificial insemination in the equine: A comparison of natural breeding and artificial insemination from six stallions. Cornell Vet., *60:*463–475, 1970.
161. Salisbury, G.W., and Flerchinger, F.H.: In vitro aging of spermatozoa and evidence for embryonic or early fetal mortality in cattle. Proceedings of the Fourth International Congress on Animal Reproduction and Artificial Insemination. Vol. 2. The Hague, 1961, pp. 601–606.
162. Salisbury, G.W.: Fertilizing ability and biological aspects of sperm storage in vitro. Proceedings of the Sixth International Congress on Animal Reproduction and Artificial Insemination. Vol. 2. Paris, 1968, pp. 1189–1204.
163. Nicolai, P., and Shaver, E.L.: The chromosome complement of rabbit blastocysts resulting from spermatozoa stored at 5° C. Biol. Reprod., *17:*640–644, 1977.
164. Maurer, R.R., Stranzinger, G.F., and Paufler, S.K.: Embryonic development in rabbits after insemination with spermatozoa stored at 37, 5 or −196° C for various periods. J. Reprod. Fertil., *48:*43–49, 1976.
165. Bell, C.L., and Shaver, E.L.: Analysis of preimplantation golden hamster conceptuses resulting from spermatozoa aged in utero. Gamete Res., *6:*199–207, 1982.
166. Hart, R.G., and Salisbury, G.W.: The effect of sperm age on embryonic mortality in the frog. Fed. Proc., *26:*645, 1967.
167. Rowson, L.E.A.: Prolonged storage of gametes in relation to fertility and progeny characteristics in farm animals. *In* Aging Gametes: Their Biology and Pathology.

Edited by R.J. Blandau. New York, S. Karger, 1975, pp. 249–264.

168. Kenney, R.M., Kent, M.G., Garcia, M.C., and Hurtgen, J.P.: The use of DNA index and karyotype analyses as adjuncts to the estimation of fertility in stallions. J. Reprod. Fertil. Suppl., *44:*69–75, 1991.

169. Flipse, R.J.: Metabolism of bovine semen. IX. Glutamic-oxaloacetic and glutamic-pyruvic transaminase activities. J. Dairy Sci., *43:*773–776, 1960.

170. Graham, E.F., and Pace, M.M.: Some biochemical changes in spermatozoa due to freezing. Cryobiology, *4:*75–84, 1967.

171. Pace, M.M., and Graham, E.F.: The release of glutamic oxaloacetic transaminase from bovine spermatozoa as a test method of assessing semen quality and fertility. Biol. Reprod., *3:*140–146, 1970.

172. Jones, R. and Mann, T.: Damage to ram spermatozoa by peroxidation of endogenous phospholipids. J. Reprod. Fertil., *50:*261–268, 1977.

173. Calamera, J.C., et al.: Effect of lipid peroxidation upon human spermatic adenosinetriphosphate (ATP). Relationship with motility, velocity and linearity of the spermatozoa. Andrologia, *1:*48–54, 1989.

174. Killian, G., et al.: Evaluation of butylated hydroxytoluene as a cryopreservative added to whole or skim milk diluent for bull semen. J. Dairy Sci., *72:*1291–1295, 1989.

175. Morrell, J.M., et al.: Sexing of sperm by flow cytometry. Vet. Rec., *122:*322–324, 1988.

176. Johnson, L.A., and Clarke, R.N.: Flow sorting of X and Y chromosome-bearing mammalian sperm: Activation and pronuclear development of sorted bull, boar, and ram sperm microinjected into hamster oocytes. Gamete Res., *21:*335–343, 1988.

177. Johnson, L.A., Flook, J.P., and Hawk, H.W.: Sex preselection in rabbits: Live births from X and Y sperm separated by DNA and cell sorting. Biol. Reprod., *41:* 199–203, 1989.

178. Johnson, L.A.: A flow cytometric/sorting method for sexing mammalian sperm validated by DNA analysis and live births. Cytometry, *4(Suppl.):*42, 1990.

179. Amann, R.P.: Treatment of sperm to predetermine sex. Proceedings of the National Association of Animal Breeders Technical Conference. Milwaukee, 1988, pp. 127–135.

180. Amann, R.P.: Treatment of sperm to predetermine sex. Theriogenology, *31:*49–60, 1989.

181. Jost, A., and Magre, S.: Testicular development phases and dual hormonal control of sexual organogenesis. *In* Sexual Differentiation: Basic and Clinical Aspects. Edited by M. Serio, M. Motta, M. Zarisi, and L. Martini. New York, Raven Press. 1984, pp. 11–15.

182. Berta, P., et al.: Genetic evidence equating SRY and the testis-determining factor. Nature, *348:*448–451, 1990.

83. Jager, R.J., Anvret, M., Hall, K., and Scherer, G.: A human XY female with a frame shift mutation in the candidate testis-determining gene SRY. Nature, *348:*452–454, 1990.

184. McLaren, A.: The making of male mice. Nature, *351:*96, 1991.

185. Koopman, P., et al.: Male development of chromosomally female mice transgenic for *Sry.* Nature, *241:*117–121, 1991.

186. Blottner, S., Böttcher, M., Schwerin, M., and Rommel, P.: Preconceptional sex determination by in vitro fertilization in cattle. Proceedings of the Seventh Annual Meeting European Embryo Transfer Association. 1991, p. 124.

187. Bradley, M.P.: Immunological sexing of mammalian semen: Current status and future options. J. Dairy Sci., *72:*3372–3380, 1989.

CHAPTER 81

SEMINAL EXTENDERS AND COOLED SEMEN

B.W. Pickett

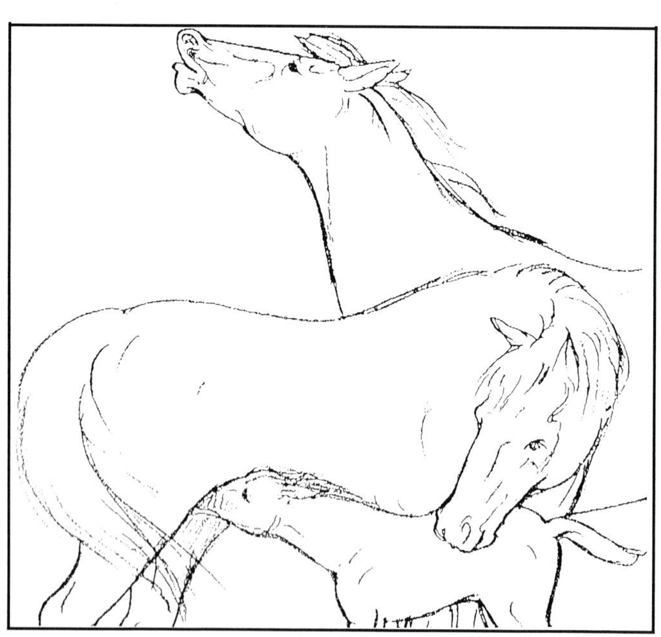

Regulations imposed by some major horse breed associations have restricted the economic incentive to develop techniques for AI, extenders, and storage systems for stallion semen. Nevertheless, numerous sound reasons exist to extend stallion semen even with existing regulations. The reasons are to:

1. Permit effective antibiotic or antibacterial treatment of semen containing pathogenic or potentially pathogenic organisms.
2. Enhance viability of spermatozoa from low-fertility stallions.
3. Prolong survival of spermatozoa.
4. Protect spermatozoa from unfavorable environmental conditions.
5. Increase volume of the inseminate.
6. Aid in proper evaluation of sperm motility.

In most studies in which extenders have been compared for their ability to prolong survival of spermatozoa, the animal was a significant source of variation.[1,2] This appears to be true regardless of species. Thus a clinician must assume that some extenders are more suitable for an individual stallion than others. Consequently, when one extender is more suitable than another, it is probably because that extender had some ingredient(s) needed by spermatozoa from that stallion or something toxic was present in the unsuitable extenders.

In general, an appropriate extender should provide:

1. An osmotic pressure compatible with spermatozoa.
2. Proper balance of mineral elements.
3. Proper combination of nutrients.
4. Chemicals for neutralizing toxic products produced by spermatozoa.
5. Materials to protect spermatozoa against changes in temperature, especially cold.
6. Materials to stabilize enzyme systems and integrity of membranes.
7. A carrier free of infectious organisms.

EXTENDERS

Numerous seminal extenders have been used to extend and/or store stallion semen. Most included egg yolk, milk, milk by-products, or chemicals to regulate osmolarity and/or pH.[3–17] Unfortunately, the majority of these studies used sperm motility as an indicator of fertility rather than pregnancy rate. Although progressive sperm motility is the seminal characteristic most highly related to fertility, some glaring exceptions are found. For example, when there was an inappropriate balance of ingredients in the extender, motility was satisfactory, but fertility was a disaster.[15,18] For fertility studies to be meaningful, appropriate controls must be included, because many factors can affect pregnancy rate.

Seventy-two mares were randomly assigned to a factorial experiment that included 3 seminal treatments, each with a dose of 500 million progressively motile spermatozoa per insemination.[13] The groups were: (1) semen plus 10 mL 2.4% TRIS extender, (2) semen plus

TABLE 81–1. THE EFFECT OF SEMINAL TREATMENTS ON PREGNANCY RATE OF MARES

	EXTENDED					
	TRIS		Cream Gel		Raw	
Cycle	Number of Mares	Pregnant (%)	Number of Mares	Pregnant (%)	Number of Mares	Pregnant (%)
1	24	37.5	24	75.0	24	75.0
2	13	38.5	5	80.0	6	66.7
3	7	57.1	1	100.0	1	0.0
Total*	24	75.0[a]	24	95.8[b]	24	91.7[b]

*Percentages within rows with different superscripts are significantly different at the 1% level of probability.
(Adapted from Pickett, B.W., Burwash, L.D., Voss, J.L., and Back, D.G.: Effect of seminal extenders on equine fertility. J. Anim. Sci., *40*:1136–1143, 1975.)

10 mL cream-gel extender,[8] and (3) raw semen. Inseminations began on May 1 and continued for three estrous periods or until pregnancy was diagnosed at 50 days postovulation. Semen was collected from three stallions every other day and all mares that had been in estrus two days or longer were inseminated.

The results are presented in Table 81–1. Fertility was significantly depressed by extension of semen in the TRIS extender,[13] probably because of the presence of glycerol.[4,18] Furthermore, Pace and Sullivan found that fertility of stallion spermatozoa was depressed almost immediately when semen was placed in hydrogen-ion extenders, such as TRIS.[18] During the first cycle, only 37.5% of the mares became pregnant when bred with spermatozoa in 2.4% TRIS extender compared with 75.0% in cream gel and raw semen, respectively. After three cycles, pregnancy rates were 75.0%, 95.8%, and 91.7% for the TRIS, cream-gel, and raw seminal treatments, respectively. Pregnancy rates of 75.0% during one cycle were higher than normally reported for nonlactating mares and would be considered excellent for other species of livestock, including cattle. Fertility has been assumed to be much lower in the equine than other species of livestock. Obviously, this is not true when AI is used under proper management conditions.

TRIS extender clearly was deleterious, because exposure of spermatozoa to this extender for less than an hour severely depressed fertility. The cream gel was obviously an excellent extender for stallion spermatozoa.[4,8] However, it is difficult and time-consuming to prepare. Furthermore, the presence of fat globules prevents microscopic observation of spermatozoa.

An experiment was conducted using 48 normally cycling, nonlactating mares to determine fertility of spermatozoa extended in heated skim milk, heated skim milk gel, or cream gel.[17] These extenders were selected for the following reasons:

1. Skim milk has been shown to be an effective extender for bovine semen,[19] and a high-quality product is easily available.
2. Gel was added to one skim milk treatment, because it was used in the half-and-half (cream gel) extender.[8]
3. Cream gel was included as a control, because it had been shown to be as good or better than spermatozoa in raw semen in promoting fertility (Table 81–1).

All mares were teased daily with one or two stallions and inseminated every other day, beginning on day 2 or 3 of estrus.[20] Each mare was bred through three cycles or until pregnant, whichever occurred first. Pregnancy was diagnosed after 50 consecutive days of diestrus by both the mare immunologic pregnancy (MIP) test and rectal palpation.

The results of that experiment by extender are presented in Table 81–2. Pregnancy rates for spermatozoa in skim milk and skim milk gel were 62.5%, while

TABLE 81–2. EFFECT OF EXTENDERS ON FERTILITY OF EQUINE SPERMATOZOA

	EXTENDER					
	Skim Milk		Skim Milk Gel		Cream Gel	
Cycle	Number of Mares	Pregnant (%)	Number of Mares	Pregnant (%)	Number of Mares	Pregnant (%)
1	16	18.8	16	18.8	16	18.8
2	13	46.2	13	38.5	13	23.1
3	7	14.3	8	25.0	10	10.0
Total	16	62.5	16	62.5	16	43.8

(Adapted from Householder, D.D., Pickett, B.W., Voss, J.L., and Olar, T.T.: Effect of extender, number of spermatozoa and HCG on equine fertility. J. Equine Vet. Sci., *1*:9–13, 1981.)

43.8% of the mares bred with spermatozoa in cream gel became pregnant. Although no significant differences in pregnancy rates were found among treatments, probably because of the small number of animals involved, spermatozoa in skim milk extenders appeared to provide as good or better fertility than spermatozoa in the cream-gel extender. Furthermore, gel did not seem particularly beneficial to fertility. Based on these results, the author recommends the skim milk extender over the cream-gel and skim milk gel extenders, because of ease of preparation and spermatozoa can be observed microscopically in skim milk extenders. Details of preparation of skim milk extenders with and without gel are presented in Table 81–3.[21]

The equine industry needs an extender that will provide maintenance of motility and fertility, permit microscopic evaluation of motility, and be easy and inexpensive to prepare. Although the skim milk extender provided some advantages over other extenders evaluated to date, the heating of milk to 92 to 95° C (~ 198 to 203° F) for 10 min is time-consuming and the procedures constitute a possible source of error. Furthermore, heating milk to 92 to 95° C (~ 198 to 203° F) becomes difficult at elevations above 5000 ft (~ 1524 m). Unheated, fresh skim milk has been shown to be toxic to equine[7] and bovine spermatozoa.[22,23] The toxic factor appears to be lactenin, an antistreptococcal agent found in milk,[22] which is inactivated in the heating process.[23]

TABLE 81–3. TECHNIQUES FOR PREPARATION OF STALLION SEMINAL EXTENDERS

1. Preparation of 100 mL of Cream-Gel Extender
   1.3 g Knox gelatin
   10 mL deionized water
   90 mL half-and-half cream
   a. Weigh out gelatin
   b. Add gelatin to deionized water.
   c. Autoclave gelatin and deionized water for 20 min.
   d. Heat half-and-half in a double boiler for 10 min at 92° C (~198° F), being sure it does not boil or exceed 95° C (203° F).
   e. Remove any scum from half-and-half after heating.
   f. Add half-and-half to the gelatin solution to make a total volume of 100 mL.
   g. Freeze in 10-mL doses and store in deep freeze until used.*
2. Skim Milk Extender
   100 mL skim milk (nonfortified)
   a. Heat skim milk in a double boiler for 10 min at 92° C. Temperature should never fall below that point or exceed 95° C.
   b. Freeze in 10-mL doses and store in a freezer until used.*
3. Skim Milk Gel Extender
   1.3 g Knox gelatin
   100 mL skim milk (nonfortified)
   a. Weigh out gelatin.
   b. Add to skim milk and agitate for 1 min.
   c. Heat mixture in a double boiler for 10 min at 92° C. Temperature should never fall below that point or exceed 95° C. Swirl mixture periodically during the heating process.
   d. Freeze in 10-mL doses and store in a freezer until used.*

*Warm frozen extender to body temperature (38° C, ~100° F) before addition of semen.

(Adapted from Voss, J.L., and Pickett, B.W.: Reproductive Management of the Broodmare. Animal Reproduction Laboratory General Series Bulletin No. 961. Fort Collins, Colorado State University, 1976.)

TABLE 81–4. COMPOSITION OF NONFAT DRIED MILK SOLIDS GLUCOSE EXTENDER

INGREDIENTS	QUANTITY
Sanalac (instant nonfat dry milk)*	2.4 g
Glucose monohydrate	4.9 g
Sodium bicarbonate (7.5% solution)	2.0 mL
Gentamicin sulfate (reagent grade, 50 mg/mL)	2.0 mL
Distilled water	92 mL
Osmolality (mOsm/kg)†	375 ± 2
pH†	6.99 ± 0.02

*The liquids should be mixed before adding powder, otherwise the acidity of gentamicin will curdle the milk powder.

†Mean ± standard error of the mean.

(Adapted from Kenney, R.M., Bergman, R.V., Cooper, W.L., and Morse, G.W.: Minimal contamination techniques for breeding mares: Technique and preliminary findings. Proc. Am. Assoc. Equine Pract., 327–335, 1975.)

Kenney et al. reported 7 of 12 mares pregnant when a simple, easy-to-prepare extender was used containing dried skim milk, glucose, sodium bicarbonate, and gentamicin (Table 81–4).[9] Province et al. included this nonfat dried milk solids (NFDMS) glucose extender as a variable into a series of studies conducted with stallion spermatozoa.[17] They found that NFDMS glucose extender was superior to skim milk for maintenance of sperm motility (Fig. 81–1). Because motility of spermatozoa in the NFDMS glucose was superior to skim milk after storage for 4 h, two small trials were conducted to compare NFDMS glucose with skim milk. In the first trial, 50 normally cycling, light horse mares were used. As they exhibited estrus, they were randomly assigned to be inseminated daily with 100 million progressively motile spermatozoa extended in either 10 mL NFDMS glucose or skim milk at 37° C (~ 99° F). A dose of only 100 million motile spermatozoa was used in this study to increase the possibilities of detecting a difference between extenders. Mares were palpated per rectum daily until ovulation was detected. Semen from one stallion was used for all inseminations. Mares were inseminated once a follicle 35 mm or larger in diameter was detected and daily thereafter until the end of estrus. Fertility was based on nonsurgical embryo recovery 6 days postovulation.

In the second study, the same extenders were compared, under similar conditions, except that 250 million motile spermatozoa were used. The mares were inseminated daily within 1 h after seminal collection, beginning on day 2 of estrus and continuing until the end of estrus. All mares were inseminated for one cycle. The results of experiments 1 and 2 are presented in Table 81–5. Six-day embryos were recovered from 40% of the 25 mares bred with 100 million spermatozoa in heated skim milk extender compared with 52% of the mares bred with spermatozoa in NFDMS glucose extender. This rate of recovery for 6-day embryos was quite satisfactory, particularly considering the mares were bred with only 100 million motile spermatozoa.[24] For experiment 2, only 6 of the 15 mares in each treatment were pregnant at 50 days postbreeding (40%). The overall low fertility of mares in this experiment, in spite of the fact that 250 million motile spermatozoa were used per insemination and inseminations were daily, was the result of their reproductive status. These 30 mares had been bred twice in another experiment and failed to become pregnant, had grade 2 or 3 uterine biopsies,[25] or had been infected. Although fertility was low in both experiments, no difference between NFDMS glucose and skim milk extended semen was found. However, decision-making is always risky when so few stallions are involved, because of the possibility of stallion by extender interactions.

Goodeaux and Kreider separated equine spermatozoa on a bovine serum albumin (BSA) column.[26] They found that spermatozoa isolated in the lower BSA fractions exhibited superior motility compared with controls. To estimate fertility, 30 Quarter Horse mares were assigned to three treatments (Table 81–6). One group was bred with spermatozoa isolated in BSA; one, with spermatozoa in Tyrode's solution; and one, in 3% BSA. Pregnancy rates at 45 days postovulation were 70%, 80%, and 80%, respectively, whereas foaling rates were 70%, 40%, and 60%, respectively. These are excellent 45-day, single-cycle pregnancy rates, considering that only 100 million live spermatozoa were inseminated. In a later study, Kreider et al. concluded, based on sperm motility, that inclusion of BSA into equine seminal extenders may prolong maintenance of sperm motility.[10]

An extender should not be used as a substitute for good management. Because NFDMS glucose is much easier to prepare, this is the type of extender currently recommended.

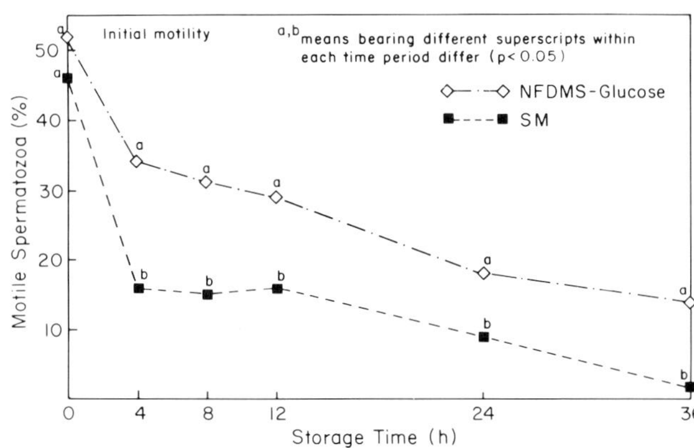

FIG. 81–1. Effect of heated skim milk (solid squares) and nonfat dried milk solids glucose (open diamonds) extender on progressive motility of equine spermatozoa stored at 20° or 15° C (68° or 59° F). Means bearing different subscripts (a, b) within each time period differ ($p < 0.05$). (Adapted from Province, C.A.: Cooling and storage of canine and equine spermatozoa. M.S. thesis. Fort Collins, Colorado State University, 1984.)

TABLE 81–5. FERTILITY OF EQUINE SPERMATOZOA EXTENDED IN NFDMS GLUCOSE OR HEATED SKIM MILK

TREATMENT	NUMBER OF MARES	FERTILITY (%)
Experiment 1*		
Skim milk	25	40
NFDMS glucose	25	52
Experiment 2†		
Skim milk	15	40
NFDMS glucose	15	40

*Fertility based on 6-day embryo recovery.
†Fertility based on 50-day pregnancy.
(Adapted from Province, C.A., Squires, E.L., Pickett, B.W., and Amann, R.P.: Cooling rates, storage temperatures and fertility of extended equine spermatozoa. Theriogenology, *23*:925–934, 1985.)

COOLING AND STORAGE

In 1776, Spallanzani, the recognized father of AI, used stallion semen to observe the effects of cooling equine spermatozoa. He found that cooling spermatozoa retarded their activity and that after rewarming, their motility returned.[27] Rapid cooling of spermatozoa can cause irreversible damage.[28] However, cooling at an appropriate rate makes it possible to store spermatozoa for extended periods. Storage temperatures of 5° C (41° F)—refrigerator temperature—and 0° C (32° F)—the temperature of iced water—are convenient temperatures to maintain and are less costly than others, with the exception of ambient temperature. Metabolic rates increase as temperature increases, unless chemicals are used to inhibit reactions. Therefore, reduced temperature has been the principal means of slowing chemical reactions, thus extending the fertile life of spermatozoa.

TABLE 81–6. PREGNANCY RATE OF MARES INSEMINATED WITH ISOLATED OR CONTROL SPERMATOZOA*

		CONTROL	
Item	Isolated	Tyrode's Solution	BSA
Number of mares per group	10	10	10
Total number pregnant†	7	8	8
Percent	70	80	80
Total number foaling	7	4	6
Percent	70	40	60

*All mares inseminated with 100 × 10^6 live spermatozoa.
†Based on rectal palpation at 45 days postovulation.
(Adapted from Goodeaux, S.D., and Kreider, J.L.: Motility and fertility of stallion spermatozoa isolated in bovine serum albumin. Theriogenology, *10*:405–414, 1978.)

Chang and Walton have suggested that the lower the storage temperature, the slower the cooling rate should be to that temperature,[29] and the rate of cooling determines subsequent active life span of spermatozoa.[30]

From a series of experiments, Province et al. concluded that an interaction between storage temperatures and extenders existed.[16,17] Based on these data, effects of extender and storage temperature on stallion spermatozoa were evaluated in several experiments using embryo recovery as a measure of fertility.[6] In the first study, semen from two stallions was used and heated skim milk was compared with E-Z Mixin (Animal Reproduction Systems, Chino, CA), a NFDMS glucose extender. The treatments were: (1) heated skim milk maintained at 37° C (~99° F) and inseminations completed within 1 h, (2) E-Z Mixin extender at 37° C and inseminations completed within 1 h, and (3) E-Z Mixin extender cooled to 20° C (68° F) and inseminations performed after storage for 12 h at 20° C (68° F). The E-Z Mixin was identical to the NFDMS glucose extender described by Kenney et al., except polymyxin B sulfate was used as the antibiotic rather than gentamicin sulfate (Table 81–4).[9] Mares for insemination were from groups of 30 to 40 normal, nonlactating animals. Each mare was teased daily, and after estrus was detected, ovaries were palpated per rectum twice a day and the day of ovulation was recorded. As mares came into estrus, they were assigned sequentially for insemination with one of the six combinations of stallion and seminal treatment. Each mare was inseminated every other day with 250 million motile spermatozoa, beginning on day 2 or 3 of estrus or after a 35-mm follicle was detected. Inseminations continued through the end of estrus. Nonsurgical embryo recovery was conducted 6.5 days postovulation.[24]

Based on embryo recovery, no difference ($p > 0.05$) among seminal treatments was found (Table 81–7). Fertility of semen extended in E-Z Mixin and used after 12-h storage at 20° C (68° F) was 50%, which was comparable with semen extended in E-Z Mixin (56.2%) or fresh, heated skim milk extender (62.5%) and used within 1 h.

A second experiment, based on the results obtained in experiment 1, was conducted to evaluate the fertility of stallion spermatozoa (1) extended in E-Z Mixin at 37° C (~99° F) and inseminated within 1 h, or (2) cooled to 20° C (68° F) and inseminated after 24-hours storage at 20° C (68° F). The insemination dose was 250 million progressively motile spermatozoa. Mares were flushed on day 6 after ovulation. Results are presented under experiment 2 in Table 81–7. Based on embryo recovery from mares bred to one of three stallions, fertility of spermatozoa extended in E-Z Mixin was not depressed by storage at 20° C (68° F) for 24 h. In fact, an embryo recovery rate of 68.1 and 61.7%, respectively, for 0 vs. 24 h storage is comparable with what is expected and is routinely attained.

An attempt was made to repeat portions (0- vs. 24-h storage) of experiment 2 and extend the observations on additional storage times and temperatures. Presented in Table 81–8 are the results of that experiment.[31] Two stallions were used and the insemination dose was 500 million progressively motile spermatozoa, determined immediately after seminal collection. In treatments 1 and 2, fertility after storage of spermatozoa for 24 h at 20° C (68° F) was compared with fertility after storage for 0 h at 37° C (~99° F). Embryos were recovered at 7 days in 75% of the flushes from mares bred with semen held at 37° C (~99° F) and used immediately compared with only 40% when semen was stored for 24 h at 20° C (68° F). The difference of 35 percentage points ($p < 0.05$) was unexpected, because a difference of only six percentage points ($p > 0.05$) between similar treatments was found in the earlier study (Table 81–7). This lack of agreement may have been the result of years, stallions, mares, and/or the inherent variation in such experiments. Obviously, some conditions exist in which stallion spermatozoa can tolerate 24-h storage and maintain excellent fertility even though motility may be depressed (experiment 2, Table 81–7), whereas under similar conditions both motility and fertility were depressed (treatment 2, Table 81–8).

Also presented in Table 81–8 is a comparison of fertility at temperatures of 20° vs. 5° C (68° vs. 41° F) after storage for 48 h. At 20° C (68° F) no embryos were re-

TABLE 81–7. THE EFFECT OF STORAGE TIME, TEMPERATURE, AND EXTENDER ON FERTILITY

TREATMENT	STORAGE (H)	TEMPERATURE (C)	MOTILITY (%)	NUMBER OF MARES	EMBRYO RECOVERY (%)
Experiment 1*					
Skim milk	0	37	57	32	62.5
E-Z Mixin	0	37	54	32	56.2
E-Z Mixin	12	20	38	32	50.0
Experiment 2†					
E-Z Mixin	0	37	54	47	68.1
E-Z Mixin	24	20	19	47	61.7

*Embryos were recovered at 6.5 days.
†Embryos were recovered at 6 days.
(Adapted from Francl, A.T., Amann, R.P., Squires, E.L., and Pickett, B.W.: Motility and fertility of equine spermatozoa in a milk extender after 12 or 24 hours at 20° C. Theriogenology, *27*:517–525, 1987.)

TABLE 81–8. EFFECT OF STORAGE TIME AND TEMPERATURE ON FERTILITY OF SPERMATOZOA IN E-Z MIXIN

TREATMENT	STORAGE (H)	TEMPERATURE (C)	MOTILITY (%)	NUMBER OF CYCLES	EMBRYO RECOVERY (%)*
1	0	37	62	40	75
2	24	20	23	40	40
3	48	20	15	16	0
4	48	5	30	34	32

*Embryos were recovered at 7 days.

(From Pickett, B.W., Squires, E.L., and McKinnon, A.O.: Procedures for Collection, Evaluation and Utilization of Stallion Semen for Artificial Insemination. Animal Reproduction Laboratory Bulletin No. 03. Fort Collins, Colorado State University, 1987.)

covered. A total of 32 embryos were recovered from mares bred with semen stored 48 h at 5° C. From data in Tables 81–7 and 81–8, equine spermatozoa apparently can be stored at 20° C (68° F) for 12 h, and in some cases 24 h, without a significant reduction in fertility. However, if semen is to be stored longer than 12 h, it should be cooled to 5° C (41° F). In the event that a storage time of 12 h or less is required, storage at 20° C (68° F) would probably permit semen from more stallions to be stored than if 5° C (41° F) were used because some stallions have spermatozoa that will not tolerate cooling to 5° C (41° F).

A similar study was conducted by Varner et al.[32] Forty-five mares were bred with 250 million progressively motile spermatozoa, from one stallion, in a skim milk glucose extender. The mares were assigned to one of three treatments: (1) insemination with fresh semen, (2) semen stored for 24 h at 20° C (68° F), or (3) semen stored for 24 h at 5° C (41° F). Mares were inseminated daily during estrus, after detection of a 35-mm follicle, until ovulation. Single-cycle, 15-day pregnancy rates were identical among treatments (73%). However, motility of spermatozoa stored at 20° C (68° F) was reduced compared with storage at 5° C (41° F).

Squires et al. conducted an additional study to compare fertility of mares inseminated with 500 million motile spermatozoa extended in E-Z Mixin cooled to either 20° or 5° C (68° or 41° F) and inseminated after 24 h of storage.[33] The control mares were inseminated with semen at 37° C (~99° F) within 1 h of collection. Semen from four stallions was utilized and the results are presented in Table 81–9. Fertility as measured by recovery of embryos was 65%, 50%, and 59% for the controls (37°) and for spermatozoa stored at 20° and 5° C, respectively.

Presented in Table 81–10 are data from all experiments conducted in our laboratory with stored semen. The controls, utilized at 37° C (~99° F), are included for comparison. Although these studies were not comparable statistically, note that as storage time increased, a trend toward some reduction in fertility occurred, particularly when semen was stored at 20° C (68° F) for longer than 12 h. Therefore, if semen is to be shipped (transported), it should be cooled to 5° C (41° F) in an E-Z Mixin extender, which contains both polymyxin B sulfate and amikacin sulfate as antibiotics. The most important factors affecting fertility under these circumstances are probably stallion and cooling rate.

A decline in percentage of motile spermatozoa with storage over time was expected. Province et al. used a NFDMS glucose extender and found that spermatozoa cooled slowly from 37° C (~ 99° F) to 20° C (68° F) and stored at 20° C (68° F) for 24 h had a mean motility of 10%.[16,17] The value of about 60% motile spermatozoa after 13 to 36 h of storage at 5° C (41° F) was reported by Douglas-Hamilton et al., also using a NFDMS glucose extender.[5] Favorable motility in their study might have been a consequence of holding the samples at 37° C (~99° F) for 10 min before evaluation. From limited observations (n = 25), percentage of motile spermatozoa seemed to be approximately 20 percentage points higher when an aliquot of the extended semen was

TABLE 81–9. FERTILITY OF EQUINE SPERMATOZOA STORED FOR 0 OR 24 H AT 37°, 20°, OR 5° C

TREATMENT	STORAGE (H)	TEMPERATURE (C)	NUMBER OF MARES	EMBRYO RECOVERY (%)
1	0	37	40	65
2	24	20	36	50
3	24	5	34	59

(Adapted from Squires, E.L., Amann, R.P., McKinnon, A.O., and Pickett, B.W.: Fertility of equine spermatozoa cooled to 5 or 20° C. Proceedings of the International Congress on Animal Reproduction and Artificial Insemination. Vol. 3. 1988, pp. 297–299.)

TABLE 81–10. EFFECT OF STORAGE TIME AND TEMPERATURE ON FERTILITY

STORAGE (H)	TEMPERATURE (C)	NUMBER OF MARES	EMBRYO RECOVERY (%)
0	37	191	65
12	20	32	50
24	20	123	51
24	5	34	59
48	20	16	0
48	5	34	32

(From Colorado State University, unpublished data.)

held at 37° C (~99° F) for 10 min before a slide was prepared for estimation of sperm motility.[6]

In general, spermatozoa are susceptible to severe damage if exposed to a sudden reduction in temperature, from 37° C (~99° F) to 0° C (32° F), commonly called cold shock. The damage manifests itself in depressed metabolism; altered membrane permeability; loss of lipids, ions, and other substances; an irreversible loss of motility; and an increase in the proportion of spermatozoa that stain with vital stains.[34] Because semen in some of these treatments (Tables 81–7, 81–8, and 81–9) was cooled to only 20° C (68° F), cold shock was not likely to be responsible for depressed motility in samples stored 12 or 24 h. Kayser has shown, in a series of well-controlled studies, that no immediate or latent damage occurs to the motility of equine spermatozoa cooled rapidly from 37° (~99° F) to 20° C (68° F).[35]

Cooling rate may be a critical factor in preservation of equine spermatozoa for transportation and subsequent maintenance of fertility. Douglas-Hamilton et al. bred mares for three cycles with semen cooled at 0.3° C per minute and stored at 4° to 6° C (~39° to 43° F), and obtained satisfactory pregnancy rates. Furthermore, using computerized equipment for analyzing motility, Kayser showed that storage at 5° C (41° F) was superior to 20° C (68° F) after 24-h storage.[35] Cooling at either 0.5° C per minute or 0.3° C per minute was inferior ($p < 0.05$) to cooling at 0.05° C per minute, considering all data over 96 h of storage at 5° C (41° F). Data for sperm motion after cooling at either 0.012° C per minute or 0.05° C per minute were similar ($p > 0.05$), and both rates were superior ($p < 0.05$) to 0.3° C per minute averaged over 96 h of storage at 5° C (41° F).

Based on motion characteristics of spermatozoa, it was concluded that stallion spermatozoa can be cooled rapidly from 37° to 20° C (~99° to 68° F), but should be cooled at ≤ 0.1° C per minute and preferably at 0.05° C per minute from 20° to 5° C (41° F) to maintain maximum sperm survival at 5° C (41° F), based on sperm motion characteristics. Optimal cooling rates for semen could easily differ from these rates because of interstallion and intrastallion and ejaculate variations.[35]

Obviously, the longer stallion semen can be stored and retain its fertility, the more flexibility stallion owners will have in collecting and shipping semen and the more flexibility mare owners will have to select sires and synchronize breeding with ovulation. Numerous investigators have stored equine semen at various temperatures and bred mares with semen after storage from 12 to 120 h.[4–6,8,36–41] Neither the concept nor the recognition of the need is new. In 1939, McKenzie et al. reported successful impregnation of 2 mares with semen stored 20 h.[39] For 1 mare, the semen was shipped 1912 mi. In the Netherlands, stallion semen is shipped and used to breed mares for up to 5 days. van der Holst reported that 87% of 68 mares bred with semen stored 4 to 5 days had foals. This is an excellent foaling rate, considering the semen was centrifuged, was cooled to 5° C (41° F), was shipped, and was 4 to 5 days old before use. I hope that these excellent results can be repeated. Unfortunately, no mention was made of number of inseminations per cycle or cycles per pregnancy. However, van der Holst stated that the insemination dose should "be at least 400 million sperms, but 500 million gave better results." Whether the number of spermatozoa was total or motile was not reported. Douglas-Hamilton et al., using three Warmblood stallions, bred 46 mares with liquid semen shipped to various parts of the United States.[5] Each shipment contained 1.0 to 1.5 billion spermatozoa. The time interval from ejaculation to insemination ranged from 6 to 23 h. Thirty-two mares were inseminated with semen 6 to 12 h after collection, and 90% became pregnant. For the 14 mares that were inseminated with semen 12 to 23 h old, 93% were reported pregnant. The per-cycle pregnancy rate at 55 days for the three stallions was 65%, 38%, and 60%, respectively. Hughes and Loy bred mares with semen extended in skim milk or cream gel stored up to 96 h and obtained a pregnancy rate of 73%.[8]

Recently, several equine breed registries have approved use of semen that has been stored. Furthermore, they have eliminated the rule that the mare and stallion must be on the same farm when insemination occurs. Some of the advantages to such a system are the following:

1. It eliminates cost and stress of shipping a mare and/or foal.
2. It increases the gene pool; minor breeds must use a local stallion or incur costs of shipment, which may increase the cost of a foal beyond economic feasibility.
3. It reduces the use of genetically inferior stallions.
4. It eliminates cash outlay for mare care; when the mare is home, many times, labor for care is supplied by family members.
5. Many young horse owners, such as 4-H members, will become involved in getting their mares bred if they have a prospect of raising a superior animal, provided the cost of getting the mare pregnant is not excessive.
6. It reduces the likelihood of disease transmission between farms.

Acceptance of stored equine semen by additional breed associations may depend on the ability to preserve semen for several days and ship it after collection without a serious reduction in fertilizing capacity of the spermatozoa or on the development of frozen semen.

REFERENCES

1. Back, D.G., Pickett, B.W., Voss. J.L., and Seidel, G.E., Jr.: Effect of antibacterial agents on the motility of stallion spermatozoa at various storage times, temperatures and dilution ratios. J. Anim. Sci., *41:*137–143, 1975.
2. Province, C.A.: Cooling and storage of canine and equine spermatozoa. M.S. thesis. Colorado State University, 1984.
3. Clay, C.M., Squires, E.L., Amann, R.P., and Pickett, B.W.: Effect of dilution, polyvinyl alcohol (PVA) and bovine serum albumin (BSA) on stallion spermatozoal motility. Proceedings of the International Congress on Animal Reproduction and Artificial Insemination. Vol. 2. 1984, pp. 187–189.
4. Demick, D.S., Voss, J.L., and Pickett, B.W.: Effect of cooling, storage, glycerolization and spermatozoal numbers on equine fertility. J. Anim. Sci., *43:*633–637, 1976.
5. Douglas-Hamilton, D.H., et al.: A field study of the fertility of transported equine semen. Theriogenology, *22:*291–304, 1984.
6. Francl, A.T., Amann, R.P., Squires, E.L., and Pickett, B.W.: Motility and fertility of equine spermatozoa in a milk extender after 12 or 24 hours at 20° C. Theriogenology, *27:*517–525, 1987.
7. Householder, D.D., Pickett, B.W., Voss, J.L., and Olar, T.T.: Effect of extender, number of spermatozoa and HCG on equine fertility. J. Equine Vet. Sci., *1:*9–13, 1981.
8. Hughes, J.P., and Loy, R.G.: Artificial insemination in the equine. A comparison of natural breeding and artificial insemination of mares using semen from six stallions. Cornell Vet., *60:*463–475, 1970.
9. Kenney, R.M., Bergman, R.V., Cooper, W.L., and Morse, G.W.: Minimal contamination techniques for breeding mares: Technique and preliminary findings. Proc. Am. Assoc. Equine Pract., 327–335, 1975.
10. Kreider, J.L., Tindall, W.C., and Potter, G.D.: Inclusion of bovine serum albumin in semen extenders to enhance maintenance of stallion sperm viability. Theriogenology, *23:*399–408, 1985.
11. McCall, J.P., Jr., and Sorensen, A.M., Jr.: Evaporated milk as an extender for stallion semen. A. I. Digest, *19*(12):8–10, 1971.
12. Nishikawa, Y.: Studies on reproduction in horses. Tokyo, Japan Racing Association, 1959.
13. Pickett, B.W., Burwash, L.D., Voss, J.L., and Back, D.G.: Effect of seminal extenders on equine fertility. J. Anim. Sci., *40:*1136–1143, 1975.
14. Pickett, B.W., et al.: Effect of centrifugation and seminal plasma on motility and fertility of stallion and bull spermatozoa. Fertil. Steril., *26:*167–174, 1975.
15. Pickett, B.W., Voss, J.L., and Demick, D.S.: Stallion seminal extenders. Proc. Am. Assoc. Equine Pract., 155–274, 1974.
16. Province, C.A., Amann, R.P., Pickett, B.W., and Squires, E.L.: Extenders for preservation of canine and equine spermatozoa at 5° C. Theriogenology, *22:*409–415, 1984.
17. Province, C.A., Squires, E.L., Pickett, B.W., and Amann, R.P.: Cooling rates, storage temperatures and fertility of extended equine spermatozoa. Theriogenology, *23:*925–934, 1985.
18. Pace, M.M., and Sullivan, J.J.: Effect of timing of insemination, numbers of spermatozoa and extender components on the pregnancy rate in mares inseminated with frozen stallion semen. J. Reprod. Fertil. Suppl., *23:*115–121, 1975.
19. Almquist, J.O.: Efficient, low cost results using milk-glycerol diluent. A. I. Digest, 7(8):11–14, 1959.
20. Back, D.G., Pickett, B.W., Voss, J.L., and Seidel, G.E., Jr.: Observations on the sexual behavior of nonlactating mares. J. Am. Vet. Med. Assoc., *165:*717–720, 1974.
21. Voss, J.L., and Pickett, B.W.: Reproductive Management of the Broodmare. Animal Reproduction Laboratory General Series Bulletin No. 961. Fort Collins, Colorado State University, 1976.
22. Flipse, R.J., Patton, S., and Almquist, J.O.: Diluters for bovine semen. III. Effect of lactenin and of lactoperoxidase upon spermatozoan livability. J. Dairy Sci., *37:*1205–1211, 1954.
23. Thacker, D.L., and Almquist, J.O.: Diluters for bovine semen. I. Fertility and motility of bovine spermatozoa in boiled milk. J. Dairy Sci., *36:*173–180, 1953.
24. Squires, E.L., Cook, V.M., and Voss, J.L.: Collection and Transfer of Equine Embryos. Animal Reproduction Laboratory Bulletin No. 01. Fort Collins, Colorado State University, 1985.
25. Shideler, R.K., McChesney, A.E., Voss, J.L., and Squires, E.L.: Relationship of endometrial biopsy and other management factors on fertility of broodmares. J. Equine Vet. Sci., *2:*5–10, 1982.
26. Goodeaux, S.D., and Kreider, J.L.: Motility and fertility of stallion spermatozoa isolated in bovine serum albumin. Theriogenology, *10:*405–414, 1978.
27. Bowen, J.M.: Artificial insemination in the horse. Equine Vet. J., *1:*98–108, 1969.
28. Watson, P.F.: The effects of cold shock on sperm cell membranes. *In* Effects of Low Temperature on Biological Membranes. Edited by G.J. Morris and A. Clark. New York, Academic Press, 1981, pp. 189–218.
29. Chang, M.C., and Walton, A.: The effect of low temperature and acclimatization on the respiratory activity and survival of ram spermatozoa. Proc. R. Soc. Lond. [Biol], *129:*517–527, 1940.
30. Salisbury, G.W.: Recent research developments in the preservation and handling of bovine semen. Cornell Vet., *31:*149–159, 1941.
31. Pickett, B.W., Squires, E.L., and McKinnon, A.O. Procedures for Collection, Evaluation and Utilization of Stallion Semen for Artificial Insemination. Animal Reproduction Laboratory Bulletin No. 03. Fort Collins, Colorado State University, 1987.
32. Varner, D.D., Blanchard, T.L., Meyers, P.J., and Meyers, S.A.: Fertilizing capacity of equine spermatozoa stored for 24 hours at 5 or 20° C. Theriogenology, *32:*515–525, 1989.
33. Squires, E.L., Amann, R.P., McKinnon, A.O., and Pickett, B.W.: Fertility of equine spermatozoa cooled to 5 or 20° C. Proceedings of the International Congress of Animal Reproduction and Artificial Insemination. Vol. 3. 1988, pp. 297–299.
34. White, I.G., and Wales, R.G.: The susceptibility of spermatozoa to cold shock. Int. J. Fertil., *5:*195–201, 1960.
35. Kayser, J.P.R.: Effects of linear cooling rates on motion

characteristics of stallion spermatozoa. M.S. thesis. Colorado State University, 1990.

36. Buiko-Rogalevic, A.N.: Storage of stallion semen for a long period. Anim. Breed. Abstr., *18:*41, 1950.

37. Ebertus, R.: The dilution of stallion semen with whole cow milk. Anim. Breed. Abstr., *31:*313, 1963.

38. Kuhr, J.: The characters of stallion semen and methods of diluting it. Anim. Breed. Abstr., *25:*236, 1957.

39. McKenzie, F.F., Lasley, J.F., and Phillips, R.W.: The storage of horse and swine semen. Am. Soc. Anim. Prod., *32:*222–231, 1939.

40. van der Holst, W.: Stallion semen production in A.I. programs in the Netherlands. *In* The Male in Farm Animal Production. Edited by M. Courot. Boston, Martinus Nijhoff, 1984, pp. 195–201.

41. Vlachos, K., and Paschaleri, E.: Research on some factors influencing fertility in solipeds. Anim. Breed. Abstr., *37:*1969.

CHAPTER 82

REPRODUCTIVE EVALUATION OF THE STALLION

B.W. Pickett

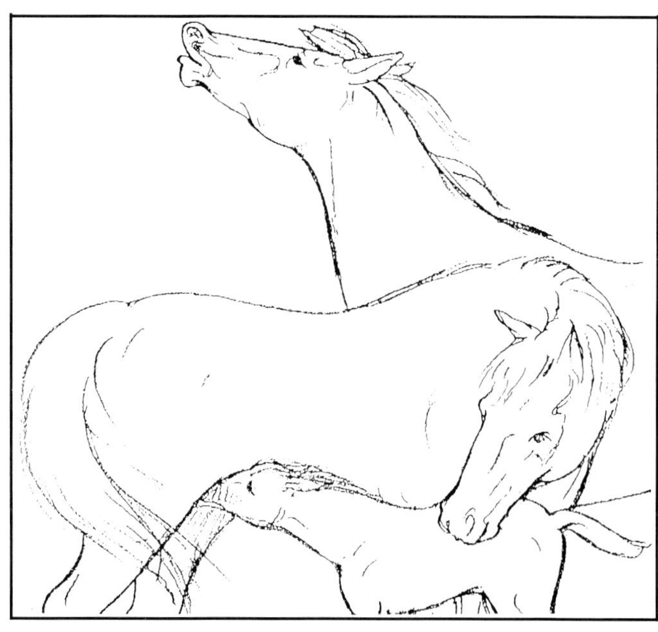

Numerous factors affect reproductive capacity, such as inherent fertility of individuals, nutrition, age, health, season, sexual behavior, and perhaps breed.[1,2,3] Clinicians must recognize that fertility is a relative term and can be markedly altered by management.[2,4,5]

Daily sperm production and output are related to testicular size and consistency and frequency of ejaculation.[6] Thus, any seminal evaluation must relate to testicular and epididymal function. An evaluation of testicular function from examination of one or more ejaculates presupposes that quality and quantity of semen obtained is an accurate reflection of testicular function.[7] This may be invalid because of the method of seminal collection, experience of the evaluator, quality and type of equipment, and techniques used for evaluation. Furthermore, all spermatozoa in an ejaculate are not functionally equivalent and differentiation between fertile and infertile spermatozoa is often difficult.[8] When all those factors are taken into consideration, to assume that an appropriate evaluation of one or even several ejaculates will be highly correlated with foaling rate is overly optimistic. Yet, an analysis of seminal characteristics of two or more ejaculates collected with an artificial vagina (AV) can be used to provide a reasonable basis to manage a stallion for maximum fertility, regardless of whether artificial insemination (AI) or natural service is utilized.

Recently, automated, computerized techniques have been developed for evaluation of sperm motion, which will result in more precise, objective measurements of sperm motion than visual observations.[8] Furthermore, these techniques may also result in a more precise relationship between spermatozoal motion and foaling rate and/or pregnancy rate, particularly for certain individual stallions, although this has not been proven. In addition, these analyses may provide some insight between pregnancy rate and foaling rate, but again for certain individuals. Unfortunately, these techniques were not used to evaluate sperm motion to obtain the results reported in this chapter.

Some situations when a stallion should have a reproductive evaluation are the following:

1. Before sale.
2. Before the breeding season.
3. To estimate the number of covers or inseminations that can be made during the season.
4. Any time lowered fertility is suspected.
5. Any time the breeder wants to increase the number of mares to be bred.
6. When abnormal sexual behavior is observed.
7. To determine if seminal quality or testicular consistency has changed since the last breeding season.
8. When the stallion is suspected of harboring a potential pathogen.

Basically, two types of reproductive evaluation are used: (1) a minimum of two ejaculates collected 1 h apart and (2) two ejaculates collected 1 h apart, then a single ejaculate collected daily for 6 or 7 days. The latter is more informative and will enable the evaluator to predict with reasonable accuracy daily sperm output and number of mares that may be bred. An appropriate AV must be used during seminal collection and semen must be adequately protected throughout collection and evaluation to ensure the stallion and the spermatozoa will not be condemned or penalized because of faulty procedures or unclean equipment.[2]

Parameters that should be included in a reproductive evaluation are:

1. Gel, gel-free, and total seminal volumes.
2. Sperm concentration (millions per milliliter of gel-free semen).
3. Spermatozoa per ejaculation (billions).
4. Percentage of progressively motile spermatozoa.
5. Sperm morphology.
6. Seminal pH.
7. Number of mounts per ejaculation and sexual behavior.
8. Cultures from at least the urethra, prepuce, and semen after the first two ejaculations.
9. Total scrotal width (TSW) and testicular consistency.

Consistency of testes is determined by palpation and descriptions should include normal, soft, firm, inconsistent, nodular, ribbed, veined, degenerating or degenerated, small, large, slick, rotated, lesions, rough, constriction, flat, irregular, high, and/or missing. The epididymides are classified as normal, large, small, uneven, irregular, hard, and/or soft.

COMPARISONS BETWEEN PASSED AND FAILED STALLIONS

Presented in Table 82–1 are the results of potential fertility evaluations of 1044 stallions.[9] In general, data on two ejaculates collected the same day, designated as first and second, were utilized and ejaculates were collected approximately 1 h apart. A total of 669 stallions (64.1%) were approved as sound breeders (passed) and 375 (35.9%) were not approved (failed). Note that these seminal collections were, for the most part, from sexually rested stallions.

The number *(n)* of stallions per characteristic that passed ranged from 417 to 664 compared with a range of 260 to 373 for stallions that failed the seminal evaluation. In many evaluations the first ejaculate was extremely good and the second extremely poor or vice versa; as a result, the clinician passed the stallion in spite of an extremely poor single ejaculate. This resulted in rather low means for sperm motility and morphology of passed stallions.

Those stallions that passed had significantly larger gel-free seminal volumes in first and second ejaculates than those that failed (45 vs. 40 mL and 42 vs. 38 mL, respectively). Volume of ejaculate has been reported to have a significant effect on fertility.[10,11] However, differences in total seminal volume between passed and failed stallions were small, 54 vs. 50 and 47 vs. 44 mL for first and second ejaculates, respectively ($p > 0.10$). Therefore, I suspect that if a true relationship between volume of ejaculate and fertility exists, it is because of the influence of volume on some other seminal characteristic. Furthermore, average insemination volumes as small as 0.6 mL with raw semen and 0.5 mL with frozen-thawed semen provided pregnancy rates equal to larger volumes, i.e., up to approximately 15 mL.[2] However, recently Rowley et al. showed that insemination volumes of 100 mL resulted in reduced fertility compared with volumes of 10 mL.[12]

A difference in sperm concentration per milliliter of gel-free semen was observed between first (335 million vs. 251 million) and second (160 million vs. 130 million) ejaculates of passed and failed stallions, respectively ($p < 0.01$). As expected, an inverse relationship existed between all measurements of seminal volumes and sperm concentration per milliliter of gel-free semen. However, all correlations were too low (range $r = -0.07$ to $r = -0.43$) to be of practical predictive value.

The number of mares that can be bred per ejaculate or per season depends on number of spermatozoa obtained,[13] percentage of those spermatozoa that are progressively motile, and inherent fertility of the stallion.[14,15] Number of spermatozoa per ejaculation depends on testicular size, age, season, and frequency of ejaculation. Therefore, the number of spermatozoa obtained per ejaculate is one of the more important criteria in determining if a stallion should be passed or failed. More spermatozoa were obtained in both first (11.9 billion vs. 8.4 billion) and second (5.6 billion vs. 4.2 billion) ejaculates from passed stallions than from those that failed ($p < 0.01$). Obviously, 8.4 billion and 4.2 billion spermatozoa, from failed stallions, were sufficient for impregnating a mare, when all other factors were normal. However, other criteria were sufficiently abnormal for clinicians to fail these stallions. Dowsett and Pattie suggested 1.3 billion total spermatozoa with 1.1 billion live spermatozoa as threshold levels for adequate fertility in the horse.[10] Assuming that live spermatozoa means progressively motile, which is not the case when spermatozoa are evaluated as live or dead based on vital staining, 500 million progressively motile spermatozoa is the recommended number for maximum reproductive efficiency in the mare.[2] Furthermore, 100 million is sufficient when the mares and stallions are highly fertile. In natural service, the number of progressively motile spermatozoa necessary for maximum reproductive efficiency probably depends primarily on frequency of breeding.[2]

The number of spermatozoa in a second ejaculate from a sexually rested stallion will usually equal approximately 50% of the number obtained in the first ejaculate.[16] The percentage was 47.1% for stallions that passed compared with 50.0% for those that failed. This is probably a function of the ejaculatory mechanism and extragonadal sperm reserves as opposed to being related to fertility. When this relationship is skewed, one or more of the following should be suspected: (1) one ejaculate was incomplete; (2) the stallion had abnormally low sperm reserves; (3) the stallion's sperm reserves had been depleted; (4) the stallion was young, immature, suffering from testicular degeneration, or had one or more rotated or missing testes; and (5) the

TABLE 82–1. MEANS AND STANDARD DEVIATIONS OF SEMINAL CHARACTERISTICS AND TOTAL SCROTAL WIDTH OF STALLIONS THAT PASSED AND FAILED A SEMINAL EVALUATION*

		PASSED		FAILED		
Variable	Ejaculate	Mean	SD ±	Mean	SD ±	Significance†
Seminal volume (mL)						
Gel	1	10	23	10	23	NS
	2	5	16	6	17	NS
Gel free	1	45	30	40	30	0.01
	2	42	28	38	28	0.05
Total	1	54	42	50	41	NS
	2	47	33	44	34	NS
Spermatozoa						
Concentration (10^6/mL)	1	335	232	251	215	0.01
	2	160	131	130	131	0.01
Total/ejaculate (10^9)	1	11.9	9.0	8.4	8.7	0.01
	2	5.6	6.7	4.2	4.9	0.01
Motile (%)	1	53	15	30	21	0.01
	2	57	15	34	22	0.01
Morphology						
Normal	1	51	15	35	18	0.01
	2	57	14	38	19	0.01
Abnormal (%)						
Neck separated	1	5	6	11	16	0.01
	2	5	6	12	19	0.01
Head	1	9	8	17	15	0.01
	2	9	7	17	16	0.01
Midpiece	1	11	11	12	12	0.05
	2	10	10	11	12	0.10
Tail	1	20	13	27	16	0.01
	2	19	12	25	15	0.01
Proximal droplet	1	3	5	3	5	NS
	2	2	3	3	4	NS
Distal droplet	1	3	4	4	7	0.01
	2	4	5	3	5	0.05
Other	1	0.14	1	0.12	1	NS
	2	0.07	1	0.15	1	NS
Seminal pH	1	7.52	0.18	7.47	0.21	0.01
	2	7.52	0.17	7.55	0.19	0.05
Total scrotal width (mm)	1	108	12	98	19	0.01

*Based on 417 to 664 observations for passed stallions and 260 to 373 for failed stallions.
†Significance, less than or equal to the number presented.
(From Pickett, B.W., et al.: Seminal characteristics and total scrotal width (T.S.W.) of normal and abnormal stallions. Proc. Am. Assoc. Equine Pract., 485–518, 1988.)

stallion was an accumulator, i.e., abnormally large extragonadal sperm reserves, resulting in abnormally high sperm numbers in the first, and sometimes the second, ejaculate.

Progressive motility of spermatozoa is essential for fertility. Spermatozoa with abnormal motility may contribute to reduced fertility by fertilizing the ovum, which then develops abnormally. Thus, extreme care should be used in this estimate.[2] Percent progressively motile spermatozoa in first and second ejaculates from passed stallions were 53 and 57%, respectively, compared with 30 and 34% in corresponding ejaculates from stallions that failed ($p < 0.01$). As expected, second ejaculates contained a higher percentage of motile spermatozoa (approximately 9%) than first ejaculates, regardless of whether the stallion passed or failed. The higher percentage of motile spermatozoa in second ejaculates was no doubt owing to the fact that these stallions were sexually rested; thus, a larger percentage of spermatozoa in the first ejaculate was stored in the ampulla and vas deferens than in the second ejaculate. In all probability, storage of spermatozoa at the higher temperature in the body cavity resulted in reduced motility.

There were more morphologically normal spermatozoa in both first and second ejaculates of stallions that passed compared with those that failed (51 and 57% vs. 35 and 38%, respectively ($p < 0.01$). Stallions that passed also had fewer abnormal spermatozoa such as neck separated, head, tail, and distal droplets. van Duijn and Hendrikse correlated percentage of morphologically normal spermatozoa with fertility of stallions in Dutch herd books.[17] They obtained a correlation of 0.25 ($p < 0.01$), which would account for approximately 6% of the variation in fertility caused by the percentage of morphologically normal spermatozoa. Although statistically significant, this correlation was quite low and would have limited or no predictive value. Voss et al. studied the relationship between seminal characteristics and fertility of Thoroughbred stallions for 2 yr.[8] During year 1, the number of matings per pregnancy was significantly related ($r = 0.53$) to midpiece abnormalities, whereas the relationship during year 2 was lower ($r = 0.01$). Dott stated that "an examination of sperm morphology alone can never justify the statement that the potential fertility of an ejaculate is high, but it is reasonable to state that potential fertility is low when a high proportion of spermatozoa have primary and secondary abnormalities."[19] Unfortunately, an ejaculate is generally inseminated before a morphologic evaluation can be conducted. However, morphology should be considered in conjunction with other seminal characteristics, TSW, and testicular consistency to predict a stallion's potential fertility.

Bielanski reported an inverse relationship ($r = -0.50$) between percentage of spermatozoa with primary abnormalities and fertility.[20] He postulated that >10% primary sperm abnormalities was always indicative of lowered fertility but that 30% secondary abnormalities was not necessarily related to fertility. Stallions that passed a seminal evaluation (Table 82–1) had a mean of 9% head abnormalities compared with 17% for those that did not pass ($p < 0.01$). Abnormalities, other than of the head, for first vs. second ejaculates, ranged from 42 and 40% compared with 57 and 54% from passed and failed stallions, respectively.

Correlations between percentages of progressively motile spermatozoa and morphology ranged from 0.29 to 0.50 in seminal samples of first and second ejaculates from passed and failed stallions ($p < 0.01$). Interestingly, the correlations were higher in samples from failed stallions than from those that passed. van Duijn and Hendrikse reported a correlation of 0.29 between percentage of progressively motile and percentage of morphologically normal spermatozoa.[17] During a 2-yr study, percentage of progressively motile spermatozoa was correlated with percentage of morphologically normal spermatozoa ($r = 0.50$ and 0.70, for years 1 and 2, respectively).[18]

The pH of second ejaculates was higher (Table 82–1)

TABLE 82–2. THE EFFECT OF BREED ON SEMINAL CHARACTERISTICS AND TOTAL SCROTAL WIDTH OF STALLIONS ACROSS MONTH AND AGE THAT PASSED A SEMINAL EVALUATION

	SEMINAL VOLUME (ML)						SPERMATOZOA										
	Gel		Gel Free		Total		Concentration per Milliliter (10^6)		Total (10^9)		Motile (%)		Normal Morphology (%)		Seminal pH		Total Scrotal Width (mm)
Breed	1*	2†	1	2	1	2	1	2	1	2	1	2	1	2	1	2	
Quarter Horse																	
Mean	12	7	43	40	55	46	309	148	10.7	5.1	55	57	53	57	7.44	7.53	106
SD±	29	20	26	25	41	32	248	110	7.5	5.6	13	14	15	14	0.18	0.19	11
Thoroughbred																	
Mean	7	4	46	44	52	48	364	164	13.0	5.9	52	57	48	54	7.42	7.52	111
SD±	21	15	29	28	39	31	227	111	6.4	4.9	15	16	14	13	0.19	0.15	11
Arabian																	
Mean	10	5	39	42	49	47	367	179	11.6	5.4	53	58	54	59	7.40	7.49	107
SD±	20	11	24	29	37	35	221	147	7.4	4.0	17	14	16	16	0.18	0.16	13
Appaloosa																	
Mean	5	4	38	35	43	39	350	161	10.3	4.1	56	61	52	58	7.43	7.57	103
SD±	11	7	26	26	33	31	245	139	5.0	2.4	14	12	15	11	0.17	0.15	7
Paint Horse																	
Mean	8	4	34	34	42	39	304	141	8.5	4.3	53	56	55	61	7.42	7.55	102
SD±	23	10	20	21	36	28	191	82	5.4	3.0	14	11	14	10	0.18	0.17	12
Overall mean																	
n	600	563	603	566	600	563	591	554	591	554	599	561	581	547	385	368	552
Mean	9	5	43	41	52	46	342	161	11.5	5.3	53	57	52	57	7.43	7.53	107
SD±	23	16	27	27	39	32	234	121	7.0	4.9	15	14	15	14	0.18	0.17	12
Significance‡	NS	NS	0.05	NS	NS	NS	0.10	NS	0.01	NS	NS	NS	0.01	0.05	NS	NS	0.01

*First ejaculates.
†Second ejaculates.
‡At least one difference at the designated level of significance exists within this column.
(From Pickett, B.W., et al.: Seminal characteristics and total scrotal width (T.S.W.) of normal and abnormal stallions. Proc. Am. Assoc. Equine Pract., 485–518, 1988.)

than pH of first ejaculates. This occurs because volumes of gel-free semen from first and second ejaculates are similar, whereas second ejaculates contain only approximately 50% of the spermatozoa found in first ejaculates and possibly a reduced quantity of fluids from the epididymides.[16] All 20 correlations between pH of gel-free semen in first and second ejaculates with all measurements of seminal volume, sperm concentrations, and total spermatozoa were negative ($r = -0.05$ to -0.23). The pH is beneficial in determining when ejaculations are complete, especially in stallions that have abnormal sexual behavior. For example, stallions with abnormal sexual behavior appear to ejaculate and may "ejaculate" relatively large volumes of semen relatively devoid of spermatozoa. In these cases, pH will approach 8.0. As previously noted, all correlations between seminal volumes and pH were negative as were those between sperm number and pH. Thus, as number of spermatozoa in an ejaculate decreases, pH increases.

The number of spermatozoa a stallion is capable of producing is directly related to grams of testicular tissue. A measurement of TSW is a reasonably good indicator of a stallion's ability to produce spermatozoa, because TSW is related to daily sperm output[21] and testicular weight.[6] In one study, daily sperm output and daily sperm production were highly correlated ($r = 0.80$) and daily sperm production and testicular weight were also highly correlated ($r = 0.77$).[13] Stallions that passed an evaluation had a TSW of 108 mm compared with 98 mm for those that failed ($p < 0.01$). This also was reflected in a lower sperm output in both first and second ejaculates of failed stallions ($p < 0.01$). Consequently, stallions with small testes are potentially poor producers of spermatozoa. Therefore, stallions with a TSW of 80 mm or less should not be approved as sound breeders.

SEMINAL CHARACTERISTICS BY BREED

Presented in Tables 82–2 and 82–3 are means and standard deviations of seminal characteristics and TSW by breed for stallions that passed or failed a seminal evaluation. Nineteen breeds were represented, but only Appaloosa, Arabian, Paint Horse, Quarter Horse, and Thoroughbred were in sufficient numbers to warrant presentation by breed.[9] For stallions that passed the examination, significant differences were found in gel-free seminal volume, sperm concentration, and total sper-

TABLE 82–3. THE EFFECT OF BREED ON SEMINAL CHARACTERISTICS AND TOTAL SCROTAL WIDTH OF STALLIONS ACROSS MONTH AND AGE THAT FAILED A SEMINAL EVALUATION

	SEMINAL VOLUME (ML)						SPERMATOZOA										
	Gel		Gel Free		Total		Concentration per Milliliter (10^6)		Total (10^9)		Motile (%)		Normal Morphology (%)		Seminal pH		Total Scrotal Width
Breed	1*	2†	1	2	1	2	1	2	1	2	1	2	1	2	1	2	(mm)
Quarter Horse																	
Mean	9	7	35	35	44	40	243	126	7.1	3.6	35	39	40	43	7.49	7.57	93
SD±	20	16	29	25	35	29	207	138	8.4	5.4	22	21	19	20	0.23	0.19	20
Thoroughbred																	
Mean	13	8	48	42	61	50	260	145	11.1	5.2	28	32	36	38	7.48	7.52	104
SD±	35	23	32	27	54	39	187	128	9.1	4.5	20	20	15	16	0.17	0.20	17
Arabian																	
Mean	8	5	33	36	42	41	300	136	7.7	4.4	20	23	23	27	7.44	7.56	101
SD±	20	12	25	24	32	28	269	132	7.7	5.0	18	20	15	17	0.20	0.16	15
Appaloosa																	
Mean	8	4	32	25	40	29	231	82	7.2	2.5	38	38	42	51	7.46	7.57	85
SD±	18	8	19	17	28	18	182	78	6.6	3.2	22	25	18	20	0.26	0.22	20
Paint Horse																	
Mean	8	2	36	36	45	38	223	205	9.3	4.5	37	45	39	44	7.37	7.53	97
SD±	11	5	32	25	41	24	190	165	11.5	3.8	28	27	15	15	0.15	0.17	18
Overall Mean																	
n	345	310	345	311	344	310	330	294	329	294	333	300	324	284	285	238	294
Mean	10	6	38	37	48	43	260	134	8.5	4.2	30	33	35	38	7.47	7.55	98
SD±	23	17	29	25	41	31	217	133	8.6	5.0	21	22	18	19	0.21	0.19	19
Significance‡	NS	NS	0.01	0.10	0.01	0.05	NS	NS	0.01	NS	0.01	0.01	0.01	0.01	NS	NS	0.01

*First ejaculates.
†Second ejaculates.
‡At least one difference exists at the designated level of significance within this column.
(From Pickett, B.W., et al.: Seminal characteristics and total scrotal width (T.S.W.) of normal and abnormal stallions. Proc. Am. Assoc. Equine Pract., 485–518, 1988.)

matozoa in first ejaculates; normal sperm morphology (%) in first and second ejaculates; and TSW. Thoroughbred stallions may have ejaculated more spermatozoa in the first ejaculate (13.0 billion) than Paint Horses (8.5 billion), which were lowest. The results of these two breeds perhaps should not be compared, because 190 Thoroughbreds and only 18 Paint Horses were used in the study. However, the sperm numbers appear to be consistent with TSW, which was 111 mm for Thoroughbreds compared with 102 mm for Paint Horse stallions.

Among stallions that failed a seminal evaluation (Table 82–3), significant differences as a result of breed were found in gel-free and total seminal volumes, total spermatozoa (first ejaculates only), motility (%), normal sperm morphology (%), and TSW. Thoroughbred stallions ejaculated 11.1 billion and 5.2 billion spermatozoa in first and second ejaculates compared with only 7.2 billion and 2.5 billion for Appaloosa stallions. Furthermore, TSW for Thoroughbred stallions was 104 mm vs. 85 mm for Appaloosas. Percent normal morphology was lowest in Arabian stallions (23 and 27%) and highest in first and second ejaculates from Appaloosa stallions (42 and 51%). In general, seminal volumes appeared to be highest among Thoroughbred and lowest among Appaloosa stallions. It is doubtful that there are sufficient differences among breeds, considering the large standard deviations, to be of major concern to the clinician.

SEMINAL CHARACTERISTICS AS AFFECTED BY SEXUAL REST AND AGE

Whenever possible, stallions were categorized as sexually rested, i.e., at least 4 days since an ejaculation. Number of spermatozoa in first ejaculates was significantly higher ($p < 0.01$) and the difference for second ejaculates approached significance from sexually rested stallions compared with non-rested stallions (12.1 billion and 5.5 billion vs. 9.0 billion and 3.6 billion, respectively). However, no difference was found in TSW between rested and non-rested stallions (108 mm vs. 111 mm, respectively). The number of spermatozoa available for ejaculation depends on reserves in the tails of the epididymides, deferent ducts, and ampullae. This number is drastically influenced by interval since previous ejaculation(s), testicular size, and age.[6,22]

Presented in Table 82–4 are means and standard deviations of seminal characteristics and TSW of stallions by age, across breed and month, that passed a seminal evaluation. Significant age differences were found for all seminal volumes, spermatozoa in both first and second ejaculates, and TSW, whereas other differences were relatively minor. Seminal volume appeared to increase until about 7 yr of age, then remained relatively constant. Sperm output and TSW appeared to increase sharply until 5 yr of age, then were essentially constant to 12 yr, after which a decline in sperm output occurred. The relationship between TSW and sperm output in first and second ejaculates appeared to be better when stallions were less than 12 yr old than after 12 yr of age (Table 82–4). This should be expected, because Amann et al. have shown that efficiency of sperm production is higher in younger than older stallions.[22] Perhaps fibrotic tissue replaces spermatogenic tissue as stallions age, resulting in reduction of efficiency.

As shown in Table 82–1, total spermatozoa in both first and second ejaculates of stallions that passed an examination was higher ($p < 0.01$) and TSW was greater ($p < 0.01$) than corresponding values for stallions that failed. The relationship between these characteristics for passed (Table 82–4) and failed (Table 82–5) stallions as a result of age was similar; however, total spermatozoa in first and second ejaculates combined were different. For example, sperm numbers from passed stallions appeared to peak at about 12 yr of age with 23.9 billion spermatozoa compared with a peak of 21.8 billion at 10 yr of age for those that failed. Similarly, TSW for passed stallions leveled off at about 11 yr of age (115 mm) and remained relatively similar until 17 to 19 yr (113 mm). More variation in TSW because of age appeared to exist in failed stallions than those that passed, probably as a result of testicular degeneration.

Woods et al. studied Standardbred stallions and found that mean testicular width of breeding stallions increased with age and, although most growth occurred by 5 yr of age, testicular size increased until 12 yr of age.[23] These workers also found that stallions on breeding farms had larger testes than stallions on race tracks. They postulated that this difference was the result of drugs received on the track. Perhaps some of the difference in testicular size could have been caused by the stress of training and racing. Also, it appeared from their study that the right testis was larger than the left,[23] which is in disagreement with other studies.[11,24,25] (R.P. Amann, E.L. Squires, and G.E. Seidel, personal communication; C.M. Clay, personal communication).

Age had a pronounced effect on seminal characteristics and TSW, which must be taken into consideration in predicting the number of mares that can be bred.[26] Testes and epididymides from stallions ≥5 yr old were heavier than those from 2- to 4-yr-olds.[22] Furthermore, the head and body of the epididymis of 10- to 16-yr-old stallions contained approximately two times more spermatozoa than those of 2- to 4-yr-old stallions, and sperm reserves of sexually rested stallions increased with age. The efficiency of sperm production was as high or higher in 2- to 4-yr-old stallions, but because of larger testes, daily sperm production was higher in older horses.[22] Ley concluded that a 3-yr-old stallion has sufficient spermatozoa to be used daily, providing testicular size is within normal ranges and sex drive adequate.[26] From these data, younger stallions seem to be more likely to be overused and older stallions underused in relation to their sperm output.

ONE FUNCTIONAL TESTIS

A cryptorchid stallion should not be approved as a sound breeder for two primary reasons: (1) the condition is probably heritable[27] and (2) eventually, they often will exhibit abnormal sexual behavior.[6] A stallion

TABLE 82–4. THE EFFECT OF AGE ON SEMINAL CHARACTERISTICS AND TOTAL SCROTAL WIDTH OF STALLIONS ACROSS BREED AND MONTH THAT PASSED A SEMINAL EVALUATION

	SEMINAL VOLUME (ML)						SPERMATOZOA										
	Gel		Gel Free		Total		Concentration per Milliliter (10^6)		Total (10^9)		Motile (%)		Normal Morphology (%)		Seminal pH		Total Scrotal Width
Age (yr)	1*	2†	1	2	1	2	1	2	1	2	1	2	1	2	1	2	(mm)
2																	
Mean	2	1	27	24	29	25	328	166	6.8	2.5	51	53	49	55	7.49	7.57	96
SD±	5	2	17	24	19	24	191	149	3.9	1.8	16	19	15	15	0.19	0.20	9
3																	
Mean	3	3	33	33	37	35	309	151	8.8	3.9	53	57	52	57	7.44	7.59	101
SD±	8	8	20	20	23	23	179	141	4.9	2.3	14	12	15	15	0.16	0.19	8
4																	
Mean	8	4	41	42	49	46	321	153	10.2	5.1	57	61	54	58	7.44	7.51	104
SD±	18	9	27	28	36	31	198	102	7.1	3.2	11	10	14	13	0.20	0.17	11
5																	
Mean	10	4	45	36	55	40	374	192	12.2	5.5	53	56	53	59	7.39	7.53	108
SD±	17	12	31	21	38	28	263	142	7.2	3.6	16	13	14	11	0.15	0.18	11
6																	
Mean	14	7	44	46	58	53	339	141	11.7	5.3	52	56	51	56	7.39	7.51	107
SD±	37	21	34	29	50	34	216	106	7.4	4.2	16	16	17	16	0.16	0.13	12
7																	
Mean	11	3	49	46	60	49	290	136	11.5	4.9	51	57	53	60	7.46	7.57	109
SD±	23	6	34	26	42	28	147	89	6.4	2.9	15	15	15	15	0.18	0.12	11
8																	
Mean	5	1	52	41	57	42	394	164	14.1	5.5	57	59	52	58	7.41	7.48	109
SD±	12	3	38	29	40	29	424	97	8.4	4.1	17	18	18	14	0.22	0.12	12
9																	
Mean	8	2	50	44	57	46	387	197	14.5	7.0	56	60	49	56	7.36	7.43	109
SD±	15	3	31	27	42	27	260	175	7.6	8.9	14	11	15	12	0.23	0.18	12
10																	
Mean	10	5	51	44	60	48	299	143	13.6	5.9	55	60	50	55	7.37	7.47	111
SD±	17	12	24	26	34	34	148	83	7.8	3.6	13	11	14	12	0.17	0.17	9
11																	
Mean	14	10	44	49	58	59	337	141	12.1	6.3	53	53	54	56	7.48	7.49	115
SD±	39	29	23	21	53	34	195	67	6.0	3.6	15	20	14	14	0.17	0.26	11
12																	
Mean	6	7	50	42	56	48	390	169	17.0	6.9	56	60	54	58	7.36	7.50	114
SD±	16	11	29	18	36	26	181	72	7.7	4.3	13	11	16	14	0.19	0.18	9
13, 14																	
Mean	20	16	49	44	65	57	352	173	12.6	6.9	50	59	51	56	7.41	7.55	114
SD±	42	35	31	28	52	43	235	96	8.1	5.4	15	13	15	13	0.16	0.17	11
15, 16																	
Mean	12	4	47	55	50	59	281	131	10.5	4.5	51	58	48	51	7.47	7.51	111
SD±	24	7	25	41	42	40	222	115	7.1	2.9	15	13	19	16	0.17	0.13	13
17–19																	
Mean	13	4	47	55	60	59	388	164	14.2	7.6	54	57	48	55	7.36	7.45	113
SD±	27	7	23	35	44	34	273	103	6.6	5.2	12	17	11	11	0.16	0.18	10
20+																	
Mean	12	18	47	42	59	60	292	184	12.1	7.6	47	55	51	53	7.41	7.49	105
SD±	23	27	32	28	44	37	240	204	10.4	14.9	18	15	12	10	0.13	0.17	12
Overall Mean																	
n	618	588	621	591	618	588	608	578	608	578	617	585	596	569	415	397	570
Mean	9	5	44	42	53	47	335	158	11.7	5.4	53	57	51	57	7.42	7.52	107
SD±	23	15	29	28	41	32	232	120	7.4	4.9	15	14	15	14	0.18	0.17	12
Significance‡	0.10	0.01	0.01	0.01	0.01	0.01	NS	NS	0.01	0.01	NS	NS	NS	NS	NS	0.05	0.01

*First ejaculates.
†Second ejaculates.
‡At least one difference exists at the designated level of significance within this column.
(From Pickett, B.W., et al.: Seminal characteristics and total scrotal width (T.S.W.) of normal and abnormal stallions. Proc. Am. Assoc. Equine Pract., 485–518, 1988.)

TABLE 82–5. THE EFFECT OF AGE ON SEMINAL CHARACTERISTICS AND TOTAL SCROTAL WIDTH OF STALLIONS ACROSS BREED AND MONTH THAT FAILED A SEMINAL EVALUATION

	SEMINAL VOLUME (ML)						SPERMATOZOA										
	Gel		Gel Free		Total		Concentration per Milliliter (10^6)		Total (10^9)		Motile (%)		Normal Morphology (%)		Seminal pH		Total Scrotal Width
Age (yr)	1*	2†	1	2	1	2	1	2	1	2	1	2	1	2	1	2	(mm)
2																	
Mean	3	1	22	20	25	20	215	140	3.7	2.4	25	31	31	34	7.57	7.65	86
SD±	6	2	20	17	22	17	195	135	3.9	3.3	19	22	16	18	0.26	0.22	17
3																	
Mean	8	3	41	36	49	39	207	96	6.5	2.6	31	30	31	34	7.50	7.60	99
SD±	18	5	39	18	41	18	174	93	5.6	2.4	20	21	19	21	0.16	0.18	18
4																	
Mean	6	4	39	31	45	35	249	155	8.6	3.3	31	34	36	39	7.42	7.52	97
SD±	16	7	26	22	30	25	188	155	9.3	3.4	22	21	18	18	0.20	0.15	17
5																	
Mean	6	2	43	36	49	39	277	127	8.3	3.6	32	37	36	38	7.54	7.61	98
SD±	15	5	33	24	37	24	233	88	7.7	2.8	24	23	18	21	0.20	0.15	16
6																	
Mean	13	10	441	31	54	41	264	142	10.0	4.3	32	33	38	41	7.41	7.50	103
SD±	22	23	31	17	43	26	265	132	10.9	4.4	28	24	20	18	0.20	0.19	18
7																	
Mean	16	3	36	37	52	40	339	155	10.6	5.9	28	32	38	48	7.45	7.53	105
SD±	26	6	23	19	47	23	242	113	8.1	5.3	23	27	22	22	0.13	0.05	19
8																	
Mean	29	18	44	39	72	57	233	114	7.3	2.5	29	31	35	37	7.47	7.55	103
SD±	44	39	39	47	55	58	234	113	8.9	2.2	21	21	20	17	0.24	0.20	13
9																	
Mean	10	7	41	41	51	47	291	120	12.4	4.2	36	43	49	49	7.38	7.51	99
SD±	14	11	24	23	29	29	120	88	10.8	3.0	21	21	23	24	0.26	0.16	20
10																	
Mean	15	17	46	45	61	62	309	145	14.9	6.9	38	39	41	36	7.46	7.52	107
SD±	18	33	22	26	27	36	150	86	10.5	4.0	21	26	18	10	0.19	0.11	18
11																	
Mean	13	11	49	47	62	58	188	132	8.3	6.7	51	41	45	47	7.44	7.48	95
SD±	19	15	22	29	35	33	160	103	8.3	6.6	15	21	16	18	0.28	0.17	25
12																	
Mean	7	7	47	56	54	63	263	102	10.1	5.7	24	30	33	42	7.47	7.50	105
SD±	11	13	28	33	33	35	232	110	8.4	5.3	17	15	14	19	0.15	0.20	25
13, 14																	
Mean	13	7	42	49	56	56	329	188	10.9	7.9	35	40	34	37	7.43	7.50	98
SD±	20	13	24	29	33	32	323	228	13.3	10.4	19	21	16	17	0.21	0.23	17
15, 16																	
Mean	14	22	47	59	61	80	156	87	7.1	3.8	24	38	41	46	7.47	7.51	101
SD±	18	56	30	32	43	78	132	75	7.6	3.6	18	20	19	17	0.18	0.11	20
17–19																	
Mean	7	3	49	51	55	54	258	108	10.7	5.5	30	39	35	38	7.37	7.41	99
SD±	9	4	27	28	27	32	293	85	8.6	4.5	23	23	20	21	0.17	0.19	23
20+																	
Mean	37	18	47	50	84	68	135	59	6.9	2.2	21	25	30	31	7.53	7.53	94
SD±	71	22	36	48	98	50	115	68	9.0	2.6	18	17	8	13	0.19	0.23	24
Overall mean																	
N	352	319	352	320	351	319	336	301	335	301	340	306	331	292	293	248	307
Mean	10	6	40	37	50	43	249	130	8.4	4.1	30	34	35	38	7.47	7.55	97
SD±	24	17	30	27	41	33	216	128	8.7	4.7	22	22	18	19	0.21	0.19	19
Significance‡	0.01	0.01	0.10	0.01	0.01	0.01	NS	NS	0.01	0.01	NS	NS	NS	NS	NS	0.05	0.05

*First ejaculates.
†Second ejaculates.
‡At least one difference exists at the designated level of significance within this column.
(From Pickett, B.W., et al.: Seminal characteristics and total scrotal width (T.S.W.) of normal and abnormal stallions. Proc. Am. Assoc. Equine Pract., 485–518, 1988.)

with only one functional testis that passes all other criteria, providing the other was removed for medical reasons, may be approved as a sound breeder, but in general, his sperm output will be approximately 50% of a normal stallion with two testes.

Presented in Table 82–6 are comparisons of seminal characteristics and TSW of stallions with one functional testis with those of stallions with two testes that passed a seminal evaluation. Seminal volumes were either larger ($p < 0.05$) or had a tendency to be larger for normal stallions. As suspected, sperm concentration and total spermatozoa were higher in both ejaculates from stallions that passed ($p < 0.01$). In addition, motile spermatozoa in the second ejaculate and percentage of morphologically normal spermatozoa in both ejaculates were lower for stallions that had one functional testis ($p < 0.05$). The TSW of stallions with only one functional testis obviously was lower than normal stallions (67 mm vs. 108 mm, $p < 0.01$).

Compensatory testicular hypertrophy occurs in some species after one testis is removed, before or near puberty.[28] If testicular hypertrophy occurred in stallions with one functional testis, it was not evident from sperm output. The combined output for first and second ejaculates from normal stallions was 17.5 billion compared with 8.8 billion; twice as many spermatozoa came from stallions with two testes. Testicular hypertrophy may not occur in cryptorchid stallions because the cryptorchid testis continues to produce inhibin or other factors. Possibly testicular hypertrophy of a descended testis would occur if the abdominal testis was removed at the appropriate age.

Of the 30 stallions (Table 82–6) in which TSW measurements were made on the functional testis, the left

TABLE 82–6. SEMINAL CHARACTERISTICS AND TOTAL SCROTAL WIDTH OF STALLIONS THAT PASSED A SEMINAL EVALUATION COMPARED WITH STALLIONS WITH ONE FUNCTIONAL TESTIS

		PASSED		ONE FUNCTIONAL TESTIS		
Variable	Ejaculate	*n*	Mean	*n*	Mean	Significance
Seminal volume (mL)						
Gel	1	661	10	32	7	NS
	2	619	5	28	6	NS
Gel free	1	664	45	32	33	0.01
	2	622	42	28	34	0.05
Total	1	661	54	32	40	0.01
	2	619	47	28	41	NS
Spermatozoa						
Concentration/mL (10^6)	1	651	335	29	184	0.01
	2	609	160	24	88	0.01
Total/ejaculate (10^9)	1	651	11.9	29	6.2	0.01
	2	609	5.6	24	2.6	0.01
Motile (%)	1	659	53	30	46	NS
	2	615	57	28	47	0.05
Morphology (%)						
Normal	1	634	51	30	43	0.05
	2	599	57	26	43	0.01
Abnormal						
Neck separated	1	633	5	29	9	NS
	2	598	5	26	10	NS
Head	1	633	9	29	13	0.10
	2	598	9	26	11	NS
Midpiece kinked,	1	633	11	29	11	NS
coiled, or irregular	2	598	10	26	12	NS
Tail reversed, coiled,	1	633	20	29	25	0.10
etc.	2	598	19	26	22	NS
Proximal droplet	1	633	3	29	2	0.01
	2	598	2	26	0.7	0.01
Distal droplet	1	633	3	29	4	NS
	2	598	4	26	2	0.05
Other	1	633	0.14	29	0	0.01
	2	598	0.07	26	0	0.05
Seminal pH	1	436	7.42	27	7.45	NS
	2	417	7.52	23	7.55	NS
Total scrotal width (mm)		605	108	30	67	0.01

(From Pickett, B.W., et al.: Seminal characteristics and total scrotal width (T.S.W.) of normal and abnormal stallions. Proc. Am. Assoc. Equine Pract., 485–518, 1988.)

testis was missing from 19 stallions (63.3%) and the right from 11 stallions (36.7%). This ratio was expected, because Bergin et al. reported that between 9 months of gestation and birth, descent of the right testis was further advanced than the left in 78% of fetuses.[29] In general, seminal characteristics and TSW were similar regardless of which testis was missing.

TESTICULAR ROTATION

A total of 37 (3.5%) of the 1044 stallions evaluated had a right testis (48.6%), left testis (51.4%), or both testes (10.8%) rotated. Stallions with at least one rotated testis had lower gel-free and total seminal volumes and fewer spermatozoa (4.2 billion vs. 5.6 billion) in second ejaculates than those that passed. Furthermore, the trend was the same for first ejaculates (10.7 billion vs. 11.9 billion) (Table 82–7). In normal stallions, the number of spermatozoa in second ejaculates should be approximately 50% of that present in first ejaculates.[16] This ratio in stallions with a rotated testis was 39.2% compared with 47.1% for passed stallions. The reason for fewer spermatozoa in the extra-gonadal sperm reserves of stallions with at least one rotated testis is unknown. However, a similar ratio of sperm number in first and second ejaculates also was observed (Table 82–6) in stallions with only one functional testis (41.9% compared with 47.1%).

Percentages of motile spermatozoa in both ejaculates and of morphologically normal spermatozoa in first ejaculates were significantly depressed (Table 82–7) in stallions with a rotated testis compared with stallions that passed a seminal examination. In addition, TSW

TABLE 82–7. SEMINAL CHARACTERISTICS AND TOTAL SCROTAL WIDTH OF STALLIONS THAT PASSED A SEMINAL EVALUATION COMPARED WITH STALLIONS WITH A ROTATED TESTIS(ES)

		PASSED		ROTATED		
Variable	Ejaculate	*n*	Mean	*n*	Mean	Significance
Seminal volume (mL)						
Gel	1	661	10	36	6	NS
	2	619	5	32	6	NS
Gel free	1	664	45	37	48	NS
	2	622	42	32	30	0.01
Total	1	661	54	36	51	NS
	2	619	47	32	36	0.05
Spermatozoa						
Concentration/mL (10^6)	1	651	335	34	291	NS
	2	609	160	30	152	NS
Total/ejaculate (10^9)	1	651	11.9	34	10.7	NS
	2	609	5.6	30	4.2	0.05
Motile (%)	1	659	53	37	43	0.01
	2	615	57	31	51	0.10
Morphology (%)						
Normal	1	634	51	35	45	0.05
	2	599	57	32	52	NS
Abnormal						
Neck separated	1	633	5	35	5	NS
	2	598	5	32	5	NS
Head	1	633	9	35	11	NS
	2	598	9	32	9	NS
Midpiece kinked, coiled, or irregular	1	633	11	35	13	NS
	2	598	10	32	11	NS
Tail reversed, coiled, etc.	1	633	20	35	21	NS
	2	598	19	32	18	NS
Proximal droplet	1	633	3	35	4	NS
	2	598	2	32	3	NS
Distal droplet	1	633	3	35	5	0.10
	2	598	4	32	4	NS
Other	1	633	0.14	35	0.07	NS
	2	598	0.07	32	0.08	NS
Seminal pH	1	436	7.42	19	7.41	NS
	2	417	7.52	17	7.53	NS
Total scrotal width (mm)		605	108	37	104	0.05

(From Pickett, B.W., et al.: Seminal characteristics and total scrotal width (T.S.W.) of normal and abnormal stallions. Proc. Am. Assoc. Equine Pract., 485–518, 1988.)

was smaller (104 mm vs. 108 mm, $p < 0.05$) when a testis was rotated. Once a testis has been observed in a rotated position, that testis seemed to remain in that position. However, one stallion was evaluated on seven occasions from 1981 through 1986. During this period, the following was observed: December 1981, right testis rotated, left testis normal; December 1982, left testis rotated, right testis normal; December 1983, September 1984, and August 1985, both testes rotated; November 1986, both testes normal.

TESTICULAR DEGENERATION

A total of 32 stallions were diagnosed by palpation as having testicular degeneration: 6 (18.7%) passed the seminal evaluation and 26 (81.3%) failed. A comparison of seminal characteristics and TSW between stallions that passed and those with degenerating testes (both passed and failed) is presented in Table 82–8. Significant differences in the following characteristics were observed between means of both first and second ejaculates in favor of those stallions that passed an evaluation: sperm concentration, total spermatozoa, percent morphologically normal spermatozoa, percent spermatozoa with neck separated in second ejaculates, percent spermatozoa with head and tail abnormalities, and percent spermatozoa with distal droplets in first ejaculates. Mean TSW was 90 mm vs. 108 mm for stallions with testicular degeneration compared with those that passed ($p < 0.01$).

Testicular degeneration was detrimental to seminal characteristics and TSW. Those stallions with degenerating testes that passed may have been in early stages of

TABLE 82–8. COMPARISON BETWEEN MEANS OF SEMINAL CHARACTERISTICS AND TOTAL SCROTAL WIDTH OF STALLIONS WITH AND WITHOUT TESTICULAR DEGENERATION

		PASSED		DEGENERATING		
Variable	Ejaculate	*n*	Mean	*n*	Mean	Significance
Seminal volume (mL)						
Gel	1	661	10	31	15	NS
	2	619	5	28	10	NS
Gel free	1	664	45	31	49	NS
	2	622	42	28	39	NS
Total	1	661	54	31	64	NS
	2	619	47	28	49	NS
Spermatozoa						
Concentration/mL (10^6)	1	651	335	29	167	0.01
	2	609	160	27	96	0.01
Total/ejaculate (10^9)	1	651	11.9	29	7.4	0.05
	2	609	5.6	27	3.7	0.05
Motile (%)	1	659	53	30	32	0.01
	2	615	57	27	34	0.01
Morphology (%)						
Normal	1	634	51	28	31	0.01
	2	599	57	27	35	0.01
Abnormal						
Neck separated	1	633	5	28	10	NS
	2	598	5	27	13	0.10
Head	1	633	9	28	17	0.05
	2	598	9	27	17	0.01
Midpiece kinked,	1	633	11	28	12	NS
coiled, or irregular	2	598	10	27	13	NS
Tail reversed, coiled,	1	633	20	28	31	0.01
etc.	2	598	19	27	27	0.05
Proximal droplet	1	633	3	28	4	NS
	2	598	2	27	3	NS
Distal droplet	1	633	3	28	5	0.10
	2	598	4	27	3	NS
Other	1	633	0.14	28	0.46	NS
	2	598	0.07	27	0.07	NS
Seminal pH	1	436	7.42	27	7.38	NS
	2	417	7.52	23	7.47	NS
Total scrotal width (mm)		605	108	29	90	0.01

(From Pickett, B.W., et al.: Seminal characteristics and total scrotal width (T.S.W.) of normal and abnormal stallions. Proc. Am. Assoc. Equine Pract., 485–518, 1988.)

testicular degeneration and evaluated before testicular degeneration was reflected in seminal characteristics. Leathem, in an excellent review, indicated that infertility was associated with degenerative changes in the testes, which was reflected in quality of ejaculate.[30] These changes included an increase in connective tissue, calcification of the tubules, and an increase in number of tubules with lowered numbers of spermatozoa. Causes of degeneration other than aging and an elevated temperature could be an autoimmune response caused by trauma, including biopsy, and migrating strongyle larvae. Indications exist that hormonal therapy may be beneficial in some cases (K. Shiner, personal communication). Therefore, hormonal imbalance may be a contributing factor.

From clinical observations in the stallion, testicular degeneration seems to follow one of two patterns: (1) testes become progressively softer than normal and may even increase in size temporarily, but eventually shrink to the point at which almost no tissue is found in the scrotum, and (2) the testes become lobulated, constricted, or both and progressively more firm and smaller until a firm, "slick" mass remains. The causes of the two courses of events probably differ. From casual observation, only one testis is initially affected then the other, thus degeneration in the first testis may be a causative factor for degeneration in the other. Once the process has been initiated, the result may be inevitable. If true, prompt removal of the affected testis may be indicated. However, if a testis is removed, it should be under general anesthesia with all vessels ligated, space obliterated, and skin sutured to prevent damage to the remaining testis caused by inflammation. Unfortunately, testicular degeneration is not confined to

TABLE 82–9. MEANS OF SEMINAL CHARACTERISTICS AND TOTAL SCROTAL WIDTH OF STALLIONS THAT PASSED COMPARED WITH THOSE THAT FAILED THE BACTERIOLOGY PORTION OF A SEMINAL EVALUATION

		PASSED		FAILED FOR BACTERIA		
Variable	Ejaculate	*n*	Mean	*n*	Mean	Significance
Seminal volume (mL)						
Gel	1	525	9	73	10	NS
	2	498	5	68	6	NS
Gel free	1	526	39	73	43	NS
	2	500	38	68	41	NS
Total	1	525	48	73	54	NS
	2	565	46	68	49	NS
Spermatozoa						
Concentration/mL (10^6)	1	515	349	72	295	0.05
	2	488	160	68	158	NS
Total/ejaculate (10^9)	1	515	11.1	72	11.6	NS
	2	488	5.2	68	5.4	NS
Motile (%)	1	523	54	72	54	NS
	2	495	58	68	59	NS
Morphology (%)						
Normal	1	508	51	72	53	NS
	2	488	57	66	57	NS
Abnormal						
Neck separated	1	507	5	72	5	NS
	2	487	4	66	5	NS
Head	1	507	9	72	10	NS
	2	487	9	66	10	NS
Midpiece kinked, coiled, or irregular	1	507	11	72	8	0.01
	2	487	10	66	8	0.05
Tail reversed, coiled, etc.	1	507	19	72	21	NS
	2	487	18	66	19	NS
Proximal droplet	1	507	3	72	3	NS
	2	487	2	66	2	NS
Distal droplet	1	507	6	72	6	NS
	2	487	4	66	4	NS
Other	1	507	0.15	72	0.04	NS
	2	487	0.09	66	0.01	NS
Seminal pH	1	358	7.42	45	7.41	NS
	2	347	7.52	43	7.51	NS
Total scrotal width (mm)		484	107	70	110	0.05

(From Pickett, B.W., et al.: Seminal characteristics and total scrotal width (T.S.W.) of normal and abnormal stallions. Proc. Am. Assoc. Equine Pract., 485–518, 1988.)

aged stallions and can occur in stallions as young as 2 yr old.

BACTERIA AND SEMINAL CHARACTERISTICS

Equine semen contains a variety of bacteria.[31–34] The majority are nonpathogenic,[32,34,35] whereas others are capable of causing infection in mares. Hughes et al. isolated Pseudomonas spp. from the urethra or semen of 25 of 70 stallions (36%), but observed no lesions of the genitalia.[34] Other bacteria isolated from semen and the genital tract of stallions in order of frequency were Proteus spp., Staphylococcus spp., Aerobacter spp., hemolytic E. coli, α-hemolytic and nonhemolytic Streptococcus spp. and β-hemolytic Streptococcus spp. Other investigators have reported similar isolations from stallion semen or genital tracts.[11,33,36] It has been shown that many of these organisms did not appear to affect fertility.[32,34,35]

A total of 73 (7.0%) of the 1044 stallions failed their seminal evaluation exclusively because a majority of culture sites were positive for one or more of the following: Klebsiella pneumoniae, Pseudomonas aeruginosa, or β-hemolytic Streptococcus spp. (Table 82–9). Of the 530 stallions that passed the bacteriologic portion of the breeding soundness examination, 29% (154) had at least one culture positive for a potentially pathogenic organism. However, frequency of isolation, perhaps from only one or two areas, or level of growth was insufficient to warrant failing those stallions. Klebsiella pneumoniae was the most commonly isolated organism. A total of 68 (12.8%) of stallions that passed had at least one positive culture for this organism compared with 72 of the 73 (98.6%) stallions that failed. For Pseudomonas aeruginosa, 58 (10.9%) of stallions that passed and 22 (30.1%) of those that failed cultured positive. β-hemolytic Streptococcus spp. were isolated from 28 (5.3%) of stallions that passed compared with 25 (34.2%) of those that failed. Some stallions were positive for more than one pathogen in one of the three culture sites and/or from one of the two ejaculates.

Presented in Table 82–9 are seminal characteristics and TSW of those stallions that passed compared with those that failed exclusively because of isolation of potentially pathogenic bacteria. Seminal characteristics of stallions that passed or failed the bacteriologic examination were similar. Only sperm concentration in first ejaculates was in favor of the passed stallions. Percentage of midpiece abnormalities and TSW was in favor of stallions that failed the examination because of bacterial isolates. Harboring potentially pathogenic bacteria obviously did not affect a stallion's seminal characteristics. Percentage of motile spermatozoa was 54% for both groups. This clearly refutes the myth that presence of potentially pathogenic bacteria in semen adversely affects sperm motility.

Seminal characteristics are related to fertility. Therefore, for maximum reproductive efficiency, the clinician must routinely and consistently characterize seminal characteristics of each stallion. Unfortunately, live foals obtained under ideal management are the best measure of fertility.[27] Stallion reproductive performance should be monitored continuously with respect to percentage of pregnancies per service[10] or cycle, number of cycles per pregnancy, number of covers or inseminations per pregnancy, and pregnancy rate (%) by month and by cycle.[2]

REFERENCES

1. Foote, R.H.: Factors influencing the quantity and quality of semen harvested from bulls, rams, boars and stallions. J. Anim. Sci., *47:*1–11, 1978.
2. Pickett, B.W., Squires, E.L., and McKinnon, A.O.: Procedures for Collection, Evaluation and Utilization of Stallion Semen for Artificial Insemination. Animal Reproduction Laboratory Bulletin No. 03. Fort Collins, Colorado State University, 1987.
3. Voss, J.L., and Pickett, B.W.: Reproductive Management of the Broodmare. University Animal Reproduction Laboratory General Series Bulletin No. 961. Fort Collins, Colorado State University, 1976.
4. Pickett, B.W., Voss, J.L., and Nelson, L.D.: Factors influencing the fertility of stallion spermatozoa in an A.I. program. Proceedings of the International Congress on Animal Reproduction and Artificial Insemination. Vol. 4. 1976, pp. 1049–1052.
5. Van der Holst, W.: Stallion semen production in A.I. programs in the Netherlands. *In* The Male in Farm Animal Production. Edited by M. Courot. Boston, Martinus Nijhoff, 1984, pp. 195–201.
6. Pickett, B.W., et al.: Management of the Stallion for Maximum Reproductive Efficiency. II. Animal Reproduction Laboratory Bulletin No. 05. Fort Collins, Colorado State University, 1989.
7. Amann, R.P.: A critical review of methods for evaluation of spermatogenesis from seminal characteristics. J. Androl., *2:*37–58, 1981.
8. Amann, R.P.: Can the fertility potential of a seminal sample be predicted accurately? J. Androl., *10:*89–99, 1989.
9. Pickett, B.W., et al.: Seminal characteristics and total scrotal width (T.S.W.) of normal and abnormal stallions. Proc. Am. Assoc. Equine Pract., 485–518, 1988.
10. Dowsett, K.F., and Pattie, W.A.: Characteristics and fertility of stallion semen. J. Reprod. Fertil. Suppl., *32:*1–8, 1982.
11. Sigler, D.H., and Kiracofe, G.H.: Ejaculate characteristics of two- and three-year old Quarter horse stallions. Proceedings of the Equine Nutrition and Physiology Symposium. 1987, pp. 291–296.
12. Rowley, H.S., Squires, E.L., and Pickett, B.W.: Effect of insemination volume on embryo recovery in mares. J. Equine Vet. Sci., *10:*298–300, 1990.
13. Gebauer, M.R., Pickett, B.W., and Swierstra, E.E.: Reproductive physiology of the stallion. II. Daily production and output of sperm. J. Anim. Sci., *39:*732–736, 1974.
14. Amann, R.P., and Pickett, B.W.: Principles of cryopreservation and a review of cryopreservation of stallion spermatozoa. J. Equine Vet. Sci., *7:*145–173, 1987.
15. Pace, M.M., and Sullivan, J.J.: Effect of timing of insemination, numbers of spermatozoa and extender components on the pregnancy rate in mares inseminated with frozen stallion semen. J. Reprod. Fertil. Suppl., *23:*115–121, 1975.
16. Pickett, B.W., et al.: Reproductive physiology of the stal-

lion. VI. Seminal and behavioral characteristics. J. Anim. Sci., *43:*617–625, 1976.

17. Van Duijn, C., Jr., and Hendrikse, J.: Rational analysis of seminal characteristics of stallions in relation to fertility. Instituut voor Veeteelkundig Onderzoek "Schoonoord" Report B97. Pretoria, 1968.
18. Voss, J.L., Pickett, B.W., and Loomis, P.R.: The relationship between seminal characteristics and fertility in Thoroughbred stallions. J. Reprod. Fertil. Suppl., *32:*635–636, 1982.
19. Dott, H.M.: Morphology of stallion spermatozoa. J. Reprod. Fertil. Suppl., *23:*41–46, 1975.
20. Bielanski, W.: The evaluation of stallion semen in aspects of fertility control and its use for artificial insemination. J. Reprod. Fertil. Suppl., *23:*19–24, 1975.
21. Gebauer, M.R., Pickett, B.W., Voss, J.L., and Swierstra, E.E.: Reproductive physiology of the stallion: Daily sperm output and testicular measurements. J. Am. Vet. Med. Assoc., *165:*711–714, 1974.
22. Amann, R.P., Thompson, D.L., Jr., Squires, E.L., and Pickett, B.W.: Effect of age and frequency of ejaculation on sperm production and extragonadal sperm reserves in stallions. J. Reprod. Fertil. Suppl., *27:*1–6, 1979.
23. Woods, G.L., Garcia, M.C., and Kenney, R.M.: Variations in testicular size of Standardbred stallions. Proc. Am. Assoc. Equine Pract., 117–121, 1980.
24. Muhe, W.: Eine Moglichkeitzur objektiven Bestimmung der Hodengrosse beim Hengst. DVM dissertation. Hannover, Tierarztliche Hochschule, 1972.
25. Nishikawa, Y.: Studies on Reproduction in Horses. Tokyo, Japan Racing Association, 1959.
26. Ley, W.B.: Method of predicting stallion to mare ratio for natural and artificial insemination programs. J. Equine Vet. Sci., *5:*143–146, 1985.
27. Leipold, H.W., et al.: Cryptorchidism in the horse: Genetic implications. Proc. Am. Assoc. Equine Pract., 579–589, 1985.
28. Schanbacher, B.D., Fletcher, P.W., and Reichert, L.E., Jr.: Testicular compensatory hypertrophy in the hemicastrated calf: Effects of exogenous estradiol. Biol. Reprod., *36:*1142–1148, 1987.
29. Bergin, W.C., Gier, H.T., Marion, G.B., and Coffman, J.R.: A developmental concept of equine cryptorchism. Biol. Reprod., *3:*82–92, 1970.
30. Leathem, J.H.: Aging and the testis. *In* The Testis. Vol. 4. Edited by A.D. Johnson and W.R. Gomes. New York, Academic Press, 1977, pp. 547–563.
31. Bain, A.M.: The role of infection in infertility in the Thoroughbred mare. Vet. Rec., *78:*168–175, 1966.
32. Burns, S.J., Simpson, R.B., and Snell, J.R.: Control of microflora in stallion semen with a semen extender. J. Reprod. Fertil. Suppl., *23:*139–142, 1975.
33. Kenney, R.M.: Clinical fertility evaluation of the stallion. Proc. Am. Assoc. Equine Pract., 336–355, 1975.
34. Hughes, J.P., Asbury, A.C., Loy, R.G., and Burd, H.E.: The occurrence of Pseudomonas in the genital tract of stallions and its effects on fertility. Cornell Vet., *57:*53–69, 1967.
35. Merkt, H., Klug, E., Bohm, K.-H., and Weiss, R.: Recent observations concerning Klebsiella infections in stallions. J. Reprod. Fertil. Suppl., *23:*143–145, 1975.
36. Crouch, J.R.F., Atherton, J.G., and Platt, H.: Venereal transmission of Klebsiella aerogenes in a Thoroughbred stud from a persistently infected stallion. Vet. Rec. *90:*21–24, 1972.
37. Kenney, R.M., et al.: Society for theriogenology manual for clinical fertility evaluation of the stallion. J. Soc. Theriol., Vol. 9, 1983.

CHAPTER 83

CRYOPRESERVATION OF SEMEN

B.W. Pickett
R.P. Amann

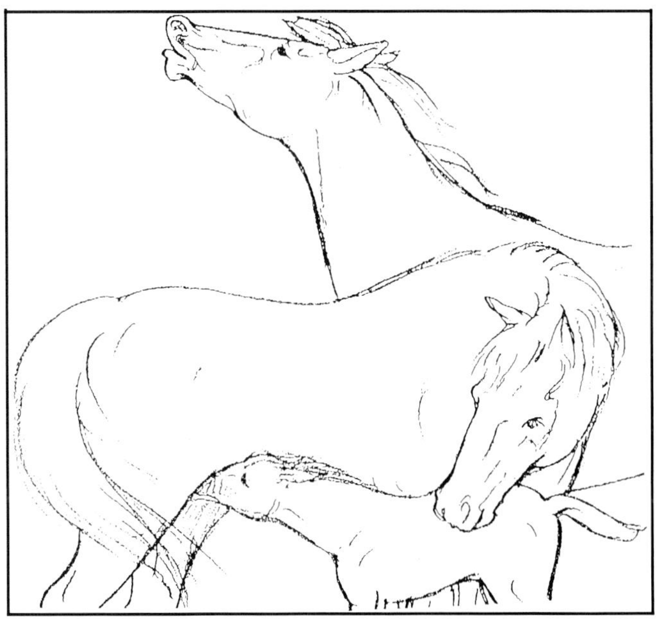

Successful cryopreservation of gametes from a variety of species was enabled by accidental discovery in 1949 that spermatozoa frozen in an extender containing glycerol were still viable after they were thawed.[1] As early as 1950, these investigators[2] noted that if stallion spermatozoa were separated from seminal plasma and resuspended in buffer containing glycerol and glucose, about 25% of the spermatozoa were motile after freezing to −79° C (−110° F) and thawing. For economic reasons, most early research focused on bull spermatozoa.[3] However, the basic procedures for successful cryopreservation of bull spermatozoa have been applied, with less success, to spermatozoa from other species.[4,5]

For successful cryopreservation of stallion spermatozoa, (1) the spermatozoa must be mixed with an appropriate extender; (2) cooled slowly, about 0.05° C/min, from at least 18° C (64° F) to near 4° C (39° F); (3) exposed to one or more cryoprotective agents in an appropriate extender; (4) packaged in an appropriate single-dose container; (5) cooled relatively rapidly, 10° to 60° C/min, from +4° C to below −100° C (−180° F); (6) stored at −196° C (−320° F); (7) warmed rapidly, about 2000° C/min, from −196° to 37° C; and (8) used for artificial insemination (AI) immediately after thawing (within 5 min). The optimal extender, cryoprotectant(s), package, cooling rate, and warming rate must be considered in total, because these factors interactively affect success.

The first pregnancy from frozen stallion semen was reported in 1957 by Barker and Gandier.[6] Spermatozoa were recovered from the cauda epididymidis and frozen in heated, whole milk extender containing 10% glycerol. Of seven mares artificially inseminated with thawed semen, one subsequently foaled. However, frozen semen has not been used widely by the horse industry because of poor pregnancy rates with many stallions as well as restrictions imposed by breed registry associations.

ADVANTAGES AND DISADVANTAGES OF FROZEN STALLION SEMEN

Several advantages and disadvantages of frozen equine semen have been noted. The relative importance of these depend on many factors. Most horse breeders should and will consider the following to be advantages:

1. It is much cheaper to ship a liquid nitrogen container across the country, or world, than to ship a horse.
2. Mares would not need to be hauled to the stallion; which would greatly reduce overall costs of breeding as well as insurance. Furthermore, the stress of hauling the mare would be eliminated, and a lactating mare's foal would not be exposed to the risks or stress of hauling. Generally, the foal would be safer and better cared for at home, and mares and foals would not be exposed to diseases often associated with large breeding farms.

3. A stallion's breeding season could continue while he is at shows or performance events or while he is recovering from an illness or injury.
4. Differences in the breeding season between northern and southern hemispheres would pose no problem for planned matings.
5. Semen from extremely valuable stallions could be stored as insurance and used later when their germ plasm was needed, even after they have been dead for many years, or in the event breed regulations changed to allow the use of frozen semen.
6. Reduce the use of genetically inferior stallions. Most likely, those who own inferior stallions will believe frozen semen to be a disadvantage.

Several disadvantages are associated with the use of frozen semen. However, several of the purported disadvantages are imaginary or are based on incomplete information. The following concerns probably are foremost in the minds of most horse owners.

1. For many stallions, techniques used for processing, packaging, freezing, and inseminating their frozen semen do not result in a satisfactory pregnancy rate. This currently is true, but lower pregnancy rates need not be an inevitable result of freezing semen. Presently, spermatozoa from perhaps one-third of all stallions will provide a pregnancy rate ≥ 60% of that achieved under comparable conditions using their fresh semen.
2. Frequently, it is stated that with availability of frozen semen, too many mares will be bred to an individual stallion. Obviously, a stallion owner can limit sales of semen. However, even with improved technology, it is unlikely that more than 35 insemination doses (straws) can be prepared from semen ejaculated by a stallion in one week, and even fewer can be prepared when semen is processed during the nonbreeding season. Furthermore, some insemination doses must be used to evaluate quality of the product and many insemination doses will be unsatisfactory and, therefore, discarded. That more than 300 to 400 insemination doses of satisfactory semen would be obtained from a normal stallion in a 12-month period is unlikely. Because most mares will be bred several times during each estrous cycle, sufficient insemination doses might be available to breed 100 to 200 mares to a stallion in 1 yr. Consequently, the number of stallions needed to breed mares will not be reduced drastically. Because of the limited number of mares that can be inseminated to a stallion annually using frozen semen, no reason exists to assume that inbreeding will occur more rapidly than through natural service; perhaps even less will occur because semen can be shipped all over the world. Thus breeders are not limited to local stallions.
3. On farms where large numbers of mares are boarded for breeding, income from mare care will be reduced.
4. Some breeders are concerned that stud fees will decline. The cost involved in collecting, processing, and storing stallion semen will increase the cost. Consequently, in addition to the regular stud fee, the cost for processing and storing a sufficient number of insemination doses to achieve one pregnancy probably will average about $100 for a mare. Addition of this amount to the regular stud fee would be necessary. Considering the limited number of doses that can be processed, and cost of processing semen, it is unlikely that availability of frozen equine semen would have a major impact on stud fees. Further, there will always be breeders who have young stallions that they feel must be proven.
5. On-the-farm freezing of stallion semen might be an advantage, but in most cases it will be a disadvantage. A portable freezing laboratory could possibly move from farm to farm, but the quality of product obtained by this approach would likely be inferior to that obtained at a permanent facility to which stallions or freshly collected semen were brought. This conclusion is based on experience with frozen bull semen. Farmers and ranchers were quick to learn that fertility of semen collected and processed by most mobile units was inferior to that processed by major bull studs. We hope that a horse breeder who stands stallions will take them to a center that has an appropriately equipped laboratory and trained personnel. Thus, stallions must be shipped to a central location for collecting, processing, and freezing of semen. Although untested, the clinician may be able to collect, centrifuge, and extend semen at the farm where a stallion is located and then transport the semen to a laboratory where processing and cryopreservation would be completed within 2 to 3 h. Such a procedure would require careful attention to detail. Obviously, a breeding farm with several valuable stallions may elect to establish its own processing laboratory, staffed with qualified personnel.
6. Some breeders are concerned that use of frozen semen would lead to errors of identity and, consequently, improper pedigrees. The integrity of the breeder, not procedure used to get mares pregnant, determines purity of a breed. However, if each stallion is carefully identified, photographed, and bloodtyped or DNA fingerprinted before semen is frozen, and if each individual insemination dose is permanently labeled with a complete identification of the semen it contains, more care will possibly be taken to identify the sire than is true on some breeding farms. Through the use of blood typing or DNA fingerprinting, of both parents and progeny, the identification of careless or dishonest individuals will be easier.

COOLING AND COLD SHOCK

Several problems are involved in freezing and thawing stallion spermatozoa that are not encountered when fresh or extended semen is held at 37° C or at room temperature (about 20° C). The first is cold shock,[5,7,8] a series of poorly understood, partially irreversible, changes in spermatozoa that occur when they are cooled rapidly from 20° to 1° C. As detailed in Chapter 80, cold shock is evidenced by increased membrane permeability and loss of intracellular molecules and ions, decreased energy production, and more obviously by the sequela of swelling of the acrosome. Cold shock can be minimized by slow cooling of extended stallion spermatozoa to 4° C, at a rate of ≤0.05° C/min from 18° to <8° C (J.-P. Kayser, personal communication). In contrast to rapid cooling, rapid warming to 37° C rarely is detrimental.

In general, injury caused by cold shock can be classified into two categories:[5,9]

1. Direct injury, which is evident shortly after reducing the temperature and depends on rate of cooling.
2. Indirect or latent damage, which sometimes is not evident until after the temperature has been reduced and is independent from the rate of cooling.

Many reactions initiated during cooling continue during freezing. The prudent clinician assumes that any change induced by cold shock or poor handling will increase damage induced by freezing and thawing. Stresses to spermatozoa often are additive. The problem in cryopreservation of spermatozoa is not ability of spermatozoa to remain viable at −196° C but rather damage resulting from cooling and warming during an intermediate zone of temperatures, about −5° to −60° C.[5,10]

PRINCIPLES OF CRYOPRESERVATION

Success in cryopreservation of stallion spermatozoa depends on a complex series of interactions among extender, cryoprotectant(s), cooling and warming rates to minimize damage from cold shock, formation of ice crystals, and dehydration. Several excellent reviews of changes in the medium and spermatozoa associated with cryopreservation are available.[5,10-13] Because cooling and warming rates are influenced by composition and dimensions of the packaging system, this factor also must be considered. Of equal importance are criteria used to evaluate success,[14,15] and degree of selection. This includes selection of stallions whose spermatozoa are known to freeze well, or against stallions whose spermatozoa are known not to remain highly motile or fertile after freezing and thawing, freezing protocol, and also the extent of selection of ejaculates from a given stallion frozen by a given procedure. Young Holstein bulls are rejected for use in commercial artificial insemination when their spermatozoa are unable to withstand cryopreservation by a fixed procedure. This is essential for economic success and has lead to a gradual, but real, improvement in average pregnancy rate.[11,15] For stallions, however, performance and emotion probably will require that spermatozoa from each valuable stallion be evaluated using several freezing protocols to identify one best for that stallion.

For a spermatozoon to fertilize an oocyte, it must retain at least four general attributes after freezing and thawing: (1) metabolism for production of energy, (2) progressive motility, (3) intact enzymes located within the acrosome that are essential for penetration of the spermatozoon through structures surrounding the oocyte, and (4) proteins on the plasma membrane that are important for survival of a spermatozoon within the female reproductive tract and for attachment of the spermatozoon to the oocyte plasma membrane at fertilization. Destruction of sperm components associated with one or more of these functions will reduce or abolish fertility. For example, motile equine spermatozoa are not always fertile. Although motile spermatozoa almost certainly have an adequate production of energy, other important aspects may have been altered.

Detailed considerations of biophysical changes in the cells and medium are available.[5,9-11,13,16-21] Briefly, when a suspension of spermatozoa is cooled below freezing, it will cool a few degrees below the freezing point of the medium, supercooling, before freezing actually is initiated. Excessive supercooling can be eliminated by "seeding" to induce ice formation. The technique of seeding is commonly used when freezing embryos, which are very complex and larger than spermatozoa. However, no evidence exists that seeding is beneficial when freezing stallion spermatozoa. With human and boar spermatozoa, no advantage is known to seeding the spermatozoal suspension as it reaches about −5° C.[22] In the absence of seeding, when the suspension reaches −6° to −15° C, extracellular ice crystals begin to form from water in the extender. This results in an increase in concentration of solutes (salt, proteins, and sugars) in the remaining fluid outside spermatozoa. Initially, water within spermatozoa does not freeze, but is cooled below the freezing point. The high extracellular concentration of solutes causes water to move from inside spermatozoa to the extracellular environment, because of osmotic pressure, and spermatozoa become progressively dehydrated. If cooling rate is very slow, sufficient water will move out of the spermatozoa so that large crystals of intracellular ice cannot form.[10,11,13] However, under these conditions, a high intracellular concentration of solutes will result, which causes cellular damage. When cooling is very rapid, water has little time to move out of the spermatozoa before actual freezing, and large intracellular ice crystals form. Large intracellular crystals of ice damage cellular compartments, although with ultrarapid cooling, intracellular solute concentration is not a problem. Thus, one must be concerned with water movement and crystallization, solute concentration inside and outside the spermatozoa, and shrinkage and swelling of the spermatozoa. An optimal cooling rate provides a compromise among these factors, and varies with composition of the extender.

To partially protect spermatozoa during freezing and thawing, cryoprotectants are included in the seminal extender. Cryoprotectants are classified as compounds penetrating the spermatozoa, which act both intracellularly and extracellularly, and nonpenetrating, which act only extracellularly. Glycerol is the most common penetrating cryoprotectant for use with spermatozoa, although dimethyl sulfoxide (DMSO) and propylene glycol have been used. Sugars that are not transported across the plasma membrane of spermatozoa (lactose, mannose, raffinose, trehalose), polyvinylpyrrolidone, and certain proteins are examples of nonpenetrating cryoprotectants. Egg yolk lipoprotein also is a nonpenetrating cryoprotectant. The exact mechanisms of cryoprotectant action are poorly understood, and may partially depend on freezing rate.

Penetrating cryoprotectants, such as glycerol, probably are beneficial because they function as a solvent with a freezing point much lower than that of water. Thus in the presence of glycerol, the proportion of solvent remaining unfrozen at any given temperature is greater than if water were the only solvent and the concentration of solutes is lower.[10,16,19] Although glycerol rapidly enters spermatozoa—probably in < 1 min, depending on the temperature of the addition (P.F. Watson, personal communication)—its primary beneficial effect probably is extracellular. By increasing the proportion of unfrozen solvent at a given temperature, inclusion of glycerol in the extender decreases solute concentrations and increases volume of "channels" of unfrozen solvent in which the spermatozoa can survive between "blocks" of ice.[16–18]

Nonpenetrating cryoprotectants, such as lactose, presumably act by osmotically drawing water from spermatozoa, as temperature is lowered, to dehydrate spermatozoa and reduce the probability that large crystals of ice will form within the cells. Such cryoprotectants also may affect the cells.[23]

There is abundant evidence that cryoprotectants, including glycerol, are toxic to spermatozoa.[24–29] Part of this toxicity is caused by biochemical injury, resulting from direct action of cryoprotectant on subcellular components, but osmotic damage also occurs. The acrosome and overlying plasma membrane may be more susceptible to cryoprotectant damage than mitochondria and structures needed for motility. Researchers have speculated that rapid egress of glycerol from spermatozoa, by diffusion down a concentration gradient to the glycerol-free environment of the female reproductive system, places physical stress on membranous compartments of the spermatozoa that induces irreversible damage.[11,12,30] The osmotic effect of glycerol on stallion spermatozoa has not been examined critically. However, any such damage might be minimized by adding glycerol judiciously before freezing (slowly and/or at 4° C) and using procedures to slow egress of glycerol from spermatozoa after thawing. Thus, the primary beneficial effect of glycerol may be extracellular and the toxic effects of glycerol may be the consequence of its entrance into cells.

The optimum concentration of cryoprotectant in an extender depends on the criteria used to evaluate sperm quality as well as procedural details. It must be a compromise to maximize beneficial effects and minimize toxic effects. For example, in one study with boar spermatozoa, use of 4% glycerol provided the highest percentage of motile spermatozoa after thawing, but use of 1% glycerol provided the highest percentage of spermatozoa with an intact acrosome.[28] The best compromise, or least damage to both systems, was use of 3% glycerol.

Ultimate success of a freezing procedure is limited by interaction of the freezing and thawing processes.[3,10–13] In general, when cooling rate is rapid, warming rate also should be rapid. Alternatively, if cooling rate is slow, warming rate must be slow.

CRITERIA OF SPERM SURVIVAL

Visual estimation of percentage of motile spermatozoa after thawing or pregnancy rate are the most common approaches to evaluate survival of stallion spermatozoa after the freeze-thaw process. Unfortunately, subjective evaluation of sperm motility is notoriously imprecise. Objective computerized methods for evaluation of sperm motion are replacing subjective evaluations in research laboratories and on large breeding farms.[31–36] Use of lectins[37] and monoclonal antibodies[38] to evaluate normalcy of the acrosome, flow cytometry,[39] hypoosmotic swelling tests,[40] column filtration tests,[41] and an in vitro oocyte penetration assay[42] may contribute to identification of procedures maximizing retention of sperm fertility.

The accuracy of data on pregnancy rates obtained with frozen stallion spermatozoa must be considered. Because of the cost of experimentation, pregnancy data for stallions usually are based on a limited number of observations.[43,44] Thus, with small numbers in an experiment or data set obtained by a clinician, inherent biologic variation can either lead one to think that a given treatment was highly effective, when in fact it had no effect, or mask the fact that a treatment really did improve fertility. This problem has been discussed in detail,[14,45] and is exemplified by data in Table 83–1. Therefore, the majority of reports on fertility of stallion spermatozoa should be interpreted with caution, because apparent differences may not be real and some real differences may not have been detected.

To achieve maximum pregnancy rates, the number of spermatozoa per insemination must exceed a "critical number." However, to increase the probability of detecting a difference between two treatments in a breeding trial, the number of spermatozoa per insemination dose should be perhaps 80% of the "critical number."[14,44] Based on data for four stallions, Pace and Sullivan concluded that 80 million spermatozoa was above the critical number using frozen-thawed semen.[46] This is a considerably smaller number of spermatozoa per insemination dose than typically used. Russian workers found no difference in fertility when doses of 100 to 800 million frozen-thawed spermatozoa were used.[47] Contrary results were reported by Volkmann and van Zyl, who found that insemination of 220 to 330 million motile spermatozoa based on post-thaw evaluations provided superior results to insemination of 140 to 210 million motile spermatozoa.[48] Pregnancy rates averaged 73 and 44%, respectively. Nevertheless, in most studies number of motile spermatozoa inseminated probably

TABLE 83–1. SELECTED 95% CONFIDENCE INTERVALS FOR A THEORETICAL BINOMIAL SUCH AS PREGNANCY*

Number Mares or Cycles	TRUE FERTILITY (%)				
	15	35	50	65	85
10	0–38	5–65	19–81	35–95	62–100
15	0–33	10–60	24–76	40–90	67–100
20	0–31	14–56	28–72	44–86	69–100
25	1–29	16–54	30–70	46–84	71–99
100	8–23	25–45	40–60	56–74	77–92

*Ranges in the body of the table are the binomial variation component of pregnancy rates that might be encountered for stallions of a known true fertility when a few mares were bred. Actual one-cycle pregnancy rate would be affected by biologic and experimental variation, as well as binomial variation, so that actual 95% confidence intervals for percentage of pregnant mares would be greater than those presented.

(From Amann, R.P., and Pickett, B.W.: An Overview of Frozen Equine Semen: Procedures for Thawing and Insemination of Frozen Equine Spermatozoa. Experiment Station Animal Reproduction Laboratory Special Series No. 33. Fort Collins, Colorado State University, 1984.)

has not been the principal factor limiting fertility of frozen-thawed equine spermatozoa.

INFLUENCE OF STALLION

Spermatozoa from individual stallions differ in their ability to survive freezing and thawing. The percentage of motile spermatozoa in 2 to 36 ejaculates from each of 7 stallions was studied.[49] For some stallions, percentage of motile spermatozoa after freezing and thawing was consistently 80 to 100% of that before freezing. Additional data have been presented based on 1 to 186 ejaculates from 21 stallions.[50–52] The percentage of motile spermatozoa, after freezing and thawing, from 7 of the 21 stallions, was at least 80% of that before freezing. However, for 6 stallions, "survival rate" of spermatozoa averaged 50% or less. For 1 stallion from which 186 ejaculates were processed, percentage of motile spermatozoa after freezing and thawing ranged from 20 to 80% (mean = 61%). Although spermatozoa in a typical ejaculate from this stallion survived freezing and thawing satisfactorily, this was not true of spermatozoa in all ejaculates.

Others studied 36 ejaculates from 16 stallions and concluded that percentage of motile spermatozoa immediately after thawing or after 24 h of subsequent storage at 5° C was influenced by both stallion and ejaculates within stallion.[53] Klug et al. reached the same conclusion after studying 40 ejaculates from 15 stallions.[54] The prefreeze and post-thaw motility of spermatozoa in 336 ejaculates from 40 stallions also were compared.[55] For 15 stallions (38%), percentage of motile spermatozoa after thawing averaged 80 to 100% of that before freezing; however, for the remaining 25 stallions (62%), the average was <65% of that before freezing.

Oshida et al. reported the first study emphasizing differences in pregnancy rate associated with stallions.[56] Semen from five stallions was frozen as pellets and used to inseminate 9 to 28 mares per stallion. Based on data from 12 and 14 mares, respectively, pregnancy rates for two stallions were 67 and 50%. However, for two other stallions whose semen was used to inseminate 25 and 9 mares, pregnancy rates were only 16 and 11%, respectively. Altogether, 34 of 98 mares became pregnant. Unfortunately, whether the reported pregnancy rate of 35% was per cycle or per season was not clear. In this study, pregnancy rate appeared to be independent of number of spermatozoa per insemination, which ranged from 0.3 to 2.1 billion, or percentage of motile spermatozoa in the thawed semen, provided it was greater than 20%. Pregnancy rates for three stallions used to inseminate 35, 67, and 243 mares with 0.3 to 1.5 billion spermatozoa per insemination were 34, 67, and 65%.[57] In this study, mares usually were not inseminated more than twice during one estrus, but pregnancy rates were based on one to three estrous cycles.

Breeding-season pregnancy rates for seven stallions whose semen had been frozen in 4-mL straws have been reported (E. Klug, personal communication). These straws have a volume of 5 mL, but typically are filled with 4 mL of extended semen and are referred to as 4-mL straws. The most extensive data were for two stallions (29 and 22 mares) whose pregnancy rates were 48 and 32%, whereas pregnancy rates of 50 to 58% were reported for three stallions (6 to 14 mares each).

In 1986, Tischner (personal communication) reported that semen from about 25% of the stallions evaluated was classified as good, 50% produced semen of moderate quality, and 25% ejaculated semen that froze unsatisfactorily. Using only semen from stallions that had more than 40% motile spermatozoa after thawing, 51% of 55 mares became pregnant. However, this was probably over the entire breeding season.

Of 341 stallions evaluated in Czechoslovakia, 35% were classified as good (i.e., initial motility more than

60%, morphologically normal spermatozoa more than 70%, and post-thaw motility 30% or more coupled with motility of some spermatozoa for at least 120 h after thawing), 25% were considered average, and 40% were classified as poor[58] (Z. Müller, personal communication). Many of the stallions classified as poor ejaculated semen containing a high percentage of abnormal spermatozoa; their classification was based on this fact rather than motility of spermatozoa after freezing and thawing. For average stallions, only 51% of the ejaculates were rated as acceptable after post-thaw evaluation. For stallions classified as good on the basis of initial evaluation of raw semen, 71% of the ejaculates were acceptable after freezing and thawing. Even after selection of stallions on the basis of post-thaw sperm motility, 1-cycle pregnancy rates differed greatly; 13, 36, and 43% for three stallions. Overall, 1-cycle pregnancy rate (for 1 or 2 cycles of breeding) averaged 42%, based on data for 1223 cycles.[58]

Extreme differences in pregnancy rate have been found at our laboratory using frozen-thawed semen from stallions selected only on the basis of normality of their semen at initial evaluation.[59–61] Even after rejecting 24 to 67% of all ejaculates frozen from a given stallion, because they contained less than 30 or 35%progressively motile spermatozoa after thawing, 1-cycle pregnancy rates ranged from 8 to 61% (Table 83–2).

Motility and fertility of frozen-thawed spermatozoa obviously differ greatly among stallions and ejaculates from the same stallion. Differences in seminal plasma could be one factor affecting sperm survival.[62] Magistrini et al. speculated that differences in composition of seminal plasma were the reason that spermatozoa collected during winter months survived cryopreservation better than those collected in the summer.[63] Based on data for boar spermatozoa, certain low molecular weight proteins in seminal plasma are rapidly bound to epididymal spermatozoa upon admixture with seminal plasma, and presumably alter sperm function.[64] No significant increase was noted in amount of protein bound by spermatozoa after exposure to seminal plasma for 10 to 30 min as compared with a few seconds. In an effort to evaluate the composition of seminal plasma with respect to differences in survival of spermatozoa after freezing and thawing, Amann et al. evaluated 136 ejaculates, 8 from each of 17 stallions.[65] It was found that 80% of the variation in percentage of progressively motile spermatozoa immediately after freezing and thawing was associated with ejaculates within stallion and 20% with stallions. Based on post-thaw sperm motility, seminal plasma from 7 stallions (2 with good, 3 with variable, and 2 with poor sperm motility) were selected for measurement of certain ions, protein concentration, and qualitative analysis of major proteins. For concentrations of protein, sodium, calcium, phosphorus, and chlorine in seminal plasma, more variation was associated with ejaculates within stallions than among stallions. A difference existed among stallions in proportion of ejaculates containing 13 of 27 proteins detected by sodium dodecyl sulfate (SDS) gel electrophoresis. However, correlations among concentrations of these components of seminal plasma, or that of potassium, and post-thaw motility of spermatozoa were too low to be of predictive value. Although an effect of a minor protein in seminal plasma cannot be excluded, variation in concentration of ions or relative amounts of major proteins in seminal plasma probably are not the cause of differences in post-thaw motility of stallion spermatozoa.

TABLE 83–2. REJECTION OF EJACULATES OF FROZEN SEMEN BECAUSE OF POOR SURVIVAL OF SPERMATOZOA AFTER FREEZING AND THAWING*

		PROGRESSIVELY MOTILE SPERMATOZOA (%)			
Stallion	Year	Initial	0-Hour Post-Thaw	Ejaculates Rejected (%)†	Fertility (%)‡
260	1982	61	41	24	10
473	1982	66	39	24	33
009	1984	55	40	29	21
298	1984	55	38	32	48
303	1983	66	43	39	56
473	1983	74	35	42	61
001	1984	58	37	45	8
002	1982	53	24	67	10

*Mean for 12 to 24 ejaculates.

†Ejaculates containing < 35% motile spermatozoa immediately after thawing (1982) or < 35% at 0 h and < 40% after 30 min (1983 and 1984) were rejected.

‡One-cycle pregnancy rate, 50 days postovulation.

(Adapted from Pickett, B.W., Squires, E.L., and McKinnon, A.O.: Procedures for Collection, Evaluation and Utilization of Stallion Semen for Artificial Insemination. Animal Reproduction Laboratory Bulletin No. 03. Fort Collins, Colorado State University, 1987.)

SEMINAL EXTENDERS

A heated, whole milk extender containing 10% glycerol was used to obtain the first pregnancy with cryopreserved stallion semen.[6] Since then, most extenders for freezing stallion spermatozoa have consisted of milk, egg yolk, various sugars, electrolytes, and glycerol.[10,44] Valid conclusions cannot be drawn by comparing data from two or more of these studies, because of confounding influences of stallion, packaging system, cooling and warming rates, and the subjective nature of visual evaluations of post-thaw sperm motility.

Japanese scientists have published numerous reports in which one of two glucose-lactose-egg yolk extenders was used.[50–52,66] The composition is provided elsewhere.[10,44] Although 2 to 5% egg yolk apparently was conventionally used in this extender, as little as 0.5% can be used.[52]

Many current procedures[32,44,48,59–61,65,67–69] are based on those described by Martin and Klug[70] and Martin et al.,[71] which, in turn, were derived from earlier research in Germany, Japan, and Russia. With their procedure,[70] and slight modifications by others,[68] a solution rich in glucose or sodium citrate dihydrate, but devoid of egg yolk, is used for initial dilution and centrifugation of semen. Centrifugation is necessary to enable resuspension of spermatozoa into a freezing extender at a concentration sufficiently high to enable packaging all spermatozoa for one insemination dose in an individual 0.5- or 4.0-mL plastic straw. Compositions of the glucose-ethylenediaminetetraacetic acid (EDTA) solution[71] and a citrate-EDTA solution serving the same function[68] are presented in Table 83–3.

Detailed procedures for preparation of these solutions and centrifugation have been presented.[67] After centrifugation at ≤400 g for 15 min, the concentrated spermatozoa should form a loose pellet, which can be easily resuspended (by swirling) in a freezing extender (Table 83–4) rich in lactose and containing EDTA, sodium bicarbonate, egg yolk, glycerol, and a small amount of a detergent (Equex STM, Nova Chemical Sales, Scituate, MA). The detergent probably alters interactions between lipoproteins in the egg yolk and the plasma membrane of spermatozoa.

Scientists in Eastern Europe use a similar extender for freezing, containing less than 5% egg yolk,[58,72–79] but have found[78,79] that substitution of mannitol for a portion of the lactose (Table 83–5) improved the percentage of motile spermatozoa after freezing and thawing (M. Tischner, personal communication). Although not reflected in publications summarizing older data,[58] an extender containing mannitol came into routine use in Poland and Czechoslovakia (M. Tischner, personal communication; and Z. Müller, personal communication) and probably in Russia.

Recognizing that centrifugation may be deleterious to stallion spermatozoa, an open artificial vagina[80] has been used to collect the sperm-rich fraction of semen.[77,81] Semen collected by this procedure is sufficiently concentrated (300 to 500 million spermatozoa per milliliter) so that semen can be extended without centrifugation, provided each insemination dose is prepared using 10 to 15 mL extender; this is a serious disadvantage with respect to storage. However, collection of only a sperm-rich fraction reduces the quantity of

TABLE 83–3. COMPOSITIONS OF THE CITRATE-EDTA CENTRIFUGATION MEDIUM AND THE GLUCOSE-EDTA SOLUTION USED DURING CENTRIFUGATION AND FOR PREPARATION OF FREEZING EXTENDER

COMPONENT	CITRATE-EDTA*	GLUCOSE-EDTA*
Glucose (g)	1.500	59.985
Sodium citrate dihydrate (g)	25.950	3.700
Disodium-EDTA (g)	3.699	3.699
Sodium bicarbonate (g)	1.200	1.200
Polymyxin B sulfate (IU)		10^6
pH	6.89	6.59
mOsm/kg	290	409

*Dilute to 1000 mL with deionized water.

(From Cochran, J.D., Amann, R.P, Froman, D.P., and Pickett, B.W.: Effects of centrifugation, glycerol level, cooling to 5° C, freezing rate and thawing rate on the post-thaw motility of equine sperm. Theriogenology, *22*:25–38, 1984.)

TABLE 83–4. COMPOSITION OF LACTOSE-EDTA-EGG YOLK FREEZING EXTENDER

Lactose solution (11% w:v) (mL)	50
Glucose-EDTA solution (Table 83-3) (mL)	25
Egg yolk (mL)	20
Glycerol (mL)	5
Equex STM (mL)	0.5

(From Cochran, J.D., Amann, R.P., Froman, D.P., and Pickett, B.W.: Effects of centrifugation, glycerol level, cooling to 5° C, freezing rate and thawing rate on the post-thaw motility of equine sperm. Theriogenology, *22*:25–38, 1984.)

TABLE 83–5. COMPOSITION OF FREEZING EXTENDERS USED IN EASTERN EUROPE

	ORIGINAL*	MODIFIED
Lactose (g)	11.0	6.6
Mannitol (g)	—	2.1
Glucose (g)	—	0.7
Disodium-EDTA (g)	0.1	0.15
Sodium citrate dihydrate (g)	0.089	0.16
Sodium bicarbonate (g)	0.008	0.015
Deionized water (mL)	100	100
Egg yolk (g)	1.6	2.5
Glycerol (mL)	3.5	3.5

*This extender also contained 50 IU penicillin and 50 mg streptomycin/100 mL of extender.

(Data from Tischner, M.: Evaluation of deep-frozen semen in stallions. J. Reprod. Fertil. Suppl., *27*:53–59, 1979; Naumenkov, A., and Romankova, N.: An improved semen diluent. Anim. Breed. Abstr., *49*:742, 1981; and Naumenkov, A.I., and Romankova, N.K.: Improving diluent composition and handling for stallion semen. Anim. Breed. Abstr., *51*:801, 1983.)

potentially deleterious seminal plasma in the ejaculate.

Extenders consisting of mixtures of skim milk or ultrahigh temperature sterilized milk, egg yolk, and nonelectrolytes have been used successfully for freezing stallion spermatozoa[63] (E. Palmer, personal communication). Extender without glycerol (Table 83–6) is used to dilute semen one part to four. The extended semen is cooled to 4° C over 1 h, then centrifuged. Spermatozoa are resuspended in a similar extender containing 2.5% glycerol, packaged in 0.5-mL straws and frozen. In contrast to the procedure developed at Colorado State University,[67,68] the contents of eight straws must be thawed and pooled to provide one insemination dose, which is inconvenient.

An extender containing sucrose has been used for freezing stallion spermatozoa in three northeastern provinces of China[82] (W.-Y. He, personal communication). Semen is diluted one to one with a solution of 11% sucrose in water and centrifuged gently (possibly 350 to 450 g) for 12 min at 20° C. The conditions of centrifugation (i.e., gravitational force and time) are adjusted for each stallion so no decrease in percentage of motile spermatozoa occurs as a consequence of centrifugation. After aspirating the supernatant, a volume of freezing extender equal to that of the loose pellet of spermatozoa is added. The freezing extender consists of 100 mL 11% sucrose solution, 45 mL skim milk, 16 mL egg yolk, and 6 mL glycerol (10% glycerol for donkey spermatozoa).[82] Apparently, starting in 1987 or 1988, semen extended as above was frozen in pellets[82] (R.P. Amann, personal observation). Initially, however, 1.0 mL extended semen at 20° C was pipetted into a 3-mL vial (W.-Y. He, personal communication). The open vials were placed in a refrigerator for about 30 min to lower the temperature to near 5° C. The vials, without being sealed, were frozen in liquid nitrogen vapor. Each dose of frozen semen was thawed by placing the pellets or open vial into 20 mL of a sucrose-milk solution at 42° C, which was prepared with 6.0 g sucrose, 3.4 g powdered skim milk, and 100 mL distilled water. As the semen thawed, spermatozoa were mixed with the thawing solution. The thawing solution was considered important.

TABLE 83–6. COMPOSITION OF A MILK EXTENDER USED IN FRANCE

Sterile skim milk (mL)*		50
Solution of salts and sugars (mL)*		50
Glucose (g)	2.5	
Lactose (g)	0.15	
Raffinose (g)	0.15	
Sodium citrate dihydrate (g)	0.03	
Potassium citrate (g)	0.04	
Water to make 50 mL		
Egg yolk (%)†		2.0
Glycerol (%)†		2.5

*Mix the skim milk and salt and sugar solutions one to one. The extender also contained approximately 5.0 mg gentamicin and 5000 IU penicillin.

†Mix 95.5 mL skim milk, salts, and sugars mixture with 2.0 mL egg yolk and 2.5 mL glycerol for the freezing extender.

(E. Palmer, personal communication.)

GLYCEROL

Glycerol is the penetrating cryoprotectant of choice when freezing stallion semen, but a sugar often is used in addition. Spermatozoa need not be exposed to glycerol for more than a few seconds before lowering the temperature.[5,83] Although glycerol rapidly enters spermatozoa, the main effect of glycerol probably is extracellular. This is supported by the observation that removal of glycerol from the medium surrounding spermatozoa lowers survival as compared with samples from which glycerol was not removed just before freezing.[50] However, these results were confounded by failure to centrifuge the control samples, and problems were also inherent in studies, with molecules rapidly crossing the plasma membrane.

Nagase et al. reported that an equilibration time of 3 to 5 h was desirable.[84] In contrast, exposure of spermatozoa to glycerol for a few seconds was equivalent to exposure for 15, 90, or 150 min when stallion spermatozoa were extended in a glucose-skim milk or a glucose-egg yolk extender and frozen in ampules.[85] Furthermore, exposure of spermatozoa, subsequently frozen in 1-mL plastic straws, to glycerol for less than 0.5 min was as effective as exposure for 2 to 3 min or 1 to 4 h, in terms of percentage of motile spermatozoa after thawing.[50,52,86] Nishikawa reported adequate fertility for stallion spermatozoa extended in a complex sugar and salt extender, containing 0.5 to 2% egg yolk, when spermatozoa were exposed to a final concentration of 10% glycerol for only a few seconds before freezing in liquid nitrogen vapor.[66] Although control data were not presented, 14 of 24 mares became pregnant. Similarly, Tischner reported that 17 of 52 mares conceived with semen frozen after equilibration of only 20 to 30 s.[87]

Nishikawa et al. reported that 5% glycerol was better than 0%, 1%, or 3% for semen in a glucose-lactose extender containing 2 to 8% egg yolk and packaged in 1-mL straws.[49,50,86] Use of 3 or 5% egg yolk was superior to 0.1%, 0.5%, or 1.0%. For semen frozen in 4-mL straws, it was found that post-thaw motility of spermatozoa and acrosin activity were higher when the extender contained 3 or 5% glycerol rather than 1%.[88]

Cochran et al. used a factorially designed experiment and 12 ejaculates to study the effects of glycerol concentration, freezing rate, and thawing temperature on motility of spermatozoa at four intervals after thawing of semen processed in 0.5-mL straws.[68] Compositions of the extenders were similar to that presented in Table 83–4. Although freezing rate did not significantly affect post-thaw sperm motility, 4% glycerol was better ($p < 0.05$) than 2 or 6% when the extender contained 20% egg yolk. Researchers have confirmed that percentage of progressively motile spermatozoa after freezing and thawing was higher for a 20% egg yolk extender containing 4 rather than 2% glycerol.[89]

For clarified extenders, use of 20 or 16% egg yolk was superior to 12%, and 4% glycerol was superior to 2%, but not 3%.[89] An interaction between concentrations of egg yolk and glycerol was not detected. Other data[61,68] support the conclusion that 4% glycerol is appropriate and superior to 2% for semen extended and processed by the method outlined by Amann and Pickett.[67]

Because addition of glycerol to extenders for stallion semen has been shown to be detrimental to fertility,[26,46] the amount to include in an extender is a trade-off between the minimal amount necessary to provide protection during freezing and thawing and the maximal concentration that is not detrimental to fertility. This is exemplified by data for ram spermatozoa.[29] A 52% lambing rate was achieved with ram spermatozoa frozen without glycerol. At least for ram spermatozoa processed by one specific procedure and used for intracervical insemination, the beneficial and contraceptive effects of glycerol were offsetting.[15,29]

CENTRIFUGATION

For semen packaged in 0.5-, 1.0-, or 4.0-mL plastic straws, as well as in 1.0-mL vials, centrifugation of semen is a routine part of the processing procedure, although centrifugation can be eliminated by collection of spermatozoa in a sperm-rich fraction.[77,81,90] Concentration of spermatozoa, regardless of method used, achieves two purposes: (1) elimination of much or virtually all seminal plasma and (2) provision of a suspension with a high concentration of spermatozoa. Seminal plasma was deleterious to stallion spermatozoa,[36,62,91] and removal of seminal plasma before cryopreservation was beneficial.[50,52,66,71,85,92] Concentration of spermatozoa is essential to permit packaging of semen for one insemination dose in a single package of reasonable size. Placement of the entire insemination dose in a small-volume, single-dose package is convenient in the field, eliminates the possibility of mixing semen from other stallions, and enables use of equipment for processing and storage that has been developed for cattle. Therefore, centrifugation appears a likely choice. Unfortunately, centrifugation is not innocuous,[93–96] although deleterious effects can be minimized by using a low centrifugal force[52,57,96] or diluting stallion semen before centrifugation[50,52,56,57,71,97] (W.-Y. He, personal communication). Even under ideal conditions, some damage is induced[36] (W.-Y. He, personal communication), although spermatozoa from certain stallions may be excessively damaged.[59]

In an early report, raw semen was layered on top of extender to allow centrifugal separation of spermatozoa from seminal plasma.[92] Since then, a range of dilutions and variety of media have been used when centrifuging stallion semen. These include a one-to-one dilution with a mixture of 5% glucose and 5% egg yolk;[56] a sugar and egg yolk solution;[92] a four-to-one dilution with a solution of 5.6% glucose;[85] a seven-to-three dilution with a mixture of electrolytes, sugars, and egg yolk (Table 83–3);[50–52,66] a solution containing EDTA and rich in glucose;[71] and a dilution to 50 million spermatozoa per milliliter with a solution containing EDTA and rich in sodium citrate (Table 83–3).[68]

Motility of stallion spermatozoa improved between 0 and 40 min after centrifugation (Fig. 83–1).[68] This improvement, 30 to 40 min after centrifugation, probably reflected recovery during incubation from transient damage caused by centrifugation. Note, however, that percentage of motile spermatozoa was still less than in raw semen. In many reports it is impossible to determine if a variable interval after centrifugation may have confounded interpretation of data, and often effects of centrifugation and other processing steps cannot be isolated.

Martin et al. compared post-thaw motility of spermatozoa centrifuged as raw semen or after one-to-one dilution with a glucose-EDTA solution[71] (Table 83–3). A higher percentage of spermatozoa was progressively motile after centrifugation of extended semen. After semiquantitative measurements of acrosin activity, Vieria et al. concluded that centrifugation by the procedure of Martin et al. did not induce damage to the acrosome, although percentage of spermatozoa with maximal acrosin activity was about 25% less in frozen-thawed samples.[98] Baumgartl et al. used transmission electron and light microscopy to study plasma membrane and acrosomal damage associated with centrifugation.[94] They concluded that even using the procedure

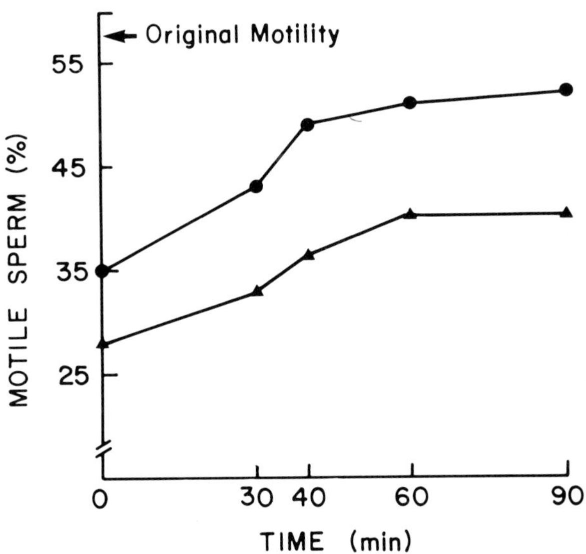

FIG. 83–1. Recovery of sperm motility after centrifugation with procedures A (circles) and B (triangles). Procedure A: semen was diluted one to one with glucose-EDTA at 37° C and incubated for 5 min at 37° C; centrifugation was 650 g for 15 min. Procedure B: semen was diluted to 50 × 10^6 spermatozoa/mL with 20° C citrate-EDTA. A 0.25-mL glucose-EDTA cushion was placed beneath the sperm suspension. Centrifugation was at 400 g for 15 min. (From Cochran, J.D., Amann, R.P., Froman, D.P., and Pickett, B.W.: Effects of centrifugation, glycerol level, cooling to 5° C, freezing rate and thawing rate on the post-thaw motility of equine sperm. Theriogenology, *22:*25–38, 1984.)

of Martin et al.,[71] dilution and centrifugation induced irreversible damage. Researchers at Colorado State University concluded that dilution with a citrate-EDTA solution (Table 83–3) was preferable to dilution with glucose-EDTA.[68] Although 15- or 50-mL centrifuge tubes are conventionally used, other scientists have reported that use of 10-mL tubes reduced sperm damage during centrifugation (W.-Y. He, personal communication). From recent data, centrifugation in clarified French extender (Table 83–6), without glycerol, appears to be a useful alternative approach (D.J. Jasko and J.K. Graham, personal communication).

Regardless of the medium used, all investigators are in agreement that minimum gravitational force necessary to pellet the majority of spermatozoa in 10 or 15 min is desirable to minimize damage to spermatozoa. Ideally, percentage of motile spermatozoa after centrifugation should be similar to that before centrifugation. When percentage of motile spermatozoa after centrifugation is significantly reduced, gravitational force, duration of centrifugation, or diluting medium should be altered.

Generally, spermatozoa have been mixed with a diluent before centrifugation and allowed to sediment to the bottom of the centrifuge tube. Cochran et al. introduced the concept of placing 0.25 mL of a dense glucose solution at the bottom of the centrifuge tube to serve as a "cushion" possibly to minimize damage to spermatozoa as they were sedimented.[68] Based on data for 11 split ejaculates, they concluded that a higher percentage of spermatozoa was progressively motile after centrifugation in aliquots diluted with a low viscosity citrate-EDTA medium and centrifuged using a cushion of glucose-EDTA than after simple dilution with glucose-EDTA and centrifugation (46 vs. 35% motile spermatozoa) (Fig. 83–1). However, based on motility of spermatozoa after freezing and thawing, Volkmann and van Zyl concluded that it was unnecessary to include a cushion at the bottom of the centrifuge tube.[48]

More recently we found (A.T. Francl and R.P. Amann, unpublished data) that regular egg yolk–containing extender (Table 83–4), without or with glycerol, provided a cushion equally as effective as the glucose solution suggested by Cochran et al.[68] As reported elsewhere, effects of concentrations of lactose (4.5 to 6.5%) and glycerol (0 or 4%) on percentage of motile spermatozoa after centrifugation were not significant nor was the interaction of these two main variables.[44] In a second study, it was concluded (also A.T. Francl and R.P. Amann, unpublished data) that use of 4% glycerol in the cushion and freezing extender may be optimum.[44] Use of regular freezing extender, rather than a glucose cushion, eliminates one source of variation (ratio of glucose solution to freezing extender) when processing semen using the method described by Amann and Pickett.[67]

There apparently is only one experiment that evaluated fertility of equine spermatozoa subjected to all steps associated with cryopreservation except actual freezing and thawing.[99] Semen from two stallions was processed for freezing, including centrifugation, and used to breed mares for attempted recovery of embryos. Control semen was extended in heated skim milk at 37° C and used to breed mares immediately. Processed semen from the same ejaculates was centrifuged in glucose-EDTA and extended in lactose-EDTA as if it were to be frozen, although it was not, and then used to breed mares. A nonsignificant difference was noted in embryo recovery of 24 percentage units between treatments in favor of the control semen (Table 83–7). Again, a substantial difference between stallions in response of their spermatozoa to processing for freezing was observed.

PACKAGING SYSTEMS

Several packaging systems have been used for freezing stallion spermatozoa.[44] Initially, glass ampules or vials were used, and ranged in volume from 1 to 10 mL or more. Plastic bags (5 × 15 cm) also have been used.[100] For some years, the potential benefits of pelleted semen were evaluated. Pelleted semen is prepared by placing small drops of extended semen into slight depressions in a block of solid carbon dioxide or a metal plate cooled below −75° C. Although pellets offer the advantage of rapid cooling rates, identification of individual pellets is impossible and some transfer of spermatozoa from one pellet to another can occur.[101,102] Both pellets and vials containing 1 mL of extended semen are used in China (W.-Y. He, personal communication and R.P. Amann, personal observation). Elsewhere, 0.5-, 1.0-, or 4.0-mL plastic straws and special 15-mL aluminum packets are used currently (Fig. 83–2).

Pace and Sullivan compared pregnancy rates obtained using semen processed in one of six extenders and frozen as pellets or in 10-mL glass ampules.[46] A significant interaction between extender and package on pregnancy rate was found. Overall, pregnancy rates were 36% for semen in pellets and 44% for semen in 10-mL ampules (n = 90 mares/package). Apparently the only fertility trials comparing semen processed as pellets or in straws were reported by Aliev.[72,103] He reported pregnancy rates, using pellets and 10-mL polypropylene straws, of 55 and 53% in one study and

TABLE 83–7. EMBRYO RECOVERY RATES FROM PROCESSED AND UNPROCESSED SEMEN

Stallion	Cycles	EMBRYO RECOVERY (%)* Control	Processed	Processed as (%) Control
480	13	69	58	84
F02	12	75	38	51
	mean	72	48	67

*See text for details of the control and processed treatments. Embryos were recovered at 8.0 days.

(From Loomis, P.R.: Survival and fertility of frozen-thawed stallion spermatozoa. M.S. thesis. Fort Collins, Colorado State University, 1982.)

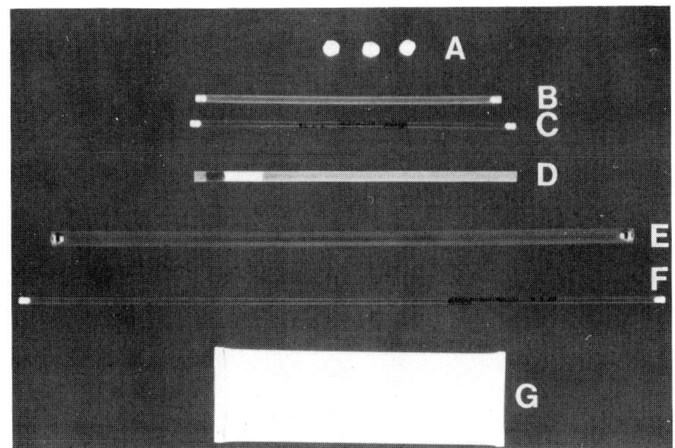

FIG. 83–2. Packaging systems for freezing stallion semen include (A) pellets, (B) 0.5-mL polypropylene straw, (C) 0.5-mL polyvinyl straw, (D) 1.0-mL plastic straw, (E) 4-mL maxitube, (F) long 1.0-mL polyvinylchloride straw of same diameter as 0.5-mL straw, and (G) 15-mL aluminum packet. (From Pickett, B.W., Squires, E.L., and McKinnon, A.O.: Procedures for Collection, Evaluation and Utilization of Stallion Semen for Artificial Insemination. Animal Reproduction Laboratory Bulletin No. 03. Fort Collins, Colorado State University, 1987.)

60 and 73% in another study. In total, 110 mares were inseminated with pellets and 90 with straws.

Other researchers used vinyl straws containing 1.0-mL.[49–52,57,66,86] Typically, each straw contained 150 to 300 million spermatozoa and semen from three to five straws was pooled after thawing in ice water and brought to 25 mL with HF-20 diluter (see composition elsewhere[10,44]) before use. Use of 0.5-mL plastic straws for stallion spermatozoa apparently was first reported by Veselinovic et al.[104] They diluted semen one to one and one to four with an extender containing 7% glycerol, 20% egg yolk, 1.3% fructose, 1.82% citric acid, and 3.03% TRIS at room temperature. Semen was frozen in straws in vapor over liquid nitrogen. After thawing at 39° C, semen was diluted to 25 mL with milk extender, and 300 to 400 million motile spermatozoa were used per insemination dose. Colorado workers (also A.T. Francl and R.P. Amann, unpublished data) have utilized this package extensively.[32,60,61,65,68,89] Volume of insemination dose has no effect on fertility.[44] Cochran et al. evaluated 1.0-mL plastic straws, identical in diameter to a 0.5-mL straw, but twice as long, and found no advantage based on motility or fertility of thawed spermatozoa.[59]

Aluminum packets, of flattened tubular material with a nontoxic lining, similar to a toothpaste tube, have been used in Russia and Europe[58,72,73,77,103,105,106] (M. Tischner, personal communication; and Z. Müller, personal communication). Similar packets have been evaluated in the United States.[81] The aluminum packet provides a container about 4 mm thick and 37 × 110 mm in width and length into which is placed 300 million motile spermatozoa in 15 mL of extender[58,73,77,81,105,106] (M. Tischner, personal communication; and Z. Müller, personal communication). The packet is sealed by folding over the ends several times (Fig. 83–2). The packets are held at 2° to 4° C or at 15° C for 90 min before freezing. Although the packets originally were laid on a grid about 1.5 cm above the surface of liquid nitrogen,[77] the packets of semen now are frozen in a slotted copper holder,[58,73,81] which is immersed about 1 cm in liquid nitrogen in a polystyrene box.

Fertility of semen frozen in aluminum packets, pellets, and 10-mL straws has been compared. Using split ejaculates from seven stallions, 1-cycle pregnancy rates of 53% were reported[105] for semen in 0.2-mL pellets and 62% for semen in aluminum packets (total of 117 mares). In two studies with 53 to 85 and 25 to 33 mares per treatment, semen in 10-mL straws, pellets, and aluminum packets provided pregnancy rates of 53%, 55%, and 47% and 73%, 60%, and 64%, respectively.[72,103] A study using spermatozoa from two stallions frozen in 4-mL plastic straws or aluminum packets revealed no significant difference in fertility associated with package.[81] Only the sperm-rich portion of each ejaculate was collected, so that centrifugation was unnecessary, and spermatozoa were extended in EDTA-lactose. Although sperm number per insemination dose favored aluminum packets (1.0 billion vs. 0.4 billion spermatozoa), 1-cycle pregnancy rates were not significantly different at 46% for spermatozoa in straws and 55% for spermatozoa in aluminum packets (26 and 20 cycles, respectively).[81]

COOLING AND WARMING RATES

Freezing rate has received little attention, perhaps because pelleted semen is difficult to measure or control, and for semen frozen in glass ampules or in 0.5-, 1.0- or 4.0-mL straws, freezing in vapor above liquid nitrogen is convenient and had proven to be successful with bull spermatozoa.[3] For semen frozen in ampules, two reports are divergent in their recommendations: Schafer and Baum recommended cooling from 6° to −79° C in 10 min (possibly 8° to 10° C/min),[107] whereas others used a slower cooling rate of 0.5° C/min to −20° C and then 3° C/min.[108] Semen frozen as 0.1-mL pellets presumably cool rapidly, probably in less than 3 min.[95] Krause and Grove reported that a temperature of −79° C was reached in less than 4 min.[109] For the aluminum packets, the cooling process required less than 7 min when the special copper holder was used.[73,106]

For semen frozen in 0.5-mL straws, Cochran et al.[68] and Cristanelli et al.[89] compared the post-thaw motility of spermatozoa cooled at about 60° C/min by placing straws horizontally in liquid nitrogen vapor at −160° C or at a controlled rate of 10° C/min from +20° to −15° C and 25° C/min thereafter (Fig. 83–3). In both studies, percentage of motile spermatozoa after thawing was not influenced by cooling rate. However, reported pregnancy rates of 30 and 72% for semen processed in thin-wall or thick-wall (0.3- and 0.8-mm) 10-mL polypro-

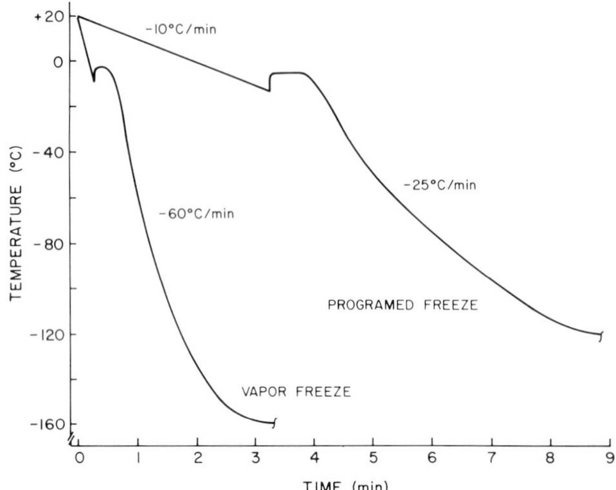

FIG. 83–3. Mean (n = 12) cooling curves for fast (vapor) and moderate (programmed) freezing rates. (From Cochran, J.D., Amann, R.P, Froman, D.P., and Pickett, B.W.: Effects of centrifugation, glycerol level, cooling to 5° C, freezing rate and thawing rate on the post-thaw motility of equine sperm. Theriogenology, *22:*25–38, 1984.)

pylene straws have been reported,[72] which may be evidence that rate of heat transfer was important.

Warming rate (thawing rate) conventionally is controlled by temperature of the water bath, package and duration of exposure to water (or diluent) of a given temperature. In addition, thermal characteristics of the package, distance to the middle of the frozen mass from the wall of the package and whether the water is stirred or quiet, influence warming rate.

Japanese investigators thawed semen packaged in 1-mL plastic straws[51,66] by immersing the straw in 4° C water for an unspecified interval. Semen in the flattened aluminum packets are thawed by immersion into 40° to 50° C water for 20 to 50 s.[58,73,77,81] Initially, researchers recommended that 4-mL plastic straws (macrotubes) be thawed by immersion into 50° C water for 40 or 45 s.[70,71] However, Vieira reported that thawing semen by immersing 4-mL plastic straws into 50° C water for 40, 50, or 60 s or in 60° C water for 30, 40, or 50 s had no significant influence on percentage of progressively motile spermatozoa after thawing or on percentage of spermatozoa that retained a high acrosin activity.[110] Thus, it was recommended to thaw semen frozen in 4-mL straws by immersion in 50° C water for 40 s.

In early research using 0.5-mL straws at our laboratory, semen was thawed by immersing a straw in 38° C water for 30 s.[59,61] This procedure is widely recommended for bovine spermatozoa and has been used[104] for equine spermatozoa frozen in 0.5-mL straws. Subsequently, Cochran et al.[68] compared the effects on motility of thawing semen processed by an older method[59,61] to a newer method by immersion of straws in 37° C water for 30 s or in 75° C water for exactly 7 s followed immediately by immersion in 37° C water for ≥ 5 s. They found that percentage of progressively motile spermatozoa was significantly higher when semen processed by the newer method was thawed by immersing 0.5-mL straws in 75° C rather than 37° C water (34 vs. 29% motile spermatozoa). Moreover, the warming rate was faster when semen had been processed in a polyvinylchloride straw than in a polypropylene straw (Fig. 83–4).[68] They stressed that although 7 s in 75° C water was appropriate for spermatozoa in a polyvinylchloride straw, a 10-s immersion was necessary for semen in a polypropylene straw. In both cases, time and temperature must be carefully controlled because a margin for error of only 1 s exists before the temperature exceeds 40° C,[67,68] which could be detrimental to pregnancy rates.

INFLUENCE OF SEASON

A goal of many interested in cryopreservation of stallion spermatozoa would be to collect and process semen during the nonbreeding season. During the nonbreed-

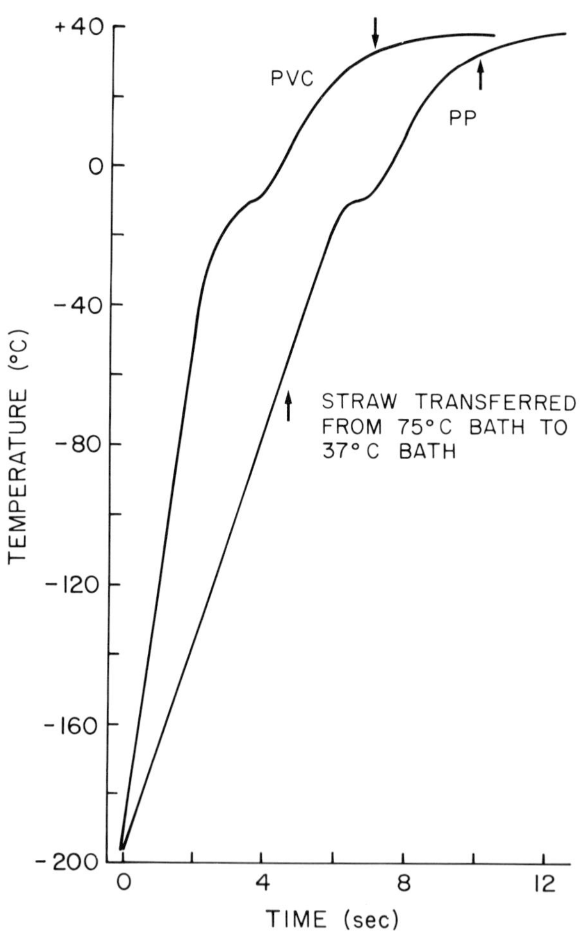

FIG. 83–4. Mean (n = 5) warming curves after transferring polyvinylchloride (PVC) and polypropylene (PP) straws from −196° C into a 75° C water bath. When the internal temperature reached 32° C, after 7 or 10 s (arrows), the straw was transferred to a 37° C water bath. (Adapted from Cochran, J.D., Amann, R.P., Froman, D.P., and Pickett, B.W.: Effects of centrifugation, glycerol level, cooling to 5° C, freezing rate and thawing rate on the post-thaw motility of equine sperm. Theriogenology, *22:*25–38, 1984.)

ing season, fewer spermatozoa can be collected for processing than can be obtained from the same stallion during the breeding season.[111,112] Originally, researchers were concerned that quality of semen cryopreserved in the nonbreeding season might not be equivalent to that processed from the same stallion during the breeding season. This probably is not the case.[44,63] (also A.T. Francl and R.P. Amann, unpublished data).

Some workers presented data on semen from four stallions that were collected in both the breeding and nonbreeding seasons.[52] For two stallions, a difference in percentage of motile spermatozoa after freezing and thawing was apparent, favoring the breeding season and for two stallions no obvious difference was noted. The researchers concluded that for some stallions, freezability of spermatozoa was slightly lower in the nonbreeding season than in the breeding season. Pregnancy rates, for two stallions from which semen was processed using 1.0-mL straws, in the breeding and nonbreeding seasons, were 70 and 62% for 33 and 40 mares, respectively.[51] They concluded that freezability and fertility of stallion spermatozoa were not greatly depressed for semen collected in the nonbreeding season.

Pickett et al. collected two ejaculates from each of five stallions about 1 h apart at weekly intervals for 13 months.[113] The percentage of progressively motile spermatozoa immediately after collection, for semen extended in a dried skim milk extender,[114] was not affected by month (season) or stallion. The semen was processed in a TRIS-based extender and frozen in 1-mL glass ampules, without centrifugation. No significant effect of month or stallion was noted on percentage of motile spermatozoa after freezing and thawing.

In other studies, semen was collected from seven stallions every other day, after depletion of epididymal sperm reserves, until eight ejaculates had been processed per month in the months of October 1984 and January, June, and October 1985.[10,44] Semen was collected and frozen using the procedures described by Cochran et al.[68] and stored at −196° C until about 2.5 months after the last samples were frozen. Samples were thawed and evaluated in a random order so that any bias toward season on the part of the observers would be eliminated. However, this introduced confounding of season with storage interval. Data from this study are summarized in Table 83–8. They concluded that no pronounced effect of season on post-thaw motility of stallion spermatozoa occurred.

Other workers studied initial quality and post-thaw motility of spermatozoa collected throughout the year from six stallions[63] (E. Palmer, personal communication). The percentage of motile spermatozoa in raw semen was higher in summer than in winter (Fig. 83–5). Surprisingly, the mean percentage of motile spermatozoa after thawing for semen collected and frozen during the summer was inferior to that for semen processed and frozen during the winter. They speculated that this was because seminal plasma was different in the summer.[63] However, the percentage of live spermatozoa with an intact acrosome, as evaluated using stained smears of spermatozoa, was highest in the summer. Differences associated with stallion were large. These workers concluded that quality of spermatozoa collected and frozen during the nonbreeding season was not inferior to that for semen collected during the breeding season and that a stallion whose semen freezes poorly would not provide better cryopreserved semen in a different season.[63]

In an early study, researchers found that percentage of second ejaculates freezing with $> 30\%$ progressively motile spermatozoa after dilution and centrifugation was less ($p < 0.05$) than for first ejaculates (66 vs. 97%).[61] Therefore, we recommend collection of one ejaculate every third or fourth day when semen is to be used for freezing. This procedure provides the maximum number of spermatozoa for processing and freezing in each collection.

INFLUENCE OF AGE OF STALLION

No convincing data exist to support or refute the concept that spermatozoa from young stallions (2 to 8 yr old) would be of higher quality after freezing and thawing, or of higher fertility, than spermatozoa from older stallions;[44] provided, of course, that motility and morphology of the spermatozoa are similar. Thus, to freeze semen from older stallions is cheaper and more effi-

TABLE 83–8. EFFECT OF SEASON OF COLLECTION AND PROCESSING ON SEMINAL CHARACTERISTICS AND POST-THAW SPERM MOTILITY*

MONTH OF COLLECTION	TOTAL SPERM/ EJACULATION (10^9)†	INITIAL MOTILITY (%)	MOTILITY (%) AFTER INCUBATION AT 37° C		
			0 h	1 h	2 h
October 1984	9.3 ± 0.7^{a}	$52 \pm 3^{a,b}$	35 ± 6^{a}	26 ± 5^{a}	13 ± 3^{a}
January 1985	9.1 ± 0.8^{a}	$54 \pm 4^{b,c}$	42 ± 4^{b}	34 ± 4^{b}	20 ± 3^{b}
June 1985	10.4 ± 0.6^{b}	51 ± 3^{a}	45 ± 4^{b}	40 ± 4^{c}	25 ± 3^{c}
October 1985	$10.2 \pm 0.7^{a,b}$	56 ± 2^{c}	43 ± 5^{b}	$36 \pm 4^{b,c}$	25 ± 3^{c}

*Mean (plus or minus standard error of the mean) number of spermatozoa in gel-free semen or percentage of motile spermatozoa for eight ejaculates from each of seven stallions.

†[a,b,c] Within a column, means with the same superscript do not differ ($p > 0.05$).

(From Amann, R.P., and Pickett, B.W.: Principles of cryopreservation and a review of cryopreservation of stallion spermatozoa. J. Equine Vet. Sci., *7*:145–173, 1987.)

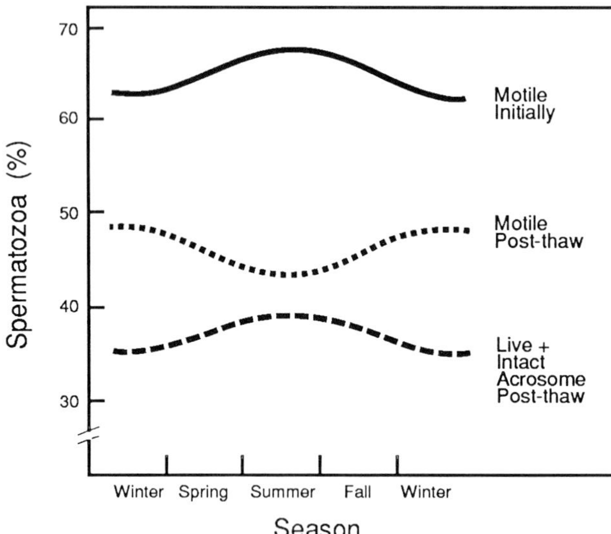

FIG. 83–5. Seasonal trends in quality of stallion spermatozoa before and after cryopreservation. (Adapted from Magistrini, M., Chanteloube, P., and Palmer, E.: Influence of season and frequency of ejaculation on production of stallion semen for freezing. J. Reprod. Fertil. Suppl., *35:*127–133, 1987.)

cient, because they generally have larger testes and ejaculate more spermatozoa with the same frequency of collection. However, the longer a stallion has lived, the greater the opportunity for that individual to have suffered an illness or injury that permanently affects his fertility. Therefore, as soon as a decision is made that an individual stallion has semen of sufficient value to be frozen, it should be done.

PREGNANCY RATES WITH CRYOPRESERVED SEMEN

Comparisons of pregnancy rates among breeding trials are invalid[10,14,45] because of (1) limited number of mares inseminated per stallion, (2) differences in number of spermatozoa per insemination dose, (3) timing of insemination(s) relative to ovulation, (4) frequent failure to stipulate number of estrous cycles per pregnancy, and (5) failure to provide data from control inseminations with fresh semen from the same stallions at the same time of year as inseminations were made with frozen semen. Several extensive early reports of pregnancy rates were made, but they do not include control data. Nishikawa and Shinomiya summarized data for semen processed in 1.0-mL straws between 1969 and 1975.[57] One to five stallions were used each year, and 359 mares were inseminated. After one to three inseminations, 65% of the mares became pregnant. Pelleted semen from one stallion was used to inseminate 105 mares between 1969 and 1979 and 61% became pregnant.[114] Based on data for 141 mares inseminated in 1982, with semen frozen in 4-mL straws, a one-cycle pregnancy rate of 22% and 45% for the breeding season was reported (E. Klug, personal communication).

In studies conducted at our laboratory (1981 through 1984), semen from 10 stallions was used in a manner that allowed direct comparisons between pregnancy rates with fresh and frozen semen,[44,59–61] but not among years. In general, stallions were selected on the basis of sexual interest and ejaculates with at least 50 million spermatozoa per milliliter of gel-free semen, of which at least 50% were progressively motile. Each year, semen from three stallions was collected every third day from late April to the end of June and frozen in 0.5- or 1.0-mL plastic straws of the same diameter. Seminal collections were continued every other day to provide fresh semen for control inseminations. Inseminations with fresh semen used 200 to 300 million spermatozoa in 10 mL skim milk extender,[115] whereas inseminations with thawed semen contained about 100 to 340 million motile spermatozoa based on sperm concentration in raw semen and evaluation of motility immediately after thawing.

One-cycle pregnancy rates, based on palpation per rectum on day 50 after ovulation, were significantly lower for mares inseminated with frozen than for fresh semen in 1981 and 1982 (Table 83–9). However, the difference between 56 and 65% in 1983 was not significant. Because procedures used for cryopreservation of spermatozoa were markedly different in 1983 than in previous years, this improvement was attributed[60] to changes in processing procedure.[68] However, when semen from three other stallions was processed by a similar procedure in 1984, the results were disappointing (30 vs. 75%).

For stallion 001 used in 1984 and stallion 002 used in 1982, one-cycle pregnancy rates using frozen semen were evidently unacceptable, even though stallion 001 was highly fertile (77%) and stallion 002 was reasonably fertile (40%) when fresh semen was used. Even allowing for the small numbers (Table 83–9), researchers noted that cryopreserved spermatozoa from these stallions was much less fertile than those from other stallions. Stallion 473 was used in 1981, 1982, and 1983. Although the actual one-cycle pregnancy rates achieved with his frozen semen were 47%, 33%, and 61%, respectively, this range probably does not represent significant differences from the results obtained with fresh semen.

Data were summarized for stallions selected because at least 40% of their spermatozoa in frozen-thawed samples were progressively motile when processed using procedures similar to those described[73,87] (M. Tischner, personal communication). Each insemination dose was prepared to contain 300 million progressively motile spermatozoa, based on initial seminal evaluation, in a volume of 12 to 18 mL. With semen from stallions whose spermatozoa were considered to freeze well and with insemination timed to ovulation, 28 of 55 mares became pregnant (51%) (M. Tischner, personal communication).

Müller (personal communication) used a procedure similar to that used in Poland. For semen that con-

TABLE 83–9. ONE-CYCLE PREGNANCY RATES AT 50 DAYS POSTOVULATION IN MARES AFTER INSEMINATION WITH FRESH OR FROZEN SEMEN*

		NUMBER OF CYCLES		PREGNANCY RATE (%)		
Year	Stallion	Fresh	Frozen	Fresh	Frozen	Fresh as Percentage of Frozen
1981†	466	17	16	71	19	27
	486	18	17	61	24	39
	473	18	15	67	47	70
	mean			*66*	*29*	*44*
1982‡	002	25	20	40	10	25
	473	26	24	62	33	53
	260	25	26	64	35	55
	mean			*55*	*27*	*49*
1983§	046	18	18	67	50	75
	303	18	18	67	56	84
	473	18	18	61	61	100
	mean			*65*	*56*	*86*
1984‖	001	13	13	77	8	10
	009	27	29	70	21	30
	298	29	27	79	48	61
	mean			*75*	*30*	*40*

*Except for 1983, the mean pregnancy rate for frozen semen was less ($p < 0.05$) than that for fresh semen. Comparisons among years are not completely valid because different processing procedures were used in 1981, 1982, and 1983; procedures in 1983 and 1984 were similar. Errors in the original publications of data for 1981 and 1982 have been corrected.

†Insemination doses for fresh and frozen semen were 250 and 100 to 130 × 10^6 progressively motile spermatozoa.

‡Insemination doses for fresh and frozen semen were 300 and 216 to 479 × 10^6 progressively motile spermatozoa.

§Insemination doses for fresh and frozen semen were 200 and 161 to 340 × 10^6 progressively motile spermatozoa.

‖Insemination doses for fresh and frozen semen were 200 and 219 to 365 × 10^6 progressively motile spermatozoa.

(From Amann, R.P., and Pickett, B.W.: Principles of cryopreservation and a review of cryopreservation of stallion spermatozoa. J. Equine Vet. Sci., *7*:145–173, 1987.)

tained at least 200 million progressively motile spermatozoa, and was inseminated when ovulation was imminent, 1-cycle pregnancy rates for three stallions were 43%, 36%, and 13%. An average of 2.2 inseminations per cycle was utilized. For 1981 through 1985, 1-cycle pregnancy rates with frozen semen were 63%, 49%, 64%, 55%, and 55% using semen from selected stallions. For the 5-yr study, 1-cycle pregnancy rates (first or second cycle) ranged from 32 to 51%, based on 69 to 413 cycles (56 to 331 mares).[58]

In another study, semen was diluted one to three immediately after collection with an extender containing skim milk, salts, sugars, and egg yolk[63] (E. Palmer, personal communication) (Table 83–6). Extended semen was cooled to 4° C over about 1 h and centrifuged. The sperm pellet was resuspended in extender containing 2.5% glycerol and packaged in 0.5-mL straws so that each straw contained 50 million spermatozoa. Only samples containing at least 35% progressively motile spermatozoa after thawing were used for insemination. For each insemination, eight straws were thawed simultaneously so that an insemination dose contained 400 million total spermatozoa. Mares were inseminated once every 48 h. The actual time of ovulation was determined by palpation per rectum. From 297 estrous cycles in which mares were inseminated 0 to 24 h before ovulation, 1-cycle pregnancy rate was 35% in contrast to 26% for 188 cycles in which the last insemination occurred 24 to 48 h before ovulation (E. Palmer, personal communication). Insemination once every 48 h, compared with once every 24 h, results in a 15% reduction of pregnancy rate, but allows insemination of twice as many mares and production of at least 1.5 times more offspring from a given stallion.

Limited pregnancy data exist for stallion semen frozen by a variety of procedures.[41,46–48,69,82] Although the numbers of stallions, ejaculates, and mares inseminated usually were limited, the results of these studies were similar to those previously discussed. In commercial operations, mares are inseminated by practicing veterinarians at various sites throughout a country. Loomis (personal communication) reported on use of semen imported from Hannover, Germany, and semen processed in Akin, South Carolina. The overall, one-cycle pregnancy rate for 116 mares inseminated 1983 through 1986 was 43%. An average of 2.3 inseminations per cycle was required in 1986 to achieve a one-cycle pregnancy rate of 45% (51 mares). One-cycle pregnancy rates from commercial use of frozen stallion semen in France in 1989 and 1990, involving 495 and 690 mares, were 38 and 40%, respectively. The number of doses of frozen semen used per pregnancy was 3.8 in 1989 and 3.9 in 1990 (A. Evain, personal communication).

TABLE 83–10. FERTILITY OF FROZEN SEMEN FROM INDIVIDUAL STALLIONS USED FOR COMMERCIAL ARTIFICIAL INSEMINATION IN FRANCE

STALLION	NUMBER OF MARES	NUMBER OF DOSES PER PREGNANCY	PREGNANT PER CYCLE (%)	PREGNANT ON OCTOBER 10 (%)
A	45	7	26	67
B	20	9	33	45
C	15	6	38	87
D	54	5	40	72
E	35	5	41	71
F	64	5	41	73
G	47	5	43	79
H	80	5	43	80
I	19	5	43	84
J	39	5	44	72
K	30	5	45	83
L	15	5	45	73
M	19	6	55	58
N	55	4	56	89
Others*	79	8	30	53

*Data for 11 other stallions whose semen was used to inseminate 2 to 14 mares, and whose apparent one-cycle pregnancy rate ranged from 11 to 75%.

(Adapted from data for 1990 provided by A. Evain of Equi-Technic, Falaise, France.)

One-cycle pregnancy rates for 25 stallions, which ranged from 11 to 75% are shown in Table 83–10. By the end of the breeding seasion, 22 to 89% of the mares bred to a stallion were pregnant. These results are similar to other data on variation in pregnancy ratės of individual stallions (Table 83–9). Age of mare apparently had little or no effect on pregnancy rate per cycle until it exceeded 15 yr old (Table 83–11). The range in pregnancy rates from 3 to 15 yr old was only 38 to 40%. However, pregnancy rate for the 273 mares 16 yr old or older was 34%.

Researchers use cryopreserved stallion spermatozoa in the three northeastern provinces of China[82] (W.-Y. He, personal communication, and R.P. Amann, personal observation). Semen is processed routinely during the nonbreeding, as well as the breeding, season using the procedures previously described. Semen from some stallions did not provide satisfactory pregnancy rates. Accurate detection of estrus is essential, and palpation of ovaries facilitates accurate timing of insemination. In 1979, the one-cycle pregnancy rate averaged 44% for 1,030 mares, which was about six percentage units lower than that obtained in the same region with fresh semen (W.-Y. He, personal communication). From 1980 through 1985, farmers in all three provinces of northeastern China have used frozen semen to inseminate a total of 110,000 mares. In 1985, frozen semen was used to inseminate 31,832 mares and a pregnancy rate of 68% was obtained for the season (W.-Y. He, personal communication). Piao and Wang reported insemination of 89,176 mares with a mean one-cycle pregnancy rate of 53%; 66% of the mares were pregnant by the end of the breeding season.[82]

TIMING OF INSEMINATION

Although mares have been inseminated daily or every other day starting on day 2 or 3 of estrus,[116] this approach requires relatively large quantities of semen. Inseminations timed by palpation of ovaries per rectum or ultrasonography should enable maximum pregnancy rates with minimum use of semen.

Pace and Sullivan extended semen in a TRIS-based diluent containing 7% glycerol and froze it in 10-mL ampules.[46] From a limited number of observations, they concluded that fertility was maximal if insemination was 0 to 12 h before ovulation, and that insemination 0 to 12 h after ovulation was somewhat lower. They also stated that insemination 12 to 36 h before ovulation was preferable to insemination 12 to 24 h after ovulation. Other investigators[117] found little difference in

TABLE 83–11. EFFECT OF AGE OF MARE ON PREGNANCY RATE WITH FROZEN SEMEN IN FRANCE

AGE	NUMBER OF MARES	PREGNANT PER CYCLE (%)
3	70	40
4	55	38
5–8	258	39
9–15	541	40
≥ 16	273	34

(Adapted from data for 1989 and 1990 provided by A. Evain of Equi-Technic, Falaise, France.)

pregnancy rates between mares inseminated 2 to 12 or 13 to 24 h after ovulation. However, that these studies were conducted before ultrasonography was a common technique to determine more precisely time of ovulation.

Aliev combined data for 198 cycles using semen processed as pellets, 10-mL straws, and aluminum packets.[103] For inseminations 2 to 12, 13 to 24, 25 to 36, and 37 to 48 h before ovulation, pregnancy rates were 62%, 72%, 33%, and 18%, respectively. Thus, pregnancy rate from inseminations within 24 h before ovulation was about twice that for inseminations 25 to 36 h before ovulation. Pregnancy rates of 35% for 0 to 24 and 26% for 24 to 48 h before ovulation (297 and 188 cycles, respectively) have been reported (E. Palmer, personal communication). Somewhat contradictory data were reported by Volkmann and van Zyl.[48] They obtained equal pregnancy rates of 55% when the last of one or two inseminations, using semen packaged in 0.5-mL straws, was 1 to 23 or 24 to 47 h before ovulation (49 and 20 cycles, respectively).

Other workers conducted a breeding trial to evaluate the effect of timing of insemination on fertility of mares bred with frozen-thawed semen.[118] Thirteen ejaculates were collected for the study, and none was discarded. Control mares were inseminated every other day during estrus, after detection of a 35-mm follicle, with 500×10^6 progressively motile spermatozoa in freshly extended semen. Frozen semen had been processed by the method of Martin et al.,[71] and each insemination dose contained 600×10^6 total spermatozoa per 4-mL straw. Two treatments were used to inseminate mares with frozen-thawed semen. They were (1) every other day during estrus after detection of a 35-mm follicle and (2) once within 6 h after ovulation. No significant difference was noted in pregnancy rates as a result of treatment (20 mares/treatment). A pregnancy rate of 70% was obtained with fresh semen and comparable inseminations every other day with frozen-thawed semen provided 60%. This treatment required 2.7 inseminations per cycle. Although insemination postovulation required only one insemination, the pregnancy rate was only 50%. Thus one must weigh the advantages of cost of semen versus number of examinations required to detect ovulation.

Considering all data from use of frozen semen,[46,48,80,103,117] maximal pregnancy rate on day ≥ 20 postovulation will likely be achieved when insemination(s) occurs 0 to 24 h before ovulation. A lower fertility might be anticipated if 24 to 36 h elapse between insemination and ovulation, although the difference may not be great. Insemination more than 6 h after ovulation will decrease fertility. The optimum time for insemination of frozen-thawed spermatozoa may include a shorter interval than if fresh semen or natural mating is used. Woods et al. presented comprehensive data on fertilization rate (embryonic vesicle detected by ultrasonography about day 12) for fresh semen.[119] Fertilization rates were similar for mares inseminated 1 to 3 days before ovulation (67% for 75 mares), and greater ($p < 0.06$) than for mares inseminated on the day of ovulation (52% for 94 mares) or the day after ovulation (6% for 70 mares). Although insemination of fresh semen 2 or 3 days before the day of ovulation need not suppress fertility with fresh semen, this procedure is not recommended with frozen semen. With frozen semen, we recommend insemination 0 to 24 h before ovulation.

EMBRYONIC DEATH

With cattle, no evidence exists that use of frozen semen resulted in a higher incidence of early embryonic death (i.e., between 3 and 60 days postovulation) than natural mating or insemination of fresh semen. However, some concern has been expressed that incidence of embryonic death might be greater in mares inseminated with frozen semen than mares inseminated with fresh semen.[120] Until the recent widespread use of ultrasonography to detect pregnancy as early as 12 or 15

TABLE 83–12. EMBRYONIC DEATH RATE BETWEEN DAYS 15 AND 50 AFTER OVULATION FOR MARES INSEMINATED WITH FRESH OR FROZEN SEMEN*

	NUMBER OF MARES PREGNANT DAY 15		NUMBER OF MARES PREGNANT DAY 50		EMBRYONIC DEATH (%)	
Year	Fresh	Frozen	Fresh	Frozen	Fresh	Frozen
1982	56	27	46	20	18	26
1983	40	36	35	30	13	17
1984	58	26	52	20	10	23
Total or mean	154	89	133	70	14	21

*Based on ultrasonography on day 15 after ovulation and palpation per rectum on day 50.

(From Pickett, B.W., Squires, E.L., and McKinnon, A.O.: Procedures for Collection, Evaluation and Utilization of Stallion Semen for Artificial Insemination. Animal Reproduction Laboratory Bulletin No. 03. Fort Collins, Colorado State University, 1987.)

days, to accurately evaluate early embryonic death was difficult.

In breeding trials conducted in 1982, 1983 and 1984, pregnancy status on day 15 was determined by ultrasonography. Data from the 3 yr are summarized in Table 83–12. For each year, and for pooled data, the apparent incidence of embryonic death was greater for mares inseminated with frozen semen than for those inseminated with fresh semen. Although relatively few embryos were involved, apparently embryonic death rate after inseminations with frozen semen might be about 1.5 times higher than obtained with fresh semen. This may be a consequence of altered sperm function resulting from cryopreservation or a consequence of attempting to minimize the interval between insemination and ovulation. The reason(s) for this difference, if it is real, are unknown. The timing of events during and after fertilization may be somehow altered by freezing and thawing or some component of the spermatozoon contributing to normal development of the embryo may be altered. Regardless of cause, the phenomenon may have similarities to the unusually high incidence of early embryonic death that occurs when spermatozoa from the proximal cauda epididymidis, rather than the distal cauda epididymidis or ejaculated semen, are used for artificial insemination of sheep, rabbits, and rats.[121,122]

The apparent high incidence of embryonic death may be a "natural" consequence of insemination near ovulation. Woods et al. studied embryonic death in 82 mares with an embryonic vesicle detected on day 12 to 14 postovulation.[119] For those inseminated before the day of ovulation, a 7% embryonic loss by day 20 was noted. However, for mares inseminated on the day of ovulation, embryonic death rate was 24%. Embryonic death rate was especially high (47%) in mares inseminated ≥ 12 h after ovulation. Time of insemination is unlikely to be the major cause of the apparently high embryonic death rate associated with use of frozen semen (Table 83–12), because timing of insemination was similar for control mares. Nevertheless, this factor cannot be ruled out. We speculate that when a fully satisfactory procedure is developed for cryopreservation of stallion spermatozoa, this difference in early embryonic death will disappear.

No procedure for cryopreservation allows spermatozoa from most stallions to achieve a pregnancy rate equal to that obtained with their fresh semen. With certain stallions, possibly 25% of those in a randomly selected population, acceptable pregnancy rates can be obtained. However, for another 30%, pregnancy rates achieved with cryopreserved spermatozoa will be extremely low.

Based on experience with cattle, selection against males whose semen does not freeze satisfactorily can lead to a gradual, but real, improvement in average pregnancy rate achieved with frozen semen. Thus, qualities of spermatozoa that enable satisfactory pregnancy rates after freezing and thawing are at least slightly heritable. Consequently, a breeder with a goal of utilizing frozen stallion semen would be advised to include among the criteria for selection of stallions the trait of sperm survival after freezing and thawing or fertility of cryopreserved spermatozoa. Obviously, this approach has limited applicability.

To assume that spermatozoa from all stallions should be frozen by the same procedure is unrealistic. At least for valuable animals, researchers want to optimize extender(s), cooling rate, and warming rate for each stallion. Although this would greatly increase cost of collection and processing ejaculates from a given stallion, this approach should be seriously considered to maximize fertility of a stallion where progeny would be valuable.

REFERENCES

1. Polge, C., Smith, A.U., and Parkes, A.S.: Revival of spermatozoa after vitrification and dehydration at low temperatures. Nature, *164*:666, 1949.
2. Smith, A.U., and Polge, C.: Survival of spermatozoa at low temperatures. Nature, *166*:668–669, 1950.
3. Pickett, B.W., and Berndtson, W.E.: Principles and techniques of freezing spermatozoa. *In* Physiology of Reproduction and Artificial Insemination of Cattle. 2nd ed. Edited by G.W. Salisbury, N.L. VanDemark, and J.R. Lodge. San Francisco, W.H. Freeman and Sons, 1978, pp. 494–554.
4. Watson, P.F.: The preservation of semen in mammals. *In* Oxford Reviews of Reproductive Biology. Vol. 1. Edited by C.A. Finn. Oxford, Clarendon Press, 1979, pp. 283–350.
5. Watson, P.F.: Artificial insemination and the production of semen. *In* Marshall's Physiology of Reproduction. Vol. 2. 4th ed. Edited by G.E. Lamming. London, 1990, pp. 747–869.
6. Barker, C.A.V., and Gandier, J.C.C.: Pregnancy in a mare resulted from frozen epididymal spermatozoa. Can. J. Comp. Med. Vet. Sci., *21*:47–51, 1957.
7. Watson, P.F.: The effects of cold shock on sperm cell membranes. *In* Effects of Low Temperatures on Biological Membranes. Edited by G.J. Morris and A. Clarke. London, Academic Press, 1981, pp. 189–218.
8. Watson, P.F., and Plummer, J.M.: The responses of boar sperm membranes to cold shock and cooling. Proceedings of the International Conference on Deep Freezing Boar Semen. Edited by L.A. Johnson and K. Larsson. Uppsala, Swedish University Agricultural Sciences, 1985, pp. 113–127.
9. Morris, G.J., and Watson, P.F.: Cold shock injury—A comprehensive bibliography. Cryoletters, *5*:352–372, 1984.
10. Amann, R.P., and Pickett, B.W.: Principles of cryopreservation and a review of cryopreservation of stallion spermatozoa. J. Equine Vet. Sci., *7*:145–173, 1987.
11. Hammerstedt, R.H., Graham, J.K., and Nolan, J.P.: Cryopreservation of mammalian sperm: What we ask them to survive. J. Androl., *11*:73–88, 1990.
12. Hammerstedt, R.H., and Graham, J.K.: Cryopreservation of poultry sperm: The enigma of glycerol. Cryobiology, *29*:26–38, 1992.
13. Mazur, P.: Basic concepts in freezing cells. Proceedings of the International Conference on Deep Freezing Boar

Semen. Edited by L.A. Johnson and K. Larsson. Uppsala, Swedish University Agricultural Sciences, 1985, pp. 91–111.

14. Amann, R.P.: Can the fertility potential of a seminal sample be predicted accurately? J. Androl., *10:*89–98, 1989.
15. Amann, R.P.: Pourquoi les spermatozoids de toutes les espèces ne donnent pas un taux élevé de fertilite après congélation? Contracept. Fertil. Sex, *19:*846–854, 1991.
16. Mazur, P.: Freezing of living cells: mechanisms and implications. Am. J. Physiol., *247:*C125–C142, 1984.
17. Mazur, P., and Cole, K.W.: Roles of unfrozen fraction, salt concentration and change in cell volumes in the survival of frozen human erythrocytes. Cryobiology, *26:*1–29, 1989.
18. Pegg, D.T., and Diaper, M.D.: The unfrozen fraction hypothesis of freezing injury to human erythrocytes: A critical examination of the evidence. Cryobiology, *26:*30–43, 1989.
19. Watson, P.F., and Duncan, A.E.: Effect of salt concentration and unfrozen water fraction on the viability of slowly frozen ram spermatozoa. Cryobiology, *25:*131–142, 1988.
20. Quinn, P.J.: A lipid-phase separation model of low-temperature damage to biological membranes. Cryobiology, *22:*128–146, 1985.
21. Koehler, J.K.: Sperm membranes: Segregated domains of structure and function. Proceedings of the International Conference on Deep Freezing Boar Semen. Edited by L.A. Johnson and K. Larsson. Uppsala, Swedish University Agricultural Sciences, 1985, pp. 37–60.
22. Fiser, P.S., Hansen, C., Underhill, K.L., and Shrestha, J.N.B.: The effect of induced ice nucleation (seeding) on the post-thaw motility and acrosomal integrity of boar spermatozoa. Anim. Reprod. Sci., *24:*293–304, 1991.
23. Crowe, J.H., Crowe, L.M., Carpenter, J.F., and Aurell, W.C.: Stabilization of dry phospholipid bilayers and proteins by sugars. Biochem. J., *242:*1–10, 1987.
24. Fahy, G.M.: The relevance of cryoprotectant "toxicity" to cryobiology. Cryobiology, *23:*1–13, 1986.
25. Fiser, P.S., and Fairfull, R.W.: The effects of rapid cooling (cold shock) of ram semen, photoperiod, and egg yolk in diluents on the survival of spermatozoa before and after freezing. Cryobiology, *23:*518–524, 1986.
26. Demick, D.S., Voss, J.L., and Pickett, B.W.: Effect of cooling, storage, glycerolization and spermatozoal number on equine fertility. J. Anim. Sci., *43:*633–637, 1976.
27. Jeyendran, R.S., Van der Ven, H.H., Perez-Pelaez, M., and Zaneveld, L.J.D.: Nonbeneficial effects of glycerol on the oocyte penetrating capacity of cryopreserved and incubated human spermatozoa. Cryobiology, *22:*434–437, 1985.
28. Fiser, P.S., and Fairfull, R.W.: Combined effect of glycerol concentration and cooling velocity on motility and acrosomal integrity of boar spermatozoa frozen in 0.5 ml straws. Mol. Reprod. Develop., *25:*123–132, 1990.
29. Abdelhakeam, A.A., Graham, E.F., and Vazquez, I.A.: Studies on the presence and absence of glycerol in unfrozen and frozen ram semen: Fertility trials and the effect of dilution methods on freezing ram semen in the absence of glycerol. Cryobiology, *28:*36–42, 1991.
30. Hammerstedt, R.H., Crichton, E.G., and Watson, P.F.: Comparative approach to sperm cryopreservation: Does cell shape and size influence cryosurvival? Proceedings of the Society of Theriogenology. San Diego, 1991, pp. 8–11.
31. Budworth, P.R., Amann, R.P., and Chapman, P.L.: Relationship between computerized measurements of motion of frozen-thawed bull sperm and fertility. J. Androl., *9:*41–54, 1988.
32. Blach, E.L., Amann, R.P., Bowen, R.A., and Frantz, D.: Changes in quality of stallion spermatozoa during cryopreservation: Plasma membrane integrity and motion characteristics. Theriogenology, *31:*283–298, 1989.
33. Amann, R.P.: Computerized evaluation of stallion spermatozoa. Proc. Am. Assoc. Equine Pract., 453–473, 1988.
34. Jasko, D.J., Lein, D.H., and Foote, R.H.: A comparison of two computer-automated semen analysis instruments for the evaluation of sperm motion characteristics in the stallion. J. Androl., *11:*453–459, 1990.
35. Varner, D.D., Vaughan, S.D., and Johnson, L.: Use of a computerized system for evaluation of equine spermatozoal motility. Am. J. Vet. Res., *52:*224–230, 1991.
36. Jasko, D.J., Moran, D.M., Farlin, M.E., and Squires, E.L.: Effect of seminal plasma dilution or removal on spermatozoal motion characteristics of cooled stallion semen. Theriogenology, *35:*1059–1067, 1991.
37. Cross, N.L., Morales, P., Overstreet, J.W., and Hanson, F.W.: Two simple methods for detecting acrosome-reacted human sperm. Gamete Res., *15:*213–226, 1986.
38. Blach, E.L., et al.: Use of a monoclonal antibody to evaluate integrity of the plasma membrane of stallion sperm. Gamete Res., *21:*233–241, 1988.
39. Graham, J.K., Kunze, E., and Hammerstedt, R.H.: Analysis of sperm cell viability, acrosomal integrity, and mitochondrial function using flow cytometry. Biol. Reprod., *43:*55–64, 1990.
40. Jeyendran, R.S., et al.: Development of an assay to assess the functional integrity of the human sperm membrane and its relationship to other semen characteristics. J. Reprod. Fertil., *70:*219–228, 1984.
41. Samper, J.C., Hellander, J.C., and Crabo, B.G.: Relationship between the fertility of fresh and frozen stallion semen and semen quality. J. Reprod. Fertil. Suppl., *44:*107–114, 1991.
42. Davis, A.P., Graham, J.K., and Foote, R.H.: Homospermic versus heterospermic insemination of zona-free hamster eggs to assess fertility of fluorochrome-labeled acrosome-reacted bull spermatozoa. Gamete Res., *17:*343–354, 1987.
43. Sullivan, J.J.: Characteristics and cryopreservation of stallion spermatozoa. Cryobiology, *15:*355–357, 1978.
44. Pickett, B.W., Squires, E.L., and McKinnon, A.O.: Procedures for Collection, Evaluation and Utilization of Stallion Semen for Artificial Insemination. Animal Reproduction Laboratory Bulletin No. 03. Fort Collins, Colorado State University, 1987.
45. Rousset, H., Chanteloube, P., Magistrini, M., and Palmer, E.: Assessment of fertility and semen evaluations of stallions. J. Reprod. Fertil. Suppl., *35:*25–31, 1987.
46. Pace, M.M., and Sullivan, J.J.: Effect of timing of insemination, numbers of spermatozoa and extender components on the pregnancy rate in mares inseminated with frozen stallion semen. J. Reprod. Fertil. Suppl., *23:*115–121, 1975.
47. Romankova, N.K., and Naumenkov, A.I.: Dosage of stallion semen. Anim. Breed. Abstr., *55:*753, 1987.
48. Volkmann, D.H., and van Zyl, D.: Fertility of stallion semen frozen in 0.5-ml straws. J. Reprod. Fertil. Suppl., *35:*143–148, 1987.
49. Nishikawa, Y., Waide, Y., and Shinomiya, S.: Studies on deep freezing of horse spermatozoa. Proceedings of the

International Congress on Animal Reproduction and Artificial Insemination. Vol. 2. 1968, 1589–1591.
50. Nishikawa, Y.: Motility and fertilizing ability of frozen horse spermatozoa. Proceedings of the International Symposium of Zootechnology. 1972, pp. 155–167.
51. Nishikawa, Y., and Shinomiya, S.: Freezability of horse semen collected during the non-breeding season. Proceedings of the International Congress on Animal Reproduction and Artificial Insemination. Vol. 2. 1972, 1539–1543.
52. Nishikawa, Y., and Shinomiya, S.: Our experimental results and methods of deep freezing of horse spermatozoa. International Congress on Animal Reproduction and Artificial Insemination. 1972, pp. 207–213.
53. Bader, H., and Mahler, R.: Tiefgefrier- und Besamungsversuche mit Hengstsperma unter Anwendung des Peletverfahrens. Zuchtygiene, *3:*6–13, 1968.
54. Klug, E., Treu, H., Hillmann, H., and Heinze, H.: Results of insemination of mares with fresh and frozen stallion semen. J. Reprod. Fertil. Suppl., *23:*107–110, 1975.
55. Nagase, H., and Tomizuka, T.: Studies on the freezing storage of horse semen. Effects of pellet freezing method on horse semen. Translated by H. Nagase. Annual Report of the National Institute of Animal Industry No. 15. Chiba-shi, 1976, pp. 133–164.
56. Oshida, H., et al.: Fertility of frozen stallion semen and some factors affecting to it. Proceedings of the International Congress on Animal Reproduction and Artificial Insemination. Vol. 2. 1968, pp. 1597–1599.
57. Nishikawa, Y., and Shinomiya, S.: Results of conception tests of frozen horse semen during the past ten years. Proceedings of the International Congress on Animal Reproduction and Artificial Insemination. Vol. 4. 1976, pp. 1034–1037.
58. Müller, Z.: Practicalities of insemination of mares with deep-frozen semen. J. Reprod. Fertil. Suppl., *35:*121–125, 1987.
59. Cochran, J.D., Amann, R.P., Squires, E.L., and Pickett, B.W.: Fertility of frozen-thawed stallion semen extended in lactose-EDTA-egg yolk extender and packaged in 1.0-ml straws. Theriogenology, *20:*735–741, 1983.
60. Cristanelli, M.J., Squires, E.L., Amann, R.P., and Pickett, B.W.: Fertility of stallion semen processed, frozen and thawed by a new procedure. Theriogenology, *22:*39–45, 1984.
61. Loomis, P.R., Amann, R.P., Squires, E.L., and Pickett, B.W.: Fertility of unfrozen and frozen stallion spermatozoa extended in EDTA-lactose-egg yolk and packaged in straws. J. Anim. Sci., *56:*687–693, 1983.
62. Corteel, J.M.: Effets du plasma seminal sur la survie et al fertilite des spermatozoides conserves in vitro. Reprod. Nutr. Dev., *20:*1111–1123, 1980.
63. Magistrini, M., Chanteloube, P., and Palmer, E.: Influence of season and frequency of ejaculation on production of stallion semen for freezing. J. Reprod. Fertil. Suppl., *35:*127–133, 1987.
64. Metz, K.W., Berger, T., and Clegg, E.D.: Adsorption of seminal plasma proteins by boar spermatozoa. Theriogenology, *34:*691–700, 1990.
65. Amann, R.P., Cristanelli, M.J., and Squires, E.L.: Proteins in stallion seminal plasma. J. Reprod. Fertil. Suppl., *35:*105–112, 1987.
66. Nishikawa, Y.: Studies on the preservation of raw and frozen horse semen. J. Reprod. Fertil. Suppl., *23:*99–104, 1975.
67. Amann, R.P., and Pickett, B.W.: An Overview of Frozen Equine Semen: Procedures for Thawing and Insemination of Frozen Equine Spermatozoa. Experiment Station Animal Reproduction Laboratory Special Series No. 33. Fort Collins, Colorado State University, 1984.
68. Cochran, J.D., Amann, R.P., Froman, D.P., and Pickett, B.W.: Effects of centrifugation, glycerol level, cooling to 5° C, freezing rate and thawing rate on the post-thaw motility of equine sperm. Theriogenology, *22:*25–38, 1984.
69. Håård, M.C., and Håård, M.G.H.: Successful commercial use of frozen stallion semen abroad. J. Reprod. Fertil. Suppl., *44:*647–648, 1991.
70. Martin, J.C., and Klug, E.: Konservierung von Hentstsperma in Kunstoffrohrchen. Anim. Breed. Abstr., *48:*9, 1980.
71. Martin, J.C., Klug, E., and Gunzel, A.R.: Centrifugation of stallion semen and its storage in large volume straws. J. Reprod. Fertil. Suppl., *27:*47–51, 1979.
72. Aliev, A.I.: A new method of freezing horse semen in polypropylene tubes. Anim. Breed. Abstr., *49:*805, 1981.
73. Müller, Z.: Fertility of frozen equine semen. J. Reprod. Fertil. Suppl., *32:*47–51, 1982.
74. Naumenkov, A.: Thawing semen. Anim. Breed. Abstr., *46:*497, 1978.
75. Naumenkov, A.I., and Romankova, N.K.: Improvement of method of long preservation of stallion sperm in deep freezing state. Proc. Fed. Eur. Zootechnol., 22–25, 1977. Cited by Müller and Rob; 117.
76. Naumenkov, A., and Romankova, N.: New composition of a semen diluent. Anim. Breed. Abstr., *49:*742, 1981.
77. Tischner, M.: Evaluation of deep-frozen semen in stallions. J. Reprod. Fertil. Suppl., *27:*53–59, 1979.
78. Naumenkov, A., and Romankova, N.: An improved semen diluent. Anim. Breed. Abstr., *49:*742, 1981.
79. Naumenkov, A.I., and Romankova, N.K.: Improving diluent composition and handling for stallion semen. Anim. Breed. Abstr., *51:*801, 1983.
80. Tischner, M., Kosiniak, K., and Bielanski, W.: Analysis of the pattern of ejaculation in stallions. J. Reprod. Fertil., *41:*329–335, 1974.
81. Love, C.C., et al.: Comparison of pregnancy rates achieved with frozen semen using two packaging methods. Theriogenology, *31:*613–622, 1989.
82. Piao, S., and Wang, Y.: A study on the technique of freezing concentrated semen of horses (donkeys) and the effect of insemination. Proceedings of the International Congress on Animal Reproduction and Artificial Insemination. Vol. 3. 1988, pp. 286a–286c.
83. Berndtson, W.E., and Foote, R.H.: Bovine sperm cell volume at various intervals after addition of glycerol at 5° C. Cryobiology, *9:*29–33, 1972.
84. Nagase, H., et al.: Studies on the freezing of stallion semen. II. Factors affecting survival rates of stallion spermatozoa after freezing and thawing and results of a fertility trial. Anim. Breed. Abstr., *35:*195, 1967.
85. Rajamannan, A.H.J., Zemjanis, R., and Ellery, J.: Freezing and fertility studies with stallion semen. Proceedings of the International Congress on Animal Reproduction and Artificial Insemination. Vol. 2. 1968, pp. 1601–1604.
86. Nishikawa, Y., Iritani, A., and Shinomiya, S.: Studies on the protective effects of egg yolk and glycerol on the freezability of horse sperm. Proceedings of the International Congress on Animal Reproduction and Artificial Insemination. Vol. 2. 1972, pp. 1545–1549.
87. Tischner, M.: Results of artificial insemination of horses in Poland in the post-war period. J. Reprod. Fertil. Suppl., *23:*111–114, 1975.

88. Oliveira, M.A.L.: Einfluss verschiedener Aufbereitungsverfahren auf Motilitat und Akrosinaktivitat in der Thermoresistenzprufung und auf das Befruchtungsergebnis von tiefgefrorenem Pferdesamen. DMV dissertation. Tierarztliche Hochschule Hannover, 1982.

89. Cristanelli, M.J., Amann, R.P., Squires, E.L., and Pickett, B.W.: Effects of egg yolk and glycerol levels in lactose-EDTA-egg yolk extender and of freezing rate on the motility of frozen-thawed stallion spermatozoa. Theriogenology, *24:*681–686, 1985.

90. Bader, H.: Zur Tiefgefrierung von Hengstsperma nach Pelletmethode. Proceedings of the Sixth International Congress on Animal Reproduction and Artificial Insemination. Vol. 2. 1968, pp. 985–988.

91. Nishikawa, Y., and Waide, Y.: Studies on the artificial insemination in horses. III. A new preservation method of the horse spermatozoa, so-called Bohen method. Jpn. J. Zootechnol. Sci., *20:*123–128, 1949.

92. Buell, J.R.: A method for freezing stallion semen and tests of its fertility. Vet. Rec., *75:*900–902, 1963.

93. Bader, H.: Weitere Erfahrungen uber die Tiefgefrierung von Hengstsperma. Zuchtygiene, *5:*87, 1970.

94. Baumgartl, C., Bader, H., Drommer, W., and Luning, I.: Ultrastructural alterations of stallion spermatozoa due to semen conservation. Proceedings of the International Congress of Animal Reproduction and Artificial Insemination. Vol. 5. 1980, pp. 134–137.

95. Hess, R., Schafer, W., Schmidt, D., and Baum, W.: Versuche zur Pelletierung von Hengstsperma. Fortpfl. Besam. Aufzucht Haust., *4:*207–214, 1968.

96. Pickett, B.W., et al.: Effect of centrifugation and seminal plasma on motility and fertility of stallion and bull spermatozoa. Fertil. Steril., *26:*167–174, 1975.

97. Oshida, H., et al.: Studies on the freezing of stallion semen. III. Pellet frozen semen preserved in liquid nitrogen. Anim. Breed. Abstr., *36:*387, 1968.

98. Vieira, R.C., Klug, E., and Rath, D.: Determination of acrosin activity using autoradiographic film plates as a control parameter for the different steps of deep-freezing stallion semen. Proceedings of the International Congress on Animal Reproduction and Artificial Insemination. Vol. 5. pp. 141–141.

99. Loomis, P.R.: Survival and fertility of frozen-thawed stallion spermatozoa. M.S. thesis. Colorado State University, 1982.

100. Ellery, J.C., Graham, E.F., and Zemjanis, R.: Artificial insemination of pony mares with semen frozen and stored in liquid nitrogen. Am. J. Vet. Res., *32:*1693–1698, 1971.

101. Merkt, H., Weitze, K.F., and Lorrmann, W.: Kapselpellets mit Deckel, eine Moglichkeit zur Vervollkommung der Pelletmethode bei der Tiefgefrierkonservierung von Bullensperma. DTW Dtsch. Tierarztl. Wochenschr., *74:*105–107, 1967.

102. Pickett, B.W., Berndtson, W.E., and Sullivan, J.J.: Influence of seminal additives and packaging systems on fertility of frozen bovine spermatozoa. J. Anim. Sci., *47 (Suppl. 2):*12–46, 1978.

103. Aliev, A.I.: The effect of Ovaritropin on reproductive function of mares, and the optimum time of insemination with frozen-thawed semen. Anim. Breed. Abstr., *49:*805, 1981.

104. Veselinovic, S., et al.: The results of application of the artificial fertilizing of mares by the use of deeply frozen semen taken from stallions in Vojvodina. Proceedings of the International Congress on Animal Reproduction and Artificial Insemination. Vol. 5. 1980, pp. 347–351.

105. Naumenkov, A., and Romankova, N.: Freezing stallion semen. Anim. Breed. Abstr., *47:*437, 1979.

106. Müller, Z., and Rob, O.: Vysledky inseminace klisen hluboce zmrazenym spermatem po spontanni a indukovane riji preparatem Alestrum inj. Spofa. Biol. Chem. Vet., *22:*259–264, 1986.

107. Schafer, W., and Baum, W.: Tiefgefrierung von Pferdsperma bei −79° C unter Verwendung von CO_2-Eis. Fortpfl. Besam. Aufzucht Haust., *1:*105–111, 1964.

108. Chao, T., and Chang, P.-H.: An experimental report of the low-temperature storage of stallion semen. Anim. Breed. Abstr., *32:*445, 1964.

109. Krause, D., and Grove, D.: Deep-freezing of jackass and stallion semen in concentrated pellet form. J. Reprod. Fertil., *14:*139–141, 1967.

110. Vieira, R.C.: Akrosinbestimmung an Pferdespermien unter Berucksichtigung bestimmter andrologischer Fragestellungen. DMV dissertation. Tierarztliche Hochschule Hannover, 1980.

111. Pickett, B.W., et al.: Reproductive physiology of the stallion. VI. Seminal and behavioral characteristics. J. Anim. Sci., *43:*617–625, 1976.

112. Clay, C.M., Squires, E.L., Amann, R.P., and Pickett, B.W.: Influences of season and artificial photoperiod on stallions: Testicular size, seminal characteristics and sexual behavior. J. Anim. Sci., *64:*517–525, 1987.

113. Pickett, B.W., Anderson, E.W., Roberts, A.D., and Voss, J.L.: Freezability of first and second ejaculates of stallion semen. Proceedings of the International Congress on Animal Reproduction and Artificial Insemination. Vol. 5. 1980, pp. 339–347.

114. Fomina, E.: Promising prospects for the storage of stallion semen. Anim. Breed Abstr., *48:*586, 1980.

115. Pickett, B.W., Burwash, L.D., Voss, J.L., and Back, D.G.: Effect of seminal extenders on equine fertility. J. Anim. Sci., *40:*1136–1143, 1975.

116. Voss, J.L., and Pickett, B.W.: Reproductive Management of the Broodmare. Experiment Station Animal Reproduction Laboratory General Series Bulletin No. 961. Fort Collins, Colorado State University, 1976.

117. Aliev, A., and Ochkin, D.: The optimum time of insemination. Anim. Breed. Abstr., *47:*576, 1979.

118. Kloppe, L.H., et al.: Effect of insemination timing on the fertilizing capacity of frozen/thawed equine spermatozoa. Theriogenology, *29:*429–439, 1988.

119. Woods, J., Bergfelt, D.R., and Ginther, O.J.: Effects of time of insemination relative to ovulation on pregnancy rate and embryonic-loss rate in mares. Equine Vet. J., *22:*410–415, 1990.

120. Baczynski, J., et al.: Artificial insemination of horses. IV. Preliminary results of inseminating mares with frozen semen. Anim. Breed. Abstr., *41:*432, 1973.

121. Fournier-Delpech, S., et al.: Epididymal sperm maturation in the ram: motility, fertilizing ability and embryonic survival after uterine artificial insemination in the ewe. Ann. Biol. Anim. Biochim. Biophys., *19:*597–605, 1979.

122. Orgebin-Crist, M.C., Danzo, B.J., and Davies, J.: Endocrine control of the development and maintenance of sperm fertilizing ability in the epididymis. *In* Handbook of Physiology. Section 7: Endocrinology. Vol. 5. Male Reproductive System. Edited by R.O. Greep and E.B. Astwood. Washington, D.C., American Physiological Society, 1975, pp. 319–338.

CHAPTER 84

ARTIFICIAL INSEMINATION

S.P. Brinsko
D.D. Varner

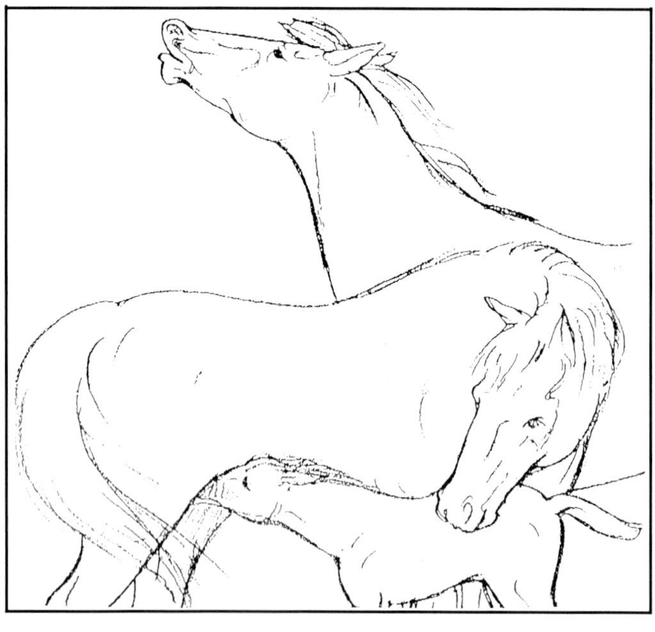

HISTORY

The first references to artificial insemination (AI) in the horse supposedly appeared in Arabic texts, and its use was reported as early as 1322. However, no evidence exists that the practice was widespread.[1] Documented scientific research in the use of artificial insemination was first reported by the Italian physiologist Spallanzani in the late 1700s, who initially investigated its use in the dog and later evaluated the procedure in horses, including the effect of cooling on equine spermatozoa.[1–3] Late in the nineteenth century, in a letter to Walter Heape, Dr. Pearson, a professor of veterinary medicine at the University of Pennsylvania stated that he and other veterinarians had successfully inseminated mares on a number of farms by artificial means.[1] European horses were first bred artificially in 1890 by the French veterinarian Repiquet who advised its use for overcoming infertility.[1,2] The supplemental use of AI following natural mating was recommended in the late 1800s by Professor Hoffman of Stuttgart. He gave a detailed description of his techniques and the instruments required.[1,2] Around the same time, Sand and Stribolt achieved four pregnancies after artificially inseminating eight mares.[1] At the 1902 Northern Livestock Conference in Copenhagen, Sand reported that the most important feature of AI was the economical use of semen from valuable stallions.

E.I. Ivanoff, the Russian investigator and leading pioneer in AI, was requested to investigate the use of AI in horse breeding by the chief of the Russian Stud in 1899.[1,2] Artificial insemination was employed at numerous studs, but the results were not consistently good. However, Ivanoff noted that when he performed the inseminations, or when they were performed under his supervision, pregnancy rates were somewhat higher than those obtained by natural service. In 1912, of 39 mares that were artificially inseminated at one Russian stud, 31 became pregnant, whereas only 10 pregnancies resulted from natural service of 23 mares.[1,2]

After World War I, a central station for experimental livestock breeding was established with Ivanoff as its director. Various investigators continued his work and developed an artificial vagina (AV) at Moscow's laboratory for AI in the 1930s.[1,2] By 1938, approximately 120,000 mares had been artificially inseminated in Russia. In other countries, AI techniques in horses also gained widespread use. A total of 323 mares were artificially inseminated in Japan between 1913 and 1917.[2] Approximately 600,000 mares were artificially inseminated in China in 1959 with an overall pregnancy rate of 61%. In 1960, semen from China's 2 most popular stallions was used to inseminate 4415 and 3093 mares with resulting pregnancy rates of 76.9 and 68.1%, respectively.[4]

In the United States, the Standardbred industry has employed widespread use of AI since the early 1950s. More than 25,000 Standardbred mares are artificially inseminated annually. Many other breed registries also allow the use of artificial insemination. In fact only three breed registries in the United States do not permit the use of artificial insemination. These are the Jockey Club (Thoroughbreds), the Standard Jack and Jennet Registry of America, and the American Miniature Horse Association. The breed registries which permit the use of AI vary considerably in their allowances and limitations regarding storage and transport of semen. The clinician should, therefore, be familiar with specific breed registry restrictions before instituting an AI program.

ADVANTAGES AND DISADVANTAGES

The use of AI in a breeding program provides numerous advantages over natural mating. Dividing an ejaculate into several insemination doses permits more efficient use of stallion semen. Several can be inseminated with a single ejaculate and the number of mares that are booked to a stallion per breeding season can be increased several fold. The addition of antibiotics to seminal extenders reduces venereal transmission of bacterial diseases to the mare where the stallion serves as a carrier. Transmission of potential pathogens from mare to stallion is also eliminated. Seminal extenders contain supportive and protective factors for spermatozoa and may improve pregnancy rates of some subfertile stallions. Artificial insemination can also be used to reinforce natural service in situations such as when a stallion may not be able to achieve full tumescence or penetration because of injury. In these instances, semen remaining in the vaginal vault after copulation can be aspirated into a syringe and then deposited in the mare's uterus via an insemination pipette. Using a breeding phantom for seminal collection greatly reduces the risk of breeding injuries. Seminal collection with an AV allows evaluation of seminal quality before insemination and assists in early detection of infertility problems in the stallion. The availability of stallion semen to mare owners is increased when extended semen can be preserved and transported from the site of collection.

A higher level of knowledge and skill are necessary for success in an AI program compared with those required for natural service. The cost of necessary equipment and supplies is also increased and the risk of human injury may be greater during the collection procedure. However, advantages gained through use of AI certainly outweigh these minor disadvantages.

SEMINAL COLLECTION

The seminal collection procedure is an essential part of the artificial insemination program. Facilities and equipment that permit safe and efficient collection and handling of the semen are mandatory for success. See Chapter 79 for detailed procedures of seminal collection for artificial insemination.

BREEDING SHED

A lighted, indoor breeding area is recommended for collection of stallion semen and AI of mares on a regular basis. This type of facility allows seminal collection and insemination to be done when it is dark and during inclement weather. Distractions the stallion may encounter during the collection procedures are reduced, and the facility provides an environment which the stallion consistently associates with breeding.

The breeding shed should provide adequate space (i.e., at least 120 to 153 m^2) so that breeding activities can proceed unimpeded. Ceiling and light fixture height should be a minimum of 3 to 4.5 m. The floor should provide good footing for the stallion during the breeding process whether it is wet or dry. A breeding phantom situated adjacent to a padded teasing rail will allow the stallion to remain in close proximity to an estrous mare while mounting the phantom for seminal collection.

An environmentally controlled laboratory should be in close proximity to the breeding area. The laboratory should be properly equipped for evaluation and processing of semen as well as preparation and maintenance of artificial vaginas.

ARTIFICIAL VAGINAS

When properly prepared and applied, using an AV with an in-line filter for seminal collection will yield consistent stallion performance and ejaculates of superior quality. The majority of stallions with average or above-average libido can be trained to use most artificial vaginas. A number of well-designed AVs are commercially available in the United States, each having distinct characteristics (Fig. 84–1). Factors to consider when purchasing an AV are its cost, maintenance requirements, ability to maintain temperature, potential for loss of spermatozoa, and ease of handling. Selection is based on personal preference and the specific requirements of the breeding program.

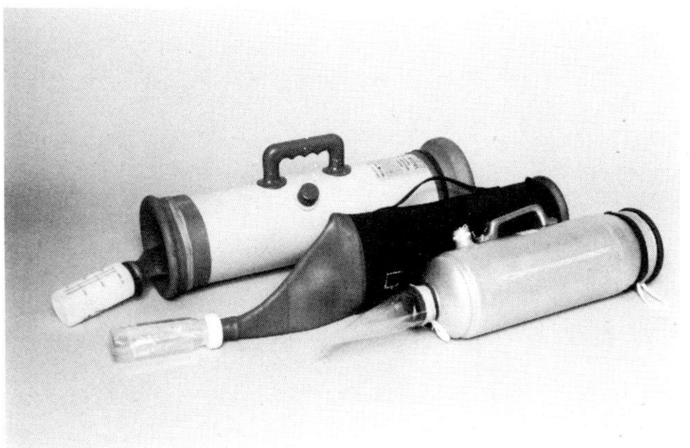

FIG. 84–1. Artificial vaginas (left to right): CSU Model, Missouri Model, and Japanese (Nishikawa) Model.

Proper preparation of an AV in regard to temperature and pressure for each stallion's preference will enhance consistent stallion performance. See Chapter 79 for preparation of the CSU Model AV; similar principles apply for other models. The preparation of the AV should be timed closely with teasing and washing of the stallion. If prepared too early the AV and seminal receptacle may cool to a less-than-satisfactory temperature and if prepared too late, the unnecessary delay can disrupt the breeding routine to which the stallion has become accustomed. Establishing and maintaining a consistent routine is important for maximizing stallion performance and the efficiency of the breeding procedure.

Artificial vaginas should be cleaned and disinfected after each use. All components which come into contact with semen must be nonspermicidal; therefore, reusable items must be chemically clean. Hot running water is usually sufficient to clean most AV liners but if the use of soap becomes necessary, it should be a nonresidual type such as Alconox (Alconox Inc., New York). Disinfectant solutions or soaps containing disinfectants (e.g., povidone-iodine or chlorhexidine) may damage spermatozoa. Povidone-iodine concentrations as low as 0.05% have been shown to render spermatozoa completely immotile within 1 min of contact.[5] After the liners have been cleaned and thoroughly rinsed with deionized water, they should be submerged in ethyl or isopropyl alcohol for 30 min and allowed to air dry in a dust-free cabinet. Gas sterilization with ethylene oxide can be used, provided that the liners are allowed to air out for 48 to 72 h before use. Sterile, nontoxic disposable liners are available, which fit most artificial vaginas. Disposable equipment simplifies cleaning and reduces risk of chemical contamination and horizontal transmission of disease with repeated use of the artificial vagina. Some stallions dislike the texture of these disposable liners and will not readily use the AV when the liners are in place.

If an AV is not available or a stallion resists using an AV, it may be necessary to use a condom for seminal collection. Novice stallions and those that are accustomed to breeding only by natural service are usually the most reluctant to use an artificial vagina. The use of a condom is a poor alternative to seminal collection in an AV, because the ejaculate is likely to be of inferior quality owing to excessive contamination with bacteria and debris. Often stallions that are reluctant to breed an AV will also not tolerate a condom. An increased risk also exists for human injury while applying the condom to a stallion's erect penis as well as in attempting its retrieval before penile detumescence.

PREPARATION OF THE STALLION

See Chapter 79 for details on preparing the stallion for seminal collection. Washing the stallion's penis with water alone reduces bacterial numbers about as effectively as washing with soap or antiseptic scrub.[6] Occasionally soap or antiseptic scrubs may be indicated for stallions that have accumulated an excessive amount of smegma or are known to harbor large numbers of pathogenic bacteria unrelated to overzealous washing procedures. The penis should be thoroughly rinsed after cleansing if this method is used, because soap residue has spermicidal properties.

Studies in the bull indicate that prolonged teasing and, in particular, false mounts before seminal collection will increase sperm output in ejaculates.[7] From existing information, no advantage has been found to sexually stimulating the stallion beyond the point necessary to achieve and maintain an erection. False mounts are likely to adversely effect ejaculations, stimulate excessive aggressiveness, and cause undesirable breeding habits in the stallion. Prolonged teasing will increase the total volume of the stallion's ejaculate but does not appear to increase spermatozoal number.[8,9]

MOUNT SOURCES

Live Mare

Either gonad-intact mares exhibiting behavioral estrus or ovariectomized mares can be used as a mount mare for seminal collection. Ovariectomized mares are generally more preferable for routine seminal collection because they are more predictable and can be used at any time. The degree of sexual receptivity exhibited while in estrus, as a gonad-intact mare, can be used to determine whether the mare will be an acceptable mount source after ovariectomy. Ovariectomized mares may, on occasions, require exogenous estrogen therapy (1 to 2 mg estradiol cypionate, IM) (ECP, Upjohn, Kalamazoo, MI) to augment signs of behavioral estrus. If the mare's behavior toward the approaching stallion is unknown or unpredictable, a relatively inexpensive or teaser stallion should be allowed to mount to see how the mare will react before permitting a more expensive stallion to mount her for seminal collection (see Chapter 79 for details on preparing the mount mare).

Breeding Phantom

Use of a breeding phantom will improve seminal collection for the majority of stallions. Most stallions will accept the breeding phantom as a sexual object and readily mount it with a minimal amount of training. Some stallions, especially novices, require an estrous mare to be in close proximity to the phantom before they will mount it; however, most experienced stallions will mount the phantom without the presence of an estrous mare.

Several advantages are obtained by using a breeding phantom in place of a live mount mare. Variability in the mount source is eliminated thereby providing more consistency in stallion performance during seminal collection. The risk of injury to the stallion is greatly reduced during the collection process as are injuries to the mare that can occur as a result of charging and biting habits of some stallions. The height of the phantom can be adjusted to meet the needs of different stallions. This attribute in conjunction with the phantom remaining stationary make it especially advantageous for collecting semen from stallions with rear limb or back problems that may limit their mobility.

GENERAL SEMEN HANDLING TECHNIQUES

Immediately after collection, semen should be quickly transported to the laboratory with minimal agitation, exposure to light, and cold shock. All materials, including the seminal extender, that will come into contact with the semen should be warmed to body temperature (37° C). If an in-line filter was not used during collection, semen should be poured through a nontoxic filter to remove the gel fraction and debris. The gel fraction can also be removed by careful aspiration with a syringe. Loss of spermatozoa tends to be greater using the latter two methods than using an in-line filter. A commercially available in-line, nylon, micromesh filter (Equine Semen Filter, Animal Reproduction Systems, Chino, CA) is preferred to minimize spermatozoal retention (loss) during filtration.[10] Spermatozoal concentration, volume and color of the gel-free semen, and percentage of progressively motile spermatozoa should be determined and recorded (see Chapter 79 for details).

Whether the semen is to be used immediately or preserved, it should always be mixed with an appropriate extender to protect spermatozoa from environmental injury before insemination. A minimum dilution ratio of 1:1 to 1:2 (semen to extender) is recommended. Warmed extender can be added to semen following its collection or placed in the seminal receptacle before collection so that the spermatozoa come into contact with this supportive medium immediately after ejaculation. To obtain accurate measurements of spermatozoal concentration in extended semen with a spectrophotometer or densimeter, extenders must be optically clear. Otherwise, a hemocytometer must be used to quantify spermatozoa in the extended semen.

Properly formulated seminal extenders improve spermatozoal survival during the interim between collection and insemination. The most commonly used equine seminal extenders are milk based (Table 84–1). The addition of appropriate antibiotics to the extender will greatly reduce the number of bacteria which inevitably contaminate the seminal sample during collection. Polymyxin B sulfate (200 to 1000 units/mL), penicillin (1000 to 1500 units/mL), gentamicin sulfate (100 to 1000 ug/mL), amikacin sulfate (100 to 1000 ug/mL), and ticarcillin (100 to 1000 ug/mL) are the most commonly used antibiotics; gentamicin and amikacin require the addition of buffer to adjust pH (see Chapter 81 for additional details).

TABLE 84–1. EQUINE SEMEN EXTENDERS

Nonfat Dry Milk Solids Glucose Extender I	
NFDMS*	2.4 g
Glucose	4.9 g
Penicillin, crystalline	150,000 units
Streptomycin, crystalline	150,000 μg
Sterile deionized water	q.s. 100 mL
Nonfat Dry Milk Solids Glucose Extender II	
NFDMS	2.4 g
Glucose	4.9 g
Gentamicin sulfate (reagent grade)	150,000 units
8.4% $NaHCO_3$	2 mL
Deionized water (sterile)	92 mL
(Mix liquids before adding NFDMS or gentamicin will curdle the milk.)	
Heated Skim Milk Extender	
Skim milk	100 mL
Polymyxin B	100,000 units
(Heat skim milk to 92° to 95° C in double boiler for 10 min; cool and add polymixin B.)	
Cream-Gel Extender	
Knox gelatin (unflavored)	1.3 g
Distilled water (sterile)	10 mL
Half-and-half cream	1 pint (475 mL)
Penicillin, crystalline	100,000 units
Streptomycin, crystalline	100,000 μg
Polymyxin B sulfate	20,000 units
(Dissolve gelatin in water and sterilize. Heat half-and-half to 92° to 95° C in double boiler for 2 to 4 min; mix 10 mL of gelatin solution with 90 mL of heated half-and-half and allow to cool; add antimicrobials.)	
E-Z Mixin Two-Way Equine Semen Extender	
Component A	Plastic bottle of distilled, deionized, water
Component B	Package containing dry powdered mixture of glucose, NFDMS, $NaHCO_3$, and polymixin B sulfate
(Add contents of component B to component A and shake well; place mixture in incubator or warm water to bring to proper temperature of 37° to 38° C before mixing with semen.)	

*NFDMS, nonfat dry milk solids.

(Adapted from Varner, D.D.: Collection and preservation of stallion spermatozoa. Proc. Soc. Theriogenology, 13–33, 1986.)

INSEMINATION TIMING AND FREQUENCY

In many AI management systems, mares are inseminated every other day beginning the second or third day of estrus until ovulation is detected or the mare no longer exhibits signs of behavioral estrus. Acceptable pregnancy rates are obtained when mares are inseminated within 48 to 72 h before ovulation with semen from fertile stallions.[11] When using semen from subfertile stallions, inseminations once or twice a day until ovulation occurs may be required to improve pregnancy rates.[12] In a recent study, a single-cycle pregnancy rate of 75% (9/12 mares) was obtained from single inseminations performed 3 days before ovulation.[13] The highest pregnancy rate (88%, 7/8 mares) in that study was in the group of mares inseminated 1 day before ovulation. In mares inseminated within 6 h of ovulation, pregnancy rates were comparable with those achieved with a single insemination before ovulation or two inseminations, one before and one after ovulation.[14] Insemination within 6 h after ovulation also resulted in pregnancy rates similar to those achieved from insemination performed 1 to 3 days before ovulation.[13] However, a high embryonic loss rate (34%) occurred in the mares inseminated after ovulation. Although good fertility has been reported when using postovulation breeding in horses,[15] this breeding protocol requires further study before it can be recommended as a routine breeding practice to improve reproductive efficiency.

Ideally, transrectal ovarian palpation and ultrasonography should be used in a breeding program to predict ovulation more accurately, so the number of inseminations required are minimized. Limiting the number of inseminations improves the overall efficiency of the breeding program and reduces the risk of iatrogenic contamination of the mare's reproductive tract. Reducing uterine contamination is especially important when breeding mares with an increased susceptibility to uterine infections.

INSEMINATION DOSE (SPERM NUMBER)

Typically, mares in an AI program are inseminated with 250 to 500 million progressively motile spermatozoa from stallions. Overall pregnancy rate for mares inseminated with 50 million motile spermatozoa (37%) was lower than for mares inseminated with 500 million motile spermatozoa (75%, $p < 0.05$).[16] Mares inseminated with 50 million motile spermatozoa also had a lower pregnancy rate ($p < 0.10$) per cycle and required more cycles per mare ($p < 0.10$) than mares inseminated with 500 million motile spermatozoa to become pregnant. Under ideal conditions, the insemination dose may be reduced to 100 million progressively motile spermatozoa without reducing fertility when using semen from highly fertile stallions.[17–19] Inseminating mares with 500 million progressively motile sperm will help ensure that acceptable pregnancy rates are achieved by allowing some margin for error in seminal evaluation and handling when conditions are less than optimal.

INSEMINATION VOLUME

The number of spermatozoa in an insemination dose appears to be more critical than the volume of the inseminate. Although smaller or larger volumes can be used successfully, typical insemination volumes for extended equine semen range from 10 to 25 mL. When timed closely with ovulation, insemination with volumes as low as 0.5 mL of frozen/thawed semen has resulted in pregnancy. Care must be taken when small volumes of highly concentrated semen are used so that a substantial portion of the inseminate and, therefore, a large number of spermatozoa do not remain in the insemination equipment. Some workers suggest that volume of inseminate within the range of 0.6 to 26.8 mL have no effect on fertility[20] but that insemination volumes ≥100 mL may be detrimental to fertility.[21] When a number of mares are to be inseminated with a single ejaculate, insemination volume can be calculated by dividing the desired number (100 to 500 million) of progressively motile spermatozoa per insemination by the product of the spermatozoal concentration in the extended semen and the percentage of progressively motile spermatozoa in the ejaculate:

$$\text{In V} = \frac{\text{desired number of pms}}{(\text{sperm concentration})(\text{percent pms})}$$

(In V = insemination volume and pms = progressively motile spermatozoa)

INSEMINATION PROCEDURE

Sterile nontoxic, disposable equipment should be used for artificial insemination procedures. Syringes with nonspermicidal, plastic plungers (Airtite, Vineland, NJ) are preferable for artificial insemination, because rubber plungers may have spermicidal properties[22–25] (D. Driscoll and D.H. Douglas-Hamilton, personal commu-

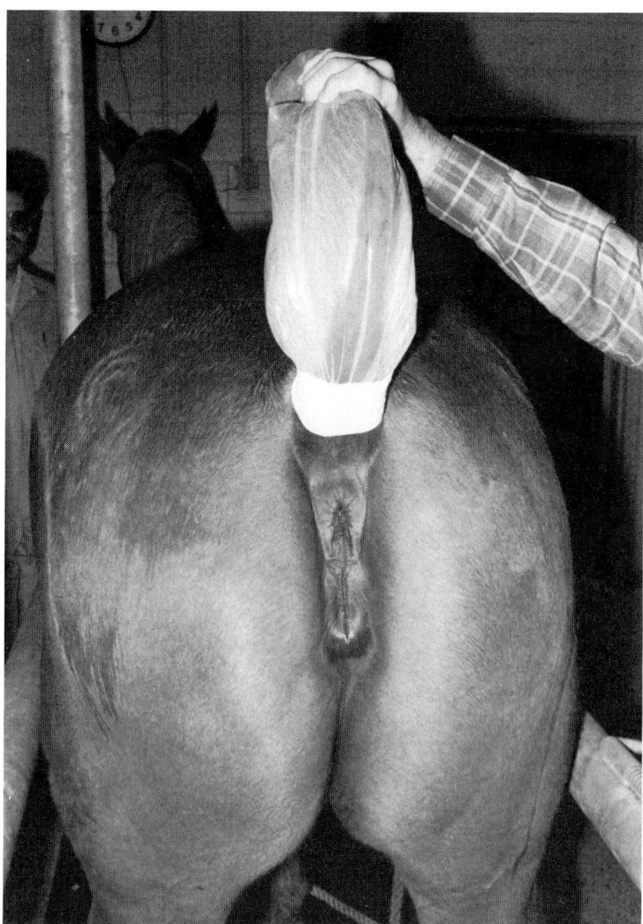

FIG. 84–2. Mare in stocks with tail wrapped and diverted.

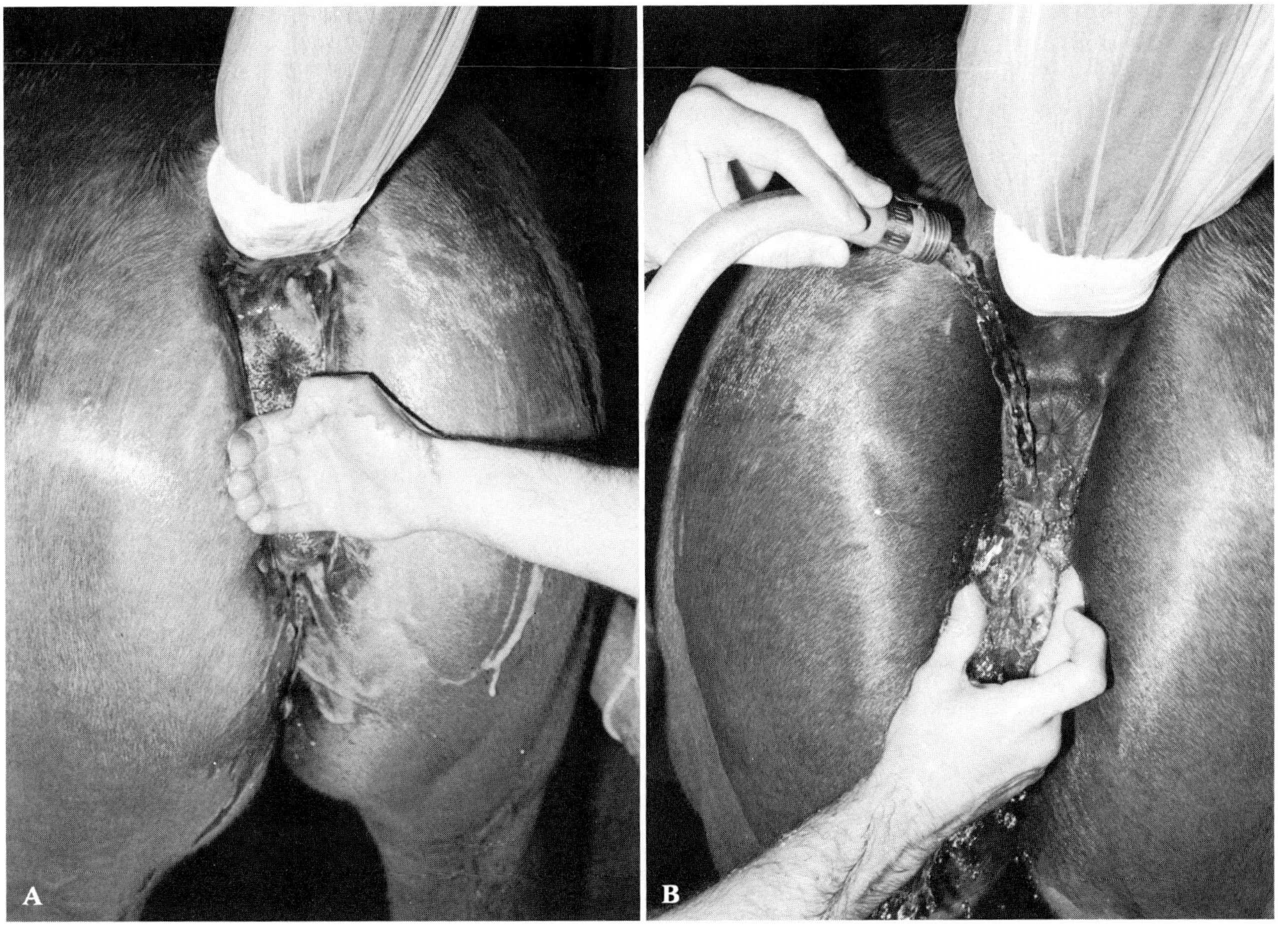

FIG. 84–3. *A*, Scrubbing the mare's perineal area. *B*, Rinsing the perineum and parting the vulvar labia to rinse the caudal vestibule free of soap and fecal contamination.

nication). Great individual stallion variation regarding spermatozoal sensitivity to the toxic effects of syringes with rubber plunger tips seems to exist. Toxic effects are apparent in semen from some stallions with as little as 1 min of contact with syringe plungers (D. Driscoll and D.H. Douglas-Hamilton, personal communication). Washing and sterilization of syringes does not appear to affect spermatozoal motility.[24]

Insemination of the mare should be performed in accordance with the minimum contamination techniques described by Kenney et al.[18] The mare should be adequately restrained with her tail wrapped and diverted either off to the side or up over her rump (Fig. 84–2). The perineal area is thoroughly scrubbed and rinsed, paying particular attention to the vulva and making sure the caudal vestibule is free of fecal contamination (Fig. 84–3). Two to three scrubs with soap or a surgical scrub are recommended. Thorough rinsing is essential to eliminate any residual soap that is spermicidal or that can irritate the mare's genitalia. Once the mare is adequately prepared, the inseminator puts on a sterile or clean plastic sleeve over which a sterile, disposable, latex glove can be worn (Fig. 84–4). The tip of the insemination pipette is covered in the gloved hand and a small amount of sterile, nonspermicidal lubricant is applied to the back of the glove (Fig. 84–5). The gloved hand and insemination pipette are passed between the vulvar lips to the cranial vaginal vault where the index finger identifies and penetrates the cervix. The insemination pipette is advanced through the cervix to uterine body where the semen is slowly deposited.

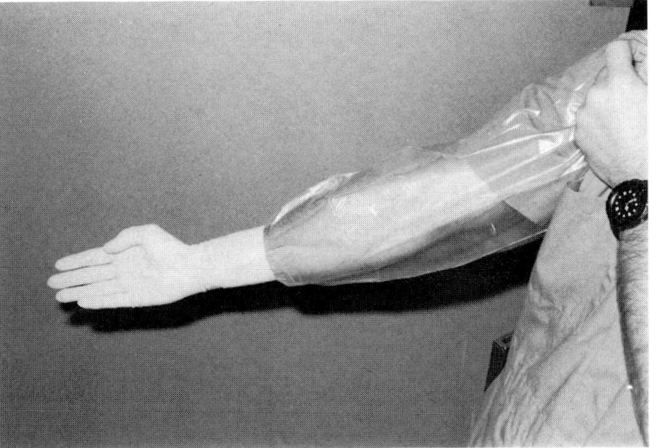

FIG. 84–4. Clean shoulder-length sleeve covered with sterile latex glove.

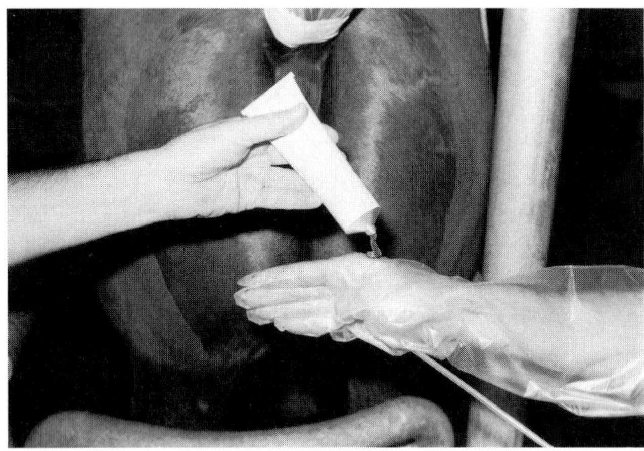

FIG. 84–5. Applying sterile nonspermicidal lubricant to sterile sleeve. Note protected position of insemination pipette tip between thumb and palm of hand.

PRESERVATION OF SEMEN

Studies regarding the effect of dilution ratio on spermatozoal motility parameters indicate that longevity of spermatozoal motility is maximized if ejaculates are diluted to a final concentration of 25 million sperm per milliliter.[26] Once extended, stallion semen tends to suffer a dramatic decrease in spermatozoal motility and longevity if it is maintained at 37° C (see Chapter 81 for details regarding extended and cooled semen). Insemination techniques for cooled, extended semen are the same as those for fresh, extended semen. Warming of the semen before insemination is not required unless the extender used forms a gel when cooled (e.g., cream-gel extender). A small drop of semen should be placed on a warmed (37° C) microscope slide to evaluate spermatozoal motility following storage. Motility estimates are made following a suitable time to warm the seminal sample but before the effects of dehydration occur. When possible, an aliquot of semen should be placed in a warm (37° C) water bath for 10 min before analyzing spermatozoal motility.

The ability to transport stallion semen to mares, rather than having to transport mares to stallions, offers numerous advantages. The most obvious advantage is the tremendous financial savings to mare owners. Bringing semen to the mare eliminates the high costs of shipping the mare, or the mare and her foal, to a distant breeding facility where boarding costs may also be high. The mare and her foal can remain in familiar surroundings thus greatly reducing the stress of transport as well as reducing the risk of illness resulting from exposure to potential pathogens to which the animals may be immunologically naive. The use of transported cooled semen is especially advantageous when the availability of a stallion for breeding is limited because of shows or other performance events. When such a stallion's collection schedule is known, the mare's estrous cycle can be manipulated with hormonal and/or prostaglandin treatments, so estrus and ovulation can be synchronized as closely as possible to the arrival of the transported semen.

When using cooled, transported semen for breeding, communication between the veterinarian and the other personnel involved in the reproductive management of both the mare and stallion is essential for success. Proper timing of insemination is critical and therefore requires accurate assessment of follicular dynamics to predict ovulation. The entire process must be well orchestrated so that once the semen is collected and packaged for shipment, the time required for seminal transport and the stage of the mare's estrous cycle are synchronized for maximum reproductive efficiency. Attempts to utilize transported semen on poorly managed farms are doomed to failure because of the complexities involved.

Development of the Equitainer system (Hamilton-Thorn Research, Danvers, MA) has greatly enhanced the successful transport of stallion semen.[27] The design of the shipment/storage container allows extended semen to be cooled slowly (−0.3° C/min) to 4° to 8° C. This temperature is maintained for up to 60 h in the durable lightweight container while it is being transported to its destination for insemination. When processed and handled correctly, semen from fertile stallions which is stored and transported with this system can achieve pregnancy rates equal to those attained by artificial breeding with fresh, extended semen.[3,27] Note that not all stallions produce semen which tolerates storage.

Development of methods to freeze bull semen effectively has revolutionized the cattle breeding industry by providing a means by which semen can be stored indefinitely and shipped worldwide. The use of frozen semen in the equine industry is becoming more popular among breeders whose registries permit its use; however, many equine breed registries in the United States strictly oppose the use of transported semen, including frozen semen. At present, more than a dozen breed registries in the United States either permit the use of frozen semen or have no stipulations forbidding its use.[3]

Unfortunately, pregnancy rates achieved by breeding mares with frozen semen are generally much lower than those obtained in the cattle industry. A marked variation is found in post-thaw spermatozoal viability among individual stallions and even between ejaculates of the same stallion.[28] Optimal pregnancy rates with frozen/thawed semen can probably be achieved when mares are inseminated within 24 h before or within 6 to 12 h after ovulation.[11,29–31] Thawing and insemination protocols are generally prescribed by the laboratory responsible for freezing the semen. Reported pregnancy rates for frozen/thawed semen range from 6 to 70%. Stallion effects certainly contribute to some of this variation; however, differences in mare fertility, insemination protocol, and cryopreservation techniques must also be considered. Simple and reliably consistent methods of freezing and thawing equine semen have yet to be obtained. Resistance by the major breed registries in the United States to accept the use of frozen semen has limited funding and greatly impaired research efforts. Despite limited support, progress in cryopreservation of stallion semen is being made. A detailed description of the principles and current techniques for cryopreservation of stallion semen can be found in Chapter 83.

REFERENCES

1. Perry, E.J.: Historical. *In* The Artificial Insemination of Farm Animals. Edited by E.J. Perry. New Brunswick, Rutgers University Press, 1945, pp. 3–8.
2. Perry, E.J.: Historical background. *In* The Artificial Insemination of Farm Animals. 4th ed. Edited by E.J. Perry. New Brunswick, Rutgers University Press, 1968, pp. 3–12.
3. Varner, D.D.: Collection and preservation of stallion spermatozoa. Proc. Soc. Theriogenology, 13–33, 1986.
4. Cheng, P.L., et al.: The present situation of artificial insemination of horses in China and some investigations on increasing conception rate of mares and breeding efficiency of stallions. Acta Vet. Zoo. Tech., Seneca, *5:*29–34, 1962.
5. Brinsko, S.P., Varner, D.D., Blanchard, T.L., and Meyers, S.A.: The effect of postbreeding uterine lavage on pregnancy rate in mares. Theriogenology, *33:*465–475, 1990.
6. Jones, R.L., et al.: The effect of washing on aerobic bacterial flora of the stallion's penis. Proc. Am. Assoc. Equine Pract., 9–16, 1984.
7. Hale, E.B., and Almquist, J.O.: Relation of sexual behavior to germ cell output in farm animals. J. Dairy Sci., *43(Suppl.):*145–169, 1960.
8. Pickett, B.W., Squires, E.L., and Voss, J.L.: Normal and Abnormal Sexual Behavior of the Equine Male. Animal Reproduction Laboratory General Series Bulletin No. 1004. Fort Collins, Colorado State University, 1981.
9. Ionata, L.M., Pickett, B.W., and Squires, E.L.: Effect of supplementary sexual preparation on stallion seminal characteristics. Proceedings of the Eleventh Symposium of the Equine Nutrition and Physiology Society. Stillwater, 1989, pp. 178–179.
10. Amann, R.P., Loomis, P.L., and Pickett, B.W.: Improved filter system for an equine artificial vagina. J. Equine Vet. Sci., *3:*120–125, 1983.
11. Palmer, E.: Factors affecting stallion semen survival and fertility. Proceedings of the Tenth International Congress on Animal Reproduction and Artificial Insemination. 1984, paper 377.
12. Varner, D.D.: Stallion utilization in artificial insemination programs. Proc. Soc. Theriogenology. 118–139, 1987.
13. Woods, J., Bergfelt, D.R., and Ginther, O.J.: Effects of time of insemination relative to ovulation on pregnancy rate and embryonic-loss rate in mares. Equine Vet. J., *22:*410–415, 1990.
14. Martin, J.C.: Untersuchungen zur zyklusteuerung, insbesondere brunstsynchronisation im rahmen der instrumentellen samenubertragung biem pferd. VMD dissertation. Veterinary College of Hannover, 1980.
15. Belling, T.H., Jr.: Postovulation breeding and related reproductive phenomena in the mare. Equine Pract., *6:*12–19, 1984.
16. Householder, D.D., Pickett, B.W., Voss, J.L., and Olar, T.T.: Effect of extender, number of spermatozoa and hCG on equine fertility. Equine Vet. Sci., *Jan./Feb.:*9–13, 1981.
17. Pickett, B.W., et al.: Effect of seminal extenders on equine fertility. J. Anim. Sci., *40:*1136–1143, 1975.
18. Kenney, R.M., et al.: Minimal contamination techniques for breeding mares: Technique and preliminary findings. Proc. Am. Assoc. Equine Pract., 327–336, 1975.
19. Demick, D.S., Voss, J.L., and Pickett, B.W.: Effect of cooling, storage, glycerolization and spermatozoal numbers on equine fertility. J. Anim. Sci., *43:*633–637, 1976.
20. Pickett, B.W., Squires, E.L., and McKinnon, A.O.: Procedures for Collection, Evaluation and Utilization of Stallion Semen for Artificial Insemination. Animal Reproduction Laboratory General Series Bulletin No. 03. Fort Collins, Colorado State University, 1987.
21. Rowley, H.S., Squires, E.L., and Pickett, B.W.: Effect of insemination volume on embryo recovery in mares. Equine Vet. Sci., *10:*298–300, 1990.
22. Peterson, M.C., et al.: Leaching of 2-(2-hydroxyethylmercapto)benzothiazole into contents of disposable syringes. J. Pharm. Sci., *70:*1139–1143, 1981.
23. Jones, W.E. (ed.): Toxic agents in equine AI procedures. Equine Vet. Data, *5:*219, 1984.
24. Shull, J.W., et al.: Spermatozoal motility parameters of equine semen stored in plastic syringes. Paper presented at the Conference of Research Workers in Animal Disease, Chicago, November 17 and 18, 1986.
25. Broussard, J.R., et al.: The effects of Monoject and Air-Tite syringes of equine spermatozoa. Theriogenology, *33:*200, 1990.
26. Varner, D.D., et al.: Effects of semen fractionation and dilution ratio on equine spermatozoal motility parameters. Theriogenology, *28:*709–723, 1987.
27. Douglas-Hamilton, D.H., et al.: A field study of the fertility of transported equine semen. Theriogenology, *22:* 291–304, 1984.
28. Amann, R.P.: Preservation of the male gamete (bull, stallion, dog). Proceedings of the Tenth International Congress on Animal Reproduction and Artificial Insemination. 1984, pp. 28–36.
29. Martin, J.C., et al.: Centrifugation of stallion semen and its storage in large-volume straws. J. Reprod. Fertil. Suppl., *27:*47–51, 1979.
30. Aliev, A., and Ochkin, D.: The optimum time of insemination. Anim. Breed. Abstr., *47:*576, 1979.
31. Kloppe, L.H., et al.: Effect of insemination timing on the fertilizing capacity of frozen/thawed semen. Theriogenology, *29:*429–439, 1988.

CHAPTER 85

NATURAL SERVICE

N.W. Umphenour
T.A. Sprinkle
H.Q Murphy

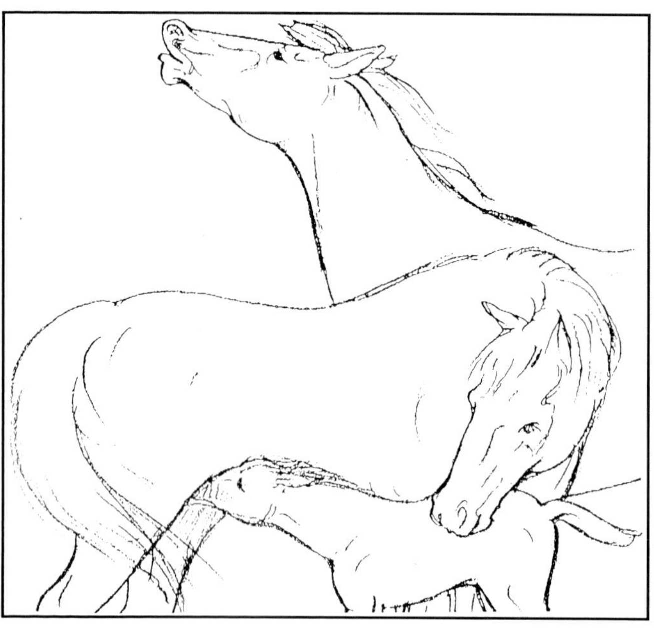

A well-managed breeding shed is much like a classic study in time and motion. The aim is to mate mares quickly and efficiently while maintaining sufficient safeguards to prevent injury to stallions, mares, and personnel. The breeding shed routine can be broken down into smaller self-contained units. Each mare must be processed in a set pattern, moving from one station to another in a specific sequence. At each step, the mare is subject to the identical requirements and policies of the mare before her and of ones to follow. This systematic approach helps to prevent many of the errors and problems that can occur in an unorganized or improperly managed breeding shed.

The assembly line analogy cannot be taken too literally, however. Both mares and stallions must be handled as individuals, and although most will fit into this system well, allowances must also be made for each animal's idiosyncracies as well as other contingencies. Some mares will not show signs of estrus; others will require more attention in the shed. Some may need additional attention after the breeding occurs. Therefore, the operation of a modern breeding shed must be managed by well-trained personnel who can adjust procedures to meet the emergencies and needs of individual mares and stallions while also being prepared for any circumstances that may arise. Although numbers may be large or small, in terms of both mares and economics, the ultimate goal is to mate each mare once, resulting in a 100% conception and foaling rate.

NATURAL SERVICE

The Jockey Club regulations state that "any foal that is the product of either artificial insemination or embryo transfer is not eligible for registration. In order to be eligible for registration, a foal must be the result of a stallion's natural service of a mare (which is the physical mounting of the mare by a stallion)."

Working under this directive, the Thoroughbred breeding shed manager must not only be cognizant of the timeliness of the breeding but also be concerned with the mares' and stallions' conduct in the breeding shed. Mares that are not receptive are difficult to breed and are a potential danger to themselves, the stallion, and the breeding shed crew; likewise an improperly or poorly handled stallion can be just as dangerous. As a result, teasing and assessment of difficult mares is an important part of breeding shed routine. Knowledgeable and skilled handling of the stallion is essential to the efficient and safe operation of the breeding shed.

Prevention of disease is another important consideration. Because the stallion and mare are in direct contact, transmission of a number of diseases is possible, in spite of rigid management practices. The outbreak of contagious equine metritis (CEM) closed the breeding sheds of Kentucky for several weeks in 1978,[1] and regulations governing its control still remain a part of breeding shed routine. Despite rigid management procedures, another outbreak of a potentially sexually transmitted disease, equine viral arteritis (EVA), occurred in Kentucky in 1984. Unfortunately, no 100% effective method exists to prevent disease in a breeding program where direct contact occurs among a large number of horses originating from a variety of farms, states, and countries. The international nature of the Thoroughbred breeding and racing industries also carries some risk of introducing new infections; consequently, the breeding shed crew and manager must be alert and attentive to signs of disease in both their mares and stallions (see Chapter 91 on sexually transmitted diseases).

In addition, some risk is always involved when a mare, even the most tractable, is bred. This risk, although small, would not exist if artificial insemination were allowed. For these and other reasons, the requirement that each mare be covered through natural service has a profound effect on how a breeding shed is managed.

THE STALLION'S BOOK

Traditionally, the number of mares that can be bred to a stallion (the book) has been held to be between 40 and 50 mares.[2] These figures were established early in the 1900s, before the advent of palpation, ultrasonography, potential fertility evaluation, and lighting programs and were based on a rule of thumb of 100 covers per stallion per breeding season, with an average of two covers per mare. Clinicians generally estimated that a stallion could make 9 covers a week, with one day off.

These figures may be satisfactory as general assumptions; however, sound criteria can be applied to a management scheme to assess more accurately the number of mares that can be bred to an individual stallion. Most normal stallions can successfully breed 40 to 55 reproductively sound and well-managed mares in a normal breeding season. However, some cannot, while others are capable of much larger books. Although these figures are reasonable rules of thumb, they are not a substitute for a prebreeding assessment of the stallion's potential capabilities and a continual review of how he is actually performing during the breeding season.

Several ways to assess the potential breeding capabilities of a stallion are known. Before the season begins, the horse should have a breeding soundness examination and one should be performed any time during the season when breeding efficiency is questioned. Accurate records of baseline seminal characteristics are invaluable for comparison during periods of poor performance and will assist in establishing a management plan for an individual stallion (see Chapters 78, 79, 82, and 86).

Along with the seminal characteristics, libido is a major factor in a stallion's breeding soundness examination. Sperm output is a function of age and testicular size;[3,4] most horses are physiologically capable of breeding larger numbers of well-managed mares.[5,6] Libido can become the limiting factor. A stallion may have excellent semen, but if his libido is subnormal, breeding him to a large number of mares may be time-consuming, tedious, and/or impossible. In such instances it is libido not seminal quality that limits the stallion's book. However, many valuable stallions are worth investing the increased time and effort to improve libido. Careful observation of a stallion's preferences and dislikes along with a good exercise program, patience, and understanding may improve a poor-performing stallion's libido.

Once the breeding season starts, an accurate record must be kept of the number of mares returning for a cover on the second estrous cycle in a given period versus the total number of mares covered during that time. This return rate should not be more than 50% if the mares are well managed. If more than 50% of a stallion's mares return for breeding in two cycles, then it is time to re-evaluate the stallion and try to determine if he has a fertility problem.

MARE MANAGEMENT

Mare management has a large influence on the success of any breeding program. Ideally, mares to be bred are maintained on the same farm as the stallion. This allows close cooperation and communication between the mare and stallion managers. Because the goal is to breed mares as close to ovulation as possible, having mares on the same farm allows each mare's status to be known well in advance of when she needs to be bred. Many mares can be efficiently handled in this situation.

However, the mare may not always be boarded at the farm where the stallion stands. In some cases, many stallions are at the same location and not enough facilities exist to handle all of the mares in their books. In areas of concentrated breeding, the mare owners may have their own preference for a boarding farm or may own farms themselves. In any event, mares can and are successfully managed in this manner. The major responsibility for the mare falls to the management of the boarding farm. There are many competent managers on these farms who, in concert with their veterinarians, can present mares to be bred that are in the proper state of estrus to optimize conception.

MANAGING THE BOOK

As the season progresses, a natural shift occurs in the profile of the mares to be bred. With the increased use of lighting programs and various medications to program mares early in the season, a significant portion of the maiden and barren mares are pregnant by the beginning of April (see Chapters 19, 38, and 39). In April, the majority of mares are foaling and they constitute the second wave of mares to be bred. Finally, the end of the season is marked by mares that have late foaling dates and racing mares that are retired late to the breeding shed, as well as problem mares who have had difficulty conceiving earlier in the season.

Most farms establish specific times of the day when they will breed mares. This usually allows each mare to be mated close to ovulation to maximize conception. Commonly, the breeding day is broken into morning and afternoon sessions, with an evening session, if demand warrants. The exception to this is in the rare case of a stallion who is encountering a fertility difficulty or is known to be subfertile. If a stallion's semen is of suspected or known poor quality, his mares may be palpated several times during the day and often bred near predicted ovulation even if late at night.

The management of breeding sessions in response to the needs of outside mares is a demanding, full-time job. The secretary or manager who is fielding phone calls needs to juggle the available sessions with the stallion as well as to make sure the necessary contracts and mare information have been completed before the mare is presented. In the case of returning mares, the secretary needs to remind the boarding farm of any cultures or paperwork that must accompany that mare for a return breeding. When more than a couple of stallions are involved, tension can be high. Because the person booking the mares has contact with many people during the course of the season, he or she must be capable of remaining calm and courteous in the face of pressure and occasional hostility.

Ideally, mares should be presented to the stallion at a constant rate throughout the breeding season. Obviously times will occur when several mares booked to the same stallion are in estrus simultaneously. The manager must then communicate with the boarding farms to try to schedule the most opportune time for each mare. Not all farms palpate mares daily during estrus. During peak booking times, an appointment may be held for a particular mare and an additional palpation may be requested before that mare is sent. This added effort and expense are often rewarded by a more accurate placement of the mare in the breeding sessions. Such cooperation is imperative in the efficient running of a large breeding shed.

Some mares, in spite of frequent palpation, need a second cover during the same estrous cycle. Some clinicians believe that mares returning for a double (second cover during the same estrous cycle) merit less consideration than a mare who is arriving for a primary cover. Another approach is to assume that the mare seeking a double is closer to ovulation and should actually merit priority over other mares. Another factor in managing doubles is to know how long the stallion's sperm is likely to live. Based on records and past experience, the clinician can usually determine if a stallion is fertile when bred to mares which ovulate 72 h (or longer) after mating. A call to the mare owner explaining that a 48-h double is not necessary, will build good working relations and confidence in the stud farm (particularly if the mare conceives).

During the busy part of the spring, a stallion may have to be bred three times a day. Some mare owners and managers will balk when they are notified that they have been offered the evening session, and they may request the following morning's first session. Such a manager's thinking is that a horse that has already made two covers before his or her mare is bred is somehow less fertile. Again, records demonstrating a particular stallion's libido, testicular size, daily sperm production, age, seminal quality, fertility results per cycle and cover, and ejaculative frequency can help alleviate the manager's apprehension. Sometimes, the evening cover is more likely to result in a conception. This may be logical if, in fact, more mares ovulate during the night. According to our records on a large number of mares over several years, no difference exists in a stallion's fertility following multiple covers.

RECEIVING AREA

The receiving area of the breeding shed should be large enough to handle the expected volume of vans arriving with mares to be bred. Some thought should be given to traffic patterns to facilitate movement of vans arriving late and allowing easy departure of mares that have already been bred. The loading and unloading area should allow for both conventional horse vans as well as trailers (Figs. 85–1 and 85–2). Unless provisions have been made for each vehicle, traffic can rapidly become congested and few horses are unloaded. The perimeter of the receiving area must be able to be secured in the event that a mare escapes or her halter breaks. Mares should be able to be unloaded as soon as possible after arriving. Because foals are not usually transported with mares to the breeding shed, a hot van is not the most desirable holding stall for a lactating mare fretting over her foal at home.

MARE RECEPTION

It is the mare's owner's responsibility (or farm manager) to send the correct mare to the breeding shed. A great deal of time and money have been spent managing the mare. The proper mare must be mated to the proper stallion. Breeding sheds should request that all mares be properly identified by name on either their

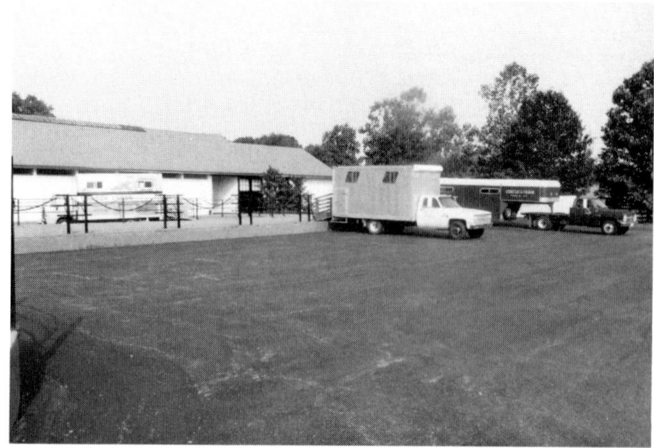

FIG. 85–1. The receiving area should have ample room to accommodate vans, trailers, and trucks of various types; an adequate number of unloading bays, and security fencing in case a mare gets loose.

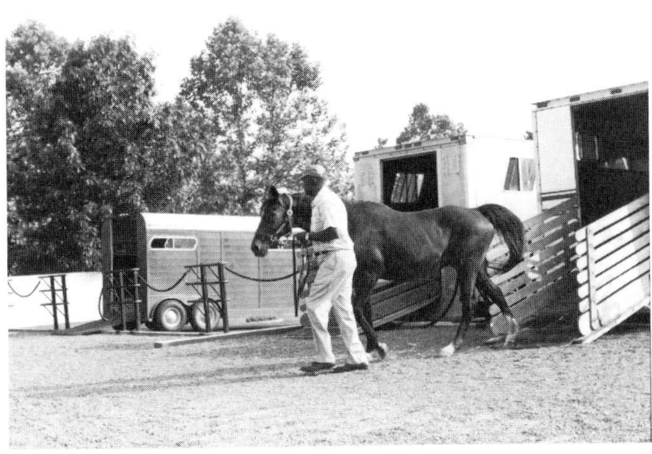

FIG. 85–2. The unloading bay should have ample room for handling horses and a variety of vans and trailers.

halters or neck straps. A specific person at the breeding shed should identify each mare and collect all paperwork arriving with the mare. At this time, some breeding sheds will also attach a tag to the halter of the mare with the name of the stallion to which she will be bred as a further safeguard against a mismating.

Paperwork arriving with each mare will vary slightly, depending on the mare's reproductive status. Breeding shed forms have proven useful as a minimum requirement for every mare bred at each visit. On such a form, the mare's name, current status, boarding farm, and veterinarian will appear as well as the stallion to which she is booked. In addition, these farms may carry general requirements for mares being bred to the farm's stallion. The requirements may vary slightly from farm to farm, but having the information recapitulated on the breeding shed form can eliminate any confusion.

Basically, mares can be divided into four broad categories. Maiden mares are those mares who have never been bred to a stallion. Mares bred the previous breeding season but that did not conceive are referred to as barren or open mares. Mares that were not bred the previous season for any reason have the same status as open mares. Mares that have foaled during the current breeding season are considered foaling or wet mares. Imported mares regardless of their category have additional requirements. Because of current CEM regulations, these mares must be bred last in line and also restricted to the last session of the day. The stallion bred to an imported mare cannot be bred to another mare until he has been treated prophylactically for CEM and sexually rested for 24 h.

Most breeding sheds require veterinary certificates attesting that a uterine culture has been performed and that the mare is clean and sound for breeding. Some may require such certificates on all mares coming to the shed for the first cover, but others may accept maiden and foaling mares, without a culture, unless they are returning to the shed for their third cycle. Regardless of the breeding shed requirements, rules must be clear to breeders when they book their mares, and someone should be at the shed to ensure that the required certificates are presented when the mares arrive and that the mares are clean and sound for breeding.

TEASING

It is important to tease every mare after she arrives at the breeding shed. In most instances, mares will exhibit classic signs of estrous behavior, a small percentage will not. This small percentage of mares will have to be handled differently.

Teasing mares is not an exact process, and because of the new environment and different teasing methods at the breeding shed, the mares may be slow to exhibit estrus. Adequate time must be allowed for the mare to respond. Some mares do not like to be teased at the head; others need to be let loose in the stall. Patience and observation will reward the handler.

A good teasing stallion is an absolute must for managing a breeding shed. He should be gentle but vocal and be aggressive enough to continue to tease day in and day out. Many mares respond quicker to a vocal teasing; some show at the first nickers of interest by the teaser. Others, who may be upset by the van ride or miss their foals, may require more intense attention. Clinicians often find it effective to turn the mare loose in a stall which is equipped with a sliding partition that allows the teaser in the adjacent stall access to the mare (Figs. 85–3 and 85–4). When the partition is lifted, the teaser can get his head and neck into the stall with the mare. Teasers quickly learn how to avoid injury and adapt well to this procedure.

In some instances, mares will not show estrus even after extensive teasing with the stallion. Some mares are merely passive, and although they do not lift the tail, urinate, or blink the vulva, they also do not fight or kick the teaser. Other mares are more adamant in their refusal and pose a real question as to whether they are suitable to be bred that day. This does not mean the

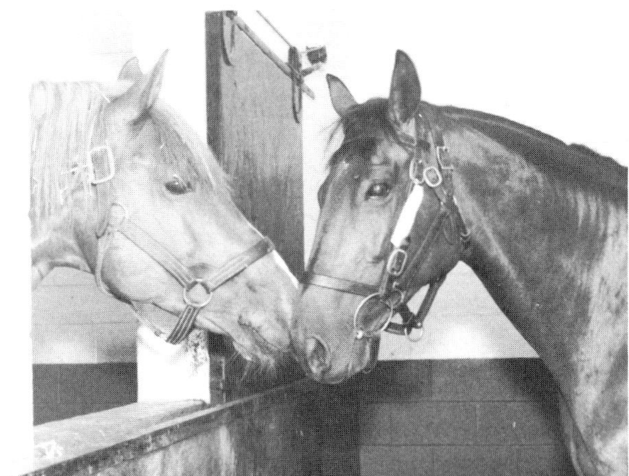

FIG. 85–3. A sliding door between stalls, controlled by a rope and pulley outside the stall, allows close contact for teasing.

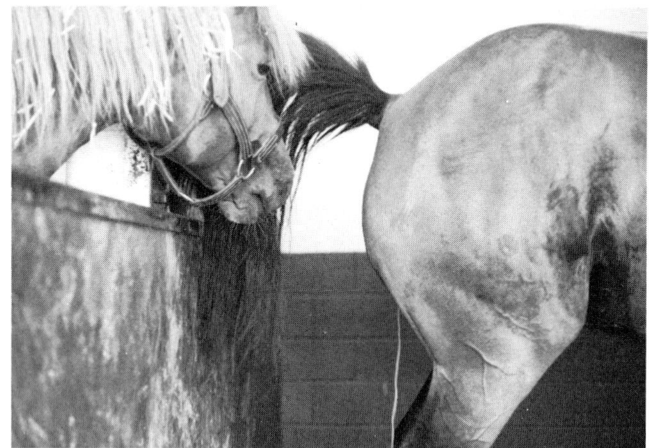

FIG. 85–4. A mare loose in an adjoining stall exhibiting signs of estrus.

boarding farm was negligent. Some mares can show well at the farm but may be intimidated in new surroundings. Others may have already ovulated and quickly gone out of heat. Some mares, particularly maiden mares on their first trip to the breeding shed, just do not show well.

In any event, the manager must ascertain whether the mare will allow herself to be covered by the stallion. The requirements of natural cover put both the stallion and his handlers (as well as the mare) at considerable risk in the event the mare chooses to respond violently. Mares can exhibit their displeasure by kicking, lunging, and even flipping over.

One way to see what a mare will do is to jump (mount) her with a teaser (Figs. 85–5 and 85–6). Although potentially as dangerous to the teaser as it would be to the stallion, teasers used for this purpose become wise in the ways of recalcitrant mares. Also the breeding crew and teaser are both aware that a mare may be nonreceptive and are prepared. In most cases, mares tend to bluff and either do not fight the teaser as anticipated or become receptive after a few jumps. Only after accepting the teaser's mounts will the mare be sent to her stallion. Even then extra care should be taken during her breeding.

PREPARATION OF THE MARE BEFORE BREEDING

After the mare has been teased and found receptive, her tail needs to be wrapped and the external genitalia and perineal area washed before breeding (Fig. 85–7). This is most safely done in a walk-in stock, which is padded to protect both the mare and person who will wash her. The floor should not become slippery when wet and should be well drained. All surfaces should be easily washed and not hold water, which will improve hygienic conditions and prevent unpleasant odors from mildew and mold. The outbreak of CEM in the late 1970s made all breeding sheds extremely aware of hygiene and the potential of cross-contamination for mares passing through the breeding shed. Before this outbreak, mares were usually washed with warm water or mild soap, such as Ivory. After CEM, many sheds experimented with a variety of stronger preparations, such as Nolvasan scrub, for washing both mare and stallion before breeding.

However, problems have occurred with this approach. Studies have shown that washing with antimicrobial compounds and even excessive scrubbing with plain water may alter the normal flora to the extent that opportunistic pathogens may colonize.[7,8] This problem is accentuated when stronger preparations are used, with a concomitant increase in incidence of Pseudomonas and other troublesome opportunistic infections. Many sheds have returned to the use of mild soaps or just warm water for cleansing mares and stallions.[9]

One result of the CEM outbreaks has been the emphasis placed on the use of disposable gloves and bucket liners. This and use of nonsterile cotton rather than sponges or towels to scrub the genitalia have proven to be effective in controlling gross contamination from mare to mare or among stallions.

The first step is to wrap the mare's tail using a disposable and inexpensive product such as 5-in. nonsterile gauze. The tail is wrapped firmly and completely from its base to the end of the tail bone. It is wrapped to minimize contamination from the mare, facilitate preparation, and prevent laceration of the stallion's penis during intromission.

The reproductive anatomy of the mare allows the perineal area to be exposed to fecal material and fluids at frequent intervals (see Chapter 2). Any attempt to sterilize the mare's genitalia before breeding is both misguided and futile. The purpose of washing the mare's vulva and perineal area before breeding is to minimize contamination from large quantities of fecal material being introduced when the mare is covered. The best cleansing agent is water. A hand-held fountain with a spray nozzle is an excellent way to dispense wa-

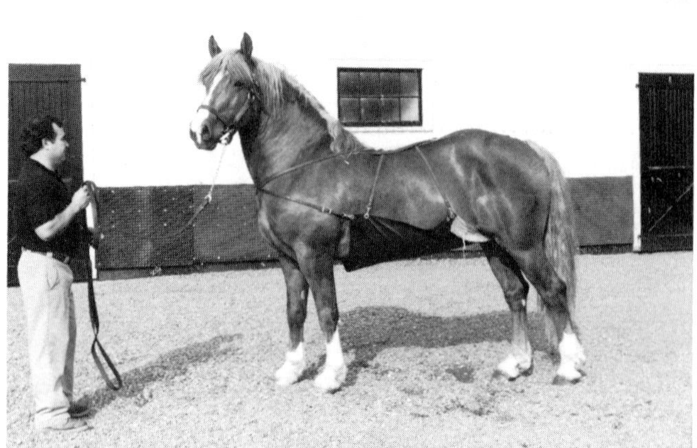

FIG. 85–5. A teaser stallion. Note special shield to prevent accidental breeding.

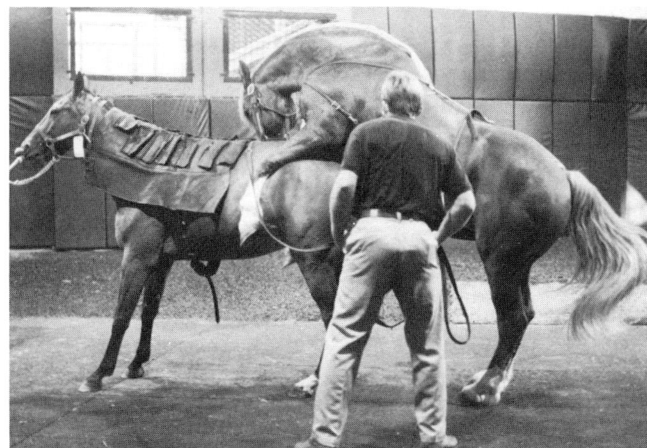

FIG. 85–6. Teaser stallion mounting mare to determine her receptivity.

ter and eliminates the need for buckets (Fig. 85–7).

If the mare has had a Caslick operation, care should be taken to wash carefully around each suture as fecal material tends to accumulate and harden there. The same is true around breeding stitches. The entire perineal area should be washed and rinsed repeatedly until wet cotton wiped on the area is no longer discolored. Care should be taken while wiping the area always to work from the vulvar lips outward, so that the center of the field, the vulva, is not repeatedly contaminated. The clitoral fossa should be averted and rinsed. Finally, a small plug of cotton should be inserted just into the lips and stroked upward, which will often dislodge any fecal material at the lowest juncture of a Caslick suture or the unsutured vulva. If the mare's rump is dirty, it too should be cleaned, as the penis often will touch it when the mare is first mounted (Fig. 85–7).

EVALUATING THE VULVA

The person washing the mare is in an excellent position to evaluate the mare's vulvar conformation. The ideal conformation has relatively vertical vulvar lips with little or no tilt and a good seal to prevent wind sucking and fecal contamination of the reproductive tract. With age and after several foalings, most mares' vulvar lips begin to tilt forward or have less than an ideal seal; a Caslick operation has proved to be an effective remedy in these cases (see Chapters 2 and 48).

Vulvar conformation changes from year to year and is affected by factors such as body weight and physical condition. Following a loss of weight or a decline in physical condition, a mare's vulva may have a greater degree of tilt than when the Caslick operation was performed the year before and, therefore, may require additional reconstructive surgery. In the event that a mare with faulty vulvar conformation may come to the shed unsutured, a reminder recommending that a Caslick operation be performed on the mare should be sent with the mare when she returns to her boarding farm.

The mare's vulva must also be evaluated from the perspective of the imminent breeding. Some mares are sutured down very low and need to be opened to permit complete penile intromission. Should this procedure be necessary, or if a mare is torn during breeding, the boarding farm must be informed so it may take appropriate and prompt action. If time and personnel allow, some mares may need to be resutured at the shed. A useful instrument to that end is the 35-mm skin stapler (Fig. 85–8). It is fast and effective, and in mares with poor vulvar conformation it may provide the extra degree of protection they need to conceive.

The position of the breeding stitch should be evaluated in terms of the stallion to which the mare is being bred. Penis size varies, and in some cases, the breeding stitch can be more of a hindrance than an advantage. Various materials are used for this stitch and care must be taken to prevent injury to the stallion's penis during breeding. The sharp edge of some of the monofilament sutures can cause a painful laceration of the dorsal surface of the penis.

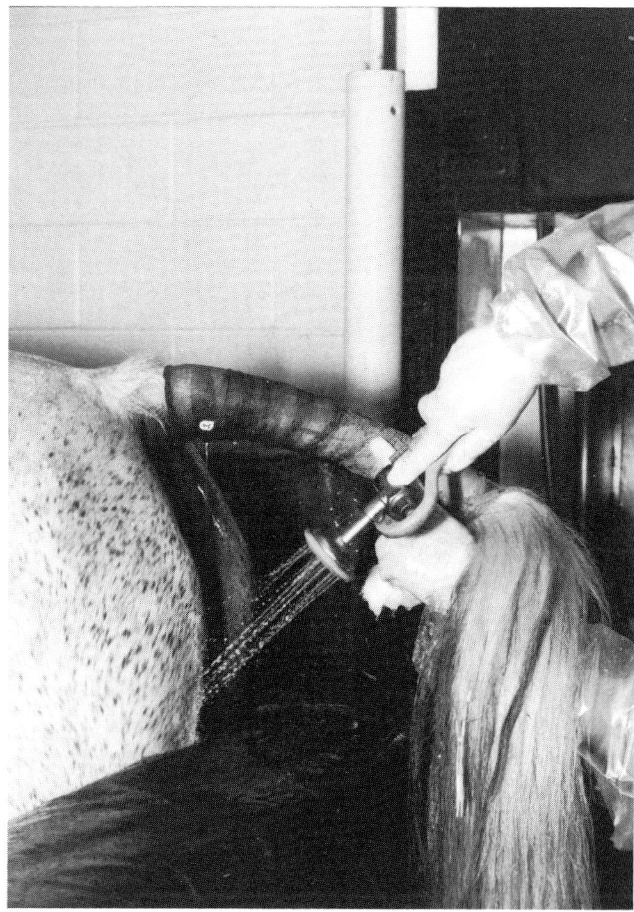

FIG. 85–7. In preparation of breeding, the mare's tail is wrapped with 5-in. nonsterile gauze and the external genitalia are cleansed. Note disposable gloves.

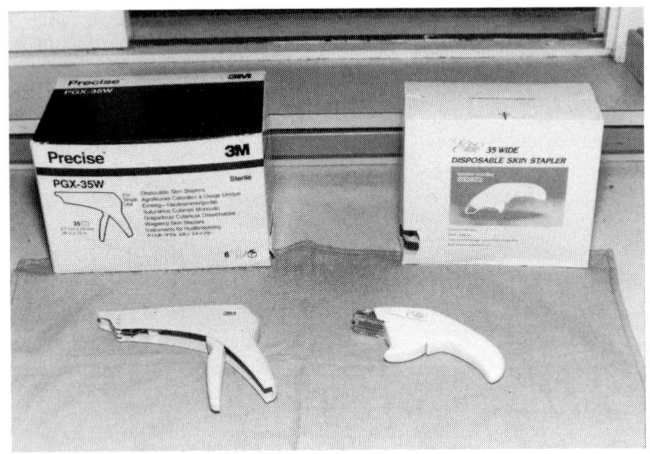

FIG. 85–8. A 35-mm stapler, which is useful for rapid repair of torn Caslick operations.

THE BREEDING SHED

The actual breeding area needs to be large enough to allow safe movement of horses and personnel. Enough room must be available so that if a mare proves difficult, the stallion can be quickly moved away from her. The ceiling needs to be sufficiently high to allow adequate clearance between the light fixtures and a mounted stallion.

The floor covering should consist of material that will provide nonslip, safe footing for the stallion, mare, and personnel. A variety of substances have been used successfully, including crushed rock, pebbles, rubber mats, and Fibar. Regardless of which is used, it should be dust free or the dust should be controllable by misting with water as necessary, allowing proper drainage following the spraying of disinfectant. Some products, such as Fibar, have the added benefit of softening a mare's or stallion's fall should that happen. This type of accident seldom occurs, but a soft floor could provide a critical difference.

Most breedings occur without problem, but some do not go exactly as planned. The mare may not stand and despite the crew's best efforts may move close to one of the walls. At these times, heavy urethane foam padding of the walls can prevent injury (Fig 85–9). Some sheds pad all walls; others, only areas where a horse is most likely to come into contact. No amount of protection is too much, particularly when handling valuable horses.

Some mares are too tall to allow easy breeding by their designated stallion. A small depression can be made in the flooring material, and the mare's hindlegs placed in it to help make up for the difference in sizes. Sometimes coconut mats (Fig. 85–10) can help raise the stallion and allow easier breeding or both methods can be used together. Trial and error will find the combination that works best for each stallion.

BREEDING SHED PROCEDURES

After the mare has been prepared, she is led into the breeding shed area where she becomes the responsibility of the breeding shed crew. The breeding shed crew should be trained to work as an efficient and experienced team. Although breeding can occur by using the boarding farm grooms, a trained breeding shed crew is far safer. Most breedings are uneventful, but sometimes difficulties arise and experienced handlers can avert a problem before an injury occurs.

The breeding shed crew consists of at least five members. After the mare is lead into the breeding area, she will be fitted with the appropriate gear, which may vary from farm to farm. Most mares will be twitched. Some farms use hindleg hobbles to prevent the mare from kicking the stallion. Others rely on a leg strap to hold up the mare's left front leg during the initial jump (Fig. 85–11) and kicking boots to lessen the chance of injury

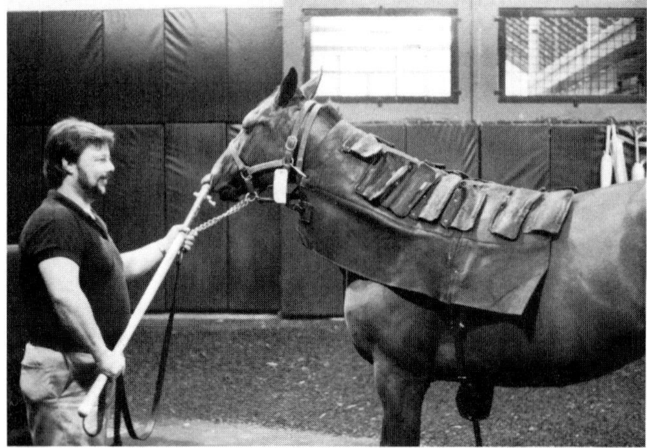

FIG. 85–9. A mare properly restrained with a twitch and fitted with a leather protective mat. The leather mat provides the stallion with something to bite on and hold onto without savaging the mare. Note padded walls.

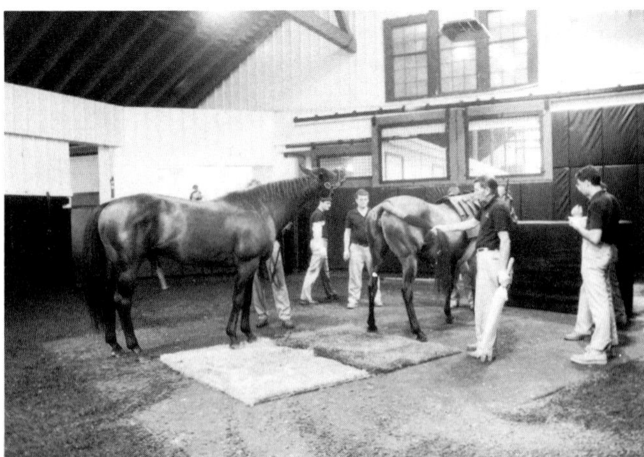

FIG. 85–10. A mare ready for breeding. The left foreleg is raised, the tail handler has pulled the tail aside, and other crew members are properly placed to do their assigned duties. Note coconut floor mats.

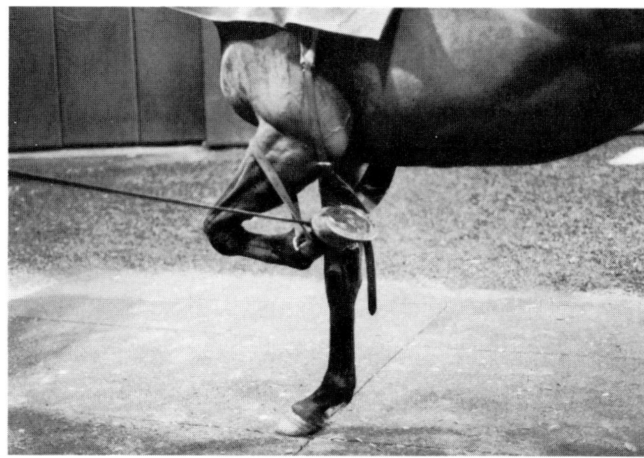

FIG. 85–11. A leg strap to hold up the left front leg to inhibit or prevent kicking. When the stallion safely enters, the strap is released, allowing the mare to stand on all four feet.

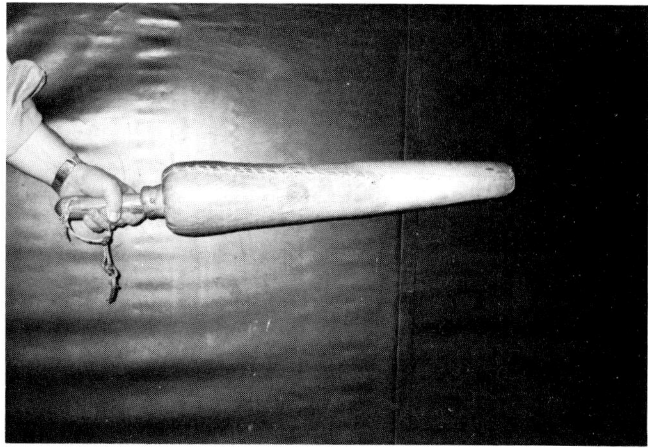

FIG. 85–12. A typical breeding roll. This long, padded, leather-covered cylinder—placed inside a clean, shoulder-length plastic disposable glove—is placed dorsal to the stallion's penis at intromission to prevent complete entry of the entire length of the penis.

to the stallion. Many farms also use a leather pad on the mare's neck to give the stallion something to hold onto with his teeth during the breeding (Fig. 85–9). Some stallions are aggressive about biting the mare's neck during mating. Some mares resent this and can suffer skin trauma and laceration.

The mare handler will hold the mare with a twitch and a leather shank (Fig. 85–9). It is his or her responsibility to control the mare during breeding. The mare handler needs to watch her reactions and warn other crew members if she appears to be about to change her attitude. The handler helps to balance the mare during breeding, which is particularly important when a leg strap is being used.

Some mares will tolerate the stallion's initial mounting only to explode later in the cover. The mare may attempt to flip or rear. Others will go down in front and try to kick. The mare handler must be sensitive to her movements and take appropriate action. At the end of the cover the handler must turn the mare's head toward the stallion so that she cannot kick the stallion as he dismounts.

The mare handler or another individual can hold the leg strap if one is used. This additional person will wait for direction from the crew member who helps the stallion enter the mare before letting the leg down. In most instances this release will be after intromission. The "leg handler" may also help the mare during the stallion's mounting thrusts. If the mare has shown an inclination to kick, she may be bred with her leg up. The stallion handler, who is in charge of the breeding, makes the decision.

The tail handler, as the title implies, pulls the mare's tail out of the way as the stallion mounts. The tail handler must take care not to be struck by the mounting stallion's hooves and yet must quickly pull the tail out of the way (Fig. 85–10). At the same time he or she can help steady the mare with a hand on her hip. When indicated, the tail handler also deals with the breeding roll (Fig. 85–12). This long, padded cylinder is placed dorsal to the stallion's penis, preventing complete entry of the entire length of the penis (Fig. 85–13). When a stallion with a long penis is bred to a small mare, the penis may penetrate the cranial vaginal wall if the breeding roll is not used.

Another individual on the near side assists the stallion with intromission. Although this might seem unnecessary in view of the intensity of the stallion's sexual drive, the prevalence of mares with Caslick operations makes this assistance imperative. Not only does the assistant help guide the stallion's penis, he or she tries to prevent unnecessary contamination of the penis and pulls the breeding stitch out of the way to prevent an injury to the penis. Once the stallion has covered the mare a dismount seminal sample is collected and examined to verify that ejaculation occurred.

The degree to which individual stallions will allow

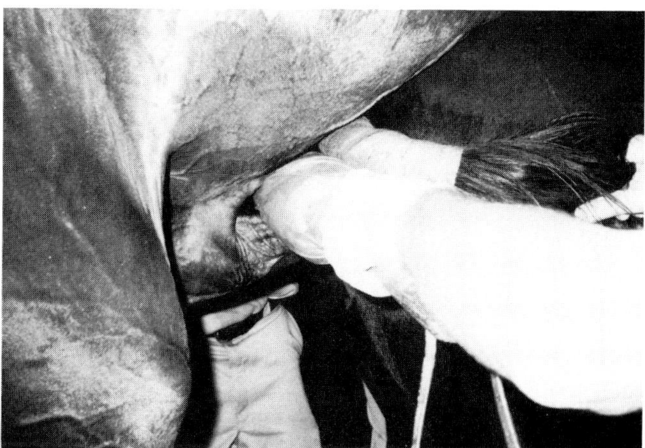

FIG. 85–13. A breeding roll inserted dorsal to the stallion's penis to prevent damage to vulvar surgery and/or rupture of vagina.

themselves to be assisted during the breeding varies. Some stallions need all the help they can get, others resent the attention and allow the handler only to help by pulling the breeding stitch up and out of the way. This illustrates the importance of knowing both the job and the stallion's habits and preferences. Each horse is an individual, and from daily exposure to the horses' habits and idiosyncrasies, the crew learns how to best assist in the breeding of each mare.

STALLION PREPARATION

Most stallions will protrude the penis and attain erection upon entering the breeding shed and seeing the mare. Later, as the breeding season progresses, a stallion may need more intense stimulation at teasing the mare; again individual reactions vary. After the penis has dropped and is fully exposed, it can be washed. As noted before, a clinician can do more harm than good in overzealous washing of the penis. Some stallions will actually be overstimulated by the prebreeding washing and bell out prematurely or produce excessive amounts of seminal gel in the ejaculate. Most stallions who are bred regularly do not accumulate visible smegma and are probably best left alone and washed only after covering a mare.

THE COVER

The stallion handler needs to know the stallion's sexual behavior. Some stallions are mild mannered, less aggressive, and mount the mare quickly and gently without unnecessary delay. Others may want to savage each mare and can upset even the most docile foaling mare, not to mention a frightened maiden mare. Other stallions may require several minutes to exhibit any sexual desire and to complete a cover. Each one must be handled differently to manage it successfully through a full and successful breeding season.

The ideal stallion would approach the mare slowly, at a slight angle, so that if she were to kick, the stallion would be out of danger. After nuzzling the mare and vocalizing quietly, he would then mount her lightly and slowly from behind, so that added weight would not throw the mare off balance and the handlers would have time to do their jobs. The ideal stallion would not try to bite the mare and would after a few thrusts clearly flag, i.e., pump the tail in the rhythmic motions that indicate ejaculation. He would then back off gently, as the dismount sample is collected (Fig. 85–14), and allow his penis to be washed without objection (Fig. 85–15).

Although not every stallion behaves in this manner, most do some or all of these things. Not all stallions are gentle, but most can be taught to behave appropriately in the breeding shed. It is the rare horse that is a constant problem.

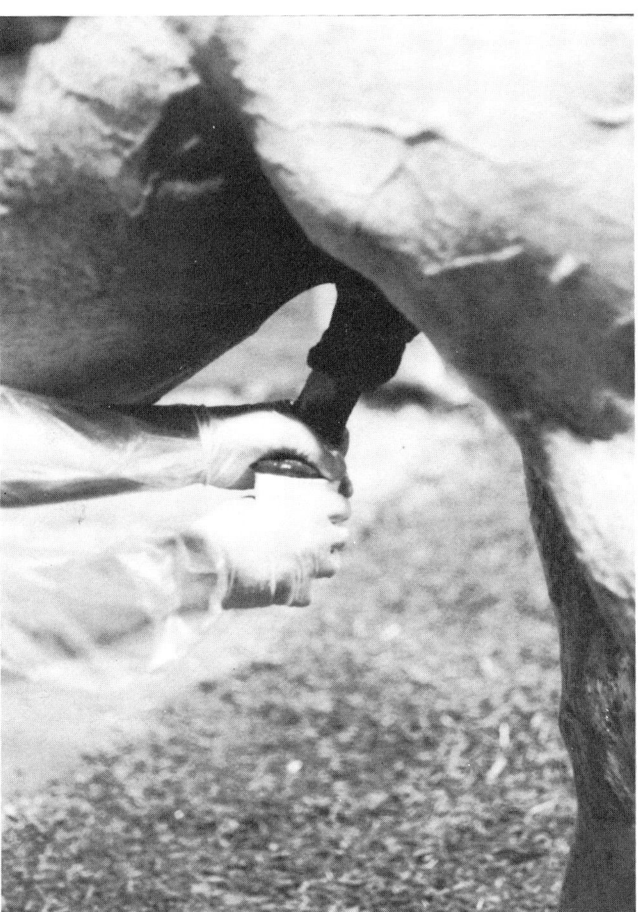

FIG. 85–14. Collection of seminal dismount sample into a polystyrene cup.

THE LABORATORY

A disposable polystyrene cup is used to collect and transport the dismount seminal sample to an adjacent laboratory. The laboratory need not be elaborate. It need only be clean, have running water, and a shelf to prepare the sample for microscopic examination (Fig. 84–16). Because spermatozoa are sensitive to changes in temperature, a slide warmer will provide a more accurate assessment of the spermatozoa, but it is not mandatory. One drop of semen is placed on a warm slide and is examined. The clinician must understand that dismount samples are used primarily to determine if the stallion has ejaculated. Material milked from the urethra plus that dragged from the mare by the penis is not representative of the seminal quality of the entire ejaculate. Some horses will flag, sigh, and give every indication of having ejaculated without actually having done so. Others will not appear to have flagged and will have ejaculated. The dismount sample helps verify the ejaculation.

Dismount samples vary widely from stallion to stallion. Horses which produce large volumes of gel may have dismount samples that seem less motile or concentrated, but may not be any less fertile than a stallion with a dismount sample containing large numbers of highly motile spermatozoa.

In addition, the dismount sample can help alert the manager to potential problems in the stallion and/or mare. If numerous red blood cells are found and the mare has not obviously been torn, hemospermia might be suspected, which warrants further investigation. White blood cells might indicate inflammation, although they may have originated in the mare. Urospermia may be suspected when the dismount sample carries a yellow tint.

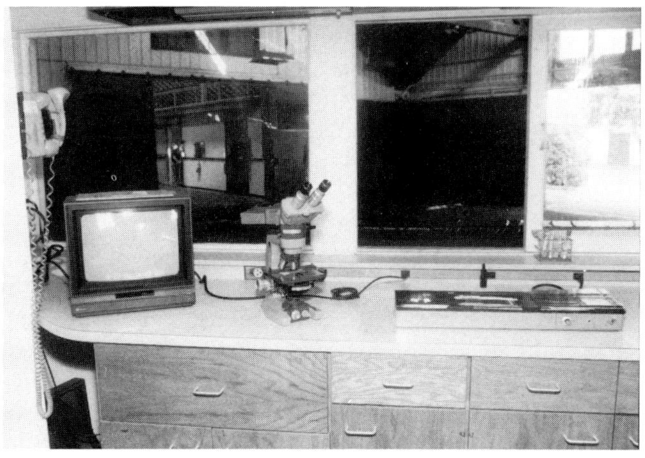

FIG. 85–16. A sufficient laboratory is dust free and has shelf space for a slide warmer, phase-contrast microscope, and other equipment. Note television monitor. All covers are recorded on videotape, providing a permanent record of mating in case of questions.

MANAGEMENT OF THE FIRST-YEAR STALLION

If possible, a new stallion should arrive at the farm long enough before the breeding season commences to allow time to complete a 4-week quarantine for a domestic stallion (45 days for imported stallions for clearance of CEM regulations), to have eating and drinking patterns and behavior characteristics monitored, to undergo complete and thorough physical and chemical examinations, and to have progress toward rehabilitating injuries assessed. During the quarantine, the stallion is able to begin to acclimate to his new environment, daily routine, and personnel. Personnel directly involved with the new stallion are the key to a smooth transition. The stallion must sense confidence and gain assurance from his groom and handlers. Handlers must recognize he is an animal and an athlete—not a machine, which means he needs to be handled and treated as an individual.

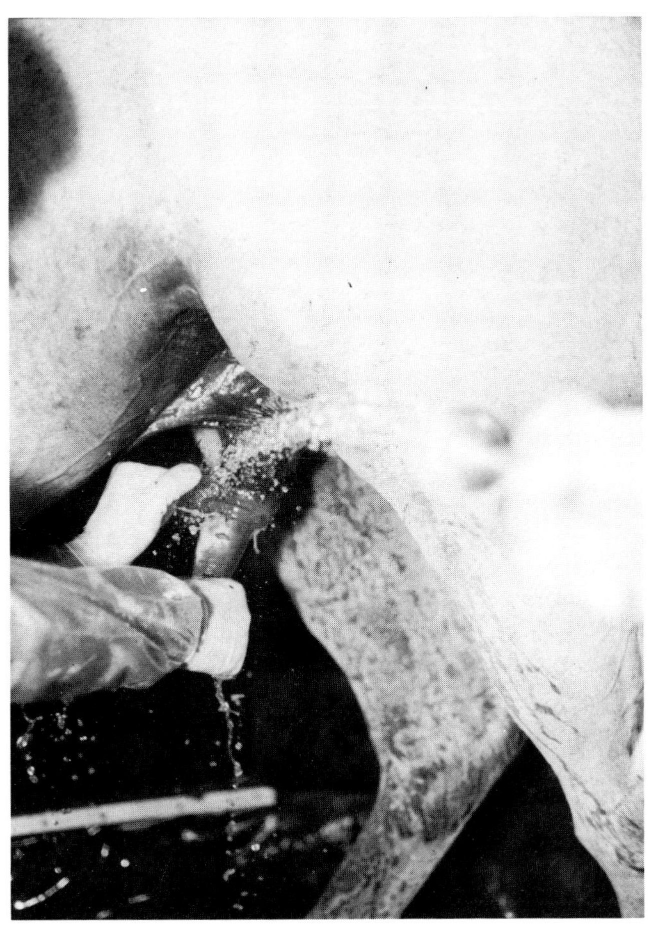

FIG. 85–15. After dismount sample is collected, the penis is rinsed with plain warm water.

When the quarantine is completed, breeding training can begin. Patience and persistence are the key words. The first step is to introduce the stallion to the breeding shed. Let him walk around the shed and become accustomed to the smells, lights, shadows, texture of the floor material, equipment, rolls, neck shields, hobbles, and pads. In some instances, depending on the horse's disposition, the horse may be turned loose in the shed to allow him to mark his territory.

Once the stallion has become familiar and comfortable with the breeding shed, bring a quiet, patient estrous mare into the shed. Under hand, the two horses should be permitted to test and tease one another. Most stallions are disciplined during their performance careers whenever they display sexual interest in a female; therefore, when confronted with a receptive mare in an environment that encourages fulfillment of sexual drive, they will not only be confused but may also be unsure of how to behave. Such stallions may be hesitant or overly aggressive. Gentle coaxing and educating by the handlers and tutoring by a patient, receptive mare can begin the foundation for a smooth, easy transition to the breeding shed. The stallion handlers must know what is and is not acceptable behavior of a breeding stallion. The handler must not misread a stallion's natural defense responses as being ill-tempered or cantankerous and, therefore, must judiciously use discipline and restraint with encouragement to maximize the stallion's normal sexual drive.

In nondomesticated horses, nuzzling, nipping, squealing, biting, and even striking are essential parts of the testing and teasing that occur between a stallion and his mares. The stallion's aggressiveness allows him to test the receptivity of the mares. With the handler's schooling, this aggression can be modulated to prompt the appropriate response by a stallion in an efficiently operated breeding shed.

In schooling the novice with his first cover, the manager may find it best not to wash the vulvar area the first time so as not to remove the natural odor of the estrous mare; the manager may also leave the external genitalia of the horse unwashed until he has made the first cover. The entire training process for some shy horses should be a positive experience, and the first ejaculation is the most significant step in the training process.

When the young stallion has completed that first ejaculation, slow adjustments and alterations in the natural breeding process (such as washing of the penis, taking penile cultures, collection in the artificial vagina, etc.) can take place so that this new stallion can become a proficient and efficient breeder.

REFERENCES

1. Bryans, J.T., and Hendricks, J.B.: Epidemiological observations on contagious equine metritis in Kentucky, 1978. J. Reprod. Fertil. Suppl., *27:*343–349, 1979.
2. Rossadole, P.D., and Ricketts, S.W.: Equine Stud Farm Medicine. 2nd ed. Philadelphia, Lea & Febiger, 1980.
3. Gebauer, M.R., Pickett, B.W., Voss, J.L., and Swierstra, E.E.: Reproductive physiology of the stallion: Daily sperm output and testicular measurements. J. Am. Vet. Med. Assoc., *165:*711–714, 1974.
4. Amann, R.P., Thompson, D.L., Jr., Squires, E.L., and Pickett, B.W.: Effect of age and frequency of ejaculation on sperm production and extrogonadal sperm reserves in stallions. J. Reprod. Fertil. Suppl., *27:*1–6, 1979.
5. Pickett, B.W., et al.: Management of the stallion for maximum reproductive efficiency, II. Colorado State University, Animal Reproduction Laboratory Bulletin No. 05. Fort Collins, 1989.
6. Ley, W.B.: Method of predicting stallion to mare ratio for natural and artificial insemination programs. J. Equine Vet. Sci., *5:*143–146, 1985.
7. Swerczek, T.W.: Contagious equine metritis—Outbreak of the disease in Kentucky and laboratory methods for diagnosing the disease. J. Reprod. Fertil. Suppl., 27:361–365, 1979.
8. Bowen, J.M., et al.: Effects of washing on the bacterial flora of the stallion's penis. J. Reprod. Fertil. Suppl., *32:*41–45, 1982.
9. Jones, R.L., et al.: The effect of washing on the aerobic bacterial flora of the stallion's penis. Proc. Am. Assoc. Equine Pract., 9–16, 1984.

CHAPTER 86

SEXUAL BEHAVIOR

B.W. Pickett

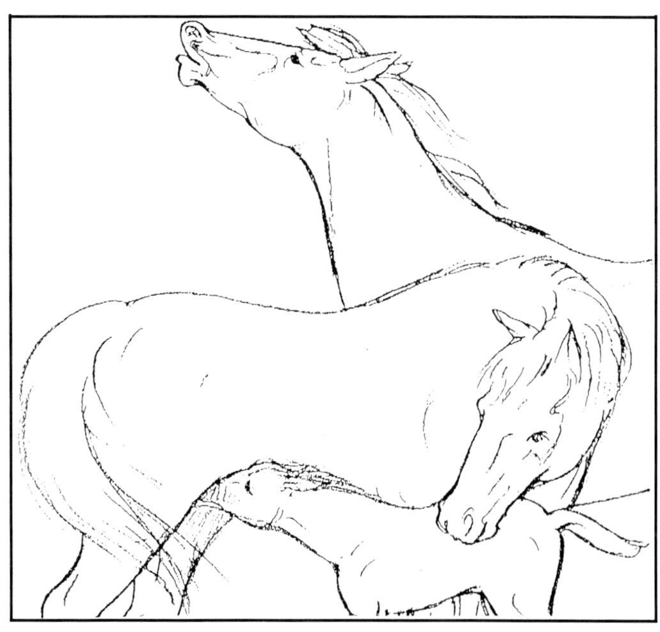

Sexual behavior and seminal characteristics of stallions are influenced by factors such as teasing, interacting with other horses, pain, fear, season, age, frequency of ejaculation, breed, testicular size, experiences during performance, management during training for breeding, health, physical condition, genetics, and blood-hormone concentrations.[1-8] The nervous system is involved to varying degrees in all aspects of the act of mating. The pattern of male sexual behavior appears to be innate, because animals reared in complete isolation generally will mate normally when introduced into the appropriate environment. Numerous factors influence impotence and sexual behavior, which can be greatly altered by psychic disturbances.[3,9-12]

Adequate expression of mating behavior by a breeding stallion is essential for maximum reproductive efficiency. The economical success of a breeding farm suffers dramatically when a stallion's behavior becomes erratic or unpredictable. More time and labor are spent for each seminal collection or breeding, and fewer mares become pregnant per cycle and for the breeding season.[12] Until stallion managers have experienced the frustration of standing a "slow" stallion at stud, they will not appreciate the ease of handling a stallion that is motivated. A responsive stallion will readily attain an erection upon presentation to an estrous mare, maintain that erection while being washed, mount immediately, copulate vigorously, and ejaculate without dismounting several times. The anxiety of an individual handling a slow stallion, or one with abnormal sexual behavior, is exceeded only by the fear that he will not become sexually aroused and thus the mare(s) will not be bred at the time appropriate for maximizing conception.

ERECTION AND EJACULATION

The stallion, like man, has a musculocavernous penis, which contains a larger amount of erectile tissue in relation to connective tissue.[13,14] The increase in size and erection of the penis is caused by a greater inflow than outflow of blood to/from cavernosus tissue, i.e., dilation of the arteries and constriction of the veins, resulting in reduced drainage of blood from the penis.[15,16] Erection occurs rather slowly in the stallion, in relation to other species of farm animals. In general, erection requires continued reception by the brain of general sexual stimuli—visual, olfactory, and auditory—derived from courtship.[3,9,15]

Ejaculation is a reflex that results in transport of components of semen from the epididymides, deferent ducts, ampullae, and accessory sex glands through the urethra. Triggering of the reflex typically is caused by stimulation of the glans penis by friction and psychic stimuli from higher brain centers.[9] Ejaculation can be divided into two parts: (1) emission, which is movement of semen into the pelvic urethra, and (2) ejaculation, which is expulsion of spermatozoa and seminal plasma (semen) from the reproductive tract. Semen is moved along the reproductive tract by a series of muscular reflex contractions. In general, seven to nine contractions are responsible for movement of semen and are accompanied by "flagging" of the tail of the stallion during ejaculation.[17] In many cases, the stallion flags without ejaculation, commonly called "cheating," which is occasionally responsible for stallion infertility. Furthermore, the stallion is one of the few species that can fractionate, no doubt unconsciously, his ejaculate, which results in incomplete ejaculation.[3]

In many cases, incomplete ejaculation is difficult to diagnose, particularly when natural service is the method of breeding. However, when artificial insemination (AI) is used, each ejaculate is evaluated. Thus, if number of spermatozoa per ejaculate varies greatly or does not increase as the season progresses, testicular dysfunction or incomplete ejaculation must be suspected. Even when AI is practiced, frequency of seminal collection must be sufficiently high, at least every other day, to ensure continued depletion of extragonadal sperm reserves, or incomplete ejaculation will be masked by spermatozoa from extragonadal sperm reserves. Other manifestations of incomplete ejaculation are (1) abnormally large variation in sperm output, (2) low libido, (3) easily distracted, (4) dismounts quickly, (5) tendency to savage mares, (6) poor pelvic thrusts, (7) generally requires multiple mounts per ejaculation, and (8) occasionally percentage of progressively motile spermatozoa and duration of sperm livability will be lowered. Unfortunately, all these signs are rarely exhibited each time an incomplete ejaculation is obtained. Therefore, diagnosis is often difficult.

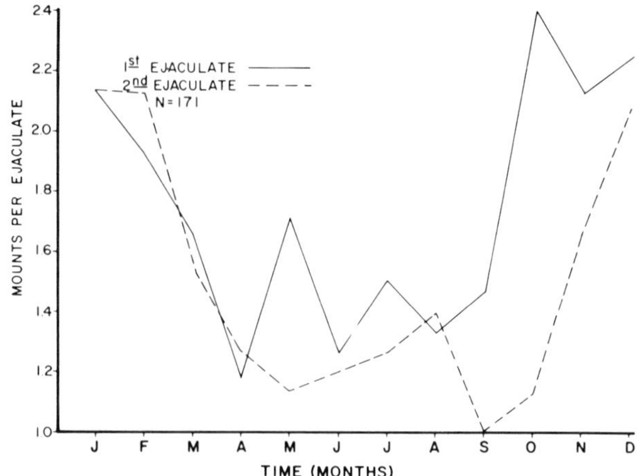

FIG. 86–1. Mean monthly variation in mounts per ejaculation. (Adapted from Pickett, B.W., Faulkner, L.C., and Sutherland, T.M.: Effect of month and stallion on seminal characteristics and sexual behavior. J. Anim. Sci., *31*:713–728, 1970.)

SEASON AND AGE

Because season has a profound effect on stallion seminal characteristics, a study was conducted to determine its effect on sexual behavior.[18] Two ejaculates of semen were collected, within 4 h of each other at approximately weekly intervals, from three (two 2-yr-old and one 3-yr-old) Quarter Horses (QH) and from two (one 4-yr-old and one 5-yr-old) Thoroughbreds (TB). The ejaculates were obtained at approximately equal intervals from December through November.

Sexual behavior as measured by reaction time (total time the stallion was in contact with the mare until beginning of copulation) was significantly affected by season. Over the 12-month period, average number of mounts required for first ejaculates was 1.8 (Fig. 86–1), ranging from 1.2 in April to 2.4 in October. The mean number of mounts per second ejaculate was 1.5; ranging from 1.0 in September to 2.1 in January. Seasonal effects were significant for both first and second ejaculates, and more mounts were required for first than for second ejaculates. Wierzbowski and Hafez reported 1.4 mounts per ejaculate in natural service.[19] This concurred with Asbury and Hughes, who reported that 1.38 mounts per ejaculate were required to collect 130 ejaculates with an artificial vagina (AV) from 52 stallions.[20] In our study, 1.4 mounts were required per first ejaculate in the spring compared with 1.5, 2.3, and 1.9 in the summer, fall, and winter, respectively.[18] The 2- and 3-yr-old stallions were responsible for shortened reaction time and fewer mounts per ejaculate for second ejaculates. The first ejaculate appeared to serve as a stimulus for the second in younger stallions. This was probably caused by a reduction in the level of anxiety.

Abnormal sexual behavior, such as biting, striking, and savaging mares, was induced by the experimental treatment. Upon completion of the study, stallions were permitted sexual rest until spring. At that time, sexual behavior of older stallions returned to pre-experimental behavior. However, the 2- and 3-yr-old stallions continued to exhibit abnormal behavior. This resulted in slow stallions that had to be muzzled during mating to prevent them from savaging mares. Thus, overuse appeared to be more detrimental to younger, inexperienced stallions than to older animals. Based on these data and clinical experience, we never recommend use of a 2-yr-old as a breeding stallion. Obviously, this is practiced routinely in the industry, primarily because of the desire to "see a few of his offspring as soon as possible." This is understandable and may be economically necessary. However, when this is done, extreme caution should be used to prevent overuse or injury, because an unfavorable experience associated with the breeding act may result in a lifetime of abnormal sexual behavior. Apparently, younger stallions are more likely to be permanently affected by an injury associated with breeding than an older stallion. Furthermore, the younger stallion is much more difficult to retrain. For example, Rasbech recorded clinical signs of 11 stallions, 4 to 16 yr old, exhibiting ejaculatory disturbances.[21] Ejaculation failure appeared to be age related. The average age of stallions that ejaculated intermittently was 11.4 yr compared with 6.0 yr for those that failed to ejaculate, indicating more pronounced abnormal behavior in younger than in older stallions.

SEXUAL PREPARATION

Although daily sperm production (DSP) and daily sperm output (DSO) are closely related in normal stallions, after extragonadal sperm reserves have been depleted,[22] only those spermatozoa obtained at collection (output) can be used to breed mares. Thus, determining the extent to which sexual preparation affects sperm output is essential for maximum utilization of any breeding male.

Numerous studies have been conducted on the effect of sexual preparation of bulls on sperm output.[23] Changing stimulus animals (teasers), moving the teaser as little as 3 feet, changing locations for seminal collection, permitting false mounts (letting the animal mount and deflecting the penis rather than allowing entry into the AV), and restraining them from mounting can influence sexual arousal and increase sperm output. Presented in Table 86–1 is a comparison of no sexual preparation with one false mount (1FM) and a comparison of 1FM with a 2-min restraint plus three false mounts (2′R + 3FM). Sperm output was increased by 72 and 64%, respectively, because of treatments.

Presented in Table 86–2 is the effect of sexual preparation on sperm output of two bulls. The sperm output of bull A was increased by 7.3 billion because sexual stimulation was augmented, whereas output from bull B was increased by only 1.9 billion spermatozoa. Differences in sperm output from these bulls may reflect differences in efficiency of individual ejaculatory mechanisms or perhaps more sexual preparation was required to maximize sperm output of bull B. Regardless, sexual preparation for bulls before collection is generally essential for maximum sperm output.[23] In the event sperm output from stallions could be influenced by sexual stimulation, the amount of sexual preparation on a particular breeding day when AI is used could be commensurate with the number of mares that needed to be bred.

A study was conducted to determine whether a stallion's sperm output could be increased by sexual stimulation.[1] Four mature QH stallions were used on even-numbered days for 1 month to tease 14 mares before preparation for seminal collection. On odd-numbered days, the stallions were used to tease 1 mare until they attained an erection. They then were washed and allowed to mount that mare for seminal collection.

Seminal and behavioral characteristics are presented in Table 86–3. Significant increases in gel volume, gel-free seminal volume, and total volume were noted. Motility also showed a small but significant increase. A decrease in spermatozoa per milliliter was observed, which usually occurs when volume is increased. No change in behavioral characteristics, as measured by reaction time and number of mounts per ejaculate, was observed. Also, spermatozoa per ejaculate did not increase on the days stallions were teased, 3.3 billion, compared with the nonteased days of 3.8 billion.

Presented in Table 86–4 are results from teasing versus nonteasing of each of the four stallions. The changes that occurred were relatively consistent among stallions, except for reaction time. Stallion 3 appeared to mount and ejaculate sooner after teasing (34 vs. 115 s). Therefore, careful use of some stallions, particularly young, shy, or slow stallions, as teasers might improve breeding behavior, providing the majority of mares are in estrus. The significant increase in seminal volume is evi-

TABLE 86–1. EFFECT OF SEXUAL PREPARATION ON SPERM OUTPUT OF BULLS

TYPE OF PREPARATION*	INCREASE IN SPERM OUTPUT (%)
None vs 1FM	72
1FM vs 2′R + 3FM	64

*FM, false mount; 2′R, 2-minute restraint.
(From Hale, E.B., and Almquist, J.O.: Relation of sexual behavior to germ cell output in farm animals. J. Dairy Sci., *43(Suppl.)*:145–169, 1960.)

TABLE 86–2. CHANGE IN SPERM OUTPUT (BILLIONS) OF BULLS CAUSED BY SEXUAL PREPARATION

	SPERMATOZOA IN TWO EJACULATES/WEEK	
	Minimum Preparation	Maximum Preparation
Bull A	12.4	19.7
Bull B	21.8	23.7

(Adapted from Hale, E.B., and Almquist, J.O.: Relation of sexual behavior to germ cell output in farm animals. J. Dairy Sci., *43(Suppl.)*:145–169, 1960.)

TABLE 86–3. THE EFFECT OF TEASING ON STALLION SEMINAL AND BEHAVIORAL CHARACTERISTICS

CHARACTERISTIC	TEASED	NONTEASED
Reaction time (s)	39.0	62.0
Mounts	1.2	1.2
Seminal volume (mL)		
Gel	23.1*	8.2
Gel-free	62.5*	37.3
Total	85.6†	45.5
Spermatozoa		
Per milliliter (10^6)	59.0*	118.4
Per ejaculate (10^9)	3.3	3.8
Motile (%)	63.0†	61.0
Seminal pH	7.57	7.59

*$p < 0.05$.
†$p < 0.01$.
(From Pickett, B.W., et al.: Management of the Stallion for Maximum Reproductive Efficiency. II. Animal Reproduction Laboratory Bulletin No. 05. Fort Collins, Colorado State University, 1989.)

TABLE 86–4. THE EFFECT OF TEASING ON INDIVIDUAL STALLION SEMINAL AND BEHAVIORAL CHARACTERISTICS

	STALLION							
	1		2		3		4	
Characteristic	T*	NT†	T	NT	T	NT	T	NT
Reaction time (s)	41.0	52.0	45.0	44.0	34.0	115.0	34.0	36.0
Mounts	1.3	1.1	1.5	1.8	1.1	1.0	1.0	1.0
Seminal volume (mL)								
Gel	22.7	5.4	5.5	0.6	18.6	4.3	45.6	22.4
Gel-free	51.1	24.7	60.5	34.2	83.5	46.5	55.1	43.9
Total	73.7	30.1	65.9	34.8	102.1	50.8	100.7	66.3
Spermatozoa								
Per milliliter (10^6)	81.5	174.8	53.0	107.9	32.9	75.5	68.5	115.5
Per ejaculate (10^9)	3.7	3.8	3.1	3.4	2.6	3.3	3.8	4.9
Motile (%)	59.0	57.0	62.0	60.0	65.0	63.0	65.0	63.0
Seminal pH	7.59	7.64	7.62	7.62	7.49	7.52	7.58	7.59

*T, teased.
†NT, not teased.
(From Pickett, B.W., et al.: Management of the Stallion for Maximum Reproductive Efficiency. II. Animal Reproduction Laboratory Bulletin No. 05. Fort Collins, Colorado State University, 1989.)

dence that the stallions were sexually stimulated. However, no increase in total spermatozoa per ejaculate was obtained. Therefore, the value of sexually stimulating a normal stallion beyond that required for washing the penis probably is unnecessary. Apparently, extra sexual preparation is not required, because more spermatozoa usually will not be obtained, excessive gel is a nuisance, and total volume is unimportant in natural service. Pickett et al. found no significant difference in gel-free seminal volume between stallions that passed compared with those that failed a potential fertility evaluation.[24] However, others reported volume of ejaculate to have a significant effect on fertility.[25,26]

The previously mentioned studies involved measuring total or gel-free seminal volumes immediately after seminal collection and relating these data to fertility.[24–26] Meanwhile, Rowley et al. found, using embryo recovery as a measure of fertility after AI, that insemination volumes of 100 mL or more decreased fertility (Table 86–5).[27] Understanding the positive relationship between volume of raw semen and fertility is difficult, particularly when researchers have found that 0.6 mL of raw semen is as effective as larger volumes in an AI program.[28]

Several horse breed associations have approved transported (shipped) semen. To obtain satisfactory fertility during cooling and shipping, the raw semen must be placed into an appropriate extender.[28] Furthermore, the extender to semen ratio should be at least 2:1.[29] Under these circumstances, insemination volume may, with some stallions, become an important factor in fertility, particularly when insemination volume exceeds 100 mL. Therefore, the stallion, particularly if he produces relatively large volumes of semen, should be managed to minimize seminal volume. For example, when stallion 3 (Table 86–4) was teased before seminal collection, gel-free seminal volume was 85.3 mL compared with 46.5 mL when he was not teased. Thus, in all probability, sexual stimulation should be minimized when semen is collected for shipment, particularly from such a stallion.

IMPOTENCE

Krane et al., in an excellent review, defined impotence as "the consistent inability to achieve or sustain an erection of sufficient rigidity for sexual intercourse."[9] These authors excluded problems associated with libido, ejaculation, and orgasm. Factors that affect sexual behavior in stallions must include disturbances in libido (sex drive), ejaculation, and orgasm, which are sometimes included in the definition of impotence.[30] Others have divided the condition into several types and/or categories.[31] For example, (1) lack of erection—no

TABLE 86–5. EFFECT OF INSEMINATION VOLUME ON PERCENTAGE OF EMBRYOS RECOVERED

	VOLUME (ML)	MOTILE SPERM (10^6)	PERCENT RECOVERY*
Experiment 1	10	100	40.0^a
	100	100	10.0
	200	100	0.0^b
Experiment 2	10	250	70.6^a
	100	250	13.0^b

*Within experiments, values with different superscripts are different ($p < 0.05$).
(Adapted from Rowley, H.S., Squires, E.L., and Pickett, B.W.: Effect of insemination volume on embryo recovery in mares. J. Equine Vet. Sci., *10*:298–300, 1990.)

erection achieved; (2) inadequate erection—complete erection cannot be achieved or, if accomplished, cannot be maintained and usually is lost without ejaculation; and (3) nonemissive erection—an erection is achieved but is not accompanied by ejaculation. Cooper divided impotence into two categories: (1) primary cases in which impotence had been present since the first attempt at intercourse and (2) secondary cases in which impotence developed after competency.[32] Cases of secondary impotence were divided further into three types: (1) constitutional—low sex drive and responsiveness, (2) organic—pathologic lesions, and (3) psychogenic—selective and transient. Many early investigators believed that approximately 90 to 95% of the causes of impotence were psychogenic.[32,33] Psychogenic factors responsible for or contributing to impotence in the human male include anxiety, fear, hostility, resentment, disgust, inhibition, insanity, ignorance, misinformation, functional psychoses, masturbation, monotony, male climacteric, homosexuality, premature ejaculation, and abstinence.[32,34,35] Others have suggested stress, depression, marriage problems, and neurosis.[16]

Spark et al.[10] showed that impotence is also caused by neurologic, vascular, and endocrine dysfunctions, which may be responsible for as much as 50% of all impotence cases.[36] Based on the earlier human data and clinical experience treating impotent stallions in our laboratory, we assumed that 90 to 95% of impotence cases in stallions were psychogenic. However, researchers have reported that impotent stallions had lower blood serum concentrations of leuteinzing hormone (LH) and estradiol-17β, whereas concentrations of testosterone were similar to normal stallions.[8] Obviously, this constitutes a physiologic basis for impotence. Whether impotence in stallions with low hormonal concentrations was caused by those hormone concentrations or whether the low hormonal concentrations were caused by impotence is not known. Clinicians note that constitutional impotence may be induced in stallions by excessive teasing, pain, fear, overuse, and poor management during training.[3,37] Irvine et al. observed two stallions with normal libido and seminal characteristics, but low LH and estradiol-17β and normal testosterone.[38] This is in contrast to those reported by Wallach et al.[8] In the human, no well-defined delineation between organic and psychogenic causes of impotence exists. In fact, numerous examples are known of an interaction between physical and psychologic factors responsible for impotence.[16] Consequently, clinicians should not assume that this interaction does not occur in the stallion. In fact, quite the contrary. Researchers have shown in humans that erections to certain stimuli are relatively independent of androgens,[39] and impotent patients can have normal concentrations of serum testosterone.[10] Thus, erection in some stallions may be relatively independent of hormones, as a result of previous psychic conditioning. Cause and effect should become much clearer in the stallion when more sophisticated diagnostic tests such as are now available for humans are used on stallions.[10,40,41]

EVALUATION AND TREATMENT OF IMPOTENCE

When a stallion is presented to the Equine Reproduction Laboratory at Colorado State University for diagnosis or treatment of abnormal sexual behavior, the following questions are asked of the handler, or the most knowledgeable individual associated with the stallion, to aid in determining factors contributing to the horse's condition.

1. What is his breeding history?
2. What type of breeding program was used, i.e., pasture, hand mating, or artificial insemination?
3. Does his sex drive appear normal?
4. What was his sexual behavior before the onset of the problem?
5. Has he been observed masturbating; if so, what type of treatment, if any, was initiated to control the problem?
6. How many mounts generally are required per ejaculation?
7. Does he dismount at onset of ejaculation?
8. Does he prefer mares of a particular color, stage of estrus, etc.?
9. Does he object to breeding certain mares; if so, what are their characteristics?
10. Has the stallion been injured or frightened during mating, teasing, or while exhibiting aggressive sexual behavior?
11. Has scrotal swelling been observed?
12. Has he exhibited pain or discomfort, particularly in the back or legs, during mounting, copulation, ejaculation, or dismounting?
13. Has he had laminitis or other forms of lameness causing difficulty in mounting?
14. Has the animal had surgery, recent illness, or displayed any type of unusual behavioral patterns?
15. Have any drugs been administered?
16. Was a tranquilizer necessary to get him into the trailer?
17. How frequently was he used as a 2 or 3 yr old, and how frequently has he been used this season, or during the season the problem first was noted?
18. What methods are used to discipline the animal and when are they used?
19. Does the glans penis become engorged with blood, i.e., "flower" when attempting to breed?
20. Is he being shown or participating in performance events and being used to breed mares during the same season?
21. Is his trainer the same person that handles him in the breeding shed?

Procedures for diagnosing and retraining a stallion generally consist of presenting the patient to a mare or variety of mares in estrus and observing his sexual behavior.[3] This generally is done immediately upon the stallion's arrival at the clinic and often in the presence of the person most familiar with the patient's behavior. Observing the stallion's reaction in the presence and absence of the routine handler and/or owner sometimes can aid in diagnosis and/or treatment. Unfortunately, many individuals handling stallions are inexperienced and/or do not understand normal breeding behavior.[42,43] For example, the objectives are different for stallions in the show ring from those in the breeding shed. Consequently, "normal" behavior in one setting will be abnormal in another. Furthermore, when the handler is the same individual, the stallion often becomes confused and develops abnormal behavior. Unless the situation is quickly rectified, the stallion may never know what behavior is expected, and the unfavorable situation is magnified. Many stallions cannot tolerate the stress of performance and/or showing and breeding during the same season. These stallions may develop abnormal behavior, and in some instances, seminal characteristics are affected in the form of lowered sperm motility and morphology. This relationship has not been proven experimentally, but such clinical observations are well known among veterinarians whose clients are primarily show-horse enthusiasts. They have estimated that approximately 20% of the stallions thus managed are affected. In the human, stress conditions may be provoked by a variety of factors, both mental and physical, and may affect some individuals and not others, or may affect individuals differently. This is believed to act through the sympathoadrenal system.[44] In all probability, this also applies to the stallion.

The stallion's behavior immediately upon arrival may change dramatically within a few days. McDonnell et al. reported that novel environment appeared to interfere with desirable sexual behavior by increasing time to erection.[45] However, a novel environment may be conducive to better behavior, particularly if the previous environment was associated with an unpleasant experience(s).

After sufficient observation, stallions are classified into one or several of the five following categories.[3]

1. *Failure to attain or maintain an erection.* Stallions with poor libido and those that have excellent libido but cannot physically attain an erection.
2. *Incomplete intromission or lack of pelvic thrusts after intromission.* Stallions with poor libido and those that were injured during breeding or associate pain with breeding.
3. *Dismounting at onset of ejaculation.* Stallions that have good libido but associate copulation with pain or a previous injury.
4. *Failure to ejaculate in spite of a complete, prolonged erection and repeated intromissions.* Stallions that have been injured by a mare during breeding or associated severe pain with the sex act.
5. *Stallions that have excellent libido can and do ejaculate normally but cannot ejaculate normally without sexual rest, although libido remains high.*

Stallions with poor sex drive are almost always slow breeders; are slow to sexual arousal; are disinterested in estrous mares; are easily distracted; fail to respond sexually to a mare in the presence of specific humans; show awkward and/or juvenile behavior; are fearful, bored, confused, and aggressive; and/or are resistant to restraint.[43] However, these stallions may show an uncommonly intense interest in a specific mare that may or may not be in standing heat. These stallions are likely psychologically impotent because of an unfavorable experience associated with breeding. However, the possibility of endocrine factors being responsible for poor sex drive cannot be ruled out,[8] particularly with older stallions suffering from testicular degeneration.[24]

Those stallions that cannot attain an erection may be suffering from endocrine, neurologic, or vascular disorders.[3,8,9,24] Wilcox et al. have suggested that psychologically inhibited stallions, which have not been observed with an erection, should be observed for masturbation after recumbent sleep.[46] This is similar to techniques used to diagnose impotence in humans.[9,16,41]

Once a category is established, patients are permitted to act as independently as possible until a given situation elicits a favorable sexual response. If the patient fails to respond favorably while under halter, he is placed in a corral adjacent to mares in estrus so his behavioral responses can be observed while unrestrained. In most cases, extreme patience is required until the desired sexual response is elicited.

Depending on the stallion's behavior, clinicians may use certain "barriers" to aid in focusing his attention. For example, when a stallion appears to be easily distracted, blinkers are used to restrict his vision. Thus, the handler can more easily keep the stallion's attention focused on the tease mare. Furthermore, when a stallion objects to and/or is unaccustomed to being collected with an AV, blinkers can prevent the stallion from being frightened when the collector approaches. Occasionally, a stallion will be easily distracted by noise. This distraction can be reduced by loud music or otherwise restricting his hearing.

When attempting to stimulate a patient sexually, one should always have a properly prepared AV, at 50° C, but not exceeding 54° C, to attempt seminal collection in the event he attains an erection. Extreme care should be exercised when attempting to collect the first few ejaculates, but particularly the first ejaculate. An AV that is too hot or cold will be a significant negative reinforcement. However, an AV too hot is much more detrimental than one too cold.

Many times a stallion, particularly an inexperienced animal, will attain an erection but will not mount an estrous mare or phantom. Efforts to collect semen from the patient should continue as long as he has an erection unless he gets mad and/or becomes vicious, then he should be placed where he can observe other stallions being collected. However, if his attitude remains "good" continue efforts to collect semen, as long as he maintains a satisfactory erection. If the patient is 15 yr old or older, he should not be allowed to get overly excited; older stallions can drop dead in the breeding shed because of an aortic rupture.

If the patient refuses to mount in spite of all inducements, he should be fitted with blinkers and maneuvered so his chest is positioned at a slightly oblique angle on the phantom or the mare's left hip. Placing an AV on the erect penis, with him in this position, will many times trigger a mounting response. If this occurs, the probability of thrusting to ejaculation is excellent.

Patients that show little or no interest in an estrous mare should not be exposed to one set of conditions for longer than 15 min. The clinician should either put the patient back in his stall, place him in a pen adjacent to estrous mares, or leave him in a pen where he can observe other stallions being collected or breeding mares rather than continue in a negative or unresponsive situation.

Occasionally, several days or weeks are required to obtain the first ejaculation. However, after this has been accomplished, all but the most severely maladjusted stallions respond favorably to continued positive reinforcement. The same techniques are used to train and/or retrain stallions that are used for natural service as those used for AI. Training or retraining a stallion with an AV is almost always easier than breeding a mare by natural service. Regardless of the situation, attempts to train or retrain stallions should be done in a calm atmosphere, free of distractions, and with no time constraints.[43] Two stallions exposed to the same traumatic experience may react differently to that trauma and require a different approach to retraining. The range of behavioral patterns may extend from complete indifference to an excessively savage attitude toward mares or even humans. To diagnose and treat cases outlined in the five categories successfully, the following are needed: (1) a variety of mares in estrus;[47] (2) other stallions, because the patient may be stimulated by observing sexual activity; (3) extreme patience, because occasionally a stallion must be observed and/or handled 4 or 5 h a day; (4) an AV that will maintain a satisfactory temperature for extended periods; and (5) equipment for seminal evaluation,[28] including a phantom[3] for extremely aggressive stallions or for stallions that are afraid of mares. Spring and summer are the best seasons for treatment.

Upon arrival at the clinic the patient may be noisy and appear confident and aggressive. Nevertheless, he is suffering some, if not a great deal of, anxiety. Therefore, if he is to remain at the clinic, a pen or stall should be selected that will remain his for the duration of treatment. Many times the first ejaculate can be collected from a shy, impotent stallion in his pen, when all other locations had failed to elicit a favorable response. Any shoeing, physical examinations, or treatments should be conducted on the patient in a designated area other than his pen. He should associate this enclosure with pleasant experiences. Generally, after the stallion has had several complete ejaculations and becomes reasonably confident that he will not be injured by a mare or personnel, limited correctional procedures can be used to alter unacceptable breeding shed behavior. Discipline must be kept to a minimum during retraining, particularly during the sexual act or any procedure that the stallion might associate with sexual activity. However, a stallion should not be allowed to endanger personnel or other horses. He should be restrained by barriers, not violence.

A virgin stallion should be introduced to the breeding program gradually over a period of weeks. This is especially important if the animal has been severely corrected or abused for showing an interest in mares while performing in shows or at the race track. This introductory period can be used effectively to train the stallion to washing, teasing, and breeding procedures. Many stallions only tolerate washing of the penis before breeding; however, this should be a sexually stimulating experience. This situation is generally induced by the breeding shed crew who look on the procedure as something that must be done before breeding or seminal collection regardless of the stallion's attitude. Training to having the penis washed should begin at least 3 weeks before the first breeding. The stallion should be presented to an estrous mare with a padded barrier between them (Fig. 86–2). When he has attained an erection, the stallion should be restrained by the handler against the barrier and the stallion's penis deflected (not grabbed) and washed with warm (42° C) water.[28] If he objects, stop the washing procedure. If this is repeated once or twice per day, it will become an enjoyable, sexually stimulating experience and will result in a sexually responsive stallion.

Racing and show stallions, regardless of breed, are presented more frequently for treatment of impotence and/or abnormal sexual behavior than stallions from any other group. Generally, a stallion susceptible to intimidation is more likely than a well-adjusted stallion to be unfavorably influenced toward the sex act by the training and discipline necessary for racing and showing. Techniques and principles used in training stallions for show and performance are opposite to those that should be used for breeding or retraining after a bad experience. When breeding and retraining, little or no force should be applied so that the sex act and associ-

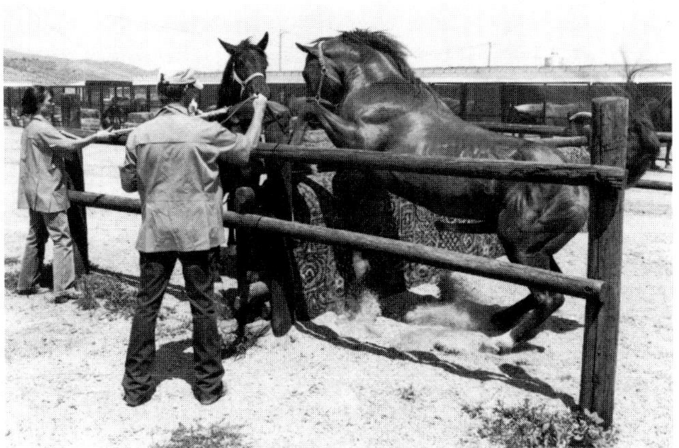

FIG. 86–2. A padded barrier to permit a stallion to tease mares safely. (From Pickett, B.W., Squires, E.L., and McKinnon, A.O.: Procedures for Collection, Evaluation and Utilization of Stallion Semen for Artificial Insemination. Animal Reproduction Laboratory Bulletin No. 03. Fort Collins, Colorado State University, 1987.)

ated procedures are pleasant experiences. Care should be taken to avoid negative factors. Identical training or retraining techniques are used for young or shy stallions as are used for impotent animals. Judicious use of a young, shy, or slow-working stallion as a teaser might improve his breeding behavior, particularly if he is allowed to tease only mares in estrus. This appears to reinforce the stallion's confidence and results in an improved behavioral pattern. However, excessive teasing, particularly of pregnant and diestrous mares, can adversely alter a stallion's attitude toward mares by inducing excessive roughness, biting, flehmen, striking, or indifference toward mares.[47–49] This may occur particularly in older stallions. Occasionally, it will induce aggressiveness toward the stallion handler. Consequently, a breeding stallion should only be used as a teaser if he enjoys teasing mares. Otherwise, a stallion should be purchased for that specific purpose. Periodically collecting semen from the teaser may be necessary to induce him to maintain interest in an unrewarding task.

Complete recovery from induced abnormal sexual behavior is most difficult in stallions injured during breeding. As safeguards, mares to be bred naturally should be hobbled and twitched, and when AI is employed, the teaser mare should be docile and restrained before seminal collection or a phantom is used.[3]

SEXUAL BEHAVIOR

Some excellent studies with bulls have aided in determining factors affecting sex drive.[23] Unfortunately, most techniques for management of stallions have been developed empirically. However, some factors affecting the animal's sex drive have been determined. Occasionally, moving a stallion to unfamiliar surroundings will influence his sexual behavior, but whether the reaction will be favorable or unfavorable cannot be easily predicted. Sexual behavior of stallions used for seminal collection throughout the year changes during the fall and winter, and number of mounts required per ejaculation and reaction time increases.[18,50,51] During the nonbreeding season, many stallions savage mares by excessive biting and striking before mounting and during copulation. Stallions that exhibit this type of behavior are those in which effect of season, as measured by reaction time and number of mounts, is most pronounced. These animals may be conditioned more quickly to a particular stimulus or to a specific procedure or may be more easily sexually satiated. Therefore, they require more stimulus pressure to maintain normal sexual behavior. The sexual behavior of 2- and 3-yr-old stallions was altered severely when semen was collected at regular intervals throughout the entire year.[18] Thus, sexual satiation, particularly in younger stallions, induced by too frequent breeding or seminal collection, can cause abnormal sexual behavior, such as slow to sexual arousal and savaging mares. Their attitude did not improve with sexual rest, and the change was believed to be permanent. In contrast, sexual behavior of older stallions returned to normal with sexual rest.

Anxiety, whether conscious or unconscious, appears to be a common cause of impotence in humans,[52,53] and may be interrelated with organic factors.[10,16] Treatment consists of providing some means for the patient to express hostility and providing an "optimal" sexual environment for changing and modifying the patient's attitude (psychotherapy). This aids the patient in developing feelings of self-confidence and self-competence.[31,52]

The situation is relatively similar for stallions. For example, impotence and abnormal sexual behavior can be induced by pain and fear. If pain persists, the stallion may become impotent and remain in that condition after the pain has subsided or totally disappeared. Under these circumstances, the cause of impotence appears to change from physiologic to psychologic. Treatment of impotence in the stallion, as with humans, also consists of providing an optimal sexual environment. The stallion should be permitted to act independently, without fear of correction, if possible. For example, many impotent stallions attempt to mount without an erection. A normal reaction of a stallion handler may be to forcibly prevent the animal from mounting or forcing the animal to dismount. This generally results in a suboptimal sexual environment. If the animal was encouraged to mount and allowed to remain, some of his fears might be dispelled. Also, maintaining a mounted position is uncomfortable, and a horse will dismount in 1 to 2 min without force being applied. Occasionally, a stallion will mount without an erection then attempt to savage the mare severely while he is mounted. Under these circumstances, the stallion handler must intervene, otherwise the stallion may be injured by the mare or otherwise exposed to a negative situation.

SEMINAL COLLECTION

As clinicians, we are occasionally requested to assist in developing procedures to collect semen from stallions that have become injured during the breeding season and either have difficulty in mounting for seminal collection or refuse to mount. Obviously, the stallion should be allowed to recover completely before any attempts are made to collect semen. As previously stated, if people persist in collecting semen or continue attempts, the stallion may become impotent and remain so even after the pain has disappeared. However, sexual rest, i.e., not breeding mares, may not be an economic option for the owners of the stallion. Therefore, procedures should be used to minimize pain during seminal collection. Techniques have been developed for collection of semen from stallions without mounting a mare or phantom, either by manual stimulation[54,55] of the penis or with an AV.[56] Apparently, these techniques do not affect seminal quality and quantity. Collection of semen while standing should, in most cases of lameness, reduce the stress and pain associated with seminal collection.

HORMONAL CONSIDERATIONS

All known effects of endogenous testosterone can be duplicated by injections of long-acting esters of testosterone into hypogonadal men, except induction and maintenance of spermatogenesis.[57] When administered in high doses, plasma testosterone is increased above the normal range and concentrations of LH and follicle-stimulating hormone (FSH), and their response to gonadotropin-releasing hormone (GnRH) are decreased, which results in a decrease in sperm production. Because sperm production is the desired result of most treatment regimens for impotent or infertile stallions, the use of testosterone is contraindicated. However, the principal aim in treatment of hypogonadal men is to restore male secondary sexual characteristics and sexual behavior and to induce normal somatic development. Therefore, use of testosterone in these subjects is relatively straightforward and generally successful.

Apparently considerable variability in plasma testosterone and human male sexual behavior exists. Similar evidence has been reported in stallions.[8,38] All stallions in both studies had normal concentrations of serum testosterone, but one group was impotent,[8] whereas the other exhibited normal sexual behavior.[38] The reason for this variability and/or inconsistency could be the result of a combination of organic factors (imbalance of other reproductive hormones) and psychic factors (impotence induced by undesirable management factors). The variability in sex drive, regardless of hormonal patterns in both species, is to be expected because of the variation in their response to psychologic factors contributing to and/or responsible for impotence.

Excellent evidence exists that sexual interest and ejaculation by hypogonadal men depended on androgen therapy. However, researchers also observed that "with the appropriate type of stimulation," erections continued regardless of the levels of androgen.[39] Thus, once the basic erectile mechanisms were established, they were no longer androgen dependent. Impotent stallions that are sufficiently stimulated to attain an erection and ejaculate will generally continue to become stimulated and exhibit reasonably normal sexual behavior accompanied by ejaculation. In most cases, the hormonal profiles have been unknown. Because these stallions' behavior becomes, if not normal, at least acceptable for breeding, clinicians have generally assumed that this type of impotence was principally, if not entirely, psychologic. However, this assumption may be as erroneous in the stallion as it has been in humans.[10,36]

In stallions, circulating concentrations of testosterone are influenced by season and are highest during the breeding season.[6,7,51,58] This fact, coupled with seasonal behavioral changes, is consistent with the hypothesis that seasonal variations in libido and spermatogenesis in stallions are mediated, at least in part, by availability of testosterone. Certain conditions, outlined in the five categories of impotence, may be endocrine mediated, but pharmacologic treatment has not been recommended. However, there is some experimental evidence that injections of GnRH may result in an increase in blood concentrations of gonadotropic hormones in stallions suffering from testicular degeneration.[59] Clinical evidence also has been presented that GnRH administered in a pulsatile fashion has, in selected cases, resulted in observable improvements in libido and seminal quality (K.A. Shiner, personal communication). Rasbech reported positive ejaculatory responses from two stallions after administration of pilocarpine or ephedrine.[21] He also suggested that administering cocaine to stallions may aid in correcting ejaculatory responses by increasing sympathetic sensitivity to norepinephrine and inactivating the enzymes that metabolize norepinephrine.

Other workers conducted a series of experiments on behavior of stallions and ponies.[45,60] These studies included (1) response-contingent aversive conditioning, (2) novel environment, and (3) continuous nonreward sexual arousal. Electric shock was used to alter sexual behavior of normal stallions. Sexual behavior of stallions was rapidly modified by the negative experience of electrical shock. Stallions could be conditioned to avoid noise or specific mares when they were associated with electric shock, even when mares were exhibiting sexual receptivity. The authors concluded that (1) perhaps stallions should be exposed to a number of novel environments, to prevent dependence on a familiar setting, and (2) continuous teasing, without the opportunity to breed mares, resulted in a decline in sexual arousal and response in about 2 weeks. These authors used psychotropic drugs to modify abnormal sexual behavior in stallions. Stallions whose previous behavior was normal but had since been modified by electric shock were treated with diazepam (Valium), which consisted of slow intrajugular injection of 0.05 mg/kg body weight. This treatment effectively reversed general and mare-specific response-contingent suppression[60] and novel environmental effects.[45] Furthermore, the drug appeared to delay suppression of sexual behavior. Apparently other drugs such as dibenzazepines, imipramine, and clomipramine were effective in eliciting erection and masturbation in some stallions.

Most stallions presented to our laboratory over the last 20 yr have responded well to retraining, and recoveries were usually complete without pharmacologic treatment. However, considering the recent evidence on the relationships between organic and psychic causes of sexual dysfunction and new diagnostic techniques in human medicine, in all probability a larger number and variety of drugs will and should be used in conjunction with creating an appropriate atmosphere to treat stallions for abnormal sexual behavior.

MASTURBATION

For many years, masturbation has been considered a vice in stallions.[61] However, recent, convincing evidence has been presented that masturbation by stallions is normal sexual behavior.[46,62] Consequently, stallions should not be discouraged from masturbating, particularly by use of antimasturbatory devices, such as rings, brushes, and/or cages. They may result in injury, hemospermia, and/or induction of abnormal sexual behavior. Masturbation appears to occur with relative frequency regardless of environmental conditions, i.e., with or without the presence of mares, in pasture or stall, and during periods of heavy breeding. Therefore, frequency of breeding does not appear to alter frequency of masturbation. Clinicians have known for some time that masturbation is rarely accompanied by ejaculation.[3] Thus, extragonadal sperm reserves are not depleted. Consequently, fertility is not affected, unless in some circumstances, stallions that are impotent because of an unpleasant sexual experience may use masturbation for sexual release rather than breed mares. In fact, Wilcox et al. suggested that observation of impotent stallions during recumbent rest may aid in diagnosis, because impotent stallions may be less likely to masturbate in the presence of humans.[46] Thus, stallions that are well-adjusted will not masturbate with sufficient frequency to reduce libido.

OTHER FACTORS AFFECTING SEXUAL BEHAVIOR

Some investigators believe a hereditary element is involved in human impotence.[53] Obvious differences exist among breeds of cattle with respect to sex drive and reaction to sexual preparation.[23,63] We have seen no striking differences among the major breeds of light horses common to the United States. However, this does not rule out hereditary influence on sexual behavior among individuals within a breed. Many knowledgeable horse owners and managers believe that stallions from some bloodlines have a tendency to be slow to sexual arousal, thus to be slow in the breeding act, while others are just the opposite.

Stallions can ejaculate normal volumes of semen that is devoid of spermatozoa.[3] Muscle contractions may be affecting only the bulbourethral, prostate, and vesicular glands. When large numbers of morphologically abnormal spermatozoa are obtained, particularly with heads separated from tails, the ampullae and deferent ducts—but not the epididymides—may be involved in the ejaculatory process. Organic as well as psychic causes may be responsible for this condition.

Our investigations during the last 20 yr with large numbers of stallions showing normal and abnormal sexual behavior have led us to believe that sex drive of the domestic stallion is the principal limiting factor in the number of mares that can be bred by a stallion in natural service. The number of breedings that have been observed by stallions and other equids in pasture[62,64] exceed the number that a stallion can breed routinely in a breeding shed environment. Therefore, conditions imposed on the stallion in the breeding shed result in a negative reaction, reducing sex drive and altering sexual behavior. Unfortunately, in the last 200 yr virtually no progress has been made to understand a breeding stallion's psyche when his sexual activities are physically directed by humans.

REFERENCES

1. Pickett, B.W., et al.: Management of the Stallion for Maximum Reproductive Efficiency. II. Animal Reproductive Laboratory Bulletin No. 05. Fort Collins, Colorado State University, 1989.
2. Nishikawa, Y.: Studies on Reproduction in Horses. Tokyo, Japan Racing Association, 1959.
3. Pickett, B.W., Squires, E.L., and Voss, J.L.: Normal and Abnormal Sexual Behavior of the Equine Male. Experimental Station Animal Reproduction Laboratory General Series Bulletin No. 1004. Fort Collins, Colorado State University, 1981.
4. Pickett, B.W., Sullivan, J.J., and Seidel, G.E., Jr.: Reproductive physiology of the stallion. V. Effect of frequency of ejaculation on seminal characteristics and spermatozoal output. J. Anim. Sci., *40:*917–923, 1975.
5. Pickett, B.W., Voss, J.L., and Squires, E.L.: Impotence and abnormal sexual behavior in the stallion. Theriogenology, *8:*329–347, 1977.
6. Berndtson, W.E., Pickett, B.W., and Nett, T.M.: Reproductive physiology of the stallion. IV. Seasonal changes in the testosterone concentration of peripheral plasma. J. Reprod. Fertil., *39:*115–118, 1974.
7. Clay, C.M., Squires, E.L., Amann, R.P., and Pickett, B.W.: Influences of season and artificial photoperiod on stallions: Lutenizing hormone, follicle-stimulating hormone and testosterone. J. Anim. Sci., *66:*1246–1255, 1988.
8. Wallach, S.J.R., Pickett, B.W., and Nett, T.M.: Sexual behavior and serum concentrations of reproductive hormones in impotent stallions. Theriogenology, *19:* 838–840, 1983.
9. Krane, R.J., Goldstein, I., and Tejada, I.S.: Impotence. N. Engl. J. Med., *321:*1648–1659, 1989.
10. Spark, R.F., White, R.A., and Connolly, P.B.: Impotence is not always psychogenic: Newer insights into hypothalamic-pituitary-gonadal dysfunction. JAMA, *243:*750–755, 1980.
11. Chenoweth, P.J., et al.: Relationships between breeding soundness and sex drive classifications in beef bulls. Theriogenology, *30:*227–233, 1988.
12. Terrell, B.A.: Effect of mount object and artificial vagina liner on stallion seminal and behavioral characteristics. M.S. thesis. Colorado State University, 1989.
13. Ashdown, R.R., and Hancock, J.L.: Functional anatomy of male reproduction. *In* Reproduction in Farm Animals. 3rd ed. Edited by E.S.E. Hafez. Philadelphia, Lea & Febiger, 1974, pp. 3–23.
14. Frandson, R.D.: Anatomy and Physiology of Farm Animals. 4th ed. Philadelphia, Lea & Febiger, 1986.

15. Chenoweth, P.J.: Libido and mating behavior in bulls, boars and rams. Theriogenology, *16:*155–177, 1981.
16. Shabsigh, R., Fishman, I.J., and Scott, F.B.: Evaluation of erectile impotence. Urology, *32:*83–90, 1988.
17. Kosiniak, K.: Characteristics of the successive jets of ejaculated semen of stallions. J. Reprod. Fertil. Suppl., *23:*59–61, 1975.
18. Pickett, B.W., Faulkner, L.C., and Sutherland, T.M.: Effect of month and stallion on seminal characteristics and sexual behavior. J. Anim. Sci., *31:*713–728, 1970.
19. Wierzbowski, S., and Hafez, E.S.E.: Analysis of copulatory reflexes in the stallion. Proceedings of the International Congress on Animal Reproduction and Artificial Insemination. Vol. 2. 1961, pp. 176–179.
20. Asbury, A.C., and Hughes, J.P.: Use of the artificial vagina for equine semen collection. J. Am. Vet. Med. Assoc., *144:*879–882, 1964.
21. Rasbech, N.O.: Ejaculatory disorders of the stallion. J. Reprod. Fertil. Suppl., *23:*123–128, 1975.
22. Gebauer, M.R., Pickett, B.W., and Swierstra, E.E.: Reproductive physiology of the stallion. II. Daily production and output of sperm. J. Anim. Sci., *39:*732–736, 1974.
23. Hale, E.B., and Almquist, J.O.: Relation of sexual behavior to germ cell output in farm animals. J. Dairy Sci., *43(suppl.):*145–169, 1960.
24. Pickett, B.W., et al.: Seminal characteristics and total scrotal width (T.S.W.) of normal and abnormal stallions. Proc. Am. Assoc. Equine Pract., 487–518, 1987.
25. Dowsett, K.F., and Pattie, W.A.: Characteristics and fertility of stallion semen. J. Reprod. Fertil. Suppl., *32:*1–8, 1982.
26. Sigler, D.H., and Kiracofe, G.H.: Ejaculate characteristics of two- and three-year old Quarter horse stallions. Proceedings of the Equine Nutrition and Physiology Symposium. 1987, pp. 291–296.
27. Rowley, H.S., Squires, E.L., and Pickett, B.W.: Effect of insemination volume on embryo recovery in mares. J. Equine Vet. Sci., *10:*298–300, 1990.
28. Pickett, B.W., Squires, E.L., and McKinnon, A.O.: Procedures for Collection, Evaluation and Utilization of Stallion Semen for Artificial Insemination. Animal Reproduction Laboratory Bulletin No. 03. Fort Collins, Colorado State University, 1987.
29. Jasko, D.J., Moran, D.M., Farlin, M.E., and Squires, E.L.: Effect of seminal plasma dilution or removal on spermatozoal motion characteristics of cooled stallion semen. Theriogenology, *35:*1059–1067, 1991.
30. Geboes, K., Steeno, O., and DeMoor, P.: Sexual impotence in man. Andrologia, *7:*217–227, 1975.
31. Proctor, R.C.: Impotence—A defense mechanism. J. Am. Geriatr. Soc., *17:*874–879, 1969.
32. Cooper, A.J.: The causes and management of impotence. Postgrad. Med. J., *48:*548–552, 1972.
33. Simpson, S.L.: Impotence. Br. Med. J., *1:*692–697, 1950.
34. Beheri, G.E.: Surgical treatment of impotence. Plast. Reconstr. Surg., *38:*92–97, 1966.
35. Finkle, A.L., and Prian, D.V.: Sexual potency in elderly men before and after prostatectomy. J. Am. Med. Assoc., *196:*139–143, 1966.
36. Karacan, I., and Moore, C.: Nocturnal penile tumescence: An objective diagnostic aid for erectile dysfunction. *In* Management of Male Impotence. Edited by A.H. Bennett. Baltimore, Williams & Wilkins, 1982, pp. 63–72.
37. McDonnell, S.M.: Stallion sexual behavior dysfunction: Experimental models and clinical considerations. Proc. Soc. Theriogenology, 1–12, 1986.
38. Irvine, C.H.G., Alexander, S.L., and Hughes, J.P.: Sexual behavior and serum concentrations of reproductive hormones in normal stallions. Theriogenology, *23:*607–617, 1985.
39. Bancroft, J., and Wu, F.C.W.: Changes in erectile responsiveness during androgen replacement therapy. Arch. Sex. Behav., *12:*59–66, 1983.
40. Slag, M.F., et al.: Impotence in medical outpatients. J. Am. Med. Assoc., *249:*1736–1740, 1983.
41. Barry, J.M., and Hodges, C.V.: Impotence: A diagnostic approach. J. Urol., *119:*575–578, 1978.
42. Marmor, J.: "Normal" and "deviant" sexual behavior. J. Am. Med. Assoc., *217:*165–170, 1971.
43. McDonnell, S.M.: Sexual behavior problems in stallions. *In* International Stockman's School Stud Managers' Handbook. Edited by L.S. Pope. 1988, pp. 179–185.
44. Von Euler, U.S.: Quantitation of stress by catecholamine analysis. Clin. Pharmacol. Ther., *5:*398–404, 1964.
45. McDonnell, S.M., Kenney, R.M., Meckley, P.M., and Garcia, M.C.: Novel environment suppression of stallion sexual behavior and effects of diazepam. Physiol. Behav., *37:*503–505, 1986.
46. Wilcox, S., Dusza, K., and Houpt, K.: The relationship between recumbent rest and masturbation in stallions. J. Equine Vet. Sci., *11:*23–26, 1991.
47. Ginther, O.J.: Reproductive Biology of the Mare: Basic and Applied Aspects. Equiservices, Cross Plaines, WI, 1979.
48. Estes, R.D.: The role of the vomeronasal organ in mammalian reproduction. Mammalia, *36:*315–341, 1972.
49. Schneider, K.M.: Das flehmen. Zool. Garten., Liepzig, *4:*183–198, 1930.
50. Pickett, B.W., et al.: Reproductive physiology of the stallion. VI. Seminal and behavioral characteristics. J. Anim. Sci., *43:*617–625, 1976.
51. Thompson, D.L., Jr., et al.: Reproductive physiology of the stallion. VIII. Artificial photoperiod, collection interval and seminal characteristics, sexual behavior and concentrations of LH and testosterone in serum. J. Anim. Sci., *44:*656–664, 1977.
52. Cooper, A.J.: A factual study of male potency disorders. Br. J. Psychiatry, *114:*719–731, 1968.
53. Strauss, E.B.: Impotence from the psychiatric standpoint. Br. Med. J., *1:*697–699, 1950.
54. Crump, J., Jr., and Crump, J.: Stallion ejaculation induced by manual stimulation of the penis. Theriogenology, *31:*341–346, 1989.
55. McDonnell, S.M., and Love, C.C.: Manual stimulation collection of semen from stallions: Training time, sexual behavior and semen. Theriogenology, *33:*1201–1210, 1990.
56. Schumacher, J., and Riddell, M.G.: Collection of stallion semen without a mount. Theriogenology, *26:*245–250, 1986.
57. Wilson, J.D., and Griffin, J.E.: The use and misuse of androgens. Metabolism, *29:*1278–1295, 1980.
58. Kirkpatrick, J.F., et al.: Seasonal variation in plasma androgens and testosterone in the North American wild horse. J. Endocrinol., *72:*237–238, 1977.
59. Blue, B.J.: Effects of pulsatile or continuous administration of GnRH on reproductive function of stallions. M.S. thesis. Colorado State University, 1990.
60. McDonnell, S.M., Kenney, R.M., Meckley, P.M., and Garcia, M.C.: Conditioned suppression of sexual behavior in stallions and reversal with diazepam. Physiol. Behav., *34:*951–956, 1985.

61. Pickett, B.W., and Voss, J.L.: Abnormalities of mating behavior in domestic stallions. J. Reprod. Fertil. Suppl., *23:*129–134, 1975.
62. McDonnell, S.M.: Spontaneous erection and masturbation in Equids. Proc. Am. Assoc. Equine Pract., 567–580, 1989.
63. Foster, J., Almquist, J.O., and Martig, R.C.: Reproductive capacity of beef bulls. IV. Changes in sexual behavior and semen characteristics among successive ejaculations. J. Anim. Sci., *30:*245–252, 1970.
64. Bristol, F.: Breeding behaviour of a stallion at pasture with 20 mares in synchronized oestrus. J. Reprod. Fertil. Suppl., *32:*71–72, 1982.

CHAPTER 87

REPRODUCTIVE ENDOCRINE FUNCTION TESTING IN STALLIONS

T.M. Nett

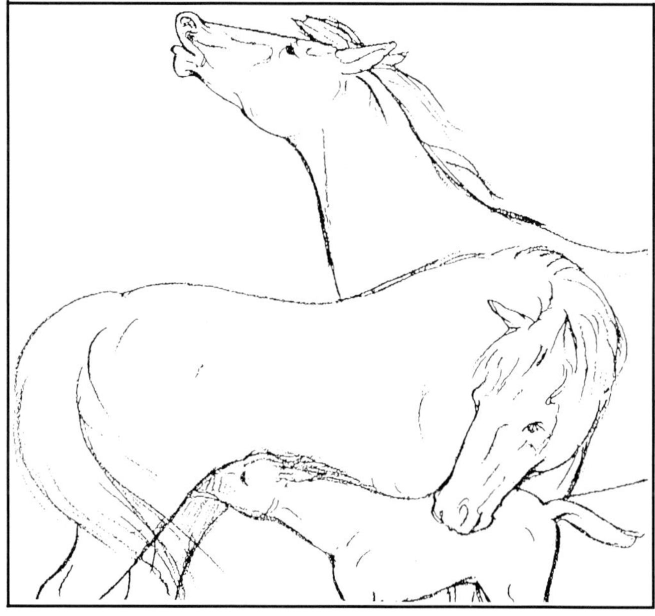

During the past several years, assays that can accurately measure a variety of hormones in biologic fluids of horses have been developed. Availability of these assays has lead to information concerning concentrations of hormones in the peripheral circulation of normal stallions. Now clinicians are able to compare concentrations of hormones in blood samples collected from stallions suspected of having an endocrine disorder with values observed in normal stallions. This has proven to be successful for diagnosis of some endocrine-related abnormalities in the stallion.

Information presented in this chapter will focus on diagnosis of endocrine disorders involving reproductive hormones in stallions. However, endocrinopathies involving nonreproductive hormones (i.e., thyroid, pancreatic, and adrenal hormones) may also lead to reproductive disorders. Therefore, when evaluating a reproductive disorder the clinician should establish that nonreproductive hormones are present at normal concentrations.

ENDOCRINE EVALUATION OF THE HYPOTHALAMIC-PITUITARY-TESTICULAR AXIS

The reproductive system of the stallion is ultimately driven by secretion of gonadotropin-releasing hormone (GnRH) from the hypothalamus. Ideally, evaluation of endocrine regulation of the reproductive system would include analysis of GnRH. However, GnRH is secreted from the hypothalamus into the hypophyseal portal vessels in small quantities and directly stimulates release of luteinizing hormone (LH) and follicle-stimulating hormone (FSH) from the anterior pituitary gland. Once the GnRH secreted into the hypophyseal portal system reaches the general circulation, it is diluted to such an extent that it is undetectable by even the most sensitive assay technique. A cannula can be inserted into the cavernous sinus via the facial vein and blood samples can be collected to monitor GnRH secretion (Chapter 4). Currently, this is considered impractical for diagnostic purposes. Normally, secretion of GnRH causes an almost immediate release of LH and/or FSH. Therefore, in most instances the clinician can infer what is happening to secretion of GnRH by monitoring the secretion of LH and FSH. An exception occurs when abnormalities are present in which the anterior pituitary gland is not responsive to GnRH. These can be diagnosed using a GnRH challenge test (see later).

The anterior pituitary hormones directly responsible for stimulation of testicular function are FSH and LH. Measurement of concentrations of these hormones in the general circulation provides an estimate of the stimulation the testis is receiving. The hormone secreted in the highest concentration by the testis is testosterone. Therefore, any evaluation of the endocrine function of the hypothalamic-pituitary-testicular axis should include measurement of testosterone.

The clinician should keep several important considerations in mind when collecting samples for evaluating the hypothalamic-pituitary-testicular axis in stallions. **First**, concentrations of these hormones are not constant in the bloodstream, but rather they appear as a series of discrete pulses.[1,2] Thus, to obtain an accurate estimate of the mean concentration of these hormones in the circulation, the clinician must collect several samples (at ~ 30-min intervals) over a period of 6 to 8 h. Evaluation of a single sample can lead to estimates that are 3- to 4-fold different from the mean concentration (Fig. 87–1). **Second**, the concentrations of circulating gonadotropins and testosterone vary with time of day. In general, concentrations of these hormones in the circulation are low early in the morning and then rise to their highest concentration around noon. **Third**, the concentrations of gonadotropins sufficient to stimulate normal testicular function vary greatly between individuals. That is, a wide range in circulating concentrations of gonadotropins has been observed in stallions having apparently normal spermatozoal production. For example, we have noted a greater than 50-fold difference in mean concentrations of LH among stallions, all of which had normal testicular function.[2] Thus, so-called normal values for concentrations of gonadotropins in individual stallions are of little merit for diagnostic purposes. In contrast, much less variation exists in circulating concentrations of testosterone among stallions. **Fourth** is a seasonal variation in concentrations of LH, FSH, and testosterone in stallions; levels are highest during the late spring and summer and lowest in the winter (Fig. 87–2).[2] **Fifth**, a universal standard is not yet available for gonadotropins in the horse. Therefore, most of the laboratories measuring gonadotropins in stallions employ a different standard, and each standard has a different purity. This means that the absolute concentrations of gonadotropins in the blood of horses reported by one laboratory may bear no relation to those reported by another laboratory; however, the patterns of change in concentrations of gonadotropins between physiologic states reported by different

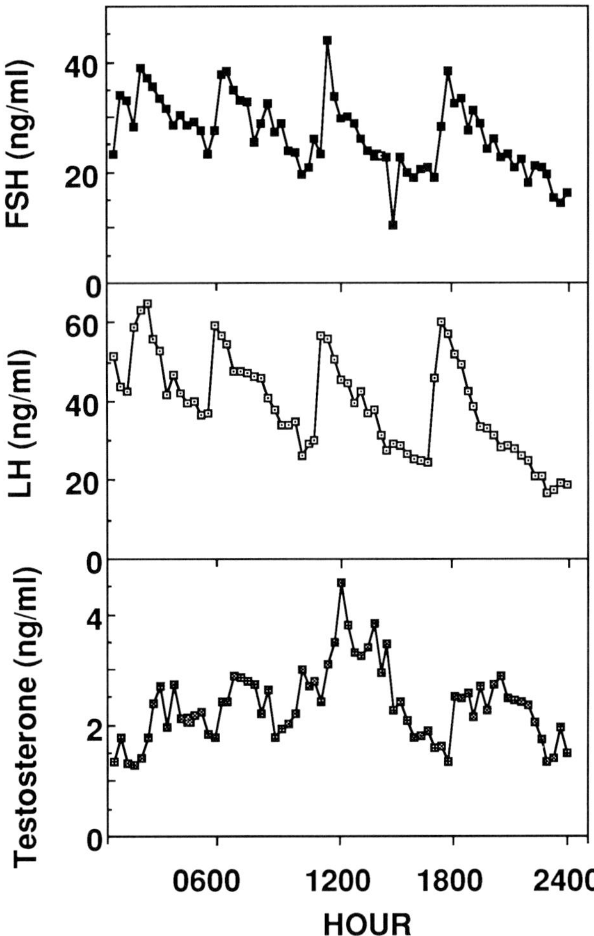

FIG. 87–1. Serum concentrations of FSH, LH, and testosterone in a stallion over 24 h. Note the pulsatile nature in which these hormones are secreted. Thus several samples must be collected over a period of at least 6 h to determine an accurate mean concentration. (Adapted from Clay, C.M., Squires, E.L., Amann, R.P., and Nett, T.M.: Influences of seasons and artificial photoperiod on stallions: Luteinizing hormone, follicle-stimulating hormone and testosterone. J. Anim. Sci., *66:*1246–1302, 1988.)

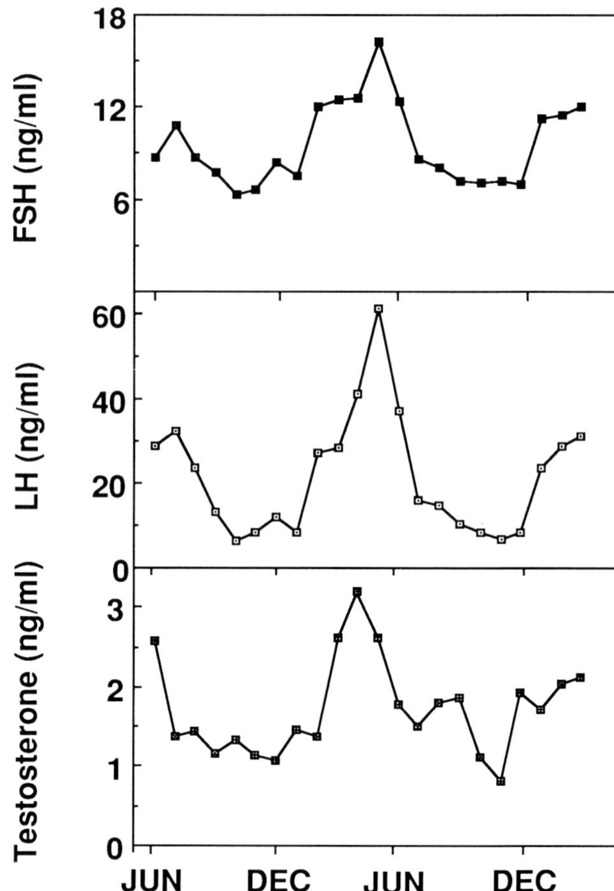

FIG. 87–2. Serum concentrations of FSH, LH, and testosterone in stallions throughout the year. Note that concentrations of each of these hormones are higher in the spring and summer than in the fall and winter. (Adapted from Clay, C.M., Squires, E.L., Amann, R.P., and Nett, T.M.: Influences of seasons and artificial photoperiod on stallions: Luteinizing hormone, follicle-stimulating hormone and testosterone. J. Anim. Sci., *66:*1246–1302, 1988.)

laboratories should be similar. In contrast, because testosterone is available in a pure form for use as a standard, the values obtained by different laboratories should be comparable.

Based on these considerations, we rely primarily on circulating concentrations of testosterone to determine if the hypothalamic-pituitary axis is functioning normally. To determine this, we recommend that blood samples be collected at 30-min intervals for 8 h beginning at 8:00 A.M. and analyzed for LH and testosterone. Data from such samples will provide information relative to the occurrence of a midday rise in secretion of LH. More importance is given to the pattern of LH secretion (i.e., being certain that the expected midday increase in secretion of LH occurs) rather than to the absolute concentrations of LH measured as a result of the high amount of variation among stallions. If the expected rise in circulating concentrations of LH occurs, then it is possible to determine if the testis responds to the rise in LH by secreting testosterone. The absolute amount of testosterone appearing in the circulation after the midday rise in secretion of LH is used to determine whether production of testosterone for testicular function is adequate.

In the event that circulating concentrations of testosterone are below the normal range for a stallion, then a GnRH challenge should be considered regardless of the concentrations of LH measured in the circulation. We utilize the GnRH challenge to determine if the pituitary gland can respond to GnRH with the subsequent release of LH and FSH, and if so, to determine if the testes respond to increased levels of gonadotropins by secreting more testosterone. We recommend that a maximally stimulatory dose of GnRH (2 μg/kg body weight) be administered to be certain that the pituitary-gonadal axis is capable of responding with increased secretion of LH and testosterone. Samples should be collected before and at 30-min intervals for 8 h after the GnRH challenge. The GnRH should be administered before 9:00 A.M. so that the increase that occurs because of the exogenous GnRH is not confused with the increase that occurs at midday in stallions. If the circulating concentration of testosterone increases into the normal range after a GnRH challenge, this indicates that both the anterior pituitary gland and testes are capable of responding to stimulation by their respective trophic hormones.

USE OF THE GNRH PUMP

As a stallion ages, an increasing likelihood exists that he will develop some degree of testicular degeneration. Many stallions undergoing testicular degeneration have subnormal circulating concentrations of testosterone, but normal or elevated concentrations of gonadotropins. Ejaculates from such stallions may have reduced numbers of spermatozoa with low motility and/or a high percentage of spermatozoa with morphologic defects. Many of these stallions respond to a challenge with GnRH by increasing their secretion of gonadotropins to even higher concentrations, and this often results in increased secretion of testosterone. A sustained increase in secretion of testosterone may improve testicular function (i.e., increase the number of sperm in the ejaculate, improve motility, and/or decrease the percentage of abnormalities). However, whether increased secretion of testosterone will have a beneficial effect in stallions undergoing testicular degeneration is unknown. Some practitioners who have stimulated testosterone secretion in stallions with a modest degree of testicular degeneration have the impression that an improvement occurs both in the percentage of morphologically normal spermatozoa and in motility. Again, this is a clinical impression developed as a result of treatment of stallions with a modest degree of testicular degeneration. In contrast, in a more rigorously designed experiment, no improvement was noted in ejaculates of stallions with advanced testicular degeneration when they were treated in such a way as to increase secretion of testosterone.[3]

As a result of the observation that circulating concentrations of testosterone are reduced in stallions undergoing testicular degeneration, considerable interest has developed in devising a treatment that will produce a sustained increase in secretion of testosterone and, it is hoped, lead to improved reproductive capacity of such stallions. In this regard, the GnRH pump has been used as a method for delivering pulses of GnRH to stallions at predetermined intervals over a prolonged period. In other species, continuous administration of GnRH results in desensitization of the anterior pituitary gland, leading to reduced secretion of gonadotropins.[4] Although clinicians do not know if the equine pituitary gland becomes desensitized to GnRH, secretion of GnRH occurs in a pulsatile manner in horses (Chapter 4). Therefore, we recommend that GnRH be administered in a manner simulating normal patterns of secretion. To this end, pumps (Pulsamat, Ferring Inc., Suffern, NY) have been used to administer pulses of GnRH to stallions.

In addition to desensitization caused by continuous administration of GnRH, too large a dose of GnRH can also cause desensitization of the pituitary gland. Therefore, even for pulsatile administration over a prolonged period the lowest dose of GnRH that will result in elevation of circulating concentrations of testosterone into the normal range should be chosen. In normal horses, administration of 10 μg GnRH is sufficient to stimulate a pulse of LH in the physiologic range and thereby induce an increase in secretion of testosterone. However, this dose may not be sufficient to increase secretion of testosterone into the normal range in stallions undergoing testicular degeneration. Thus, circulating concentrations of LH and testosterone should be monitored in each stallion to be treated with GnRH. Initially, 10 μg GnRH should be administered before 9:00 A.M., and blood samples collected at 30-min intervals for 8 h for analysis of LH and testosterone. If this dose of GnRH stimulates secretion of LH, which in turn increases circulating concentrations of testosterone into the normal range, then this dose of GnRH should be administered via the pump. If this dose of GnRH is not sufficient, then the test should be repeated with twice the amount of GnRH. This approach is continued until a dose of GnRH that increases circulating concentrations of testosterone into the normal range is found. This is the dose of GnRH that should be delivered in a pulsatile manner using the pump.

If a GnRH pump is to be used on a stallion, treatment should ideally begin approximately 2 months before the breeding season so that the elevated concentrations of testosterone have sufficient time to influence testicular function. Moreover, blood samples for analysis of LH and testosterone should be collected at 30-min intervals for 6 to 8 h once each month during treatment so that the dosage of GnRH can be altered in the event the stallion's sensitivity to GnRH changes.

DETERMINING COMPLETENESS OF CASTRATION

Owners frequently complain that males that were supposedly castrated still demonstrate stallion-like behavior. Such males often have an absence of scrotal testes. Thus, the possibility arises that the animal is a cryptorchid or that some testicular tissue remained after castration. Frequently, the clinician can determine if castration of a stallion was complete by measuring circulating concentrations of testosterone and LH.

To determine whether testicular tissue is present, a blood sample for analysis of testosterone should be collected in the early afternoon. Because this is the time of day when circulating concentrations of testosterone are highest, it constitutes the best time to determine if any testicular tissue remains to secrete testosterone. A concentration of testosterone of less than 100 pg/mL is indicative of complete castration. A concentration of greater than 200 pg/mL indicates that functional testicular tissue may still remain. If the concentration of testosterone is between 100 and 200 pg/mL the test is inconclusive and further analysis is necessary.

Normally, testosterone exerts a negative feedback on secretion of LH. Thus, in geldings, circulating concentrations of LH should be elevated compared with stallions.[5] Therefore, when circulating concentrations of testosterone are between 100 and 200 pg/mL, analysis of LH in the blood sample may help determine if functional testicular tissue is still present. If concentrations of LH are higher than those found in normal stallions, testicular tissue is absent. However, if circulating concentrations of LH are within the normal range, then functional testicular tissue quite likely still remains. Normal values for LH in stallions and geldings will vary greatly between laboratories, and clinicians using circulating concentrations of LH to determine the completeness of castration must rely on normal values provided by the laboratory they use.

A second method to confirm the presence (or absence) of testicular tissue when analysis of testosterone gives inconclusive results is the hCG stimulation test. Human chorionic gonadotropin (hCG) is a hormone that has LH-like activity, and when administered, it should stimulate secretion of testosterone if functional testicular tissue is present. The test is most diagnostic when administered in the morning, before the midday rise in LH and testosterone. A blood sample should be collected; then 2500 IU of hCG should be administered intravenously. An additional blood sample should be collected 90 min after the hCG injection. An increase in circulating concentrations of testosterone to greater than 200 pg/mL in the second blood sample is indicative of the presence of testicular tissue.

REFERENCES

1. Thompson, D.L., Jr., St. George, R.L., Jones, L.S., and Garza, F., Jr.: Patterns of secretion of luteinizing hormone, follicle-stimulating hormone and testosterone in stallions during the summer and winter. J. Anim. Sci., *60:*741–748, 1985.
2. Clay, C.M., Squires, E.L., Amann, R.P., and Nett, T.M.: Influences of seasons and artificial photoperiod on stallions: Luteinizing hormone, follicle-stimulating hormone and testosterone. J. Anim. Sci., *66:*1246–1302, 1988.
3. Blue, B.J., et al.: Effects of pulsatile or continuous administration of GnRH on reproduction function of stallions. J. Reprod. Fertil. Suppl., *44:*145–154, 1991.
4. Nett, T.M., Crowder, M.E., Moss, G.E., and Duello, T.M.: GnRH-receptor interaction. V. Down-regulation of pituitary receptors for GnRH in ovariectomized ewes by infusion of homologous hormone. Biol. Reprod., *24:*1145–1155, 1981.
5. Thompson, D.L., Jr., Pickett, B.W., Squires, E.L., and Nett, T.M.: Effect of testosterone and estradiol-17β alone and in combination of LH and FSH concentrations in blood serum and pituitary of geldings and in serum after administration of GnRH. Biol. Reprod., *21:*1231–1237, 1979.

CHAPTER 88

PHARMACOLOGIC MANIPULATION OF SEXUAL BEHAVIOR

S.M. McDonnell

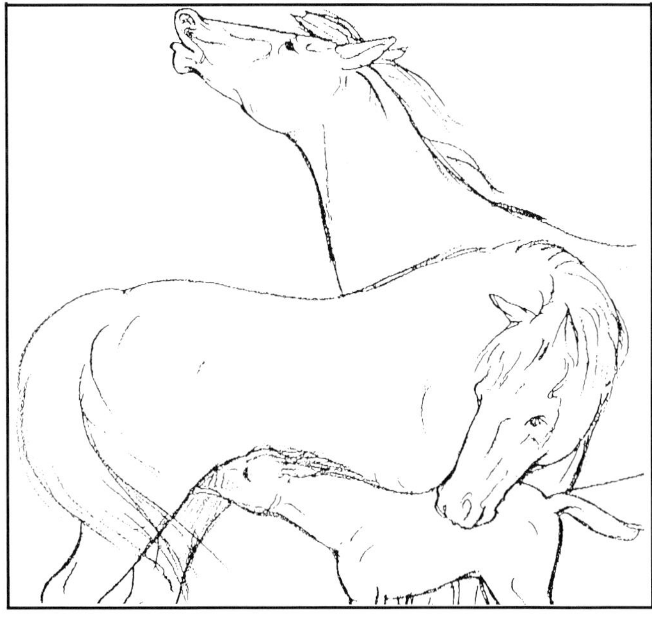

The quest for pharmacologic methods of enhancing or suppressing sexual behavior has a long and colorful history.[1] In the last decade, the medical and scientific communities began to accept and actively investigate methods of pharmacologically manipulating sexual behavior.

Sexual behavior involves a variety of interdependent components,[2,3] including precopulatory motivation and arousal, erection, copulatory function (mounting, insertion, thrusting), and ejaculation. Sexual motivation, interest, and arousal comprise the component of sexual behavior commonly referred to in humans and farm animals as libido. This aspect of sexual behavior is usually assessed in terms of the animal's speed and vigor in achieving erection, mounting, and ejaculating as well as breeding stamina and perseverance. Sexual motivation and arousal are known to be affected by genetic, social, hormonal, sensory, and experience factors. The erection component of sexual behavior requires both parasympathetic and sympathetic coordination of pelvic vascular events and basic integrity of the vascular supply to the penis. Copulation requires reasonable levels of musculoskeletal and proprioceptive function to attain and maintain appropriately oriented mount, intromission, thrusting, and dismount. Presumably, afferents via the pudendal nerve provide feedback, maintaining intravaginal thrusting and leading to the emission and ejaculation reflexes. Emission is the deposition of the spermatozoa from the epididymis and ampullae as well as the contents of the vesicular glands, prostate gland, and bulbourethral glands into the pelvic urethra. Current evidence indicates that emission is an α-androgenic-mediated reflex, possibly with cholinergic modulation. Ejaculation is the forceful expulsion of jets of semen from the urethra, resulting from rhythmic contractions of the bulbocavernosus and ischiocavernosus muscles. The bladder neck closes tightly simultaneously with emission and ejaculation, thus preventing passage of semen into the bladder as well as preventing expulsion of urine with the ejaculate. Specific types of ejaculatory dysfunction as well as side effects of pharmacologic agents indicate that emission, ejaculation, and bladder neck closure, while occurring contemporaneously, are independent reflexes. The event known as orgasm in humans is believed to be a cerebral event associated with emission and ejaculation and related pelvic muscular contraction.

Pharmacologic manipulation of sexual behavior has proven to be a complex undertaking. Almost all psychoactive, neuroactive, and vasoactive drugs, or even simple hormones, have dose-dependent positive and negative effects on the various components of sexual behavior. Effective dose ranges for facilitation of any specific component are usually remarkably narrow and frequently species or individual specific. Pharmacologic enhancement of one component may result in impairment of another component or of the general sensory and musculoskeletal competence necessary for mating. Nevertheless, the number of potential pharmacologic approaches to sexual behavior modification grows steadily with advances in psychopharmacology and neuropharmacology. In stallions, the principal focus of clinical and experimental work has been on developing therapies for sexual behavior dysfunction. Methods of suppressing undesirable sexual behavior of stallions and geldings have also been explored.

PRELIMINARY EVALUATION

The consensus among clinics and laboratories working with stallions has been to use pharmacologic agents as a last resort aid to traditional methods of sexual behavior modification. Accordingly, consideration of pharmacologic aids is usually preceded by a thorough evaluation of the horse and its breeding environment to understand the specific components of sexual behavior involved in the dysfunction, to identify and treat or accommodate physical deficits that may contribute to the dysfunction, and to identify environmental conditions that optimize the particular stallion's sexual performance. Typically, this requires 1 to 10 days of sessions once or twice a day with the horse and its handlers. In most instances, the behavioral problem is resolved during this initial systematic evaluation, usually with traditional behavior modification or simple management changes. In my experience, most cases of sexual behavior dysfunction are primarily attributable to management factors that can be modified to accommodate the individual stallion. Even when the primary cause of dysfunction is organic, the behavior of most stallions can be affected positively or negatively by management factors. Knowledge of a stallion's idiosyncrasies regarding management and sexual behavior can be useful even if drug therapies are eventually utilized.

ENHANCING GENERAL SEXUAL INTEREST AND AROUSAL

ANDROGENS

Testosterone and other androgens have been used to increase sexual interest and arousal of stallions with low libido. Moderate increases in circulating androgens may be useful for novice breeding stallions with slow or no arousal, however, moderate to high levels of androgens often result in an increase in the aggressive components (biting and striking) rather than the copulatory (erection and mounting) elements of sexual behavior.[4] Although the stallion may appear to exhibit increased libido, the aggressive behavior may further complicate dysfunction by eliciting an aggressive rather than solicitous response from the mare or by eliciting harsh discipline from the handler, either of which may inhibit precopulatory behavior. These complications, together with known side effects of androgens on endocrine function and spermatogenesis, make androgen therapy for sexual arousal in stallions controversial.

If androgens are used, high levels should be avoided. For slow-starting stallions for which more conservative approaches have failed, I have found that administering small amounts of testosterone (testosterone propionate in oil, 50 to 200 μg/kg SC every other day) is effective. To avoid reaching undesirably high circulating androgen concentrations (higher than 4 ng/mL), plasma testosterone can be measured every other day while the stallion is receiving treatment, and the dose adjusted accordingly. Increased sexual interest can be expected within 10 days of initial treatment. Recent experimental work indicated sexual behavior can be affected by relatively small increases in androgen levels.[5] In slow novice breeders, further androgen treatment is usually not required after the first ejaculation, because the positive reinforcement of ejaculation seems to result in more goal-directed and organized sexual response.

GONADOTROPIN-RELEASING HORMONE

Gonadotropin-releasing hormone (GnRH) has been shown to affect male sexual behavior via increased circulating testosterone as well as by extraendocrine (possibly direct central nervous system) effects on sexual behavior. Experimental evidence indicates that GnRH given in a pulsatile fashion (25 μg SC every 3 h) has direct facilitatory effects on precopulatory and copulatory behavior of pony geldings given a fixed low-level testosterone replacement.[6] Several different GnRH treatment regimens and routes (pulsatile pumps, subcutaneous frequent injections, continuous release implants) have been used for improving libido of stallions. Methods of measuring sexual behavior have also varied. In general, results can be interpreted as inconsistent. GnRH, whether administered by pulsatile pump (releasing 10 μg every 2 h SC) or by continuous-release subcutaneous implants, had no measurable effect on behavior of stallions with or without behavioral abnormalities.[7] Similarly, I have found no effects of continuous-release subcutaneous GnRH implants (5 μg/h) on any of 20 measures of precopulatory, copulatory, and postcopulatory sexual behavior of stallions with low libido. In contrast, a regimen of 50 μg SC GnRH (Cystorelin, CEVA) administered 2 h and again 1 h before breeding sometimes increases arousal of slow-starting novice stallions and mature breeding stallions that have soured and may superarouse a stallion with normal libido that has specific erection or ejaculatory dysfunction.[8] This regimen is typically associated with a doubling of resting testosterone levels, which may, in part, mediate the behavioral response.

PAIN MEDICATION

The effects of pain on sexual behavior seem to vary considerably among stallions. With retired performance horses, clinicians often reasonably suspect that unidentified physical pain may be interfering with sexual arousal or, more commonly, copulatory function. Phenylbutazone treatment (1 to 2 g orally bid for at least 10 days) often results in marked improvement within 10 to 14 days.[8] In a recent study, no adverse effects of a 30-

day course of phenylbutazone treatment (1 g orally bid) on semen of stallion were found.[9]

ANXIOLYTIC AGENTS

Anxiolytic compounds have proven useful in stallions with experience-related suppressed sexual interest or arousal.[10] Most widely used has been diazepam. Slow, novice breeding stallions, particularly those exhibiting signs of anxiety, often respond favorably with a single dose of diazepam. After one ejaculation, libido of the novice usually remains adequate and further treatment is not required. Diazepam has also been useful for treating specific aversions, for example, to an artificial vagina, a specific handler, a dummy mount, or a particular mare. Novel environment has a transient adverse effect on sexual arousal in stallions, which can be blocked by diazepam treatment.[11]

YOHIMBINE

Yohimbine, an indolalkylamine similar to reserpine, is one of the oldest purported aphrodisiacs. Controlled studies in rats have recently demonstrated effects on mating behavior, erection, and ejaculation. Acute yohimbine treatment increases mounting behavior and decreases intercopulatory interval in several models of low sexual arousal or motivation, including normal mature rats with the penis anesthetized, spontaneous noncopulators, and novice breeders.[12] Whether this is the result of effects on the sexual motivation component of sexual behavior or direct effects on erection is unclear. In those studies, effects indicating increased arousal have been observed for a period of 5 to 75 min following intraperitoneal injection of yohimbine hydrochloride across a dose range of 1 to 4 mg/kg. Effects on erection, presumably caused by selective α-2 receptor blockade, have also been demonstrated in controlled animal studies.[13] I have evaluated the effects of yohimbine at a variety of doses (0.05 to 0.5 mg/kg) and routes of administration (IV, IM, and SC) in pony stallions with normal sexual arousal and response, pony stallions with spontaneously sluggish breeding behavior, and in pony geldings with low-level testosterone replacement resulting in sluggish breeding behavior. The effects of these doses on the sexual refractory period of normal intact pony stallions have also been evaluated. Thus far, the studies have shown that yohimbine generally induces hyperexcitability and a panic state in horses that confound any facilitatory effects on sexual function. Nevertheless, at low doses (0.05 to 0.10 mg/kg IM), yohimbine has had positive effects on arousal, with no observable change in erection or ejaculatory function. Midrange doses appeared to reduce ejaculatory threshold (number of thrusts required to achieve ejaculation). This may have been confounded by apparent adverse effects on erection and arousal and the emergence of oral stereotypies (lip licking and yawning) and mild panic behavior that appeared to momentarily distract the animals during heterosexual interaction, prolonging the precopulatory phase. In geldings with low-level testosterone replacement, a midrange dose (0.15 mg/kg SC) of yohimbine had no measurable effect on sexual behavior. Those animals exhibited stereotypies and mild hyperexcitability similar to those observed in intact stallions at this dose. High doses (greater than 1 mg/kg IM or IV) of yohimbine have caused a severe panic state that is incompatible with sexual interaction.

OPIATE ANTAGONISTS

Naloxone and other opiate antagonists have been found to have facilitatory effects on male sexual motivation and copulatory behavior in several species.[14] Similar effects in pony stallions have not been demonstrated.

DOPAMINERGICS

Apomorphine and other selective dopamine type 2 receptor agonists stimulate copulation in noncopulator male rats and enhance ejaculatory function in normal rats.[15] In horses, apomorphine at relatively low doses (2 to 5 mg, SC) induces a panic state, characterized by increased locomotion, hypersensitivity to environmental stimuli, and apparent anxiety. These properties have purportedly been exploited in race horses.[16] In experiments with horses, I have tried several low doses of apomorphine as well as LY163502, a preparation of apomorphine and bromocriptine; no dose has yet been found at which sexual behavior is measurably enhanced.

INADEQUATE ERECTION

A relatively uncommon problem in the stallion is true impotence, that is, inadequate erection in spite of otherwise normal sexual arousal. One type of erection dysfunction involves what appears to be adequate erection during precopulatory interaction until mounting and insertion, at which time erection subsides. In most cases, the horse discontinues thrusting and dismounts soon after the erection subsides. Sometimes thrusting continues and ejaculation occurs in spite of erection failure. The cause of such failure is not well understood. A similar phenomenon has been described in humans, where it has been traditionally viewed as psychogenic. Erection failure during intromission and thrusting is a part of a syndrome known as pelvic steal, seen in men suffering vascular disease.[17] Upon exertion of the extremities, blood supply to the pelvic organs is compromised.

Inadequate rigidity of erection, though not common, has been seen in stallions. Often the problem is in association with, and difficult to distinguish from, inadequate libido. It does tend to occur in shy, novice stallions and in aged stallions with reduced libido. It is also a common problem in stallions that appear to have recovered from paralysis of the penis. The problem can also occur in horses with normal sexual interest and arousal and apparently normal penile function. Evaluation of spontaneous erection and masturbation in the stallion may help in determining whether the erection problem is specific to the copulatory situation.[18,19] Erection often shows marked improvement with androgen or GnRH therapy, as described earlier. Although improved erection may simply be the result of increased motivation and arousal, the degree of tumescence, as well as responsiveness of the penis to tactile stimulation, appears to be improved by these treatments.

Pharmacologically induced erection has become an accepted method for management of neurovasculogenic erection dysfunction in men.[20] Similar methods have not been reported in the stallion. In preliminary work in stallions, erections have been experimentally produced with intracorporal injection of imipramine hydrochloride. Penile paralysis and paraphimosis resulted in all instances. No method has been developed in the horse for reducing erections produced by intracorporal injection so as to avoid paraphimosis.

SPECIFIC EJACULATORY DYSFUNCTION

Ejaculation is principally an α-adrenergic mediated reflex event. Certain regimens for treating ejaculatory dysfunction are based on selectively enhancing α-adrenergic and/or blocking β-adrenergic transmission.

ADRENERGIC AGENTS

A treatment regimen developed by Klug for enhancement of ejaculatory function in copula involves administration of an α agonist (L-norepinephrine, 0.01 mg/kg IM, 15 min before breeding) followed by a β antagonist (carazolol, 0.015 mg/kg 10 min before breeding).[21] This method was successful in 17 of 24 stallions suffering ejaculatory failure. Ephedrine sulfate has been used to enhance ejaculatory function in copula.[22] The β-antagonists bunitrolol and propranolol have also been tested[23] (R.M. Kenney, personal communication).

Xylazine has been used to induce ejaculation ex copula in stallions unable to mount or to ejaculate in copula.[24] Xylazine has α_1- and α_2-adrenergic effects, both centrally and peripherally,[25] but has been viewed as predominantly promoting α_2 events. In normal horse and pony stallions, ejaculation occurs approximately 25% of the time following injection of 0.66 mg/kg IV with the horse standing quietly and undisturbed. The ejaculate can be collected in a plastic bag attached over the prepuce by a girth strap.

TRICYCLIC ANTIDEPRESSANTS

Widely used for alleviation of depression, anxiety, and obsessive-compulsive disorders in humans, the tricyclic antidepressant drugs have been known to affect ejaculatory function. Most well known are their adverse effects at antidepressant dose levels.[26] Among the side effects reported by men treated for depression with these agents are delay or failure of emission and ejaculation, emission without ejaculation (semen dribble), ejaculation without emission (dry ejaculation), and retrograde ejaculation (semen into bladder because of failure of bladder neck closure). Also reported are effects on ejaculation that may indicate enhancement, including spontaneous ejaculation and orgasm associated with yawning[27] and defecation.[28] Patients experiencing delayed or absent ejaculation sometimes improve function when treated with low doses of tricyclic antidepressants.[29] The mechanism of action is not clearly understood; however, these compounds and their metabolites promote α-adrenergic activity by inhibiting norepinephrine reuptake.

In horses, imipramine at relatively low doses (500 to 800 mg IV) induces erection and masturbation in both stallions and geldings and also appears to reduce the threshold for ex copula ejaculation in stallions.[30] At this dose, the animal is drowsy if undisturbed. Imipramine (100 to 500 mg orally bid) has also appeared to enhance ejaculation during copulation in stallions suffering long-term ejaculatory dysfunction. This regimen has also been useful in treating urine spillage into the ejaculate.

PROSTAGLANDINS

In other species, positive effects of prostaglandins (PG), both $PGF_2\alpha$ and PGE, on sexual behavior and ejaculation have been demonstrated. In horses, studies of effects of prostaglandins on reproductive behavior have been limited. In a preliminary study, 10 mg $PGF_2\alpha$ administered subcutaneously 2 to 5 min before breeding caused muscle weakness that was judged incompatible with safe breeding of the stallion (P.L. Sertich and M.C. Garcia, personal communication). In other work, stallions treated with 10 mg IM 1 h before collection of semen apparently exhibited no changes in copulatory behavior.[31] During the hour following treatment, some of the stallions were observed to have an extended flaccid penis, with fluid dripping from the penis.

OXYTOCIN

Oxytocin has also been investigated for its role in copulatory behavior. In other species, it has been demonstrated that oxytocin levels rise in association with copulation.[32] In rats, oxytocin induces a syndrome of yawning and erection in a nonsexual context.[33]

PHARMACOLOGIC AIDS TO SUPPRESS EXCESSIVE OR UNDESIRED SEXUAL BEHAVIOR

In general, overt sexual response is considered undesirable for colts, geldings, and stallions in racing, performance, or work situations. Even in breeding stallions, excessive sexual behavior may preclude safe management. Most horses can be trained to refrain from sexual interaction in performance situations and moderate their behavior in the breeding shed. Yet individuals or situations exist for which traditional methods fail and owners request pharmacologic aids to temporarily suppress stallion sexual behavior. Similarly, owners of geldings with residual stallion-like behavior request treatment.

ENDOCRINE APPROACHES

The most common endocrine approach to quieting sexual or aggressive behavior of stallions or geldings is administration of progestins. Progestins may work via antiandrogenic as well as general tranquilizing properties. Several forms of natural and synthetic progestins have been used.[34] Clinically, injectable forms produce more consistent results than oral forms.

TRANQUILIZERS AND OTHER NEUROLEPTICS

Although considerable anecdotal evidence indicates that tranquilizers are widely used to quiet undesired sexual or aggressive behavior of stallions and geldings, little systematic study of the drugs' efficacy or safety has been conducted. In stallions, phenothiazine tranquilizers have been associated with paralysis of the penis and paraphimosis. A long-acting phenothiazine agent, fluphenazine decanoate (Prolixen decanoate), has also been used, although its potential for inducing paralysis has not been studied. Similarly, reserpine has been used as a long-acting tranquilizer to calm horses. In stallions, it too has been associated with penile paralysis and paraphimosis[35,36] as well as hyperactivity and apparent psychotic behavior. Accordingly, these agents are no longer recommended for use in breeding stallions.

REFERENCES

1. Taberner, P.V.: Aphrodisiacs, The Science and the Myth. Philadelphia, University of Pennsylvania Press, 1985.
2. Sachs, B., and Meisel, R.L.: The physiology of male sexual behavior. *In* The Physiology of Reproduction. Edited by E. Knobil and J.D. Neill. New York, Raven Press, 1988, pp. 1393–1485.
3. Benson, G.S.: Male sexual function: Erection, emission, and ejaculation. *In* The Physiology of Reproduction. Edited by E. Knobil and J.D. Neill. New York, Raven Press, 1988, pp. 1121–1139.
4. McDonnell, S.M.: Precopulatory behavior of pony stallions. MS thesis. West Chester (Pennsylvania) University, 1981.
5. Pozor, M.A., McDonnell, S.M., Tischner, M., and Kenney, R.M.: GnRH facilitates copulatory behavior in geldings treated with testosterone. J. Reprod. Fertil. Suppl., *44:*666–667, 1991.
6. McDonnell, S.M., Diehl, N.K., Garcia, M.C., and Kenney, R.M.: Gonadotropin releasing hormone (GnRH) affects precopulatory behavior in testosterone-treated geldings. Physiol. Behav., *45:*145–149, 1989.
7. Blue, B.J., et al.: Effect of pulsatile and continuous administration of GnRH on reproductive function of stallions. J. Reprod. Fertil. Suppl., *44:*145–154, 1991.
8. McDonnell, S.M., et al.: Ejaculatory failure in association with aortic-iliac thrombosis in two stallions. J. Am. Vet. Med. Assoc., 200:954-957, 1992.
9. McDonnell, S.M., Love, C.C., Pozor, M.A., and Diehl, N.K.: Phenylbutazone treatment in breeding stallions: preliminary evidence for no effect on semen and testicular size. Theriogenology. In press.
10. McDonnell, S.M., Kenney, R.M., Meckley, P.E., and Garcia, M.C.: Conditioned suppression of sexual behavior in stallions and reversal with diazepam. Physiol. Behav., *34:*951–956, 1985.
11. McDonnell, S.M., Kenney, R.M., Meckley, P.E., and Garcia, M.C.: Novel environment suppression of sexual behavior in stallions and effects of diazepam. Physiol. Behav., *37:*503–505, 1988.
12. Clark, J.T., Smith, E.R., and Davidson, J.M.: Enhancement of sexual motivation in male rats by yohimbine. Science, *235:*847–849, 1984.
13. Goldberg, M.R., and Robertson, D.: Yohimbine: A pharmacological probe for study of the alpha2-adrenoreceptor. Pharmacol. Rev., *35:*143–180, 1983.
14. Sachs, B.D., Valcourt, R.J., and Flagg, H.C.: Copulatory behavior and sexual reflexes of male rats treated with naloxone. Pharmacol. Biochem. Behav., *14:*251–253, 1981.
15. Foreman, M.M., and Hall, J.L.: Effects of D2 dopaminergic receptor stimulation on male rat sexual behavior. J. Neural Transm., *68:*153–170, 1987.
16. Tobin, T.: Drugs and the Performance Horse. Springfield, IL, Charles C Thomas, 1981.
17. Lakin, M.M.: Diagnostic assessment of disorders of male sexual function. *In* Disorders of Male Sexual Dysfunction. Edited by D.K. Montague. Chicago, Yearbook Medical, 1988, pp. 26–43.
18. McDonnell, S.M.: Spontaneous erection and masturbation in equids. Proc. Am. Assoc. Equine Pract., 567–580, 1989.
19. McDonnell, S.M., Henry, M., and Bristol, F.: Spontaneous erection and masturbation in equids. J. Reprod. Fertil. Suppl., *44:*664–665, 1991.
20. Brindley, C.G.: Cavernosal alpha-blockade: A new technique for investigating and treating erectile impotence. Br. J. Psychiatry, *143:*332–337, 1983.
21. Klug, E.: Ejaculatory failure. *In* Current Therapy in Equine Medicine—2. Edited by N.E. Robinson. Philadelphia, W.B. Saunders, 1987, pp. 562–563.
22. Rasbech, N.O.: Ejaculatory disorders of the stallion. J. Reprod. Fertil. Suppl., *23:*123–128, 1975.
23. Klug, E., et al.: Effect of adrenergic neurotransmitters upon the ejaculatory process in the stallion. J. Reprod. Fertil. Suppl., *32:*31–34, 1982.
24. McDonnell, S.M., and Love, C.C.: Xylazine-induced ex copula ejaculation in stallions. Theriogenology, *36:*73–76, 1991.
25. Adams, H.R.: Adrenergic and anti-adrenergic drugs. *In* Veterinary Pharmacology and Therapeutics. 6th ed. Edited by N.H. Booth and L.E. McDonald. Ames, Iowa State University Press, 1988, pp. 91–116.
26. Mitchell, J.E., and Popkin, M.K.: Antidepressant drug therapy and sexual dysfunction in men: A review. J. Clin. Psychopharmacol., *3:*76–79, 1983.
27. McLean, J.D., Forsythe, R.G., and Kapkin, I.A.: Unusual side effects of clomipramine associated with yawning. Can. J. Psychiatry, *28:*569–570, 1983.
28. Breier, A., Ginsberg, E.M., and Charney, D.S.: Seminal

emission induced by tricyclic antidepressant. Am. J. Psychiatry, *141*:610–611, 1984.

29. Segraves, R.T.: Effects of psychoactive drugs on human erection and ejaculation. Arch. Gen. Psychiatry, *46*:275–284, 1989.

30. McDonnell, S.M., Garcia, M.C., Kenney R.M., and Van Arsdalen, K.N.: Imipramine-induced erection, masturbation, and ejaculation in male horses. Pharmacol. Biochem. Behav., *27*:187–191, 1987.

31. Kreider, J.L., Ogg, W.L., and Turner, J.W.: Influence of prostaglandin F_2 alpha on sperm production and seminal characteristics of the stallion. Theriogenology, *22*:903–913, 1981.

32. Carmichael, M.S., et al.: Plasma oxytocin increases in the human sexual response. J. Clin. Endocrinol. Metab., *64*:27–31, 1987.

33. Argiolas, A., Melia, M.R., and Gessa, G.L.: Oxytocin: An extremely potent inducer of penile erection and yawning in male rats. Eur. J. Pharmacol., *130*:265–272, 1986.

34. Roberts, S.J., and Beaver, B.V.: The use of progestins for aggressive and for hypersexual horses. *In* Current Therapy in Equine Medicine—2. Edited by N. E. Robinson. Philadelphia, W.B. Saunders, 1987, pp. 129–131.

35. Memon M.A., et al.: Penile paralysis paraphimosis associated with reserpine administration in a stallion. Theriogenology, *30*:411–419, 1988.

36. Lloyd, K.C.K., Harrison, I., and Tulleners E.: Reserpine toxicosis in a horse. J. Am. Vet. Med. Assoc., *186*:980–981, 1985.

CHAPTER 89

EFFECTS OF DRUGS OR TOXINS ON SPERMATOGENESIS

R.P. Amann

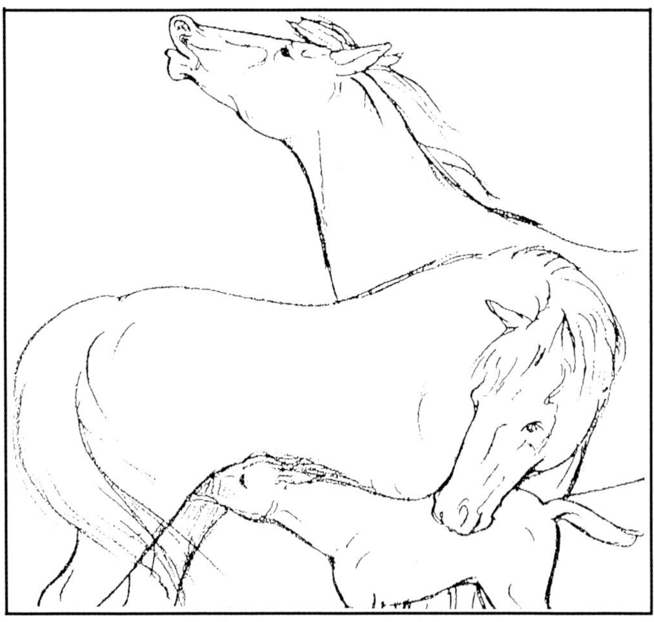

Spermatogenesis and endocrine regulation of spermatogenesis are discussed in Chapter 77 and that information should be reviewed, if necessary, to understand the material in this chapter more clearly. Spermatogenesis is the most conspicuous aspect of testicular function, because disturbances of spermatogenesis often will be reflected in obvious changes in characteristics of semen from a stallion inadvertently or intentionally exposed to some noxious agent. Changes in spermatogenesis could be manifested as a reduction in number of spermatozoa produced, alteration of an attribute(s) of some or all of the spermatozoa produced, or concurrent changes of both types. Alternatively, the agent might affect epididymal function or pass into semen via secretions of the accessory sex glands and hence alter quality of the spermatozoa ejaculated without directly affecting the testes. Unfortunately, a change in seminal characteristics may not occur until 4 to 7 weeks after occurrence of a deleterious event, because of the time required for spermatogenesis and epididymal transit of sperm (Fig. 89–1). Because spermatogonia or primary spermatocytes usually are affected once the agent is removed and normal primary spermatocytes are formed, an additional 4 to 6 weeks pass before normal spermatozoa can be ejaculated.[1]

Circumstances on many breeding farms will preclude detection of all disturbances of spermatogenesis. In severe cases, abnormal spermatogenesis will be evidenced by a reduction in size of one or both testes or an unusually firm or flaccid parenchyma. Both are detectable by palpation, provided earlier measurements or palpations of the testes of that stallion have established a baseline. Frequently, the first evidence of altered spermatogenesis will be a change in seminal characteristics. However, if seminal collections are infrequent or procedures used to evaluate seminal quality are insensitive, seminal changes may remain undetected. Failure to detect an obvious change of seminal characteristics, testicular size or consistency, or hormone concentrations in blood serum does not mean that potential fertility has not changed. No laboratory test or combination of laboratory tests provides an accurate prediction of fertility of spermatozoa from a given male when they are used to inseminate a particular group of mares, either by natural mating or artificial insemination.

The apparent fertility of a male is the product of his true fertility and that of the females with which he is mated. The implication of this fact is evident in several hypothetical cases (Table 89–1), in which fertility is expressed as a decimal fraction (0.64) rather than a percentage (64%). A 50% reduction in apparent fertility of a stallion (0.32 vs. 0.64) could be caused by a decline in his true fertility (case A) or to an unknown change in the population of mares to which he was bred (case B). In either case, to have a 90% probability of reaching the right conclusion that fertility was actually reduced, for whatever reason, each fertility estimate should be based on > 35 cycles in which timely inseminations occurred. The initial 25% reduction in fertility illustrated in case C might go undetected until the severity of the problem became worse. Detection of a decrease in fertility might

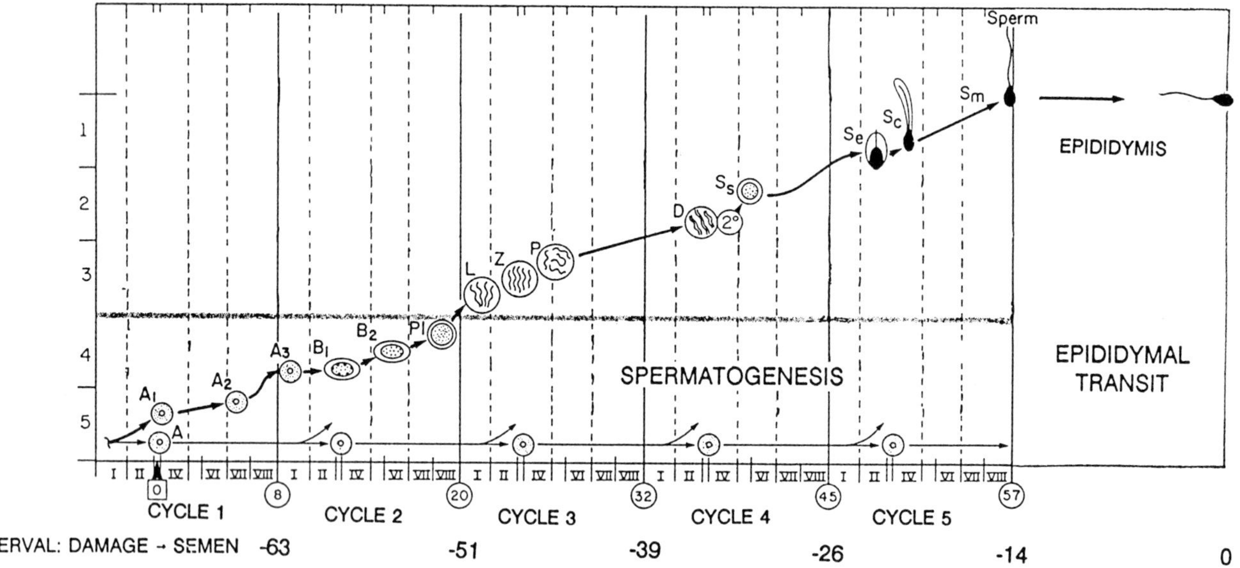

FIG. 89–1. A skeleton diagram of spermatogenesis in the stallion (see Fig 77–10 for details) to illustrate the intervals from death of specific types of germinal cells and when the effect might be anticipated in ejaculated semen. Cells designated A_1, A_2, A_3, B_1, and B_2 are spermatogonia; Pl, L, Z, P, and D are primary spermatocytes; 2° is a secondary spermatocyte; and S_s, S_e, S_c, and S_m are spermatids. An agent altering production of preleptotene spermatocytes (Pl) will be detectable in terms of a decreased number of spermatozoa ejaculated, or altered spermatozoa, about 51 days later. However, an agent affecting newly formed spherical spermatids (Ss) might be detectable by altered seminal quality 34 days later. Similarly long intervals will be the minimum needed for restoration of normal spermatozoa once action of the agent stops. The duration of spermatogenesis is 57 days and it is assumed that 14 days are required for transport of spermatozoa through the epididymis.

be partially masked by insemination of an excessive number of spermatozoa.[1,2] On the other hand, insemination of an unusually high number of spermatozoa usually will not solve the problems of reduced fertility.[3]

Spermatogenesis places unique demands on the testis. A high rate of cell proliferation occurs in spermatogonia undergoing mitosis and spermatocytes undergoing meiosis. This imposes high demands for delivery of glucose, amino acids, and lipid precursors to the interior of the seminiferous tubule, for energy and formation and remodeling of the germinal cells. Spermatogonia are in the basal compartment of the seminiferous tubule, and hence have relatively easy access to substrates in the interstitial fluid. However, more differentiated germinal cells must rely on Sertoli cells to provide all substrates and oxygen. Although data are not available for stallions, in rams a testis extracts about 15% of the glucose in testicular arterial blood and most of this is utilized by Sertoli cells.[4] Much of this glucose is metabolized to lactate or pyruvate which, in turn, is oxidatively metabolized by the developing germinal cells to provide the energy necessary for their development.

TABLE 89–1. ROLE OF THE TRUE FERTILITY OF GROUPS OF MARES ON THE APPARENT FERTILITY OF STALLIONS AND THE APPROXIMATE NUMBERS OF MARES NEEDED TO DETECT CHANGES IN TRUE FERTILITY OF A STALLION

Case	TRUE FERTILITY Stallion	TRUE FERTILITY Mares	Apparent Fertility*	Difference	Number of cycles to Detect Decreased Fertility†
A	0.80	0.80	0.64		
	0.40	0.80	0.32	0.32	35
B	0.80	0.80	0.64		
	0.80	0.40	0.32	0.32	35
C	0.80	0.70	0.56		
	0.60	0.70	0.42	0.14	100
	0.30	0.70	0.21	0.35	33

*Apparent fertility is the product of true fertility of the stallion and the mares to which he is mated: (0.40)(0.80) = 0.32.

†The approximate number of cycles required to have a 90% chance of detecting this difference in apparent fertility is shown. This number of inseminations is necessary for establishing initial fertility and for determining if a reduction of fertility of the magnitude indicated has occurred.

The testis also has a high demand for oxygen, and the normal oxygen tension in the seminiferous tubule is relatively low. Thus, agents or events which depress delivery of glucose or oxygen to the seminiferous tubules will have a deleterious effect, even though general bodily functions remain unimpaired.

Reproductive toxins may act by virtue of structure similar to an endogenous hormone, growth factor, or other compound involved in reproduction, because of their chemical reactivity to alkylate or chelate, because a metabolite of the agent exerts a toxic effect such as inhibiting or inducing an enzyme, or by a combined action.[5] For a stallion, perhaps agents that mimic endogenous hormones are the greatest problem, because of intended administration. However, other types of agents should be considered in cases where administration of exogenous hormones can be excluded. Agents affecting delivery of spermatozoa, rather than production of normal spermatozoa and accessory sex gland fluids, should not be ignored. For example, drugs with α-adrenergic-blocking properties can result in failure of seminal emission or retrograde ejaculation in humans.[6] However, combined administration of a β-adrenergic receptor blocker and an α agonist to stallions can induce emission in otherwise impotent stallions.[7]

Agents affecting spermatogenesis might act directly on the germinal cells by interfering with synthesis or function of microtubules or microfilaments.[8] Such drugs will block cell division, so that primary spermatocytes are not formed, or differentation of spermatids, so that any spermatozoa produced are malformed. Other drugs or reprotoxins alter function of Sertoli cells, and the lesion(s) on germinal cells are secondary to abnormal Sertoli cell function.[1] Perhaps the most common clinical cause of abnormal spermatogenesis is a secondary response to abnormal function of the hypothalamic-hypophyseal-testes axis. Insufficient luteinizing hormone (LH) for stimulation of Leydig cells to secrete sufficient testosterone and to maintain the high concentration around the seminiferous tubules essential for normal Sertoli cell function, or insufficient follicle-stimulating hormone (FSH) to maintain Sertoli cell function will adversely affect spermatogenesis. Little information exists on effects of drugs or other agents on testicular function in stallions. Hence, the following discussion is based mainly on data for humans, mice, rats, and other animals. Data for stallions are identified when presented.

AGENTS THAT MIGHT ACT DIRECTLY ON GERMINAL CELLS

Germinal cells are actively dividing, and hence are susceptible to any drug which blocks cell division. Clearly γ radiation or x rays can directly affect spermatogenesis, and the spermatogonia are much more sensitive to radiation than spermatocytes or spermatids.[9,10] Antineoplastic drugs (e.g., chlorambucil, cyclophosphamide, doxorubicin, and procarbizine) are selected because they kill rapidly dividing cells in tumors, but this property also targets them against spermatogonia. A decrease in number of spermatozoa ejaculated will be evident several weeks after initial treatment and the last spermatozoa produced may be malformed. The reserve spermatogonia are often spared because they rarely divide, and in many cases surviving reserve spermatogonia ultimately can repopulate the seminiferous epithelium. Alkylating agents (e.g., dibromochloropropane and ethylene dibromide, both used as pesticides or fumigants, or methyl chloride), colchicine, or the fungicide methyl 2-benzimidazolecarbamate (Carbendazim) all block division of germinal cells in several species.

AGENTS THAT MIGHT ACT ON SERTOLI CELLS

During the evolution of most mammals, the Sertoli cells developed so that they produce necessary amounts of molecules needed by developing germinal cells only at a temperature 3° to 6° C below core body temperature. This is clearly evident from studies with cultured Sertoli cells, which have reduced secretory capacity at 37° C compared with that at 32° C.[11] Studies are beginning to provide a molecular basis for the well-known, and clinically important, sensitivity of the seminiferous epithelium to elevated testicular temperature. Although pachytene spermatocytes and B-spermatogonia are the germinal cells most sensitive to elevated testicular temperature,[4] the primary lesion causing their death and degeneration may be in Sertoli cells. In any case, summer heat or febrile conditions can induce a transitory decrease in number and quality of spermatozoa produced.

Chemicals also can alter Sertoli cell function, and this probably is a common primary site of action for reprotoxins, the effect of which is seen secondarily by a decrease in number of normal spermatozoa ejaculated. For example, both di(2-ethylhexyl) phthalate and 1,3-dinitrobenzene act directly on Sertoli cells,[12] and vacuolation of the cytoplasm and exfoliation of germ cells are characteristic sequelae. Di(2-ethylhexyl) phthalate is converted to an active ester by Sertoli cells, and this compound decreases response of Sertoli cells to FSH.[12] Dinitrobenzene suppresses production of lactate and pyruvate by Sertoli cells, and this compromises the ability of Sertoli cells to nurture germinal cells.[13] Pachytene spermatocytes and spermatids undergo degeneration. Drugs which modify hepatic function also might alter Sertoli cell function, because both hepatocytes and Sertoli cells secrete many transport proteins (e.g., transferrin and ceruloplasmin). Those produced by Sertoli cells are essential for spermatogenesis.

AGENTS THAT MIGHT ACT ON LEYDIG CELLS

Most alterations of Leydig cell function are a consequence of a change in the hypothalamic-hypophyseal-testes axis (as discussed in the next section), but some reprotoxins act directly on Leydig cells. For example, 2,3,7,8-tetrachlorodibenzo-*p*-dioxin blocks production of pregnenolone by Leydig cells,[14] and hence testosterone cannot be produced (see steroidogenic pathway depicted in Fig. 77–15). Ethane dimethanesulfonate apparently has a similar action.[8,15] In addition to environmental toxins, such as in the two examples, steroids or other drugs affecting androgen or estrogen synthesis can act directly on Leydig cells.

AGENTS THAT MIGHT AFFECT THE HYPOTHALAMIC-HYPOPHYSEAL-TESTES AXIS

Normal spermatogenesis depends on the negative feedback regulation of the hypothalamic-hypophyseal-testes axis (Fig. 89–2 A). This provides sufficient FSH and testosterone to the seminiferous epithelium for maximum production of normal spermatozoa; testosterone in amounts necessary for normal function of accessory sex glands; steroids for expression of sexual behavior and achievement of erection of the penis at copulation; and negative feedback of testosterone, estradiol, and inhibin on the central nervous system, hypothalamus, and adenohypophysis (anterior pituitary gland). Unfortunately, both natural events and human intervention can alter this delicate hemostatic balance.

ANDROGENS

The most common pharmacologic manipulation of spermatogenesis probably is the unintended side effect of administration of testosterone esters or anabolic steroids to stallions. Although the intent is to raise the concentration of androgen circulating in the blood and available to muscle tissue and bone, this therapy also raises the concentration of androgen impinging on the hypothalamus and anterior pituitary gland. As depicted in Figure 89–2 B, the high concentration of androgen in systemic blood causes a depression or cessation of secretion of gonadotropin-releasing hormone (GnRH) and LH and probably a decrease in secretion of FSH. Because of unavailability of LH, secretion of testosterone by Leydig cells is decreased and the concentration of testosterone in the interstitial fluid bathing the seminiferous tubules is reduced to a concentration insufficient for normal spermatogenesis. In many cases, Leydig cells would produce no testosterone and the concentration of testosterone in interstitial fluid would be equal to that in peripheral blood rather than 20 to 100 times greater. Testicular production of estrogens also would be reduced or eliminated.

This is not just a hypothetical scenario. Countless clinical observations and direct experimentation show the severity of the problem in stallions[16–20] and the potential for reversibility or restoration of normal spermatogenesis. In stallions receiving testosterone propionate intramuscularly (200 μg/kg every other day) for 88 days,[17] a gradual decrease in testicular size was noted, determined as total scrotal width (Fig. 89–3). Concentrations of LH in serum from treated stallions averaged approximately 50% of the values for control

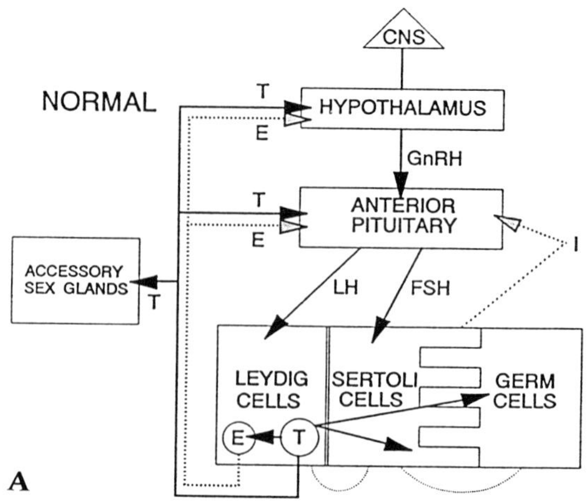

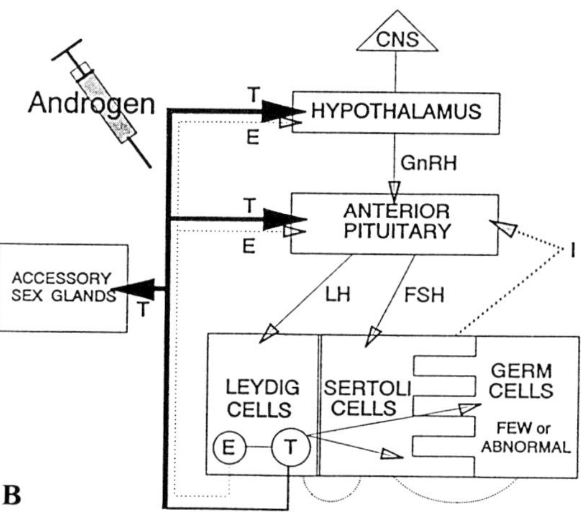

FIG. 89–2. The hypothalamic-hypophyseal-testes axis in a normal stallion *(A)* and a stallion receiving an injection(s) of androgen *(B)*. Injection of androgen elevates (larger solid arrow) the concentration of androgen (T) in the blood, and this suppresses (smaller open arrow) secretion of GnRH by the hypothalamus and FSH and LH by the anterior pituitary gland. Secretion of testosterone and estrogens (E) declines. The effect on concentration of inhibin (I) is unknown, but an increase might occur. Although blood concentration of androgen is high, the intratesticular concentration of androgen is low, and Sertoli cells will receive insufficient stimulation of androgen and FSH. Consequently, with prolonged administration of androgen, a decrease or cessation of spermatogenesis will occur.

stallions. By 74 to 90 days after the start of treatment, spermatozoal concentration in ejaculated semen, total number of spermatozoa per ejaculate, percentage of motile spermatozoa, and percentage of normal spermatozoa were reduced from their pretreatment values; volumes of gel or gel-free semen were not significantly altered. The adverse effect of testosterone propionate is evident in data comparing the control and treated stallions (Table 89–2). Some of the stallions were castrated 90 days after starting the treatment and the remaining stallions were allowed 92 days to recover; semen was collected between days 166 and 180 when these stal-

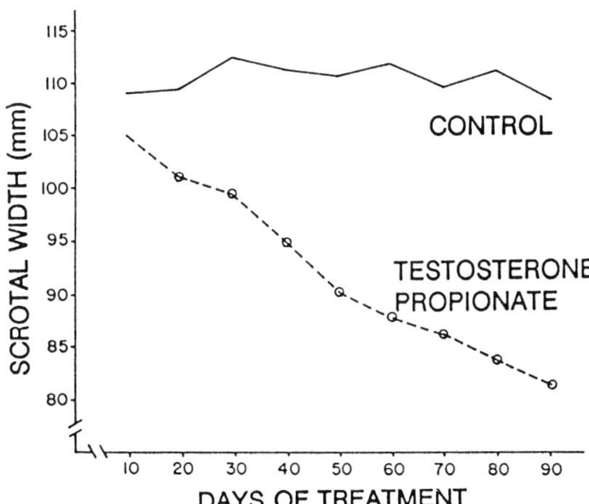

FIG. 89–3. Total scrotal width in control stallions and in stallions receiving testosterone propionate (200 μg/kg). (Modified from Pickett, B.W., et al.: Management of the Stallion for Maximum Reproductive Efficiency. II. Animal Reproduction Laboratory Bulletin No. 05. Fort Collins, Colorado State University, 1989.)

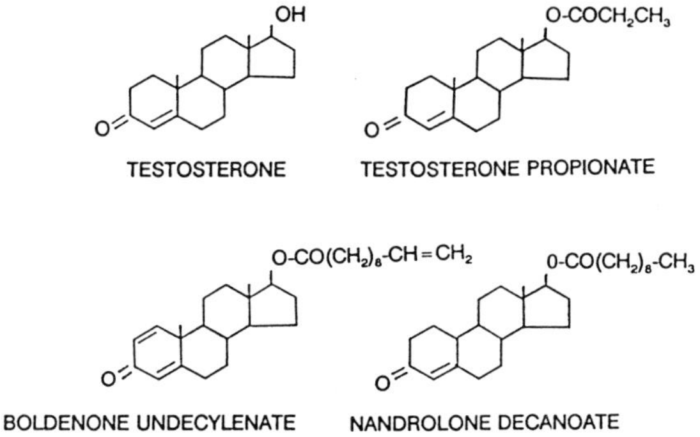

TESTOSTERONE — TESTOSTERONE PROPIONATE — BOLDENONE UNDECYLENATE — NANDROLONE DECANOATE

FIG. 89–4. Structures of testosterone and related steroids sometimes administered to stallions, although administration of these compounds to stallions is not a recommended practice or an approved use. All have androgenic effects, and boldenone undecylenate and nandrolone decanoate have enhanced anabolic activity.

lions were castrated.[18] Total sperm per ejaculate and testicular weight as well as spermatozoal production (data not shown) had recovered, because characteristics for stallions receiving 200 μg/kg testosterone propionate were similar to those for untreated (control) stallions (Table 89–2). Thus, although recovery from suppression of spermatogenesis occurred in stallions receiving 200 μg/kg testosterone propionate every other day, treatment for a longer interval or at a higher dose might have more severe or longer lasting effects.

Anabolic steroids rather than testosterone esters frequently are administered to stallions, although this is not an approved use. Anabolic steroids have structures similar to those of testosterone or testosterone propionate (Fig. 89–4), and thus they might be expected to affect spermatogenesis adversely. This was shown to be the case in a comprehensive study[19] which compared changes in stallions treated with boldenone undecylenate (Equipose) (0.23 or 0.91 mg/kg body weight) or nandrolone decanoate (Deca-Durabolin) (0.23 mg/kg body weight) by intramuscular injection once every third week for 15 weeks. Eight stallions received each treatment, and the experiment was conducted with three replicates, staggered so that the 15-week treatment period ended in September, October, or November. For all three groups of treated stallions, total scrotal width decreased compared with that for untreated (control) stallions (Fig. 89–5). Characteristics of semen collected during weeks 13 through 15 of treatment were compared with pretreatment values. Total spermatozoa per ejaculate, percentage of motile spermatozoa, and percentage of normal spermatozoa all were greatly suppressed in the treated stallions, and these changes

TABLE 89–2. EFFECT OF TREATMENT OF STALLIONS WITH TESTOSTERONE PROPIONATE FOR 90 DAYS

	DAYS 74 TO 90 (N = 8)			DAYS 166 TO 180 (N = 4)		
	Control	TP*	Difference (%)	Control	TP	Difference (%)
Gel-free semen (mL)	35	40	+14	43	51	+19
Spermatozoa/mL (10^6)	230	87	−62	104	64	−38
Spermatozoa/ejaculate (10^9)	6.7	3.3	−51	3.5	3.2	−8
Motile spermatozoa (%)	58	50	−14	63	60	−5
Normal spermatozoa (%)	53	39	−26	—	—	—
Testes weight (g)	338	219	−35	283	365	+29

*Treated stallions received 200 μg/kg testosterone propionate (TP), intramuscularly every other day for 88 days. Four stallions per treatment group were castrated on day 90 and four were allowed to recover until day 180. Semen was collected every other day from days 74 to 90 and 166 to 180, after depleting extragonadal spermatozoal reserves.

(Adapted from Hoyer, J.H.: The effect of testosterone on reproductive function in stallions. M.S. thesis. Colorado State University, 1978; and Squires, E.L., et al.: Restoration of reproductive capacity in stallions after suppression with exogenous testosterone. J. Anim. Sci., *53:*1351–1359, 1981.)

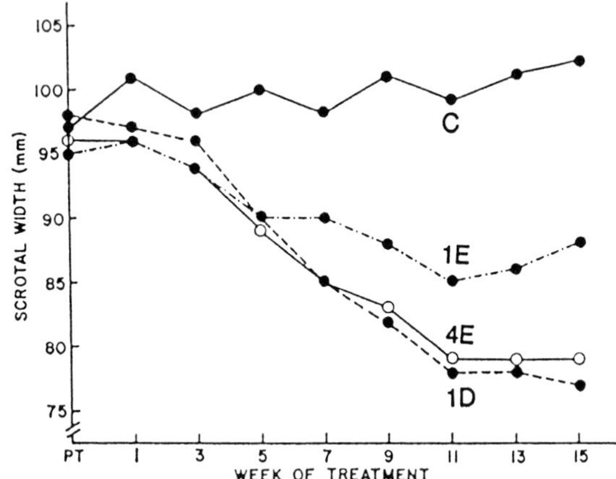

FIG. 89–5. Total scrotal width in control stallions and stallions receiving anabolic steroids before treatment (PT) and during the treatment period. Groups are designated as: C, control; 1E, 0.23 mg/kg boldenone undecylenate; 4E, 0.91 mg/kg boldenone undecylenate; and 1D, 0.23 mg/kg nandrolone decanoate. Stallions received steroid every 3 weeks. (Modified from Pickett, B.W., et al.: Management of the Stallion for Maximum Reproductive Efficiency. II. Animal Reproduction Laboratory Bulletin No. 05. Fort Collins, Colorado State University, 1989.)

were greater than those attributable to season in the untreated stallions (Table 89–3).

Severity of the damage induced by these anabolic steroids was evident in comparisons of testicular weight after 15 weeks of treatment (Table 89–3). Similar data were reported by Blanchard et al., who studied pony stallions treated with stanozolol (Winstrol-V) or boldenone undecylenate (each tested at 0.55 or 1.11 mg/kg) for 13 weeks.[20] Testes weight was reduced in all treated stallions, relative to the untreated (control) group, except those receiving 0.55 mg/kg stanozolol.

As discussed elsewhere, administration of testosterone propionate or anabolic steroids appeared to have no beneficial effect on sexual behavior of stallions or growth rate of healthy geldings.[16] Because such compounds do have adverse effects on spermatogenesis, androgenic compounds should not be administered to healthy stallions to be used for breeding.

HUMAN CHORIONIC GONADOTROPIN

Occasionally a horse owner or veterinarian will consider administration of human chorionic gonadotropin (hCG) to a stallion, in the belief that an increase in testosterone might help some reproductive function. Concentration of testosterone in peripheral blood is doubled in < 1 h after intravenous injection of hCG, and increased secretion of testosterone may continue for several days.[21] Although both LH and hCG bind to LH receptors on Leydig cells, the two hormones are chemically and biologically different. Because hCG is more glycosylated, it is cleared more slowly from the blood and available to LH receptors on target cells far longer than LH. Target cells, and presumably stallion Leydig cells, process hCG-receptor complexes differently from LH-receptor complexes, further prolonging the stimulatory effect and interval of increased steroid secretion. Because concentration of testosterone in peripheral blood may be increased for days rather than hours after a single injection, changes in endocrine homeostasis may occur (Fig. 89–6), especially with a series of injections of hCG. Assuming that the endocrine profiles of a stallion are reasonably normal, injection of hCG causes increased production of testosterone by Leydig cells and abundant testosterone is available to the seminiferous epithelium; this is not deleterious to spermatogenesis. Secretion of estrogens by Leydig cells also increases. The increased concentrations of testosterone and estradiol impinging on the central nervous system and hypothalamus cause suppression of GnRH secretion. The anterior pituitary gland, in turn secretes less LH and FSH. The lack of LH is not a problem because the Leydig cells are receiving stimulation of hCG. However, the lack of FSH available to Sertoli cells could have deleterious effects on spermatogenesis if administration of hCG was prolonged. Both number of spermatozoa produced and spermatozoal structure could be affected, although no valid data exist for stallions showing sequelae of chronic administration of hCG. Repeated injection of a stallion with hCG is not recommended.

GONADOTROPIN-RELEASING HORMONE

Use of GnRH to stimulate secretion of LH by the anterior pituitary gland and, thereby, secretion of testosterone by Leydig cells is more biologically normal than administration of hCG to stimulate secretion of tes-

TABLE 89–3. EFFECT OF TREATMENT OF STALLIONS WITH ANABOLIC STEROIDS FOR 15 WEEKS*

	C†	1E‡	4E§	1D‖
Gel-free volume	30	22	17	20
Spermatozoa/mL (10^6)	226[a]	117[b]	60[c]	30[c]
Spermatozoa/ ejaculate (10^9)	5.0[a]	2.5[b]	1.4[b]	0.5[b]
Motile spermatozoa (%)	55[a]	34[b]	34[b]	21[c]
Normal spermatozoa (%)	68	63	62	53
Testes weight (g)	285[a]	176[b]	128[c]	114[c]

*Means for eight stallions per group. Treated animals were injected intramuscularly every 3 weeks. Semen was collected every other day for the last 22 days of the experiment.

†, control stallions.

‡, stallions received 0.23 mg/kg boldenone undecylenate.

§, stallions received 0.91 mg/kg boldenone undecylenate.

‖, stallions received 0.23 mg/kg nandrolone decanoate.

(Adapted from Squires, E.L., Todter, G.E., Berndtson, W.E., and Pickett, B.W.: Effect of anabolic steroids on reproductive function of young stallions. J. Anim. Sci., *54*:576–582, 1982.)

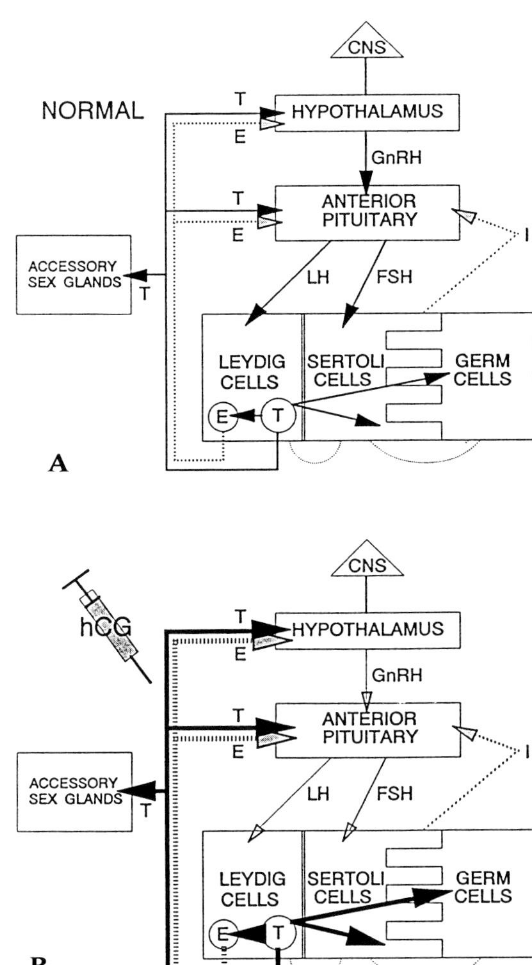

FIG. 89–6. The hypothalamic-hypophyseal-testes axis in a normal stallion *(A)* and in a stallion receiving an injection(s) of hCG *(B)*. Injection of hCG stimulates (larger solid arrow) Leydig cells to secrete testosterone (T), and the high concentration of testosterone in blood reaching the hypothalamus and anterior pituitary gland suppresses (smaller open arrow) secretion of GnRH, FSH, and LH. Although there may be adequate testosterone and estrogens (E) secreted by Leydig cells, Sertoli cells will be deprived of FSH. Concentration of inhibin (I) probably would not change following a single injection of hCG. Consequently, with repeated administration of hCG, the seminiferous epithelium receives insufficient stimulation of FSH for normal spermatogenesis.

tosterone. In a normal stallion, and many stallions with changes in the homeostatic balance of the hypophyseal-hypothalamic-testes axis, intravenous or subcutaneous injection of a bolus of GnRH is followed by increased secretion of FSH and especially LH. Availability of a transitory rise in LH impinging on the Leydig cells results in temporary elevations of concentrations of testosterone and estrogens in the interstitial fluid and blood. Thus, in contrast to injection of hCG, injection of GnRH results in an elevation of both FSH and, at least under some conditions, testosterone in fluid bathing the seminiferous tubules, rather than only testosterone. Furthermore, assuming appropriate dosage of GnRH is used (Chapter 87), the probability of down regulating LH or testosterone receptors on Leydig cells or Sertoli cells, respectively, is low whereas it is a virtual certainty after administration of hCG. The short interval of elevated blood concentrations of testosterone and estrogens after GnRH administration provides a relatively normal negative drive to the hypothalamic-hypophyseal axis.

In theory, pulsatile administration of GnRH could be

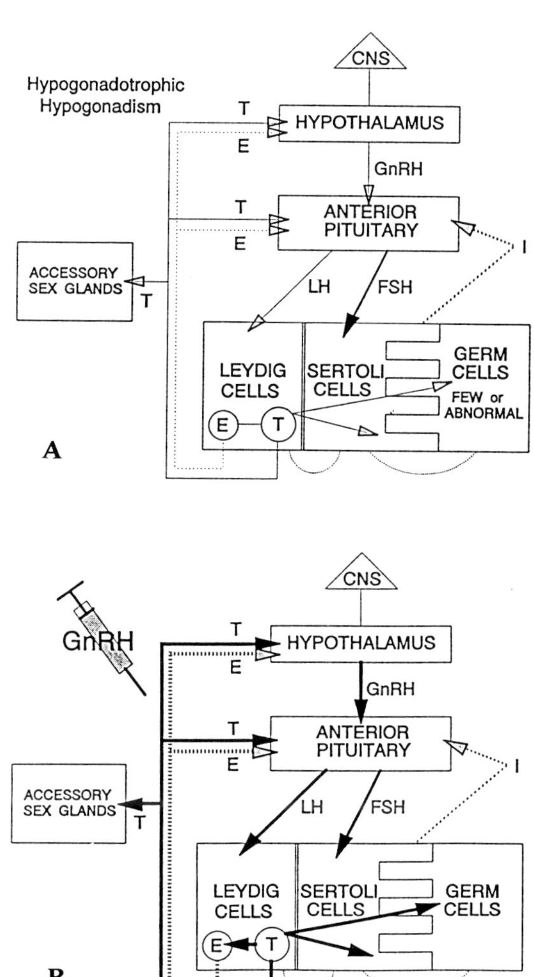

FIG. 89–7. The hypothalamic-hypophyseal-testes axis in an abnormal stallion, with a central nervous system or hypothalamic abnormality resulting in a lack (small open arrow) of GnRH secretion *(A)* or a similar abnormal stallion receiving injections of GnRH *(B)*. Pulsatile injection of GnRH stimulates the anterior pituitary gland to secrete LH and FSH (larger solid arrow). The LH, in turn, stimulates Leydig cells to secrete testosterone (T) in a pulsatile manner. Thus adequate amounts of FSH and testosterone might reach the seminiferous epithelium to stimulate restoration of spermatogenesis, and sufficient testosterone and estrogens (E) might reach other organs for normal expression of feedback regulation and other reproductive functions or behaviors. Although not studied, concentration of inhibin (I) might decline, especially if it had been elevated initially. Such GnRH therapy would have to continue for several months, because it might take several weeks of GnRH stimulation before normal function of Sertoli cells was restored, and the duration of spermatogenesis is 57 days in stallions.

used to mimic the endogenous secretion of GnRH and hence drive a stallion's endocrine system. Effects of this treatment have been studied in normal stallions.[22,23] As anticipated, pulsatile injections of GnRH (1.25 to 5.0 μg/kg each 0.5 h or 10 μg/kg each 2 h, in the two experiments) resulted in pulsatile discharge of LH and FSH. However, in normal stallions the effect on testosterone secretion is more pronounced during the winter than summer,[22] and this may explain why Blue et al. found no increased blood concentration of testosterone in normal stallions receiving pulsatile injections of GnRH.[23] Pulsatile injection of GnRH into an abnormal stallion (with low serum concentrations of LH and testosterone similar to those of a normal stallion in the winter) probably would result in pulsatile secretion of LH and testosterone even in the spring or summer.

Some stallions may have clinical symptoms of adult-onset hypogonadotropic hypogonadism, namely, reduced production of normal spermatozoa and low concentrations of LH and especially testosterone in peripheral blood (Fig. 89–7 A); blood concentration of FSH might be normal or elevated. In these stallions, the testicular malfunction is secondary to an insufficiency of GnRH. Diagnostic use of GnRH to distinguish these stallions from others with advanced or irreversible testicular degeneration is discussed in Chapter 87. In stallions where the primary problem is insufficient secretion of GnRH, the anterior pituitary gland should respond to an injection of GnRH with increased secretion of LH, and increased secretion of testosterone by Leydig cells is likely (Fig. 89–7 B); this indeed happens (T.M. Nett, personal communication). Appropriate pulsatile injection of GnRH (Chapter 87) may result in an improvement in spermatozoal production or quality after 1 to 2 months of treatment. Anecdotal reports of clinicians with an equine practice and published reports by physicians provide evidence that this treatment can be effective in some individuals, although others with an apparently similar clinical picture will not benefit.[24–26]

REFERENCES

1. Amann, R.P.: Detection of alterations in testicular and epididymal function in laboratory animals. Environ. Health Perspect., *70:*149–158, 1986.
2. Amann, R.P.: Can the fertility potential of a semen sample be predicted accurately? J. Androl., *10:*89–98, 1989.
3. Pickett, B.W., Squires, E.L., and McKinnon, A.O. Procedures for Collection, Evaluation and Utilization of Stallion Semen for Artificial Insemination. Animal Reproduction Laboratory Bulletin No. 03. Fort Collins, Colorado State University, 1987.
4. Waites, G.M.H., and Setchell, B.P.: Physiology of the mammalian testis. *In* Marshall's Physiology of Reproduction. 4th ed. Edited by G.E. Lamming. London, Churchill Livingstone, 1990, pp. 1–105.
5. Mattison, D.R., and Thomford, P.J.: Mechanism of action of reproductive toxicants. *In* Toxicity of the Male and Female Reproductive Systems. Edited by P.K. Working. New York, Hemisphere Publishing, 1989, pp. 101–129.
6. Benson, G.S.: Male sexual function. *In* The Physiology of Reproduction. Vol 1. Edited by E. Knobil and J.D. Neill. New York, Raven Press, 1988, pp. 1121–1139.
7. Klug E., et al.: Effect of adrenergic neurotransmitters upon the ejaculatory process in the stallion. J. Reprod. Fertil. Suppl., *32:*31–34, 1982.
8. Klinefelter, G., and Gray, L.E. Jr.: The clinical relevancy of animal models: Animal studies which assess the potential for drugs and environmental agents to cause reproductive disorders in man. Fundam. Appl. Toxicol., in press.
9. Meistrich, M.L. Interspecies comparison and quantitative extrapolation of toxicity to the human male reproductive system. *In* Toxicity of the Male and Female Reproductive Systems. Edited by P.K. Working. New York, Hemisphere Publishing, 1989, pp. 303–321.
10. Oakberg, E.F.: Irradiation damage to animals and its effect on their reproductive capacity. J. Dairy. Sci., *43(Suppl.):*54–64, 1960.
11. Hagenas, L., Ritzen, E.M., and Suginami, H.L.: Temperature dependence of Sertoli cell function. Int. J. Androl. Suppl., *2:*449–458, 1978.
12. Chapin, R.E., and Foster, P.M.D.: Testis *en plastique:* Use and abuse of in vitro systems. *In* Toxicity of the Male and Female Reproductive Systems. Edited by P.K. Working. New York, Hemisphere Publishing, 1989, pp. 273–284.
13. Williams, J., and Foster, P.M.D.: The production of lactate and pyruvate as sensitive indices of altered rat Sertoli cell function in vitro following the addition of various testicular toxicants. Toxicol. Appl. Pharmacol., *9:*160–170, 1988.
14. Kleeman, J.M., Moore, R.W., and Peterson, R.E.: Inhibition of testicular steroidogenesis in 2,3,7,8-tetrachlorodibenzo-*p*-dioxin-treated rats: Evidence that the key lesion occurs prior to or during pregnenolone formation. Toxicol. Appl. Pharmacol., *106:*112–125, 1990.
15. Klinefelter, G.R., Laskey, J.W., and Roberts, N.L.: In vitro/in vivo effects of ethane dimethanesulfonate on Leydig cells of adult rats. Toxicol. Appl. Pharmacol., *107:*460–471, 1991.
16. Pickett, B.W., et al.: Management of the Stallion for Maximum Reproductive Efficiency. II. Animal Reproduction Laboratory Bulletin No. 05. Fort Collins, Colorado State University, 1989.
17. Berndtson, W.E., Hoyer, J.H., Squires, E.L., and Pickett, B.W.: Influence of exogenous testosterone on sperm production, seminal quality and libido of stallions. J. Reprod. Fertil. Suppl., *27:*19–23, 1979.
18. Squires, E.L., et al.: Restoration of reproductive capacity in stallions after suppression with exogenous testosterone. J. Anim. Sci., *53:*1351–1359, 1981.
19. Squires, E.L., Todter, G.E., Berndtson, W.E., and Pickett, B.W.: Effect of anabolic steroids on reproductive function of young stallions. J. Anim. Sci., *54:*576–582, 1982.
20. Blanchard, T.L., et al.: The effects of stanozolol and boldenone undecylenate on scrotal width, testis weight, and sperm production in pony stallions. Theriogenology, *20:*121–131, 1983.
21. Amann, R.P., and Ganjam, V.K.: Effects of hemicastration or hCG-treatment on steroids in testicular vein and jugular vein blood of stallions. J. Androl., *3:*132–139, 1981.
22. Roser, J.F., and Hughes, J.P.: Prolonged pulsatile admin-

istration of gonadotrophin-releasing hormone (GnRH) to fertile stallions. J. Reprod. Fertil. Suppl., *44:*155–168, 1992.

23. Blue, B.J., et al.: Effect of pulsatile and continuous administration of GnRH on reproductive function of stallions. J. Reprod. Fertil. Suppl., *44:*145–154, 1992.

24. Baker, H.W.G., and Kovacs, G.T.: Spontaneous improvement in semen quality: regression towards the mean. Int. J. Androl., *8:*421–426, 1985.

25. Wagner, T.O.F.: Pulsatile LHRH Therapy of the Male. Hameln, TM-Verlag. 1985.

26. Winter, S.J.: Evaluation and management of hypogonadotropic hypogonadism. Serono Symp. Rev., *20:*93–102, 1989.

CHAPTER 90

FEEDING THE STALLION

H.F. Hintz

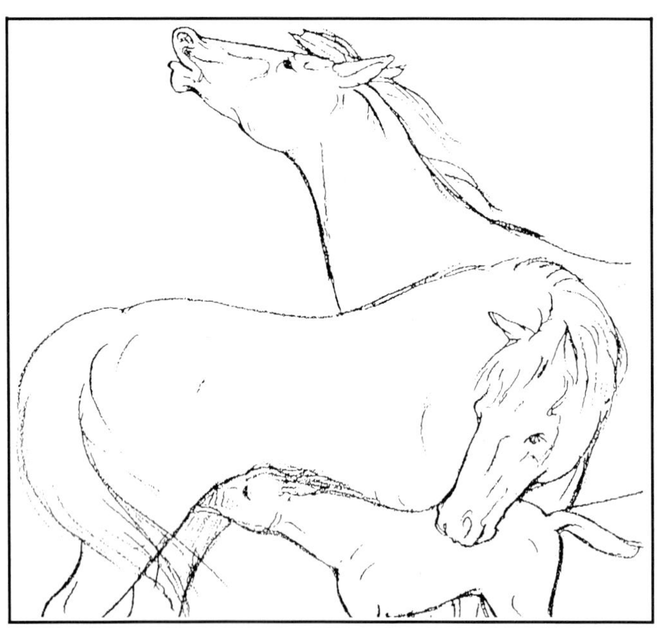

Relatively few studies have been conducted on the nutrient requirements of the stallion. In early editions of the National Research Council's (NRC) *Nutrient Requirements of Horses,* no values were given for the stallion. In the 1989 edition, values are given but they are primarily derived from observation and studies with other classes of horses rather than from experiments with stallions (Table 90–1).[1] In most textbooks on horse production or horse nutrition, discussion of the feeding of the stallion is limited to one page or less. The most common recommendation is that stallions should not be too fat or too thin. Ironically, the most valuable animal on the horse farm has received the least amount of attention from experimental nutritionists. Perhaps lack of research is related to the commonly held theory that if the male is fed a balanced ration that will maintain normal health reproduction will not suffer because of nutritional deficiency.[2]

ENERGY

REQUIREMENTS

For stallions, as for mares, energy is of the greatest concern. It has long been held that underfeeding can result in stallions that are too thin and lack sex drive. Columella, in A.D. 50, stated that stallions should be fattened on barley before the breeding season so that they could be equal to "the fatigues of breeding." According to Jeremiah 5:8, well-fed stallions have a greater sex drive than poorly fed horses.

Overfeeding is more likely to be a problem than underfeeding in current management of stallions. Overfeeding can be harmful for several reasons. One potential problem is that severe obesity has been shown to reduce sperm production in some species. Another factor is that excessive energy intake can predispose a stallion to laminitis. The lameness and associated pain of chronic laminitis could decrease libido. Acute laminitis could terminate the stallion's career. Overfeeding could predispose to laminitis by two routes. Excessive weight would cause greater stress on the digit. Excessive carbohydrates could cause endotoxemia as a result of changes in the bacterial population of the digestive tract.

Thus the level of feed intake should be consistent with activity and body condition. Rapid increases of intake should not be allowed if the feed has a high soluble carbohydrate content. Corn and barley would, therefore, require more careful feeding management than oats, which contains less soluble carbohydrate and more fiber. Stallions and mares are considered to be at greater risk of developing laminitis than geldings.[3] Stabling on concrete surfaces is also a risk factor.[3]

The NRC suggested that stallions during the breeding season require about 25% more digestible energy (DE) than for maintenance.[1] A 545-kg stallion requires 17.8 Mcal of DE for maintenance; a 25% increase would be 4.45 Mcal. This increase is equivalent to 2.3 kg hay or 1.5 kg grain. Note that the estimated energy increase for

TABLE 90–1. DAILY NUTRIENT REQUIREMENTS OF STALLIONS BASED ON EQUATIONS DEVELOPED BY THE NRC.

	STALLION WEIGHT (KG)		
	450	500	550
Digestible energy (Mcal)*	18.6	20.5	22
Crude protein (g)	745	820	895
Calcium (g)	23	25	27
Phosphorus (g)	16	18	19
Magnesium (g)	8	9	10
Potassium (g)	28	31	34
Zinc (mg)	310	345	375
Copper (mg)	77	86	95
Magnesium (mg)	310	345	375
Selenium (mg)	0.8	0.9	1.0
Iodine (mg)	0.8	0.9	1.0
Vitamin A (IU)	20	22.5	25
Vitamin E (mg)	385	425	470
Thiamin (mg)	23	26	28
Riboflavin (mg)	15	17	19

*Assuming 1.9 Mcal per kilogram hay and 3 Mcal per kilogram grain, the values for 450-, 500-, and 550-kg stallions would be 6.4:2.2, 6.7:2.6, and 7:3 kg hay to grain, respectively.

the stallion during the breeding season is greater than the estimated increase (20%) for the mare in the last month of gestation. The Institut National de la Recherche Agronomique (INRA) suggests that the energy requirements for stallions during the breeding season may be 30% higher than for geldings at maintenance.[4] The INRA also based its recommendations on observation rather than research. According to Morrison, during the breeding season some stallions will need as much grain as a horse at hard work.[5]

Of course, as stressed in Chapter 75, the important factor is the body condition of the animal. Energy requirements, however, may vary greatly among animals because of differences in metabolism, temperament, and environment. Therefore, all stallions should be weighed monthly or the weight should be estimated with a weight tape during off-season; weight should be taken weekly during the breeding season. Body score or condition should also be recorded. Feed intake could then easily be adjusted.

Body weight and condition also can be regulated by exercise. Moreover, some farm managers believe that exercise has a benefit above that of weight control. Many stallion managers believe exercise may affect attitude and/or boredom, which in turn can affect behavior-causing problems such as incomplete ejaculation, impotence, savaging mares, etc. Cahill suggested that exercise helps keep a proper mental attitude and is one of the most important management tools that can be used to maintain libido.[6] The Standardbred stallions of Armstrong Brothers Farm in Canada are exercised on a slow-speed treadmill for 20 min per day (T. Morley, personal communication). Morley suggested that exercise improved the attitude of the stallions and that the treadmill was useful because some of the stallions (particularly the older ones) would not voluntarily exercise when turned out in a paddock. Crawford and Kirkham suggested that turning the stallion out on grass or changing the routine or environment may improve vigor and attitude.[7]

Not everyone agrees that exercise is of value. Dinger and Noiles studied eight sexually inexperienced 2-yr-old Morgan stallions using a reversal design in which half of the animals were exercised (24 min per day) and half were not.[8] Exercise did not increase libido. In fact, libido decreased in the exercised group. They concluded that less sexually aggressive stallions may have their libido increased over a period of time by decreasing or eliminating regular exercise. They also pointed out, however, that hard-to-handle stallions may become easier to control if placed on a regular exercise program.

PROTEIN

Severe protein deficiency could cause reduced feed intake and, therefore, reduce body condition and decrease libido. No controlled studies exist indicating that high levels of protein are beneficial. The NRC uses the same ratio of protein to energy for breeding stallions as for maintenance.[1] That is, 40 g crude protein/1 Mcal DE-/day is considered adequate. Thus a 450-kg stallion needs 745 g crude protein daily (Table 90–1). The NRC further suggested that a ration containing 8.6% protein (90% dry matter basis) should be adequate.[1]

MINERALS

Few studies have been conducted on the mineral requirements of stallions. The NRC suggested that diets containing 0.26% calcium, 0.19% phosphorus, 0.10% magnesium, 0.33% potassium, 9 mg/kg copper, 36 mg/kg zinc, 0.09 mg/kg selenium, and 0.09 mg/kg iodine (90%) (dry matter basis) should be adequate.[1] Some of those concentrations are slightly above that required for maintenance, because the stallion diet may have a greater energy density (more digestible energy per kilogram of dry matter) than diets for maintenance. Thus, to keep nutrients to digestible ration the same, the concentration of the nutrients must be increased.

VITAMINS

Vitamins have received some attention. The NRC suggested that the vitamin A requirement for maintenance should be 1650 IU per kilogram feed.[1] Ralston et al. concluded that 17 to 19 mg β-carotene per kilogram dry matter in grass hay was adequate for seminal production and to maintain libido in stallions.[9] This would be equivalent to 7200 IU of vitamin A activity per kilogram feed, assuming 1 mg β-carotene results in 400 IU vitamin A. They also pointed out that the 17 to 19 mg value should not be used as a requirement but rather to illustrate that vitamin A supplements are not usually necessary, because the vitamin A activity can be supplied by the forage.

As mentioned in Chapter 75, considerable attention has recently been focused on vitamin E nutrition in several species. However, no studies have clearly demonstrated that supplementation of the conventional diet with vitamin E improves reproductive performance in the horse. Rich et al. fed 20 stallions 7 to 9 kg grass hay and 2 to 4 kg of a grain mixture daily.[10] A total of 10 stallions also received 5000 IU of *dl*-α-tocopherol acetate daily. This amount of supplemental vitamin E would provide about 5.5 times the NRC requirement. No information was given about the amount of vitamin E provided in the basal ration. No difference was found in reaction time of the stallion, number of mounts per ejaculate, seminal volume, motility or total spermatozoa per ejaculate between treatments. The authors concluded that high levels of vitamin E supplementation were not necessary.

The NRC stated that experiments in the 1940s suggested that supplementary vitamin C improved the sperm quality of stallions.[1] However, other workers have not been able to repeat their results. The NRC concluded that insufficient evidence exists to establish a vitamin C requirement for horses and that horses synthesize vitamin C in the liver.[1] Evidence does not show that the stallion's requirement for the other water-soluble vitamins is significantly greater than that for maintenance.

RATION FORMULATION

When formulating a ration, the clinician should remember that the important factor is supplying all the needed nutrients in a readily accepted form. Many different feeds can be used to supply the nutrients. The grain to forage ratio should also be considered. As mentioned earlier, an excessive intake of soluble carbohydrate such as found in grains can predispose to obesity and founder. Stallions should usually be fed at least an amount of roughage equivalent to 1.5 kg per 100 kg body weight. In general, the same grain mixture that is formulated for mares can be fed to stallions. The body condition of the stallion should be evaluated to determine how much grain should be fed. Guidelines of 0.5 to 1 kg grain per 100 kg body weight during breeding season are sometimes used.[11,12] Thus a 500-kg stallion would be fed 2.5 to 5 kg grain daily. This would be equivalent to 4 to 8 qt of grain daily if the grain weighs approximately 0.6 kg/qt. Of course, the amount of grain needed depends on the energy density and the individuality of the stallion. Harvey reported that he usually fed Standardbred stallions about 10 qt of oats daily during the breeding season but that some stallions required as much as 16 qt daily.[13] If the clinician assumes that oats weigh 36 lb per bushel, 10 qt would be about 11 lb (5 kg) and 16 qt would be 18 lb (8.2 kg). Further evidence of the variation among stallions is supplied by Hatch who surveyed four farms (two Standardbred and two Thoroughbred) involving a total of 18 stallions.[14] All stallions were fed a commercial concentrate (sweet feed, pelleted feed, or extruded feed). The average amount of concentrate fed daily was 4.6 kg but the range was 1.8 to 8.2 kg per day. Daily hay intake was estimated to be about 9 to 10 kg (half a bale).

REFERENCES

1. National Research Council: Nutrient Requirements of Horses. Washington, DC, National Academy of Science, National Research Council, 1989.
2. Roberts, S.J.: Veterinary Obstetrics and Genital Diseases. 3rd ed. Woodstock, VT, published by the author, 1986.
3. Dorn, C.R., et al.: Castration and other factors affecting the risk of equine laminitis. Cornell Vet., *65:*57–64, 1975.
4. Martin-Rosset, W. (ed.): L'Alimentation des Chevaux. Paris, Institut National de la Recherche Agronomique, 1990.
5. Morrison, F.B.: Feeds and Feeding. 22nd ed. Ithaca, NY, Morrison Publishers, 1957.
6. Cahill, C.: Stallion management. Paper presented at the New York Horse Breeders Conference, Albany, 1981.
7. Crawford, B., and Kirkham, W.: Care and management of the stallion. Thoroughbred Rec. Suppl., n.d.
8. Dinger, J., and Noiles, E.: Effect of controlled exercise on libido in 2-year-old stallions. J. Anim. Sci., *62:*1220–1223, 1986.
9. Ralston, S., et al.: Effect of vitamin A supplementation on the seminal characteristics and sexual behavior of stallions. Proceedings of the Equine Nutrition and Physiology Symposium. 1985, pp. 74–76.
10. Rich, G., et al.: Effect of vitamin E supplementation on stallion seminal characteristics and sexual behavior. Proceedings of the Equine Nutrition and Physiology Symposium. College Station, TX, 1983, pp. 85–87.
11. Frape, D.: Equine Nutrition and Feeding. London, Longman, 1986.
12. Cunha, T.: Horse Feeding and Nutrition. New York, Academic Press, 1980.
13. Harvey, H.M.: Stock farm management. *In* Care and Training of the Trotter and Pacer. Edited by J.C. Harrison. Columbus, United States Trotting Association, 1968, pp. 920–1001.
14. Hatch, W.: Survey of Feeding Practices for Stallions on Four Farms. Elmira, Ontario, Martins Feeds, 1991.

SECTION C

DISEASES OF THE STALLION'S REPRODUCTIVE TRACT

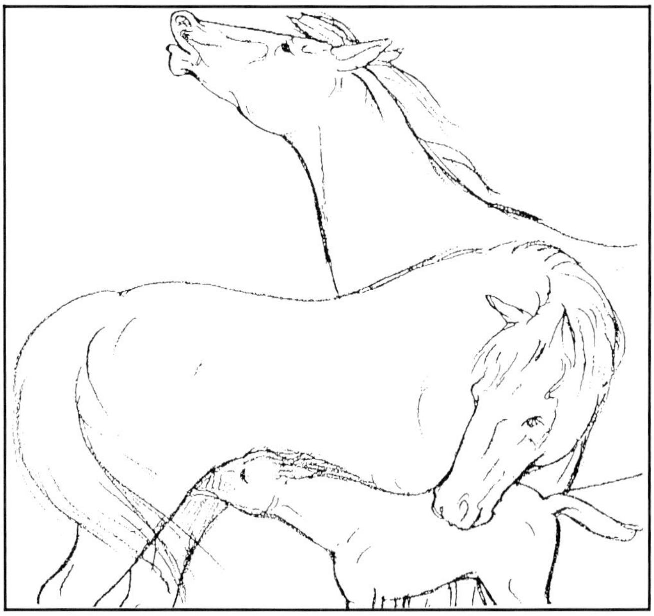

CHAPTER 91

SEXUALLY TRANSMITTED (VENEREAL) DISEASES OF HORSES

M.A. Couto
J.P. Hughes

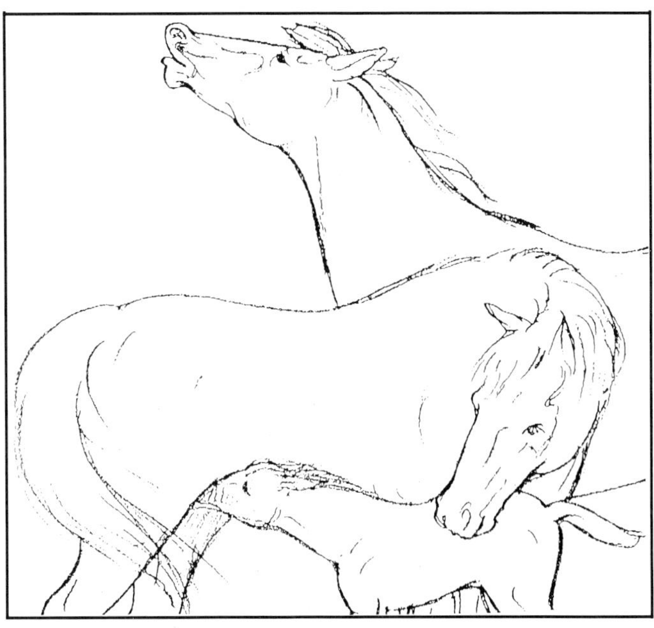

Sexual transmission of genital infections among horses can lead to infertility caused by endometritis, early embryonic death, abortion, or the birth of weak and diseased foals which die during the neonatal period. Certain sexually transmitted diseases (STDs) cause clinical systemic illness among mares and stallions, whereas others may, in addition, restrict the export of breeding stock from countries in which these diseases are prevalent.

Based on their causes, STDs of horses can be categorized as bacterial, viral, and protozoal. Depending on the sex of the affected individual, infections can be clinical or subclinical. With few exceptions, bacterial infections are apparent only in the mare. Viral diseases, on the other hand, vary in their clinical manifestations. While signs of coital exanthema (equine herpesvirus type 3) are readily noticeable in both mares and stallions, equine viral arteritis (EVA) can be sexually transmitted by asymptomatic carrier stallions. Dourine, the only recognized protozoal venereal disease of horses, affects mares and stallions, causing obvious clinical signs in both.

Fortunately, though, STDs are not as prevalent as other sporadic infections of the genital tract. This is largely the result of early recognition of these disease entities with consequent sexual rest of affected stallion(s) as well as stringent codes of practice implemented following outbreaks of these conditions.

BACTERIAL INFECTIONS

Although bacterial infections of the genital tract, such as those caused by Taylorella equigenitalis, Pseudomonas aeruginosa, Klebsiella pneumoniae, and possibly Streptococcus zooepidemicus and Escherichia coli are frequently transmitted through coitus, these infections are by no means strictly venereal. In fact, most if not all of these infections may also be spread by mechanical means, such as contaminated instruments and supplies. Sexually transmitted diseases are more prevalent in pasture breeding or hand breeding operations utilizing natural service. The overall prevalence of bacterial STDs could be reduced or eliminated altogether by the use of artificial insemination (AI) with antibiotic-containing seminal extenders.

As a general rule, only mares display clinical signs of bacterial STD. These include failure to conceive, endometritis, pyometra, and placentitis. The latter may lead to early embryonic loss or abortion, as well as the development of septicemia in newborn foals.[1] Many of the signs, however, are not pathognomonic of any specific genital infection; therefore, an etiologic diagnosis cannot be made on clinical grounds alone. Affected mares frequently exhibit signs of nonspecific genital inflammation, such as discharge of exudate through the vulva, hyperemia of the cervix and vagina, and abnormal numbers of neutrophils on endometrial cytology and biopsy. Indirect manifestations of genital inflammation include shortening of the luteal phase and failure to conceive after mating to a normal fertile stallion. Venereal transmission is strongly suggested when most of the affected mares can be traced to a recent mating by natural service with a particular stallion.

Most mares with functional uterine defenses (i.e., resistant) eliminate the invading pathogens inoculated by the stallion at coitus spontaneously and rather promptly allowing the pregnancy to become established. On the other hand, mares with compromised uterine defense mechanisms (i.e., susceptible) remain persistently infected. The inflammatory reaction usually lingers into early or mid-diestrus stimulating the release of endogenous prostaglandin $F_2\alpha$ ($PGF_2\alpha$) which, in turn, shortens the luteal phase.

Only rarely do stallions show clinical signs of genital bacterial infection. When they do, the signs generally consist of abnormal seminal characteristics.[2]

CONTAGIOUS EQUINE METRITIS

The first reported outbreak of contagious equine metritis (CEM) occurred in the Newmarket area of England during the 1977 breeding season. The causal agent, a gram-negative microaerophilic coccobacillus, was initially identified as Haemophilus equigenitalis and later renamed Taylorella equigenitalis.[3] Since the original outbreak, the disease has been diagnosed among horses in numerous countries (Table 91–1), including the United States, where the importation of two carrier stallions from France was followed by an outbreak of CEM affecting several breeding farms in Kentucky in 1978. At that time, two strains of T. equigenitalis were isolated, one sensitive to and the other resistant to streptomycin. The streptomycin-resistance trait was effectively utilized in the isolation of T. equigenitalis from contaminating commensal and environmental bacteria. Comprehensive reviews regarding the historic and etiologic aspects of CEM are available.[4–6]

Pathogenesis

The transmission of CEM is mainly effected through coitus, although careless handling of the genitalia of both mares and stallions as well as use of contaminated instruments (e.g., specula) can also contribute to spread of the disease. Although most mares recover spontaneously from this condition, a small proportion become carriers of T. equigenitalis. The ubiquity and persistence of T. equigenitalis in the genital tract of diseased animals may greatly enhance its transmissibility. The organism is readily isolated from the clitoral sinuses of carrier mares and the urethral fossa of positive stallions.[6] The organism has also been recovered from the placenta of positive mares[7] and from the genitalia of colts and fillies.[8] In the latter, the infection had been acquired in utero or at the time of parturition.

In an attempt to elucidate further the pathogenesis of CEM, a study was conducted whereby a group of mares was experimentally infected by intrauterine inoculation of T. equigenitalis and subsequently necropsied at various intervals after inoculation.[9,10] During the first 2 weeks postinfection, the organism was isolated from the uterine and cervical lumen and less frequently from the vagina, vestibule, clitoral fossa, clitoral sinuses, and oviducts. Between 3 weeks and 4 months following inoculation, T. equigenitalis was only occasionally recovered from the ovarian surface, oviducts, uterus, cervix, and vagina, but more frequently from the clitoral sinuses and fossa. This study stressed the importance of the clitoral sinuses and fossa as harboring sites for organisms in the chronic carrier state.

Natural or experimental CEM does not afford absolute protection from subsequent infectious episodes. Both local immunization by intrauterine instillation of killed T. equigenitalis and experimental infection with viable organisms evoke an antibody response in serum. In one study, the intrauterine immunization with killed T. equigenitalis stimulated systemic immunoglobulin (Ig) G titers and elevated IgA and IgM levels in uterine and vaginal secretions.[11] Subsequent intrauterine challenge of these mares with live T. equigenitalis resulted in development of a characteristic metritis in both control and vaccinated mares. A second experimental challenge, following natural resolution of the initial infection and a period of reimmunization, resulted in reduced clinical signs and bacterial isolation rates from both control and vaccinated mares.[11] The presence of a local IgA and IgM response, as well as a systemic elevation of IgG titers seemed to point to the profound and abiding effect of T. equigenitalis on the equine immune system. This was in marked contrast to another study which evaluated the immune response of the mare's genital tract to experimentally inoculated S. zooepidemicus.[12] In this investigation, increased local titers of specific IgA, IgM, and IgG were detected 7 days postexperimental infection; a systemic antibody response, however, was not observed.

The absence of significant local IgG titers in response to the T. equigenitalis challenge underscores the importance of phagocytosis of microorganisms by neutrophils within the uterus. However, for the neutrophils to execute their phagocytic function successfully, they require participation of other components of the immune system, mainly opsonins. Thus, absence of a local IgG response, a presumed major opsonin in uterine secretions, suggests that phagocytosis of T. equigenitalis by uterine neutrophils is performed inefficiently in the absence of opsonins. Alternative opsonizing molecules (possibly complement and/or fibronectin) may contribute to elimination of bacteria from the genital environ-

TABLE 91–1. COUNTRIES IN WHICH CASES OF CEM HAVE BEEN REPORTED AND ARE CURRENTLY SUBJECT TO QUARANTINE BEFORE BEING ADMITTED TO THE UNITED STATES

Austria	France	The Netherlands
Belgium	Germany	Norway
Czechoslovakia	Ireland	Sweden
Denmark	Italy	Switzerland
England	Japan	

ment. The first hypothesis seems to be supported by the demonstrated ability of the T. equigenitalis to avoid phagocytosis,[13,14] a factor that may conceivably account for the persistence of this organism in the equine genital tract. The second hypothesis, in turn, stems from the finding, in one study, that depletion of complement from uterine washings significantly reduces bactericidal activity against S. zooepidemicus.[15] Furthermore, phagocytosis of yeasts by uterine-derived neutrophils is complement dependent.[15] Thus phagocytosis of T. equigenitalis by uterine neutrophils may depend on the presence of complement or other opsonizing molecules. However, different microorganisms likely elicit and require different immune responses; one response being entirely dependent on the presence of opsonins (S. zooepidemicus) and the other being opsonin independent (T. equigenitalis). Pereira and Hosking have shown that, although neutrophils are able to engulf certain bacteria in the presence of complement alone, maximal phagocytosis appears to require the participation of both antibody and complement.[16] Detectable serum antibodies have not been demonstrated in the carrier stallion.[17]

Clinical Signs

The most consistent clinical finding in mares infected with CEM is a copious, grayish vulvar discharge. Signs usually develop 8 to 10 days after being covered by a carrier stallion and persist for 13 to 17 days. Other mares fail to show outward signs of disease, although they may exhibit a shortened luteal phase. No systemic involvement occurs and most mares recover spontaneously, although the microorganism may persist in the genital tract for several months following clinical recovery. Recurrences of the disease have not been reported. Stallions do not show any clinical signs; however, many remain asymptomatic carriers.

Diagnosis

A diagnosis of CEM can be made on the basis of the isolation of T. equigenitalis or by means of serologic tests.

Bacteriologic Method. Currently, the most reliable means of diagnosis of CEM is the bacteriologic examination of swabs from the genitourinary tract of infected animals.[18] This method consists of recovering the organism from swabs collected from all accessible sites of infection (i.e., endometrium, cervix, clitoral fossa, and sinuses) in the estrous mare. The samples for culture must be placed in a liquid transport medium (Amies with charcoal) immediately after collection and kept refrigerated until delivered to the laboratory. On arrival, the specimens should be streaked onto a solid culture medium (chocolate agar plus 10% horse blood) as quickly as possible if false negative results are to be avoided. Rapidly developing commensal bacteria, notably Proteus spp., may quickly outgrow T. equigenitalis, obscuring its presence. Selective media containing antibiotics (streptomycin and clindamycin), trimethoprim, and fungistatic compounds (amphotericin B) have been used successfully to suppress Proteus spp and other contaminants. Plates are incubated at 37° C in an atmosphere of 5 to 10% carbon dioxide. Growth is enhanced in an atmosphere of 90% H_2 and 10% CO_2.[17] Within 48 h, T. equigenitalis colonies appear grayish, small, pinpoint in size, and smooth in outline. Beginning at 72 h, colonies become raised and shiny, with elevated, opaque centers. Organisms isolated from carrier mares grow more slowly than those obtained from field cases.[19]

For screening purposes, a swab of the clitoral sinuses offers the advantage of allowing samples to be obtained from the nonpregnant mare at any stage of the cycle and from the pregnant mare at any stage during gestation.

The stallion or colt should be sampled with the penis in the extruded position.[6] Samples should be obtained from the urethral fossa, urethra, preputial folds and skin of the penis, and if possible, pre-ejaculatory fluid. Specimens are delivered to the laboratory and processed as described previously. A major disadvantage of the bacteriologic method is frequent extended cultivation time, resulting in considerable delays before a diagnosis can be confirmed.[18]

Serologic Methods. All serologic tests for diagnosis of CEM are based on detection of antibodies against T. equigenitalis in serum.

Complement Fixation Tests. Various complement fixation (CF) tests for CEM have been developed.[20,21] Although CF tests have been used successfully to diagnose chronically infected mares, these tests are not reliable for identification of carrier animals.[17] Because CF test titers in affected mares are detectable 10 days after infection, recent cases of CEM may go undetected.[4]

Serum Agglutination Test. A rapid microtitration serum agglutination test (SAT), based on that used for brucellosis, was recently described.[22] This assay was introduced as a backup serologic test to supplement and cross-check results of the CF test and to minimize the incidence of false negatives caused by recent infections. The SAT was found to be one of the most useful tests for diagnosing acute cases of CEM.[4] No false positive or false negative reactions were associated with this test.

Enzyme-Linked Immunosorbent Assay. A reliable technique for the diagnosis of CEM by the micro-enzyme-linked immunosorbent assay (ELISA) method employing rabbit anti–T. equigenitalis antiserum has been utilized.[23] In this study, immunoglobulin binding to the CEM organism was strongest for IgG and less for IgM, whereas IgA did not bind.

Passive Hemagglutination. A passive hemagglutination (PHA) test for the diagnosis of CEM has also been developed.[24] It employs an antigen prepared from sonicated hyaluronidase-treated T. equigenitalis and equine red blood cells (RBC) fixed with glutaraldehyde.

Immunofluorescence. An indirect immunofluorescence test was recently described.[25] The authors emphasized the usefulness of this technique in circumventing the problem of autoagglutination of isolates of T. equigenitalis.

Miscellaneous Methods. Examination of Gram- or Giemsa-stained endometrial smears has been used for diagnostic purposes in cases of acute CEM.[6] Appearance of numerous neutrophils together with gram-negative coccobacilli, free or engulfed by polymorphonuclear leukocytes (PMNs) should be considered only as a presumptive indication of the presence of CEM. Specific tests are required to make an assertive diagnosis.

The intrauterine inoculation of test mares using smegma from a suspect CEM carrier stallion has been recommended in cases in which T. equigenitalis has been impossible to isolate.[26]

A more sophisticated method of diagnosis employed gas-liquid chromatography in the identification of T. equigenitalis.[27]

Treatment

The most efficacious, albeit not infallible, treatment for mares affected with CEM is the intrauterine instillation of antibiotics. The daily infusion of 5 to 10 million units of penicillin for 5 to 7 days has been successful in eliminating T. equigenitalis. An important consideration is the thorough cleansing of the clitoris, clitoral fossa, and median and lateral clitoral sinuses. Vigorous scrubbing of these areas using a 4% solution of clorhexidine followed by packing with a nitrofurazone or clorhexidine ointment has proved adequate to this end. This procedure should be repeated daily for a total of 5 days. In cases in which the successful elimination of the CEM organism is in doubt, the suspect mares should have this treatment performed on each of 3 consecutive days in early estrus before breeding. For those mares in which the elimination of the organism has proved unsuccessful after several courses of intrauterine and topical therapy, the clinician might have to remove the clitoral sinuses surgically (clitoral sinusectomy).[28] According to one study, only the median clitoral sinus is involved in the pathogenesis of CEM.[29] Although the lateral sinuses trap smegma, they are too shallow to support the anaerobic growth of T. equigenitalis.

Stallions are treated topically by thoroughly washing the external genitalia (penis and prepuce) with a 4% clorhexidine solution followed by a nitrofurazone dressing. The penis must be cleansed in the extruded position with special attention to the fossa glandis (urethral fossa) and skin folds of the prepuce. When this treatment is repeated for 5 consecutive days, it is highly successful.

Control

The successful identification and treatment of positive mares and stallions effectively reduces the prevalence of CEM among the susceptible equine population. Implementation of the codes of practice by the affected countries contributed to bringing the epidemic to a halt. In fact, the prompt recognition of clinical signs of CEM, together with stringent hygienic measures, such as the greater use of disposable and sterile equipment and supplies, together with sound bacteriologic screening policies constituted the mainstay of the control program. The original code of practice was introduced in the United Kingdom in 1977, and since then similar plans were implemented in countries such as the United States, France, Ireland, Italy, Sweden, and Germany. The few outbreaks that occurred since the enforcement of the codes were limited to a small number of animals and invariably were caused by the introduction of a carrier mare.[6] These mares with a known history of CEM infection were categorized as high-risk animals and were required to produce at least three negative cultures from the endometrium, clitoris, and clitoral sinuses before they could be admitted to the breeding shed. In an attempt to avoid the false negative carrier state, countries such as the United States have required that, in addition to a period of quarantine and cleansing of the clitoral harboring sites, a sinusectomy be performed on mares imported from countries in which the disease had been reported.

As indicated above, immunization of mares against CEM has heretofore been unsuccessful. In spite of the development of high levels of circulating immunoglobulin, the antibody did not protect the animals against subsequent bacterial challenge.

PSEUDOMONAS AERUGINOSA, KLEBSIELLA PNEUMONIAE, STREPTOCOCCUS ZOOEPIDEMICUS, AND ESCHERICHIA COLI INFECTIONS

A true venereal route of transmission has been strongly suggested for both P. aeruginosa and K. pneumoniae. While other pathogenic organisms residing on the stallion's external genitalia (i.e., S. zooepidemicus and E. coli) are in a position to be transmitted via natural service, their venereal transmission has not been adequately documented. In fact, no reports are available on the occurrence of outbreaks of STD caused by either S. zooepidemicus or E. coli among mares mated to the same stallion. Because S. zooepidemicus and E. coli are part of the equine normal external genital and fecal flora, respectively, identifying the source of the organism in any given case is difficult. Furthermore, the establishment and severity of the infections, as well as their consequences on fertility, are determined by both individual host susceptibility and intrinsic pathogenicity of the particular strain involved.

Pathogenesis

The sexual transmission of bacterial infections largely depends on the delicate balance between normal microflora and the coexisting population of pathogenic bacteria residing on the external genitalia of stallions. Most bacteria present on the penis and prepuce are innocuous skin commensals related to the local environment, mainly the horse's fecal microflora and stall bedding material. The microflora, which generally has no harmful effects on fertility, thrives in the smegma of the stallion's external genitalia, restricting or discouraging the growth of potentially pathogenic organisms. Although P. aeruginosa, K. pneumoniae, S. zooepidemicus, and E. coli are often associated with reduced fertility caused by endometritis, their mere presence on the external genitalia and/or in the semen does not necessarily result in infertility.[30] On the other hand, the uncommon occurrence of active infection of the stallion's urogenital tract (i.e., urethritis, cystitis, seminal vesiculitis, and ampullitis) may interfere with normal fertility.[2,31–33] Although S. zooepidemicus and E. coli are most often associated with endometritis in the mare, P. aeruginosa and K. pneumoniae are more frequently involved in apparent venereal disease outbreaks. The reason for this differential response is not at all clear. The fact that the latter are more apt to cause clinical endometritis when transmitted during coitus from an infected or carrier stallion might be explained on the basis of a greater intrinsic pathogenicity. Paradoxically, P. aeruginosa organisms exhibit a typically low pathogenicity toward humans, becoming established only when a breakdown of the local defense mechanism occurs in the skin and subcutaneous tissues (e.g., burn patients), pulmonary alveolar epithelium (cystic fibrosis), and cornea and conjunctiva (keratitis and conjunctivitis). In horses, however, differences in pathogenicity among strains of Pseudomonas spp. were suggested by the fact that some stallions harboring the organism in their genital tracts were associated with low conception rates, whereas most stallions harboring Pseudomonas organisms exhibited normal fertility.[1]

The persistence and recurrence of certain P. aeruginosa and K. pneumoniae infections in mares may be the result of harboring of these organisms in the clitoral sinuses, similar to the case of T. equigenitalis.

Because S. zooepidemicus and E. coli are mostly responsible for cases of uterine infection, the establishment of endometritis in these instances is likely the result of individual mare susceptibility. S. zooepidemicus is the most common and ubiquitous microorganism residing on the mare's external genitalia and caudal vagina, whereas E. coli is a prominent member of the equine fecal flora. Clinicians recognized that the prevalence of endometritis caused by E. coli and S. zooepidemicus is highly correlated with a marginal to poor perineal and/or vulvar conformation. Clearly, mares are continually exposed to both β-streptococci and E. coli. However, a proportionately modest number of (susceptible) mares become infected with these organisms. While E. coli are commonly recovered from the smegma of stallions, as well as from isolated cases of endometritis, they seldom if ever produce true outbreaks of venereal disease.[34]

Heavily encapsulated strains of K. pneumoniae (capsule types K1, K2, and K5) have been implicated in the venereal transmission of infection from stallion to mare. However, other strains, such as K7, frequently isolated from stallion genital swabs, were not associated with outbreaks of sexually transmitted endometritis.[30,35] Strains of K. pneumoniae, found predominantly in feces (90.5% of all isolates), were less frequently recovered from cervical swabs (8%) in metritis cases or from semen (36.8% of the isolates).[35]

Many strains of P. aeruginosa form part of the normal genital flora of the stallion's penis and prepuce, whereas other strains are venereal pathogens. Unfortunately, because of the difficulty of categorizing the different P. aeruginosa strains, the clinician must consider all isolates as potentially pathogenic.

Clinical Signs

As indicated previously, the clinical signs exhibited by affected mares are common to most endometritides (see Chapter 43 for details).

Diagnosis

As mentioned previously, the diagnosis of the presence of STD is mainly based on the history and clinical signs. A specific diagnosis can only be made by bacteriologic culture of the uterus and clitoral sinuses in the mare and the urethral fossa, urethra, and ejaculate in the stallion. In addition, capsule typing in the case of K. pneumoniae may aid in distinguishing pathogenic from nonpathogenic strains.

Treatment and Prophylaxis

The therapeutic considerations of endometritis in the mare are discussed in Chapter 43. This chapter will discuss those aspects directly relevant to the venereal transmission of genital disease.

A strict prebreeding bacteriologic screening program is crucial if the spread of STD is to be avoided. If an outbreak of venereal disease is diagnosed or suspected, the implicated stallion(s) and/or mare(s) should be immediately withdrawn from mating until the condition is confirmed and adequately treated.

A strict hygiene before and during the service are of the essence in preventing the venereal spread of disease. A set of guidelines termed "minimal contamination techniques" was introduced to minimize the transmission of pathogens from the stallion to the mare at mating.[36] These techniques emphasize the use of AI, employing antibiotic-containing seminal extenders. The use of small seminal volumes reduces the number of potentially pathogenic bacteria deposited in the mare's uterus, thereby lowering the challenge to her local immune system. The use of postovulatory uterine lavage followed or not by an antibiotic intrauterine infusion may also be a useful adjunct to the minimal contamination techniques.

Contrary to the expected effect, vigorous scrubbing of the penis with potent antiseptic cleansers, such as povidone-iodine and clorhexidine, widely practiced after the CEM outbreak, actually may increase the incidence of penile contamination with K. pneumoniae and Ps. aeruginosa. Vigorous antiseptic washing removes the normal penile skin commensal flora and allows resistant organisms to proliferate in a competition-free environment. Thus, at mating, large numbers of K. pneumoniae and P. aeruginosa may be deposited in the mare's uterus. Washing the stallion's penis with only water had little effect on its bacterial environment and is a preferred method for cleaning the penis before mating.[39] Jones et al. suggested that, regardless of the use of antiseptics, a more gentle wash technique (i.e., pouring water on the penis vs. vigorous scrubbing) preserves the "deep-skin" resident bacterial flora while removing transient skin bacterial population.[38] The deep-skin flora might play a role in reducing colonization of the penis by potential pathogens.

VIRAL INFECTIONS

EQUINE VIRAL ARTERITIS

Equine viral arteritis (EVA), also known as pinkeye and epidemic cellulitis is a multifaceted acute, contagious, communicable viral disease of horses causing fever, ocular and respiratory signs, edema of the limbs, and abortion. The etiologic agent is a RNA pestivirus of the Togaviridae family. This disease was first recognized in the United States in the 1950s following an outbreak of abortion and systemic illness among horses on a Standardbred stud farm in Bucyrus, Ohio. After successful control of the initial outbreak, the disease was not reported again until the summer of 1984 when a limited outbreak among Thoroughbred horses developed in central Kentucky. Since then, clinical EVA has been infrequently diagnosed in the United States, although isolated cases have been documented in Arizona, California, Colorado, Indiana, Kentucky, New York, Ohio, and Pennsylvania. Seroepidemiologic studies have revealed a widespread prevalence of antibodies against the equine arteritis virus (EAV) worldwide. A significantly higher proportion of Standardbreds tested positive for EAV antibodies than any other breed. In one study, up to 85% of the Standardbred population was seropositive for this disease, followed by American Saddlebred Horses as a distant second with 25% of seropositivity. Quarter Horses (12%) and Thoroughbreds (2%) exhibit the lowest incidence of positive sera.[39] The reason for the remarkably high prevalence in Standardbreds is unknown.

Pathogenesis

The virulence of the various field strains of virus appear to vary considerably. The disease is rarely fatal except for experimental infections. The incubation period ranges from 3 to 8 days. The virus tends to occur in an epidemic form usually attributable to the movement of horses, especially on racetracks and stud farms. In the latter, carrier/shedder stallions play a central role in the spread of the virus.[40] About 34% of the stallions recovering from EVA shed virus in the semen for a long time (up to years) after the original infectious episode.

The spread of EVA is achieved through contaminated secretions, mainly respiratory aerosols. Venereal transmission occurs owing to the presence of infective virus in the semen of carrier stallions.[41] Experimentally, EAV can be recovered from the nasopharynx, serum, and buffy coat during the initial 3 weeks of infection.

Abortion storms may affect up to 80% of pregnant mares, especially in late gestation. However, abortions occurring as early as 60 days of pregnancy have been documented. Invariably the aborting mare is febrile and shows clinical signs of the disease with the abortion occurring during or shortly after the acute febrile phase. Interestingly, and in contrast to some stallions, mares recovered from the disease no longer shed virus.

Clinical Signs

Subclinical EVA poses a great danger to breeding animals, because the presence of the virus may remain unnoticed for a great length of time before abortions occur. Unfortunately, subclinical EVA appears to be the rule except in pregnant or stressed horses. Clinical signs of EVA vary greatly among individuals ranging from a mild fever and conjunctivitis to severe depression and illness. These signs must be differentiated from those of rhinopneumonitis and influenza. The occurrence of abortion during or just following illness is a valuable diagnostic feature. Although mares rarely abort subsequent to a bout with influenza, abortions as a result of rhinopneumonitis usually occur in the absence of any clinical signs. Moreover, in these cases fetuses present characteristic lesions and inclusion bodies.

Stallions may, on occasion, exhibit clinical signs of genital disease such as scrotal and preputial edema. After a rest period of several weeks, most infected animals recover spontaneously from the disease.

Diagnosis

The diagnosis of EVA is based on clinical signs, virus isolation (nasal secretions, semen, urine, and aborted fetuses), and serologic tests. Although EAV can be isolated from the sperm-rich fraction of most stallions, virus isolation is not considered to be absolutely reliable. The successful virus isolation can vary with the capabilities of the laboratory and the handling of the sample obtained for culture. Therefore, antibody titers from paired serum samples taken 2 weeks apart is considered an important diagnostic test. Subclinical infections can only be detected by serology.

Several serologic tests are available, including virus neutralization (VN), CF, and ELISA. In acute or recent cases, CF is superior to other tests, whereas VN and ELISA are useful in the detection of more chronic cases. Complement-fixating antibodies, primarily IgM, tend to decline rapidly. Virus-neutralizing antibody is also present in horses that have been exposed either by vaccination or natural infection. The disadvantage of the VN test is that it takes 4 to 5 days to yield a result, whereas CF assays can be read the next day. On the other hand, the CF test may exhibit false positive results when used on serum from animals recently vaccinated. This is because CF antigen preparations contain bovine serum products as stabilizers which may interfere with the test.

Seroconversion of mares from negative to positive following mating is considered evidence of a shedder stallion. Caution must be exercised when evaluating serum samples with low or stable titers. Whereas rising titers in paired samples is an unequivocal indication of disease, a low titer may reflect use of the modified-live EVA vaccine.

Treatment

As indicated, most horses recover spontaneously. However, good nursing care as well as the use of antimicrobials may conceivably reduce the incidence and severity of secondary bacterial infections.

Control

Because the EVA virus can be recovered from secretions for up to 3 weeks following experimental infection, a quarantine period of at least 3 weeks for newly arrived horses has been suggested as a satisfactory control measure. The screening of carrier/shedder stallions cannot be overemphasized. Kentucky has introduced a control program indicating that the owner/agent of mares booking to known shedding stallions must be notified in writing by the owner/agent of the stallion and a copy must be sent to the chief livestock sanitary official. Shedder stallions are allowed to mate only seropositive mares from prior vaccination or exposure or mares that have been vaccinated against EVA at least 21 days before mating. The serologic testing of positive mares must have been conducted on or after November 1 of the previous calendar year. All shedding stallions must be housed, handled, and bred in a facility isolated from nonshedding stallions.

All mares bred to shedding stallions are classified as either category 1 or category 2 mares for the breeding season based on the following criteria. Category 1 includes mares bred to a shedding stallion for the first time, whereas category 2 refers to mares previously bred to shedding stallions. A detailed description of this classification system is available from the State Veterinarian of the Commonwealth of Kentucky. The guidelines also state that the chief livestock sanitary official and the stallion owner/manager are responsible for determining whether a stallion is shedding the virus before breeding. Seropositive vaccinated stallions never associated with the transmission of EVA must have been seronegative before vaccination and/or must have had no known contact with EVA-infected and/or -exposed horses before vaccination or during the 21 days postvaccination. Stallions and mares becoming infected during the breeding season must be removed from the breeding program immediately and reported to the sanitary officials. All owners/agents having mares booked or previously bred to such stallions must be immediately notified in writing by the stallion owner/agent and a copy must be sent to the sanitary officials. Stallions becoming infected during the breeding season are classified as shedders and handled accordingly. All horses vaccinated against EVA for the first time must have a negative EVA test before vaccination.

A modified-live virus vaccine, based on the Bucyrus strain of EVA, was successfully employed to elicit the development of long-lived protective antibodies.[42,43] This vaccine has been available commercially for intramuscular administration since 1985. However, its use is controlled by state regulatory officials. The disinfection of equipment and facilities can easily be achieved by the use of antiseptic detergents which dissolve the lipid envelope of the equine arteritis virus.

EQUINE COITAL EXANTHEMA

Equine coital exanthema (ECE), or equine herpesvirus type 3 (EHV 3), is a benign viral disease of horses affecting both sexes and primarily transmitted at coitus. Its causative agent was originally presumed to be a single virus (EHV 3), although present evidence indicates a combination of small and large plaque variant viruses is involved in the development of this disease.[44]

Although the primary route of transmission is venereal, passive transfer by contaminated supplies and instruments during gynecological manipulations is also possible.[45] Two outbreaks of ECE, each comprising more than 20 mares, were observed in which the only stallion present was demonstrably a nonshedder of the virus. Because the affected mares had been subjected to multiple palpations per rectum using the same glove, the spread of the virus was determined to be iatrogenic in nature (A.O. McKinnon, personal communication). The virus has also been isolated from nonbreeding animals.[46]

Clinical signs in mares develop 4 to 7 days after sexual contact and are manifested by the appearance of multiple circular nodules up to 2 mm in diameter on the vulvar mucosa and perineal skin. The lesions progress to vesicles and pustules that eventually rupture leaving naked ulcerated areas approximately 3 to 10 mm in diameter. The affected areas are painful on touch. Unless seriously complicated by secondary bacterial infection, the lesions granulate and heal in 2 to 3 weeks leaving unpigmented areas. Clitoral ulcers heal more slowly. When severe bacterial contamination is present, the pustules tend to coalesce and exude a thick mucopurulent discharge. Edema may be quite prominent extending to the perineal region and inner thighs.

Vesicles progressing to pustules and ulcers also develop on the shaft of the penis and on the prepuce of affected stallions which, in the acute stages of the disease, may be justifiably reluctant to mate. Infrequently, edema of the prepuce, scrotum, and perineal region extending to the belly is found.

Extragenital lesions are uncommon, although, on occasion the lips and nasal mucosa may be affected. The only systemic sign of ECE consists of a temporary depression with variable pyrexia. The disease can only be transmitted during the acute stages (first 10 to 14 days). After ulcers have healed the condition is no longer contagious. The diagnosis of ECE is based on the clinical signs.

Treatment consists of the institution of immediate sexual rest for 3 weeks. This allows the ulcers to heal and prevents the spread of disease. The use of a demulcent antibiotic-containing ointment for at least 3 consecutive days is useful to discourage the development of secondary bacterial infections. Topical therapy also aids in preventing development of rare preputial adhesions. Because of the benign nature of this condition, the use of antiviral preparations is not warranted. A carrier state has not been reported.

Control of the disease is clearly achieved by withholding mating of all horses affected as well as the use of disposable equipment when handling these animals.

PROTOZOAL INFECTIONS

The only recognized venereal condition caused by protozoa is dourine. Dourine (mal de coit) is a chronic, protozoal disease affecting horses, mules, and donkeys of either sex. The etiologic agent is Trypanosoma equiperdum, and the disease is characterized by low morbidity but high mortality which, in untreated cases may reach 50 to 70%. This condition is currently prevalent in the Middle East, North and South Africa, and Central and South America; it has been eradicated from Europe and North America. The onset is slow with an incubation period of 1 to 2 weeks and an extremely protracted clinical course extending over a period of weeks or months. In mares, the early signs include mild recurrent fever, edematous swelling of the external genitalia, and a mucopurulent vulvar discharge. Later, typical cutaneous lesions develop consisting of raised plaques 2 to 10 cm in diameter. Parenthetically, the aspect of the cutaneous lesions gave origin to the name of the disease, because they were initially described in Spain as resembling a local coin known as *duro*.

In the stallion, initial signs consist of a mucopurulent discharge from the urethra; mild pyrexia; and nonpainful edema of penis, prepuce, and scrotum. A serious sequela of this disease includes paralysis of the penis. Both affected mares and stallions become progressively emaciated exhibiting lameness and hindlimb incoordination. Note that asymptomatic positive stallions may become lifelong carriers.[47]

Diagnosis of dourine is made on the basis of the clinical signs and the demonstration of the causal agent from urethral and vaginal exudates, skin lesions, and buffy coat from peripheral blood samples. Centrifugation of the material (2500 × g for 20 min at 4° C) before microscopic observation enhances the demonstration of the parasite. Positive identification of T. equiperdum involves serologic testing by CF, immunofluorescent antibody, ELISA, or card agglutination tests. When a comparison among tests was conducted, CF emerged as the most reliable technique for the diagnosis of dourine.[48] Nonspecific or anticomplementary reactions were found occasionally with horse sera and frequently when testing mule or donkey sera. Cross-reactivity with T. evansi and T. brucei as a result of shared antigens may give rise to ambiguous results if the agents are also present in the particular geographic region.

Affected horses may be treated with quinapyramine sulfate in endemic areas, although it is not known whether such treated and recovered stallions are safe for breeding purposes. Thus the strict screening (by CF test) and slaughter of positive animals, and institution of quarantine programs are the preferred methods of control for this disease.

REFERENCES

1. Hughes, J.P., Loy, R.G., Asbury, A.C., and Burd, H.E.: The occurrence of Pseudomonas in the reproductive tract of mares and its effect on fertility. Cornell Vet., *56:*595–610, 1966.
2. Blanchard, T.L., et al.: Bilateral seminal vesiculitis and ampullitis in a stallion. J. Am. Vet. Med. Assoc., *192:*525–526, 1988.
3. Sugimoto, C., Isayama, Y., Sakazaki, R., and Kuramochi, S.: Transfer of Haemophilus equigenitalis Taylor et al. 1978 to the genus Taylorella gen. nov. as Taylorella equigenitalis comb. nov. Curr. Microbiol., *9:*155–162, 1983.
4. Brewer, R.A.: Contagious equine metritis: A review/summary. Vet. Bull., *53:*881–891, 1983.
5. Platt, H., and Taylor, C.E.D.: Contagious equine metritis. *In* Medical Microbiology. Vol 1. Edited by C.S.F. Easmon and J. Jeljaszewicz. New York, Academic Press, 1983, pp. 149–196.
6. Powell, D.G.: Contagious equine metritis. *In* Current Therapy in Theriogenology 2. Edited by D.A. Morrow. Philadelphia, W.B. Saunders, 1986, pp. 786–792.
7. Powell, D.G., and Whitwell, K.: The epidemiology of contagious equine metritis (CEM) in England 1977–1978. J. Reprod. Fertil. Suppl., *27:*331–335, 1979.
8. Timoney, P.J., and Powell, D.G.: Isolation of the contagious equine metritis organism from colts and fillies in the

United Kingdom and Ireland. Vet. Rec., *111*:478–482, 1982.

9. Acland, H.M., and Kenney, R.M.: Lesions of contagious equine metritis in mares. Vet. Pathol., *20*:330–341, 1983.

10. Strezmienski, P.J., Benson, C.E., Acland, H.M., and Kenney, R.M.: Comparison of uterine protein content and distribution of bacteria in the reproductive tract of mares after intrauterine inoculation of Haemophilus equigenitalis or Pseudomonas aeruginosa. Am. J. Vet. Res., *45*:6, 1109–1113, 1984.

11. Widders, P.R., Stokes, C.R., David, J.S., and Bourne, F.J.: Specific antibody in the equine genital tract following local immunization and challenge infection with contagious equine metritis organism (Taylorella equigenitalis). Res. Vet. Sci., *40*:54–58, 1986.

12. Watson, E.D.: The influence of estrogen and progesterone on antibody synthesis by the endometrium of the mare. *In* Equine Infectious Diseases V: Proceedings of the Fifth International Conference of Equine Infectious Diseases. Edited by D.G. Powell. Lexington, University Press of Kentucky, 1988, pp. 181–185.

13. Bertram, T.A., Coignoul, F.L., and Jensen, A.E.: Phagocytosis and intracellular killing of the contagious equine metritis organism by equine neutrophils in serum. Infect. Immun., *37*:1241–1247, 1982.

14. Bertram, T.A., Coignoul, F.L., and Jensen, A.E.: Phagocytosis and intracellular killing of the contagious equine metritis organism by equine neutrophils in genital secretions. Am. J. Vet. Res., *44*:1923–1927, 1982.

15. Watson, E.D.: Opsonins in uterine washings influencing in vitro activity of equine neutrophils. Equine Vet. J., *20*:435–437, 1988.

16. Pereira, H.A., and Hosking, C.S.: The role of complement and antibody in opsonization and intracellular killing of Candida albicans. Clin. Exp. Immunol., *57*:307–314, 1984.

17. Timoney, J.F.: The genus Taylorella. *In* Hagan and Bruner's Microbiology and Infectious Diseases of Domestic Animals. 8th ed. Edited by J.F. Timoney, J.H. Gillespie, F.W. Scott, and J.E. Barlough. Ithaca, NY, Comstock Publishing Associates, 1988, pp. 100–103.

18. Brown, B.S., and Timoney, P.J.: Contagious equine metritis and fluorescence [letter]. Vet. Rec., 123:39, 1988.

19. Swerczek, T.W.: Contagious equine metritis. Outbreak of the disease in Kentucky and laboratory methods for diagnosing the disease. J. Reprod. Fertil. Suppl., *27*:361–365, 1979.

20. Croxton-Smith, P., Benson, J.A., and Dawson, F.L.M.: A complement fixation test for antibody to the contagious equine metritis organisms. Vet. Rec., *103*:270–278, 1978.

21. Gummow, B., Herr, S., and Brett, O.L.: A short, reliable, highly reproducible complement fixation test for the serological diagnosis of contagious equine metritis. Onderstepoort J. Vet. Res., *53*:241–243, 1986.

22. Gummow, B., Herr, S., and Brett, O.L.: A rapid microtitration serum agglutination test for the detection of contagious equine metritis antibodies. Onderstepoort J. Vet. Res., *54*:97–98, 1987.

23. Widders, P.R., Stokes, C.R., Newby, T.J., and Bourne, F.J.: Nonimmune binding of equine immunoglobulin by the causative organism of contagious equine metritis. Infect. Immun., *48*:417–421, 1985.

24. Eguchi, M., Kuniyasu, C., and Kishima, M.: Passive hemagglutination test for detection of antibodies against Taylorella (Haemophilus) equigenitalis in sera of mares. Vet. Microbiol., *18*:155–161, 1988.

25. Ter Laak, E.A., Fennema G., and Jaartsveld F.H.: Contagious equine metritis in the Netherlands. Tijdschr. Diergeneeskd., *114*:189–201, 1989.

26. Swerczec, T.W.: Contagious equine metritis: Tests for suspect carriers. Vet. Rec., *108*:420–421, 1981.

27. Neill, S.D., et al.: Contagious equine metritis: Use of gas-liquid chromatography in identifying the causal agent. Equine Vet. J., *16*:430–434, 1984.

28. Swerczek, T.W.: Elimination of CEM organisms from mares by excision of clitoral sinuses. Vet. Rec., *105*:131–132, 1979.

29. McAllister, R.A., and Sack, W.O. Identification of anatomic features of the equine clitoris as potential growth sites for Taylorella equigenitalis. J. Am. Vet. Med. Assoc., *196*:1965–1966, 1990.

30. Dowsett, K.F.: Seminal Abnormalities. *In* Current Therapy in Equine Medicine. 2nd ed. Edited by N.E. Robinson. Philadelphia, W.B. Saunders, 1987, p. 564–566.

31. Klug, E., et al.: The effect of vesiculectomy on seminal characteristics in the stallion. J. Reprod. Fertil. Suppl., *27*:61–66, 1979.

32. Johnson, T.L., et al.: Pseudomonas infection in a stallion: A case report. Proc. Am. Assoc. Equine Pract., 111–116, 1980.

33. Sojka, J.E., and Carter, G.K.: Hemospermia and seminal vesicle enlargement in a stallion. Compend. Contin. Educ. Practicing Vet., *7*:S587–S588, 1985.

34. Bowen, J.M.: Venereal Diseases of Stallions. *In* Current Therapy in Equine Medicine. 2nd ed. Edited by N.E. Robinson. Philadelphia, W.B. Saunders, 1986, pp. 508–511.

35. Kikuchi, N., Iguchi, I., and Hiramune, T.: Capsule types of Klebsiella pneumoniae isolated from the genital tract of mares with metritis, extra-genital sites of healthy mares and the genital tract of stallions. Vet. Microbiol., *15*:219–228, 1987.

36. Kenney, R.M., et al.: Minimal contamination techniques for breeding mares: Techniques and preliminary findings. Proc. Am. Assoc. Equine Pract., 327–336, 1975.

37. Bowen, J.M., et al.: Effects of washing on the bacterial flora of the stallion's penis. J. Reprod. Fertil. Suppl., *32*:41–45, 1982.

38. Jones R.L., et al.: The effect of washing on the aerobic bacterial flora of the stallion's penis. Proc. Am. Assoc. Equine Pract., 9–16, 1984.

39. Vander Schalie, J., and Evermann, J.: Equine viral arteritis alert—Status in the Northwest. Equine Vet. Sci., *10*:14–15, 1989.

40. Timoney, P.J., et al.: The carrier state in equine arteritis virus infection in the stallion with specific emphasis on the venereal mode of virus transmission. J. Reprod. Fertil. Suppl., *35*:95–102, 1987.

41. Timoney, P.J., and McCollum, W.H., The epidemiology of equine viral arteritis. Proc. Am. Assoc. Equine Pract., 545–551, 1985.

42. McCollum, W.H.: Development of a modified virus strain and vaccine for equine viral arteritis. J. Am. Vet. Med. Assoc., *155*:318–322, 1969.

43. McKinnon, A.O., et al.: Vaccination of stallions with a modified live equine viral arteritis virus. J. Equine Vet. Sci., *6*:66–69, 1986.

44. Jacob, R.J., et al.: Molecular pathogenesis of equine coital exanthema: Identification of a new equine herpesvirus isolated from lesions reminiscent of coital exanthema in a donkey. *In* Equine infectious diseases V: Proceedings of the Fifth International Conference of Equine Infectious

Diseases. Edited by D.G. Powell. Lexington, University Press of Kentucky, 1988, pp. 140–146.

45. Krogsrud, J., and Onstad, O.: Equine coital exanthema—Isolation of a virus and transmission experiments. Acta Vet. Scand., *12:*1–14, 1971.

46. Crandell, R., and Davis, E.R.: Isolation of equine coital exanthema virus (equine herpesvirus 3) from the nostril of a foal. J. Am. Vet. Med. Assoc., *187:*503–504, 1985.

47. Robertson, A.R. (ed.): Handbook of Animal Diseases in the Tropics, 3rd ed. London, British Veterinary Association, 1976.

48. Williamson, C.C., et al.: An investigation into alternative methods for the serodiagnosis of dourine. Onderstepoort J. Vet. Sci., *55:*117–119, 1988.

CHAPTER 92

TESTICULAR DEGENERATION

T.L. Blanchard
D.D. Varner

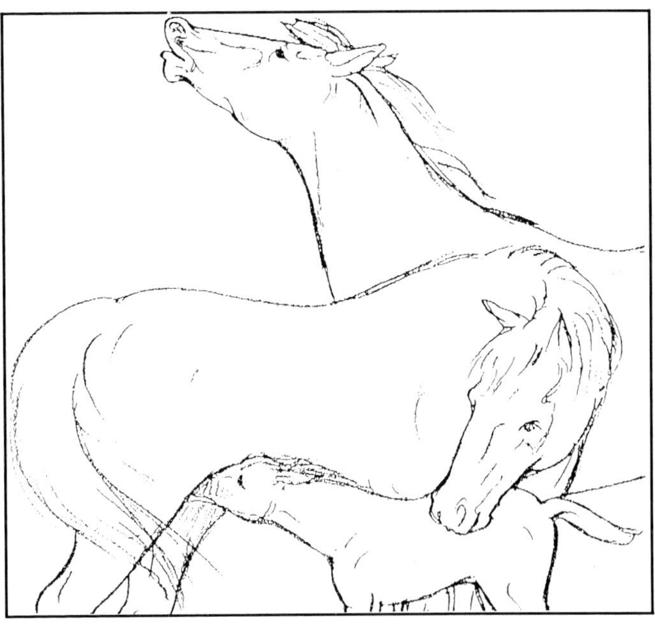

Testicular degeneration is a major cause of infertility and subfertility in stallions. Despite the variable nature of insults to the testis, responses of the seminiferous epithelium appear similar histologically, varying only according to severity of the condition. Thus testicular degeneration can be slight to severe. Gross anatomic and histologic appearance, as well as seminal characteristics, are similar to those seen in stallions with testicular hypoplasia, and the two conditions can only be clinically differentiated if evidence shows that testicular size and function were once normal.[1]

Testicular degeneration is strictly an acquired condition as opposed to testicular hypoplasia, which can be congenital or acquired. Hypoplastic testes, however, have an increased susceptibility to degenerative changes.[2,3] The condition can be unilateral or bilateral, depending on whether the causative factor is localized, as with an invading tumor, or generalized, as with a fever associated with systemic illness.[4] The condition can be temporary or permanent, depending on the severity and duration of injury. Late-generation spermatogonia, spermatocytes, and spermatids are more susceptible to injury than are mature spermatozoa or early-generation spermatogonia. Though the germinal epithelium is quite susceptible to injury, the degeneration created is often temporary, because of the resistant nature of the stem-cell spermatogonia and Sertoli and Leydig cells. The comparatively more resistant nature of those cells may permit restoration of normal spermatogenic function once the insult to the testis is removed.[1]

CAUSES OF TESTICULAR DEGENERATION

Testicular degeneration has a multitude of causes, of which thermal injury is common. Maintenance of the testes at a temperature lower than normal body temperature is necessary for normal spermatogenic function in stallions. Testicular degeneration associated with thermal factors may follow elevation of body temperature from systemic infections; prolonged increase in ambient temperature; scrotal insulation from edema, dermatitis, or hemorrhage;[1,4] or possible conformation factors, resulting in an incompetent heat exchange system.[5]

Injury to essential vasculature may precipitate testicular degeneration. Strongyle larvae, viruses (e.g., equine arteritis virus), and other unknown agents may produce inflammation of the testicular artery, resulting in areas of testicular degeneration.[4] Occlusion of testicular vasculature may occur with torsion of the spermatic cord, resulting in degeneration and necrosis of dependent structures.[6] Varicocele of the spermatic vein occurs sometimes in stallions and may interfere with thermal regulation.[2]

Systemic and/or local infections often produce testicular degeneration, though the relative damage produced by thermal versus toxic effects is poorly understood. Infectious or traumatic orchitis may progress to permanent degenerative atrophy.

Malnutrition, ingestion of toxic plants, testicular tumors, efferent/epididymal duct obstruction, production of antisperm antibodies or intratesticular hemorrhage can also lead to testicular degeneration.

Age-related testicular degeneration has been documented in other species and may also occur in stallions. Gradually developing degenerative vascular lesions within the testis have been postulated to be a cause of senile changes in testicular parenchyma.

Certain chemicals, heavy metals, rare earth salts, and ionizing radiation are capable of inducing testicular degeneration by a variety of mechanisms, including induction of vascular damage (e.g., cadmium chloride), reduction of amino acid uptake by spermatogonia (e.g., organomercurial), destruction of spermatogonia (e.g., busulfan and ionizing radiation), destruction of spermatocytes or spermatids (e.g., nitrofuran), and damage to Sertoli cells (e.g., o-pthalic acid).[1,4] Administration of steroid hormones may induce testicular degeneration by inhibiting production of gonadotropins.[7,8] The effects of most drugs and chemicals on spermatogenic function are largely unexplored and they should be used as if they are potentially toxic to the seminiferous epithelium.

DIAGNOSIS

Diagnosis of testicular degeneration is based on physical examination and semen evaluation. Without an accompanying history of normal testis size, texture, and function at some time before atrophy, differentiation from hypoplasia is usually not possible. If an identifying cause is noted, such as adhesions of the testicular tunics, the acquired nature of degeneration can be confirmed. Discrepancies between testicular size, measured by calipers or ultrasound examination, and daily spermatozoal output may suggest the diagnosis of testicular degeneration.[9] Testes with only mild degenerative changes may be of normal size or slightly small, with a slightly turgid or soft consistency. Marked reduction in testicular size is associated with severe degenerative changes. Proportional displacement of testicular parenchyma with connective tissue results in a firm consistency. As testicular parenchymal volume decreases, the tunica albuginea sometimes becomes palpably wrinkled. With advanced degeneration and diminished testicular size, the epididymis feels more prominent and may seem disproportionately large. Some clinicians use the relative size of the epididymis as an indication of whether the associated testis was once of normal size and function, because the epididymides tend not to be as well developed in animals with testicular hypoplasia. Depending on the extent and number of seminiferous tubules affected with degeneration, ejaculates will contain a low concentration of spermatozoa, often with a high percentage of morphologic defects (Figs. 92–1 and 92–2). Experimentally elevating the scrotal temperature of stallions ~2° to 3° C for 24 or 48 h results in an increase in spermatozoal morphologic abnormalities and a corresponding decrease in spermatozoal motility, concentration and number in ejaculates.[10] Deterioration in semen quality is most apparent 10 to 40 days following elevation of scrotal temperature. Return of semen quality to pretreatment values occurs by 54 to 80 days

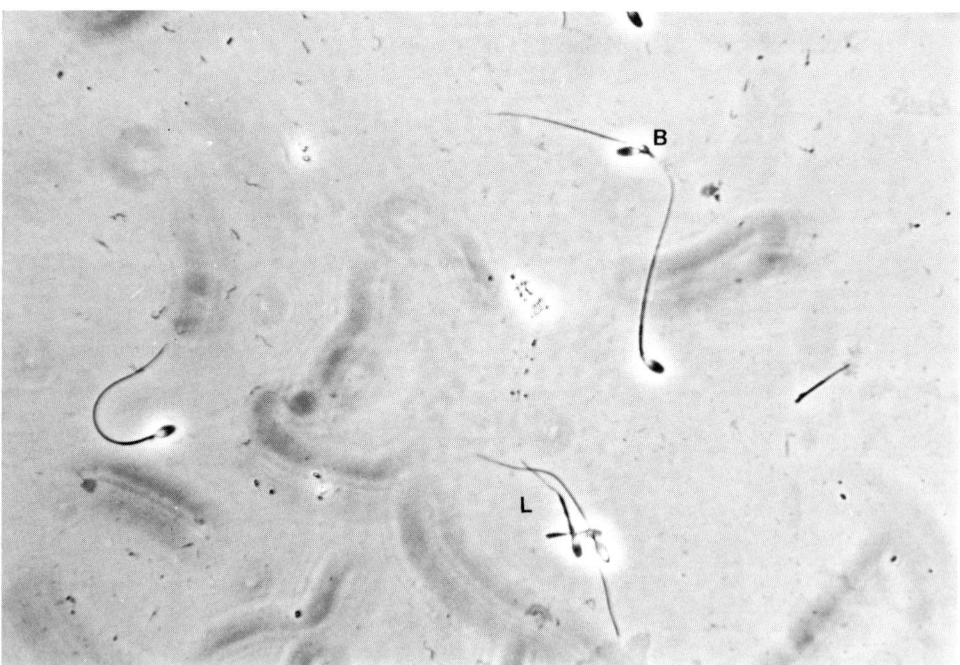

FIG. 92–1. Phase contrast photomicrograph of spermatozoa from a stallion with testicular degeneration resulting from traumatically induced bilateral hematocele. Seminal sample was collected approximately 1 month after injury. Spermatozoal defects include bent midpiece (B) and looped, irregular midpiece (L).

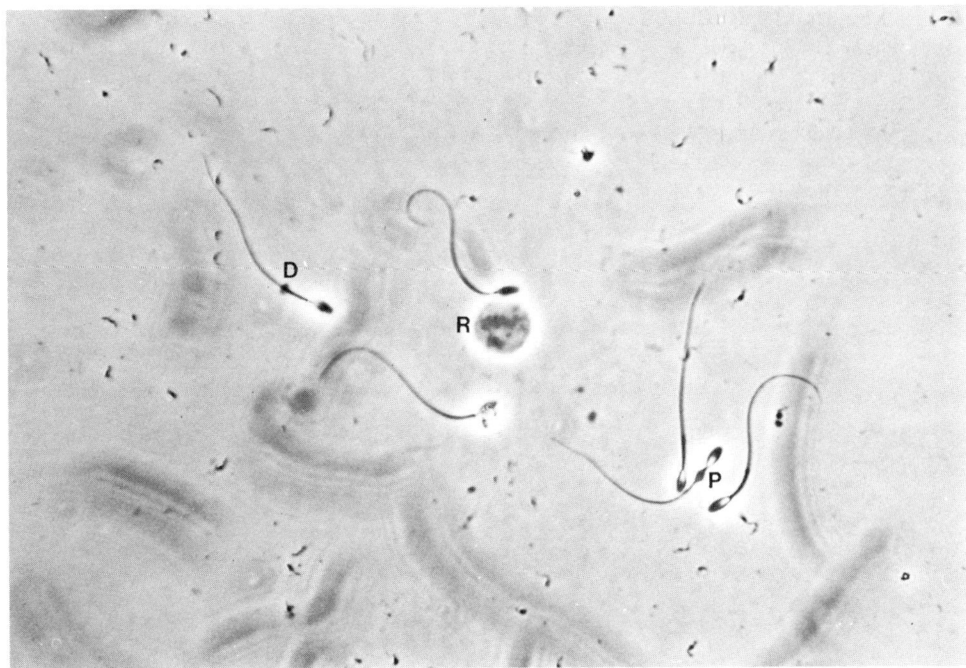

FIG. 92–2. Phase contrast photomicrograph of spermatozoa from semen of stallion illustrated in Figure 92–1. Spermatozoal defects include distal droplet (D), proximal droplet (P), and round spermatogenic cell (R).

following thermal injury. In severe testicular degeneration, azoospermia may occur. Round spermatogenic cells of varying sizes appear (Fig. 92–2) along with giant and medusa cells in the ejaculate. Multinucleated giant cells may be present as a result of incomplete cytoplasmic divisions in spite of nuclear division.[1,2,4]

Testicular biopsy may provide evidence of degeneration, but is not widely used in the horse and is not without risk[11] (see Chapter 104 for details). To obtain sufficient testicular parenchyma for adequate histologic evaluation, open surgical techniques are preferred to obtain biopsies. Excision of this amount of parenchyma from stallion testes often results in considerable hemorrhage, attendant pressure degeneration and necrosis (R.M. Kenney, personal communication). Decrease in sperm counts and formation of antisperm antibodies are among the reported complications in men.[12] Interest in obtaining testicular tissue from stallions for histologic evaluation has resulted in the recent resurgence of the use of aspiration cytology or needle biopsies.[13] While these techniques may seem more appealing, they are discouraged in men, because results obtained may not be representative and testicular damage may still occur.[12] The authors believe that further research is required before widespread use of testicular biopsy can be recommended for stallions.

Histologic evidence of testicular degeneration (Fig. 92–3) includes cytoplasmic vacuolation, germinal-cell desquamation, decreased thickness of the seminiferous epithelium, decreased cross-sectional diameter of the seminiferous tubules, pyknosis of spermatocyte nuclei, intratubular giant cell formation, spermiostasis, mineralization of inspissated tubular elements, diminished tubule size, fibrosis, and apparent interstitial-cell hyperplasia.[1,4] Leydig cell atrophy occurs in some cases of androgen induced degeneration.[8] Hyaline thickening of the basement membrane may be wave-like as a result of buckling following the collapse of the seminiferous tubules. With prolonged testicular insult, the only remaining cells may be the Sertoli cells which are more resistant to injury.[1]

TREATMENT

While testicular degeneration may be reversible, once it has occurred, treatment is usually of no benefit. Inciting causes that contribute to degeneration should be corrected. The cause of febrile conditions, such as systemic illness, requires diagnosis and rapid resolution to minimize the degree of, if not the potential for, degeneration. Antipyretics may be of use in this respect. With preputial and scrotal injuries, immediate antiphlogistic and anti-inflammatory therapy may speed resolution of local swelling and inflammation, facilitating an earlier return to normal spermatozoal production and concurrent improvement in semen quality. With scrotal injury and resultant increase in scrotal temperature, azoospermia may occur within 1 to 2 weeks, with a gradual return of semen quality over a few months. Spermatozoal numbers may not return to preinjury levels in the ejac-

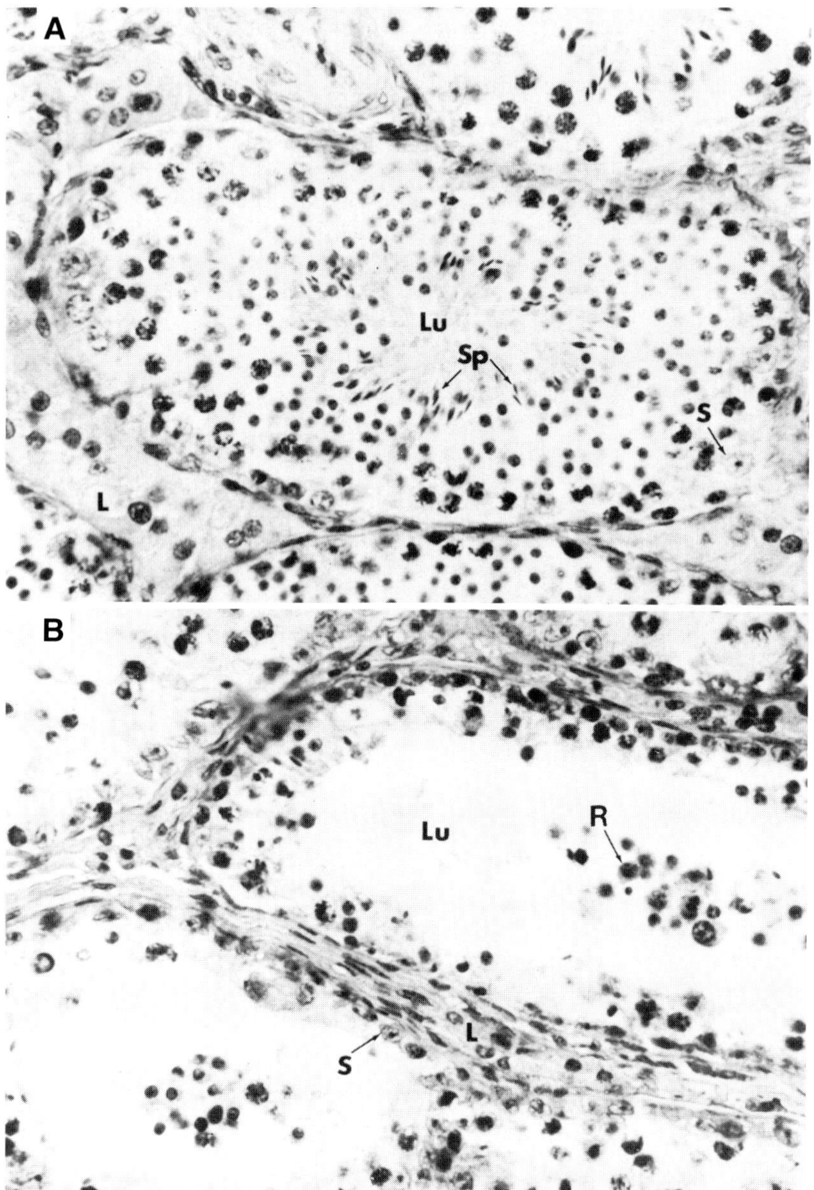

FIG. 92–3. *A,* Histologic section taken from the testis of a pony stallion with normal spermatogenesis (× 385). Daily spermatozoal production per gram of testicular parenchyma was 14.5×10^6. L, Leydig cells; Lu, lumen of seminiferous tubule with elongating spermatids (Sp); S, Sertoli cells on the basement membrane. *B,* Histologic section taken from the testis of a pony stallion with reduced spermatozoal production (× 385). Testicular degeneration was induced by administration of an anabolic steroid. Daily spermatozoal production per gram of testicular parenchyma was 0.3×10^6. Few Leydig cells (L) are present. Lu, lumen of seminiferous tubule with few elongating spermatids; R, round spermatogenic cells present in the lumen. (Photos by D.A. Kinden.)

ulate for 4 to 5 months after injury if scrotal thickening from edema is protracted (Fig. 92–4).

If permanent damage results and atrophy and fibrosis occur in a testis, the uninjured testis may hypertrophy and produce an increased number of spermatozoa. Spermatozoal numbers per ejaculate then usually plateau at a level somewhat below the number produced when the horse had two normal scrotal testes. Whether a permanently injured testis should be surgically removed is a matter of debate. Support for this approach stems from possible antibody production against an injured testis which could eventually interfere with function of the remaining uninjured testis. Studies in men with unilateral testicular torsion suggest that when surgical correction is delayed more than 8 h, spermatogenesis in the contralateral testis is frequently adversely affected, sometimes permanently.[14] The detrimental effect is thought to be caused, in part, by a breakdown in

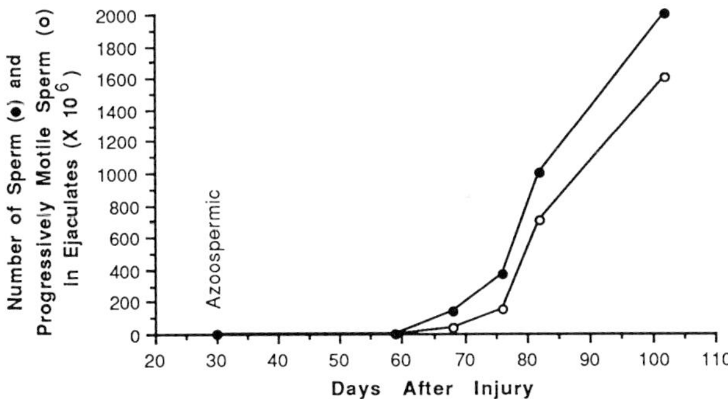

FIG. 92–4. Reappearance of spermatozoa and progressively motile spermatozoa in ejaculates of a stallion with transient testicular degeneration induced by traumatic preputial and scrotal edema.

the blood-testis barrier. Spermatozoa are liberated, resulting in production of antispermatozoal antibodies.[15] However, we have observed a number of fertile stallions that ejaculate semen of acceptable quality in spite of having traumatically induced unilateral testicular atrophy.

Investigation of hormone concentrations in subfertile stallions has demonstrated that serum gonadotropin concentrations, while often within normal limits, are sometimes abnormally low or high.[16] Such findings have stimulated an interest in gonadotropin replacement therapy, including the use of gonadotropin-releasing hormone (GnRH). This treatment is likely to be of most benefit in cases of hypogonadotropic-hypogonadism (i.e., suboptimal testicular function associated with low concentrations of circulating gonadotropins) (R.H. Douglas, personal communication). Aged stallions with high serum follicle-stimulating hormone (FSH) concentrations, which is thought to be associated with seminiferous epithelial damage, are probably less likely to respond to treatment with GnRH. In men, replacement therapy with GnRH is only effective when both the pituitary and gonads are functional.[17] In addition, dose and frequency of administration must mimic physiologic pulsatile release characteristics to avoid desensitizing the human pituitary to the GnRH.[17] Few controlled studies have been made to evaluate effectiveness of this therapy in stallions. Pulsatile administration of GnRH subcutaneously every 30 min for 5 days consistently increased plasma concentrations of LH, FSH, and testosterone in normal stallions treated during the winter, yet treatment actually decreased the total amount of LH released per pulse.[18] Responses achieved by treating the same stallions during the summer were more variable, with exogenous GnRH failing to elevate consistently plasma gonadotropin and testosterone concentrations. Pulsatile or constant administration of GnRH for 20 weeks did not significantly elevate secretion of testosterone, enhance growth of testes or alter spermatozoal output in reproductively sound or unsound stallions;[19] however, considerable variation in testosterone response occurred among reproductively unsound stallions. For a stallion to respond to treatment with GnRH with an improvement in fertility, it must first have a deficiency in GnRH synthesis or release while the pituitary-testicular axis remains functional. Further research in this area is indicated to determine optimal diagnostic and therapeutic strategies for gonadotropin replacement in stallions.

Effective management of stallions with testicular degeneration that are producing low numbers of progressively motile, morphologically normal spermatozoa is predicated on limiting the mare book sufficiently to maintain an optimal number of normal motile spermatozoa per breeding. Breeding only those mares near ovulation and use of a suitable semen extender in an artificial breeding program may improve pregnancy rates.

REFERENCES

1. Ladds, P.W.: The male genital system. *In* Pathology of Domestic Animals. 3rd ed. Edited by K.V.F. Jubb and P.C. Kennedy. New York, Academic Press, 1985, pp. 428–432.
2. Roberts, S.J.: Veterinary Obstetrics and Genital Diseases. 3rd ed. North Pomfret, VT, published by the authors, 1986.
3. Veeramachaneni, D.N.R., et al.: Pathophysiology of small testes in beef bulls: Relationship between scrotal circumference, histologic features of testes and epididymides, seminal characteristics, and endocrine profiles. Am. J. Vet. Res., *47:*1988–1999, 1986.
4. McEntee, K.: The male genital system. *In* Pathology of Domestic Animals. 2nd ed. Edited by K.V.F. Jubb and P.C. Kennedy. New York, Academic Press, 1970, pp. 450–454.
5. Rossdale, S.D., and Ricketts, S.W.: Equine Stud Farm Medicine. 2nd ed. Philadelphia, Lea & Febiger, 1980.
6. Threlfall, W.R., et al.: Recurrent torsion of the spermatic cord and scrotal testis in a stallion. J. Am. Vet. Med. Assoc., *196:*1641–1643, 1990.
7. Squires, E.L., Todter, G.E., Berndtson, W.E., and Pickett, B.W.: Effect of anabolic steroids on reproductive function of young stallions. J. Anim. Sci., *54:*576–582, 1982.
8. Garcia, M.C., et al.: The effects of stanozolol and boldenone undecylenate on plasma testosterone and gonadotropins and on testis histology in pony stallions. Theriogenology, *28:*109–119, 1987.
9. Thompson, D.L., Jr., Pickett, B.W., Squires, E.L., and Amann, R.P.: Testicular measurements and reproductive characteristics in stallions. J. Reprod. Fertil. Suppl., *27:*13–17, 1979.
10. Friedman, R., et al.: The effects of increased testicular temperature on spermatogenesis in the stallion. J. Reprod. Fertil. Suppl., *44:*127–134, 1991.
11. Smith, J.A.: Biopsy and the testicular artery of the horse. Equine Vet. J., *6:*81–83, 1974.
12. Glezerman, M.: Testicular biopsy. *In* Disturbances in Male Fertility. Edited by K. Bandhauer and J. Frick. New York, Springer-Verlag, 1982, pp. 215–223.
13. Threlfall, W.R., and Lopate, C.: Testicular biopsy. Proceedings of the Annual Meeting of the Society of Theriogenology. 1987, pp. 65–73.

14. Bartsch, G., et al.: Testicular torsion: Late results with special regard to fertility and endocrine function. J. Urol., *124:*375–378, 1980.
15. Merimsky, E., et al.: Assessment of immunologic mechanism in infertility of the rat after experimental testicular torsion. Urol. Res., *12:*179–182, 1984.
16. Burns, P.J., and Douglas, R.H.: Reproductive hormone concentrations in stallions with breeding problems: Case studies. Equine Vet. Sci., *5:*40–42, 1985.
17. Spratt, D.I., Hoffman, A.R., and Crowley, W.F., Jr.: Hypogonadotropic hypogonadism and its treatment. *In* Male Reproductive Dysfunction: Diagnosis and Management of Hypogonadism, Infertility, and Impotence. Edited by R.J. Santen and R.S. Swerdloff. New York, Marcel Dekker, 1986, pp. 227–249.
18. Roser, J.F., and Hughes, J.P.: Prolonged pulsatile administration of gonadotrophin-releasing hormone (GnRH) to fertile stallions. J. Reprod. Fertil. Suppl., *44:*155–168, 1991.
19. Blue, B.G., et al.: Effect of pulsatile or continuous administration of GnRH on reproductive function of stallions. J. Reprod. Fertil. Suppl., *44:*145–154, 1991.

CHAPTER 93

SEMINAL VESICULITIS

D.D. Varner
T.S. Taylor
T.L. Blanchard

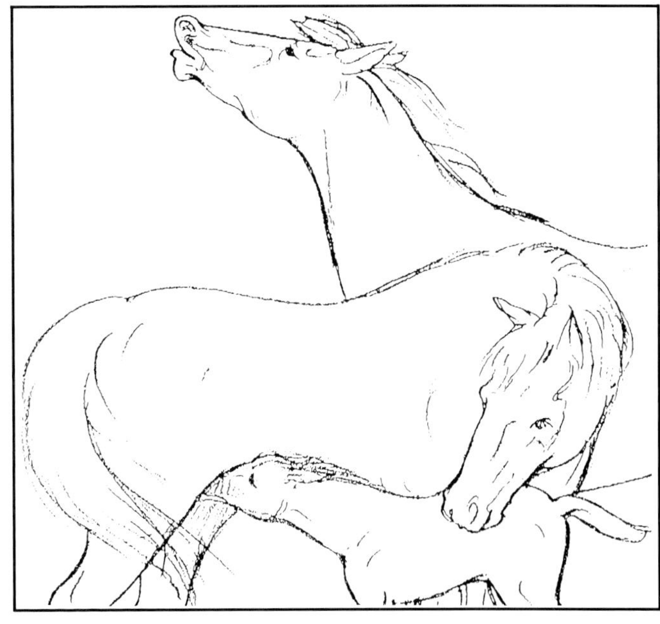

The stallion has four distinct accessory genital glands: (1) the paired seminal vesicles, or more appropriately, vesicular glands; (2) the paired ampullae, which surround the terminal segment of each deferent duct; (3) the bilobed prostate gland; (4) and the paired bulbourethral glands (see Chapter 76 for detailed description). The vesicular glands are slightly pyriform sacs which are situated on either side of bladder neck and extend craniolaterad into the posterior abdomen. These thin-walled elongated glands can reach 15 to 20 cm in length and 5 cm in diameter when their lumina are fully distended following sexual stimulation. Each vesicular gland lies just lateral to the ipsilateral ampulla. The base (or fundus) is covered by the genital fold, hence the vesicular glands are in a retroperitoneal position. Each gland cones into a singular excretory duct which communicates with the lumen of the proximal urethra via a protuberance on its dorsal surface, the seminal colliculus.[1]

The precise roles of accessory genital gland secretions remain unclear. Although the secretions contain a number of physiologically active substances, they are not essential to the fertilization process in man and domestic animals, except as a vehicle for spermatozoal transport to the uterus during coitus.[2,3]

INCIDENCE AND PATHOGENESIS

Seminal vesiculitis (also termed vesicular adenitis) is quite uncommon in stallions; however, it is a noteworthy disorder because of its persistent nature and interference with fertility. Reported etiologic agents include Pseudomonas aeruginosa, Klebsiella pneumoniae, Streptococcus spp., Staphylococcus spp., and Brucella abortus. Although mycoplasmata, ureaplasmata, chlamydia, protozoa, and viruses have been incriminated in seminal vesiculitis involving other animal species, these microorganisms have not been isolated from vesicular glands of affected horses. Noninfectious seminal vesiculitis has not been described in stallions.

The precise pathogenesis of seminal vesiculitis remains an enigma. Potential routes for infection of the vesicular glands include (1) ascent through the urethra, (2) descent from the upper genital or urinary tract, (3) lymphogenous or hematogenous spread, and (4) direct invasion from periglandular tissues.

CLINICAL FEATURES AND DIAGNOSIS

Characteristically, seminal vesiculitis in stallions is not manifested by overt clinical signs. In general, affected horses are afebrile and do not exhibit signs of pain at time of urination, defecation, or breeding. Presumptive diagnosis of seminal vesiculitis is usually made through gross and microscopic analysis of semen. Semen of stallions with seminal vesiculitis has varying quantities of neutrophils. It may be blood-tinged and contain numerous clumps of purulent material. Large numbers of bacteria may also be detectable microscopically. Spermatozoal quality is usually unaffected when observed immediately on ejaculation, but longevity of spermatozoal viability may be reduced.

Clinicians may have difficulty determining the site of inflammation if neutrophils are detected in semen, because they may arise from lesions involving the exterior of the penis, urethra, upper urinary tract, deferent ducts, epididymides, testes, or any of the accessory genital glands. An internal genital infection is suspected if no lesions are observed on the penile integument or urethral process.

A comparison of bacterial types and numbers recovered from the exterior of the penis, urethra, and semen can be used to help localize an infectious process. Culture swabs of the unwashed penis and preputial cavity are first obtained to determine the bacterial flora in these areas. The penis is then washed with a bactericidal soap, thoroughly rinsed and dried, in preparation for further cultures. Additional swabs are obtained from the distal urethra, both before and immediately after ejaculation, and semen. Semen is collected using an artificial vagina. The liner and semen receptacle of the artificial vagina should be sterilized before use to ensure that any microorganisms recovered are not contaminants from an improperly maintained artificial vagina. A heavy pure growth of bacteria in the postejaculate urethra and semen are consistent with an internal genital infection.

Culture and cytologic evaluation of expressed secretions of the vesicular glands aids in diagnosis of seminal vesiculitis. To fill the vesicular gland lumina with secretions, the stallion is first stimulated sexually (teased) for approximately 15 min by exposure to a mare in estrus. The distal penis is then washed, rinsed, and dried and a sterile 100-cm rubber catheter with an inflatable cuff is passed into the urethra until its tip is immediately caudal to the seminal colliculus (where the ducts of the vesicular glands enter the urethra). Proper placement of the catheter tip is aided by palpation per rectum. After the cuff is inflated, either vesicular gland is identified, and the contents removed by manual compression of the gland. Fluid is collected for culture and cytology, using a sterile container attached to the catheter opening at the urethral orifice.[4]

Palpation of the vesicular glands is usually not rewarding diagnostically in stallions with seminal vesiculitis. Typically, no changes are detected in size, shape, and consistency of affected glands, although they may occasionally be enlarged, firm, and lobulated. Pain may be elicited on palpation if the infection is accompanied by acute inflammatory changes.[5,6] Abscessation of vesicular glands is reported to occur rarely in stallions.[7] Such lesions may be detectable by palpation per rectum.

Transrectal ultrasonography has been used to evaluate the accessory genital glands of normal stallions; however, we found no reports in the literature regarding its use in the diagnosis of seminal vesiculitis.[8–10] The technique has been described for diagnosis of seminal vesiculitis in bulls.[9]

We have recently used a flexible endoscope for definitive diagnosis of seminal vesiculitis in two stallions. A small-diameter (7-mm) fiberoptic or video endoscope can be passed directly into the vesicular gland lumina, via the duct openings at the seminal colliculus. Care should be taken to prevent undue trauma to the duct openings when the endoscope is inserted into each vesicular gland. The gland lumina can be directly visualized and swabs and aspirates can be obtained for culture and cytology, respectively. Culture instruments or catheters designed for endoscopes can be passed into position via the biopsy channel for acquisition of samples.

TREATMENT

Treatment of seminal vesiculitis in stallions has generally consisted of systemic antibiotic therapy, with selection of antibiotics based on in vitro sensitivity patterns of the causative bacteria. This therapeutic approach is unlikely to be rewarding because most antibiotics are incapable of reaching therapeutic concentrations in the lumen of the accessory genital glands when administered parenterally.[11,12] Features of antibiotics which permit easy passage across the epithelial membranes of the accessory genital glands include (1) high lipid solubility, (2) low molecular size, (3) low binding affinity with plasma proteins, and (4) high pKa to increase the fraction of unionized antibiotic.[13] Unfortunately, most antibiotics do not possess these characteristics and thus are pharmacodynamically inappropriate for parenteral use. Studies in other species have revealed that trimethoprim passes readily into the prostate gland; hence, this may be the antibiotic of choice for parenteral therapy of bacterial-induced seminal vesiculitis in stallions, provided the causative bacteria is susceptible to trimethoprim.[13]

Antibiotics have been directly deposited into the vesicular glands of a stallion with seminal vesiculitis by passing a catheter via the urethra to the level of the seminal colliculus.[12] By manipulation of the catheter tip per rectum, efforts were made to direct the catheter blindly into each vesicular duct. When successful, antibiotics were directly infused into the glandular lumen. When attempts at duct cannulation were unsuccessful, the bladder orifice was occluded by the hand in the rectum and antibiotic was ejected from the preplaced catheter into the proximal urethra. Subsequently, transrectal ultrasonography was used to verify filling of the vesicular glands with antibiotic solution. However, seminal vesiculitis was not corrected in this stallion, after using this approach.[12]

A flexible endoscope was used for treatment of two stallions. Each vesicular gland was cannulated via its duct opening at the seminal colliculus by passing a catheter through the biopsy channel of an endoscope preplaced in the pelvic urethra so that the seminal colliculus could be easily visualized. The affected glands were first lavaged with large quantities of saline, then antibiotics (ticarcillin disodium or ampicillin sodium) were instilled directly into the gland lumina. This protocol was repeated for 5 consecutive days. In both instances, the seminal vesiculitis was resolved. Because other accessory genital glands may be infected concomitantly and are not amenable to this treatment approach, success may be limited to cases with involvement only of the vesicular glands.

Surgical removal of affected vesicular glands has been performed in bulls that did not respond favorably to medical therapy.[14,15] However, the surgical procedure is rather difficult, and several postoperative complications have been observed, including severe postsurgical hemorrhage, postoperative infection, and damage to the intrapelvic nerves, which subsequently prevented ejaculation.

Using a surgical technique that was developed for use in bulls, unilateral seminal vesiculectomy was reportedly successful when performed on a stallion with purulent seminal vesiculitis.[16] Seminal vesiculectomy when performed on reproductively normal stallions does not suppress spermatozoal motility and may actually improve this parameter.[16,17] The postsurgical complications described above for the bull are also applicable to the stallion.

We have modified the surgical procedure for seminal vesiculectomy in the stallion to permit improved surgical exposure. With the stallion standing in stocks, under sedation and caudal-epidural anesthesia, and appropriately draped, a midline incision is made along the caudal 8 to 10 cm of the rectal floor and perineal body. Tissues underneath the rectum are then dissected bluntly to the level of the seminal vesicles and the rectum is elevated to improve exposure of the surgical site. Accurate identification of the vesicular glands is dependent on prior catheterization and distention with fluid, using a flexible endoscope as described above. Once identified, vesicular glands are freed from the surrounding tissues by blunt and sharp dissection. Penetration of the genital fold and entry into the abdominal cavity are required. The freed vesicular glands are directed posteriorly, then ligated and transected near the duct opening into the pelvic urethra. During closure of the surgical site, the peritoneum (genital fold) is not repaired, but the other tissues are carefully apposed to prevent postsurgical infection. Lobes of the prostate gland and the bodies of the bulbourethral glands may also be removed by this surgical approach. The effects of removal of these glands on subsequent fertility of the stallion have not been investigated.

If seminal vesiculitis cannot be corrected in a stallion, the horse's breeding life may be extended by the use of minimum contamination breeding techniques (see Chapter 84). For artificial insemination programs, semen is placed in a seminal extender containing antibiotics to which the bacteria from the vesicular glands are susceptible. Samples of extended semen can be swabbed for bacterial culture after 15 to 30 min to ensure that all bacteria are eliminated. Mares are bred with the extended semen. For natural service programs, seminal extender (100 to 150 ml) can be instilled into the uterus immediately before breeding. These protocols have restored fertility of a stallion with seminal vesiculitis caused by Pseudomonas aeruginosa.[18]

REFERENCES

1. Nickel, R., Schummer, A., Seiferle, E., and Sack, W.O.: The Viscera of the Domestic Mammals. New York, Springer-Verlag, 1973.
2. Mann, T., and Lutwak-Mann, C.: Male Reproductive Function and Semen. New York, Springer-Verlag, 1981.
3. Posakoski, K.L., and Kopta, M.: Seminal plasma. *In* Biochemistry of Mammalian Reproduction. Edited by L.J.D. Zaneveld and R.T. Chatterton. New York, John Wiley & Sons, 1982, pp. 89–115.
4. Cooper, W.C.: Methods of determining the site of bacterial infections in the stallion reproductive tract. Proceedings of the Society of Theriogenology, 1–4, 1979.
5. Neely, D.P.: Physical examination and genital diseases of the stallion. *In* Current Therapy in Theriogenology. Edited by D.A. Morrow. Philadelphia, W.B. Saunders, 1980, pp. 694–706.
6. Hurtgen, J.P.: Stallion genital abnormalities. *In* Current Therapy in Equine Medicine 2. Edited by N.E. Robinson. Philadelphia, W.B. Saunders, 1987, pp. 558–562.
7. Ladds, P.W.: The male genital system. *In* Pathology of Domestic Animals. 3rd ed. Edited by K.V.F. Jubb and P.C. Kennedy. New York, Academic Press, 1985, pp. 409–459.
8. Little, T.V., and Woods, G.L.: Ultrasonography of accessory sex glands in the stallion. J. Reprod. Fertil. Suppl., *35:*87–94, 1987.
9. Weber, J.A., and Woods, G.L.: Ultrasonographic studies of accessory sex glands in sexually rested stallions and bulls, sexually active stallions, and a diseased bull. Proceedings of the Society of Theriogenology, 157–165, 1989.
10. Weber, J.A., Geary, R.T., and Woods, G.L.: Changes in accessory sex glands of stallions after sexual preparation and ejaculation. J. Am. Vet. Med. Assoc., *196:*1085–1089, 1990.
11. Blanchard, T.L., et al.: Bilateral seminal vesiculitis and ampullitis in a stallion. J. Am. Vet. Med. Assoc., *192:*525–526, 1988.
12. Strzemienski, P.J., Benson, C.E., Blanchard, T.L., and Love, C.C.: Failure of gentamicin sulfate to enter stallion accessory fluids. Proceedings of the International Congress of Equine Infectious Diseases. 1987.
13. Meares, E.M.: Prostatitis and related disorders. *In* Campbell's Urology. 5th ed. Edited by P.C. Walsh, R.S. Gittes, A.D. Perlnutter, and T.A. Stamey. Philadelphia, W.B. Saunders, 1986, pp. 868–887.
14. Dargatz, D.A., Mortimer, R.G., and Ball, L.: Vesicular adenitis of bulls: A review. Theriogenology, *28:*513–521, 1987.
15. Linhart, R.D., and Parker, W.G.: Seminal vesiculitis in bulls. Compend. Contin. Educ. Practicing Vet., *10:*1428–1432, 1988.
16. Klug, E., et al.: The effect of vesiculectomy on seminal characteristics in the stallions. J. Reprod. Fertil. Suppl., *27:*61–66, 1979.
17. Webb, R.B.: Effects of vesiculectomy and bulbourethralectomy on stallion spermatozoa. M.S. thesis. Texas A&M University, 1988.
18. Blanchard, T.L., et al.: Use of a semen extender containing antibiotic to improve the fertility of a stallion with seminal vesiculitis due to Pseudomonas aeruginosa. Theriogenology, *28:*541–546, 1987.

CHAPTER 94

HEMOSPERMIA AND UROSPERMIA

J.L. Voss
A.O. McKinnon

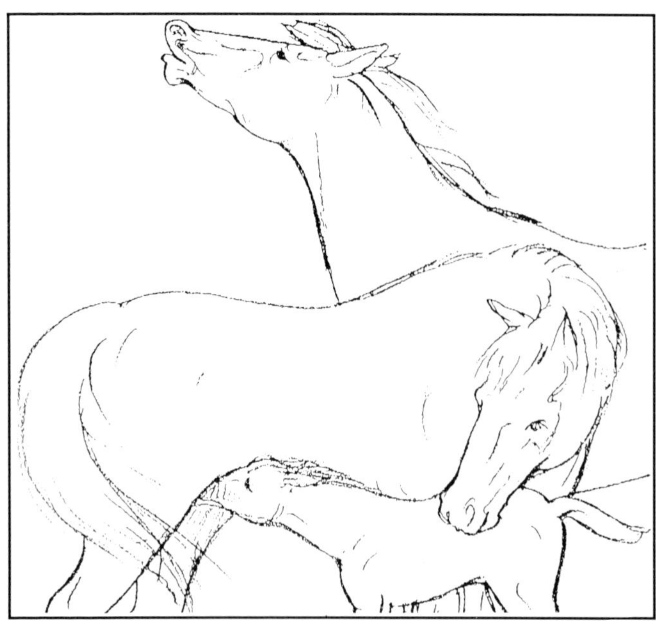

Abnormal ejaculations caused by hemospermia and urospermia (urination during ejaculation) are uncommon but can be highly detrimental to breeding efficiency. Stallions that have overt hemorrhage in each ejaculate are usually infertile.[1–3] In affected stallions, hemospermia may be seen occasionally or be present in each ejaculate. When hemospermia occurs as an isolated event, fertility is affected in that ejaculate only. Urospermia usually occurs sporadically and is generally noted in about 30 to 40% of ejaculates from affected stallions.

Blood-containing ejaculates are easily detected by their pink to reddish color. Less obvious contamination can be detected by microscopic evaluation. Semen containing a small amount of blood may be compatible with fertility, especially if the semen is diluted immediately with a seminal extender. In natural service, seminal extender placed in the uterus before breeding may help prevent adverse effects on fertility. Affected stallions often have a history of a high frequency of ejaculation. Thus, the condition is most often seen in heavily booked horses whose owners do not or cannot utilize artificial insemination. Affected stallions frequently require several mounts to ejaculate and often exhibit pain on ejaculation. Occasionally in natural service, it may be difficult to determine whether the blood is originating from the stallion or mare. Diagnosis of hemospermia is simplified when semen is collected with an artificial vagina.

Urine is infrequently observed in ejaculates from most species from which semen is routinely collected. Urine has adverse effects on spermatozoal motility and fertility. The concentration of urine required to affect seminal quality is unknown but is presumed to be quite low. The reason for urination during ejaculation is unknown. Although contamination of an ejaculate with urine is uncommon, it can be a perplexing disorder. Affected stallions usually have normal libido and sexual behavior and in only a few cases will urospermia be seen at each ejaculation. In one report involving only three stallions, each experienced urospermia during ejaculation approximately 30% of the time.[4] Because of the tendency for stallions to ejaculate urine in their semen only sporadically, treatment models are difficult to evaluate and often inconclusive.

HEMOSPERMIA

The effects of hemospermia in a breeding program are devastating, and stallions with overt hemorrhage into each ejaculate are considered infertile or highly subfertile. The mechanism of how blood in an ejaculate renders spermatozoa infertile is unknown. Spermatozoal motility, morphology and number of spermatozoa per ejaculate are generally unaffected. Voss et al. reported that erythrocytes rather than serum appear to be responsible for the marked disruption in fertility.[2] In their experiment, 24 nonlactating, clinically normal mares of mixed breeds were artificially inseminated every other day beginning on day 2 or 3 of estrus with 500 million

TABLE 94–1. PREGNANCY RATES OF MARES INSEMINATED WITH RAW SEMEN OR SEMEN CONTAINING 20% SERUM OR 20% WHOLE BLOOD

	TREATMENT					
	Raw Semen		Serum		Whole Blood	
Cycle	Mares	Percent	Mares	Percent	Mares	Percent
1	8 (1)*	12.5	8 (2)	25.0	8 (1)	12.5
2	6†(3)	50.0	6 (5)	83.3	5‡(0)	0.0
Total pregnant		57.1		87.5		12.5

*Numbers in parentheses are the number of mares that became pregnant.
†One mare died.
‡Two mares never returned to estrus.
(From Voss, J.L., Pickett, B.W., and Shideler, R.K.: The effect of hemospermia on fertility in horses. Proceedings of the Eighth International Congress on Animal Reproduction and Artificial Insemination. Vol. 4. Krakow, 1976, pp. 1093–1095.)

progressively motile spermatozoa from one stallion. Mares were randomly divided into three groups: (1) mares (controls) inseminated with raw semen, (2) mares inseminated with raw semen plus 20% serum from the stallion, and (3) mares inseminated with raw semen plus 20% whole blood from the stallion. All mares were inseminated within 1 h of seminal collection. Serum was collected from the stallion by harvesting jugular blood 2 to 3 h before seminal collection and allowing it to clot for 30 min and then separating the serum by centrifugation. Whole blood for inclusion in the inseminate was obtained from the stallion by jugular venipuncture immediately after seminal collection. The volume of whole blood or serum was calculated as a percentage (20%) of the insemination volume. Fertility results are presented in Tables 94–1 and 2. A total of 7 of 8 mares became pregnant when inseminated with semen containing 20% serum whereas only 1 of 8 (12.5%) became pregnant when inseminated with semen containing 20% whole blood. Consequently, they concluded that infertility associated with hemospermia appeared to be caused by the presence of the red blood cells.

TABLE 94–2. REPRODUCTIVE PERFORMANCE OF MARES INSEMINATED WITH RAW SEMEN OR SEMEN CONTAINING 20% SERUM OR 20% WHOLE BLOOD

	TREATMENT		
Variables	Raw Semen	Serum	Whole Blood
Number of mares	8	8	8
Number pregnant	4	7	1
Number of mare cycles	15	14	13
Pregnant/cycle (%)	28.6	50.0	7.7

(Adapted from Voss, J.L., Pickett, B.W., Shideler, R.K.: The effect of hemospermia on fertility in horses. Proceedings of the Eighth International Congress on Animal Reproduction and Artificial Insemination. Vol. 4. Krakow, 1976, pp. 1093–1095.)

ETIOLOGY

Causes of hemospermia are variable and the condition occurs in all breeds. In a survey of 18 cases, stallions averaged 7.1 yr of age at onset of signs (with a range of 3 to 18 yrs).[5] The average number of successful breeding seasons before onset of clinical signs was 3.7 yr (ranging from 0 to 13 yr).

One of the most common causes of hemospermia is association with bacterial urethritis. The most commonly isolated bacteria have been Streptococcus spp., E. coli, and Pseudomonas aeuroginosa.[5] The pelvic urethra from the ischial arch to the colliculus seminalis appears to be more commonly affected than the penile urethra. Dilation and trauma to the inflamed epithelial lining of the urethra associated with erection and muscular contractions of ejaculation are most likely responsible for hemospermia. Other specific causes of hemospermia include lacerations on the exterior penis, cutaneous habronemiasis of the urethral process or glans penis, and urethral lacerations. Damage to the urethra from continual pressure of a stallion ring can result in scar tissue strictures. Increased urethral pressure during urination or erection while the stallion ring is in place can apparently cause splitting of the epithelium and protrusion of underlining blood vessels (Fig. 94–1). A stallion ring is generally used to prevent masturbation. Because of the association with penile damage and hemospermia, it is not recommended. Infrequent masturbation without ejaculation appears to be normal behavior. Even if a stallion masturbates, he is not likely to deplete his extragonadal spermatozoal reserves.[3]

When the penis becomes erect, the urethral process becomes engorged with blood and can protrude beyond the glans penis. It can be easily lacerated by tail hairs during intromission and is one reason the mare's tail should be wrapped during breeding or seminal collection. Lacerations on the urethral process can become infected from bacterial contamination and form ulcerative lesions (Fig. 94–2) which bleed profusely during ejaculation. Continued irritation may result in calcifica-

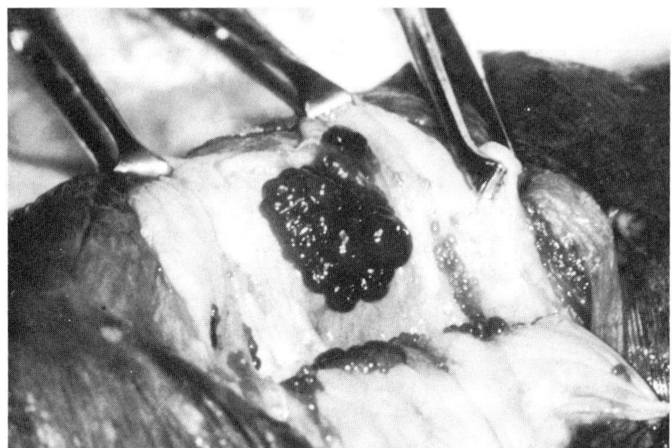

FIG. 94–1. Protrusion of blood vessels into the urethra, which was believed to be caused from a stallion ring. Constriction of urethra and contractions during urination and ejaculation cause splitting of mucosa with prolapse of underlying vessels.

tion and even varicosities of the urethral process. Habronemiasis of the urethral process is also a potential cause of hemospermia. This condition is caused by invasion of a wound by stomach worm larvae (Habronema spp.) that are transmitted by flies. Involved tissues become swollen, irritated, and friable and can split easily during ejaculation (Fig. 94–3). This condition is usually seen during the warmer months because of association with the fly season. Without early treatment, the lesions may become chronic, mineralized, and require surgical removal.

Viral urethritis has also been suspected as a cause of hemospermia.[6] Urethritis characterized by an inflammation typical of viral infection was observed in a Thoroughbred stallion with a history of no sexual experience. This stallion hemorrhaged from the urethra at each seminal collection. Upon visual examination of the urethra, it was observed that the epithelium covering the small vesicles had sloughed and coalesced, resulting in ulcerations. Cells with inclusion bodies indicative of a viral infection were observed in cells from urethral smears although attempts to culture a virus from the urethra were unsuccessful.

Infection or inflammation of the accessory sex glands can be associated with hemospermia.[7] Seminal vesiculitis, although uncommon, has also been observed in stallions with hemospermia.[7,8] The advent of ultrasonography as a diagnostic aid has added a dimension of new diagnostic capabilities for evaluating accessory sex glands in the stallion. With time, this technology will allow researchers to provide meaningful information on problems associated with these organs.

Small quantities of blood can be observed in the gel fraction of semen after collection in an artificial vagina. In one instance at our laboratory, this was apparently associated with a larvae of Strongylus endenatus migrating through the vesicular glands and producing sporadic irritation.[9]

Lacerations and penetrating wounds to the glans penis may result in hemorrhage during erection and ejaculation as a result of increased vascular pressure and enlargement of the glans. A breeding stitch of inflexible material (vetifill or monofilament nylon) apparently caused penetrating wounds to the glans penis in a stallion on pasture (Fig. 94–4).

Presently unrecognized causes of hemospermia may exist in the horse. In man, some reported causes of hemospermia are varicosities in the pelvic urethra, hypertension, prostatitis, vesiculitis, tuberculosis, urethritis, seminal calculi, neoplasia, and trauma.[10–13]

DIAGNOSIS

Diagnosis of hemospermia is easy when semen is collected with an artificial vagina. The first step in evaluation of hemospermia is external examination of the stallion's penis and urethral process for signs of trauma, irritation, proliferations, and abnormalities. The examination is best performed while washing the stallion's penis. Direct visual examination of the stallion's urethra with a fiberoptic endoscope is often useful in identifying causes of hemospermia. The procedure should be performed while the stallion is standing and tranquilized. Promazine tranquilizers are contraindicated because of occasional development of priapism, or penile paralysis. Air is used to dilate the urethra and when necessary, saline can be infused to permit a clear view of the entire lumen. Conditions such as urethritis, strictures, growths, ulcers, fissures, and prolapsed subepithelial vessels can be observed. In addition, the neck of the bladder, opening of the deferent ducts, and colliculus seminalis can be visualized. When vesiculitis is sus-

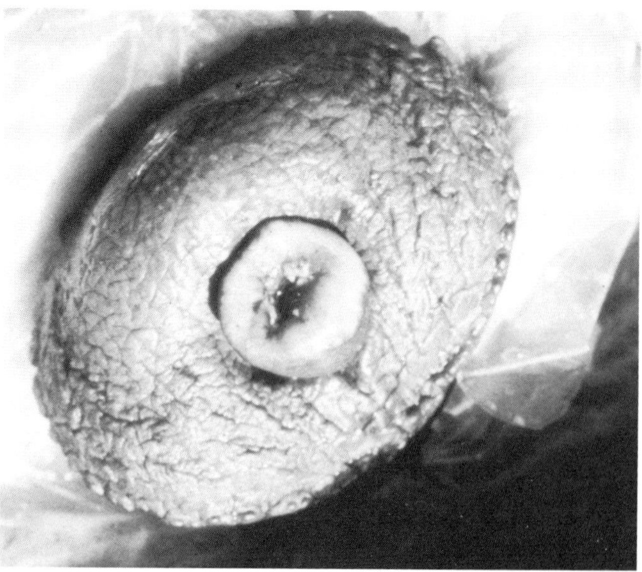

FIG. 94–2. Lesions on the urethral process caused by lacerations by hairs from the mare's tail are frequently invaded by bacteria and hemorrhage easily.

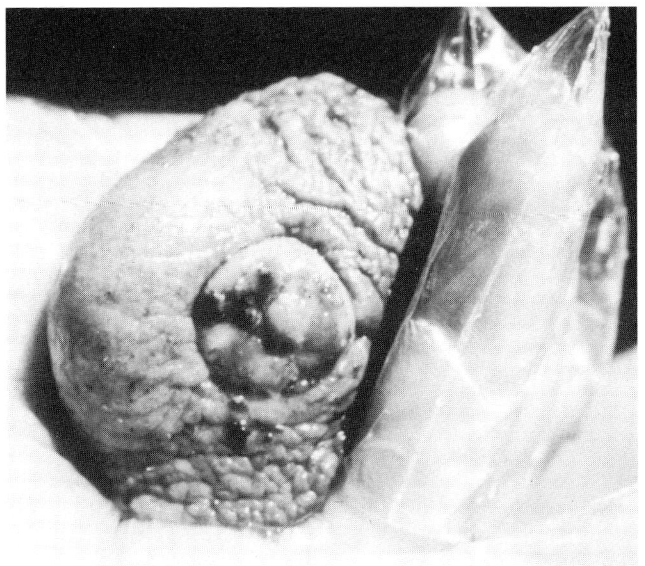

FIG. 94–3. Habronemiasis of the urethral process.

pected, the ejaculatory ducts and fluid extruded from the accessory sex glands should be observed while individually massaging each gland per rectum. Observed lesions can be biopsied with small forceps passed through the fiberoptic endoscope.

Radiographic examination of the urethra may also be a valuable procedure for diagnosing urethral disorders. Six ounces (180 mL) of a suspension of barium sulfate are injected into the urethra, and a radiographic plate is exposed. The barium is allowed to drain from the urethra and air infused and another plate exposed to provide a double-contrast effect. The testis should be shielded from the x-ray beam. This technique allows strictures, space-occupying lesions, ulcerations, pseudomembranous urethritis, fistulas, and vessels prolapsing into the lumen of the urethra to be visualized (Figs. 94–5 and 94–6).

Exfoliative examination of cells can also be used to diagnose a stallion with hemospermia. Cells are collected immediately after ejaculation from the distal urethra with a plastic, disposable spatula. The cells are spread onto a glass slide and fixed immediately with a suitable fixative (Spray—Cite, Primary Care Diagnostics, Powson, MD). Viral inclusion bodies, neoplastic cells, and other abnormal cells may be identified with this technique. Ultrasonography also can be used to evaluate accessory sex glands, blood-filled seminal vesicles, neoplasia, and other lesions.

TREATMENT

Many traumatic lesions to the glans penis will heal spontaneously with sexual rest. Cleansing with water and applying chemotherapeutic agents may prevent infection and aid healing. Also, cases of urethritis may heal following 2 to 4 weeks of sexual rest. During the period of sexual rest, broad-spectrum antibiotics as dictated by culture and sensitivity results can be administered. After sexual rest, endoscopic examination of the urethra should be performed before seminal collection with an artificial vagina and before the stallion is returned to a heavy breeding schedule. Hemospermia caused by urethral strictures, prolapsed subepithelial vessels, neoplasia, habronemiasis, or lesions on the urethral process, may be corrected with surgery.

Treatment with formalin intravenously has been reported but the problem recurred when treatment was withdrawn.[6] This treatment should be used only as a last resort. Drugs that acidify and sterilize the urine also have been used as treatment for hemospermia. Urinary acidifiers can be given alone or in combination with antibiotics. To acidify the urine, 60 to 100 g ammonium chloride must be ingested daily. The drug can be given for as long as necessary. Ammonium chloride alone was used successfully for treatment of hemospermia in six stallions.[6] Methenamine, a urinary disinfectant, also has been advocated for treatment of hemospermia.[6] To be effective, the drug must be absorbed through the lining of the small intestine. These forms of medication are not used frequently because of the difficulty of administration.

Before flexible endoscopy became available, surgical exploration of the pelvic urethra via a subischial urethrostomy was initiated to make a visual diagnosis. Early reports addressing hemospermia reported use of a rigid endoscope.[1] In early studies following urethrostomy, successful recovery was observed with twice daily installation of furacin/hydrocortisone suppositories through the urethrostomy site. The suppositories (no longer commercially available) consisted of a base of polyethylene glycol which melted slowly at body tem-

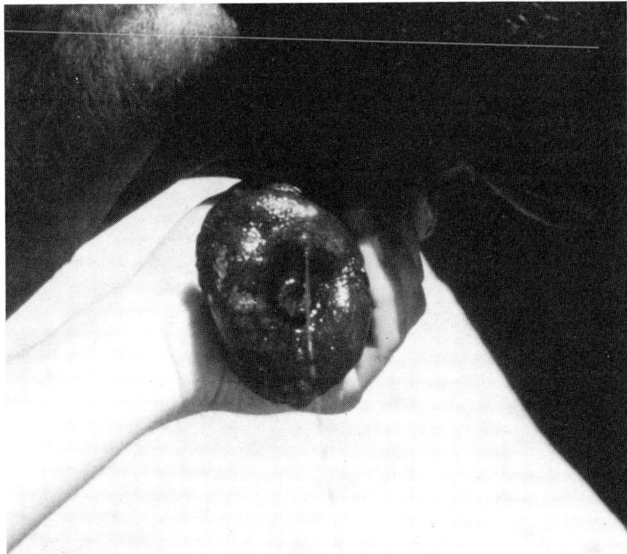

FIG. 94–4. Trauma (puncture wound) to the glans penis resulting in hemospermia.

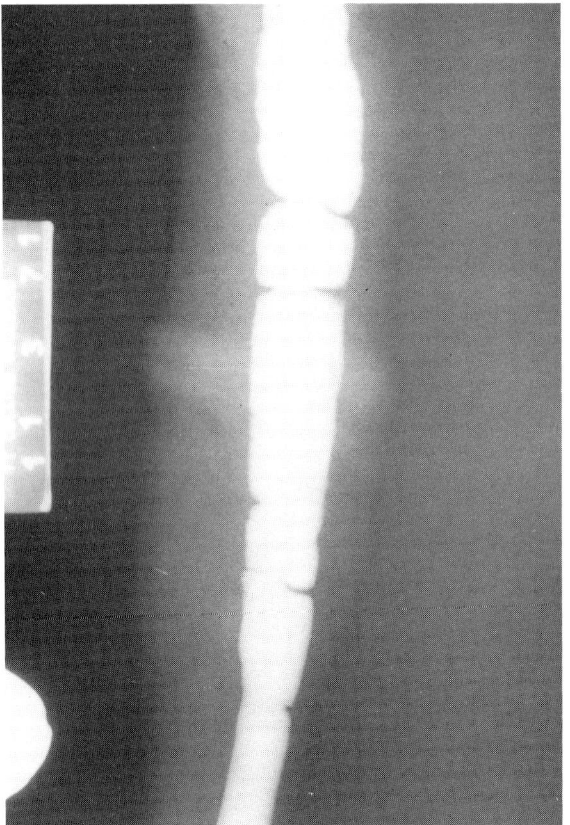

FIG. 94–5. A urethrogram of a stallion with strictures.

perature. When it became possible to diagnose urethritis as a cause of hemospermia using a flexible endoscope, similar therapy was attempted (without urethrotomy) by infusion of furacin/hydrocortisone suspension in glycerine into the pelvic urethra via a stallion catheter. This treatment was not as effective even when associated with extended sexual rest and prolonged antibiotic administration. Thus, the effect of a subischial urethrotomy may have been beneficial in the treatment of hemospermia. Subischial urethrotomy may be the most successful method of therapy of hemospermia in stallions.[5] Stallions that were successful breeders before the onset of hemospermia usually returned to breeding soundness. Most patients that were infertile before the onset of hemospermia did not become fertile after recovery. In a retrospective study by Sullins et al. two of six horses returned to breeding soundness after sexual rest.[5] Three of the stallions that did not recover after conservative treatment recovered after urethrotomy. Although the reasons are not clearly understood, the success of urethrostomy may be the result of a counterirritant effect, temporary diversion of urine, or to other factors.

Sexual rest with concurrent antibiotic administration resulted in approximately 40% of stallions returning to normal within 2 weeks.[14] Approximately 80% of those stallions with urethritis that did not respond to sexual rest and antibiotic administration returned to normal ejaculations after subischial urethrotomy. Although there have been few complications with this procedure, occasional, excessive postsurgical bleeding and urethral fistula have been observed. Insertion of suppositories or other forms of medication is possible for approximately 15 days after which time granulation tissue seals the urethra from the cutaneous perineum.

UROSPERMIA

ETIOLOGY

A possible explanation for urospermia in the stallion is a functional disturbance of the neuromechanism that controls the normal pattern of ejaculation.[15–18] Under some circumstances, stimulation of this nerve can induce contraction of the bladder. In the stallion, hypogastric fibers serving the ejaculatory mechanism and the bladder might be stimulated simultaneously, and if the bladder were full, urine could contaminate the ejaculate. Apparently this condition is different from retrograde ejaculation in man in which there is ejaculation into the bladder.[19–22] Because closure of the bladder sphincter and seminal emission are controlled by the α-adrenergic sympathetic nervous system, a disturbance in this nervous pathway might be involved in the pathogenesis of this disorder.[18] Neuropathies causing

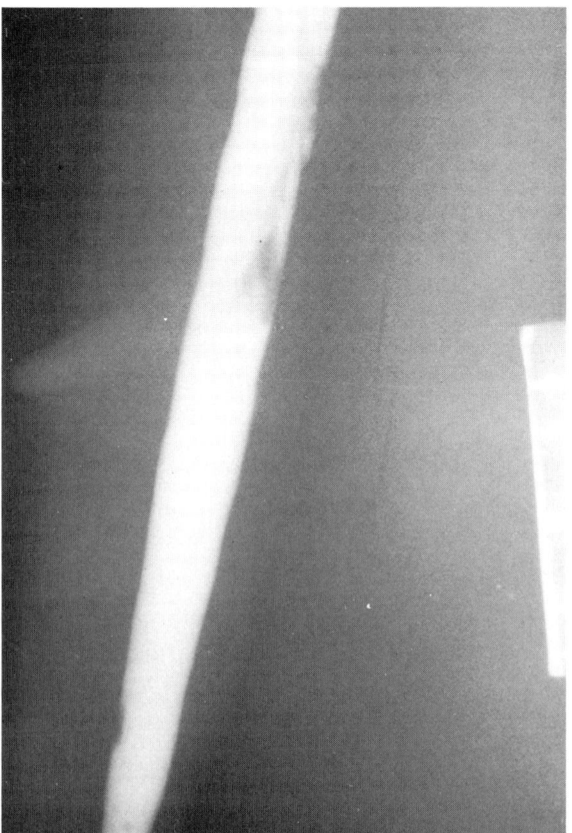

FIG. 94–6. A urethrogram of a stallion with a space occupying lesion (exuberant granulation tissue).

bladder paralysis such as cauda equina neuritis, nerve damage secondary to equine herpesvirus type 1 (EHV 1) infection, or sorghum/Sudan grass poisoning could create urinary incontinence during ejaculation. Most stallions with urospermia do not exhibit signs of neurologic defect other than urinating during ejaculation.

DIAGNOSIS

Diagnosis of urospermia is relatively simple. Gross contamination of ejaculated semen with urine is easily detected by the seminal sample's color and odor. Microscopically, crystals commonly associated with urine can be observed. Spermatozoal motility is generally severely depressed or absent in semen containing large quantities of urine. In contrast, motility and ejaculates from the same stallion that contain no urine usually have normal spermatozoal motility.

Other than the commonly observed characteristic odor and color of ejaculates containing urine, elevated seminal concentrations of urea nitrogen or creatinine also serve to diagnose urospermia. Seminal samples containing as little as 10% urine can be readily confirmed in the field by using commercially available test strips for either urea nitrogen or creatinine.[17,23] Urea nitrogen strips (Azostix, Miles, Inc., Ag Vet., Shawnee, KS) should be fully emerged in the seminal sample, then removed and held horizontally for 10 s before examination.

Samples positive for urine turn the reagent pad from yellow to green. False positive readings are likely if the reagent pad is evaluated for color change after the recommended 10-s exposure period. Nitrate reagent pads (Multistix, Miles, Inc., Ag. Vet., Shawnee, KS) also can be used in a similar manner. Best results with this test are achieved if the sample is elevated 3.5 min after immersion in the suspect sample. The color change for urine contamination with this test is from yellow to radiant orange.

Stallions tend to ejaculate in series of jets associated with urethral contraction and a system for seminal collection without the gel fraction has been described.[24,25] The sperm-rich fraction is ejaculated primarily in the first three to four jets and the gel fraction in the last two to three jets. For observation of urination during ejaculation, a similar system was developed with an artificial vagina that was shortened to 7.5 cm.[4] Thus the glands could protrude through the apparatus and allowed a round container (2.5 cm in diameter) with the bottom removed and the edges protected by a smooth, soft rubber flange to be used to collect separate jets of semen during ejaculation. A clear plastic tube (8 cm long, inside diameter 2.5 cm) was attached to the mouth of the container with a radiator hose clamp. When the stallion obtained an erection and was allowed to mount the mare, the AV was placed over the glans onto the shaft of the penis. The collector placed one hand on the ventral aspect of the penis to palpate the urethral pulsations during the onset of ejaculation. When ejaculation commenced, the plastic tube was directed toward a rack containing 10 plastic bottles (500 mL each). Using this technique, it was determined in one horse that urination occurred inconsistently in all of the various jets of semen. After fractionating ejaculates of several stallions associated with urospermia, it was noted that urination was not a leakage from the bladder but an all or none phenomenon.[4]

TREATMENT

Because little is known about the causes of urospermia, treatment varies and often tends to be unrewarding. Urospermia can best be controlled or decreased through management. Delaying seminal collection (or breeding) until immediately after the stallion has urinated is helpful as urospermia is less likely if the bladder is empty. Consequently, management techniques that allow collection of semen immediately after urination should be established. Many stallions will urinate if presented with a fecal pile of other stallions or feces of estrous mares. This behavior appears to be an inherent natural marking system in stallions. As a last resort, the bladder can be catheterized to evacuate urine before ejaculation. Unfortunately, subsequent development of urethritis or cystitis is an obvious drawback to routine catheterization. Urination can also be stimulated by diuretic administration such as furosemide.

Drugs such as bethanechol chloride or flavoxate hydrochloride have been used to treat urospermia in stallions but their effectiveness is questionable.[17] Alpha-sympathomimetic drugs have been used to prevent retrograde ejaculation in men by stimulating bladder neck closure.[22] Similar therapeutic regimens have not been reported for urospermia in stallions. Other drugs such as oxytocin and those that may have a constricting effect on the musculature of the neck of the bladder have been administered as a treatment in clinical cases. Results with these drugs have been unrewarding and the effect is difficult to determine because urospermia generally occurs sporadically. Obviously, much must be learned about the mechanisms of ejaculation in the stallion before a consistent treatment can be established.

REFERENCES

1. Voss, J.L., and Wotowey, J.L.: Hemospermia. Proc. Am. Assoc. Equine Pract., 103–112, 1972.
2. Voss, J.L., Pickett, B.W., and Shideler, R.K.: The effect of hemospermia on fertility in horses. Proceedings of the Eighth International Congress of Animal Reproduction and Artificial Insemination. Vol. 4. Krakow, 1976, pp. 1093–1095.
3. Pickett, B.W., et al.: Hemospermia. *In* Management of the Stallion for Maximum Reproductive Efficiency, II. Animal Reproduction Laboratory Bulletin No. 05. Fort Collins, Colorado State University, 1989, pp. 121–125.
4. Nash, J.G., Jr., Voss, J.L., and Squires, E.L.: Urination during ejaculation in a stallion. J. Am. Vet. Med. Assoc., *176*:224–227, 1980.

5. Sullins, K.E., Bertone, J.J., Voss, J.L., and Pederson, S.J.: Treatment of hemospermia in stallions: A discussion of 18 cases. Compend. Contin. Educ. Practicing Vet., *10:* 1396–1403, 1988.
6. Voss, J.L., and Pickett, B.W.: Diagnosis and treatment of hemospermia in the stallion. J. Reprod. Fertil. Suppl., *23:*151–154, 1975.
7. Sojka, J.E., and Carter, G.K.: Hemospermia in seminal vesicle enlargement in a stallion. Compend. Contin. Educ. Practicing Vet., *7:*S587–S588, 1985.
8. Blanchard, T.L., et al.: Use of semen extender containing antibiotic to improve the fertility of a stallion with seminal vesiculitis due to Pseudomonas aeruginosa. Theriogenology, *28:*541–546, 1987.
9. Pickett, B.W., Voss, J.L., Squires, E.L., and Amann, R.P.: Management of the stallion for maximum reproductive efficiency. Animal Reproduction Laboratory, General Series Bulletin No. 1005. Fort Collins, Colorado State University, 1981.
10. Cattolica, E.V.: Massive hemospermia: A new ideology and simplified treatment. J. Urol., *128:*151–152, 1982.
11. Eliasson, R.B., et al.: Biochemical and morphological changes in semen from men with diseases in the accessory genital glands. Proceedings of the World Congress on Fertility and Sterility. 1966, pp. 625–627.
12. Hamburger, S.: Hemospermia and hypertension in two case reports. J. Kan. Med. Soc., *81:*459–460, 1980.
13. Murphy, N.J., and Weiss, B.D.: Hemospermia. Am. Fam. Physician, *32:*167–171, 1985.
14. McKinnon, A.O., et al.: Hemospermia of the stallion. Equine Pract. *10:*17–23, 1988.
15. Gennser, G., et al.: Significance of adrenergic innervation of the bladder outlet during ejaculation. Lancet, *1:*154, 1969.
16. Rasbech, N.O.: Ejaculatory disorders of the stallions. J. Reprod. Fertil. Suppl., *23:*123–128, 1975.
17. Varner, D.D., Schumacher, J., Blanchard, T.L., and Johnson, L.: Diseases and Management of Breeding Stallions. Goleta, CA, American Veterinary Publishers, 1990, pp. 337–340.
18. Kaufman, D.G., and Nagler, H.M.: Male infertility. Urol. Clin. North Am., *16:*489–498, 1987.
19. Stewart, B.H., and Bergant, J.A.: Correction of retrograde ejaculation by semipathomimetic medication: Preliminary report. Fertil. Steril., *25:*1073–1074, 1974.
20. Stockamp, K., Schreiter, F., and Altwein, J.E.: α-adrenergic drugs in retrograde ejaculation. Fertil. Steril., *25:*817–820, 1974.
21. Glezerman, M., et al.: Retrograde ejaculation: Pathophysiologic aspects and report of two successfully treated cases. Fertil. Steril., *27:*796–800, 1976.
22. Schram, J.D.: Retrograde ejaculation: A new approach to therapy. Fertil. Steril., *27:*1216–1218, 1976.
23. Althouse, G.C., Seager, S.W.J., Varner, D.D., and Webb, G.W.: Diagnostic aids for the detection of urine in the equine ejaculate. Theriogenology, *31:*1141–1148, 1989.
24. Ellery, J.C.: A modified equine artificial vagina for the collection of gel-free semen. J. Am. Vet. Med. Assoc., *158:*765–766, 1971.
25. Tischner, M., Kosiniak, K., and Bielanski, W.: Analysis of the pattern of ejaculation in stallions. J. Reprod. Fertil., *41:*329–335, 1974.

CHAPTER 95

NEOPLASIA OF THE STALLION'S REPRODUCTIVE TRACT

J. Schumacher
D.D. Varner

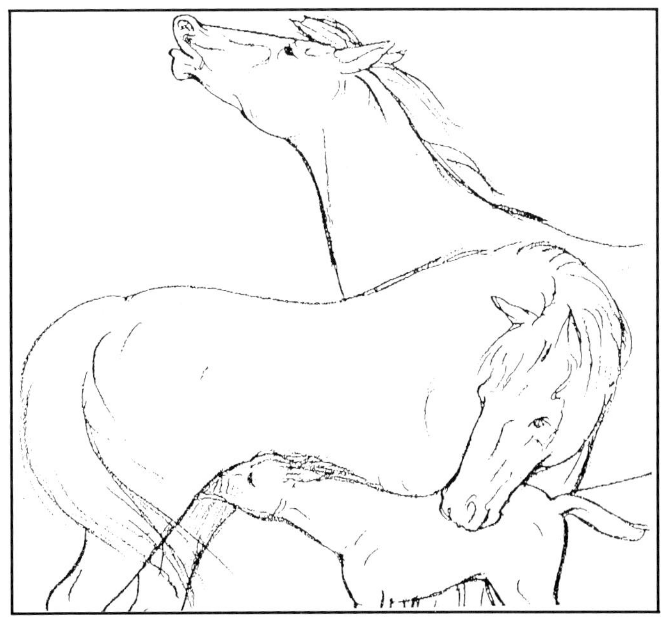

NEOPLASIA OF THE PENIS, PREPUCE, AND SCROTUM

GENERAL CONSIDERATIONS

The most common neoplasms of the penis, prepuce, and scrotum are squamous papillomas, squamous cell carcinomas, melanomas, and sarcoids, but any neoplastic disease of skin can affect the external genitalia.[1] Cutaneous neoplasms of the external genitalia are frequently found on the penis and prepuce but occur less commonly on the scrotum.[2]

The penis, prepuce, and scrotum should be examined for neoplasia by inspection and palpation. The scrotum and external lamina of the prepuce of most horses are easily and quickly examined, but because the penis is easily retracted into the preputial cavity, examination of the free part of the penis and the internal lamina of the prepuce may be more difficult. The penis and internal lamina of the prepuce can be palpated by inserting a lubricated, gloved hand into the preputial cavity. To inspect the free part of the penis and the internal lamina of the prepuce, the penis must be withdrawn from the preputial cavity. Traction is usually resented by the horse, and overzealous traction can damage the penis.

A stallion can be sexually stimulated with a mare to induce penile protrusion. A horse can also be induced to protrude its penis, at least partially, by stimulating urination. Urination can be stimulated by placing the horse in a freshly bedded stall or by administering a diuretic such as furosemide. The horse can also be induced to protrude its penis by administering sedatives such as xylazine. Use of phenothiazine-derivative tranquilizers on stallions should be avoided because these tranquilizers can, on rare occasions, cause priapism, or penile paralysis. Occasionally, large neoplasms of the internal preputial lamina or free body of the penis hinder protrusion of the penis.

Differentiation among exuberant granulation tissue, neoplasia, and verminous lesions is not always possible without cytologic or histologic examination. Carcinomas, for instance, often require microscopic differentiation from granulomas caused by larvae of Habranema spp.[2] Excisional biopsy should be performed on isolated lesions, and histologic examination of multiple areas of a tumor is advisable.[3]

Treatment of scrotal, penile, and preputial neoplasia includes application of 5-fluorouracil, surgical excision, or destruction by cryotherapy, radiofrequency-induced hyperthermia or carbon dioxide laser. Extensive involvement may require preputial reefing, or phallectomy. Regional lymph nodes should first be carefully examined for metastases. Lymphatic fluid from the scrotum, penis, and prepuce passes through the superficial and deep inguinal lymph nodes.[4] The superficial inguinal lymph nodes can be palpated lateral to the penis. Deep inguinal lymph nodes are found in the femoral canal around the femoral artery and vein. Enlarged lymph nodes may be the result of secondary infection, so the lymph nodes should be reassessed after the local neoplastic lesion has been removed. The horse's general body condition should be noted because a horse in poor condition may be systemically affected by neoplasia.

SQUAMOUS PAPILLOMA

Squamous papillomas, or warts, are benign, keratinizing, epithelial neoplasms with little fibrous stroma.[5] Papillomas appear as multiple, small (1 to 2 mm), gray, cauliflower-like, cutaneous growths.[6] They have no known predisposition for breed or gender.[7] Papillomas occur most commonly on the nose, muzzle, and lips of young horses 6 months to 3 yr of age but occasionally can be found on the external genitalia.[3] They may stretch and hemorrhage during erection and ejaculation causing hemospermia (T.L. Blanchard, personal communication).

Histologically, papillomas are characterized by benign hyperplasia of stroma and epithelium that can, under certain circumstances, undergo malignant change.[3] They may be caused by a papillomavirus; antigens of a papilloma virus were isolated from 3 to 17 genital papillomas.[7]

Treatment of nongenital papillomas is optional because active acquired immunity to the papilloma virus is usually sufficient to effect spontaneous cure usually after 1 to 3 months.[3,6,7] Nongenital papillomas have been successfully treated with 0.1% retinoic acid cream,[3] castor oil, glacial acetic acid, or a mixture of salicylic acid and podophyllin cream.[3,6] Treatment of genital papillomas is generally less successful.

SQUAMOUS CELL CARCINOMA

Squamous cell carcinoma is the most common neoplasm of the horse's penis and prepuce.[2,8] The lesions may be multiple and arise mostly from the glans penis and internal lamina of the prepuce.[5,7] Although papillomaviruses are increasingly implicated in the pathogenesis of squamous cell carcinomas of many species including man,[9] they have not been identified in penile or preputial carcinomas of horses.[10] Genital squamous cell carcinomas of the horse may be associated with smegma formed by the secretion of sebaceous material from the penis and the desquamation of epithelial cells from the prepuce.[11,12]

Carcinomas occur more frequently in aged geldings, perhaps because they produce more smegma.[13] Because unpigmented or lightly pigmented skin appears to be more commonly affected, genital carcinomas are most commonly seen on Appaloosas, American Paint Horses, palominos, and cremellos.[7,8,13]

Precancerous lesions appear as small (< 5 mm), white, slightly raised plaques, occasionally with soft horny growths. Cancerous lesions may be productive or erosive.[7] Productive lesions are papillary growths of varying size, many of which have a cauliflower-like appearance. The erosive type often appears as a shallow, crusted, painless ulceration that fails to heal. As the lesion increases in diameter, the center usually ulcerates and develops a necrotic, secondarily infected base with a ragged, raised margin (Fig. 95–1). A persistent penile or preputial lesion should be considered a squamous cell carcinoma until proven otherwise.

Squamous cell carcinoma is derived from stratified squamous epithelium.[5,7] Histologically, squamous cell carcinoma of the penis or prepuce is well differentiated and is characterized by irregular masses or cords of epidermal cells that proliferate downward to invade the dermis and subcutis. Because the cell of origin is the keratinocyte, these neoplasms are characterized by formation of keratin and epithelial pearls. Infiltration of inflammatory cells, especially eosinophils, around the neoplasm is common, and foci of necrosis and calcification are frequent.

Squamous cell carcinomas of the penis and prepuce of the horse are often of low-grade malignancy and tend to remain localized until lymphatic spread occurs.[5,7] Extension of neoplasia occurs either by infiltration into the corpus cavernosum or by metastasis, especially to the superficial and deep inguinal lymph nodes and less frequently to other organs such as lung or liver.

Cryotherapy has been recommended for early lesions of squamous cell carcinoma.[14,15] Lesions are frozen to $-20°$ to $-30°$ C, usually with liquid nitrogen administered as a spray or with a cryoprobe. Depth and degree of freezing can be monitored with thermocouples. Two or three freeze-thaw cycles, with fast freezes and slow thaws, are most effective.

Radiofrequency-induced hyperthermia has been recommended for treatment of ocular squamous cell carcinoma of horses and cattle,[16,17] but its use for treatment of squamous cell carcinoma of the genitalia has not been evaluated. Small lesions can be treated by applications of an antimetabolite, 5-fluorouracil, and/or local excision.

Horses with extensive lesions of squamous cell carcinoma of the genitalia require resection of a circumferential segment of internal preputial lamina (i.e., reefing) or phallectomy. Reefing is indicated if preputial neoplasms are so extensive that simple excision of lesions is

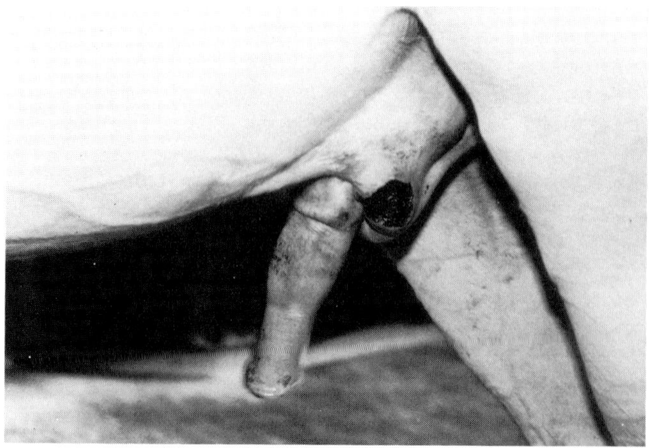

FIG. 95–1. Erosive squamous cell carcinoma of the external lamina of the prepuce. (Photo courtesy of W.C. McMullan.)

impossible. Phallectomy is indicated when neoplasia has invaded the tunica albuginea or is so extensive that treatment by cryosurgery, hyperthermia, local excision, or reefing is impossible. Phallectomy of stallions is performed to salvage the horse for purposes other than breeding. Penile amputation can be performed using Vinsot's,[18] Williams's,[19] or Scott's[20] techniques. Rarely, prescrotal urethrostomy combined with en bloc resection of the penis, prepuce, and superficial inguinal lymph nodes may be required[21] (see Chapter 103 for details of reproductive surgery in stallions).

MELANOMA

Melanomas in horses generally originate in the skin.[7,22,23] They are usually multiple and may develop on the body, head, neck, or limbs, and occasionally on the genitalia, but by far the most frequent site of primary tumors is on the ventrum of the tail near the anus. Melanomas are generally smooth, round neoplasms ranging from 0.5 to 2.0 cm in diameter. The skin over a dermal melanoma may ulcerate, but generally it remains intact. The tumors are darkly pigmented and hairless and on a cut surface are well defined although seldom encapsulated.

For reasons not understood, melanomas appear more frequently on old gray horses and may occur with greater frequency in some families of gray horses.[22,23] When they occur on horses of other colors, they tend to be more aggressive.[3,23–25] Lerner and Cage suggested that Arabian horses are predisposed to melanomas, but this may be a reflection of the high incidence of grays in the breed.[24]

Because melanomas may undergo transformation with accelerated growth, any melanoma should be regarded as potentially malignant. Malignant melanomas initially spread by way of lymphatics, but the final involvement of the internal organs is mainly by hematogenous spread.[23]

Histologic appearance of melanomas is variable. Some melanomas may produce so much melanin that it appears in the blood and urine.[25] Some melanomas are so amelanotic that the diagnosis must be made by use of special stains. Cytologically, neoplastic cells are medium to large, round or oval, and characteristically many of them are multinucleated with up to 20 nuclei.[22]

Genital melanomas are generally not treated because these neoplasms develop slowly, are nonulcerative, and do not interfere with coitus.[26] Small isolated tumors, however, can be removed surgically or with cryotherapy. Melanomas too numerous to remove or treat with cryotherapy can be treated with cimetidine (2.5 mg/kg, PO, q 24 h).[27] Cimetidine appears to stop progression and decrease number and size of the neoplasms by approximately half after 3 to 4 months of treatment. Effects of cimetidine on fertility of the stallion have not been evaluated, but men treated with cimetidine may develop decreased concentration of sperm.[28]

SARCOID

Sarcoids are nonmalignant, fibroblastic cutaneous neoplasms peculiar to equidae.[29] The sarcoid is the most common neoplasm of horses.[29,30] It has no predilection for color, breed, gender, or geographic area but does have a definite tendency to occur in horses 6 yr of age or younger.[3,30,31] A familial tendency to develop sarcoids has been reported.[32] No seasonal incidence has been noted.[31] Sarcoids appear anywhere on the body but are found most commonly on the head, limbs, and ventral midline. Because they often arise from wounds, sites predisposed to trauma have a higher incidence for occurrence. The scrotum and external lamina of the prepuce are occasionally affected.

Evidence indicates that the tumor has an infectious and presumably a viral cause.[3,33] Electron microscopic examination of a cell line derived from a sarcoid revealed intracytoplasmic oncornavirus-like particles.[34] The etiologic agent of sarcoids may be a papovavirus closely related to the bovine papilloma virus (BPV).[31,33] Intradermal inoculation of horses with BPV has produced tumors, but these tumors are not identical to naturally occurring sarcoids.

The term "sarcoid" was applied to the neoplasm by Jackson, who first described it to distinguish it from sarcomas, which it closely resembles.[35] Sarcoids are usually composed of epidermal and dermal tissue, but the epidermal component of some fibroblastic sarcoids may be minimal or nonexistent.[7,31] The epidermis is acanthotic, hyperkeratotic, and hyperplastic with irregular bands of epidermal cells (rete pegs).[33] The dermal component consists of fibroblasts and varying amounts of collagen fibers arranged in whorls or tangles.[7] The fibroblasts have increased mitotic figures and nuclei of variable size. Sarcoids extend only into the dermis; underlying tissue is not involved, and metastasis to internal organs has not been reported.[30,31]

A large percentage of sarcoids spontaneously regress, but this may take years.[31] Sarcoids are characteristically resistant to therapy, especially if rapidly growing or multiple, and those on the extremities are said to be more resistant to all types of therapy than those on the trunk.[3,36] Treatments have included chemical cautery with escharotic agents such as podophyllin,[36] topical antimetabolites such as 5-fluorouracil,[36] surgical excision,[37] cryotherapy,[38] intratumoral hyperthermia,[39] radiation therapy,[40,41] and nonspecific local immunostimulation.[42]

NEOPLASIA OF THE TESTES

GENERAL CONSIDERATIONS

Testicular neoplasia of the horse is rare,[1,43–46] but its true incidence cannot be estimated because most male horses are castrated at an early age. The incidence of the various types of equine testicular neoplasms is difficult to determine because many early reports of testicular neoplasia provide no histologic description.[46]

Although rare, primary testicular neoplasms of horses are much more common than secondary neoplasms. Primary testicular neoplasms are generally divided into germinal and nongerminal types.[47] As in dogs and man, germinal neoplasms are, by far, the most common neoplasms of horses and include seminomas, teratomas, teratocarcinomas, and embryonic carcinomas.[5] Nongerminal neoplasms arise from testicular stromal cells.[47,48] Reported nongerminal neoplasms of the horse include the Leydig cell tumor and the Sertoli cell tumor.[2,48,49]

Combinations of common types of testicular neoplasia occur in about 25% of neoplastic testes of dogs and in about 62% of neoplastic testes of men.[2,47] Combinations of testicular neoplasms of horses have not been reported except for a teratocarcinoma (a combination of embryonic carcinoma and teratoma).[50] Approximately 1 to 3% of primary testicular tumors in man are bilateral, occurring either simultaneously or successively.[47] Willis and Rudduck reported multicentric development of teratomas in the testes of a horse,[46] and Gibson reported a seminoma in both testes of a pony.[51]

Cryptorchidism of dogs and man is associated with a high incidence of testicular neoplasia.[43,47] Epidemiologic studies have reported the relative risk of testicular neoplasia in cryptorchid men to be 3 to 14 times the normal expected incidence.[47] Factors that may initiate tumorigenesis of a cryptorchid testis are abnormal structure of germ cells, elevated temperature, interference with blood supply, hormonal dysfunction, and gonadal dysgenesis. In man, orchiopexy of a cryptorchid testicle does not prevent neoplasia from developing in that testis.

Horses with neoplasia of a scrotal testis are usually presented because of painless, insidious enlargement of the affected testis.[49] Occasionally, the stallion may show signs of tenderness at service or on palpation of the testis.[52] Horses with neoplastic abdominal testes may also be presented because of weight loss,[53,54] dyspnea,[51] or colic.[54–56] Because most neoplasms of the equine cryptorchid testis are teratomas (which are benign), neoplasia of an abdominal testis is usually discovered during routine cryptorchid castration[57] (Fig. 95–2).

Neoplastic enlargement of the testis must be differentiated from enlargement of the scrotum caused by orchitis, epididymitis, torsion of the spermatic cord, thrombosis of the testicular artery, hematocele, hydrocele, varicocele, inguinal and scrotal herniation, hematoma of the testicular parenchyma, and spermatocele. Acute pain in the scrotal area is more likely to be caused by inflammation (e.g., orchitis and epididymitis) or ischemia (e.g., torsion or thrombosis of the cord and herniation) than testicular neoplasia. Palpation alone may be insufficient to determine the nature of scrotal enlargement, and in these cases, diagnosis may be aided by biopsy, ultrasonography, or measurement of serumal tumor markers.

Punch or incisional biopsy of the testis has been used only to a limited extent in horses, perhaps because of reports of harmful consequences in other species[58] (see Chapter 104). Biopsy of testes of bulls causes a decrease

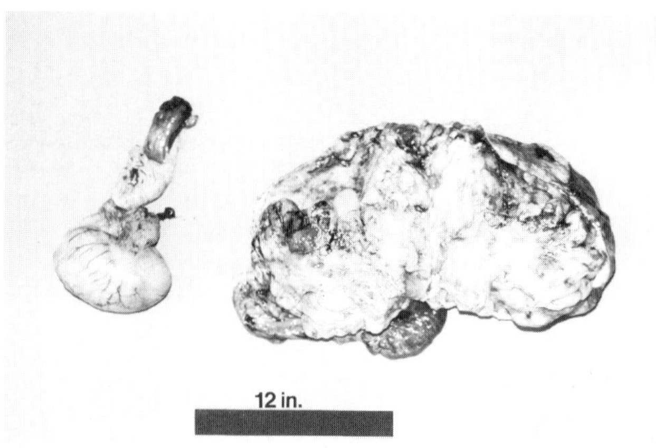

FIG. 95–2. Normal scrotal testis (left) and teratomatous abdominal testis (right) discovered during routine cryptorchid castration. (Photo courtesy of H.D. Moll.)

in numbers of spermatozoa in ejaculates, although generally this decrease is transient. Taking punch biopsies from 20 stallions, however, caused no decrease in number of sperm in ejaculates.[59] Occasionally, decrease in testicular size has followed punch biopsy of bulls, probably from hemorrhage and subsequent deposition of connective tissue at the biopsy site.[58] Other detrimental effects include adhesions between the vaginal tunics, infection, and hematoma. Biopsy of neoplastic testes of man is contraindicated because biopsy has been associated with a high incidence of local recurrence, which is otherwise rare.[60,61] If testicular neoplasia is strongly suspected, the horse's entire testis should be removed.

Aspirational biopsy can also be performed. The aspirate is usually sufficient to differentiate inflammatory from noninflammatory disease and may allow diagnosis of neoplasia by an experienced cytologist. Decreased spermatogenesis following aspiration is unlikely.

Using ultrasonography, intrascrotal masses can be identified as intratesticular or extratesticular and can be characterized as solid or cystic.[62] Normal testicular parenchyma is evenly echogenic, whereas testicular neoplasia produces areas of decreased echogenicity.[63] Decreased echogenicity within the parenchyma, however, is not specific for neoplasia, because benign conditions such as abscessation, hematomas, seromas, and cysts may be hypoechogenic. The contralateral testis should be ultrasonographically examined for comparison and to identify multicentric, occult neoplasia. A 5-mHz, high resolution, real-time system usually provides sufficient imaging.

Concentrations of α-fetoprotein (α-FP) and β fraction of human chorionic gonadotropin (hCG) have been used to diagnose and stage germinal testicular neoplasms of men and to monitor therapeutic response.[47] Persistence of these markers 1 week after removal of a neoplastic testis indicates metastasis. Similar use of marker proteins in horses has not been reported.

Removal of an affected scrotal testis and its cord, using a closed technique, is the treatment of choice if neoplasia has not metastasized. If the neoplasm has metastasized, hemiorchiectomy is useless. Some large cystic abdominal testicular neoplasms (e.g., teratomas) can be removed with an inguinal approach through the vaginal ring by draining the cyst with a needle.[57] Removal of some neoplastic cryptorchid testes may require a parainguinal or flank approach. Primary closure of the scrotal incision is recommended to minimize postoperative swelling and inflammation that may affect fertility of the remaining testis.[49] Cross sections of spermatic cord adjacent to the plane of excision should be histologically examined for neoplastic emboli.[5] Radiation and chemotherapy of horses for treatment of metastatic testicular neoplasia are impractical and have not been described.

Fertility is generally maintained following hemiorchiectomy.[64] Neoplasia of one testis may cause temperature-induced dysfunction of spermatogenesis in the other testis, but removal of the neoplastic testis may cause the remaining testis to undergo compensatory hyperplasia and may allow the testis to regain normal spermatogenesis.[64]

SEMINOMA

Seminomas arise from germinal cells of the seminiferous tubules. They are probably the most frequently observed testicular neoplasm of horses and, as in dogs and man, appear with greatest frequency in cryptorchid testes.[43,47,65] Although most seminomas of horses are relatively benign, they seem to progress more rapidly and have a higher degree of malignancy and invasiveness than those reported for other domestic species.[43,54,66] Occasionally, they metastasize (Fig. 95–3).

Seminomas are soft to moderately hard, and on cut section are gray-white and glistening (Fig. 95–4); when squeezed, the cut surface may exude milky fluid.[2,43,52,67] Thick, fibrous trabeculae divide the seminoma into multiple large lobules. Microscopically, seminomas are largely monocellular. They are composed of

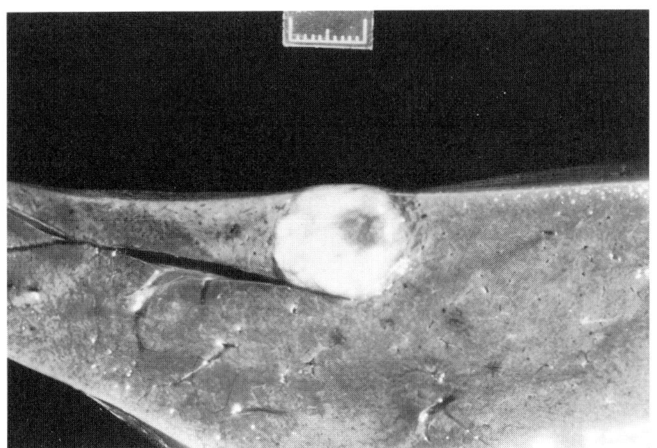

FIG. 95–3. Cut surface of liver containing a metastatic seminoma. (Photo courtesy of B.L. Smith.)

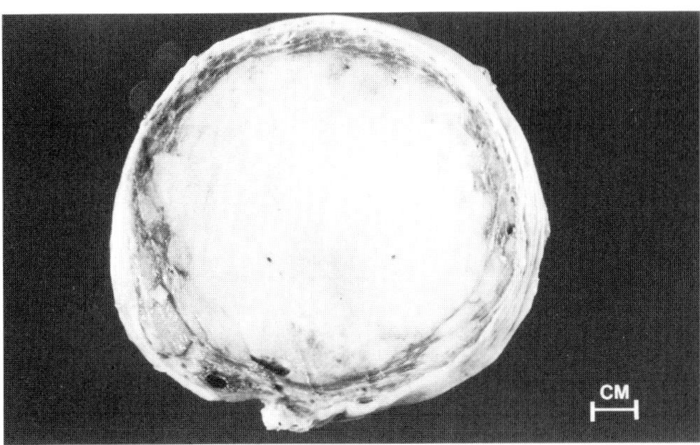

FIG. 95–4. Cut surface of a primary testicular seminoma. The neoplasm (white) compressed normal testicular parenchyma to a thin rim. (Photo courtesy of L.A. Hanrahan.)

cords of round or polygonal cells with large nuclei and prominent nucleoli.[52,55,68] Normal and bizzare mitotic figures may be numerous.

TUMORS OF PLURIPOTENTIAL CELLS

Teratomas, teratocarcinomas, and embryonic carcinomas are germinal neoplasms that arise from pluripotential stem cells of the seminiferous tubules.[47,69] The pluripotential stem cells are capable of differentiating into the three primary germ layers: endoderm, mesoderm, and ectoderm.

Teratomas are composed of multiple, differentiated, nonmalignant tissues of different embryologic origin from the tissue in which they arise.[2,46,47,69] Although teratomas can be found in any location, those of horses are most frequently located in the gonads.[29] Teratocarcinomas resemble teratomas, but have undifferentiated tissue (embryonic carcinoma cells) interspersed in the mix of differentiated tissues, whereas embryonic carcinomas are composed entirely of this undifferentiated tissue.[47,50,69] Continued proliferation of undifferentiated tissue is responsible for the malignant properties of teratocarcinomas and embryonic carcinomas.[69]

Teratomas are found more frequently in horses than in other animals, but equine teratocarcinomas and embryonic carcinomas are evidently quite rare. We have found only one report of equine teratocarcinoma[50] and one report of equine embryonic carcinoma.[70]

Teratomas are usually spherical or ovoid, with an irregular surface. They are covered by a tunica albuginea, and most are composed of solid areas and multiple fluctuant cysts filled with viscous brown fluid.[56,57,71] Some large cysts may contain semisolid greasy material, hair, and teeth. Solid parts of teratomas are usually grayish white, and often contain yellow, fatty areas. Normal testicular tissue may be present.[56,71] Testicular teratomas are found predominantly in abdominal testes, but they are also found in scrotal testes.[46]

SERTOLI CELL TUMOR

The Sertoli cell tumor (sustentacular cell tumor) is a nongerminal neoplasm of the testis that arises from primitive gonadal mesenchyme.[47] It is rarely encountered in horses and man, even though it is the most common testicular neoplasm of dogs.[43,47,72] Because so few equine Sertoli cell tumors have been reported, their biologic behavior is unknown. Only approximately 10% of Sertoli cell tumors of man, and 10 to 14% of those in dogs metastasize.[43,47] The feminizing effect of these neoplasms in dogs is caused by their high content of estrogen.[5]

LEYDIG CELL TUMOR

Although the Leydig cell tumor (interstitial cell adenoma) of dogs is common,[43] it is a rare testicular neoplasm of horses. In contrast to germinal neoplasms, Leydig cell tumors of man are unassociated with cryptorchidism;[47] although these neoplasms are occasionally found in retained testes of dogs, they are not as commonly associated with cryptorchidism as are other canine testicular neoplasms.[43] The authors found only one report of a Leydig cell tumor in a horse, and this horse's affected testis was abdominally located.[73]

REFERENCES

1. Baker, J.R., and Leyland, A.: Histological survey of tumours of the horse, with particular reference to those of the skin. Vet. Rec., *96:*419–422, 1975.
2. Jubb, K.V.F., and Kennedy, P.C. (eds.): Pathology of Domestic Animals. Vol. 1. 2nd ed. New York, Academic Press, 1970.
3. Montes, L.F., and Vaughan, J.T.: Atlas of Skin Diseases of the Horse. Philadelphia, W.B. Saunders, 1983.
4. Schummer, A., Wilkens, H., Vollmerhaus, B., and Habermehl, K., (eds.): The Circulatory System, the Skin and the Cutaneous Organs of the Domestic Mammals. Berlin, Paul Parey, 1981.
5. Ladd, P.W.: The male genital system. *In* Pathology of Domestic Animals. Vol. 3. 3rd ed. Edited by K.V.F. Jubb, P.C. Kennedy, and N. Palmer. New York, Academic Press, 1985, pp. 409–459.
6. Pascoe, R.R.: Equine Dermatoses. New South Wales, University of Sydney, Post-Graduate Foundation in Veterinary Science, 1981.
7. Stannard, A.A., and Pulley, L.T.: Tumors of the skin and soft tissues. *In* Tumors of Domestic Animals. 2nd ed. Edited by J. Moulton. Berkeley, University of California Press, 1978, pp. 16–74.
8. Vaughan, J.T.: Surgery of the penis and prepuce. *In* Bovine and Equine Urogenital Surgery. Edited by D. F. Walker and J.T. Vaughan. Philadelphia, Lea & Febiger, 1980, pp. 125–175.
9. McCance, D.J., et al.: Human papillomavirus types 16 and 18 in carcinomas of the penis from Brazil Int. J. Cancer, *37:*55–59, 1986.
10. Junge, R.E., Sundberg, J.P., and Lancaster, W.D.: Papillomas and squamous cell carcinomas of horses. J. Am. Vet. Med. Assoc., *185:*656–659, 1984.
11. Plaut, A., and Kohn-Speyer, A.C.: The carcinogenic action of smegma. Science, *105:*391–392, 1947.
12. Pratt-Thomas, H.R., et al.: The carcinogenic effect of human smegma: An experimental study. Cancer, *9:*671–680, 1956.
13. Akerejola, O.O., Ayivor, M.D., and Adam, E.W.: Equine squamous-cell carcinoma in northern Nigeria. Vet. Rec., *103:*336, 1978.
14. Stick, J.A., and Hoffer, R.E.: Results of cryosurgical treatment of equine penile neoplasms. J. Equine Med. Surg., *2:*505–507, 1978.
15. Joyce, J.R.: Cryosurgical treatment of tumors of horses and cattle. J. Am. Vet. Med. Assoc., *168:*226–229, 1976.
16. Grier, R.L., Brewer, W.G., Paul, S.R., and Thielen, G.H.: Treatment of bovine and equine ocular squamous cell carcinoma by radiofrequency hyperthermia. J. Am. Vet. Med. Assoc., *177:*55–61, 1980.
17. Kainer, R.A., Stringer, J.M., and Leuker, D.C.: Hyperthermia for the treatment of ocular squamous cell tumors in cattle. J. Am. Vet. Med. Assoc., *176:*356–360, 1980.
18. Frank, E.R.: Veterinary Surgery. 7th ed. Minneapolis, Burgess, 1964.
19. Williams, W.L.: The Diseases of the Genital Organs of Domestic Animals. 3rd ed. Worcester, MA, Ethel Williams Plimpton, 1943.
20. Scott, E.A.: A technique for amputation of the equine penis. J. Am. Vet. Med. Assoc., *168:*1047–1051, 1976.
21. Markel, M.D., Wheat, J.D., and Jones, K.: Genital neoplasms treated by en bloc resection and penile retroversion in horses: 10 cases (1977–1986). J. Am. Vet. Med. Assoc., *192:*396–400, 1988.
22. Garma-Avian, A., Valli, V.E., and Lumsden, J.H.: Cutaneous melanomas in domestic animals. J. Cutan. Pathol., *8:*3–24, 1981.
23. McFadyean, J.: Equine melanomatosis. J. Comp. Pathol., *46:*186–204, 1933.
24. Lerner, A.B., and Cage, G.W.: Melanomas in horses. Yale J. Biol. Med., *46:*646–649, 1974.
25. Runnells, R.A., and Benbrook, E.A.: Malignant melanomas of horses and mules. Am. J. Vet. Res., *2:*340–344, 1941.
26. Neely, D.P.: Physical examination and genital diseases of the stallion. *In* Current Therapy in Theriogenology. Edited by D.A. Morrow. Philadelphia, W.B. Saunders, 1980, pp. 694–706.
27. Goetz, T.E., Ogilvie, G.K., Keegan, K.G., and Johnson, P.J.: Cimetidine for treatment of melanomas in three horses. J. Am. Vet. Med. Assoc., *196:*449–452, 1990.
28. McClure, R.D.: Endocrine investigation and therapy. Urol. Clin. North Am., *14:*471–488, 1987.
29. Smith, H.A., Jones, T.C., and Hunt, R.D. (eds.): Pathology. 4th ed. Philadelphia, Lea & Febiger, 1972.
30. Strafuss, A.C., Smith, J.E., Dennis, S.M., and Anthony, H.D.: Sarcoid in horses. Vet. Med. Small Anim. Clin., *68:*1246–1247, 1973.
31. Ragland, W.L., Keown, G.H., and Spencer, G.R.: Equine sarcoid. Equine Vet. J., *2:*2–11, 1970.
32. James, V.S.: A family tendency to equine sarcoids. Southwest Vet., *21:*235–236, 1968.
33. Voss, J.L.: Transmission of equine sarcoid. Am. J. Vet. Res., *30:*183–191, 1969.
34. England, J.J., Watson, R.E., and Larson, K.A.: Virus-like particles in an equine sarcoid cell line. Am. J. Vet. Res., *34:*1601–1603, 1973.
35. Jackson, C.: The incidence and pathology of tumors of

domesticated animals in South Africa. Onderstepoort J. Vet. Sci. Anim. Ind., *6:*378–385, 1936.

36. Roberts, D.: Experimental Treatment of Equine Sarcoid. Vet. Med. Small Anim. Clin., *65:*67–73, 1970.

37. Brown, M.P.: Surgical treatment of equine sarcoid. *In* Current Therapy in Equine Medicine. Edited by N.E. Robinson. Philadelphia, W.B. Saunders, 1983, pp. 537–539.

38. Joyce, J.R.: Cryosurgery for removal of equine sarcoids. Vet. Med. Small Anim. Clin., *70:*200–203, 1975.

39. Hoffman, K.D., Kainer, R.A., and Shideler, R.K.: Radiofrequency current-induced hyperthermia for the treatment of equine sarcoid. Equine Pract., *5:*24–31, 1983.

40. Lewis, R.E.: Radon implant therapy of squamous cell carcinoma and equine sarcoid. Proc. Am. Assoc. Equine Pract., 217–220, 1964.

41. Wyn-Jones, G.: Treatment of equine cutaneous neoplasia by radiotherapy using iridium 192 linear sources. Equine Vet. J., *15:*361–365, 1983.

42. Wyman, M., Rings, M.D., Tarr, M.J., and Alden, C.L.: Immunotherapy in equine sarcoid: A report of 2 cases. J. Am. Vet. Med. Assoc., *171:*449–451, 1977.

43. Moulton, J.E.: *In* Tumors in Domestic Animals. Edited by J.E. Moulton. Berkeley, University of California Press, 1978, pp. 309–320.

44. Sundberg, J.P., et al.: Neoplasms of Equidae. J. Am. Vet. Med. Assoc., *170:*150–152, 1977.

45. Cotchin, E., and Baker-Smith, J.: Tumors in horses encountered in an abattoir survey. Vet. Rec., *97:*339, 1975.

46. Willis, R.A., and Rudduck, H.B.: Testicular teratomas in horses. J. Pathol. Bacteriol., *55:*165–171, 1943.

47. Morse, M.J., and Whitmore, W.F.: Neoplasms of the testis. *In* Campbell's Urology. Vol. 2. 5th ed. Edited by P.C. Walsh, R.F., Gittes, A.D. Perlmutter, and T.A. Stamey. Philadelphia, W.B. Saunders, 1986, pp. 1535–1575.

48. Gonzalez-Crussi, F.: Testicular and paratesticular tumors of childhood. *In* Pathology of the Testis and Its Adnexa. Edited by A. Talerman and L.M. Roth. New York, Churchill Livingstone, 1986, pp. 131–153.

49. Caron, J.P., Barber, S.M., and Bailey, J.V.: Equine testicular neoplasia. Compend. Contin. Educ. Practicing Vet., *7:*53–59, 1985.

50. Shaw, D.P., and Roth, J.E.: Testicular teratocarcinoma in a horse. Vet. Pathol., *23:*327–328, 1986.

51. Gibson, G.W.: Malignant seminoma in a Welsh Pony stallion. Compend. Contin. Educ. Practicing Vet., *6:*296–298, 1984.

52. Knudsen, O., and Schantz, B.: Seminoma in the stallion. A clinical, cytological, and pathologicoanatomical investigation. Cornell Vet., *53:*395–403, 1963.

53. Trigo, F.J., Miller, R.A., and Torbeck, R.L.: Metastatic equine seminoma: Report of two cases. Vet. Pathol., *21:*259–300, 1984.

54. Vaillancourt, D., Fretz, P., and Orr, J.P.: Seminoma in the horse: Report of two cases. J. Equine Med. Surg., *3:*213–218, 1979.

55. Smith, B.L., et al.: Malignant seminoma in a cryptorchid stallion. J. Am. Vet. Med. Assoc., *195:*775–776, 1989.

56. Parks, A.H., Wyn-Jones, G., Cox, J.E., and Newsholme, B.J.: Partial obstruction of the small colon associated with an abdominal testicular teratoma in a foal. Equine Vet. J., *18:*342–343, 1986.

57. Stick, J.A.: Teratoma and cyst formation of the equine cryptorchid testis. J. Am. Vet. Med. Assoc., *176:*211–214, 1980.

58. Galina, C.S.: An evaluation of testicular biopsy in farm animals. Vet. Rec., *88:*628–631, 1971.

59. Threlfall, W.R., and Lopate, C.: Testicular biopsy. Proceedings of the Annual Meeting of the Society for Theriogenology. Austin, TX, 1987, pp. 65–73.

60. Vogelzang, N.J.: Clinical management of patients with testicular tumors. *In* Pathology of the Testis and Its Adnexa. Edited by A. Talerman, and L.M. Roth. New York, Churchill Livingstone, 1986, pp. 207–209.

61. Mostofi, F.K., and Davis, C.J.: Male reproductive system and prostate. *In* Anderson's Pathology. Vol. 1. 8th ed. Edited by J.M. Kissane and W.A.D. Anderson. St. Louis, C.V. Mosby, 1985, pp. 791–832.

62. Nachtsheim, D.A., Scheible, F.W., and Gosink, B.: Ultrasonography of testis tumors. J. Urol., *129:*978–981, 1983.

63. Leopold, G.R., Woo, V.L., Scheible, F.W., Nachtsheim, D., and Gosink, B.B.: High resolution ultrasonography of scrotal pathology. Radiology, *131:*719–722, 1979.

64. Hoagland, T.A., et al.: Effects of unilateral castration on morphological characteristics of the testis in one-, two-, and three-year-old stallions. Theriogenology, *26:*397–405, 1986.

65. Reif, J.S., and Brodey, R.S.: The relationship between cryptorchidism and canine testicular neoplasia. J. Am. Vet. Med. Assoc., *155:*2005–2010, 1969.

66. Pandolfi, F., and Roperto, F.: Seminoma with multiple metastases in a zebra (Equus Zebra) × mare (Equus caballus). Equine Vet. J., *15:*70–72, 1983.

67. Galofaro, V., and Di Guardo, G.: Spontaneous seminoma in a mule. Equine Vet. J., *18:*218–219, 1986.

68. Schonbauer, M., and Schonbauer-Langle, A.: Seminome beim pferd eine retrospektivuntersuehung. Zentrablbl. Veterinarmed. [A], *30:*189–198, 1983.

69. Martin, G.R.: Teratocarcinomas and mammalian embryogenesis. Science, *209:*768–775, 1980.

70. Valentine, B.A., and Weinstock, D.: Metastatic testicular embryonal carcinoma in a young horse. Vet. Pathol., *23:*92–96, 1986.

71. Conway, D.A.: A teratoma in the undescended testicle in a horse. Ir. Vet. J., *20:*226–228, 1966.

72. Rahaley, R.S., Gordon, B.J., Leiopold, H.W., and Peter, J.E.: Sertoli cell tumor in a horse. Equine Vet. J., *15:*68–69, 1983.

73. Smith, H.A.: Interstitial cell tumor of the equine testis. J. Am. Vet. Med. Assoc., *124:*356–357, 1954.

CHAPTER 96

DISEASES OF THE TESTES, PENIS, AND RELATED STRUCTURES

P.J. De Vries

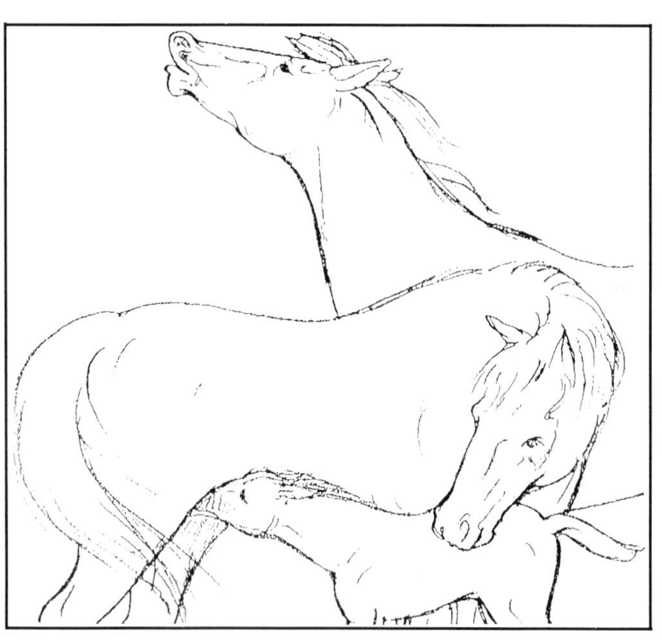

Diseases of the testes, penis, and related structures are relatively common causes of fertility problems in the stallion. These diseases can be disruptive during the breeding season and have adverse effects on breeding efficiency and management. Some diseases have a temporary and minor effect while others can have a serious and permanent adverse impact on fertility. Sexual behavior and libido can also be influenced by some diseases. A rapid and correct diagnosis can lead to prompt and effective therapy. This is the best guarantee for a fast recovery. The risk of irreparable damage to the male reproductive tract by the disease is thus diminished.

INFLAMMATION OF THE PENIS AND PREPUCE

The most common disease of the penis is inflammation or balanitis. This inflammation may also include the prepuce, in which case, balanoposthitis is the appropriate term. The characteristic appearance of this disease is the predominance of lesions and reddening of the penis, sometimes together with swelling and/or an abnormal odor. In cases of a balanitis in a gelding or stallion without sexual experience, or after an extended period of sexual rest, the diagnosis may be hindered by excessive smegma on the penis. Balanitis may lead to painful intromission and a reluctance to mount and ejaculate. This is often the first sign of the problem in pasture breeding.

Balanitis may be caused by a viral, bacterial, protozoal, or parasitic infection or may result from an injury or a neoplasm. Some causes of balanitis are sexually transmitted (see Chapter 91).

VIRAL INFECTION

Equine herpes virus 3 (EVH 3) is the cause of coital exanthema (equine venereal balanitis or genital horse pox) (see Chapter 91). The virus is spread by coitus and can also cause infection in the mare (Fig. 96–1). About 1 week after infection, small vesicles of about 2 to 3 mm are visible on the penis and/or prepuce. In 2 to 7 days, these vesicles exude serum that dries and forms crusts. The crusts will fall off a few days later, leaving a nonpigmented small ulcer (Fig. 96–1). In this stage, secondary bacterial infection, usually with Streptococci spp. may occur, resulting in an extended healing period. The ulcers soon heal, but the discoloration may remain for much longer, demonstrating previous infection.

During the acute stages of the infection, the stallion may be reluctant to copulate because of painful intromission. The disease is highly contagious and infection triggers an immune response, but as with most herpes viruses, the immunity is not permanent. However, stallions remain resistant to reinfection at least through the breeding season during which the condition was diagnosed.

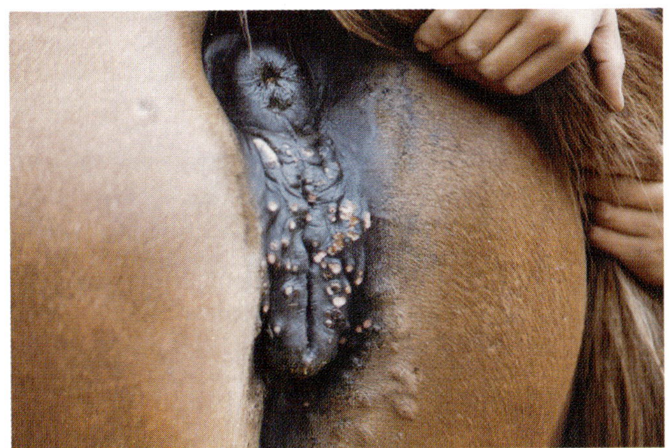

FIG. 96–1. Coital exanthema in a mare. Resulting nonpigmented ulcers heal but may remain as discolorations for an extended time.

The disease is diagnosed by the typical lesions. Virologic confirmation can be made by isolation of the virus from the lesions or by demonstration of the typical herpesvirus intranuclear inclusion bodies from cytologic smears, or histologic studies. Serologic studies such as virus neutralization or complement fixation tests on serum samples taken at 2 to 3 week intervals can also be diagnostic.

Because no vaccine is available, prevention must be carried out by eliminating contact between affected animals. Artificial insemination can be used to avoid the infection if an infected mare is noticed before breeding. In cases of a viral balanitis, sexual rest until the lesions have healed is necessary to prevent spread of the infection. Local treatment with an antibiotic-containing ointment may prevent secondary bacterial infection.

BACTERIAL INFECTION

A balanitis caused by bacteria is rare and usually occurs secondarily to viral infection or injury. Bacteria frequently isolated from a balanitis are Streptococci spp., Klebsiella spp. and Pseudomonas spp. (see Chapter 91). However, these bacteria may also be cultured from the penis of stallions without noticeable balanitis and are potential pathogens that could possibly infect mares at breeding. It has been shown that stallions with Pseudomonas on their penises have reduced fertility.[1–3] Taylorella equigenitalis, the causative organism of contagious equine metritis (CEM) can also be cultured from the penis of stallions but has never been reported as a cause of balanitis. This organism appears to be harmless to the stallion. However, the stallion can serve as a major source of disease spread.

The disease is diagnosed on clinical appearance and bacterial culture. Prevention is based on reducing primary causes of balanitis (viral or traumatic) and cleansing the penis and prepuce regularly with clean water and, if necessary for the removal of excessive smegma, a mild soap. Disinfectants or antibiotics should not be used routinely. These treatments may select bacteria that are resistant to the agent that is used. These bacteria may then replace the normal penile bacterial flora.[4]

In mild cases of confirmed bacterial balanitis, daily cleansing of the penis with clean water or with mild soap may be useful. In more severe cases, treatment with an antibiotic-containing ointment after cleansing, may be necessary. Choice of antibiotic should be based on bacterial sensitivity testing. The clinician may also try to re-establish a normal bacterial flora on the stallion's penis by topical application of petroleum jelly that contains smegma from an untreated normal stallion.[2] During treatment, sexual rest is necessary to promote fast recovery.

PROTOZOAL INFECTION

In several countries in Asia, Africa, and South America, the protozoa Trypanosoma equiperdum causes the infection dourine (see Chapter 91). This highly contagious disease is transmitted during coitus. Weeks to months after infection, fever and general sickness develop, accompanied by swelling of the penis and prepuce. This swelling can be followed by a mucopurulent discharge from the urethra and small lesions occurring on the penis leaving depigmented spots after healing. Typical plaques varying in size between 2 to 10 cm may appear in the skin, mainly on neck and shoulders.

The diagnosis is based on clinical appearance and can be confirmed by demonstration of trypanosomes in discharges or by complement fixation test.[5] For disease prevention, isolation of affected and suspect animals is necessary. Treatment is impractical and usually not attempted, but quinapyramine sulfate has been used.[6]

PARASITE INFECTION

In some areas, especially in warm, humid climates, flies can spread the larvae of the large stomach worms: Habronema muscae, Habronema microstoma, and Draschia megastoma. These larvae may cause cutaneous habronemiasis. Small granulomatous swellings, "summer sores," may occur on the limbs, penis, or prepuce. On the penis, the predominating spots are around the preputial ring and the urethral process. These spots may produce intense pruritus and an abnormal odor.[7]

The diagnosis of cutaneous habronemiasis is made from the clinical appearance and by demonstrating larvae in scrapings of the lesions. A biopsy may be necessary to differentiate habronemiasis from equine sarcoid or squamous cell carcinoma. Prevention of infection is by the use of insecticides or fly repellents for fly control. Regular collection and treatment of manure will also help to control habronemiasis.

Treatment with ivermectin at an oral dose of 0.2 mg/kg will give clear improvement of the condition in 1 to 2 weeks in cases of small sores, although a second treatment may be necessary after about 1 month.[8] For

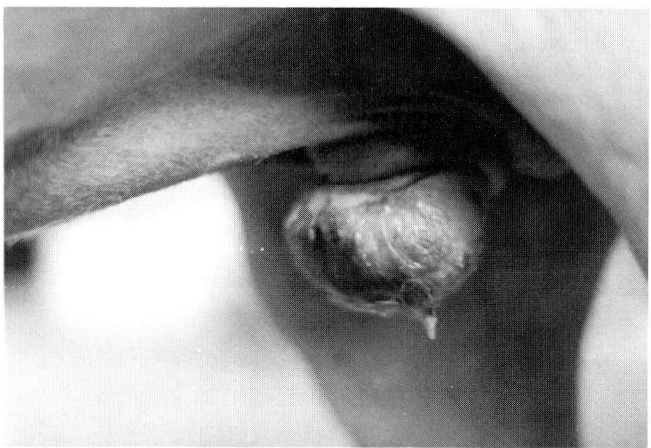

FIG. 96–2. A traumatic penile wound resulting from a kick by a mare during breeding.

supplementary local treatment, daily application of an ointment containing an anti-inflammatory drug and a larvicidal ingredient can be used.[9] Systemic organophosphate treatment has given precarious responses. Surgery or cauterization may be necessary in the case of a larger lesion, and if the lesion affects the urethral process, amputation of the urethral process is an alternative.[10] Cryosurgery using a double freeze-thaw cycle has been used with excellent results for the treatment of habronemiasis lesions on legs.[11] This is a relatively simple and cost-effective method of treatment. A combination of surgery and cryosurgery will generally resolve the problem.

TRAUMA

Trauma—for example, from kicks by a mare (Figs. 96–2 through 4), a mare's tail hairs stretched across the vulvar lips during coitus, improperly fitted stallion rings or brushes, rubber bands that slip off an artificial vagina (Fig. 96–5), broken fences, and loose wires in stable or field—can result in injury to the penis. As a result, severe, acute swelling of penis and prepuce (Fig. 96–6) may occur. Trauma is a common cause of balanitis/balanoposthitis. If the cause of the swelling is unknown, a thorough examination must be performed, if necessary with the help of a sedative. Some phenothiazine-derived tranquilizers have been reported to be associated with penile paralysis in geldings and stallions.[7,12]

Treatment of balanitis caused by trauma is dependent on the underlying cause, but reducing swelling by cold water therapy, massage, exercise, and diuretics is essential to minimize further damage. Cold water therapy should be frequent but no longer than 15 min. Increased testicular temperature, as a result of preputial and scrotal edema, may cause testicular degeneration or a transitory reduction of seminal quality.[13] Therefore, treatment should start as early as possible after injury. Local and parenteral antibiotics can be used to prevent secondary bacterial infection. During treatment, sexual stimulation should be avoided. Penile wounds must be treated by proper wound care and measures should be taken to prevent adhesions, although uncommon in the stallion.

For a penile prolapse resulting from an injury, the clinician may have to use a suspensory apparatus on the stallion to prevent further damage to the penis. Penile paralysis can result from swelling and edema and the increased weight on the penile structures. As swelling and weight increase and gravitate toward the glans penis, it becomes part of a vicious circle producing further trauma. If the penis can be returned into the preputial cavity, a purse string suture in the preputial orifice will give temporary retention, reduce swelling, and prevent further damage.[14] In very serious cases of penile trauma, penile amputation may be required.[14–16]

Prevention of penile trauma is important. Both breeding hobbles and a nose twitch should be used on a mare to prevent her from kicking and injuring the stallion before, during, or after mating. A mare's tail should be wrapped before mating to prevent laceration from tail hairs. If a stallion ring or a brush is absolutely necessary to prevent a stallion from masturbating, it should be used with care and removed and cleaned daily.

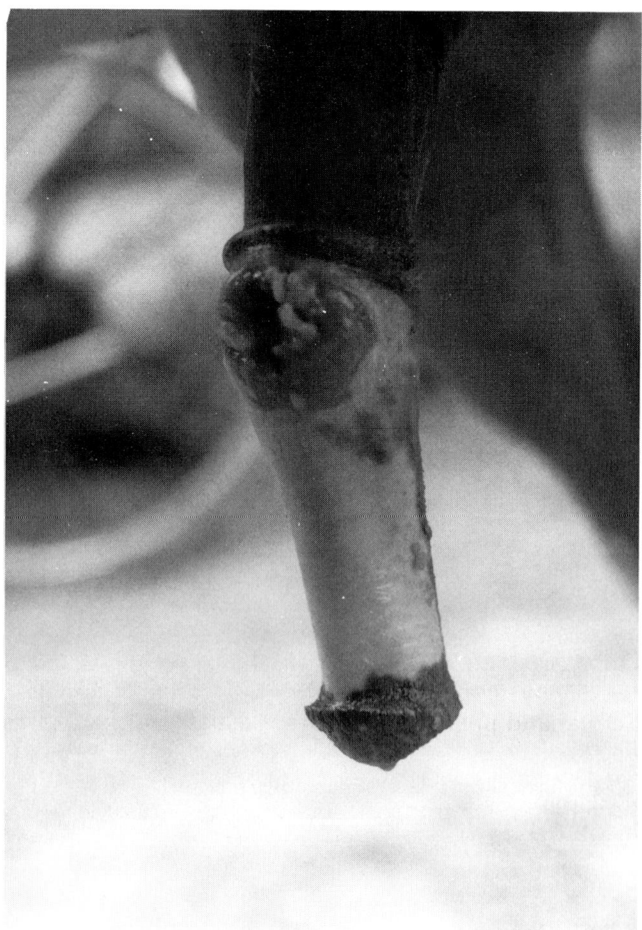

FIG. 96–3. A penile injury several days after being kicked by a mare.

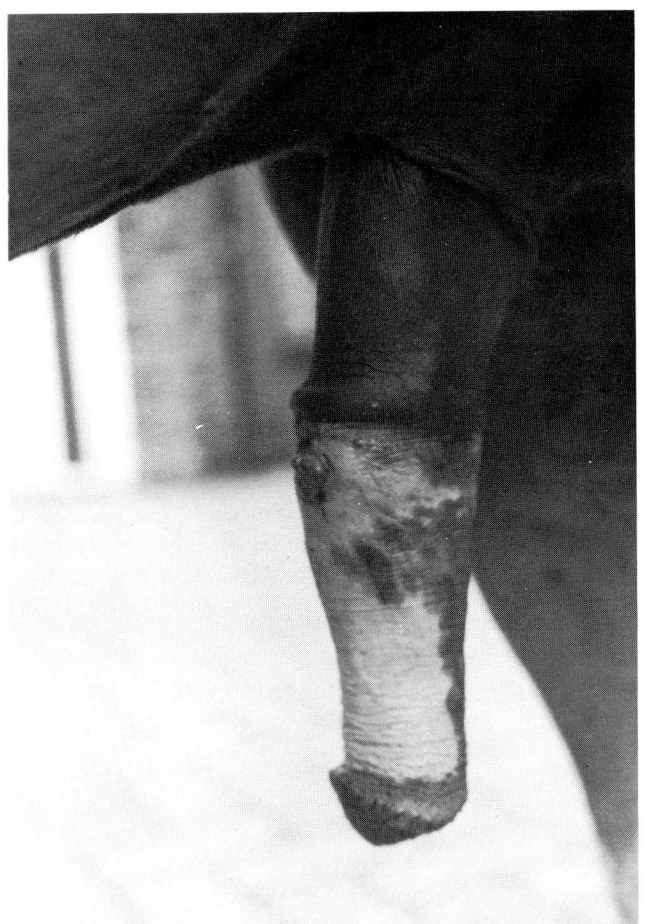

FIG. 96–4. Same lesions presented in Figure 96–3 after 2 weeks.

NEOPLASIA

Squamous cell carcinomas, fibropapillomas, sarcoids, and melanomas will lead to a balanoposthitis (see Chapter 95). Treatment of this balanoposthitis must start with the elimination of the underlying cause.[17,18]

DISEASES OF TESTES AND RELATED STRUCTURES

ORCHITIS

Orchitis is an inflammation of the testis and is characterized by a painful and warm swelling of the testis. Scrotal and preputial edema are usually present. Orchitis may be unilateral or it may affect both testes. Inflammation of the epididymis is usually a complication of orchitis, and a primary epididymitis is rare.[19] Orchitis can be caused by trauma, infection and parasites or it can have an autoimmune origin.

Trauma to the scrotal area from a kick before, during, or after mating or during teasing is the most common cause of orchitis. If no penetrating wound results, the orchitis will usually remain noninfectious.

Orchitis from an infectious organism can be caused by a systemic infection with hematogenous spread of the causative organism, or it may result from a local penetrating wound. Known bacterial causes are Streptococcus equi (strangles) and Streptococcus zooepidemicus and, less frequently, Pseudomonas mallei (glanders), Salmonella abortus equi, and Klebsiella pneumoniae. Viral causes of orchitis include equine viral arteritis, equine infectious anemia, and equine influenza viruses.[7,20] An orchitis caused by an infection, usually involves both testes and epididymides.

Strongylus edentatus larvae have also been reported as a cause of orchitis.[7,17] These larvae can produce small inflammatory lesions in the testis during their migration. Most infections will remain imperceptible, only in the case of a large number of larvae in the testicle will swelling become obvious.

An autoimmune orchitis is triggered by a damaged blood-testis barrier caused by trauma. This stimulates the stallion's immune system to produce antisperm antibodies.[21,22]

The diagnosis of orchitis is based on case history, clinical appearance, careful palpation, and ultrasonographic evaluation. If testicular trauma is known (visible or suspected), the cause will be clear. If the stallion is still willing to breed, seminal collection and evalua-

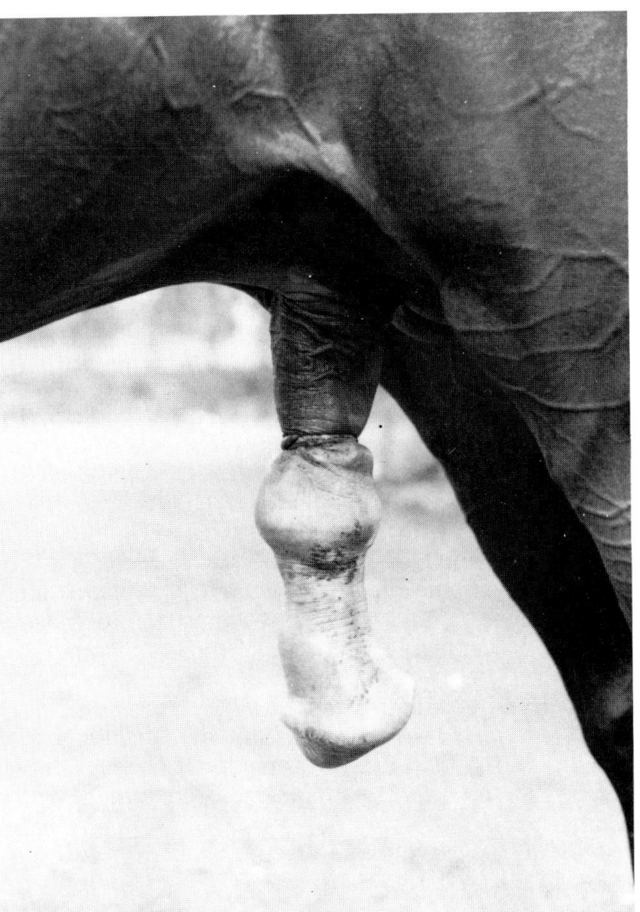

FIG. 96–5. Penile swelling from a rubber band that slid off the artificial vagina during seminal collection.

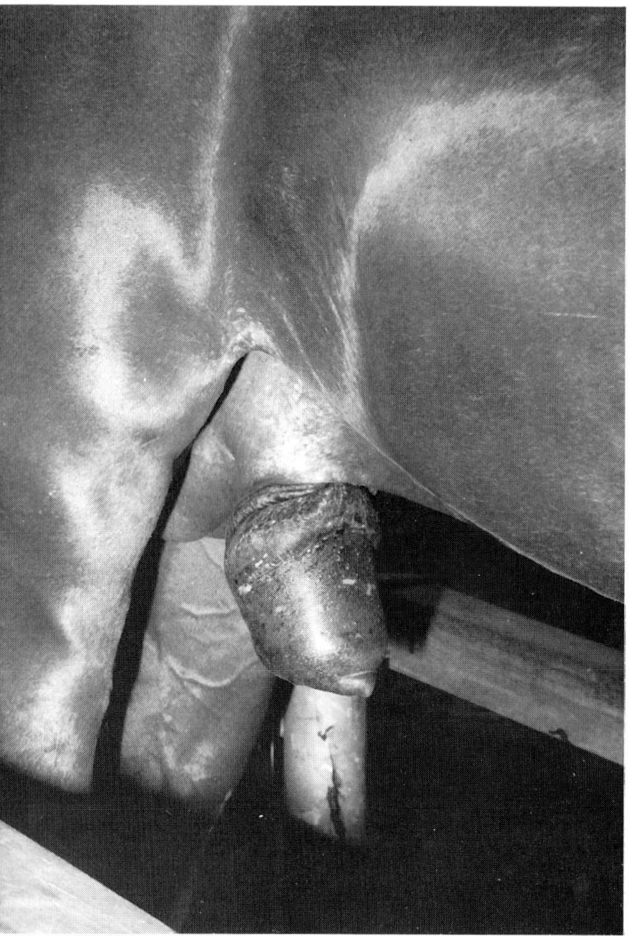

FIG. 96–6. Swelling of the preputial and scrotal areas resulting from a kick by a mare.

tion may also be helpful. An aspiration biopsy may help reveal the cause of testicular swelling.[17] A biopsy of the affected testes can provide a definitive diagnosis of orchitis, but not without great danger (see Chapter 104).

The clinical appearance of an acute orchitis can be confused with several other diseases. In case of an orchitis, a firm, swollen, painful testicle can be palpated and the stallion may have an increased temperature. However, a thorough palpation can be hindered by presence of scrotal edema. In severe cases, the stallion will exhibit a rise in body temperature, anorexia, and hindlimb lameness. Because testicular hormone production is relatively independent from testicular temperature, the stallion's libido may be unaffected. Ultrasonography using an at least 5-Mhz transducer can give detailed information on the size and structure of the affected testis and on the possible presence of testicular lesions.[23,24]

If seminal evaluation can be performed, large numbers of white blood cells and sometimes bacteria can be found. Spermatozoal concentration, motility, and morphology will be abnormal after the acute phase of orchitis. Primary spermatozoal morphologic defects will be more predominant than secondary defects.[7]

Treatment of acute orchitis is based on the necessity to prevent degeneration and permanent damage to the affected testis. The clinician must start treatment as soon as possible. Increased testicular temperature (caused by inflammation and edema) is a serious threat to seminal quality.[13] A fast restoration to the normal situation is the best guarantee for a minimal effect on fertility. Frequent hydrotherapy (15 min every 2 to 3 h) or ice packs to cool the testis and broad-spectrum antibiotics to prevent infection can be accompanied by nonsteroidal anti-inflammatory drugs (e.g., flunixin meglumine). If the orchitis is caused by bacteria and the agent is known, the choice of antibiotic will depend on a sensitivity test. If the causative organism is unknown, broad-spectrum antibiotics should be used. In cases with large swelling, support of the scrotum may be indicated. The use of diuretics can be considered. In cases of unilateral orchitis, castration of the affected testes is often indicated to prevent the formation of antitesticular antibodies.[20–22] Corticosteriod treatment has proven useful to suppress the inflammation and in cases of an autoimmune orchitis.[21,22]

Because most cases of orchitis are caused by trauma at breeding, proper management and restraint of the mare are important when collecting semen or in natural breeding (see Chapter 85). Breeding hobbles and a nose twitch used routinely during breeding will prevent many cases of traumatic orchitis. Although not given specifically to prevent orchitis, vaccination and deworming programs can also serve as preventive measures. Vaccination programs that immunize against some of the common bacterial isolates (Streptococcus spp.) and viral agents (equine viral arteritis virus, equine influenza virus, etc.) may help in preventing orchitis. Parasite control programs, especially those incorporating ivermectin, will reduce the possibility of Strongylus edentatus larvae migrating into testicular tissue and causing orchitis.

The prognosis for orchitis is guarded. Acute orchitis can become chronic, which may lead to degeneration and fibrosis (see Chapter 92). In less severe cases, granulomas may result from a spermatozoal extravasation from seminiferous tubules. Only rarely will a total restoration of sperm-producing capacity occur. Prompt, vigorous treatment is essential.

SCROTAL HERNIA

Scrotal hernia (Fig. 96–7) can be differentiated from orchitis by careful palpation, ultrasonographic examination of the contents of the scrotum, and by lack of a temperature rise. A rectal exam may reveal presence of abdominal contents entering the internal inguinal ring (for an in-depth discussion, see Chapter 102).

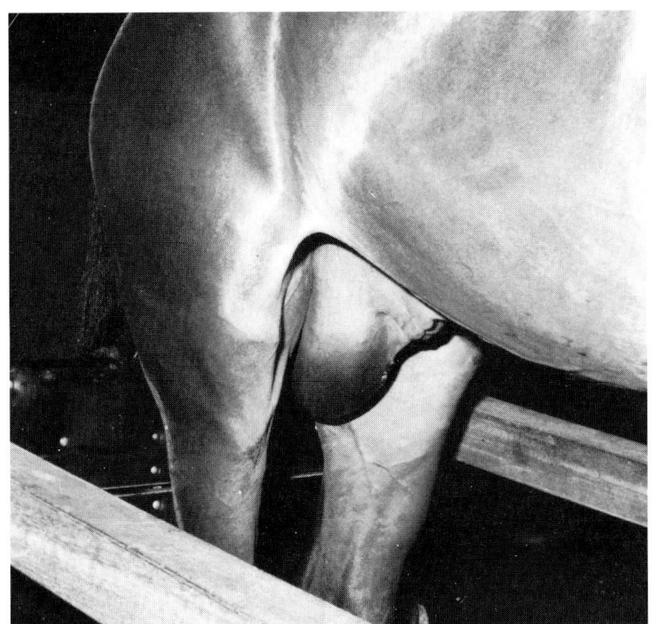

FIG. 96–7. A right-sided scrotal hernia in a stallion.

TESTICULAR TORSION

The acute form of testicular torsion, which is in fact torsion of the spermatic cord, can result in symptoms comparable to orchitis. Colic, scrotal swelling caused by vascular disturbances, and a slight to moderate rise in temperature caused by discomfort are typical symptoms of acute testicular torsion. The torsion can be 360° or, more frequently, 180°. Usually diagnosis of testicular torsion can be established during careful palpation (in case of a 180° torsion, the tail of the epididymis can be palpated anteriorly). The symptoms can be diminished by rotation of the testicle in the opposite direction. The chronic form of a testicular torsion can occur without any clinical symptoms (Fig. 96–8) and some testicular torsions seem to be transient.[25,26]

TESTICULAR HEMATOMA

A testicular hematoma can result from trauma. The rise in testicular temperature is not as predominant as in the case of orchitis. Ultrasonographically, the acute stage reveals an intratesticular hypoechoic or anechoic area.[23] A definite diagnosis can be made after testicular biopsy, though this procedure may be risky. Cold water therapy several times a day and other anti-inflammatory therapies are recommended.

VARICOCELE

Varicocele, a disease of the spermatic vein, has been reported in the stallion.[7,17,27] It may lead to testicular swelling and scrotal edema caused by an effect on circulation. This may interfere with the temperature-regulating mechanism of the pampiniform plexus and thus with seminal quality. This condition seems to be congenital and is not painful. Varicoceles can be palpated and visualized with ultrasonography, if they are situated close to the testicle. If therapy is desired, castration seems to be the only option.

HYDROCELE

In stallions with a hydrocele, transudate is present in the vaginal cavity and the scrotum is enlarged. The disease can cause discomfort and a temperature rise. Several parasites (Strongylus edentatus and Fasciola hepatica) have been suggested as well as a congenital cause.[27] Hydroceles may also be induced by a high ambient temperature.[17] By palpation and the use of ultrasonography, the clinician can differentiate hydrocele from orchitis. The presence of fluctuating fluid and a small- to normal-sized testis in the scrotal cavity indicate a hydrocele. The diagnosis can be confirmed by centesis of the vaginal space. A serous amber-colored fluid is collected. Castration with resection of the vaginal cavity has been suggested as a therapy. If the fluid present in the vaginal cavity is blood, hematocele is the proper term for the condition. This can arise as a result of testicular trauma.[27]

NEOPLASIA

Testicular neoplasia has been reported but is uncommon (see Chapter 95). Patient history usually rules out suspicion of orchitis. Neoplasia usually cause a gradual increase in testicular size; they are not painful, and stallions do not show a rise in temperature.

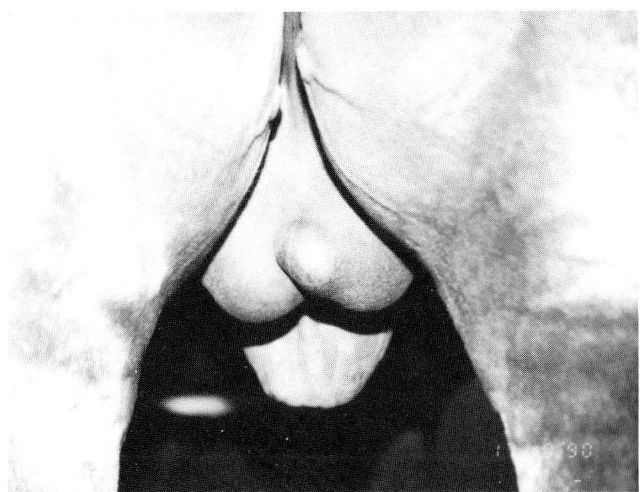

FIG. 96–8. A chronic left-sided testicular torsion. No signs of discomfort were noted and excellent breeding results were obtained. Note the absence of the tail of the epididymis on the left testis (it is rotated to front of the scrotum).

REFERENCES

1. Hughes, J.P., Asbury, A.C., Loy, R.G., and Burd, H.G.: The occurrence of Pseudomonas in the genital tract of stallions and its effect on fertility. Cornell Vet., *57:*53–59, 1967.
2. Swerczek, T.W.: Aggravation of strangles, equine clostridial typhlocolitis (colitis X) and bacterial venereal diseases in the horse by antibacterial drugs. Proc. Am. Assoc. Equine Pract., 305–311, 1979.
3. Johnson, T.L., Kenney, R.M., McGee, W.R., and Polk, H.C.: Pseudomonas infection in a stallion. A case report. Proc. Am. Assoc. Equine Pract., 111–116, 1980.
4. Bowen, J.M., et al.: Effect of washing on the bacterial flora of the stallion's penis. J. Reprod. Fertil. Suppl., *32:*41–45, 1982.
5. Barrowman, P.R.: Observations on the transmission, immunology, clinical signs and chemotherapy of dourine Trypanosoma equiperdum infection in horses, with special reference to cerebrospinal fluid. Onderstepoort J. Vet. Res., *43:*55–56, 1976.
6. Bowen, J.M.: Venereal diseases of stallions. *In* Current Therapy in Equine Medicine 2. Edited by N.E. Robinson. Philadelphia, W.B. Saunders, 1987; pp. 567–571.
7. Robert, S.J.: Veterinary Obstetrics and Genital Diseases (Theriogenology). 3rd ed. North Pomfret, VT, published by the author, 1986.
8. Bridges, E.R.: The use of ivermectin to treat genital cutaneous habronemiasis in a stallion. Compend. Contin. Educ. Practicing Vet., *7:*S94–S97, 1985.
9. Larsen, R.E.: The stallion. *In* Equine Medicine and Surgery. 3rd ed. Edited by R.A. Mansmann and E.S. McAllister. Santa Barbara, American Veterinary Publications, 1982, pp. 1384–1396.
10. Stick, J.A.: Amputation of the equine urethral process affected with habronemiasis. Vet. Med. Small Anim. Clin., *74:*1453–1457, 1979.
11. Migiola, S.: Cryosurgical treatment of equine cutaneous habronemiasis. Vet. Med. Small Anim. Clin., *73:*1073–1076, 1978.
12. Pearson, H., and Weaver, B.M.Q.: Priapism after sedation, neuroleptanalgesia and anaesthesia in the horse. Equine Vet. J., *10:*85–90, 1978.
13. Friedman, R., et al.: The effects of increased testicular temperature on spermatogenesis in the stallion. J. Reprod. Fertil. Suppl., *44:*127–134, 1991.
14. Kersjes, A.W., Nemeth, F., and Rutgers, L.J.E.: Atlas of Large Animal Surgery. Utrecht, Bunge Wetenschappelijke Uitgeverij, 1985.
15. Walker, D.F., and Vaughan, J.T.: Bovine and Equine Urogenital Surgery. Philadelphia, Lea & Febiger, 1980.
16. Cox, J.E.: Surgery of the Reproductive Tract in Large Animals. 3rd ed., Liverpool, Liverpool University Press, 1987.
17. Varner, D.D., Schumacher, J., Blanchard, T.L., and Johnson, L.: Diseases and Management of Breeding Stallions. Goleta, CA, American Veterinary Publications, 1991.
18. Howarth, S., Lucke, V.M., and Pearson, H.: Squamous cell carcinoma of the equine external genitalia: A review and assessment of penile amputation and urethrostomy as a surgical treatment. Equine Vet. J., *23:*53–58, 1991.
19. Van der Schaaf, A., and Hendrikse, J.: Infection of the internal genital organs of a stallion with Str. zooepidemicus. Tijdschr. Diergeneeskd., *88:*834–835, 1963.
20. Rossdale, P.D., and Ricketts, S.W.: Equine Stud Farm Medicine. 2nd ed. London, Bailliere Tindall, 1980.
21. Zhang, J. Ricketts, S.J., and Tanner, S.J.: Antisperm antibodies in the semen of a stallion following testicular trauma. Equine Vet. J., *22:*138–141, 1990.
22. Papa, F.O., et al.: Infertility of autoimmune origin in a stallion. Equine Vet. J., *22:*145–146, 1990.
23. Miskin, M., and Bain, J.: Use of diagnostic ultrasound in the evaluation of testicular disorders. Prog. Reprod. Biol., *3:*117–130, 1978.
24. Cartee, R.E., et al.: Preliminary implications of B-mode ultrasonography of the testicles of beef bulls with normal breeding soundness evaluation. Theriogenology, *31:*1149–1157, 1989.
25. Kenney, R.M.: Clinical fertility evaluation of the stallion. Proc. Am. Assoc. Equine Pract., 336–355, 1975.
26. Threlfall, W.R., et al.: Recurrent torsion of the spermatic cord and scrotal testis in a stallion. J. Am. Vet. Med. Assoc., *196:*1641–643, 1990.
27. Dietz, O., and Wiesner, E. (eds.): Handbuch der Pferdekrankheiten fur Wissenschaft und Praxis. Basel, Karger, 1982.

CHAPTER 97

PENIS AND PREPUCE

J.T. Vaughan

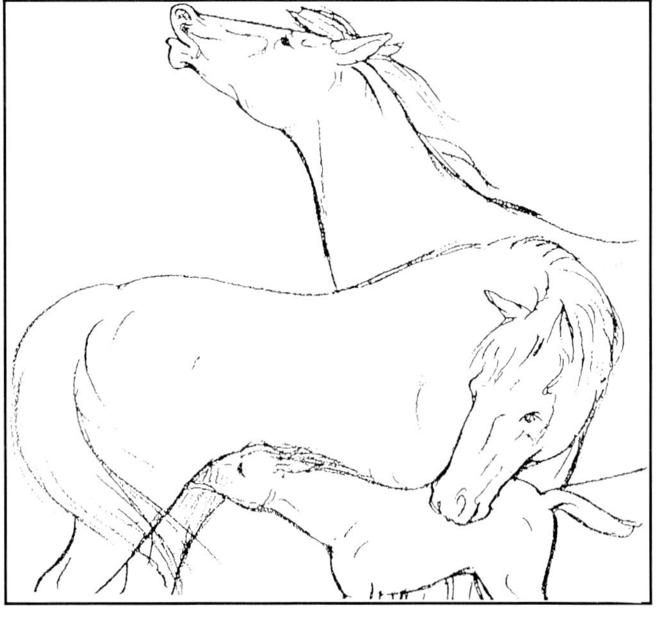

Injuries, phimoses, paraphimoses and priapisms, obstructions, parasitisms and infections, neoplasms, and anomalies constitute the majority of problems affecting the external genitalia of stallions. The seven categories and their variations and complications provide an appropriate etiologic outline for study. As with diseases of the skin or eye, for example, the disorders of the penis and prepuce may be entirely local or else local manifestations of regional, systemic, or general disease. Therefore, the doctor is reminded to examine the whole patient before reaching any conclusions. Overlap of cause and effect is inevitable in contiguous tissues and structures, so conveniently drawn lines of division are apt to become blurred before the ink is dry.

Although disorders of the penis and prepuce do not account for an impressive percentage of the medical problems of horses, their importance assumes larger proportions when they threaten the essential functions of urination and (although of slightly less consequence in the entire stallion) of copulation. For the blood horse whose value rests on his performance in the breeding shed, any interference compromises that worth.

Experience in medicine usually supports the principle of timing that says it is better to err on the early side. Problems that may become life or career threatening can often be prevented or controlled as minor ailments while still in the acute stage. Thus, a horse treated promptly for a kick in the act of breeding may be sidelined for only a week or so. Better yet that the mare be restrained by hobbles or have a front foot tied up. If this seems too elementary for discussion, remember that most of the problems addressed in this chapter could be avoided by applying well-known principles of good husbandry.

However, causes are not always apparent or anticipated. Chronic diseases may be occult until they progress to the point of acute clinical signs. This justifies the presumptive diagnosis and symptomatic treatment until definitive decisions can be made. Familiarity with the normal state and the common pathologies facilitates early recognition and treatment. For these reasons, it is appropriate to discuss general aspects of examination and treatment that have broad application and, with modification, may satisfy specific requirements.

GENERAL ASPECTS OF EXAMINATION

Pertinent information in the medical case history includes fertility rates over time, general management practices and breeding shed procedures (such as use of the stallion to tease), pasture breeding, use of stallion rings or other devices, use of breeding stitches in mares with Caslick operations, breeding shed accidents, patterns of urination, characteristics of urine and semen (gross appearance as well as laboratory analysis), unusual discharges or secretions, wounds, irritations, swellings, any unexplained phenomena, and previous medical attention. All specimens should be submitted for laboratory examination, including cytology, microbiology, chemistry, and others so indicated.

Physical examination of the external genitalia of the adult horse, jack, or mule should commence with observation of the undisturbed patient under normal conditions. If possible, this would include the unprovoked act of urination, upon which a naturally voided sample of urine could be caught in a long-handled cup readied for this purpose. Patients hauled to the clinic will oftentimes oblige the receiving clinician with this if led to a freshly bedded box stall immediately upon arrival. Missing this opportunity, the normal act may be provoked by administration of a diuretic such as intravenous furosemide. However, it results in a diluted specimen. This also provides a timely view of the protruded penis and inner laminae of the prepuce in the unexcited state that does not require either tranquilization or physical manipulation. Any disturbances of form or function may be judged and noted for future reference. The general physical examination and registration of all baseline data should follow (Fig. 97-1).

Continuing on the theme of natural observations at the outset, the intact male should, when appropriate, be allowed to demonstrate his behavior around mares, especially one in heat. In addition to libido and manners, observers should note the physical characteristics of the tumescent penis and prepuce and analyze semen collected either naturally or artificially as conditions might dictate. The natural act of breeding may constitute the most important part of the examination when considering such complaints as faulty performance (e.g., premature dismounts, failure to ejaculate, hemospermia, or evidence of pain or timidity). Horses and jacks behave in individual ways that are subject to psychic, as well as physical, disturbances. Although the target organ system may be urogenital, the cause could be neural, musculoskeletal, or other; hence the need always to regard the total patient.

The final phase of the physical examination involves direct palpation, manipulation, and close inspection of the external genitalia, first in the relaxed, detumescent state and subsequently in the extended or exposed state. With the patient appropriately restrained, the genitalia and surrounding regions are carefully explored for lesions, scars, and other physical evidence, including pain or hypersensitivity; anesthesia; local temperature; secretions and discharges; and alterations of color, consistency, or form. The manual examination of the retracted penis and access all the way into the preputial fornix is facilitated by the use of an examination glove lubricated with obstetrical jelly. Afterward, the penis can be withdrawn from the prepuce manually or allowed to protrude under the influence of a tranquilizer for further inspection. Because phenothiazine-derivative tranquilizers have been incriminated in some cases of paralytic paraphimosis, an alternative method

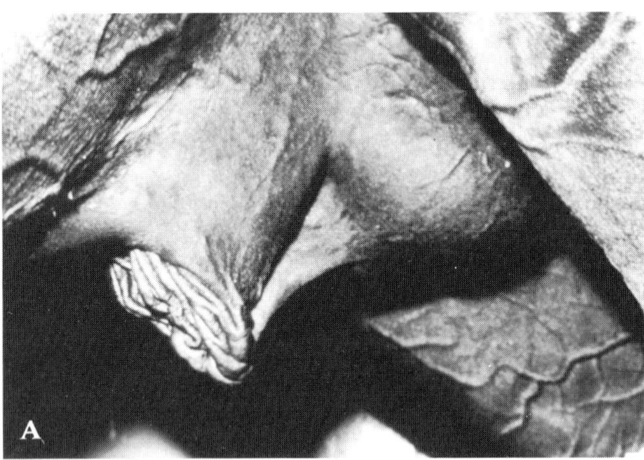

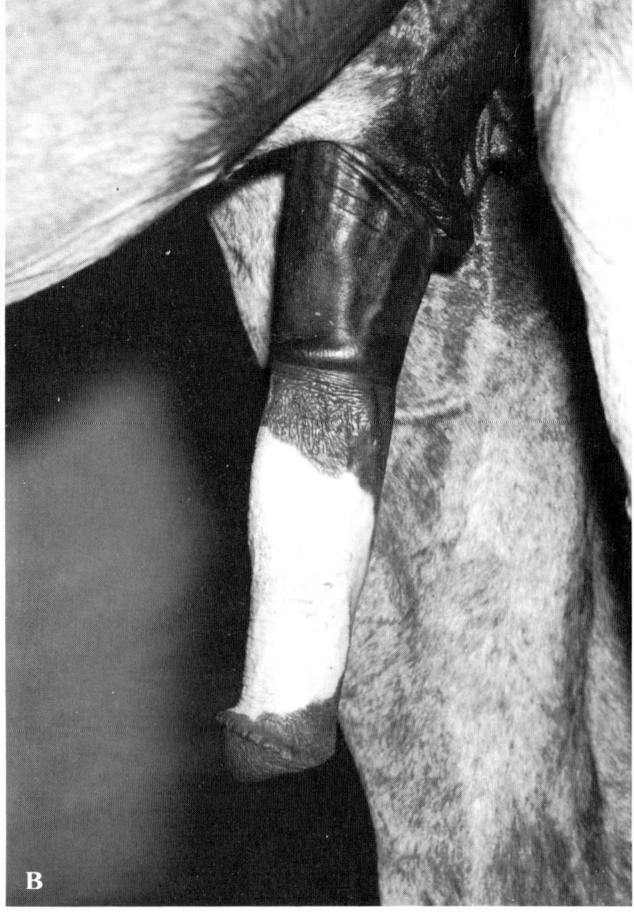

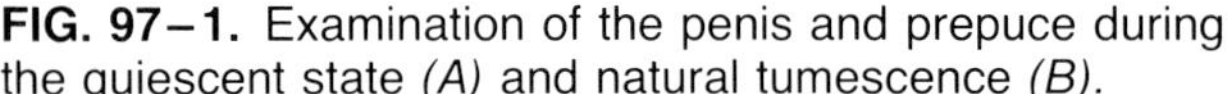

FIG. 97–1. Examination of the penis and prepuce during the quiescent state *(A)* and natural tumescence *(B)*.

in the valuable stallion is to rely on psychic stimulation by the presence of a mare. The exposed penis is cleansed of smegma and associated detritus to permit better visualization, inspection of lesions, biopsies, swabs, etc. Good illumination at the floor level is essential, as is good restraint, because the examination is usually done on the standing patient who may be unaccustomed to such advances. Stocks are ideal; however, the corner of a box stall may suffice. Be sure to close the door to remove the temptation to escape. Hindleg hobbles or a tied-up forefoot may be necessary at times but are not standard procedures.

Certain dysfunctions such as a restricted urine stream, abnormal discharges, and encroachments on the urethra may dictate catheterization, pelvic examination per rectum, endoscopy, and/or a choice of imaging techniques including ultrasonography and contrast radiography. Congenital anomalies are usually self-evident but require interpretation, which may call for techniques ranging from pelvic examinations and endocrine assays to cytogenetic analysis. All tissues in question should be biopsied, infections should be cultured, fluids should be analyzed, and baseline data and vital signs should be regularly monitored for the patient's overall well-being.[1–4]

GENERAL ASPECTS OF TREATMENT

Injuries are varied; nearly always are attended by inflammation, edema, and/or extravasation of blood; and often are complicated by infection and necrosis. Space-occupying swellings and granulomatous reactions necessitate differentiation from neoplasms and other neoformations.

Medical treatment is intended to contain and reverse acute problems and to obviate the need for surgery. For disruptions of tissue, however, operative management may be the first course. Chronic problems such as paralytic paraphimosis may require extended periods of nursing care that strain resources. Management and control measures can be classified as follows:

1. Ensure patency of the urethra and integrity of the urinary system.
2. Control edema, both gravitational and inflammatory.
3. Promote circulation, especially venous and lymphatic drainage.
4. Protect against extremes of temperature (e.g., frostbite), desiccation, maceration, insects, self-irritation, psychic stimulation, and competition with other horses (i.e., provide physiologic rest).
5. Expose the disease and provide ventral drainage.
6. Provide continuous hygiene and wound toilet, while combating inflammation and infection.
7. Correct anatomic defects and physiologic dysfunction.

These principles apply, with appropriate modification, to the treatment of any organ system. Special methodologies are discussed under their respective subject headings.

INJURIES

Contusions, abrasions, punctures, lacerations, ruptures, displacements, strangulations, infarctions, frostbite, photosensitization, toxic and chemical irritations, and a few iatrogenic mistakes make up a representative list of injuries. Examples of blunt injuries include kicks from the mare during breeding, fighting with other horses across fences or stall partitions, abrasions from loose breeder's stitches in mares with Caslick operations, kicks from behind that can rupture the corpus spongiosum penis and cause hematomas that occlude the urethra, and falls on top of jumps or fences.

Sharp or penetrating wounds have been caused by accidents with automobiles, wire fences, sheet metal edges, disk plows, tree limbs, splintered planks, and surgeon's scalpels (e.g., misdirected dissections for incompletely descended testes during castration).

Penetrating wounds of uncertain origin, especially in the inguinal regions, should be explored for foreign bodies. These are oftentimes wood splinters or fragments of tree limbs which, if undetected, will result in abscess. Also at risk are the deep, contaminated wounds that are not provided adequate ventral drainage. Similarly, fistulous tracts, pyogenic membranes, and areas of necrosis must either be debrided or allowed uninhibited opportunity to slough.

Rupture of the suspensory ligament of the penis results in a bowing of the shaft of the penis away from the body wall in the inguinal region. Displacements are mainly prolapses of penis and/or prepuce that result in paraphimosis. Strangulations may result from well-intentioned use of ill-fitting stallion rings or rubber bandages used to reduce edematous swellings. Infarctions may be caused by anything that compromises circulation including hematomas, abscesses, neoplasms, and necrotizing cellulitis.

Frostbite and photosensitization are the results of exposure to the elements, but may be precipitated by complicating factors. Excoriation and ulceration may result from prolonged exposure of paraphimosis with desiccation of the skin, or from overzealous hydrotherapy and maceration of tissues in attempts to promote circulation and control edema. Irritating chemicals may be caused by improper choice or strength of insecticides, medicinals, or accidental contact with strong liniments and vesicants.

The use of pursestring sutures to retain the penis in the prepuce commonly results in stitch abscesses and worse swelling in the prepuce. Unattended slings and suspensories may aggravate matters because of accumulation of exudate, serum, and urine or may even obstruct urination. Injudicious use of catheters may provoke ascending urethritis and inoculate the bladder with opportune pathogens. Complications of castration such as edema and wound infections are frequent sequelae that extend by gravity drainage into the prepuce and penis. Puncture wounds and foreign bodies of the inguinal region and ventral body wall may similarly invade or drain into the prepuce. Urine scald of the prepuce that results from chronic failure or inability to protrude the penis before urination is seen in the neonate with a congenital anomaly, the chronic cystitis case with or without vesical calculus, phimosis from any cause, and the aged or debilitated individual with general constitutional distress.

These varied injuries and associated problems are accompanied by conspicuous disturbances of tissue and the cardinal signs of inflammation, notably heat, pain, redness, swelling, and interference with function. The complications of infection result in more inflammation and necrosis as well as regional sepsis and lymphangitis. Systemic illness and constitutional distress may follow from spread of septic emboli and obstruction of the urinary tract. Certain infections, especially staphylococcosis and the parasitisms such as habronemiasis, provoke intense granulomatous reactions and space-occupying lesions that require differentiation from neoplasms, hematomas, and similar masses.[1,2,4–7]

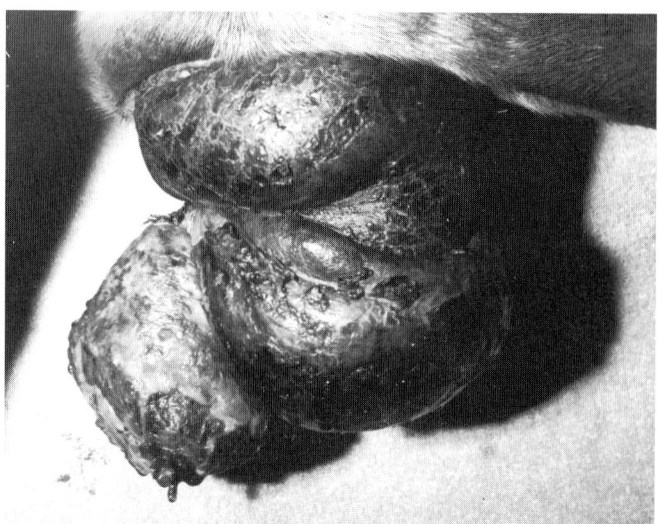

FIG. 97–2. Traumatic balanoposthitis with secondary ulceration of indurated tissues.

PHIMOSIS

The definition of *phimosis* in the equine species is more useful if expanded beyond the classic condition in man. The closest example is the congenital stricture of the preputial ring which causes retention of the penis from birth. Despite these origins, the patient may not be presented until much later for the problem of dribbling urine and its consequence, urine scald of the prepuce. Correction requires a simple transection of the circular muscular band, described in Chapter 103.

Other conditions causing confinement of the penis in the prepuce are congenital abbreviation of the penis and phallocrypsis caused by locally invasive processes, either inflammatory or neoplastic, in which the penis is entrapped. Surgery is usually indicated in both instances and is described in Chapter 103.

PARAPHIMOSIS AND PRIAPISM

Paraphimosis and priapism, which have varied causes, require special attention. As the term has come to be used in veterinary medicine, *paraphimosis* should properly refer to an inflamed prepuce which has displaced or prolapsed in the only direction it can go—ventrad. Under the weight of pendent edema, with or without hemorrhage, the penis is pulled along with it. However, no such clear-cut line of demarcation need exist between the primary and secondary involvements, because the penile tissues often have been injured by the inciting cause, such as a kick to the erect penis during the act of breeding. Therefore, instead of a simple posthitis, the problem may become a balanoposthitis. In fact, the balanitis may precede involvement of the prepuce (Fig. 97-2).

The classical hematoma of the penis of the bull that results from spontaneous rupture of the tunica albuginea of the corpus cavernosum penis is rare in the horse; the more common occurrence is from the rich blood supply located in the subcutaneous fascia superficial to the tunica albuginea. Other instances have been reported, however, of hematomas originating in the corpus cavernosum and the corpus spongiosum.[8–11]

Now the lines begin to blur. Priapism, a morbid engorgement of the corpus cavernosum and the resultant intractable erection, has historically been associated with satyriasis. However, it has also been attributed in the human to diseases and injuries of the spinal cord, vesical calculus, and injuries to the penis. In the horse, particularly (but not exclusively) in the intact stallion, a comparable distress has been reported in a number of instances following the use of phenothiazine-derivative tranquilizers. Clinicians have rationalized it as a failure of the reciprocal waxing and waning of the cholinergic-adrenergic control of blood flow to the corpus cavernosum with resultant stasis and sludging of blood in the cavernous spaces and eventual trabecular fibrosis leading to irreversibility.[6] To further confuse the issue, paraphimosis has also been recognized as a complication of castration (with or without wound infection or associated use of tranquilizers), neoplasia, parasitisms, and aging and debilitation.[12–16]

For these reasons, the clinical management of paraphimosis, balanoposthitis, paralysis, and priapism must be approached on the basis of cause. Medical treatment should still adhere to the principles discussed under general aspects. Examination should rule out urolithiasis and obstruction. If catheterization becomes necessary, the options of periodic recatheterization or use of an indwelling catheter exist. In the latter case, care should be taken to apply a one-way exit valve to prevent retrograde aspiration of contaminants into the bladder, a sure invitation to secondary cystitis. Self-retaining features may be by use of a human balloon catheter or by suturing the mouth of a horse catheter to the urethral orifice.

If caught in the early stages, gravitational edema can be reduced by massage, pneumatic bandage, careful application of an elastic bandage, ice packs, hydrotherapy by shower head or nozzle, and judicious exercise—walking or jogging. The exposed skin surfaces should be protected against friction, desiccation, or maceration with petrolatum-base emollients such as A and D Ointment. Anti-inflammatories, diuretics, topical osmotic applications, and antibiotics are also useful when indicated.

As soon as the prolapsed structures can be replaced by passive manipulation, venous and lymphatic drainage is greatly facilitated and edema controlled. The passive mechanical return to the retracted, detumescent state precedes the patient's ability to retract the penis voluntarily, but recovery of this function too is favored by retention of the penis in the retracted state. This can be best accomplished by the use of a sling or suspensory of nylon or polyester net such as that used for laundry bags to wash socks or lingerie. The material is inexpensive and allows for unobstructed drainage of urine and body secretions away from the affected tissues, thereby preventing maceration. The used suspensory is quickly cleansed and dried for reuse. It is easily adjusted and held in place over the preputial orifice by a surcingle and crupper, both readily accessible pieces of tack, or they can be conveniently fashioned from leather or web

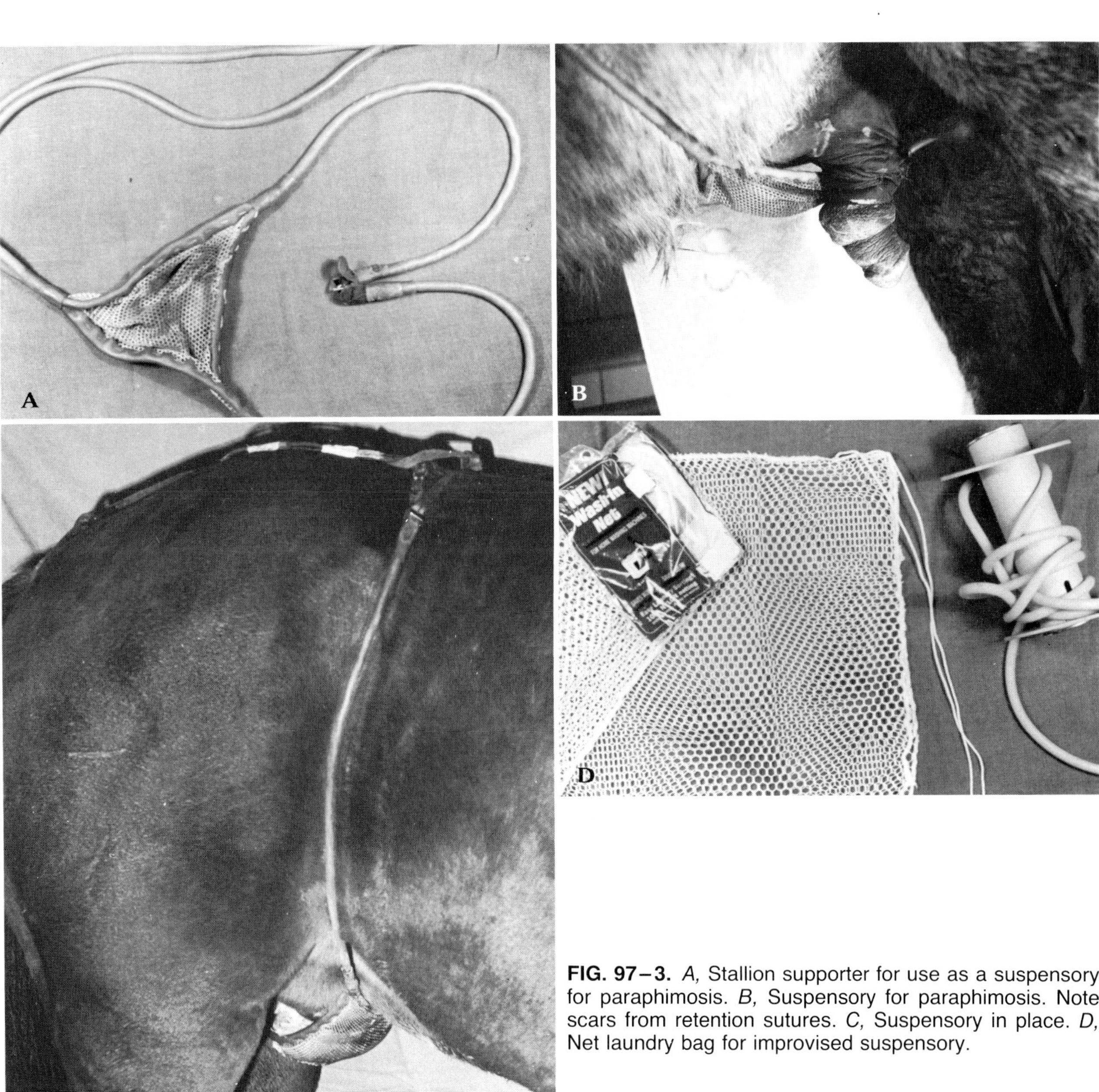

FIG. 97–3. *A*, Stallion supporter for use as a suspensory for paraphimosis. *B*, Suspensory for paraphimosis. Note scars from retention sutures. *C*, Suspensory in place. *D*, Net laundry bag for improvised suspensory.

straps, gum rubber tubing, etc. Buckles make adjustments easier. Alternatives include cylindric pessaries and pursestring sutures, which often lead to other problems (Fig. 97-3).

Hematomas and seromas will complicate the early resolution of acute swellings and may require drainage or open evacuation once the threat of hemorrhage is past. This is a judgment call on the part of the surgeon who must weigh the consequences of uncorrected paraphimosis during the early states against the possibility of further bleeding or infection. Small accumulations of blood or serum should be left to reabsorb if they cause no mechanical interference to function. Extravasated blood and serum are ideal culture media for opportune pathogens accidentally introduced by the well-meaning effort to drain or evacuate such accumulations.

When acute paraphimosis is unresolved, the chronic pathologic process advances to include excoriation and ulceration of the skin surfaces and fibrosis of the deeper layers. The products of inflammation undergo consolidation, circulation is compromised, and the elasticity and retractility of the tissues are lost. The result is intractable paraphimosis, and although some few may be successfully nursed through this, surgery offers the usual recourse. Several alternatives exist: circumcision (the reefing operation) for minor paraphimosis, the Bolz technique of penis retraction when amputation is not required, and finally amputation at the preputial level (as distinguished from the prepubic or ischial sites).[3–6] These procedures are discussed in Chapter 103.

PRIAPISM

Unnatural penile tumescence in the horse has been attributed to injuries and inflammations of the spinal cord, certain diseases such as purpura hemorrhagica, severe constitutional distress, complications of castration, and use of phenothiazine tranquilizers—an interesting variety of causes that curiously omits satyriasis. The common denominator of these pathophysiologic problems has been ascribed to an unexplained failure of the reciprocal sympathetic to parasympathetic stimulation of blood flow to the cavernous spaces of the penis. Researchers have proposed that when the adrenergic stimulation necessary for detumescence fails, vascular stasis and increased carbon dioxide tension of the stagnant blood cause a sickling of the erythrocytes and occlusion of the veins that drain the corpus cavernosum. Fibrosis of trabeculae and regressive changes in the arteriolar-venous system result in impotence.[6]

Extrapolating from the human, use of the cholinergic blocker benztropine mesylate has been suggested at the dosage rate of 8 mg intravenously within the first 24 h, because its success depends on potency of the venous drainage system. This failing, the corpus cavernosum can be flushed with heparinized saline (10 units sodium heparin per milliliter saline) to evacuate the sludged blood. Under general anesthesia and asepsis, the corpus cavernosum is flushed through 12-gauge needles inserted proximal to the corona glandis and 10 to 15 cm caudal to the base of the scrotum. A small stab incision through the tunica albuginea can also be used as an exit but must be closed under suture. Appearance of fresh blood in the irrigation is a good sign; however, the converse warrants a poor prognosis.[6]

If the problem persists after 4 days or three irrigations, according to Schumacher and Vaughan, the creation of a shunt between the corpus cavernosum and the corpus spongiosum should be considered to provide an anatomic exit for the arterial blood in the corpus cavernosum.[6] A description of the surgery is given in Chapter 103.

OBSTRUCTIONS

The importance of patency and integrity of the greater length of the urethra distal to the perineum must be emphasized. Interruptions of the external urethra beyond this point may range from injuries as conspicuous as lacerations to obscure obstructions from urethral calculi or dissecting hematomas. Failure to recognize such problems can result in rupture of the urethra or bladder and consequent urine cellulitis or peritonitis, thus the imperative always to ensure patency of the urinary tract.[9,16,17] Any surgery of the penis and prepuce may approximate, if not involve, the urethra, hence the need for positive identification usually by catheter placement.

Maintenance of patency during the healing process may require catheterization either repeated or indwelling; both increase the risk of ascending tract infection. In fact, obstruction and infection frequently coexist and may change places in precedence. Urethral surgery is discussed in Chapter 103.

PARASITISMS AND INFECTIONS

The extensive hairless and thin-skinned areas in proximity to the ground, tendency toward moisture, accumulations of smegma, and frequent excretions attractive to insects all predispose the external genitalia of equidae to varied irritations which often result in infections and parasitisms.

HABRONEMIASIS

The most common habronemiasis is the summer sore (swamp cancer, bursatti, or esponja), or cutaneous habronemiasis, caused by invasion of the skin by larvae of Draschia spp. and Habronema spp. This is a parasite of minor consequence in the stomach until infective larvae passed out in the feces are picked up by flies serving as intermediate hosts and transmitted to moist or irritated skin surfaces. The larvae, harbored primarily in the heads of the flies, are deposited on attractive sites where they migrate into the tissues causing an intense eosinophilic inflammation attended by itching, self-irritation, and severe granulomatous reaction. Skin surfaces become ulcerated, exudative, and thickened. Sites of predilection are the urethral process and the preputial ring, although other areas may be affected. Lesions on the urethral process can be a cause of hemospermia in breeding stallions (Chapter 94). On lower extremities, these lesions often result in exuberant granuloma, or proud flesh. The reaction may subside spontaneously in the winter in temperate climates, but the chronic fibrosis and deformity remain. On the penis and prepuce, this interferes with function and may necessitate surgical revision even in the absence of active parasitism[18,19] (Fig. 97-4).

Cut surfaces of the granuloma yield calcareous nodules referred to as kunka, or Bollinger's granules, described histologically as caseous masses of dead eosinophils. Larvae can be demonstrated on biopsy of fresh tissues scraped or excised from the lesion and examined on slide preparations under low power magnification. Although not essential, habronemiasis should be distinguished from look-alikes such as phycomycosis and staphylococcosis, as well as less frequently tumors. Most cases, however, are diagnosed and treated on the basis of their clinical appearances.[20]

Treatment of the acute parasitism is often successful with the use of systemic anthelmintics, including the organophosphates and ivermectin, given in pharmacologic doses. The older method of parenteral injections of trichlorfon (22 mg/kg body weight) by slow intravenous drip in 1 to 2 L sterile saline was proven effective but not without risk of clinical toxicity. Local treatment is advantageous in the acute stages and may consist of topical use of organophosphate parasiticides or simply glycerine-based medicants such as the combination recommended by Georgi: 85 parts of glycerine, 10 parts of oil of tar, and 5 parts of phenol. Glycerine is larvacidal as well as osmotic, and the combination repels insects and suppresses pruritus. Local treatment should be administered daily in conjunction with wound toilet and fly control, including manure disposal and fresh bedding. Rigorous husbandry is the best prevention against recurrence.[20,21] Chronic scar tissue may require extirpation described in Chapter 103.

OTHER PARASITISMS

Other parasitisms of lesser consequence include the microfilariasis caused by Onchocerca spp. and Setaria spp., characterized by swollen genitals and erysipelatoid le-

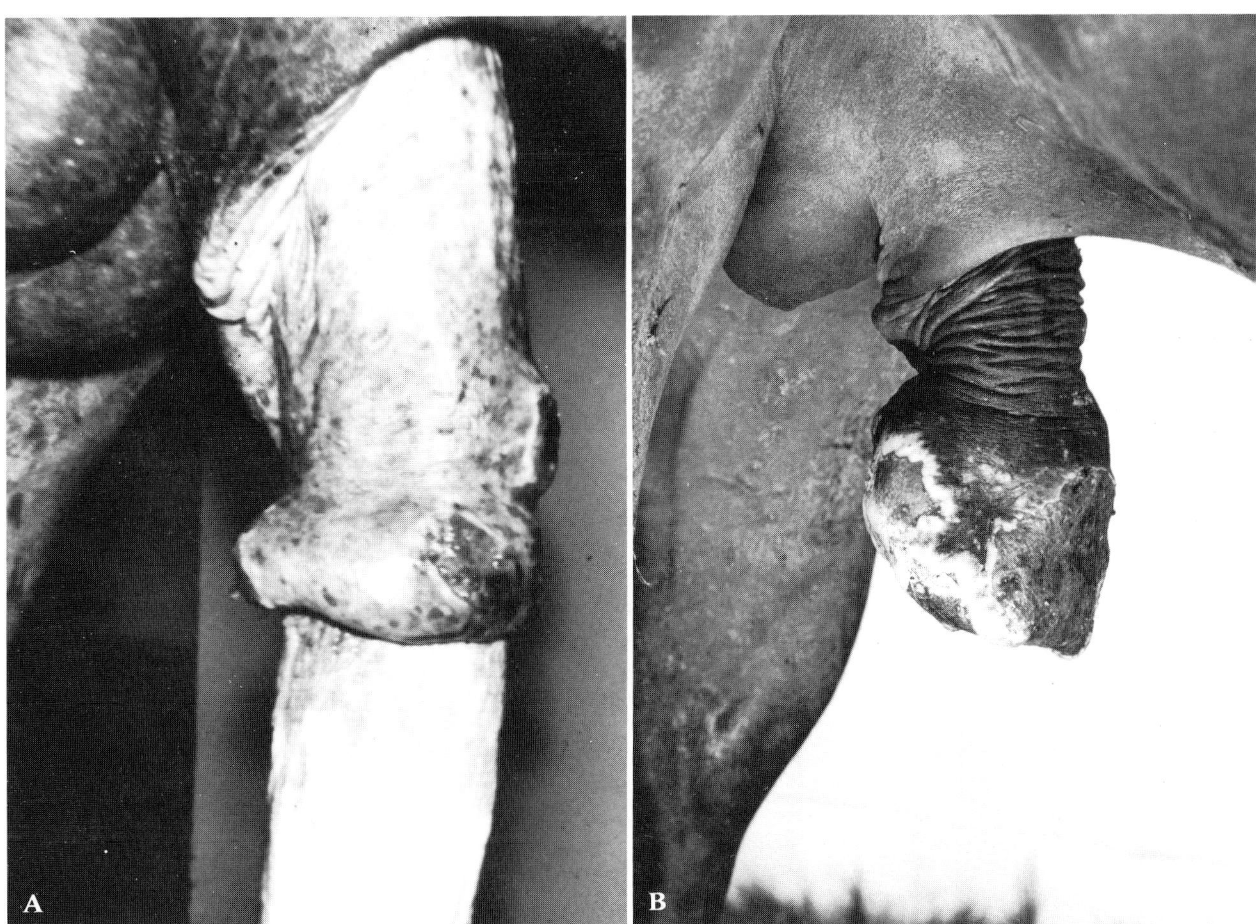

FIG. 97–4. *A*, Acute habronema lesions on the preputial ring and lamina. *B*, Chronic habronemiasis with proliferation of scar tissue and paraphimosis.

sions of the prepuce. Thomas described dry, crusted, and fissured skin and firm, pendulous swellings of the prepuce.[22] Treatment of onchocerciasis (and possibly other microfilariases) has been effective with oral administration of diethylcarbamazine citrate (DEC), 6.6 mg/kg daily mixed with the feed for 21 days, together with dexamethasone given on feed, 10 mg (total daily dose) for 3 days and 5 mg for 4 days of the first week of treatment.[20] An alternative regimen recommended by Schumacher and Vaughan was to administer by mouth DEC 1.5 mg/kg twice a day for 7 to 14 days and prednisolone orally 1.5 mg/kg once daily for 10 to 14 days.[6]

A more current treatment of choice is ivermectin given by mouth in the paste formulation at recommended pharmacologic dosage rates of 200 mg/kg and repeated at monthly intervals as needed (2 or 3 times). The alternative route of intramuscular injection has been discontinued because of too many adverse reactions.[23]

Spirochete infections caused by Treponema were described as multiple circumscribed gummatous lesions and irregular shallow ulcers through the external and internal folds of the prepuce and extending onto the free body of the penis.[24] Spirochetes were also found in the semen and pathologic alteration of the left testis was observed. Still a problem in regions of Latin America, especially south of the Darien Gap, and in other subtropic and tropic climates in the world are members of the family of Sarcophagidae and Calliphoridae, notably Cochliomyia hominivorax, the screwworm, and its Old World relatives. The wound myiasis caused by the larvae of this obligate parasite of living tissue affects many species and is a problem of serious consequence where widescale control measures are not in force. Wound treatment consists of direct applications of larvacides (ranging from benzene to organophosphates), removal of the larvae from the recesses of the wound, subsequent treatment as indicated, and prevention of reinfestation.[21]

OTHER INFECTIONS

Other infections which may confuse diagnosis include the phycomycosis (leeches) caused by Hyphomyces destruens and botryomycosis, an old synonym for staphylococcosis. A case of phycomycosis was diagnosed as involving an inguinal lymph node in a Thoroughbred filly that had a refractory lesion on the hindlimb.[25] Successful treatment for phycomycosis usually requires perseverance in addition to systemic and local fungicides (e.g., amphotericin) and cryosurgery performed on the granuloma and its borders with healthy tissue.[20]

Staphylococcus infection may attend not only any or all of the foregoing but also squamous cell carcinoma. Kunka, or Bollinger's granules, are virtually indistinguishable from those seen in botryomycosis or, for that matter, phycomycosis. Treatment of such lesions involves much of the same: exposure of the disease by debridement and excision, sterilization of pyogenic linings and cavities, ventral drainage, conscientious wound hygiene, and vigorous contrasepsis against extension to regional or systemic status.

Streptococcus is an unusual infection of the penis and prepuce, but it does cause metastatic abscess of the superficial inguinal lymph nodes associated with Streptococcus equi infections that commonly spread from the respiratory tract (strangles). These abscesses should be included in differential diagnosis.

Equine coital exanthema is a contagious disease caused by an equine herpesvirus transmitted venereally. In the stallion, papules, pustules, and ulcers appear on the free body of the penis, and healing may leave vitiligoid patches of skin. Control requires isolation of affected animals and symptomatic treatment for a month or so until healed. Affected animals may remain as asymptomatic carriers.[1,26]

Dourine is an infectious disease caused by Trypanosoma equiperdum, and is important in parts of the Mediterranean, Africa, and South America. It is sexually transmitted and manifests itself in the stallion as edematous swellings of penis and prepuce (including paraphimosis) as well as the scrotum. Inguinal lymphadenopathy may also be a feature. Although treatment can be attempted with quinapyramine sulfate (3 mg/kg subcutaneously), preference is expressed for control by eradication.[1,27]

The importance of this discussion is to emphasize that more than a few conditions exist that may masquerade as space-occupying or other lesions and require careful identification for diagnosis.

NEOPLASMS

Neoplasms of the penis and prepuce may be organized into epithelial and mesenchymal origins. Epithelial tumors of the haired portions of the prepuce reflect the same distribution as tumors elsewhere on the skin surfaces of the body: sarcoids, melanoma, mastocytoma, hemangioma, and squamous cell carcinoma. The last mentioned is the most common of both the external and internal surfaces of the prepuce as well as of the penis[20,27–31] (Fig. 97-5).

SQUAMOUS CELL CARCINOMAS

Squamous cell carcinomas present in a variety of forms ranging through the following.

1. Flat, white, premalignant leukoplakia on mucous membranes and mucocutaneous junctions.
2. Phagedenic, ulcerous kissing lesions on opposing surfaces of the preputial laminae.
3. Quiet, uneroded sessile lesions that invade deeper layers and metastasize to regional lymph nodes.
4. Pedunculated, single tumor in situ.
5. Verrucous lesion confused with warts.
6. Exuberant, granulomatous cauliflowers that must be differentiated from summer sores.
7. Large, malodorous, open sores.

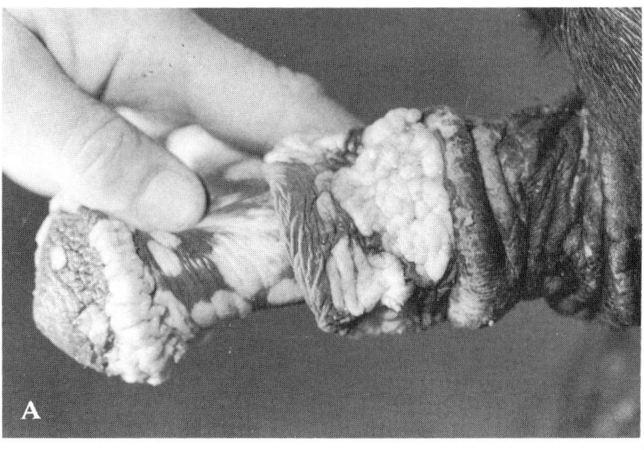

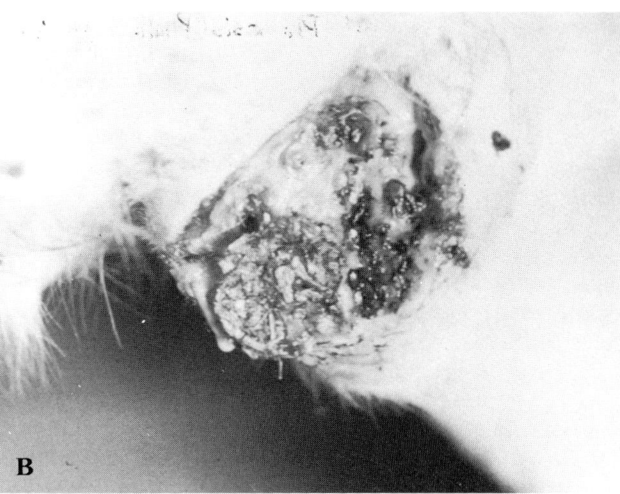

FIG. 97–5. *A*, Squamous cell carcinoma of penis and prepuce. *B*, Invasive squamous cell carcinoma with deep ulceration of the external prepuce.

The third example, quiet, uneroded sessile lesions, is a particularly troublesome one in that it may be described as an iceberg process, presenting an innocuous lesion on the surface while undermining and extending itself deeply. In the course, it may cause edema, abscess, multiple draining sinuses, and lymphadenopathy, confusing the diagnosis all the while. Shallow biopsy specimens may be unrevealing, which only emphasizes the importance of clinical hunches. In one such case, the presenting complaint was phimosis (phallocrypsis) in which the penis was transfixed in retraction by the invading tumor.

Lesions tend to be slow-growing at the outset and late to metastasize. This favors surgical management and prognosis, whether it be the simple excision of an individual tumor in situ or a more extensive resection of the prepuce. Occasionally, amputation of the penis is required, and once in a while the radical en bloc resection of penis and prepuce as a lifesaving measure (Chapter 103).

Nonoperative treatment includes radiation therapy in the form of either radon seeds implanted in the tumor bed (which may require prior surgical debulking) or conventional radiation teletherapy from a source of γ rays such as 60 cobalt. No reports were found on the use of chemotherapy. Techniques employing cryosurgery and laser surgery are discussed in Chapter 103.

SARCOIDS

The second most common neoplasm is the benign cutaneous tumor attributed to a virus similar to that incriminated in bovine papilloma. Grossly, the lesion is elevated above the epidermis, has a broad sessile base, and has a rough, often eroded surface. It may invade deeply into the dermis especially on recurrence, for which it shows a strong tendency. This and its benignity and accessibility have accounted for a variety of treatments, including the following.

1. Chemical cautery with escharotic agents such as podophyllum 20 to 50% in compound benzoin tincture.
2. Topical antimetabolites such as 5-fluorouracil in propylene glycol applied daily for 3 to 4 weeks to the tissue bed following surgical excision.
3. Local immunotherapy by weekly infiltrations of the tumor base with bacille Calmette-Guérin (BCG) vaccine, tuberculin, or bovine transfer factor.
4. Electrofulguration.
5. Radiation therapy.
6. Cryosurgery.
7. Laser surgery.
8. Conventional surgical excision.

Each modality has enjoyed its enthusiastic advocates at one time or another. Suffice it to say that most still have certain individual advantages.[20] The surgical methods are discussed in Chapter 103.

The rare instance of tumors of mesenchymal origin are represented by fibrosarcoma and lymphosarcoma, distinguishable on biopsy, necessary for all such diagnoses. Note that in a series of 10 cases treated by radical resection Markel et al. confirmed lymphosarcoma in 1 case and squamous cell carcinoma in the other 9.[28]

ANOMALIES

The most prevalent of an uncommon lot is the male pseudohermaphrodite, demonstrating the outward physical characteristics of a mare and the behavior of a stallion. The prominent features of the external genitalia are a vulva and clitoris which may be overdeveloped to resemble more closely the glans penis. The location of the urethra is variable from the floor of the incomplete vagina to a deformed penile structure in the inguinal region. The subject is genetically a female and the gonads are typically testes, virtually always abdominal cryptorchids. The behavior may be that of a cryptorchid stallion or a nymphomanic mare, dictating castration if the animal is to be kept. Surgical revision of the external genitalia and urethral orifice may be attempted for aesthetic reasons.[3]

Less common are the female pseudohermaphrodite, with a reversal of features, and the true hermaphrodite with vestiges of ovarian and testicular tissue. External characteristics may resemble those of the incompletely developed male. Confirmation of all cases of intersex is made on the basis of cytogenetic examination.[3]

Other reported examples of developmental disorders include abbreviated penis, aplasia or dysgenesis of the corpus spongiosum glandis, ejaculatory dysfunction, hypospadias, and preputial aplasia with penile retroversion and bilateral cryptorchidism. As with pseudohermaphroditism, some cases lend themselves to surgical revision which, together with castration, can salvage these individuals for useful purposes.

REFERENCES

1. Cox, J.E.: Surgery of the Reproductive Tract in Large Animals. 3rd ed. Liverpool, Liverpool University Press, 1987.
2. Hurtgen, J.P.: Stallion genital abnormalities. *In* Current Therapy in Equine Medicine. 2nd ed. Edited by N.E. Robinson. Philadelphia, W.B. Saunders, 1987, pp. 558–562.
3. Walker, D.F., and Vaughan, J.T.: Examination of the stallion. *In* Bovine and Equine Urogenital Surgery. Philadelphia, Lea & Febiger, 1980, pp. 105–114.
4. Vaughan, J.T.: The male genital system (horse). *In* Textbook of Large Animal Surgery. 2nd ed. Edited by F.W. Oehme. Baltimore, Williams & Wilkins, 1974, pp. 511–526.
5. Vaughan, J.T.: Surgery of the prepuce and penis. Proc. Am. Assoc. Equine Pract., 19–40, 1972.
6. Schumacher, J., and Vaughan, J.T.: Surgery of the penis and prepuce. Vet. Clin. North. Am. Equine Pract. *4:*473–493, 1988.
7. Walker, D.F., and Vaughan, J.T.: Surgery of the penis and prepuce. *In* Bovine and Equine Urogenital Surgery. Philadelphia, Lea & Febiger, 1980, pp. 125–144.
8. Pascoe, R.R.: Rupture of the corpus cavernosum penis of a stallion. Aust. Vet. J. *47:*610, 1971.
9. Firth, E.C.: Dissecting hematoma of corpus spongiosum and urinary bladder rupture in a stallion. J. Am. Vet. Med. Assoc., *169:*800–801, 1976.
10. Pascoe, R.R.: A Colour Atlas of Equine Dermatology. London, Wolfe Publishing, 1990.
11. Memon, M.A., McClure, J.J., and Usenik, E.A.: Preputial hematoma in a stallion. J. Am. Vet. Med. Assoc., *191:*563–564, 1987.
12. Clem, M.F., and DeBowes, R.M.: Paraphimosis in horses—Part I. Compend. Contin. Educ. Practicing Vet., *11:*72–75, 1989.
13. Clem, M.F., and DeBowes, R.M.: Paraphimosis in horses—Part II. Compend. Contin. Educ. Practicing Vet., *11:*184–187, 1989.
14. Carr, J.P., and Hughes, J.P.: Penile paralysis in a Quarter horse stallion. Calif. Vet., *13:*16, 1984.
15. Simmons, H.A., et al.: Paraphimosis in seven debilitated horses. Vet. Rec., *116:*126–127, 1985.
16. Yovich, J.V., and Turner, A.S.: Treatment of a postcastration urethral stricture by phallectomy in a gelding. Compend. Contin. Educ. Practicing Vet., *8:*S393–S399, 1986.
17. Dyke, T.M., and Maclean, A.A.: Urethral obstruction in a stallion with possible synchronous diaphragmatic flutter. Vet. Rec., *121:*425–426, 1987.
18. Stick, J.A.: Surgical management of genital habronemiasis in a horse. Vet. Med. Small Anim. Clin., *76:*410–414, 1981.
19. Deppe, R., Munzenmayer, W., and Sepulveda, O.: Fimosis debido a un granuloma prepucial en un potro. Arch. Med. Vet. (Chile), *20:*69–72, 1988.
20. Montes, L.F., and Vaughan, J.T.: Atlas of Skin Diseases of the Horse. Philadelphia, W.B. Saunders, 1983.
21. Georgi, J.R.: Parasitology for Veterinarians. 2nd ed. Philadelphia, W.B. Saunders, 1974.
22. Thomas, D.D.: Microfilariasis in the horse. J. S. Afr. Vet. Med. Assoc., *34:*17, 1963.
23. Scott, D.W.: Large Animal Dermatology. Philadelphia, W.B. Saunders, 1988.
24. Osborne, V.E.: Genital infection of a horse with spirochaetes. Aust. Vet. J., *37:*190–191, 1961.
25. Murray, D.R., Ladds, P.W., Johnson, R.H., and Pott, B.W.: Metastatic phycomycosis in a horse. J. Am. Vet. Med. Assoc., *172:*224, 1980.
26. Simpson, D.J.: Venereal diseases of mares. *In* Current Veterinary Therapy in Equine Medicine. 2nd ed. Edited by N.E. Robinson. Philadelphia, W.B. Saunders, 1987, pp. 513–516.
27. Bowen, J.M.: Venereal diseases of stallions. *In* Current Veterinary Therapy in Equine Medicine. 2nd ed. Edited by N.E. Robinson. Philadelphia, W.B. Saunders, 1987, pp. 567–570.
28. Markel, M.D., Wheat, J.D., and Jones, K.: Genital neoplasms treated by en bloc resection and penile retroversion in horses: 10 cases (1977–1986). J. Am. Vet. Med. Assoc., *192:*396–400, 1988.
29. Vaughan, J.T.: Surgery of the male equine reproductive system. *In* Current Therapy in Theriogenology. 2nd ed. Edited by D.A. Morrow. Philadelphia, W.B. Saunders, 1986, pp. 740–745.
30. Vaughan, J.T.: Surgery of the male equine reproductive system. *In* The Practice of Large Animal Surgery. Vol. 2. Edited by P.B. Jennings, Jr. Philadelphia, W.B. Saunders, 1984, pp. 1083–1105.
31. Strafuss, A.C.: Squamous cell carcinoma in horses. J. Am. Vet. Med. Assoc., *168:*61–62, 1976.

CHAPTER 98

DEVELOPMENTAL ABNORMALITIES OF THE MALE REPRODUCTIVE TRACT

J.E. Cox

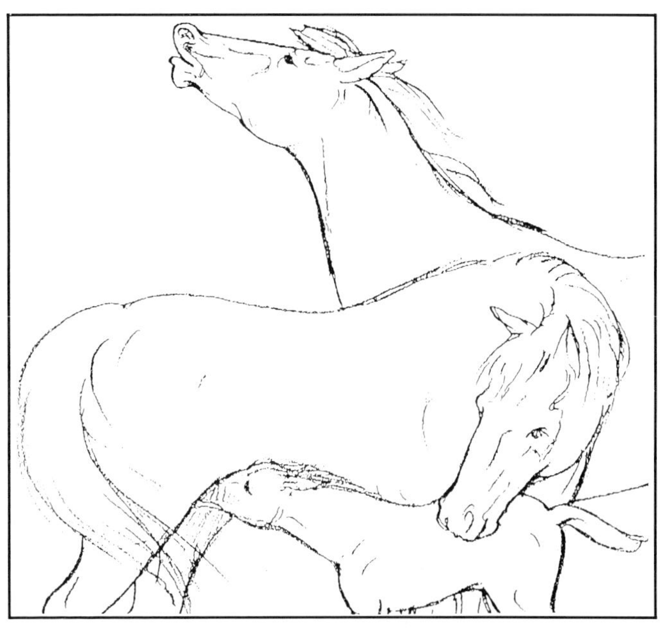

TESTICULAR DESCENT

The gonad differentiates in the early embryo in the sublumbar region and migrates from this position to descend through the inguinal canal into the scrotum. Relevant details of embryologic differentiation related to descent of the testis are discussed here as they help to elucidate cryptorchidism.

EARLY DIFFERENTIATION

Gonadal differentiation begins with the formation of a gonadal ridge at approximately day 27 of gestation with sexual differentiation occurring by day 40.[1] The fetal testis is suspended from the dorsal body wall by a double fold of peritoneum, the mesorchium, in the cranial edges of which runs the suspensory ligament of the testis. A cord of mesenchyma, the gubernaculum, connects the testis to the abdominal wall at a point ventral and lateral to the developing pelvis. The mesonephric duct (which eventually differentiates into epididymis and ductus deferens) lies initially lateral to the developing gonad and passes through the gubernacular cord near the testis to pass mediad toward the developing bladder. This effectively divides the gubernaculum into a shorter proximal part (joining the caudal pole of the gonad to the mesonephric duct) and a longer distal part (running from the mesonephric duct to the blastema of the pelvis). The tail of the epididymis will eventually develop at the point where the mesonephric duct crosses the gubernaculum, the body and head will develop from that part lateral to the developing gonad, and the ductus deferens will develop from that part of the mesonephric duct which passes from the gubernaculum to the developing bladder (see Fig. 100–1).

FORMATION OF THE VAGINAL PROCESS

At about 45 days of gestation an invagination of the peritoneum, called the vaginal process, forms in the inguinal region and pushes its way into the extra-abdominal part of the distal part of the gubernaculum. The part of the gubernaculum distal to the invading vaginal process is called the infravaginal gubernaculum. A few elementary fibrous strands connect the infravaginal part of the gubernaculum to the rudimentary scrotum. As the vaginal process in cross section is C-shaped, it divides the remainder of the extra-abdominal portion of the gubernaculum into an outer, annular, shaped part called the vaginal part of the gubernaculum and an inner cylinder shaped part called the gubernaculum proper. The gubernaculum proper is, therefore, suspended within the vaginal process by a fold of peritoneum continuous cranially with the fold of peritoneum which suspends the intra-abdominal part of the gubernaculum and the testis. The C-shaped opening of the vaginal process into the peritoneal cavity is called the vaginal ring, even though it is not circular.

This opening is not to be confused with the deep inguinal ring, a larger opening bounded cranially by the caudal edge of the internal oblique muscle and caudally by the caudal edge of the external oblique muscle. The caudal edge of the external oblique muscle is sometimes mistakenly called the inguinal ligament by analogy with the human, but in animals, it is not a ligament.

INGUINAL PASSAGE

By day 150 of gestation, the tail of the epididymis is close to, if not within, the vaginal ring and deep inguinal ring, and the gubernaculum proper thickens. Where the gubernaculum lies within the inguinal canal, the effect is to dilate the inguinal canal in preparation for inguinal passage of the testis. Where enlargement occurs extra-abdominally, the result is a swelling called the gubernacular bulb. Inguinal passage, however, does not occur at this time, because prominent testicular enlargement has begun between 100 to 120 days of gestation which precludes passage.[2] The testis reaches maximum size at approximately 210 to 240 days and thereafter shrinks until about approximately 300 days of gestation. Inguinal passage of the testis, therefore, occurs during the last month of pregnancy, with the testis changing to a more cylindrical shape for this passage. The gubernacular bulb continues to enlarge, and this appears to draw the testis out of the abdomen.

Both hormonal and mechanical factors have been deemed responsible for co-ordinated descent of the testis, but the precise mechanism remains incompletely understood. Inguinal passage has often been attributed to shortening of the gubernaculum, but this cannot be the case. First, the gubernaculum does not shorten significantly until after inguinal passage of the gonad, and second, the gubernaculum does not have strong enough distal connections for gubernacular contraction to be meaningful in testicular descent. Inguinal passage must, therefore, depend on other factors. Movement of the testis is probably achieved by a combination of factors. One factor is the extra-abdominal expansion of the gubernacular bulb, and respiratory and other movements of the fetus may increase abdominal pressure and so facilitate expulsion of the testis. Once the testis has passed through the inguinal canal, the gubernaculum shortens and shrinks, but recent work has emphasized that the gubernaculum is compressed below a descending testis rather than its contractions actually pulling the testis distad.

LATER GROWTH

The infravaginal part of the gubernaculum becomes the scrotal ligament, which joins the distal part of the vaginal tunic to the scrotum. The distal portion of the gubernaculum becomes the ligament of the tail of the epididymis running from epididymal tail to the distal part of the vaginal tunic, and the proximal part of the gubernaculum becomes the proper ligament of the testis (Fig. 98–1).

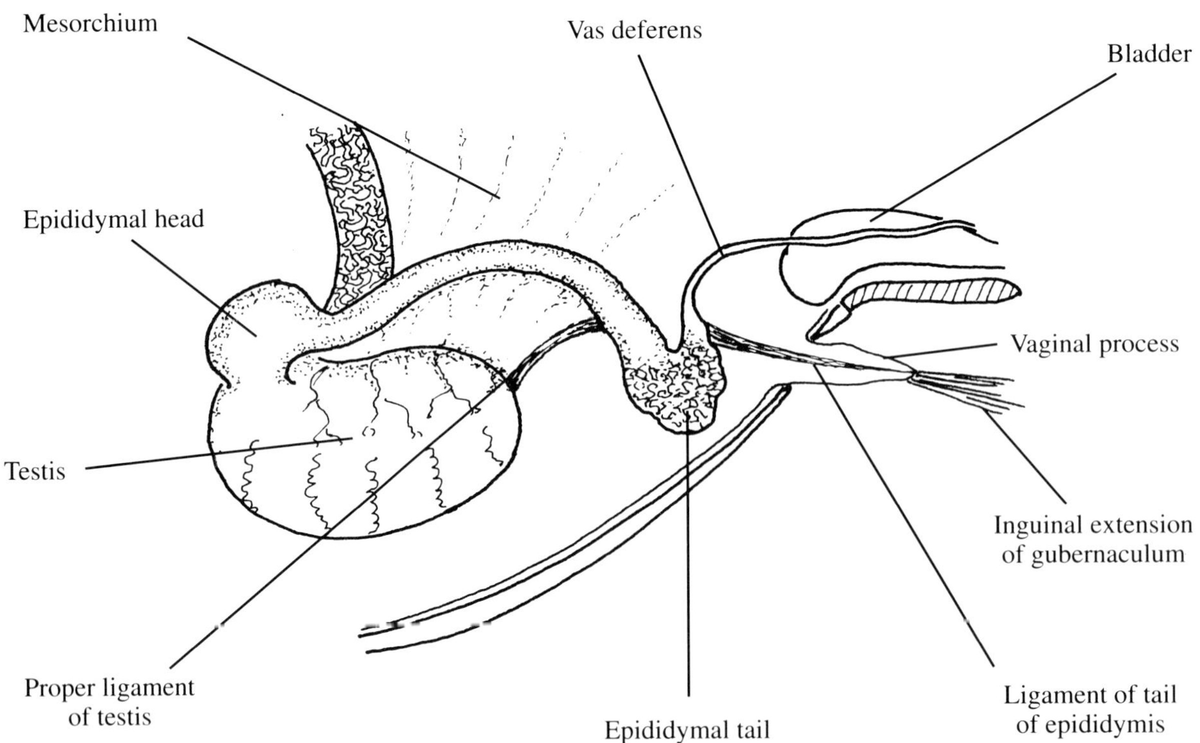

FIG. 98–1. Abdominal testis and epididymis completely retained in the abdomen. The small vaginal process contains the ligament of tail of epididymis.

After inguinal passage is complete, continued growth in length of the mesorchium, blood vessels and the deferent duct allow the testis to move into and occupy the scrotum. Testis growth is probably the final determining factor in ensuring that the testis reaches the scrotum, because congenitally hypoplastic testes or testes with delayed growth do not occupy the scrotum.

The earliest complete descent of both testes is reported as 315 days.[1] Descent of the right testis usually precedes that of the left whereas by birth both testes are usually within or through the inguinal canal. During the first 2 weeks of neonatal life, the vaginal rings contract and become sufficiently fibrous to prevent descent of an abdominal testis. However, some testes that are inguinally located at this time may subsequently descend into the scrotum.

SIGNIFICANCE

The normal process of descent and the anatomy of aberrations in that process are of great importance for the surgeon. Despite differences in size and shape, all structures described as involved in testicular descent are present in normal adult horses and in cryptorchid horses. Their correct isolation and identification by the surgeon is a necessary prelude to successful cryptorchid surgery or probable identification of monorchidism or other developmental abnormality.

CRYPTORCHIDISM

A cryptorchid testis may be retained within the deep inguinal ring, called abdominal, or external to that ring, called inguinal. In each case, two types of retention occur.

TEMPORARY INGUINAL RETENTION

Temporary inguinal retention occurs predominantly, but not entirely, in ponies and is characterized by small testes weighing less than 40 g. The larger testis can generally be palpated in the inguinal region of the quiet standing horse, and testes of all sizes are usually readily palpable in (and can be readily removed from) the anesthetized horse in dorsal recumbency. If not removed, the testes grow and descend into the scrotum usually before the animal is 3 yr old. This type of retention should be distinguished from cases in which testes are temporarily retracted because of fear or resistance to inguinal palpation. The condition is usually unilateral and is predominantly (> 75%) right sided.

The testis has the relationships and the macroscopic appearance of a normal scrotal testis. Because the testis is smaller than most scrotal testes, it appears to have a relatively large epididymis—especially in the older and larger horse.[3]

The microscopic appearance of the testis is that of an immature testis from a 9- to 12-month-old foal with spermatogenic tubules occupying most of the substance of the testis and with few interstitial cells.[4] The spermatogenic tubules contain supporting cells and spermatogonium-like germ cells which fill the tubules. However, the nearer the testis gets to the scrotum, the more mature and normal its appearance becomes. Testes which are almost scrotal may produce spermatozoa in some tubules.

PERMANENT INGUINAL RETENTION

Permanent inguinal retention occurs in all types of horse and is characterized by testes which generally weigh more than 40 g and may be misshapen. The testes cannot always be palpated readily in the standing horse and may sometimes be palpable only with difficulty in the anesthetized horse in dorsal recumbency. Deep palpation may reveal a tail of epididymis within a vaginal process, but this structure may also be present in incomplete abdominal retention. The testis must, by definition, have passed through the deep inguinal ring, but it may still be retained partly within the inguinal canal (Fig. 98–2). The testis usually has a short vaginal tunic and can be brought outside the skin only with difficulty. Animals with this type of retention are sometimes called high-flankers. The condition is usually unilateral and the left or the right testis is retained with equal frequency. Occasionally, the contralateral testis may be abdominally retained.

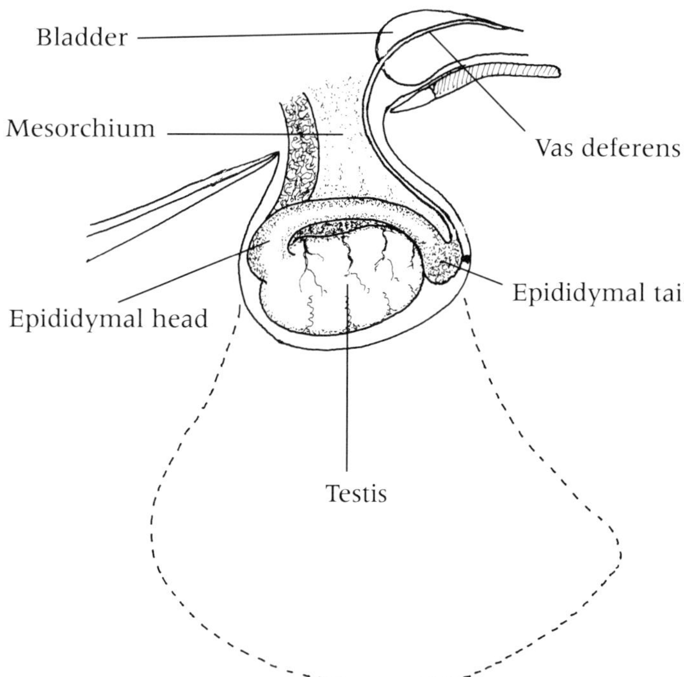

FIG. 98–2. Inguinal testis retained just outside the inguinal canal. The dotted line shows the approximate size and position of the vaginal tunic of a scrotal testis. The mesorchium suspends the vascular cone and deferent duct, the latter passing onto the dorsal surface of the empty bladder.

In the young horse, the microscopic appearance of the testis is similar to a temporarily retained testis, but in the older horse, the number of interstitial cells increases and the tubules show evidence of degeneration, e.g., the supporting cells become vacuolated and the cells aggregate around the periphery of the tubule.

COMPLETE ABDOMINAL RETENTION

In complete abdominal retention, both the testis and epididymis are completely retained within the abdomen (Fig. 98–1). The testis itself is suspended in the abdominal cavity from the sublumbar region by a fold of peritoneum reaching from just caudal to the kidney. The cranial edge of this fold contains the testicular vessels which pass dorsad and craniad from the testis. This fold is then occupied, in succession, passing caudad by (1) the testis, (2) the remains of the proximal part of the true gubernaculum joining testis to epididymal tail (proper ligament of the testis), (3) the epididymal tail itself, and (4) the deferent duct. The proper ligament of the testis is usually longer than that in a scrotal testis, thus separating the epididymal tail from the testis. The body of the epididymis is supported in a minor lateral fold of the peritoneum, thus creating an epididymal sinus similar to that of a normally descended testis. Another small fold of peritoneum passes from the epididymal tail to the area of the deep inguinal ring. This small fold contains the remains of the distal part of the true gubernaculum (ligament of the tail of the epididymis). A small vaginal process with a cremaster muscle develops in the inguinal canal, and only a small fold of peritoneum containing the ligament of the tail of the epididymis enters the inguinal canal within the vaginal process. A few fibrous strands can usually be found in the inguinal region, running distad from the tip of such a vaginal process. These are strands associated with the remains of the infravaginal part of the gubernaculum and are sometimes called the inguinal extension of the gubernaculum. The similarity between all these structures and their relationships and those of the fetal gonad is striking.

The abdominally retained testis, therefore, is somewhat mobile within the abdomen. Although the testis usually lies close to the deep inguinal ring, it may become mixed up with coils of intestine and may lie dorsal to the rectum or lateral to the bladder. In exceptional cases it is adherent to the wall of the abdomen or to other organs, such as the spleen, and may then be exceedingly difficult to identify.[5]

The abdominally retained testis is usually small—normally weighing only between 10 and 20 g—and is characteristically flabby. Occasionally, however, it is grossly enlarged, as a result of teratoma formation, which in some cases is cystic. The testis parenchyma resembles that of a 3- to 4-month-old foal, but with increasing age takes on the appearance of islands of spermatogenic tubules with associated interstitial cells in a sea of loose connective tissue. The spermatogenic cells rarely progress beyond primary spermatogonia (although spermatozoa were reported in one case).[6] The proportion and density of the fibrous tissue increase with age.

INCOMPLETE ABDOMINAL RETENTION

In incomplete abdominal cryptorchidism, the vaginal process is well developed. It has an attached cremaster muscle and contains the epididymal tail as well as part of the deferent duct and part of the body of the epididymis (Fig. 98–3). These latter two structures each have a fold of peritoneum and pass proximally through the vaginal ring toward the bladder and testis, respectively. The length of vaginal tunic is variable, sometimes not extending beyond the limits of the inguinal canal and at others, reaching the scrotum. The vaginal tunic and contents can sometimes be palpated in the standing horse and can often be felt in the inguinal region of the anesthetized horse in dorsal recumbency, when they may be mistaken for a small inguinal testis. The testis is within the abdomen but usually close to the deep inguinal ring and has less potential mobility than found with complete abdominal retention. Its texture and microscopic structure are similar to that of a complete abdominal cryptorchid.

BILATERAL OR UNILATERAL, LEFT OR RIGHT?

In an individual animal, either only one or both testes may be retained and abdominal or inguinal retention can occur on either side.

TABLE 98–1. CRYPTORCHID HORSES SEEN AT THE UNIVERSITY OF LIVERPOOL VETERINARY SCHOOL BETWEEN 1955 AND 1989, INCLUSIVE, CLASSIFIED BY SIDE AND TYPE OF RETENTION

	Position of the Right Testis			
Position of the Left Testis	Scrotal	Inguinal	Incomplete Abdominal	Complete Abdominal
Scrotal	—	208	59	67
Inguinal	104	37	2	3
Incomplete abdominal	22	—	11	1
Complete abdominal	106	5	2	34

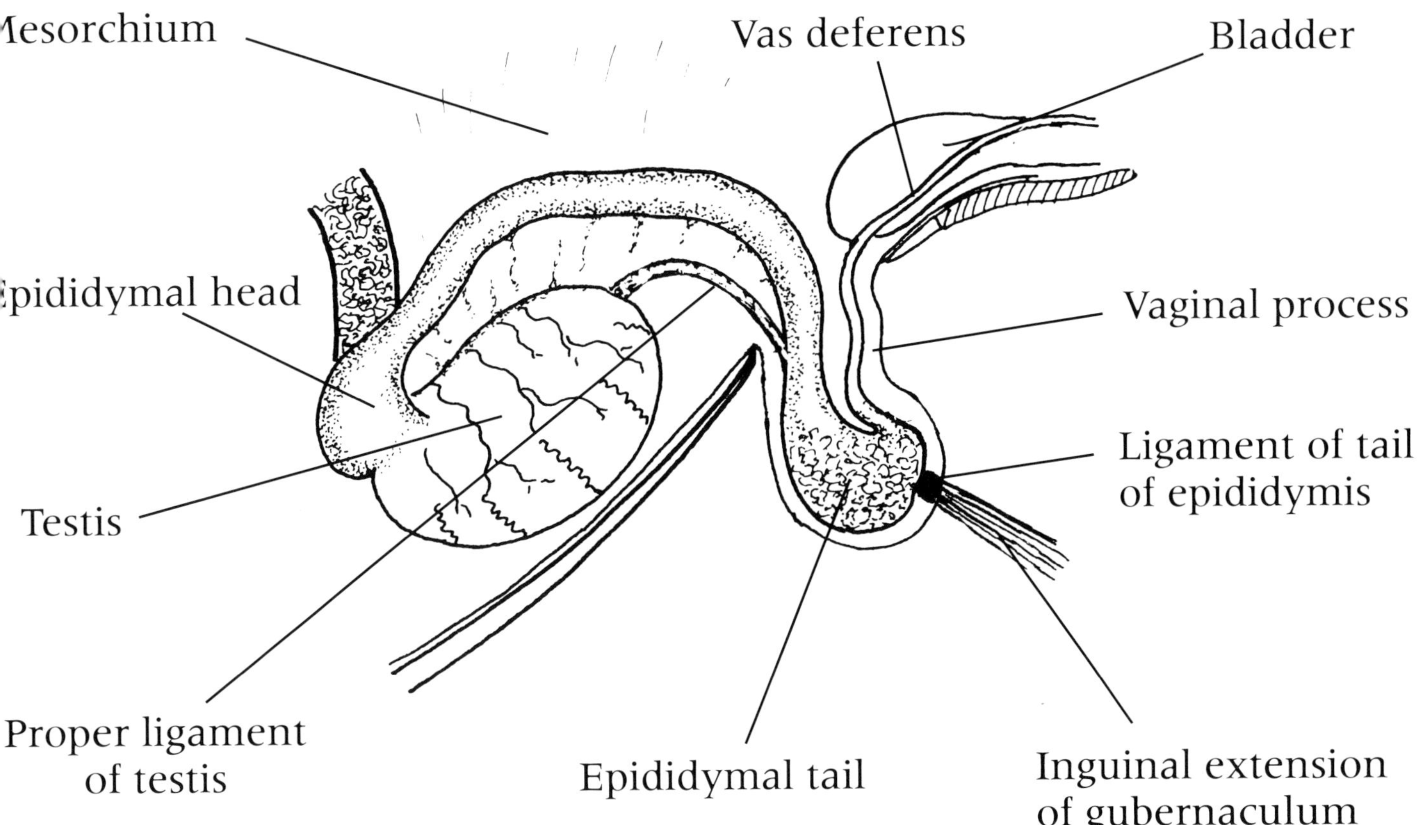

FIG. 98–3. Incomplete abdominal retention with testis in the abdomen, but the epididymal tail has descended through inguinal canal. The vaginal process contains epididymal head, part of epididymal body, and part of deferent duct.

Table 98–1 summarizes information on more than 600 cryptorchid horses castrated at Liverpool since 1955. The table does not distinguish between temporary and permanent inguinal retention, but the high proportion of right-sided unilateral retention is primarily caused by the large number of ponies in the sample.

Incomplete retention occurs in about 50% of cases of unilateral, right-sided abdominal retention but in only about 15 to 20% of unilateral, left-sided cases. In cases with bilateral retention both testes are usually complete or both are incomplete—only three cases of bilateral abdominal retention have been seen at the Liverpool Veterinary School since 1955 in which one side was complete and one incomplete. Irrespective of whether the epididymal tail is or is not descended, in ponies, the left testis is abdominally retained as frequently as the right. However, in Thoroughbreds, Quarter Horses, Trotters, and larger horses such as Cobs and Shires left-sided abdominal cases outnumber right-sided cases by a 2:1 ratio. These findings are discussed elsewhere.[7]

RELATIVE RISK

The spread and control of the condition has been studied.[8] An especially higher relative risk of cryptorchidism occurs in Percherons and an increased relative risk occurs in American Saddle horses, Quarter Horses, and ponies. A noticeably lower relative risk has been found in Thoroughbreds, Standardbreds, Morgans, and Tennessee Walking Horses.

In contrast to other species, developmental defects in the horse such as umbilical and inguinal hernia were significantly less common in cryptorchids than expected. A higher prevalence of "hypoplastic testes" has been recorded in cryptorchid horses,[8] but this is almost certainly an artificial deduction because the majority of cryptorchid testes are naturally hypoplastic.

CAUSES AND GENETICS OF CRYPTORCHIDISM

No good studies of the genetics of cryptorchidism in horses have been conducted, although anecdotal stories of cryptorchid stallions which have thrown cryptorchid colts are widespread, and statements are often made that the condition is the result of an autosomal recessive allele. Extensive studies in pigs, however, have failed to identify either a single gene or polygenes, and no clear-cut pattern of inheritance can be discerned.[9] Nevertheless, decreased prevalence of cryptorchidism in certain breeds (such as Thoroughbreds) and increased prevalence in others (particularly American Quarter

Horses) suggests strongly that the selection processes can exert some control over the condition.

The general premise, in the absence of proof that the condition is caused solely by maternal environment, has been that both inguinal and abdominal cryptorchids should be considered genetically unsound and should not be bred. Two reviews are available.[8,10]

Speculation exists about the mechanism of failure of descent. Hormonal imbalance in the dam and/or fetus has been held to be the primary factor, but because current evidence cannot describe a definite hormonal influence on gubernacular growth, this theory remains speculative. Moreover, the protracted nature of testicular descent in equidae, preparation beginning some 9 months before descent takes place, makes a single explanation unlikely.

The testis must be small enough to descend, and some equine testes may not adequately shrink from their fetal maximum. Increased size probably explains why most teratomas are abdominal, although the clinician should note that some teratomas do reach the scrotum.

The testis must be free to move. Cases have been described in which persistence of a substantial suspensory ligament precluded descent[11] or in which splenic-gonadal fusion occurred.[5]

The role of the gubernaculum is crucial, and—in theory at least—failure or misdirection of gubernacular outgrowth or failure of gubernacular expansion could result in cryptorchidism. Some of these failures have been demonstrated in fetal pigs,[12] but they have not been described in horses.

In the pig, an association exists between inguinal hernia and cryptorchidism—perhaps congenital enlargement of the canal, which then fills with intestine, precludes testicular descent.[13] No such association occurs in horses, and the single most significant factor in causing cryptorchidism in horses seems to be the inordinate growth of the fetal gonad.[2]

SIGNIFICANCE

Unilateral cryptorchid horses, ones with one testis scrotal, will be fertile. A reduction in fertility is only likely to occur if the animal has a large book of mares. However, the condition is no doubt hereditary, and cryptorchid horses should not be used as breeding stallions. Bilaterally cryptorchid horses (or unilateral cryptorchids which have had their scrotal testis removed) will be infertile unless the retained testis (or testes) are temporarily retained in the inguinal region—such testes will produce sperm as they near the scrotum.

Although sperm production is impaired or abolished by cryptorchidism, hormone production is not as drastically curtailed. Testosterone production continues, though a difference of opinion exists as to whether production is impaired[14] or not.[15] Estrone sulfate production, however, does seem to depend not only on age[16] and season[17] but also on testis weight. Because cryptorchid testes are smaller than normal, reduced conjugated estrogen production occurs.

OTHER ABNORMALITIES ASSOCIATED WITH THE TESTIS

ANORCHIDISM

An anorchid is an animal in which neither testis has developed. It does not mean an animal with no scrotal testes. Anorchidism is extremely rare.

MONORCHIDISM

A monorchid is an animal with only one testis, the second not having developed. It does not mean an animal with only one scrotal testis—an animal with one testis scrotal and one retained is a unilateral cryptorchid. A series of cases has recently been described.[18] The authors speculated that some cases of equine monorchidism were acquired (because the vaginal process could usually be readily identified), whereas other cases appear to be primary testicular agenesis. Positive diagnosis rests on finding at surgery (or postmortem) all structures normally associated with the testis in the correct location but no testis. Presumptive diagnosis can be made in a horse, known not to have been castrated previously, in which only one testis is located and for which a later blood test shows to be a gelding.

ECTOPIC TESTIS

An ectopic testis is one which has deviated from the normal pathway of descent. Such testes may lie alongside the penis cranial to the scrotum but are unusual in the horse.

POLYORCHIDISM

A polyorchid is an animal with more than two testes. Although such animals have been described,[19,20] certain diagnosis requires the finding of three testes at the same time, otherwise the possibility of wrong identification of the animal cannot be ruled out. Other possible explanations of apparent polyorchidism are that the epididymis and testis have been mistaken for separate glands, most likely to happen if the animal is an incomplete abdominal cryptorchid. Other possible explanations of polyorchidism are that a hard cyst on the spermatic cord has been diagnosed as an extra testicle.

TERATOMA

A teratoma is a tumor which contains tissue derived from more than one of the three primary germ layers: ectoderm (often neurectoderm), mesoderm, and endoderm. Teratomas occur more commonly in the cryptorchid testis but can occur in scrotal testes.[21] Teratomas appear to be more common in the heavy draft breeds and possibly in Arabs than in other breeds and are probably well established at an early age. Sometimes they are grossly cystic, and the cystic structure appears to be lined by an ependymal epithelium similar to choroid plexus,[22] perhaps induced to develop by the presence of neural elements. At other times they are more solid with lumps of cartilage or bone and may contain either teeth or hair.[23]

In contrast to the situation in humans, teratomas are rarely (if ever) malignant and are, generally speaking, symptomless, only arising as incidental findings at castration. Sometimes they cause problems at cryptorchid castration, because the surgeon is expecting a small flabby testis. Most abdominal teratomas are of a size to preclude removal through the inguinal canal.

HYDROCELE

Hydrocele is an excess of peritoneal fluid in the lumen of the vaginal process. If blood is mixed with the fluid, it is called a haematocele. Although hydrocele may accompany ascites (and the older literature attributes it to a chronic vaginalitis following injury to the scrotum), the cases I have seen have all been congenital and in Shire horses.

Hydrocele is characterized by soft, fluctuating scrotal swelling and is sometimes bilateral. Palpation of the scrotum and inguinal area fails to reveal the presence of intestine or omentum, although in my experience in Shires the inguinal canal is larger than normal. The presence of fluid can make it difficult to palpate the testis, especially in young animals in which the testes are small. The condition does not usually affect the animal, although that pressure from the fluid may cause atrophy of the testis and reduced spermatogenesis.

Diagnosis is usually easy on clinical grounds but may be confirmed by exploratory puncture under surgically clean conditions or by ultrasonography. In animals with hydrocele, a serous, amber-colored fluid escapes. The condition has a superficial resemblence to inguinal hernia and to varicocele and must be distinguished in the gelding from cystic ends to cords.

Medical treatment is unlikely to be of lasting benefit. If the animal is to be castrated this should be done by a "closed" method, because the inguinal canal is probably larger than normal.

INGUINAL HERNIA AND RUPTURE

DEFINITIONS

A hernia or rupture is a protrusion of an organ or part of an organ or other structure through the wall of the cavity normally containing it. A hernia or rupture consists of three parts: (1) the ring is that opening in the cavity wall through which the hernia or rupture occurs, (2) the sac encloses the contents of the hernia or rupture, and (3) the contents of a hernia or rupture involving the abdominal wall are usually intestine and mesenteric support or omentum.

The words *hernia* and *rupture* are often considered to be synonyms, but a clinically useful distinction can be drawn between them.[24] *Rupture* can be used to describe a situation in which discontinuity of tissue has occurred to form an unnatural ring. *Hernia* can be used when the defect forming the ring is natural, even if only in the fetus. Usually, therefore, a hernia has a sac of which the innermost layer is peritoneum, whereas in a rupture, the peritoneal continuity is disrupted and the sac is formed solely by local fascia.

Hernias and ruptures may be classified as reducible or irreducible. The latter may be incarcerated by distension, incarcerated by adhesion, or strangulated.

CONGENITAL INGUINAL HERNIA

In the horse, the commonest form of inguinal hernia forms through the vaginal ring, which is thus the hernial ring (Fig. 98–4A and B). The sac of the hernia is the vaginal tunic, the contents of the hernia occupying its lumen. The terms "direct" and "indirect" as appellations of hernia are confusing because the "direct hernia" that occurs in man (Fig. 98–4C) does not occur in domestic animals (see Chapter 102).

Evidence shows that congenital inguinal hernia is inherited. The condition is extremely rare in horses in the UK, almost certainly because the Horse Breeding Acts in force until the late 1960s forbade the licensing of a stallion with the condition. In the author's opinion, animals with congenital hernia should always be destined for castration and should not be used as breeding animals.

The development of inguinal hernia in the pig has been shown to be closely related to the extent to which the gubernaculum dilates the inguinal canal during the process of testicular descent.[13] One reason, therefore, why congenital inguinal hernia may occur in the horse is because in this species the testis has descended only just before birth, in the process of which the inguinal canal has been dilated by the gubernaculum. In some cases the internal oblique muscle does not completely underlie the superficial inguinal ring. Whether this anatomical abnormality is caused by abnormal gubernacular development or not is unknown, but it clearly predisposes to inguinal hernia.

The presenting sign in the foal is unilateral (or rarely bilateral) scrotal swelling. The swelling may not be large and may not inconvenience the foal. Provided the foal remains fit and continues to grow well, the hernia may be left, and in the great majority of cases, spontaneous resolution will have occurred by 6 to 12 months of age. As the foal and his intestines grow larger, the inguinal canal becomes smaller, the mesentery apparently becomes shorter, and the intestines are gently, but inexorably, returned to the abdominal cavity by peristaltic activity. Sometimes, however, the swelling may be large

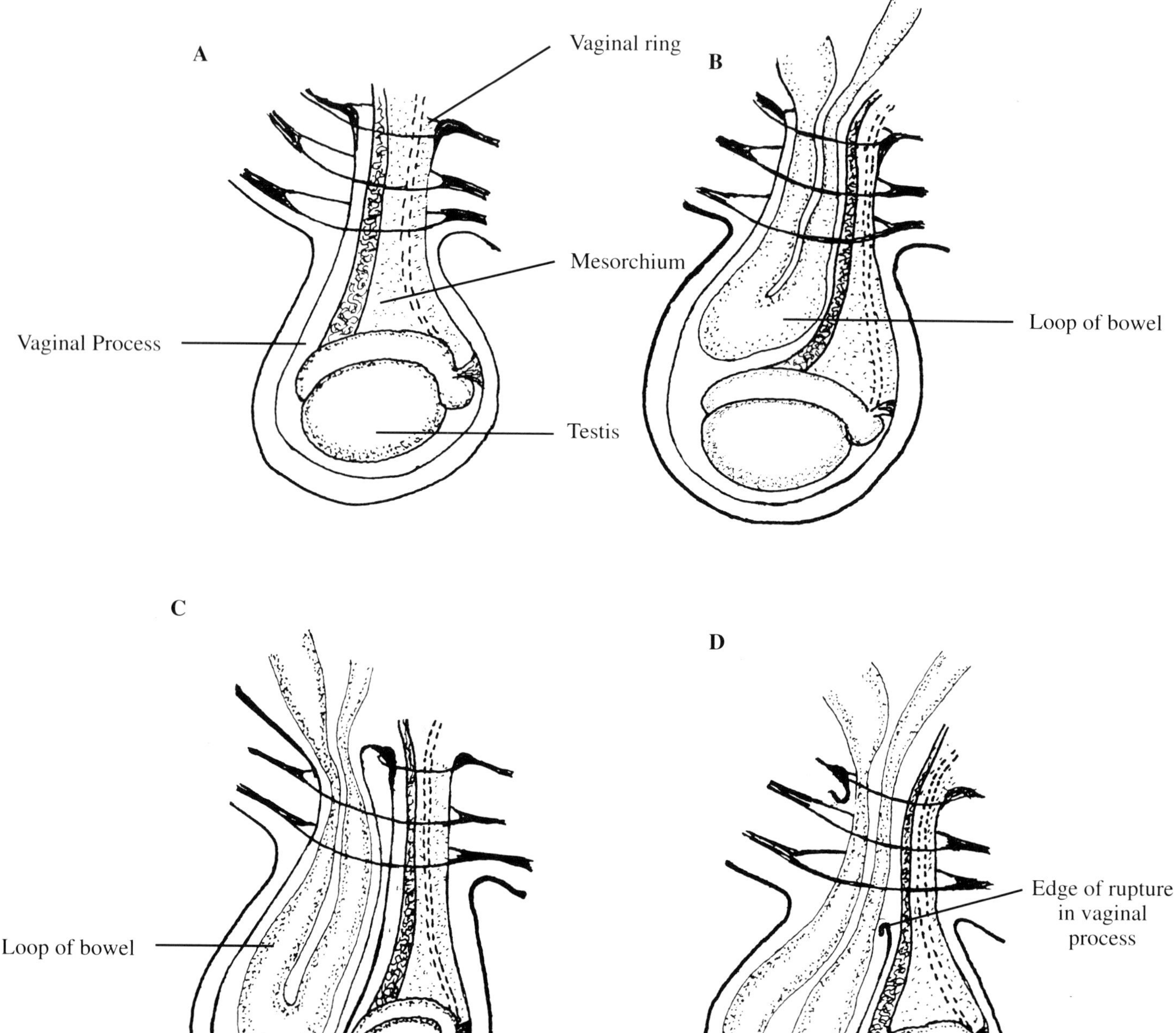

FIG. 98–4. Diagrams of different types of hernia and rupture in the inguinal region. *A,* Normal anatomy of vaginal process showing testis suspended by mesorchium. *B,* Inguinal hernia (indirect) showing loop of intestine within vaginal process. *C,* Inguinal hernia (direct) showing loop of intestine within peritoneal pouch independent of the vaginal process—this type of hernia does not occur in the domestic animal. *D,* Diagram of inguinal rupture with loop of intestine ruptured through vaginal tunic and lying outside the vaginal process.

enough to interfere with walking or galloping or so large as to impede lymphatic drainage from the preputial area, which thus becomes edematous. In such a case, or if deterioration is noted in the foal's condition or if he fails to grow as quickly as normal, the hernia should be repaired immediately (see Chapter 102). Although the condition may possibly resolve completely and the inguinal rings may become normal in size, in some cases the inguinal rings remain slightly enlarged and the abdominal contents herniate more readily when the animal is castrated. Care should always be taken, therefore, to perform a "closed" castration on a horse with a history of inguinal hernia as a foal.

INGUINAL RUPTURE

In inguinal rupture, prolapse of intestinal contents occurs through a rupture in the parietal layer of the vaginal tunic (Fig. 98–4D), usually just external to the deep inguinal ring but sometimes involving the vaginal ring itself.[25] The prolapsed intestine comes to lie cranial to the spermatic sac in the loose fascia without a peritoneal sac. With the passage of time, a fibrous sac may develop, with or without adhesions between the intestine and sac.

The foal with this condition may have had a congenital hernia or the foal may have been normal at birth but was kicked or otherwise injured immediately before the development of scrotal swelling. Van der Velden believes the rupture actually occurs at parturition.[25] Clinicians may have difficulty distinguishing rupture from hernia in the early stages, though in the former the swelling does not resolve and the contents are not usually totally reducible. In some cases, the extent of the prolapse results in disruption of subcutaneous tissues over a wide area and the blood supply of the skin is compromised. The skin then becomes edematous, macerated, or even necrotic and may not heal well after surgery.

In other cases, the disruption is less severe and the foal may not grow as well as expected or may actually deteriorate. Actual colic, except briefly after the original traumatic incident, is unusual, which is radically different from the comparable situation in the older horse in which intestine becomes strangulated in the inguinal canal. In the newborn foal the canal is so large, because it is dilated by the gubernaculum and testis, that strangulation is unlikely. Discomfort, however, is more marked than with congenital hernia. Any apparently congenital hernia which is not readily reducible or which does not progress toward spontaneous resolution should be investigated surgically.

ABNORMALITIES ASSOCIATED WITH THE PENIS

Rare congenital anomalies of the penis include congenitally short penis, retroverted penis, aplasia or dysgenesis of the corpus spongiosum glandis, aplasia of the prepuce, hypospadias (in which the urethra opens on the ventral surface of the penis or in the perineal region), and epispadias (in which the urethra opens on the dorsal surface of the penis).[26]

Varying types of intersex (Chapters 30 and 47) are also present with abnormalities of the penis and prepuce. The true hermaphrodite, with both male and female external genitalia and both ovarian and testicular tissue (either conjoined or separate) is rare, but a case has been described.[27] Although a yearling, the animal showed no sexual desire. The penis was incomplete and, though the urethral opening was in the normal place, urination in the sheath caused chronic urine scald. Subsequent surgery revealed both ovarian and testicular tissues in vestigial gonads at the ends of uterine tubes. The female pseudohermaphrodite, with ovaries but external genitalia which are primarily male, is also rare.[28]The male pseudohermaphrodite is more common, often presenting as a mare with an enlarged clitoris or, if old enough, with stallion-like behavior. These animals are genetic females (XX) but usually have cryptorchid (inguinal or abdominal) testes. Internally, although a uterus-like structure in the genital fold is often found, the vestibule is blind and terminates at the level of the urethral opening. Externally, the udder is sometimes enlarged and a penis-like structure (of varying size and capable of erection) with a urethral opening is enclosed in a vulva-like prepuce anywhere between the anus and the umbilicus.

Horses with these congenital deformities usually require castration for behavioral reasons. Imaginative plastic reconstruction is possible.[29,30] The animals are unlikely to be fertile.

REFERENCES

1. Bergin, W.C., Gier, H.T., Marion, G.B., and Coffman, J.R.: A developmental concept of equine cryptorchidism. Biol. Reprod., *3*:82–92, 1970.
2. Cole, H.H., Hart, G.H., Lyons, W.R., and Catchpole, H.R.: The development and hormonal content of fetal horse gonads. Anat. Rec., *56*:275–289, 1936.
3. Bishop, M.W.H., David, J.S.E., and Messervey, A.: Some observations on cryptorchidism in the horse. Vet. Rec., *76*:1041–1048, 1964.
4. Arighi, M., Singh, A., and Bosu, W.T.K.: Histology of the normal and retained equine testis. Acta Anat., *129*:127–139, 1987.
5. Noakes, D.E., and White, R.A.S.: Splenic gonadal fusion in the horse. Vet. Rec., *98*:382–383, 1976.
6. Hobday, F.T.G.: Castration (Including Cryptorchids and Caponing) and Ovariotomy. Edinburgh, W. Johnston, 1914.
7. Cox, J.E., Edwards, G.B., and Neal, P.A.: An analysis of 500 cases of equine cryptorchidism. Equine Vet. J., *11*:113–116, 1979.
8. Hayes, H.M.: Epidemiological features of 5009 cases of equine cryptorchidism. Equine Vet. J., *18*:467–471, 1986.
9. Mikami, H., and Fredeen, H.T.: A genetic study of cryp-

torchidism and scrotal hernia in pigs. Can. J. Genet. Cytol., *21*:9–19, 1979.

10. Leipold, H.W., et al.: Cryptorchidism in the horse: Genetic implications. Proc. Amer. Assoc. Equine Pract., *31*:579–590, 1986.

11. Wilson, D.G., and Nixon, A.J.: Case of equine cryptorchidism resulting from persistence of the suspensory ligament of the gonad. Equine Vet. J., *18*:412–413, 1986.

12. Wensing, C.J.G.: Testicular descent in some domestic mammals. II. The nature of the gubernacular change during the process of testicular descent in the pig. Proc. Konige Nederland. Akad. Wetenschaft, *C76*:190–195, 1973.

13. Wensing, C.J.G., and Colenbrander, B.: Cryptorchidism and Inguinal Hernia. Proc. Konige Nederland. Akad. Wetenschaft, *C76*:489–494, 1973.

14. Cox, J.E.: Testosterone concentrations in normal and cryptorchid horses. Response to human chorionic gonadotrophin. Anim. Reprod. Sci., *18*:43–50, 1989.

15. Ganjam, V.K., and Kenney, R.M.: Androgens and oestrogens in normal and cryptorchid stallions. J. Reprod. Fertil. Suppl., *23*:67–73, 1975.

16. Velle, W.: Urinary oestrogens in the male. J. Reprod. Fertil., *12*:65–73, 1966.

17. Raeside, J.I.: Seasonal changes in the concentration of oestrogens and testosterone in the plasma of stallions. Anim. Reprod. Sci., *1*:205–212, 1978.

18. Parks, A.H., Scott, E.A., Cox, J.E., and Stick, J.A.: Monorchidism in the horse. Equine Vet. J., *21*:215–217, 1989.

19. Foster, A.E.C.: Polyorchidism. Vet. Rec., *64*:158, 1952.

20. Earnshaw, R.E.: Polyorchidism. Can. J. Comp. Med., *23*:66, 1959.

21. Willis, R.A., and Rudduck, H.B.: Testicular teratomas in horses. J. Comp. Pathol. Bacteriol., *55*:165–171, 1943.

22. Parks, A.H., Wyn-Jones, G., Cox, J.E., and Newsholme, B.J.: Partial obstruction of the small colon associated with an abdominal testicular teratoma in a foal. Equine Vet. J., *18*:342–343, 1986.

23. Cotchin, E.: Equine testicular teratoma. *In* Tumours of early life in man and animals, Proceedings of the Sixth Perugia Quadrennial International Conference on Cancer, Perugia, Italy. Edited by L. Severi. 1978, p. 20.

24. Cox, J.E.: Hernias and ruptures: Words to the heat of deeds. Equine Vet. J., *20*:155–156, 1988.

25. Van der Velden, M.A.: Ruptured inguinal hernia in newborn colt foals: A review of 14 cases. Equine Vet. J., *20*:178–181, 1988.

26. Vaughan, J.T.: Surgery of the prepuce and penis. Proc. Am. Assoc. Equine Pract., *18*:19–40, 1972.

27. Walker, D.F., and Vaughan, J.T.: Bovine and Equine Urogenital Surgery. Philadelphia, Lea & Febiger, 1980.

28. Roberts, S.J.: Veterinary Obstetrics and Genital Diseases. Ithaca NY, published by the author, 1971.

29. Bracken, F.K., and Wagner, P.C.: Cosmetic surgery for equine pseudohermaphrodism. Vet. Med. Small Anim. Clin., *78*:879–884, 1983.

30. Trotter, G.W.: Normal and Cryptorchid Castration. *In* Urogenital Surgery. Vet. Clin. North Am.: Equine Practice, *4*:493–513, 1988.

SECTION D

REPRODUCTIVE SURGERY OF THE STALLION

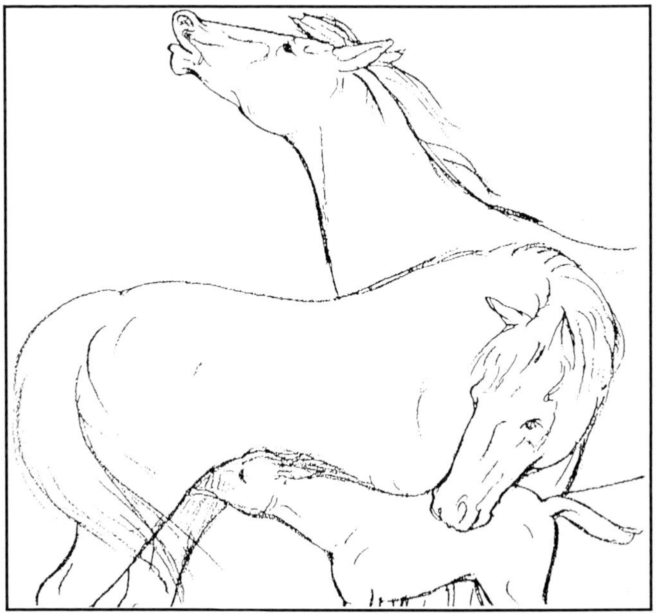

CHAPTER 99

CASTRATION

G.W. Trotter

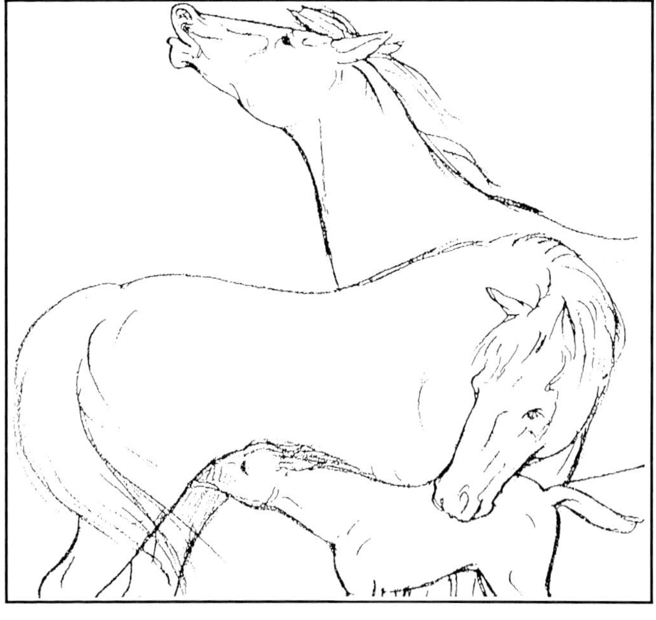

Castration is one of the most common surgical procedures performed in horses. Although it is a relatively simple procedure to complete, some basic preoperative and postoperative guidelines should be followed to ensure success and minimize complications. Most male horses are castrated to eliminate aggressive male behavior in animals not intended to become breeding stallions. Other indications for castration include tumors, varicocele, hydrocele, testicular trauma, orchitis/periorchitis, spermatic cord torsion, and most cases of scrotal hernia.[1–5]

The age at which a horse should be castrated is optional. Traditionally, most horses are castrated near 1 yr of age. Some prefer to delay castration until the horse is 2 yr old so that masculine traits develop more fully. Support for this contention is largely subjective. Others prefer to castrate when the animal is a few weeks to a few months old to avoid the nuisance of masculine behavior as the animal becomes more sexually mature.

Castration is effective to eliminate male behavior, but persistent mounting, with copulatory and ejaculatory behavior can persist in some geldings.[6,7] Such horses are referred to as being proud cut or as false rigs, the inference being that castration was not properly completed.[8,9] Some geldings also display aggressiveness toward other horses and people.[8,9] In a study in which the behavior of geldings was compared after castration, no significant difference was noticed in sexual and aggressive behaviors whether colts were castrated prepuberally (< 2 yr of age) or as stallions (> 3 yr of age).[8] The authors did not indicate whether any horses were castrated at or less than 1 yr of age or whether any of the horses that still displayed aggressive behavior had been castrated at less than 1 yr. However, 20 to 30% of geldings displayed stallion-like sexual behavior and aggression toward other horses, and 5% were aggressive toward people. Therefore, sexual behavior in male horses seems to be only partially dependent on the presence of testosterone or may be related to steroid metabolites originating endogenously or exogenously.

Technically, to castrate a horse and not to remove the entire testis and epididymis is difficult. Furthermore, the epididymis is incapable of producing testosterone, and proud-cut horses produce no more testosterone than normally behaved geldings.[9,10] The presumption that behaviorally aggressive geldings may have an abnormally high adrenal source of androgens has also been disproven by finding that proud-cut horses respond the same as normal geldings to exogenous adrenocorticotropic hormone.[9] Some anecdotal reports describe improvement in the behavior of some aggressive geldings after reoperation and removal of a segment of the remaining spermatic cord.[7] Success with this approach more likely reflects altered training or handling after surgery than any real benefit from further cord excision. Some proud-cut horses are possibly unilateral cryptorchids and perhaps only the tail of the epididymis was removed from the cryptorchid side at previous castration.[11] Cryptorchidectomy is required in such cases.

Spermatozoa may remain in the ampulla and ductus deferens for many months after castration. However,

Shideler et al. have shown that spermatozoa in ejaculates collected 7 to 8 days after castration are nonmotile and unlikely to result in fertilization.[12]

ANESTHESIA

For standing castration, a combination of chemical sedation and local infiltration anesthesia is usually used. Some prefer to not use chemical sedation but to complete surgery using local anesthesia and the aid of a twitch or a lip chain. Detomidine has also been used successfully for standing castration without needing further local anesthetic.[13]

Anesthesia of the testis and spermatic cord can be achieved in many ways. Some prefer to inject local anesthetic into the spermatic cord at the level of the superficial inguinal ring.[1] Others inject anesthetic directly into the testicular parenchyma, presumably gaining cord anesthesia by diffusion from the pampiniform plexus.[14] Anesthesia of the scrotal skin is gained by local infiltration on either side of the midline raphe or by depositing a small volume of anesthetic subcutaneously as the needle is withdrawn after intratesticular anesthetic administration.[1]

Numerous drugs or drug combinations have been used for castration under general anesthesia.[15,16] Xylazine (1.1 mg/kg) followed by ketamine (2.2 mg/kg) is a commonly used anesthetic regimen.[15,17] Xylazine (0.55 mg/kg) followed by thiopental or thiamylal sodium (6.6 mg/kg) has also been recommended. Acepromazine or xylazine followed by a guaifenesin-barbiturate mixture is also used.[17] A recommended dose is 0.04 mg/kg promazine, 100 mg/kg guaifenesin, and 4 mg/kg thiopental.[17] Most of these combinations give 15 to 20 min of operative time. Succinylcholine has been popular as an immobilizing agent used for castration. Castration could be completed, and the animal was able to stand soon after surgery.[18] Succinylcholine is a neuromuscular blocking agent and has no anesthetic properties. Respiratory failure, tachycardia, hypertension, dysrhythmias, and direct myocardial damage are reported complications associated with the use of succinylcholine. With the excellent short-acting anesthetic regimens currently available, no justification remains for the use of succinylcholine in equine castration.

METHODS OF CASTRATION

ANATOMIC CONSIDERATIONS

For all surgical techniques, tissue layers encountered at surgery are the same. Starting at the skin, the tissue layers in sequence are the dartos, external spermatic fascia, cremasteric fascia and cremaster muscle, internal spermatic fascia, parietal layer of vaginal tunic, visceral layer of vaginal tunic, and tunica albuginea. When the tunic-contained testis and spermatic cord are stripped free of surrounding tissues at surgery, the blunt dissection occurs between the external spermatic and the cremasteric fascia.[1]

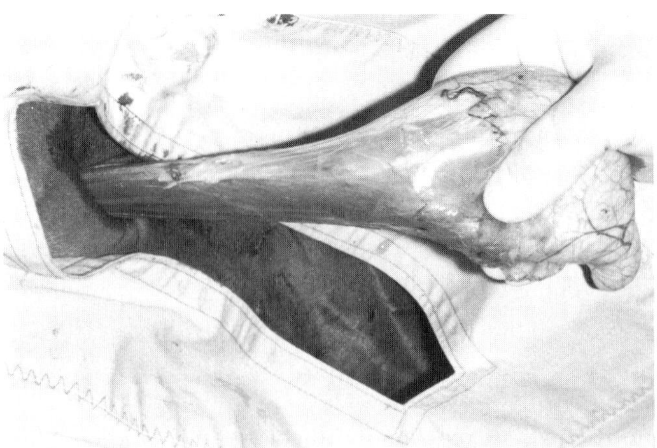

FIG. 99–1. Removal of the right testis from a horse in dorsal recumbency. Unless the testis is rotated within the scrotum, the cremaster muscle should lie on the lateral aspect of the parietal layer of the vaginal tunic. The tail of the epididymis forms a bulge at the caudal pole of the testis.

Over most of the scrotum, the dartos is closely attached to the scrotal skin. The dartos forms the scrotal septum, and at the caudoventral aspect of the scrotum, the scrotal ligament attaches the dartos to the parietal layer of the vaginal tunic. The cremaster muscle also attaches to the lateral aspect of the parietal layer of the vaginal tunic (Fig. 99–1). This muscle orientation will differ only in those unusual cases in which the testis is rotated 180° within the scrotum. The epididymis is located on the proximal and lateral aspect of the testis; the head is cranially located and the tail is caudally located. The epididymal sinus is the cavity formed between the loosely attached body of the epididymis and the testis. The proper ligament of the testis connects the tail of the epididymis to the testis, and the ligament of the epididymis connects the tail of the epididymis to the parietal layer of the vaginal tunic. The mesorchium supports the structures of the spermatic cord, including the neurovascular structures cranially and the ductus deferens caudally (Fig. 99–2).

OPEN VERSUS CLOSED CASTRATION

Definitions differ regarding what represents an open or closed castration. Some consider a closed castration to be one for which the parietal layer of the vaginal tunic is never opened before transfixation ligature placement around the cord with emasculation just distal to the ligature.[1] Others consider open versus closed to refer to whether the parietal layer of the vaginal tunic is incised and the testis prolapsed before ligation and/or emasculation of the spermatic cord.[19] The term half-closed has also been used to describe the technique where the vaginal tunic is initially opened but is subsequently closed by crushing, with or without the use of a ligature.[20] In cases for which intraoperative pull of the cremaster muscle is excessive, opening the vaginal tunic and prolapsing the testis gives relatively relaxed access to the testis and vascular portion of the spermatic cord. Care must be taken during open castration that excessive tension is not placed on the neurovascular portion of the cord leading to rupture of the spermatic artery. Traction that is required should be placed on the caudal musculofibrous portion of the cord (Fig. 99–3).

STANDING CASTRATION

Both testes should be well descended into the scrotum, and the patient reasonably tractable and handled by an experienced handler. The right-handed surgeon is positioned on the left side of the horse as is the handler. The left hand grasps the scrotum from in front and the testes are tensed distally into the scrotum. Two parallel incisions are made equidistant from the median raphe and in a cranial to caudal direction for the length of the testis. These incisions extend through the skin and dartos.[21] Some prefer to make an initial bold incision that extends from the skin through the parietal layer of the vaginal tunic; this prolapses the testis out of the tunic but makes subsequent separation of the tunic from surrounding fascia more difficult.[1,17] Blunt dissection is used to free the testis and spermatic cord contained within the vaginal tunic from the surrounding fascia. An incision is then made through the tunic at or proximal to the cranial pole of the testis and the testis is prolapsed from the tunic. Tunic incision near the cranial pole allows for eversion of the parietal layer of the vaginal tunic to form a cul-de-sac that can be used as a finger hold or handle for further manipulation (Fig. 99–4). It also eliminates much of the pull of the cremaster muscle on the testis and allows removal of a longer portion of the spermatic cord.[21] The emasculator is then placed proximal to the testis, advanced toward the scrotum, and applied to the cord at its most proximal extent. In mature stallions, the mesorchium should be perforated above the epididymis and the cord separated into its cranial neurovascular and caudal musculofibrous portions before emasculation. The emasculator is applied first to the neurovascular portion before removing the musculofibrous (cremaster muscle, vaginal tunic, and ductus deferens) portion. Alternatively, the neurovascular portion of the cord can be independently ligated before emasculating the rest of the cord (Fig. 99–5). The emasculator should be applied directly transversely rather than obliquely and should remain in place for at least 1 min. After both testes are removed, any loose tags of fascia or fat that could protrude from the incision should be removed.

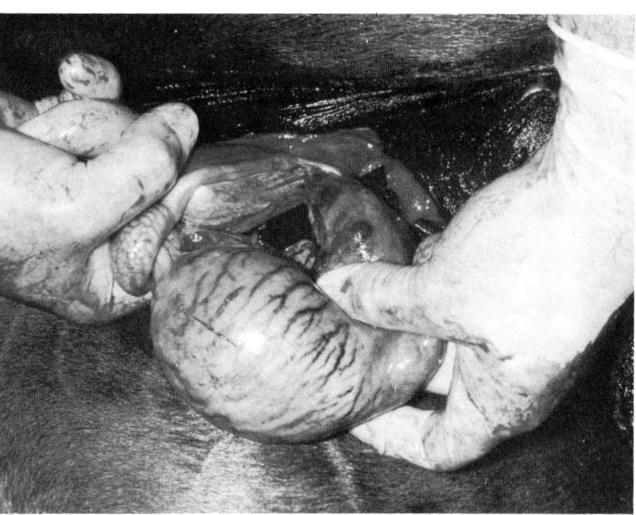

FIG. 99–3. Removal of the left testis from a horse in left lateral recumbency. The mesorchium has been penetrated to divide the spermatic cord into its cranial neurovascular component and its caudal musculofibrous component.

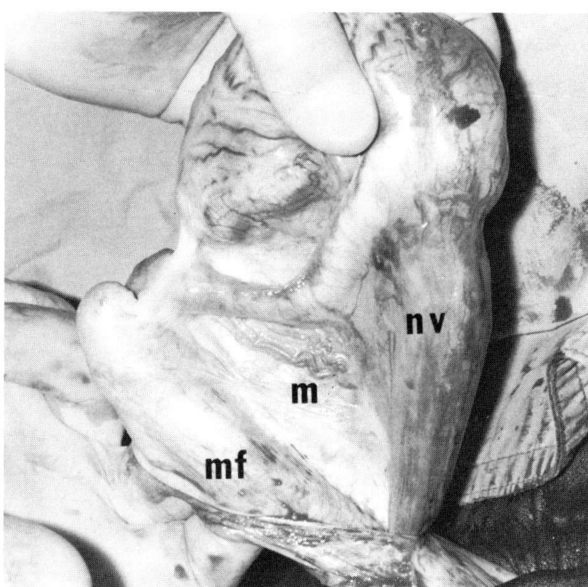

FIG. 99–2. The mesorchium (m) connects the neurovascular cranial portion of the spermatic cord (nv) and the more musculofibrous caudal portion of the spermatic cord (mf). The ductus deferens courses with the caudal portion of the cord (left testis from a horse in dorsal recumbency).

CASTRATION IN LATERAL RECUMBENCY

For right-handed operators, the horse should be positioned in left lateral recumbency. A cotton rope preplaced around the neck helps with guiding the horse into left recumbency, and it is then conveniently in place for securing the upper hindlimb forward and out of the operative field. Once the horse is recumbent, the horse handler should be situated behind the horse's head. The surgical techniques that are used are the same as or similar to those used for standing castration. Some prefer to use transfixation ligatures in conjunction with emasculation (Fig. 99–6).[1] Although this procedure takes somewhat longer to complete, the liga-

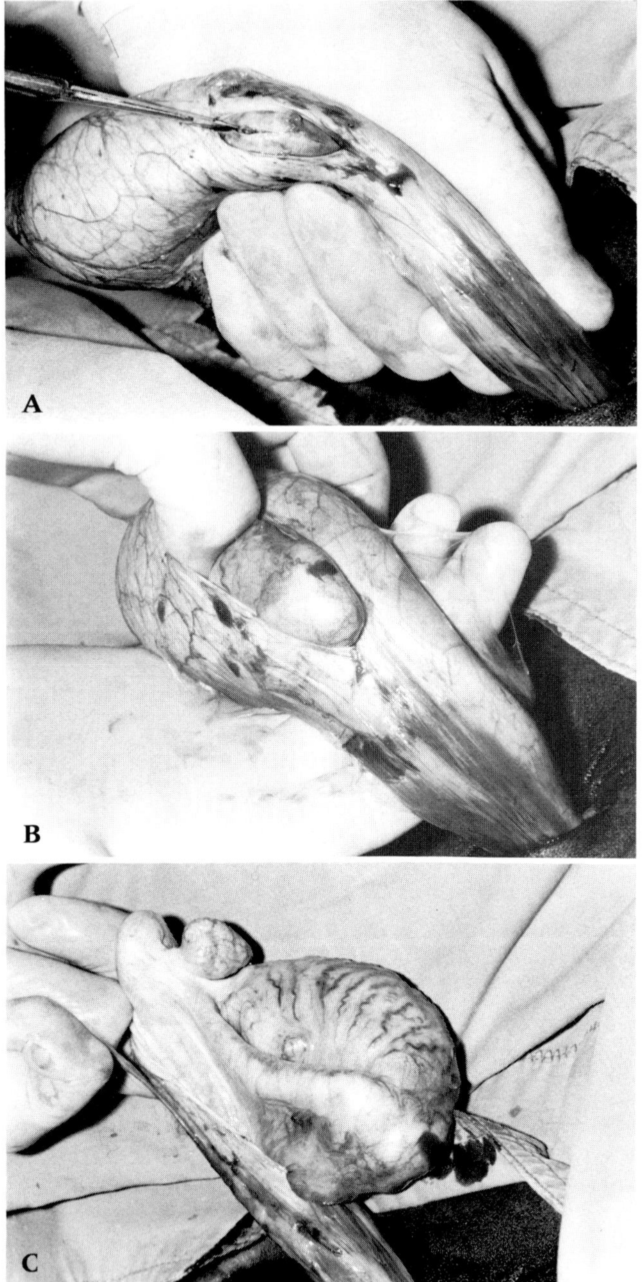

FIG. 99–4. *A,* Removal of left testis from a horse in dorsal recumbency. For an open castration, the incision through the parietal layer of the vaginal tunic should be made near the cranial pole of the testis. *B,* The testis is then prolapsed through the tunic incision. *C,* The reflected vaginal tunic can be used as a finger hold for traction.

ture would obviously prevent any viscera from descending through the remaining vaginal tunic once the horse stands. Others complete the castration procedure using the open or closed techniques as previously described. Another procedure combines ligation of the spermatic cord with transection of the scrotal ligament; the vaginal tunic is allowed to retract into and remain in the inguinal canal.[22] Although this technique does

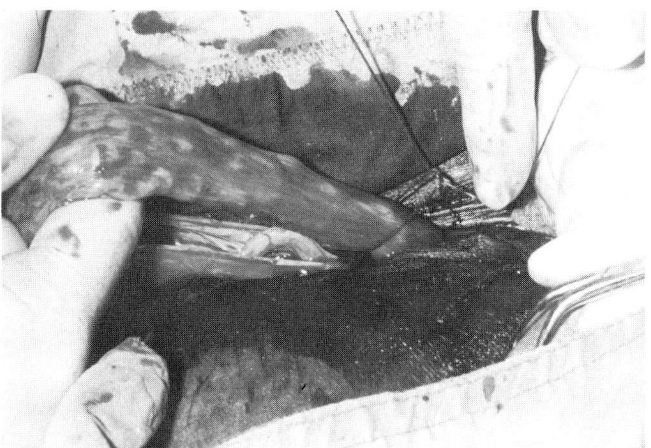

FIG. 99–5. The neurovascular portion of the cord can be ligated independently from the rest of the cord. In mature stallions with a large spermatic cord, separate vessel ligation may be indicated.

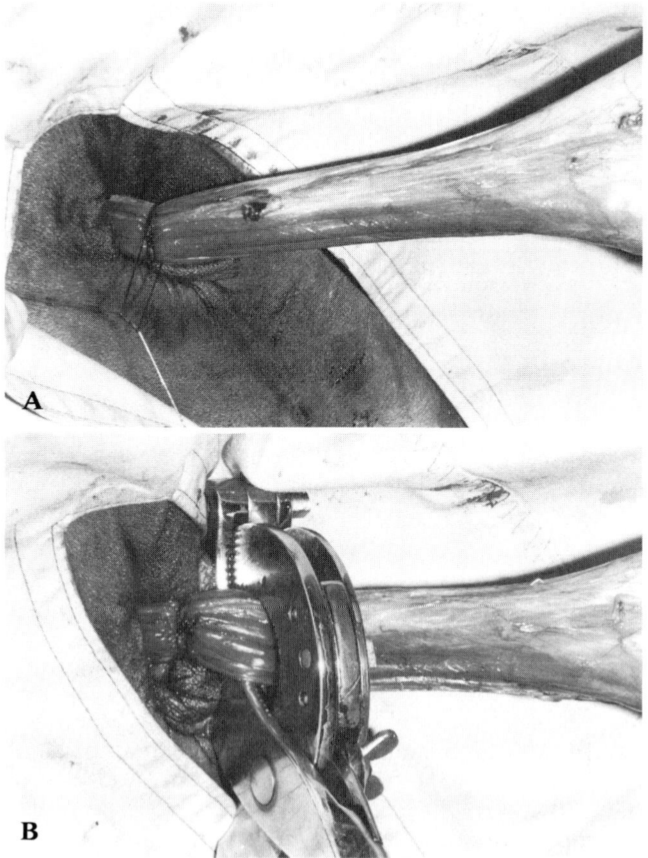

FIG. 99–6. *A,* A transfixation ligature has been secured and looped around the entire spermatic cord and vaginal tunic. Large-diameter suture material is used, and it must be secured tightly to avoid loose application (right testis with horse in dorsal recumbency, cranial is left). *B,* The cord is then emasculated distal to the transfixation ligature. Care should be taken to apply the emasculator transversely rather than obliquely.

not use emasculation and crushing of tissues, little else exists to recommend it, and the retained cremaster muscle and vaginal tunic could contribute to local or ascending infection in certain cases.[23]

Removal of the scrotal septum is an option for castration using any of the described procedures in which the scrotal wound(s) is left open. Advocates of the technique believe better postoperative drainage is provided if the septum is removed.

CASTRATION WITH PRIMARY CLOSURE

Traditional castration techniques allow second intention healing of the scrotal wounds. Numerous reports also advocate primary closure with first intention healing.[24–28] Although most of the techniques are not routinely suited for field use, they can be of benefit in certain cases in which castrations are done in other than field conditions. Reported advantages include early return to work, ease of postoperative management, more favorable early cosmetic result, fewer postoperative complications, and no possibility of eventration.[24] Disadvantages include longer surgery time, the increased cost, and the need, in most cases, for a suitable facility where the surgery can be completed. Other indications for primary closure include cases for which eventration is more likely after surgery, castration when insect populations are high, castration of the unilateral cryptorchid, castration when postoperative management of the patient will be difficult, castration associated with scrotal hernias, and castration done in conjunction with another procedure for which stall rest is necessary. In breeding stallions for whom unilateral elective castration is indicated, primary closure should also be used to keep perioperative swelling to a minimum.[24] Such a unilateral castration can be done with minimal interruption to a normal breeding schedule.

Dorsal recumbency is recommended when primary closure will be used. Operative conditions also need to be of a higher standard than when castration wounds will be allowed to heal by second intention. Lowe and Dougherty,[27] and later Hoffman,[28] described a technique in which skin incisions were made midway between the scrotum and the superficial inguinal ring. The parietal layer of the vaginal tunic was incised, the scrotal ligament was incised, and the contents of the vaginal tunic were removed. Spermatic cord vessels were ligated, and the vaginal tunic incisions closed. The loose spermatic fascia was apposed, and subcuticular sutures were used to appose the skin. Surgery time was more protracted than for conventional castration, and transient scrotal swelling developed in a number of cases. Cox later described a primary closure technique that he believed was adapted to field use.[25] Patients were positioned in dorsal recumbency, and the testes were isolated as they would be for a closed castration. Either emasculation alone or emasculation plus ligation was used on the spermatic cord. Closure was simply a continuous horizontal mattress suture pattern in the skin using absorbable suture material. Surgery time was sufficiently short to make the technique potentially useful in the field, but a stricter standard of asepsis than what is often available under field conditions was necessary.

Other reports documented varying degrees of scrotal ablation in conjunction with closure of the deeper fascial tissue layers for castration with primary closure (Fig. 99–7).[24,26] With these techniques, less postoperative scrotal region swelling was seen than with some of the other primary closure techniques.

POSTOPERATIVE MANAGEMENT

All horses should receive or be current regarding tetanus immunization. Regulated exercise is recommended for the first 7 to 10 days to help minimize postoperative swelling and stiffness. Perioperative antibacterial therapy is unnecessary unless the conditions under which the procedure was completed were less than optimal.

COMPLICATIONS OF CASTRATION

Complications after castration represent one of the major categories of malpractice claims in equine surgery.[23,24] The most frequently reported complications include hemorrhage, eventration, edema, and infection.[23] Less frequently reported complications include unaltered behavior, hydrocele, varicocele, peritonitis, penile trauma, penile paralysis, and injuries to personnel during induction or recovery.[23,24]

Significant postoperative hemorrhage usually originates from the testicular artery. Other potential sources of hemorrhage include the scrotal skin or the large pudendal vessels that may have been damaged by overzealous dissection in the inguinal region. If hemorrhage of testicular artery origin is present, the patient may need to be reanesthetized to allow definitive hemostasis.

In one study, eventration was reported in 11 of 371 horses that were castrated.[29] More recently, an incidence of 0.4 to 0.8% was reported for eventration after castration in larger groups of horses.[20] Factors such as intra-abdominal pressure, position of the animal, and size of the vaginal ring have all been incriminated in the development of eventration.[20] The inguinal canal is also thought to open when the hindlimb is flexed, making the period of time associated with assumption of sternal recumbency and standing particularly prone to eventration.[20] Some recommend that a transfixation ligature should always be used at castration to prevent this possibility.[20] Eventration has also occurred in some cases where the scrotal wound was closed primarily but the vaginal tunic had not been closed.[20]

Most horses that eventrate intestine do so within the first few hours after surgery, and their early detection and immediate treatment is vital to a successful outcome. The offending viscera is usually the small intestine, and it needs to be adequately cleaned and protected until it can be replaced. Omentum also prolapses through the inguinal canal, but its presence may not be

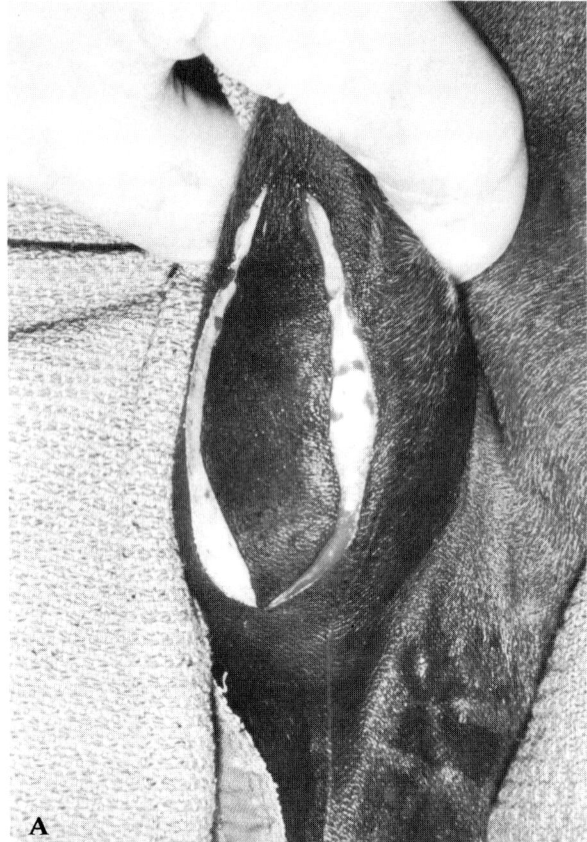

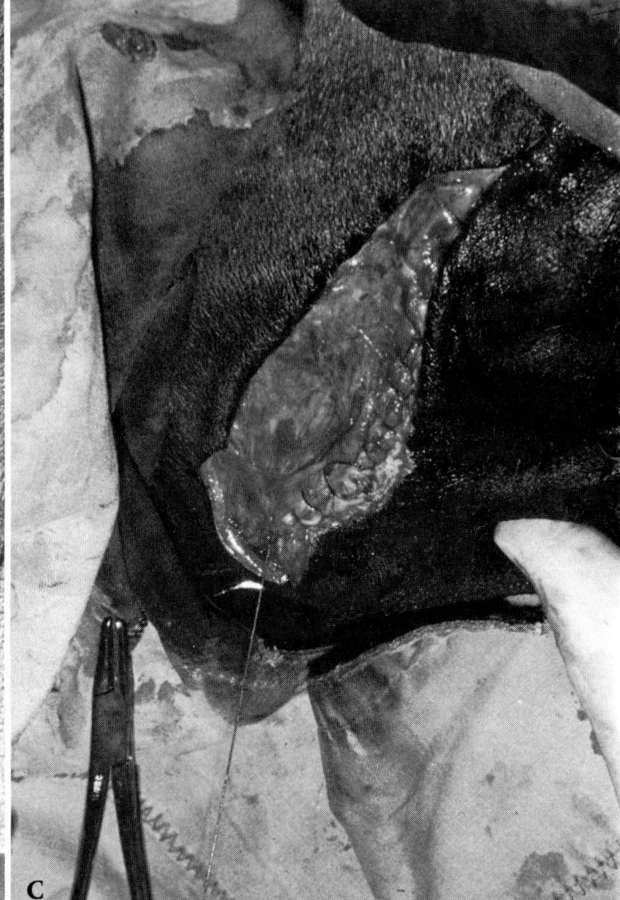

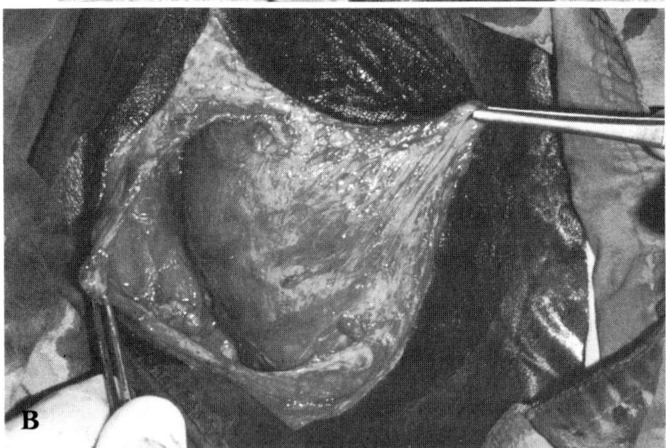

FIG. 99–7. *A*, Excision of an elliptical piece of scrotal skin minimizes the chances of redundant skin hanging from the scrotal region. In mature stallions, this excised piece of skin can be quite large. The horse pictured was a unilateral cryptorchid. *B*, Appearance of the scrotal wound after ligation and emasculation and just before closure. The penis is bulging into the surgical field. *C*, Closure of the superficial fascia is completed. The deep fascia has already been apposed in a separate layer. A subcuticular layer of sutures will complete the closure.

apparent for a few days after surgery.[20] The patient needs to be supported with fluids and antibiotics, and visceral replacement must be done with the patient under general anesthesia. Referral to a facility where adequate intraoperative support can be given is recommended versus attempting quick replacement of viscera under short-acting anesthesia in the field. In some cases, resection and anastomosis of affected intestine will be necessary. The mortality rate in affected cases can be minimal if early recognition and support are given.[20]

Some degree of edema and swelling is common after castration. With atraumatic technique, proper patient preparation, and clean surroundings, postoperative swelling can be minimized. Liberal postoperative exercise is also necessary to minimize this complication. If early sealing of open scrotal wounds is a cause of inadvertent swelling, these wounds must be opened to facilitate drainage.

Infection occasionally complicates the postoperative period. Local minor wound infections are often self-limiting, but more severe infections can be life threatening. Peritonitis occurs in some horses after castration, bacteria presumably gaining access to the peritoneal cavity through the vaginal tunic.[30] Abdominal paracentesis is recommended to aid with the diagnosis in any horse

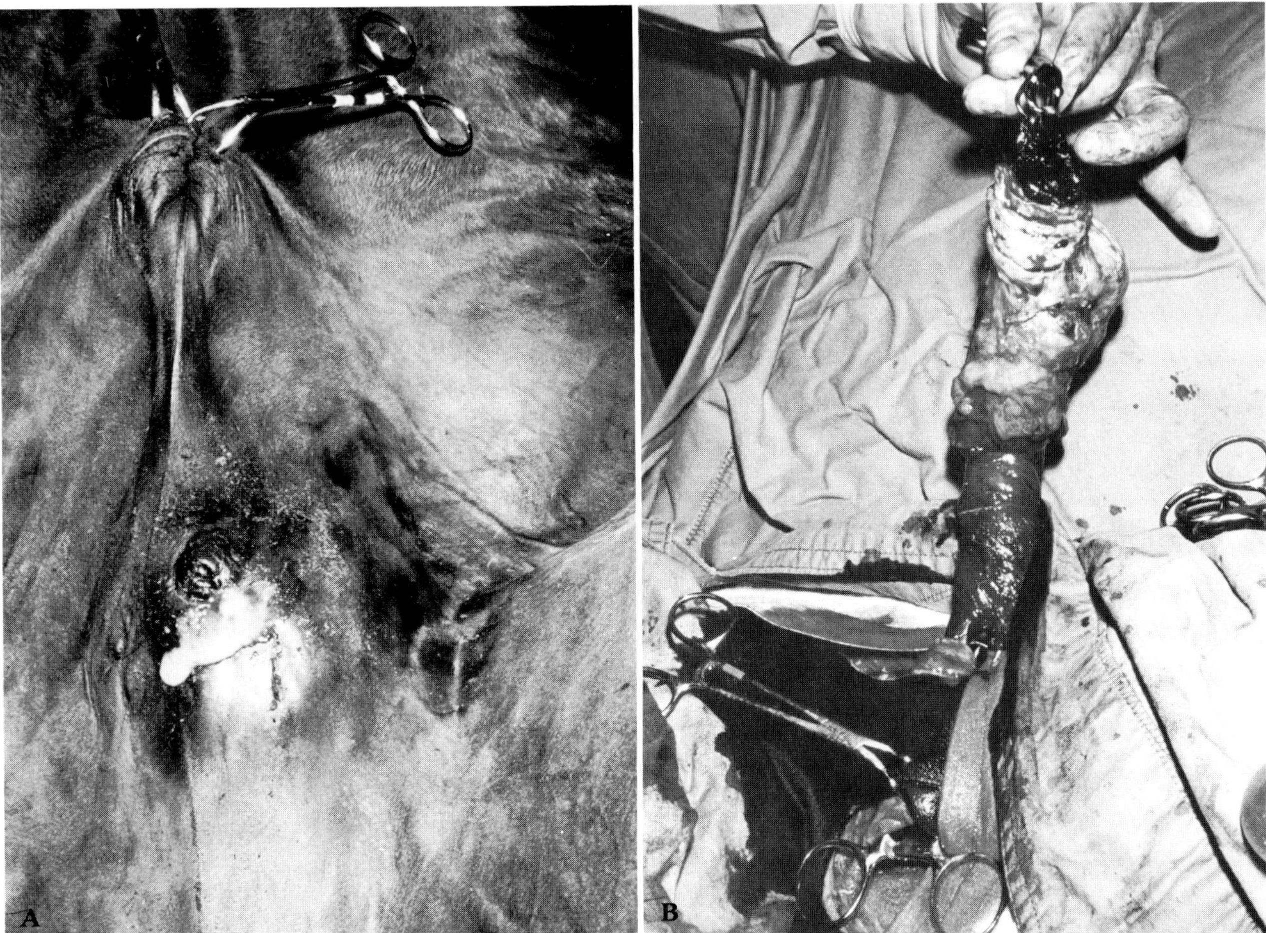

FIG. 99–8. *A,* Purulent drainage from the left scrotal region of a gelding with fever, and left hindlimb lameness. The castration wounds have healed except for this persistent unilateral drainage. *B,* The indurated and swollen spermatic cord has been dissected free from surrounding tissues and has been excised.

showing signs of systemic disease after castration. Wound botulism was also reported in the infected castration wound of a horse after surgery.[31] "Champignon" refers to a spermatic cord infection caused by streptococcal organisms. This complication seemed to occur more frequently when silk or whip cord ligatures were used in open castrations.[23] Scirrhous cord is caused by a chronic, low-grade staphylococcal infection of the spermatic cord (Fig. 99–8).[1,23] Microabscesses and extensive fibrous tissue are associated with this condition. With both of these conditions, clinical signs may not become apparent for weeks to months after surgery. Surgical excision of affected tissues is necessary for a successful outcome.

An intraoperative complication that can obviously lead to severe postoperative problems is mistaking the penis for a testis and lacerating the urethra.[1,32,33] Early recognition of this error allows for the best resolution of the problem. Suturing of the urethral mucosa was done successfully in one case, but phallectomy was required to resolve another case.

REFERENCES

1. Cox, J.E.: Surgery of the Reproductive Tract in Large Animals. 3rd ed. Liverpool, Liverpool University Press, 1987.
2. Belknap, J., Arden, W., and Yamini, B.: Septic periorchitis in a horse. J. Am. Vet. Med. Assoc., *192:*363–364, 1988.
3. Horney, F.D., and Milne, F.J.: Thrombosis of the spermatic artery resembling torsion of the spermatic cord in a stallion. Can. Vet. J., *5:*88–90, 1964.
4. Pascoe, J.R., Ellenburg, T.V., Culbertson, M.R., and Meagher, D.M.: Torsion of the spermatic cord in a horse. J. Am. Vet. Med. Assoc., *178:*242–245, 1981.
5. Threlfall, W.R., et al.: Recurrent torsion of the spermatic cord and scrotal testis in a stallion. J. Am. Vet. Med. Assoc., *196:*1641–1643, 1990.
6. Voith, V.L.: Effects of castration on mating behavior. Mod. Vet. Pract., *60:*1040–1041, 1979.
7. Smith, J.A.: Masculine behavior in geldings. Vet. Rec., *94:*160, 1973.

8. Line, S.W., Hart, B.J., and Sanders, L.: Effect of prepubertal versus postpubertal castration on sexual and aggressive behavior in male horses. J. Am. Vet. Med. Assoc., *186:*249–251, 1985.
9. Cox, J.E.: Behavior of a false rig: Causes and treatments. Vet. Rec., *118:*353–356, 1986.
10. Crowe, C.W., et al.: Plasma testosterone and behavioral characteristics in geldings with intact epididymides. J. Equine Med. Surg., *1:*387–390, 1977.
11. Trotter, G.W., and Aanes, W.A.: A complication of cryptorchid castration in three horses. J. Am. Vet. Med. Assoc., *178:*246–248, 1981.
12. Shideler, R.K., Squires, E.L., Pickett, B.W., and Anderson, E.W.: Disappearance of spermatozoa from the ejaculates of geldings. J. Reprod. Fertil. Suppl., *27:*25–29, 1979.
13. Parnakivi, H.: Use of domosedan in standing castration of the horse. Acta Vet. Scand., *82:*203, 1986.
14. Vaughan, J.T.: Surgery of the testes. *In* Bovine and Equine Urogenital Surgery. Edited by D.F. Walker and J.T. Vaughan. Philadelphia, Lea & Febiger, 1980, pp. 145–156.
15. Geiser, D.R.: Practical equine injectable anesthesia. J. Am. Vet. Med. Assoc., *182:*574–577, 1983.
16. Turner, A.S., and McIlwraith, C.W.: Techniques in Large Animal Surgery. 2nd ed., Philadelphia, Lea & Febiger, 1989.
17. Vaughan, J.T.: Surgery of the male equine reproductive system. *In* Current Veterinary Therapy in Theriogenology. Edited by D.A. Morrow. Philadelphia, W.B. Saunders, 1986, pp. 783–801.
18. Newberry, W.E., Garrett, E.D., and Alkire, L.T.: Use of succinylcholine in castration of horses. J. Am. Vet. Med. Assoc., *164:*1161–1162, 1974.
19. Heinze, C.D.: Surgery of the male genitalia. *In* Equine Medicine and Surgery. 3rd ed. Edited by R.A. Mansmann and E.S. McCallister. Santa Barbara, CA, American Veterinary Publications, 1982, pp. 1396–1402.
20. Van Der Velden, M.A., and Rutgers, L.: Visceral prolapse after castration in the horse: A review of 18 cases. Equine Vet. J., *22:*9–12, 1990.
21. Vaughan, J.T.: The male genital system. *In* Textbook of Large Animal Surgery. 2nd ed. Edited by F.W. Oehme. Baltimore, Williams & Wilkins, 1988, pp. 511–526.
22. Bergevin, J.D., Merritt, F.D., and Schoenberg, R.A.: Field-adapted equine castration technique with ligation of spermatic vessels and vaginal tunics left in place. Proc. Am. Assoc. Equine Pract., 193–197, 1977.
23. Nickels, F.A.: Complications of castration and ovariectomy. Vet. Clin. North Am., *4:*515–523, 1988.
24. Palmer, S.E.: Castration of the horse using a primary closure technique. Proc. Am. Assoc. Equine Pract., 17–20, 1984.
25. Cox, J.E.: Castration of horses and donkeys with first intention healing. Vet. Rec., *115:*372–375, 1984.
26. Barber, S.M.: Castration of horses with primary closure and scrotal ablation. Vet. Surg., *14:*2–6, 1985.
27. Lowe, J.E., and Dougherty, R.: Castration of horses and ponies by a primary closure method. J. Am. Vet. Med. Assoc., *160:*183–185, 1972.
28. Hoffman, P.E.: Castration of normal and cryptorchid horses by a primary closure method. Proc. Am. Assoc. Equine Pract., 219–223, 1973.
29. Hutchins, D.R., and Rawlinson, R.J.: Eventration as a sequel to castration of the horse. Aust. Vet. J., *48:*288–291, 1972.
30. Schumacher, J., Scrutchfield, W.L., and Martin, M.T.: Peritonitis following castration in 3 horses. J. Equine Vet. Sci., *7:*220–221, 1987.
31. Bernard, W., et al.: Botulism as a sequel to open castration in a horse. J. Am. Vet. Med. Assoc., *191:*73–74, 1987.
32. Todhunter, R.J., and Parker, J.E.: Surgical repair of urethral transection in a horse. J. Am. Vet. Med. Assoc., *193:*1085–1086, 1988.
33. Yovich, J.V., and Turner, A.S.: Treatment of a postcastration urethral stricture by phallectomy in a gelding. Compend. Contin. Educ. Practicing Vet., *8:*S393–S399, 1986.

CHAPTER 100

CRYPTORCHID CASTRATION

J.E. Cox

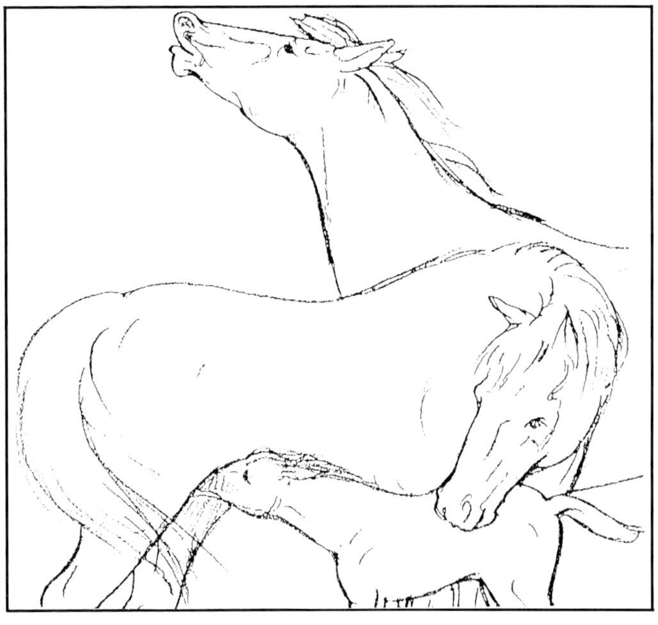

DIAGNOSIS

HISTORY

Most cryptorchid horses will have a history either of never having been castrated or of having only had one testis removed. Some, however, may have been sold as geldings (perhaps several times) before an owner has decided to seek veterinary opinion.

CLINICAL EXAMINATION

The horse's scrotal area can be viewed from a position about level with the front legs but far enough away to avoid being kicked. Vision alone is inadequate, however, because the horse can temporarily retract the testes (particularly smaller ones) into the inguinal region under the influence of its powerful cremaster muscles.

External palpation is best performed with the palpator standing at the left shoulder of the horse with the left arm round the neck in the case of a smaller pony or holding onto the withers. The right arm is used for palpation while the head remains high and out of reach of a kick. Slide either hand along the body wall toward the scrotum (though some horses resent this as tickling) or the scrotum may be palpated directly. If only one testis is palpable, its side can be ascertained by its relationship to the penis, which is readily palpable in the midline. If no testis is palpable on any particular side, then the extended fingers of the flat hand should be used to push up alongside the penis toward the superficial inguinal ring. Testes retained just above the scrotum will usually be palpated readily in this way, provided the horse is reasonably relaxed. Alternatively, "something" may be palpated higher up in the groin or just within the canal—this may be either a testis or a spermatic sac, containing the epididymal tail, or a spermatic sac from a previous castration. Occasionally, contents of the inguinal canal can be "milked" into the scrotum by deep digital pressure applied craniad to caudad, starting just in front of the superficial ring.

A technique to locate the deep inguinal ring at rectal palpation has been described.[1] The left hand is put into the rectum to palpate the right ring, and vice-versa. The lateral aspect of the wrist is rested on the pelvic rim with the fingers pressed against the abdominal wall laterally. The middle finger is flexed and then, as it is extended, it should enter the vaginal ring. A flap of peritoneum will cover the entrance to the ring, rendering it impalpable if the fingers are drawn backward over it.

In theory, in a case of inguinal retention, the vas deferens would be found passing through the ring, accompanied by the testicular artery and vein. However, the vessels are impossible to palpate.[2] Moreover, the same structures would be felt in a case in which a scrotal or inguinal testis has been previously removed, and only surgical exploration of the inguinal region can discriminate absolutely between these two possibilities. In a case of incomplete abdominal retention, the vas deferens again passes through the deep ring but is accompanied by the body of the epididymis. This latter structure is not easy to palpate, so incomplete abdominal retention cannot be readily distinguished from inguinal retention. In a case of complete abdominal retention, the vaginal opening is usually small and the ligament of the tail of the epididymis passes through it, but it is unlikely that this will be palpated. The abdominally retained testis itself can rarely be palpated, so a negative finding at rectal palpation is not particularly helpful.

Rectal palpation alone is, therefore, of little value in differentiating the variety of types of cryptorchidism. However, ultrasonography offers the possibility of an almost ideal form of diagnosis, once sufficient experience is gained in the interpretation of the picture. Trans-scrotal scanning can be rewarding, especially in cases of incomplete retention, and transrectal scanning offers positive identification of an abdominal testis. Such preoperative examination can eliminate surgical surprises and may be useful in allocating surgical time and the planning of a surgical approach.

BLOOD TESTS

A number of studies have established the usefulness of blood tests in diagnosing cryptorchidism in horses without scrotal testes.[3–6] The current recommendation is that in horses 2 yr old and younger (and in donkeys of any age) the testosterone concentrations in a pair of plasma or serum samples—one taken before and the other 30 to 120 min after the intravenous injection of at least 6000 IU of human chorionic gonadotropin (hCG)—prove useful. Geldings and false rigs have concentrations of less than 40 pg/mL, whereas cryptorchids have concentrations of testosterone in excess of 100 pg/mL, though occasionally an overlap exists between the two groups. Animals with an abdominal testis respond poorly to the hCG; the testosterone concentration in the second sample is rarely more than twice that in the first. Those horses with inguinal testes usually show a rise greater than twofold.[7] In horses 3 yr old or over, simply measure estrone sulfate (or conjugated estrogen but not free estrogen[4]) in a single sample of blood. Concentrations in geldings are usually less than 40 pg/mL, whereas cryptorchid horses generally have concentrations exceeding 400 pg/mL. In older horses or in those instances in which the result of one test is inconclusive or appears to contradict a good history, both tests should be run.[2]

A word of warning—the samples must be analyzed by a laboratory used to measuring testosterone or estrone sulfate in equine plasma. Assays tuned for measuring these hormones in other species can give false readings and, especially in the case of testosterone, false positives.

PRESURGICAL CONSIDERATIONS

To attempt artificially to make an undescended testis descend or to implant a testicular prosthesis to give the horse the appearance of normality is unethical. Both options could be considered fraud with intent to deceive.

The objective in operating on a cryptorchid is, therefore, to castrate it by removing both testes, which must be presumed to be present until proved otherwise. However, no attempt should be made to castrate a cryptorchid horse unless the surgeon is prepared to search for an abdominal testis and has the surgical knowledge and expertise and anesthetic support to carry it through.

The horse should be starved of food for 24 h before anesthesia. That procedure reduces the bulk of abdominal contents, making a search for an abdominal testis easier. Furthermore, the danger of the intestine becoming trapped in a laparotomy repair, if a laparotomy should prove necessary, is reduced.

ANESTHESIA AND RESTRAINT

The horse should be placed in dorsal recumbency, a position far superior to semidorsal recumbency. The hindlegs should be left completely free, but covered to prevent dirt falling off them onto the operation site.

PREOPERATIVE OBSERVATIONS

Examination of the inguinal region under anesthesia may show the presence of scars. The mere presence of a scar may indicate nothing more than an incision had been made, though a puckered scar almost invariably indicates a scrotum was at one time incised and, by implication, that a scrotal testis has been removed.

Palpation of the inguinal region with the animal in dorsal recumbency may reveal a testis which was not previously palpable. Palpation is best carried out by pushing the fingers of the outstretched hand into the scrotal area, dorsad, laterad, and slightly craniad toward the superficial inguinal ring. By pushing hard and deeply, if necessary, the structures inside the superficial ring can often be palpated by the fingertips. Surgical exploration of the inguinal area is, however, always imperative.

SURGICAL TECHNIQUE—INGUINAL EXPLORATION

The surgeon stands or kneels behind the horse. If a testis can be brought to and held against the scrotal area it may be removed by any appropriate technique for castration. Otherwise, an incision about 10 cm long is made through the skin in the area where the scrotum should be. This approach has two advantages over an incision made over the superficial inguinal ring: (1) it results in less hemorrhage from skin vessels and (2) the inguinal fat does not have to be displaced or incised to locate the superficial inguinal ring. After incising the skin, the scalpel is laid aside immediately to avoid cutting the sometimes large tributaries of the external pudendal vein. Dissection is continued toward the superficial ring with the fingers.

During dissection down to the inguinal canal, a search is made for structures other than fat and blood vessels. Four possible things may happen. First, a testis enveloped in a vaginal tunic may be found (Fig. 98–2). It may then be brought to the exterior and removed.

Second, a vaginal tunic without a testis may be found. This may vary in thickness from a fine pencil to a fat thumb and in length from short and retained within the inguinal canal to long enough nearly to reach the scrotum. It can be recognized by the whiteness of its fascial structure and by the attached cremaster muscle. In the horse in which a scrotal testis has been previously removed by an open castration technique, the distal end of the vaginal tunic is usually adherent to the scrotal scar. In cases in which no surgical interference has been made, the vaginal tunic will only have tenuous fibrous connections with the scrotum. The vaginal tunic is in any case opened, and its contents inspected.

In the horse in which a testis has been previously removed, the deferent duct and remains of spermatic vessels will be found and will usually terminate in a fibrous nubbin in the region of the scrotal scar. It may be desirable to remove a section of the spermatic sac for histologic identification of remains of blood vessels and the deferent duct, in which case a 5-cm length may be readily obtained by use of the emasculator.

In the horse which is an incomplete abdominal cryptorchid, the deferent duct will again be found inside the vaginal tunic, but the duct will be seen to become epididymal tail distally and this in turn returns up the lumen of vaginal tunic as the epididymal body (Fig. 98–3). The latter two structures can be recognized because they consist of coiled tubes: the tail of the epididymis consists of a large loosely coiled tube and the body of the epididymis consists of a fine tightly coiled tube, which is recognizable only on close inspection. In such a case, traction may be applied to the body of the epididymis, and the clinician may be able to deliver the testis through the vaginal ring and then sever its blood

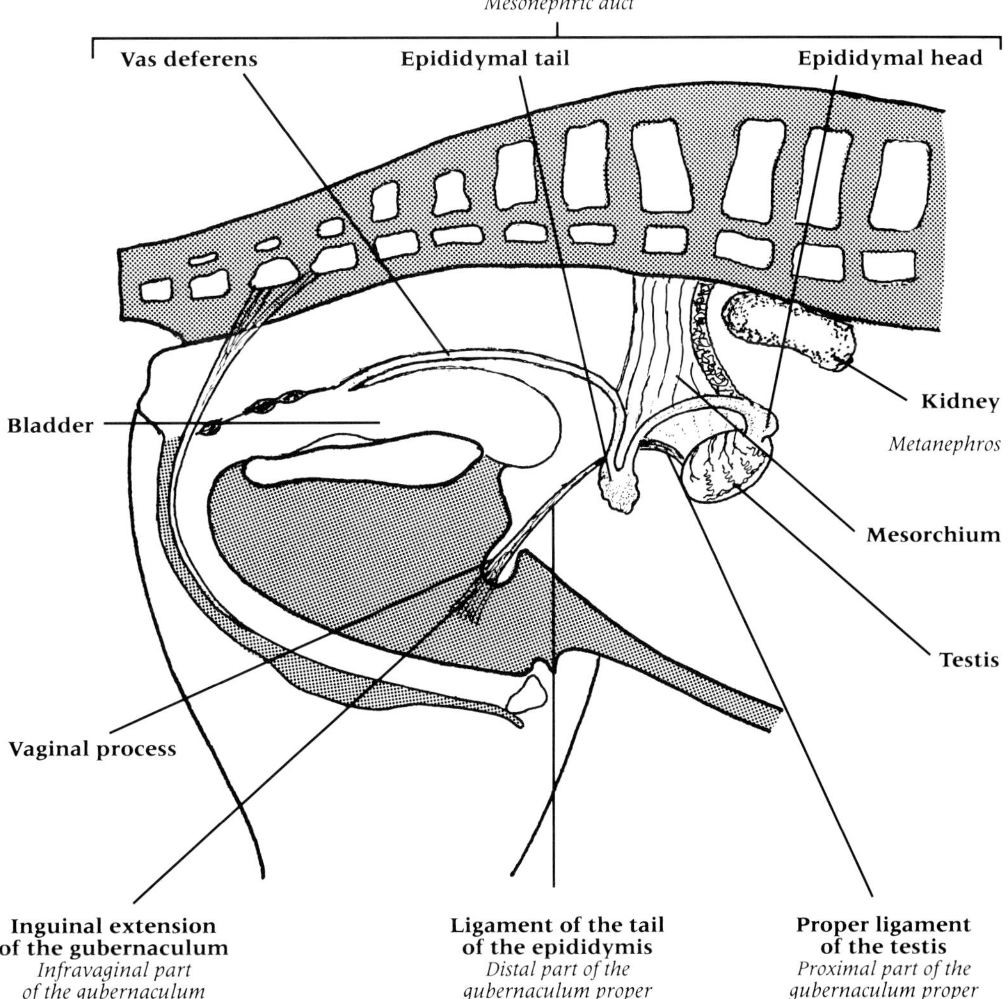

FIG. 100–1. Approximate location and connections of an abdominally retained testis. The mesorchium suspends the testis from the dorsal body wall as shown. Other folds of peritoneum suspend the vas deferens and the ligament of the tail of the epididymis but are omitted for clarity. Labels in boldface type are for adult structures; those in italics are for the fetal structures from which they are derived (see Chapter 98).

supply and attachments with the emasculator. Sometimes it is necessary to incise the vaginal tunic up to the level of the vaginal ring at the top of the inguinal canal before the testis can be procured. The clinician will rarely be able to deliver an abdominal testis in this way from a horse whose contralateral testis has been previously removed. If the testis cannot be delivered by traction, laparotomy is indicated.

Rarely, the surgeon will find a case of incomplete abdominal cryptorchidism in which the tail of the epididymis has been previously removed in the mistaken belief that it was a malformed testis. In such a case, the vaginal tunic will contain deferent duct and body of epididymis, both passing distad to enter a nub of fibrous tissue. Positive identification of the body of the epididymis (by tissue examination, if necessary) allows this condition to be distinguished from the remains of the spermatic vessels. Traction on the body may again deliver the testis from the abdomen, but if it does not, laparotomy is indicated.

In a case of complete abdominal retention, another tenuous structure, the so-called inguinal extension of the gubernaculum, will be found (Fig. 100–1). It will be attached to a small vaginal tunic which contains only a single cord of fibrous tissue (Fig. 98–1). This cord is the remains of the distal part of the gubernaculum and is equivalent to the ligament of the tail of the epididymis in the normal adult. The way in which these structures can be used to deliver the abdominal testis is described later in this chapter.

The third possibility during dissection is that no vaginal tunic is found (particularly by the inexperienced operator) even though adequate exposure of the superficial ring is obtained. The ring should be readily defined by its straight solid caudolateral edge and its crescent-shaped, softer but still tendinous mediocranial edge. Two fingers should be inserted deep into the inguinal canal, which passes laterad, dorsad, and slightly craniad, to ensure that no vaginal tunic is present within the canal. In such a case, the testis will be intra-abdominal, and an immediate exploratory laparotomy is indicated.

Fourth, fibrosis from previous interference may sometimes make dissection impossible. In such a case, either an immediate exploratory laparotomy is indicated or a blood test for cryptorchidism should be performed to confirm or refute the presence of a testis.

If a scrotal testis is present on the opposite side, it should be removed before proceeding to a laparotomy. If no scrotal testis is present on the opposite side, then exploration of the inguinal area should proceed along the lines outlined above.

SURGICAL APPROACHES TO AN ABDOMINAL TESTIS

Approaches to an abdominal testis can be classified as invasive inguinal, noninvasive inguinal, and body wall invasive.

INVASIVE INGUINAL

There are two invasive inguinal techniques, usually called the Belgian and the Danish methods.[8] Both techniques require the horse to be anaesthetized in dorsal or semidorsal recumbency and in both cases an incision is made in the scrotum or over the superficial inguinal ring, as described for surgical exploration of the inguinal region. In the Belgian method, either the whole hand is formed into a cone or two fingers are used.[9] A path is forced up through the superficial inguinal ring, into the inguinal canal, and through the fascia of the deep inguinal ring until the fingers enter the abdomen. The fingers can then be hooked round the testis, its appendages or its blood vessels and the testis exteriorized.[10] The hole made by this approach cannot be sutured.

The Danish method involves puncturing the body wall medial and slightly cranial to the superficial inguinal ring. The rent has been pinpointed at 1 to 2 cm medial to the superficial ring and centered on the cranial aspect of it.[11] The fingers are passed through the external and internal oblique muscles, admitting two fingers (or, if necessary, the whole hand) into the abdomen to hook testis or blood vessels. Although this incision, or more accurately, this rent, can be sutured, the procedure is not easy.

Both techniques were particularly in vogue around the turn of the century and remained popular throughout the heyday of the heavy working horse. However, a retrospective study showed that the invasive inguinal approach—particularly if the whole hand is introduced—has a significant risk of bowel prolapse and death.[12] Moreover, the level of postoperative discomfort experienced by horses operated on in this way has received unfavorable comment.

NONINVASIVE INGUINAL

Studies of normal testicular descent in horses and other animals[13] and the development of better anaesthetics, which enabled the inguinal region to be seen and not simply palpated, combined in the 1960s in the development of noninvasive inguinal techniques for the procurement of abdominal testes. The first of these involved introducing a pair of sponge forceps through the superficial inguinal ring and up the inguinal canal to locate the inverted vaginal process just within the deep ring.[14] Traction on the forceps delivered the vaginal tunic, in which could be located the ligament of the tail of the epididymis. Traction on this ligament delivered the epididymal tail and then the testis. However, the technique is based on a misconception. The vaginal tunic is not inverted (Fig. 98–1 and 100–1).

Later, a technique was described which relied on locating the remains of the infravaginal part of the gubernaculum (called the inguinal extension of the gubernaculum) in the inguinal region and following this to the distal end of the vaginal tunic.[15] Trotter pointed out, however, that identification of the inguinal extension of the gubernaculum is not essential if the vaginal process itself can be identified, though this lies deeper.[2] If the process is well developed, it may be retrieved with the fingers. Alternatively, a curved sponge forceps may be introduced into the canal, gently opened and closed until the vaginal process is grasped. The vaginal tunic, once identified and brought within view, is then incised to reveal the ligament of the tail of the epididymis (Fig. 100–1). Traction on this will usually deliver, in succession, the epididymal tail, proper ligament of testis, and finally the testis, perhaps after dilation or incision of the vaginal process up to the level of the vaginal ring. If the vaginal process cannot be found, either the abdomen must be penetrated through or close to the inguinal canal or a body wall invasive approach must be adopted.

The inguinal extension is a structure consisting of a tissue band, which is sometimes slightly pink and varies in size, shape, and consistency. Because this tenuous structure is not easily located, the technique has a significant rate of technical failure, a retrospective study quoting a failure rate of 30%, often caused by either failure to identify the vaginal process or the occurrence of adhesions in the inguinal region.[12] Although the failure rate falls as the operator gains experience in identifying the inguinal extension of the gubernaculum testis or vaginal process, other situations exist in which failure to locate the structure is almost axiomatic. In cases in which previous surgical interference has led to the deposition of fibrous tissue, the infravaginal gubernacular remnant will not be identifiable. In cases of large abdominal testes, traction may fail to deliver the testis even if the vaginal process is dilated manually. Large abdominal testes can be found as a result of hypertrophy because of removal of the contralateral scrotal testis. Most such testes are twice the size of normal ones, and I have encountered one weighing 365 g, nearly 20 times normal size. Teratomas, particularly cystic ones, can weigh more than 1 kg and should be removed via a body wall invasive approach.

Difficulties can also be encountered in which only part of the epididymis, particularly the tail in a case of incomplete testicular descent, has been removed at previous surgery. In other cases, appropriate landmarks will be absent.[16] Postoperatively, the inguinal canal is traditionally packed with sterile gauze or a sterile towel for 24 to 48 h to prevent bowel prolapse.

BODY WALL INVASIVE

Although often grouped with the invasive inguinal techniques, body wall invasive techniques have the significant advantage of making controlled and readily repairable incisions. They also have the advantage over noninvasive inguinal techniques of a lower rate of technical failure, because they do not rely on identifying the rather nebulous inguinal extension of the gubernaculum testis or a small vaginal process. Moreover, they can be adapted to deal with larger testes. They do, however, have the disadvantage of prolonging surgical preparation and anesthetic time, because they require a second site to be prepared for surgery. Absolute prerequisites are that inguinal exploration must have been thorough and that the presence of an inguinally retained testis must have been eliminated. All inguinal structures associated with testicular descent should be identified.

The flank approach to the abdomen, while well suited to cattle which have a large sublumbar fossa, is less ideal in horses with their 18 pairs of ribs. It also involves rolling the horse from dorsal to lateral recumbency following inguinal exploration.[17] Some clinicians have advocated that the flank incision can be done standing. However, inguinal cryptorchidism must be eliminated for a standing flank cryptorchidectomy to be successful, and because inguinal cryptorchidism can only be satisfactorily eliminated by surgical exploration of the inguinal region or transrectal ultrasonography, the concept of a standing flank laparotomy has little to commend it. However, standing flank laparotomy has been recommended as a last resort after failed inguinal and paramedian exploration.[2] In such a case, the mesorchium supporting the testicular vessels may be more readily located as the weight of the testis stretches the peritoneal fold and palpation from the kidney caudad is said to locate this structure more readily.

The suprapubic paramedian laparotomy, originally described by Marrell in 1838 in the first recorded description of an abdominal cryptorchidectomy, was rediscovered by Wright,[18] was further described by Lowe and Higginbotham,[19] and was reviewed by Cox et al.[20] The technique involves making a skin incision about 10 cm long parallel to and about 15 cm away from the midline at the level of the sheath opening. The subcutaneous fat is incised to expose the yellow abdominal tunic which, together with the adherent tendons of external and internal oblique muscles, is cut along the line of the skin incision to expose the straight abdominal muscle. This muscle can be split along the line of its fibers (caudocraniad) and the tendon of the transverse muscle exposed. This tendon can then also be cut along the line of incision or, preferably, split along its fibers at right angles to the incision, thus creating a grid approach to the abdomen. The hand is inserted into the abdomen and initially kept close to the body wall. Most testes are located just inside the deep inguinal ring and can be exteriorized from both sides of the abdomen through the one incision. If the testis is not found close to the ring, then the vas deferens is located at the bladder neck (Fig. 100–1) and followed to the epididymal tail, which is connected to the testis by the proper ligament of the testis.[21]

Technical failures are few (2 cases out of 214 in my hands plus 6 other cases, which blood tests showed to be monorchids). Postoperative complications have also been insignificant. One horse in the series died during recovery from anesthesia (no cause was found), and another horse, operated on in the early days, had bowel trapped in the suture repair.

SUMMARY

Cryptorchid surgery is an essay in applied anatomy. A systemic surgical exploration and a thorough knowledge of the possible anatomical variations in the positions and size and shape of the testis and its appendages are essential. Nevertheless, no hard-and-fast rules are applicable to every case. An accurate history of the animal can be helpful; a partial one, positively misleading, especially when an epididymal tail has been removed and mistakenly identified as a small testis. The introduction of diagnostic blood tests has been a significant advance and the advent of transrectal ultrasonography promises to be another. Each surgeon will have, or will develop, a preferred technique, but a knowledge of the experiences of others will sometimes prove invaluable. No one person will likely meet every eventuality, and the words of Degive (the great cryptorchid operator of the last century) remain as true today as in 1880—"When one has done one's hundredth cryptorchidectomy, one hasn't done one's hundred and first."[22]

REFERENCES

1. O'Connor, J.P.: Rectal examination of the cryptorchid horse. Ir. Vet. J., *25:*129–131, 1971.
2. Trotter, G.W.: Normal and cryptorchid castration. Vet. Clin. North Am., *4:*493–514, 1988.
3. Cox, J.E., Williams, J.H., Rowe, P.H., and Smith J.A.: Testosterone in normal cryptorchid and castrated horses. Equine Vet. J., *5:*85–90, 1973.
4. Cox, J.E.: Experiences with a diagnostic test for equine cryptorchidism. Equine Vet. J., *7:*179–183, 1975.
5. Ganjam, V.K., and Kenney, R.M.: Androgens and oestrogens in normal and cryptorchid stallions. J. Reprod. Fertil. Suppl., *23:*67–73, 1975.
6. Cox, J.E., Redhead, P.H., and Dawson, F.E.: A comparison of the measurement of plasma testosterone and plasma oestrogens for the diagnosis of cryptorchidism in the horse. Equine Vet. J., *18:*179–182, 1986.
7. Cox, J.E.: Testosterone concentrations in normal and cryptorchid horses. Response to human chorionic gonadotrophin. Anim. Reprod. Sci., *18:*43–50, 1989.
8. O'Connor, J.J.: Dollar's Veterinary Surgery. General, Operative and Regional. 4th ed. London, Bailliere, Tindall and Cassell, 1950.
9. Walker, D.F., and Vaughan, J.T.: Bovine and Equine Urogenital Surgery. Philadelphia, Lea & Febiger, 1980.
10. Berge, E., and Westhues, M.: Veterinary Operative Surgery. Copenhagen, Medical Book, 1966.
11. Wilson, D.G., and Reinertson, E.L.: A modified parainguinal approach for cryptorchidectomy in horses. An evaluation in 107 horses. Vet. Surg., *16:*1–4, 1987.
12. Stickle, R.L., and Fessler, J.F.: Retrospective study of 350 cases of equine cryptorchidism. J. Am. Vet. Med. Assoc., *172:*343–346, 1978.
13. Gier, H.T., and Marion, G.B.: Development of mammalian testes and genital ducts. Biol. Reprod., *1:*1–12, 1969.
14. Adams, O.R.: An improved method of diagnosis and castration of cryptorchid horses. J. Am Vet. Med. Assoc., *145:*439–446, 1964.
15. Valdez, H., Taylor, T.S., McLaughlin, S.A., and Martin, M.T.: Abdominal cryptorchidectomy in the horse, using inguinal extension of the gubernaculum testis. J. Am Vet. Med. Assoc., *174:*1110–1112, 1979.
16. Trotter, G.W., and Aanes, W.A.: A complication of cryptorchid castration in three horses. J. Am. Vet. Med. Assoc., *178:* 246–248, 1981.
17. Arthur, G.H.: The surgery of the equine cryptorchid. Vet. Rec., *73:*385–389, 1961.
18. Wright, J.G.: The surgery of the inguinal canal in animals. Vet. Rec., *75:*1352–1363, 1963.
19. Lowe, J., and Higginbotham, R.: Castration of abdominal cryptorchid horses by a paramedian laparotomy approach. Cornell Vet., *59:*121–126, 1969.
20. Cox, J.E., Edwards, G.B., and Neal, P.A.: Supra-pubic paramedian laparotomy for abdominal cryptorchidism in the horse. Vet. Rec., *97:*428–432, 1975.
21. Cox, J.E.: Surgery of the Reproductive Tract in Large Animals. Liverpool, Liverpool University Press, 1987.
22. Degive, A.: De la castration de, animaux cryptorchides. Ann. Med. Vet., *11:*629–647 and 693–720, 1875.

CHAPTER 101

UNILATERAL CASTRATION

G.W. Trotter

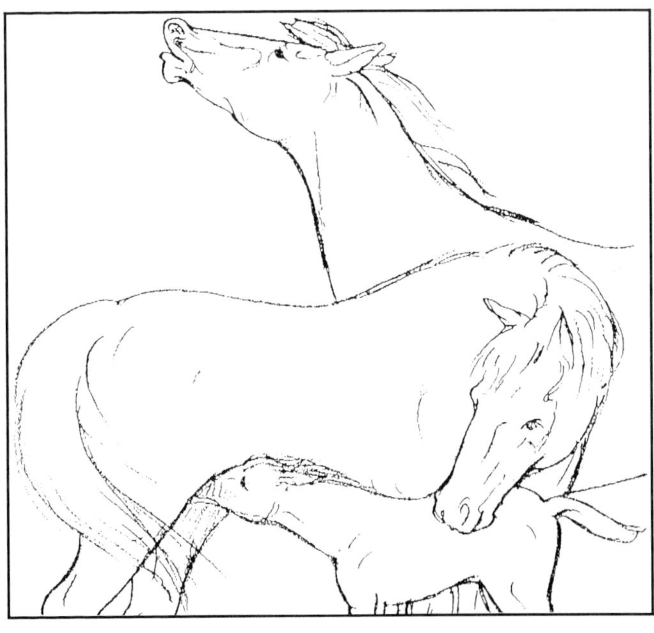

Occasionally, one testis needs to be removed from a breeding stallion or from a foal destined to become a breeding stallion. Surgery may be completed as either an elective procedure (certain tumors, sperm granuloma, nonspecific testis degeneration, orchitis/periorchitis, varicocele, hydrocele, and epididymitis)[1–9] or as an emergency procedure (testicular torsion, hematoma, and inguinal/scrotal hernia).[10–12] The surgical technique that will be used is partially dictated by the clinical indication for surgery and partially by the surgeon's preference. Unilateral castration can also be useful in certain research protocols where both testicular structure and sequential seminal analyses are parameters that need to be evaluated.[13–15]

Hoagland et al. have shown that unilateral castration of stallions at either 1, 2, or 3 yr of age results in compensatory hypertrophy of the remaining testis.[14,15] This hypertrophy included both the epithelial and interstitial components of the testis.[14] Serum testosterone concentrations were also similar between intact and unilaterally castrated stallions.[15]

INDICATIONS

Elective unilateral castration may be necessary in some stallions following testicular trauma. Stallions can incur trauma to one or both testes that is self-limiting and only temporarily affects fertility,[3] but researchers also believe that in some cases trauma with swelling and degeneration involving one testis can sufficiently affect local thermoregulatory mechanisms such that spermatogenesis in the opposite testis may be affected.[3,16] Although this proposed phenomenon remains speculative, unilateral castration is sometimes recommended to remove any potential negative influence of the damaged testis. Even in some chronic cases, removal of a fibrotic testis and associated scar tissue can result in compensatory hypertrophy and increased sperm production in the remaining testis.[3,16]

Some chance exists that immune-related infertility and testicular degeneration can develop after unilateral testicular trauma.[17,18] Specific spermalozoal surface antigens do not form until spermatogenesis starts at puberty. The blood-testis barrier normally sequesters spermatozoa in the seminiferous tubules and away from the general circulation.[17,18] If this barrier is lost (trauma, infection, or testicular torsion) after spermatogenesis starts, immune cells can gain access to the spermatozoa and antisperm antibodies may be formed. This is a well-recognized cause of infertility in people; increased levels of antisperm antibodies are seen in two-thirds of men having vasectomies.[19] Degenerative changes in the contralateral testis have also been seen experimentally in rabbits within 24 h of inducing testicular torsion in one testis.[20] Complement-dependent sperm immobilizing factors, which were assumed to be antisperm antibodies, were demonstrated in two stallions using a complement-dependent sperm immobilizing assay.[17,18] Both stallions had improved fertility after receiving corticosteroid therapy for 2 to 3 weeks.

Torsion involving the scrotal testis and spermatic cord or thrombosis of the spermatic artery can cause sufficient tissue compromise to necessitate castration.[10–12] If torsion is of short duration, surgical replacement with orchiopexy may be successful.[12] With more severe soft tissue damage in a stallion which has limited future breeding potential, bilateral castration should be considered. Unilateral castration is required when future breeding potential is important.

The surgical wound may be closed primarily or be left open to heal by second intention. This decision is based on the degree of soft tissue compromise that is encountered at surgery. In one report, satisfactory semen quality was present by 60 days after unilateral castration for torsion of the spermatic cord and scrotal testis when the surgical wound was allowed to heal by second intention.[12]

Unilateral castration is also usually required in the surgical management of inguinal/scrotal hernia in the stallion (see Chapter 102). Unilateral castration may also be necessary in certain cases of epididymitis and/or sperm granuloma when sperm production is abnormal or when inflammation is causing lameness and/or reluctance to ejaculate.[2,4,5,7] Diagnostic ultrasonography can be a useful adjunct in diagnosis of some of these conditions and may detect some testicular or epididymal changes that are not detectable by palpation.[3] In most cases, castration with primary closure can be used.

Testicular neoplasia is uncommon in horses; seminoma is the most common testicular neoplasm.[1] Malignancy is uncommon and most tumors can involve both normally descended testes as well as cryptorchid testes. Tumors involving descended testes often cause nonpainful scrotal enlargement; the testis usually remains freely movable within the scrotum (Fig. 101–1). Neoplasms must be differentiated from other causes of scrotal enlargement; ultrasonography again is a useful diagnostic tool.[3] The specific diagnosis of neoplasia is usually made by histopathologic examination of tissues removed at surgery.[1,6] Unilateral casration with primary closure is recommended as is radical removal of spermatic cord.[3] Radical scrotal ablation is also recommended if the tumor has involved adjacent tissues.[3]

Orchitis and periorchitis are uncommon in stallions. Unilateral septic periorchitis of hematogenous origin requiring castration was reported in a 2-month-old foal; bilateral castration was performed.[8] Unilateral castration was also used to remove an infected testis and testicular prosthesis, the prosthesis having originally been placed to fill the scrotum when the testis could not be located.[9] Subsequent fertility of the stallion was not described. With unilateral orchitis of any cause, appropriate medical and symptomatic therapy should be utilized to try to minimize local heat and swelling. However, prompt unilateral castration should be considered if early improvement is not seen, to minimize damage to the opposite testis.

METHODS

The surgical approach and technique used depends on the clinical indication(s) for surgery. For cases in which preoperative soft tissue is compromised and swelling has been excessive, the postcastration wound may best be managed using temporary packing and allowing healing by second intention. Otherwise, a primary closure technique is recommended to minimize local inflammation and swelling and thereby minimize any effect this may have on the remaining testis.[16] General anesthesia with the patient in dorsal recumbency is required. Care should be taken to avoid incising into testicular parenchyma during castration and strict attention should also be paid to local hemostasis. The neurovascular portion of the spermatic cord can be ligated independently by making a small incision in the vaginal tunic and elevating the vessels from the tunic. A separate transfixation ligature can then be placed around the musculofibrous portion of the cord before

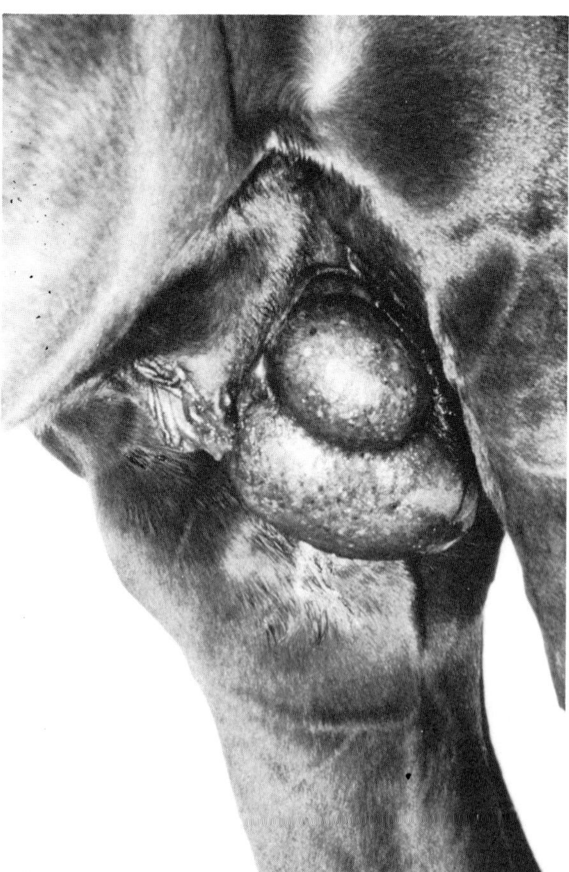

FIG. 101–1. Right-sided scrotal enlargement associated with a seminoma. (Courtesy of T. Stashak.)

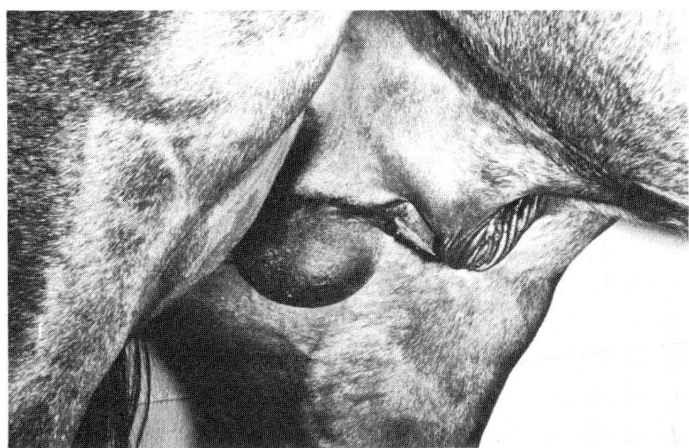

FIG. 101–2. Appearance of the inguinal region 3 days after right-sided unilateral castration with primary closure in a mature stallion.

distal emasculation or transection (see Chapter 99). Closure of the superficial inguinal ring is optional, but partial or total ablation of the scrotum on the affected side should be used to help eliminate local dead space. The spermatic fascia is closed in two or more layers using small-diameter absorbable suture material, and the same material is used to complete a subcuticular skin closure.

An alternate technique is to position the horse in dorsal oblique recumbency with the body tilted away from the affected side.[21] The surgical approach is through an 8- to 10-cm skin incision made 2 cm axial to and parallel with the superficial inguinal ring, rather than through the scrotum. Sharp dissection through the spermatic fascia is used to expose the tunic-enclosed testis. After exteriorization of the testis from the tunic, the ductus deferens is doubly ligated and transected. The mesorchium is then sharply divided; electrocautery or ligation is used as needed for hemostasis. The spermatic artery is then isolated and doubly ligated separately from the veins. The distal ligature in each case is a transfixing ligature; the end is left long and tagged so that the tissues are easily retrieved later during surgery. After ligating the veins, the external cremaster muscle is elevated from the cord portion of the tunic, and a serrated clamp is applied across the muscle. The muscle is then sectioned across its crushed portion, and the remaining crushed muscle is oversewn using adjacent intact vaginal tunic. The tunic is then sectioned distal to this site, and the testis and its appendages are discarded. Sectioning of spermatic cord structures and vaginal tunic is at the approximate level of the superficial inguinal ring (see Fig. 102–1). The sectioned ductus deferens, spermatic artery, and veins are then elevated and incorporated into the closure of the vaginal tunic. Inguinal fascia is then apposed to eliminate local dead space.

Hand walking exercise is provided for 10 to 14 days after surgery, but with appropriate attention paid to local hemostasis and to closure of dead space, postoperative swelling is usually minimal (Fig. 101–2). Semen collection can be considered in as little as 48 h after surgery and natural service is usually possible by 3 weeks after surgery.

REFERENCES

1. Caron, J.P., Barber, S.M., and Bailey, J.V.: Equine testicular neoplasia. Compend. Contin. Educ. Practicing Vet., *7:*S53–S62, 1985.
2. Held, J.P., et al.: Sperm granuloma in a stallion. J. Am. Vet. Med. Assoc., *194:*267–268, 1989.
3. Varner, D.D., and Schumacher, J.: Diseases of the reproductive system: The stallion. *In* Equine Medicine and Surgery. 4th ed. Edited by P.T. Colahan, I.G. Mayhew, A.M. Merritt, and J.N. Moore. Goleta, American Veterinary Publications, 1991, pp. 847–948.
4. Held, J.P., et al.: Bacterial epididymitis in two stallions. J. Am. Vet. Med. Assoc., *197:*602–604, 1990.
5. Traub-Dargatz, J.L., et al.: Ultrasonographic detection of chronic epididymitis in a stallion. J. Am. Vet. Med. Assoc., *198:*1417–1420, 1991.
6. Barber, S.M.: Castration of horses with primary closure and scrotal ablation. Vet. Surg., *14:*2–6, 1985.
7. Blue, M.G., and McEntee, K.: Epididymal sperm granuloma in a stallion. Equine Vet. J., *17:*248–251, 1986.
8. Belknap, J., Arden, W., and Yamini, B.: Septic periorchitis in a horse. J. Am. Vet. Med. Assoc., *192:*363-364, 1988.
9. Hinrichs, K., Gentile, D.G., Hurtgen, J.P., and Richardson, D.W.: Complications from a testicular prosthesis in a stallion. J. Am. Vet. Med. Assoc., *186:*390–391, 1985.
10. Pascoe, J.R., Ellenburg, T.V., Culbertson, M.R., and Meagher, D.M.: Torsion of the spermatic cord in a horse. J. Am. Vet. Med. Assoc., *178:*242–245, 1981.
11. Horney, F.D., and Milne, F.J.: Thrombosis of the spermatic artery resembling torsion of the spermatic cord in a stallion. Can. Vet. J., *5:*88–90, 1964.
12. Threlfall, W.R., et al.: Recurrent torsion of the spermatic cord and scrotal testis in a stallion. J. Am. Vet. Med. Assoc., *196:*1641–1643, 1990.
13. Amann, R.P., et al.: Reproduction function in stallions treated with cambendazole. J. Am. Vet. Med. Assoc., *170:*730–732, 1977.
14. Hoagland, T.A., et al.: Effects of unilateral castration on morphologic characteristics of the testis in one, two and three year old stallions. Theriogenology, *26:*397–405, 1986.
15. Hoagland, T.A., et al.: Effects of unilateral castration on serum luteinizing hormone, follicle stimulating hormone and testosterone concentrations in one, two and three year old stallions. Theriogenology, *26:*407–418, 1986.
16. Neeley, D.P.: Physical examination and genital disease of the stallion. *In* Current Therapy in Theriogenology. Edited by D.A. Morrow. Philadelphia, W.B. Saunders, 1980, pp. 694–706.
17. Zhang, J., Ricketts, S.W., and Tanner, S.J.: Antisperm antibodies in the semen of a stallion following testicular trauma. Equine Vet. J., *22:*138–141, 1990.

18. Papa, F.O., Alvarenga, M.A., Lopes, M.D., and Compos Filho, E.T.: Infertility of autoimmune origin in a stallion. Equine Vet. J., *22:*145–146, 1990.
19. Hofmeyr, G.J., and Robson, A.R.: Prevention of antisperm autoantibody response in vasectomized Swiss white mice by infusion of heterologous antisperm serum. Br. J. Urol., *56:*418–421, 1984.
20. Cerasaro, T.S., Nachtsheim, D.A., Otero, F., and Parsons, C.: The effect of testicular torsion on contralateral testis and the production of antisperm antibodies in rabbits. J. Urol., *132:*577–579, 1984.
21. Stashak, T.S.: Indications and technique for primary closure of castration. Proceedings of the Third European American College of Veterinary Surgeons Surgical Forum, Munich, 1989, pp. 56–58.

CHAPTER 102

INGUINAL HERNIA

T.S. Stashak

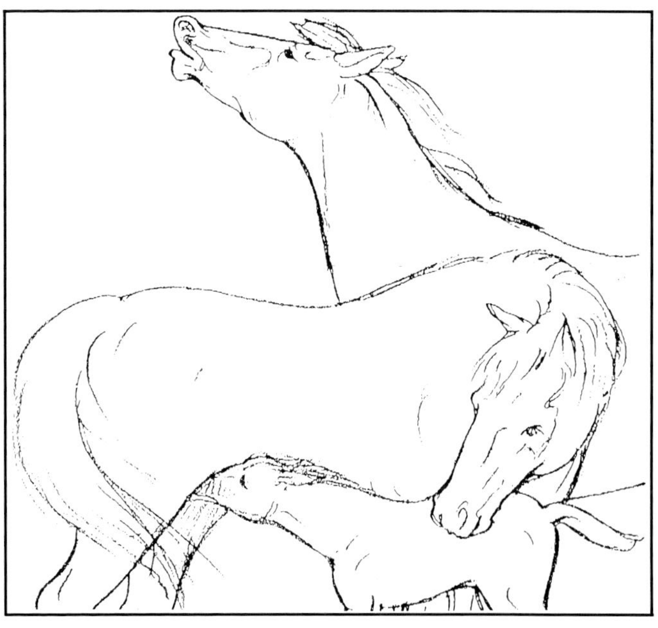

The term inguinal hernia describes the passage of abdominal contents from the abdomen into the inguinal canal. If the contents pass through the superficial (external) inguinal ring and enter the scrotum, the condition may be described as scrotal hernia; however, the term inguinal hernia is often used to describe both conditions.[1,2] Although inguinal hernia may be seen in either sex, it is most commonly seen as a congenital condition in colts and in adult stallions as an acquired condition. Rarely is the condition seen in mares or geldings, because the tunica vaginalis is almost nonexistent. Although the hernia may involve the bladder, small colon, omentum, or pelvic flexure of the large colon, the jejunum and ileum are most frequently involved.[3,4] The incidence of congenital inguinal hernia in the colt is reported to be 1.13 cases per 1000 admissions.[5,6] The prevalence of acquired inguinal hernia ranges from 2 to 10% of those horses presenting for colic.[7–9] The Arabian, Tennessee Walking Horse, Standardbred, and American Saddlebred breeds appear to be at higher risk for the acquired inguinal hernia.[6,10,11] and the congenital condition may be heritable.[5,12]

DIRECT VERSUS INDIRECT HERNIA

Inguinal hernia may be described as either indirect or direct.[4,7,13–17] In an indirect hernia, the abdominal viscera enter the vaginal ring and are located within the vaginal cavity (Figs. 102–1 and 102–2). In a direct hernia, viscera are located in the inguinal-scrotal region outside the vaginal cavity (Figs. 102–3 and 102–4).[7,12,17] The latter condition develops if a rent occurs in the peritoneum and transverse fascia or in the vaginal tunic. If the rent develops in the peritoneum and transverse fascia overlying the deep (internal) inguinal ring, it usually occurs just medial or craniomedial to the vaginal ring. The abdominal viscera herniate through the rent and descend through the inguinal canal outside the vaginal tunic through the superficial inguinal ring, finally reaching the scrotal region where they are located subcutaneously[15] (Fig. 102–3). If the rent develops in the vaginal tunic it is usually craniolateral, the vaginal ring may not be involved and the abdominal viscera follow the same route and reside in the subcutaneous tissue as just described (Fig. 102–4).[17,18]

Although the term "direct herniation" comes from human medicine, the condition in the horse is different from that described in humans. In people, the transverse fascia beside the vaginal ring becomes weakened after which it protrudes along with the peritoneum through the inguinal canal. Thus, a real hernia sac with a peritoneal lining develops. Because the intestines in the equine direct inguinal herniation are not surrounded by peritoneum, van der Velden suggested that the term "inguinal rupture" or "ruptured inguinal hernia" be adopted.[17] This has merit because it is more descriptive. The term inguinal rupture indicates a rupture of the peritoneum and transverse fascia adjacent to the vaginal ring (Fig. 102–3), whereas the term ruptured inguinal hernia indicates a rent in the vaginal tunic,

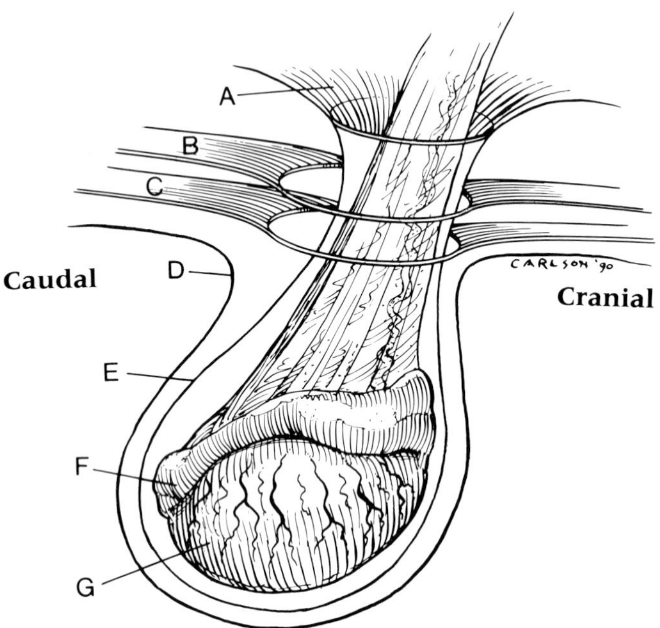

FIG. 102–1. Lateral view of a normal inguinal canal, scrotum and right testicle. A, peritoneum, transverse fascia, and vaginal ring; B, internal abdominal oblique muscle and deep inguinal ring; C, external abdominal oblique muscle and superficial inguinal ring; D, skin; E, vaginal tunic; F, epididymis; G, testis.

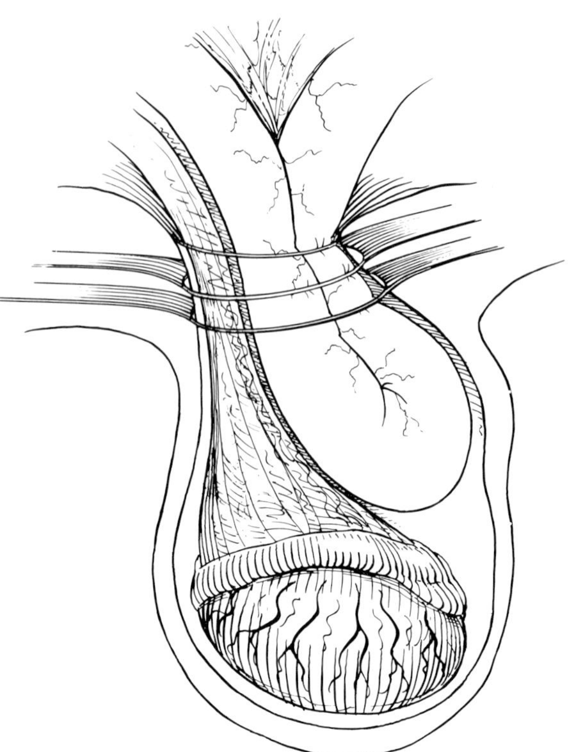

FIG. 102–2. Indirect inguinal hernia. The intestine descended to the scrotum and the vaginal ring and tunic are intact.

usually within the inguinal canal with or without tearing of the vaginal ring (Fig. 102–4). This is particularly descriptive of what occurs in the colt with a congenital inguinal hernia that ruptures the vaginal tunic because of increased abdominal compression at delivery.

CONGENITAL INGUINAL HERNIA

Congenital inguinal hernia can be indirect or direct (inguinal rupture or ruptured inguinal hernia). Generally the indirect hernia is recognized shortly after birth. It is easily reduced because of the large inguinal canal diameter, and it often resolves spontaneously in 3 to 4 months.[12,17] Daily manual reduction of the indirect hernia may enhance spontaneous resolution, and it ensures that an incarceration of the bowel will not be missed.[17] Occasionally, colic signs develop and the hernia may become irreducible, necessitating immediate surgery (Fig. 102–5). Surgery should also be considered if the hernia is large or has not resolved after 4 months. If the indirect inguinal hernia is large (10 to 12 cm), surgical intervention should be considered because chances of spontaneous resolution are remote.

Direct inguinal hernia probably results from a scrotal hernia that was present at delivery. The increased pressure of delivery may cause a rupture of the vaginal tunic and abdominal viscera may enter the subcutaneous tissue adjacent to the vaginal tunic. This hernia is recognized by depression and colic.[17,19] Intestinal contents can usually be palpated, but they often cannot be re-

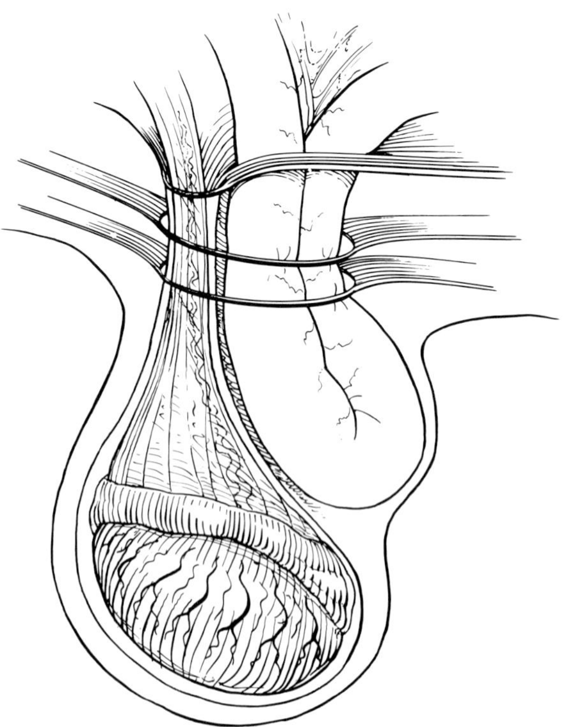

FIG. 102–3. Direct inguinal hernia (inguinal rupture). The intestine has herniated through a rent in the peritoneum and transverse fascia adjacent to the vaginal ring. The intestine is outside the vaginal cavity.

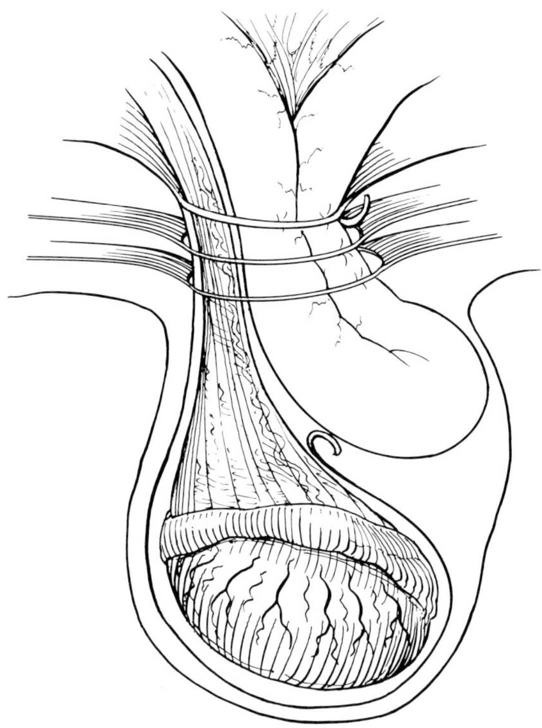

FIG. 102–4. Direct inguinal hernia (ruptured inguinal hernia). The intestine has herniated through a rent in the vaginal tunic in the inguinal canal and the vaginal ring remains intact.

duced. In contrast to the indirect hernia, the skin often feels cool and edematous, and transudation and skin erosion may be observed.[7] In addition, the swelling is often more pendulous, extending from the inguinal region to the cranial aspect of the prepuce and occasionally into the medial aspect of the thigh.[19] When clammy, edematous skin is encountered, attempts to reduce the direct hernia manually are discouraged because of the risk of further trauma to the soft tissues surrounding the herniated viscera. Surgical intervention is recommended as soon as possible.

ACQUIRED INGUINAL HERNIA

Acquired inguinal hernia can be indirect (most common) (Fig. 102–6) or direct (inguinal rupture or ruptured inguinal hernia). The hernia is usually unilateral; however, one case of bilateral hernia has been observed.[7] Although many causes have been implicated, including recent breeding, external abdominal trauma (falls and failure to clear fences or gates while jumping), strenuous work and a history of congenital inguinal hernia, spontaneous development of an inguinal hernia has been observed.[8]

Colic signs may range from mild to severe, depending on the duration of the hernia. On palpation, the inguinal scrotal region usually feels enlarged and firm and occasionally cool. Other considerations that must be differentiated include testicular torsion, thrombosis of the spermatic artery, testicular abscess, neoplasia, and testicular hematoma. If the hernia is recent or it remains inguinal, scrotal enlargement may not be present. With a direct hernia, the testicle on the affected side may appear enlarged, but it may also be pulled proximad because of the contraction of the cremaster muscles. On auscultation of the inguinal and scrotal regions, intestinal sounds may be heard. Rectal examination usually reveals a loop of small intestines entering the vaginal ring and distended loops of jejunum. Nasogastric reflux after intubation may also be seen. In most cases of indirect inguinal hernia, the intestine is strangulated.[4,11] Peritoneal fluid may have increased white blood cells and protein, and the packed cell volume and total solids become elevated with dehydration. Strangulation occurs at the vaginal ring and not at the deep or superficial inguinal rings. Thus, at surgery only the vaginal ring needs to be enlarged, either bluntly or by incision to allow reduction of the intestines.

To differentiate the direct inguinal hernia from indirect inguinal hernia on clinical findings alone is often difficult, and ultrasonographic examination of the scrotal and inguinal regions may help with the diagnosis. The need to examine every stallion with colic for inguinal hernia is illustrated by a review that reported only 50% of the cases of inguinal hernia were diagnosed be-

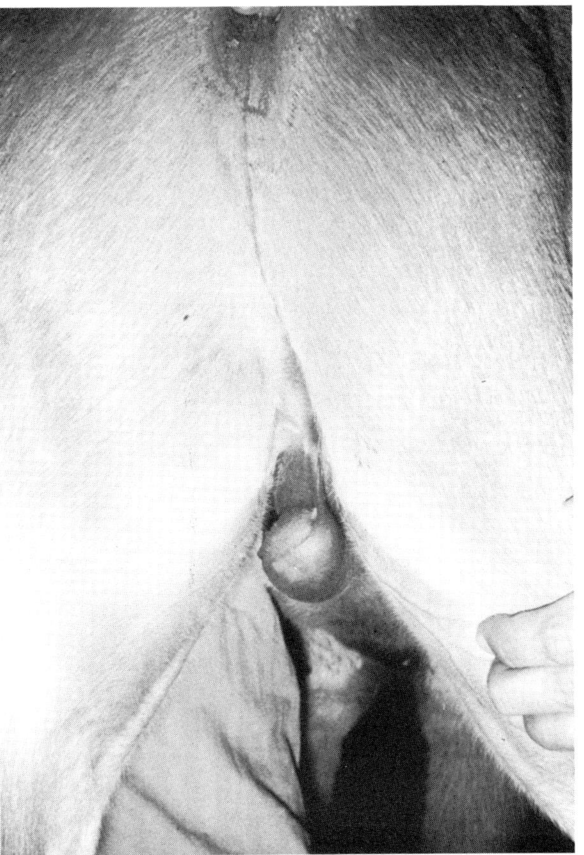

FIG. 102–5. A unilateral congenital indirect inguinal hernia in a 2-week-old foal. Reportedly, the hernia was becoming more difficult to reduce and intermittent signs of colic were observed. Surgery was indicated at this time.

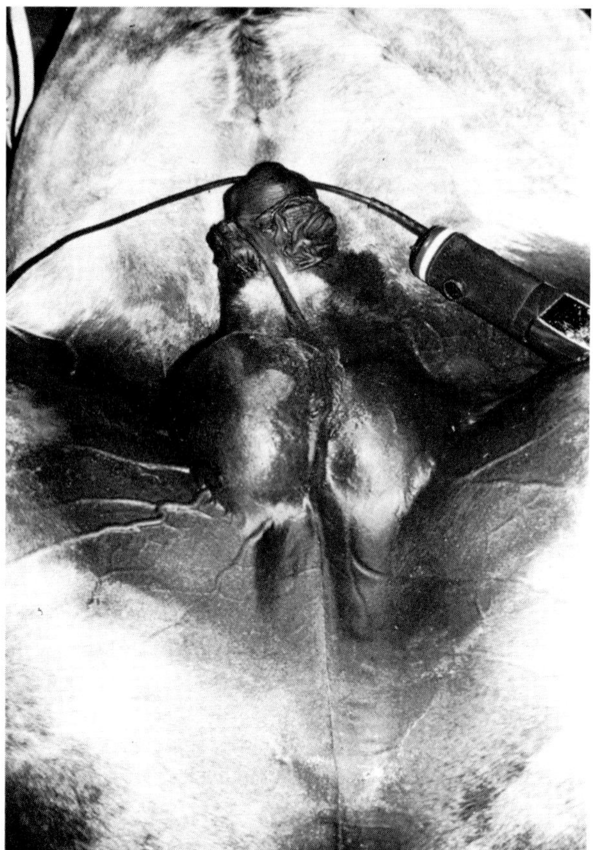

FIG. 102–6. An example of a unilateral indirect inguinal hernia in a stallion. Note enlargement of the right scrotal contents. This horse had a history of placing his forefeet on a wooden rail to look over the top of an enclosure. Clippers were used to remove the hair from the ventral abdominal region.

fore referral.[4] Although rectal taxis assisted by external manipulation have been used successfully in a limited number of early cases, it is difficult to recommend because of the risk of tearing the intestine or rectum and the increased chances of recurrence of hernia. With a diagnosis of acquired inguinal hernia, surgical exploration should follow as soon as possible. The discussion and treatment of acquired inguinal hernia and evisceration that develops after normal or cryptorchid castration are reviewed in other chapters.

SURGICAL PREPARATION AND ANESTHESIA

Administration of intravenous balanced electrolyte solutions should commence before surgery. For the incarcerated inguinal hernia, broad-spectrum antibiotics and flunixin meglumine are recommended because septicemia and toxemia are often associated with intestinal strangulation. In addition, they appear most effective in reducing adhesions of the small intestine after vascular compromise. A nasogastric tube should be passed before induction of anesthesia, and lavage and siphoning should be attempted to reduce fluid accumulation in the stomach.

Induction of anesthesia is by personal choice, yet a regimen that minimizes cardiovascular and respiratory depression is recommended. Although maintenance of anesthesia has been done in the past with intravenous agents, gas anesthesia is strongly recommended. Positive pressure ventilation may also be needed in cases in which severe small intestinal distention is a problem (Fig. 102–7). The patient is placed in dorsal recumbency and tilted slightly away from the affected side. However, before aseptic preparation commences, the prepuce should be packed with a 4 × 4 gauze, after which the opening of the prepuce is clamped shut with towel clamps or closed with a pursestring suture. Alternatively, the penis and sheath can be aseptically cleansed and a urinary catheter placed to divert urine flow. Inguinal, scrotal, and ventral abdominal regions in the adult are prepared simultaneously for sterile surgery. These regions are draped in anticipation that both inguinal exploratory and ventral midline laparotomy will be performed. My preference in the adult is to do both. Even though hernia reduction and intestinal resection and anastomosis of the jejunum can be accomplished through an inguinal laparotomy, a second abdominal incision (ventral midline) is necessary to complete the examination of the intestines and perform an ileal resection and jejunoceceal anastomosis if necessary. In support of this concept, 33 of 50 cases[7] and 14 of 24 cases[4] operated for inguinal hernia required a ventral midline laparotomy. Furthermore, the ventral midline laparotomy can facilitate reduction of herniated intestine, and it allows the surgeon to decompress the markedly distended small intestines (Fig. 102–7). In one case, a volvulus of the small intestine approximately 4 meters cranial (oral) to the strangulated inguinal hernia was present, and two intestinal resections and anastomoses were required. In a report on acquired

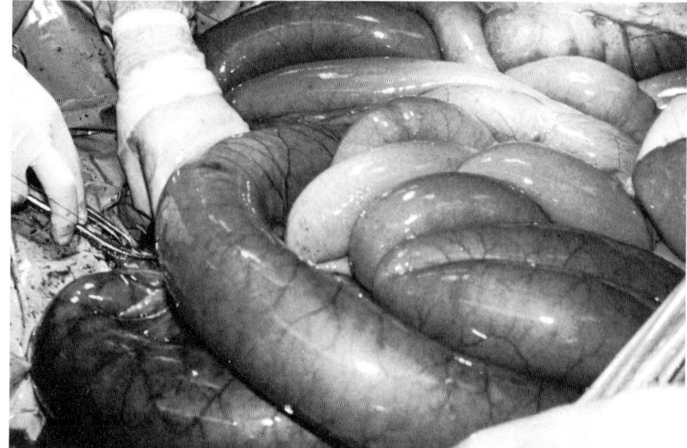

FIG. 102–7. Small intestinal distention cranial (oral) to the incarcerated inguinal hernia. The small intestines were exteriorized through a ventral midline laparotomy. They were decompressed by finger stripping of the fluid from the resected end of the intestine into a container adjacent to the surgical table. After this, an intestinal anastomosis was performed.

inguinal hernia in two horses, volvulus of the jejunum cranial to the herniated incarcerated intestines was observed.[20]

SURGERY

If rectal examination revealed markedly distended small intestines, the inguinal exploration and ventral midline incisions can be made simultaneously when two surgeons are available. If the small intestines were minimally distended on rectal examination, the inguinal exploratory may proceed first and the ventral midline follows if needed. The ventral midline laparotomy is generally not needed in the newborn colt when the small intestines are not incarcerated.

A straight 10-cm-long incision in foals and a 15- to 20-cm-long incision in adults is made directly over the external inguinal ring. Larger hernias may require longer incisions. The incision is made carefully so that intestines in the subcutaneous tissues outside the vaginal tunic will not be damaged. If the hernia is indirect, the incision is extended through the tunica dartos, inguinal subcutaneous tissue, and fascia until the vaginal tunic is exposed. Using a combination of scissor and blunt dissection, the vaginal tunic surrounding the testicle and herniated intestines is freed from scrotal fascia.

INGUINAL HERNIORRHAPHY IN THE FOAL

Surgery for nonincarcerated indirect congenital hernia in a foal can be handled in one of two ways. The intestines can be returned to the abdominal cavity by hand stripping the intestines within the tunics toward the abdominal cavity while traction is placed on the testis, vaginal tunic, and spermatic cord. Twisting the vaginal tunic and cord may also facilitate the reduction of the intestines. Once the intestines are reduced, a transfixation ligature of #1 synthetic absorbable suture is placed as close to the vaginal ring as possible, after which the vaginal tunic and spermatic cord are transected distal to the ligature.

The second approach (my preference) is to open the vaginal tunic so the intestines within the cavity can be examined. If the intestine appears reddened and fibrin is present on the surface, resection and anastomosis of the involved segment should follow. In most cases, the bowel will appear normal and the loops of small intestines can be replaced into the abdominal cavity using a single digit. Once the intestines are reduced, the spermatic cord is ligated with a transfixation ligature of #1 synthetic absorbable suture. The spermatic cord is then transected distal to the ligature. Following this, the vaginal tunic is trimmed close to the vaginal ring and is sutured to the stump of the spermatic cord (distal to the ligature) to obliterate completely the vaginal cavity.

No matter which method is selected, the superficial inguinal ring is sutured with 1-0 or #1 synthetic absorbable suture in a simple interrupted or continuous suture pattern. Adduction of the hindlimb will facilitate this. Following closure of the superficial inguinal ring, subcutaneous tissues are apposed to obliterate any remaining dead space. Several rows of 3-0 synthetic absorbable suture in a simple continuous pattern are used to appose the subcutaneous tissues. A continuous subcuticular suture using similar suture material is placed to appose the skin, and no skin sutures are used (my preference). Alternatively, the subcutaneous space can be left unsutured and packed with gauze or drained with a Penrose drain. The skin is usually partially sutured in the latter case so the gauze pack or drain can be removed.

If the hernia is direct (ruptured inguinal hernia), the intestines or abdominal contents and occasionally the testicle will be found in the subcutaneous tissues. After the viability of the intestine is ascertained (usually viable), the rent in the tunic is identified. In most cases, the rent is found in the inguinal canal.[17] The loops of intestine are returned to the abdominal cavity one by one using one or two digits. Once the intestines are reduced, the spermatic cord is ligated with transfixation ligatures of #1 synthetic absorbable suture, after which the spermatic cord is transected distal to it. Following this, the vaginal tunic is sutured with simple continuous sutures of 2-0 synthetic absorbable as close to the vaginal ring as possible so the vaginal cavity is completely obliterated; the stump of the spermatic cord distal to the ligature may be included in the suture. The superficial inguinal ring is then sutured with 1-0 or #1 synthetic absorbable suture in a simple interrupted or simple continuous suture pattern. Subcutaneous tissues are apposed with continuous sutures as previously described for an indirect hernia. If the intestinal herniation is quite large, dissecting on the medial side of the thigh, complete subcutaneous closure is unlikely and drainage of the dead space should be considered. If intestines within the hernia appear inflamed and edematous and fibrin adhesions have developed, resection and anastomosis of the small intestine should be done. Removal of the unaffected testicle at the time of surgery is by personal choice and discussion should include client input. In all cases, however, heritability should be discussed and a promise made to return the horse as a yearling for castration of the remaining testicle.[16]

INGUINAL HERNIORRHAPHY IN THE ADULT

The indirect hernia in the adult is managed by opening the vaginal tunic and examining the testes and intestines (Fig. 102–8A). In most cases, the herniated small intestine will be strangulated, requiring resection and anastomosis. If only one surgeon is available and the jejunum is involved, the small intestines can be further exteriorized and the resection anastomosis can be accomplished through the inguinal incision after unilateral castration. However, the vaginal ring may have to be enlarged to allow further exteriorization of the procedure. The vaginal ring may be enlarged by cutting it at its cranial limits with scissors (Fig. 102–8B) or utilizing a blunt bistoury. Once the vaginal ring is cut, the

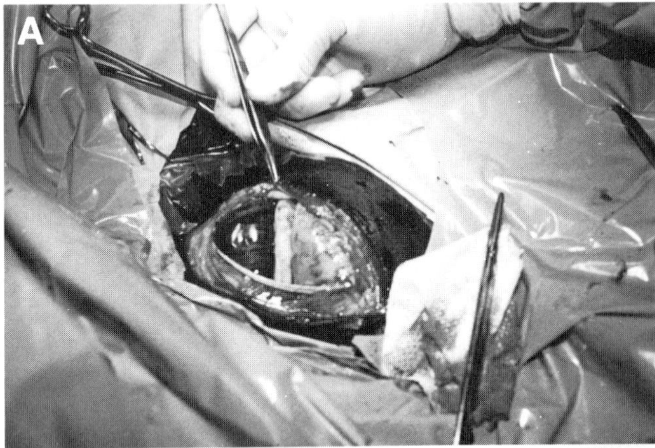

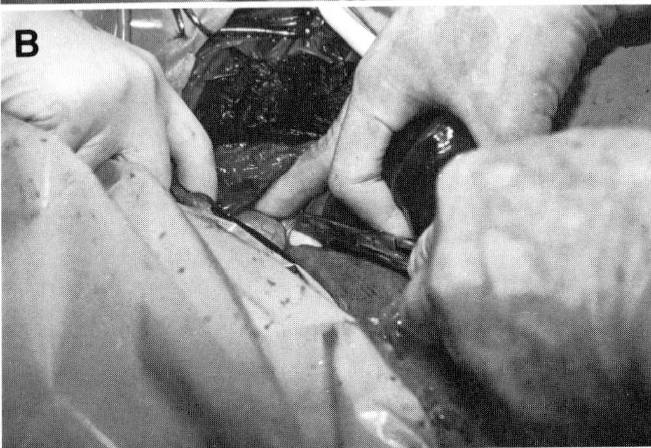

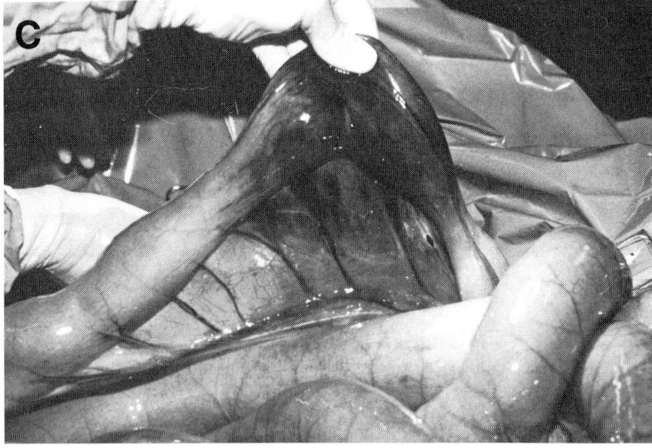

FIG. 102–8. *A*, Indirect hernia in a stallion. The vaginal tunic has been incised and the incarcerated small intestines (left) and testicle (right) can be seen. *B*, Scissors are being used to cut the vaginal ring. This was done so the intestines could be retracted into the abdominal cavity. The right hand is being used to retract the incarcerated intestines. Note the antimesenteric band between the thumb and forefinger of the right hand, indicating the ilium was involved. *C*, The incarcerated ilium was retracted into the abdominal cavity and exteriorized through a ventral midline laparotomy. Note the distended small intestines cranial (oral) to the incarceration.

intestines can be more easily manipulated and exteriorized if needed. After the resection anastomosis is complete, the bowel can be returned to the abdominal cavity. A short ventral midline incision should be made so the intestines can be pulled through the inguinal canal into the abdominal cavity. The rent in the mesentery can be sutured at this time and the distended loops of small intestines cranial (oral) to the resection anastomosis can be examined and decompressed (Figs. 102–7 and 102–8C).

If two surgeons are available, the ventral midline and inguinal incisions can be made simultaneously. Once the vaginal tunic is open, the strangulated intestines can be managed in one of several ways. If the jejunum is involved, the bowel is exteriorized further (a small incision in the vaginal ring may be required to do this) (Fig. 102–8B) so ligatures can be placed at the extremities of the strangulation. Alternatively, the intestine can be resected with stapling equipment or resected sharply and oversewn with sutures. The intestines can be returned to the abdominal cavity by applying traction from within the abdominal cavity. If the ligature method is used, the strangulated bowel may have to be decompressed by needle suction before attempting to reduce it. The intestine is then exteriorized from the abdominal incision and the anastomosis is completed by the assistant.

If the ileum is involved, exteriorization of the small intestine cannot be accomplished, and the bowel will have to be reduced into the abdominal cavity without placing ligatures or accomplishing resection (Fig. 102–8C). While the assistant is performing the anastomosis and bowel decompression, unilateral castration can commence.

In the mature breeding stallion, separate ligation of the vas deferens, and testicular vessels is preferred to placing a transfixation ligature that incorporate all these tissues (Fig. 102–9). Separate ligatures are placed as close to the vaginal ring as possible. After ligature is complete, the cremaster muscle is clamped with crushing forceps (Oschner) after which the crushed tissue is incised. This is done to minimize bleeding from the musculature, though individual cautery of small leaking vessels may be required. The vaginal tunic is then incised in a circular fashion as close to the vaginal ring as possible. Incorporating the distal extremity of the separately ligated structures of the spermatic cord, including the fascia surrounding the transected cremaster muscles in the suture closure of the vaginal tunic, will ensure obliteration of the inguinal canal. The external inguinal ring may then be sutured with simple interrupted sutures of #2 synthetic absorbable. The subcutaneous and subcuticular tissues are sutured as was described for closure of congenital inguinal hernia.

A direct hernia resulting from a ruptured inguinal hernia can be surgically managed in a manner similar to that described in the foal. However, if the direct hernia is a result of inguinal rupture (Fig. 102–3), an attempt should be made to repair the rent in the abdominal wall fascia by suturing it after the intestine has been replaced in the abdominal cavity.

Although inguinal herniorrhaphy techniques to salvage the testes and prevent reherniation have been described, they are not recommended unless unique circumstances exist. One such case may be the valuable breeding stallion that has lost the function of the other

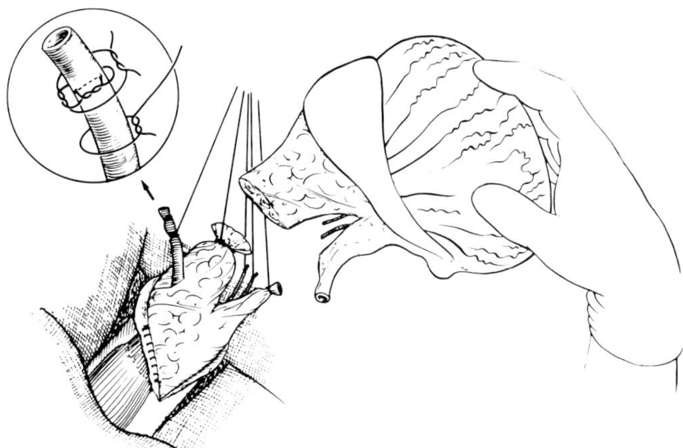

FIG. 102–9. Separate ligation of the vas deferens and testicular vessels. Note the testicular artery is isolated and double ligated. The ligature closest to the cut end of the artery is a transfixation ligature (circle upper left).

testis. In this situation, an encircling (pursestring) ligature can be placed around the spermatic cord as close to the vaginal ring as possible. After the intestines are reduced, it is then tightened just enough so not to occlude the vascular supply to the testis but prevent reherniation of intestines. If the hernia is from an inguinal rupture, the rent in the abdominal wall fascia should be sutured appropriately. Unfortunately, in most cases of strangulated inguinal hernia, the impaired venous return to the testis will often result in testicular degeneration.

POSTOPERATIVE CARE

Postoperative care should include continued intravenous fluids, antibiotics, and nonsteroidal anti-inflammatory drugs in the adult. Intensive postoperative monitoring will be required for several days. If colic and ileus occur, rectal examination should be performed to identify small intestinal distention or adhesions or to rule out a reherniation of the intestines. Laparotomy should also be considered if colic persists. Treatment of colic and ileus in the postoperative period is often needed. Gastric decompression via a nasogastric tube is often required until bowel function returns to normal. If gauze packs or Penrose drains were used, they are usually removed within 48 h.

PROGNOSIS

Generally a good prognosis can be given for congenital indirect inguinal hernias if they are repaired within a few hours after colic signs commence. The longer the duration, the worse the prognosis for life. In one case series of ruptured inguinal hernias in 14 colts, 7 survived.[17] Causes for death or euthanasia included pneumonia, recurrence of the hernia and colic because of persistent ileus, and necrotic intestines. In another case series of 5 colts with ruptured inguinal hernia, all survived 12 months and the colts appeared to be developing normally.[19] Because adhesions appear to be a problem in foals, the prognosis should be reduced appropriately if the intestines are strangulated and a resection and anastomosis is required.

Because the majority of acquired inguinal hernias are strangulated, the prognosis is generally adjusted according to the duration of the incarceration and the clinical signs of colic; the longer the duration the poorer the prognosis. In three case series, complete recovery with long-term followup was achieved in 6 of 9 cases (67%),[8] 20 of 27 cases (74%),[4] and 38 of 50 cases (76%),[7] respectively. Reasons for death postoperatively were unresponsive shock and ileus, adhesive peritonitis, gastric rupture, reherniation, and postoperative myositis.[7,8] The prognosis for reproductive soundness remains favorable as long as the remaining testicle is normal.

REFERENCES

1. Cohrs, P.: Nieberle and Cohrs' Textbook of Special Pathological Anatomy of Domestic Animals. Translated by R.Crawford. Oxford, Pergamon Press, 1967.
2. Goetz, T.E., Boulton, C.H., and Coffman, J.R.: Inguinal hernias in stallions and colts. Compend. Contin. Educ. Practicing Vet., *3:*S272–S276, 1981.
3. Noone, J.P.: Scrotal herniation of the urinary bladder in the horse. Ir. Vet. J., *20:*11, 1966.
4. Schneider, R.K., Milne, D.W., and Kohn, C.W.: Acquired inguinal hernia in the horse: A review of 27 cases. J. Am. Vet. Med. Assoc., *180:*317–332, 1982.
5. Hayes, H.M.: Congenital umbilical and inguinal hernias in cattle, horses, swine, dogs and cats: Risk by breed and sex among hospital patients. Am. J. Vet. Res., *35:*839–842, 1974.
6. Sembrat, R.F.: The acute abdomen in the horse. Epidemiologic considerations. Arch. Am. Col. Vet. Surg., *4:*34–39, 1975.
7. Van der Velden, M.A.: Surgical treatment of acquired inguinal hernia in the horse: A review of 51 cases. Equine Vet. J., *20:*173–177, 1988.
8. Weaver, D.A.: Acquired incarcerated inguinal hernia: A review of 13 horses. Can. Vet. J., *28:*195–199, 1987.
9. White, N.A., Moore, J.N., Cowgil, L.M., and Brown, J.: Epizootiology and risk factors in colic at university hospitals. Proceedings of the Second Equine Colic Research Symposium. Vol. 2. Athens, GA, Veterinary Learning Systems, 1986, pp. 26–29.
10. Livesey, M.A.: Inguinal hernia. *In* Current Practice of Equine Surgery. Edited by N.A. White and J.N. Moore. Philadelphia, J.B. Lippincott, 1990, pp. 321–327.
11. White, N.A.: Inguinal hernia. *In* The Equine Acute Abdomen. Edited by N.A. White. Philadelphia, Lea & Febiger, 1990, pp. 349–351.
12. Cox, J.E.: Hernias and ruptures of the inguinal region. *In* Surgery of the Reproductive Tract in Large Animals. 3rd ed. Liverpool, Liverpool University, Press, 1987, pp. 53–69.
13. Ashdown, R.R.: The anatomy of the inguinal canal in the domestic animals. Vet. Rec., *75:*1345–1351, 1963.

14. McIlwraith, C.W., and Turner, A.S.: Inguinal herniorrhaphy. *In* Equine Surgery Advanced Techniques. Philadelphia, Lea & Febiger, 1987, pp. 333–338.
15. Vasey, J.R.: Simultaneous presence of a direct and an indirect inguinal hernia in a stallion. Aust. Vet. J., *57:*418–421, 1981.
16. Vaughan, J.T.: Surgery of the male reproductive system. *In* Textbook of Large Animal Surgery. Edited by P. Jennings. Philadelphia. W.B. Saunders, 1984, pp. 1101–1102.
17. Van der Velden, M.A.: Ruptured hernia in newborn colt foals: A review of 14 cases. Equine Vet. J., *20:*178–181, 1988.
18. Moore, J.N., et al.: A case report of inguinal herniorrhaphy in a stallion. J. Equine Med. Surg., *1:*391–394, 1977.
19. Spurlock, G.H., and Robertson, J.T.: Congenital inguinal hernias associated with a rent in the common vaginal tunic in five foals. J. Am. Vet. Med. Assoc., *193:*1087–1088, 1988.
20. Moll, H.D., et al.: Small intestinal volvulus as a complication of acquired inguinal hernia in two horses. J. Am. Vet. Med. Assoc., *198:*1413–1414, 1991.

CHAPTER 103

SURGERY OF THE PREPUCE AND PENIS

J.T. Vaughan

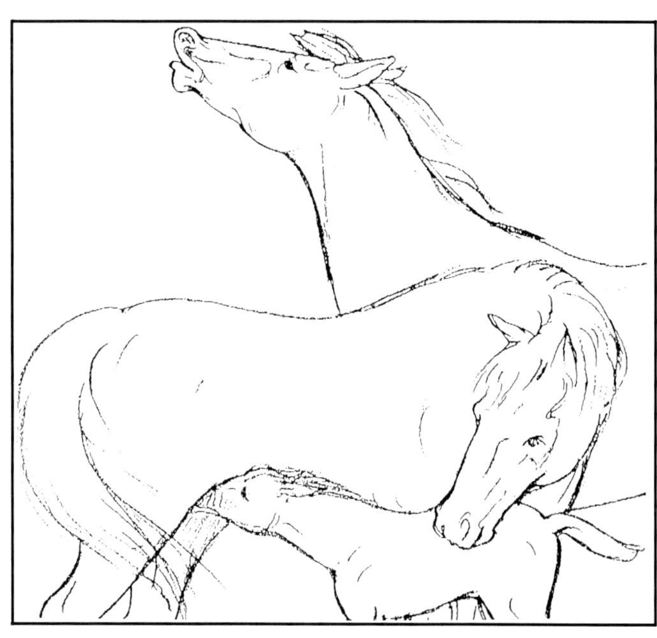

GENERAL SURGERY

Welch and Powers classified four major categories of operative surgery which embrace essential principles: (1) treatment of wounds, (2) extirpative surgery, (3) reconstructive surgery, and (4) physiologic surgery.[1] Each specialty of surgery, regardless of the system, is composed of operative procedures that involve one or more of these four principal types.

WOUND CARE

The importance of urinary patency and the control of inflammation and infection, including tetanus immunization, cannot be overemphasized. The rewards are the minimization of deformity and the early return of function. See Chapter 97 for the methods of examination and the treatment of wounds.

EXTIRPATION

The classic example of extirpative surgery is the resection of a neoplasm. Such lesions frequently involve infectious processes when the tumor ulcerates on the surface or abscesses in the interior. Resections run the gamut from the simple wedge excision of a superficial tumor in situ to the en bloc resection of prepuce, penis, and regional lymphatics for an invasive malignancy. Not all lesions require the knife. Effective extirpation may be accomplished by the use of cryosurgery and the laser.

RECONSTRUCTION

Examples of the restoration of disturbed architecture include the revision of scars left in the wake of injury and infection, the creation of new stoma, and general wound repair. Posthioplasty alone falls into at least three categories of wedge excision, circumcision, and ablation of the prepuce for neoplastic disease, parasitisms, intractable infections, and congenital anomalies. Relocation of the urethral orifice may be necessitated by obstructions and disruptions of a varied nature.

PHYSIOLOGIC SURGERY

Physiologic surgery is any surgery which has the purpose of restoring or altering function or behavior, such as with spay and castration. Thus the Bolz technique of penis retraction seeks to return the function lost as a result of paralytic paraphimosis,[2] as does the corpus shunt for priapism.[3] Provision of physiologic rest for the injured part may require castration as well as separation from outside sources (other horses) of psychic stimulation.

Obviously, most instances involve components of two or more of these cardinal types of operative surgery and the approximation, if not the full return, of both structure and function are the ultimate objectives.

SPECIAL SURGERY

Special surgery is arbitrarily divided into 10 categories for convenience of discussion in addition to the appropriateness of classification. All of these should stand on the foundations of wound care and general surgery. Indeed, the success of special surgical methods, no matter how innovative, can never be separated from an absolute dependence on thoughtful preoperative preparation; a reverence for atraumatic, hemostatic, and aseptic techniques; and conscientious aftercare.

PREPARATION

Because of the relative inconvenience of the location, as well as the liability of hemorrhage, the patient preferably should be restrained in dorsal recumbency with the pelvic limbs abducted. Ischial urethrotomy for urolithiasis and small superficial lesions that can be removed by wedge excision or treated by cryosurgery under local anesthesia by infiltration are the exceptions. In the main, dorsal recumbency under general anesthesia permits more careful attention to dissection, better delineation of the disease, more effective hemostasis and asepsis, and more accurate reconstruction.

In all cases where decompression of the urinary bladder and positive identification of the urethra are desirable, an indwelling catheter should be in place before dissection is commenced. This is doubly important if a tourniquet is to be used. Drainage of urine should exit remote to the surgical field to obviate wetting of the drapes. The presence of infective discharges (such as exudative ulcers, fistulous tracts, or wounds) justify the additional use of impervious drapes and packing off (isolating) sources of contamination in close proximity to the field.

Tourniquets may be of the pneumatic type but are most commonly gum rubber tubing. Control of hemorrhage by interlocking pedicle suture as well as point ligation is required when invading sinusoidal vascular spaces. Healing by primary intention of any surgery on such tissues places a premium on leaving a hemostatically dry field upon closure. A dissecting hematoma postoperative virtually ensures dehiscence and healing by granulation, which is also a frequent cause of urethral stenosis.

A further word of caution is in order concerning positioning of the patient. Lateral support of the pelvic limbs in the form of cushions or overhead support by suspension should be provided to prevent the strained position of unsupported abduction, especially for procedures that are apt to require more than 30 minutes. The stretching that occurs to the obturator nerves during prolonged abduction in dorsal recumbency is theorized to be the cause of what appears in such patients upon recovery as a classical obturator paralysis. The principal loss of function occurs in the adductor muscles of the thigh, and the pelvic limbs of patients so affected spread-eagle during abortive attempts to stand. The result is either a coxofemoral luxation or fracture with rupture of muscle insertions on the pelvis. The patient invariably must be destroyed.

In addition to emptying the urinary bladder, the rectum should be evacuated manually so the pelvic canal be as free of contents as possible. Elective cases may benefit from further preparation by diet, fasting, and premedication. Other preoperative preparations are standard procedure in stabilization of the patient, contraseptic management of existing infections, preparation of the field, and induction of anesthesia.

URETHROTOMY

The principal indication is the re-establishment of patency interrupted by obstructions from urinary calculi in the bladder or the urethra,[4,5] from cicatricial stenosis usually caused by surgical or accidental wounds of the distal urethra,[6] and from compression of encroaching disease, such as neoplasia or hematoma,[7] that occludes the urethra. An occasional reason is to examine, debride, or otherwise treat chronic lesions of the urethra as may be the cause of hemospermia.[8]

The ischial approach is done on the standing horse under local anesthesia, usually local infiltration, although the epidural block can be used. The rectum and bladder are emptied and a catheter is left in place. A longitudinal skin incision of 8 cm is made on the median raphe just ventral to the sphincter ani and directly over the ischiatic arch. The incision is deepened by sharp dissection between the retractor penis muscles and through the bulbospongiosus muscle, the corpus spongiosum, and the urethra, in that order. Accuracy of incision on the median raphe is aided by stabilizing the penis and the catheterized urethra between the fingers of the free hand, placing the tissues under tension. This also minimizes the hemorrhage that occurs upon incision of the corpus spongiosum (which otherwise obscures the field of dissection) until the incision can be extended to the lumen of the urethra. Active hemorrhage thereafter requires both compression sutures and ligatures.[4]

The incision is lengthened dorsally as needed for access to the horizontal pelvic urethra. Small calculi that lodge in the neck of the bladder can be removed either intact by patiently dilating and lubricating the pelvic urethra or by fragmenting the calculus with a lithotrite. This is done with greater facility in the mare because of the short and comparatively more distensible urethra, as well as the option of performing a sphincterotomy in the female. The alternative, of course, is laparocystidotomy, covered elsewhere in this volume.[4]

After removal of all fragments has been confirmed, the bladder must be irrigated more or less continually until all sand and detritus are eliminated and hemorrhage within the bladder has ceased. Otherwise, clots form and reobstruct the urethra.

Resumption of normal evacuation may be delayed for hours or days, and the urinary tract is vulnerable to ascending infections during that time. The urethrotomy wound is best left to heal by second intention, which capacity the urethra has to a gratifying degree. It does benefit, however, from obliterating by finely placed sutures (delayed absorbable) any pocket or dead space in the ventral end of the incision.

The aftercare consists of regular wound toilet, confirmation of unrestricted urine flow, periodic urinalysis and hemogram, good hydration, and medication with urinary antiseptics and antibiotics as determined by diagnostic microbiologic and clinical pharmacologic data. Inasmuch as the chronic cystitis that almost always attends urolithiasis can be obstinate, the use of the laboratory from the outset is time-saving and economic in such cases.

The use of urine acidifiers such as ammonium chloride can be effective in producing an environment inhospitable to even the most resistant bacteria. It may also be helpful in dissolving (or preventing recrystallization) of urine salts, which tend to be favored by the alkaline urine of herbivores.

Urethrotomy in more distal locations may be indicated by urethral calculi or lesions elsewhere along the course of the external urethra. The procedure is the same except that positioning of the patient would revert to dorsal recumbency under general anesthesia.

Where obstruction by small urethral calculi is of recent duration and when the site can be palpated, the stone may possibly be dislodged by infusion of lubricants through the urethral orifice to facilitate the distal movement of the calculus by both distention of the urethra and progressive massage (E. Kincaid, personal communication).

URETHROPLASTY

The indications for urethroplasty are acute wound repair, relocation of the urethral orifice, and correction of chronic deformities such as parasitisms of the urethral process, stenosis and fistula. Acute wounds are represented by both blunt and sharp injuries. Horses in a kicking duel may sustain trauma to the corpus spongiosum of the root of the penis with compressive hematoma that occludes the urethra and necessitates urethrotomy to relieve obstruction of urine.[7] Sharp and penetrating wounds of the urethra may require plastic reconstruction to restore essential architecture for healing by either primary or secondary intention.[6] As long as urine is not allowed to accumulate at the site or to suffuse into the tissues, it does not appreciably retard healing by granulation and epithelialization. This relives some of the burden of providing a leakproof repair. In fact, overzealous attempts to do so may predispose to resultant stenosis. It does not, however, reduce the need for daily nursing care to ensure unobstructed urine flow and a healthy wound. Tendency toward cicatricial stricture can be dealt with by daily bougienage with soft, flexible catheters that match the size of the normal urethra.[4] Again, this must be done with a strict regard for hygienic technique. Relocation of the urethral orifice (urethrostomy) is discussed later in this chapter.

Deformities of the urethral process are usually caused by parasitisms, neoplasms, and anomalies, in descending order. Lesions that involve the glans penis may require more extensive amputation; however, lesions limited to the urethral process, most commonly habronemiasis, can be effectively removed by circumscribed amputation. Suture closure by finely placed interrupted sutures is necessary to control hemorrhage.

Minor stenosis may be approached by linear release incisions and bougienage or by revisions of the orifice to permit spatulation of the urethra. More extensive stenosis caused by abortive wound repair, neoplasia, and so forth may require amputation.

PREPUTIOTOMY

Constriction of the preputial ring is usually a congenital problem that manifests itself as phimosis, urination within the prepuce, and chronic ulceration of the preputial orifice (urine scald). Surgical correction is easily accomplished by percutaneous transection of the muscular ring in its dorsal aspect through a stab incision in the skin of the preputial ring where the inner lamina reflects on the outer lamina. Hemorrhage is inconsequential and the skin incision is closed with one or two interrupted mattress sutures. Although present at birth, the complaint may not be registered until months later.[9]

POSTHIOPLASTY

Limited to only the superficial planes of tissue, posthioplasty finds indication for resection of superficial lesions, revision of scar, relief of minor prolapse, and correction of anomalies. It ranges from wedge excisions of discrete tumors in situ to total ablation of refractory and widespread dermatosis of the entire prepuce, as exemplified by the case of chronic seborrhea.

Excisional Posthetomy

The best example of posthioplasty is the single, isolated carcinoma, or the indurated mass of scar tissue that remains in the site of an old summer sore. Such lesions can be removed under local infiltration anesthesia in the standing patient. An elliptical skin incision is made to girdle the base of the lesion in normal skin. The plane of dissection is the subcutaneous fascia, which, if separated by blunt scissor dissection with Mayo scissors, causes little hemorrhage. Suture repair should be in two layers, the skin closure supported by a subcuticular suture. Healing, in the absence of hemorrhage or infection, is uneventful.[10]

Circumcision

Commonly known as the reefing operation, circumcision is indicated for the superficial pathologies of the prepuce (neoplasia, parasitism, and scar) as well as minor prolapse. Circumferential posthetomy differs from the excisional posthetomy only in extent. The preputial ring and a variable amount of the adjacent internal and external preputial laminae, as determined by the disease, are removed intact by two girdling incisions proximal and distal to the surgical specimen. A tourniquet is usually unnecessary. As in the foregoing description, the disease is confined for the most part to the skin, and the plane of dissection is the subcutaneous fascia. Blunt scissor dissection is employed with Mayo scissors, inserting the closed blades into the fascial plane and then spreading them to open up the space. Sharp scissor dissection is alternated as bleeders are identified and avoided until clamped. In this way, the pathologic tissue is separated from the normal until freed of all underlying attachment. Bisecting the specimen may ease dissection.

After removal of the diseased tissue, hemostasis is confirmed by ligation or electrofulguration of small bleeders and ligation of larger ones as needed. To pre-

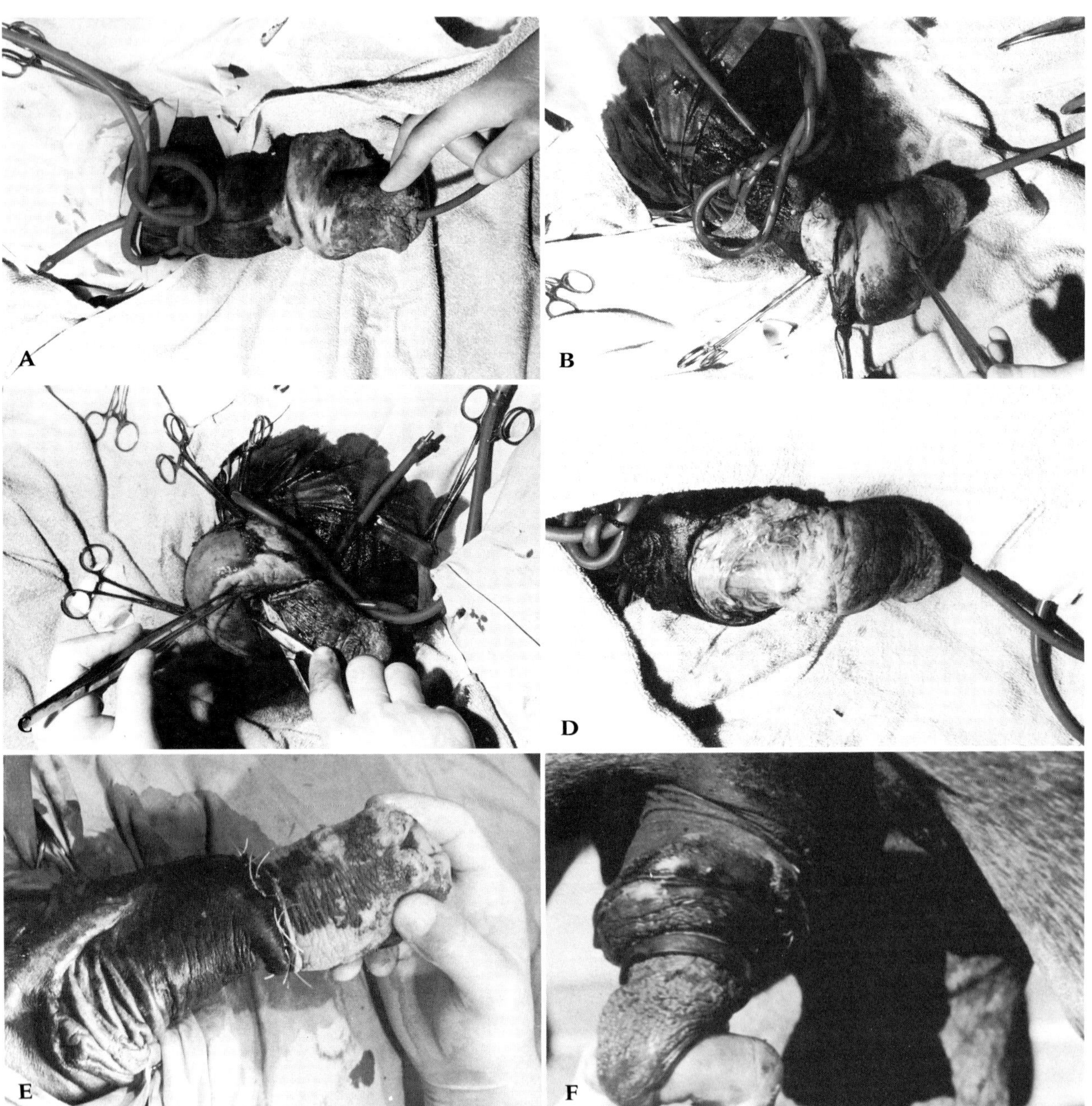

FIG. 103–1. Reefing operation. *A*, The surgical field prepared. Note the urethral catheter and tourniquet. *B*, Dissection of the disease. *C*, Dissection continued. *D*, Pathologic process resected. *E*, Tourniquet and catheter removed. *F*, Stallion ring as a postoperative precaution.

serve the sliding planes of tissue, suture closure is limited to the incised edges in a two-layer pattern of interrupted subcuticular and cutaneous sutures of either vertical or horizontal mattress type. Dead space seems not to be a problem as long as seroma or hematoma are averted. As with all surgery of the external genitalia, sexual rest by isolation from psychic stimulation is essential[3,10–14] (Fig. 103-1).

The objective of the reefing operation, other than removal of disease and revision of scar, is the abbreviation of the function of protrusion and the assistance of retraction. From least to greatest, the three alternatives to interferences of retraction that result from paraphimosis, paralysis, or space-occupying lesions are posthioplasty (reefing), surgical retraction (the Bolz technique), and amputation. Although the reefing operation seems like a small weapon, the results can be dramatic and quite satisfying in such instances as when the natural return of the penis to the sheath is impeded by a large, fibrous mass or other lesion that, by its size and weight alone, effectively nullify retraction. In such cases, even horses at stud can be returned to service.

Ablation

In the infrequent case of widespread dermatosis of the prepuce that is refractory to treatment, such as chronic seborrhea, kissing lesions of carcinoma, and precancerous plaques, posthetomy may extend to resection of virtually the entire hairless laminae of the prepuce, leaving just enough to serve as a recess for the quiescent free body and glans of the penis. Of course, this is indicated only in geldings or requires gelding in advance of the posthetomy.

The surgical technique differs from that described for circumcision only in extent. The hazard in both procedures is contamination of the surgical field by the pathologic tissue being resected. This increases the need for careful preoperative preparation and isolation of the pathology during dissection (Fig. 103-2).

PENIS RETRACTION

As described by Berge and Westhues, the operation for prolapse of the penis is indicated in cases of paralysis.[2] The exposure and gravitational edema complicating chronic prolapse result in desiccation, excoriation and ulceration of the skin surfaces, and indurated thickening of subcutaneous fascia. The sinusoidal vascular spaces fill with sludged blood and, if untreated, resultant disease perpetuates itself in a vicious circle. This emphasizes the importance of a period of several days devoted to preoperative treatment of the prolapse by suspensory bandage, protectant and osmotic agents, massage, and fomentation to reduce the edema and inflammation and to promote healthy epithelialization. Contraseptic treatment of infection, control of irritation, and progressive attempts to return the prolapse to the natural retracted state by manipulation all contribute to the success of surgery. Refractory lesions or scars of the prepuce that interfere with function should be excised by wedge or circumferential incision.[2,3,14]

Castration of the intact male is thought to be advisable if penile tumescence and priapism are apt to be complicating factors. If this is judged not to be the case, alternatives may include use as a teaser. I know of no cases of return to service as a stallion. Orchiectomy may be staged before, during, or after the retraction operation, and aseptic technique with primary closure should be used to minimize postoperative complications in consideration of the precipitating complaint.

With the patient in dorsal recumbency under general anesthesia and catheterized, a 6- to 10-cm skin incision is made longitudinally on the median raphe just caudal to the castration scar or behind the base of the scrotum (Fig. 103-3). A laudable precaution for all sharp dissection in regions of rich superficial vasculature or other vital anatomy is to tent the skin and subcutaneous fascia when making the incision, so as to avoid accidental injury to unexposed underlying structures. Afterward, the field may be extended by blunt dissection through the elastic fascia surrounding the penis so as to permit exteriorization of a loop of the penis sufficient to reach

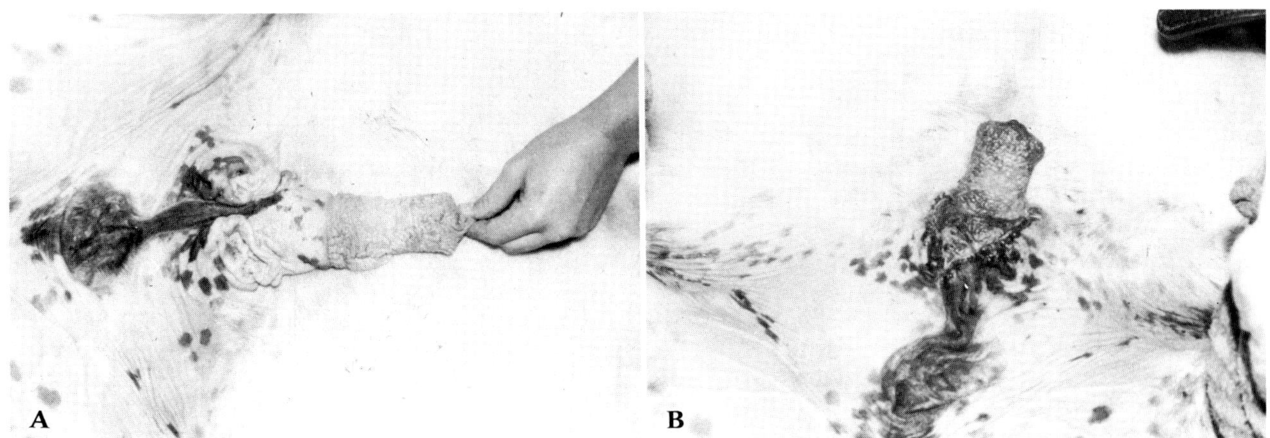

FIG. 103–2. Ablation of the prepuce. *A*, Preoperative view of the chronic posthitis. *B*, Postoperative view following ablation.

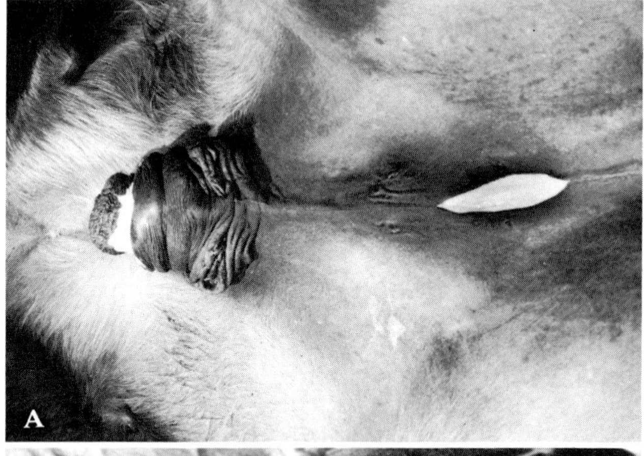

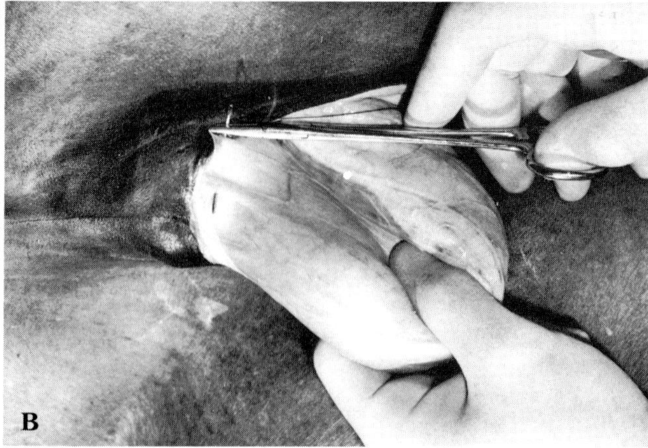

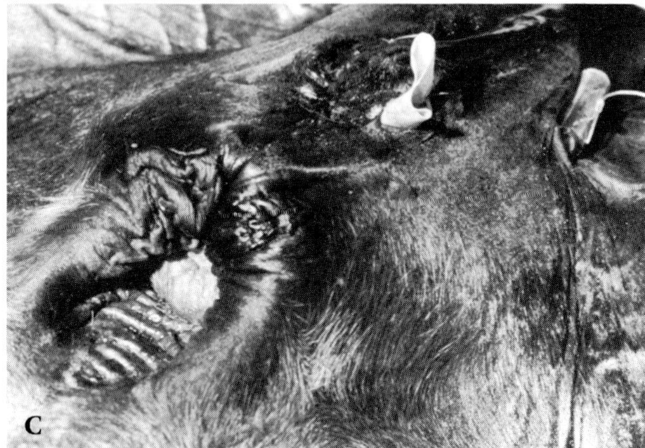

FIG. 103–3. Penis retraction. *A,* The postscrotal incision site. *B,* Traction suture placement in annular thickening of preputial reflection. *C,* Retracted penis with Penrose drains in the dissection site.

the annular thickening (in the cranial end of the incision) where the prepuce reflects onto the free body of the penis.[2]

A mattress suture is placed on each side of the penis through this thickened ring in such a way as to provide a secure anchor for traction to be maintained during the subsequent healing period for at least 14 days. A large-diameter suture is less likely to cut out through the tissues. Stitch abscesses can be prevented by using noncapillary nonabsorbable material, and by avoiding perforation through the skin of the prepuce on the other side. This can be accomplished by having an assistant palpate the interior of the preputial cavity during suture placement. Care should also be taken to position the sutures well to the side of the urethra so that no compression from suture tension occurs.[2,3,14]

The paired long ends of the two traction sutures are then armed with needles and passed to the outside through the skin of the inguinal region on each side at least 5 cm lateral to the skin margins so as to complete the mattress suture. They are tightened over stents just enough to retract the glans penis even with the external orifice of the prepuce. The use of large-diameter, thick-walled plastic tubing as stents will minimize the pressure necrosis often associated with tension sutures.[2,3,14]

The exteriorized loop of penis is returned to the wound and fascial spaces are apposed with a few interrupted absorbable sutures to minimize pockets of serum. The slight sigmoiding of the penis has not been known to interfere with either blood supply or urination. The subcutaneous fascia and skin are apposed with a conventional two-layer closure. Drains and stent bandages are discretionary as are postoperative antibiotics, diuretics, and anti-inflammatories.

The traction sutures should be clamped or secured in a bow versus a hard knot until the patient recovers and regains his feet, at which time tension on the sutures can be adjusted to position the end of the penis properly. If it protrudes, the glans can become dessicated or irritated from exposure to sunlight, cold, or insects. If recessed too far, urination inside the sheath causes urine scald.[14]

The horse should be cross-tied standing for 48 h, bedded on clean straw, and hand walked regularly to aid circulation and minimize edema. Sutures can be removed in 2 weeks and work resumed thereafter, depending on the progress of healing. Isolation from mares and other stallions should be maintained for at least 1 month.[14]

AMPUTATION

The last resort for invasive disease and refractory prolapse is amputation. The indications are straightforward, the only decision being the site. Lesions of the glans or distal penis that exceed circumscribed excision or cryosurgery may be amputated along the free body of the penis, and this is the classic procedure that leaves the abbreviated penis recessed in the preputial cavity with no other disturbance of the normal architecture. In those cases where the disease involves the prepuce and/or the more proximal penis, amputation may be required at almost any level. Common examples are neoplasia, infections, and parasitisms; complications of urethral obstruction (such as urine cellulitis); congenital anomalies; and injuries, including iatrogenic surgical misadventures. Thus, discussion of the subject must range from the simple amputation along the free body to the en bloc resection of the prepuce, penis, and regional lymphatics. Relocation of the urethra and reconstruction of supporting components of the penis in unorthodox ways that are compatible with structure and function require innovation.

Preputial Amputation

The patient is prepared in dorsal recumbency under general anesthesia and catheterized. The penis must be mobile to facilitate dissection under tourniquet and the abnormality must be isolated from the field by drapes.

Several variations of technique exist.[3] The procedure as done according to the Williams technique provides positive control of hemorrhage, reconstruction by primary closure under full epithelial surface, and gored spatulation of the urethra to prevent stenosis and direct the urine stream properly downward[10,14,15] (Fig. 103-4).

With the penis placed under forward traction, the plane of amputation is identified, the tourniquet is tightened, and a section of skin and subcutaneous tissue in the shape of an isosceles triangle is removed over the ventral aspect of the urethra. The base of the triangle (3 cm) coincides with the plane of amputation. The sides of the triangle (4 cm) extend caudad over the urethra and outline the gore of the subsequent repair. The section of tissue includes fascia, the retractor penis and bulbospongiosus muscles, and the corpus spongiosum, the last being the principal source of hemorrhage at this point. When the urethra has been exposed by removal of all overlying tissues, it is incised lengthwise from apex to base along the midline. The catheter is removed, and the margins of the urethral incision are sutured to the margins of the skin incision along the sides of the triangle with fine monofilament of either nylon, polypropylene, or a long-duration absorbable suture. The suture line controls hemorrhage from the sinusoidal spaces of the corpus spongiosum.[10,14,15]

At this time, the penis is amputated by sharp dissection along a plane angled slightly forward from the base of the triangle at the urethra to the dorsum of the penis. In addition to facilitating closure, this plane ensures that the urine stream is directed downward rather than forward, wetting the forelimbs and feet. The cut extends through the urethra and surrounding corpus spongiosum, the urethral groove, the tunica albuginea and corpus cavernosum, the multiple branches of dorsal veins and arteries, and nerves and lymphatics in the fascial planes that surround the tunica albuginea and underlie the skin.[10,14,15]

Pathologic engorgement of vessels requires individual ligation. The sinusoidal spaces of the corpus cavernosum are compressed by radial sutures in the tunica albuginea. These consist of 10 to 12 or more interrupted nonabsorbable sutures preplaced to bridge the cut surface of the corpus cavernosum from the urethra and urethral groove to the outer curvature of the tunica albuginea and then the skin of the penis. The first suture bisects the cut surface with a bite in the urethra, then the urethral groove of the tunica, the midpoint of the dorsal curvature of the tunica, and the fourth bite in the skin. The two suture ends are clamped together with hemostats for later tying. The two halves of the cut surface are then bisected the same way, the four quarters likewise, and so on until a series of sutures are preplaced in a radiating pattern. Then the sutures are tightened and tied in the same order as placed so as to prevent puckering. When all sutures are tied, the tourniquet is loosened to test the security of hemostasis. Additional sutures are placed as needed. A stent bandage of sterile gauze sponges is applied until the horse recovers from anesthesia and regains his feet. The bandage should be removed at this time to avoid interference with urination.[10,14,15]

Some slight bleeding may occur at intervals during the first few days, especially during urination, but this should cease spontaneously with healing. Hematomas occurring beneath the suture line should be evacuated. Dehiscence can be treated as an open wound with conscientious nursing care in the hope that healing by second intention will not be complicated by urethral stenosis. Antibiotics are advisable as is tetanus immunization. Skin sutures can be removed in 14 days and physiologic rest by isolation from mares and stallions should be provided for up to 1 month.

Perineal Amputations

Interruptions of the penis from the regio pubica to the ischiatic arch are occasioned by malignancies and anomalies for the most part. The separate classification provides some distinction from the previous category of limited amputations of the free body of the penis, still within the confines of the prepuce, and the radical en bloc resection required by metastatic disease.

The anatomic boundaries are ill-defined and the techniques as varied as the disease. At the discretion of the surgeon, the prepuce may or may not be removed. The relocated urethral orifice may exit anywhere from the prepuce to the ischiatic arch, supported by the amputated stump of the penis. Commonalities of dissection include rigorous attention to hemostasis, careful creation of the urethrostomy, and direction of the urine stream so that the feet and legs are neither soiled nor scalded. The more cranial the site, i.e., prepubic, the more the urine stream is directed forward. In the perineal region, the stump of the penis and the urine stream are retroverted. The latter technique has been well described by Markel et al.[16] in a series of 10 cases.[6]

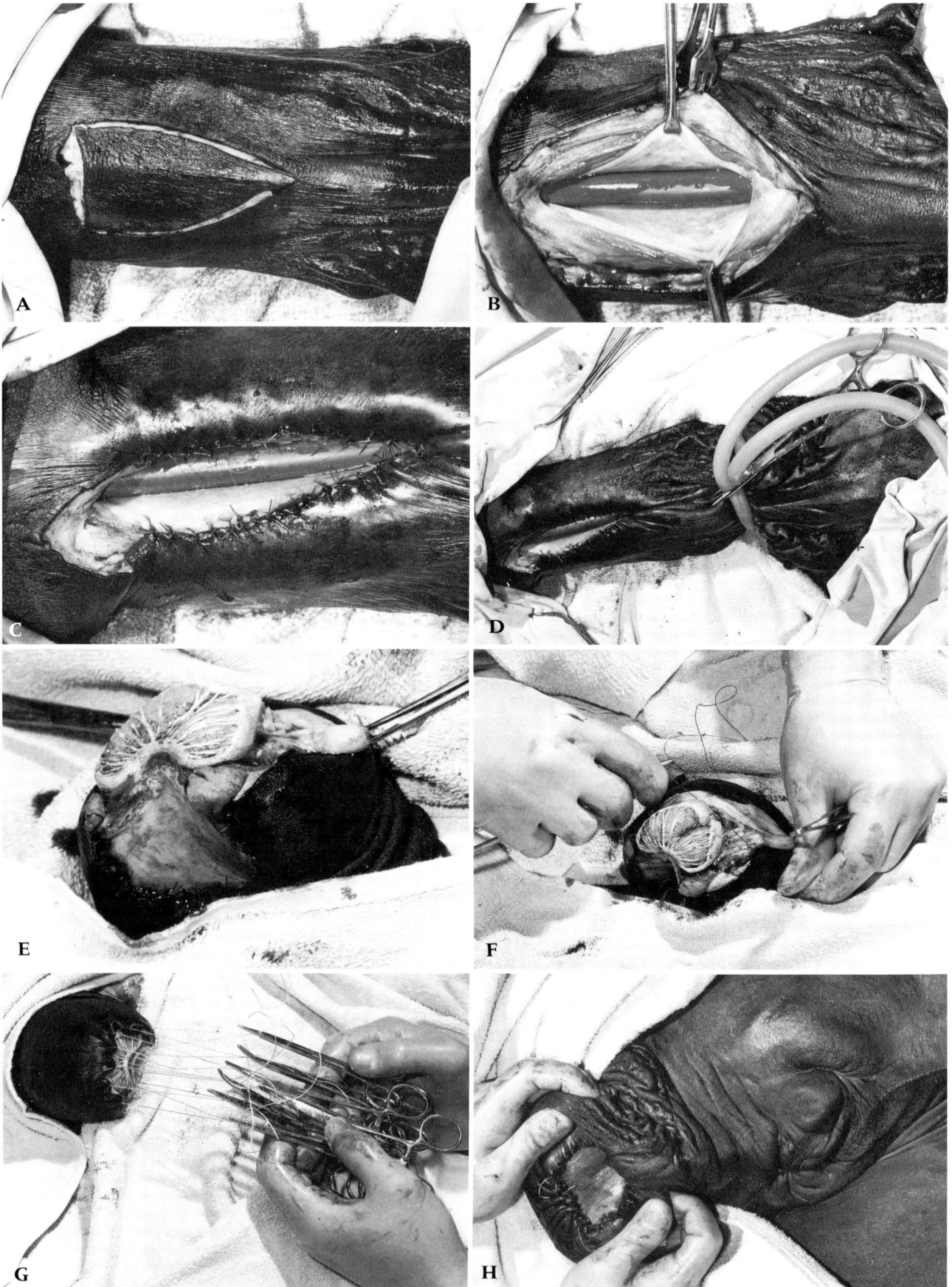

FIG. 103–4. Amputation of the penis. *A,* Triangular section of tissue to be removed to expose the urethra (base of triangle craniad). *B,* Urethra incised. Base of triangle craniad, catheter exposed. *C,* Interrupted sutures to appose skin to the urethra. *D,* Tourniquet tightened in preparation for amputation. *E,* Amputation complete. *F,* Ligation of all bleeding vessels external to the corpus cavernosum penis. *G,* Preplacement of sutures in the corpus cavernosum penis. *H,* Operation complete.

EN BLOC RESECTION

The rationale for radical dissection is invasive and regionally metastatic malignancy. Retrospective studies have supported the assumption that squamous cell carcinoma, the principal offender, spreads slowly and that surgical treatment is statistically justified even in the presence of regional lymphadenopathy. What was once considered as a somewhat heroic procedure for a guarded prognosis has been upgraded to a rational procedure for a better prognosis. Moreover, the alternative technique of penile retroversion through a subischial urethrostomy has been demonstrated to its advantage. Therefore, en bloc resection of the prepuce, penis, and regional lymphatics takes its place among other legitimate and recognized operative surgeries.[16]

A diseased organ should be removed in its entirety if it is expendable, and this is doubly so in the case of cancer. The concept of resection en bloc is based on the surgical removal of the tumor with a wide margin of grossly unaffected tissue together with regional lymphatics, all in one piece. This is to minimize the seeding of dislodged tumor cells and to bracket safely any inapparent microscopic metastases. A further precaution is to ligate the major venous drainage of the tumor site before mobilization and handling of the disease to prevent dissemination of neoplastic emboli[1] (Fig. 103-5).

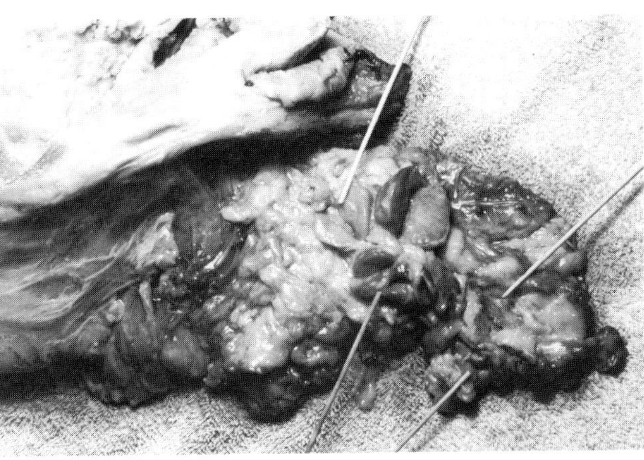

FIG. 103–5. En bloc resection of the pathologic specimen. Note the loose aggregation of superficial inguinal lymph nodes.

In accordance with these principles, the dissection commences with an elliptical skin incision encompassing the external preputial orifice and extending backward along the midline as far as needed to fully expose the superficial inguinal lymph glands and external pudendal arteries and veins in that same vicinity of the superficial inguinal ring. Identification of the normal as well as the pathologic anatomy requires good retraction, illumination, hemostasis, and familiarity with the regional architecture. The collateral branches of the external pudendal vein draining the intended field of dissection are ligated along with the arteries. The inguinal lymph nodes are dissected free and mobilized with the tissue contiguous to the penis and prepuce. The natural plane of dissection is the superficial abdominal and inguinal fascia. A complicating factor is the rich plexus of large veins located above and along the sides of the penis and prepuce that drain into the external pudendal vein before it passes through a foramen in the gracilis tendon. Furthermore, just in front of the vein, the external pudendal artery (a branch of the prepubic artery) emerges at the medial angle of the superficial inguinal ring to divide into the subcutaneous abdominal artery and the anterior dorsal artery of the penis; its many branches supply the superficial inguinal lymph glands, prepuce, penis, and scrotum. Collateral branches to the corpus cavernosum also pass backward and anastomose with the obturator artery.[17,18] Blunt and sharp dissection proceed apace with hemostasis by ligation and electrofulguration until the entire pathologic specimen has been mobilized and isolated. The penis is amputated well proximal to visible or palpable disease, in the vicinity of the pubis, according to Markel et al.,[16] or alternatively, perineal. The stump of the penis is closed with long-duration absorbable sutures in the tunica albuginea to compress the corpus cavernosum, and the urethra, in its sheath of corpus spongiosum, is dissected free for a distance of 4 cm beyond the amputated stump in preparation for subsequent urethrostomy.[16]

A median skin incision (6 to 8 cm) is made in the lower perineum, described as subischial or postpubic, through which the fascia is tunneled sufficiently distad to retract the stump of the penis, now retroverted.[16] The dissection should be regarded as an extensile incision in that some adjustment may be required for a proper match. The amputated stump is sutured in place, fascia to fascia and tunica albuginea to fascia with the urethra oriented dorsally and the dorsal corpus cavernosum directed ventrally. The urethral projection is split lengthwise along its ventral aspect (opposite the urethral groove) and spatulated to the skin edges of the incision with fine simple interrupted sutures placed closely to control hemorrhage from the corpus spongiosum and to ensure primary healing of the urethrostomy. All dead space and excessive incision must be closed. The urine stream should be directed downward and backward on a median plane to avoid soiling the hocks.[16] A protectant dressing on the dependent skin surfaces may be indicated for a time until this can be confirmed.

The ventral abdominal wound is reconstructed with an effort to obliterate as much dead space as possible, leaving drains where needed in the depths of the wound, especially where the extirpation of suspect and diseased tissue has been most extensive and where blood and serum are apt to accumulate. Drains should be exited away from the primary skin closure along the midline.

Postoperative care should include antibiotic therapy and general support as indicated. The extensive dissection predisposes to complications ranging from hematoma, seroma, and edema to dehiscence and infection. Of course, more distant concerns include ascending tract urinary infections and recurrence of tumor.

CORPUS SHUNT

In addition to the irrigation technique described in Chapter 97, a vascular shunt can be created for an anatomic exit for the arterial blood sequestered in the corpus cavernosum penis. With the patient under general anesthesia and in dorsal recumbency, the urethra is catheterized for ease of identification during dissection. Through a longitudinal skin incision on the midline 5 cm caudal to the scrotum, a 3-cm incision is made through the tunica albuginea of the corpus cavernosum adjacent and parallel to the bulbospongiosus muscle, which must be elevated from the tunica to expose the corpus spongiosum. The medial edge of the incision into the corpus cavernosum is sutured with #2-0 gut (or equivalent) to the tunica of the corpus spongiosum. Then a companion incision is made into the corpus spongiosum, and the resulting stoma is created by joining the lateral edges of the opposing incisions. The dissected structures and tissue planes are reapposed to complete the operation. This technique has been used with some success in the human. Further evaluation in the horse is warranted.[3]

CRYOSURGERY

The efficacy of cryosurgery on sarcoids, fungal granulomas, and squamous cell carcinomas justifies consideration of this method as an alternative to conventional dissection for extirpative operational surgery. It should be evaluated whenever preservation of a breeding stallion is an objective.[19–21]

The technique advocated is the double– or triple–freeze-thaw cycle using a liquid nitrogen spray and an imbedded needle thermocouple to measure subsurface temperatures from −20° to +30° C. The treatments can be repeated at 21-day intervals.[19–21] Wound care is necessary during the period of sloughing and subsequent healing by second intention. Other treatment includes anti-inflammatory medication, tetanus immunization, and antibiotics.

LASER SURGERY

One report reviewed the use of the carbon dioxide laser in 30 operations on 25 horses with sarcoids in various locations.[22] The tumors were classified according to four types: I, alopecia and hyperkeratosis; II, verrucous and sessile; III, nodular, sessile, and nonulcerated; and IV, nodular, sessile or pedunculated, and ulcerated. The prepuce was most affected by type III. Three surgical procedures were used according to size and type: (1) simple vaporization; (2) excision and vaporization; and (3) excision, vaporization, and suturing of the resultant wound. The laser beam potency in the tissues varied from 800 to 50,000 W/cm^2. Wound healing by both primary and secondary intention was good. Other advantages included precision, speed, and patient comfort. Recurrence was seen in 7 of 25 cases.[22] Further use of this modality by transurethral applications of the argon laser for internal lesions would seem to be warranted.

REFERENCES

1. Welch, C.S., and Powers, S.R.: The Essence of Surgery. Philadelphia, W.B. Saunders, 1958.
2. Berge, E., and Westhues, M.: Veterinary Operative Surgery. Translated by W.G. Siller, and J.A. Fraser. Baltimore, Williams & Wilkins, 1966.
3. Schumacher, J., and Vaughan, J.T.: Surgery of the penis and prepuce. Vet. Clin. North Am. Equine Pract. *4:*473–493, 1988.
4. Walker, D.F., and Vaughan, J.T.: Surgery of the urinary tract. *In* Bovine and Equine Urogenital Surgery. Philadelphia, Lea & Febiger, 1980, pp. 170–182.
5. McCue, P.M., Brooks, P.A., and Wilson, W.D.: Urinary bladder rupture as a sequela to obstructive urethral calculi. Vet. Med., *84:*912–914, 1989.
6. Yovich, J.V., and Turner, A.S.: Treatment of a postcastration urethral stricture by phallectomy in a gelding. Compend. Contin. Educ. Practicing Vet., *8:*S393–S399, 1986.
7. Firth, E.C.: Dissecting hematoma of corpus spongiosum and urinary bladder rupture in a stallion. J. Am. Vet. Med. Assoc., *169:*800, 1976.
8. Voss, J.L., and Pickett, B.W.: Diagnosis and treatment of hemospermia in the stallion. J. Reprod. Fertil. Suppl., *23:*151–154, 1975.
9. Frank, E.R.: Veterinary Surgery. 6th ed. Minneapolis, Burgess Publishing, 1959.
10. Turner, A.S., and McIlwraith, C.W.: Circumcision and amputation of the penis (reefing). *In* Techniques in Large Animal Surgery. 2nd ed. Philadelphia, Lea & Febiger, 1989, pp. 204–210.
11. Clem, M.F., and DeBowes, R.M.: Paraphimosis in horses—Part II. Compend. Contin. Educ. Practicing Vet., *11:*184–187, 1989.
12. Peyton, L.C.: The reefing operation in large animals. Vet. Med. Small Anim. Clin., *75:*112, 114–117, 1980.
13. Taylor, N.R.: Traumatic balanoposthitis in a yearling Appaloosa colt. Vet. Rec., *107:*154–155, 1980.
14. Walker, D.F., and Vaughan, J.T.: Surgery of the penis and prepuce. *In* Bovine and Equine Urogenital Surgery. Philadelphia, Lea & Febiger, 1980, pp. 125–144.
15. Danks, A.G., and Frost, J.N.: Williams' Surgical Operations. Ithaca, NY, published by the authors, 1943.
16. Markel, M.D., Wheat, J.D., and Jones, K.: Genital neoplasms treated by en bloc resection and penile retroversion in horses: 10 cases (1977–1986). J. Am. Vet. Med. Assoc., *192:*396–400, 1988.
17. Sisson, S.: The Anatomy of the Domestic Animals. 3rd ed. Philadelphia, W.B. Sanders, 1950.
18. Nickel, R., Schummer, A., Seiferle, E., and Sack, W.O. (eds.): The Viscera of the Domestic Mammals. Berlin, Verlag Paul Parey, 1973.
19. Montes, L.F., and Vaughan, J.T.: Atlas of Skin Diseases of the Horse. Philadelphia, W.B. Sanders, 1983.
20. Stick, J.A., and Hoffer, R.E.: Results of cryosurgical treatment of equine penile neoplasms. J. Equine Med. Surg., *2:*505–507, 1978.
21. Fretz, P.B., and Barber, S.M.: Cryosurgery as the sole treatment for equine sarcoids. Vet. Clin. North Am., *10:*847–859, 1980.
22. Vingerhoets, M., et al.: Traitement de la sarcoide equine au laser a gaz laser carbonique. Schweiz. Arch. Tierheilk., *130:*113–126, 1988.

CHAPTER 104

TESTICULAR BIOPSY

W.R. Threlfall
C. Lopate

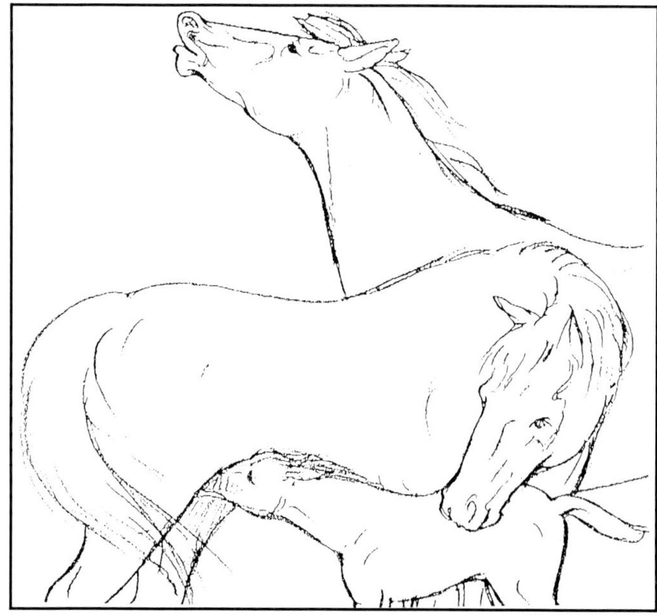

Reports on the causes of infertility of a general nature are not available for most domestic species. However, in the human, Tomaszewski reported that 40% of infertility problems are of male origin; 50%, female origin, and 10%, a combination of male and female disorders.[1] The percentage of domestic animal infertility caused by the male is more variable and depends on the male to female ratio.

Many factors can cause infertility in the male. One method of classification is by pretesticular, testicular, and post-testicular causes.[2–4] Examples of pretesticular causes include hypogonadotropism, excessive estrogen, excessive androgen, glucocorticoid excess, and hypothyroidism. Testicular causes include maturation arrest, hypospermatogenesis, chromosomal abnormalities, cryptorchidism, and orchitis. Post-testicular causes include blockage of ducts leaving the testis, defective spermatozoal maturation or storage in the epididymis, and biochemically abnormal seminal plasma. The closer to the testis a blockage occurs, the more severe the lesion will be.[5] In addition, extratesticular causes of infertility can occur, which include infections, excessive heating of the genital tract, and toxic chemicals.[2,3]

Veterinarians are generally asked to examine infertile stallions following failure of bred mares to conceive. The sequence of the evaluation involves obtaining a complete history and then performing a breeding soundness or fertility examination. Medical history includes viral and bacterial infections, traumatic injury, and general health status (past and present). History of fertility includes past pregnancy rates, seminal evaluations, and libido. Medications administered include those related to past or present fertility treatment, systemic or localized body infections, and the use of androgenic steroids. Palpation of the testes, epididymides, vas deferentia, spermatic cords, accessory sex glands, and penis should be performed. Seminal analysis should be performed on more than one occasion; blood chemistries and hormonal concentrations if indicated should be performed. The seminal examination includes spermatozoal motility, concentration, morphology and volume of the ejaculate. Depending on the results of this examination and the endocrine profiles, sequential examinations over as long as a 2-month period, testicular ultrasonography, spermatozoal antibody titers, karyotyping, and testicular biopsy may be indicated. Any of the aforementioned tests may be indicated either individually or in combination, depending on the abnormalities found.

METHODS OF EVALUATION

ENDOCRINE PROFILES

Endocrine profiles should include multiple samples for quantitative assays for testosterone, luteinizing hormone (LH), follicle-stimulating hormone (FSH), and thyroid hormones. Serum concentrations of FSH provide the most useful information regarding testicular disorders. In cases of azoospermia in man, FSH concentrations are elevated in patients exhibiting signs of tubular hyalinization and Sertoli cell only syndrome and in 50% of patients showing maturation arrest. In azoospermatic human patients with normal testicular biopsies and FSH concentrations, complete ductular obstruction is suspected.[6,7] Partial excurrent duct obstruction is likely if FSH levels and the testicular biopsy are normal in an oligospermic patient.[6,7] In cases of severe oligospermia (<5 million cells/mL) with elevated FSH concentrations, severe hypospermatogenesis is the most frequently seen lesion and the prognosis is poor.[6–9] Obstructive causes of infertility in the human can often be surgically repaired.[7] The lack of commercially available FSH assays for most domestic species is a definite disadvantage in male fertility examinations; however, these determinations are available at some diagnostic and teaching institutions.

ULTRASONOGRAPHY

The use of ultrasonography to delineate lesions within the testis has been described and may be beneficial in the stallion. Lesions such as sperm granulomas, spermatoceles, and neoplasia are easily visualized with B-mode ultrasonography.

SPERMATOZOAL ANTIBODY DETERMINATION

If autoimmune orchitis is suspected, spermatozoal antibody titers should be determined.

KARYOTYPING

If genetic mutation is suspected, then karyotyping is indicated (see Chapter 30).

TESTICULAR BIOPSY

Testicular biopsy has been used with seminal evaluation to help diagnose and classify human males with varying degrees of testicular failure.[10–12] This combination is especially useful in veterinary medicine, because the commercial availability and economic practicality of hormonal assays is often limited. Testicular biopsy was first recommended in man to diagnose cases of obstructive versus nonobstructive aspermia, to classify oligospermia, and to aid in the determination of treatment and prognosis. The first clinical testicular biopsy in man was performed by Hotchkiss in 1944.[13] Testicular biopsy can aid in the determination of many disorders, including but not limited to germinal cell aplasia, germinal cell arrest, hypogonadotropic eunuchoidism, hypospermatogenesis, Klinefelter's syndrome, and hypogonadotropism.[2,5,10,13] Biopsy can also help discriminate among inflammatory disorders, noninflammatory disorders, and neoplasia.[2,14] Biopsy may be indicated in cases of cryptorchidism, because testes allowed to remain retained tend to become dysfunctional and often fibrotic or neoplastic.[2] For this reason, in man, at the time of orchiopexy, biopsy is often recommended. Although orchiopexy is not recommended in the stallion because of the possible inheritance of cryptorchidism, biopsy should also be performed to determine the probability of future testicular function if this surgical procedure is to be practiced.

Many researchers have reported that if the testes are of equal size and consistency, unilateral biopsy is sufficient.[5,12,15–17] In such cases in man, biopsy specimens as small as 10 mg from the right testis have provided representative quantitative values for both testes, and the quality and quantity of sperm production was found to be uniformly distributed throughout the testicular parenchyma.[18] Shakkebaek and Heller found no significant difference between left and right testes in man with quantitative histologic analysis.[19] Unilateral biopsy of the left testis has provided accurate information in 85% of the men regarding sperm production in the opposite testis because of the uniformity of spermatogenesis from one testis to the other, if size and consistency are similar.[5] Therefore, a biopsy sample from one testis may provide an accurate histologic diagnosis that represents the status of both testes in appropriate situations.[18] However, bilateral biopsy provides the pathologist with an idea of the generalization or focality of a lesion.

Histometric Analysis

The use of quantitative histometric analysis with testicular biopsy has shown significant positive correlation between the number of germ cells per seminiferous tubule or the number of Sertoli cells per tubule and the sperm concentration in the human ejaculate.[18–20] There are two methods whereby histomorphometrics can be utilized. The first is the Sertoli cell ratio method and allows quantification by comparison of the germinal epithelium to a reference cell, the Sertoli cell.[19] The number of Sertoli cells per tubule rarely changes because of tissue fixation or preparation or because of pathologic or therapeutic circumstances (i.e., hormone treatment or irradiation). In laboratory animals and man, Sertoli cells do not divide after sexual maturity. Therefore, comparison of germ cell to Sertoli cell numbers can provide an indication of dysfunction in spermatogenesis or spermiogenesis. In situations in which tubules are so severely damaged that Sertoli cells are also damaged, this method provides less accurate results.[19,20]

The second method is the cell association method and permits quantification of germinal epithelium compared with seminiferous tubular circumference.[20] This method can be used in the more severely damaged tubules with greater precision than can the Sertoli cell ratio. Comparison of numbers of each type of germ cell (and Sertoli cells) present with known standards of germ cells present in normal testes has permitted localization of a lesion to a specific cell type in the tubular epithelium. Correlations between spermatozoal output and patterns of spermatogenesis can also be made.

Value of Testicular Biopsy

Biopsy has been shown to be of value in the determination of the cause, severity, and prognosis of a low spermatozoal count.[10,19,20] In cases of blockage or varicocele, biopsy has helped to determine whether normal spermatogenic activity is present.[19,20] If so, the procedures should be performed to relieve the cause of the blockage.[10,19,20] Blockage may also be the cause of spermiostasis in stallions. Normal spermatogenesis in a tissue sample does not reflect on spermatozoal count.[2,16,19,20] In man, normal spermatogenesis to Sertoli cell only syndrome was observed in tissue sections of patients clinically demonstrating conditions from aspermia to oligospermia.[16,19,20] Normal spermatogenesis can also be seen with surrounding abnormal supporting tissue.[15]

The relationship of testicular biopsy to stallion fertility has not been reported. In mink, testicular palpation, seminal examination, and testicular biopsy were all found to be practical and suitable methods of assessing male reproductive capacity. Serum testosterone quantities were found to be poorly correlated.[21]

Biopsy Techniques

Three different biopsy techniques are used commonly in man and certain domestic and laboratory animals.

Incisional or Open. The first and most common technique in human medicine is the incisional or open biopsy.[2,10,20] This technique is also commonly used in small animals. The scrotal area is clipped and scrubbed. Anesthesia is accomplished by infiltration of the skin and subcutaneous tissue only with a locally acting anesthetic agent (Fig. 104–1). An incision is made through the scrotum and tunica albuginea. The incision into the tunic should not be larger than 0.5 cm to minimize the trauma to the testis and its vasculature (Fig. 104–2).[12] The internal pressure pushes a small section of testicular tissue through the incision in the tunic. This tissue is gently cut with a razor blade and placed immediately into a fixative solution (Fig. 104–3). The tunic and scrotum are closed with an appropriate suture (Fig. 104–4).

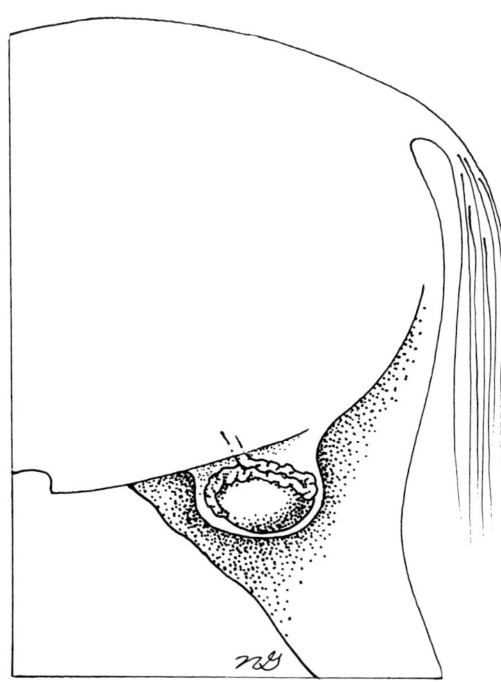

FIG. 104–1. Position of testicle within scrotum.

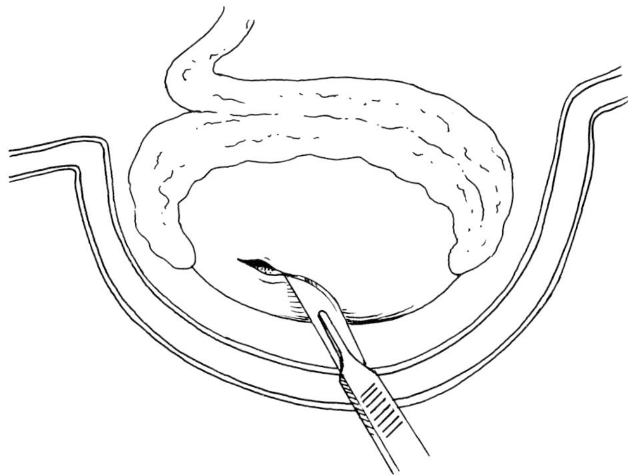

FIG. 104–2. Incision of tunica propria.

Split Needle. The second type of biopsy is the split needle method.[11,22] The scrotal area is clipped (optional) and scrubbed. In this procedure local anesthesia is appropriate for the scrotal skin and subcutaneous tissue only. The skin incision is 0.5 cm in length. The scrotum is incised with the point of a #10 blade, and the split needle is gently pushed through the tunic albuginea and into the testicular tissue (Figs. 104–5 and 104–6). Puncture of the tunic is painless because no sensory neural pain fibers normally exist between the dermal layer and the tunica albuginea.[13] In addition, extraction of the testicular tissue sample is also relatively painless because of the lack of innervation within the testicular parenchyma. The testicular tissue is obtained with the split needle and immediately and care-

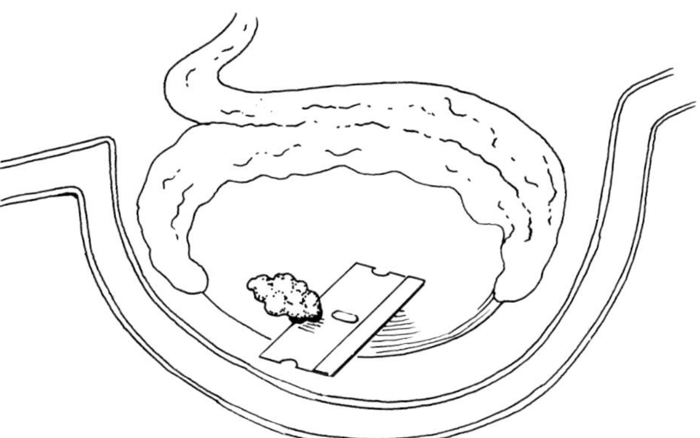

FIG. 104–3. Removal of testicular tissue that bulges through tunica propria incision.

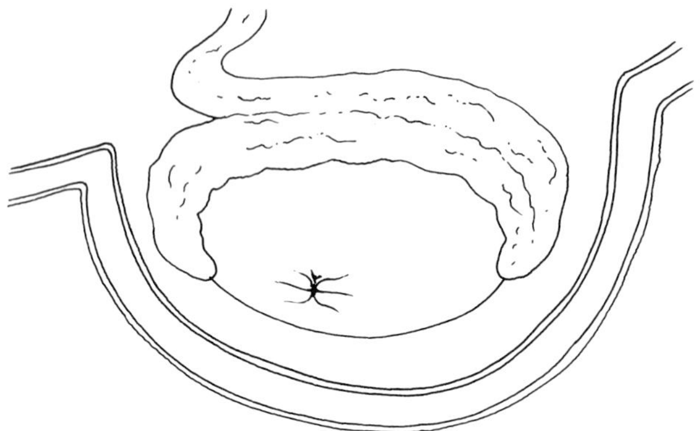

FIG. 104–4. Surgical closure of tunica propria.

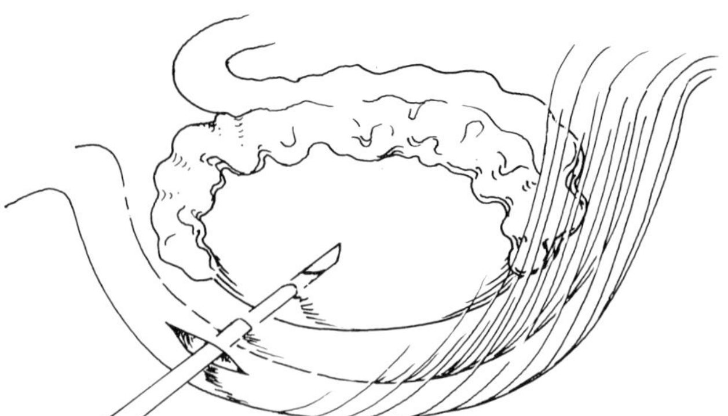

FIG. 104–6. Placement of split needle biopsy instrument into testicle.

fully placed in fixative (Figs. 104–7 and 104–8). The scrotal incision is medicated with a topical antibiotic, but not sutured. No systemic antibiotics are necessary after this procedure if asepsis was maintained. The split needle biopsy will provide tissue samples of approximately 1.0 mm in diameter and between 2.0 to 6.0 mm in length.[13]

Fine Needle Aspiration. The third type of biopsy is known as fine needle aspiration biopsy. It is the most recently described technique and is currently used in human medicine clinically and in veterinary medicine experimentally.[10,14,23] After surgical preparation and anesthesia, the testis is percutaneously punctured with a 20- or 23-gauge needle.[23,24] A small portion of tissue is aspirated into a 5-mL syringe. The aspirate can be placed on a slide for cytologic examination or placed in a fixative for histologic examination.

Technique Summary. The open biopsy technique provides the most tissue and, therefore, the most tubules for examination.[5,14] The split needle biopsy usually provides adequate tissue; however, the interstitium may be disrupted.[5,13,14] The fine needle aspiration biopsy will usually provide few intact tubules; however, this technique provides germinal cells of all types, including Sertoli cells, and allows the diagnosis of the conditions of normal spermatogenesis and spermatogenic arrest.[10,14,23,24] A high correlation exists between the results of cytologic examination and histologic examination in regard to spermatogenic activity.[24] Histologic examination allows the distinction of interstitial changes whereas cytologic examination does not.[24] Fine needle aspiration biopsy is the least invasive of the three techniques, split needle biopsy is mildly invasive, and open biopsy is moderately invasive.

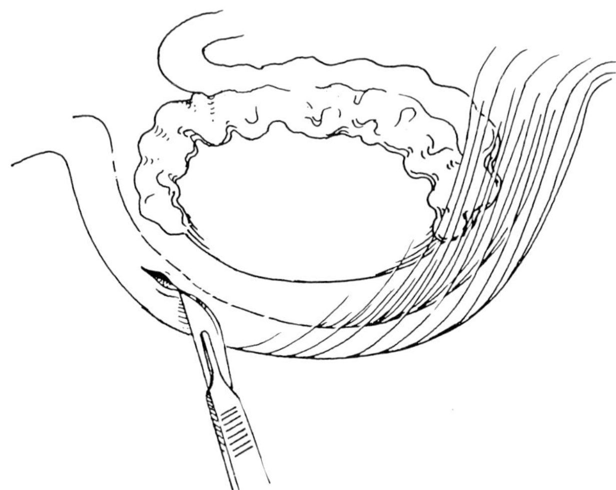

FIG. 104–5. Scrotal skin incision for passage of split needle.

The testicular biopsy technique that we recommend for use in the stallion is as follows. The stallion is first tranquilized intravenously with 0.8 mg/kg of xylazine. Approximately 5 min after this administration, 0.66 mg/kg of morphine or 0.22 mg/kg of torbugesic is administered intravenously. The primary consideration of a testicular biopsy in any species is that of asepsis. Proper preparation of the surgical site is of extreme importance such that no bacteria are introduced into the testicle. The surgical area is prepared by first thoroughly cleansing with a detergent, cotton, and clean water. Because the procedure is performed in the standing position, the clinician must thoroughly cleanse the entire scrotum and the inner surfaces of the legs in the inguinal area. After cleansing, a surgical scrub is performed using povidine-iodine or a similar product and cotton. After an approximate 10-min scrub of the area, it is rinsed thoroughly with clean water, then rinsed a final time with an alcohol solution. The testicle to be biopsied is isolated within the scrotum and grasped firmly with a gloved hand so that the skin over the testis is tight. The area of the skin incision, which generally is in the midportion of the testis on the free or most ventral border, is infiltrated with 2 to 3 mL of a local anesthetic. Anesthetic is placed in the skin and subcutaneous area, with a 23- to 25-gauge needle. No anesthetic should be placed within the testicle, because doing so can cause testicular degeneration.

Once the anesthetic has been administered, the point of a #10 surgical blade is used to incise the anesthetized skin (Fig. 104–5). The approximate length of the incision is 0.5 cm. A Tru-Cut (Travenol Laboratories, Inc.,

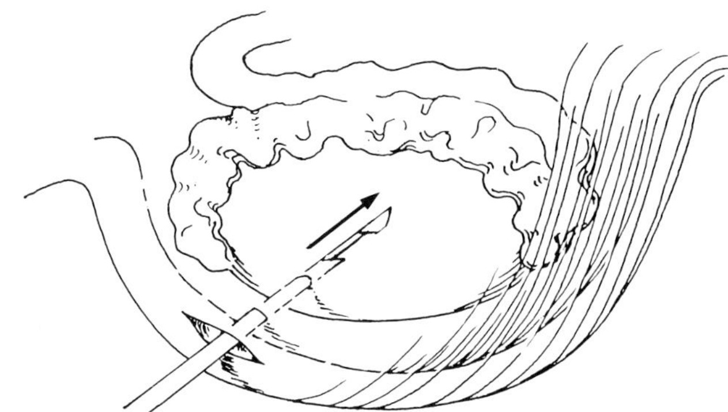

FIG. 104–7. Advancement of inner needle into testicular tissue.

Deerfield, IL) or a Monoject (Sherwood Medical, St. Louis, MO) split needle biopsy instrument is used. The needle is inserted through the skin incision and forced with sharp pressure through the tunica albuginea surrounding the testis. The biopsy instrument will pop through the tunic and then progress inward easily (Fig. 104–6). The inner portion of the needle is advanced deeper into the posterior portion of the testis, away from the anterior aspect and the area of the head of the epididymis (Fig. 104–7). Then the outer portion of the biopsy instrument is advanced to cover the inner needle, which provides the biopsy sample (Fig. 104–8). The instrument is removed with the outer portion closed over the inner needle. The biopsy sample must be gently teased off the instrument into the fixative.

COMPLICATIONS

Early reports in the bull indicated that incisional biopsy induced a decrease in spermatozoal count, an increase in the number of abnormal spermatozoa, tubular degenerative changes, adhesions between the tunics (which was believed to deleteriously affect spermatogenesis), and hemorrhage for 2 weeks to 4 months postbiopsy.[25] In 1960, clinicians reported that split needle biopsy of the bull testis did not produce any long-term effect on the testis, although a transient decrease in spermatozoal number occurred. More recently, Galina evaluated the effects of split needle biopsy in the boar, bull, ram, and stallion.[25] In the boar, no significant differences in spermatozoal counts were found. In the bull, the ejaculate had a transient discoloration 1 week after biopsy, but within 3 weeks, the color had returned to normal. Two of four bulls had a line of fibrotic demarcation within the testes. The volume and motility of the bulls with normal fertility before biopsy were normal after biopsy. Rams had no histologic change or alteration in spermatozoal count. In the horse, no histologic lesions were found after biopsy. This has also been reported by Threlfall and Lopate.[26] Seminal evaluation was not performed in any of the stallions used in the previous two reports. Because open biopsy may temporarily be detrimental to spermatogenesis in some species, split needle biopsy may be a more desirable and effective method to evaluate abnormalities of the testes in these animals.[25]

Considerable research has been conducted in man and little in the domestic species on the effect of biopsy on seminal quality and output. Although conflicting results have been reported, a transient decrease in spermatozoal output for several weeks to months after incisional biopsy seems likely, but seminal values return to normal given adequate time.[3,9,14,15,17,18,25,27] In man, spermatozoal counts were decreased (42% average median) by 3 weeks after a biopsy and had returned to normal within 10 to 18 weeks.[27] In the same study, researchers found that the higher the spermatozoal count was before biopsy, the more profound the decrease in number after biopsy. In the dog, heat and swelling lasted for more than a week after incisional biopsy, and these signs were associated with decreased concentration and increased morphologically abnormal spermatozoa. How long these signs will persist or if these effects are permanent is unknown.[10] The transient decrease in spermatozoal counts can be attributed to several factors: (1) inflammation induced by the procedure, (2) heating of the testis as a result of the inflammatory response, or (3) autoimmune reaction to spermatozoa.[14]

Careful handling of testicular tissue prevents artifacts in the histologic preparation.[10,12,13,28] Clinicians have reported that the reason testicular biopsy was slow to gain universal acceptance in human medicine was because of the poor quality of the tissue sample slides. Excessive pressure on the testis must be avoided. The surgeon must handle the testis gently so as not to disrupt normal tissue architecture. Trauma can be inflicted on the tissue by using a blade that is too thick or dull. The tissue sample should be gently nudged into the fixative utilizing a fine-gauge needle. If the specimen is manipulated excessively, the tubular and interstitial architecture will be disrupted. The tissue should never be handled by forceps or placed onto any surface before fixation to prevent crush artifact.

The choice of fixative will also determine the quality of the histopathologic slide. Bouin's solution is the preferred fixative, because it causes the least tissue shrink-

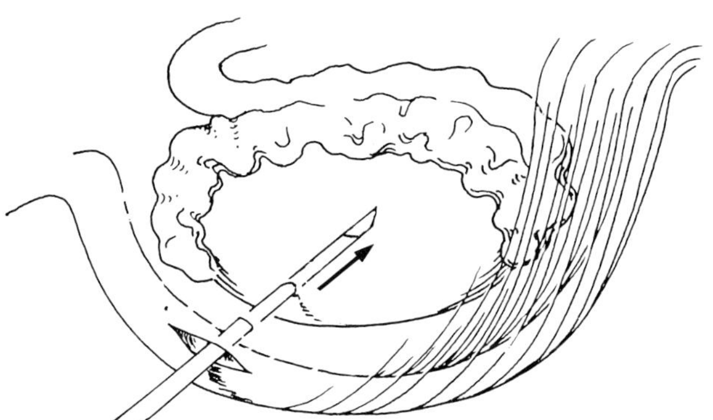

FIG. 104–8. Advancement of outer needle to separate biopsy sample and maintain in biopsy instrument channel.

age and preserves the greatest nuclear detail.[12,13,28] Markewitz et al. recommend that the sample be allowed to fix for 6 to 12 h before further processing.[28] The sample cannot be left in Bouin's fixative longer than 24 h because it will become too hard to cut with the microtome. Zenker's formol is also an acceptable fixative.[12,13] However, it causes the dissociation of architecture between tubules, which may be mistakenly interpreted as sloughing.[28] A less desirable choice is 10% formalin, because it causes tissue shrinkage, provides poor nuclear images, and can result in a loss of mature spermatozoa.[2,11,12,28]

Many authors allude to the disadvantages or complications of testicular biopsy but have presented little evidence to justify this concern. Cahill reported that testicular biopsies were not considered by owners of famous Kentucky stallions with infertility problems to aid in the diagnosis of the problem "for obvious reasons."[29] We believe these reasons are not obvious, and if in fact they do exist, they should be elucidated. If the reasons do not exist, factual information should be presented.

Several considerations are necessary before testicular biopsy. Hematomas occurring between the testicular tissue and the tunics, or between the tunics and scrotum, are the most common complication.[12] They usually result from vigorous manipulation of the testicle. The biopsy must be performed gently without excessive tension or torsion on the testicle, the spermatic cord, or the vasculature to the testicle. In most cases, during incisional or split needle biopsy, hemorrhage can be controlled by exerting gentle pressure on the tunic with a sterile sponge for 1 to 2 min.[12,14,17] If the surgeon is sure that bleeding is controlled, then hematomas rarely result. The testicular artery partially embedded in the tunica albuginea passes around the caudal pole of the testis and then branches on the ventral surface into a medial and lateral branch.[30] These branches then pass craniad. In addition, lateral branches may originate dorsally to the testis from the testicular artery and pass ventrad. Approximately 30% of stallions have these lateral branches. The lateral branches supply the cranial portion of the testis and head of the epididymis, whereas the termination of the testicular artery (medial and lateral branches) supplies the posterior portion of the testicle. Biopsy should be taken to avoid the main branches of testicular artery. No permanent side effects as a result of testicular biopsy in the stallion have been reported. However, in one case in which a large hematoma between testicle and vaginal tunic occurred as a result of a lateral approach in a pony stallion, it resolved without adverse effects on that stallion's fertility.[25]

Adhesions are seen commonly between the two tunics as a sequelae to incisional biopsy of the canine testicle.[10] The adhesions are not related to hemorrhage but rather to apposition of the incised tunics during healing.[10] Careful suturing of the tunica vaginalis will reduce the probability of adhesions. Adhesions between the tunica vaginalis and tunica albuginea have been rarely observed in the human, but when present were asymptomatic in regard to testicular function.[12] Other possible complications induced by biopsy are inflammation, increased intratesticular pressure, and the induction of an immune reaction against the sperm.[9,10,13] These are uncommon problems in most species and can usually be prevented by using a careful technique and by maintaining sterile conditions.[10,13] A decrease in testicular size has been noted following incisional biopsy.[31] This decrease may be the result of hemorrhage and connective tissue deposition at the site of the biopsy.[14,31] The formation of a connective tissue reaction to the tissue insult results in a contraction of the tissue, which in turn causes a decrease in testicular size. In the rat, both split needle and fine needle aspiration biopsy induced secondary lesions in the testicle.[32] Tubules with degenerate germinal epithelium were found to be focally located at the biopsy site and in the surrounding parenchyma. These lesions were found 8 weeks after biopsy at which time the rats were castrated. This finding indicates that the biopsy procedure may damage the testis. If a tumor or abscess is suspected, removal of the affected testis is advised and biopsy is contraindicated.

In a study consisting of eight serial split needle biopsies on Beagle dogs,[33] slight scrotal swelling and polycythema vera (primary increase in red blood cells in the circulating blood) were noted for 3 days after biopsy. In addition, at 3 days, cellular degeneration and necrosis were present at the biopsy site. This condition had changed to focal interstitial fibrosis and tubular atrophy 2 weeks later. The adjoining tissue was histologically normal. Testicular size and/or seminal characteristics did not change overall. The researchers concluded that serial split needle biopsy had no effect on reproductive functionability of these dogs.

Clearly, differences between species concerning the method of biopsy that will provide the most valuable information and the least detrimental effects on the testicle must be considered. The majority of the research has been done in man. This emphasis has resulted in a large population of patients from which to evaluate data and techniques. In domestic and laboratory animals, accurate information regarding the effects of each type of biopsy on the different species is scarce.

SUMMARY

The following information is a summary of data collected through the use of split needle testicular biopsy on client-owned and research stallions over the past 17 yr. Split needle biopsies have been performed on research stallions and have indicated no decrease in total spermatozoa per ejaculate following biopsy. The lesions induced to the testis also have not appeared to affect adversely the functional capability of the biopsied testis. Biopsies performed on client animals have been beneficial in the diagnosis and prognosis of many infertility conditions affecting the stallion.

Biopsies from 50% of the infertile stallions indicated testicular degeneration had occurred. The remainder of the stallions had normal testicular tissue present. Stallions with severe disruption or no normal germinal epithelium remaining within the tubules are candidates for retirement from breeding. These animals cannot respond to any type of current therapy and to attempt such is economically unrewarding to the owners. Animals with normal germinal epithelium in the absence of mature spermatozoal production or with low sperm production may be candidates for attempted hormonal therapy. These animals may respond to therapy. The use of testicular biopsy is advocated in the human male to have complete obtainable information on the patient and to determine which patients are potentially treatable. Stallions with normal germinal epithelium and spermatozoal production but with no spermatozoa in the ejaculate should be examined for obstruction of spermatozoal transports.

In conclusion, testicular biopsy is not without disadvantages. However, the clinical significance of the trauma induced to the testis appears to be insignificant in regard to the total productivity of that testis when the split needle biopsy technique is utilized. Testicular biopsy may be useful in clinical situations when it can provide the clinician with additional information about the spermatogenic state of an infertile stallion that otherwise would not be possible. Testicular biopsy can be used to help determine the cause, the prognosis and the potential for therapy of infertile stallions when used with fertility records and other diagnostic techniques.

REFERENCES

1. Tomaszewski, J.E.: Male and female infertility. Paper presented at the Seventy-sixth Annual Meeting of the International Academy of Pathology, Short Course #25. Chicago, March, 1987.
2. Levin, H.S.: Testicular biopsy in the study of male infertility. Hum. Pathol., *10:*569–584, 1979.
3. Scott, R., et al.: The results of 100 small tissue biopsies of testis in male infertile patients. Postgrad. Med. J., *52:*693–698, 1976.
4. Wong, T.W., et al.: Pathological aspects of the infertile testis. Urol. Clin. North Am., *5:*503–509, 1978.
5. Larsen, R.E.: Evaluation of fertility problems in the male dog. Vet. Clin. North Am., *7:*735–745, 1977.
6. Anthony, S., Leong, Y., and Matthews, C.D.: The role of testicular biopsy in the investigation of male infertility. Pathology, *14:*205–209, 1982.
7. de Kretser, D.M.: Testicular biopsy in the management of male infertility. Int. J. Urol., *5:*449–456, 1982.
8. Curtis, D., et al.: Cytogenetic and histological studies in a series of subfertile males. Int. J. Urol., *5:*113–119, 1982.
9. Hjort, T., Linnet, L., and Shakkebaek, N.E.: Testicular biopsy: Indications and complications. Eur. J. Pediatr., *138:*23–31, 1982.
10. Larsen, R.E.: Testicular biopsy in the dog. Vet. Clin. North Am., *7:*747–755, 1977.
11. Netto, N.R.: Needle method of testicular biopsy. Int. Surg., *59:*172–180, 1974.
12. Rowley, M.J., and Heller, C.G.: The testicular biopsy: Surgical procedure, fixation, and staining techniques. Fertil., Steril., *17:*177–186, 1966.
13. Cohen, M.S., et al.: Testicular needle biopsy in diagnosis of infertility. Urology, *24:*439–451, 1984.
14. Finco, D.R.: Biopsy of the testicle. Vet. Clin. North Am., *4:*377–381, 1974.
15. Brannen, G.E., and Roth, R.R.: Testicular abnormalities of the subfertile male. J. Urol., *122:*757–762, 1979.
16. Meinhard, E., McRae, C.U., and Chisholm, G.D.: Testicular biopsy in evaluation of male infertility. Br. Med. J., *3:*577–581, 1973.
17. Paufler, S.K., and Foote, R.H.: Semen quality and testicular function in rabbits following repeated testicular biopsy and unilateral castration. Fertil. Steril., *20:*618–625, 1969.
18. Johnson, L., Petty, C.S., and Neaves, W.B.: The relationship of biopsy evaluations and testicular measurements to over-all daily sperm production in human testes. Fertil. Steril., *34:*36–40, 1980.
19. Shakkebaek, N.E., and Heller, C.S.: Quantification of human seminiferous epithelium. I. Histological studies in twenty-one fertile men with normal chromosome complements. J. Reprod. Fertil., *32:*379–389, 1973.
20. Zukerman, Z., et al.: Quantitative analysis of the seminiferous epithelium in human testicular biopsies, and the relation of spermatogenesis to sperm density. Fertil. Steril., *30:*448–455, 1978.
21. Sundquist, C., et al.: Elimination of infertile male mink from breeding using sperm test, testicular palpation, testosterone test and fine needle aspiration biopsy of the testis. Anim. Reprod. Sci., *11:*295–305, 1986.
22. Wilson, G.P.: Surgery of the male reproductive tract. Vet. Clin. North Am., *5:*537–550, 1975.
23. Nseyo, U.D., et al.: Aspiration biopsy of testis: Another method for histologic examination. Fertil. Steril., *42:* 281–284, 1984.
24. Persson, P.S., Ahren, C., and Obrant, K.D.: Aspiration biopsy smear of testis in azoospermia. Scand. J. Urol. Nephrol., *5:*22–29, 1971.
25. Galina, C.S.: An evaluation of testicular biopsy in farm animals. Vet. Rec., *88:*628–631, 1971.
26. Threlfall, W.R., and Lopate, C.: Testicular biopsy. Proc. Soc. Theriogenol., 65–73, 1987.
27. Rowley, M.J., O'Keefe, K.B., and Heiler, C.G.: Decreases in sperm concentration due to testicular biopsy procedure in man. J. Urol., *101:*347–356, 1969.
28. Markewitz, M., et al.: Testicular biopsy artifacts resulting from improper tissue processing. J. Urol., *100:*44–51, 1968.
29. Cahill, C.: Immature spermatozoa in Thoroughbred stallion. Southwestern Vet., *28:*13–17, 1975.
30. Smith, J.A.: Biopsy and the testicular artery of the horse. Equine Vet. J., *6:*81–83, 1974.
31. Lopate, C., Threlfall, W.R., and Rosol, T.J.: Histopathologic and gross effects of testicular biopsy in the dog. Theriogenology, *32:*585–602, 1989.
32. Schwedes, U., et al.: Morphologic testicular changes in rats after biopsy or puncture. Acta Endocrinol., *173:*149, 1973.
33. James, R.W., Heywood, R., and Fowler, D.J.: Serial percutaneous testicular biopsy in the Beagle dog. J. Small Anim. Pract. *20:*219–228, 1979.

PART III

THE NEONATE

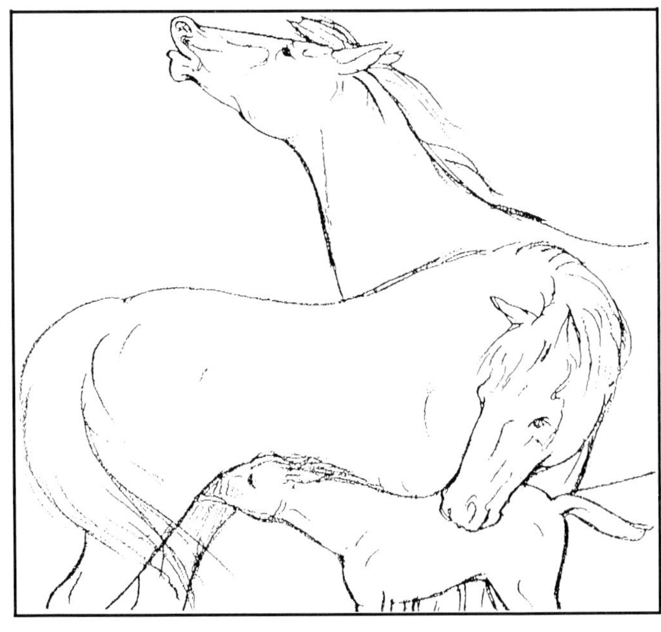

SECTION A

CARE OF THE MARE AND FOAL IN THE NEONATAL PERIOD

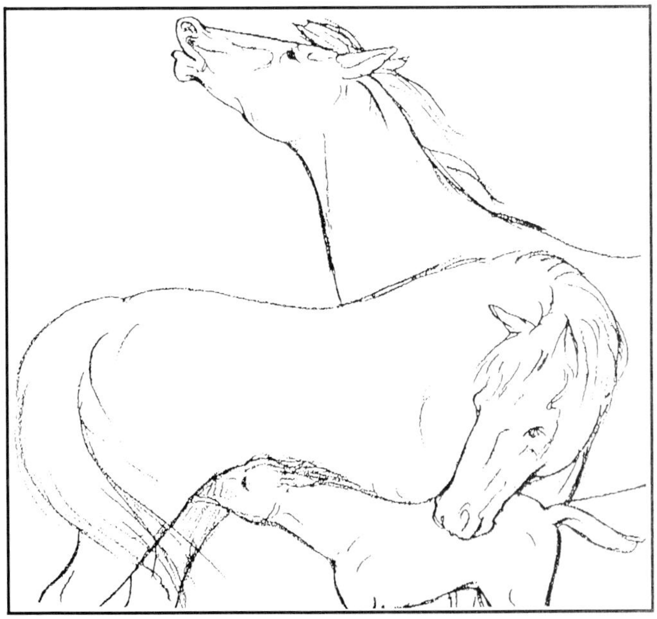

CHAPTER 105

THE PREFOALING PERIOD

R.K. Shideler

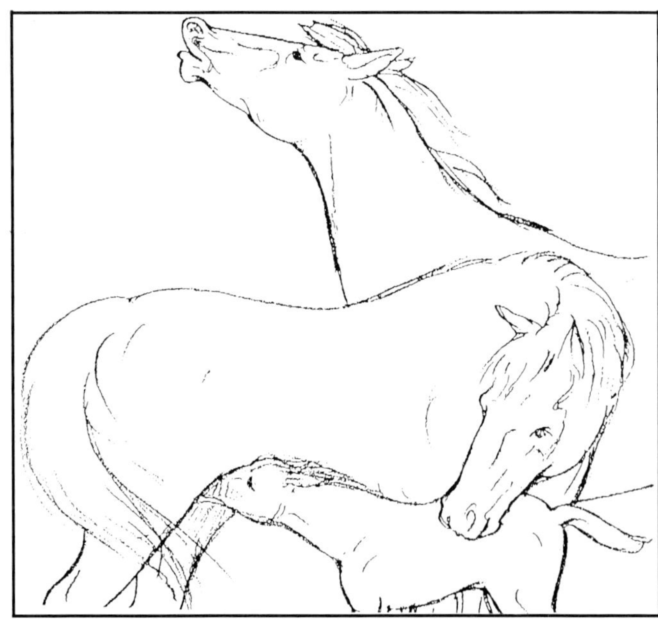

The horse is frequently described as having the lowest reproductive efficiency of all domestic animals. Burns has estimated that only 55 to 60% of mares bred annually produce live foals.[1] Sound management practices are necessary to maintain optimal health for maximum reproductive efficiency. The mare must be maintained on a balanced ration during gestation. The average mare will consume 1.5 to 2.0% of its body weight each day in feed. An excellent reference regarding this subject has been published.[2] The clinician must keep the mare in a nutritional state that will allow her to be healthy, active, alert, and vigorous. Care should be taken to protect the mare from excessive weight gain or loss. The clinician should be able to palpate the ribs, but they should not be visible on a well-conditioned horse (Chapter 75). Heavy work, including racing, may be accomplished during early pregnancy (up to 5 months); moderate activity and exercise are recommended during later gestation. The purpose of prenatal care, therefore, is to provide sufficient care for the mare that will result in a viable and healthy full-term foal.

DISEASE PREVENTION AND IMMUNIZATIONS FOR THE PREGNANT MARE

The goal in disease prevention in the pregnant mare is obviously to prevent illness that will adversely affect development of the fetus and delivery of a full-term, normal foal. The objectives in a health care plan include (1) eliminating exposure of the pregnant mare to infectious diseases capable of affecting the fetus and ultimately cause abortion and (2) using immunizing agents that will be most effective in preventing disease in the mare and concurrently result in antibody formation for colostral transfer to the foal.

A vaccination program must be used that protects the brood mare and stimulates her to produce antibodies that will be transferred in her colostrum for protection of the foal. For maximum effect, vaccinations should be given 1 month before foaling. Antibodies helpful to the neonatal foal are also produced from antigens encountered in the dam's environment. In deficient geographical areas, nutritional supplementation with vitamin E and selenium appears to produce humoral immune response to antigens such as tetanus toxoid and equine influenza virus.[3] In the event the mare is to foal in an area or farm away from her natural quarters, she should be moved to the foaling area no later than 1 month before term. This allows the mare, through natural exposure, to build antibodies associated with antigens of infective organisms present in the new environment. Consequently, at birth the foal, through colostrum, develops a passive immunity to these potential disease factors. A suggested schedule for vaccination of the brood mare is listed in Table 105–1.[4] This schedule may have additions or deletions depending on the advice of the veterinarian familiar with each farm or local circumstance.

Obviously, selection of actual dates for vaccinations

TABLE 105–1. SUGGESTED PROGRAM OF IMMUNIZATION FOR THE PREGNANT MARE

VACCINE	DATE
Tetanus toxoid; equine influenza	4 to 6 weeks before foaling
Eastern and western equine encephalomyelitis	Late spring to early summer
Equine influenza	Fall
Rhinopneumonitis (Pneumobort-K)	5, 7 and 9 months of pregnancy (other options may be considered utilizing MLV)*
Strangles vaccine	Optional, depends on individual farm disease problems

*From Witherspoon, D.M.: Preventative medicine at Spendthrift Farm, Inc. Proc. Am. Assoc. Equine Pract., 345–347, 1984.

in pregnant mares will hinge on foaling dates and will proceed through the year according to the individual's schedule and needs. The clinician should keep in mind that under circumstances of severe repeated exposure, most vaccines provide immunity for the horse no longer than 6 months. Therefore, booster injections at 3- or 6-month intervals may be recommended for many farms.

Planning an immunization schedule for the pregnant mare incorporates a knowledge of the action of the vaccine and the duration of immunity produced. Tetanus toxoid stimulates antibody protection for at least a year. Viral vaccines (influenza, rhinopneumonitis, and eastern and western encephalomyelitis) allow protective immunity for 4 to 6 months. Strangles vaccine also appears to provide an equally short period of immunity. The clinician must know the vaccination status of each mare and her proximity to parturition when planning a program. In the event booster immunizations are necessary, they are best given approximately 30 days before foaling to allow adequate time for antibody production and successful colostral immunoglobulin transfer.

NUTRITION FOR THE PREGNANT MARE

Nutritional requirements of the pregnant mare in the first and second trimesters of gestation differ little from the normal adult. An effort should be made to maintain visually adequate body condition and a bright, alert individual. Traditionally, the pregnant female depends on nutritional intake to supply her needs as well as those of the developing fetus. In addition, however, the mare will withdraw from her own body reserves of carbohydrates, protein, calcium, phosphorus, and other minerals to supply adequately the needs of the fetus when an intake deficiency develops (Chapter 75). Calcium nutrition has been the subject of interest and research, most particularly in recent years, as it relates to osteochondrosis in foals. Hintz et al. reported on the effect of overfeeding calcium to pregnant mares with the resulting increased incidence of osteochondrosis in their foals.[5] Other reports indicate deficiencies in calcium intake might also contribute to osteochondrosis in foals.[6] Further studies are needed to determine the effect of calcium intake by the mare on the incidence of skeletal disease in the foal.

The addition of copper to the diet of mares did not significantly influence milk copper.[7] Dietary deficiencies did not cause the production of low copper milk. While the copper concentration of milk decreases dramatically during the first few weeks of lactation, no external influence of excess or deficiency in the mare's diet on copper concentration in the milk appears to exist.[7,8]

The effect of energy intake on reproductive performance has been the subject of speculation, clinical impression, and in the last decade, some research. Flushing, or increasing energy intake just before the breeding season, has been reported to hasten regular cycling and to cause ovulation to occur earlier in the breeding season.[9] Supplementing the diet of mares already receiving a balanced ration is not beneficial to conception rate.[10]

A study was conducted to determine if ovarian activity and other parameters of reproductive performance are affected by the amount of digestible energy in the diet during the last 90 days of gestation and during lactation.[11] Energy restrictions during gestation resulted in an average weight loss of 26.3 kg per mare but had no effect on gestational duration or weight of the foal at birth. Free-choice fed mares gained weight (53.4 kg); however, no difference was noted for foal weights between groups at 75 days of age. No difference was found between groups in estrous cycle duration, estrous periods, or number of ovulations per cycle. These parameters were within the range of previously reported values.[12] Conception rates for the first cycle breeding and overall conception rates were 71 and 86%, respectively, for free-choice fed mares versus 83.3 and 100% for the restricted-energy group. These values are higher than those reported in a later study.[9] Energy restriction during the last 90 days of gestation appeared to have no effect on foal birth weight. The development and growth rate of the foal was, however, at the body condition expense of the mare. Postpartum energy restriction did not adversely affect reproductive efficiency nor did free choice feeding or flushing of the lactating mare enhance reproductive performance.[11]

PARASITES IN THE PREGNANT MARE

Parasites remain one of the great health threats to all horses, including the pregnant mare. Most horses harbor internal parasites. Where infected animals are found and favorable temperature and moisture conditions exist, pastures will eventually become infested. Once a pasture has become infested, the parasites are virtually impossible to eradicate. Thus the problem of horse infection is constant, requiring the attention of the horse owner and veterinarian. Parasite control is an important management factor relating not only to the general condition of the mare but also to the unborn foal. The most common internal parasites have widely varying adverse effects, depending on (1) pathogenic potential of the invading species, (2) number of parasites involved in the infection, (3) duration over which infection is acquired, (4) age of the horse, and (5) resistance of the horse.

Injurious effects such as blood loss, tissue destruction, mechanical obstruction, intoxication, and competitive food utilization result from infections of various parasites. These effects can be caused by immature or larval stages, as well as the adult or mature parasite. Parasites are destructive in all horses regardless of age; however, the most serious damage occurs in young horses, during their first 2 yr of life. Numerous methods exist to detect infections of internal parasites and to estimate the worm burden. Direct microscopic examination of feces is a quick method to identify parasite eggs (Fig. 105–1). Negative findings are inconclusive as egg shedding occurs in cyclic patterns; however, positive results indicate infection. Intestinal worms have varying egg-laying rates. Some female worms, such as the ascarid, may lay 100,000 eggs per day, while others produce significantly less. Parasites also may lay eggs in cycles, producing more at one time than another. Egg counts are usually lower in older animals' feces than in the young's, and counts may also be lower when the horse is on a high-energy ration. Low egg counts may fail to reflect the presence of a large number of immature female worms that are not producing eggs. Because of these factors, repeated counts or examinations of feces from several horses on the same premises are necessary to evaluate the parasite burden of the farm. Culturing infective larvae in feces is also a method of identifying a parasite. This may be necessary in some herds to differentiate microscopically between the eggs of large and small strongyles.

LARGE STRONGYLES

Large strongyles, also known as blood worms, are the most dangerous parasites infecting the horse. They are especially destructive because the larvae migrate extensively in several of the internal organs. Severe tissue damage may result from only small numbers of such larvae. Adult strongyles damage the large colon and cecum while sucking blood.

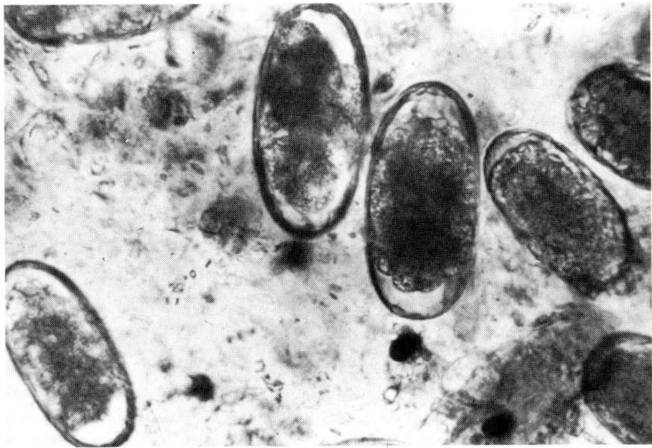

FIG. 105–1. Strongyle spp. eggs seen through a microscope in a routine fecal examination.

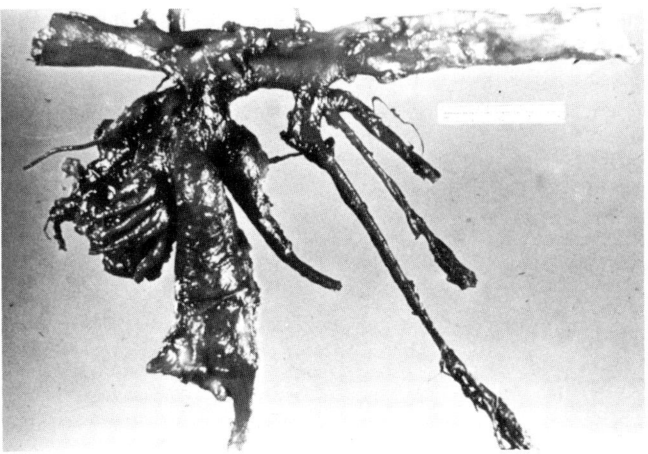

FIG. 105–2. Damaged mesenteric arteries (aneurysms) resulting from larvae of Strongylus vulgaris (blood worms).

Strongylus Vulgaris

The larval development of Strongylus vulgaris is a prolonged process, requiring six months for completion. When the larvae are ingested by the horse with feed or grass, they penetrate the intestinal mucosa. This usually occurs in the cecum and ventral colon. After penetration of the intestinal wall, the larvae enter the small arteries and migrate upstream within the walls until they reach the anterior mesenteric artery. They usually remain in this artery, where they mature and then return to the intestine. The fourth stage larvae cause an inflammation, thrombosis, and aneurysm within the anterior mesenteric artery and may eventually partially or totally obstruct the vessel (Fig. 105–2). This is particularly dangerous because this artery supplies blood to a large segment of the bowel. Decrease or loss of the blood flow to a section of intestine will result in death of tissue and severe colic in the horse. Strongylus vulgaris has been estimated to be the cause, directly or indirectly, of 90% of the colic episodes in horses *where effective parasite control measures are not practiced.*[13] The adult strongyles are active blood suckers and in heavy infections may cause anemia, weakness, weight loss, and diarrhea.

Strongylus Edentatus

The migration pattern of this large strongyle differs from that of the Strongylus vulgaris in that after penetration of the intestinal wall, it travels through the portal vein to the liver. In heavy infections, considerable damage to the liver may result. From the liver, Strongylus edentatus migrates to the peritoneal cavity and eventually back to the intestine where the cycle is completed. This process takes approximately 11 months, nearly twice as long as that of Strongylus vulgaris.[14]

SMALL STRONGYLES

Small stronglyle parasites essentially spend their lives and migratory phases within the intestine itself. While their numbers may be extremely high, actual damage to the horse is considerably less than that of the large strongyles. In heavy infections, digestive function of the large intestine may be impaired, causing colic, intermittent diarrhea, and constipation.

ASCARIDS

Large roundworm infections are common, especially in the foal and young horse (Fig. 105–3). Mature horses appear to acquire a resistance to ascarids. Therefore, only an occasional mature horse is infected. No evidence exists that intrauterine infection occurs, but foals become infected soon after birth.[15]

PINWORMS

The pinworm Oxyuris equi can occur in horses of all ages but appears to be present more commonly in the young. Pinworms develop entirely within the intestine. Eggs are deposited on the perianal area by adult females which die without re-entering the rectum (Fig. 105–4). The principal effect of pinworm infection is anal irritation caused by females protruding from the anus and the adherence of the eggs. The irritation and itching may be intense and can result in tail rubbing and scratching the rear quarters.

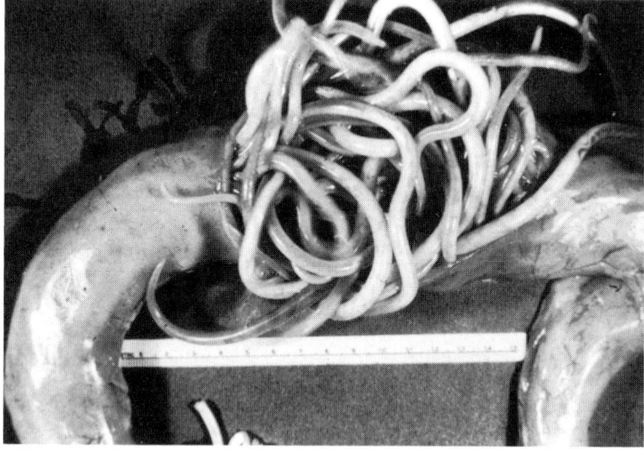

FIG. 105–3. Mass of ascarids emerging from rupture of small intestine.

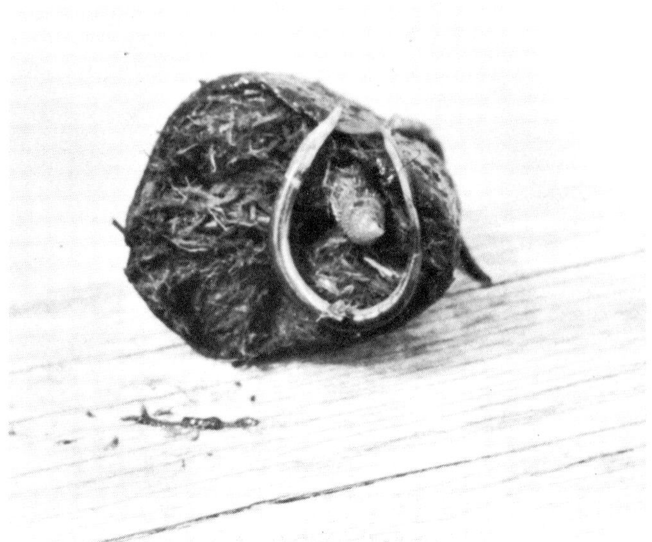

FIG. 105–4. Adult pinworm and bot larva on a fecal ball.

BOTS (GASTROPHILUS)

The larvae of botflies are found in the stomachs of horses of all ages. The damage they cause is not as severe as that caused by Strongylus vulgaris. However, the potential for gastritis exists. Eggs produced by the adult female fly are deposited on individual hairs on the legs, neck and throat. Eggs of Gastrophilus intestinalis are laid on the hair of the legs and do not hatch spontaneously, but must be stimulated by warmth, moisture, and the action of the horse's lips. Eggs laid by Gastrophilus nasalis on the neck and face hatch after 1 week into infective first in-star larvae. In either case, these first in-star larvae invade the mouth tissues and can cause oral ulcers. Three weeks later these larvae emerge and pass to the stomach as second in-star larvae. Further development to the third stage takes 3 to 4 weeks. They remain in the stomach up to 10 months before detaching and then passing in the feces. Once expelled, the bot burrows into the ground, pupates, and within 1 to 2 months, becomes an adult botfly. Bot larvae in the stomach form clusters and produce deep pits at the point of attachment (Fig. 105–5). Occasionally they may perforate the wall resulting in fatal peritonitis. Stomach rupture has also been attributed to heavy bot infection. Other adverse effects such as digestive disturbances and colic have been attributed to bot infections.

CONTROL AND TREATMENT

Sanitation and Management

Pasture management can be an important part of parasite control. Certain pastures should be designated for brood mares, others for mares with foals, and still oth-

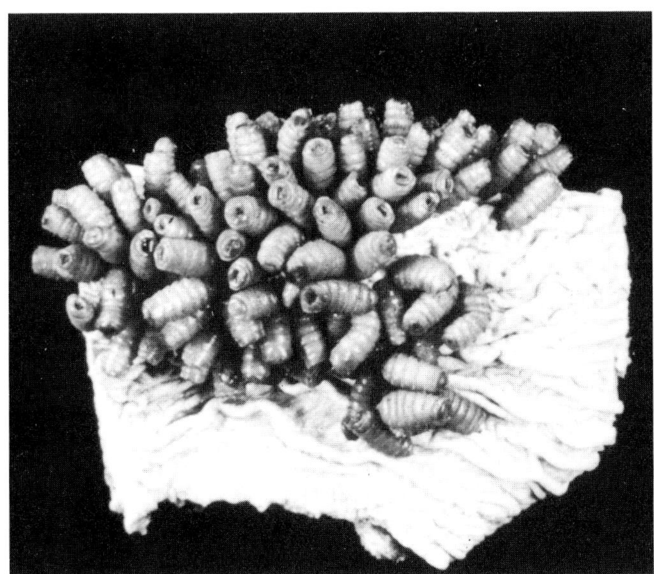

FIG. 105–5. Bot larvae attached to a portion of a horse's stomach.

ers for yearlings. Most authorities emphasize that pastures should be rotated at intervals of approximately 2 months. Between rotations, pastures should be chain harrowed and mowed to aerate the soil, reduce weed growth, and level the pastures to eliminate standing contaminated water. Pastures can be fertilized during this fallow period. An orderly biologic sequence of pasture rotation, parasite treatment, and general horse management exists that fits into the practical logistics of raising horses. The horse owner, farm manager, and veterinarian should adopt a program that will be most effective for their area. From studies done over a 6-yr period, parasite larvae survived on pastures at a consistent rate under natural factors related to alterations of heat and cold, sunlight and darkness, and periods of wetness and dryness.[16] During hot, rainy weather, infective strongyle larvae are stimulated to start their migration up grass blades; as the weather cools or as it becomes dry during the day, the larvae move down the blades of grass. This back and forth movement consumes energy. Because these ensheathed infective larvae cannot feed, they deplete their energy supply and die. This is natural biologic decontamination. In hot, wet summer weather and particularly in late spring or early fall, pastures can become practically decontaminated within an 8-week period. However, in cool weather or when it becomes quite cold or with the arrival of more stable temperatures, parasite larvae live longer because they are not stimulated to utilize their energy. Under these circumstances, natural decontamination requires approximately 6 months. In frigid weather, infective larvae will survive even longer. Infective larvae of Strongylus vulgaris that were refrigerated at 5° C, removed a year later, and administered to foals via stomach tube, were still infective enough to kill the foals.

Parasite control should be continued on a regular basis throughout the year. Research over several years has shown that pasture rotation and administration of antiparasitic drugs given at 2-month intervals will reduce potential contamination by almost 90%. This 2-month interval of anthelmintic treatment coincides well with the 2-month pasture rotation to take advantage of biologic decontamination. In addition to effectively managing the pasture, the clinician must prepare the nursery in which foals will be born. Stalls should be disinfected by first stripping them to their base. If the stall has a clay base, then all material above it should be removed. Stalls should then be scrubbed as high as the horse can reach with hot solutions of povidone-iodine (Betadine) or Lysol and allowed to dry thoroughly. There is no hard-and-fast rule regarding how frequently stalls should be disinfected.

In summary, a crucial factor determining the amount of contamination is the stocking rate of any particular area, or the number of horses using a particular paddock. Good pasture management is as important to parasite control as use of therapeutic agents such as anthelmintics.[16]

Rationale for Treatment

A control program should prevent or minimize infections through long-term sustained efforts. Unfortunately, many of the parasites, especially the large strongyles, produce their primary damage during larval migration through tissue. The migrating larvae are in tissues outside the intestinal lumen and are often not affected by anthelmintics whose principal effect is on adults in the digestive tract. However, removal of those in the gut lumen relieves the horse of certain damage, such as blood losses, and temporarily stops or reduces contamination of the environment with eggs or larvae.

General Features of a Control Program

Several universally applicable measures should be practiced to control parasites successfully.

1. All horses on the farm should be included in the program.
2. Transient, boarded, or any newly acquired horses should be dewormed and isolated for 4 to 7 days before they are turned out with resident horses.
3. Foals can be protected against infection, particularly from strongyles, by regular treatment of mares.
4. Laboratory examinations of fecal samples should be done periodically (three to four times a year) to maintain surveillance on the effectiveness of the drug program.
5. No single drug or mixture should be used exclusively, especially for strongyle control. Alternating drugs may help prevent or delay the development of drug-resistant strains of parasites.
6. The directions on the label of the anthelmintic should be read and completely understood before the drug is administered; all dosage recommendations and special preparatory procedures should be followed.

7. An appropriate time should be reserved for deworming such as the first day of every other month.

The effectiveness of a good worming program depends on efficacy of the drug against the parasites and treatment at appropriate intervals. Both serve to keep the number of parasites in the intestinal lumen at minimal levels. Little is to be gained from a single treatment once or twice a year because reinfection will quickly restore worm burdens to pretreatment levels in 8 to 12 weeks.

Anthelmintic Treatment

An ideal antiparasitic drug should have high efficacy and a wide therapeutic range and be easily administered. If a single anthelmintic is used continuously, drug resistance may occur. A recommended treatment system is to alternate classes of anthelmintics (for example, benzimidazoles followed by pyrantel for strongyle and ascarid removal). Bots are removed by ivermectins and organophosphate drugs (such as dichlorvos or trichlorfon). Generally, mares should not be treated past midgestation for bots. The mare may be wormed after foaling and before rebreeding. The antiparasitic agent ivermectin (Eqvalan) is effective in treating nearly all the internal parasites affecting the horse. According to the manufacturer, all horses may be included in a regular parasite control program. Directions for use and dosage must be followed. Followup fecal examination is recommended to determine the presence and degree of ascarid infection. Oral use of piperazine or a benzimidazole in appropriate dose is also effective for ascarid removal. The veterinarian is best qualified to develop a program for each farm that will be most beneficial to the health of the brood mare and foal.

Suggested Medication for Parasite Control in Pregnant Mares

For strongyles: benzimidazoles (Telmin, Anthelcide EQ, etc.), pyrantel (Strongid T or P), or ivermectin (Eqvalan). For bots: ivermectin or organophosphates such as trichlorfon (Combot). **Caution:** Do not use organophosphate boticide drugs after midgestation in the pregnant mare. If stage of pregnancy dictates bypassing bot worming, worm the mare within the first 4 days after foaling. Table 105–2 contains a summary of the common parasites of the horse and their effects.

PREPARATION FOR FOALING

Gestational length should be documented, because it is common in subsequent foalings for the mare to repeat a similar gestational schedule. Consequently, any marked variation in anticipated foaling could be cause for concern and should be investigated. Normal gestation requires 335 to 345 days and any birth under 325 days is classified as premature. Foals born before day 300 of gestation usually will not survive, because of various deficiencies in organ system development. In preparation for foaling, take the mare to the farm and/or foaling area 4 to 6 weeks before parturition. This gives her an opportunity to adjust to the environment and management practices. The mare will have time to adjust psychologically to this change and will also be exposed to local bacterial and viral antigens. This allows her to produce antibodies to these organisms, which will be passed on to the foal in her colostrum.

The area selected for the mare in the last 4 to 6 weeks of gestation should be sufficient in size to allow her room for self-exercise during the day. The mare should be kept in the foaling stall at night. This will permit her

TABLE 105–2. COMMON HORSE PARASITES AND THEIR EFFECTS

PARASITE	SIGNS	DAMAGE
Large strongyles S. vulgaris (blood worm) S. edentatus S. equinus S. vulgaris	Fluctuating low-grade fever, depression, intermittent inappetence, constipation, leukocytosis, anemia, unthriftiness, colic, anorexia, malaise, soft feces; in long-standing infections, legs and abdomen may swell	The most harmful of internal parasites; adults suck blood, cause ulcers on mucosa; larvae cause severe tissue damage, including thrombosis, embolisms, and aneurysms of anterior mesenteric artery and its branches
Small strongyles Triodontrophorus Poteriostomun Cyathostomum and others	Anemia, anorexia, dark or black feces, soft feces with a foul odor	Irritate intestinal wall causing thickening and nodules with larvae in them
Large white worms Parascaris equorum	Flatulence, diarrhea, rough hair coat, "pot belly," more common in young horses	Irritate intestinal wall, possible obstruction or rupture
Pinworm Oxyuris equi	Restlessness, irregular feeding with consequent loss of condition—dull hair coat, tail rubbing	Adults feed on gut contents; larvae feed on mucosa
Gastrophilus G. intestinalis G. nasalis	Digestive upsets, bowel irritations, periodontal ulcers	Inflammation, perforation of stomach wall, gum irritation

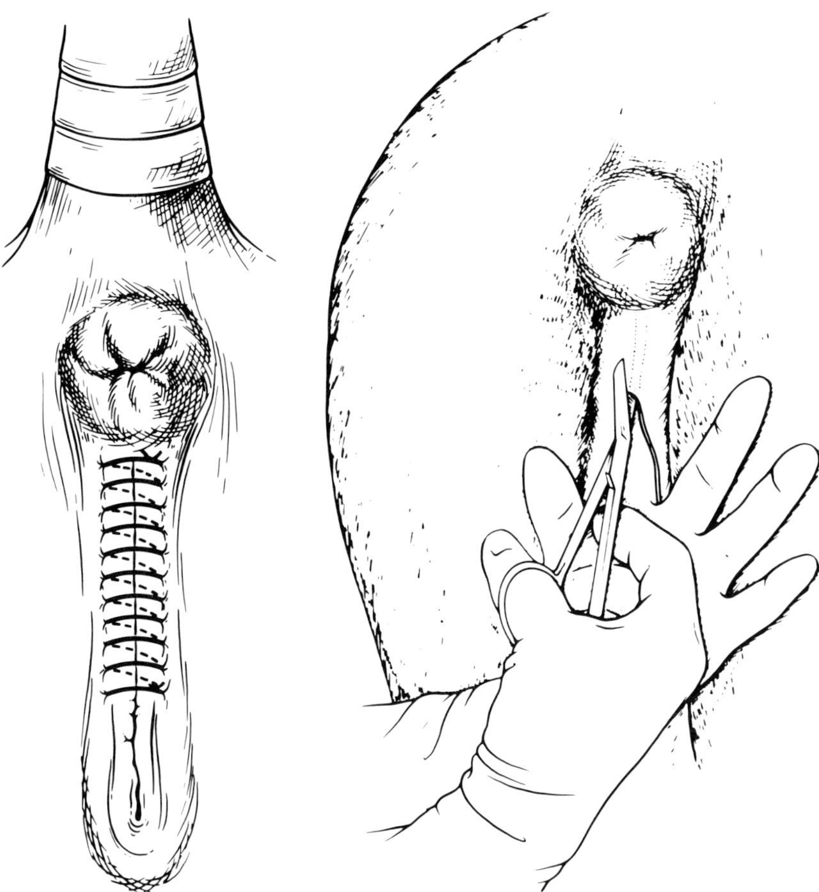

FIG. 105–6. Caslick operation—suturing of vulvar labia to prevent aspiration of air into vagina.

FIG. 105–7. Removing Caslick operation with scissors before foaling.

to acclimate to a routine and serve as a precaution, because the majority of mares foal at night. Before foaling, thoroughly clean the foaling stall or area. The ideal stall is 16 × 16 ft. A viewing window is helpful to avoid disturbing the mare during parturition. Cleanliness and good hygiene are essential to reduce the incidence of foal septicemia, which can be acquired via the umbilical stump or by aerosol or by mouth during or after foaling. With this in mind, cleansing of the perineal area of the mare is desirable and includes wrapping the tail.

Tamed iodine solutions, such as povidone-iodine, are acceptable antiseptics for disinfecting the walls and floor of the foaling stall. Dirt or clay floors may be limed between foalings as an aid in reducing bacterial numbers. Bedding for the foaling stall may be varied according to available material, however clean wheat straw is probably the best choice. Wood shavings are satisfactory, although shavings from walnut wood have been identified as toxic to horses.[17,18]

A large number of young performance mares and older subfertile mares will have the vulvar labia partially sutured with the Caslick operation (Fig. 105–6). This is done to prevent the aspiration of air into the vagina, which is a potential cause of endometritis or infection in the uterus. Likewise, many brood mares are also

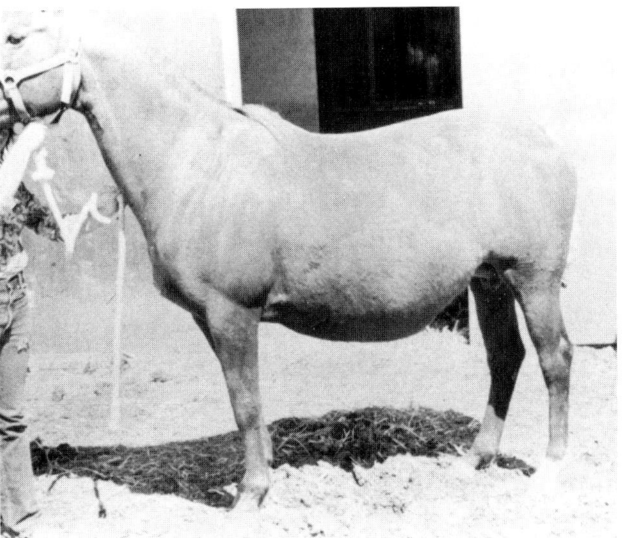

FIG. 105–8. Pregnant mare near foaling. Enlarged and dropped abdomen.

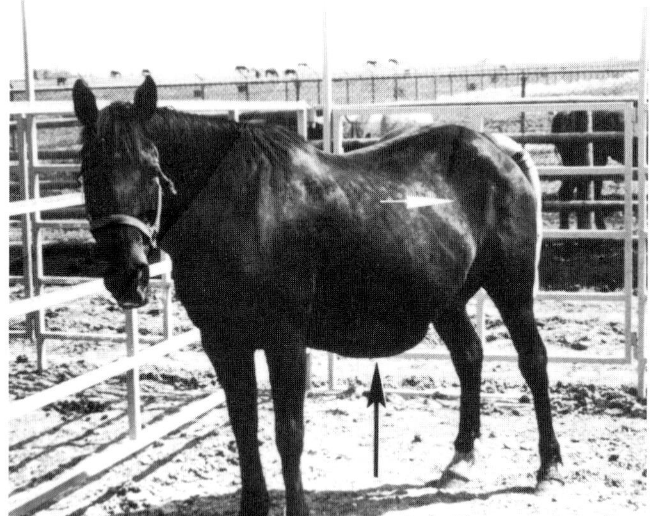

FIG. 105–9. Hollowing of paralumbar fossa (white arrow). Note ventral edema (black arrow).

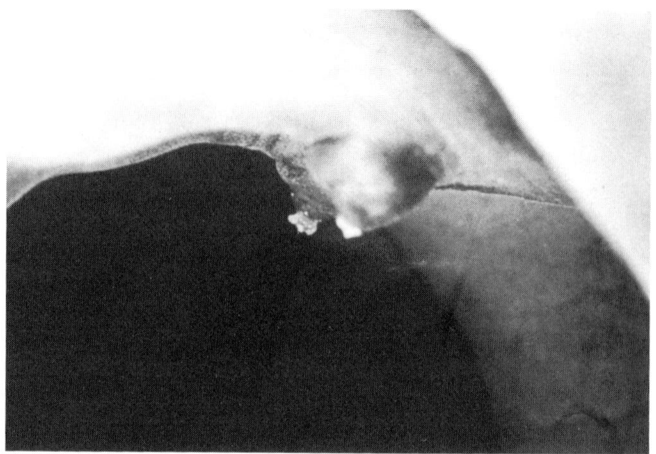

FIG. 105–11. Waxing of teats.

"closed down" (sutured or Caslick operation) after breeding for the same reason. The vulvar lips must be opened before foaling. This will prevent undesirable tearing of the vulva during foaling. The sutured vulva should be opened about 1 week before foaling (Fig. 105–7). The Caslick operation may be replaced immediately after foaling, after breeding, or after pregnancy verification and remain intact until the next prefoaling period. The timing for replacement of the vulvar closure is based on the needs of the individual mare and her potential for pneumovagina.

The mare in the latter stages of pregnancy will naturally show an enlarged abdomen and a decrease in normal activity. In the last 2 to 3 weeks, additional signs are noted that include a relaxation of the abdominal muscles and a "dropping" of the abdomen (Fig. 105–8). The degree will vary with each mare and will be more pronounced as the mare advances in age. Approximately 2 weeks before foaling, the paralumbar fossa becomes more evident and "hollows" (Fig. 105–9). Sequentially, in another week the gluteal muscles and area lateral to the tail head noticeably soften and relax in preparation for parturition (Fig. 105–10).

The average mare will begin to show enlargement and some edema of the udder 2 to 4 weeks before term. The process continues with the teats or nipples filling out 4 to 7 days before foaling. A clear serous or watery secretion will be present in the udder 4 to 5 days before foaling and is sometimes seen as a clear droplet on the teat.

The secretion gradually thickens and becomes sticky. A color change to cloudy or smoky usually occurs 24 to 48 h before parturition. Many mares will show a milk-like secretion 12 to 24 h before foaling, indicating the concentrating of colostrum in the mammary gland. A thick, waxy exudate visible on the nipples is termed waxing (Fig. 105–11) and may be interpreted as an indicator of probable parturition within 24 to 48 h. Use of laboratory tests to determine proximity to parturition has been reported by Ley et al.[19] In these studies on

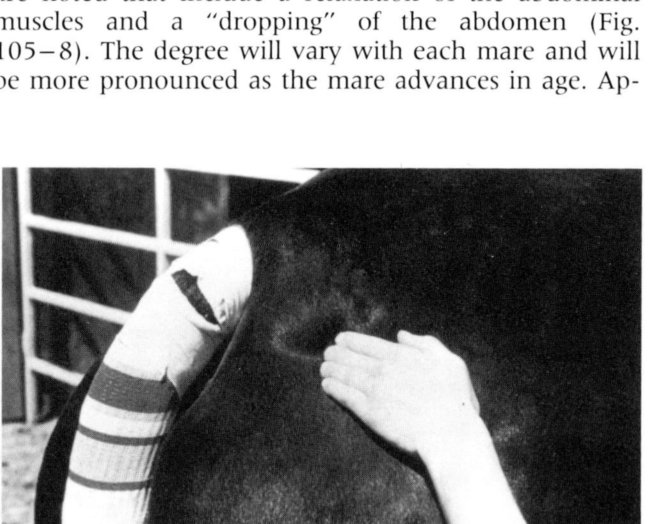

FIG. 105–10. Softening and relaxing of muscle area lateral to tail head.

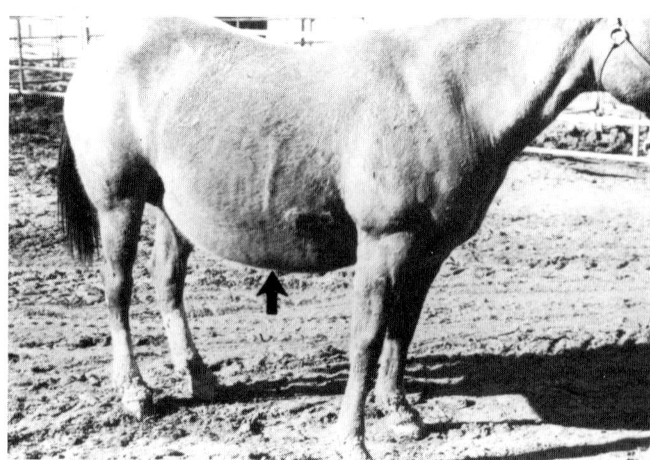

FIG. 105–12. Enlargement and swelling of abdomen (arrow) caused by fluid accumulation (ventral edema).

prefoaling mammary secretion, electrolyte changes have demonstrated the ability to predict foaling time to within 24 to 48 h. These tests essentially measure calcium content in the mammary secretion and its rise in concentration before parturition. At 12 h before foaling in spontaneously foaling mares, 95% of all mares tested were within the range of 180 to 280 ppm (water hardness) using the Sofchek Water Hardness Test Strip (Environmental Test Systems, Elkhart, IN). Additional studies have addressed the importance of mammary secretion as an indicator of fetal readiness for birth. Admittedly, these signs are variable, but do serve as a guide to pending parturition. Commonly, confined mares show ventral edema; increasing exercise will usually eliminate this fluid accumulation under the skin of the ventral abdomen (Fig. 105–12). This may be accomplished by placing the mare in a larger paddock or exercise area during the day. In case of the older, heavier, or more severely affected mare, 15 to 20 min of hand walking twice a day will often provide marked regression of the edema.

REFERENCES

1. Burns, S.J.: The barren mare. Equine Vet. Data, *4:*65–75, 1983.
2. Lewis, L.D.: Feeding and Care of the Horse. Philadelphia, Lea & Febiger, 1982.
3. Baalsrud, K.J., and Overnes, G.: Influence of vitamin E and selenium on antibody production in horses. Equine Vet. J., *18:*472–474, 1986.
4. Witherspoon, D.M.: Preventive medicine at Spendthrift Farm, Inc. Proc. Am. Assoc. Equine Pract., 345–347, 1984.
5. Hintz, H.F., Schryver, H.F., and Lowe, J.E.: Calcium for pregnant mares and growing horses. Equine Pract., *8:*5–10, 1986.
6. Knight, D.A., et al.: Correlation of dietary minerals to incidence of severity of metabolic bone disease in Ohio and Kentucky. Proc. Am. Assoc. Equine Pract., 445–461, 1985.
7. Baucus, K.L., et al.: The effect of dietary copper and zinc supplementation on composition of mare's milk. Proc. Equine Nutr. Physiol., 179–181, 1987.
8. Kincaid, R.L., Hodgson, A.S., Riley, R.E., and Conrath, J.D.: Supplementation of diets for lactating cows with zinc as zinc oxide and zinc methionine. J. Dairy Sci., *67:*103, 1984.
9. Van Niekirk, C.H., and Van Heerden, J.S.: Nutrition and ovarian activity of mares early in the breeding season. J. S. Afr. Vet. Assoc., *43:*355, 1972.
10. Voss, J.L., and Pickett, B.W.: Effect of a nutritional supplement on pregnancy rate in nonlactating mares. J. Am. Vet. Med. Assoc., *165:*702–703, 1974.
11. Banach, M.A., and Evans, J.W.: Effects of inadequate energy during gestation and lactation on the estrous cycle and conception rates of mares and their foal weights. Proc. Equine Nutr. Physiol., 92–100, 1981.
12. Hughes, J.P., Stabenfeldt, G., and Evans, J.W.: Clinical and endocrine aspects of the estrous cycle of the mare. Proc. Am. Assoc. Equine. Pract., 119–151, 1972.
13. Drudge, J.H., and Lyons, E.T.: The chemotherapy of migrating strongyle larvae. *In* Equine Infectious Disease II. Edited by J.T. Bryans and H. Gerber. Basel, S. Karger, 1970, pp. 310–322.
14. Round, M.C.: The development of strongyles in horses and the associated serum protein changes. *In* Equine Infectious Disease II. Edited by J.T. Bryans and H. Gerber. Basel, S. Karger, 1970, pp. 290–303.
15. Levine, N.D.: Nematode Parasites of Domestic Animals and Man. Minneapolis, Burgess, 1968.
16. Bello, T.R.: The Control and Treatment of Internal Parasites. Somerville, American Hoescht Corp. Animal Health Division, 1978.
17. Ralston, S.L., and Rich, V.A.: Black walnut toxicosis in horses. J. Am. Vet. Med. Assoc., *183:*1095, 1983.
18. Ulinger, C.: Black walnut toxicosis. J. Am. Vet. Med. Assoc., *193:*343–344, 1989.
19. Ley, W.B., et al.: Daytime management of the mare. 1: Prefoaling mammary secretion testing. J. Equine Vet. Sci., *9:*88–94, 1989.
20. Leadon, D.P., Jeffcott, L.B., and Rossdale, P.D.: Mammary secretions in normal spontaneous and induced premature parturition in the mare. Equine Vet. J., *16:*251–259, 1984.
21. Ousey, J.C., Dridan, F., and Rossdale, P.D.: Preliminary studies of mammary secretions in the mare to assess foetal readiness for birth. Equine Vet. J., *16:*259–263, 1984.
22. Peaher, M., Rossdale, P.D., Forsyth, I.A., and Falk, M.: Changes in mammary development and the composition of secretion during late pregnancy in the mare. J. Reprod. Fertil. Suppl., *27:*555–561, 1979.

CHAPTER 106

ASSESSMENT OF FETAL WELL-BEING

H.C. Schott II

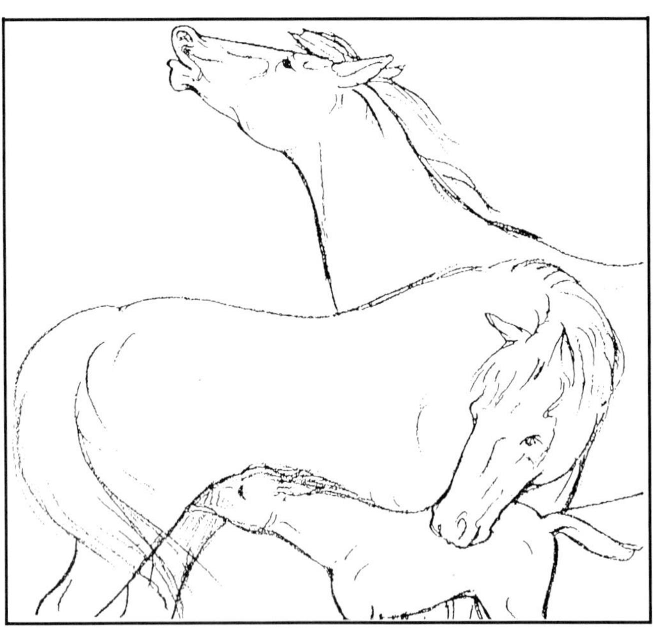

In comparison with advances made over the past few years in the ability to improve conception rates and care for sick neonatal foals, knowledge of the physiologic development of the equine fetus has progressed slowly. Assessment of the foal in utero is not a new area of interest as fetal electrocardiograms were recorded in horses as early as 1921.[1] Nevertheless, monitoring of fetal well-being has only recently regained attention, as equine neonatologists have realized the importance of being able to predict when a high-risk pregnancy may result in delivery of a compromised neonate.

Antepartum evaluation of the equine fetus is not routinely considered unless the pregnant mare develops a vaginal discharge, exhibits premature mammary gland development and lactation, the gestation length is prolonged, and a history of an abnormal gestation or neonatal foal exists, or the mare develops a serious medical or surgical problem in the latter stages of gestation. In such instances, a variety of techniques are available to assess fetal development and viability, which range from simple, noninvasive techniques (including palpation per rectum and collection of blood for hormone or fetal protein analyses) to more sophisticated or invasive techniques (such as fetal electrocardiography, fetal ultrasonography, and amniocentesis). Although use of the latter techniques has largely been limited to university hospitals and research centers, several investigations have provided a substantial data base such that use of some of these techniques is beginning to extend into the realm of clinical practice. This chapter discusses the techniques which are available to assess fetal development and well-being in the pregnant mare.

NONINVASIVE TECHNIQUES

PALPATION PER RECTUM

The most commonly used technique for assessment of fetal viability during gestation is palpation per rectum. Although it is actually an invasive technique, rectal palpation is discussed here because it is a routine procedure. From about 200 days to term, the fetus is readily palpable directly or by ballottement. As gestation advances, tension of the uterine wall decreases and the fetus passes upward toward the pelvic inlet. In mares that are pregnant for the first time, the uterine contents are usually nearer the pelvic inlet in comparison with multiparous mares, and the clinician can often palpate the fetal head in the pelvic canal.[2] Palpation of a thickened, doughy uterus and decreased uterine fluids may indicate a compromised or dead fetus and would be an indication for further evaluation of fetal viability. In addition to palpation of uterine contents, active movement by the fetus should be felt in the latter stages of gestation to ensure that the foal is alive. Unfortunately, episodes of fetal activity are intermittent and normally developing foals may be unresponsive during the examination. Periods of inactivity for the equine fetus are rarely longer than 10 to 15 min although "sleep" periods approaching 1 h have been described.[3] If activity is not apparent, further manipulation of the fetus during palpation is often, but not always, a sufficient stimulus to induce fetal movement. Asphyxia, however, also leads to a decrease in fetal movement;[4] thus, a lack of fetal activity during palpation does not differentiate between a normal or a compromised fetus. Consequently, palpation per rectum is an insensitive method of assessing fetal well-being.

HORMONAL, MAMMARY SECRETION, AND FETAL PROTEIN SCREENING

A relatively simple technique to assess fetal well-being is the assay of maternal blood or mammary secretions for changes in concentrations of hormones or specific molecules associated with pregnancy.

Maternal plasma progesterone and chorionic gonadotropin concentrations are elevated during the first half of pregnancy but are unreliable for assessing fetal well-being in midgestation because both hormones undergo a natural decline after about 150 days. Furthermore, progesterone levels may remain elevated and chorionic gonadotropin concentrations routinely follow a normal pattern with fetal loss before 150 days of gestation.[5] In the last month of gestation, the total concentration of progesterone metabolites (total progestogens) in maternal plasma rises from 10 ng/mL or less to about 20 ng/mL in the week before parturition. Persistently low or rapidly declining maternal plasma progestogen concentrations in the last month of gestation were valuable in predicting abortion in a limited number of late gestational mares with serious medical or surgical problems.[6] In addition, premature increases in plasma progestogen concentration (before 310 days of gestation) appear to be an indicator of fetal stress and cortisol production, possibly as a consequence of placental pathology.[7]

Maternal plasma concentrations and urinary excretion of estrogens fall rapidly after fetal loss.[8,9] After day 40 of pregnancy, the placenta is the primary source of estrogens, but continued production requires an adequate supply of the precursor dehydroepiandrosterone (DHA) from fetal gonads.[10] Beyond 280 days of gestation, the fetal gonads begin to regress with a concomitant decrease in DHA production. This leads to a natural decline in maternal plasma concentration of estrogens. In addition to a fall in maternal plasma estrogen concentrations, fetal gonadectomy resulted in growth retardation, weak expulsive efforts by the mare, and death during or shortly following parturition in three of four fetuses, suggesting that placental estrogen is important for fetal development (the fourth gonadectomized foal was delivered prematurely but went on to develop normally).[10] Placental estrogen enhances uterine and placental blood flow and the dysmaturity observed in gonadectomized foals may have resulted from decreased blood flow to the uteroplacental unit. Declining estrogen concentrations should be a sensitive indicator of fetal compromise before 280 days of gestation; however, fetal death could not be accurately predicted with maternal estrone sulfate concentrations in the series of late gestational mares described previously (the two mares which aborted maintained normal levels of estrone sulfate).[6] In another report,[11] maternal plasma concentrations of estrone sulfate and equilin fell prior to abortion, but in contrast, estrogen concentrations were found to remain elevated until the time of abortion in mares infected with equine herpesvirus type 1.[12] Consequently, the usefulness of measuring estrogen concentration to assess fetal well-being in the pregnant mare remains uncertain.

The concentrations of several electrolytes (calcium, potassium, and sodium) in pre- and full-term mammary secretions appear to be good indicators of impending parturition and readiness for birth. Specifically, calcium concentration is low (less than 4 mmol/L) in preterm secretions but increases to greater than 10 mmol/L during the 24 to 48 h before parturition.[13] Furthermore, premature increases in colostral calcium concentration (i.e., to greater than 10 mmol/L by 310 days of gestation) have been suggested to indicate placental pathology and fetal compromise.[14]

A rapid screening test has recently been promoted for early detection of twinning, early embryonic death, and placentitis in the mare.[15] The test is an enzyme-linked immunosorbent assay of maternal serum for a glycoprotein (molecular weight 70,000) produced by the fetus. The protein, equine α-fetoprotein, is undetectable in the serum of nonpregnant mares but is routinely found in low concentrations in the serum of healthy pregnant mares. Newborn foals have serum concentrations of the protein which are substantially greater than maternal serum concentrations, supporting the notion that the protein is of fetal origin. In serum samples collected from problem mares (twins, early embryonic death, or placentitis), increased levels of the equine fetal protein were found. Greater production of the protein was suggested to occur in twin pregnancies, whereas elevated maternal serum concentrations of the fetal protein in cases of early embryonic death or placentitis were considered to result from increased vascular permeability of the placenta.

Although these biochemical tests have been performed only in a limited number of problem mares, extension of such testing to a larger population of normal and diseased late gestational mares and availability of rapid field assay kits may be of great value in screening for high-risk pregnancies in the future.

FETAL HEART RATE MONITORING

Monitoring heart rate of the developing foal has received greatest attention as a technique to assess fetal well-being, largely because fetal heart rate (FHR) patterns have been used to indicate fetal "distress" in women for many years.[16–18] With further experience, however, documentation of fetal well-being on the basis of alterations in FHR alone has been found to be unreliable, because considerable variability exists in fetal heart rate. In women, abnormalities in FHR include fetal tachycardia, fetal bradycardia, and a loss of FHR

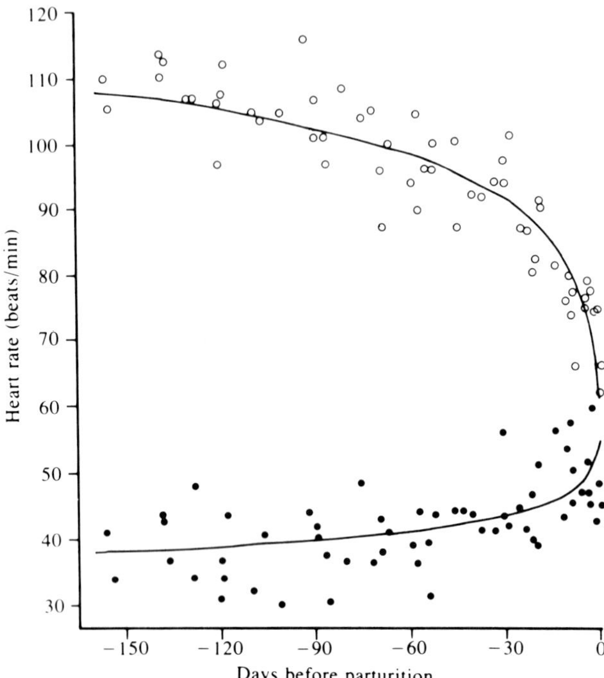

FIG. 106–1. Changes in fetal (○) and maternal (●) heart rates during gestation. (From Matsui, K., Sugano, S., and Masuyama, I.: Changes in the fetal heart rate of Thoroughbred horse through gestation. Jpn. J. Vet. Sci., *47*:597–601, 1985.)

variability. Fetal tachycardia may be found during periods of maternal fever or dehydration, with fetal anemia, or with fetal/placental infection and is usually associated with a favorable outcome unless infection is present.[18] Bradycardia and a loss of FHR variability are usually a consequence of asphyxia. Asphyxia (insufficient gas exchange leading to fetal hypoxemia, hypercapnia, and acidemia) may result from a decrease in uterine blood flow (with maternal disease) or a decrease in placental blood flow and exchange (placental insufficiency). Fetal bradycardia is mediated by a vagal response to the hypoxemia sensed by peripheral chemoreceptors. Asphyxia also results in a redistribution of fetal cardiac output to maintain blood flow to vital organs, central nervous system (CNS), and myocardium. However, if these fetal compensatory responses are insufficient to maintain oxygenation of these vital tissues, CNS depression will ensue and be reflected by a loss of normal FHR variability.[19]

In horses, the basal FHR declines and maternal heart rate increases as gestation advances[20,21] (Fig. 106–1). A progressive increase in parasympathetic tone in the developing fetus has been suggested to explain this FHR decrease.[22] As in women, episodes of FHR variability (accelerations and decelerations) increase in frequency with advancing gestation and transient (15 to 30 s) accelerations usually coincide with periods of fetal activity. Abnormal FHR patterns in foals include persistent fetal tachycardia and arrhythmias (premature wave forms), which have been observed preceding abortion in several instances. Fetal bradycardia has also been observed in the hour before death in abortions that were monitored throughout.[20]

Fetal heart rate can be detected by fetal electrocardiography,[3,20–27] transabdominal Doppler ultrasonography,[3,28–30] or by direct visualization of the heart via transabdominal or transrectal real-time ultrasonography.[31,32] All three techniques have limitations caused by fetal size and mobility, but fetal electrocardiography (FECG) is the most practical technique available.

The FECG can be recorded in the majority of pregnant mares from 150 days of gestation to term. The recording is made with a bipolar lead system with the positive electrode (LL) placed on the dorsal midline in the midlumbar region and the negative electrode (RA) placed on the ventral midline about 15 cm in front of the udder (Fig. 106–2). Recording is performed in lead II (using LA as the negative electrode and recording in lead III gives an identical configuration). A separate ground electrode is not required. This electrode and lead arrangement is most consistent in yielding maximal tracing deflections but moving the negative electrode to either side of midline and recording in alternate leads may be required if no FECG is observed with the standard lead placement.[27] Unfortunately, successful recording of FECG often requires a recording device for which the sensitivity can be adjusted. Many recording devices do not have this capability, limiting their use for fetal electrocardiography. Sensitivity should be set at the highest available setting (4 to 8 cm/mV desired). The FECG will appear as a regular sharp deflection with only the fetal QRS complex being routinely recognized (Fig. 106-3). Clipping small patches of hair for placement of adhesive electrodes or use of needle electrodes is usually necessary to record successfully the small fetal

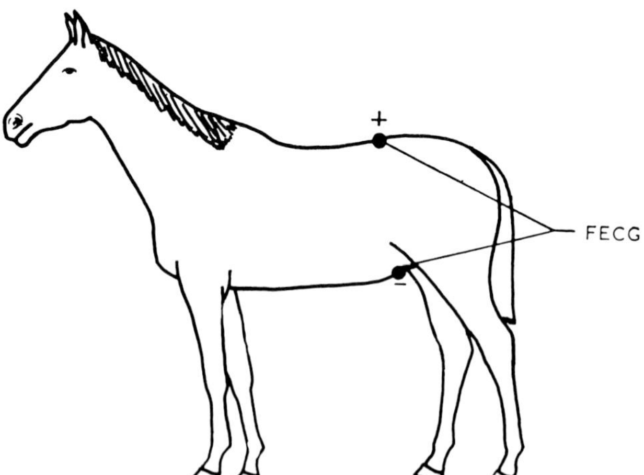

FIG. 106–2. Sites of attachment of electrodes for recording fetal electrocardiogram. The positive electrode (RA) is placed on the dorsal midline in midlumbar region and the negative electrode (LL) is placed in front of the mammary gland for recording in lead II. (From Holmes, J.R. and Darke, P.G.G.: Feotal electrocardiography in the mare. Vet Rec., *82*:651–655, 1968.)

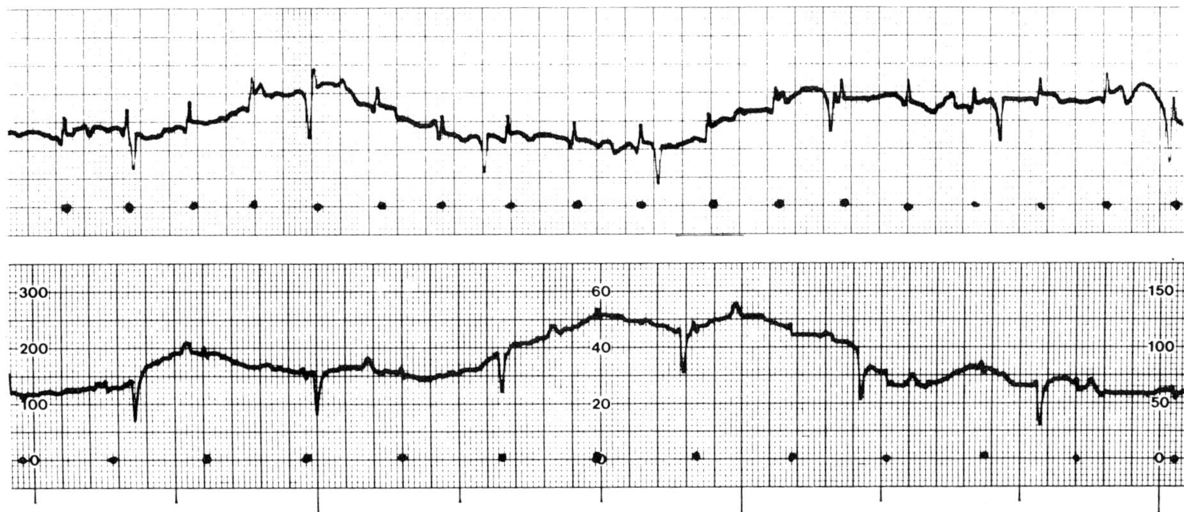

FIG. 106–3. Fetal electrocardiographic tracings from two pregnancies recorded at about 290 (top) and 280 (bottom) days of gestation. The maternal complexes are the regular large negative deflections in the baseline, and fluctuation of the baseline is commonly observed with respiration. The fetal complexes are marked on the tracings and reveal a FHR of about 80 beats/min (top) and 54 beats/min (bottom). The fetal bradycardia on the bottom strip was a consequence of maternal sedation with xylazine hydrochloride 20 min before recording. The two tracings also demonstrate the variation in FECG amplitude which is commonly observed between fetuses of similar gestational age or between tracings recorded from the same fetus over a period of a few minutes. This variation in amplitude is a consequence of changes in fetal position.

complexes. Needle electrodes have the further advantage of ease of repositioning. Collection and interpretation of the FECG may seem difficult at first until the clinician becomes familiar with changes in amplitude of the FECG with fetal movement, intermittent superimposition of fetal complexes on the maternal ECG, and artifacts from abdominal wall motion. Furthermore, electrical interference must be kept to a minimum as the FECG can be completely obscured by 60-cycle interference. With limited experience, however, FHR can be consistently and accurately determined by counting number of fetal complexes, at a regular RR interval, during a 6-s interval and multiplying by 10 (Fig. 106–3). The FHR may vary considerably over a short time; consequently, several repeated tracings at 10-min intervals are recommended for accurate assessment of basal FHR and FHR variability.

Primary indication for FECG in clinical practice is rapid determination of fetal viability (live or dead fetus) when rectal palpation is inconclusive. The FECG has also been valuable in detection of twins in later stages of pregnancy (Fig. 106–4), but a single FECG does not rule out possibility of a dead twin or a smaller twin from which the FECG is not recorded.[30,34] Another application of FECG is in investigation of fetal responses to administration of pharmacologic agents to pregnant mares[35,36] (Fig. 106–5).

Because of the large variation in basal FHR and FHR variability (Table 106–1), FHR monitoring alone is not a sensitive method of documenting fetal distress or asphyxia. To improve the sensitivity of FHR monitoring for assessment of fetal well-being, perinatologists perform nonstress and stress tests on humans.[16–18,37] The nonstress test is a prolonged monitoring period for observation of normal FHR variability. The nonstress test is considered normal (a reactive nonstress pattern) when at least two episodes of FHR acceleration of 15 or more beats per minute (for at least a 15-s duration) are found in association with fetal movements during a 20- to 30-min monitoring period. An abnormal nonstress test (a nonreactive nonstress pattern) is reported when FHR accelerations are absent or when spontaneous decelerations (not immediately following an acceleration) are observed. Such findings usually indicate asphyxia. Because the FHR accelerations should coincide with fetal activity during the nonstress test, ultrasonography is generally used for FHR monitoring during this procedure. The stress test is performed to assess uteroplacental function and reserve and consists of monitoring the FHR response to uterine contractions induced by massage of the mammary glands or an infusion of oxytocin. A normally functioning uteroplacental unit should have sufficient reserve to maintain adequate gas exchange across the placenta during the induced uterine contractions. Consequently, a normal FHR is maintained. However, if placental insufficiency exists, fetal hypoxemia and acidosis may develop. A transient bradycardia, termed a late deceleration, is subsequently observed. Some perinatologists consider the stress test to be more sensitive than the nonstress test because it frequently becomes positive (late decelerations apparent) before the nonstress test becomes nonreactive. The

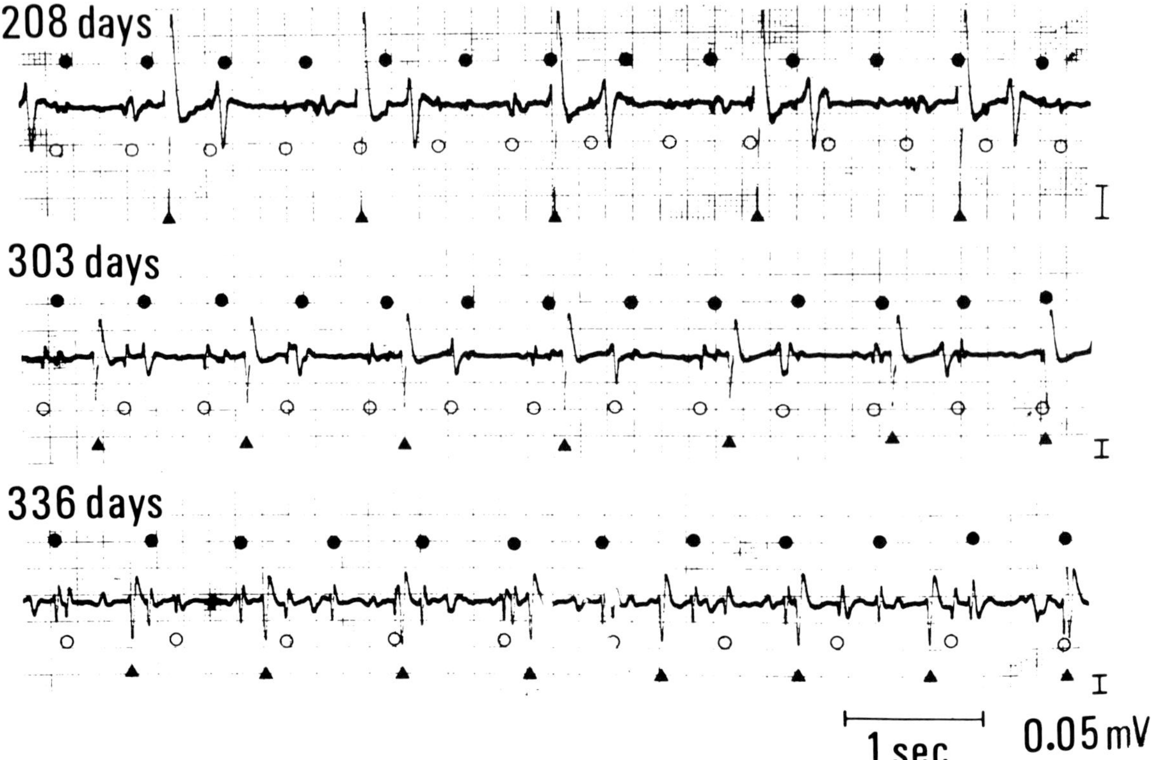

FIG. 106–4. Characteristic FECG tracings in a twin pregnancy recorded at 208, 303, and 336 days of gestation. The maternal QRS complex is most prominent and represented by the filled triangles (▲). The two series of fetal complexes, represented by filled (●) and open (○) circles above and below the tracing are readily detectable in the 336-day recording. With experience, the presence of two fetal heart rate patterns may be detected as early as 150 to 200 days of gestation. (From Matsui, K.: Fetal and maternal heart rates in a case of twin pregnancy of the Thoroughbred horse. Jpn. J. Vet. Sci., *47:*817–821, 1985.)

stress test can be performed with electrocardiographic or ultrasonographic monitoring devices, but induction of labor is a potential adverse effect.

Nonstress testing has been performed in a limited number of pregnant mares with transabdominal Doppler ultrasonographic recording of the FHR.[3,30] The normal or reactive pattern shows more frequent and prolonged FHR accelerations (>10 accelerations in a 10-min period with durations of 20 to 40 s) in comparison with human fetuses. In addition, fetal movements without FHR accelerations were also observed, suggesting that equine fetuses may be more active than human fetuses during the nonstress test. Recently, stress testing also has been performed in the pregnant mare by the intravenous administration of oxytocin or by use of a vibroacoustic device placed in proximity to the fetal head during rectal palpation. Preliminary findings suggest that stress testing may be of value in the assessment of fetal well-being.[7]

FETAL ULTRASONOGRAPHY

Transabdominal ultrasonographic examination of the fetus is routinely performed in women to determine gestational age, evaluate developmental anomalies, and detect fetal asphyxia.[4,18] The equine fetus can be imaged with both transrectal and transabdominal ultrasonography; the latter approach is more commonly employed because of the close proximity of the fetus to the

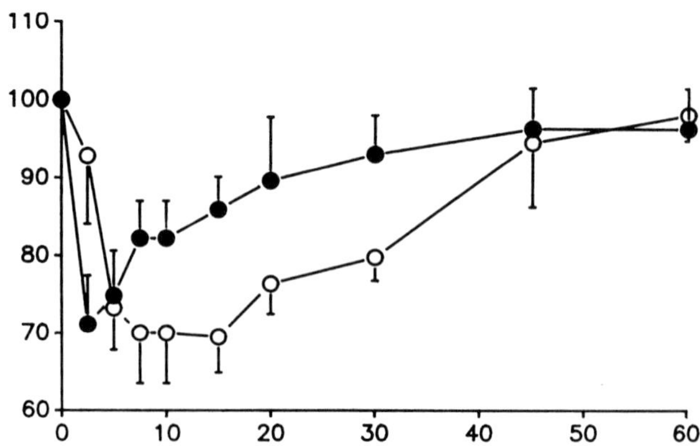

FIG. 106–5. Maternal (●) and fetal (○) heart rates expressed as a percentage of basal heart rate (on the vertical axis) after administration of xylazine hydrochloride (0.5 mg/kg) to pregnant mares. From the horizontal axis (representing time in minutes following xylazine administration) note that FHR is suppressed to a much greater extent and duration than is maternal heart rate.

TABLE 106–1. REPORTED VALUES FOR HEART RATE OF THE EQUINE FETUS AT VARIOUS GESTATIONAL AGES

RECORDING METHOD AND REFERENCE NUMBER	OBSERVATIONS
FECG[23]	120 at 6 months
FECG[24]	Range of 84 to 114 in 17 Percheron mares recorded between 272 and 342 days
FECG[25]	Range of 62 to 140 in 14 mares with progressive decrease from 144 days to term
Doppler ultrasound[28]	Range of 100 to 180 in 70 mares with progressive decrease from 3 months to term
Doppler ultrasound[29]	Range of 100 to 160 in 311 recordings with a linear decrease from 40 days to term
FECG[20]	Range of 90 to 120 in 595 recordings; linear decrease from 5 months to term; variability noted
FECG[27]	109 ± 15.4 (SD) in 45 mares at 235 ± 45 (SD) days of gestation; great variability emphasized
Transabdominal ultrasound[32]	Range of 60 to 80 to 180 observed in 50 mares from 100 days to term; FHR increases with activity
FECG[21]	Mean of 110 at 6 months with a logarithmic decrease to 75 at term; FHR accelerations noted
Doppler ultrasound[30]	76 ± 8 (SD) in 108 recordings from 14 mares near term; 25 to 40 beat/min; increases with activity

ventral abdominal wall (by as early as 60 days of gestation).[3,30–32,38,39] In addition, because a complete examination often requires 15 to 30 min, the transabdominal approach is safer. The mare is restrained in stocks, and the ventral abdomen is clipped or shaved. Sedation is avoided owing to possible suppression of FHR and fetal activity which are important observations to record during examination. Transabdominal scanning can be performed with the same equipment used for routine transrectal ultrasonographic pregnancy detection, but use of lower frequency transducers (2.5 to 5 MHz) allows deeper tissue penetration and more complete examination. Both linear array and sector scanners may be used; the primary advantages of the latter are ease of directing the beam and ability to image deeper structures through small acoustic windows. After application of contact gel to the abdominal wall, the transducer is oriented longitudinally a few inches in front of the mammary gland with the end of the transducer directed caudad (Fig. 106–6). The transducer is moved abaxially to either side until the anechoic allantoic fluid and hyperechoic fetus are found. Examining cranially and caudally allows determination of fetal presentation. Typically, the late gestational fetus is found lying in an oblique ventrodorsal position (lying slightly tilted on its back) in an anterior presentation (fetal head toward mare's pelvis). In early gestation (60 to 120 days), the transducer may need to be placed farther caudad in the inguinal areas to image the fetus, while in late gestation, the fetus may extend as far craniad as the mare's xiphoid.

In women, crown-rump length, biparietal diameter, femur length, and head and abdominal circumference are measured to determine fetal size and weight for comparison with expected values for reported age of the fetus.[4] Inconsistencies in ages determined from history and the sonogram may indicate intrauterine growth retardation caused by developmental anomalies or placental insufficiency. As a result of the large size of the equine fetus, imaging of anatomical structures for correlation of size and fetal age is limited to smaller structures which can be consistently visualized in their entirety. Structures which have been measured sequentially include fetal eye size and fetal aortic diameter.[3,30,40] Fetal eye size (measured as sum of length and width) increases from ~4 cm at 180 days of gestation to ~6 cm at term, but 95% confidence intervals are

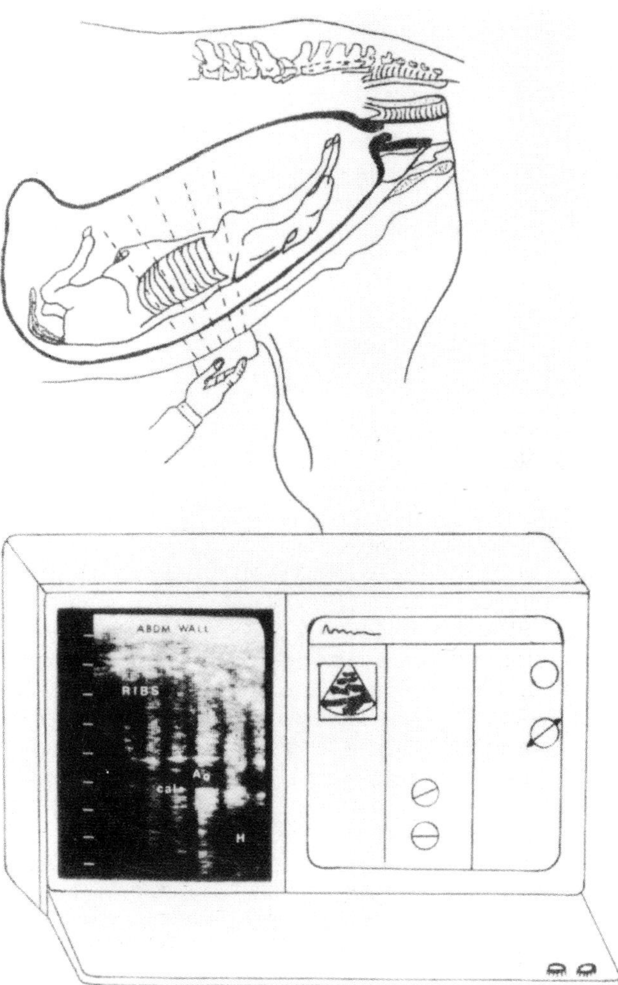

FIG. 106–6. Schematic representation of a linear-array transducer used for transabdominal ultrasonography of the developing foal. (From Pipers, F.S., and Adams-Brendemeuhl, C.S.: Techniques and applications of transabdominal ultrasonography in the pregnant mare. J. Am. Vet. Med. Assoc., *185*:766–771, 1984.

±0.5 cm (or ± 40 days) making fetal eye size an insensitive estimator of fetal age.[40] Fetal aortic diameters measured during systole in Thoroughbred mares in the week before parturition correlated well with weight, circumference at the girth, and hip height of newborn foals (Fig. 106–7).[3,30] Aortic diameter increased from ~2.1 cm at 300 days gestation to ~2.7 cm at term in fetuses examined serially; consequently, aortic diameter increases at ~1 mm per 5 days in late gestation. Similar measures of systolic aortic diameter performed in Arabian and draft breed fetuses revealed breed variation. Unfortunately, aortic diameter measured during fetal ultrasonography in high-risk pregnancies correlated poorly with birth weight. In addition, in many pregnancies which resulted in the delivery of emaciated or dysmature foals, transabdominal ultrasonographic measurement of aortic diameter was normal.[3,30]

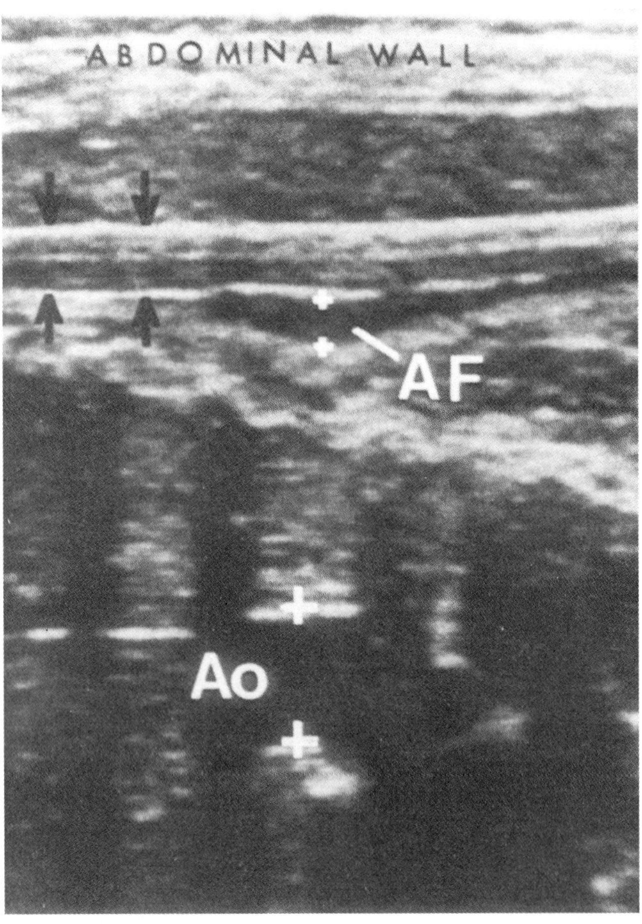

FIG. 106–7. Transabdominal ultrasonograph of an equine fetal thorax imaged with a 4-MHz linear-array transducer. The image is a transverse section revealing (from top) the abdominal wall, uterus and allantiochorion (between black arrows), and fetal thorax. The ribs are readily visualized. The systolic aortic diameter (Ao) as well as the distance between the placenta and fetal scapulohumeral joint (which represents an estimate of allantoic fluid volume, AF) can be determined with this orientation. (From Adams-Brendemeuhl, C., and Pipers, F.S.: Antepartum evaluations of the equine fetus. J. Reprod. Fertil. Suppl., *35:*565–573, 1987.)

Consequently, before transabdominal ultrasonography becomes useful for determination of fetal age or size in horses, further morphometric studies, such as a recent report detailing cardiac growth in the equine fetus,[41] will need to be performed in conjunction with ultrasonographic measurements to identify appropriate anatomical structures to measure.

Transabdominal ultrasonography can be used to assess integrity of the placenta and volume and character of fetal fluids. When imaging the uterine wall and placenta, a transducer with greater resolution (5.0 to 7.5 MHz) may be needed to distinguish between the two layers. In late gestational mares, the uterine wall and chorioallantoic membrane of the normal gravid horn are ~1 to 1.5 cm thick.[3,30] Increased uteroplacental thickness (greater than 1.75 to 2.0 cm) is usually consistent with placentitis. With chronic placental thickening, highly echogenic foci (confirmed to be placental mineralizations at parturition) have been found in some mares. Both the allantoic and amniotic cavities can be seen to contain hypoanechoic to anechoic fluid via ultrasonography. Allantoic fluid is usually evident in all fields imaged. Separation between the allantoic and amniotic cavities is visualized as a thin sheet of tissue representing the amnion. This membrane lies in close contact with the fetus, and most of the free amniotic fluid is found around the head, neck, and forelegs.[3,30,32]

The fetal fluids are recycled several times a day via placental and transcutaneous exchange, fetal swallowing, and fetal urine production. In women, amniotic fluid volume is routinely assessed because both increased (polyhydramnios) and decreased (oligohydramnios) amounts of amniotic fluid suggest a compromised fetus.[4,18,19] Polyhydramnios is commonly associated with esophageal atresia, while oligohydramnios is found with renal agenesis. Oligohydramnios is also an important sign of fetal asphyxia (in the absence of renal anomalies), because decreased fetal urine production is consistent with a decrease in fetal renal blood flow as a consequence of asphyxia. In horses, abnormalities in volume of fetal fluids are rare with only one well-documented case of polyhydramnios in a triplet pregnancy,[42] while excess accumulation of allantoic fluid has been recognized in several instances.[42,44] Developmental anomalies or twins were found in the majority of such cases. An ultrasonographic method to estimate amniotic fluid volume has not been described for mares, but an attempt to estimate allantoic fluid volume has been made by measuring the vertical distance of allantoic fluid observed on a frontal view of the fetus at the level of the scapulohumeral joint (Fig. 106–7). The distance in normal mares from 300 days of gestation to term was about 2 cm.[3,30]

In women and horses, echogenic material termed vernix or free-floating particles (FFPs) are commonly visualized during late gestation in amniotic and allantoic fluids.[3,4,30] These FFPs are composed of desquamated epithelial cells and secretions from sebaceous glands in the fetal skin. They may also contain urinary crystals. Presence of FFPs has been suggested to correlate with pulmonary maturity in human fetuses but premature appearance or an increased quantity of FFPs may also represent passage of meconium, hemorrhage, or accumulation of septic debris in the amniotic cavity. In horses, FFPs are observed in allantoic fluid as early as 40 days before parturition and by 10 days before foaling, FFPs are found in the allantoic fluid of most mares.[3,30] The significance of FFPs in equine allantoic fluid and their possible relation to pulmonary maturity are unknown. The hippomanes, commonly found with the placenta after parturition, are likely composed of FFPs which have coalesced into a larger mass.

The primary applications of ultrasonography in the pregnant mare are for pregnancy diagnosis and the detection of twins in early gestation (via a transrectal approach). As gestation advances past 60 to 90 days, transabdominal ultrasonography becomes more useful and allows documentation of fetal orientation and twins which escaped earlier detection. In select cases, transabdominal ultrasonography may be used to evaluate fetal well-being, to support a diagnosis of placentitis (by visualization of placental thickening), or to determine the site of excess fluid accumulation (amniotic or allantoic cavity). Transabdominal ultrasonography also allows visualization of the amniotic cavity for amniocentesis.

FETAL BIOPHYSICAL PROFILING

Placental insufficiency leading to asphyxia is a major cause of morbidity and mortality among perinates.[4,18,19,45] Consequently, antepartum recognition of asphyxia is of great benefit in identifying which fetuses are likely to have greater difficulty in adapting to extrauterine life. Immediate physiologic responses of the fetus to episodes of asphyxia are well characterized and include selective vasoconstriction and redistribution of cardiac output to maintain oxygenation of vital organs, a decrease in fetal activity, and changes in FHR patterns. These responses allow the fetus to tolerate substantial reductions in oxygen delivery and consumption for periods up to 45 min (as routinely occurs during labor). Prolonged asphyxia, however, may lead to oligohydramnios, intrauterine growth retardation, permanent neurologic damage, or death with the severity of fetal compromise paralleling the degree of asphyxia.

Many parameters have been measured to assess the degree of fetal "distress" resulting from asphyxia, but no individual factor has proven to be sensitive. This lack of sensitivity, however, has been overcome by grouping several measurements into a fetal biophysical profile.[4,46] Biophysical profiling is successfully used in women to decide when premature delivery of a "distressed" fetus is indicated. Although premature delivery is rarely a viable option for the compromised equine fetus,[47] recognition of fetal asphyxia would ensure appropriate foaling management or possible referral to a hospital where neonatal intensive care would be available immediately after foaling.

In high-risk pregnancies in women, ultrasonographic examination in concert with FHR monitoring are used to construct the biophysical profile.[4,46] Five parameters are evaluated: fetal breathing movements, body movements, fetal tone, FHR variability (nonstress test), and an estimate of amniotic fluid volume (Table 106–2). If a parameter is normal, a score of 2 is given but if the parameter is abnormal, a value of 0 is assigned. The scores are summed and a total of 8 or 10 is considered

TABLE 106–2. BIOPHYSICAL PROFILE SCORING OF THE HUMAN FETUS: TECHNIQUE AND INTERPRETATION

BIOPHYSICAL VARIABLE	NORMAL*	ABNORMAL†
Fetal breathing movements	At least one episode of FBM‡ of at least 30 s duration in 30 min of observation	Absent FBM or no episode of ≥30 s in 30 min
Gross body movement	At least three discrete body or limb movements in 30 min (episodes of active continuous movement considered a single movement)	Two or fewer episodes of body or limb movements in 30 min
Fetal tone	At least one episode of active extension with return to flexion of fetal limb(s) or trunk; opening and closing of hand considered normal tone	Either slow extension with return to partial flexion or movement of limb in full extension or absent fetal movement
Reactive FHR§	At least two episodes of FHR acceleration of ≥15 bpm and of at least 15 s duration associated with fetal movement in 30 min	Less than two episodes of acceleration of FHR or acceleration of <15 bpm in 30 min
Qualitative AFV‖	At least one pocket of AF# that measures at least 1 cm in two perpendicular planes	Either no AF pockets or a pocket <1 cm in two perpendicular planes

*Score = 2.
†Score = 0.
‡FBM = Fetal breathing movement.
§FHR = Fetal heart rate.
‖AFV = Amniotic fluid volume.
#AF = Amniotic fluid.
(From Manning, F.A., et al.: Fetal assessment based on fetal biophysical profile scoring: Experience in 12,620 referred high-risk pregnancies. Am. J. Obstet. Gynecol., *151*:343–350, 1985.)

normal. A value of 6 or less is consistent with asphyxia and if the profile is not improved on repeat examination several hours later, delivery is recommended (depending on gestational age). Use of the biophysical profile to decide when intervention (delivery) was indicated resulted in a substantial decrease in perinatal mortality in a large prospective study of high-risk pregnancies in women.[48]

A similar concept of biophysical profiling developed for use in late gestational mares involved measurement of six parameters: fetal size (based on aortic diameter), FHR, fetal movement, placental thickness, qualitative allantoic fluid appearance (presence of FFPs), and an estimation of allantoic fluid volume.[3,30] If all parameters were normal, the biophysical profile was considered negative but if one or more of the parameters were abnormal, the profile was positive. Application of biophysical profiling to 17 mares (ranging from 270 to 346 days of gestation) with suspected obstetrical complications yielded a negative (normal) profile in 9 mares, and 7 (78%) delivered healthy foals. Of the two foals which had an unfavorable outcome despite a negative (normal) profile, one died after premature delivery at 291 days of gestation and the other foal died because of a lack of rupture of the amnion during an unattended foaling. Of 8 mares with a positive (abnormal) profile, seven (88%) of the fetuses had poor outcomes (Table 106–3). These preliminary findings suggest that biophysical profiling of equine fetuses in high-risk pregnancies has merit. However, indications for biophysical profiling and parameters which should be measured in such a profile need further investigation. If a standardized fetal biophysical profile could be further developed for the equine fetus, detection of fetal asphyxia or placentitis could be of practical value in predicting which foals are likely to be compromised and to require immediate attention at birth.

INVASIVE TECHNIQUES

AMNIOCENTESIS

Amniocentesis is routinely performed in women for collection of amniotic fluid for biochemical and cytogenetic testing.[18,45] Biochemical testing includes evalua-

TABLE 106–3. ANTEPARTUM BIOPHYSICAL PROFILES AND OUTCOMES IN 17 HIGH-RISK PREGNANCIES IN LATE GESTATIONAL MARES

MARE NUMBER	PRESENTING COMPLAINT	GESTATIONAL AGE (DAYS) IN UTERO	BIOPHYSIC PROFILE	FETAL OUTCOME	MARE PROBLEMS POSTPARTUM
1	Udder development	291	Negative	Negative (foal small, weak; died day 5)	Placentitis
2	Lactating	310	Positive (FHR 48)	Negative (pneumonia, recovered)	Focal placentitis
3	Twins (1 dead), udder development, laminitis	322	Positive (FHR 58)	Negative (dystocia, stillborn, necrotizing twin)	Diffuse placentitis
4	Lactating	280	Positive (placenta 0.5 cm)	Negative (weak, pneumonia, recovered)	Placentitis
5	Rapid abdominal, enlargement	236	Positive (posterior presentation particles)	Negative (aborted)	Placentitis
6	Udder development	291	Positive (FHR 48, no activity)	Negative (seizures, killed)	Unknown
7	Vaginal discharge	270	Positive (arrhythmia, bradycardia)	Negative (stillborn)	Placentitis, calcifications
8	Lactating, cervix relaxed	315	Negative	Positive	Focal placentitis
9	Colic	335	Negative	Positive	None
10	MHR 100 beats/min, jugular pulse, ventral oedema	335	Negative	Positive	Uterine haemorrhage
11	Uterine torsion	338	Negative	Positive	None
12	Udder development, laminitis	327	Positive (FHR 56)	Positive	None
13	Rapid abdominal, enlargement	338	Negative	Positive	None
14	Udder development	335	Negative	Positive	None
15	Udder development	346	Negative	Positive	None
16	Udder development	280	Positive (placenta 3.4 cm)	Negative (stillborn)	Unknown
17	Discharge	320	Negative	Negative (unattended foaling, foal retained in amniotic membrane)	Diffuse placentitis

(From Adams-Brendemuehl, Co., and Pipers, F.S.: Antepartum evaluations of the equine fetus. J. Reprod. Fertil. Suppl., *35*:565–573, 1987.)

tion of fetal and pulmonary maturity and specific assays for inherited defects such as increased amniotic fluid α-fetoprotein with neural tube defects. Assessment of pulmonary maturity is usually performed only after intrauterine growth retardation or asphyxia have been demonstrated on biophysical profiling. Parameters assessed include lecithin to sphingomyelin ratio (L:S ratio) or phosphatidyl glycerol (PG) content of amniotic fluid. When used in conjunction with the biophysical profile, these tests have substantially reduced fetal morbidity and mortality from neonatal respiratory distress (hyaline membrane disease) associated with preterm delivery. The tests are not without problems, however, and improved assessment of fetal well-being with noninvasive methods (as a consequence of further experience with and advances in technology of transabdominal ultrasonography) is reducing the indication for amniocentesis to assess pulmonary maturity. In women, amniotic fluid analysis is of greater value for the diagnosis of cytogenetic defects. When grown in tissue culture, the desquamated fetal cells collected during amniocentesis of high-risk pregnancies allow karyotyping and extensive assays to be performed to screen for chromosomal abnormalities and inborn errors of metabolism.

Amniocentesis has been performed experimentally in the pregnant mare, but it will likely remain primarily a research tool because normal laboratory parameters for equine amniotic fluid are not well established and the clinical indications for amniocentesis are limited.[48–53] Screening for inherited defects in horses is probably not practical because such disorders are uncommon and antepartum detection is not as great a concern as in women (perhaps with the exception of combined immunodeficiency of Arabian foals). To date, investigations of amniotic fluid L:S ratios and PG content in horses have yielded inconsistent results. This may be attributed to differences in assay technique as well as species differences. Remember that assessment of pulmonary maturity in women is performed to determine the best time to intervene and deliver an already compromised fetus. Because preterm delivery of premature foals is not often an option in equine medicine, antepartum assessment of pulmonary maturity would rarely be indicated. Furthermore, neonatal respiratory distress is much less commonly observed in premature or sick foals in comparison with premature infants. For all of these reasons, amniocentesis is not likely to become a commonly used procedure in clinical practice.

The technique for amniocentesis in the mid- to late gestational mare has been described. Briefly, after locating an area of contact of the uterus and the ventral abdominal wall with ultrasonography (where a pocket of amniotic fluid can also be visualized), the abdominal wall is locally anesthetized and aseptically prepared. A 22-cm 18-gauge spinal needle is passed via a skin incision through the abdominal and uterine walls and into the amniotic sac with the assistance of a sterile biopsy guide attached to the ultrasound probe. This method was reported to have an 85% success rate in collection of amniotic fluid.[50]

In women, amniocentesis is a relatively safe procedure with a complication rate of 0.5%.[45] In horses, the complication rate in preliminary investigations has been much higher. Unintentional collection of allantoic fluid occurred in up to 33% of the attempts in one study when amniocentesis was attempted without continuous ultrasound guidance.[49] More significant, abortion or stillbirth occurred in 25% of the mares in which the technique was repeated serially. This unacceptably high fatality rate may be a result of the repeated amniocenteses. As greater experience was gained, the complication rate decreased substantially.[50] In another investigation in which a single amniocentesis was performed during the second trimester of pregnancy for determination of fetal sex and amniotic fluid hormone concentrations, no complications were reported despite the use of blind needle passage after localization of a pocket of amniotic fluid via transabdominal ultrasound.[52] Interestingly, analysis of metaphase chromosomes for determination of fetal sex was accurate in only 15 of 19 mares (80%).

Other parameters of equine amniotic fluid which have been investigated as indicators of fetal well-being include gross contamination of the fluid with blood or meconium (which may be detected via ultrasonography) and urea nitrogen, creatinine, and cortisol concentrations.[45] Urea nitrogen and creatinine concentrations are elevated to about 40 and 10 mg/dL, respectively, in normal equine amniotic fluid at parturition.[51] Such increases are consistent with leakage of fetal urine into the amniotic cavity in late gestation. Serial measurement of these parameters in amniotic fluid during the last 4 weeks of pregnancy revealed no increase toward term; consequently, amniotic fluid urea nitrogen and creatinine concentrations do not appear to provide an indication of fetal maturity (similar findings have been reported in women).[53] Amniotic fluid cortisol concentration, on the other hand, increases at term consistent with maturation of the fetal hypothalamic-pituitary-adrenal axis.[48] Assay of amniotic fluid cortisol concentration may be of value in select cases in which induction of parturition is contemplated (in mares with orthopedic problems or when the gestation length is prolonged). However, because the rise in amniotic fluid cortisol precedes natural parturition by less than a week, risks of amniocentesis must be weighed against advantages of delivery.

Bacterial culture of equine amniotic fluid collected via amniocentesis[50] or via puncture of the amnion at parturition has yielded positive results in 20 to 30% of samples collected. The majority of isolates have been nonpathogenic aerobic organisms commonly considered to be contaminants. The significance of these positive amniotic fluid cultures is not known, but similar results were found when fluid was collected either after brief antiseptic swabbing of the amnion before puncture or via amniocentesis performed with aseptic technique.

CHORIONIC VILLUS SAMPLING

Chorionic villus sampling is an invasive technique used to collect tissue samples for cytogenetic or biochemical testing in high-risk pregnancies (i.e., a history of inherited diseases).[45] The advantage over amniocentesis is that chorionic villus sampling can be performed much earlier in gestation to diagnose serious genetic disorders. Consequently, decisions concerning maintenance of pregnancy can be made when elective termination would be safer to the mother. Clinical application of this technique has not been investigated in the horse. In the future, it may provide a method of sample collection for early determination of fetal sex or diagnosis of genetic diseases such as combined immunodeficiency (CID) by cytogenetic or molecular biologic techniques.

FETOSCOPY AND FETAL BLOOD SAMPLING

Fetoscopy is used when the fetus must be visualized for collection of fetal blood samples or for therapeutic intervention.[45,54] The technique gained popularity in human perinatologic practice when clinicians discovered that many biochemical disorders which could not be diagnosed with amniotic fluid analysis could be determined by fetal blood sampling or biopsy of fetal organs. Furthermore, fetoscopy has proved a valuable technique to visualize the fetus for blood transfusions in treatment of isoimmunization syndromes. Transcervical fetoscopy (with resultant fetal death) has been used in first trimester mares, but the purpose of the investigation was to study early embryonic development rather than assess fetal well-being.[55]

All invasive techniques employed for the assessment of fetal well-being carry the risk of inducing abortion, but as the techniques become more invasive, complication rate increases. Abortion rate following fetoscopy in women was initially ~10%, but with further experience the complication rate has decreased to 2 to 3%. As with amniocentesis, the complication rate with fetoscopy is related to the experience of the individual performing the technique.

REFERENCES

1. Norr, J.: Fotale elektiokardiogramme vom pferd. Z. Biol., *73:*123–128, 1921.
2. Rossdale, P.D., and Ricketts, S.W.: Equine Stud Farm Medicine. 2nd ed. Philadelphia, Lea & Febiger, 1980.
3. Adams-Brendemuehl, C.: Fetal assessment. *In* Equine Clinical Neonatology. Edited by A.M. Koterba, W.H. Drummond, and P.C. Kosch. Philadelphia, Lea & Febiger, 1990, pp. 16–33.
4. Manning, F.A.: Ultrasonography in perinatal medicine. *In* Neonatology: Pathophysiology and Management of the Newborn. 3rd ed. Edited by G.B. Avery. Philadelphia, J.B. Lippincott, 1987, pp. 110–129.
5. Roberts, S.J.: Gestation and pregnancy diagnosis in the mare. *In* Current Therapy in Theriogenology 2. Edited by D.A. Morrow. Philadelphia, W.B. Saunders, 1986, pp. 670–678.
6. Santschi, E.M., LeBlanc, M.M., and Rossdale, P.D.: Preliminary investigation of progestogen and oestrone sulphate concentrations in the serum of late pregnant mares during severe medical and surgical stress. Equine Vet. J., *5(Suppl.):*62, 1988.
7. Rossdale, P.D., and McGladdery, A.J.: Perinatology: a clinical concept. Equine Vet. Educ., *3:*208–214, 1991.
8. Jeffcott, L.B., et al.: Changes in maternal hormone concentrations associated with induction of fetal death at day 45 of gestation in mares. J. Reprod. Fertil. Suppl., *35:*461–467, 1987.
9. Kasman, L.H., et al.: Estrone sulfate concentrations as an indicator of fetal demise in horses. Am. J. Vet. Res., *49:*184–187, 1988.
10. Pashen, R.L., et al.: The role of the fetal gonads and placenta in steroid production, maintenance of pregnancy, and parturition in the mare. J. Reprod. Fertil. Suppl., *27:*499–509, 1979.
11. Parkes, R.D., et al.: Plasma concentrations of equilin and oestrone in the assessment of fetoplacental function in the mare. Vet. Rec., *100:*511–512, 1977.
12. Ousey, J.C., et al.: Plasma concentrations of progestagens, oestrone sulfate and prolactin in pregnant mares subjected to natural challenge and equine herpesvirus 1. J. Reprod. Fertil. Suppl., *35:*519–528, 1987.
13. Ousey, J.C., Dudan, F., and Rossdale, P.D.: Preliminary studies of mammary secretions in the mare to assess foetal readiness for birth. Equine Vet. J., *16:*259–263, 1984.
14. Rossdale, P.D., et al.: The effects of placental pathology on maternal plasma progestagen and mammary secretion calcium concentrations and on neonatal adrenocortical function in the horse. J. Reprod. Fert. Supplil., *44:*579–590, 1991.
15. Sorensen, K., et al.: Measurement and clinical significance of equine fetal protein in pregnant mare's serum. J. Equine Vet. Sci., *10:*417–420, 1990.
16. Freeman, R.K., and Garite, T.J.: Fetal Heart Rate Monitoring. Baltimore, Williams & Wilkins, 1981.
17. Parer, J.T.: Fetal heart rate. *In* Maternal Fetal Medicine: Principles and Practice. Edited by R.K. Creasy and R. Resnick. Philadelphia, W.B. Saunders, 1984, pp. 285–319.
18. Andolsek, K.M.: Obstetric Care: Standards of Prenatal, Intrapartum and Postpartum Management. Philadelphia, Lea & Febiger, 1990.
19. Parer, J.T., and Livingston, E.G.: What is fetal distress? Am. J. Obstet. Gynecol., *162:*1421–1427, 1990.
20. Colles, C.M., Parkes, R.D., and May, C.J.: Foetal electrocardiography in the mare. Equine Vet. J., *10:*32–37, 1978.
21. Matsui, K., Sugano, S., and Masuyama, I.: Changes in the fetal heart rate of Thoroughbred horse through the gestation. Jpn. J. Vet. Sci., *47:*597–601, 1985.
22. Matsui, K., et al.: Alterations in the heart rate of Thoroughbred horse, pony, and Holstein cow through pre- and post-natal stages. Jpn. J. Vet. Sci., *46:*505–510, 1984.
23. Larks, S.D., Holm, L.W., and Parker, H.R.: A new technic for the demonstration of the fetal electrocardiogram in the large domestic animal (cattle, sheep, horse). Cornell Vet., *50:*459–468, 1960.
24. Kanagawa, H., et al.: Fetal electrocardiogram at late gestational stages in horses: Preliminary study. Jpn. J. Vet. Res., *15:*15–20, 1967.
25. Holmes, J.R., and Darke, P.G.G.: Foetal electrocardiography in the mare. Vet. Rec., *82:*651–655, 1968.
26. Schott, H.C., and Morley, P.S.: Fetal electrocardiography revisited. Int. Soc. Vet. Perinatol. Newslett., *2:*1–12, 1989.
27. Buss, D.D., Asbury, A.C., and Chevalier, L.: Limitations

in equine fetal electrocardiography. J. Am. Vet. Med. Assoc., *177:*174–176., 1980.

28. Fraser, A.F., Keith, N.W., and Hastie, H.: Summarised observations on the ultrasonic detection of pregnancy and foetal life in the mare. Vet. Rec., *92:*20–21, 1973.

29. Mitchell, D.: Detection of foetal circulation in the mare and cow by Doppler ultra-sound. Vet. Rec., *93:*365–368, 1973.

30. Adams-Brendemuehl, C., and Pipers, F.S.: Antepartum evaluations of the equine fetus. J. Reprod. Fertil. Suppl., *35:*565–573, 1987.

31. O'Grady, J.P., et al.: In utero visualization of the fetal horse by ultrasonic scanning. Equine Pract., *3:*45–49, 1981.

32. Pipers, F.M., and Adams-Brendemuehl, C.S.: Techniques and applications of transabdominal ultrasonography in the pregnant mare. J. Am. Vet. Med. Assoc., *185:*766–771, 1984.

33. Parkes, R.D., and Colles, C.M.: Fetal electrocardiography in the mare as a practical aid to diagnosing singleton and twin pregnancy. Vet. Rec., *100:*25–26, 1977.

34. Matsui, K.: Fetal and maternal heart rates in a case of twin pregnancy of the Thoroughbred horse. Jpn. J. Vet. Sci., *47:*817–821, 1985.

35. McGladdery, A.J., Cotrill, C.M., and Rossdale, P.D.: Effects upon the fetus of sedative drugs administered to the mare. Proceedings of the Second International Conference of Veterinary Perinatology. Edited by P.D. Rossdale, Newmarket, Equine Veterinary Journal, 1990, p.14.

36. Smith, L.J., and Schott, H.C.: Xylazine-induced fetal bradycardia. Proceedings of the Second International Conference of Veterinary Perinatology. Edited by P.D. Rossdale. Newmarket, Equine Veterinary Journal, 1990, p. 36.

37. Killam, A.P.: Management of the high-risk pregnancy. *In* Neonatology: Pathophysiology and Management of the Newborn. 3rd ed. Edited by G.B. Avery. Philadelphia, J.B. Lippincott, 1987, pp. 147–158.

38. Fraser, A.F., et al.: An exploratory ultrasonic study on quantitative foetal kinesis in the horse. Appl. Anim. Ethol., *1:*395–404, 1975.

39. Kahn, W., and Leidl, W.: Die ultraschall biometrie von pferdefeten in utero und die sonographische darstellung ihrer organe. DTW Dtsch. Tierarztl. Wochenschr., *94:*497–540, 1987.

40. McKinnon, A.O., Squires, E.L., and Pickett, B.W.: Equine Reproductive Ultrasonography. Fort Collins, Colorado State University Animal Reproduction Laboratory, 1988.

41. Machida, N., Yasuda, J., and Too, K.: A morphometric study of foetal and newborn cardiac growth in the horse. Equine Vet. J., *20:*261–267, 1988.

42. Allen, W.E.: Two cases of abnormal equine pregnancy associated with excess foetal fluid. Equine Vet. J., *18:*220–222, 1986.

43. Vanderplassche, M., et al.: Dropsy of the fetal sacs in mares: Induced and spontaneous abortion. Vet. Rec., *99:*67–69, 1976.

44. Blanchard, T.L., et al.: Management of dystocia in mares: Examination, obstetrical equipment, and vaginal delivery. Compend. Contin. Educ. Practicing Vet., *11:*745–753, 1989.

45. Evans, M.I., and Schulman, J.D.: Prenatal diagnosis: Invasive techniques and alpha-fetoprotein screening. *In* Neonatology: Pathophysiology and Management of the Newborn. 3rd ed. Edited by G.B. Avery. Philadelphia, J.B. Lippincott, 1987, pp. 130–146.

46. Manning, F.A., Platt, L.D., and Sipos, L.: Antepartum fetal evaluation. Development of a fetal biophysical profile score. Am. J. Obstet. Gynecol., *136:*787–795, 1980.

47. Juzwiak, J.S., et al.: Cesarean section in 19 mares: Results and postoperative fertility. Vet. Surg., *19:*50–52, 1990.

48. Manning, F.A., et al.: Fetal assessment based on fetal biophysical profile scoring: Experience in 12,620 referred high-risk pregnancies. Am. J. Obstet. Gynecol., *151:*343–350, 1985.

49. Williams, M.A., et al.: Preliminary report of transabdominal amniocentesis for the determination of pulmonary maturity in an equine population. Equine Vet. J., *20:*457–458, 1988.

50. Schmidt, A.R., et al.: Evaluation of transabdominal ultrasound-guided amniocentesis in the late gestational mare. Equine Vet. J., *23:*261–265, 1991.

51. Schott, H.C., and Mansmann, R.A.: Biochemical profiles of normal equine amniotic fluid at parturition. Equine Vet. J., *5(Suppl.):*52, 1988.

52. Bennett, S.D., et al.: Equine amniocentesis. Equine Vet. J., *8(Suppl.):*86, 1989.

53. Williams, M.A.: Amniotic fluid analysis for evaluation of equine foetal development. Proceedings of the Second International Conference of Veterinary Perinatology. Edited by P.D. Rossdale. Newmarket, Equine Veterinary Journal, 1990, p. 38

54. Daffos, F.: Fetal blood sampling. Annu. Rev. Med., *40:*319–329, 1989.

55. Ginther, O.J., and Adams, G.P.: Equine fetal mobility as observed by video-imaging endoscopy. Compend. Contin. Educ. Practicing Vet., *11:*1275–1281, 1990.

CHAPTER 107

CARE OF THE MARE AFTER FOALING

A.C. Asbury

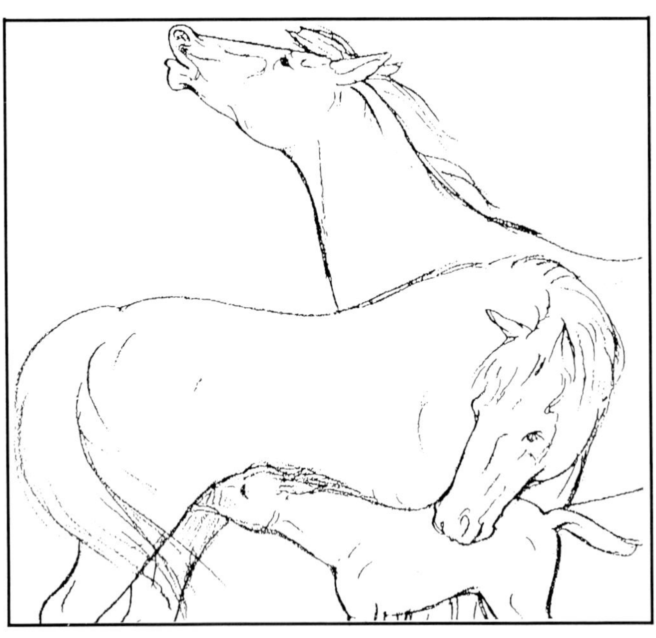

The great majority of mares deliver their foals without incident, suffer no adverse consequence of the foaling process, and initiate normal maternal behavior promptly. However, when problems occur, they tend to develop rapidly and have a major impact on both dam and neonate. For these reasons, veterinarians tend to overexamine and overtreat mares in the early postpartum period.

Too much medical management carries a risk for the normal mare. Unnecessary handling can jeopardize bonding between mare and foal, unnecessary clinical procedures risk contamination of the reproductive tract, and unnecessary medications can disturb the delicate balance of health of both mare and foal.

The willingness of the veterinarian to let nature take its course depends greatly on his or her experience, familiarity with the behavior of the postfoaling mare, and confidence in detection of real problems early in their course. The competence of the attending personnel is another important factor.

The objective of this chapter is to review normal and abnormal behavior of mares who have recently foaled, with emphasis on the criteria for decisions on when to intensify diagnostic and therapeutic management. Major traumatic complications are treated from a diagnostic perspective, and general management and preventive medicine practices are reviewed.

THE NORMAL MARE AFTER FOALING

The evaluation of mares after foaling is most relevant when the examiner is familiar with the foaling process and with the normal postpartum reactions and behavior of mares. The veterinarian's experience with normal foaling may be limited, because practice involvement in the foaling process is usually limited to crises such as dystocia and management of serious complications. Knowledge of the normal reactions may have to be supplemented by other means. Excellent descriptions of the foaling process and the postpartum period have been published.[1–3] Other information is available in publications targeted toward the horse-owning public. An excellent video—*Foaling* (The Blood Horse, Inc., Lexington, KY)—is recommended to those who desire a general review.

NORMAL POSTPARTUM BEHAVIOR

Mares naturally deliver foals while they are lying down, with the active expulsive efforts applied while in lateral recumbency. As soon as the foal's hips clear the pelvic canal the mare will cease major abdominal pressure and relax. She will usually roll into a sternal position and look for and nicker to the foal within a few minutes. If undisturbed, most mares undergo a period of tranquility for up to 20 min after delivery. Often they will pick at hay or grass, depending on the location, and seem relatively uninterested in the foal until it becomes active.

The usual incentive for the mare to rise is activity on the part of the foal, both movement and vocalization. As soon as the mare stands, she will usually turn to the foal and begin to lick it. Nickering softly is common behavior at this point.

Occasionally, the intact placenta will fall from the mare as she rises for the first time, but in most mares, the membranes remain attached for 30 min to several hours. Some degree of abdominal discomfort is usually evident soon after the mare rises. Mild intermittent pain is most likely associated with the normal uterine contractions of third-stage labor (delivery of the placenta) and initial uterine involution. The pain may be intense enough to cause the mare to lie back down and roll intermittently. Contractions may persist until the membranes are delivered, but in most cases, this pain decreases markedly in 30 to 40 min.

The behavior of the mare toward her foal can be quite varied and still be classified as normal. The great majority of mares are somewhat protective, considerably concerned with the well-being of the foal and helpful during the first hours of its life. These mares will help direct the foal to the best alignment for nursing, will stand over it while it is resting, and are generally aware of the location of the foal, while taking care not to step on it or knock it down.

One variation on this ideal behavior is the overprotective mare. She anticipates that any person or any other animal constitutes a threat to her foal and will stop at nothing to eliminate that threat. Some of these mares are truly dangerous and should be handled only by experienced personnel. Unfortunately, in their role as protector, the mares may injure their own foals. This behavior may persist for a few weeks, at most. Such mares are best isolated from other horses until the excessive protective behavior stops.

In contrast to the overprotective mare, occasional mares are totally unconcerned with their foals. They seem not to understand the problems the foal must overcome to learn routines for nursing, rising, and lying down. They will wander away with no regard to the foal's needs. This behavior is most common in primiparous mares and can usually be reversed in a short time by keeping the pair in tight confinement and holding the mare while the foal nurses. Bonding and maternal concern follows a few serious nursing sessions.

Fear of the foal or aggressive behavior toward it is another variation which is a rare, but significant behavior pattern. Again, this reaction is typical of, but not unique to, primiparous mares. The usual reaction is observed when the mare has stood and the foal begins vigorous movements. Striking, biting, or kicking attacks represent the extreme of this attitude and must be dealt with by prompt intervention and restraint. Usually once the mare has allowed the foal to nurse a few times, the hostility wanes. Close supervision is indicated until clear signs are noted that the mare has accepted her foal. Tranquilization delays the acceptance and will cause sedation in some foals when they nurse.

Perhaps at this most extreme degree, aggressiveness toward an offspring cannot be called normal. It is probably a function of human intervention and domestication of the horse. Mares foaling in a more natural environment, such as in a range setting, either do not experience this reaction, or it is brief and inconsequential. My impression is that this behavior is most common in those breeds with the highest degree of inbreeding. An excellent discussion of mare behavior related to foal rejection has been published.[4]

EXAMINATION OF THE NORMAL POSTPARTUM MARE

When the postfoaling mare is judged to be normal in behavior and attitude and is showing proper maternal interaction with the foal, the clinical examination should be as simple as possible to avoid unneccesary disturbance. An impression of the mare's general condition—including character of pulse and respiration, color of mucous membranes, degree of alertness, and responsive reaction to stimuli—should be noted. Further evaluation of the systemic condition, such as blood counts and clinical chemistry tests are not indicated unless a specific problem is suspected based on the general examination.

Careful evaluation of the udder is always important, assessing the texture and uniformity of all portions of the mammary gland, the patency of the teats, and the character of the secretions. The perineal area should be inspected for evidence of trauma during parturition and for the necessity of a Caslick operation.

Routine reproductive examinations such as palpation of the tract per rectum or vaginoscopic exam are contraindicated in mares that have recently foaled, unless a clear indication of a problem exists. Intervention beyond absolute necessity may disrupt the critical processes of adaptation that are underway during this time. Furthermore, the dilation of the vaginal tract by a speculum will allow large volumes of air to rapidly enter the uterus.

CARE OF THE NORMAL POSTPARTUM MARE

The general approach to husbandry of the mare after foaling should be to achieve the most natural environment and management conditions in as short a time as possible. The ideal place for a mare and a new foal is outside, in a clean pasture or paddock, with some shelter from sun and the elements. This allows for exercise, a key factor in promoting uterine involution, stimulation of appetite, and improved gastrointestinal function. Furthermore, the mare should not be subject to competition from other foaling mares until she has established satisfactory bonding with the foal. Constraints of weather and available facilities will obviously modify these goals. Feeding should be light to moderate for the first few days after foaling, and laxative feeds such as bran mashes are appropriate to reduce the incidence of constipation.

Routine care of the mare postpartum should include essential preventive medicine procedures. In the ideal situation, mares will have received routine vaccinations for the common infectious diseases during the last month of gestation (Chapter 105). This allows maximum protection for the foal by way of colostrum. When vaccination history is vague or absent, the first priority should be tetanus prophylaxis, because parturition renders the mare particularly susceptible to tetanus. If any documented history of tetanus toxoid administration within the previous 5 or 6 years exists, a tetanus toxoid booster is indicated. If no valid history is available, the mare should be simultaneously vaccinated with tetanus antitoxin and toxoid, at different sites.[5]

Control of internal parasites in foaling mares should be directed at minimizing the contamination of foals. Mares with an inadequate history of deworming should be treated immediately after foaling with a broad-spectrum vermifuge. Then, intensive parasite control programs should be implemented (Chapter 105).

If the postpartum examination indicates that the mare would benefit from measures to reduce pneumovagina, some immediate steps may be indicated. Mares with a history of a Caslick operation as an essential part of infertility management, should be resutured as soon as practical. If the procedure will upset the relationship between mare and foal, wound clips can be used to appose the vulvar lips for a few days until proper suturing can be completed. In cases of extremely poor vulvar conformation, the clips should be applied immediately after the foal is delivered. Local anesthesia of the vulvar lips is not necessary within the first 15 min of foaling.

CARE OF MARES SUBSEQUENT TO POSTPARTUM COMPLICATIONS

Problems arising as a result of abnormal parturition present diagnostic and management challenges to the practitioner. Variations from normal postpartum behavior and specific clinical signs provide the material for problem solving that leads to the diagnosis of the disorder. Commonality of signs between several clinical entities demands a careful diagnostic effort to separate them and to achieve success in their treatment.

The balance of this chapter is a consideration of the major complications seen in mares after foaling, grouped by their principal presenting signs. The important diagnostic criteria and the elements of successful management are discussed.

PROBLEMS CHARACTERIZED BY ABDOMINAL PAIN

Because some degree of abdominal pain has been described as occurring normally as a result of uterine contractions, the distinction between this pain and that associated with a more serious cause is an important step in evaluating the mare in pain. The duration, intensity, and time of occurrence of the pain are important considerations.

Severe Pain Related to Uterine Contractions

Extreme increase in the degree of abdominal pain caused by uterine contraction is encountered occasionally, particularly in primiparous mares. Lack of pain tolerance or inexperience are probably involved in the cause of the problem rather than some abnormality. The onset of pain is similar to the normal postpartum contractions as described, and the pain tends to be intermittent. The severity of the reaction is alarming in some cases, as mares may throw themselves to the ground and roll violently. Running in the stall or paddock are possible manifestations, and the safety of the foal must be considered.

Systemic signs in these cases are limited to moderate elevations in heart rate and sweating. Moderate doses of analgesics such as xylazine or detomidine hydrochloride are usually quite effective in reducing the degree of this pain. Once the mare's pain is under control, palpation of the uterus per rectum is indicated to rule out more serious problems. Finding no area of the uterus that causes undue reaction to palpation, the mare is best managed by continuing the analgesics as indicated. This problem rarely persists beyond 1 or 2 h.

Inversion of the Uterine Horn

With inversion of the uterine horn, pain begins suddenly and is steady and of considerable magnitude. Analgesics and sedatives are not effective in relieving the problem. The onset is usually within the first few hours of foaling when, in the process of involution, the ovary and tip of one horn become inverted and trapped within the uterine lumen by a ring of myometrial spasm. Because the onset of this condition is much earlier than the other causes of severe and unrelenting abdominal pain, the clinician can logically suspect the problem based on symptoms alone and proceed to confirm and correct it. Sedation is imperative to further examination and correction, and if necessary, general anesthesia should be employed.

Confirmation of the entrapment may be possible by palpation per rectum, but correction will require manual reduction with the hand in the uterine lumen. Overcoming the spasm of the uterine muscle may require a sustained, firm manual pressure. The ovary is grasped through the uterine wall and the fist is applied to the area of resistance until it gives way and allows the ovary and tip to be reduced. If reduction is impossible with the analgesic drug–treated mare, anesthesia with halothane is the next logical choice. The muscle relaxation achieved with halothane should result in prompt correction. Followup care for mares subjected to this treatment should include lavage with large volumes of hot saline to encourage involution and to reduce the uterine contamination.[6]

Hemorrhage into the Broad Ligament

Uterine artery hemorrhage is a problem of older mares and a frequent cause of death in aged mares that continue to produce foals.[7] When bleeding occurs into the broad ligament, a progressively dissecting hematoma occurs below the serosal surface of the uterus. The pain which results from the stretching of the serosa is localized to the side of the hemorrhage and is seldom evident before 12 h after foaling. Reactions of the mare mimic those of colic caused by gastrointestinal lesions that are localized.

Concurrent signs of anemia are typical, including pale membranes and rapid thready pulse. Sweating is common, with localization to the affected side. Confirmation is by palpation or ultrasonography of the affected area of the uterus, per rectum. Considerable discomfort is induced by palpation of the affected ovary and uterine horn. The hematoma may be palpable if the mare will tolerate the examination.

Treatment is aimed at minimizing any stress or excitement until clotting has occurred. The mare is best confined to a dark, quiet stall with or without her foal, depending on her temperament. Minimal interference will enhance her chances for survival. Blood transfusions, fluid therapy or any upsetting procedures are contraindicated. Tranquilization may depress blood pressure to dangerous levels, but in some mares, that may be a better choice than allowing continued sustained excitement. Bleeding into the peritoneal cavity and death are the consequences of rupture of the serosa that contains the hematoma.

Once a clot forms in the uterine artery and the hematoma is contained, recovery from dangerous anemia takes 7 to 10 days. The hematoma will require months for resolution.

Pain Caused by Gastrointestinal Damage

Mild to moderate abdominal pain, beginning about day 2 after foaling, may indicate trauma to the small colon.[7] When a portion of the small colon is pinched between the fetus and the pelvis during parturition, serious damage to that organ may occur. Vascular compromise or direct trauma to the colon wall results in leaking of the gut contents, usually slowly. The resultant peritonitis is local at first, but then becomes generalized.

Small bowel injury is confirmed by palpation per rectum. The lesion is usually identified as a distinct swelling in the small colon, which has been described as sausage shaped.[7] Immediate surgical intervention is the appropriate course of action to correct the problem.

PROBLEMS CHARACTERIZED BY DEPRESSION

Profound and deep depression, usually accompanied by signs of shock, vascular compromise, or toxemia, are indicators of grave complications after foaling. Clinical signs do not help to separate the following three catastrophic problems, but uterine lavage or paracentesis may be useful.

Acute Metritis with Toxemia

Acute metritis with toxemia is discussed in detail in Chapter 70. Suspicion of the condition based on the clinical signs described is an indication for large volume uterine lavage.[6] The fluid recovered from the uterus, dark red-brown and fetid, will confirm the diagnosis.

Uterine Rupture

During difficult delivery, or occasionally without obvious cause, the uterus may rupture, allowing escape of its contents into the peritoneal cavity. If the rupture is unsuspected, clinical signs are apparent from shortly after the incident to several hours, depending on the size of the tear and degree of contamination. A detailed discussion of uterine rupture is presented in Chapter 70.

Rupture of the Large Colon or Cecum

Abdominal pressure generated during second-stage labor in mares is sufficient to rupture portions of the large colon or cecum in certain circumstances.[8] The resulting overwhelming peritonitis produces signs within a few hours of the accident. In such a case of depression and toxemia, paracentesis will usually confirm the cause of the problem, which is a clear indication for euthanasia.

Because treatment of colon or cecal rupture is impossible, the clinician would be wise to consider means of minimizing its incidence. Mares typically reduce their feed intake during the last few days before foaling. This behavior obviously favors reduction of the mass of ingesta in the colon. Management systems that ensure a reduction in available roughage to these mares are logical in reducing the incidence of colonic or cecal rupture. If mares are pastured in groups, individuals that are competitive at feeding time should be identified. These mares may not voluntarily cut back on dietary intake because of herd pressures. Separation of these mares when parturition is close will facilitate proper feeding.

SIGNS OF PELVIC OR PERINEAL DISORDER

Evidence of physical trauma or suggestions of discomfort and straining are clues to injury or dysfunction of pelvic or perineal structures, which demands careful evaluation.

Constipation

The combination of pain and inflammation of pelvic structures and a decrease in water consumption often results in constipation in the first few days after foaling. Feces impact in the caudal small colon and rectum, indicated by tail elevation, occasional straining and absence of fresh feces in the stall or paddock. After relieving the problem by manual evacuation of the impaction, treatment with nonsteroidal anti-inflammatory drugs is indicated in addition to mineral oil per os and enemas when needed.

Rectovaginal Laceration and Perineal Lacerations

During the expulsive stage of parturition, the feet of the foal may become trapped by the ring of tissue cranial to the vestibulovaginal junction, including the vestibular sphincter and the hymenal fold. In primiparous mares this tissue may be quite resistant to stretching and when the foal is impelled by strong expulsive efforts, the tissues in the dorsal vagina may be torn. When the tear occurs through the vaginal wall and through the ventral rectal wall, a rectovaginal defect occurs. If the foal's feet are repelled or fall back into the birth canal and the foal is delivered vaginally, a rectovaginal defect may persist, allowing fecal material to drop into the vagina.

If labor continues with the foal's feet through the rectovaginal defect, all the tissues of the ventral rectum, dorsal vagina, perineal body, and anal sphincter are lacerated to allow the delivery. The lesion produced is a third-degree perineal laceration. Second-degree lacerations occur when the foal's feet pass through the vestibulovaginal junction and lacerate the dorsal vestibular mucosa and the perineal body. First-degree lacerations involve dorsal mucosa of the vestibule and the skin of the dorsal commissure of the vulva, with no other damage. All of these injuries occur most commonly in primiparous mares.

All degrees of the perineal laceration will be evident to the examiner conducting a routine perineal inspection after foaling. The rectovaginal defect, or fistula, will often not be suspected on routine examination. Fecal material in the vestibule may be the first evidence of the problem.

Because the vestibulovaginal junction is located well caudad to the peritoneal reflection in the mare, rectovaginal damage and third-degree lacerations rarely open the peritoneal cavity to contamination. Therefore, no threat exists to the mare's health by the fecal contamination of the involved tissues. Time is needed for resolution of the edema and inflammation that accompany these accidents before surgical repair is possible. Care of these mares during that period should include keeping the affected areas clean. Antibiotics and uterine treatments are not necessary. Because these problems most commonly involve young, primiparous mares, uterine defenses will invariably resolve any endometritis once the lesions are repaired. Surgical approaches to the correction of the injuries described appear in Chapter 48.

COMPLICATIONS WITH NO PRESENTING SIGNS

During foaling, and particularly if dystocia occurs, the cervix may become overstretched or lacerated to the degree that the future fertility of the mare is compromised. Generally no external signs exist of this damage, and often the problem is not evident until the cervix has returned to relatively normal size and the mare is cycling. For these reasons, the clinician should perform a manual evaluation of the cervix of all foaling or aborting mares, before their next breeding.

The vagina may also be traumatized during parturition. If the vaginal wall is lacerated incompletely, scarring will result, which will be evident after a variable period of time. Vaginal trauma, especially that occurring during manual intervention in dystocia, may also produce serious vaginal adhesions, which if severe, may occlude the cranial vaginal tract. These vaginal lesions are most easily detected by manual examination of the area during the evaluation of the cervix, as described. If the cranial vagina is lacerated through to the peritoneal cavity, the signs will mimic those of uterine rupture.

REFERENCES

1. Arthur, G.H.: Veterinary Reproduction and Obstetrics. 4th ed. London, Bailliere Tindall, 1975.
2. Roberts, S.J.: Veterinary Obstetrics and Genital Diseases. 2nd ed. Ithaca, NY, published by the author, 1971.
3. Rossdale, P.D., and Ricketts, S.W.: Equine Stud Farm Medicine. 2nd ed. London, Bailliere Tindall, 1980.
4. Haupt, K.A.: Foal rejection. *In* Current Therapy in Equine Medicine. 2nd ed. Edited by N.E. Robinson. Philadelphia, W.B. Saunders, 1987, pp. 126–128.
5. Johnston, J.: Tetanus. *In* Current Therapy in Equine Medicine. 2nd ed. Edited by N.E. Robinson. Philadelphia, W.B. Saunders, 1987, pp. 370–373.
6. Asbury, A.C.: Large volume uterine lavage in the management of endometritis and acute metritis in mares. Compend. Contin. Educ. Practicing Vet., *12:*1477–1479, 1990.
7. Zent, W.W.: Postpartum complications. *In* Current Therapy in Equine Medicine. 2nd ed. Edited by N.E. Robinson. Philadelphia, W.B. Saunders, 1987, pp. 544–547.
8. Voss, J.L.: Rupture of the cecum and ventral colon of mares during parturition. J. Am. Vet. Med. Assoc., *155:*745–747, 1969.

CHAPTER 108

POSTNATAL CARE OF THE FOAL

J.L. Traub-Dargatz

The role of the veterinarian in the immediate postnatal period will vary with training and experience of the foaling attendants. The veterinarian is seldom present for a normal foaling because of the rapidity with which the mare delivers (Chapter 66). Whether or when the newborn foal is examined by a veterinarian will be determined by several factors, such as (1) the value of the foal, (2) the experience of the foaling attendant, (3) complications during pregnancy and/or the foaling process itself, and (4) the foal's adaptation to the extrauterine environment.

At birth, the foal must make several adjustments to the extrauterine environment, including (1) initiation of respiration, (2) clearing the respiratory tract of fluid, (3) establishment and maintenance of a normal body temperature, (4) development and coordination of the musculoskeletal system, and (5) ability to nurse. The foaling attendant must recognize when any of these adaptations have not occurred within the appropriate times (Table 108–1) and initiate some lifesaving support and alert the veterinarian. Unless a problem with parturition or adaptation of the foal was anticipated, the veterinarian may not generally be present to assist at foaling. Thus, the inexperienced foaling attendant may contact a veterinarian with a perceived emergency which is a normal adaptive process or fail to recognize an emergency and contact the veterinarian when the foal is moribund. An effort should be made to educate the foaling attendant by talking with the veterinarian before foaling, providing educational material on the normal adaptive processes of the foal, and offering initial training with an experienced foaling attendant.

OBSERVATION OF THE NEONATE'S BEHAVIOR AND INITIAL TREATMENTS

In most instances, when the veterinarian examines the foal for the first time, it will have established a normal respiratory pattern, stood, nursed, and passed meconium. Additional treatments commonly include treatment of the naval with iodine and an enema. The foaling attendant must be able to recognize if the foal is having problems within the first hour after birth. The attendant must be able to recognize when the foal is not adapting properly to the extrauterine environment and contact the veterinarian for immediate care of the foal. If the foal is having difficulty breathing, the attendant should have the training to assist it with respiration until a veterinarian arrives. The attendant should frequently observe the foal for normal foal criteria, which include a gradual gain of strength and stamina with each hour. Normal foals nurse frequently and keep the mare's udder drained, urinate small amounts of near colorless urine frequently, and pass feces without a great deal of straining or discomfort. If the attendant has any doubts about the foal's condition or is unsure of his or her ability to evaluate the foal's condition, a veterinarian should be contacted to examine the foal on an emergency basis. If no doubt exists that the foal is behaving normally, then the complete examination by

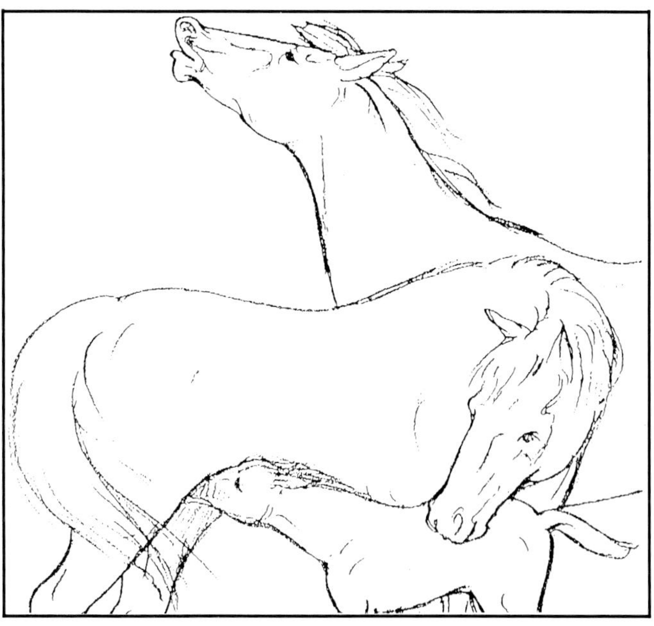

TABLE 108–1. ROLES OF FOALING ATTENDANT AND VETERINARIAN

FOALING ATTENDANT	VETERINARIAN
1. Attend mare during parturition, being sure all stages (I, II, III) of parturition proceed normally 2. Be sure foal begins respiration on delivery, sternal recumbency within minutes of delivery, and stands within 1 h; if foal fails to breathe normally, resuscitate foal (see Chapter 110); if fails to become sternal or stand, call veterinarian immediately 3. Treat naval with iodine, give enema 4. Be sure foal nurses within 2 h of birth 5. Monitor foal's vigor, willingness to nurse, etc. critically during the neonatal period (7 days)	1. Assist at parturition if high-risk mare, dystocia, or premature placental separation occurs 2. Attend foal if it fails to adapt to initial extrauterine life 3. Attend foal if it fails to nurse or if mare does not have adequate colostrum 4. Test foal for passive transfer of immunoglobulins and conduct physical examination on foal at 12 h of age

the veterinarian can wait until the earliest appropriate time, usually early morning.

EXAMINATION OF THE NEONATE

The first examination of the foal by a veterinarian should include observation of the foal from a distance to determine its behavior, ability to rise, coordination and strength, ability and willingness to nurse, attitude, and response to external stimuli. The actual physical examination should be brief but complete. The eyes, oral cavity, and nasal openings should be examined and the color of the mucous membranes noted. The neck, chest wall, and limbs should be observed and palpated for evidence of trauma, swellings, or conformational problems. The navel should be examined to be sure it has been treated with iodine and is beginning to dry and that no pain or swelling is present.

The veterinarian should auscultate the lungs and heart. Respiratory rate and effort and heart rate and regularity should be determined. Rate of both respiration and heartbeat can be influenced by excitement, thus the pattern, effort, regularity, and lack of pathologic murmurs will be of more value in evaluating the foal than will the actual heart and respiratory rate. Normal respiratory rate ranges from 60 to 80 breaths per minute for the first few hours following delivery to 20 to 40 breaths per minute during the first few weeks of life.[1] Any deviation from the normal, smooth respiratory pattern should be reason for concern. The normal heart rate is quite variable and ranges from 40 to 80 beats per minute with an average of 70 immediately following birth. As the foal attempts to stand, heart rate increases to 130 to 150 and higher.[1] Over the first few days of life, heart rate ranges from 70 to 100 beats per minute and can go higher because of excitement.[1] A holosystolic grade I to IV murmur is often heard at the left heart base for up to 1 week in some foals. Louder murmurs with palpable thrills may be pathologic and associated with congenital anomalies.[2]

The foal's rectal temperature should be determined and should be between 38.5° and 37.5° C (100.5° and 99.5° F). A deviation of 0.55° C (1° F) or more from this normal range in either direction is reason for concern. Neonatal foals may become hypothermic even with infection, especially if the ambient temperature is low. The foal's perineum should be checked for evidence of fecal staining, and the patency of the anus determined by the fact that the thermometer can be passed into the rectum.

The foal's strength should be assessed by its ability to rise and resist restraint. The strength and straightness of the limbs should be noted, and if the limbs appear weak or deviated, discretion is advised as many of these problems will resolve in the first few days of life. However, do not assume this will occur. The foal should be reevaluated a few days later to ensure that the legs are strong and straight before the mare and foal are turned out. Generally, mares and newborn foals are confined to a large box stall and run for 2 to 3 days to allow bonding before they are turned out with other mares and foals.

PROPHYLACTIC TREATMENTS OF NEONATES

Prophylactic treatment of a normal foal with antibiotics and vitamin supplements is controversial. Antibiotics such as penicillin and streptomycin have been proposed to prevent infection and disease while the navel is closing and the foal is adjusting to the outside world.[3] Certainly, if such treatments could ensure that the foal would not develop infection or nutritional imbalances, no question would exist as to the need for their use. However, the efficacy of such treatments has not been established and, in fact, has been challenged.[4,5] Use of such prophylactic treatments has been associated with an increased occurrence of diarrhea in foals in one study, but a cause-and-effect relationship was not determined.[4] Tetanus prophylaxis can be accomplished either by immunizing the mare before foaling and ensuring passive transfer or by injecting the foal with 1500 units of tetanus antitoxin.

SCREENING TESTS FOR NEONATES

Use of screening tests to determine better the normalcy of the foal is another important but controversial issue.[6] Certainly, no laboratory tests can take the place of good husbandry and the need for continued experienced observation in the postnatal period. Several tests, which if properly interpreted, may allow early detection of disease or of increased susceptibility to disease, but the clinician must interpret the results with the individual foal and the type of farm management in mind. Some veterinarians feel the time and expense incurred by use of these tests are unwarranted. Tests include determination of red blood cell count, white blood cell count and differential, and determination of serum immunoglobulin concentration. These tests are usually performed when the veterinarian does the initial physical examination, generally within the first 12 h after birth.

The necessity of such tests on foals that appear clinically normal is debated. The reason for controversy is multifactorial; some of the factors are differences in level of observation and management of newborn foals between farms compared with the situation of a single foaling mare and inaccuracies in the tests. The level of observation on some intensively run farms is such that an alteration in a foal's nursing frequency and vigor will be detected before any detectable change in the hemogram, but this is not true for care of foals on all farms. Also, if disease occurrence in all horses on a particular farm is low, the occurrence of disease in neonatal foals on this same farm may be low even if the foals do not receive adequate passive transfer.[7] Also, some tests of serum immunoglobulin concentration in the foal have been unreliable (zinc sulfate turbidity test) or not immediately available (radioimmunodiffusion test).[8–11] Quick and reasonably reliable tests of immunoglobulin concentration are available. The test kit used should be relatively reliable, easy to perform, test up to an immunoglobulin concentration of 800 mg/dL, and be inexpensive.[11] The CITE test (Enzyme Immunoassay IgG Test Kit, Portland, ME) tests up to 800 mg/dL of Ig and has been found to be reasonably accurate, but it is relatively expensive.[11] Some of the quick test kits only have tests up to 400 mg/dL of Ig.[11]

Another debatable issue regarding need for evaluation of immunoglobulin concentration is that not all foals that have a low immunoglobulin concentration, indicating a failure of passive transfer, become ill[6] nor has an increased risk for development of infection been clearly demonstrated in one study.[7] Thus, if results of immunoglobulin determination indicate the foal has a low immunoglobulin concentration, the time postfoaling the immunoglobin should be considered low is a matter of debate. The veterinarian is left with the decision as to need to supplement the immunoglobulin level with plasma.[6] Debate also exists as to the efficacy of the administration of plasma from just one horse with a typical vaccination history.[12] Researchers have suggested that if plasma is given, it should be obtained from horses that have been hyperimmunized against endemic infections which occur on the farm where the foal is located or that pooled plasma should be used to try to provide many specific antibodies.[12,13] For optimum foal management, the serum immunoglobulin concentration of the neonatal foal should be determined at 12 h of age. If the immunoglobin concentration is below 200 mg/dL at 12 h or older, the foal should be supplemented with a plasma transfusion. If the foal is less than 12 h old, colostrum, if available, should be given. The foal should be retested for immunoglobin concentration within 12 h. The concentration should then be re-evaluated within 12 h. If the foal's immunoglobulin concentration is then between 200 mg/dL and 800 mg/dL, the occurrence of disease in horses and foals on the particular farm, past foaling history of the mare, and value of the foal will be used to determine how to manage the foal. If the initial concentration was greater than 200 mg/dL but less than 800 mg/dL, the aforementioned aspects must be considered in regard to the need to supplement.

SUMMARY

The foal must be observed frequently and by a knowledgeable attendant in the first 7 to 10 days postfoaling. Note that just because the foal appeared normal in the immediate postfoaling period and to the veterinarian on the initial examination, no guarantee exists that the foal will stay normal in the following few days. Time should be spent observing the foal's behavior with emphasis on regularity of nursing, physical activity, frequency of urination, and regularity of defecation. The most important thing to remember is that any foal affected by any problem, regardless of cause, first suffers from weakness and depression, which will be reflected as a decrease in amount of milk consumed. Foals can quickly go from normal to moribund within hours, so recognition of early signs of disease is important. One of the most reliable ways to determine if the foal is nursing adequately is to examine the mare's udder. Most normal foals will keep the mare's udder drained of milk at all times. If the foal appears to have milk on the muzzle or face, a good chance exists that it is not nursing adequately. As the foal approaches the mare's distended udder but does not adequately nurse, the mare will let down milk, and it will run onto the foal's face. An important aspect of recognizing an ill foal is knowing what is normal behavior for a neonatal foal. The normal neonatal foal should gradually spend more time investigating its surroundings. It should gradually become stronger and jump up if approached while lying down. The normal foal is usually confined to a stall with the mare until it gains strength, coordination, visual acuity, and bonds to the mare. When first turned out in a small paddock, the normal foal will play and easily follow the mare. If a foal does not appear to be adapting normally (e.g., is depressed or decreases its nursing) a veterinarian should be contacted.

REFERENCES

1. Koterba, A.M.: Physical examination. *In* Equine Clinical Neonatology. Edited by A.M. Koterba, W.H. Drummond, and P.C. Kosch. Philadelphia, Lea & Febiger, 1990, pp. 71–87.

2. Madigan, J.E.: Physical exam of the equine neonate. *In* Manual of Equine Neonatal Medicine. Edited by J.E. Madigan. Woodland, CA, Live Oak Publishing, 1987, pp. 38–46.
3. Lose, M.P.: Blessed Are the Foals. New York, Macmillan, 1987.
4. Madigan, J.E.: Post foaling procedures—Routine. *In* Manual of Equine Neonatal Medicine. Edited by J.E. Madigan. Woodland, CA, Live Oak Publishing, 1987, pp. 19–21.
5. Traub-Dargatz, J.L., et al.: Epidemiological survey of diarrhea in foals. J. Am. Vet. Med. Assoc., *192:*238–239, 1986.
6. Brewer, B.D., and Mair, T.S.: Failure of passive transfer: To treat or not to treat? Equine Vet. J., *20:*394–396, 1988.
7. Baldwin, J.L., Vanderwall, D.K., Cooper, W.L., and Erb, H.N.: Immunoglobulin G and early survival of foals: A three year field study. Proc. Am. Assoc. Equine Pract., 179–187, 1989.
8. Jeffcott, J.B.: Immune passive transfer to foals: Sixty years on. Equine Vet. J. *17:*162–163, 1985.
9. Rumbaugh, G.E., et al.: Measurement of neonatal equine immunoglobulins for assessment of colostral immunoglobulin transfer: Comparison of single radioimmunodiffusion with zinc sulfate turbidity test, serum electrophoresis, refractory for total serum protein and sodium sulfite precipitation test. J. Am. Vet. Med. Assoc., *172:*321–325, 1978.
10. Bertone, J.J., and Jones, R.L.: Evaluation of a field test kit for determination of serum IgG concentration in foals. J. Vet. Int. Med., *2:*181–183, 1988.
11. LeBlanc, M.M.: Immunologic considerations. *In* Equine Clinical Neonatology. Edited by A.M. Koterba, W.H. Drummond, and P.C. Kosch. Philadelphia, Lea & Febiger, 1990, pp. 275–296.
12. White, S.L.: The use of plasma in foals with failure of passive transfer. Proc. Am. Assoc. Equine Pract., 215–218, 1989.
13. Green, E.M., Loch, W.E., Hook, R.R., and Olsen, R.: Colostral transfer of equine endotoxin core antigen antibodies from mare to foal. Proc. Am. Assoc. Equine Pract., 187–197, 1989.

CHAPTER 109

IDENTIFICATION OF THE MARE AND FOAL AT HIGH RISK FOR PERINATAL PROBLEMS

R. Adams

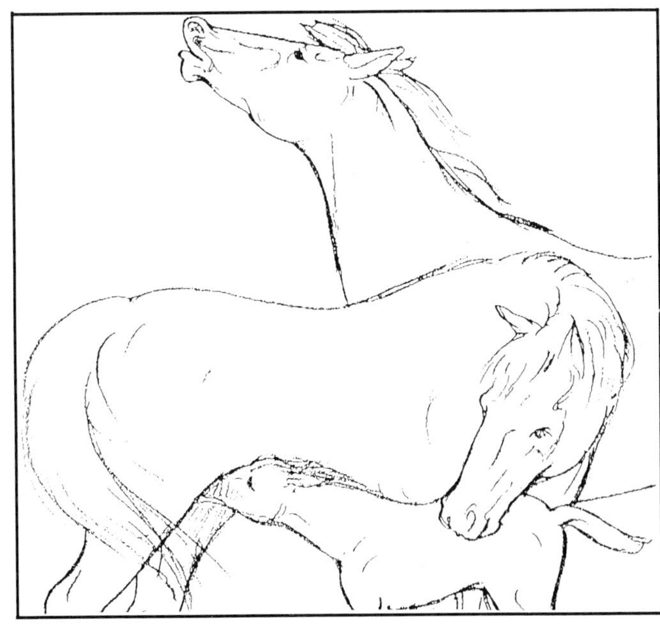

In human medicine, prenatal health care for the mother is well recognized as the most effective means of reducing health risks in the newborn. Based on both the mother's medical history and clinical signs observed during pregnancy, the fetus and newborn at risk for having or developing medical problems is identified. Survival rates improve when problems are identified early and treated immediately. Medical expenses are lowered when prepartum assessment of the pregnancy is made and abnormalities which might harm the developing fetus are identified and corrected. Although technology to monitor the fetus during gestation and knowledge about the fetoplacental unit are more advanced for the human than the horse, the principle that events of gestation directly affect the newborn's health status is well accepted by clinicians caring for both species.

Among equine neonatal care specialists, the importance of disease diagnosis in early stages and the tendency for sick foals to result from abnormal pregnancies are accepted axioms. Investigating the relationship between the dam and fetus during gestation is a target research area. Some new information in this area is reported in Chapters 67 and 106. However, major advances should be anticipated in the coming years. This chapter presents warning signs of when health of the newborn foal is in jeopardy. Because of the intimate relationship between dam and fetus throughout gestation, events starting before conception that potentially affect the fetus and newborn are discussed. Evaluation of the compromised foal, a standard diagnostic protocol, instructions for transportation if referral is chosen, and resuscitation procedures are reviewed.

HIGH-RISK PREGNANCY

Significant advances have been made in the last 20 yr in treating equine venereal diseases, improving fertility, and maintaining pregnancy. In contrast, measures to evaluate and optimize the quality of uterine environment during gestation remain rudimentary. Because of the cost and labor involved in keeping a pregnant mare and caring for a foal, attention should be paid to details which enhance the well-being of the offspring from the time breeding is first contemplated. Breeders take pains to calculate the optimal match of bloodlines and conformation for performance, and the veterinarian offers suggestions which maximize reproductive efficiency.

ASSESSMENT OF THE BREEDING OPERATION

Before breeding the mare, education of the owner and attendant(s) on the proper care of the brood mare and newborn foal is an essential step to avoiding unnecessary disease in the newborn. The facilities, dam, and stallion should also be examined.

The Facilities

Review of the suitability of the facilities for foaling is the first step to avoiding problems with the neonate. If this is not possible before breeding and the veterinarian is called to evaluate a sick neonate, information about the organization of these facilities may lend insight into the cause of neonatal disease.

Ample room is needed to isolate the pregnant mare(s) and the postpartum mare and foal from other horses in the stable. Although recent evidence concerning equine herpesvirus type 1 (EHV 1) discounts the belief that respiratory infection in young horses may cause a threat of abortion in mares, peripartum mares and foals should not be exposed to infectious diseases (brought to the farm by horses in transit) to which the foals or pregnant mares may be susceptible.[1] Conversely, horses in training need not be exposed to infectious diseases of young foals, especially strangles and infectious causes of diarrhea.

The knowledge and experience of the foaling attendants should be established prepartum so the veterinarian can provide supplemental information or accurately evaluate the attendant's interpretation of a particular situation (Chapters 105 and 108).

The foaling area should be clean, well drained, and large enough that the mare and foal do not get trapped in an awkward position during parturition. Several types of areas are suitable: a large stall, clean pen, or a grassy pasture. If more than one mare will be foaling in a confined area, it should be completely disinfected between uses. Thorough disinfection between foalings minimizes the bacteria to which the newborn is exposed before absorbing maternal immunoglobulins. Results from an epidemiologic study on foal diarrhea indicate that measures to ensure basic hygiene at foaling (washing the mare's udder, wrapping the tail, and disinfecting the foaling stall) were associated with a reduced number of foals developing diarrhea.[2]

A warm, dry, clean area is needed to house the foal and mare postpartum. The thermoneutral range of the 2- to 3-day-old foal is 20° to 35° C.[3] Out of that range, the foal must expend excessive energy to maintain body temperature. This excessive stress can be avoided by providing an appropriate maternity area.

The Mare

A thorough history of the mare's past breeding experiences should be taken. If a problem occurred with foaling previously, some problems may be more likely to occur again unless extra precautions are taken. A history of infertility or uterine infection is an indication that the mare may be more difficult to get in foal and to keep in foal and produce a normal foal. Placental insufficiency and placentitis are causes of fetal growth retardation, which can result in abortion, stillbirth, or a weak foal. If a suspicion of neonatal isoerythrolysis exists in previous foals, late-term prepartum blood samples from the mare should be tested for antibodies to the stallion's red blood cells (Chapter 111).

Before breeding the mare, a specific examination of the reproductive tract as well as a complete physical examination should be performed. A breeding prospect is routinely evaluated for pelvic conformational faults that increase the likelihood of dystocia; caudal tract deformities that may lead to wind sucking, urine pooling, or ascending infections; uterine disease; and mammary defects. Because of the relationship between the systemic health of the mare and the fetus, the thorough examination extends beyond the reproductive tract to include the whole horse (Chapter 105).

The Stallion

The stallion has a genetic and not a nurturing influence on the developing fetus. Therefore, once the stallion is deemed fertile, free of venereal disease, and in some breeds, able to impregnate the mare, further examination of the stallion is not usually a critical part of preventive neonatal health care.

THE MARE DURING PREGNANCY

The well-being of the fetus is influenced by the general health of the mare from time of implantation, but precise information on this influence remains a black box in the specialty of equine reproduction. The person directly responsible for the mare(s) must be able to recognize warning signs shown by the dam which may cause or be a sign that a problem exists with the pregnancy. Technologic advances, such as transabdominal ultrasonography, fetal electrocardiography, and amniocentesis, enable more precise measurements of equine fetal well-being, but interpretation of these tests in the horse is still naive (Chapter 106). Many aspects of pregnant brood mare management deserve investigation and could improve reproductive efficiency by increasing survival of the newborn. Many recommendations for care of the pregnant mare that affect the fetus are empirical rather than the result of rigorous scientific testing. The following aspects of the mare's health and care are reviewed because they affect the health of the fetus and, in turn, the newborn.

Diet

The National Research Council has recommended diets for pregnant mares, but the effects of these diets on the vigor and growth rate of the equine newborn have not been tested rigorously.[4] The effects of feed micronutrients, protein, and carbohydrate concentration during late gestation on the ability of offspring to survive in beef cattle have been investigated.[5] More specific recommendations for the horse are needed.[4] For example, some evidence suggests deprivation or imbalance of micronutrients (copper, zinc, and manganese in particular) in the diet of the dam during late gestation and lactation may affect the incidence of metabolic bone disease in the developing fetus and newborn foal.[6] However, the concentrations of these nutrients in the feed of the pregnant mare required to optimally nurture the fetus have not yet been carefully defined.[4] Baucus et al. reported no difference in copper or zinc concentrations in the dam's milk, the blood of dams and foals, or the growth rate of their foals when lactating mares were fed two different concentrations of copper and zinc for 4 weeks postpartum.[7] More research of this type is needed.

More rigorous guidelines are needed on the optimal body condition of brood mares.[8] In beef cattle, a body condition score is recommended, which results in optimal calving ease yet enables the cow to breed back quickly and support lactation.[9] Because the mare is treated as an individual and not managed in a herd situation with large numbers of genetically similar animals, such studies are difficult to perform with the horse.

Preventive Health Care

The pregnant mare must be on a preventive health care program that addresses adequate parasite control and regular vaccinations (Chapter 105). Inadequate parasite control may lead to colic in the dam, inadequate nourishment for the fetus, and contamination of the mare's milk and newborn's environment with a large parasite load. One of the numerous avoidable causes of neonatal diarrhea is Stronglyloides westeri infection.[10] A current vaccination program in the pregnant mare is also important. Adequate circulating immunoglobulins in the dam are the only way to promote adequate immunoglobulin levels in the colostrum.

Stress

One reaction to stress is alteration of the neuroendocrine system, affecting the mare's metabolism and altering reproductive events. Common sense dictates that the pregnant mare should be subjected to the least possible stress. When the effect of long periods of transportation during the first trimester of gestation on the abortion rates and serum hormone concentrations in pregnant mares was studied, serum progesterone and cortisol levels varied but abortion rates did not increase.[11]

Systemic Disease

Any systemic disease in the mare may adversely affect the fetus. The signs of systemic disease may go undetected (equine herpesvirus type 1 infection) yet cause abortion, stillbirth, or a weak foal itself systemically infected. Acute but severe disease such as colic, endotoxemia, and diarrhea may lead to fetal asphyxia, acidosis, endotoxemia, or infection, which can result in abortion or premature delivery. Metabolic, respiratory, renal, or gastrointestinal disease causing persistent maternal acidosis is recognized clinically to affect human fetuses adversely and experimentally to affect the offspring of rats, guinea pigs, and cattle.[12] Offspring of acidotic dams are born either acidotic or, soon after birth, develop severe metabolic acidosis which can lead to death if left uncorrected.

Systemic or Focal Infection

Systemic or focal infection in the dam may lead to infection of the fetus in utero. Vaginal discharge anytime during gestation may be a sign of placentitis. Chronic placentitis can result in growth retardation of the newborn or death of the fetus.[13] Acute placentitis may cause abortion or premature birth with or without infection of the newborn.[13] Optimal treatment of uterine infections during pregnancy is not known, because many drugs can adversely affect the fetus. For example, a pregnant mare with signs of equine protozoal myelitis was treated with pyrimethamine and sulfonamides during late gestation. The foal was born weak and severely leukopenic, although hematologic side effects of the drug therapy were not recognized in the mare.

General Anesthesia

General anesthesia of a pregnant mare should be undertaken with care.[14] The pathophysiologic state of this stress is not clearly defined, but during general anesthesia, especially when the dam is placed in dorsal recumbency, blood flow to the uterus may be sufficiently decreased to cause intrauterine fetal asphyxia. If this insult is sufficient, the fetus may die in utero and abort, be born dead, or be born weak and die. Even the live foal born to a mare undergoing general anesthesia during late gestation has been subjected to stress in utero and should be assessed carefully. When dam's serum progestagen and estrone sulfate concentrations were measured to assess fetal viability in late gestation, low (< 2 ng/mL) or rapidly falling progestagen levels, but not estrone sulfate, were associated with late-term abortion.[15] Further documentation of maternal serum hormone levels may provide a better understanding of how the types and timing of various stresses, including anesthesia, affect the fetus.

Abdominal Contour

Any abnormal abdominal contour in the late-term pregnant mare is cause for concern. Conditions to be considered include edema of late pregnancy, abdominal wall herniation, prepubic tendon rupture, hydroallantois, and hydroamnios[16] (Chapter 70). Physical examination and ultrasonography may be used to differentiate these conditions. In the case of excessive edema, abdominal wall herniation, and prepubic tendon rupture, the fetus may not necessarily be compromised at the time of evaluation. However, hydroallantois, fetal giants, or twins may lead to abdominal wall herniation or prepubic tendon rupture. These cases are managed by alleviating the weight of the pregnant uterus on the supporting structures. Induction of parturition is a treatment option which includes the risk of delivering a premature foal. As described in Chapter 67, accurate prediction of the maturity of the fetus in utero is difficult.

Hydroamnios is an accumulation of fluid in the amniotic cavity and is usually associated with a congenitally abnormal fetus. Because of overdistention of the uterus, dystocia often occurs.[17] Hydroallantoisis is caused by excessive allantoic fluid and is differentiated from hydroamnios by a more rapid onset, characteristic tense and rounded abdomen, and large distended uterus. The defect, more common in cattle, is caused by an abnormal chorioallantois.[17] The fetus is often growth retarded and may abort or be born small and weak. The care of a foal born to a mare with hydroallantois and chronic placentitis has been described.[18] The mare was induced, the foal born small and weak, but survived with intensive care initiated immediately after birth.

Premature Lactation

The causes of premature lactation are not well understood but this is considered a sign that the pregnancy is abnormal. Health risks for the newborn foal are increased for several reasons: uterine environment may be abnormal, having an adverse effect on the fetus; the foal may be deprived of valuable colostrum from the mare; and if sufficiently stressed in utero, the newborn may not absorb supplemental colostrum.

UTERINE ENVIRONMENT AND FETAL WELL-BEING

Considerable advances evaluating the fetus and placenta have been made in the last 10 yr. Pregnancy can be diagnosed using intrarectal ultrasonography at 14 days with greater than 95% accuracy, and during mid- and late gestation, fetal size, position, development, and well-being may be assessed using transabdominal ultrasonography[19] (Chapter 106).

Recognition of Placental Abnormalities In Utero

For mares carrying twins, which represents one type of chronic placental insufficiency, the high risk of perinatal morbidity and mortality is well appreciated. More subtle causes of placental abnormalities, resulting in stressed fetuses and abnormal newborns, are being discovered as technologic developments improve. If the foal attendants, owners, and attending veterinarians are forewarned of placental abnormalities before parturition, they can optimize the chance of survival of affected foals by watching the mare closely at the time of parturition and thoroughly evaluating the foal after birth.

Fetal well-being and survival depend on uterine environment and proper function of the placenta. Normal structure and function of the placenta are discussed in Chapter 60. The pathophysiologic condition of equine placental disease and how it affects the fetus are not yet well understood because of the complexities of placental function and the technical difficulties of instrumenting the pregnant mare. Placental disease may be acute or chronic, infectious or noninfectious. Regardless of the cause, if the disease is sufficiently severe, it results in fetal deprivation.

Infectious Placentitis

Most cases of equine infectious placentitis are caused by bacterial organisms that presumably gain access to the uterus through the cervix.[13] However, the placenta can also become infected with fungi, by bloodborne organisms, or from latent foci of endometritis. The infection spreads from the placenta to the allantoic and amniotic fluid or through the umbilical vein into the fetus.[13] The outcome of fetal infection may be death and abortion, growth retardation, or premature delivery. Growth retardation secondary to placentitis is probably the result of the chronic fetal infection and/or inadequate fetal nourishment. Bacterial organisms cultured from the reproductive tracts of barren mares, infected placentas, aborted fetuses, and the blood of foals believed to be born with infection acquired in utero are similiar: Streptococcus spp., Escherichia coli, Klebsiella spp., Actinobacillus spp., Salmonella spp., Staphylococcus spp., and Pseudomonas spp.[13] The fetus may not be infected even though the placenta appears so grossly, and a normal placenta does not guarantee that the newborn has not acquired an infection in utero. Equine herpesvirus type 1, which is the most common viral cause of equine abortion, may also result in an infected weak or premature foal that is likely to die soon after birth if not supported. In these cases, the placenta may be grossly normal. The suspicion that a foal has acquired a bacterial infection in utero is based on a high sepsis score in the first 12 h of life (Chapter 111).

Noninfectious Placental Disease

Noninfectious placental disease can cause a functional abnormality which results in inadequate nourishment of the fetus. The placental abnormality may be obvious to the naked eye, like avillous atrophy or edema, or subtle enough to elude histologic examination.[20] Placental insufficiency may be chronic, as is suspected with twins, or it may be acute as occurs with asphyxia caused by prolonged labor.

Acute Placental Insufficiency. Umbilical cord twisting, premature placental separation, or prolonged delivery result in insufficient blood flow to the placenta and fetus and acute placental insufficiency. If the severity and duration of such an incident is sufficient, in utero or birth asphyxia can result.[21] The sequelae of acute asphyxia in utero range from stillbirth to a newborn showing subtle signs or multiorgan failure.

Chronic Placental Insufficiency. The most common example of chronic placental insufficiency condition in the horse occurs with twins, resulting in increased incidence of perinatal morbidity and mortality. Twins are aborted or born dead, small, or premature. The condition is also suspected when large areas of the chorion are avillous and probably unable to support the fetus. If the foal is born alive with numerous signs of prematurity, it is susceptible to a wide array of neonatal diseases.

Intrauterine Growth Retardation. Symmetrical and asymmetrical intrauterine growth retardation (IUGR) of the human fetus have been defined.[22] Both types of IUGR are believed to be the result of an abnormality of the fetoplacental unit. If the cause of the growth retardation inhibits mitotic division of cells, as in viral infection, prolonged toxin exposure, or severe nutritional deprivation, the fetus will be small but symmetrically proportioned. If the growth-retarding insult occurs more acutely in late gestation, the fetus tends to be asymmetrically affected, with a large head, long frame and little subcutaneous fat. The fetus which suffers mitotic inhibition is more likely to have congenital defects, but if not life threatening, the foal may survive.

These growth-retardation patterns are believed to occur in the foal.[23] A foal with symmetrical IUGR, exposed to chronic stress in utero, tends to survive parturition better than the asymmetrically growth retarded fetus. If both types of foals survive parturition, the asymmetric foal tends to grow to normal size, but the symmetrical foal will likely remain small for age and breed.

HIGH-RISK NEWBORN

The veterinarian may be introduced to the foal at one of four times during the breeding season: as an embryo or fetus when the mare is confirmed pregnant, as a newborn when assisting delivery, as an apparently healthy newborn for physical examination, and as a sick foal at the request of the attendant. In the latter case, signs of disease are obvious and other chapters discuss neonatal disease. In the first three cases, the veterinarian has the opportunity to assess impending catastrophe by recognizing the warning signs that the newborn is at risk of developing disease. Identification of the high-risk pregnancy was discussed previously. The high-risk newborn foal can appear normal on physical examination but either have a disease, which is not readily apparent, or have been subjected to circumstances that make it more susceptible to acquiring disease.

THE ADAPTIVE PERIOD

To appreciate how vulnerable the newborn foal is to disease, the clinician must understand the dynamic transition the normal-term newborn undergoes at birth in adapting to extrauterine life. The magnitude of this physiologic transition is easily overlooked, because the foal is precocious at birth and normally stands and suckles within the first 2 h. Detailed description of the physiologic events which occur at birth are available, but are beyond the scope of this chapter.[24] The most well-recognized component of the changes which occur in the neonatal period is the transfer of maternal immunoglobulins to protect the newborn from infection while the immune system matures. However, all major body systems, including the cardiovascular, respiratory, endocrine, renal, nervous, musculoskeletal, and gastrointestinal systems, must adapt to extrauterine life and undergo maturational changes during the neonatal period. The newborn in the neonatal adaptive period, which is generally accepted to be the first 7 days of life, should be approached diagnostically or therapeutically differently from the adult horse or even the foal several weeks of age.

The Stress of Parturition

Serum catecholamine levels in healthy human newborns delivered vaginally are four times that of an adult man during exercise.[25] The stress response to parturition aids the newborn in the transition to extrauterine life. The most life-threatening adaptation which the newborn must undergo at birth involves the cardiopulmonary system. Ironically, this transition is often not as well appreciated as that of the immune system, because it is not as well understood. A succinct explanation of these events is available.[24]

During gestation, the fetus depends on the placenta for oxygen and carbon dioxide exchange, waste removal, nutrients, and metabolic regulation. The placental-dependent oxygen delivery system may be compromised during gestation and parturition causing hypoxemia and/or ischemia. If these are severe enough, the fetus develops metabolic acidosis, asphyxial damage, and may die. With the rupture of the umbilical cord this dependency is severed, and all systems of the foal must function autonomously. If the newborn does not make the transition to independent cardiopulmonary function rapidly, it is also subject to asphyxia. The sequelae to intrauterine or extrauterine asphyxia in the live foal depend on the duration and severity of the insult, and the presentation of affected individuals varies from mild subclinical disease to severe multiorgan failure[21] (Chapter 110).

If the fetus has been stressed acutely or chronically in utero, the stress of parturition and adaptation to extrauterine life may be too taxing. For example, depletion of glycogen stores during gestation or a prolonged delivery may lead to myocardial infarctions and in utero acquired bacterial pneumonia may compromise pulmonary function. Premature birth because of an abnormal uterine environment (placentitis or placental insufficiency) may produce a newborn who is severely or subtley handicapped. Surfactant deficiency and respiratory distress syndrome are obvious debilitating results of prematurity, but incomplete ossification of the skeletal system, which is less readily apparent at birth, may limit the foal's career as a performance horse. If historic information about the pregnancy includes evidence that the fetus was stressed in utero, delivery should be attended and the foal carefully assessed.

EXAMINATION OF THE FOAL

The following discussion reviews some observations that will forewarn the veterinarian that the foal is at high risk of having or developing neonatal disease. A complete discussion of the physical examination of the newborn foal is presented in Chapter 108.

Historical Information

If this is a first visit to the farm, information discussed in the section on the high-risk pregnancy should be obtained (Fig. 109–1). Because many equine births are not witnessed, information about parturition is often not available.

General Appearance

The general health status of the foal should immediately and quickly be assessed by evaluating the respiratory rate and pattern, mucous membrane color, heart rate, and peripheral perfusion. If the foal needs resuscitation, refer to that section of this chapter. Care of the foal that is seizuring, in respiratory distress, or showing signs of an abdominal crisis is discussed in the appropriate chapters on neonatal diseases. If the foal is stable, the examination proceeds systematically to evaluate each body system in turn as discussed in Chapter 108.

Special attention is paid to signs of difficult parturition, such as trauma to the foal or to the dam's reproductive tract and meconium staining of the placenta or foal. If any evidence of difficult parturition is found, the foal is considered to be at risk of having perinatal asphyxia and is more susceptible to developing neonatal disease regardless of how apparently healthy it may appear soon after birth. Immediately after birth, newborns look suprisingly vigorous and alert. This state may deteriorate as the high serum catecholamine levels of parturition decline.[25]

Foals which are small for gestational age, asymmetrically or symmetrically growth retarded, premature, or from a twin birth deserve special thorough evaluation regardless of their apparent health because abnormal influences in utero are suspected.

Petechiation or schleral injection unassociated with eye trauma may be an early sign of septicemia and should be noted. Fever and abnormal thoracic auscultation are often not present even if the foal is actively suffering from pneumonia or generalized infection.

Foals which exhibit any odd or abrupt change in behavior or lack of vigor are candidates for neonatal disease (Chapter 112). Foals which are inappetent, will not stand, or cannot nurse should be examined thoroughly and treated immediately. The physiologic nature of the neonate contests the wait-and-see approach to foal care and supports prompt diagnostic and therapeutic action to optimize the high-risk foal's chance of survival. Because the signs of illness are so vague in the early stages of neonatal disease, a complete diagnostic workup is recommended if the foal is considered high risk. The testing may seem excessive, but the prognosis for survival is better if the foal is treated before obvious clinical signs are present. If the owner has any interest or investment in the foal, the clinician should seek permission to pursue this protocol rather than wait. Because the foal can look deceptively healthy although suspicion of compromise is high, this urgency should be carefully explained to the owner.

REFERRAL CLINICS

Treatment of neonatal foals is time-consuming and labor intensive. In the best interest of the patient and the ambulatory veterinarian, consider referring the foal to a facility specifically equipped to care for the foal 24 h a day. The costs and benefits of early referral should be explained to the owner when a high-risk foal is first identified. Because of the nature of disease in neonatal foals, status of the foal may change rapidly making it difficult for the ambulatory clinician to respond to changing needs of the patient.

Transportation of the Critical Newborn to an Intensive Care Unit

A few simple measures taken to stabilize the foal before shipping to a referral center will enhance its chance of survival and response to treatment. Table 109–1 lists recommendations for transport of the compromised neonate. The veterinarian must make arrangements with the referral clinic before shipping the foal.

DIAGNOSTIC PROTOCOL TO EVALUATE A HIGH-RISK NEONATAL FOAL

If the foal stays on the farm or is transported to a referral clinic, the thorough diagnostic protocol listed in Table 109–1 (developed through experience at the University of Florida Equine Neonatal Intensive Care Unit) should be performed. Because neonatal foals present with subtle signs of disease, the clinician must perform all of the tests to evaluate the foal thoroughly, develop an inclusive therapeutic plan, and project a realistic prognosis and cost estimate for the owner.

Generalized infections are common in neonatal foals, yet difficult to identify in the early stage. A weighted score to estimate the likelihood that a neonatal foal is septicemic has been developed based on historic, clinical, and pathologic data.[26] The "sepsis score" and further information on septicemia is presented in more detail in Chapter 111. Broad-spectrum antibiotics are best initiated during the early stage of the infection.

Serum immunoglobulin and whole blood glucose levels can conveniently be tested at stallside. An immediate assessment will allow the veterinarian to proceed with therapy. Although foals with low serum immunoglobulins do not necessarily get sick, foals with high serum immunoglobulins are less likely to die of infection, if they do get sick.[27] The high-risk newborn foal is more likely to succumb to the stresses of extrauterine life, in-

FOAL NAME: ________ CLINIC NUMBER: ________ DATE: ________
MARE NAME: ________ SIRE NAME: ________ BREED: ________
AGE OF MARE: ____ # OF PREVIOUS FOALINGS: ____ # OF PREVIOUS ABORTIONS: ____

PREVIOUS PROBLEMS

1. History of infertility or uterine infection? ________ Negative culture pre-breeding? ____
   Comments ________
2. Problems with other foals? ________ Still births? ________ Dystocia? ____
   NMS foals? ________ NI foals? ________ Premature foals? ________
   Twins? ________

PRESENT FOAL

1. Is the foal insured? ________ If so, by whom? ________
2. Breeding dates of mare: ________ Expected foaling date: ________
   Actual foaling date: ________ Time: ________ Calculated gestational age: ____

PROBLEMS DURING GESTATION

1. Vaccinated for rhino? ________ Full series? ________ Tetanus toxoid during gestation? ____
2. Any exposure to infectious diseases during gestation? ________
3. Did mare drip milk prior to foaling? ________ How long? ________
4. Other problems? (e.g., fevers, vaginal discharges, cough, colic, and laminitis) ________

PROBLEMS DURING FOALING

1. Was foaling observed? ____ Delivery was (circle one): Faster than normal Normal Dystocia
   Comments: ________
2. Early cord rupture? ________ Meconium stained? ________ Resuscitation? ____
   Placenta intact? ________ Normal appearance? ________ Premature separation? ____
   Comments ________

PROBLEMS AFTER FOALING

1. Time to get up: ________ Time to nurse: ________ Colostrum quality? ____
2. Normal behavior post foaling? ________
3. TAT given? ________ Umbilicus treated? ________ Meconium observed? ____
4. Normal urination observed? ________

CLINICAL COMPLAINT(S)

1. Time of onset of clinical signs: ________
2. Previous treatment: ________
3. Clinical course: ________

FIG. 109–1. Neonatal history form: University of Florida. (From Koterba, A.M.: Diagnosis and management of the normal and abnormal neonatal foal: General considerations. *In* Equine Clinical Neonatology. Edited by A.M. Koterba, W.H. Drummond, and P.C. Kosch. Philadelphia, Lea & Febiger, 1990, p. 9.)

cluding infection, and may benefit from high circulating immunoglobulin concentrations.

Samples which must be submitted to a clinical pathology laboratory include hemogram and plasma fibrinogen concentrations, which provide information on the likelihood of infection. The clinician must have a total and differential neutrophil count performed as well as cytologic evaluation of the cells. A left shift or any sign of toxic neutrophils is a strong indication that the foal has an infection. Serum chemistry measurements are necessary because accurate prediction of these concentrations in ill neonates is impossible. Anaerobic and aerobic blood cultures taken aseptically can definitively diagnose septicemia and provide information on the most effective antibiotics. Arterial blood gas measurements—which are taken anaerobically, capped, and stored in ice water for measurement within 4 h—and thoracic radiographs are more reliable methods of judging cardiopulmonary function than auscultation and mucous membrane color. These physical findings often appear normal in an abnormal foal. Successful care of the sick neonate is based on meticulous concern for detail, proactive identification of disease, and complete nursing care.

EMERGENCY CONDITIONS IN NEONATAL FOALS

If the subtle signs of neonatal disease are not appreciated early in the disease course, the veterinarian is likely to be called later for a life-threatening emergency. Management of the foal with seizures, respiratory distress, acute abdominal distention, septic shock, and/or pain are covered in other chapters. However, if the pregnancy has been followed, as suggested above, and parturition attended when difficulties are suspected, foals can be saved by providing support early in the adaptive neonatal period before the onset of an emergency.

TABLE 109–1. TRANSPORT INSTRUCTIONS AND ADMISSION PROTOCOL

Transport instructions

1. Administer colostrum before shipping the foal and send colostrum with foal; 1 L is preferred, if possible
2. Send placenta, if available, and for information regarding the labor and delivery, as well as the perinatal condition of mare
3. If the foal is too weak to stand, check whole blood glucose with strip; If value <40 mg/dL, administer 5 to 10% glucose IV (500 to 1000 mL). Continue the infusion during the trip, if possible.
4. Check body temperature before transport; if <37.8° C (100° F), make every attempt to keep foal warm during the trip; use a heated van or station wagon, do not wait for mare transport
5. If foal is in respiratory distress, send E-tank of oxygen to provide nasal insufflation; at a flow rate of 5 L/min, one tank should last about 2 h

General comments

1. All initial workup should be done on foal bed, transport cart, or thick pad in stall; if foal cannot stand unassisted or nurse from the mare, place it in a controlled environment
2. Keep supplies needed for initial workup packaged together in a "catheter kit"
3. Be sure to perform a complete physical examination to rule out the presence of congenital abnormalities

Evaluation of foal

1. Assess immediate needs: evaluate breathing pattern, respiratory rate, heart rate, and mucous membrane perfusion; perform resuscitation procedures or begin oxygen therapy before proceeding with further diagnostic tests
2. If body temperature <37.8° C (100° F), apply heat lamps and heating blankets of <40° C (103° F)
3. Draw EDTA and clot blood tubes for:
   a. whole blood glucose determination
   b. complete blood count and differential; look for band neutrophils and evidence of toxicity such as vacuoles, granular material, and cell disruption as soon as possible (ASAP)
   c. serum electrolytes, calcium, and rapid IgG test (ASAP)
   d. chemistry panel and quantitative IgG test
4. Draw aerobic and anaerobic blood cultures
5. Assess fluid balance and insert intravenous catheter, if indicated
6. Attempt to acquire sample for arterial blood gas analysis; if the pulse quality is excessively poor, obtain a venous sample for metabolic evaluation
7. When condition is stabilized, radiograph the thorax, and if indicated, the abdomen
8. In any down or dehydrated foal, take indirect blood pressure and record it
9. Compute sepsis score as soon as laboratory data are available
10. Start frequent observation charting
11. Weigh foal
12. Evaluate laboratory data, physical examination, and history and decide on appropriate antibiotic, plasma, fluid therapy, tetanus prophylaxis, and umbilical care

(From Koterba, A.M.: Diagnosis and management of the normal and abnormal neonatal foal: General considerations. *In* Equine Clinical Neonatology. Edited by A.M. Koterba, W.H. Drummond, and P.C. Kosch. Philadelphia, Lea & Febiger, 1990, pp. 12–13.)

RESUSCITATION OF THE NEWBORN FOAL

Very ill foals and those born from dystocia present unpredictably for resuscitation. In contrast, a foal from an induction or caesarian section is likely to need resuscitation and a team can be ready to provide this support. Prompt action can make the difference between life and death or a normal foal and a permanently debilitated foal. If engaged in any type of brood mare practice, the equipment and drug doses for resuscitation of a foal should be close at hand. The practitioner may carry an emergency box or convince the brood mare operation to have the equipment on the farm. The basic procedures of resuscitation follow.[28]

1. Establish a patent airway by cleaning debris from the nares and using suction. If suction is not available, hold the foal upside down to drain out amniotic fluid or meconium.

2. The breathing rate should be given at 15 to 25 breaths per minute with the expiratory pause two to four times the duration of inspiration. Foals can benefit from ventilation, even if they are breathing independently, because positive pressure ventilation enhances gas exchange, thus providing oxygen and removing carbon dioxide. Mouth to nose resuscitation is rational but not successful unless an endotracheal tube is passed. Oral intubation is easiest in the comatose foal, but nasotracheal intubation is best for the conscious foal. An endotracheal tube must be passed to ventilate a foal effectively. Silicone rubber tubes that are 45 to 50 cm long and 7 to 10 mm in internal diameter (ID) are best for nasal intubation and 9- to 11-mm ID tubes are used for oral intubation. Ventilation can be provided using an Ambu bag, oxygen demand valve, anesthetic machine, or by blowing down the endotracheal tube. Although humidified oxygen is optimal for long-term therapy, room air will suffice for short periods. Doxapram or other pharmacologic respiratory stimulants should not be used in place of ventilation. They may be effective in primary apnea but have only a transient effect, are ineffective in secondary apnea, and increase oxygen consumption. Assume the foal is in secondary apnea if any delay occurs in initiating therapy.

3. Establish effective cardiac function. To perform ex-

ternal cardiac massage, place the foal in right lateral recumbency with a sandbag under the sternal end of the thorax and place the hands over the ventricles between ribs 4 and 5. Compress the thorax 60 to 70 times a minute, giving one breath for each of 3 compressions. A total of 75 pounds of pressure is necessary, and mean rather than peak pressure is important. Epinephrine is given intravenously (IV), intracardiac (IC), or intratracheal (IT) for cardiac standstill at 0.1 to 0.2 mL/kg of a 1:10,000 solution. For sinus bradycardia, atropine (0.01 to 0.03 mg/kg IV or IT) is used.

Effective therapy can be judged by return of pupil constriction, corneal sensation, palpable pulses, muscle tone, and spontaneous cardiac activity. Complications of external massage include regurgitation, rib fractures, liver lacerations, impaired lung function, and pneumothorax.

To establish peripheral circulation, place an intravenous catheter and begin fluid therapy with a buffered-balanced electrolyte solution. Administration of sodium bicarbonate and calcium are no longer routinely recommended during resuscitation by the American Heart Association (AHA).[29] Sodium bicarbonate may cause metabolic alkalosis, hypernatremia, hyperosmolarity, paradoxic central nervous system acidosis, or respiratory acidosis. The efficacy and safety of calcium has been questioned. The AHA recommends its use only if the patient is hyperkalemic, hypocalcemic, or has calcium channel blocker drug toxicity.

Once the foal is stabilized, the whole blood glucose concentration should be determined and 5 to 10% dextrose solutions given if the foal is hypoglycemic. For treatment of severe hypoglycemia, 5 to 10 mL/kg of 10% dextrose may be needed rapidly. The rate is then reduced to 4 to 8 mg/kg/min. Do not use bolus doses of concentrated hypertonic glucose solutions, because the foal may suffer central nervous system hyperosmolarity or develop a rebound hypoglycemia. Keep the foal warm using blankets, a heat lamp, and/or a hot water pad.

Monitoring blood pressure and cardiac electrical activity will probably not be possible in the field, although this would be the next important step before administering drugs for cardiac inotropic support.

The crisis is not over when the foal responds, because it will likely need aggressive followup care. After the foal stabilizes, referral to a clinic which specializes in intensive care should be considered. Foals suffering from an asphyxial incident can develop a wide spectrum of neonatal diseases which are usually impractical for the practitioner to manage on the farm, including failure of passive transfer, septicemia, gastrointestinal disease, renal tubular necrosis, and cardiopulmonary disease. Details of intensive care of the neonatal foal, are available.[30]

REFERENCES

1. Powell, D.G.: Viral respiratory disease. *In* Current Veterinary Therapy in Equine Medicine. 2nd ed. Edited by N.E. Robinson. Philadelphia, W.B. Saunders, 1987, pp. 581–590.
2. Traub-Dargatz, J.L., et al.: Epidemiologic survey of diarrhea in foals. J. Am. Vet. Med. Assoc., *192*:1553–1556, 1988.
3. Ousey, J.C., Murgatrotd, P.R., Stewart, J.H., and Rossdale, P.D.: Thermoregulation in the neonatal pony foal. Equine Vet. J., *5(Suppl.)*:50, 1988.
4. Donoghue, S., Meacham, T.N., and Kronfeld, D.S.: A conceptual approach to optimal nutrition of broodmares. Vet. Clin. North Am. Equine Pract., *6*:373–391, 1990.
5. Perry, T.W.: Beef Cattle Feeding and Nutrition. San Diego, Academic Press, 1980.
6. Knight, D.A., et al.: Correlation of dietary mineral to incidence and severity of metabolic bone disease in Ohio and Kentucky. Proc. Am. Assoc. Equine Pract., 445–461, 1985.
7. Baucus, K.L., Ralston, S.L., Rich, G.A., and Squires, E.L.: Effect of copper and zinc supplementation on mineral content of mare's milk. J. Equine Vet. Sci., *9*:206–209, 1989.
8. Kowalski, J., Williams, J., and Hintz, H.F.: Weight gains of mares during the last trimester of gestation. Equine Pract., *12*:6–10, 1990.
9. Odde, K.G.: Survival of the neonatal calf. Vet. Clin. North Am. Food Anim. Pract., *4*:501–508, 1988.
10. Di Pietro, J.A.: A review of Strongyloides westeri infection in foals. Equine Pract. *11*:35–40, 1989.
11. Baucus, K.L., Squires, E.L., Ralston, S.L., and McKinnon, A.O.: Effect of transportation on the estrous cycle and concentrations of hormones in mares. J. Anim. Sci., *68*:419–426, 1990.
12. Szenci, O., Kutas, F., and Haraszti, J.: Influence of induced maternal acidosis on the acid-base balance of the newborn calf. Acta Vet. Acad. Sci. Hung., *30*:71–77, 1982.
13. Koterba, A.M.: Prenatal influences on neonatal survival in the foal. Proc. Am. Assoc. Equine Pract., 139–152, 1983.
14. Brock, K.A.: Anesthesia of the late-term mare. *In* Equine Clinical Neonatology. Edited by A.M. Koterba, W.H. Drummond, and P.C. Kosch. Philadelphia, Lea & Febiger, 1990, pp. 87–105.
15. Santschi, E.M., Slone, D.E., LeBlanc, M.M., and Juzwiak, J.S.: The effect of maternal colic on the equine fetus. Proc. Am. Assoc. Equine Pract., 79–83, 1990.
16. Hansen, R.R., and Todhunter, R.J.: Herniation of the abdominal wall in pregnant mares. J. Am. Vet. Med. Assoc., *189*:790–793, 1986.
17. Roberts, S.J.: Veterinary Obstetrics and Genital Disease. Ithaca, NY, published by the author, 1971.
18. Koterba, A.M., Haibel, G.K., and Grimmet, J.B.: Respiratory distress in a premature foal secondary to hydrops allantois and placentitis. Compend. Contin. Educ. Practicing Vet., *5*:S121–S125, 1983.
19. Adams-Brendemuehl, C., and Pipers, F.S.: Antepartum evaluations in the equine fetus. J. Reprod. Fertil. Suppl., *35*:565–573, 1987.
20. Naeye, R.L., Kissane, J.M., and Kaufman, N.: Perinatal Diseases. Baltimore, Williams & Wilkins, 1981.
21. Drummond, W.H., and Koterba, A.M.: Neonatal asphyxia. *In* Equine Clinical Neonatology. Edited by A.M. Koterba, W.H. Drummond, and P.C. Kosch. Philadelphia, Lea & Febiger, 1990, pp. 125–135.
22. Lockwood, C.J., and Weiner, S.: Assessment of fetal growth. Clin. Perinatol., *13*:3–35, 1986.
23. Koterba, A.M.: Intrauterine growth retardation. Proceedings of the Seventh Annual Meeting of the American College of Internal Medicine. San Diego, 1989, pp. 413–415.
24. Randall, G.C.B.: Perinatal mortality: some problems of

adaptation at birth. Adv. Vet. Sci. Comp. Med., *22:*53–81, 1978.

25. Lagercrantz, H., and Slotkin, T.A.: The "stress" of being born. Sci. Am., *254:*100–107, 1986.

26. Brewer, B.D., and Koterba, A.M.: Development of a scoring system for the early diagnosis of equine neonatal sepsis. Equine Vet. J., *20:*18–22, 1988.

27. Koterba, A.M., Brewer, B.D., and Tarplee, F.A.: Clinical and clinicopathologic characteristics of the septicemic neonatal foal. Equine Vet. J., *16:*376–383, 1984.

28. Webb, A.I.: Neonatal resuscitation. *In* Equine Clinical Neonatology. Edited by A.M. Koterba, W.H. Drummond, and P.C. Kosch. Philadelphia, Lea & Febiger, 1990, pp. 136–150.

29. American Heart Association: Standards and guidelines for cardiopulmonary resuscitation and emergency cardiac care. J. Am. Med. Assoc., *255:*2905–2989, 1986.

30. Koterba, A.M., Drummond, W.H., and Kosch, P.C. (eds.): Equine Clinical Neonatology. Philadelphia, Lea & Febiger, 1990.

SECTION B

DISEASES OF FOALS DURING THE NEONATAL PERIOD

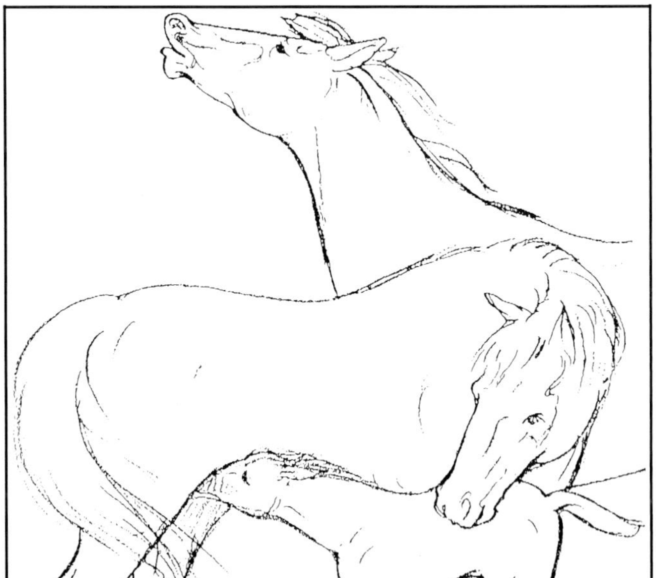

CHAPTER 110

NEONATAL DISEASE: AN OVERVIEW

R. Adams

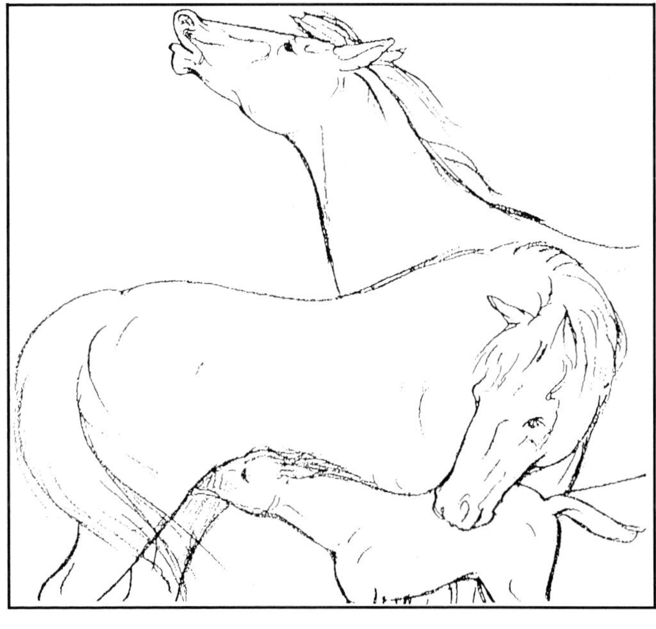

Evaluation of reproductive performance in domestic species raised for food and fiber is based on the production of healthy offspring. In the beef cattle industry, reproductive performance is calculated by the number of calves weaned per dam exposed to the bull.[1] In the equine industry, the definition of reproductive performance is less clear because there is no single goal and, therefore, no specific criteria on which to measure success. Generally, the goal of the horse breeder is to produce a healthy foal which performs athletically. Jeffcott estimated overall wastage in English Thoroughbred racehorses from conception to 4 y of age to be 72.8%.[2] This loss was subdivided into categories: 22.5% failed to conceive, 10.1% aborted or had a nonsurviving foal, 13.9% had a live foal which was not named, 20.1% had a named foal that did not race, and 6.2% were trained animals that did not race. Thus, almost half (32.6%) of the total loss (72.8%) could be categorized as unsatisfactory reproductive performance.

Successful solutions to problems which arise during the perinatal period require expertise in two specialty areas: theriogenology centers on the physiologic and pathologic aspects of conception and pregnancy, and neonatology encompasses the physiologic state of the newborn and disease accompanying the transition from fetal to extrauterine life. Understanding the complex events affecting the mare and foal during the perinatal period requires information from both of these specialties. Reproductive performance can be enhanced by improving the survival of the young.

Many sections of this volume are devoted to fertilization, the diagnosis and maintenance of pregnancy, and parturition. Other sections focus on the foal and mare during the perinatal period, presenting advances of the last decade in the understanding of equine neonatal disease. The material presented here summarizes information available in more detail elsewhere.[3]

The precise definition of the perinatal period varies between authors but always includes some portion of late gestation through the first several days or weeks of the newborn's life. Chapters 105 to 109 divide the perinatal period into discrete time segments (fetus, newborn foal, prefoaling mare, and postpartum mare) but continuity underlies these subdivisions. Two examples help illustrate this: (1) when treating disease in a brood mare, the short- and long-term effects of both disease and treatment on the fetus must be considered, and (2) delivery of a premature foal raises questions about the mare's general health, the intrauterine environment, and the gestational events which led to premature parturition.

In the following chapters in this section, the diseases of the foal are presented by organ system. Despite this manner of organization, note that disease in newborn foals may initially show signs specific to a single organ system, but usually involve, or progress to involve, multiple systems. A complete evaluation of the foal is necessary before making a final diagnosis and formulating a realistic prognosis. Consider the foal which presents with signs of a ruptured bladder. If the foal has only a ruptured bladder of relatively short duration, it has a relatively good prognosis. However, if the foal also presents with common complications such as severe electrolyte imbalances, failure of passive transfer (FPT), bacteremia, pneumonia, and peritonitis, the prognosis is grave. The distinction between these two scenarios often cannot be made on physical examination alone.

ASPECTS OF NEONATAL DISEASE

Information gained retrospectively from equine neonatal intensive care hospitals has revised the manner in which neonatal equine disease conditions are evaluated.[4] A study based on followup of the first foals treated at the University of Florida concludes that foals ill as neonates can perform well as adults.[5] The rewarding lesson learned from treating newborn foals during the 1980s is that medical ignorance rather than equine genetic inferiority doomed most sick newborn foals to die.[6]

The dramatic improvement in recovery rates of sick neonatal foals is in part caused by the recognition that disease in the neonate does not present, progress, or respond to therapy exactly like diseases in the juvenile or adult.[4] Closer assessment of the newborn foal has resulted in the development of principles on which diagnostic and therapeutic decisions are made.

DISEASE ORIGIN—EXTRAUTERINE VERSUS INTRAUTERINE

Disease processes that affect the newborn foal can develop during gestation (congenital defect, in utero growth retardation, infection, or asphyxia), parturition (trauma, acute asphyxia, or rupture of the urinary tract), or extrauterine life (FPT, bacteremia, pneumonia, diarrhea, intestinal accident, trauma, etc.). Insults to the fetus in utero or during parturition may result in an aborted fetus, a stillborn, or a neonate that shows abnormal clinical signs in the first few days of life. Although these insults to the fetus within the uterus and during parturition may be unapparent at first in the live foal, they can hamper its ability to adapt successfully to extrauterine life. Diagnostic techniques that identify abnormal intrauterine events are not well developed in the horse, although recent research has added greatly to the knowledge of physiologic aspects of the fetomaternal unit and gestational events as well as the effect of these on the fetus and the neonate's ability to adapt to extrauterine life.[7]

PRESENTING SIGNS

Early signs of disease in a newborn foal are often subtle and nonspecific. When the foal becomes disinterested in the dam, inappetent, or lacks curiosity and vigor, diagnostic testing to identify the early stages of disease is warranted. If appropriate therapy is initiated at that time, chances for survival increase. A standard diagnostic protocol has been suggested, because of the inability to recognize disease based on the physical examination alone[3] (Chapter 109). Briefly, this protocol uses (1) routine measurement of serum immunoglobulins as a measure of passive transfer of maternal immunoglobulins; (2) measurement of plasma fibrinogen and total white blood cell count, including differential and cell structure, to identify focal or widespread infection; (3) aerobic and anaerobic blood cultures to identify causative organism(s) and determine appropriate antibiotic therapy; (4) arterial blood gas analysis and thoracic radiographs to diagnose respiratory disease for which auscultation alone is unsatisfactory; (5) abdominal radiographs to evaluate foals with signs of pain and/or abdominal distension; and (6) serum chemistry panels to identify unpredictable variations in serum electrolyte and glucose concentrations, common in sick foals.

CLINICAL COURSE

Newborn foals succumb to disease rapidly. If the foal is dull because of hypoglycemia, in only a few hours it may develop seizures or become comatose. A foal with diarrhea can rapidly become dehydrated and succumb to hypovolemic shock.

MULTISYSTEMIC NATURE OF DISEASE

Disease in the newborn foal is unlikely to be limited to one organ system as is the common presentation in an older foal or adult horse. The septic foal may have one or two obviously septic joints on physical examination, but necropsy often reveals widespread osteomyelitis and septic arthritis, pneumonia, and umbilical infection. The premature foal with lax ligamentous structures and respiratory compromise necessitating supplemental oxygen, may also have FPT and incomplete ossification of bones. An asphyxiated foal which has signs of neurologic damage is likely to have renal tubular necrosis, necrotizing enterocolitis, and pulmonary hypertension as well. The foal with colic is just as likely to be septicemic with peritonitis, ileus, diarrhea, pneumonia, and septic arthitis/osteomyelitis as to have a discrete surgical lesion. Therefore, the clinical diagnostic challenge is to identify all organ systems involved. A complete examination must be performed on the foal and all organ systems assessed before formulating a realistic prognosis. Anything less is a disservice to the patient and client.

Because of the expense and labor necessary to care for an ill newborn foal, efforts have been made to predict the likelihood that the patient with a particular set of clinical problems will survive and lead a productive career.[8,9] After treating newborn foals in an intensive care unit from 1982 to 1987, Koterba summarized the outcome of selected conditions, including the average days of hospitalization and cost of treatment for various conditions.[10] Results will vary between clinics based on the available expertise, technical support, and level of nursing care provided, but this general information is helpful for counseling clients.

The percent of newborn foals (less than 2 weeks of age) discharged improved from 40% in 1981 to 64% in 1982 when the intensive care unit opened. In 1987, discharge rate increased to 75%. Each year, approximately 12% of the treated foals died or were euthanatized following discharge, usually because of complications of chronic infection and/or musculoskeletal abnormalities. In general, from 1982-1986, the best prognosis was for foals with focal infections (76% discharged) and the worst for septicemic foals (43% discharged). A total of 55% of the premature foals and 66% of the foals with neonatal maladjustment syndrome (NMS) were discharged (Chapter 112). Foals treated for uroperitoneum or surgical gastrointestinal disease were discharged at a rate of 50% and 56%, respectively. In 1986, the average cost for treatment varied with the disease: (1) $1680 ($230/day) for foals with NMS (100% discharge), (2) $2250 ($310/day) for term septicemic foals (83% discharged), (3) $3675 ($245/day) for premature foals born from mares with placentitis (100% discharge), and (4) $996 ($498/day) for premature foals with other problems (0% discharge).

GENERAL THERAPEUTIC CONCERNS

Because of the nature of equine neonatal disease (subtle initial clinical presentation, rapid time course of disease, and multisystemic involvement), therapeutic plans are formulated differently from those for older foals and adults. These decisions are often difficult. Additional clinical problems may be induced iatrogenically because of lack of knowledge about disease processes, pharmacokinetics of drugs, and nutritional requirements of the newborn. Medical therapy is directed toward all problems identified and anticipated as likely to develop. For example, when presented with a premature foal, consideration must be given to the likelihood that the foal either is also septicemic or will develop generalized infection.

Supportive nursing care is usually the most time-consuming and labor intensive part of any therapeutic regimen. Clinical experience with the care of foals has proven that attention to these details improves survival rate dramatically. The following are just a few areas to which the clinician must direct attention: (1) keep the foal warm, dry, and clean; (2) provide adequate nutrition orally or parenterally; (3) position in sternal recumbency to maximize efficiency of ventilation; (4) prevent self-trauma (corneal and decubital ulcers); (5) maintain the integrity and cleanliness of intravenous catheters; and (6) provide sufficient exercise, either passively or actively, to prevent limb deformities.

GENERALIZED PROBLEMS OF NEONATAL FOALS

Any attempt to classify diseases of the newborn is artificial and frought with limitations of oversimplicity. The following is an overview of four conditions which affect the foal in the perinatal period. The overlap inherent in these divisions must be stressed. For example, prematurity may be caused by in utero infection or in utero asphyxia. In turn, the premature foal may be more susceptible to asphyxia or acquisition of infection postpartum.

PREMATURITY

There are two principal reasons to characterize the stage of development of the newborn at birth: first, the underdeveloped newborn is less likely to readily adapt to extrauterine life and, second, the disturbance of the normal fetomaternal relationship which triggered premature parturition indicates a maternal, placental, or fetal abnormality. Early identification of this problem might prompt lifesaving therapy.

The full-term gestational length of the Thoroughbred is defined by a wide range of days (320 to 370) with a mean of 340 days.[7] Measurement of equine fetal development using gestational age, birth weight, and crown-rump length is prone to inaccuracies because of inexact breeding dates and inherent size variation between breeds. In human medicine, the guidelines for fetal development also vary based on the criteria used (birth weight, gestational age, bone development, or neurologic development) and the socioeconomic group measured. The availability of noninvasive ultrasonography has improved the estimation of fetal development because it enables the fetus to be visualized throughout gestation. Ultrasonographic measurements have been used to generate in utero growth curves for human babies. The large size of the equine fetus makes whole body measurements by ultrasonography difficult. Discussion of techniques used to evaluate fetal well-being and growth can be found in Chapter 106. The shortcomings of assessment of fetal development by birth weight, size, and gestational age include miscalculation of gestational length, difficulties establishing true normal standard birth weight information, and potential disregard for physiologic parameters that may be more important to survival of the newborn.

Presently, gestation duration is the most commonly used criterion by which to evaluate equine fetal development. The newborn Thoroughbred foal is considered premature if born at less than 320 days of gestation. Premature foals have several distinctive physical features that are readily identifiable: silky hair coat, floppy ears, soft lips, lax flexor tendons, thin body condition, and low birth weight. The premature foal may also be recognized by certain physiologic characteristics: adrenocortical function, carbohydrate metabolism, and the renin-angiotensin-aldosterone axis do not respond as in the full-term newborn foal.[7] Other researchers have noted different responses to neurologic testing and a predisposition to incomplete ossification of the skeletal system in premature versus term foals.[11,12]

Premature foals show problems during transition to extrauterine life when compared with normal-term foals. Even if the premature foal appears healthy on initial physical examination, the attending veterinarian must keep in mind that it is likely abnormal. The clinician may have difficulty distinguishing the origin of clinical disease. An abnormality may be the result of inherent prematurity of the newborn or may represent an acquired disease state. Ability of the premature newborn to survive depends on the stage of development at which the foal is born, reason the foal was born prematurely, and level of intensive care available to support the newborn through the adaptive period.

Hospital discharge rates for premature foals presented for treatment have improved with establishment of equine neonatal care units, but the hospitalization time and cost are greater than the average for disease syndromes in full-term foals.[10] The best prognosis is for premature foals born spontaneously with abnormal placental changes such as villous atrophy or placentitis. Koterba et al. have developed a predictive score for survival in premature foals.[9] The prognosis for survival of premature foals is based on six historic or measurable parameters: (1) fibrinogen < 400 mg/dL, (2) white blood cell count < 5000 cells/μL, (3) neutrophil to lymphocyte ratio < 3:1, (4) arterial pH < 7.30, (5) problems during parturition, and (6) a normal-appearing placenta. Death is predicted if the premature foal has three or more of these.

Dysmaturity is a confusing term used to describe a newborn foal which physically and physiologically resembles the premature foal but for which gestational age is within the range considered to be term. Miscalculation of the breeding date and a poor-quality intrauterine environment are possible causes for this state. Despite duration of gestation, the foal must be treated and supported like a premature foal.[7]

INTRAUTERINE GROWTH RETARDATION

Human babies that are small for gestational age (SGA) are thought to suffer from intrauterine growth retardation (IUGR). Normal rate and pattern of growth can be disturbed by abnormal hormonal, nutritional, genetic, or infectious conditions. The onset of IUGR can be acute or caused by chronic fetal deprivation through gestation. Severity varies and can result in a newborn with no obvious clinical problems but affected by subtle handicaps at time of birth. For example, if IUGR is caused by uteroplacental vascular insufficiency, the fetus may have diminished energy reserves with which to endure parturition and the immediate postnatal period.

Presently, the two classifications of IUGR used for children are also used to subjectively assess foals because an equine-specific classification based on intrauterine growth curves has not been established.[13] Researchers speculate that foals that are SGA but that have a symmetrical, well-proportioned shape suffer mitotic inhibition. This effect may result from viral infections, congenital abnormalities, toxin exposure, or chronic nutrient deprivation. Newborns that have a normal crown-rump length and head size but that are very thin exhibit asymmetrical IUGR. A retrospective study of premature foal mortality sought to identify characteristics that distinguished survivors from nonsurvivors. Foals that seemed to suffer chronic intrauterine growth retardation (symmetrical IUGR) were more likely to survive the stress of parturition than those that suffered acute intrauterine insults in late gestation (asymmetrical IUGR).[9] Although newborn foals with symmetrical IUGR were more likely to survive the immediate postpartum period, they were also more likely to have congenital defects and less likely to grow to normal size. Foals with asymmetrical IUGR, although more stressed at birth, could compensate and grow to normal size if they survived.

PERINATAL ASPHYXIA

Throughout the following chapters on neonatal disease, mention will be made of conditions believed to be sequelae to asphyxial damage (IUGR, necrotizing enterocolitis, persistent pulmonary circulation and hypertension, renal tubular necrosis, and cerebral hemorrhages). The following is a brief review of the condition.

Asphyxia is defined as impaired oxygen delivery to cells caused by hypoxemia and/or ischemia. The fetus in utero and during parturition, and the newborn as well, are at risk of asphyxial injury. Asphyxia can result in an array of clinical signs ranging from subtle loss of neurologic function to multisystem organ compromise and death.[14]

The fetus in utero is adapted to resist injury from some degree of asphyxia. Such adaptations include the greater oxygen affinity of fetal versus adult hemoglobin, greater tissue oxygen extraction capabilities, preferential perfusion of vital organs, and alteration of activity and growth rate to match nutrient supplies. Despite these fetal protective mechanisms, in utero asphyxia may be sufficient in duration and severity to compromise the well-being of the fetus. Conditions affecting the circulatory or oxygen delivery capacity of the dam, placenta, or fetus can lead to asphyxia. Some examples include cardiopulmonary disease in the dam or fetus, umbilical cord occlusion during dystocia, placentitis, premature placental separation, and placental insufficiency.

At parturition the newborn must make the sudden transition to independent existence, and the fetal adaptations are no longer effective. Transition to extrauterine life involves major physiologic changes: (1) establishment of systemic and pulmonary blood flow and circulation patterns, (2) aeration of the lungs, (3) metabolic autonomy including the need to supply nutritional requirements, (4) maintainance of fluid and electrolyte balance, and (5) independent thermoregulation. The most obvious cause of asphyxia in the neonate is failure of the cardiovascular or pulmonary systems to support systemic perfusion and oxygenation. Sequelae to neonatal asphyxia are wide ranging, depending on duration and severity, and include subclinical damage, failure of a single organ, or severe multisystem disease. The onset of clinical signs may be immediately obvious at birth or develop gradually over the first several days of life. The organ damage is believed to be caused by a combination of direct asphyxial damage and by superoxide radicals generated following reperfusion.

INFECTIOUS DISEASE

Any discussion of diseases of the neonatal foal must emphasize the susceptibility of the neonate to infection and its devastating consequences. Generalized infections can cause or complicate the problems of individuals that also suffer from prematurity, dysmaturity, IUGR, and/or perinatal asphyxia. The pathogenesis of neonatal infections is not well defined, but the clinical syndrome and its invasive nature are well appreciated. In 1984, Koterba et al. reported the clinical characteristics of septicemia in 38 neonatal foals.[15] This retrospective report drastically revised the classic description of generalized infection in newborn foals by using diagnostic techniques (blood cultures, thoracic radiographs, and arterial blood-gas analysis) to identify the presence of infection in its early stages. The following observations on neonatal infection are currently considered valid:

1. Septicemic foals generally have a poor survival rate.
2. Survival rate can be improved if the disease process is identified early in its course and appropriate treatment initiated immediately.
3. Clinical signs may be subtle and fever need not be present. Clinicopathologic results vary early in the course of infection, but a left shift in white cell population and toxic changes in neutrophils are useful indicators. Affected foals are often hypoglycemic, hypoxemic, and have a metabolic and/or respiratory acidosis.
4. No single diagnostic criterion can be used to establish immediately and conclusively the presence of infection in its early stages. A sepsis score has been developed that evaluates numerous clinical parameters concurrently and predicts the likelihood that a patient is septicemic at the first examination.[8] Broad-spectrum antibiotic therapy can be initiated promptly before final receipt of blood culture results. Therapy may be altered later based on antibiotic minimum inhibitory concentration (MIC) information necessary to overcome the offending organism.
5. Blood cultures are a useful diagnostic tool and provide essential information on which to base appropriate antimicrobial therapy. Gram-negative bacteria, especially Escherichia coli and Klebsiella spp., comprise the majority of isolates.
6. Acquisition of an infection in utero is suggested when the following are found: evidence of chorioamnionitis, vaginal discharge from the mare before foaling, foal weak at birth, positive blood cultures at less than 6 h of age, elevated fibrinogen levels at less than 12 h of age, and/or abnormal white blood cell counts in the newborn foal.
7. The route of infection in foals less than 7 days of age is most likely the respiratory and gastrointestinal tracts. At the time the foal is likely to be septicemic based on positive blood cultures, signs of omphalophlebitis are uncommon.
8. Foals presenting with omphalophlebitis and septic arthritis/osteomyelitis are usually several days to weeks old. In this stage of generalized infection, blood culture results are often negative. Umbilical infection can be successfully treated by surgical excision, but treatment of the skeletal infection is usually unrewarding because of the insidious nature.
9. Although not all foals with low serum immunoglobulins die of generalized infection, foals with elevated immunoglobulins (> 800 mg/dL) generally have a better chance of survival, when faced with a bacterial challenge.

Despite advances made in the diagnosis and treatment of neonatal infection, numerous clinical dilemmas remain unsettled. Following are three topics of concern. First, management of the foal with septic arthritis/osteomyelitis is still disheartening. When infection involves the skeletal system, the prognosis for recovery as a successful athlete is diminished. A primary cause of late deaths or elective euthanasia in foals which have recovered from systemic neonatal infections is degenerative arthritis or recurrence of septic arthritis (Chapter 116). Second, the complexities of the neonatal immune system must be further investigated. Important unanswered questions include: (1) what kind of evaluation of serum immunoglobulins will predict adequate passive transfer against infectious disease, (2) which foals need immunoglobulin supplementation; and (3) what is the best method of and product for supplementation? Finally, the pathogenesis, identification, treatment, and prevention of infection acquired in utero and perinatal asphyxia are not well understood because of technical difficulties in performing equine fetal research. The events of late gestation and the effect of these events on the newborn foal's ability to survive need to be better described.

Earlier recognition and treatment of infectious disease in foals has reduced the associated mortality and morbidity. The attending veterinarian must be alert to signs that a foal is at risk of developing infection and to historic or early behavioral evidence that a foal may not be normal. Prompt referral to a treatment center or initiation of comprehensive treatment at the time these signs are first seen will increase chances of survival and development into a normal athletic adult. Prophylactic use of broad-spectrum antibiotics in newborn foals is discouraged because this management procedure increases the risk of patient infection and the appearance of resistant bacterial organisms, may lead to colonization of the gastrointestinal and respiratory tract of the newborn with potential pathogens, and may expose the newborn to unnecessary toxic side effects associated with antibiotic therapy.[16,17]

REFERENCES

1. Odde, K.G.: Survival of the neonatal calf. Vet. Clin. North Am. Food Anim. Pract., *4:*501–508, 1988.
2. Jeffcott, L.B. et al.: An assessment of wastage in Thoroughbred racing from conception to 4 years of age. Equine Vet. J., *14:*185–198, 1982.
3. Koterba, A.M., Drummond, W.H., and Kosch, P.C. (eds.): Equine Clinical Neonatology. Philadelphia, Lea & Febiger, 1990.
4. Koterba, A.M., and Drummond, W.H.: Equine clinical neonatology in the USA: Past, present and future. Equine Vet. J. *5(Suppl.):*6–10, 1988.
5. Baker, S.M., Drummond, W.H., Lane, T.J., and Koterba, A.M.: Follow-up evaluation of horses after neonatal intensive care. J. Am. Vet. Med. Assoc., *189:*1454–1457, 1986.
6. Brewer, B.D.: Equine neonatal intensive care: success or failure? Compend. Contin. Educ. Practicing Vet., *12:*415–418, 1990.
7. Rossdale, P.D.: Perinatology: An end and a beginning. Equine Vet. J. *5(Suppl):*19–24, 1988.
8. Brewer, B.D., and Koterba, A.M.: Development of a scoring system for the early diagnosis of equine neonatal sepsis. Equine Vet. J., *20:*18–22, 1988.
9. Koterba, A.M., Chase, J.P., and Bain, F.T.: Development and evaluation of a scoring system predicting mortality in premature and immature equine neonates undergoing intensive care. Equine Vet. J. *5(Suppl.):*56, 1988.
10. Koterba, A.M.: Equine neonatal intensive care at the University of Florida 1982–1987: An update. Proc. Am. Assoc. Equine Pract., 805–816, 1987.
11. Adams, R., and Mayhew, I.G.: Neurologic examination of the newborn foal. Equine Vet. J., *16:*306–312, 1984.
12. Adams, R., and Poulos, P.: A skeletal ossification index for neonatal foals. Vet. Radiol., *29:*217–222, 1988.
13. Koterba, A.M.: Intrauterine growth retardation. Proceedings of the American College of Veterinary Internal Medicine Forum. 1989, pp. 413–415.
14. Drummond, W.H.: Acute asphyxia in the newborn: Effects and management. Proceedings of the American College of Veterinary Internal Medicine Forum. 1989, pp. 421–425.
15. Koterba, A.M., Brewer, B.D., and Tarplee, F.A.: Clinical and clinicopathological characteristics of the septicemic neonatal foal: Review of 38 cases. Equine Vet. J., *16:*376–383, 1984.
16. Kaufman J.: Nosocomial infections: Klebsiella. Compend. Contin. Educ. Practicing Vet., *6:*303–310, 1984.
17. Koterba, A.M., et al.: Nosocomial infections and bacterial antibiotic resistance in a university equine hospital. J. Am. Vet. Med. Assoc., *189:*185–191, 1986.

CHAPTER 111

THE IMMUNE SYSTEM

J.J. McClure

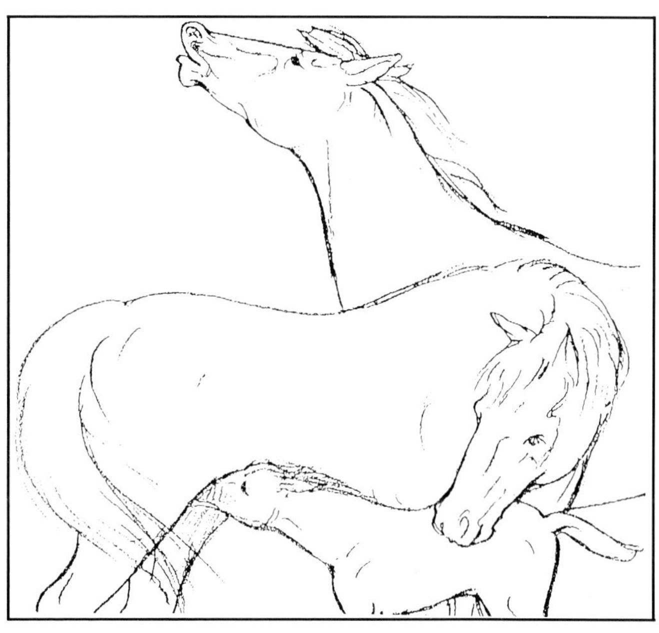

DISORDERS OF PASSIVE IMMUNITY

The neonatal foal is thrust from a sterile, protected environment into a hostile, contaminated world in an instant. While the foal's immune system is functional and able to respond to external challenges at birth, it is totally (immunologically) naive and vulnerable to the challenges of the outside world.

To protect neonates under these circumstances, nature has devised ways of temporarily providing protection against external challenges of the environment until the foal's own immune system matures sufficiently to assume that task. These mechanisms are considered passive immunity.

The most significant component of passive immunity in foals is colostral immunoglobulins.[1–3] In horses, the diffuse epitheliochorial form of placentation prevents transplacental passage of large molecules such as immunoglobulins from mare to foal during pregnancy under usual circumstances. For this reason, the normal foal is born essentially devoid of immunoglobulin except for a small amount of IgM, which it synthesizes itself in utero.[4] Before parturition, large quantities of immunoglobulins are secreted into the milk from the blood of the mare, forming one component of colostrum. When ingested and absorbed by the foal, the preformed antibodies in this colostrum help provide temporary protection against microbial invaders until autogenous production of immunoglobulin by the foal, which begins at birth, reaches protective concentrations.

Two disorders of passive immunity in foals have been recognized. These can be characterized as resulting from either the presence of a harmful antibody in the colostrum (e.g., neonatal isoerythrolysis [NI]) or deficiencies of colostral antibody (e.g., failure of passive transfer [FPT]).

NEONATAL ISOERYTHROLYSIS

Neonatal isoerythrolysis (NI) has also been known as hemolytic disease of the newborn foal (HDNF) and hemolytic icterus.[5,6]

PATHOGENESIS

Neonatal isoerythrolysis results from the destruction of the foal's red blood cells (RBCs) by colostral maternal antibody. Offending antibody is produced by the mare on exposure to red blood cells (often the foal's) which are of an antigen type different from its own. The most likely natural sources of exposure of the mare to incompatible blood cells are retroplacental hemorrhages during pregnancy and hemorrhage present at parturition.[5,6] Exposure can also result from blood transfusion. Historically, tissue vaccines containing RBC antigens were notorious for sensitizing mares; however, this has not been a problem recently.[6] Most cases of NI occur in multiparous mares, although NI can occur during the first pregnancy.

When a mare produces anti–red blood cell antibody, it is secreted and concentrated in the colostrum near parturition just as are all other antibodies. When the foal nurses, these antibodies are absorbed and enter its circulation. If the foal's RBCs have the antigen against which the antibodies are directed, the antibodies will react with the RBCs and result in either their premature removal by the reticuloendothelial system or their intravascular lysis.[6] The accelerated destruction and/or removal of RBCs may result in anemia with subsequent decreased oxygen carrying capacity of the blood and/or pigment nephropathy.

Although more than 30 different RBC antigens have been characterized in horses, most cases of NI have been associated with antibody directed against *Aa* and *Qa*.[5–9] Rarely, NI may result from incompatibilities in other factors in horses. Different factors may be involved in NI in mules. Red blood cell factors are inherited as codominant traits.[6,9,10] That is, a foal will exhibit both the allele inherited from the sire and the allele inherited from the dam on its red blood cells. In almost all pregnancies, some degree of incompatibility between the mare and stallion is present; however, the vast majority of these are clinically inconsequential in regard to disease.[7,8] Some factors are virtually absent in certain breeds (e.g., *Qa* in Standardbreds) and, therefore, NI caused by incompatibilities between the stallion and mare for these factors does not occur.[7,8] The frequency with which offending factors occurs varies among breeds.[10]

A number of conditions must be met for NI to naturally occur. Only mares which do not have a factor on their RBCs can make antibodies against that factor. An at risk mare must become sensitized to the factor which she lacks (meaning that she must somehow be exposed to the RBC antigen) and must make antibodies against it. The mare must then be bred to a stallion that has the antigen that the mare lacks). The foal must then inherit the incompatible blood factor from the sire. The antibody must subsequently be concentrated in the colostrum, and the foal must ingest sufficient colostrum that contains the offending antibody.

CLINICAL SIGNS

Clinical syndromes associated with NI can be peracute (occurring within a matter of hours after birth) to acute (occurring over several days), depending on the particular antibody involved and the amount ingested. Classically, foals develop clinical signs within the first 24 to 48 h, characterized by icterus or pallor and tachypnea.

Hemoglobinuria and hemoglobinemia (pinkish discoloration of the serum) may be evident in these foals. The packed cell volume (PCV) and other indicators of RBC status such as the RBC count and hemoglobin, will be decreased. Foals initially are bright and alert and afebrile. Clinical signs may progress to depression and lethargy, and the foal may eventually collapse and seizure if the anemia is severe. In some cases, RBC destruction is slower and few clinical signs except icterus may occur. The onset of icterus in these cases is often several days after birth.

In peracute cases, lysis of RBCs may occur so quickly that icterus does not have time to develop by the onset of other clinical signs. These foals' mucous membranes are generally pale as opposed to yellow. Because of this, NI is sometimes erroneously left off a differential list because of the absence of icterus. This form of NI is highly fatal, and death often occurs before the disease can be recognized and treated. Neonatal isoerythrolysis should be suspected clinically based on either the presence of icterus in a foal less than 7 days of age or a foal with extreme pallor less than 24 h of age.

A complete blood count will show the presence of anemia. The degree of anemia is variable, depending on the strength and amount of offending antibody. The PCV in most cases will be less than 22%, and in severe cases may be less than 10%. Serial PCV evaluations are extremely useful in evaluating the course of disease and determining need for therapy.

Other blood biochemical parameters may be altered as a result of RBC destruction. Bilirubin is generally increased. Serum potassium may be increased because of RBC destruction. Abnormalities of glucose, blood gases, and electrolytes may accompany the disease as the foal becomes more stressed.

DIAGNOSIS

Specific diagnostic tests for NI all share the characteristic that they demonstrate the presence of maternal anti-RBC antibody. Maternal anti-RBC antibody can be detected in the mare's plasma, serum, or colostrum or attached to the RBC of the affected foal.

Routine cross-matching agglutination tests which use the mare's serum or colostrum and the foal's RBC are useful in detecting some cases of NI; however, they do not allow detection of all cases of NI.[5,6,11] This is related to the fact that most offending antibodies are IgG rather than IgM, and IgG is less efficient at causing agglutination. The jaundiced foal agglutination (JFA) test is an improved crossmatching test which employs a centrifugation step.[7] Results of the JFA test compare well with results of standard saline agglutination and complement-mediated hemolytic tests. The JFA test is rapid and simple and can be performed using the mare's colostrum and her foal's RBC before allowing the foal to nurse.

The presence of potentially offending antibody in mare's serum and/or colostrum can also be detected by standard saline agglutination and complement-mediated hemolytic activity using a panel of RBCs from horses with different blood types.[5–8] Using this approach, the specificity of an antibody can generally be determined (e.g., which specific factor the antibody is directed against). Because this method does not consider the blood type of the foal, it only predicts the possibility of a problem if the foal has the blood type against which the antibody is directed.

A direct Coombs' antiglobulin test can be performed

to detect the presence of antibody on the foal's RBCs.[5] Specific equine reagents must be used as human Coombs' reagents will not work. Free circulating antibody directed against the RBCs is not usually present in the foal's serum, because it attaches to the RBC factors making the foal's serum a poor place to look for offending antibody. Indirect Coombs' tests using sera from the mare and a panel of RBCs from horses representing a variety of blood groups can also be done.[5]

THERAPY

Therapy for affected foals may include both nonspecific support and specific provision of RBCs. Nonspecific therapy may include fluids and electrolytes, antibiotics, and nursing care. Limitation of exercise with stall confinement is important in the management of foals with NI because they may collapse with even limited exertion. Administration of intravenous fluids containing balanced electrolytes and, in some cases, glucose solutions may be indicated to treat dehydration and to induce diuresis particularly in cases where pigment nephropathy is of concern.

In cases for which anemia is severe, additional RBCs should be provided by transfusion. If the PCV remains above 15% and is stable, transfusions are probably not necessary if exercise is restricted and other supportive care is given. However, if the PCV is between 20 and 15% and falling, provision should be made for transfusion.

The major consideration in the selection of a RBC donor is that the foal needs RBCs which will not be destroyed by the maternal anti-RBC antibody present. Cells from the foal's sire are not the ideal RBC because they will have the same RBC factor as the foal and will be subject to destruction the same as the foal's cells.

The ideal RBCs would be those from the mare, because obviously they do not react with her own antibodies. However, because the mare's plasma contains antibodies which are harmful to the foal's cells, whole blood should not be used without washing the RBCs free of plasma before administration to avoid compounding the problems.

Any horse which lacks the factor to which the anti-RBC antibodies are directed (usually *Aa* or *Qa*) is potentially a suitable donor. These individuals can be identified by standard blood typing or by cross matching the donor RBCs with the questionable sera or colostrum from the mare. Standard blood typing is seldom available on an emergency basis; however, prospective donors can be screened in advance to identify those horses which are negative for both factors *Aa* and *Qa* and lack anti-RBC antibody in their sera for use in situations in which laboratory support is unavailable.

Based on the frequency with which factors *Aa* and *Qa* (the most frequently offending factors) occur in the population, most horses, depending on breed, will have these factors on their RBCs.[7,10] This means that the odds of randomly selecting a horse which is negative for the factor causing the problem, regardless of sex, breeding, or transfusion history of the prospective donor, are not good and such transfusions should not be done without performing a cross match between donor cells and the mare's serum or colostrum.

Mare's RBCs can be washed using the following procedure. Blood is collected (4 to 8 L can generally be collected from a full-size horse) in 3.8% sodium citrate (w/v) or acid citrate dextrose (ACD) using one part sodium citrate or ACD for each nine parts blood. If a large-volume centrifuge is available, the procedure can be done quite rapidly by centrifugation; however, the process can also be done by gravity sedimentation. Using sedimentation, the blood is allowed to settle several hours until the RBCs and plasma have separated. The plasma is then removed by aspiration from the RBCs, and a volume of sterile, room temperature 0.9% NaCl sufficient to produce a 50% suspension of RBCs is added. The RBCs and NaCl are mixed, and the suspension is allowed to settle again. The RBCs do not sediment as rapidly or as completely in the NaCl as they do in plasma. When the RBCs have sedimented, the NaCl is removed and the RBCs are again suspended to approximately 50%. This process can be repeated again; however, even a single wash will generally dilute out the offending antibody sufficiently for use. Because the sedimentation process requires a minimum of several hours, the clinician must start the procedure early based on anticipated need.

Approximately 1 to 4 L of the washed RBC suspension administered intravenously may be needed to supply adequate RBCs for the foal. Half of the volume can be given quite rapidly (within a 30- to 60-min period) and the other half can be given slowly over several hours with care taken not to volume overload the foal.[5] A blood administration set with a filter must be used to administer the washed RBCs. The transfused RBCs will be quickly removed from the foal's circulation, and the PCV drops gradually over several days after the transfusion before stabilizing. Transfusion may sensitize the foal to any factors which are present on the donor's RBCs and absent on its own cells, but this is of little consequence in the immediate transfusion period.

PREVENTION

Neonatal isoerythrolysis is a preventable disease with proper management. Those mares which are at risk (e.g., negative for factors *Aa* and/or *Qa*) can be identified by blood typing. These mares can then be screened for the production of anti-RBC antibody late in pregnancy by a blood typing laboratory or the colostrum can be tested for the presence of antibody which reacts with the foal's RBCs using the JFA test before allowing the foal to nurse.

Selection of a stallion which lacks the same RBC factor(s) as the mare, thereby eliminating the possibility of an incompatibility between the mare and foal, can also be done. However, identification of a stallion which has a compatible blood type and also meets other breeding criteria is often difficult because the number of compatible horses may be significantly less than those which are incompatible.[7]

JAUNDICED FOAL AGGLUTINATION TEST (JFA)

Materials

1. Centrifuge capable of centrifuging blood tubes at moderate speeds (300 to 600 g).[7]
2. Test tube rack.
3. Test tubes, either 13 × 100 mm disposable tubes or blood collection tubes.
4. Pasteur pipettes and rubber bulbs or other pipette system to deliver 1.0 mL volumes.
5. Room temperature 0.9% NaCl.
6. Serum or colostrum from mare and blood from mare and foal, preferably in EDTA anticoagulant.

Methods

1. Collect colostrum from mare.
2. Collect blood in anticoagulant from the foal.
3. Make serial dilutions of the colostrum with 0.9% NaCl solution as follows: 1:2, 1:4, 1:8, 1:16, and 1:32; total volume in each tube is approximately 1 mL.
4. Add one drop of the foal's whole blood to each tube and mix.
5. Centrifuge the tubes for 2 to 3 min at medium speed (300 to 500 g).
6. Invert each tube, one at a time, pouring out the liquid contents; observe the status of the button of the RBCs at the bottom of the tube (Fig. 111–1).

Complete agglutination causes the cells to remain tightly packed in the button; strong agglutination causes the cells to remain in large clumps; for weaker agglutination, the cells are in smaller clumps as they run down the side of the tube. When no agglutination exists the cells easily flow down the side of the tube.

Two controls should also be run when a positive reaction to the JFA test occurs. The blood should be tested with 0.9% NaCl alone to be certain the cells do not agglutinate by themselves. Colostrum should be tested with the dam's own cells to be certain that it is not the conditions of the test or viscosity of the colostrum which is causing the agglutination.

Positive reactions at 1:16 or greater are considered significant. At concentrations of 1:16 or greater, this test correlates well with the standard hemolytic assay. At dilutions less than 1:16, the correlation is not as strong and more false positives will be recorded. Other factors such as colostral viscosity make less diluted samples more difficult to read at lower dilutions.

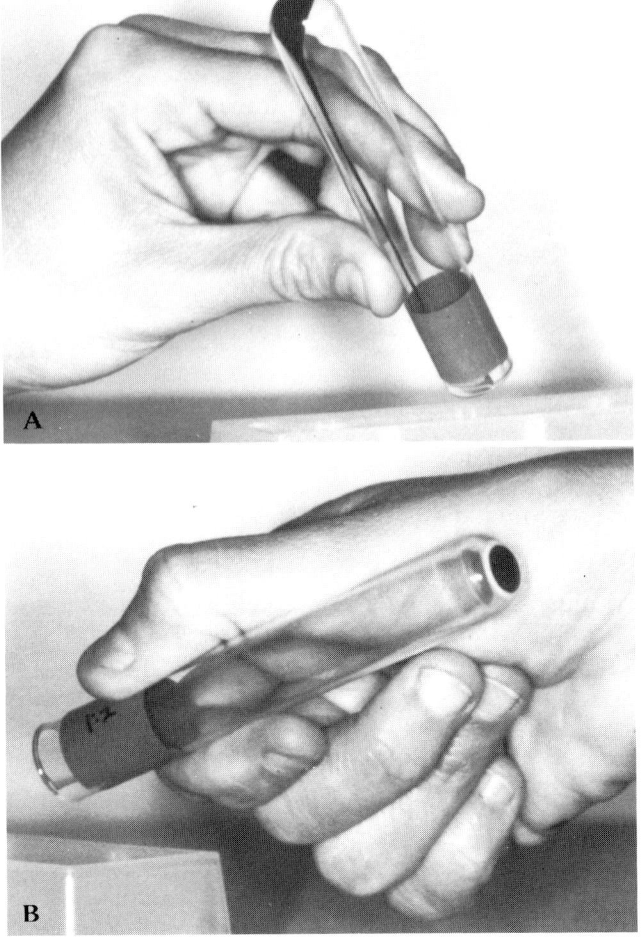

FIG. 111–1. Jaundiced foal agglutination test. *A*, The pelleted red blood cells flow smoothly down the side of the tube in negative samples (no offending antibody) when the tube is inverted. *B*, In strongly positive samples (offending antibody present), the red blood cell pellet remains in the bottom of the tube when the tube is inverted.

FAILURE OF PASSIVE TRANSFER AND FOAL SEPTICEMIA

Foals are devoid of immunoglobulins at birth except for a small amount of IgM produced in utero.[4] Significant amounts of IgG and IgG(T) and lesser amounts of IgM and other immunoglobulin classes are normally absorbed by the foal from colostrum and provide significant, transient protection against infectious agents.[4,12] The minimum concentration of IgG considered to be adequate passive transfer (achieved within 24 h of birth) ranges from 400 to 800 mg/dL in the foal's serum.[3,13] The lower range may be adequate to maintain health in foals in relatively clean environments and not heavily exposed to pathogens, but it is not considered adequate in foals showing evidence of infection.

Failure of the foal to achieve adequate concentrations of maternal immunoglobulin transfer can occur as a result of low immunoglobulin content of colostrum caused by premature lactation or failure of the mare to secrete immunoglobulin into the colostrum, failure of the foal to ingest colostrum because of weakness, death or disability of the mare, or failure of the foal to absorb colostrum within the period of time following birth before gut "closure."[1,14]

Colostrum is produced during the final weeks of pregnancy. The foal is capable of nonselective absorption of proteins from colostrum, including immunoglobulins, within the first 8 to 12 h after birth. Both the production of colostrum and absorption by the foal taper off rapidly from birth to 12 h.

The quality of colostrum in regard to immunoglobulin content can be evaluated based on specific gravity using a modified hydrometer (Equine Colostrometer, Lane Manufacturing, Inc., Denver, CO) or by measurement of IgG by radial immunodiffusion (Fig. 111–2). Good-quality colostrum should have a specific gravity of at least 1.060, which corresponds to an immunoglobulin content of approximately 3000 mg/dL.[15,16]

CLINICAL SIGNS

Failure of passive transfer (FPT) has no primary symptoms apart from the development of infections. It is a major underlying factor in most neonatal septicemias and bacterial infections.[1–3,13] Neonatal sepsis can be surprisingly difficult to recognize in early stages, because affected foals may not show the expected signs of infection such as fever or leukocytosis. Recognition of historical and environmental factors which predispose to septicemia in addition to those which suggest the possibility of FPT can help identify high-risk individuals for early intervention. Foals born in unsanitary, overcrowded, or poorly ventilated conditions receive a higher exposure to potential pathogens. Foals born of mares with chronic health problems or poor nutritional status are also at higher risk for septicemia. Foals born of mares transported long distances within 30 days of foaling also seem to be at increased risk.[13,17,18]

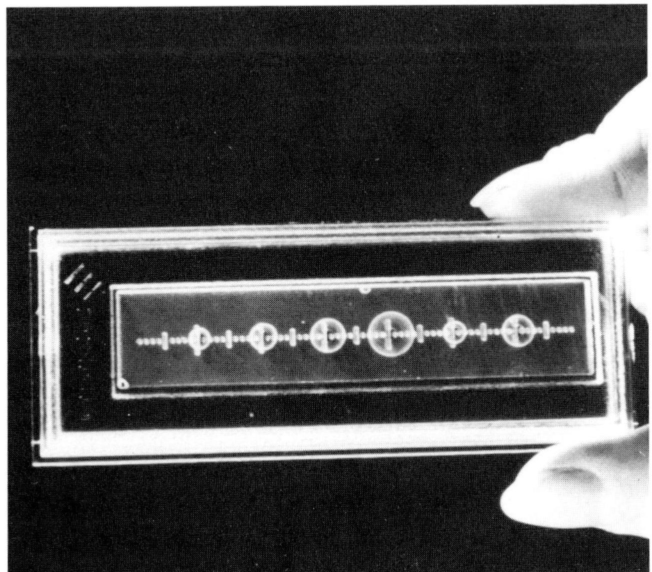

FIG. 111–2. Radial immunodiffusion test (Equine R.I.D. Test) for equine IgG. The diameter of the precipitation circle which develops in the reagent-impregnated gel is directly proportional to the amount of IgG in the sample. IgG can be accurately quantitated by comparing the patient's value with known standards.

Problems encountered during labor and delivery (dystocia, premature placental separation, induction of parturition, and twins) and placental abnormalities (placentitis, villus atrophy, and edema) seem to predispose a foal to infections. Premature foals, small for gestational age foals, postmature (> 365 days) foals, and foals which fail to show normal behavior after birth (delayed suckle reflex, maladjustment, and colic) are also considered at risk.[13,18,19] The presence of any of these factors should heighten the awareness of possible neonatal septicemia and prompt particular attention to detection of early signs.

Infections may be acquired in utero, during delivery, or after delivery. In utero acquired infections may ascend from the vagina, arrive hematogenously, or invade directly through the uterine wall. Placental disease may be present; however, the severity of placentitis does not accurately predict the severity of illness in the newborn foal. Signs of in utero acquired infection usually occur within 24 h of life.[17] Any weak or depressed foal after delivery should be considered at risk for septicemia.

Infection during the birth process or in the neonatal period may be acquired via the oral, respiratory, or umbilical routes. Perinatal stress (dystocia) and meconium staining of the foal signal an increased risk of infection by these routes. Infections acquired after delivery frequently result from FPT, poor environmental conditions, or endemic pathogens on the farm. Foals with disease conditions requiring medical intervention are at risk for iatrogenic introduction of infection (catheter, ventilator, and nosocomial agents).[17] Postnatally acquired infections generally first manifest themselves between 2 and 4 days of age. Sites of focal infection associated with neonatal septicemia most commonly include the lungs, joints, intestinal tract, and umbilicus.

Early recognition of problems and prompt initiation of treatment is imperative to achieve successful clinical outcomes. Severe disease may be present before any clinical signs are observed. The early signs of neonatal septicemia are subtle but rapidly progressive. They are often not referable to any particular system or anatomic area. Early signs include slight lethargy, weakening suckle reflex, diminishing appetite, and increased time spent in lateral recumbency. Observation of these signs in a foal, particularly one deemed to be at risk based on historical or environmental factors, should prompt a thorough examination. Signs of septicemia may parallel those of other diseases, including trauma (lameness), neonatal maladjustment (seizures), and foal heat diarrhea.

A host of abnormal findings may be present in septicemia; however, none is either consistently present or constant in character.[13,18] Body temperature may be elevated, depressed, or normal. Mucous membranes may be congested, mottled, pale, cyanotic, or muddy. Petechiation of the pinnae of the ear, sclera, and other mucous membranes suggest septicemia but are not consistently present. Localization of infection in the lungs may be characterized by tachypnea, respiratory distress, or apnea. Gastrointestinal manifestations may include diarrhea, ileus, abdominal distention, colic, and inappetence. Increased heart rate (> 120 beats per minute) and prolonged capillary refill (> 2 s) suggest cardiovascular compromise but may also reflect pain and excitement or blood loss, respectively. Ocular changes including hypopyon and uveitis suggest systemic or focal disease. Lameness with or without joint enlargement or focal pain may be present and mistaken for traumatic injury in the absence of generalized signs early in the course of sepsis. Enlargement of, discharge from, or heat in the umbilicus is suggestive of infection; however, at times the umbilicus may be infected with no externally clinically obvious signs. Seizures suggestive of neonatal maladjustment syndrome may also characterize septicemia. Septicemia should be assumed if any of these signs are present until proven otherwise.

DIAGNOSIS OF SEPTICEMIA

Laboratory tests which are of value in detection of septicemia include a complete blood count (CBC), which includes fibrinogen, blood glucose, and blood gases.[13,17] Of the white blood cell (WBC) parameters, the number of band neutrophils and the presence or absence of toxic changes (Döhle inclusion bodies, toxic granulation, basophilic cytoplasm, and cytoplasmic vacuolization) within neutrophils are significant indicators of sepsis. The total WBC count and total number of neutrophils show no constant trend and can be either elevated or depressed. Fibrinogen is generally increased in septic foals, suggesting active inflammation. Hypoglycemia (< 90 mg/dL glucose) and metabolic acidosis are present in a large portion of septic foals.[17,18] Evaluation of passive transfer by measurement of IgG concentrations is also important because a large proportion of the FPT foals become septicemic.[13,18]

No single sign or laboratory finding confirms the presence of septicemia and no individual sign is consistently present in all cases. For these reasons, the sepsis score, which evaluates a number of discriminating factors, is a useful aid in diagnosis and evaluation of septicemia in foals less than 14 days of age (Table 111–1).[17,20,21] The sepsis score assigns a value to each significant variable evaluated from 0 to 4. The scores for each item for the patient are then totaled up, and if the sum equals or exceeds a certain level (11 for the modified sepsis score of Brewer[17] and Brewer et al.[21]), the foal is considered infected. The scoring system is not perfect, and if a high clinical suspicion of infection exists, treatment should be initiated regardless of the sepsis score.

Positive blood cultures are the only definitive antemortem proof of bacteremia. However, culture results take time, even for preliminary results, and treatment should not be delayed pending results.

DIAGNOSIS OF FAILURE OF PASSIVE TRANSFER

The diagnosis of FPT is based on the demonstration of serum immunoglobulin concentrations less than 800 mg/dL in the foal at 18 to 24 h of age. An immunoglobulin concentration of 400 mg/dL may be adequate in healthy foals; however, in foals showing signs of infectious disease, a concentration of 800 mg/dL is felt to be the minimum acceptable concentration.[3,13] The amount of circulating immunoglobulin varies with age and the amount of maternal immunoglobulin absorbed within the first 24 h. The half-life of maternal IgG is approximately 3 weeks. As maternal immunoglobulin declines, the concentration of immunoglobulin produced by the foal increases such that the immunoglobulin concentrations normally do not fall to dangerously low concentrations. Older foals (up to several weeks of age) with immunoglobulin concentrations less than 400 to 800 mg/dL may benefit from plasma transfusion, particularly if evidence of sepsis is present or the environment is heavily contaminated.

Numerous semiquantitative test kits are available to measure plasma immunoglobulin concentrations (Table 111–2) including zinc sulfate turbidity (Fig. 111–3), latex agglutination, enzyme-linked immunosorbent assay (ELISA) (Fig. 111–4), and hemagglutination inhibition tests (Fig. 111–5). These kits have the advantage of speed, economy, and convenience. IgG can be quantitated more precisely by radial immunodiffusion (RID) (Fig. 111–2); however, the test requires 18 to 24 h for results.

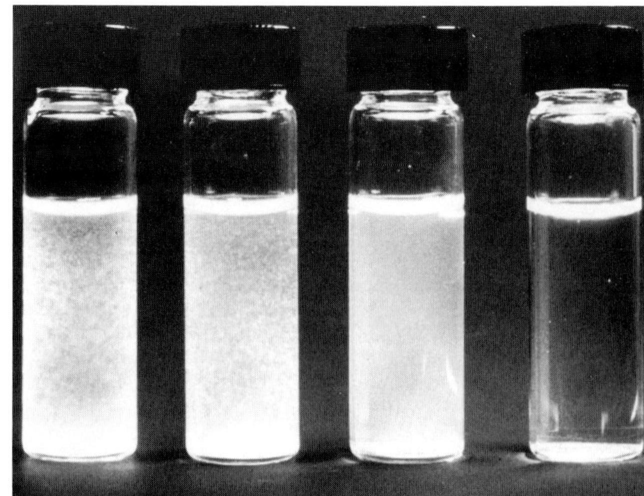

FIG. 111–3. Zinc sulfate turbidity test (Equi-Z) of IgG. The degree of turbidity which develops in test solutions is directly proportional to the amount of IgG in the test serum.

TABLE 111–1. SEPSIS SCORE (MODIFIED)

INFORMATION COLLECTED	NUMBER OF POINTS TO ASSIGN	4	3	2	1	0	THIS CASE
CBC							
Neutrophil count/mm³ (not total WBC)	Record exact number		< 2,000	2,000–4,000 or > 12,000	8,000–12,000	Normal	
Band neutrophil count/mm³			> 200	50–200		< 50	
Doehle bodies, toxic granulation, or vacuolization in neutrophils		Marked	Moderate	Slight		None	
Fibrinogen (mg/dL)				> 600	410–600	≤ 400	
Other laboratory data							
Hypoglycemia (mg/dL)				< 50	50–80	> 80	
Zinc sulfate turbidity test (ZST) (or other IgG test) (mg/dL)*		< 200	200–400	410–800		> 800	
Clinical examination							
Petechiation or scleral injection not secondary to eye disease or trauma			Marked	Moderate	Mild	None	
Fever				> 38.9° C	< 37.8° C	Normal	
Hypotonia, coma, depression, convulsions				Marked	Mild	Normal	
Anterior uveitis, diarrhea, respiratory distress, swollen joints, open wounds			Yes			No	
Historical Data							
Placentitis, vulvar discharge prior to delivery, dystocia, long transport of mare, mare sick, foal induced			Yes			No	
Prematurity			< 300 days	300–310	311–330	> 330	
Total points†							

*If a foal is older than 12 h, compute the ZST score using the actual serum immunoglobulin concentration. If less than 12 h, give 2+ for ZST if history of nursing what appeared to be good colostrum. Give the foal a 4+ if it has not nursed or if in doubt.

†A score of 11 or higher correctly predicts sepsis > 90% of the time. A score of 10 or less predicts nonsepsis correctly > 85% of the time.

(Adapted from Brewer, B.D.: Neonatal infection. *In* Equine Clinical Neonatology. Edited by A.M. Koterba, W.H. Drummond, and P.C. Kosh. Philadelphia, Lea & Febiger, 1990, pp. 295–316. Brewer, B.D., and Koterba, A.M.: Development of a scoring system for the early diagnosis of equine neonatal sepsis. Equine Vet. J., *20:*18–22, 1988. Brewer, B.C., Koterba, A.M., Carter, R.L., and Rowe, E.D.: Comparison of empirically developed sepis score with a computer generated and weighed scoring system for the identification of sepsis in the equine neonate. Equine Vet. J., *20:*23–24, 1988.)

MANAGEMENT OF FPT

Anticipated FPT—Foal Less Than 12 h Old

Failure of passive transfer may be anticipated if the mare experiences premature lactation, colostrum specific gravity is < 1.060, or the foal does not nurse adequately because of disability of the mare or foal. In these cases, an alternate source of colostrum should be provided as soon as possible within the first 12 h after birth. A total of 2 to 3 L of colostrum divided into three or four doses at hourly intervals should be provided if available. The colostrum can be administered via nasogastric tube or by allowing the foal to suck a bottle. Lyophilized equine IgG (Foal-Aide, Equilab, Rockville, MD) may also be administered orally. Doses as high as 40 to 60 g IgG are needed to raise plasma IgG concentrations from 0 to > 400 mg/dL in an average-size foal.[22] If colostrum or lyophilized IgG is not available, serum or plasma can be fed orally, although volumes as large as 6 to 9 L of plasma may be required for adequate transfer.[14] Serum immunoglobulin concentrations in the foal should be measured at 18 to 24 h of

TABLE 111–2. COMMERCIALLY AVAILABLE TEST KITS FOR DETECTION OF FAILURE OF PASSIVE TRANSFER IN HORSES

TEST	SOURCE	SAMPLE TYPE	COMMENTS
Radial immunodiffusion (Equine R.I.D. Test)	VMRD, Inc., Pullman, WA	Serum	Accurate, but takes 18 to 24 h for results
Zinc sulfate turbidity (Equi-Z)	VMRD, Inc., Pullman, WA	Serum	Quantitative
Latex agglutination (FoalChek)	Haver Mobay Corp., Shawnee, KS	Serum, whole blood	Semiquantitative
ELISA (CITE Foal IgG Test)	AgriTech Systems, Inc., Portland, ME	Serum, whole blood	Semiquantitative, 400 to 800 mg/dL
Hemagglutination inhibition (One-Step IgG Screen)	Hamilton-Thorn Research, Danvers, MA	Whole blood	Semiquantitative 400 to 800 mg/dL

age to determine if adequate concentrations have been obtained. Administration of an alternate colostrum source is generally safe with the exception of overloading the stomach, producing colic, or administering colostrum that contains anti-RBC antibody which might react with the foal's RBCs.

Bovine colostrum has been used as an alternate source of colostrum for foals.[23,24] Bovine immunoglobulins are absorbed by the foal in the immediate perinatal period and reach significant concentrations in the blood. The half-life of bovine immunoglobulins is much shorter in horses than that of equine immunoglobulins and the antibody specificity may not be ideal. However, some beneficial effect may be achieved, and bovine colostrum is generally more readily available than equine colostrum. Kits available for equine IgG quantitation cannot be used to assess the adequacy of colostral transfer of bovine immunoglobulin.

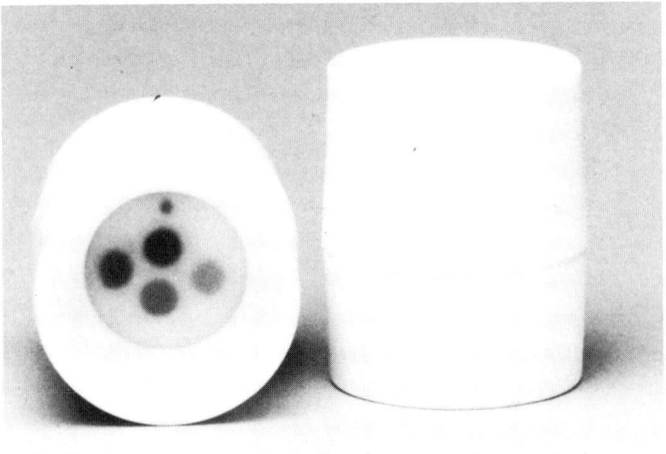

FIG. 111–4. Enzyme-linked immunoassay test (CITE Foal IgG Test) for equine IgG. The color development (darkness) of the dot representing patient IgG (top center dot below the small dot) is compared with the dots representing 200 (right), 400 (bottom), and 800 (left) mg IgG/dL.

Unanticipated FPT—Foal More Than 12 h Old

If serum immunoglobulin concentrations are found to be deficient after 18 to 24 h of age, then oral supplementation with colostrum or serum will be ineffective because of the closure of the gut to immunoglobulin transfer. Depending on the level of transfer, age at diagnosis and environment, plasma (or serum) transfusion may be indicated. Foals with less than 200 mg/dL of IgG at any age or foals 1 week old or younger with less than 400 mg/dL should always be treated. Foals younger than 6 weeks of age with less than 400 mg/dL IgG should be treated if they show evidence of sepsis or are maintained in contaminated conditions or are moved to new environments. If evidence of sepsis is present or if environmental exposure to pathogens appears excessive, the aim of transfusion should be to provide concentrations of at least 800 mg/dL IgG.

The volume of normal plasma required to raise plasma IgG to adequate concentrations is variable. Formulas based on degree of passive transfer, weight of the foal, and the concentration of IgG in the donor plasma have been suggested to determine the quantity of plasma for transfusion.[14,25,26] However, expected results in terms of final plasma concentration of immunoglobulin in the transfused foal are frequently not achieved. A standard dose of plasma for a foal with FPT has been suggested to be 20 mg/kg, which is equivalent to 1 to 1.5 L of normal plasma.[14,25,26] However, this dose is generally inadequate and often 2 to 4 L of normal plasma (IgG concentration between 1000 and 2000 mg/dL) are required to achieve desired concentrations of immunoglobulin in the foal. Normal equine plasma may be purchased commercially (Foalimmune, Lake Immunogenics, Inc., Ontario, NY; Equine Plasma, Veterinary Dynamics, Inc., Chino, CA) or prepared on site. Commercial plasmas are screened for presence of anti-RBC antibodies, are produced for hyperimmunization against various equine diseases, and are convenient to use. They are, however, quite expensive; the cost to the veterinarian is generally more than $100 per liter. The donors of locally prepared plasma should be free of dis-

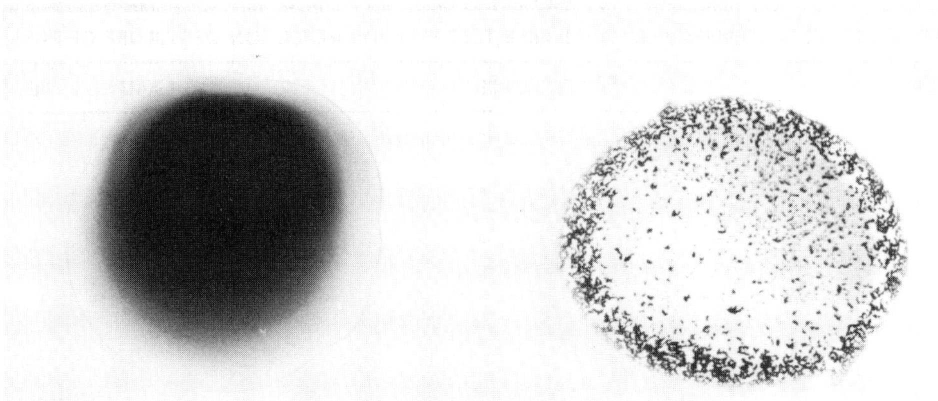

FIG. 111–5. Hemagglutination inhibition test (One-Step IgG Screen) for equine IgG. The presence of IgG in a sample inhibits the agglutination of patient RBCs used in the test. Agglutination of the sample means that the IgG level is below the labeled concentration of the test (either 400 or 800 mg/dL).

ease, test negative for equine infectious anemia, and be screened for the presence of anti-RBC antibody in their serum. Concentrated immunoglobulin products are commercially available; administration of a smaller volume of those products may provide adequate immunoglobulin concentrations (HiGamm-Equi, Lake Immunogenics, Inc.; Amer-Vet Serum, Amer-Vet Labs, Addison, IL). Because of the variability observed in final IgG concentrations regardless of the type of product used, the clinician is advised to recheck the immunoglobulin concentrations after transfusion to ensure that sufficient concentrations have been achieved.

Additional Considerations in Management of Neonatal Sepsis

Antibiotic therapy should be instituted as soon as sepsis is suspected without waiting for culture results. Gram-negative infections are common;[13,18] therefore, the clinician must select broad-spectrum agents pending actual culture results. A combination of penicillin and an aminoglycoside (gentamicin or amikacin) generally provides adequate antimicrobial coverage. The susceptibility of microbial agents to trimethoprim-sulfa and ampicillin is quite variable, and use of these and other antimicrobial agents should be guided by culture and sensitivity testing. Prophylactic use of antibiotics on a farm encourages development of resistant strains, and any antimicrobial agent used under these circumstances should be avoided as a first-use drug.

The duration of antimicrobial treatment is variable but in all circumstances should probably be at least 7 to 10 days. Patients with documented septicemia based on blood culture with no evidence of localized infections should probably be treated for a minimum of 2 weeks. The development of localized infections often requires 3, 4 or more weeks of treatment. Fibrinogen concentration is a good indicator of active inflammation process, and as a rule of thumb, antimicrobial treatment should be continued as long as the fibrinogen is elevated. Blood cell counts can return to normal in the face of continued infection; thus, fibrinogen is more useful than WBC count as an indicator of active inflammation.[13,17]

Hypoglycemia, if present, can be treated by administration of 5 to 10% dextrose solutions intravenously (4 to 8 mg/kg/min). This dosage of glucose will help correct hypoglycemia but does not meet the foal's daily nutritional caloric requirement. Continuous infusion is preferred to bolus dosing of hypertonic (25 to 50%) dextrose. Administration of a bolus of hypertonic dextrose may aggravate central nervous system damage and frequently results in rebound hypoglycemia within an hour after administration.

Metabolic acidosis may complicate sepsis because of an accumulation of acid owing to poor tissue perfusion resulting from decreased cardiac output, asphyxia, pulmonary disease, or anemia. Acidosis may also occur because of loss of buffer from the body associated with diarrhea or renal dysfunction. In cases of poor tissue perfusion, volume expansion with intravenous fluids without sodium bicarbonate supplementation is preferable, particularly if pulmonary function is compromised. In the face of severe presumed bicarbonate losses, intravenous fluids supplemented with sodium bicarbonate may be used.

Good nursing care is important. Restraint and handling should be minimized by performing treatments in groups. General cleanliness is important to minimize iatrogenic infections. Recumbent foals must be kept clean and dry to prevent decubitus ulcers. If a foal has a poor suckle reflex and will not nurse from the mother or bottle, pan or nasogastric tube feeding must be substituted. Body temperature should be monitored and maintained using heat lamps, heat pads, hot water bottles, or blankets. Recumbent foals must be turned regularly.

DISORDERS OF ACTIVE IMMUNITY

The active immune response is incredibly complex, and many sites exist wherein defects can occur and result in a failure of the final response. Failure of the immune system leaves an individual vulnerable to a host of outside infectious invaders. Defects in the immune response can be characterized as primary or secondary. Primary defects are those for which a genetic basis is proven or suspected. Secondary defects are those for which the animal was initially capable of producing normal defense responses.

There have been numerous primary immunodeficiencies described in horses. Most are characterized by abnormalities in humoral immunity (immunoglobulin production), but this is because the tools exist to characterize antibody by class and quantity, whereas the clinician has more difficulty characterizing cellular aspects of the immune response.

In a sterile world, animals with immunodeficiencies would probably live an uneventful life or meet their demise as a result of noninfectious diseases. In the real world, animals affected with immunodeficiencies are constantly bombarded with external challenges against which they are unable or only partially able to defend themselves. These animals clinically encounter chronic, recurring nonresponsive infections caused by a variety of organisms and involving numerous body systems.

No external physical signs allow the identification of horses with primary immunodeficiencies or differentiate among the various immunodeficiencies. Affected animals, regardless of underlying defect, develop clinical signs which are the result of external infections.

The time of onset of infections associated with immunodeficiencies relates in large measure to the degree of passive transfer which the foal obtained and the type of defect. Adequate passive transfer confers a measure of protection until the maternal antibody is metabolized and will mask other immunodeficiencies for varying periods. Thus, in contrast to FPT in which clinical signs can occur within hours, clinical signs associated with most other immunodeficiencies appear at a later age of perhaps weeks to months.

COMBINED IMMUNODEFICIENCY

Combined immunodeficiency (CID) is a lethal genetic disease of Arabian and part-Arabian horses characterized by failure of the immune system.[27–30] Affected foals succumb to a variety of infectious agents and do not survive beyond 4 months of age. A similar condition has been reported in other breeds on rare occasions.[31] The condition is inherited as an autosomal recessive trait.[32,33] Both the sire and dam of an affected foal are carriers of the trait. As many as 25% of the Arabian horses in the United States may be carriers of the trait and the prevalence of CID in Arabian and part-Arabian foals may be between 2 and 3%.[28,34] At present, no way is known to identify carrier animals other than the production of an affected foal.

Foals affected with CID appear outwardly physically normal at birth. All clinical signs of CID which develop are referable to secondary infections. Bronchopneumonia is common, however; infectious lesions in other systems are also frequently found including arthritis, colitis, hepatitis, dermatitis, septicemia, and central nervous system infections. Pneumonia is often the result of infection with opportunistic agents such as adenovirus or Pneumocystis carinii. The age of onset of clinical infections varies with the degree of environmental exposure to organisms and the level of passive transfer achieved from the dam.

Combined immunodeficiency foals lack both humoral and cellular responses, such that many immunologic tests will be abnormal including lymphocyte blastogenesis,[35] skin testing,[36] quantitation of T cells and B cells by surface markers,[35] and immunoglobulin quantitation.[37] Two prominent diagnostic features of CID include an absolute lymphopenia ($< 1000/mm^3$) and the absence of serum IgM. Affected foals can be identified before onset of infectious disease and as early as immediately after birth if presuckle blood samples are collected and analyzed for absolute lymphocyte count and IgM. Less than 1000 lymphocytes/mm^3 and absence of IgM in presuckle serum are suggestive of combined immunodeficiency. The clinician must not base a diagnosis solely on lymphocyte count, because other conditions such as septicemia may be accompanied by lymphopenia in unaffected foals.

Affected foals which receive adequate colostral immunoglobulin transfer will have circulating maternal IgM for up to 3 weeks. [4] The absence of IgM in the face of adequate maternal transfer cannot be evaluated until after that time.

Histologic changes in lymphoid organs are fairly characteristic for CID and provide a third criterion for diagnosis in addition to lymphopenia and absence of IgM. The thymus of affected foals is hypoplastic with a scarcity of lymphocytes and is composed mostly of fat. The organ can be difficult to identify grossly at the time of necropsy. The spleen has an absence of germinal centers and periarteriolar lymphocyte sheaths. The lymph nodes are devoid of germinal centers and lymphocytes are scarce.[38,39] Because a diagnosis of CID implicates both the sire and dam as carriers of the CID trait,[32] diagnosis should only be made if lymphopenia, absence of IgM, and histologic evaluation confirm the diagnosis.

Although successful reconstitution of immunity in a CID foal using compatible bone marrow from an unaffected full sibling has been accomplished under experimental circumstances,[40] no treatment for the condition exists in a practical sense. Early diagnosis can save clients the expense of treatment and allow for appropriate genetic counseling.

SELECTIVE IGM DEFICIENCY

Selective IgM deficiency is characterized by a decrease or absence of IgM in the serum. As the name implies, foals affected with this condition selectively fail to produce IgM although they produce other classes of immunoglobulins in apparently normal or increased amounts.[41,42] Foals affected with this condition tend to suffer from respiratory infections, frequently caused by Klebsiella spp., as well as septic arthritis and enteritis. This condition is usually always fatal before 10 months of age, although recovery in one case has been reported.[42] Affected animals often have a long course of illness and debilitation with only transient responses to therapy.

Two other selective IgM deficiency syndromes have been described. One is associated with stunted growth and recurrent infections in young animals; death usually occurs between 1 and 2 y of age. The other syndrome occurs in horses usually between 2 and 5 y of age and is often associated with the presence of lymphosarcoma.[43]

Diagnosis of the condition is based on demonstration of low or undetectable concentrations of serum IgM in conjunction with normal lymphocyte counts and normal concentrations of IgG, IgA, and IgG(T). The normal concentration of IgM in the serum varies with age; however, in foals, a concentration less than 15 mg/dL should be considered significantly decreased. In case of adequate passive transfer of colostral immunoglobulin, maternal IgM may be present for up to 3 weeks and this must be considered when making a diagnosis.

Whether selective IgM deficiency is a primary or secondary (acquired) condition is not known; however, in foals a genetic basis is suspected, although the mode of inheritance is not clear. The condition has been reported to occur in several breeds, including Quarter Horse and Arabian.[41,42]

AGAMMAGLOBULINEMIA

Agammaglobulinemia is a rare primary immunodeficiency of horses. Foals with agammaglobulinemia have a defect somewhere in the early stages of immunoglobulin production which prevents the production of any class of immunoglobulin. Cell-mediated responses are relatively normal.[44–46]

Diagnosis is based on the absence of serum immunoglobulins. Some immunoglobulins may be present during the first few months of life, if passive transfer occurred, but in this case, serial evaluations should demonstrate the decreasing concentrations of immunoglobulin. Affected horses fail to respond to vaccination by production of specific antibody. The condition is ultimately fatal, although affected horses may live to be more than 1 yr of age. This condition has only been reported in males, suggesting an X-linked mode of inheritance.[44–46] A similar X-linked condition has been reported in humans.

TRANSIENT HYPOGAMMAGLOBULINEMIA

Transient hypogammaglobulinemia is a rare disorder characterized by the delayed onset of immunoglobulin synthesis by the foal.[2,42] Normally, the onset of production of immunoglobulins begins at birth when the foal is exposed to foreign antigens. In transient hypogammaglobulinemia, the onset is delayed, sometimes for as long as 3 months, although eventually production does occur. This condition can only be documented by serially monitoring immunoglobulin concentrations to demonstrate the decline in maternal antibody followed by the eventual increase in autologous immunoglobulin concentrations. Affected foals usually have low, but detectable, concentrations of IgM and IgA, which help differentiate the condition from agammaglobulinemia, which usually has no detectable concentrations. Lymphocyte counts are normal. This condition appears to be quite rare, although because it is not easily documented, the actual prevalence is unknown. The condition has been reported primarily in Arabians, but it also occurs in other breeds. Affected animals suffer from recurrent episodes of bacterial and viral infections during the period of hypogammaglobulinemia. Management includes antimicrobial therapy and plasma transfusions to minimize infections until such time as the foal's immune system begins to respond normally.

UNCLASSIFIED IMMUNODEFICIENCY DISEASES

Dozens of different immunodeficiency syndromes have been characterized in children based on the site of the defect in the immune response. Definitive tests for analogous conditions in horses are not generally available, particularly in regard to cellular immune responses. Therefore, identification and diagnosis of these conditions is not yet possible. Most foals with evidence of immunologic defects do not fit into any of the recognized immunodeficiency syndromes thus described.

Immunodeficiency Associated with Oral Candidiasis and Bacterial Septicemia

A group of foals has been described with oral candidiasis and bacterial septicemia which had laboratory and/or histologic evidence of immunodeficiency but did not fit into any recognized category of primary immunodeficiency.[47] Affected foals ranged from several days of age to 4 months. Lymphocyte counts were variable but persistent lymphopenia was not a feature. Serum IgM and IgG concentrations were variable but tended to be low. These cases differed from previously described immunodeficiencies involving immunoglobulin defects in that tests for cellular immunity were also abnormal. The thymus could not be identified in most of the cases and lymphoid depletion was present in the spleen and lymph nodes. A variety of different bacterial organisms were associated with the septicemia, many of which are usually considered to be limited pathogens. Affected foals did not respond to therapy with antimicrobials and plasma. From what is known, the prognosis for foals manifesting oral candidiasis and associated bacterial septicemia is guarded to poor.[47]

TABLE 111–3. DIAGNOSTIC FEATURES OF IMMUNODEFICIENCY DISEASES

CONDITION	LYMPHOCYTES/MM³	IgG	IgM	OTHER
Combined immunodeficiency	< 1000	Absent*	Absent*	Negative skin tests, depressed lymphocyte blastogenesis, thymic hypoplasia, lymphoid tissue depletion
Agammaglobulinemia	> 1000	Absent*	Absent*	Normal cellular immune responses
Selective IgM deficiency	> 1000	Normal	< 15 mg/dL	Normal cellular immune responses
Transient hypogammaglobulinemia	> 1000	Decreased for age	Present	Normal cellular immune responses
Oral candidiasis with bacterial septicemia	Variable, but not consistently lymphopenic	Variable, but often low	Variable, but often low	Depressed cellular immune responses
EHV 1 induced immunodeficiency	Decreased	Probably varies with passive transfer	Unknown	Lymphoid tissue necrosis

*Depends on level of passive transfer at time of sampling.

Perinatal Infection with Equine Herpesvirus Type 1

Perinatal infection with equine herpesvirus type 1 (EHV 1) has been shown to cause lymphoid tissue necrosis, which results in a secondary immunodeficiency syndrome. The functional immune status of affected foals has not been well characterized based on laboratory testing. However, histologic lesions include variable degrees of necrosis of lymphoid tissue. Immunodeficiency secondary to the marked lymphoid damage induced by the virus is credited with allowing secondary bacterial infections to establish. A variety of infectious bacterial diseases have been associated, including colibacillosis, streptococcal septicemia, salmonellosis, and Tyzzer's disease. Equine herpesvirus type 1 can be isolated from the nasal passages in about 30% of the cases.[48]

DIFFERENTIAL DIAGNOSES

A complete blood count (absolute lymphocyte count) and serum concentrations of IgG and IgM are minimal essential tests for diagnosis and differentiation of various immunodeficiencies. Serial quantitation of various immunoglobulin classes may be necessary to confirm a diagnosis in some conditions.

Skin testing with phytohemagglutinin (PHA) can be performed as an assessment of cellular immunity in the field to aid in diagnosis.[36] A total of 50 μg PHA in 0.05 mL volume is injected intradermally into a shaved area of the neck. A similar volume of 0.9% NaCl is injected into an adjacent site as a negative control. Thickening of the skin is normally detectable within 4 h and maximal by 24 h.

Other immunologic diagnostics are largely limited to specialized laboratories or to the evaluation of necropsy material. Table 111–3 compares features of immunodeficiency diseases which have been described in neonates in regard to various immunologic parameters. Early diagnosis of immunodeficiency diseases is important so an accurate prognosis can be made in regard to treatment of secondary infections and appropriate genetic counseling can be done if indicated.

At present, no practical treatments for any type of recognized immunodeficiency exist. Immunoglobulin supplementation and antimicrobial drugs may prove transiently beneficial, but they do not correct underlying problems. Immunostimulants which are currently being marketed are not effective, because most work as adjuvants, which means they require an intact immune system to produce an effect. Procedures such as bone marrow transplantation are not clinically practical at this time.

REFERENCES

1. Jeffcott, L.B.: Some practical aspects of the transfer of passive immunity to newborn foals. Equine Vet. J., *6:*109–115, 1974.
2. McGuire, T.C., Poppie, M.J., and Banks, K.L.: Hypogammaglobulinemia predisposing to infection in foals. J. Am. Vet. Med. Assoc., *166:*71–75, 1975.
3. McGuire, T.C., Crawford, T.B., Hallowell, A.L., and Macomber, L.E.: Failure of colostral immunoglobulin transfer as an explanation for most infections and deaths of neonatal foals. J. Am. Vet. Med. Assoc., *170:*1302–1304, 1977.
4. McGuire, T.C., and Crawford, T.B.: Passive immunity in the foal: Measurement of immunoglobulin classes and specific antibody. Am. J. Vet. Res., *34:*1299–1303, 1973.
5. Scott, A.M., and Jeffcott, L.B.: Haemolytic disease of the newborn foal. Vet. Rec., *103:*71–74, 1978.
6. Stormont, C.: Neonatal isoerythrolysis in domestic animals: A comparative review. Adv. Vet. Sci. Comp. Med., *19:*23–45, 1975.
7. Bailey, E., and Albright, D.G.: Equine neonatal isothyrolysis: Evidence for prevention by maternal antibodies to

the Ca blood group antigen. Am. J. Vet. Res., *49:*1218–1222, 1988.
8. Bailey, E.: Prevalence of anti-red blood cell antibodies in the serum and colostrum of mares and its relationship to neonatal isoerythrolysis. Am. J. Vet. Res., *43:*1917–1921, 1982.
9. Bell, K.: The blood groups of domestic mammals. *In* Red Blood Cells of Domestic Mammals. Edited by N.S. Agar and P.G. Board. New York, Elsevier Science, 1983, pp. 133–164.
10. Bowling, A.T., and Clark, R.S.: Blood group and protein polymorphism gene frequencies for seven breeds of horses in the United States. Anim. Blood Grp. Biochem. Genet., *16:*93–108, 1985.
11. Becht, J.L., and Page, E.H.: Neonatal isoerythrolysis in the foal: An evaluation of predictive and diagnostic field tests. Am. Assoc. Equine Pract., 247–259, 1979.
12. Jeffcott, L.B.: The transfer of passive immunity to the foal and its relation to immune status after birth. J. Reprod. Fertil., *23:*727–733, 1975.
13. Koterba, A.M., Brewer, B., and Drummond, W.H.: Prevention and control of infection. Vet. Clin. North Am. Equine Pract., *1:*41–50, 1985.
14. Kruse-Elliot, K., and Wagner, P.C.: Failure of passive antibody transfer in the foal. Comp. Contin. Educ. Practicing Vet., *6:*S702–S707, 1984.
15. Leblanc, M.M., McLaurin, B.I., and Boswell, R.: Relationships among serum immunoglobulin concentration in foals, colostral specific gravity, and colostral immunoglobulin concentration. J. Am. Vet. Med. Assoc., *189:*57–60, 1986.
16. LeBlanc, M.M.: Use of a modified hydrometer to assess immunoglobulin content in mare colostrum. Am. Assoc. Equine Pract., 157–162, 1985.
17. Brewer, B.D.: Neonatal infection. *In* Equine Clinical Neonatology. Edited by A.M. Koterba, W.H. Drummond, and P.C. Kosch. Philadelphia, Lea & Febiger, 1990, pp. 295–316.
18. Koterba, A.M., Brewer, B.D., and Tarplee, F.A.: Clinical and cliniopathological characteristics of the septicaemic neonatal foal: A review of 38 cases. Equine Vet. J., *16:*376–383, 1984.
19. Firth, E.C., et al.: Polyarthritis and bone infection in foals. Zentralbl. Veterinarmed. [B], *27:*102–124, 1980.
20. Brewer, B.D., and Koterba, A.M.: Development of a scoring system for the early diagnosis of equine neonatal sepsis. Equine Vet. J., *20:*18–22, 1988.
21. Brewer, B.C., Koterba, A.M., Carter, R.L., and Rowe, E.D.: Comparison of empirically developed sepsis score with a computer generated and weighted scoring system for the identification of sepsis in the equine neonate. Equine Vet. J., *20:*23–24, 1988.
22. Shideler, R.K., Squires, E.L., Mifflin, R.E., and Lance, W.R.: Evaluation of lyophilized IgG as an oral supplement for failure of passive transfer in foals. Am. Assoc. Equine Pract., 763–767, 1987,
23. LeBlanc, M.M., and Pritchard, E.L.: Effects of bovine colostrum, foal serum immunoglobulin concentration and intravenous plasma transfusion on chemiluminescence response of foal neutrophils. Ann. Genet., *19:*435–445, 1988.
24. Lavoie, J-P., Spensley, M.S., and Smith, B.P.: Use of bovine colostrum in newborn foals. Proceedings of the American College of Veterinary International Medical Forum. 1988, pp. 342–344.
25. Rumbaugh, G.E., Ardans, A.A., Ginno, D., and Trommershausen-Smith, A.: Identification and treatment of colostrum deficient foals. J. Am. Vet. Med. Assoc., *174:*273–275, 1979.
26. Perryman, L.E., and Crawford, T.B.: Diagnosis and management of immune system failures in foals. Am. Assoc. Equine Pract., 235–244, 1979.
27. Magnuson, N.S., Decker, D.M., and Perryman, L.E.: Increased susceptibility of fibroblasts from horses with severe combined immunodeficiency to growth inhibition by 2′-deoxyadenosine. Clin. Immunol. Immunopathol., *29:* 391–402, 1983.
28. Splitter, G.A., Perryman, L.E., Magnuson, N.A., and McGuire, T.C.: Combined immunodeficiency of horses: A review. Dev. Comp. Immunol., *4:*21–32, 1980.
29. Snyder, S.P, England, J.J., and McChesney, A.E.: Cryptosporidiosis in immunodeficient Arabian foals. Vet. Pathol., *15:*12–17, 1978.
30. Tarr, M.J., and Olsen, R.G.: Suppression of the cell-mediated immune system of the horse by systemic corticosteroid administration. J. Equine Med. Surg., *2:*129–134, 1978.
31. Perryman, L.E., Boreson, M.W., Conaway, M.W., and Bartsch, R.C.: Combined immunodeficiency in an Appaloosa foal. Vet. Pathol., *21:*547–548, 1984.
32. Perryman, L.E., and Torbeck, R.L.: Combined immunodeficiency of Arabian horses: Confirmation of autosomal recessive mode of inheritance. J. Am. Vet. Med. Assoc., *176:*1250–1251, 1980.
33. Thompson, D.B., Studdert, M.J., Beilharz, R.G., and Littlejohns, I.R.: Inheritance of a lethal immunodeficiency disease of Arabian foals. Aust. Vet. J., *51:*109–113, 1975.
34. Poppie, M.J., and McGuire, T.C.: Combined immunodeficiency in foals of Arabian breeding: Evaluation of mode of inheritance and estimation of prevalence of affected foals and carrier mares and stallions. J. Am. Vet. Med. Assoc., *170:*31–33, 1977.
35. McGuire, T.C., Banks, K.L., and Poppie, M.J.: Combined immunodeficiency in horses: Characterization of the lymphocyte defect. Clin. Immunol. Immunopathol., *3:*555–566, 1975.
36. Hodgin, E.C., McGuire, T.C., Perryman, L.E., and Grant, B.D.: Evaluation of delayed hypersensitivity responses in normal horses and immunodeficient foals. Am. J. Vet. Res., *39:*1161–1167, 1976.
37. McGuire, T.C., Poppie, M.J., and Banks, K.L.: Combined (B- and T-lymphocyte) immunodeficiency: A fatal genetic disease in Arabian foals. J. Am. Vet. Med. Assoc., *164:*70–75, 1975.
38. McGuire, T.C., Banks, K.L., and Davis, W.C.: Alterations of the thymus and other lymphoid tissue in young horses with combined immunodeficiency. Am. J. Pathol., *84:*39–53, 1976.
39. McGuire, T.C., and Poppie, M.J.: Hypogammaglobulinemia and thymic hypoplasia in horses: A primary combined immunodeficiency disorder. Infect. Immun., *8:* 272–277, 1973.
40. Bue, C.M., et al.: Correction of equine severe combined immunodeficiency by bone marrow transplantation. Transplantation, *42:*14–19, 1986.
41. Perryman, L.E., McGuire, T.C., and Hilbert, B.J.: Selective immunoglobulin M deficiency in foals. J. Am. Vet. Med. Assoc., *170:*212–215, 1977.
42. Perryman, L.E., and McGuire, T.C.: Evaluation for immune system failures in horses and ponies. J. Am. Vet. Med. Assoc., *176:*1374–1377, 1980.
43. Dopson, L.C., et al.: Immunosuppression associated with lymphosarcoma in two horses. Am. J. Vet. Res., *182:*1239–1241, 1983.

44. Banks, K.L., and McGuire, T.C.: Absence of B lymphocytes in a horse with primary agammaglobulinemia. Clin. Immunol. Immunopathol., *5:*282–290, 1976.

45. McGuire, T.C., Banks, K.L., and Evans, D.R.: Agammaglobulinemia in a horse with evidence of functional T lymphocytes. Am. J. Vet. Res., *37:*41–46, 1976.

46. Deem, D.A., Traver, D.S., and Thacker, H.L.: Agammaglobulinemia in a horse. J. Am. Vet. Med. Assoc., *175:* 469–472, 1979.

47. McClure, J.J., Addison, J.D., and Miller, R.I.: Immunodeficiency manifested by oral candidiasis and bacterial septicemia in foals. J. Am. Vet. Med. Assoc., *186:*1195–1197, 1985.

48. Bryans, J.T., Swerczek, T.W., Darlington, R.W., and Crowe, M.W.: Neonatal foal disease associated with perinatal infection by equine herpesvirus I. J. Equine Med. Surg., *1:*20–26, 1977.

CHAPTER 112

THE NEUROLOGIC SYSTEM

B.B. Welsch

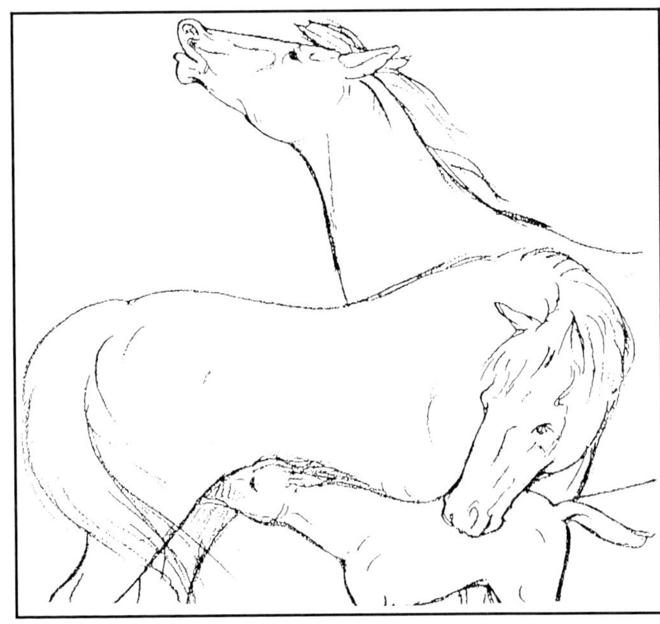

Most diseases of neonatal foals, neurologic or otherwise, begin insidiously with similar signs: less suckling activity, depression, decreasing affinity for the mare, and more time spent in recumbency. Familiarity with normal neonatal behavioral patterns will allow for early diagnosis and, therefore, more successful treatment of foal problems.

The average foal will have a suckle reflex present within 20 min of birth, can right itself, will stand and nurse within the first hour or two following birth, is alert and visual, responds to its environment, and follows its dam. Absence of any of these predictable behaviors mandates the need for a thorough physical examination and collection of a minimum data base: a complete blood count and a chemistry profile, including fibrinogen and immunoglobulin levels, arterial blood gas, and blood culture.[1]

Neurologic examination of the newborn foal is performed and interpreted in a manner similar to the neurologic evaluation of a large dog.[2,3] The newborn foal carries its head in a fixed, angular position and has abrupt, jerky head movements. Stimulation of the foal may cause jaw chomping, and attempts to restrain the foal may cause it to relax (collapse slowly). Reflexes obtained (particularly the patellar reflex) are brisker than would be expected from an adult dog and far easier to elicit than from an adult horse. Passive manipulation of the limbs reveals a wide range of motion. Foals lack the menace response for the first days to weeks of life, although they have good vision, normally have a crossed extensor reflex, and may have a dysmetric gait. Some normal foals will pace, rather than trot.

For the purposes of this chapter, neurologic diseases of newborn foals have been divided into three categories (Table 112–1): those resulting in altered states of consciousness, paroxysmal disorders, and those causing an inability to stand or an abnormal gait.

ALTERED STATES OF CONSCIOUSNESS

Depression is typically a component of all neonatal diseases. Depressed foals should not be dismissed as maladjusted foals merely needing to be watched closely, because time is critical in successful treatment of newborns. Infectious conditions, electrolyte or osmolality imbalances, acid-base disturbances, and hypoglycemia are disorders which cause depression and warrant immediate treatment. Foals with ruptured urinary tracts or neonatal isoerythrolysis will also appear depressed before other signs become evident. Every effort to rule out these and other non-neurologic diseases must be made before a foal is diagnosed as suffering from a neurologic problem.

NEONATAL MALADJUSTMENT SYNDROME

Neonatal maladjustment syndrome (NMS) refers to a noninfectious condition of newborn foals characterized by gross behavioral disturbances with onset in the first

TABLE 112–1. NEUROLOGIC DISEASES OF NEONATAL FOALS BY PRESENTING PROBLEM

I. Altered states of consciousness	III. Inability to stand/abnormal gait
Neonatal maladjustment syndrome	Contracted foals
Prematurity, asphyxiation	Vascular accidents
Skull trauma	Vertebral trauma
Bacterial meningitis	Epidural abscess; osteomyelitis
Heat stroke	Occipito-atlanto-axial malformation
II. Paroxysmal disorders	Foaling injury
Seizures	White muscle disease
Narcolepsy	Equine degenerative myelopathy
Cerebellar abiotrophy	Botulism
	Tetanus

24 h of life.[4] These abnormal behaviors can include unusual vocalization (barking), aimless wandering, excessive sleepiness, odd posturing, teeth grinding, constant licking, or generalized seizures. The term was not intended to be applied to premature or dysmature foals (foals of normal gestational length which appear premature) or foals with developmental or immunologic conditions.[4] Unfortunately, NMS has sporadically been used to refer to young foals with any neurologic disease, foals older than 24 h at the onset of signs, or premature or dysmature foals. Depressed foals in early stages of other diseases have been mislabeled NMS foals, leading to an often fatal delay in appropriate treatment.

Researchers have been able to identify two distinct types of neurohistopathologic conditions in the brains of foals with tentative diagnoses of NMS: necrosis or hemorrhage (with or without edema).[5,6] These lesions are similar to those caused by the effects of acute total or prolonged partial asphyxia on the central nervous system (CNS) of fetal and neonatal rhesus monkeys.[7]

Often foals have signs compatible with NMS but no CNS lesions are detected at necropsy. Furthermore, foals that have died without neurologic signs have had CNS hemorrhage and necrosis. Clearly the term NMS does not describe one single specific etiologic or pathologic entity.

The foal with NMS is frequently reported as having been born quickly and without complications. Most are said to have appeared completely normal for the first hours of life. Other foals that have been classified with the same syndrome are foals which have been induced or are the product of dystocia or premature placental separation or caesarian section. Typically, these foals were never normal, although their condition deteriorated further with the passage of time.

Because our clinical experience is that the prognosis is different for these two groups, the second group should not be classified as NMS foals. This observation was confirmed in a recent international survey.[8] A total of 91% of 23 foals with signs of NMS which were normal at birth and had suffered no known perturbation during birth survived, whereas only 42% of 19 foals with similar clinical signs but which were abnormal at birth and had experienced an intrapartum difficulty survived.

The diagnosis of NMS is a diagnosis of exclusion. Sepsis and septicemia must be ruled out (normal physical examination and complete blood count, negative blood cultures, negative bacterial cultures of suspicious organ systems, or normal thoracic radiographs), and metabolic abnormalities (normal serum chemistry panel and blood gases) must also be ruled out. Clinicians must keep in mind that infection is the usual cause of depression and other alterations in behavior in foals older than 24 h. Serum immunoglobulin levels should be determined in these foals, because failure of passive transfer (FPT) is a frequent sequela to neonatal maladjustment syndrome. If FPT is untreated, NMS is likely to become complicated by septicemia, the signs of which typically become evident on day 3 of life.

Treatment of NMS is directed at immediately controlling seizures, if present, and supportive care. While the labor involved (and/or the cost) may be substantial for the first 24 to 48 h, foals usually recover quickly and completely if no complications ensue. Assessment of respiratory rate and effort and mucous membrane color (as well as temperature, heart rate, and fluid balance) should be performed periodically. Nasal oxygen insufflation and fluid therapy may be indicated and are not too difficult to accomplish in field situations. If the foal's body temperature falls below 38° C (100° F), efforts are needed to raise it. Heat lamps, blankets, warm water beds, and water-circulating heating pads prove useful. The foal, if down and thrashing, may need to be manually restrained on as soft a surface as possible. The recumbent eye must be protected and both eyes frequently stained to check for corneal ulceration. If entropion is present, the lower eyelid should be everted using a suture or a bleb of procaine penicillin. Again, FPT must be treated as soon as possible. Dimethyl sulfoxide (DMSO) (1 g/kg bid diluted to 20% in dextrose) has been used intravenously in foals with neurologic dysfunction for 1 to 3 days, but its efficacy is unproven. The author does not routinely recommend its use. Antiulcer medication can be administered empirically.

PREMATURE FOALS, ASPHYXIATED FOALS, AND FOALS UNREADY FOR BIRTH

Prematurity is discussed in Chapter 110 but is mentioned here because many premature foals exhibit alterations in consciousness. Foals which have been delivered by cesarian section or induced prematurely exhibit abnormal mentation and follow a similar clinical course as some premature foals. The first 12 to 18 h after birth are deceptively uneventful, occasionally with a slight improvement noted.[9] This grace period is followed by loss of the suckle reflex, a decline in consciousness, the onset of seizure activity, and failure of many body systems, often terminating in death. Hypoglycemia, iatrogenic hyperglycemia, respiratory and metabolic acidosis and iatrogenic hyperosmolarity will exacerbate the neurologic signs accompanying this condition. Close monitoring is crucial. Postmortem examination of the brain in these cases often reveals no histologic abnormalities; occasionally, hemorrhage or necrosis is present.

SKULL TRAUMA

Traumatic injury is another common cause of abnormal behavior in newborn foals and may have occurred in absence of visible signs of trauma. An acute onset of signs of cerebral disease (blindness, circling, seizures, and dementia) and/or vestibular disease or facial paralysis may be noted. Other cranial nerve deficits in conjunction with ataxia and weakness suggest brain stem involvement. Bleeding from the ear canal is pathognomonic for skull fracture.

Swollen eyelids attributable to facial trauma incurred during a seizure episode may often make cranial nerve evaluation difficult. A good effort must be made, however, because skull trauma should be treated with DMSO, and the prognosis is favorable, although return to complete normalcy may require many months.

Diagnosis is by properly positioned skull radiographs and a cerebrospinal fluid (CSF) tap. The CSF may reveal intact red blood cells and xanthochromia with no bacteria and few white blood cells present. These foals should also be treated with antibiotics to prevent CNS infection.

Cerebrospinal fluid can be easily collected at the atlanto-occipital site, frequently without tranquilization in depressed foals (5 to 10 mg intravenous diazepam can be used if needed). The tap site (the area directly between the cranial edges of the wings of the atlas) is surgically prepared and blocked with a local anesthetic. The foal's reaction to the anesthetic injection will be predictive of its response to the tap itself. A 20-gauge 3.8 cm (1.5-in.) disposable needle is inserted slowly on the midline between the cranial edges of the wings of the atlas, directed at the mandible. Cerebrospinal fluid will drip freely from the hub when the subarachnoid space is penetrated about 2.5 cm (1 in.) below the skin, approximately 1 to 2 mL are collected and examined.

BACTERIAL MENINGITIS

Fortunately, meningitis is a rare sequela to septicemia in newborn foals. Agents which have been incriminated include Escherichia coli, Actinobacillus equuli, and Streptococcus spp., Staphylococcus spp., Klebsiella spp., Salmonella spp., and Pasteurella spp. Septicemic foals developing neurologic signs should be considered likely candidates for meningitis. Cerebral signs include blindness with responsive pupils, abnormal mentation and behavior, and seizures. Other signs are neck pain, hyperesthesia, hyper-reflexia, tetraplegia, and coma. Diagnosis is confirmed by presence of numerous bacteria and neutrophils on an atlanto-occipital CSF tap.

Third-generation cephalosporins are the drugs of choice for gram-negative meningitis in human infants and most likely are the optimal drug for this condition in foals. However, the cost can be prohibitive. As in human infants, antibiotic therapy can appear to be successful in that subsequent CSF taps become culture negative and cell counts return to normal; however, periventricular abscesses and ventriculitis are sequelae which are difficult to treat successfully. The prognosis is considered poor for foals with confirmed meningitis.

HEAT STROKE

Neonatal foals are prone to heat stroke on hot, humid days when they have no shelter, or are, for other reasons, unable to reach a shelter. Mild signs include ataxia and depression, progressing to recumbency, coma, and/or seizures. Physical examination reveals a high temperature, dehydration, hyperventilation, tachypnea, and tachycardia. Electrolyte abnormalities may be present.

Treatment is directed at cooling the body (cool water and alcohol bath with a rectal enema with cool water), replacing fluid and electrolyte losses and controlling seizures with anticonvulsant therapy. Acute renal failure can be seen as a sequela to heat stroke.

PAROXYSMAL DISORDERS

SEIZURES

Correctly identifying presence of seizure activity in the newborn can be more difficult than would at first be imagined. Behavior in two situations can be mistakenly attributed to seizure activity: movements noted in the sleeping premature foal (rapid eye movements, chewing, and paddling of limbs) and the thrashing and extensor rigidity noted in foals which are unable to rise because of musculoskeletal abnormalities. In both cases, foals are easily aroused, respond to noxious stimuli, and do not urinate or defecate during the apparent seizure.

Seizure activity in neonatal foals can run the gamut from abnormal jaw movements, salivation, and flemen accompanied by facial grimacing and muscle twitching, to generalized seizures with nystagmus, paddling, extensor rigidity, and/or opisthotonos. Foals must be protected from traumatic injury while experiencing seizures, and prolonged seizures with accompanying hyperthermia can cause further neurologic damage.

Once the presence of seizures has been ascertained, a cause must be sought. Metabolic abnormalities (including hypoglycemia, acidosis, hyponatremia, hypocalcemia, and hypochloremia) must be eliminated as a cause, and septicemia with or without meningitis must be considered. As indicated earlier, foals which have suffered an anoxic or traumatic insult may develop seizures. Benign epilepsy occurs in young foals and is particularly common in the Arabian breed.[10] If the foal is 24 h old or younger, NMS needs to be considered. These latter two diagnoses are made only after all others have been ruled out.

Generalized seizures should be controlled immediately. Diazepam is the initial drug of choice, because its onset is rapid and it is relatively safe. Approximately 5 to 10 mg/45 kg are administered intravenously (IV), slowly. This dose can be repeated as necessary. Resuscitation equipment must be readily available, because diazepam may cause respiratory depression or arrest. Rapid administration can cause cardiac arrest.

Should two or three doses of diazepam fail to control the seizures, phenobarbital or phenytoin can be used. The loading dose of phenobarbital is 10 to 20 mg/kg diluted in saline and administered over 15 min IV. Maintenance dose is 5 to 10 mg/kg IV or orally, two to three times a day. Abrupt withdrawal of phenobarbital can precipitate seizures, so the dose should be tapered over 7 to 10 days before discontinuation. Phenytoin can be administered 5 to 10 mg/kg IV, alone or in combination with phenobarbital, should either drug fail to control the seizures when used alone. Maintenance dosage of phenytoin is 1 to 5 mg/kg every 4 to 6 h.

NARCOLEPSY

Newborn foals, particularly pony and miniature horse foals, may suffer from classic narcolepsy, which is narcolepsy (sleep attacks) with cataplexy (muscular weakness usually brought on by excitement). A typical episode begins with the foal buckling at the knees, and falling into recumbency. Flaccid paralysis (as opposed to the extreme extensor tone and paddling seen with seizures) then follows. Rapid eye movement may be present, and the foal is momentarily unarousable and still. Shetland Pony foals may be narcoleptic for life, but the problem rarely persists beyond several weeks of age in other foals. No treatment is necessary.

CEREBELLAR ABIOTROPHY

Cerebellar abiotrophy is an inherited disorder of Arabian foals, which is not usually diagnosed in the first weeks of life, because jerky head movements and a dysmetric gait are normally prominent in many newborn foals. At first, the disorder may be reported as paroxysmal, because the head tremors, wide-base stance, and ataxia may only be noted occasionally, particularly when the foal is approached from the front, or its head is raised. However, careful evaluation will reveal a persistence of signs at all times. Foals are not weak, but fall over backward when they are asked to back up or raise their heads, and they often paddle while struggling to rise. The menace response is absent.

Diagnosis is by signalment and clinical signs. Cerebrospinal fluid frequently has a mildly elevated white blood cell count. The prognosis is hopeless for recovery, and most foals are euthanatized as they become dangerous to themselves or their handlers.

INABILITY TO STAND/ABNORMAL GAIT

The inability to stand and abnormal gait category includes foals that are ataxic, weak, or are unable to stand, but which have normal mentation and no cranial nerve deficits. Foals which are not weak but which have abnormal gaits (which can be difficult to distinguish from ataxia) should be evaluated for infection and joint pain. Pelvic osteomyelitis, in particular, can be difficult to diagnose clinically and can produce a stiff, stilted gait in foals. Plasma fibrinogen levels are usually quite high in these cases and radiographs can help to confirm the diagnosis.

CONTRACTED FOALS (ARTHROGRYPOSIS)

Varying degrees of tendon contracture in one to four limbs occur in newborn foals. The contractures can be mild to severe and occasionally the vertebral column will be concurrently deformed. Despite the frequency of mild forms of the problem and the knowledge that a similar syndrome occurs in calves (genetic, toxic, and viral causes have been incriminated), the cause in the foal remains unexplained. Malpositioning or restricted movement in utero is a possible factor which merits consideration along with the ingestion of certain feeds.

Treatment with splints, braces, casts, surgery, and physical therapy has resulted in complete recovery in some cases. Milder cases frequently resolve as the foal bears weight on its limbs. Because these foals may not have nursed vigorously early in life, special attention to passive immunity is crucial. These foals, as mentioned earlier, can become so frustrated at their inability to stand that they appear to be convulsing.

VASCULAR ACCIDENTS

Vascular accidents in the CNS of newborn foals are quite common, and subarachnoid hemorrhage in the spinal cord seems to predominate.[11] Typically, foals do not show clinical signs, but, again, mild ataxia may be missed because the newborn foal's gait is dysmetric. In foals exhibiting signs of spinal cord disease, reflexes may be depressed and/or asymmetrical. Cerebrospinal fluid xanthochromia confirms a previous bleed in these cases, but foals showing no neurologic signs may also have xanthochromic cerebrospinal fluid. Furthermore, because not all bleeds are subarachnoid, the lack of xanthochromic CSF does not rule out a vascular accident as a cause of spinal ataxia.

VERTEBRAL TRAUMA

Vertebral fracture or luxation as a result of a fall or other traumatic event can result in ataxia or paresis. Approximate location of the lesion is usually readily ascertained by careful neurologic examination, and diagnosis can be confirmed with appropriate radiographs. Occasionally, small fracture lines will not be evident until repair begins to occur. Vertebral trauma resulting in spinal cord injury can occur with a temporary luxation which leaves no radiographic evidence. Treatment is usually medical management with DMSO as described for head trauma and attention to nursing care to prevent further injury or illness.

EPIDURAL ABSCESSATION/OSTEOMYELITIS

Epidural abscessation and osteomyelitis are rare sequelae to septicemia and would be unusual in a foal under 2 weeks of age. Typical offending agents are Corynebacterium equi, Salmonella spp., and Actinobacillus equuli. Other signs of infection usually are (or were) present, but may have gone unnoticed. Localization of the lesion is by careful neurologic examination; radiographs will confirm osteomyelitis, and CSF tap is usually abnormal in cases of abscessation.

OCCIPITO-ATLANTO-AXIAL MALFORMATION

Developmental anomalies of the occiput, atlas, and axis occur in all breeds, but are most commonly noted in Arabians. Foals may be born dead or may be ataxic at birth and may not show clinical signs until later in their first year of life. Physical and neurologic examination may reveal an abnormal head posture, "clicking" sounds on manipulation of the atlanto-occipital joint, or asymmetric palpation of the atlas or axis. A diagnosis of occipito-atlanto-axial malformation can be readily confirmed radiographically.

FOALING INJURIES

Foals which are products of dystocia may have sustained damage to the brachial or lumbar plexus or to a peripheral nerve. Clinical signs would, of course, depend on the site and severity of injury, but neurologic examination would reveal depressed reflexes in the affected limb(s). Treatment consists of intravenous DMSO and bandaging or splinting to protect the limb from injury.

WHITE MUSCLE DISEASE

White muscle disease is a myodegeneration resulting from selenium deficiency, which can affect foals from birth throughout the first year of life. It is particularly common in the United States on the East and West Coasts as well as the northern Midwestern states.

Clinical presentation can range from mild stiffness and reluctance to walk, with or without painful muscles, to weakness and inability to rise. Dysphagia, manifested by nasal regurgitation of milk, and dyspnea or rapid respiration may be present. Foals may be reluctant or unable to nurse, presumably because of neck pain, and repeated attempts to rise may be misinterpreted as colic or seizure episodes.

Serum creatine kinase and serum aspartate aminotransferase levels are usually markedly elevated, and myoglobinuria may be present. Electromyography (EMG) will confirm the presence of a myopathy but is not diagnostic.

Treatment with a vitamin E–selenium preparation (1 mg/45 kg) has been advised.[12] This should be repeated in 3 days and again in 10 days. Such therapy resulted in recovery of 5 of 11 foals treated.[12] Physical exertion should be minimized to avoid further muscle damage, and complete diagnostic workups should be performed on these foals, because they may suffer concurrent infection, failure of passive transfer, or electrolyte abnormalities, all of which require conscientious treatment. Good nursing care is critical.

EQUINE DEGENERATIVE MYELOPATHY

Equine degenerative myelopathy is thought to be a familial disease which becomes clinically apparent in horses during the first 2 years of life. Rarely it is noted in the neonatal period. This disease is characterized by onset of mild to moderate, slowly progressive (in most cases) ataxia and weakness, affecting all four limbs or initially just the hindlimbs. Hyporeflexia of local cervical and cervicofacial reflexes is usually noted. Cerebrospinal fluid and EMG studies are within normal limits. The diagnosis can only be confirmed at necropsy.

BOTULISM (SHAKER FOAL SYNDROME)

Botulism, a neurologic syndrome caused by the exotoxin produced by Clostridium botulinum, is common in certain areas of the United States. The form seen in foals is referred to as toxicoinfectious botulism. It is a result of infection with the clostridial organism which then continues to produce exotoxin, rather than ingestion of preformed toxin as is seen in adult horses. Affected foals are usually 2 to 8 weeks of age, but the disease has been seen during the first week of life. Clinical signs include dysphagia, weakness of the muscles of the head, and dilated, unresponsive pupils; rapid progression to generalized weakness and inability to stand follow. Foals will tend to tremble violently before collapsing. Untreated, foals will die from respiratory arrest in 1 to 3 days.

Treatment consists of intravenous potassium penicillin, polyvalent equine type B antitoxin, and supportive care, including artificial ventilation and provision of nutrition. Vaccination of pregnant mares with botulism type B toxoid and yearly vaccination of all adults on problem farms is recommended.

TETANUS

Tetanus, caused by Clostridium tetani, can occur in neonatal foals which have suffered failure of passive transfer, or foals from dams which were not vaccinated for tetanus in the last trimester. The bacteria can enter via wounds or the umbilical stump.

Presenting signs include hyperesthesia, exaggerated responses to external stimuli, and progressive muscle rigidity. Before becoming extremely rigid and completely recumbent, foals may assume a sawhorse stance with elevation of the tail and rigid extension of the head and neck. Terminally, tetanic spasms, convulsions, and respiratory paralysis occur.

Treatment consists of debridement of wounds and infiltration with penicillin, high doses of potassium and procaine penicillin administered intravenously and intramuscularly, respectively, and administration of 10,000 IU tetanus antitoxin qid for several days. Intrathecal instillation of antitoxin has been recommended.[13] Muscle spasms are controlled using diazepam or glycerol guaiacolate.

The prognosis is poor once the animal is recumbent, but fair if the diagnosis is made early. Supportive care and astute observation for signs of other problems are critical to a favorable outcome.

Prevention is best accomplished by vaccinating pregnant mares with tetanus toxoid 3 to 4 weeks before foaling. Newborn foals from unvaccinated dams should be passively immunized with 1500 units tetanus antitoxin. Active immunization during the neonatal period is not recommended for the foal of a properly vaccinated mare who has adequate passive transfer of immunity, because passively derived antibodies interfere with the immune response.

REFERENCES

1. Koterba, A.M.: Diagnosis and management of the normal and abnormal neonatal foal: general considerations. *In* Equine Clinical Neonatology. Edited by A.M. Koterba, W.H. Drummond, and P.C. Kosch. Philadelphia, Lea & Febiger, 1990, pp. 3–15.
2. Chrisman, C.L.: Problems in Small Animal Neurology. Philadelphia, Lea & Febiger, 1982, pp. 39–58.
3. Adams, R., and Mayhew, I.G.: Neurologic diseases. *In* Veterinary Clinics of North America, Equine Practice, Neonatal Equine Disease. Edited by J. Beech. Philadelphia, W.B. Saunders, 1985, pp. 209–234.
4. Rossdale, P.D.: Abnormal perinatal behavior in the Thoroughbred horse. Br. Vet. J., *124:*540–553, 1968.
5. Palmer, A.C., and Rossdale, P.D.: Neuropathology of the convulsive foal syndrome. J. Reprod. Fertil. Suppl., *23:*691–694, 1975.
6. Mayhew, I.G.: Neurological and neuropathological observations on the equine neonate. Equine Vet. J. Suppl., *5:*28–33, 1988.
7. Brann, A.W.: Effects of acute total and prolonged partial asphyxia on the central nervous system of the foetal neonatal and juvenile rhesus monkey: A review. Equine Vet. J., *5(Suppl.):*25–28, 1988.
8. Cudd, T.A., and Koterba, A.M.: Results of the 1988 ISVP member survey of equine neonatal disease. Int. Soc. Vet. Perinat. Newslett. *3:*2–3, 1990.
9. Koterba, A.M.: Prematurity. *In* Equine Clinical Neonatology. Edited by A.M. Koterba, W.H. Drummond, and P.C. Kosch. Philadelphia, Lea & Febiger, 1990, pp. 55–70.
10. Mayhew, I.G.: Large Animal Neurology: A Handbook for Veterinary Clinicians. Philadelphia. Lea & Febiger, 1989.
11. Mayhew, I.G.: Observations on vascular accidents in the central nervous system of neonatal foals. J. Reprod. Fertil. Suppl., *32:*569–575, 1982.
12. Dill, S.G., and Rebhun, W.C.: White muscle disease in foals. Compend. Contin. Educ. Practicing Vet., *7:*5627–5631, 1985.
13. Green, S.L., and Mayhew, I.G.: Neurologic disorders. *In* Equine Clinical Neonatology. Edited by A.M. Koterba, W.H. Drummond, and P.C. Kosch. Philadelphia, Lea & Febiger, 1990, pp. 496–530.

CHAPTER 113

DISORDERS OF THE DIGESTIVE TRACT

J.L. Traub-Dargatz

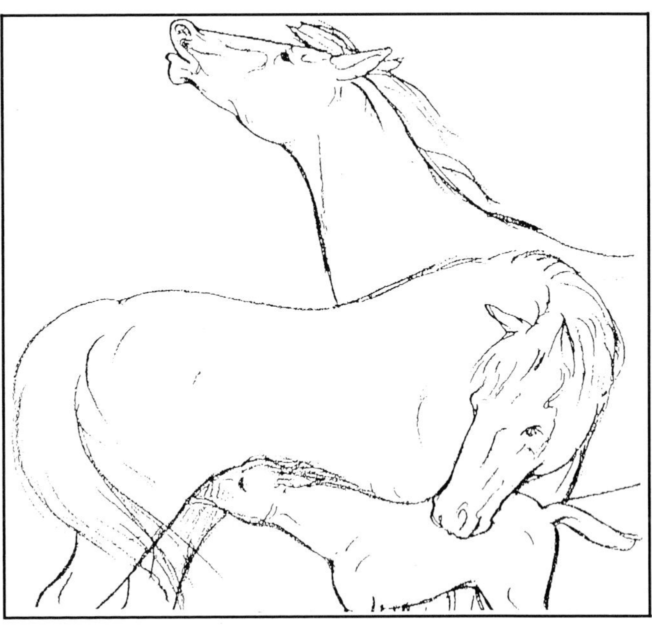

Foals that develop signs of abdominal pain in the neonatal period are a most frustrating problem. These cases present several problems for the attending clinician and include the following: (1) diagnostic techniques available to the veterinarian when evaluating the neonatal foal with colic are more limited than in the adult, (2) most veterinarians have less experience in managing neonatal foals with colic than in adult horses, and (3) many neonatal foals with abdominal pain often manifest severe, unrelenting pain, thus creating a feeling of urgency and helplessness for all involved. A painful foal can make execution of diagnostic tests and administration of therapy difficult. Also, because colic is a nonspecific symptom, it can have multiple potential causes that are not always obvious from history and physical examination, and in some cases are still elusive after multiple diagnostic procedures have been performed. The potential causes of colic in the neonatal foal include ileus with or without evidence of enterocolitis, meconium impaction, gastroduodenal ulcers, intussusception, volvulus of the intestine, atresia of the anus or a portion of the colon, aganglionosis and strangulation/obstruction of the intestine by external forces such as the ovarian pedicle, or rents in the diaphragm or mesentery.[1–3] Rupture of the urinary bladder with subsequent uroperitoneum can result in abdominal distention, decreased frequency of nursing, and mild signs of abdominal pain and is a differential diagnosis in foals showing signs of abdominal discomfort. The clinician should also be aware that rupture of the urinary bladder can occur concurrently with disease of the intestinal tract.[4]

Diarrhea in foals is a common occurrence. When outbreaks of foal diarrhea occur on farms during spring and the height of the breeding season, financial and labor-intensive impacts occur. Epizootics of foal diarrhea have been reported from densely populated equine centers from around the world.[5]

MECONIUM IMPACTION

Clinical signs of meconium impaction are generally recognized in foals from 6 to 24 h of age and include restlessness, reduced frequency of nursing, attempts to defecate, swishing of the tail, walking around the stall with the tail elevated, and straining with kyphosis (Fig. 113–1). More advanced signs include colic pain evidenced by rolling, lying in dorsal recumbency, and getting up and down frequently. Meconium, which is a combination of the digested amniotic fluid, mucous, bile, and epithelial cells, is black to dark brown, has a tarry to rock hard consistency, and normally begins to be passed in the first 3 h after birth. Meconium can be retained in either the large colon or rectum and male foals seem to be predisposed to meconium impaction, possibly because they have a narrower pelvis than fillies.[6] The diagnosis of meconium impaction is based on the presence of the above described clinical signs and the digital palpation of meconium in the terminal rectum. If the area of meconium retention is in the large

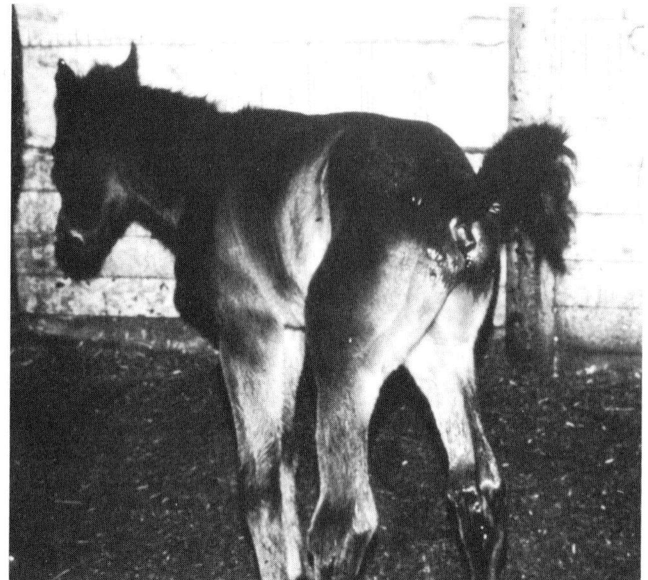

FIG. 113–1. Foal straining to pass meconium. Note kyphosis when straining.

intestine, the diagnosis is more difficult and may require abdominal radiography. However, radiography may not lead to a definitive diagnosis. Certainly, the resolution of clinical signs associated with passage of meconium would be diagnostic. Differentials would include those listed earlier as potential causes of colic. Treatment of meconium impaction in the foal includes use of soapy water enemas (0.5 to 1 L warm soapy water). The clinician must be gentle when administering the enema and avoid traumatizing the rectal mucosa. Thus the enema should be given with a soft flexible tube by gravity flow. Forceps or firm metal instruments to grasp the meconium are not recommended.[6] Simple digital extraction may work in some foals. Some clinicians use a fecal loop to remove retained fecal balls.[7] If a loop is used, adequate restraint and a gentle approach are essential to avoid trauma to the rectal wall.[7] Treatment of high meconium impaction includes the administration of mineral oil (240 mL or 8 oz.) via nasogastric tube and administration of intravenous electrolyte solutions. Isotonic fluids infused at a rate that supplies more than maintenance requirements are given in an effort to increase intraluminal fluid content. All electrolyte and volume deficits should be replaced. Daily maintenance fluid requirements of an equine neonate have been estimated to be 80 to 120 mL/kg/day.[8] A constant infusion of maintenance fluids is preferred via an indwelling catheter, however many foals tolerate bolus dosing (total maintenance volume divided into several separate infusions, particularly if the cardiovascular and renal systems are not compromised).[8] A total volume of 1 to 2 L of warm lactated Ringer's injection (IV) has been suggested as an initial fluid therapy.[6] Controlling the foal's pain should be a consideration, but it is vital that the drug given does not mask a worsening of the foal's condition. Drugs such as pentazocine (Talwin, Upjohn, Kalamazoo, MI), xylazine (Rompun, Haver Lockhart, Shawnee, KS), and flunixin meglumine (Banamine, Schering-Plough Corp., Kenilworth, NJ), have been advocated.[6] The use of xylazine in neonatal foals can result in marked respiratory and cardiac suppression and should be avoided if at all possible, especially in compromised individuals. Diazepam (Valium, Roche Laboratories, Nutley, NJ) has been utilized to restrain neonatal foals but is expensive and short acting. Meconium impaction is best managed medically, but a small percentage of foals fail to respond to the above described medical therapy and may require surgery to relieve the impaction, especially when the impaction is located in the large colon.[1,3]

Postoperative peritoneal adhesions do occur in some foals following gastrointestinal surgery and result in abdominal pain. The cause of these adhesions has not been adequately discerned. Efforts to avoid septic adhesions by aggressively treating septicemia, proper care of exposed bowel during surgery, and minimal trauma to the bowel at surgery may minimize adhesion formation.[9]

OBSTRUCTION OR TORSION OF THE INTESTINE

Obstruction or torsion of the intestine of the neonatal foal is uncommon but does occur and should be included in the differential diagnosis of foals with colic and/or abdominal distention.[3] The decision to explore the abdomen of the foal is not an easy one. Measuring the circumference of the foal's abdomen when initial colic is noted and monitoring for worsening of distention can be helpful. If the foal has gradually worsening distention with continued pain, it would be one criterion to consider exploration of the abdomen. Abdominal radiographs will aid the veterinarian in localizing the area of intestinal distention but will not in all cases differentiate between gas accumulation because of ileus and that caused by obstruction or torsion of the bowel[3,10] (Fig. 113–2). In one report, neonatal foals were passing diarrheic feces at the time they were sent to surgery and were found to have a torsion of the colon; therefore, even when a foal is passing feces, an obstruction or torsion and the need for exploratory laparotomy are not ruled out.[3] Hematologic results were not helpful in a series of 20 foals in determining the need for surgical intervention.[3] The most consistent clinical signs in foals requiring surgical intervention in this series of 20 foals were severe abdominal pain and/or abdominal distention, but not all of the foals had what have classically been considered lesions requiring surgery, such as strangulation obstruction. In some cases all that was found was ileus. The authors believed ileus cases may have benefited from surgical decompression.

Abdominal ultrasonography has been utilized in the neonatal foal to evaluate the umbilical structures, abdominal fluid, liver, spleen, urinary bladder, and kidneys (Chapter 118). Diagnostic ultrasonography has been reported to aid in the diagnosis of intussusception

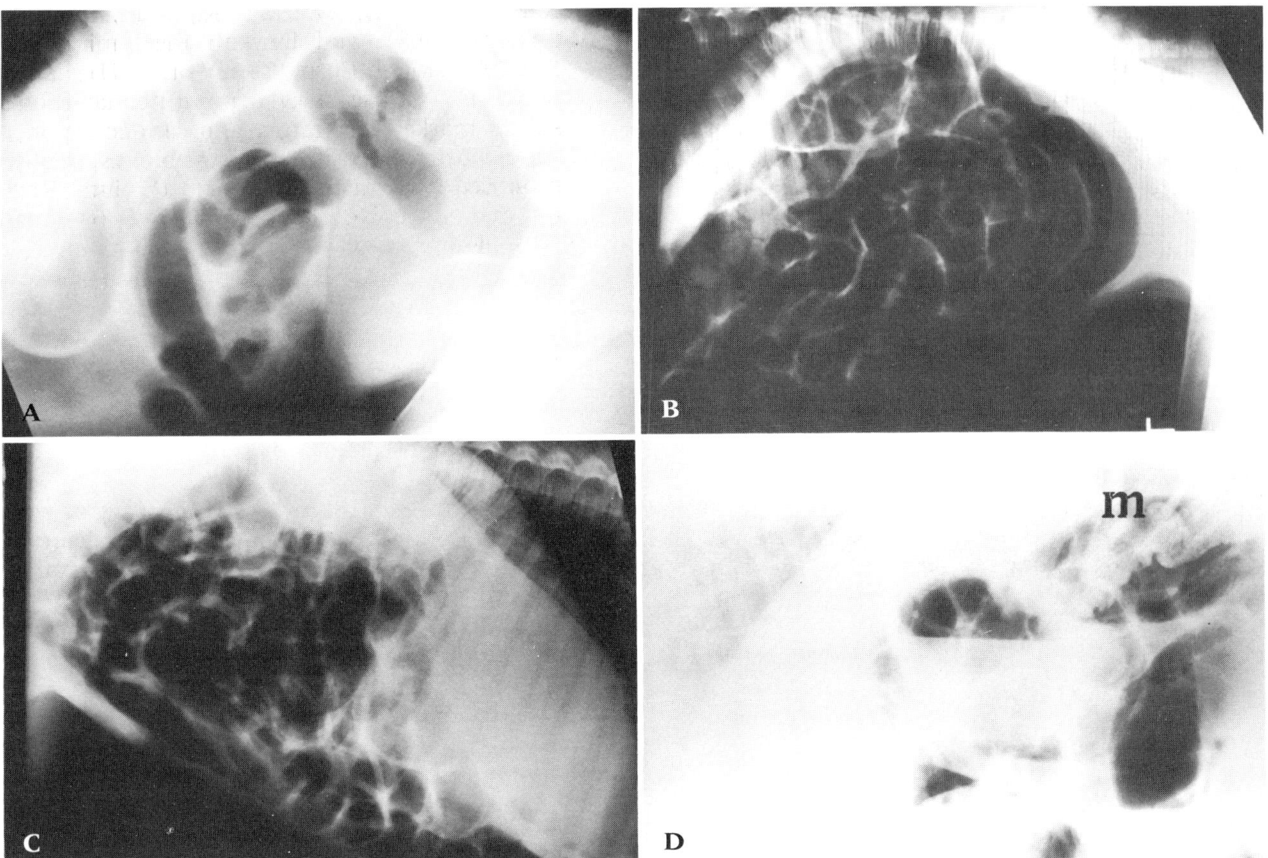

FIG. 113–2. *A*, Distention of small intestine on radiograph. Note multiple loops of black tubular structures. Intestinal obstruction is difficult to differentiate from ileus. This foal had enteritis and septicemia but no intestinal obstruction. *B*, Distention of small intestine and large intestine. This foal had a volvulus of the small intestine. *C*, Gas in both small and large intestine but no significant distention of bowel. This foal had a meconium impaction. The meconium is not visible in this figure. *D*, Meconium visible in large intestine (m) because of distention of surrounding bowel with gas.

in three foals.[12] Because the abdomen of the foal is smaller than that of the adult, these authors report that fluid-filled large and small intestine can be seen with ultrasonography as well as abnormal intestinal wall thickness, intussusception, and excess peritoneal fluid. The wall of the intussusception of one of these foals was thick, with echogenic intussusception eccentrically located within a sonolucent core. In a second foal, multiple loops of distended small intestine with an echogenic center surrounded by fluid was seen ultrasonographically. Multiple cross sections of affected intestine were visualized, indicating one extensive intussusception or multiple lesions.

ILEUS

Ileus with gas accumulation in the intestinal lumen can result in colic in the neonatal foal. Ileus can occur secondarily to electrolyte imbalance, sepsis, asphyxia, hypoxia, and enteritis. The pathogenic mechanism of ileus includes impaired innervation, electrolyte imbalance, or intestinal inflammation. The diagnosis of ileus in the foal can be challenging. Foals with ileus may develop abdominal distention, are often intolerant of oral feeding, and have signs of abdominal pain that may progress to depression.[7] Radiographic examination of the abdomen may reveal multiple gas distended loops of small or large intestine. Differentiation of intestinal gas distention caused by ileus or strangulation obstruction is difficult and in some cases impossible.[7] Ultrasonography of the abdomen can be used to rule out free abdominal fluid as the cause for abdominal distention.[12] Abdominocentesis in the presence of distended bowel carries a higher risk of enterocentesis.[7] The results of peritoneal fluid analysis will vary with the cause of the ileus (e.g., if caused by sepsis or enteritis, it may be suppurative; if caused by an electrolyte imbalance or asphyxia, the fluid would likely be normal). Management of foals with ileus would include reducing or discontinuing enteral feeding, meeting the foal's fluid and energy needs via parenteral route, and correcting the underlying cause if possible.[7] Also correction of electrolyte imbalances, supplementation with oxygen if hypoxic, and light exercise if mobile may help. If sepsis is suspected, antimicrobial therapy is indicated. Use of analgesics may be necessary to prevent self-trauma, but use should be limited because most analgesic drugs reduce intestinal motility.[12] Surgical decompression may ultimately be required.[7] Ileus was an intraoperative diagnosis in 9 of 20 foals that had exploratory celiotomy.[3] Ileus is not generally considered to be an abdominal condition requiring surgical intervention. However, because of the difficulty in differentiating ileus from intestinal obstruction preoperatively, 9 foals in this series had surgery. The authors indicated the foals with ileus may have actually benefited from surgical decompression of the bowel at surgery.[3] Certainly, any foal with a continuing abdominal crisis should have a hemogram, biochemical profile, blood culture, and an arterial blood gas analysis performed as well as an evaluation of its immunoglobulin level to help determine its potential for having or developing septicemia and to manage more accurately its anesthetic and perioperative care.

AGANGLIONOSIS OR ATRESIA

Foals with aganglionosis or atresia of a portion of the bowel will present like foals that have colic from another source. Ileocolonic aganglionosis occurs in foals that are completely white who are born to ovaro spotted parents.[13] Atresia ani and coli have been reported in foals, and atresia ani may occur along with defects in the urinary tract of the foal.[14,15] Heritability of atresia coli or ani has not been fully defined in the foal and no breed predilection has been reported. Unlike foals with meconium impaction, ileus, or torsion of the colon, these foals will never have passed feces. No fecal staining will be noted in the perineum, and no history will exist of feces being passed. These foals generally develop colic between 12 to 36 h of age and progressively worsen because of inability to pass feces. Ileocolonic agangliosis is not a treatable condition. Atresia coli and ani require surgical intervention.

DIARRHEA, ENTEROCOLITIS

Diarrhea in foals is a common occurrence. In one prospective study, 50% of foals developed diarrhea.[16] Most of these foals did not have other clinical signs of disease. In certain cases, diarrhea in the neonatal foal can lead to colic, severe dehydration, and electrolyte abnormalities and be associated with subsequent septicemia.[17] The etiologic agents associated with diarrhea in foals are many, including viruses such as rotavirus,[18–21] coronavirus,[22,23] and adenovirus;[24] bacteria such as Escherichia coli,[25,26] salmonellae,[27–30] Clostridium per fringens,[31,32] and Clostridium difficile;[33] parasites; consumption of fibrous feeds, sand, or manure; foal heat diarrhea; and idiopathic agents.

The cause of diarrhea in the foal cannot generally be determined from clinical signs alone. However, foals with diarrhea caused by salmonella and clostridia are generally systemically ill. Clostridial organisms can result in severe enterocolitis with resultant colic and bloody, foul-smelling diarrhea.[31–33] Foal heat diarrhea is a term used for diarrhea that develops in foals 6 to 10 days of age when the mare is in estrus, and generally, the foal has no other abnormal clinical signs.[34] However, diarrhea in foals 6 to 10 days of age has been recognized in foals removed from the mare soon after birth and reared on artificial supplements.[35] Therefore, whatever the cause of this form of diarrhea, it is not the influence of the mare or her milk. Researchers have proposed that foal heat diarrhea is the result of a change in intestinal microbial flora and/or an inability to deal with the need for increased electrolyte and fluid absorption.[36]

Identification of a causative agent is not necessary to initiate effective therapy of the foal with diarrhea. But if a cause is known, more directed therapy can occur as soon as possible and preventive measures on a farm basis may be developed. For example, rotavirus can survive in the environment for months.[5] Rotavirus concentration in the neonatal calf with diarrhea can be up to 1×10^7 infective doses of rotavirus per gram of feces, so environmental contamination and subsequent exposure of the susceptible neonate to the environment is the proposed means of infection of the neonate.[5] Dwyer et al. reported that quarantine, routine cleaning of stalls with phenol disinfectant, and use of protective clothing proved effective in controlling and preventing rotavirus diarrhea on 19 farms.[5] Feces should be collected as early in the course of the diarrhea as possible, because viral agents in the feces of foals with diarrhea are often present only early in the course of the disease. Feces submitted for viral identification should be examined via electron microscopy and enzyme-linked immunosorbant assay for rotavirus (Rotazyme, Abbott Diagnostics, Chicago, IL) or latex agglutination test (Virogen Rotatest, Wampole Laboratories, Cranbury, NJ). Feces should also be submitted for aerobic and anaerobic culture.

The veterinarian must consider the significance of each agent identified in the diarrheic feces. A heavy growth of Salmonella spp. or Clostridium perfringens from the feces of a foal which is systemically ill and has diarrhea is likely associated with the disease process. However, a heavy growth of E. coli in a mixed enteric population recovered from feces would be more debatable as a cause of the foal's illness. Rotavirus has been recovered from feces of foals with diarrhea and foals that did not have diarrhea; however, an association was noted of rotavirus in fecal samples and a high occurrence of diarrhea in foals on a particular farm.[5] Some foals with enterocolitis do not develop diarrhea but have abdominal distention, ileus, abdominal pain, melena, gastric reflux, and sepsis. Necrotizing enterocolitis has been documented in foals that were hospitalized for serious illnesses.[7] An incident that results in bowel ischemia is followed by bacterial colonization of ischemically damaged bowel wall. Pneumatosis intestinalis is recognized radiographically as gas lucency within the bowel wall.

Therapy and diagnostic tests performed on a foal with diarrhea depends on the severity of clinical signs. If the foal has diarrhea alone but appears normal in all other respects, is 6 to 10 days of age, and has had evaluation of passive transfer, then close observation along with cleaning and protection of the perineum with a petroleum jelly may be all that is necessary. If the foal appears depressed or has reduced frequency of nursing, then a hemogram, plasma fibrinogen, chemistry profile, immunoglobulin evaluation, and blood glucose test along with fecal and blood cultures should be submitted. Blood for culture should be collected aseptically from the jugular vein and submitted to the laboratory in blood culture media (BBL Microbiology Systems, Cockeysville, MD). If septicemia is suspected, a broad-spectrum antibiotic should be initiated.[37] If the foal is azotemic, electrolyte depleted, hypoglycemic, or clinically dehydrated, appropriate intravenous fluids should be initiated until laboratory results are available.

Loss of fluid and electrolytes in diarrhea can be substantial and in the face of disease, the foal's caloric needs are increased. The choice of fluids should be based on electrolyte, glucose, and acid-base values and the clinical condition and state of hydration of the foal.[8] A fluid should be chosen that most closely meets the particular needs of the individual. Specific deficits of glucose, potassium, or bicarbonate may require further addition of one or more of these to commercial fluids. In the majority of situations, a balanced crystalloid fluid that is approximately isotonic is suitable. A reasonable initial replacement fluid would be 0.45% NaCl with 2.5% dextrose, because it would provide electrolytes, fluid, and glucose and is isotonic. The clinician should not assume this fluid is appropriate for sustained therapy because it will not correct acidosis, hypokalemia, or severe hypoglycemia. Continuous fluid infusion is preferred over bolus infusion, thus necessitating the sterile placement of an indwelling intravenous catheter. A general rule of thumb on fluid rates is to replace 50% of the calculated deficit in the first 6 to 12 h and complete correction over the next 12 to 24 h. Too rapid an infusion can overload the vascular system. Compromised neonates may have difficulties eliminating excess fluid. In an attempt to quantitate fluid loss, several parameters can be used and include clinical signs, skin turgor, capillary refill, heart rate, peripheral pulse quality, packed cell volume and total protein, serum urea nitrogen, and creatinine. In a 50-kg neonate, estimates of 5%, 10%, and 15% dehydration represent a 2.5 L, 5 L, and 7.5 L fluid deficit, respectively (body weight [kg] × percent deficit estimate = water deficit in liters).[8] Mild signs of dehydration are associated with 5% (of total body weight) fluid deficit, 10% moderate signs, and 15% severe compromise and impending cardiovascular collapse.[8] Oral electrolyte/glucose fluids may be of benefit to the foal with diarrhea with minimal signs of dehydration but should not be relied on to correct moderate to severe dehydration and should not be used in foals with gastric reflux or abdominal pain.

Limiting milk consumption has been advocated and is a debatable aspect of management of the foal with diarrhea. If the foal has colic or if viral diarrhea is suspected, then limited milk consumption for a short time may be beneficial. To ensure parenteral caloric support is critical if the foal is withheld from milk for 24 h or more.

Antibiotic therapy in foals with diarrhea of unknown cause is controversial. In neonatal foals, the risk of untreated, generalized gram-negative infection usually outweighs the potential side effects of antibiotic therapy. A combination of penicillin with an aminoglycoside is often used.[7] The foal should be well hydrated and efforts made to monitor renal function when using an aminoglycoside. Orally administered potentiated sulfa drugs have both a gram-positive and gram-negative spectrum, but in a foal that has diarrhea absorption may be unpredictable. Intestinal protectants such as bismuth subsalicylate have been used in foals with diarrhea with an improvement in fecal consistency.[7] No established dosage exists in the neonatal foal, and constipation and a discoloration of the feces may occur. If a favorable response is obtained, the foal should gradually be weaned off treatment. A dosage that has been used is 0.5 to 1.0 mL/kg several times a day. Low dose nonsteroidal anti-inflammatory drug (NSAID) therapy should be considered if signs of endotoxic shock exist (e.g., flunixin meglumine 0.25 mg/kg bid or tid). Gastrointestinal ulceration and renal damage can be sequelae of NSAID therapy, especially in dehydrated foals.[7]

Plasma transfusion would be indicated in foals with hypoproteinemia or failure of passive transfer.[7] Prevention of gastrointestinal ulceration in foals with diarrhea is frequently attempted. Therapy has included hydrogen antagonists or sucralfate. The efficacy of prophylactic treatment is unknown. If the foal has diarrhea as well as colic, then ileus, necrotizing enterocolitis, gastric ulceration, or intestinal accident could be occurring concurrent with the diarrheic state, and diagnostics and therapy should be directed accordingly.

Prevention of foal diarrhea outbreaks includes isolation of affected foals and hygiene to reduce traffic between sick and susceptible foals. Hygiene at the time of foaling (disinfection of the foaling stall, wrapping the mare's tail, and washing the mare's udder) has been associated with a lower occurrence of foal diarrhea.[16] Avoiding overfeeding of foals and limiting their access to foreign material such as sand would be indicated.

GASTRODUODENAL ULCERATION AND GASTRIC OUTFLOW PROBLEM

Gastroduodenal ulceration may result in a variety of clinical signs, ranging from no abnormal signs to hypophagia, bruxism, diarrhea, and colic. The best antemortem means of diagnosing gastric ulceration in foals is endoscopy. Gastric ulceration was diagnosed in 25% of foals necropsied during a survey.[38] In this study, approximately half of the foals had abnormal clinical signs attributed to the gastroduodenal ulceration. In a prospective study of gastric ulceration in foals without clinical signs attributable to gastric ulceration but detected via endoscopy of the stomach, 51% had gastric ulceration.[39] The most commonly affected age groups were foals 21 to 30 days of age, with 11 to 20 and 0 to 10 days, respectively, being the next most frequently affected age groups. Thus gastric ulceration may occur in the neonatal foal.

Clearly, not all foals with gastric ulceration will have signs of colic, hypophagia, or bruxism. The location of the gastric ulceration is an important factor. Lesions in the nonglandular stomach were common in foals in two prospective studies.[38,39] The significance of these lesions in the nonglandular stomach are difficult to interpret because they were common in foals with no abnormal clinical signs, yet this was the most common site for fatal ulcer perforation.

The cause of gastric and duodenal ulceration is unknown other than in cases which have received large doses or prolonged therapy with drugs such as phenylbutazone or flunixin meglumine.[40,41] Proposed causes include stress,[42] infectious agents,[43] altered motility,[44] epithelial desquamation, and significant weather and barometric changes.[38] Gastric ulceration can occur in outbreaks on a particular farm, but the reason for this has not been determined.[45] Because the cause of gastric ulceration in foals is unknown, prevention of the problem is difficult.

Researchers have suggested that foals stressed because of other illnesses be treated prophylactically to prevent gastric ulceration with drugs like cimetidine (Tagamet, Smith Kline & Beecham, Bristol, TN), ranitidine (Zantac, Alaxo Inc., Research Triangle Park, NC), and/or sucralfate (Carafate, Marion Labs, Inc., Kansas City, MO). The dosage of each of these drugs in the neonatal foal is still under investigation.[46] Concern exists that the recommended human dose of cimetidine is inadequate in the foal.[44,46] Ranitidine and cimetidine are histamine inhibitors and act to reduce gastric acid production. Ranitidine appears to be more effective than cimetidine in the treatment of gastric ulcers in foals 7 to 12 months of age.[7] Suggested dosage of ranitidine is 0.5 to 1 mg/kg qid IV or 4 to 8 mg/kg tid orally for foals up to 12 months of age. However no controlled studies have been performed in young foals, thus dosage may not be appropriate in young suckling foals.[7] A suggested dosage of cimetidine is 4 mg/kg qid IV or 8 to 16 mg/kg qid orally in foals 7 to 12 months of age; again the appropriate dosage in neonatal foals has not been determined.[7] Sucralfate is a gastric protectant. No clinical efficacy trial for this drug is available as of this writing.[7] A suggested dosage is 20 to 40 mg/kg qid orally.[7] Antacids may be of some benefit but can result in constipation (dosage of aluminum hydroxide 15 to 60 mL orally every 2 to 4 h).[7] Omeprazole (Losec, Merck, Sharp, and Dohme, West Point, PA) is a recently approved drug for use in humans which is a potent inhibitor of gastric acid secretion.[47] Preliminary investigation in the horse of intravenous omeprazole shows it to be an inhibitor of gastric acid secretion. No form of omeprazole is approved for use in the horse or foal at this time.

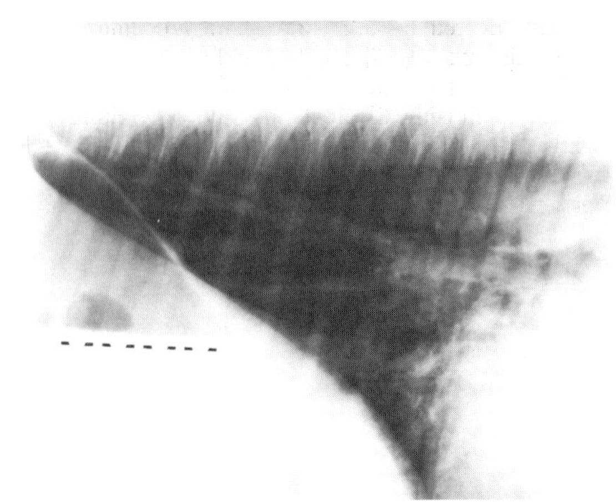

FIG. 113–3. Barium still present in stomach after 12 h indicates gastric emptying or outflow problem. Fluid line in stomach, which is the barium/air interface, is highlighted with a dotted line.

If a mechanical gastric outflow problem exists because of duodenal stricturing, clinical signs will be present in the form of colic, lying on the back in dorsal recumbency, bruxism, and hypophagia. Double contrast gastrogram will demonstrate an outflow problem[10,44] (Fig. 113–3) but will not always differentiate a mechanical from physiologic problem. As well as a dilated stomach with prolonged to no emptying of barium into the duodenum, these foals may have a dilated air-filled esophagus and air or contrast material in the hepatic duct.[46,48] If an outflow problem exists, surgical intervention is the only effective treatment if the foal fails to improve with intensive medical therapy,[48,49] but the prognosis remains guarded to poor. Medical therapy consists of gastric decompression, parenteral H_2-receptor antagonist, intravenous fluids with electrolytes and possibly parenteral nutrition.[44]

REFERENCES

1. Madigan, J.E.: Manual of Equine Neonatal Medicine. Woodland, CA, Live Oak Publishing, 1987.
2. Becht, J.L., and Semrad, S.D.: Gastrointestinal diseases of foals. Compend. Contin. Educ. Practicing Vet., *8:*S367–S375, 1986.
3. Adams, R., et al.: Exploratory celiotomy for gastrointestinal disease in neonatal foals. Equine Vet. J., *20:*9–12, 1988.
4. Adams, R., Koterba, A.M., Cudd, T.C., and Baker, W.A.: Exploratory celiotomy for suspected urinary tract disruption in neonatal foals: A review of 18 cases. Equine Vet. J., *20:*13–17, 1988.
5. Dwyer, R.M., et al.: Infectious foal diarrhea: A three year study of epidemiology and prevention. Proc. Am. Coll. Vet. Int. Med., *8:*569–571, 1990.
6. Madigan, J.E.: Meconium impaction. *In* Manual of Neo-

natology. Edited by J.E. Madigan. Woodland, CA, Live Oak Publishing, 1987, pp. 113–116.

7. Wilson, J.H., and Cudd, T.A.: Common gastrointestinal diseases. *In* Equine Clinical Neonatology. Edited by A.M. Koterba, W.H. Drummond, and P.C. Kosch. Philadelphia, Lea & Febiger, 1990, pp. 412–430.
8. Spurlock, S.L., and Furr, M.: Fluid therapy. *In* Equine Clinical Neonatology. Edited by A.M. Koterba, W.H. Drummond, and P.C. Kosch. Philadelphia, Lea & Febiger, 1990, pp. 671–700.
9. Adams, R.: Gastrointestinal surgery. *In* Equine Clinical Neonatology. Edited by A.M. Koterba, W.H. Drummond, and P.C. Kosch. Philadelphia, Lea & Febiger, 1990, pp. 430–443.
10. Cudd, T.A., Toal, R.L., and Embertson, R.M.: The use of clinical findings, abdominocentesis and abdominal radiographs to assess surgical versus nonsurgical abdominal disease in the foal. Proc. Am. Assoc. Equine Pract., 41–53, 1987.
11. Cudd, T.A., and Wilson, J.H.: Diagnostic techniques for abdominal problems. *In* Equine Clinical Neonatology. Edited by A.M. Koterba, W.H. Drummond, and P.C. Kosch. Philadelphia, Lea & Febiger, 1990, pp. 412–430.
12. Bernard, W.V., et. al.: Ultrasonographic diagnosis of small-intestinal intussusception in three foals. J. Am. Vet. Med. Assoc., *194:*395–397, 1989.
13. Hultgren, B.D.: Ileocolonic aganglionosis in white progeny of overo spotted horses. J. Am. Vet. Med. Assoc., *180:*289–292, 1982.
14. Kingston, R.S., and Park, R.D.: Atresia ani with an associated urogenital tract anomaly in foals. Equine Pract., *4:*32–34, 1982.
15. Schneider, J.E.: Agenesis or atresia of the colon of newborn foals. Proc. Am. Assoc. Equine Pract., 285–290, 1981.
16. Traub-Dargatz, J.L., et al.: Epidemiologic survey of diarrhea in foals. J. Am. Vet. Med. Assoc., *192:*1553–1556, 1988.
17. Koterba, A.M., Brewer, B.D., and Tarplee, F.A.: Clinical and clinicopathological characteristics of septicemic neonatal foals: Review of 38 cases. Equine Vet. J., *16:*312–318, 1984.
18. Tzipori, S., and Walker, M.: Isolation of rotavirus from foals with diarrhea. Aust. J. Exp. Biol., *56:*453–457, 1978.
19. Eugster, A.D., Whitford, H.W., and Mehr, L.E.: Concurrent rotavirus and salmonella infections in foals. J. Am. Vet. Med. Assoc., *173:*857–858, 1978.
20. Studdert, M.J., Mason, R.W., and Patten, B.E.: Rotavirus diarrhea in foals. Aust. Vet. J., *54:*363–364, 1978.
21. Conner, M.E., and Darlington, R.W.: Rotavirus infection in foals. Am. J. Vet. Res., *41:*1699–1703, 1980.
22. Bass, E.P., and Sharpee, A.L.: Coronavirus and gastroenteritis in foals. Lancet, *2:*822, 1975.
23. Ward, A.C.S., Evermann, J.F., and Reed, S.M.: Presence of coronavirus in diarrheic foals. Vet. Med. Small Anim. Clin., *78:*563–565, 1983.
24. Studdert, M.J., and Blackney, M.H.: Isolation of an adenovirus antigenically distinct from equine adenovirus type I from diarrheic foal feces. Am. J. Vet. Res., *43:*543–544, 1982.
25. Ward, A.C.S., et al.: Isolation of piliated Escherichia coli from diarrheic foals. Vet. Microbiol., *12:*221–228, 1986.
26. Sriranganathan, N., and DuPont, L.: Isolation of enterotoxigenic Escherichia coli from a foal with diarrhea. J. Am. Vet. Med. Assoc., *194:*389–391, 1989.
27. Carter, M.E., Deines, H.G., and Griffiths, O.V.: Salmonellosis in foals. J. Equine Med. Surg., *3:*78–83, 1979.
28. Smith, B.P., Reina-Guerra, M., and Hardy, A.J.: Prevalence and epizootiology of equine salmonellosis. J. Am. Vet. Med. Assoc., *172:*353–356, 1978.
29. Trauer, D.S., Trimmel, B.J., and Armstrong, C.: Salmonellosis in foals. Proc. Am. Assoc. Equine Pract., *25:*225–234, 1979.
30. Smith, B.P., et al.: Equine salmonellosis: Experimental production of 4 syndromes. Am. J. Vet. Res., *40:*1072–1081, 1979.
31. Dickie, C.W., Klinkerman, D.L., and Petrie, R.J.: Enterotoxemia in two foals. J. Am. Vet. Med. Assoc., *173:*306–307, 1978.
32. Niilo, L., and Chalmers, G.A.: Hemorrhagic enterotoxemia caused by Clostridium perfringens type C in a foal. Can. Vet. J., *23:*299–301, 1982.
33. Jones, R.L., et al.: Hemorrhagic necrotizing enterocolitis associated with Clostridium difficile infection in four foals. J. Am. Vet. Med. Assoc., *193:*76–79, 1988.
34. Palmer, J.E.: Gastrointestinal diseases of foals. Vet. Clin. North. Am. Equine Pract., *1:*151–169, 1985.
35. Stowe, H.D.: Automated orphan foal feeding. Proc Am. Assoc. Equine Pract., *13:*65–75, 1967.
36. Masari, M.D., Gronwall, M.R., and Burrows, C.F.: Fecal composition in foal heat diarrhea. Equine Vet. J., *18:*301–306, 1986.
37. Brewer, B.D., and Koterba, A.M.: Development of a scoring system for the early diagnosis of equine neonatal sepsis. Equine Vet. J., *20:*18–22, 1988.
38. Wilson, J.H.: Gastric and duodenal ulcers in foals: A retrospective study. Proceedings of the Second Equine Colic Symposium. Edited by J.N. Moore, N.A. White, and J.L. Becht. Trenton, Veterinary Learning Systems, 1986, pp. 126–129.
39. Murray, M.J., Hart, J., and Parker, G.A.: Equine gastric ulcer syndrome: Endoscopic survey of asymptomatic foals. Proc. Am. Assoc. Equine Pract., 769–776, 1987.
40. Traub, J.L., et al.: Phenylbutazone toxicosis in the foal. Am. J. Vet. Res., *44:*1410–1418, 1983.
41. Traub-Dargatz, J.L., et al.: Chronic flunixin meglumine therapy in foals. Am. J. Vet. Res., *49:*7–12, 1988.
42. Furr, M.D.: The effects of stress on gastric ulceration and serum T3, T4, rT3 and cortisol in neonatal foals. Proc. Am. Assoc. Equine Pract., 517, 1989.
43. Becht, J.L., and Byars, T.D.: Gastroduodenal ulceration in foals. Equine Vet. J., *18:*307–312, 1986.
44. Gross, T.L., and Mayhew, I.G.: Gastroesophageal ulceration and candidiasis in foals. J. Am. Vet. Med. Assoc., *182:*1370–1373, 1983.
45. Campbell-Thompson, M.L.: Diagnosis and treatment of gastroduodenal ulceration in foals and adults. Proc. Am. Assoc. Equine Pract., 57–71, 1989.
46. Campbell-Thompson, M.L., and Merritt, A.M.: Gastroduodenal ulceration in foals. Proc. Am. Assoc. Equine Pract., 29–40, 1987.
47. Jenkins, C.J., and DeNovo, R.C.: Omeprazole: An overview of experience in the dog and horse. Proc. Am. Coll. Vet. Int. Med., *8:*437–439, 1990.
48. Orsini, J.A., and Donawick, W.J.: Surgical treatment of gastroduodenal obstruction in foals. Vet. Surg., *15:*205–213, 1986.
49. Campbell-Thompson, M.L., et al.: Gastroenterostomy for treatment of gastroduodenal ulcer disease in 14 foals. J. Am. Vet. Med. Assoc., *188:*840–844, 1986.

CHAPTER 114

THE URINARY SYSTEM

K.L. Seltzer
T.J. Divers
W.E. Vaala
T.D. Byars
and J.L. Rubin

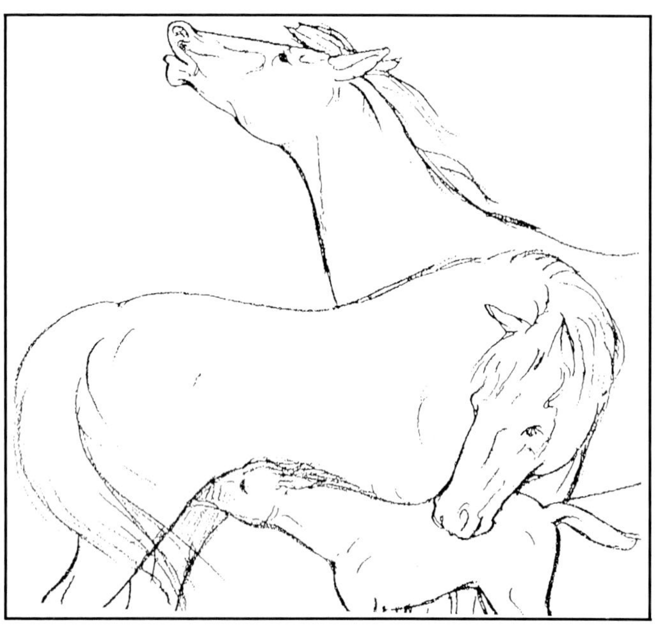

ACUTE RENAL FAILURE

K.L. Seltzer
T.J. Divers

Intrinsic renal failure in foals can be divided into three causative groups: ischemic (hemodynamic), toxic, and septic. Renal failure, patent urachus, rupture of the urinary tract, cystitis, and urachal abscess are common diseases in the equine neonatal period. Ectopic ureter is a more sporadic condition affecting foals. This chapter is intended to provide up-to-date information on causes, clinical signs, laboratory findings, and diagnosis and treatment of these conditions. Normal values for serum chemistries (e.g., creatinine, calcium, and α-glutamyl-transferase) in foals can vary from those of the more mature equine. The high values of serum creatinine, which may be spurious elevations in many foals, is also discussed.

CAUSES OF ACUTE RENAL FAILURE

HEMODYNAMIC

The most frequent causes of acute renal failure (ARF) in foals are hemodynamic events that affect normal blood flow to and/or within the kidney. Foals that become hypovolemic, hypotensive, or hypoxic have a high risk of developing renal dysfunction and failure. If such conditions persist, irreversible renal failure may result. Foals with diarrhea and dehydration, or septicemic foals that advance into septic shock are at highest risk of developing acute renal failure. Some positive correlation also exists between foals with respiratory acidosis and central nervous system (CNS) depression and the subsequent development of hypotension, hypoglycemia, and hypothermia which can contribute to the onset of renal dysfunction and/or failure. Foals with hemodynamic induced renal failure may have histopathologic changes of severe tubular nephrosis, or only minimal changes in the kidney are noticed on light microscopic exam.

TOXIC

Drug-induced toxicities (aminoglycosides are the most frequent offenders) are the second most common cause of renal dysfunction/failure in the foal. Aminoglycoside toxicity, as in hemodynamic-induced renal failure, manifests as acute tubular necrosis. Hypovolemic and/or hypotensive foals are more susceptible to the toxic effects of aminoglycosides. These are most often foals with diarrhea and/or those unable to nurse adequate volumes, e.g., maladjustment foals or foals with musculoskeletal problems.

Term foals are reported to have glomerular filtration rates (GFR) similar to adults.[1] Although not proven, the feeling among some practicing veterinarians is that neonatal foals are more predisposed to aminoglycoside toxicity than the more mature equine. If this predisposition exists, it may be the result of the foal being less efficient than adults at conserving water and compensating for changes in body fluid and electrolyte balance (e.g., sodium and potassium) which may occur with disease (e.g., diarrhea and septicemia).[2] Normal physiologic changes in extracellular fluid volume of the foal could also influence risks of aminoglycoside toxicity.[3] Premature foals should not be assumed to have normal GFR at birth.

SEPTIC

Less frequently, acute renal failure in the foal may be attributable to septic nephritis. Actinobacillus is the most common causative organism of septic renal failure in foals. Most foals with actinobacillus septicemia die before uremia has time to develop. Septic shock resulting from any agent would have hemodynamic alterations that affect renal function.

CONGENITAL

Although rare, congenital disorders (e.g., renal glomerular hypoplasia) may also cause renal failure in foals. This is more likely though to result in a chronic condition of poor growth.

CLINICAL SIGNS AND DIAGNOSIS

Foals with renal failure show depression and deterioration in physical condition and mental awareness. Oral plaques and oral ulcers may occasionally be seen with uremia. Clinical evidence of dehydration or hypovolemia may exist such as sunken eyeballs, poor pulse quality, and a prolonged capillary refill time. Blood pressure values may also be markedly decreased. In acute renal failure of hemodynamic origin, foals are often anuric or oliguric. A generalized edema that develops with fluid therapy is strongly suggestive of severe, acute oliguric renal failure. Foals with acute renal failure caused by aminoglycoside toxicity are usually polyuric.

CLINICAL LABORATORY DATA

The most common electrolyte abnormalities in foals with acute renal failure are hypochloremia, hyponatremia, and elevated serum creatinine and urea nitrogen ($>$ 20 mg/dL). Serum creatinine, as an indicator of renal function, may be difficult to interpret in the neonatal foal because elevated serum creatinine (up to 15 mg/dL) in clinically normal and healthy neonatal foals is not rare. However, successive samples should decrease to normal range by day 5 of life in those foals. Urine specific gravity and urinary proteins may also be difficult to interpret in the equine neonate. This is because the foal normally produces hyposthenuric or isothenuric urine and a mild proteinuria may commonly be found in healthy foals 24 to 36 h of age, caused by gut-absorbed and renal-filtered colostral microglobulins.[4,5] Granular and renal tubular casts and microscopic hematuria in the urine sediment are other abnormal clinical laboratory findings of foals with acute renal failure. Urine volume in normal healthy foals has been recently reported to be about 148 mL/kg/day.[4]

Foals with acute renal failure as a result of hemodynamic causes often show a worsening metabolic and respiratory acidosis. These foals are most often oliguric or anuric and hyperkalemia is common. When hyperkalemia is present in foals, severe acidosis and/or oliguric renal failure or urinary tract rupture should be considered.

TREATMENT

Treatment of renal dysfunction/failure should be instituted immediately and is aimed at improving renal blood flow and nephron function and preventing further renal damage before the onset of irreversible renal failure occurs. In general, fluid deficits should be restored by intravenous (IV) fluid therapy and electrolyte imbalances should be corrected according to measured serum abnormalities. Choice and type of fluids should be based on acid base and electrolyte abnormalities.

The IV fluids used should be nearly isotonic, because foals normally have a lower serum osmolality than the adult horse.[4] During administration of IV fluids, the clinician must monitor urine output versus fluid input. This is of most importance in the oliguric or anuric patient. With oliguric and/or anuric renal failure, the clinician may have to slow fluid administration rates to prevent formation of extensive generalized edema until further pharmacologic intervention allows urine production to increase.

In foals with acute renal failure resulting from hemodynamic causes, the primary goals of therapy are to increase blood volume, increase systemic blood pressure and renal perfusion, and promote diuresis. In the anuric, oliguric, or extremely hypotensive patient pharmacologic agents are often necessary and beneficial in addition to IV fluid therapy. Pharmacologic agents of choice for foals with oliguric or anuric acute renal failure are dopamine, dobutamine, mannitol, and furosemide. A dopamine drip at 3 to 8 μg/kg/min or mannitol administered at 0.25 mg/kg is recommended to aid in the improvement of renal blood flow and renal function. Slightly higher concentrations of dopamine may be used as long as systemic hypertension does not occur. During administration of dopamine and/or mannitol, furosemide should be given at 25 to 50 mg IV every hour for two to three injections or until urine output increases. If the foal is hypotensive, dobutamine should be given in addition to the foregoing at the rate of 3 to 10 μg/kg/min in hopes of returning system blood pressure to the normal range.

In cases of aminoglycoside toxicity or in cases where aminoglycoside therapy is thought to be contributing to the renal dysfunction, the aminoglycoside therapy should be discontinued or the dosage and/or the dosing interval adjusted. These adjustments should be made based on serum creatinine concentration and clinical condition of the patient.

Septic renal failure should be managed similarly to renal failure as a result of hemodynamic causes with addition of appropriate antibiotic therapy. Antimicrobials without nephrotoxic properties (e.g., timentin and ceftiofur) are preferred.

Treatment of all cases of acute renal failure in foals and especially those owing to hemodynamic causes should be prompt, aggressive, and persistent. Premature foals with respiratory distress and/or central nervous signs that have been treated for concurrent acute renal failure and progressed from anuria/oliguria to polyuria have been noted to relapse back into hypotension and oliguric renal failure if therapy or supportive fluid therapy is discontinued too abruptly. Therapy should persist well beyond start of polyuria to ensure hemodynamic stability and continued renal function in those foals. Foals that relapse into a second episode of oliguric renal failure may be harder to convert back into polyuric states for a second time.

When treating any foal with ARF, the clinician must monitor urine output, serum creatinine and urea nitrogen, urinalysis, and the foal's general attitude and appearance, because these are important indicators as to response to and effectiveness of treatment. Peritoneal dialysis is an additional treatment that has been beneficial in reducing azotemia and removing aminoglycosides from the body, but it has been noted to be more mechanically difficult in foals because of omental plugging of peritoneal catheters.[6]

PROGNOSIS

Renal dysfunction caused by hemodynamic alterations and aminoglycoside toxicity that can be readily reversed with intravenous fluid therapy and/or dopamine, dobutamine, and diuretics hold a good prognosis for renal recovery. Polyuria, decrease in azotemia, resolution of metabolic acidosis, correction of electrolyte abnormalities, and a general attitude improvement are good prognostic findings.

However, foals with anuria or oliguria that does not progress to polyuria or begin producing adequate amounts of urine after aggressive diuresis with IV fluids, diuretics, and dopamine/dobutamine have a poor to grave prognosis. Development of anasarca during fluid therapy is a poor prognostic sign. Foals with anuric renal failure and edema will usually die despite pharmacologic intervention. On rare occasions, foals may survive an acute episode of renal failure but acquire sufficient renal fibrosis that normal growth is disrupted.

PREVENTION

Early and appropriate treatment for dehydration and severe hypotension in foals is important in preventing hemodynamic ARF or aminoglycoside induced nephrotoxicity. Foals given aminoglycoside treatments and having a possible predisposition for aminoglycoside toxicity (e.g., diarrhea and prematurity) should have serum creatinine and/or aminoglycoside troughs concentration performed every 2 to 3 days. The aim of trough measurements is to allow for adjustment of dosage/dosing intervals before progression of nephrosis occurs. Gentamicin trough levels should remain <2.0 μg/mL. Amikacin levels should remain < 6 μg/mL. Urinary enzymes, e.g., α-glutamyltransaminopeptidase (GGT) are increased in the urine of foals with tubular nephrosis, but the degree of elevation of GGT to creatinine ratios may not correlate with GFR and renal function. Foals treated with aminoglycosides for extended periods (>10 days) or those with possible predisposition for aminoglycoside toxicity should have serum creatinine measured not only during aminoglycoside therapy but also 2 to 3 days after therapy is discontinued. Aminoglycoside toxicity may continue during this time in spite of discontinuation of therapy.

Metaclopramide may possibly contribute to or incite renal dysfunction or failure. Metaclopramide, commonly used to treat gastrointestinal ileus, is an antagonist to dopamine,[7] which means that metaclopramide may interfere with and inhibit both endogenous and exogenous dopamine, thereby possibly reducing renal plasma flow. Therefore, when using metaclopramide concurrently with dopamine as a treatment in foals with renal failure, the clinician may have to increase the dosage of dopamine. The clinician also may have to monitor renal parameters (serum creatinine, blood urea nitrogen, and urinalysis) in foals receiving metaclopramide. If renal dysfunction or failure occurs during metaclopramide therapy—and especially if not explainable by another cause such as hypotension, hypovolemia, dehydration, or aminoglycoside toxicity—metaclopramide should be discontinued or the dosage should be reduced.

PATENT URACHUS

W.E. Vaala

The umbilical cord develops from expansion of fetal membranes around the vestige of the yolk sac and vitelline duct.[8] The cord contains two arteries, a vein, and the urachus. The urachus is derived from the allantois and cloaca. In utero, it is a thin-walled structure extending beyond the amniotic portion of the cord and serving as the excretory conduit for urine between the fetal bladder and allantoic cavity. Spontaneous closure of this portal occurs at birth or shortly thereafter with rupture of the cord. Normally, within 24 h of birth, the umbilical remnant is a dry, shriveled structure. The urachus atrophies to become a fibrous scar on the apex of the bladder. If urachal patency occurs, the umbilicus remains moist because of continuous or intermittent urine dribbling.

CAUSES

Failure of the urachus to close postpartum is termed congenital patency and can result from excessive torsion of the umbilical cord in utero or during parturition.[8] Unusually long cords seem predisposed to excessive twisting which threatens the integrity of umbilical vessels and urachus. Cord torsion results in urachal dilatation and urine pooling proximal to lumen narrowing or obstruction. Urachal overdistention prevents normal sealing between the bladder apex and urachus at birth resulting in patency.[8] Other possible sequelae of urachal overdistention include persistent urachus and peripartum rupture of the bladder and/or urachus. Excessively traumatic cord rupture postpartum can also prevent normal closure of the urachus.

Acquired patency, the most common form, describes reopening of the urachus during the early neonatal period and is usually associated with secondary inflammation of the umbilicus.[9,10] Acquired urachal patency often coincides with sloughing of the necrotic umbilical stump and is frequently observed in recumbent, debilitated foals with urine scalding and umbilical inflammation. Umbilical cords that are cut or tied at parturition are more likely to reopen, especially following ligature removal. Any neonatal condition producing increased intra-abdominal pressure may also result in reopening of the urachus. Foals with tenesmus caused by meconium impaction or dysuria associated with cystitis, uroperitoneum, or bladder catheterization are candidates for acquired urachal patency. After prolonged bladder catheterization, many foals strain excessively to urinate because of catheter-related inflammation and/or infection. These same foals often develop a pervious urachus within 24 to 48 h of catheter removal.

Persistent urachus exists when the external urachus is sealed distal to the abdominal wall but remains patent between the bladder apex and abdominal wall.[11] This condition is normal in foals up to 10 days old but can also be associated with secondary inflammation. Affected foals strain and make frequent attempts to urinate while voiding only small volumes of urine. This condition may resolve uneventfully or lead to complete patency.

CLINICAL SIGNS AND COMPLICATIONS

The relationship between urachal patency and umbilical vessel infection is unclear. A pervious urachus can occur without infection of surrounding structures. However, an increased incidence of acquired patency exists in foals with concurrent umbilical remnant disease. This observation suggests local extension of inflammation and necrosis of umbilical vessels contributes to reopening of the urachus. Urachal patency may also predispose to umbilical remnant disease. Among one group of foals with umbilical infections, the urachus was the most frequently affected structure.[10]

The role urachal patency plays in development of neonatal sepsis remains controversial.[12–15] "Navel-ill," an older term used to describe systemic bacterial infection in young foals complicated by septic arthritis, implicated the umbilicus as the primary portal of entry for bacterial pathogens.[9,13] The description of this syndrome suggests patent urachus predisposes to umbilical infection followed by bacteremia. More recent reports emphasize the importance of respiratory and gastrointestinal tracts as primary routes of bacterial infection in neonatal foals.[14] Supporting this concept is the observation that many critically ill foals acquire urachal disease days or weeks following clinical confirmation of septicemia. However, once patent, the urachus represents another potential avenue of ascending infection.

If a patent urachus occurs, the umbilicus remains moist because of continuous or intermittent discharge of urine. In young colts, who often urinate in their sheath, urine streams down the ventral body wall and drips off the umbilicus. Careful inspection is required to distinguish this event from true urachal patency. A pervious urachus often results in a thicker than normal umbilicus, which may be warm and painful if inflammation is present.

DIAGNOSIS

Diagnostic ultrasonography can help identify infection of internal umbilical structures that is not evident by external palpation. Umbilical remnants are best visualized using a 7.5-mHz ultrasonographic transducer (linear array or sector scanner).[16] The urachus is located along the ventral midline next to the umbilical arteries and appears as an echogenic structure that is poorly defined unless it is persistent and fluid filled.[16] Communication between the urachus and bladder apex is best seen in the longitudinal view. Occasionally, a thumbprint-shaped urachal diverticulum is visualized, originating from the apex of the bladder (Fig. 114–1). In some foals, this proximal urachal dilatation is asymptomatic and closes uneventfully. Other foals with the condition strain frequently to urinate and develop true urachal patency.

Contrast radiographs can help demonstrate some urachal disorders. A persistent urachus produces a triangular appearance to the bladder apex which may extend

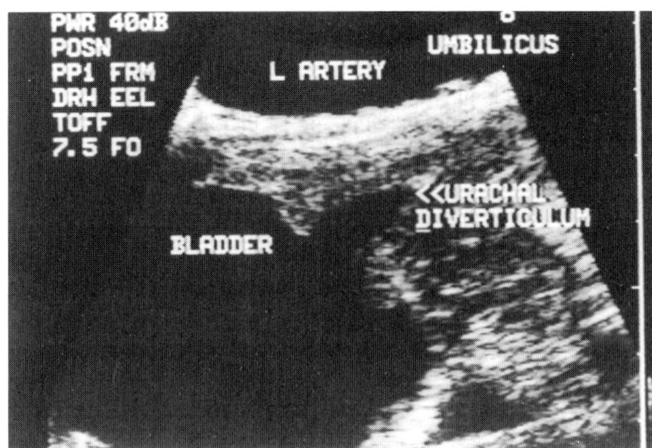

FIG. 114–1. Sonogram of a foal's bladder containing a thumbprint-shaped urachal diverticulum.

to the ventral body wall. After 1 week of age, the normal urachus can not be seen radiographically. Contrast material, infused into the bladder via a urethral catheter or via the urachus, can be used to delineate urachal patency, persistence and dilatation between the bladder and ventral body wall (Fig. 114–2). Urachal rupture can be demonstrated by leakage of contrast into the peritoneal cavity.

THERAPY

A patent urachus that occurs in the absence of concurrent umbilical remnant infection often resolves within 5 to 7 days with conservative therapy.[11] The umbilicus should be kept as clean and dry as possible. Recumbent foals should be kept on absorbent bedding that can be changed frequently. Use of strong chemicals to cauterize a patent urachus is controversial and may produce undesirable inflammation of already irritated tissues. Strong cauterants such as 7% tincture of iodine should be avoided and milder disinfectants such as 2% tincture of iodine used instead. Silver nitrate applicators, inserted 1 to 3 cm up into the urachal lumen, have produced beneficial results but should not be used more than two to three times a day for several days and should not be inserted too deeply.

Excessive straining associated with bladder catheterization may respond to oral administration of phenazopyridine (Pyridium, Parke-Davis, Morris Plains, NJ). This compound is an azo dye employed in people as a urinary tract analgesic to reduce irritation and straining caused by cystitis. The drug will result in orange discoloration of the urine. Dosed at 200 mg orally three times a day, Pyridium did reduce straining in a foal following removal of a urinary catheter. In humans, other side effects of the drug include methemoglobinemia and, rarely, hemolytic anemia.

All neonatal foals should have serum immunoglobulin concentrations measured to ensure sufficient absorption of colostral antibodies. Because of the threat of ascending infection, foals with patent urachus should receive broad-spectrum antibiotics until urachal closure has occurred.

Surgical excision of the umbilical remnants combined with systemic antibiotic therapy is recommended for foals with patent urachus that fails to respond to local cautery within 5 to 7 days or is associated with discrete abscessation of other umbilical structures. Antimicrobial therapy is crucial for cases of patent urachus associated with fever, leukocytosis, hyperfibrinogenemia, and other localized signs of bacterial infection. Choosing the most appropriate antibiotic regimen is difficult, because umbilical remnant infections frequently involve a mixed bacterial population that includes gram-positive and -negative aerobes and anaerobes and occasional yeast organisms.

Surgical resection of the umbilical remnants is performed through a ventral midline elliptical skin incision around the umbilicus. Details of the surgical procedure are described elsewhere.[12,17,18] Ligation of infected umbilical vessels is made proximal to infected segments. With urachal patency, the transition area between the urachus and bladder is usually thickened and necessitates amputation of the apex of the bladder.[18] Stay sutures are placed through the muscular portion of the bladder wall on either side of the apex and proximal to the intended line of resection. Following placement of an intestinal clamp across the apex, the abnormal bladder is amputated. Tension on the stay sutures elevates the apex of the bladder to prevent urine spillage into the peritoneal cavity. Prior placement of a urinary catheter helps minimize risk of urine leakage. A two-layer closure of the bladder apex is performed using absorbable suture with a continuous pattern in the mucosa and an interrupted or continuous Lembert pattern in the seromuscular layer. Umbilical remnants should be cultured and foals maintained on antibiotics for a minimum of 3 days postoperatively. Prolonged antibiotic therapy is indicated if other areas of infection exist.

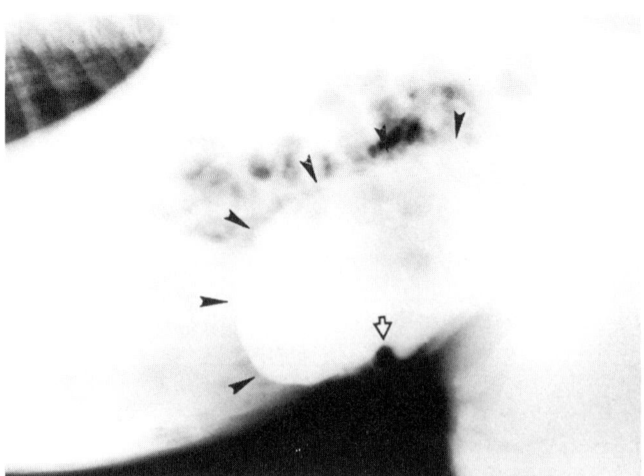

FIG. 114–2. Foal bladder filled with contrast material introduced with a teat cannula inserted up through the patent urachus. Solid arrows identify bladder margins. The open arrow marks the site of urachal attachment. No evidence of urachal rupture exists.

The uninfected, congenitally patent urachus is most likely to respond to local therapy. More aggressive treatment is warranted for the acquired patent urachus complicated by patient recumbency, infection of umbilical structures, and/or evidence of systemic infection.

UROPERITONEUM

T.D. Byars

Rupture of the urinary tract in foals has traditionally been regarded as a clinical entity in colts, 3 to 5 days of age, and considered to be a congenital bladder defect or rupture secondary to compression during birth. These clinical scenarios have been joined by recognition of an almost equal proportion of fillies and some older foals (up to 1 month of age) with uroperitoneum and an appreciation for defects of the ureters and urachus as sources of urine contamination within the abdomen. The role of sepsis in the pathogenesis of necrotic defects has not been adequately determined, but with increased case loads occurring in neonatal facilities, necrosis of the bladder or urachus is not infrequently discovered as sequelae in septic foals. Infection, infarction, and necrosis of the urachus and/or bladder often appear to be a sequelae to septicemia, rather than the result of ascending infections.

UROGENITAL TRACT LESIONS

The anatomic site of postrenal urinary tract lesions varies but includes ureteral, bladder, and urachal developmental or acquired defects. Urethral defects are not described in foals, and ectopic ureters are discussed elsewhere in this chapter. Causes of lesions are believed to be congenital defects of the ureters or bladder wall or acquired lesions secondary to sepsis infarction and necrosis.

Ureteral defects have been described and the precise cause is not known, although they are considered to be congenital.[19] Bladder lesions are more commonly encountered and may be aseptic defects primarily noted on the dorsal wall, or septic lesions more commonly associated with or near the urachus. Urachal lesions are usually the results of septic necrosis and may involve either the peritoneal cavity or extraperitoneal subcutis.[20] In some cases of peritoneal urachal openings, omentum may be observed exiting from the umbilicus (Fig. 114–3). In these cases, both anatomic site and presence of uroperitoneum can be clinically confirmed by this omental exteriorization.

A persistent urachus is a relatively common urogenital tract lesion observed in foals and is most often self-limiting. These and umbilical abscesses are discussed elsewhere in this chapter.

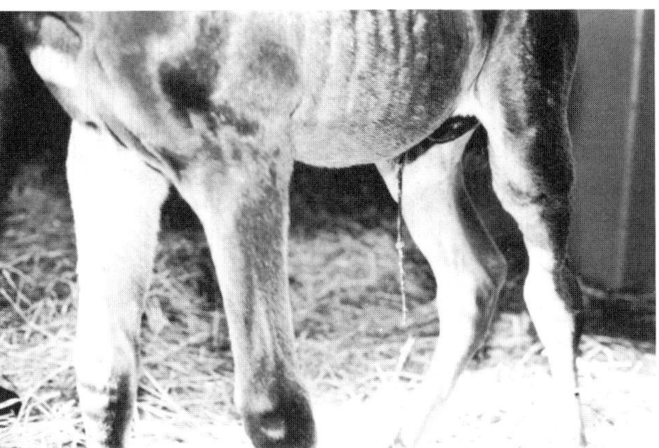

FIG. 114–3. Foal with omentum through the urachus.

CLINICAL SIGNS OF UROPERITONEUM

Age at which foals may be recognized as having urine accumulation within the peritoneal cavity is usually within the first few days of life, with the majority at 2 to 5 days. A history of abnormal urination (dysuria, stranguria, and pollakiuria) is characteristic of a defective urinary tract in either colts or fillies but is not always present. The clinical sign of stranguria in a young foal is suggestive of a urinary tract defect or colonic impaction (e.g., meconium impaction). Depending on the degree of clinical compromise, some foals may continue to nurse while others become depressed and anorectic, lose their suckle response, and are confused or associated with the neonatal maladjustment syndrome. Colic may be encountered in the history.

Mucous membranes of foals with uroperitoneum vary from pale to normal to toxic. Vital signs are also inconsistent, although tachycardia occurs more frequently than the bradycardia expected with hyperkalemia. Shock and muscle fasciculations may be observed in prolonged cases. Foals with uroperitoneum are usually noted to have an enlarged abdomen which appears pendulous. Ballottement of the abdomen may produce a "fluid wave" and "tinkling sound."

Foals with a ruptured urachus beneath the abdominal subcutis can demonstrate large amounts of ventral abdominal or preputial edema.[20] A persistent urachus presents as a free flow of urine from the umbilicus and may develop a few days to 2 weeks after birth. Urine scalding is minimal in foals with a persistent urachus as opposed to colts having ectopic ureters.[21]

LABORATORY DIAGNOSIS

Blood work can strongly suggest the presence of uroperitoneum. In the author's practice, a more rapid blood evaluation is obtained by the use of lithium heparin tubes, which allow plasma to be analyzed for hematology, and specific chemistry analyses—i.e., blood urea nitrogen (BUN), creatinine (Cr), and electrolytes—without having to await clot formation for serum analysis. Typically, moderate dehydration may be observed by elevations in the packed-cell volume (PCV) and total proteins, although anemia (PCV ranges of 24 to 29%) may also be found with normal to elevated total protein (TP) levels. The BUN or serum urea nitrogen (SUN) may be normal or modestly elevated, because urea nitrogen diffuses readily between the abdominal urine and body spaces. Creatinine levels are also elevated but usually not to the extremes seen with neonatal renal disorders. Creatinine ranges for uroperitoneum foals usually are between 2.5 to 4.5 mg percent. Serum or plasma electrolytes typically demonstrate hyponatremia and hyperkalemia. Blood gases and TCO_2 and chloride levels may also be abnormal but are usually less consistent because of the presence of concurrent gastrointestinal dysfunction (i.e., hypochloremic metabolic alkalosis in foals with ileus or gastric reflux). Low sodium and high potassium concentrations are caused by osmotic transport of higher plasma sodium and higher urinary potassium equilibrating between the plasma and a relatively large volume of urine within the abdominal cavity. Table 114–1 shows typical laboratory findings of a foal with uroperitoneum. A comprehensive review of uroperitoneum along with normal hematology and clinical chemistry values of the neonatal foal is available.[22]

An abdominal paracentesis can be performed to assist or confirm the diagnosis. This procedure should be performed in neonates using a teat canula and not a hypodermic needle as used in older foals and adults, because the visceral wall of neonatal and perinatal foals is thinner and can be more easily penetrated resulting in fecal peritonitis. Once the teat canula is in place (the foal may be recumbent or standing), clear to straw-colored urine readily flows from the abdomen unless the canula becomes clogged by the foal's omentum. Suction can make the clogging worse. When the canula is withdrawn, the omentum usually is attached. The omentum should be cut free with sterile scissors and an alternate abdominal paracentesis site can be chosen for a subsequent paracentesis procedure. Ultrasonographic evaluation of the abdomen can aid in identifying the most appropriate site for obtaining a paracentesis sample. Once a sample has been obtained, it should be submitted for Cr analysis. A ratio of at least 2:1 of abdominal fluid Cr to plasma or serum Cr is a consistent feature of uroperitoneum and should be considered diagnostic. This ratio occurs because the large molecular size of creatinine prevents its diffusing across membranes which divide the abdomen from the general circulation. As much of the abdominal fluid as possible should be removed during the paracentesis procedure if the abdomen is markedly distended.

ANCILLARY DIAGNOSTIC FEATURES

If laboratory analysis is not available to the practitioner, ancillary diagnostic procedures may be performed. The use of dyes such as intravenous Neoprontosil followed by an abdominal paracentesis may reveal red staining to the abdominal urine. Colt or filly bladders can be catheterized and infused with sterile fluids which have had sterile fluorescein ophthalmic dye strips or dilute povidone-iodine (Betadine) solution added. In these cases, the subsequent abdominal paracentesis may reveal the greenish hue typical of fluorescein or a purple discoloration on sheet cotton from betadine solution.

Ultrasonographic evaluation with either linear or sector scanners has become the premier ancillary diagnostic method for cases of uroperitoneum. Presence of a free fluid within the abdomen is suggestive of uroperitoneum. If the volume of free fluid is large enough that abdominal viscera are not touching each other (i.e., spleen, bowel, omentum, etc. are free floating), a presumptive diagnosis of uroperitoneum or peritonitis can be made. In uroperitoneum, the fluid is usually black, noncellular and may occasionally demonstrate sparse echogenic particles which appear bright within the dark fluid (Fig. 114–4); with peritonitis, the abdominal fluid is more cellular (grayish) with a greater incidence of fibrin noted floating in the exudative fluid. Ultrasonographic findings in conjunction with typical uroperitoneal blood chemistry results are usually sufficient for a diagnosis of uroperitoneum; however, in doubtful situations an abdominal paracentesis for the purpose of obtaining creatinine ratios would provide diagnostic confirmation. In cases of ureteral defects, accumulation of urine is often retroperitoneal and ultrasonography reveals excessive amounts of fluid surrounding the kidneys or paralumbar subcutaneous regions. Subcutaneous accumulation of fluid in the ventral abdominal region can indicate a urachal defect.[20] Lower urinary tract endoscopy can be used to localize lesions before surgery, although those procedures require small endoscopes not commonly available in exclusively large animal practices.

TABLE 114–1. TYPICAL LABORATORY FINDINGS IN A FOAL WITH UROPERITONEUM

	VARIABLE							
	PCV	TP	BUN	Cr*	Na	K	Cl	TCO_2
Value	29%	6.1 g/dL	35 mg/dL	4.1 mg/dL	119 mEq/L	5.7 mEq/L	92 mEq/L	32 mEq/L

*The abdominal fluid will have a creatinine ratio of at least 2:1 measured against the plasma or serum Cr (i.e., 10.4 mg/dL versus 4.1 mg/dL from the blood sample).

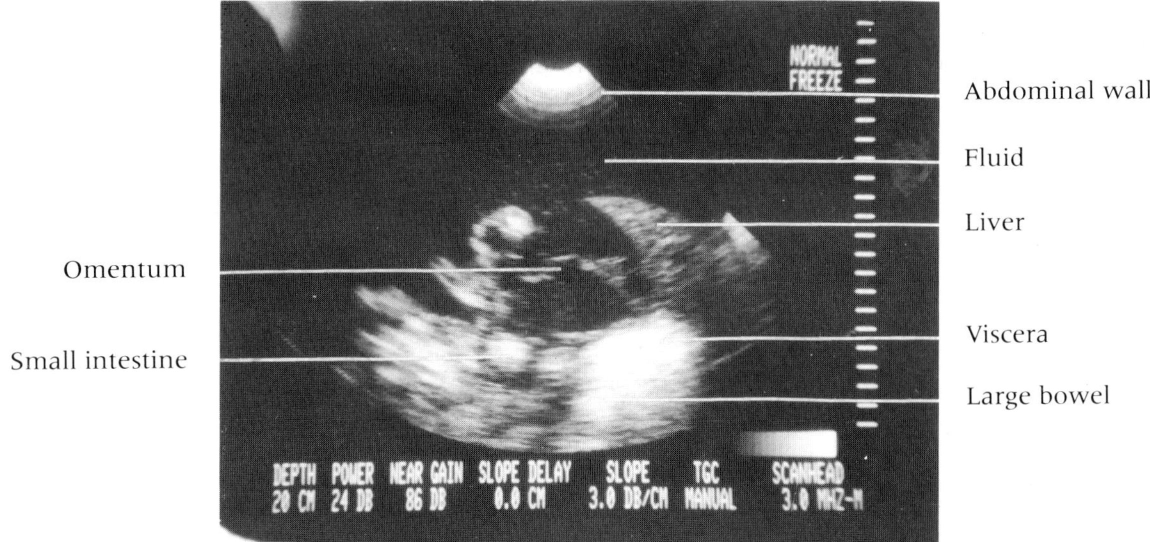

FIG. 114–4. Ultrasonogram of a 4-day-old colt with uroperitoneum. Note the fluid margins and displacement of abdominal viscera, which results in the various abdominal organs not being in contact with each other.

TREATMENT

Definitive treatment of uroperitoneum is to repair surgically the urinary tract defect. If the foal's vital signs and electrolyte changes are not largely altered from normal, anesthesia and surgery need not be delayed. In severe cases exhibiting extreme depression, shock, muscle fasciculations, cardiac arrhythmias or tachycardia, blood chemistry analysis will usually reveal severe hyperkalemia with associated anesthetic risks. The increased potassium level should be treated by intravenous fluid therapy (correction of bicarbonate deficits in 5% dextrose or the empirical use of 50 to 100 mEq of bicarbonate in 5% dextrose regardless of the acid-base status), the oral administration of sodium polystyrene as a potassium chelating agent (30 mL in tap water), or by enema if gastric refluxing is present, and the concurrent removal of abdominal urine by teat canula paracentesis. Once stabilized, the foal should undergo surgical correction with appropriate anesthesia. If the foal has obvious cardiovascular and/or respiratory compromise, special consideration should be given to the induction procedure and pharmacologic intervention. When repairing the defect, stainless steel staples should not be used because they can result in bladder stone formation at a later date. Necrotic lesions should be cultured during surgery to provide appropriate postoperative antibiotic treatments. Postoperative care may include Foley catheter placement in fillies and catheters in colts to bypass the possibility of increased urinary sphincter tone contributing to an increased tension on bladder repair sites. This is a controversial and still debated issue. In some cases, especially bladder surgeries dealing with necrotic repair, sites may break down and a second or even a third surgery may be required before permanent repair is achieved. The overall prognosis for bladder or urachal surgeries with minimal sepsis is reasonably good, and unlike colic surgery in foals, the postoperative development of intestinal adhesions are uncommon. The prognosis for ureteral defects is less well defined because the condition is relatively rare.[23]

DYSURIA, STRANGURIA, AND POLLAKIURIA

J.L. Rubin

Foals may present for dysuria, stranguria, or pollakiuria because of a number of underlying causes. A primary congenital neurologic deficit or more likely an infectious process (i.e., abscessation) involving the lumbosacral spinal cord could alter normal urination. Bacterial infection of the urachus (discussed elsewhere in this chapter) can also result in pollakiuria and dysuria.[24] Likewise, cystitis and urethritis (often associated with urachal infection or catheterization) may also result in abnormal urination. Cystic calculi and neoplasia though less common in the foal than the adult should also be considered. Ureteral ectopia must also be included in a list of differential diagnoses for urinary incontinence. Because of a lack of a consolidated reference on ureteral ectopia the remainder of this section will be devoted to this particular condition.

Occurrence of ureteral ectopia has been reported in many species, including the horse, human, dog, cat, pig, and ox, and is considered the most important ureteral anomaly in domestic animals.[25,26] Mammalian embryogenesis involves development of the pronephric, mesonephric, and metanephric systems; detailed reviews have been published.[26–28] The metanephric duct ultimately forms the ureter as it migrates craniad to the kidney and the caudad end joins the area of the urogenital sinus, which will become the trigone of the bladder. Abnormal formation/migration of the metanephric duct—or abnormal urogenital sinus, uterine—or vaginal development may result in aberrant entry of the ureter into the urogenital system.

TABLE 114–2. URINARY EXCRETED DYES

DYE	DOSE
Sodium fluoroscein	11 mg/kg BW* IV
Neoprontosil	10 mL IV
Phenolsulphonopthalein	0.01 mg/kg BW IV
Indigo carmine	0.25 mg/kg BW IV

*BW, body weight.

CLINICAL SIGNS

Although the incidence is low, ureteral ectopia should be considered in foals which present with a history of urinary incontinence since birth. Evidence of urine scalding of the perineal area and medial aspects of the thighs in females or the abdomen in males is also characteristic. Ectopic ureters may terminate caudal to the internal urethral sphincter in the dorsal aspect of the urethra or in females in the vagina. Affected animals typically urinate small amounts frequently and dribble urine, but intermittently urination may occur normally. No apparent breed predilection exists. The abnormality has more frequently been reported in females. The incidence is presumably similar, but a competent external urethral sphincter in the male may result in urethral-vesicular reflux and normal filling of the bladder. Males identified as having an ectopic ureter frequently present for persistent urinary tract infections rather than incontinence.

DIAGNOSIS

Physical examination of the foal with urinary incontinence should include a thorough neurologic examination to rule out a potential neurogenic basis. A minimum data base should also include a white blood cell count and differential, fibrinogen, creatinine, urinalysis and culture of urine obtained via catheterization.

Further evaluation of the urogenital tract can be accomplished with endoscopic and/or radiographic studies. Endoscopic examination is performed most easily under general anesthesia. However, adequate examination can be performed under sedation while standing.[29] Examination is facilitated by removal of urine and mild distention of the bladder with air, utilizing the endoscope to perform both tasks. Advancing the endoscope to the apex of the bladder and retroflexing it dorsocaudad allows examination of the trigone region and identification of the urethral openings. Identification of the openings is aided by intravenous injection of any of a number of dyes excreted via the urine[21,30] (Table 114–2). If two normal openings are not visualized, attempts should be made to visualize the location of the entry by thorough examination of the urethra and in females, the vagina. Once again, mild distention with air and use of urine excreted dyes aids identification of the ectopic ureteral opening.

Radiographic evaluation of the urogenital system should be performed under general anesthesia to be of greatest benefit. Plain lateral and ventrodorsal radiographs as well as pneumocystograms are often unrewarding. Contrast pneumocystograms/urethrograms allow evaluation of the urethra, bladder, and potentially the ureters if reflux of contrast material occurs. Concurrent intravesical pressure measurement can assess bladder capacity, sphincter competency, and detrusor muscle function in response to distention.[25]

Intravenous pyelography is an effective manner of assessing the renal pelvis and ureters for distention. In some instances, entry of the ureters can be identified; however, frequently a definitive diagnosis of ureteral ectopia cannot be accomplished.

THERAPY

Having diagnosed ureteral ectopia, the clinician has surgical intervention as the only avenue for resolution. Two main options exist: either unilateral nephrectomy or ureterovesicular anastomosis. The latter procedure is preferred in unilaterally affected animals with no signs of infection or in those affected bilaterally. Several techniques for anastomosis have been described, some of which have incorporated submucosal tunneling of the ureter.[21,25,31] Increased intravesicular pressure during micturition theoretically compresses the submucosal segment of ureter decreasing reflux of urine into the ureter.[25] Prevention of reflux of urine may in turn decrease occurrence of pyelonephritis from an ascending infection. Success of the anastomosis has been related to meticulous fine dissection, thereby minimizing vascular damage.[25] Nephrectomy is recommended in unilaterally affected animals with evidence of infections but normal renal function.[32] Unfortunately, the current number of reported cases is too small to assess accurately which techniques are most successful.[21] Regardless, early recognition of urinary incontinence and diagnosis of ureteral ectopia may decrease the likelihood of developing pyelonephritis and identifies affected animals as neonates when surgical access is greatest.[17]

SPURIOUS ELEVATIONS IN SERUM CREATININE

T.J. Divers

Glomerular filtration rate (GFR) in the healthy term foal is thought to be equal to that of the adult.[1] Regardless, serum creatinine concentrations in newborn foals are normally 30 to 40% above their dams' creatinine concentrations for the initial 24 to 72 h of life. To distinguish between spurious elevation of serum creatinine and diminished GFR in some foals is difficult. If the foal appears ill and/or septic then diminished GFR resulting from acute tubular nephrosis should be considered more likely. No single laboratory test exists that would readily distinguish between the two. If the foal is azotemic and hyperkalemic and/or hyponatremia and/or hypochloremia are present, acute renal failure and uroperitoneum are more likely because these electrolyte abnormalities are not usually present with spurious elevations in serum creatinine. If the foal in question has a urine specific gravity less than 1.006 or greater than 1.02, the azotemia is probably a result of spurious elevation or dehydration. Normal foals commonly void hyposthenuric urine. Marked elevation in urinary GGT may also be supportive of acute tubular necrosis.

Many premature foals and some term foals with neonatal maladjustment syndrome have much higher serum creatinine concentrations. These elevations in serum creatinine concentration occur both with the modified Jaffé method and Lloyd's reagent, suggesting that the elevation is truly creatinine rather than interfering substances (Table 114–3). In the neonate, the placenta is primarily responsible for fluid and electrolyte homeostasis and excretion of nitrogenous wastes.[5] The cause of elevated creatinine in some newborn foals is unclear but the author believes it is related to the inability of creatinine to equilibrate across placental membranes. Blood urea nitrogen concentration is usually abnormally high but does not have as marked an elevation above normal as does serum creatinine.[5] If the mare's placenta is diseased or has dysfunction, marked elevations in the foal's serum creatinine may occur, which often correlates with the finding of prematurity and/or maladjustment.

TABLE 114–3. COMPARISON OF THE MODIFIED JAFFE METHOD AND LLOYD'S REAGENT IN MEASURING SERUM CREATININE IN FIVE FOALS BELIEVED TO HAVE SPURIOUS ELEVATION IN SERUM CREATININE

FOAL NUMBER	JAFFE METHOD (mg/dL)	LLOYD'S REAGENT (mg/dL)
1	4.9	4.68
2	6.0	6.35
3	9.7	7.16
4	8.2	7.3
5	4.1	3.6

TREATMENT

If a newborn foal is found to have an elevated creatinine concentration (> 2.2 mg/dL) but appears clinically normal, no treatment is usually needed. If the foal is suffering from neonatal maladjustment, treatment should be directed toward the maladjustment. In both of these situations the creatinine should return to normal within 72 to 96 h. Marked elevations in serum creatinine in foals should not be assumed to be entirely spurious elevations. If the foal is or has been hypotensive or septic, treatment should be instituted to establish normal blood pressure, renal blood flow, and urine production.

REFERENCES

1. Brewer, B., Clement, S., Lotz, W., and Gronwall, R.: A comparison of inulin, para-aminohippuric acid and endogenous creatinine clearances as measures of renal function in neonatal foals. J. Vet. Int. Med. *4:*301–305, 1990.
2. Pipkin, F.B., Ousey, J.C., Wallace, C.P., and Rossdale, P.D.: Studies on equine prematurity 4: Effect of salt and water loss on the renin-angiotensin-aldosterone system in the newborn foal. Equine Vet. J., *16:*292–297, 1984.
3. Spensley, M., Carlson, G.P., and Harrold, D.: Plasma, red blood cell, total blood, and extracellular fluid volumes in healthy horse foals during growth. Am. J. Vet. Res., *48:*1703–1707, 1987.
4. Brewer, B., Clement, S., Lotz, W., and Gronwall, R.: Renal clearance, urinary excretion of endogenous substances and urinary diagnostic indices in healthy neonatal foals. J. Vet. Intern. Med., *5:*28–33, 1991.
5. Koterba, A.M., Adams, R., McClure, J.R., and Cudd, T.: Renal and urinary tract function and dysfunction in the neonatal foal. Proc. Am. Assoc. Equine Pract., 659–671, 1985.
6. Divers, T.J.: Disorders of the urachus, bladder, and kidneys of the neonatal foal. Paper presented at the Eightieth Annual Conference for Veterinarians, New York State College of Veterinary Medicine, Ithaca, NY, 1988.
7. Gerring, E.E.L., and Hunt, J.M.: Pathophysiology of equine postoperative ileus: Effect of adrenergic blockade, parasympathetic stimulation and metoclopramide in an

experimental model. Equine Vet. J., *18:*249–255, 1986.
8. Whitwell, K.E.: Morphology and pathology of the equine umbilical cord. J. Reprod. Fertil. Suppl., *23:*599–603, 1975.
9. Turner, T.A., Fessler, J.F., and Evert, K.M.: Patent urachus in foals. Equine Pract., *4:*24–31, 1982.
10. Adams, S.B., and Fessler, J.F.: Umbilical cord remnant infections in foals: 16 cases (1975–1985). J. Am. Vet. Med. Assoc., *190:*316–318, 1987.
11. Murray, M.J.: Diagnosis and therapy of umbilical and urachal disorders in the foal. Proceedings of the Fifth Annual Veterinary Medical Forum. Madison, WI, Omni Press, 1987, pp. 459–461.
12. Adams, R.: Urachal and umbilical disease. *In* Equine Clinical Neonatology. Edited by A.M. Koterba, W.H. Drummond, and P.C. Kosch. Philadelphia, Lea & Febiger, 1990, pp. 482–487.
13. Platt, H.: Septicemia in the foal. A review of 61 cases. Br. Vet. J., *129:*221–229, 1973.
14. Koterba A.M., Brewer B.D., and Tarplee F.A.: Clinical and clinicopathological characteristics of the septicaemic neonatal foal: Review of 38 cases. Equine Vet. J., *16:*376–383, 1984.
15. Van Pelt, R.W., and Riley, W.F.: Clinicopathologic findings and therapy in septic arthritis in foals. J. Am. Vet. Med. Assoc., *155:*1467–1480, 1969.
16. Reef, V.B.: Ultrasonographic diagnosis of umbilical infections in the foal. Proceedings of the Fifth Annual Veterinary Medical Forum. Madison, WI, Omni Press, 1987, pp. 462–465.
17. Robertson, J.T., and Embertson, R.M.: Surgical management of congenital and perinatal abnormalities of the urogenital tract. Vet. Clin. North Am. Equine Pract., *4:*359–379, 1988.
18. McIlwraith, C.W. and Turner, A.S.: Surgery of the urogenital system. *In* Equine Surgery Advanced Techniques. Edited by C.N. McIlwraith and A.S. Turner. Philadelphia, Lea & Febiger, 1987, pp. 346–372.
19. Divers, T.J., Byars, T.D., and Spirito, M.: Correction of bilateral ureteral defects in a foal. J. Am. Vet. Med. Assoc., *192:*384–386, 1988.
20. Robertson, J.T., et al.: Repair of a ureteral defect in a foal. J. Am. Vet. Med. Assoc., *183:*799–800, 1983.
21. Pringle, J.K., Ducharme, N.G., and Baird, J.D.: Ectopic ureter in the horse: Three cases and a review of the literature. Can. Vet. J., *31:*26–30, 1990.
22. Koterba, A.M., Drummond, W.H., and Kosch, P.C. (eds.): Equine Clinical Neonatology. Philadelphia, Lea & Febiger, 1990.
23. Lees, M.J., et al.: Subcutaneous rupture of the urachus, its diagnosis and surgical management. Equine Vet. J., *21:*462–464, 1989.
24. Dean, P.W., and Robertson, J.T.: Urachal remnant as a cause of pollakiuria and dysuria in a foal. J. Am. Vet. Med. Assoc., *192:*375–376, 1988.
25. Christie, B., et al.: Surgical correction of bilateral ureteral ectopia in a male Appaloosa foal. Aust. Vet. J., *57:*336–340, 1981.
26. Jubb, K.V.F., Kennedy, P.C., and Palmer, N.: Pathology of Domestic Animals. 3rd ed. Orlando, FL, Academic Press, 1985.
27. Dean, P.W., et al.: Canine ectopic ureter. Compend. Contin. Educ. Practicing Vet., *10:*146–157, 1988.
28. Owen, R.R.: Canine Ureteral ectopia—A review 1. Embryology and aetiology. J. Small Anim. Prac., *14:*407–417, 1973.
29. MacAllister, C.G., and Perdue, B.D.: Endoscopic diagnosis of unilateral ectopic ureter in a yearling filly. J. Am. Vet. Med. Assoc., *197:*617–618, 1990.
30. Sullins, K.E., McIlwraith, C.W., and Yovich, J.V.: Ectopic ureter managed by unilateral nephrectomy in two female horses. Equine Vet. J., *20:*463–466, 1988.
31. Modransky, P.D., et al.: Surgical correction of bilateral ureteral ectopia in two foals. Vet. Surg., *12:*141–147, 1983.
32. Houlton, J.E.F., Wright, I.M., Matic, S., and Herrtage M.E.: Urinary incontinence in a shire foal due to ureteral ectopia. Equine Vet. J., *19:*244–247, 1987.

CHAPTER 115

THE CARDIAC AND RESPIRATORY SYSTEMS

W.E. Vaala

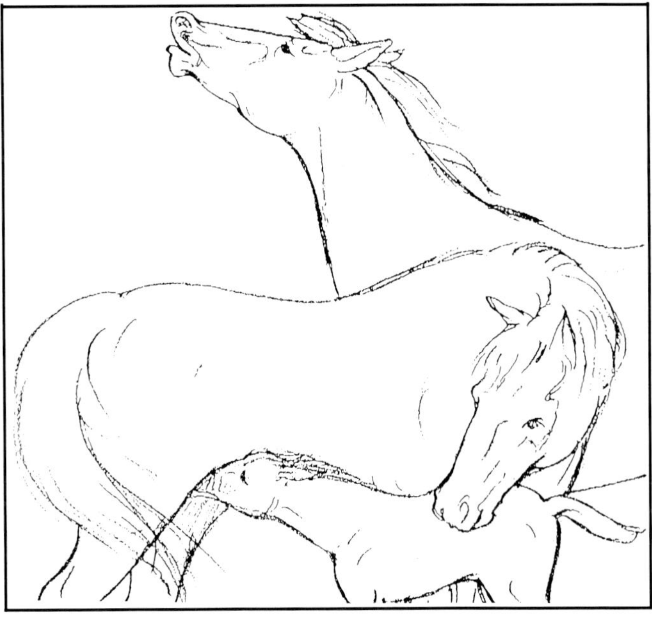

The transformation of a fetus into a neonate depends on a series of physiologic adaptations that must occur during the perinatal period. Successful cardiopulmonary adaptation to extrauterine life is essential for neonatal survival. Causes of cardiac dysfunction during the early neonatal period include congenital malformations, persistent fetal circulation, arrhythmias secondary to severe metabolic disturbances and/or hypoxia, and myocardial disease associated with septicemia or severe peripartum hypoxia. Respiratory disorders include respiratory distress caused by lung immaturity and/or surfactant deficiency, bacterial/viral pneumonia, aspiration of meconium or milk, and ineffectual control of breathing as a result of prematurity or severe hypoxia. Clinical evaluation of the foal's cardiopulmonary system is discussed followed by a description of the more common disorders affecting the neonate's heart and lungs during the early postnatal period. Therapeutic intervention is discussed briefly when appropriate.

TRANSITION FROM FETAL TO NEONATAL CIRCULATION

In the fetus, the placenta serves as the primary site for oxygen and carbon dioxide exchange. Two fetal shunts, the foramen ovale and ductus arteriosus, exist as bypass channels to divert blood away from the constricted pulmonary circulation. Oxygenated blood returning from the placenta via the umbilical vein enters the posterior vena cava and flows into the right atrium (RA). Approximately two-thirds of this blood will pass out of the RA across the foramen ovale into the left atrium (LA) to be delivered preferentially to the heart, head, and upper torso. The remaining blood passes through the right ventricle (RV) and is shunted across the ductus arteriosus into the descending aorta to perfuse abdominal viscera and the lower extremities. During fetal life, pulmonary vascular resistance is higher than systemic vascular resistance. Both ventricles work in parallel, with the RV dominating in both size and cardiac output. Fetal and neonatal circulatory patterns are illustrated in Fig. 115–1.

As the neonate takes its first few breaths following delivery, the collapsed, liquid-filled alveoli expand with air. In mature lungs, surfactant acts to reduce surface tension, stabilize alveoli, and prevent complete alveolar collapse during expiration.[1,2] Pulmonary vascular resistance declines rapidly, accompanied by a dramatic increase in pulmonary blood flow. The placental circulation is eliminated and systemic vascular resistance increases. As systemic vascular resistance becomes higher than pulmonary vascular resistance, blood returning to the right atrium now flows through the pulmonary circulation rather than across the ductus. Left atrial pressure rises as a result of increased blood flow from the lungs. The foramen ovale closes once left atrial pressure exceeds right atrial pressure. Blood leaving the left ventricle (LV) via the aortic root encounters the still-patent ductus arteriosus. Some blood flows prefer-

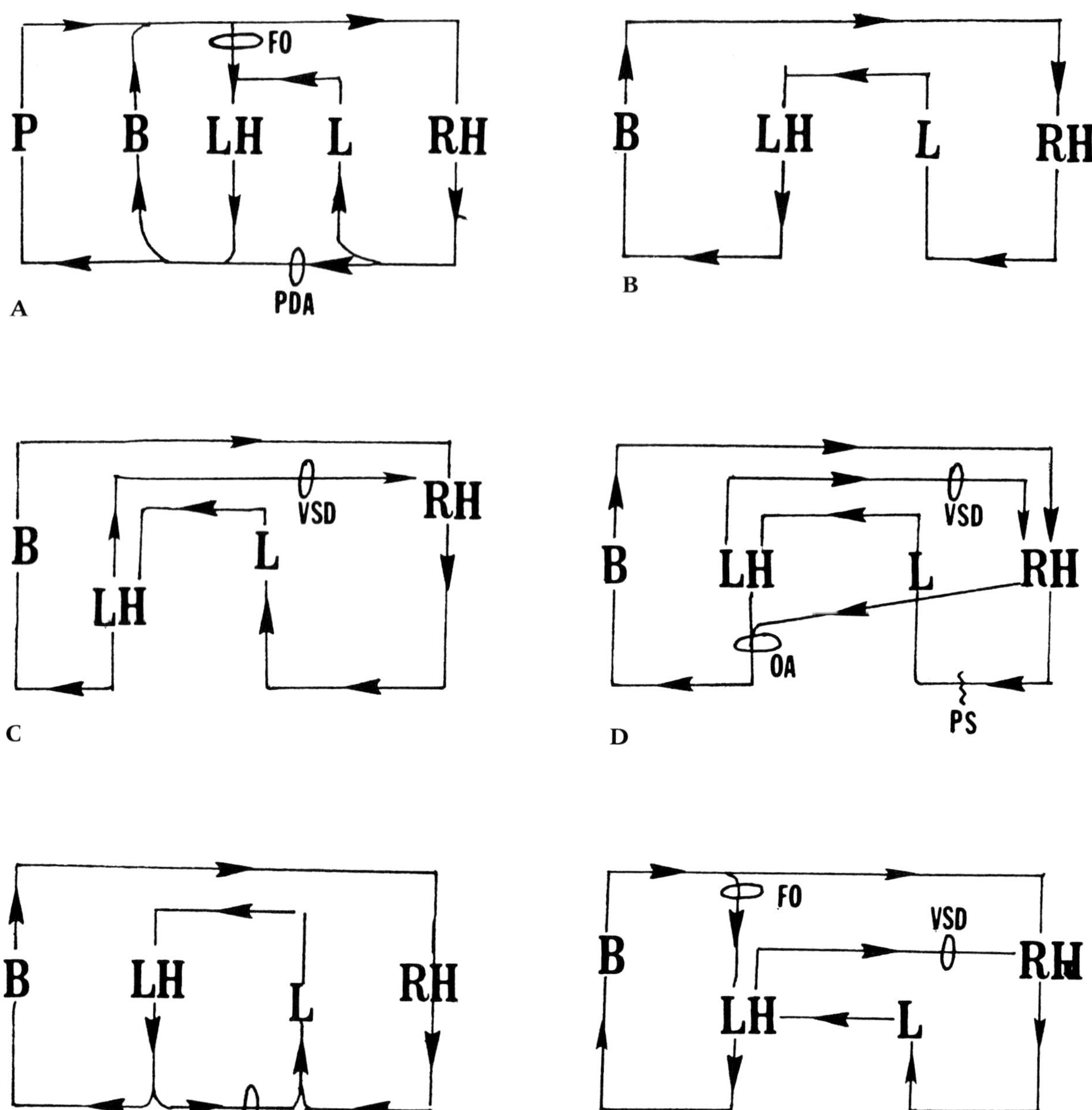

FIG. 115–1. Fetal and neonatal circulation in health and disease. *A,* Normal fetal circulatory pattern. *B,* Normal neonatal circulation following closure of all prenatal shunts. *C,* Ventral septal defect. *D,* Tetralogy of Fallot. *E,* Patent ductus arteriosus. *F,* Tricuspid atresia. P, Placenta; B, body; LH, left heart; L, lungs; RH, right heart; PDA, patent ductus arteriosus; FO, foramen ovale; VSD, ventral septal defect; OA, over-riding aorta; PS, pulmonic stenosis.

entially across the ductus (left to right) to recirculate through the lungs.

In most foals, the ductus arteriosus closes by day 4 of life.[3,4] Closure of this fetal channel is mediated by decreasing concentrations of tissue and blood prostaglandins and by rising oxygen tensions. Until complete anatomic closure occurs, the ductus arteriosus can reopen in response to severe hypoxemia, resulting in persistent fetal circulatory patterns.

EVALUATION OF THE CARDIOVASCULAR SYSTEM

PHYSICAL EXAMINATION

A healthy newborn foal should have pink, moist mucous membranes with a capillary refill time of 1 to 2 s. Remember that visible cyanosis appears only when arterial oxygen pressure drops below 35 to 40 mm Hg. Arterial pulses should be strong and easily palpable at the facial, brachial, and great metatarsal arteries. Extremities should be warm. The jugular veins should not be distended but should fill readily when occluded near the thoracic inlet. Pulse abnormalities suggestive of cardiac dysfunction are listed in Table 115–1.

A newborn's heart rate ranges from 40 to 80 beats per minute (BPM) immediately following birth and increases to 120 to 150 BPM during the first few postnatal hours. The heart rate then plateaus between 80 and 100 BPM during the first week of life.[3–5] Immediately following birth, a sinus arrhythmia may be present, but this should disappear during the first 24 h. The most intense apex beat is palpable over the left fifth intercostal space in the ventral third of the thorax. The pulmonic valve area is located in the left third intercostal space just below the point of the shoulder. Just above this location in the fourth intercostal space is the aortic valve area. The mitral valve area is located in the fifth intercostal space halfway between horizontal lines drawn from the point of the olecranon and point of the shoulder. The tricuspid valve area is in the right third and fourth intercostal spaces in the ventral third of the thorax. A foal's heart sounds are quite loud because of the thin chest wall.

The closing ductus arteriosus gives rise to a systolic murmur that may range from a grade I to IV in intensity with a point of maximal intensity over the left heart base. In most foals, the murmur disappears during the first week postpartum. In some foals a soft systolic murmur over the left heart base may persist for 1 to 2 months without evidence of underlying heart disease.[5]

TABLE 115–1. PULSE ABNORMALITIES SUGGESTIVE OF CARDIAC DYSFUNCTION

Jugular venous distension/jugular pulsations
Tetralogy of Fallot
Tricuspid atresia
Right-sided congestive heart failure
Weak arterial pulses
Left ventricular failure
Hypovolemic or septic shock
Tricuspid atresia
Left heart obstruction
Aortic malformation
Bounding (hyperkinetic) arterial pulses
Large interventricular septal defect
Patent ductus arteriosus
Aortic insufficiency

ELECTROCARDIOGRAPHY

Electrocardiograms (ECGs) can be obtained with the foal standing or in lateral recumbency. A base-apex lead is satisfactory for routine monitoring of cardiac rate and rhythm disturbances. Use of electrocardiography to evaluate chamber enlargement or pressure/volume overload requires more meticulous and consistent lead placement using both elbows and stifles.

Using electrodes attached to alligator clips or adhesive patches, a base-apex lead is formed as follows: right leg lead (green) on right side of neck or right stifle; right arm lead (white) on right scapular spine; left arm lead (black) in the left sixth intercostal space level with the point of the elbow. Most ECGs are recorded at a paper speed of 50 mm/s. Ultrasonic coupling gel or alcohol is used to improve contact between the electrode and skin. The ECG reflects the electrical activity of the heart and is most useful for documenting T-wave changes and sinus tachyarrhythmias.

An ECG from a normal foal has a PR interval of approximately 0.12 to 0.18 s, a QRS complex duration of 0.05 to 0.08 s, and a QT interval of 0.19 to 0.35 s. Detailed reviews of electrocardiography in the foal have been published.[3,5]

RADIOLOGY

Two lateral thoracic views should be obtained, preferably with the foal in lateral recumbency and the forelimbs extended as far forward as possible. Dorsoventral positioning is possible only with anesthetized or depressed foals. Cardiomegaly is characterized by caudodorsal tracheal displacement, straightening of the caudal heart border, and increase in the craniocaudal heart dimension. Pulmonary hypoperfusion is recognized by diminished pulmonary vascular markings. Left-to-right shunts, producing increased pulmonary blood flow may result in hypervascular lung fields.[4]

ECHOCARDIOGRAPHY

Two-dimensional echocardiography is most useful for anatomic diagnosis of a variety of cardiac malformations. M-mode techniques are used primarily for obtaining cardiac measurements. Echocardiograms can be recorded with the foal standing or laterally recumbent. The right thoracic approach with the transducer placed in the third or fourth intercostal space near the costochondral junction is the most commonly used view.[4,5]

Nonselective contrast echocardiography is performed using microbubbles formed when 5 to 10 mL of carbon dioxide is added to 5 to 10 mL of the patient's blood, which is then agitated in a syringe before injection into a peripheral vein. The bubbles produce a "white out" of the right atrium and ventricle during normal circulation. The microbubble technique can be used to detect atrial and septal defects. More complex malformations require contrast echocardiograms.

CARDIAC CATHETERIZATION AND OXIMETRY

Right heart catheterization is performed using a Swan-Ganz, balloon-tipped, flow-directed catheter inserted via the jugular vein into the right atrium and ventricle and pulmonary artery. During the procedure, pressures can be recorded using a pressure transducer and blood samples can be obtained for oximetry (i.e., measurement of oxygen saturation).[4–6]

CONGENITAL HEART DISEASE

The incidence of congenital heart disease in foals is low. In one survey of 2500 equine necropsies only 4 cases were reported.[7] In another survey of 8954 necropsies of foals from central Kentucky a 2.3% incidence of congenital cardiac malformations was found.[8] However, because some foals with severe congenital cardiac disease die during the perinatal period without diagnosis, the true incidence is probably higher than reflected by most surveys.

The cause of most equine congenital heart diseases is unknown. Genetic factors likely play a role in the cause. This theory is supported by the over-representation of purebred and half-bred Arabian foals among neonates with congenital heart disease. Viral infection and teratogen exposure during the early prenatal period of organogenesis are also possible causes. Morphogenesis of the equine heart is complete by day 49 of gestation. Therefore, potential teratogens or prenatal infection would have to be active before this time to induce such heart malformations as tetralogy or pentalogy of Fallot.[9] Other congenital disorders, such as persistent foramen ovale and persistent patent ductus arteriosus, occur when fetal shunts fail to close during the early postnatal period. Events occurring late in gestation or immediately postpartum may disturb the transition from fetal to neonatal circulatory flow patterns.

Congenital cardiac anomalies reported in the foal include interventricular septal defect, tetralogy and pentalogy of Fallot, tricuspid valve atresia, persistent foramen ovale, persistent ductus arteriosus, persistent right aortic arch, persistent truncus arteriosus, and other malformations of the valves and great vessels.[4,7–10] Clinical signs and characteristic murmurs associated with the more common heart defects are listed in Table 115–2.

INTERVENTRICULAR SEPTAL DEFECT

Interventricular septal defect (VSD) is the most common congenital cardiac disorder in the foal and may occur alone or in conjunction with other defects such as tetralogy of Fallot and tricuspid atresia. The VSD in horses is usually located in the upper third of the septum in the membranous portion and opens under the septal leaflet of the tricuspid valve on the right and just below the aortic valve on the left.[9,11]

With a VSD, the blood flow pattern is from the LV to the RV, resulting in overperfusion of the pulmonary circulation and volume overload of both ventricles. Clini-

TABLE 115–2. CONGENITAL DISORDERS OF CARDIAC BLOOD FLOW

ANOMALY	CLINICAL SIGNS	CHARACTERISTIC MURMUR(S)*
Interventricular septal defect (VSD)	No abnormalities with small defect; large defect results in exercise intolerance, weakness, poor growth, and heart failure	Grade III to V/V, harsh-, band-, or diamond-shaped holosystolic murmur with PMI over R ICS 3 to 4; similar murmur with PMI over L heart base; murmur radiates widely and has precordial thrill
Patent ductus arteriosus (PDA)	Congestive heart failure develops if PDA persist; hyperkinetic (bounding) arterial pulses	Occasionally a continuous machinery murmur, but more commonly a holosystolic murmur grade I to IV/V with PMI over L ICS 3 to 4
Tetralogy of Fallot VSD Pulmonic stenosis Dextroposition of aorta with overriding R Ventricular hypertrophy	Severity of signs depend on size of VSD and degree of RV outflow obstruction; exercise intolerance, weakness, cyanosis, and poor growth	Grade IV to V/V coarse, band-shaped pansystolic murmur with PMI over L heart base
Tricuspid atresia Atrial septal defect VSD R ventricular hypoplasia	Cyanosis caused by R to L shunting; severe exercise intolerance weakness, respiratory distress, weak arterial pulses, and poor growth	Grade IV to V/V crescendo-decrescendo pansystolic murmur with PMI over L heart base
Persistent foramen ovale	Clinical signs are rare unless other cardiac defects are present; closure often occurs between 15 days and 9 weeks postpartum	

*PMI, point of maximal intensity; R, right; ICS, intercostal space; L, left.

cal signs of VSD in foals depend on the defect's size and location. Small defects (less than 5.0 mm in diameter) are well tolerated and, except for an incidental systolic murmur, cause no significant clinical abnormalities.[4] Larger defects result in weakness, exercise intolerance, stunted growth, and failure to thrive.[11] Severe VSD leads to congestive heart failure[4,11] with accompanying pulmonary edema characterized by fine crackles on thoracic auscultation and labored breathing. If, on rare occasions, severe pulmonary hypertension accompanies the VSD, a right-to-left shunt develops, resulting in pulmonary hypoperfusion, hypoxemia, and cyanosis.[4]

The murmur associated with a VSD is a harsh, grade III to V/V holosystolic, band or diamond-shaped murmur with its point of maximal intensity (PMI) over the right third to fourth intercostal spaces above the sternal border.[4,10] A similar murmur is usually heard over the left heart base with a PMI over the pulmonic valve area. The murmur radiates widely and has a precordial thrill. Unless the foal is already in congestive heart failure, arterial pulses, capillary refill time, and mucous membrane color are normal, as is the ECG. Lateral thoracic radiographs are normal if the defect is small. Larger defects result in generalized cardiomegaly, increased pulmonary vascular markings, and increased prominence of the main pulmonary artery.

Two-dimensional echocardiography is the diagnostic method of choice. The defect is best visualized in the right parasternal long axis view[4] (Fig. 115–2). The left ventricle and atrium are either normal or enlarged. A larger VSD can be recognized on M-mode echocardiograms as septal or aortic root drop-out.[4] Doppler echocardiography can be used to demonstrate turbulent blood flow during systole in the RV along the septum near the defect.[4] Turbulent blood flow in that area helps document a left-to-right shunt across the VSD.

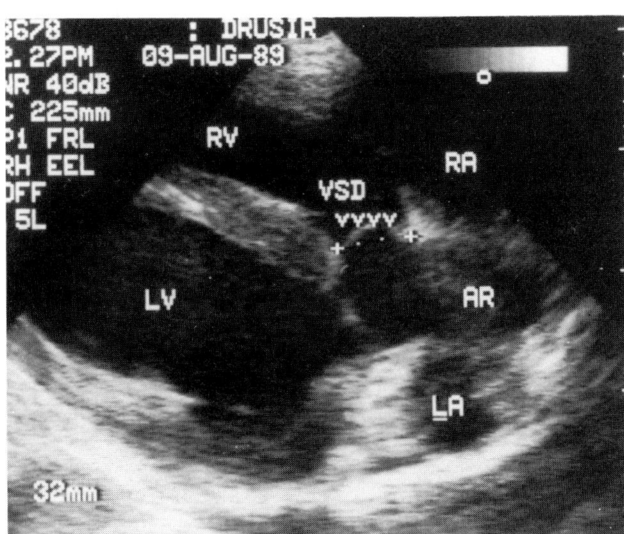

FIG. 115–2. Two-dimensional echocardiogram demonstrating a ventral septal defect (VSD) in a weanling. The scan was obtained using a 2.5-MHz transducer. RV, right ventricle; RA, right atrium; AR, aortic root; LA, left atrium; LV, left ventricle. Arrows indicate location of the VSD; 0, artifact (no significance); plus signs, width of the VSD.

Diagnosis can be confirmed by cardiac catheterization. Right heart catheterization demonstrates greater oxygen saturation in the pulmonary artery (PA) and RV than in the RA or great veins. Pulmonary arterial and right ventricular pressure may be elevated. A left ventricular angiogram confirms the presence of a ventral septal defect. Injection of radiopaque contrast medium into the left ventricle results in simultaneous opacification of both ventricles provided the shunt is from left to right. This technique permits subjective assessment of the VSD size.

Foals with an isolated VSD 5 to 6 mm in diameter or smaller have a good prognosis for a normal life.[4] Any foal with an uncomplicated VSD should be monitored at regular intervals to assess cardiac function, because pulmonary hypertension and subsequent shunt reversal (i.e., right to left) may develop at a later date. Foals with large defects have a poor prognosis for survival and are at risk for left heart failure.

PATENT DUCTUS ARTERIOSUS

In the fetus, the ductus arteriosus shunts blood from the pulmonary artery to the aorta. During the early postnatal period, a decrease in pulmonary vascular resistance accompanied by an increase in systemic vascular resistance results in reversal of the shunt. Physiologic closure of the ductus occurs in most foals by approximately 4 days of age.[4,9]

In the neonate during the transitional stage, the usual left-to-right shunting of blood from the aorta through the patent ductus arteriosus (PDA) into the PA results in pulmonary hyperperfusion (Fig. 115–1) and volume overload of both ventricles. If pulmonary hypertension develops, blood flow across the PDA may decrease and even revert to the right-to-left fetal circulatory pattern resulting in respiratory distress.

Auscultation reveals a continuous, machinery murmur loudest over the left heart base in the third and fourth intercostal spaces. The murmur frequently radiates widely and may be accompanied by a palpable thrill. The diastolic component of the murmur is often located in the left third to fourth intercostal spaces and may become less distinct as pulmonary arterial pressures increase.[9] Arterial pulses are hyperkinetic or bounding. Mucous membranes are pink. Affected individuals usually fail to thrive and exhibit exercise intolerance. Older animals with a PDA may develop pulmonary hypertension.[9]

Right heart catheterization may reveal increased PA and right ventricular pressures. Oxygen saturation in the PA exceeds that in the RV, RA and great veins.[9] Injection of radiopaque contrast medium at the aortic root results in opacification of the aorta and pulmonary artery, provided the shunt is left to right.[9] Echocardiographic documentation of a PDA is difficult. Left atrial and ventricular enlargement may be detected.

The degree of shunting for foals with PDA dictates

the prognosis. The younger the age at which the affected foal becomes symptomatic, the poorer the prognosis. No case reports could be found in the equine literature of successful PDA repair. Rupture of one of the pulmonary artery branches secondary to pulmonary hypertension is a potential and lethal complication associated with a PDA.[9]

TETRALOGY OF FALLOT

The four defects comprising tetralogy of Fallot (TOF) are a VSD, dextroposition of the aorta overriding the VSD, pulmonic stenosis, and secondary right ventricular hypertrophy. Pentalogy of Fallot includes the aforementioned defects in addition to a PDA.[4,9]

In TOF, pulmonary stenosis and the VSD result in right ventricular hypertension and hypertrophy.[4,11] During systole, most of the combined ventricular output is ejected into the over-riding aorta, resulting in aortic dilatation and pulmonary hypoperfusion (Fig. 115–1). Arterial hypoxemia and cyanotic mucous membranes are observed in severe cases of pulmonary hypoperfusion.[9] Foals with TOF are likely to exhibit poor growth, weakness, marked exercise intolerance, dyspnea, and cyanosis.[11] Some affected foals experience syncope following exertion. A coarse, grade IV to V/V pansystolic murmur associated with pulmonic stenosis is heard best over the left heart base and radiates widely.[10] The systolic murmur corresponding to the VSD is loudest over the left heart base and right sternal border.

Polycythemia may develop in response to hypoxemia. Lateral thoracic radiographs reveal varying degrees of cardiomegaly with right ventricular enlargement, increased prominence of the ascending aorta, and hypoperfusion of the pulmonary vasculature. The electrocardiogram is not a reliable diagnostic aid, but may reveal a large QRS complex (more than 2.5 mV) suggestive of ventricular hypertrophy.[9] Cardiac catheterization abnormalities include a distinct pressure gradient across the area of pulmonic arterial stenosis; right ventricular hypertension with values approaching systemic pressures; the recording of similar pressures in the RV, LV, and aorta; and the recording of normal pressures in the RA and pulmonary artery.[9] Echocardiography reveals right ventricular dilatation, free-wall hypertrophy, a VSD, and over-riding aorta. Pulmonic stenosis is difficult to visualize. Contrast echocardiography with microbubbles or contrast medium injected into the RV demonstrates simultaneous clearance by way of the PA, LV, and aorta.[4]

The prognosis for survival for foals with TOF is poor. With pentalogy of Fallot and the presence of a PDA aortic blood shunts into the pulmonary artery via the ductus, thereby reducing the degree of pulmonary hypoperfusion and the tendency to develop cyanosis. But even these foals have a poor long-term prognosis for survival, and euthanasia is probably the most rational recommendation. Attempts have been made to dilate the pulmonic valve with balloon catheters to reduce the stenosis and degree of right-to-left shunting.[4]

TRICUSPID ATRESIA

Tricuspid atresia (TA) is a relatively uncommon, complex malformation consisting of an enlarged RA, a hypoplastic RV, a patent foramen ovale (PFO) or atrial septal defect, tricuspid valve atresia, an enlarged left atrium and ventricle, and a ventral septal defect.[4,9] The PA may be normal or stenotic and the pulmonic valve may be abnormal.

In TA, blood flows from an enlarged RA through the PFO into the LA and then into the LV. During systole, blood is ejected from the LV partly through the aorta and partly via the VSD into the RV and PA (Fig. 115–1). Pulmonary hypoperfusion is common and results in varying degrees of cyanosis. A small VSD allows little blood to reach the lungs and cyanosis is more pronounced. A large atrial septal defect and VSD may be associated with excessively high pulmonary blood flow with mild cyanosis and signs of congestive heart failure. Other clinical signs associated with TA include stunted growth, severe weakness, exercise intolerance, respiratory distress, and generalized venous distension with weak arterial pulses.[4,9] Polycythemia may develop secondary to hypoxemia.

A full range of diagnostic aids is employed to confirm the diagnosis antemortem.[4] Electrocardiogram abnormalities include tall, wide P waves and increased QRS complex amplitudes. Echocardiography is used to detect abnormal cardiac chamber dimensions and the ventral septal defect. Contrast echocardiography has been used to demonstrate the right-to-left shunt across the atrial septal defect. The prognosis for survival is grave. Euthanasia of affected foals is recommended.

ACQUIRED HEART DISEASE

Acquired heart disease is uncommon in neonatal foals. Inflammatory or degenerative myocardial changes are often recognized only at necropsy and may be associated with toxemia, infection, uremia, hypoxia, drugs, or nutritional deficiencies.

WHITE MUSCLE DISEASE

Dystrophic myodegeneration is seen in foals from selenium-deficient areas. Affected foals are usually less than 5 to 6 months of age and may exhibit a stiff gait, acute recumbency, tachycardia, dyspnea, and sudden death.[12] Cardiac arrhythmias have been associated with cardiac muscle degeneration. Necropsy reveals pale streaks in the myocardium and cardiac hypertrophy with or without pulmonary edema. Serum creatine kinase concentrations are elevated and glutathione peroxidase levels are low. Vitamin E and selenium therapy is beneficial in milder cases. Foals with myocardial involvement have a grave prognosis.[12]

RUPTURED BLADDER

Uroperitoneum occurs most commonly in equine neonates, usually colts, less than 5 to 7 days of age (Chapter 114). Affected foals experience severe electrolyte imbalances (e.g., hyponatremia, hypochloremia, and hyperkalemia) and may exhibit a variety of arrhythmias that can be exacerbated by general anesthesia. Rhythm disturbances associated with this condition include sinus tachycardia, third-degree atrioventricular block, ventricular arrhythmias, and cardiac arrest.[10,13] Intravenous administration of 0.9% sodium chloride, isotonic bicarbonate, dextrose, and insulin is recommended to help correct metabolic abnormalities and stabilize the foal preoperatively. Because halothane is arrhythmogenic, isoflurane is the preferred anesthetic agent for these foals.[13]

OTHER ACQUIRED CARDIAC DISEASES

Persistent pulmonary hypertension (PPH) or persistent fetal circulation (PFC) is a syndrome characterized by elevated PA pressure and cyanosis associated with right-to-left shunting through the ductus arteriosus and foramen ovale.[14] Severe hypoxemia is the primary stimulus for pulmonary vasoconstriction. Concurrent acidosis accentuates the pulmonary vascular response. Treatment includes administration of high oxygen concentrations and correction of existing acid-base abnormalities.[14]

Severe perinatal hypoxemia may also lead to left or right ventricular dysfunction. Foals suffering from severe asphyxia should have their cardiac function closely monitored. Serum concentrations of cardiac isoenzymes [creatine kinase-myocardial band (CK-MB) and hydroxybutyrate dehydrogenase (HBDH)] can also be monitored to detect myocardial damage.

Septic foals may also experience myocardial dysfunction. Septic shock has been associated with decreased myocardial contractility, altered systemic resistance, pulmonary hypertension, decreased coronary perfusion, and altered myocardial metabolism.[15] Mediators of sepsis-induced cardiac dysfunction include thromboxane, platelet-activating factor, serotonin, myocardial depressant factor, and circulating endotoxin. Cardiovascular support of affected neonates requires careful monitoring of cardiac function and blood pressure, judicious fluid therapy, and positive inotrope administration (e.g., dobutamine: 3 to 15 μg/kg/min). Premature foals may require higher infusion rates.

ESTABLISHMENT OF PULMONARY RESPIRATION

The first few breaths following delivery result in expansion of fluid-filled alveoli, removal of pulmonary fluid, and creation of an air-blood interface at the alveolar level. Changes in systemic and pulmonary vascular resistances and closure of prenatal shunts result in redirection of blood flow through the pulmonary vasculature allowing the neonate's lungs to replace the placenta as the primary site of gas exchange.

Successful establishment of respiration depends on functional and structural maturation of the lung. Lung expansion is facilitated by surfactant-mediated reduction in alveolar surface tension. Surfactant, a complex lipoprotein substance, provides alveoli with a surface film to reduce surface tension and prevent transudation and lung collapse at end expiration.[1,2] Composed primarily of dipalmitoyl phosphatidylcholine (DPPC) and phosphatidylglycerol (PG) and other surfactant-associated proteins, surfactant is produced by the type II alveolar pneumocytes. Lung surfactant reduces work of breathing by improving lung compliance, stabilizing alveoli, and enhancing lung liquid clearance.[1,2,14] Maturation of the type II pneumocyte occurs during the last quarter of gestation. In the foal, surfactant maturation occurs at or after 300 days of gestation and is not always fully complete even in term foals.[16] The phospholipids DPPC and PG are secreted into alveolar fluid and from there transported into amniotic fluid. In humans, stage of fetal lung maturation can be predicted based on assay of selected phospholipids in amniotic fluid obtained via amniocentesis. Corticosteroids and thyroxine enhance maturation of the surfactant system.[17]

Lung maturation also involves thinning of the alveolar capillary barrier, reduction in alveolar epithelial permeability, and maturation of the chest wall.[18] The immature chest wall is highly compliant and predisposes

TABLE 115–3. CAUSES OF NEONATAL RESPIRATORY DISTRESS

Airway obstruction
Choanal atresia
Stenotic nares
Nasal edema
Collapsed trachea
Laryngeal paralysis
Subepiglottic cyst
Collapsed trachea
Space occupying lesions
Pneumothorax
Diaphragmatic hernia
Pulmonary lesions
Pneumonia (bacterial, viral)
Hyaline membrane disease (respiratory distress syndrome)
Aspiration syndromes (meconium and milk)
Transient tachypnea of the newborn (delayed lung liquid absorption)
Metabolic causes
Hypothermia
Metabolic acidosis
Hypoglycemia
Nonpulmonary causes
Anemia, acute blood loss
CNS lesions
Persistent fetal circulation
Birth asphyxia

to low end expiratory tidal volumes even in the present of surfactant.

Postpartum, lung liquid is removed by several mechanisms. Some is expelled forcefully from the mouth during vaginal delivery as the thorax is compressed in the birth canal. Fluid remaining in the alveoli must be removed gradually by evaporation, through the pulmonary capillaries, or via the pulmonary lymphatics.

Most respiratory disorders in the newborn foal are characterized clinically by respiratory distress (not to be confused with respiratory distress syndrome, a specific condition associated with surfactant dysfunction). Respiratory distress simply describes increased respiratory rate and effort of breathing. Some causes of neonatal respiratory distress are listed in Table 115–3. Periparturient events associated with respiratory distress are described in Table 115–4.

CLINICAL EVALUATION OF THE RESPIRATORY SYSTEM

PHYSICAL EXAMINATION

A foal's respiratory rate, effort, and pattern are best observed from a distance. Handling or restraining the foal quickly alters resting respiratory parameters. Immediately following delivery the newborn's respiratory rate increases to between 60 and 80 breaths/min. During the first few weeks of life the normal respiratory rate is between 20 and 40 breaths/min. Awake, full-term foals should have a regular breathing pattern. During sleep, breathing patterns may change to include brief periods of apnea followed by rapid, shallow breathing. Respiratory effort should be minimal for a healthy foal.

Signs of increased work of breathing include nostril flaring, exaggerated abdominal effort, rib retractions, and expiratory grunting. Foals with severe lung disease will display more labored breathing when recumbent and will often rest with head and neck extended. Premature and immature foals may display paradoxical breathing (i.e., chest wall moves in and abdomen moves out on inspiration). Foals with brain stem damage associated with peripartum hypoxia/ischemia may exhibit irregular respiratory patterns with prolonged periods of apnea.

Lung sounds are normally easier to hear in the foal than in the adult horse because of the thin neonatal chest wall. Air moving in the larger airways frequently obscures or obliterates subtle changes occurring in the small airways. Thoracic auscultation is not a reliable means of assessing pulmonary disease in the neonatal foal. Atelectasis and interstitial lung disease may not produce detectable auscultatory abnormalities. Likewise, nasal discharge and spontaneous coughing are frequently absent in newborn foals with severe underlying lung disease. In the foal, respiratory rate and effort remain two of the more reliable indicators of pulmonary disease.

RADIOGRAPHY AND BLOOD GAS ANALYSIS

Because of the limitations of physical examination in the detection of neonatal lung disease, other diagnostic aids must be employed. Lateral thoracic radiographs can be obtained with the foal standing or laterally recumbent. If recumbent, the foal should have its forelegs extended as far forward as possible to improve visualization of the cranioventral lung field. Normal foal lungs have prominent vascular markings over the caudal dorsal lung fields. Good vascular clarity of vessels should exist posterior to the heart. The posterior vena cava and aorta should be clearly defined. A dark triangle comprising the caudoventral lung fields should be visible posterior to the caudal border of the heart,

TABLE 115–4. PERIPARTURIENT EVENTS ASSOCIATED WITH NEONATAL RESPIRATORY DISTRESS

CONDITION	RESULT
Premature placental separation (partial or complete)	Decreases effective area of gas exchange; diminishes fetal respiration
Dystocia (prolonged uterine contractions)	Contractions disrupt uterine blood, contributing to fetal hypoxia
Umbilical cord compression	Reduces or abolishes umbilical blood flow; diminishes fetal respiration; more common with posterior presentation.
Caesarean section	Maternal dorsal recumbency compresses the vena cava, increases pressure in uterine vein, and retards uterine blood flow; absence of vaginal delivery removes thoracic compression and other stimuli responsible for inducing spontaneous respiration maternal anesthesia/drug therapy further depress fetal respiration
Maternal hyperventilation (pain-induced or iatrogenic during anesthesia)	Decreases Pa_{CO_2} to produce respiratory alkalosis; shifts maternal Hb_{O_2} dissociation curve to the left and increases maternal Hb's affinity for O_2; decreases O_2 diffusion across placenta

ventral to the posterior vena cava, and cranial to the diaphragm. A thymic shadow may be visible cranial to the heart base. Early signs of ventral consolidation may involve the lung overlying the heart base. Ribs are examined carefully for fractures associated with birth trauma.

Pulmonary infiltrates are classified according to the type (alveolar, interstitial, or nodular) and location (diffuse, cranioventral, caudoventral, or caudodorsal). Diffuse pulmonary infiltrates have been described with bacterial/viral pneumonia (Fig. 115–3) and atelectasis (Fig. 115–4). Interstitial lung disease (Fig. 115–5) has been associated with both viral and bacterial infections. Caudoventral and cranioventral pulmonary infiltrates are seen with aspiration pneumonia (Fig. 115–6) and some cases of bacterial pneumonia (Figs. 115–7 and 115–8). Nodular infiltrates are suggestive of discrete abscessation such as that seen in slightly older foals with Rhodococcus equi pneumonia (Fig. 115–9).

Arterial blood gas analysis helps determine type and severity of pulmonary dysfunction present and allows respiratory therapy to be tailored to the individual's specific needs. Arterial blood gas analysis provides a more critical assessment of changes in respiratory condition that may be missed by physical examination and thoracic radiography. The great metatarsal artery is the preferred site for arterial puncture. Other sites include the brachial, facial, and femoral arteries. The carotid artery, although easily palpated in the jugular furrow, is a less desirable site, because hematoma formation is common and inadvertent trauma to the closely associated jugular vein destroys a valuable route of venous access. A small 25-gauge needle attached to a heparinized 1 or 3 mL Luer's slip syringe is used to obtain the sample. Once obtained, any air bubbles should be removed promptly from the sample and the syringe sealed with a cork and kept on ice until analysis is performed. The foal should be kept as sternal as possible during the

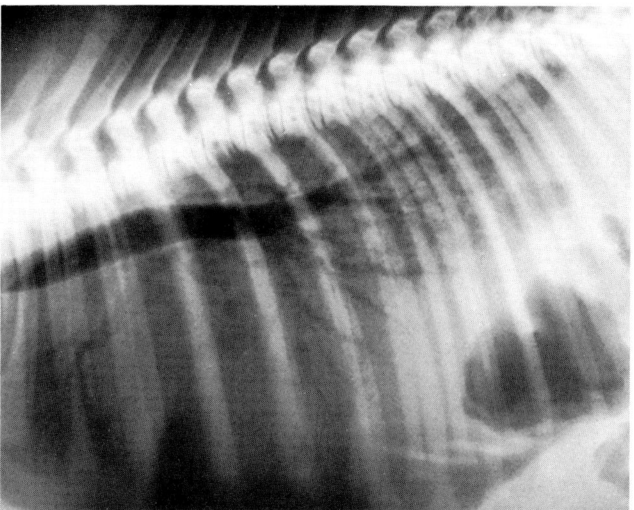

FIG. 115–4. Recumbent lateral thoracic radiograph of a premature foal 2 h following cesarean section delivery. The filly was the product of a 322-day gestation and had severe bradycardia and no spontaneous respiration at delivery. After vigorous resuscitation procedures, the filly was unable to maintain normal tidal volumes. A diffuse alveolar pattern is seen in all lung fields compatible with diffuse pulmonary atelectasis.

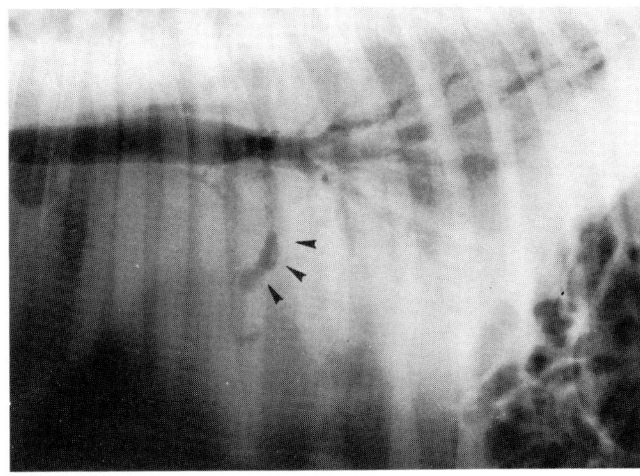

FIG. 115–3. Standing lateral thoracic radiograph of a 3-day-old, full-term foal with septicemia. The foal developed signs of progressive respiratory distress during the first 48 h of life, accompanied by high fevers and dyspnea. The radiograph reveals a diffuse alveolar pattern consistent with consolidation. Note the focal accumulations of gas in the cranial and midthoracic lung fields compatible with trapped air or pulmonary bullae (arrows). Air bronchograms are present in the ventral lung region. Necropsy revealed diffuse, severe, and suppurative bronchopneumonia with a fibrinous pleuritis and pericarditis. Tissue cultures were positive for β-Streptococci sp.

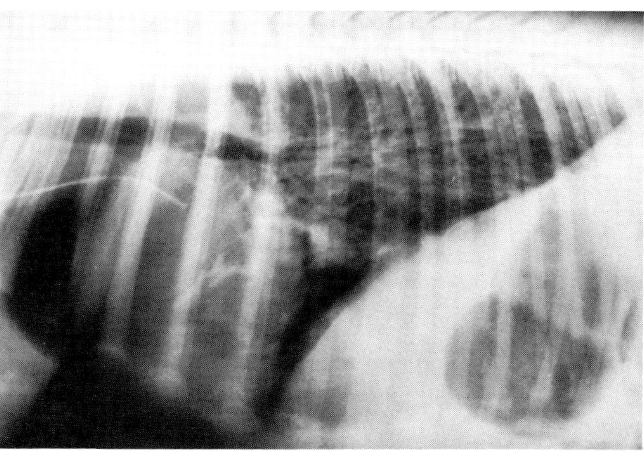

FIG. 115–5. Recumbent lateral radiograph of a 7-day-old, full-term filly; the foal was a twin. The radiograph shows a diffuse increase in interstitial density primarily in the caudodorsal lung field. A nonconsolidating alveolar pattern in the ventral lung field is represented by a wispy, reticulated pattern superimposed over the caudal aspect of the heart and ventral diaphragm. Note the radiopaque intravenous catheter extending down the jugular vein into the right atrium.

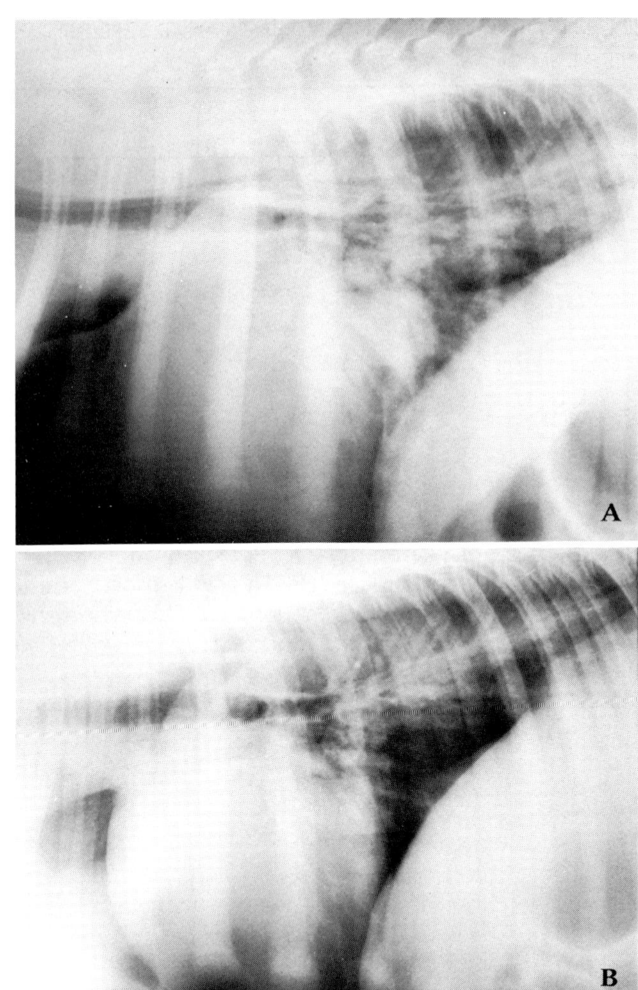

FIG. 115–6. Recumbent lateral radiographs of a full-term, 12-h old foal. Periparturient complications included premature placental separation and meconium aspiration. *A,* The radiograph reveals a mixed interstitial and alveolar infiltrate. The increased interstitial density in the caudodorsal and caudoventral lung fields is compatible with incomplete insufflation, interstitial edema, and/or inflammatory infiltrate associated with meconium aspiration and atelectasis. Note the nasogastric tube in the esophagus. *B,* Lateral thoracic radiograph of the same foal 8 days later, following intravenous antibiotic therapy and positive pressure ventilation. The lung and pulmonary vasculature are within normal limits.

sampling procedure because lateral recumbency and dependent lung atelectasis contribute to the development of hypoxemia.

Normal arterial blood gas values are presented in Table 115–5 and are published.[19,20] Intranasal oxygen therapy is recommended when arterial oxygen pressure decreases below 70 mm Hg. Mechanical ventilatory support is required to treat respiratory failure (i.e., $Pa_{CO_2} \leq 60$ mm Hg, $Pa_{CO_2} \geq 70$ mm Hg). Some causes of a low Pa_{O_2} and high Pa_{CO_2} are listed in Table 115–6. Oximetry and capnography are noninvasive techniques

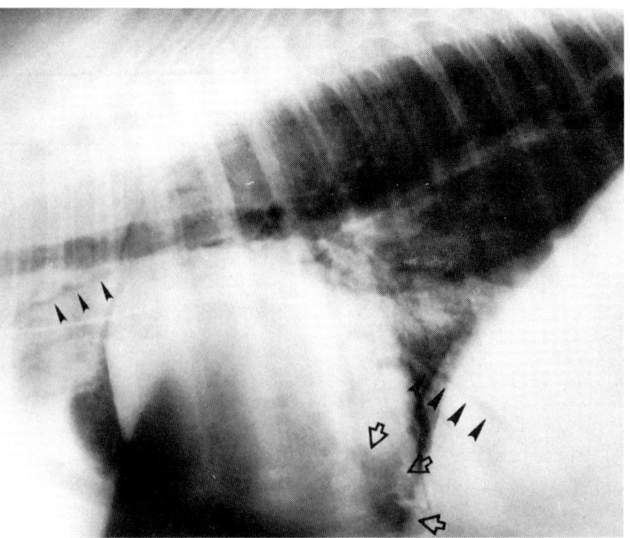

FIG. 115–7. Lateral thoracic radiograph of a 7-day-old, full-term foal delivered via cesarean section. The radiograph demonstrates a prominent alveolar pattern throughout the ventral lung field. Note the air bronchograms in the cranial lung fields and superimposed over the heart base and diaphragm (solid arrows). Small bullae are seen ventrally, adjacent to the cardiac apex (open arrows). Consolidation of the ventral lung field is compatible with bronchopneumonia. A radiopaque jugular catheter is visible.

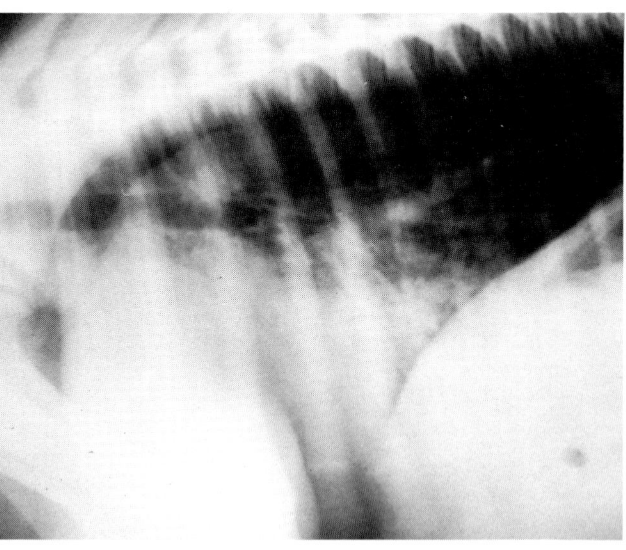

FIG. 115–8. Lateral thoracic radiograph of a 5-day-old, premature colt. The foal was the product of a 315-day gestation. The mare had a vaginal discharge and diffuse placentitis. The colt had an infected umbilical remnant and history of fevers. Blood cultures were positive for Klebsiella pneumoniae. The radiograph demonstrates a marked alveolar infiltrate involving the caudal and ventral lung fields compatible with consolidation secondary to bronchopneumonia.

TABLE 115–5. NORMAL ARTERIAL BLOOD GAS VALUES IN NEONATAL FOALS

POSTNATAL AGE	POSITION	PH	PA_{CO2} (mm Hg)	PA_{O2} (mm Hg)
Birth	Lateral	7.413 ± 0.019	45.7 ± 1.1	39.7 ± 2.1
2 min	Lateral	7.312 ± 0.016	54.1 ± 2.0	56.4 ± 2.3
30 min	Lateral	7.354 ± 0.010	51.5 ± 1.5	57.0 ± 1.8
12 h	Lateral	7.357 ± 0.024	44.3 ± 1.2	73.5 ± 3.0
48 h	Lateral	7.396 ± 0.008	46.1 ± 1.1	74.9 ± 3.3
4 days	Lateral	7.396 ± 0.012	45.8 ± 1.1	81.2 ± 3.1

(Adapted from Stewart, J.H., et al.: Respiratory studies in foals from birth to seven days old. Equine Vet. J., *16*:323–328, 1984.)

used to monitor arterial oxygen saturation and end tital carbon dioxide concentration, respectively.[19]

CULTURES

Transtracheal aspirates can be obtained in cases of suspected bacterial pneumonia. In young foals exhibiting signs of respiratory distress, however, this procedure is often too stressful and can seriously compromise respiratory function. Blood cultures help identify pulmonary pathogens when pneumonia is associated with septicemia and complete or partial failure of passive transfer or immunoglobulins or when lung infection is acquired hematogenously.

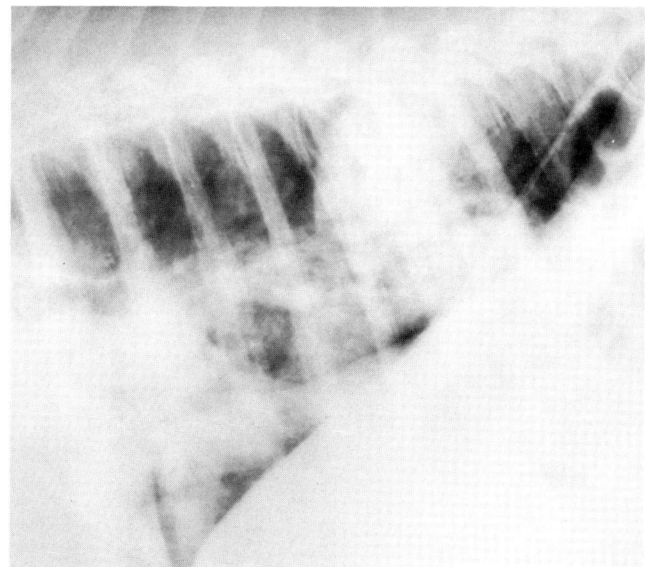

FIG. 115–9. Recumbent lateral thoracic radiograph of a 5-week-old Arabian foal with a 2.5-week history of recurrent respiratory disease and persistent lymphopenia. The final diagnosis was combined immunodeficiency disease (CID). Culture of a transtracheal aspirate produced a moderate growth of Rhodococcus equi and Nocardia sp. The radiographs reveal a patchy pattern of alveolar consolidation seen within the caudal and perihilar lung fields. These findings are consistent with areas of pneumonia and focal abscessation.

RESPIRATORY DISTRESS SYNDROME

Surfactant deficiency is the main factor contributing to development of respiratory distress syndrome (RDS) or hyaline membrane disease (HMD) and is most common among premature/immature neonates. This syndrome is defined as progressive respiratory failure caused by surfactant dysfunction and is characterized by tachypnea, cyanosis, rib retractions, and expiratory grunting.[2] Greatly increased work of breathing and poor gas exchange are the result of poor lung compliance and a compliant, immature chest wall. Hypoxia and acidosis develop. Pulmonary overperfusion occurs secondary to left-to-right shunting.

Hyaline membrane formation is the typical histopathologic lesion associated with RDS and is created by aggregations of cellular debris and plasma protein within the alveoli secondary to increased alveolar and capillary permeability.[14] These protein aggregates also serve to inactivate surfactant. The result is atelectatic and diffusely edematous lungs.

Surfactant deficiency may be primary caused by lung immaturity or may be secondary to other pulmonary and systemic diseases. Conditions known to interfere with surfactant activity and/or production include asphyxia, hypercapnia, acidosis, sepsis, toxemia, hypoperfusion, shock, and pulmonary edema.[21] Prematurity appears to increase the lung's susceptibility to these perinatal insults. Birth asphyxia enhances the risk of RDS although the precise mechanism is unclear. Asphyxia may interfere with alveolar stability and/or pulmonary perfusion by causing a decrease in surfactant production and vasoconstriction of the pulmonary arterioles.

A neonate afflicted with RDS may show only mild signs of respiratory distress immediately postpartum. During the next 24 to 48 h signs of severe respiratory distress develop as the work of breathing increases dramatically. Radiographically the lungs display a diffuse, ground-glass appearance with prominent air bronchograms (Fig. 115–4). Clinical signs of RDS in foals have been associated with peripartum asphyxia, prematurity/immaturity, and shock. In humans, a lecithin to sphingomyelin ratio of $< 2:1$ and an absence of phosphatidylglycerol in amniotic fluid are highly suggestive of

TABLE 115–6. SOME CAUSES OF A LOW PA_{O_2} AND A HIGH PA_{CO_2}

Hypoventilation
- Inadequate respiratory effort
  - CNS depression caused by asphyxia, trauma, hemorrhage, or drug administration
  - CNS immaturity resulting in apnea of prematurity
  - Neuromuscular disease, such as botulism, resulting in generalized muscle weakness and decreased chest excursions with secondary lung atelectasis
- Upper airway obstruction
  - Choanal atresia
  - Meconium aspiration
  - Blocked or kinked nasotracheal tube
  - External compression of airway
- Decreased lung compliance
  - Pneumothorax
  - Respiratory distress syndrome
  - Interstitial edema/fibrosis

Ventilation/perfusion mismatching
- Small airway obstruction (meconium aspiration)
- Atelectasis (RDS and pneumothorax)
- Alveolar infiltrate (pneumonia)
- Pulmonary edema (heart disease)

fetal lung immaturity and surfactant deficiency.[22,23] Limited studies with equine amniotic fluid have provided conflicting results.[24]

Depending on the severity of RDS, affected neonates may require a combination of oxygen administration, continuous positive airway pressure (CPAP), or mechanical ventilation with positive end expiratory pressure (PEEP). Complications associated with assisted ventilation include secondary lung infections and air leaks. Chronically ventilated neonates may suffer from barotrauma and oxygen toxicity resulting in conditions such as bronchopulmonary dysplasia (BPD). In human neonates, surfactant replacement therapy for RDS has been highly effective. Artificial surfactants and natural surfactants (harvested from bovine, porcine, and human amniotic fluid) have been instilled endotracheally in premature infants at risk for RDS during the first few breaths of life with dramatic improvement in pulmonary function.[2,25,26] More recent work suggests surfactant replacement therapy may also help treat conditions associated with secondary surfactant deficiency.

In pregnant women, maternally administered corticosteroids have been used to enhance fetal lung maturation in certain high-risk pregnancies. Although prepartum steroid administration has been used in pregnant mares, no documentation exists of its efficacy in accelerating fetal lung maturation. Prevention of peripartum birth asphyxia is probably more important in helping prevent RDS than maternal steroid administration.

PERIPARTUM ASPHYXIA

Asphyxia is caused by impaired oxygen delivery to cells and usually results from a combination of hypoxemia and ischemia. Hypoxemia is defined as decreased oxygen in the blood. Ischemia denotes decreased tissue perfusion. Specific peripartum causes of neonatal asphyxia are listed in Table 115–7.

Neonatal asphyxia affects multiple organ systems in addition to the lungs. The nature and extent of tissue injury depends on the age of the neonate (full term or premature) and the duration and severity of asphyxia (acute or chronic, partial or complete). These differences are illustrated in the wide variation in central nervous system (CNS) damage associated with peripartum hypoxia. Mature fetuses dying of severe asphyxia dem-

TABLE 115–7. CAUSES OF PERIPARTUM ASPHYXIA

Prepartum conditions
- Placentitis
- Premature placental separation
- Chronic placental insufficiency
- Twinning
- Severe maternal disease
- Maternal drug therapy (e.g., prostaglandin inhibitors, sedatives, and analgesics)

Intrapartum condition
- Dystocia
- Cesarean section
- Umbilical cord compression
- Uterine inertia

Postpartum neonatal conditions
- Airway obstruction
- Pneumonia (bacterial and viral)
- Hyaline membrane disease
- Meconium aspiration syndrome
- Central nervous system lesions
- Anemia
- Persistent fetal circulation
- Congenital malformations

onstrate hemorrhagic softening involving primarily the cerebral cortex and hemispheral white matter.[27,28] Immature fetuses dying of asphyxia experience brain damage involving structures deep within the hemispheres, namely the periventricular white matter.[27,28] Partial prolonged asphyxia results primarily in hemispheral injury patterns often accompanied by brain swelling. Acute total asphyxia tends to damage structures in the brain stem and spinal cord and is less commonly associated with brain swelling.

PHYSICAL EXAMINATION

Peripartum hypoxia can produce a wide range of clinical signs, depending on which organ systems are involved. A foal suffering from mild asphyxia may be hyperalert and hyperesthetic with a diminished suckle reflex and inappropriate nursing behavior. More severe episodes of asphyxia produce profound hypotonia, coma, seizures, central blindness, abnormal vocalization, and abnormal spinal reflexes accompanied by oliguria or anuria, gastrointestinal disturbances, respiratory distress, and myocardial dysfunction.

During hypoxia, hypercarbia, and/or acidosis in the newborn, a circulatory redistribution is found, resulting in increased blood flow to the heart, brain, adrenal glands, and liver and diminished blood flow to the kidneys, gastrointestinal tract, lung, and muscle.[29] Clinical signs associated with hypoxia-induced multisystem damage and therapeutic protocols are listed in Table 115–8.

Postasphyxial CNS dysfunction is usually characterized by depression followed by a hyperalert state. If cerebral edema develops, seizures appear within 48 h postpartum.[30] Therapy includes cautious fluid administration to avoid overhydration and hyperosmolar states. Intravenous dimethyl sulfoxide (DMSO) (0.5 to 1.0 gm/kg body weight) given slowly as a 20% solution has been used to reduce cerebral edema and to scavenge free oxygen radicals generated during reperfusion of ischemic tissues. Brief, transient seizures are controlled with intravenous diazepam (0.11 to 0.44 mg/kg). Prolonged or recurrent seizures may require phenobarbital (3 to 10 mg/kg) given as a slow intravenous infusion. The use of corticosteroids to reduce cerebral edema remains controversial and can produce significant immunosuppression. Mannitol (0.25 g/kg) given slowly as a 20% solution has also been used, but is contraindicated when cerebral hemorrhage is suspected or confirmed, because extravascular leakage of this osmotic diuretic may exacerbate cerebral edema.

Ischemic myocardial damage has been associated with A-V valve regurgitation, decreased cardiac output, cardiac enlargement, ventricular dysfunction, cardiac arrhythmias, and pulmonary edema.[31,32] Management includes cautious fluid therapy and careful monitoring of heart rate and rhythm, peripheral pulse quality, and blood pressure. Severe cardiac dysfunction may require administration of inotropic agents, dopamine (2 to 10 μg/kg/min), and dobutamine (2 to 20 μg/kg/min). Furosemide (1 to 2 mg/kg) is effective in reducing pulmonary edema.

TABLE 115–8. SEQUELA TO PERIPARTUM ASPHYXIA AND RECOMMENDED THERAPY

ORGAN SYSTEM/ DISEASE	SIGNS	THERAPY
Cardiovascular	Decreased cardiac output, weak pulses, arrhythmias, hypotension, generalized edema, and increased cardiac isoenzymes	Cautious fluid therapy, dopamine, dobutamine, furosemide
Respiratory	Respiratory distress, surfactant deficiency, pulmonary hypertension, and hypoxemia	Oxygen therapy, positive pressure ventilation, surfactant administration
Nervous	Hypotonia, abdominal respiratory pattern, loss of suckle, seizures, abnormal vocalization, blindness, and abnormal spinal reflexes	Cautious fluid therapy IV DMSO (1 g/kg), IV mannitol (0.5 to 1.0 g/kg), diazepam (0.1 to 0.25 g/kg), phenobarbital (3 to 10 mg/kg)
Hepatic	Icterus and increased hepatic enzymes	Monitor hepatic function
Renal	Oliguric/anuric renal failure	Dopamine (2 to 10 μg/kg/min), fluid therapy
Gastrointestinal	Dysmotility, ileus, colic, gastric reflux, abdominal distention, and necrotizing enterocolitis	NPO*, parenteral nutrition, antibiotics, metoclopramide
Metabolic	Hypoglycemia, hypercalcemia, and acidosis	IV dextrose, IV calcium, IV fluids, isotonic bicarbonate

*NPO, Nulla per os (nothing by mouth).

Increased pulmonary vascular resistance and pulmonary vasoconstriction may occur in response to acidosis and hypoxemia associated with asphyxia. If pulmonary arterial pressure exceeds systemic pressure, right-to-left shunting occurs and blood is diverted away from the lungs through the ductus arteriosis and foramen ovale. This condition, termed persistent fetal circulation, exacerbates existing hypoxemia. Therapy includes supplemental oxygen, mechanical ventilation, and correction of existing metabolic and respiratory acidosis.

Compromised pulmonary blood flow impedes substrate delivery to type II pneumocytes, resulting in decreased surfactant production, progressive atelectasis, and development of respiratory distress. Effective treatment requires lung expansion using positive pressure ventilatory support. Intratracheal instillation of artificial or bovine-origin surfactant is still investigational, but may prove beneficial. Thoracic radiography, serial arterial blood gas sampling and capnography help monitor efficacy of treatment.

In utero asphyxia may stimulate prepartum meconium passage. Hypoxia-induced fetal gasping results in aspiration of meconium-stained fetal fluids. Meconium filling only the nasopharynx and oropharynx can be removed by immediate postpartum suctioning of the nasal passages and pharynx. Meconium aspirated into the lower airways produces mechanical airway obstruction associated with local atelectasis, chemical pneumonitis, and surfactant dysfunction.

Asphyxia and associated hypercapnea and acidosis, reduces renal blood flow and produces acute tubular necrosis, oliguria/anuria, and azotemia.[33] Dopamine administration (2 to 10 μg/kg/min) and small intravenous doses of furosemide (1 to 2 mL of a 20% solution) improve renal blood flow and urine output. Fluid therapy should be carefully balanced with urine output to prevent fluid overload and edema formation.

Mesenteric hypoperfusion leads to gut ischemia with loss of mucosal integrity. A serious sequela is necrotizing enterocolitis characterized by gastrointestinal dys-

TABLE 115–9. GUIDELINES FOR RESUSCITATION*

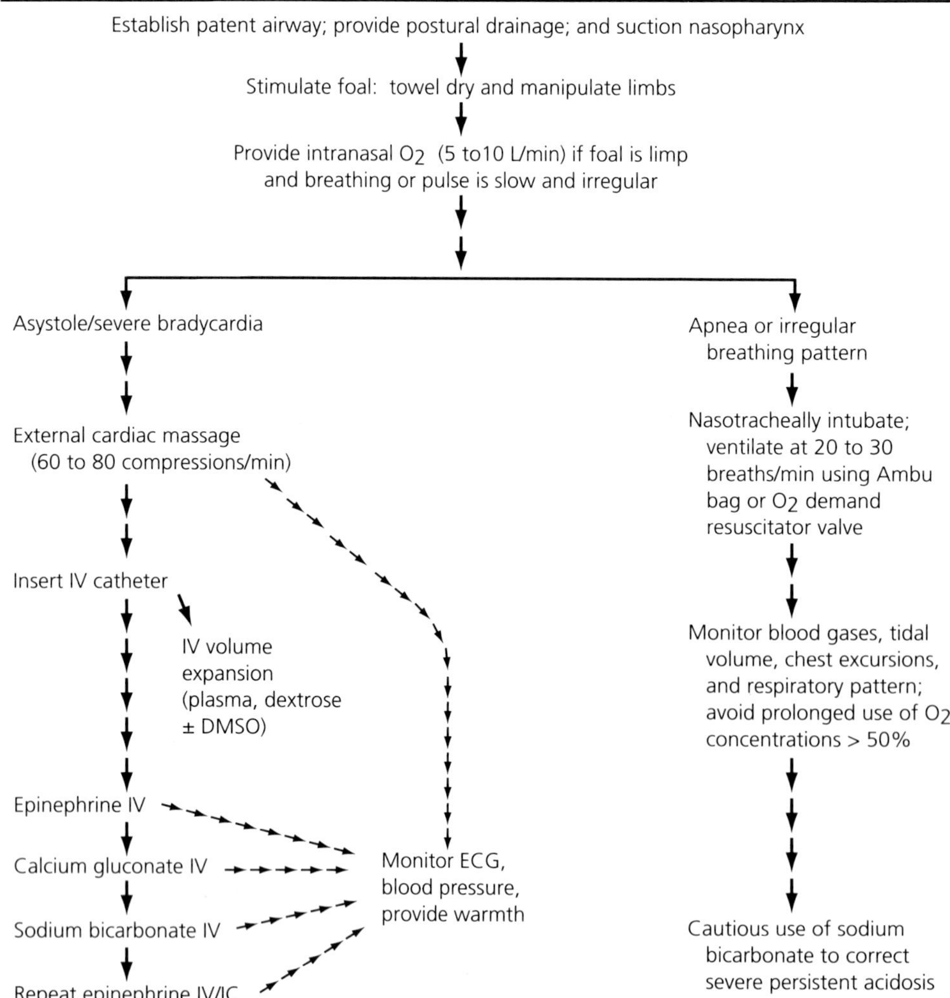

*Small arrow, improvement; large arrow, no improvement.

motility, malabsorption, colic, bloat, gastric reflux, bloody diarrhea, and septicemia secondary to absorption of bacteria across the disrupted gastrointestinal mucosal barrier. Severe hypoxia, hypothermia, hypotension, and immaturity/prematurity increases a foal's risk for necrotizing enterocolitis. Therapy includes withholding oral feeds, the use of parenteral nutrition, and administration of broad-spectrum antibiotics. Enteral feeding should be reinstituted slowly once vital parameters are stable. Gastric reflux and small intestinal dysmotility may respond to metoclopramide therapy (0.6 mg/kg orally q 4 to 6 h; 0.25 to 0.30 mg/kg IV as a slow 1-h infusion repeated q 4 to 6 h).

RESUSCITATION PROCEDURE

Aggressive treatment of neonatal asphyxia serves to reduce the severity of postpartum complications. Signs of respiratory arrest are cyanosis and apnea. Absence of a heartbeat and palpable pulses denote cardiac arrest. Causes of primary respiratory arrest include airway obstruction and CNS depression. Circulatory arrest includes asystole, ventricular fibrillation, and cardiovascular collapse. General resuscitation guidelines are presented in Table 115–9 and dosages of commonly used drugs are listed in Table 115–10.

Airway

Immediately following delivery, the foal's airway should be cleared of fetal fluids using postural drainage and nasopharyngeal suctioning (Laerdal Compact Suction Unit, Laerdal Medical Corp., Armonk, NY). Rubbing the foal with dry towels and extending the limbs helps stimulate initiation of respiration. Within 5 min of birth, normal foals should quickly establish a regular heart rate greater than 60 beats/min and a rapid respiratory rate of at least 40 to 50 breaths/min. The foal should be able to maintain sternal recumbency with minimal assistance and should grimace in response to nasal stimulation.

Ventilation

The absence of regular or adequate respiration requires nasotracheal intubation using a long (45 to 55 cm), silicone cuffed nasotracheal tube 7 to 10 mm in internal diameter (Air Cuf, Bivona, Inc., Gary, IN). Ventilation is begun using a self-inflating resuscitation bag (Laerdal Silicone Adult Respirator, Laerdal Medical Corp., Armonk, NY) or an oxygen demand valve resuscitator (AIRCO, Huntingdon Valley, PA). Although mouth-to-nose resuscitation can be attempted, the technique is usually inadequate to provide uniform lung expansion. Assisted ventilation is essential to remove carbon dioxide, which in turn helps correct respiratory acidosis, reduce pulmonary hypertension, and normalize cerebral blood flow. A breathing rate of 15 to 25 breaths/min is usually adequate. The expiratory pause should be at least twice as long as inspiration.

The use of doxapram, a respiratory stimulant, should not be used in place of positive pressure ventilation. Doxapram is a CNS stimulant with an affinity for the respiratory center. Doxapram may help reverse respiratory depression associated with inhalant anesthesia and primary apnea, but is ineffective during secondary apnea when the respiratory center becomes refractory to chemical stimuli.[34]

TABLE 115–10. DOSAGES OF DRUGS USED FOR RESUSCITATION

DRUG	CONCENTRATION	DOSE	ROUTE*	INDICATIONS
Atropine	1 mg/mL	0.01 to 0.03 mg/kg	IV	Bradycardia
Bretyllium tosylate	50 mg/mL	5 to 10 mg/kg	IV	Fibrillation
Calcium chloride	10% solution, 100 mg/mL, 1.4 mEq Ca^{++}/mL	20 mg/kg 0.3 mEq/kg	IV	Asystole, hypocalcemia
Calcium gluconate	23% solution, 20 mg/mL, 1 mEq Ca^{++}/mL	0.6 mg/kg 0.3 mEq/kg	IV	Asystole, hypocalcemia
Doxapram	20 mg/mL	0.5 to 2.5 mg/kg	IV	Anesthesia induced respiratory depression, ineffective during secondary apnea
Epinephrine	1:1000 (1.0 mg/mL), 1:10,000 (0.1 mg/mL)	0.01 to 0.02 mg/kg	IV IT IC	Asystole, severe bradycardia, fibrillation
Naloxone	0.4 mg/mL	5 to 10 μg/kg	IV	Narcotic-induced respiratory depression
Sodium bicarbonate	5% solution (0.6 mEq HCO_3/mL), 8.4% solution (1 mEq HCO_3/mL)	1 to 2 mEq/kg	IV	Metabolic acidosis with adequate ventilation

*IV, intravenous; IT, intratracheal; IC, intracardiac.

Circulation

If a pulse is absent or severe bradycardia exists closed-chest cardiac massage is begun at a rate of 60 to 80 compressions/min. The foal should be in lateral recumbency with a sandbag or board placed under the thorax to provide the firm support required to achieve effective cardiac compression. If ventilation and cardiac massage are effective, peripheral pulses become palpable, pupils begin to constrict, and mucous membrane color improves.

Drugs

Drug administration begins once positive pressure ventilation and cardiac massage are established. A 14- or 16-gauge jugular catheter should be inserted and volume expansion begun using a balanced electrolyte solution and/or isotonic dextrose-containing fluids. Plasma, if available, is an ideal volume expander. During initial resuscitation, fluid rates of 10 to 20 mL/kg/h may be required. Drugs can be injected directly into the IV line while fluids are running.

Epinephrine should be administered if effective circulation has not been established within 2 to 3 min of initiating artificial ventilation and chest massage. Epinephrine improves myocardial contractile force. If no improvement in circulation occurs, calcium should be administered followed by sodium bicarbonate. Sodium bicarbonate infusions should be given slowly and cautiously and only after adequate ventilation is established. Overzealous administration of sodium bicarbonate has been associated with metabolic alkalosis, decreased tissue oxygenation, hyperosmolality, hypernatremia, and paradoxic myocardial and CNS acidosis.

Once a regular heartbeat and spontaneous ventilation have been established, careful monitoring of vital signs, including blood pressure, should be continued. The foal should be kept warm, because hypothermia adversely affects cardiovascular stability. Blood glucose concentrations should be measured to avoid hypoglycemic and hyperglycemic states. Urine output and gastrointestinal function should be monitored closely. Postresuscitation administration of DMSO should be considered to minimize possible reperfusion injury of ischemic tissue beds. Detailed reviews of neonatal asphyxia and resuscitation guidelines have been published.[32,34]

PNEUMONIA

BACTERIAL

Bacterial infections are a common cause of respiratory disease in the neonate. Bacterial pneumonia frequently occurs as one component of generalized neonatal sepsis. In utero acquired infections may occur hematogenously or via an infected placenta. During the birth process, fetal aspiration of vaginal bacteria represents a third route for infection. Postpartum infection occurs via the umbilicus or by ingestion or inhalation of potential pathogens. An immature immune system, inadequate absorption of colostral immunoglobulins, and lung immaturity are factors predisposing to neonatal pneumonia.

Bacteria responsible for neonatal pneumonia are essentially the same as those pathogens causing foal septicemia. Common pathogens include gram-negative enteric bacteria (e.g., Escherichia coli, Klebsiella spp., Salmonella spp.), Actinobacillus spp., Pasteurella spp., and Streptococcal spp.[35] Fungal and yeast pathogens may become secondary invaders in chronically debilitated foals receiving long-term parenteral nutritional support and broad-spectrum antibiotic therapy.

The clinical presentation of pneumonia is nonspecific and includes fever, depression, and the previously described signs of respiratory distress. If systemic sepsis is present, other sites of infection (e.g., polyarthritis and uveitis) may be apparent. Diagnosis is frequently based on thoracic radiography (Figs. 115–3, 115–7, 115–8, and 115–10). Radiographically, pneumonia may be associated with alveolar, interstitial, or mixed pulmonary infiltrates. In the newborn foal, atelectasis is often difficult to distinguish from consolidation caused by pneumonia. Radiographic changes often lag behind changes in clinical condition.

During the initial stages of acute sepsis, the neonate frequently develops leukopenia and neutropenia with a degenerative left shift. Once localized sites of infection (e.g., pneumonia) become established, the leukogram often shows a leukocytosis and neutrophilia and is ac-

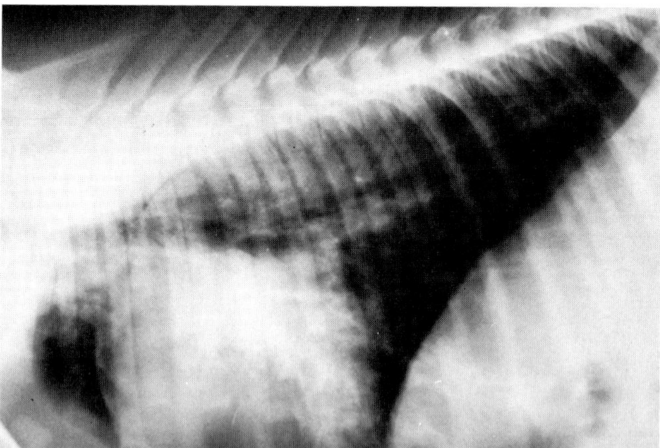

FIG. 115–10. Recumbent lateral thoracic radiograph of a 16-day-old foal hospitalized at 1 day of age for septicemia and neonatal maladjustment syndrome. Therapy included broad-spectrum antibiotics, positive pressure ventilation, and parenteral nutrition. An increase exists in interstitial pulmonary infiltrates overlying the heart base and evidence is found of consolidation involving the ventral aspects of the caudal and hilus regions of the lung. These changes are consistent with a diagnosis of pneumonia. Cultures of urine, blood, and a transtracheal aspirate were all positive for Candida albicans. Numerous other bacterial pathogens were also cultured from the transtracheal aspirate.

TABLE 115–11. DOSAGE RECOMMENDATIONS FOR ANTIMICROBIAL DRUGS USED IN FOALS

DRUGS	DOSE	ROUTE	DOSING INTERVAL
Procaine penicillin G	20,000 to 50,000 μ/kg	IM	12 h
Potassium/sodium penicillin	20,000 to 50,000 μ/kg	IV	6 h
Sodium ampicillin	20 to 50 mg/kg	IM	6 h
Gentamicin sulfate	1 to 2 mg/kg	IM/IV	8 h
Amikacin sulfate	6.6 mg/kg	IM/IV	8 h
Trimethoprim sulfa	25 to 30 mg/kg	IV/PO	12 h
Erythromycin estolate	20 to 30 mg/kg	PO	6 h
Rifampin	5 to 10 mg/kg	PO	12 to 24 h
Timentin	50 to 75 mg/kg	IV	6 h

companied by a hyperfibrinogenemia. Blood and tracheal aspirates can be cultured to try to identify specific pathogens.

Therapy should begin by ensuring that the foal has adequate passive immunity. Foals with serum IgG concentrations below 800 mg/dL are treated intravenously with hyperimmune plasma (20 to 50 mL/kg). Broad-spectrum, bactericidal antibiotic therapy is essential. Dosages are listed in Table 115–11. Ampicillin or penicillin and an aminoglycoside (amikacin or gentamicin) are a reasonable empiric treatment pending culture results. Aminoglycoside administration—in particular, gentamicin—should be avoided in dehydrated foals because of the risk of nephrotoxicity. Third-generation cephalosporins and extended spectrum antibiotics such as ticarcillin with clavulanic acid (e.g., timentin) are other more expensive alternatives. Potentiated sulfa derivatives are appropriate when microbial sensitivity exists. Antibiotic therapy should be continued until the leukogram, plasma fibrinogen concentration, and chest radiographs are within normal limits. If a positive blood culture is obtained, a minimum of 2 weeks of therapy is recommended. Cases of established pneumonia with abscessation may require a minimum of 3 to 5 weeks of antibiotic therapy.

Rhodococcus equi causes pneumonia with abscessation in slightly older foals (≥2 weeks of age). Erythromycin and rifampin are particularly effective against this intracellular pathogen. Foals suffering from R. equi pneumonia often require a minimum of 4 to 8 weeks of antibiotic therapy.

Respiratory physiotherapy is an often overlooked treatment. Laterally recumbent foals should be turned frequently and propped into sternal recumbency to minimize dependent lung atelectasis. Chest coupage can be performed using electric percussionators or a cupped hand positioned over the intercostal space. Exercise and maintenance of adequate hydration promote improved clearance of tracheobronchial secretions. Nebulization of mists, containing bronchodilators (isoproterenol and aminophylline), mucolytic agents (bicarbonate and acetylcystine), saline, and antibiotics may also help alleviate signs of respiratory distress. Intranasal oxygen therapy and mechanical ventilatory support are required in cases with more severe and/or diffuse lung involvement.

VIRAL

Viral pathogens causing pneumonia in foals include equine herpesvirus type 1 (EHV 1), influenza virus, adenovirus, and equine arteritis virus.[35] Equine herpesvirus can cause interstitial pneumonia or bronchopneumonia in neonatal foals. Maternal EHV 1 infection may result in abortion or the birth of a live—healthy or weak—neonate. Foals born alive develop signs of respiratory distress within the first few hours or days of life. Fetuses aborted following EHV 1 infection contain intranuclear inclusion bodies in the lung and liver. However, inclusion bodies cannot always be demonstrated in infected fetuses born alive.

Influenza virus has also been reported as a less common cause of severe interstitial pneumonia in neonatal foals.[35] Adenovirus pneumonia is usually associated with combined immunodeficiency (CID) syndrome observed in Arabian and part-Arabian foals. Equine arteritis virus has also been incriminated as a cause of severe interstitial pneumonia in newborn foals. Affected foals may be born weak or may be born healthy and develop respiratory signs within the first 48 h of life.

Virus isolation is the definitive way to confirm viral infection. However, many laboratories cannot perform virus isolation, and specimen mishandling during shipping often results in failure to isolate the virus. In one foal infected with equine arteritis virus, the virus was cultured from amniotic fluid collected at the time of delivery and stored frozen for 2 weeks. Viral infections are often associated with lymphopenia and lymphoid depletion. Unfortunately, these conditions are not pathopneumonic for viral infections and can be observed in foals debilitated by bacterial infections and poor nutrition as well.

Serologic studies are also unreliable in diagnosing perinatal viral infections in the foal. Passively derived colostral immunoglobulins produce erroneous antibody titer results in the neonate. Presuckle serum samples are more useful.

MECONIUM ASPIRATION SYNDROME

In utero asphyxia or umbilical cord compression can result in fetal evacuation of meconium into the amniotic fluid. Fetal meconium staining is recognized as an indicator of fetal stress and asphyxia. Fetal gasping before and/or during delivery results in varying degrees of meconium aspiration. Obstructive, aspiration pneumonia develops if meconium moves down into the lower airways. Meconium aspiration can produce mechanical obstruction, air trapping and local atelectasis, chemical irritant bronchopneumonia, alveolar edema, ventilation-perfusion abnormalities, and increases in pulmonary vascular and airway resistance.[36]

Foals at risk for meconium aspiration are stained with yellow-brown amniotic fluid at delivery. Nasal secretions may be brown tinged. The degree of respiratory distress is related to the severity of aspiration. Blood gas analysis may be normal or may indicate profound hypoxemia with metabolic acidosis. Thoracic radiography may demonstrate a caudoventral infiltrate (see Fig. 115–6). Hyperluscent areas of lung may be observed along the periphery caused by meconium obstruction of small airways during expiration resulting in air trapping.

Careful nasotracheal suctioning of the upper airways should be performed as soon as meconium aspiration is recognized. Excessive suctioning must be avoided to prevent exacerbation of existing hypoxia. Large-bore suction cannulas inserted through a nasotracheal tube are required when thick meconium is present distal to the nasopharynx. The foal should be ventilated mechanically or with a hand-held oxygen demand valve between suctioning attempts. Continued oxygen therapy or mechanical ventilatory support may be indicated, based on serial blood gas results. Because of the focal pattern of obstruction, meconium aspiration predisposes to the development of pneumothorax. The use of mechanical ventilation increases this risk. Antibiotic therapy is initiated to help prevent secondary bacterial pneumonia associated with the chemical pneumonitis and nasotracheal intubation and suctioning procedures.

Early recognition of cardiopulmonary dysfunction in the newborn is essential so treatment can be initiated before irreversible damage occurs. A comprehensive physical examination followed by frequent observation are required to detect trends in the patient's status.

REFERENCES

1. Kullander, S., et al.: A review of surfactant principles in the fetal physiology of man and animals. J. Reprod. Fertil. Suppl., *23:*659–661, 1975.
2. Reynolds, M.S., Wallander, K.: Use of surfactant in the prevention and treatment of neonatal respiratory distress syndrome. Am. J. Hosp. Pharm., *46:*1902–1907, 1989.
3. Rossdale, P.D.: Clinical studies in the newborn Thoroughbred foal. II. Heart rate, auscultation and electrocardiogram. Br. Vet. J., *123:*521–532, 1967.
4. Lombard, C.W.: Cardiovascular diseases. *In* Equine Clinical Neonatology. Edited by A.M. Koterba, W.H. Drummond, and P.C. Kosch. Philadelphia, Lea & Febiger, 1990, pp. 240–261.
5. Lombard, C.W., et al.: Blood pressure, electrocardiogram and echocardiogram measurements in the growing pony foal. Equine Vet. J., *16:*342–347, 1984.
6. Vaala, W.E., and Webb, A.I.: Cardiovascular monitoring of the critically ill foal. *In* Equine Clinical Neonatology. Edited by A.M. Koterba, W.H. Drummond, and P.C. Kosch. Philadelphia, Lea & Febiger, 1990, pp. 262–272.
7. Rooney, J.R., and Franks, C.W.: Congenital cardiac anomalies in horses. Pathol. Vet., *1:*454–464, 1964.
8. Crowe, M.W., and Swerczek, T.W.: Equine congenital defects. Am. J. Vet. Res., *46:*353–358, 1985.
9. Button, C.: Congenital disorders of cardiac blood flow. *In* Current Therapy in Equine Medicine 2. Edited by N.E. Robinson. Philadelphia, W.B. Saunders, 1987, pp. 167–170.
10. Reef, V.B.: Cardiovascular disease in the equine neonate. Vet. Clin. North Am. Equine Pract., *1:*117–129, 1985.
11. Fregin, G.F.: The cardiovascular system. *In* Equine Medicine and Surgery. 3rd ed. Edited by R.A. Mansmann, E.S. McAllister, and P.W. Pratt. Santa Barbara, CA, American Veterinary Publications, 1982, pp. 645–704.
12. Wilson, T.M., et al.: Myodegeneration and suspected selenium and vitamin E deficiency in horses. J. Am. Vet. Med. Assoc., *169:*213–217, 1976.
13. Richardson, D.W., and Kohn, C.W.: Uroperitoneum in the foal. J. Am. Vet. Med. Assoc., *182:*267–271, 1983.
14. Koterba, A.M., and Paradis, M.R.: Specific respiratory conditions. *In* Equine Clinical Neonatology. Edited by A.M. Koterba, W.H. Drummond, and P.C. Kosch. Philadelphia, Lea & Febiger, 1990, pp. 177–199.
15. Carmana, R.H., et al.: Myocardial dysfunction in septic shock. Arch. Surg., *120:*30–38, 1985.
16. Pattle, R.E., et al.: The development of the lung and its surfactant in the foal and in other species. J. Reprod. Fertil. Suppl., *23:*651–657, 1975.
17. Coustan, D.R.: Clinical aspect of antenatal enhancement of pulmonary maturation. Clin. Perinatol., *14:*697–703, 1987.
18. Jobe, A.: Respiratory distress syndrome—New therapeutic approaches to a complex pathophysiology. Adv. Pediatr., *30:*93–98, 1988.
19. Koterba, A.M.: Respiratory disease: Approach to diagnosis. *In* Equine Clinical Neonatology. Edited by A.M. Koterba, W.H. Drummond, and P.C. Kosch. Philadelphia, Lea & Febiger, 1990, pp. 153–176.
20. Stewart, J.H., et al.: Respiratory studies in foals from birth to seven days old. Equine Vet. J., *16:*323–328, 1984.
21. Kotas, R.V.: Surface tension forces and liquid balance in the lung. *In* Neonatal Pulmonary Care. Edited by D.W. Thibeault and G.A. Gregory. Menlo Park, Addison-Wesley, 1979, pp. 35–53.
22. Gluck, L., et al.: The diagnosis of respiratory distress syndrome (RDS) by amniocentesis. Am. J. Obstet. Gynecol., *109:*440–445, 1971.
23. Kulovich, M.V., Hallman, G.B., and Bluck, L.: The lung profile. I. Normal pregnancy. Am. J. Obstet. Gynecol., *135:*57–63, 1979.
24. Paradis, M.R.: Lecithin/sphingomyelin ratios and phos-

phatidylglycerol in term and premature equine amniotic fluid. Proceedings of the Fifth Annual Forum of the American College of Veterinary Internal Medicine. Madison, WI, Omnipress, 1987, pp. 789–792.

25. Enhorning, G., et al.: Prevention of neonatal respiratory distress syndrome by tracheal instillation of surfactant: A randomized clinical trial. Pediatrics *76:*145–153, 1985.

26. Kwong, M.S., et al.: Double-blind clinical trial of calf lung surfactant extract for the prevention of hyaline membrane disease in extremely premature infants. Pediatrics, *76:*585–592, 1985.

27. Brann, A.W.: Effects of acute total and prolonged partial asphyxia on the central nervous system of the foetal neonatal and juvenile rhesus monkey: A review. Equine Vet. J., *5*(Suppl.):25–27, 1988.

28. Brann, A.W., and Myers, R.E.: Central nervous system findings in the newborn monkey following severe in utero partial asphyxia. Neurology, *25:*327–338, 1975.

29. Patton, J.B., et al.: Umbilical blood flow, cardiac output, and organ blood flow in the miniature baboon fetus. Am. J. Obstet. Gynecol., *117:*560–566, 1973.

30. Drummond, W.H.: Neonatal maladjustment syndrome: Its relationship to perinatal hypoxic-ischaemic insults. Equine Vet. J., *5*(Suppl.):41–43, 1988.

31. Drummond, W.H.: Acute asphyxia in the newborn: Effects and management. Proceedings of the Seventh Forum of the American College of Veterinary Internal Medicine. Edited by G. Pidgeon. Madison, WI, Omnipress, 1989, pp. 421–425.

32. Drummond, W.H., and Koterba, A.M.: Neonatal asphyxia. *In* Equine Clinical Neonatology. Edited by A.M. Koterba, W.H. Drummond, and P.C. Kosch. Philadelphia, Lea & Febiger, 1990, pp. 124–135.

33. Dauber, I.M., et al.: Renal failure following perinatal anoxia. J. Pediatr., *88:*851–855, 1976.

34. Webb, A.I.: Neonatal Resuscitation. *In* Equine Clinical Neonatology. Edited by A.M. Koterba, W.H. Drummond, and P.C. Kosch. Philadelphia, Lea & Febiger, 1990, pp. 136–150.

35. Beech, J.: Respiratory problems in foals. Vet. Clin. North Am. Equine Pract., *1:*131–149, 1985.

36. Holtzman, R.B., et al.: Perinatal management of meconium staining of the amniotic fluid. Critical issues in intrapartum and delivery room management. Clin. Perinatol., *16:*825–838, 1989.

CHAPTER 116

THE MUSCULOSKELETAL SYSTEM

R. Adams

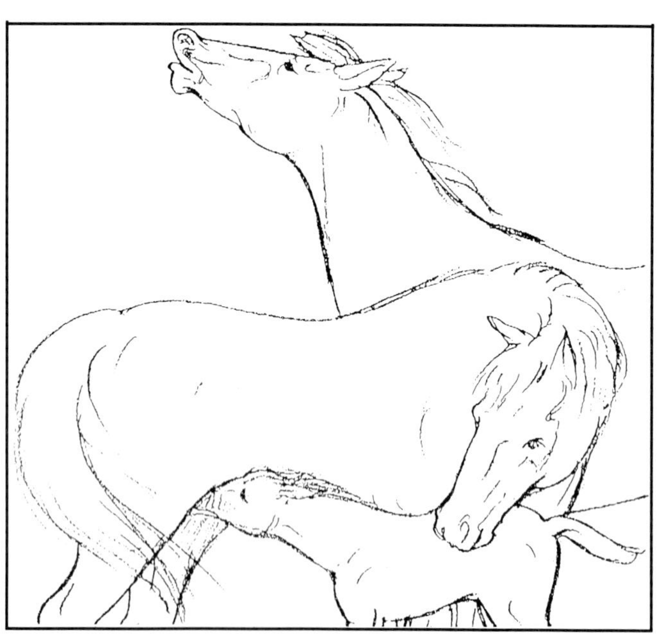

Diseases involving the musculoskeletal system of the newborn foal are usually not immediately life threatening but have great potential to affect detrimentally the animal's future athletic ability. Sequelae to polyarthritis/osteomyelitis and incomplete ossification of the skeletal system are common causes of euthanasia of foals after discharge from neonatal intensive care units.[1] Two major types of orthopedic problems occur in neonatal foals: infectious (polyarthritis/osteomyelitis complex) and noninfectious (incomplete ossification of the bones, angular limb deformities, flexural deformities, and traumatic sprains and fractures.)

INFECTIOUS DISEASE: POLYARTHRITIS AND OSTEOMYELITIS

Firth classified equine neonatal infectious polyarthritis and osteomyelitis into four types (S, E, T, and P) according to the clinical signs, history, radiographic findings, bacterial culture results, and necropsy lesions[2] (Table 116–1). Distinction between the four types can be difficult on physical examination alone but is necessary in order to devise a rational course of therapy for the patient and a realistic prognosis for the owner.

DIAGNOSIS

Foals with a history of failure of passive transfer, prematurity, and adverse prepartum events are at high risk for developing generalized infection. Signs of bone and joint involvement may be present when systemic disease is first noticed or develop several weeks after apparent recovery.

Lameness and intra-articular or focal periarticular swellings of the distal limbs are obvious clinical signs associated with infection. Infection of the axial skeleton is suspected if the foal has an abnormal gait, reluctance to move, or muscle soreness. Frequently, these abnormalities are mistakenly believed to be caused by trauma or are masked by weakness in the septicemic foal.

Bone infection may be the most prominent clinical sign of disease in the foal. Before aggressive diagnostic or therapeutic action, the foal's general condition should be closely assessed. If dehydration and septic shock are present but unnoticed, the foal can die during therapy for the skeletal disease. Because bone infection is usually a sequelae of septicemia, the foal should be carefully examined for umbilical, gastrointestinal, and respiratory disease. Once the general condition of the foal has been attended, diagnosis and treatment of the bone infection must begin immediately.

Radiographs are the first essential diagnostic procedure when polyarthritis/osteomyelitis is suspected.[3] They help rule out other causes of lameness and detect bony lesions associated with infection which may significantly alter the prognosis. The S and E types of infection cannot be distinguished via clinical examination alone (Table 116–1). If bone lesions are identified indi-

TABLE 116–1. POLYARTHRITIS AND OSTEOMYELITIS SYNDROMES

PARAMETER	S TYPE	E TYPE	P TYPE	T TYPE
Age of foal	A few days old or older	Slightly older than S-type foal	9 to 90 days	<1 month
History	Acute onset lameness, systemically ill	Acute onset lameness, may appear only to have orthopedic problems; may have had previous illness	Variable degree of lameness; past history of diarrhea, pneumonia	Previous history of systemic disease, prematurity, twin birth
Clinical signs	One or several joints distended, warm, and painful	Joint distention; warm, painful in two or more joints	Swelling over physis, painful on palpation, ± joint distention	Usually multiple joints affected; moderate to severe lameness; both tibial tarsal and small tarsal joint capsules distended
Common sites	Any or all joints	Medial and lateral femoral condyles; tibial tarsal condyle; lateral styloid process of the distal radius; distal tibia, patella	Distal radial physes; distal tibial physes; metacarpal/tarsal physes	Small tarsal bones
Radiographic impression	Soft tissue swelling, joint distention, impression of increased joint space	Lucencies in the epiphyses; cuboidal bones may be involved	Lucencies in the metaphyses, physes, epiphyses; sequestra may be evident	Lucencies in third and central tarsal bones and proximal metatarsus; apparent collapsed third tarsal bone
Synovial fluid analysis	Purulent, increased protein and white blood cell count, Gram stain positive	Purulent, increased protein and white blood cell count, Gram stain positive	± abnormal ± increased protein, white blood cells ± positive Gram stain	Abnormal in small tarsal joints; ± abnormal in tibial tarsal joint
Bacterial culture	±	±	±	±
Bacteria commonly cultured	Escherichia coli, Klebsiella, Actinobacillus, Streptococcal spp.	Escherichia coli, Streptococcus, Salmonella spp.	Salmonella spp., Klebsiella spp., Streptococcal spp. Rhodococcus equi	Escherichia coli, Salmonella spp.
Necropsy lesions of affected areas	Primarily synovial membrane, superficial cartilage loss; subchondral bone usually not affected	Fibrinopurulent arthritis; purulent bone lesions corresponding to radiographic lucencies	Osteomyelitis of physes, metaphyses, epiphyses; infectious arthritis and subcutaneous abscess may or may not be present	Fibrinopurulent arthritis; cartilage may be cracked and bone shape irregular or fractured
Prognosis	Often die early in life because of medical problems	Often poor prognosis because of widespread osteomyelitis and septic arthritis	Aggressive surgical curettage may help with well-localized lesions; poor prognosis because of physeal damage and extent of bone destruction	Poor prognosis because of multiple joint involvement and degenerative arthritis that may develop in hock even if infection is controlled

S Type = Infectious synovitis without bone involvement; E Type = Infection of the joint and adjacent epiphysis; P Type = Bone infection adjacent to the metaphyseal growth plate of the physis; T type = Infection of the small tarsal bones that may also occur with infections in other joints.

(From Adams, R.: Polyarthritis/osteomyelitis. *In* Equine Clinical Neonatology. Edited by A. Koterba, W.H. Drummond, and P.C. Kosch. Philadelphia, Lea & Febiger, 1990, pp. 318–319.)

cating E-type infection, the prognosis diminishes. Distinguishing the incomplete ossification of skeletal immaturity from lysis secondary to bone infection may be difficult, and both may occur simultaneously[4] (Fig. 116–1). Comparison of radiographs from the contralateral but unaffected joint can be helpful to distinguish the two conditions.

Bacterial culture and cytologic analysis of the synovial fluid is the next diagnostic step.[3] The fluid sample should be taken under strict sterile conditions to avoid skin contamination and faulty culture results. Part of the sample is collected in an EDTA tube for cytologic analysis, and the remaining portion is transported in a culture medium or in a capped syringe to a microbiology laboratory. Use of a culturette transport system is not recommended. Failure to culture bacteria from joints that are suspected of being infected is common and may be the result of several factors: prior antibiotic therapy, mishandling of the sample, inadequate laboratory techniques, and defense mechanisms within the joint. Adherence to the principles of aseptic sampling technique and submission of a large quantity of fluid

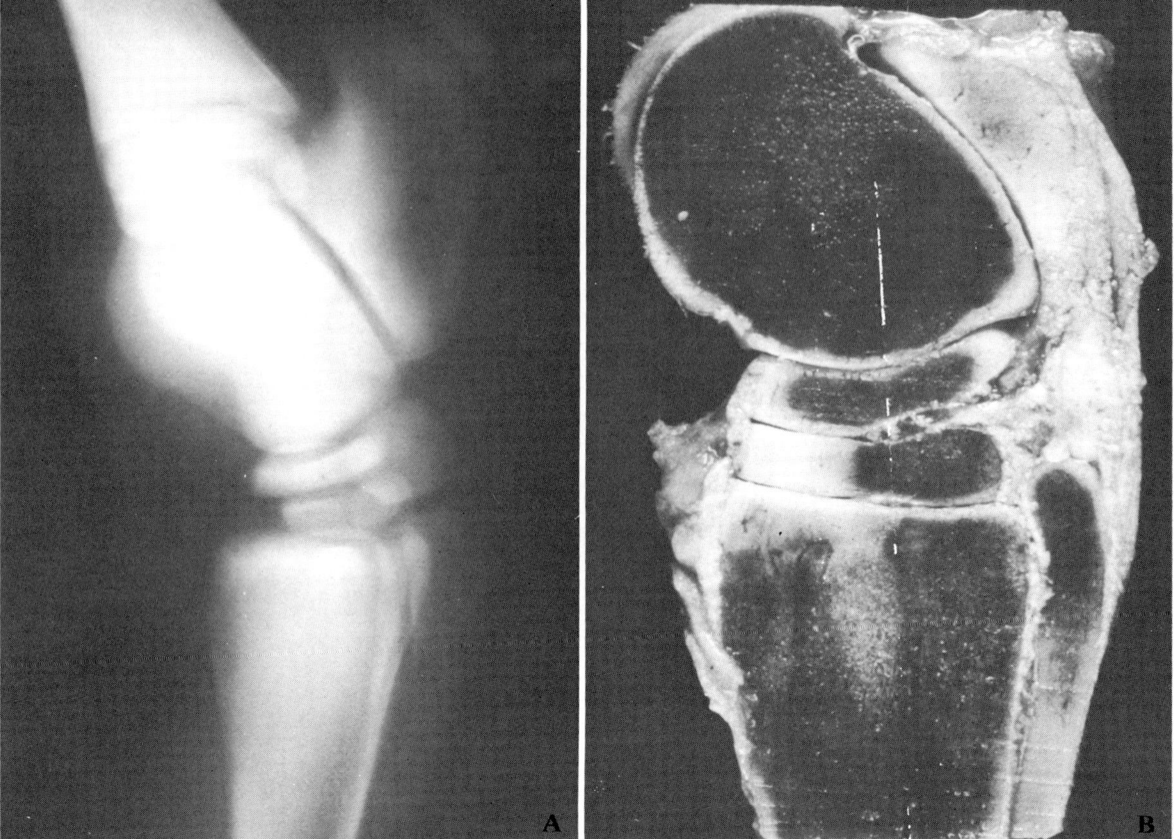

FIG. 116–1. *A*, Lateral radiograph of the tarsus of a 5-day-old foal. The tarsus was swollen and painful. The foal was lame. Radiographic diagnosis was septic arthritis, type T, with lysis of the cranial aspects of the third tarsal and proximal third metatarsal bones. *B*, Slab section of the same tarsus. Complete cartilage template of the cranial aspects of the central and third tarsal bones are present. Sepsis is not apparent. The lucency in proximal third metatarsus is caused by incomplete ossification as well as lysis secondary to bone infection. The two processes may be difficult to differentiate radiographically.

will improve the yield of positive cultures, which accurately represent the pathogenic organism.

Samples for synovial fluid analysis should be transported in an EDTA tube. Normal synovial fluid contains only a few hundred leukocytes per microliter, predominately mononuclear cells, and a total protein concentration less than 2.0 g/dL. If the fluid is turbid, is discolored, has a low viscosity, has a poor mucin clot, and has an elevated total white cell count or total protein concentration, infection is suspected. Total white cell counts are occasionally normal in infected joints due to dilution by excessive synovial fluid effusion or sequestration of the cells in fibrin clots. A predominance of neutrophils, presence of intracellular bacteria or toxic neutrophil changes are also evidence of infection, regardless of the total cell count.

Diagnostic arthroscopy may be used to evaluate the joint further for bone lesions and to obtain synovial membrane and subchondral bone samples for culture. Therapeutic joint flushes and synovectomy may also be performed with the arthroscope. However, if bone lesions are not identified with arthroscopy, they may still be present.[5]

TREATMENT

Therapy for infectious arthritis/osteomyelitis must begin immediately if a chance of reversing the disease process is to exist. By the time the diagnosis is made, the infection is often widespread and the prognosis poor. Most foals less than 2 weeks of age with joint effusions have concurrent osteomyelitis, even if signs are absent on the radiographs at the time clinical manifestations are first apparent. Because treatment of multifocal bone infections are usually unsuccessful and costly, the owner must make a real commitment to proceed with treatment. Euthanasia may be a viable alternative.

If treatment is pursued, broad-spectrum parenteral antibiotics in adequate doses should begin immediately after synovial fluid and blood samples are taken for culture.[3,5] Blood and synovial fluid culture results can be used to modify the antibiotic regimen, but initial therapy should provide coverage for gram-negative aerobic as well as anaerobic organisms. Exercise restriction is recommended to minimize the potential damage of excessive weight bearing on inflamed articular surfaces. The usefulness of heavy bandages to further protect the joint is unconfirmed. Passive manipulation of the limb four to six times a day may prevent formation of fibrinous adhesions within the joint. Administration of nonsteroidal anti-inflammatory drugs may minimize synovial inflammation and subsequent cartilage damage. The disadvantage of these drugs are twofold: they will eliminate the clinician's ability to evaluate the patient's response to other therapeutic regimens and they can cause gastrointestinal irritation and ulceration.

Removal of the products of inflammation from the septic joint is a rational component of therapy and recommended if the infection is limited to one or two joints and no bony lesions are apparent radiographically. The options for joint drainage include simple drainage, distention-irrigation, through and through lavage, arthrotomy, and arthroscopy and synovectomy.[3] The more invasive techniques are more effective at clearing the joint, but each technique also has its drawbacks, which include the potential to introduce infection, the possibility of fibrous damage to the joint capsule, and the expense. If the infection involves the long bones, repeated joint drainage is ineffective because it does not address the primary focus of infection. If the infection is a type P and involves only the physis of the long bone, effective but expensive treatment that includes administration of systemic antibiotics and the curretage and lavage of the physis is recommended.

If the joint infection does respond to therapy, a prolonged course of antibiotics should be administered because relapse is common. Hyaluronic acid and/or polysulfated glycosaminoglycans may be administered to help prevent or treat degenerative joint disease.[3,5]

PROGNOSIS

If no bony lesions exist on the radiographs, the foal probably has the type-S syndrome and the best prognosis.[2] However, absence of bone lesions early in the course of the disease does not rule out their development later. Foals with the E and T syndromes have bone lesions in the epiphyses and often multiple sites of osteomyelitis as well as infectious polyarthritis. Even if such an animal survives, it has a poor prognosis as a performance animal. Foals with type-P osteomyelitis must be examined closely to define the extent of the disease. If the infection is localized to the physis and does not involve the adjacent joint, the prognosis is better. Although curretage, lavage, and systemic antibiotics are expensive and the recovery period is long, some foals respond to therapy and can develop into sound, performance animals (J. Foerner, personal communication).

NONINFECTIOUS ORTHOPEDIC DISEASES

Noninfectious musculoskeletal abnormalities of the young foal such as osteochondrosis, angular limb deformities, physitis, juvenile osteoarthritis, incomplete skeletal ossification, and tarsal collapse are collectively referred to as developmental orthopedic diseases.[6] The cause and pathogenesis of these diseases remain inadequately defined despite extensive research. Evidence is available for genetic, nutritional, traumatic, toxic, and metabolic causes; detailed reviews have been published.[7]

At the initial examination of the neonate, the musculoskeletal system should be carefully appraised for congenital or traumatic defects. Assessing newborn foals for conformational faults may be difficult, because most at birth have a base wide stance and a hypermetric gait. This changes rapidly in the first few days of life. Evaluation of the skeletal system must begin at birth to avoid missing flaws that are correctable early yet are potentially detrimental to later performance.

INCOMPLETE OSSIFICATION OF THE SKELETON

The most easily overlooked musculoskeletal defect is that of incomplete ossification of the skeletal system. Newborns which are twins, premature (<320 days gestational age), small for gestational age or growth retarded in utero, and/or those born with an in utero acquired infection are more likely to have incomplete ossification of the cuboidal bones at birth, even if their conformation is apparently normal.[8]

Incomplete ossification is a vague term which encompasses a wide range of radiographic patterns, indicating different degrees of skeletal ossification. In the fetus, the skeleton begins as a cartilage template which ossifies throughout gestation. The exact gestational age at which each bone develops sufficient density to bear weight at birth is not known. Ossification of the carpal and tarsal regions accelerates in late gestation, and these regions are more likely to be incompletely ossified at birth than other components of the skeleton.[9] Because the carpus and tarsus are easily radiographed in the equine neonate, they are commonly used to evaluate ossification of the skeleton.

To categorize better the radiographic impression of skeletal ossification in the foal's carpus and tarsus at birth, a skeletal ossification index (SOI) has been proposed.[8] This index divides ossification patterns into four grades based on dorsopalmar and lateromedial radiographic views of the carpus and tarsus taken soon after birth (Table 116–2 and Figs. 116–2 to 116–5). The significance of subtle variations in bone shape and density on the radiographs cannot be interpreted reliably until radiographic and histopathologic studies of many more individuals are performed. Depending on the severity of the variation in question, the foal should be reexamined and followup radiographs taken at regular in-

TABLE 116–2. SKELETAL OSSIFICATION INDEX

GRADE	CRITERIA
One	Some cuboidal bones show no radiographic evidence of ossification
Two	All cuboidal bones show some radiographic evidence of ossification; first carpal and tarsal bones are not included in this assessment
	The proximal epiphysis of either the third metacarpal or metatarsal bones is present and either physis is open
	The lateral styloid process of the distal radius and the malleoli of the distal tibia are absent or just barely visible
Three	Cuboidal bones are small with rounded edges
	Joint spaces appear wide
	Lateral styloid process of the distal radius and malleoli of the distal tibia are distinct
	Proximal physes of the third metacarpus and metatarsus are closed radiographically
Four	Cuboidal bones are appropriately ossified, reminiscent of the shape of their adult counterpart
	Joint spaces are of expected width

(From Adams, R., and Poulos, P.: A skeletal ossification index for neonatal foals. Vet. Rad., *29*:217, 1988.)

tervals until the area in question resolves or becomes clearly pathologic.

The carpal and tarsal areas of foals born with incomplete ossification (grades 1 to 3) ossify surprisingly rapidly postnatally. Ossification patterns of the epiphysis and cuboidal bones do not proceed from a central focus in a uniform manner.[10] More commonly, numerous initial ossifying foci are found with irregular borders that later fuse. A diagnosis of osteochondrosis is tempting but not appropriate for these normal, but irregular, patterns of ossification.

Patient Evaluation

To obtain diagnostic radiographs of the carpus and tarsus of neonatal foals, special attention must be paid to positioning and exposure. The uncooperative nature of neonates and the soft tissue laxity of their joints can make positioning difficult. To distinguish true bony abnormalities from artifacts caused by positioning, the foal may be placed in lateral recumbency and the limb straightened by distraction.

The clinical diagnosis of neonatal foal orthopedic diseases is based not on radiographs alone but on all of the information (history, physical examination, laboratory results, and radiographs) available on the patient. Distinctly different bone abnormalities can have a similar radiographic appearance. Conditions which can be easily confused radiographically include incomplete ossification and bone lysis associated with infection, secondary centers of ossification and fractures, incomplete ossification and tarsal collapse, normal ossification patterns, and osteochondrosis.[3] Followup radiographs are taken at frequent intervals after the initial diagnosis of incomplete ossification is made to assess the progression of skeletal ossification.

Treatment

Because of the many unknowns of skeletal development of the neonatal foal, appropriate treatment or need for treatment of incomplete ossification is made empirically based on clinical and radiographic signs. Postnatal ossification in other species is affected by weight bearing, nutritional status, and systemic health, and all of these facets should be evaluated. To avoid excessive weight bearing on incompletely ossified bones, various regimens ranging from restricted exercise to application of tube casts have been suggested, but each of these treatments has its drawbacks. Repeated radiographs (taken at regular intervals to assess the progress of ossification) and clinical examination of the foal (paying close attention to lameness, limb deformities, and joint effusions) influence the type of therapy chosen. If the clinical and/or radiographic signs deteriorate, a more aggressive treatment regimen is instituted or the foal euthanitized.

Prognosis

A guarded prognosis must be given for any foal with incomplete skeletal ossification because of the incomplete knowledge of postnatal bone ossification and the medical and musculoskeletal problems which often develop in these immature foals. Incomplete ossification of bones in the carpal and tarsal regions has been sited as the cause of many common foal orthopedic problems, including tarsal and carpal collapse, angular limb deformities, etc. However, until foals are routinely radiographed at birth to determine the degree of bony ossification before developing orthopedic problems, a causal relationship cannot be confirmed nor can a reliable prediction of future athletic soundness for foals born with different degrees of incomplete ossification be formulated.

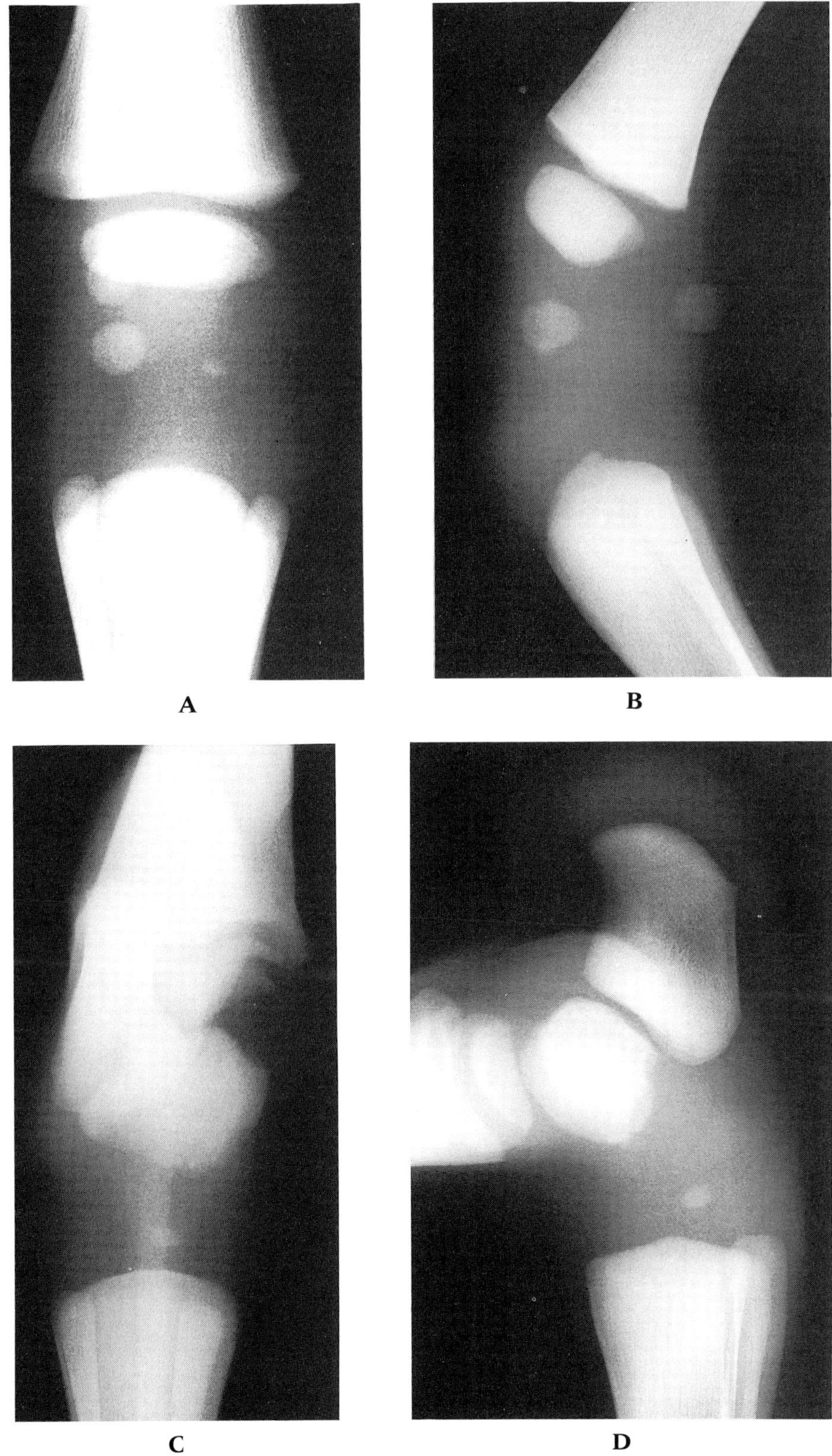

FIG. 116–2. Skeletal ossification index grade I. Dorsopalmar *(A)* and lateromedial *(B)* radiographs of the carpus and dorsoplantar *(C)* and lateromedial *(D)* radiographs of the tarsus of a 1-day-old Thoroughbred cross filly born at 307 days of gestational age. The dam had severe chronic/active placentitis, and the foal died shortly after birth. Note the lack of ossification of most cuboidal bones and the absence of the lateral styloid process of the radius, the malleoli of the tibia, and the proximal epiphyses of MC3 and MT3. (From Adams, R., and Poulos, P.: A skeletal ossification index for neonatal foals. Vet. Radiol., *29:*218, 1988.)

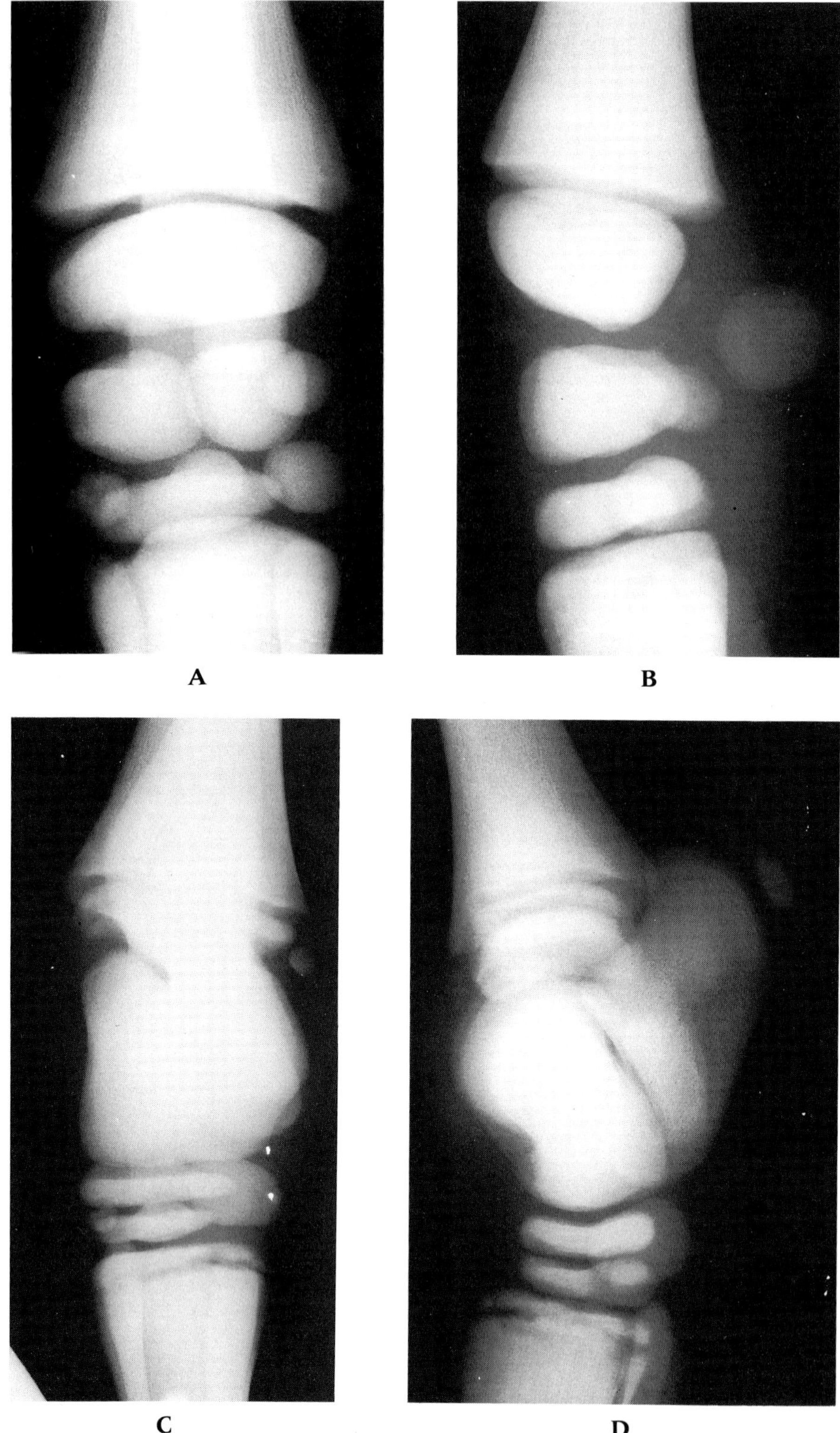

FIG. 116–3. Skeletal ossification index grade II. Dorsopalmar *(A)* and lateromedial *(B)* radiographs of the carpus and dorsoplantar *(C)* and lateromedial *(D)* radiographs of the tarsus of a 2-day-old Thoroughbred filly born with a gestational age of 297 days. The mare had placentitis and the foal was born weak, small (27 kg), and septicemic. Some degree of ossification of each of the cuboidal bones exists *(A)*. Although the lateral styloid process does not appear ossified on this view, it can be seen faintly in the lateromedial view. The proximal physis of MC3 is closed. Some ossification of each of the primary tarsal bones is seen *(C)*. The lateral malleolus is small. The proximal physis of MT3 is open, as seen best in the lateromedial radiograph. (From Adams, R., and Poulos, P.: A skeletal ossification index for neonatal foals. Vet. Radiol., *29*:218, 1988.)

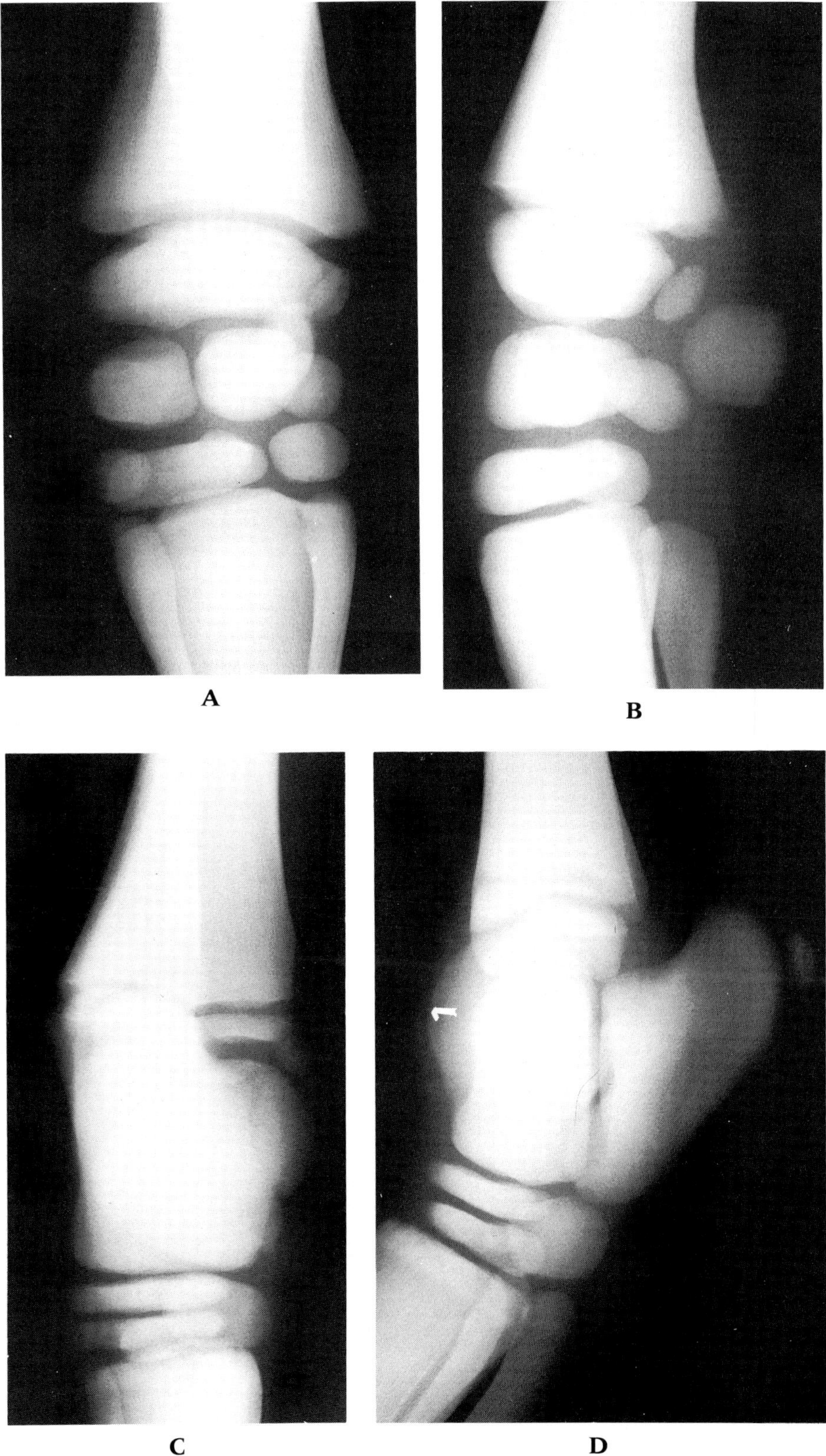

FIG. 116–4. Skeletal ossification index grade III. Dorsopalmar *(A)* and lateromedial *(B)* radiographs of the carpus and dorsoplantar *(C)* and lateromedial *(D)* radiographs of the tarsus of a 1-day-old Thoroughbred filly born with a gestational age of 309 days and presented with pneumonia, presumedly acquired in utero. The small round appearance of the carpal bones characterize this grade and is best depicted in the dorsopalmar view of the carpus. The lateral styloid process is clearly visible in both dorsopalmar and lateromedial views. The tarsal bones also appear small, especially as seen in the lateromedial radiograph. The lateral malleolus is present, but small, as seen in the dorsoplantar radiograph of the tarsus. The proximal physis of MT3 is closed. (From Adams, R., and Poulos, P.: A skeletal ossification index for neonatal foals. Vet. Radiol., *29:*219, 1988.)

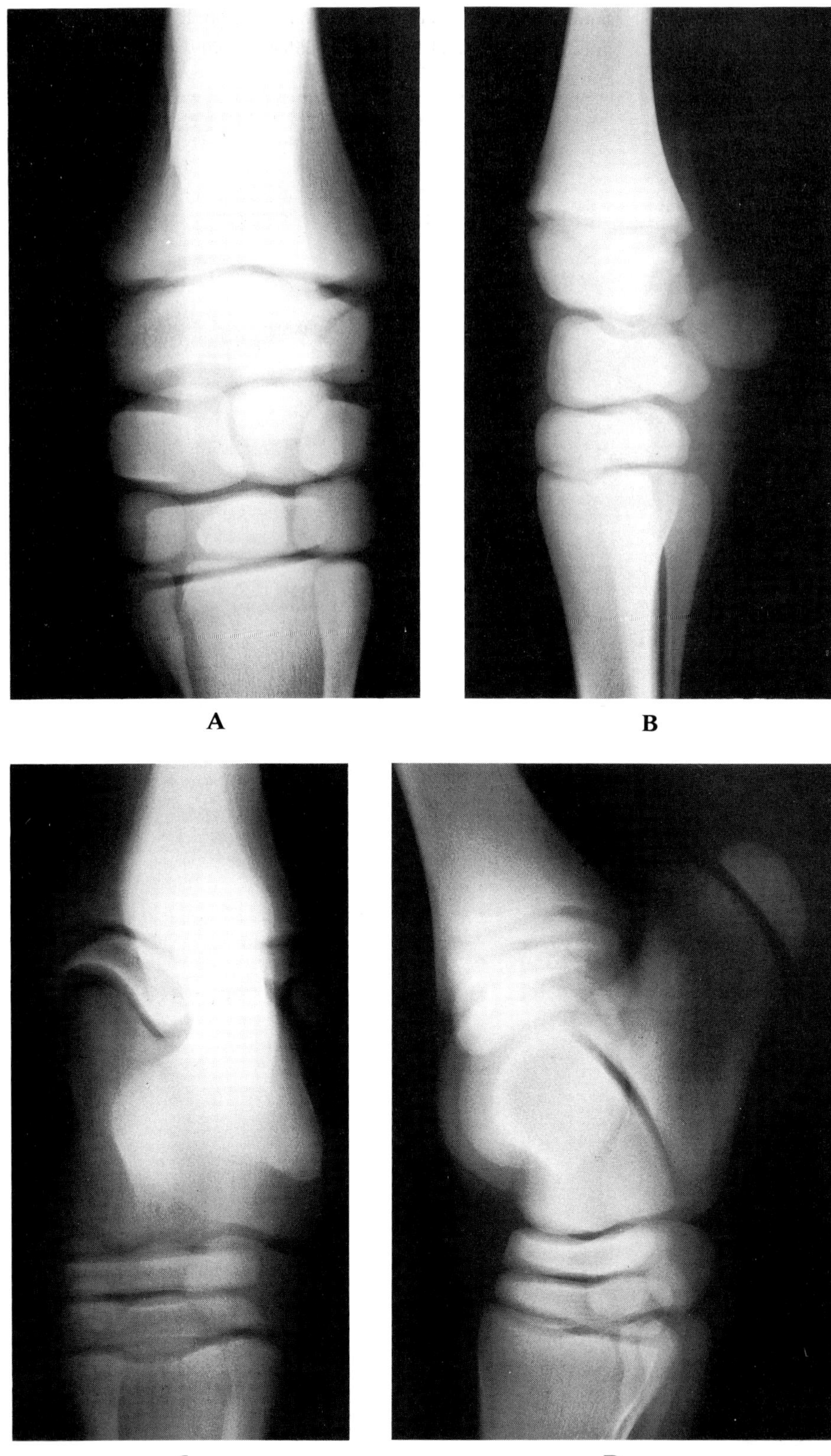

FIG. 116–5. Skeletal ossification index grade IV. Dorsopalmar *(A)* and lateromedial *(B)* radiographs and dorsoplantar *(C)* and lateromedial *(D)* radiographs of a healthy 3-day-old Appaloosa colt born with a gestational age of 342 days. The carpal bones in the dorsopalmar and lateromedial views appear well formed and resemble the shape of the adult counterpart. The joint spaces are of normal width and the lateral styloid process is triangular. Dorsoplantar and lateromedial views of the tarsus illustrate well-ossified tarsal bones. (From Adams, R., and Poulos, P.: A skeletal ossification index for neonatal foals. Vet. Radiol., *29:*219, 1988.)

ASSESSMENT AND CORRECTION OF ANGULAR LIMB DEFORMITIES IN THE FRONTAL PLANE (VARUS OR VALGUS)

Most foals that are born with crooked legs correct spontaneously in the first few days after birth. Thorough examination and, perhaps, corrective therapy are warranted for those foals which do not show signs of improvement in the first few days of life or those foals which develop angular limb deformities (ALD) after birth and become worse with time. Treatment for each manifestation of the ALD syndrome remains empirical because definitive biomechanical studies on the limbs of the growing foal have not been conducted. Therefore, therapeutic recommendations may vary. Treatment regimens available include time-tested therapies of exercise restriction, hoof trimming, splints and casts, transphyseal bridging surgeries, periosteal stripping surgery, and newer techniques using dynamic modification with orthotic braces. Combinations of any of the foregoing are also used.

Patient Evaluation

History. The patient evaluation begins with an accurate history on the mare and foal to elucidate the type of ALD (congenital versus acquired) as well as speculate on cause. Numerous factors have been incriminated as the cause of both types of ALD.[7,11]

Congenital ALD is not necessarily inherited. Factors associated with congenital ALD include (1) abnormal uterine positioning, which is most common in overweight mares; (2) ingestion of toxins by pregnant mares; (3) incomplete ossification of the cuboidal bones; (4) joint laxity caused by weakness of the supporting structures; and (5) endocrine and metabolic imbalances.[7,11] Mild to moderate angular deformity at the carpus, tarsus, and/or fetlocks are common in newborn foals, and these deviations usually improve dramatically during the first few days of life without intervention. The improvement is attributed to developing muscle tone and strengthening of the ligaments.

Acquired ALD is most often associated with skeletal abnormalities (including disproportionate growth of the long bones, mishapen epiphyses and cuboidal bones) discovered radiographically after the ALD is present.[12] Nutrition, toxins, trauma, rapid growth, and excessive weight bearing as a result of contralateral limb lameness are considered causes.[7,11]

Physical Examination. The limb conformation of all newborn foals should be evaluated on a regular basis. A reasonable schedule involves careful assessment at birth, weekly examinations until 1 month of age, and then monthly examinations until 6 months. Polaroid-type snapshots provide an excellent record of the deviation for future comparison. The foal should be watched as it moves freely on a flat surface, and the legs should be thoroughly palpated.

Table 116–3 lists a series of questions which should be answered by conducting a thorough examination to devise appropriate and properly timed therapy. The goal of the examination is to determine the limbs involved, the pivot point of the deformity, the severity, the cause, and the change since the last examination. ALDs are classified as valgus if the limb distal to the pivot point or origin of the deformity deviates laterad and varus if the limb deviates mediad (Fig. 116–6). If rotational deformities are present, they must be carefully assessed and differentiated from angular deformities. Rotational deformities often improve as the foal's chest expands but are not corrected by surgeries recommended for ALD. Flexural and extensor deviations should also be noted and appropriate action taken. To monitor the progression or resolution of the ALD, the angle, which can change with the foal's stance and level of fatigue, must be precisely characterized. Palpation of the limbs will reveal stability or laxity of soft tissue structures, pain associated with trauma or infection, and/or structural congenital defects.

TABLE 116–3. PHYSICAL ASSESSMENT OF THE FOAL WITH ANGULAR LIMB DEFORMITIES

Watch the foal as it moves freely on a flat surface.

1. Where is the pivot point of the deviation: at the proximal limb, carpus or tarsus, or fetlock?
2. What is the angle of the deviation while standing?
3. Does the deviation change with increased weight bearing when the foal is running?
4. Is the deviation symmetrical, involving both forelimbs or hindlimbs? Is it unilateral? If unilateral, is the foal lame in the contralateral limb?
5. If the ALD is severe in the hindlimbs, does a forelimb lameness exist causing excessive weight bearing behind?

Palpate the limb(s) while the foal is standing and in lateral recumbency.

1. Are there any signs of infection (pain, heat, or swelling) or trauma (pain, swelling, or crepitation)?
2. Are the ligaments of the joints lax and thus allow cranial/caudal or lateral/medial manipulation? Is the joint stable and the deviation appears to come from disproportionate growth at the associated physis?
3. Is there a flexor/extensor deviation as well?
4. Is the hoof balanced or does it show signs of abnormal shape or wear?
5. Although far less common, could a congenital limb abnormality exist such as hypoplasia of the phalanx or osteopetrosis?

Radiographs. The limb(s) involved must be radiographed to identify skeletal abnormalities which coexist with the ALD: degenerative joint disease, infection, fractures, congenital anomalies, and/or abnormal bone shape. Identification of the pivot point of the ALD is made to recommend the appropriate treatment and a reasonable prognosis for correction.[11] For example, young foals with joint laxity and abnormal carpal bones are treated with external support whereas foals with disproportionate growth of a long bone are surgical

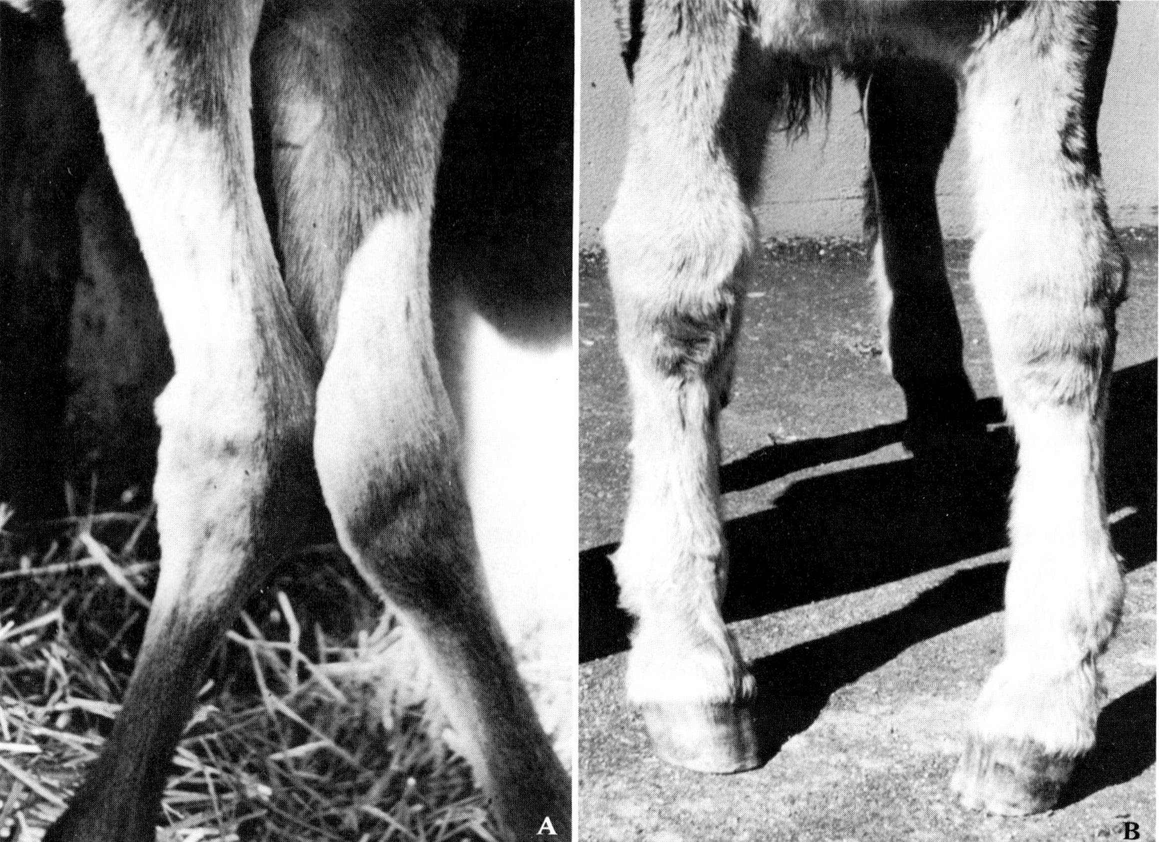

FIG. 116–6. *A*, Example of carpus valgus deformity. Distal limb (third metacarpus) deviates laterally from pivot point (carpus). (Courtesy of J. Traub-Dargatz). *B*, Example of varus deformity of both front fetlocks. Distal limb (phalanges 1, 2, and 3) deviates medial from pivot point (fetlock). (Courtesy of G. Trotter).

candidates. More than one area of the limb may contribute to the ALD, and this will influence treatment and prognosis. A method for identification of the radiographic center of a carpal deviation by geometric analysis has been described.[11] When evaluating the radiographs, factors influencing the evaluation include the angle of the radiographic projection, the degree of weight bearing on the limb when the radiograph was taken, and the estimated central axis of the long bone.

Correction of Angular Limb Deformities

The appropriate treatment for ALD depends on the severity and location of the deformity and age of the foal. General opinion suggests that an ALD of greater than 15° is severe and warrants immediate, aggressive action. Some therapy is instituted for any deviation over 6°. Conservative treatment procedures, such as hoof trimming, exercise restriction, and external supports may be initiated soon after birth. Sufficient noninvasive intervention provided early in life may circumvent the need for more aggressive therapy later.

The timing of surgical procedures is based on the growth patterns of the various anatomic locations and the surgical procedure used (growth stimulating versus growth retarding). The current tendency is to perform periosteal stripping surgery earlier and perhaps more frequently than required, because the technique is so easy and the premium for straight-legged foals so high. Generally, periosteal stripping on fetlocks is performed at 2 to 4 weeks and on the carpus or tarsus at 4 weeks to 4 months of age, depending on the severity of the condition.[13] Surgery may always be performed at later times, but the prognosis for correction is less favorable as the growth potential of the physis wanes. If surgery is performed late in the growth period of a particular physis, more aggressive techniques such as transphyseal bridging or a combination of transphyseal bridging and periosteal stripping might be tried. Wedge osteotomies may be performed in foals with diaphyseal angulation or older horses in which the physes are closed.[13]

Nonsurgical Treatment. Nonsurgical treatment, consisting of hoof trimming, exercise restriction, splints, casts, and braces, is recommended as initial therapy for a foal born with congenital ALD which does not improve within a few days after birth or a foal with a mild/moderate acquired ALD. This treatment option is not always the most conservative route, because of the morbidity associated with improperly applied casts and splints compared with the relatively uncomplicated surgical procedure of periosteal stripping.

Hoof Trimming. Considerable clinical success has been attributed to early and regular corrective hoof trimming. The goal of this procedure is to maintain or obtain a balanced foot to distribute the compressive forces across the growth plates evenly. Aggressive trimming which seeks to counter the abnormal forces of a deviated limb is no longer advocated, because severe abnormal axial alignment will cause unequal weight distribution and may lead to future lameness.

The theory that hoof balance can affect the forces on the limb is challenged by a study on the compressive and tensile strains on the third metacarpus (MC3) and distal radius of newborn foals.[14] In the foal with normal conformation, the compressive strain on the medial side of MC3 is twice that of the lateral side. After application of a lateral wedge (12 to 15°) to the hoof sole, lateral surface compressive strain increased by 100% as medial strain decreased. However, over 10 days relative strains returned to prewedge values. In this model, abnormal hoof balance had no lasting effect on compressive forces up the limb as has been speculated. Further investigations with strain gauges are needed to evaluate if balancing the feet of foals that have an ALD really has a beneficial effect.

The goal of corrective hoof trimming of a young foal is to balance the foot and only calls for a few passes with the hoof rasp. As soon as the foot gets tough enough to accept a rasp, the pointed toe should be squared to encourage even break over and rounding of the foot. Trimming is repeated at regular intervals according to the rate of hoof growth (weekly, biweekly, or monthly).

The balanced hoof is characterized by a round shape with the frog centrally placed and the walls of equal dimension. In the unbalanced foot, the frog will be asymmetric: one wall will be short and under-run and the other wall, longer and flared. The hoof of a foal with a carpus valgus deviation often needs lowering of the outside or lateral wall to encourage even breakover of the foot. In the hindlimb, the toe is usually squared to improve the tracking of the cow-hocked foal. Often foals that stand base narrow appear to have outward rotation of their whole limb although all of the joints are properly aligned. In these foals, this ALD appearance will correct as the chest develops and the elbows spread apart. The foot should be rasped regularly to maintain the balanced foot.

Exercise Restriction. Exercise restriction of an active foal with mild/moderate ALD is recommended to minimize the axial compressive forces on the growth plate and to prevent remodeling of the epiphyses or damage to hypoplastic cuboidal bones, which may cause skeletal deformation. Studies on the ability of exercise restriction to eliminate disproportionate forces on the limbs (measured by strain gauges) are needed. Until that time, recommendations for exercise restriction remain empirical.

The degree of confinement varies from complete box stall rest to restriction to a small paddock. The regimen appropriate for an individual foal is dictated by the severity of ALD, radiographic abnormalities, and associated problems (flexural laxity and weakness) of that individual. Once a certain degree of exercise restriction is begun, the ALD should be assessed daily, and if the condition worsens, restriction should be more limiting. If the ALD becomes worse when the foal is stalled, more aggressive therapy must be instituted.

External Supports. When joint instability (secondary to soft tissue laxity, cuboidal bone hypoplasia or collapse, or metacarpal bone anomalies) is the cause of the ALD, external supports are recommended.[13,15] Tube casts or splints have been used to support the skeletal structures until bone ossification is complete; they straighten the limb by maintaining it rigidly in proper alignment. Newer braces have recently been marketed which employ modifications of the orthotic principles and materials developed for humans.

Of the supports commonly used, a tube cast provides the strongest, most rigid form of support. It can be molded to the foal's limb, minimizing the chance of pressure sores. Fiberglas-type material is lightweight while being strong, water resistant, and quick drying. The disadvantages include all those inherent in a cast, the need for anesthesia during application, initial cost, and the static leverage which the cast applies. Splints, regardless of the material of which they are composed, are less rigid than casts, are more likely to cause pressure sores, need daily resetting, and are of questionable effectiveness in larger and heavier foals. The advantage of splinting is that the material is readily available, the expense is initially less than a cast, anesthesia is not required for application, and the position may be changed daily as the correction progresses.

The future for more effective and less risky nonsurgical correction of mild/moderate ALD as well as effective support for newborn foals with incomplete ossification of the cuboidal bones may well lie in the field of equine orthotics. Two orthotic braces with different principles of action are available. One type of brace applies counterpressure only above and below the knee while allowing joint flexion (Carpus Valgus/Varus Brace, Smith & Nephew Roylan, Inc., Menomonee Falls, WI). The brace is applied for 12 h and then removed for 12 h. The other type of brace is designed to align the whole leg (Farlay Brace, Equine Orthotics of Florida, Ocala, FL). The foot is placed in a cup and then the fetlock and carpus are brought into alignment by application of a few pounds of pressure. The service of a trained technician applying the brace is marketed, rather than selling just the brace, which may cause problems if improperly used.

Surgical Treatment of ALD. Surgical procedures which stimulate or retard bone growth are used to correct ALD caused by unequal bone growth at the physis. Foals with other skeletal abnormalities causing the ALD should not logically respond to manipulation of growth at the physis. However, successful correction of such problems with periosteal stripping, a growth-promoting technique, has been reported.[16,17] The explanation for the effectiveness of this treatment deserves further investigation.

Growth-Stimulating Procedure: Hemicircumferential Transection and Periosteal Stripping. Periosteal stripping has revolutionized the treatment of ALD in foals since its introduction in the early 1980s by Auer.[13] Transection of the periosteum at the physis "releases" the physis from restrictive forces generated by the fibroelastic periosteum. Vascular changes identified at the physis are presumably caused by the increased metabolic rate in this area. The exact procedure is described in surgery texts.[18] Followup studies have confirmed that the technique is relatively easy and overcorrection does not occur.[16,17] Surgery may be repeated if sufficient correction does not occur with the first transection. Treatment response has been noted even in older animals when the growth potential of the normal physis is minimal and in some cases when the deviation has involved the intra-articular structures. Recently, Bramlage observed that periosteal stripping of the fetlocks to correct a mild valgus deformity in young foals may lead to varus fetlock deformities in yearlings and older horses.[19] The later conformational defect is more stressful to the athlete than a mild valgus deformity. This relationship emphasizes the need to judiciously evaluate young foals for the severity of the deformity and time surgical corrections appropriately.

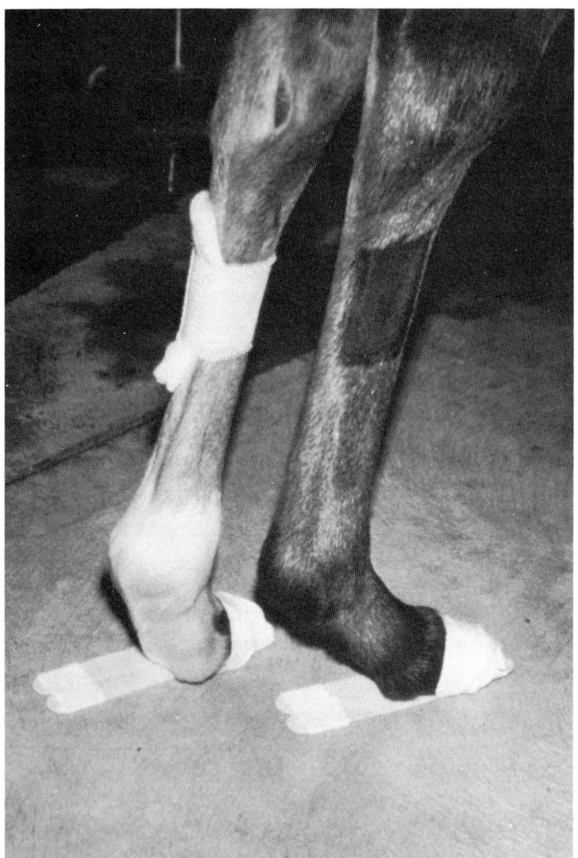

FIG. 116–7. Two-day-old premature foal with heel extensions taped to front feet to correct flexor tendon laxity. (Courtesy of J. Traub-Dargatz).

Growth-Retardation Technique: Transphyseal Bridging of the Physis with Screws and Wire. The transphyseal bridging technique involves placement of screws and wires, plates, or staples across the physis to retard growth asymmetrically.[18] The success of the technique depends on compensatory growth on the contralateral side of the physis and thus must be performed while the physis still has sufficient growth potential. If carpal joint instability is also present, an external support is applied. If the ALD is severe, a combination of transphyseal bridging and periosteal stripping may be used. Success of the operation includes timely removal of the implants postoperatively. The implants must be removed as soon as the limb has straightened even if one limb corrects before the other. In such cases the implants must be removed in two stages.

ASSESSMENT AND CORRECTION OF FLEXOR-EXTENSOR LIMB DEFORMITIES

The flexor-extensor limb deformities are those that exist in the cranial-caudal plane at the carpus, fetlock, or pastern. The pathophysiologic nature of these deformities is not well understood and treatment is primarily empirical.

Flexor Tendon Laxity in the Neonatal Foal (Less than 2 Weeks of Age)

Foals born prematurely or small for gestational age are most often affected with flexor tendon laxity. Various degrees of deformity exist, ranging from a foal with a slightly dropped fetlock to one that walks with the palmar/plantar surface of the fetlock on the ground. This deformity tends to respond to exercise which strengthens the tendons rather than supports which allow further weakening. Exercise, proper nutrition, and nursing care are the best therapies for mild cases. More severe cases respond surprisingly well to exercise and shoes with a heel extension which can be tapped, wired, or glued on (Fig. 116–7). These shoes reposition the weight-bearing surface of the foot on the ground and thus change the angle of the fetlock. Response to treatment should be rapid, within 1 to 2 weeks, and surgical correction by shortening the tendons is rarely necessary.

Flexor Tendon Laxity in the Older Foal (1 to 6 Months of Age)

Older foals with flexor tendon laxity usually have badly under-run heels. Like the newborn foal with tendon laxity, the aim of treatment is to restore weight bearing on the flat surface of the hoof. Trimming the heels can make spectacular improvement in the limb angle but complete correction may take several weekly trimmings. If trimming does not correct the problem, a shoe with extended heels may be used. Older foals with these shoes must be supervised closely when they exercise, because they may pull off the shoe by over reaching with the hindfeet and/or hurt themselves.

Flexor Contraction Deformities in the Neonatal Foal

Flexor contraction deformities include deformities of the carpus, tarsus, fetlock, and pastern characterized by a flexed position and an inability to straighten the joint. If apparent at birth, these deformities could be considered a form of arthrogryposis, which is a well-defined severe flexural deformity in cattle. This type of severe arthrogryposis is less common in foals, thus the disease and its cause are not well understood. Mild to moderate congenital flexural deformities, present at birth may be caused by malpositioning of the fetus in utero or simply persistence of the uterine position. Herd outbreaks of flexural deformities in foals and fetuses of mares that ingested astragalus spp. (locoweed) or hybrid Sudan grasses during gestation have also been reported.[7,20] Congenital spinal cord lesions have been described in a foal with severe contraction of the tarsus and fetlock at birth.[21] Various degrees of these deformities present: (1) mild cases include foals which stand with elevated pasterns and very straight limbs, (2) in moderate cases the foal knuckles over occasionally when standing, and (3) in severe cases the limb is so contracted the foal must be assisted to rise.

Usually contracture deformities result from soft tissue structure abnormality. If the contracture is not corrected, irreversible damage to the bony structures can occur because of inappropriate weight bearing. Treatment varies with the severity of the condition and the joint involved[22] (Table 116–4). The pathophysiologic nature of flexural deformities is not clearly understood, so if the foal is not making progress with a particular therapy, re-evaluate and institute a more aggressive therapy.

Acquired flexural deformities can develop in young foals that are recumbent for long periods or are weak. Attention must be paid to these musculoskeletal deformities while the medical problems of these foals are treated. The clinician must encourage the patients to exercise, or at least stand periodically through the day. Passive manipulation of the limbs to discourage flexor contracture should be performed every few hours in a foal that is recumbent and developing flexor contractures. Asymmetric flexor contracture can occur in a foal that is painful or nonweight bearing on a limb. Resolution of the primary cause of the pain is the prime goal of therapy and moderate doses of analgesic medication may be necessary to encourage sufficient weight bearing to prevent further flexor tendon contraction. In contrast, symmetric flexural deformities develop in older foals that are growing rapidly or may be exercising excessively. In these cases, exercise should be restricted; toe extensions, splints, or casts should be applied; or surgery should be performed in accordance with the severity of the deformity.

TABLE 116–4. THERAPEUTIC PRINCIPLES FOR NEONATAL FOAL FLEXURAL DEFORMITY

SEVERITY	SUGGESTED TREATMENT
Mild: foal with straight fetlocks and pasterns; distal joints begin to knuckle	If the foal is recumbent because of systemic illness: passive manipulation and massage of legs and frequent weight bearing; if the foal is ambulatory, bandage limbs or splint to relax tendons; toe extensions with acrylic or small rim pads can be applied to stretch the tendons and to prevent wearing of the toe
Moderate: foal knuckles over when standing	Splint, cast, or brace to apply countertension to the contraction; alternating splint application with periods of physical therapy may speed results; casting with the feet incorporated may cause the muscle and tendons to lose tone; if the condition is treated with orthopedic devices bilaterally, the foal must be watched carefully to be sure it can stand to nurse; pressure sores are devastating complication of these correctional devices
Severe: foal cannot stand unassisted	Surgery to transect the soft tissue structures until a normal posture can be obtained; often the joint capsule must be incised, which may lead to intra-articular infection; euthanasia is a viable alternative.

Rupture of the Common Digital Extensor Tendon

Rupture of the common digital extensor tendon is characterized by swelling over the dorsolateral aspect of one or both carpi of the neonatal foal.[23] The ruptured ends of the tendons may be palpable if excessive synovial fluid has not accumulated. Flexor contractures of the carpus and/or fetlock may also be present.

The cause is unknown. When associated with flexural contractures, tendon rupture appears to occur secondary to the tension created by the contracture. The contracture may also occur secondary to the extensor rupture although experimental denervation of the lateral and common digital extensor muscles of normal weanling foals does not result in contracture.[24] Trauma or congenital weakness of the tendons may be another contributing factor.

If contracture is not present, therapy may only consist of stall rest and light bandaging to protect the dorsum of the fetlock. If contracture is present, the limb should be splinted, cast, or braced to treat the contracture. Surgical repair of the tendon is not necessary for return to function, but at least 3 weeks are required for the tendon to heal with a fibrous scar. The prognosis for a sound horse is good if flexor contracture is not present. But if it is, the prognosis deteriorates, depending on the severity of the associated contracture.

TRAUMATIC FRACTURES

Traumatic fractures in newborn foals are usually caused by the mare's mistep, rough handling, or vigorous play. If the mare stepped on the foal, the question should arise and the answer pursued as to why the foal allowed this to happen. Most bright, active, healthy foals do not get stepped on.

The physis is the weakest part of the long bone of an immature animal and is thus susceptible to trauma-induced fracture.[25] Pressure physes which contribute to longitudinal bone growth are usually under compressive force and more susceptible to trauma in the young foal. Traction physes are points of muscle attachment, determine bone shape, and are subject to distractive forces. The configuration of the physeal fracture depends on the magnitude and type of force applied, the site of application, and whether the limb is weight bearing at the moment of force application. The most common type of pressure physeal fracture is the Salter type II (through the physis and metaphysis).

The diagnosis is based on radiographs, including stress films if compression of the physis, a Salter type V physeal fracture, is suspected.[26] When a mare steps on her foal, Salter type II fractures of the distal limb physes usually occur. Foals with a history of rearing back and flipping over likely fracture the proximal femoral physis (Salter type I or II). The fractures should be reduced and stabilized internally for the best chance of healing as a functional, straight, and sound limb.[27] Epiphysiodesis, or bone formation across the physis, usually occurs radiographically but clinical impairment related to early closure of the physis is less common. The pressure physeal fracture repair most frequently reported in the foal is the proximal tibial physis which consistently presents as a Salter type II with a lateral metaphyseal corner and moderate displacement.[26] Repair techniques described include use of a bone plate, cancellous bone screws, and modified external fixator.

The prognosis for physeal fractures is based on all of the common factors which affect the prognosis of equine long bone fractures (fracture opened or closed; fracture duration before treatment; method and exactness of stabilization; and age, temperament, and weight of the patient). In addition, the type of physeal fracture, the severity of trauma sustained by the physis, the integrity of the epiphyseal vasculature, and the physis affected are considered influencial on the successful outcome of a physeal fracture.[27] Better fracture stabilization can usually be achieved in younger foals (<4.5 months) because of their smaller size. Tension physeal fractures have a better prognosis for soundness than pressure physeal fractures. Proximal femoral physeal fractures and distal third metacarpal/metatarsal physeal fractures heal best if internal fixation is used. Foals with distal humeral and distal femoral physeal fractures have a poor prognosis. At any site, articular disruption reduces the prognosis for athletic ability because of the likelihood that degenerative joint disease will develop.

REFERENCES

1. Koterba, A.M.: Equine neonatal intensive care at the University of Florida 1982–1987: An update. Proc. Am. Assoc. Equine Pract., 805–816, 1987.
2. Firth, E.C.: Current concepts of infectious polyarthritis in foals. Equine Vet. J., *15:*5–9, 1983.
3. Adams, R.: Polyarthritis/osteomyellitis. *In* Equine Clinical Neonatology. Edited by A.M. Koterba, W.H. Drummond, and P. Kosch. Philadelphia, Lea & Febiger, 1990, pp. 318–330.
4. Adams, R., and Poulos, P.W.: Radiographic evaluation of the carpal and tarsal regions of neonatal foals. Proc. Am. Assoc. Equine Pract., 677–682, 1987.
5. Firth, E.C.: Hematogenous osteomyelitis in the foal. Proc. Am. Assoc. Equine Pract., 795–804, 1987.
6. Gabel, A.A., et al.: Comparison of incidence and severity of developmental orthopedic disease on 17 farms before and after adjustment of ration. Proc. Am. Assoc. Equine Pract., 163–170, 1987.
7. Stashack, T.S. (ed.): Adams' Lameness in Horses. 4th ed. Lea & Febiger, Philadelphia, 1987.
8. Adams, R., and Poulos, P.W.: A skeletal ossification index for neonatal foals. Vet. Rad., *29:*217–222, 1988.
9. Kupfer, M.: Beitrage zum modus der ossifikation svorgange in der anlage des extremitatenskelettes bei den equiden. Denkschr. d. Schweiz. Naturf. Ges., *67:*1–352, 1931.
10. Firth, E.C., and Poulos, P.W.: Development of the epiphysis, metaphysis and diaphysis in the foal. Proc. Am. Assoc. Equine Pract., 787–794, 1987.
11. Caron, J.P.: Angular limb deformities in foals. Equine Vet. J., *3:*225–228, 1988.
12. Pharr, J.W., and Fretz, P.B.: Radiographic findings in foals with angular limb deformities. J. Am. Vet. Med. Assoc., *179:*812–817, 1981.
13. Auer, J.A.: Current treatment methods for angular limb deformity problems in foals. Proc. Am. Assoc. Equine Pract., 263–282, 1988.
14. Firth, E.C., Schamhardt, H.C., and Hartman, W.: Measurements of bone strain in foals with altered foot balance. Am. J. Vet. Res., *49:*261–265, 1988.
15. Adams, R.: Non-infectious orthopedic problems. *In* Equine Clinical Neonatology. Edited by A.M. Koterba, W.H. Drummond, and P. Kosch. Philadelphia, Lea & Febiger, 1990, pp. 317–330.
16. Bertone, A.L., Turner, A.S., and Park, R.D.: Periosteal transection and stripping for treatment of angular limb deformities in foals: Clinical observations. J. Am. Vet. Med. Assoc., *187:*145–152, 1985.
17. Bertone, A.L., Park, R.D., and Turner, A.S.: Periosteal transection and stripping for treatment of angular limb deformities in foals: Radiographic observation. J. Am. Vet. Med. Assoc., *187:*153–156, 1985.
18. McIlwraith, C.W., and Turner, A.S.: Equine Surgery Advanced Techniques. Philadelphia, Lea & Febiger, 1987.
19. Bramlage, L.R., and Embertson, R.M.: Observations on the evaluation and selection of foal limb deformities for surgical treatment. Proc. Am. Assoc. Equine Pract., 273–279, 1990.
20. Prichard, J.T., and Voss, J.L.: Fetal ankylosis in horses associated with hybrid Sudan pasture. J. Am. Vet. Med. Assoc., *150:*871–873, 1967.

21. Mayhew, I.G.: Neuromuscular arthrogryposis multiplex congenita in a Thoroughbred foal. Vet. Pathol., *21:*187–192, 1984.
22. Wagner, P.C.: Flexural limb deformities. *In* Large Animal Internal Medicine. Edited by B.P. Smith. St. Louis, C.V. Mosby, 1990, pp. 1181–1185.
23. Yovich, J.V., Stashak, T.S., and McIlwraith, C.W.: Rupture of the common digital extensor tendon in foals. Compend. Contin. Educ. Practicing Vet., *5:*373–378, 1984.
24. Firth, E.C.: Thoracic limb digital extensor denervation in young horses. Am. J. Vet. Res., *47:*43–45, 1986.
25. Watkins, J.P., and Auer, J.A.: Physeal injuries. Compend. Contin. Educ. Practicing Vet., *6:*S26–S35, 1984.
26. Embertson, R.M., Bramlage, L.R., Herring, D.S., and Gabel, A.A.: Physeal fractures in the horse. I. Classification and incidence. Vet. Surg., *15:*223–229, 1986.
27. Embertson, R.M., Bramlage, L.R., and Gabel, A.A.: Physeal fractures in the horse. II. Management and outcome. Vet. Surg., *15:*230–236, 1986.

CHAPTER 117

OCULAR DISORDERS

S.M. Roberts

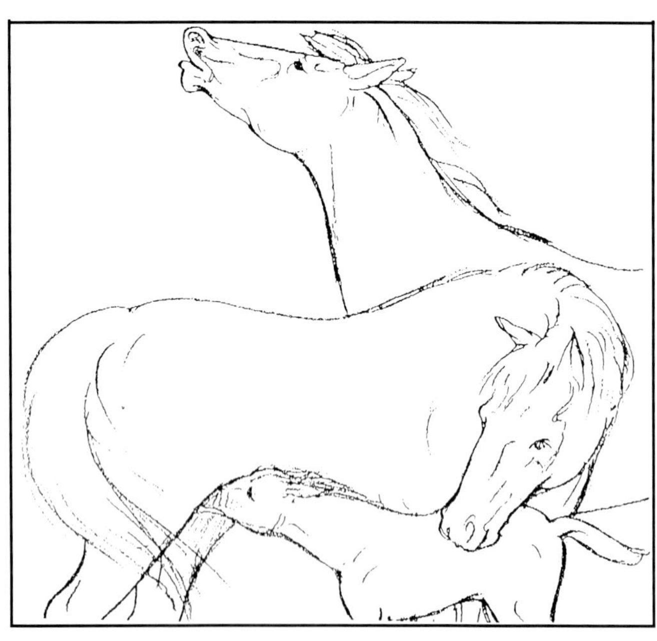

Neonatal ocular disorders in horses, while not reported as frequently as in dogs or cats, encompass a surprising array of conditions. Broadly classified, these disorders are either inherited, congenital, or acquired. Survey articles, review articles, and textbooks describe normal equine ocular appearance, variations of normal, and many specific ocular abnormalities.[1–8] Several good anatomic reviews also help develop an understanding of normal ocular anatomy and disease conditions.[9–13]

A variety of people perform ocular examinations, including laypeople, health care professionals, and veterinarians with variable experience with horses and ocular conditions. As a result, questions frequently arise. Questions about examination findings vary, depending on the background and training of the horse owner, handler, and examiner. Frequent questions include the following. Is the condition a normal variation or disease state? Is it inherited? Is it correctable? Will the condition affect performance?

To put equine neonatal ocular diseases in perspective, this chapter includes a review of the Colorado State University—Veterinary Teaching Hospital (CSU—VTH) medical records from January 1972 through June 1990. The study population does not precisely represent the overall equine population, but some noteworthy comparisons and observations surfaced. In general, neonatal ocular disease occurred in 113 of 2137 ocular diagnoses (5.3%). The survey included 92 diagnoses of congenital and 21 diagnoses of acquired disorders (retinal detachment and uveitis). This chapter includes pertinent data regarding these diagnoses and reviews the literature of the more common abnormalities.

The purpose of this chapter is to inform the busy veterinary practitioner and veterinary medical student of common ocular disorders documented in the foal. It will provide a basis for answering questions, improving advice, treating, and making a prognosis.

NORMAL EYE IN THE NEONATE

The horse is precocious at birth; the eyelids are open, the eyes are fully developed, and good functional vision exists. The open eyelids and lack of a learned menace response until about 5 days of age predisposes the globe to trauma. At birth, the pupil, moderately dilated and circular, has a sluggish pupillary light response. The pupil becomes more adult-like, taking on the shape of a horizontal oval by 3 to 5 days of age. It displays a pupillary light response typical of the adult horse by 5 days of age.[1–3,6,7] Vibrissae are abundant below the lower eyelid and sparse above the upper eyelid. Long cilia (eye lashes) are characteristic along the margin of the upper eyelid, but absent from the lower. Usually the nictitating membrane margin contains pigment,[5,6] but nonpigmentation also occurs normally.

A well-developed caruncle is present at the nasal canthus, anterior to the nictitans. The cornea should be clear, horizontally oval, and broader nasally. The average corneal dimensions in the foal are 26.1 mm horizontally and 19.8 mm vertically.[5] In the adult horse, measurements are 34 mm and 26.5 mm, respectively.[9] The sclera overhangs the cornea at the superior and inferior aspects, thus masking visualization of the iridocorneal angle. The angle is visible at the temporal and nasal aspects of the corneoscleral junction and appears as a fine, gray line composed of a porous meshwork of mesenchymal tissue.

Use a penlight, ophthalmoscope, or transilluminator to examine the intraocular structures. Typically the iris is dark brown, unless heterochromia iridis is present. The color lightens to tan or gray toward the iris base. Heterochromia iridis is considered a normal variation and does not adversely effect vision or predispose to ocular disease. Granula iridica are prominent on the superior edge of the pupil, but are small and variably present on the inferior pupil margin.[4,5]

The normal lens is transparent, although close viewing will reveal a bluish gray discoloration along the pathway of the examining beam. This color is caused by slight changes in the refractive index of the various lens layers, thus causing light refraction and scatter. Lens structures often confused with cataracts include the lens suture lines at the anterior and posterior surfaces and hyaloid remnants. The anterior lens suture appears as an upright *Y* and the posterior is an inverted *Y* or stellate shape.[5,11] The posterior surface of the lens capsule commonly has a hyaloid remnant. This is normal and easily seen during the first 24 h of life. Some hyaloid remnants appear as black or blood-filled curvilinear fine lines traversing the vitreous. The remnants extend from the axial posterior lens surface toward the physiologic cup of the optic disc. Within a few days to weeks after birth, the hyaloid remnants in horses rapidly regress.

The ocular fundus of the horse, unique among common domestic animals, has only a few retinal blood vessels leaving the optic disc; this condition is called a paurangiotic vascular pattern. Arteries and veins, indistinguishable from one another, appear as 40 to 60 vessels radiating from the optic nerve for a radius of one to two disc diameters.[4,6,14] The optic disc, located in the nontapetal fundus, may be round, oval, or football shaped.[5] Within 24 h of birth, the optic disc is pale pink to red in color, but changes to salmon pink soon after birth. The ventral portion of the optic disc often appears as an elevated white rim.

The tapetum lucidum is a roughly triangular area encompassing most of the superior fundus. It varies in color from yellow to blue-green; yellow-green is most common.[6] Tapetal coloration is variable in the horse. Tapetal color of horses with light hair coats is more yellow, while chestnut to bay hair coats are more yellow-green. Tapetal color in black or gray hair coats is more blue-green in color.[2,6] The choroidal blood vessels penetrate the tapetum lucidum, creating a brown to black peppered appearance over the tapetum lucidum called stars of Winslow.

Striking fundus color patterns of both the tapetal and nontapetal portions occur in partially to totally albinotic individuals; commonly red or blue choroidal patches and streaks are seen. Other albinotic horses have a light yellow to pale cream colored fundus or a decreased tapetum size. In normally pigmented horses, the junction between the tapetal and nontapetal fundus is prominent and irregular. Islands of either tapetal coloration or pigment occur along the transition zone between the tapetum and nontapetum.

A challenge faced by all veterinarians, is differentiating normal variations from abnormalities. Despite the array of normal variations, with practice, recognition of normal variations becomes easier. As the veterinarian gains confidence, the diagnostic accuracy of the ophthalmic examination increases. For more information, consult one of several reviews on examination methods and findings for a thorough coverage of this subject.[1,6–8,14,15]

CONGENITAL ABNORMALITIES

Many case reports of congenital defects in a wide range of domestic animal species abound in the literature. Liepold et al. reviewed the literature and, in table format, reported congenital defects, including ocular disorders of foals.[16] The overall prevalence of congenital equine ocular defects is low (0.5%).[17] Large case studies show cataracts and microphthalmia among the most common ocular defects.[4,5,15,18,19] Congenital cataracts occurred in 0.5 to 35.3% and microphthalmia, in 4.6 to 14.7% of the foals examined.[18,19] The CSU—VTH medical record data base documented a similar prevalence of both conditions. Cataracts represented 33.7% (31/92) and microphthalmia, 8.7% (8/92) of the congenital ocular diagnoses (Table 117–1). Entropion and persistent pupillary membranes occurred, each representing 8.7% of the diagnoses.

The following disordered cell mechanisms cause teratogenesis: impaired cell proliferation, disrupted cell migration, and failure of cell differentiation. Most likely, multiple causes interact and could include genetic defects, extraneous teratogenic substances, infections, or trauma.[19] Extraneous teratogenic substances encompass drugs, toxins, vitamin deficiencies or excesses, and ionizing radiation. Idiopathic defects also occur, actually representing the largest etiologic group. Congenital ocular defects occur sporadically, thus diminishing awareness of these disorders. The common ocular congenital defects presented in this chapter will help maintain awareness of these and other congenital conditions. Table 117–2 lists reported ocular defects of foals, along with the associated breeds, proposed causes, essential features, and management methods.

CATARACTS

The normal lens is biconvex and suspended behind the pupil. It is transparent, although appearing slightly bluish gray as viewed along an examining light beam pathway. The lens is unique in that it represents surface ectoderm sequestered within the globe and enclosed by a basement membrane. Lens cells and fibers, retained

TABLE 117–1. NEONATAL OCULAR DIAGNOSES JANUARY 1972 TO JUNE 1990 AS RETRIEVED FROM THE COLORADO STATE UNIVERSITY—VETERINARY TEACHING HOSPITAL MEDICAL RECORDS.*

	BREED								
DISORDER	AMERICAN PAINT	AMERICAN SADDLE HORSE	APPALOOSA	ARABIAN	MIXED	MORGAN	QUARTER HORSE	THOROUGHBRED	TOTAL
Amaurosis				1/0†			1/0	1/0	3/0
Amblyopia							0/1		0/1
Aniridia							0/1		0/1
Cataract *(Y)*		1/0		1/0			3/2	1/0	6/2
Nuclear		1/0	1/0	1/1			6/5		9/6
Hyaloid				1/0			1/1		2/1
Mature		0/1		3/2			1/5		4/8
Coloboma Eyelid			0/1						0/1
Lens							1/0		1/0
Entropion			1/0		0/2	1/0	1/1	1/1	4/4
Dermoid							1/1		1/1
Nasolacrimal atresia				1/1		0/1	1/2		2/4
Nasal									
Palpebral	1/0		0/1				1/0		2/1
Microphthalmia				2/2			2/2		4/4
Microphakia			1/0						1/0
Persistent pupillary membrane			1/2			1/2	1/1		3/5
Optic nerve				1/0			0/1		1/1
Coloboma									
Hypoplasia							0/1		0/1
Retinal detachment		0/1					4/2		4/3
Retinal dysplasia		0/1					2/1		2/2
Stationary night blindness			1/3						1/3
Uveitis							9/4	0/1	9/5
Total	1/0	2/3	5/7	11/6	0/2	2/3	35/31	3/2	59/54
Total of breed seen, male	439	133	937	1,082	1,229	205	7,195	1,743	12,963
Total of breed seen, female	356	111	640	1,018	1,102	201	4,885	1,206	9,519

*A total of 1183 cases having at least one abnormality were identified, representing 2137 ocular diagnoses. Neonatal disorders occurred in 113 of these diagnoses (5.3%); 92 represented congenital abnormalities (4.3%) and 21 represented acquired conditions (0.98%).

†The first number represents males and the second, females.

throughout life, react to insult by cell death, abnormal cell proliferation, and loss of osmotic homeostasis. The result is vacuolation and loss of transparency and thus cataract formation. A cataract may partially or totally involve the lens capsule, cortex, or nucleus. Different portions of the lens often become involved to different degrees. Thus one part of the cataract is immature, while another part is mature. More information about the lens is available elsewhere.[6–9,14,20,21]

Complete congenital cataracts are totally opaque and termed a mature cataract. The term immature cataract describes partially opaque lenses. Depending on the severity or degree of maturity, a cataract can impair vision slightly or result in total blindness. Cataracts represent an unsoundness, whether or not inherited. Excluding external traumatic injuries, congenital cataracts represent the most common cause of blindness or vision impairment in foals. Owners and handlers frequently complain that the affected foal displays visual deficits, clumsiness, and repeated tendency toward traumatic injuries. Congenital cataracts occur with other ocular defects such as aniridia and microphthalmos.[4,22–27] In most instances, the cause of congenital cataracts remains unknown. Potential causes include faulty in utero nutrition, genetic factors, ocular inflammation occurring in utero, radiation, and prenatal trauma.[28–30] Rarely is heredity documented in the horse.[22,31,32]

By definition, a congenital cataract is present at birth, developing during fetal life. Usually, both eyes have cataracts. The four basic types of congenital cataracts in the horse include (1) a completely mature cataract, (2) nuclear cataract, (3) *Y* suture type cataract, and (4) cataract associated with persistent hyaloid vasculature.[6,7,14] A total of 38 congenital cataract diagnoses (31 cases) occurred in the CSU—VTH medical record data base. The distribution by type included 15 nuclear, 12 ma-

TABLE 117–2. NEONATAL OCULAR DISORDERS IN FOALS

DISORDER	BREEDS	CAUSES	ESSENTIAL FEATURES AND MANAGEMENT
Microphthalmia			
May be associated with other ocular defects, e.g., multiple ocular defect syndrome, cataracts, and retinal detachments	All breeds; Thoroughbreds have higher incidence	Not established; most cases are idiopathic, some caused by toxic, infectious, or nutritional episodes	Small eyes, prominent third eyelid; no treatment; lid surgery for secondary entropion
Strabismus	Appaloosa		Rare; usually convergent; some patients have compensatory head deviation; surgery to straighten eyes has been described
Eyelid coloboma			Defects in eyelid margin; surgery, depending on extent of other problems
May be associated with multiple ocular anomalies			
Ankyloblepharon congenita			Partial fusion of upper and lower lids; surgery
Entropion			
Primary		Some patients have oversize palpebral fissures	Inturned eyelids, epiphora, corneal ulceration; manual eversion of the eyelids;
Secondary		Prematurity or illness	palpebral injections or horizontal mattress sutures or surgery to turn out the eyelids; treatment of underlying cause, then surgery
Nasolacrimal			Absence of nasal opening; watery eye; some patients have mucopurulent discharge
Atresia of nasolacrimal meatus			Dacrocystorhinography may aid in diagnosis; surgery to create new opening
Misplaced punctum			Surgery to enlarge punctum
Atresia of punctum			Surgery to create new punctum
Cornea			
Microcornea; may be associated with microphthalmia syndromes			Small cornea; no treatment
Corneal melanosis			Superficial axial nonprogressive pigment; superficial keratectomy
Dermoid; probably most common congenital anomaly		Not known to be inherited	Lateral or ventral corneal conjunctival masses containing hair and sebaceous glands; surgical removal
Aniridia			
May be associated with cataracts	Belgian Draft horse	Autosomal recessive	Complete absence of iris tissue
Uveal Cysts			
May be associated with heterochromia iridis			Pigmented cysts in anterior chamber or pupillary edge; can be transilluminated; aspiration if large and vision obstructed
Heterochromia iridis	Many color-dilute breeds	Pigment failure in one iris or part of one iris	Tapetum may be absent; iris can be hypoplastic
Cataracts			
Some associated with microphthalmia syndromes	Arabian, Belgium Draft, Morgan, Thoroughbred, Quarter Horse	May be inherited	Spontaneous resorption can offer useful vision in stud animals; consider surgery if the cataracts interfere with vision

Continued

TABLE 117–2. NEONATAL OCULAR DISORDERS IN FOALS—CON'T

DISORDER	BREEDS	CAUSES	ESSENTIAL FEATURES AND MANAGEMENT
		Other cataracts can be caused by trauma (prenatal and foaling), poor nutrition, metabolic abnormalities, or toxic sources	Note: Need to differentiate from prominent posterior *Y* sutures, which are present in the majority of foals
Persistent Papillary Membranes May be associated with other ocular anomalies			Strands of iris tissue that can run to iris; cornea (opacity) or lens (cataracts); may continue to atrophy during the first year of life
Vitreous			
Remnants of hyaloid tissue			Visible behind the lens; present in most foals and will atrophy by 6 to 9 months
Persistent hyperplastic primary vitreous			Uncommon; fibrovascular membrane behind the lens
Retina			
Retinal hemorrhages		Mostly incidental; difficult birth	
Retinal dysplasia; may be associated with other defects	Thoroughbred may have higher incidence		Bilateral retinal disorganization; may also have retinal detachment
Retinal detachment; may be associated with dysplasia			Complete retinal detachment
Coloboma of the fundus			Corioretinal defect
Retinal aplasia		Possibly autosomal recessive	Absence of the retina
Stationary night blindness	Appaloosa and other breeds	Autosomal recessive defect in neuroretinal transmission	No lesions visible on ophthalmoscopic examination; some patients have microphthalmia or dorsal strabismus/nystagmus
Optic Nerve			
Optic nerve hypoplasia (congenital optic atrophy); may be associated with other defects			Small optic nerve heads either unilateral or bilateral; slow or absent pupillary light reflex; searching nystagmus
Papilledema		Maladjustment	Swelling of optic nerve associated with cerebral edema

(Adapted from Slatter, D.: Fundamentals of Veterinary Ophthalmology. Philadelphia, W.B. Saunders, 1990, pp. 554–555. Table by R.G. Stanley and J.R. Blogg.)

ture, 8 *Y* suture, and 3 hyaloid-related cataracts. In 7 cases, two different types of cataract occurred in each eye. Breeds represented included the American Saddlebred, Arabian, Quarter Horse, and Thoroughbred (Table 117–1). Cataracts secondary to a persistent hyaloid artery and *Y* suture type cataracts did not affect vision. Complete cortical or nuclear congenital cataracts were more serious, with a potential for vision loss. Heritable, congenital cataracts occur in the Belgian,[22] Morgan,[32] and Thoroughbred[8] breeds. Cataracts in the Morgan are typically bilateral, nonprogressive, nuclear cataracts that do not seriously interfere with vision. Noninherited nuclear cataracts occur in the Morgan breed.[33] Recently, congenital nuclear cataracts occurred in three related Quarter Horses, at CSU—VTH. The mode of inheritance is unknown.

The genesis of congenital cataracts is not simply a matter of untoward genetic or environmental influences; complex developmental issues become involved. Lens development takes place in four stages: (1) formation of the lens plate, (2) formation of the lens vesicle, (3) formation of the primary lens fibers, and (4) formation of the secondary lens fibers.[34] Early in fetal development, induction of lens formation results from the primordial neural retina. The resulting lens placode undergoes cellular division to form the lens cup with an initial hollow lumen. The lumen becomes sealed off and surrounded by the epithelial basement membrane, thus preventing mixture with other cell types. Thus, the lens tissue has limited permeability. Extrinsic factors transform the lens vesicle into a mature lens. Influence of a healthy, developing neural retina is necessary,[34,35] as is a proper conformation between the lens and the rim of the optic cup.

The posterior lens epithelial cells elongate to form primary lens fibers which obliterate the lumen of the lens vesicle. Anterior epithelial cells begin to divide, migrating in an equatorial fashion and elongate in an anterior-posterior direction to form secondary lens fibers. The primary lens fibers become crowded centrally to form the fetal nucleus. As lens fibers elongate, the cell nuclei and organelles undergo dissolution. Only the anterior capsule epithelial cells and superficial, equatorial lens cortex fibers keep organelles and nuclei. The secondary lens fibers become closely associated with neighboring cells by gap junctions, desmosomal attachments, and ball-and-socket interdigitations.[8,9] No exfoliation of the secondary lens cells or fibers occurs. Because the lens retains cellular material for the life of the animal, cataract formation eventually occurs.

Congenital nuclear cataracts seen frequently in the horse are a lamellar (zonular) type. They involve the lens portion immediately external to the fetal nucleus (the inner part of the adult nucleus). The cataract occurs as newly developed lens fibers become subjected to a cataractogenic influence for a limited period, thus resulting in a circumscribed zone of opacity. The time during lens formation at which the cataractogenic influence occurs, determines the location of the opacity. Lens fibers that form before or after the influence are transparent. Many horses that show moderate to severe vision impairment early, undergo clinical improvement because normal lens fibers form around the abnormal. The overall effect is a relative decrease in size of the cataract as the lens continues to grow. On occasion, the adjacent normal lens fibers become opaque over time, leading to progression of the cataract. Similar and frequently inherited cataracts occur in humans[36] (transmitted by an autosomal dominant mode) and in dogs.[37]

If a congenital cataract is causing vision loss, the only recourse for improved vision is surgical removal. Many reports describe removal of cataracts in the horse and the paper by Whitley and Meek is a good overview.[38] In general, cataract extraction in the horse is not as successful as in the dog. Medical treatment before and after surgery is logistically difficult, vision after surgery may not allow the horse to return to a normal level of performance, and the horse is more sensitive to developing chronic uveitis. Deprivation amblyopia is a potential in foals with congenital cataracts. Deprivation amblyopia results from inadequate visual stimulation to the central nervous system, producing irreversible functional and structural abnormalities in the lateral geniculate nuclei and visual cortex.[8] Thus, successful cataract surgery in a 6-month-old foal may not improve visual abilities of the animal. Foals with a searching, wandering type nystagmus should be suspected of having deprivation amblyopia.

MICROPHTHALMIA

Normally, the globe fills the orbit, thus maintaining the palpebral fissure and providing a curved surface for the eyelids to move across. Microphthalmia or nanophthalmia, one of the more common ocular developmental abnormalities, ranges from a minimal to severe reduction in globe size. Confusion is frequent between severe microphthalmia and anophthalmia. True anophthalmia is rare.[14] Foals with microphthalmia show a smaller than normal palpebral fissure and a protruded nictitating membrane, which may be unilateral or bilateral. Ocular discharge is common, because of a poorly functioning lacrimal drainage system caused by the abnormal ocular and orbital anatomy. The cornea is often opaque or pigmented, and the affected eye is usually blind. Microphthalmic globes often have cataracts as noted in five of eight microphthalmia cases at CSU—VTH (Table 117–1). One case also had a corneal dermoid associated with microphthalmia (Fig. 117–1). As the foal grows, the orbit may fail to grow, resulting in asymmetry of the periocular region.

Microphthalmia results from defective organogenesis. The factors determining the final globe size are complex and closely interrelated. Embryologically, the primary optic vesicle buds from the forebrain and differentiates to form the eye. Retarded growth of the optic vesicle and associated degeneration or atrophy results in microphthalmia. The three classes of microphthalmia are (1) pure microphthalmia (nanophthalmos) with a small but otherwise normal eye, (2) colobomatous microphthalmia with a defect associated with failure of the optic vesicle to involute or the embryonic fissure to close, and (3) complicated microphthalmia in which anomalous development occurs independent of fissure closure.[39] In addition, microphthalmia as reported in humans, is the result of a variety of ocular and systemic diseases or syndromes.[40] The severity of microphthalmia depends on the time of gestation at which the insult occurred. Severe changes result when the defect occurs early in gestation, at the time of optic vesicle and lens formation.[40] If the tip of the optic vesicle makes contact with surface ectoderm over less than the normal area, a perfectly formed microphthalmic eye results.[35,41] In humans, most examples of microphthalmos relate to defective closure of the embryonic fissure.[34]

Reports of microphthalmia in the horse suggest that

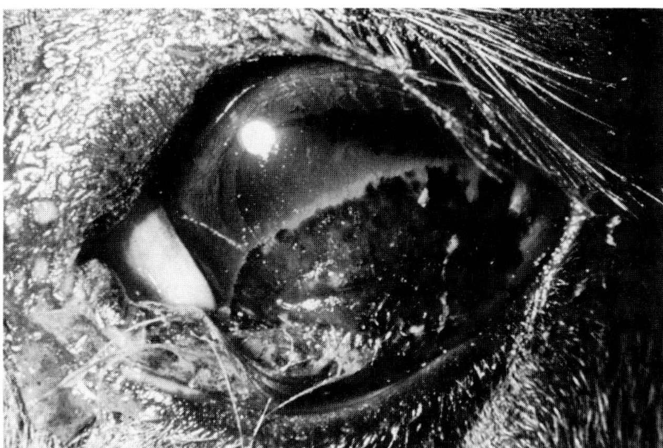

FIG. 117–1. Mild microphthalmos (nanophthalmos) and corneal dermoid. Notice the slightly protruded nictitans caused by enophthalmos. Surgical removal of this dermoid, by superficial keratectomy, allowed retention of functional vision.

the optic vesicle degenerates because the affected globes contain intraocular tissue remnants showing wide morphologic variation, faulty formation, and disorganization.[3,4,18,19,25–27,42–44] In the horse, colobomatous microphthalmia accurately describes the condition. In association with microphthalmia, the orbit forms, but has a reduced volume. The optic nerves are hypoplastic or atrophic.

Various bacterial, fungal, parasitic, and viral infections during organogenesis produce microphthalmia in people. Causes in animals include bovine viral diarrhea-mucosal disease (BVD-MD) (cattle),[45,46] mechanical trauma,[47] hypervitaminosis A,[48] hypovitaminosis A,[49] maternal griseofulvin administration,[50] and heredity (rodents, dogs, and cattle).[51–57] Incriminated causes of microphthalmia in people include a variety of vitamin deficiencies, hypoxia, insulin, sulfonamides,[34,38,57] and heredity.[34] A case of equine microphthalmia associated with a history of maternal sulfadimethoxine administration during week 6 of gestation[25] raises the question of a teratogenic effect similar to that seen in humans. Most equine cases occur sporadically with an unknown cause. No genetic association is known in horses.

No correction is possible for microphthalmia. In unilateral cases, enucleation is helpful in preventing secondary problems associated with abnormal ocular discharge. Secondary entropion that develops requires surgical correction. Usually, foals with unilateral involvement adapt with maturity. Bilateral disease causes blindness, and those foals may have to be euthanatized. Microphthalmia handicaps horses and, depending on the intended use, represents an unsoundness.

NASOLACRIMAL ATRESIA

Congenital anomalies of the nasolacrimal excretory system reported in the horse include atresia of the eyelid punctum, atresia of the nasal meatus punctum, and ectopic eyelid puncta. The most common anomalies are atresia of the nasal meatus puncta.[6–8,14,58–61] Atresia of the nasal meatus occurred in six CSU—VTH cases. Atresia of the proximal bony portion occurred in two horses, and one case had atresia of the bony portion and canaliculi. Thus involvement of all portions of the nasolacrimal outflow pathway occur. To date, no evidence supports an inherited basis in the horse.

In humans, congenital atresia of the nasolacrimal duct is common and potentially familial.[39] The lacrimal passages form in people as epithelial cords beneath the cleft between the nasal and maxillary processes. Canalization begins by the end of the first trimester of gestation. Communication exists between the eye and nose by the end of the second trimester. Patency of the canaliculi lumina develops during midgestation. The eyelid puncta open onto the eyelid margins early during the third trimester of gestation. A mucosal membrane often covers the nasal meatus puncta at birth.[34] This developmental process is likely quite similar in the horse.

Clinical signs of atresia of the nasolacrimal system consist of epiphora and mucopurulent ocular discharge, the latter secondary to dacryocystitis.[60,61] Sometimes a delay in the onset of symptomatic epiphora occurs until the horse is several months of age. Explanations for this phenomenon include a lower tear volume in neonates,[14] distention of the existing nasolacrimal duct portion, [7] and transmucosal absorption of tears across the duct wall.[61] Commonly, confusion between nasolacrimal obstruction and chronic conjunctivitis occurs; however, the quantity of ocular discharge is profuse with nasolacrimal obstructions.

Diagnosis is by (1) examination and palpation of the floor of the nasal vestibule for a distended structure, (2) irrigation of the proximal nasolacrimal duct with saline solution through the palpebral puncta, and (3) radiographic contrast studies.[1,2,6,61–63] During irrigation procedures look for abnormal material refluxing from the puncta, a change in size of the fluctuant swelling in the nostril, and the reduction or lack of irrigating solution exiting the nasal meatus puncta. Treatment requires placement of a retention tube for 3 to 8 weeks[7,58–61,64,65] and use of a topical antibiotic or antibiotic-corticosteroid preparation for several weeks. Surgery is successful in most instances.

Atresia or ectopic placement of the eyelid puncta occur, but both conditions are less common than nasal meatus problems. If epiphora results from either condition, surgical intervention to open, slightly enlarge, or move the puncta is possible. If correction of atresia or agenesis is not possible, create an alternative nasolacrimal outflow pathway or conjunctivorhinostomy.[6,14] All nasolacrimal anomalies represent an unsoundness until corrected surgically.

MISCELLANEOUS CONDITIONS

A wide range of rare conditions, some occurring more frequently than others, exist. For further information about such congenital abnormalities, refer to published review articles,[1,2,6,14,16] survey articles,[3–5,16,19] and textbooks.[7,8,14]

Aniridia

Aniridia means absence of the iris. However, common usage also includes iris hypoplasia in which a rudimentary iris bud is present. True aniridia, with total absence of the iris, is rare in all species. The anomaly arises from a third-wave mesenchyme failure of in-growth and disorderly differentiation. Rarely are the first and second mesenchyme waves, which form the corneal endothelium and stroma, involved in congenital defects. At least 16 theories have been proposed to explain aniridia.[39] The major flaw is a maldevelopment of capsulopupillary vessels of the tunica vasculosa lentis, thus preventing growth of the iris.

A single family of Belgian Draft horses[22] and Jersey cattle[66] exhibited anirida, however many years have passed since these reports. Presumably, the defect has not persisted in the gene pools. More recent reports document sporadic aniridia in a Quarter Horse stallion[23] and a Welsh/Thoroughbred filly.[24] Aniridia is usually bilateral and is frequently confused with an abnormally large pupil. In distinction from simple mydriasis, aniridia allows visualization of the lens equator and ciliary processes. Associated clinical signs may include: blepharospasm, cataracts,[22,24] ocular discharge, perilimbal keratitis,[23] photophobia, and reduced vision. No specific treatments exist for aniridia, and symptomatic supportive measures must deal with any associated signs.

Coloboma

Coloboma, meaning mutilation and first coined in 1821,[39] describes a missing part of an ocular structure, resulting from a failure of the optic fissure to close. Colobomas are either typical and positioned along the line of closure of the optic fissure or atypical and positioned outside the line of closure. Involved ocular structures include the eyelids,[1,7] iris,[1,2] ciliary body, lens,[1-3,7] retina-choroid,[8] optic disc,[7] and optic nerve.

All forms of coloboma are rare in the horse and frequently associated with concomitant ocular disorders. The cause of colobomata in domestic animals is usually unknown. Typical coloboma of the posterior pole may result from abnormal eversion of the neurosensory retina through the embryonic fissure.[39] This theory, supported by work in the Collie dog, suggests that defective neurosensory retinal differentiation is responsible for optic disc coloboma formation.[67]

Eyelid colobomas, usually termed eyelid agenesis, do not result from embryonic fissure abnormalities. Experimental work suggests that ischemia to a rapidly developing embryonic eyelid could cause infarction of the lid farthest from the blood supply,[34] thus resulting in a focal defect. Repair of eyelid colobomata requires blepharoplastic surgery. Such surgery also corrects exposure keratopathy and other associated problems. Defects located within the globe are not amenable to surgical correction. A coloboma that directly or indirectly causes vision loss represents an unsoundness, unless surgery resolves the problem.

Dermoid

A dermoid is a choristoma, representing normal tissue elements located at an abnormal site. It is basically a congenital tumor of skin and related appendage tissues. Tissues involved include the cornea, conjunctiva, nictitating membrane, eyelids, and anterior segment. Most commonly, the temporal limbus and adjoining cornea show involvement.[2,7,14,43,44,68] Corneal and scleral dermoids involve the superficial tissue layers. Deeper tissue involvement is possible and epibulbar dermoids in man can reportedly involve the full corneal thickness and intraocular structures.[39] No genetic association is known in horses.

If hair is a part of the dermoid, mechanical irritation of the cornea usually results. Visual impairment results from corneal involvement or secondary disease. Dermoids can involve the globe and adnexa and, cause corneal opacity, nictitans deformity, eyelid disfigurement, and nasolacrimal punctal occlusion. Large lesions such as depicted in Figure 117–1 require surgery, although small lesions may go untreated.[7] To avoid dermoid regrowth, remove completely while avoiding globe perforation. Corneal wounds created during surgery require treatment as an ulcer. If needed, provide corneal mechanical support by conjunctival flap grafts, nictitans flaps, collagen shields, or tarsorrhaphies. Some degree of permanent corneal scarring results following surgical removal.

Entropion

Inversion of the eyelid margin, termed entropion, usually involves the lower eyelid. It occurs infrequently in neonates as either a congenital defect or an early acquired problem.[4-6,14] The problem, reportedly inherited in Thoroughbreds,[2] actually may relate to weakness of the tarsal plate, position of the globe, and spasm of the orbicularis oculi muscle.[69] Painful conditions of the conjunctiva and cornea frequently lead to or exacerbate entropion caused by the associated blepharospasm. Similarly, enophthalmia resulting from debilitation or dehydration can lead to entropion.

Six CSU–VTH entropion cases occurred in debilitated foals: three suffering from failure of passive transfer, two with septicemia and uveitis, and one with an intestinal impaction (Table 117–1). Clinical signs develop when facial hair contacts the cornea and conjunctiva, causing increased lacrimation, blepharospasm, conjunctivitis, and keratitis. Ulcerative keratitis directly threatens vision. Severe vision-threatening corneal ulceration occurred in one of the CSU–VTH cases.

Treatment varies with both severity and chronicity and includes manual repositioning of the lids several times a day, subcutaneous injection of procaine penicillin G,[70] placement of repositioning sutures,[4,6-8,14,71-73] and excision of skin next to the lid margin.[6,14,64,74] Topical antibiotic ointments serve as adjunct treatment with the above techniques. Do not inject materials, such as mineral oil or paraffin,[75] that cause a foreign body reaction. Entropion is a blemish, not an unsoundness.

Night Blindness

Congenital stationary night blindness is an incompletely understood condition reported in Appaloosa horses of the United States[76-79] It occasionally affects other breeds.[76] Visual disturbances range from poor vision during reduced lighting conditions to poor vision during the day and blindness at night. Proposed inheritance modes include autosomal recessive,[76] and sex-linked recessive with the defect on the X chromosome.[77] The CSU–VTH data may support a sex-linked recessive mode of inheritance, since three of four affected Appaloosa horses were female (Table 117–1).

Definitive diagnosis by electroretinography shows a characteristic large negative wave form. A history of poor vision, observing behavior associated with poor vision, and a normal ocular fundus allow presumptive diagnosis.[76–79] Other clinical signs include having subtle microphthalmia, holding the head in a star gazing position when visualizing objects, seeking lighted conditions, and displaying a dorsomedial strabismus. Histologic examination did not explain this functional disorder.[78] The disorder may result from abnormal neural transmission between the photoreceptor and inner nuclear layers of the retina. No treatment is available and the condition is nonprogressive. Affected horses are unsound and thus unsuitable for breeding. Using a mildly affected horse for riding requires that the people involved understand the degree of visual impairment. The clinician should issue a written statement to avoid medicolegal liability.

Rare Conditions

Other reported congenital conditions include glaucoma,[1,6,63,80] lens luxation,[6,26,44,81] lenticonus,[7,44] lentiglobus,[7,44] microphakia,[7,44] optic nerve hypoplasia/atrophy,[44,82,83] persistent pupillary membranes,[3,5,7,14,44] retinal cysts,[14] retinal dysplasia,[1,2,7,44] retinal detachment,[2,7,84] and strabismus.[6,7,85] Conditions such as persistent pupillary membranes, retinal cysts, mild retinal dysplasia, and strabismus do not interfere seriously with vision. These represent blemishes rather than actual unsoundness, which are conditions that directly threaten vision. Four cases of retinal dysplasia in the CSU–VTH data showed severe bilateral involvement, with either poor vision or no vision. Two had cataracts and one had retinal detachments and lens luxations (Table 117–1).

ACQUIRED ABNORMALITIES

INFLAMMATORY AND INFECTIOUS DISEASES

Systemic or local inflammatory and infectious diseases may result in conjunctivitis, iridocyclitis, or chorioretinitis in the neonate. Systemic bacterial and viral infections are especially prone to causing uveal inflammation. Local primary intraocular inflammatory and infectious diseases may also result in uveal inflammation. In many instances, the problem is one of extraocular disease spreading to an intraocular site, such as mycotic keratitis resulting in endophthalmitis. Whether local or systemic disorders cause an ocular inflammatory disorder is not always clear. Consider bilateral ocular involvement as a systemic disease with ocular involvement until shown otherwise. To preserve ocular function, start treatment rapidly and aggressively. Otherwise, ocular inflammation quickly builds in intensity, threatening vision. Despite efforts at treatment, successful return to function is not always possible. Excellent discussions of inflammatory ocular conditions are available.[1,6–8,14,65,86–88]

The most common ocular disorder of foals is conjunctivitis (usually caused by microbial infection), environmental irritants, and injury. Neonatal trauma or systemic infectious agents frequently cause intraocular inflammation. The CSU–VTH data contained nine septicemic and three failure of passive transfer cases with intraocular inflammation (Table 117–1). Table 117–3 lists reported infectious causes of conjunctivitis, iridocyclitis, and chorioretinitis. Despite the wide variety of infectious agents known to cause ocular disease, most cases remain idiopathic. A sterile inflammatory reaction may develop and become self-perpetuating.

Clinical signs of ocular inflammation are not unique in the neonate or in the horse. Evidence of conjunctivitis includes increased lacrimation; catarrhal to mucopurulent discharge; conjunctival injection, especially the bulbar conjunctiva; chemosis; and signs of ocular discomfort such as squinting, rubbing, and blinking. In contrast, clinical signs of anterior uveitis include increased lacrimation, photophobia, conjunctival and episcleral injection, hypotony, corneal changes such as edema and vascularization, flare, miosis, iris congestion, hypopyon, cataracts, and synechia. Chorioretinitis cases do not necessarily show anterior segment abnormalities. Fundus changes could include loss of the normal tapetal reflectivity, grayish areas in the nontapetal fundus, optic neuritis, optic disc atrophy, and pigment proliferation or destruction.

TRAUMA ASSOCIATED PROBLEMS

A wide variety of traumatic insults can result in direct injury to the globe and periocular tissues. Blunt trauma and lacerating injuries occur in foals and require conventional surgical and medical treatments. Compressive trauma associated with parturition commonly causes conjunctival and subconjunctival hemorrhage. This type of hemorrhage is not serious, unless caused by a systemic problem such as a bleeding disorder. With or without treatment, subconjunctival hemorrhage resolves in 7 to 10 days, although some cases take several weeks.

Retinal hemorrhage, a nonspecific lesion, occurs with trauma of parturition. Uveal inflammation and systemic disorders such as septicemia, bleeding disorders, or neonatal maladjustment syndrome, also may have retinal hemorrhage. Severe retinal hemorrhage may involve the vitreous and choroid in addition to the retina. If caused by birth trauma, retinal hemorrhage usually resolves quickly over the course of 7 days. Most instances of retinal hemorrhage do not result in permanent vision loss.

OPHTHALMIC UNSOUNDNESS OF THE NEONATE

Unfortunately, no strict criteria exist for ophthalmic unsoundness. The basic principles presented in this chapter and elsewhere serve as a starting point.[6] At the root level, classification of a horse as having ocular unsoundness hinges on loss of visual function. The visual acuity required by horses is variable, depending on their use. While performance horses need optimal vision, in-

TABLE 117–3. COMMON INFECTIOUS AGENTS ASSOCIATED WITH CONJUNCTIVITIS, IRIDOCYCLITIS, AND CHORIORETINITIS IN NEONATAL AND OLDER FOALS

AGENT	CONJUNCTIVITIS	IRIDOCYCLITIS	CHORIORETINITIS
Bacteria	Actinobacillus spp. Chlamydia psittici Moraxella spp. Rhodococcus equi Streptococcus equi	Actinobacillus spp. Brucella spp. Escherichia coli Leptospira spp. Rhodococcus equi Salmonella spp. Streptococcus equi	Streptococcus equi
Viral	Adenovirus Equine influenza Equine viral arteritis Herpesvirus Rhinovirus	Adenovirus Equine viral arteritis	
Parasitic	Habronema spp. Onchocerca cervicalis Thelazia lacrymalis	Onchocerca cervicalis	Onchocerca cervicalis Sarcocystis spp. Toxoplasma gondii
Mycotic	Aspergillus spp. Histoplasma fariminosus Rhinosporidium seeberi		

frequently used horses may function well with a minor vision deficit. Superior athletic ability of the horse or excellent rider skill may overcome suboptimal vision, but minor vision loss creates an unsafe situation for the average horse or inexperienced rider.

Any congenital ocular defect or neonatal-acquired eye problem represents an unsoundness if one or both eyes are blind. Likewise, partial loss of vision as a result of stationary night blindness makes the horse unsound. In this later situation, some horse owners may be able to use the horse if they implicitly understand the ramifications of the abnormality. Corneal disease causing small focal opacities usually does not seriously interfere with functional vision. Large opacities on the other hand can result in near blindness or functional blindness. Some corneal problems represent a blemish, and others, an unsoundness. Most inflammatory lesions of the eye are blemishes, pending resolution or determination of the degree of visual interference. Inactive chorioretinitis lesions, if associated with clinically normal vision, thus represent blemishes. If intraocular inflammation is likely to become chronic or recurrent, then the horse is unsound. Vitreous opacities such as persistent hyaloid remnants would represent blemishes unless they were large or caused a cataract.

In most situations, cataracts make a horse unsound. While some cataracts result in minimal vision impairment, the tendency of many cataracts to progress and the behavioral characteristics of the horse make classification of affected horses as unsound the most prudent and safest approach. Cataract extraction is capable of improving vision loss, but the postoperative suboptimal visual function raises serious questions about the safety of using such a horse.

Rarely are real-life situations black or white. Thus the horse owner may have difficulty understanding and accepting some statements about the use of his or her animal. The decision on unsoundness versus blemish must incorporate the veterinarian's knowledge about the condition, the horse in general, and specifics about individual circumstances of the horse and owner. The previous information should help stimulate dialogue between all parties involved in the diagnosis, management, and decision-making processes regarding horses, thus overcoming a major barrier. The overall goal is to improve the well-being of horses and their respective owners.

REFERENCES

1. Latimer, C.A., and Wyman, M.: Neonatal ophthalmology. Vet. Clin. North Am. Equine Pract., *1*:235–259, 1985.
2. Munroe, G.A., and Barnett, K.C.: Congenital ocular disease in the foal. Vet. Clin. North Am. Large Anim. Pract., *6*:519–539, 1984.
3. Barnett, K.C.: The eye of the newborn foal. J. Reprod. Fertil. Suppl., *23*:701–702, 1975.
4. Koch, S.A., et al.: Ocular disease in the newborn horse: A preliminary report. J. Equine Surg., *2*:167–170, 1978.
5. Latimer, C.A., Wyman, M., and Hamilton, J.: An ophthalmic survey of the neonatal horse. Equine Vet. J., *2(Suppl. 2)*:9–14, 1983.
6. Gelatt, K.N.: The eye. *In* Equine Medicine and Surgery. 3rd ed. Edited by R.A. Mansmann and E.S. McAllister. Santa Barbara, CA, American Veterinary Publishers, 1982, pp. 1295–1296.
7. Lavach, J.D.: Large Animal Ophthalmology. St. Louis, C.V. Mosby, 1990.
8. Slatter, D.H.: Fundamentals of Veterinary Ophthalmology, Philadelphia, W.B. Saunders, 1990.
9. Samuelson, D.A.: Ophthalmic embryology and anatomy.

In Veterinary Ophthalmology. 2nd ed. Edited by K.N. Gelatt. Philadelphia, Lea & Febiger, 1991, pp. 3–123.

10. Diesem, C.: Gross anatomic structure of equine and bovine orbit and its contents. Am. J. Vet. Res., *29:*1769–1781, 1968.

11. Wyman, M., and Anderson, B.G.: Anatomy of the equine eye and orbit: Gross anatomy of the lids. J. Equine Med. Surg., *2:*307–311, 1978.

12. Anderson, B., and Wyman, M.: Anatomy of the equine eye and orbit: Histological structure and blood supply of the eyelids. J. Equine Med. Surg. *3:*4–9, 1979.

13. Peiffer, R.L.: Foundations of equine ophthalmology: Clinical anatomy and physiology. Equine Pract., *1:*39–46, 1979.

14. Davidson, M.G.: Equine ophthalmology. *In* Textbook of Veterinary Ophthalmology. 2nd ed. Edited by K.N. Gelatt. Philadelphia, Lea & Febiger, 1991, pp. 576–610.

15. Glaze, M.B.: Examination of the eye. *In* Current Therapy in Equine Medicine. 2nd ed. Edited by N.E. Robinson and M.B. Glaze. Philadelphia, W.B. Saunders, 1987, pp. 427–433.

16. Leipold, H.W., Saperstein, G., and Woollen, N.E.: Congenital defects in foals. *In* Large Animal Internal Medicine. Edited by B.P. Smith. St Louis, C.V. Mosby, 1990, pp. 1567–1597.

17. Walde, I.: Some observations on congenital cataracts in the horse. Equine Vet. J. *15:*27–28, 1983.

18. Priester, W.A.: Congenital ocular defects in cattle, horses, cats, and dogs. J. Am. Vet. Med. Assoc., *160:*1504–1511, 1972.

19. Crowe, M.W., and Swerczek, T.W.: Equine congenital defects. Am. J. Vet. Res., *46:*353–358, 1985.

20. Kunze, D.J.: Cataracts. *In* Current Therapy in Equine Medicine. Edited by N.E. Robinson and G.M. Schmidt. Philadelphia, W.B. Saunders, 1983, pp. 390–393.

21. Whitley, R.D.: Cataracts. *In* Current Therapy in Equine Medicine. 2nd ed. Edited by N.E. Robinson and M.B. Glaze. Philadelphia, W.B. Saunders, 1987, pp. 456–458.

22. Ericksson, K.: Hereditary aniridia with secondary cataract in horses. Nord. Vet. Med., *7:*773–793, 1955.

23. Joyce, J.R.: Aniridia in a Quarter Horse. Equine Vet. J., *15:*21–22, 1983.

24. Irby, N.L., and Aquirre, G.D.: Congenital aniridia in a pony. J. Am. Vet. Med. Assoc., *186:*281–283, 1985.

25. Dziezyc, J., Kern, T.J., and Wolf, E.D.: Microphthalmia in a foal. Equine Vet. J., *15:*15–17, 1983.

26. Garner, A., and Griffiths, P.: Bilateral congenital ocular defects in a foal. Br. J. Ophthalmol., *53:*513–517, 1969.

27. Mosier, D.A., Engleman, R.W., Confer, A.W., and McCarroll, G.D.: Bilateral multiple congenital ocular defects in Quarter Horse foals. Equine Vet. J., *15:*18–20, 1983.

28. Rathbun, W.B.: Biochemistry of the lens and cataractogenesis. Curr. Concepts Vet. Clin. North. Am. Small Anim. Pract., *10:*377–398, 1980.

29. Morris, D.A.: Cataracts and systemic disease. *In* Clinical Ophthalmology. Vol. 5. Edited by T.D. Duane. Philadelphia, J.B. Lippincott, 1984, pp. 1–10.

30. Luntz, M.H.: Clinical types of cataracts. *In* Clinical Ophthalmology. Vol. 1. Edited by T.D. Duane. Philadelphia, J.B. Lippincott, 1984, pp. 1–20.

31. Weber, W.: Hereditary cataract, a recessive character in the horse. Schweiz. Arch. Teirheilkd, *89:*397, 1947.

32. Beech, J., and Irby, N.: Inherited nuclear cataracts in the Morgan horse. J. Heredit., *76:*371–372, 1985.

33. Beech, J., Aquirre, G., and Gross, S.: Congenital nuclear cataracts in the Morgan horse. J. Am. Vet. Med. Assoc., *184:*1363–1365, 1984.

34. Mullaney, J.: Normal development and development anomalies of the eye. *In* Pathobiology of ocular disease. Edited by A. Garner and G.K. Klintworth. New York, Marcel Dekker, 1982, pp. 443–522.

35. Coulombre, A.: The eye. *In* Organogenesis. Edited by R. DeHaan and H. Ursprung. New York, Holt, Reinhart and Winston, 1965, pp. 219–251.

36. Marner, E.: A family with eight generations of hereditary cataract. Acta Ophthalmol., *27:*537–551, 1949.

37. Gelatt, K.N.: Lens and cataract formation in the dog. Compend. Contin. Educ. Practicing Vet., *1:*175–180, 1979.

38. Whitley, R.D., and Meek, L.A.: Cataract surgery in horses. Compend. Contin. Educ. Practicing Vet., *11:* 1396–1401, 1989.

39. Duke-Elder, S.: Congenital deformities. *In* Duke-Elder System of Ophthalmology. Vol. 3. Part 2. St Louis, C.V. Mosby, 1963.

40. Apple, D.J., and Naumann, G.O.H.: Malformations and anomalies of the eye. *In* Pathology of the Eye. New York, Springer-Verlag. 1986, pp. 63–97.

41. Coulombre, A.J.: Experimental embryology of the vertebrate eye. Invest. Ophthalmol. Vis. Sci., *4:*411–419, 1965.

42. Trapp, C.W.: Congenital maldevelopment of the eyes of a colt. Cornell Vet., *47:*467–468, 1957.

43. Saunders, L.Z., and Rubin, L.F.: Ophthalmic Pathology of Animals. New York, S. Karger, 1975.

44. Wilcock, B.P.: Ocular anomalies. *In* Comparative Ophthalmic Pathology. Edited by R.L. Peiffer. Springfield, C.C. Thomas, 1983, pp. 3–46.

45. Bistner, S.I., Rubin, L.F., and Saunders, L.Z.: Ocular lesions of bovine viral diarrhea-mucosal disease. Pathol. Vet., *7:*275–286, 1970.

46. Kahrs, R.F., Scott, F.W., and de Lahunta, A.: Congenital cerebellar hypoplasia and ocular defects in calves following bovine viral diarrhea-mucosal disease infection in pregnant cattle. J. Am. Vet. Med. Assoc., *156:*1443–1450, 1970.

47. Limborg, J., and Tonneyck-Muller, I.: Experimental studies on the relationships between eye growth and skull growth. Ophthalmologica, *173:*317–325, 1976.

48. Shenefelt, R.E.: Gross congenital malformations. Animal model: Treatment of various species with large doses of vitamin A at known stages in pregnancy. Am. J. Pathol. *66:*589–592, 1972.

49. Bendixen, H.C.: Littery occurrence of anophthalmia or microphthalmia together with other malformations in swine—presumably due to vitamin A deficiency of the maternal diet. Acta Pathol. Microbiol. Scand., *54(Suppl.):* 161–179, 1944.

50. Scott, F.W., et al.: Teratogenesis in cats associated with griseofulvin therapy. Teratology, *11:*79–86, 1974.

51. Browman, L.G.: Microphthalmia, prolactin and fertility in rats. J. Reprod. Fertil., *24:*353–360, 1971.

52. Oda, S., Watanabe, K., Fujisawa, H., and Kameyamo, Y.: Impaired development of lens fibers in genetic microphthalmia, eye lens obscolescence, Elo, of the mouse. Exp. Eye Res., *31:*673–681, 1980.

53. Jackson, C.G.: Prenatal development of the microphthalmic eye in the golden hamster. J. Morphol., *167:*65–90, 1981.

54. Roberts, S.R.: The collie eye anomaly. J. Am. Vet. Med. Assoc., *155:*859–878, 1969.

55. Laratta, L.J., Kern, T.J., and Koch, S.A.: Multiple congenital ocular defects in the akita dog. Cornell Vet., *75:*381–392, 1985.

56. Rupp, G.P., and Knight, A.P.: Congenital ocular defects in a crossbred beef herd. J. Am. Vet. Med. Assoc., *184:*1149–1150, 1984.
57. Wilson, J.G.: Present status of drugs as teratogens in man. Teratology, *7:*3–15, 1973.
58. Hjorth, P.: Atresia of the nasolacrimal duct in a horse. Nord. Vet. Med., *23:*260–262, 1971.
59. Lundvall, R.L., and Carter, J.D.: Atresia of the nasolacrimal meatus in the horse. J. Am. Vet. Med. Assoc., *159:*289–291, 1971.
60. Mason, T.A.: Atresia of the nasolacrimal orifice in two Thoroughbreds. Equine Vet. J., *11:*19–20, 1979.
61. Latimer, C.A., and Wyman, M.: Atresia of the nasolacrimal duct in three horses. J. Am. Vet. Med. Assoc., *184:*989–992, 1984.
62. Latimer, C.A., Wyman, M., Diesem, C.D., and Burt, J.K.: Radiographic and gross anatomy of the nasolacrimal duct of the horse. Am. J. Vet. Res., *45:*451–458, 1984.
63. Said, A.H., Shorky, M., Saleh, M.A., and Hegazi, A.A.: Contribution of the nasolacrimal duct of donkeys in Egypt. Anat. Histol. Embryol., *6:*347–350, 1977.
64. Frank, E.R.: Veterinary Surgery. 7th ed. Minneapolis, Burgess Publishing, 1964.
65. Roberts, E.J.: Some modern surgical operations applicable to the horse. Vet. Rec., *76:*137–147, 1964.
66. Saunders, L.Z., and Fincher, M.G.: Hereditary multiple eye defects in grade Jersey cattle. Cornell Vet., *41:*351–366, 1951.
67. Latshaw, W.K., Wyman, M., and Venzke, W.G.: Embryonic development of an anomaly of the ocular fundus in Collies. Am. J. Vet. Res., *30:*211–217, 1969.
68. McLaughlin, S.A., and Brightman, A.H.: Bilateral ocular dermoids in a colt. Equine Pract., *5:*10–12, 1983.
69. Peiffer, R.L., Jr., Williams, R., and Schenk, M.: Correction of congenital entropion in a foal. Vet. Med. Small Anim. Clin., *72:*1219–1224, 1977.
70. Senk, G.W.: Ocular discharge in young horses. *In* Current Therapy in Equine Medicine. Edited by N.E. Robinson and G.M. Schmidt. Philadelphia, W.B. Saunders, 1983, pp. 385–388.
71. Nicolas, E.: Veterinary and Comparative Ophthalmology. Translated and edited by H. Gray. London, H&W Brown, 1914.
72. Bullard, J.F.: Entropion operation in foals. J. Am. Vet. Med. Assoc., *82:*927–928, 1933.
73. Severin, G.A.: Veterinary Ophthalmology Notes. 2nd ed. Fort Collins, Colorado State University, 1976.
74. Vestre, W.A., and Brightman, A.H.: Correction of cicatricial entropion and trichiasis in the horse. Equine Pract., *2:*13–16, 1980.
75. Craven, J.R.: Significance of lesions of the cornea and lens in the examination of horses for soundness. Equine Vet. J., *3:*141–143, 1971.
76. Witzel, D.A., Joyce, J.R., and Smith, E.L.: Electroretinography of congenital night blindness in an Appaloosa filly. J. Equine Med. Surg., *1:*226–229, 1977.
77. Witzel, D.A., Riis, R.C., Rebhun, W.C., and Hillman R.B.: Night blindness in the Appaloosa: Sibling occurrence. J. Equine Med. Surg., *1:*383–386, 1977.
78. Witzel, D.A., Smith, R.D., Wilson, R.D., and Aguirre, G.D.: Congenital stationary night blindness: An animal model. Invest. Ophthalmol. Vis. Sci., *17:*788–795, 1978.
79. Rebhun, W.C., Loew, E.R., Riis, R.C., and Laratta, L.J.: Clinical manifestations of night blindness in the Appaloosa horse. Compend. Contin. Educ. Practicing Vet., *6:*S103–S106, 1984.
80. Gelatt, K.N.: Glaucoma and lens luxation in a foal. Vet. Med. Small Anim. Clin., *68:*261, 1973.
81. Mathews, A.G., and Handscombe, M.C.: Bilateral cataract formation and subluxation of the lenses in a foal: A case report. Equine Vet. J., *2(Suppl 2):*23–24, 1983.
82. Gelatt, K.N., Leipold, H.W., and Coffman, J.R.: Bilateral optic nerve hypoplasia in a colt. J. Am. Vet. Med. Assoc., *155:*627–631, 1969.
83. Gelatt, K.N.: Ophthalmoscopic studies in the normal and diseased ocular fundi of horses. J. Am. Anim. Hosp. Assoc., *7:*158–167, 1971.
84. Rebhun, W.C.: Equine retinal lesions and retinal detachments. Equine Vet. J. Suppl. 2, *2:*86–90, 1983.
85. Gelatt, K.N., and McClure, J.R.: Congenital strabismus and its correction in two Appaloosa horses. J. Equine Med. Surg., *1:*240–244, 1977.
86. Rebhun, W.C.: Diagnosis and treatment of equine uveitis. J. Am. Vet. Med. Assoc., *175:*803–808, 1979.
87. Bistner, S., and Shaw, D.: Uveitis in the horse. Compend. Contin. Educ. Practicing Vet., *2:*S35–S43, 1980.
88. Kern, T.J.: Intraocular inflammation. *In* Current Therapy in Equine Medicine. 2nd ed. Edited by N.E. Robinson and M.B. Glaze. Philadelphia, W.B. Saunders, 1987, pp. 445–450.

CHAPTER 118

DIAGNOSTIC ULTRASONOGRAPHY OF THE FOAL'S ABDOMEN

V.B. Reef

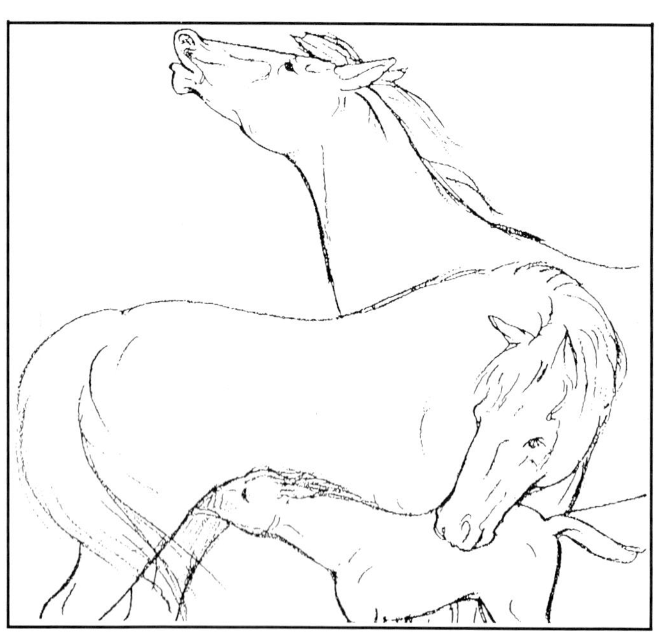

Ultrasonography is a noninvasive diagnostic technique which provides the veterinary clinician with a window through which the intra-abdominal structures and organs can be evaluated. The foal abdomen is better suited to ultrasonographic investigation than in adults because of the overall smaller size of the abdomen, better visualization of the liver and bladder during the neonatal period, relatively small size of the gas-filled large colon, and ability to position the foal (lateral recumbency or standing).[1] The preponderance of small intestinal disorders in foals presenting with colic also enables the veterinary ultrasonographer to assess many different gastrointestinal lesions.[1,2]

Sedation is usually not necessary for patient preparation except in unusually fractious foals. The foal should be prepared by clipping the hair over the portion of the abdomen under investigation with a #40 surgical clipper blade, cleaning the skin, and applying an ultrasonographic coupling jelly. Transducer selections should be based on use of the highest frequency transducer which will penetrate adequately to the area under investigation and yield optimal image quality. In most instances a 7.5- or 5.0-MHz straight linear, curved linear, or sector scanner transducer will be sufficient to perform the abdominal ultrasonographic investigations; a 3.0- or 3.5-MHz may be needed for particularly large foals. Better contact between the patient and the transducer will usually be obtained with the curved linear or sector scanner transducer, except on the ventral midline because of the abdominal curvatures. A built-in fluid bath or hand-held stand-off pad is often necessary to evaluate adequately superficial structures (umbilical remnants, bladder, and portions of the gastrointestinal tract).

GASTROINTESTINAL TRACT

Ultrasonographic evaluation of the foal abdomen and gastrointestinal tract should begin with a 7.5-MHz transducer containing a built-in fluid bath (see Figs. 118–1 to 118–5, 118–7, and 118–8) or using a hand-held stand-off pad. Ultrasonographic evaluation of the normal foal abdomen reveals little or no peritoneal fluid. Visualization of fluid with cellularity (echogenicity) is consistent with a diagnosis of peritonitis.[1–3] Fibrin strands may be imaged between the serosal surface of the bowel and other intra-abdominal structures in foals with peritonitis. Maturing adhesions appear as echogenic, thick bands between the serosal surface of the bowel or other intra-abdominal organs. Adhesions may also be suspected when no movement is detected between a portion of bowel and adjacent structures. A hemoperitoneum may be suspected if homogeneous echogenic fluid is seen within the peritoneal cavity, often with a swirling pattern caused by movement of the diaphragm and intra-abdominal structures. Flocculent echogenic fluid with free gas echoes within the peritoneal cavity should suggest a ruptured viscus (Fig. 118–1) or the possibility of a bacterial peritonitis with anaerobic involvement.[1,3] If a peritoneal fluid sample is

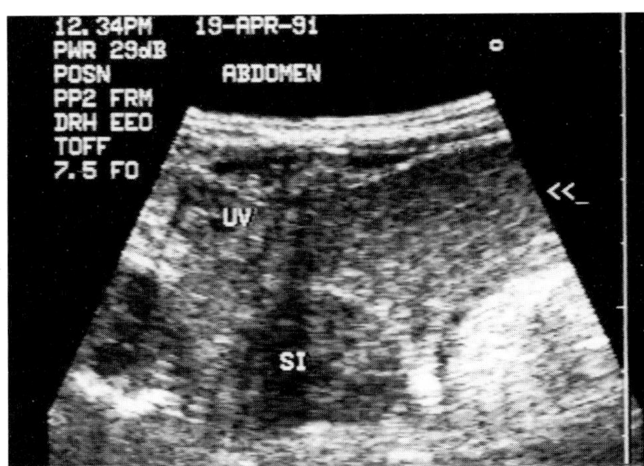

FIG. 118–1. Transverse sonogram from a 2-day-old Standardbred colt with atresia coli and a ruptured viscus. Notice the echogenic fluid in the abdomen (arrows) which is similar in echogenicity to the intestinal contents. This sonogram was obtained with a 7.5-MHz sector scanner transducer containing a built-in fluid bath. UV, Umbilical vein; SI, small intestine.

desired, the ultrasonographic examination can be used to localize fluid, minimizing risk of accidental gastrointestinal perforation from needle insertion.

SURGICAL DISORDERS

Ultrasonography has become an important part of the diagnostic workup of foals with colic. Ultrasonography can also be used to select a site for abdominal paracentesis. The higher incidence of small intestinal disorders in foals makes them uniquely suited to ultrasonographic evaluation of the gastrointestinal tract.[1] A 7.5-MHz sector scanner transducer containing a built-in fluid bath or a hand-held stand-off pad with a 7.5-MHz curved or straight linear transducer should be the choice for initial ultrasonographic evaluation of the abdomen. Edematous compromised loops of intestine are heavier, fall to the ventral aspect of the abdomen, and are readily imaged. After thorough investigation of the abdomen with this probe, a 7.5-MHz sector, curved or straight linear transducer may be used to image the deeper abdominal structures, followed by a 5.0-MHz transducer, if needed. Ultrasonographic evaluation of the gastrointestinal tract is easier with the foal standing, as gas rises dorsad and any free fluid in the abdomen provides an acoustic window through which the sonographic evaluation can be performed.

Detection of a target or bull's-eye appearance to the small intestine is diagnostic of a small intestinal intussusception[4] (Fig. 118–2). This appearance is caused by the relative different tissue densities of the central edematous intussusceptum, the outer edematous intussuscipiens, and the interposed fluid. Distention of the more proximal portions of small intestine with fluid is imaged in foals with intussusceptions or other types of strangulating obstructions.[1,3,4] Fluid and gas distention of the stomach can be visualized from the left cranial abdomen in the 7th through 9th or 10th intercostal spaces or from the ventral abdomen (neonates only) caudal to the liver.[1,3,4] Compromised intestine has thickened, hypoechoic, edematous walls with little or no detectable peristaltic activity. With complete volvulus of the small intestine the entire abdomen is filled with thickened, edematous, hypoechoic, distended loops of small intestine with no visible peristaltic activity.[1] Intramural masses and intestinal strictures have been detected ultrasonographically in foals.[1] Infection, microabscesses, and hematomas of the intestinal wall are possible causes of intramural masses in young foals; neoplasms are rare. Intraluminal masses such as ascarid and meconium impactions (Fig. 118–3) may also be visualized ultrasonographically.[1] Ascarids may be visualized within the lumen of the intestinal tract, as individuals or as a mass of echogenic curvilinear parasites. Meconium impactions may be visualized as hypoechoic to echogenic masses within the lumen of the small colon. Distention of the intestine proximal to the impaction with fluid and gas is common and may aid in the visualization of the intraluminal mass.

Large bowel displacements or torsions are difficult to diagnose ultrasonographically, but may be suspected in a foal with much gaseous distention of the large bowel and persistent unrelenting pain. Many foals with gaseous distention of the large bowel have spasmodic colic which resolves with symptomatic therapy. Displacement of gastrointestinal viscera into another body cavity, such as in a diaphragmatic hernia, may be diagnosed ultrasonographically if the edge of the diaphragm is involved, enabling direct visualization of the diaphragmatic defect. Gastrointestinal viscera are visualized in the thorax with dorsal displacement of thoracic viscera. Hernias involving the central portion of the diaphragm are not visible ultrasonographically although

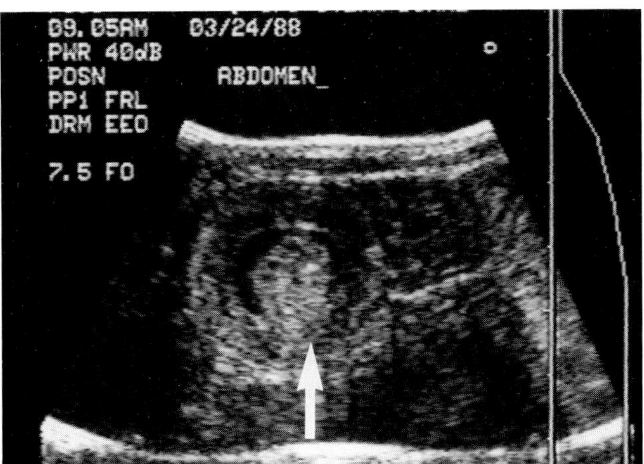

FIG. 118–2. Transverse sonogram from a 7-day-old Thoroughbred filly with an intussusception. Notice the echogenic thickened intussusceptum (arrow) surrounded by fluid and the outer hypoechoic edematous intussuscipiens. This sonogram was obtained from the ventral abdomen with a 7.5-MHz sector scanner transducer containing a built-in fluid bath.

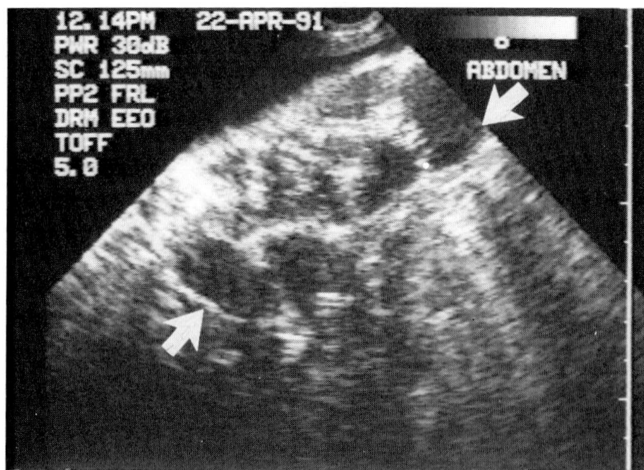

FIG. 118–3. Sagittal sonogram obtained from a 2-day-old Standardbred colt with a meconium impaction. Notice the cluster of ingesta-filled small colon in the caudal abdomen (arrows). This sonogram was obtained with a 7.5-MHz sector scanner transducer containing a built-in fluid bath. Cranial is to the right of the scan and the bladder is at the top of the scan (ventral abdomen).

gastrointestinal viscera may be imaged in the thoracic cavity. Atresia coli may be suspected if gas and fluid distention of the more proximal portions of the intestine are visualized in the absence of edematous, hypoechoic, and distended bowel. Visualization of the caudal portion of the gastrointestinal tract is usually difficult in these foals, because of the large amount of distention in the more proximal intestine. If visualized, the caudal portion of the gastrointestinal tract should appear empty. Direct ultrasonographic visualization of the atretic portion of the gastrointestinal tract has not been performed successfully in foals.

MEDICAL DISORDERS

Medical colics can often be distinguished ultrasonographically from surgical colics based on the ultrasonographic appearance and motility of the gastrointestinal tract. Fluid-filled small or large intestines with normal to increased motility are consistent with an enteritis.[1] The wall of the affected portion of the intestine may be thicker than normal, hypoechoic, and edematous if severe inflammatory bowel disease is present. Shreds or fragments of intestinal mucosa may be seen floating within the gastrointestinal contents, particularly in foals with severe necrotizing enterocolitis (Fig. 118–4). Gas echoes in the wall of the gastrointestinal tract and along the mucosal surface have been seen in foals with clostridial enteritis. Intra-abdominal abscesses have also been diagnosed ultrasonographically.[2,5] Clinical findings, clinical pathologic data, and ultrasonographic findings can complement each other and aid the clinician in arriving at or refining a diagnosis of surgical or medial colic.

URINARY TRACT

LOWER URINARY TRACT

Ultrasonographic evaluation of the neonatal bladder may be performed from the ventral abdomen using a 7.5-MHz sector scanner transducer containing a built-in fluid bath or using a curved or straight linear transducer and hand-held stand-off pad until the foal is 4 to 8 weeks old.[1,2,6] At that time, gastrointestinal viscera becomes superimposed between the bladder and ventral abdominal wall. Omphaloarteritis or urachitis may result in persistent visualization of the bladder in older foals.

The neonatal bladder is usually round or oval and filled with sonolucent fluid. This is in contrast to adult horse urine which is often echogenic, because of the large amount of mucus and calcium carbonate

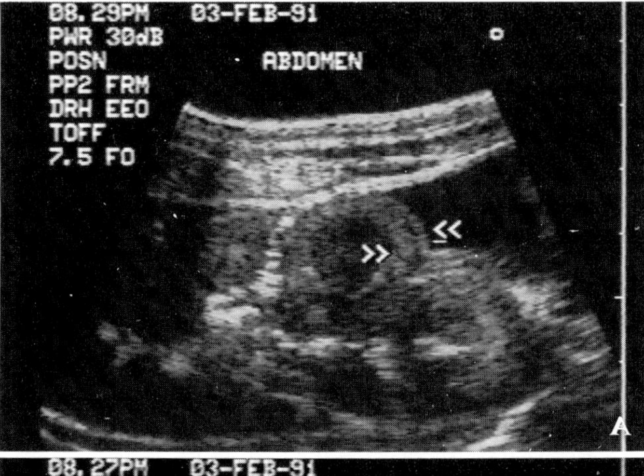

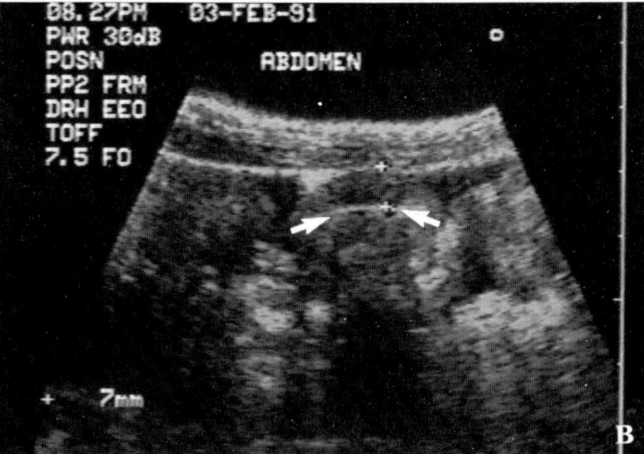

FIG. 118–4. Transverse sonogram from a 3-day-old Thoroughbred colt with colic and abdominal distention. This sonogram was obtained from the ventral abdomen with a 7.5-MHz sector scanner transducer containing a built-in fluid bath. *A*, Arrowheads point to the thickened wall of the jejunum. Notice the anechoic peritoneal fluid surrounding the jejunum. *B*, Cursors measure the thickened jejunal wall (7 mm). Notice the hyperechoic gas echo (arrows) lining the jejunal mucosa. The thickened fluid-filled jejunum and gas lining the mucosa are suggestive of a necrotizing enterocolitis. The colt subsequently developed bloody diarrhea.

crystals. Distortion of the intact neonatal bladder most commonly occurs in foals with large amounts of gastrointestinal distention. Homogeneous, echogenic to hypoechoic intraluminal masses have been seen in several foals associated with a blood clot in the bladder.[1]

Defects of the bladder wall may be visible ultrasonographically or the appearance of the bladder may suggest uroperitoneum.[1] With a bladder rupture, the bladder appears collapsed ultrasonographically. It may be folded on itself or the rent in the bladder wall may be visualized with fluid communicating between the bladder and the peritoneal cavity (Fig. 118–5). Large amounts of anechoic fluid are visible within the peritoneal cavity, and the gastrointestinal viscera float in this free fluid. Thickened edematous hypoechoic to anechoic bladder wall has been seen in a foal with a necrotic bladder and uroperitoneum, while gas echoes in the bladder wall have been imaged in foals with an emphysematous bladder and uroperitoneum. Rents in the urachus or ureters may also cause uroperitoneum. Tears in the ureter or urachus are difficult to visualize directly, but may be suspected because of the ultrasonographic appearance of the surrounding structures and the bladder. With a urachal tear, the bladder may be filled with anechoic fluid. Fluid may be imaged dissecting retroperitoneally along the urachus and falciform ligament, or the defect in the urachus may be visualized communicating with the peritoneal cavity. Ureteral ruptures are more difficult to diagnose, because the ureter is not normally visible. Accumulation of anechoic fluid around the kidney in the retroperitoneal space would indicate this possibility. The bladder of the foal with a ureteral rupture will appear intact, but may contain less urine than that of the foal with the urachal defect. This diagnosis should be suspected in foals with a large amount of anechoic fluid visible in the peritoneal cavity, an intact bladder and a normal urachus.

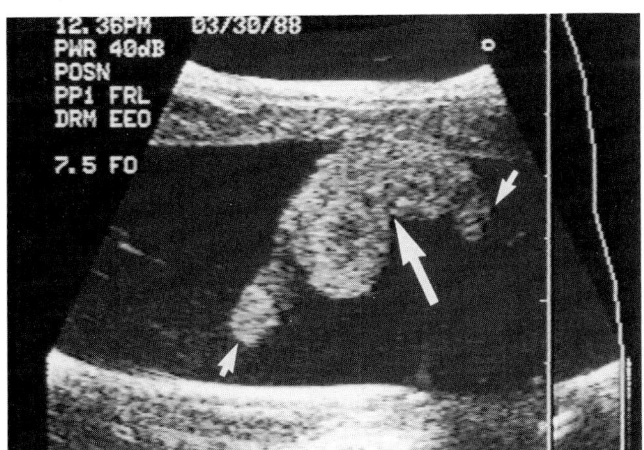

FIG. 118–5. Transverse sonogram of a collapsed bladder from a 6-day-old Thoroughbred filly with a ruptured bladder. Notice the collapsed bladder folded on itself (large arrow), the left and right umbilical arteries (small arrows), and the large quantity of anechoic fluid. The right side of the sonogram is to the left side of the foal's abdomen and the top of scan is the foal's ventral abdomen. This sonogram was obtained with a 7.5-MHz sector scanner transducer containing a built-in fluid bath.

Persistent patent urachus is visible ultrasonographically in the neonatal foal as a fluid communication extending from the bladder apex cranially to the external umbilical remnant.[1] The urachus is normally a hypoechoic area between the two umbilical arteries from the umbilicus to the bladder apex and is a potential space. A urachal diverticulum may form at the bladder apex with closure of the patent urachus. Serial evaluation of these foals is important because they are more likely to have urachitis.

UPPER URINARY TRACT

Evaluation of the foal kidneys can easily be performed from the flank area using a 7.5- or 5.0-MHz sector scanner or curved linear transducer, depending on the size of the foal and the kidney under investigation.[1,7–9] The right kidney is normally found in the dorsal portion of the abdomen between the 14th and 16th intercostal spaces in a cranial to caudal plane and between the dorsal and ventral aspects of the tuber coxae in a dorsal to ventral plane. Ultrasonographic evaluation of the right kidney can be performed with a 7.5-MHz transducer in the small foal, whereas a 5.0-MHz transducer may be needed in a larger, older individual. The left kidney is more caudal and slightly more ventral in the abdomen and is found between the 17th intercostal space and the paralumbar fossa in a cranial to caudal plane, and the dorsal aspect of the tuber coxae and the tuber ischii in a dorsal to ventral plane. This kidney is medial to the spleen and farther away from the abdominal wall. Therefore, a 5.0-MHz transducer is needed to evaluate this kidney ultrasonographically in all but the neonatal foal. Older foals may require a 3.5-MHz transducer (weanlings and yearlings).

The kidney is the least echogenic abdominal organ with a relatively anechoic medulla, echogenic renal pelvis, and hypoechoic cortex which is less echogenic than the adjacent hepatic parenchyma.[1,10] An ultrasonographic-guided biopsy can be performed if indicated.[1,11] Congenital renal anomalies are rare in foals, but cystic areas may be detected as anechoic fluid-filled portions of the kidney with acoustic enhancement of the far wall (typical of a cystic structure). Acute renal failure is most commonly seen and often results in large, swollen sonolucent kidneys (more anechoic than normal).[1,10,12,13] Echogenic kidneys are more commonly seen with any type of cellular infiltrate (inflammatory, granulomatous, and fibrotic) and often indicate chronicity.[1,10,13–15] Ultrasonographic visualization of the ureter suggests ureteral obstruction and hydroureter. Perirenal edema is rarely seen, but may be detected in foals with a ruptured ureter or renal failure (usually acute).

LIVER

The liver can be imaged from both sides of the abdomen ventral to the ventral most lung margin as well as from the cranial ventral abdomen in the neonatal foal.[1,8,9,16,17] Ultrasonographic evaluation of the foal liver is performed with a 7.5-MHz transducer in the neonate or a 5.0-MHz transducer in the older foal. Once the foal reaches 4 to 8 weeks of age, gastrointestinal viscera become interposed between the ventral abdominal wall and the liver, preventing its visualization from the cranial ventral abdomen. Hepatic parenchyma can normally be visualized on the right side of the foal abdomen from the 6th to the 15th intercostal spaces ventral to the ventral most lung margins and similarly in the left cranial abdomen from the 6th to the 9th intercostal spaces. Between 4 and 8 cm of hepatic parenchyma may normally be visualized. The entire liver is not accessible for ultrasonographic evaluation in the normal foal because of superimposed aerated lung in the thoracic cavity and gastrointestinal viscera in the cranial ventral abdomen. The caudal vena cava can often be visualized in the neonatal foal, but cannot normally be visualized in the older individuals. Estimations on hepatic size are therefore based on the amount of hepatic parenchyma that can be visualized ventral to the ventral most lung margin and are only relative estimates at best.

The hepatic parenchyma is intermediate in echogenicity between the kidney and spleen.[8,9,16,17] Visualization of the portal vein and hepatic veins is easily accomplished, whereas bile ducts are not visible in normal foals. Increased sonolucency and collapse of the hepatic parenchyma with a smaller than normal liver would suggest acute hepatocellular necrosis.[1,17] Increased echogenicity of the hepatic parenchyma can be seen with inflammatory, granulomatous, fatty, or fibrotic infiltrates in the liver but is most commonly associated with an inflammatory cell infiltrate in the young foal.[1,17,18] Foals with a marked inflammatory cell infiltrate in the liver will often have livers which appear larger than normal with a relatively diffuse increase in echogenicity of the hepatic parenchyma. Tyzzer's disease should be suspected in a foal with this ultrasonographic appearance, if the age and clinical signs are compatible. Ultrasonographic-guided biopsies can be performed to assess the area of hepatic parenchyma histopathologically.[1,11]

Miliary echogenic areas in the hepatic parenchyma have been imaged in several neonatal foals associated with microabscesses. Biliary distention with sludging of bile (echogenic debris within the biliary tree) has been detected ultrasonographically in foals with proximal duodenitis[1] (Fig. 118–6). The biliary tree has thick echogenic walls and when distended, parallel channel signs can be seen associated with the distended bile duct adjacent to the hepatic vein. The fluid within the biliary tree is more echogenic than blood in the hepatic vessels and lacks the rapid flow seen in the hepatic veins.

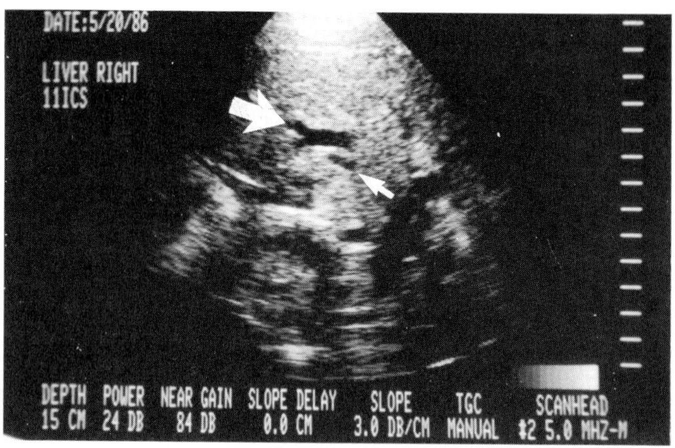

FIG. 118–6. Sagittal sonogram of the right lobe of the liver from a 3-month-old Standardbred filly with proximal duodenitis and elevated biliary enzymes. A gastrojejunostomy had been performed, and a dilated common bile duct was detected at surgery. Notice the echogenic hepatic parenchyma and parallel channel sign [dilated bile duct (small arrow) adjacent to the hepatic vein (larger arrow)]. This sonogram was obtained in the 11th intercostal space with a 5.0-MHz sector scanner transducer. Dorsal is to the right of the sonogram and ventral is to the left.

UMBILICUS

UMBILICAL REMNANTS

Umbilical remnants are visualized ultrasonographically from the ventral abdomen with a 7.5-MHz transducer containing a built-in fluid bath or using a hand-held stand-off pad (Fig. 118–7). The umbilical remnants have a characteristic size and appearance and atrophy as the foal ages.[1,6] The umbilical vein is a small, thin-walled structure usually with a fluid lumen. It may have an echogenic core associated with clot formation. The umbilical vein normally measures 6 ± 2 mm in diameter and can be followed craniad to the liver. Umbilical arteries are thicker-walled structures and usually contain an echogenic core (clot) with little or no fluid visible in the lumen. Umbilical arteries alongside the bladder usually measure 8.5 ± 2 mm in normal foals. The urachus is a potential space between the two umbilical arteries and is imaged as a small amount of hypoechoic tissue between the two arteries. The urachus with both umbilical arteries at the bladder apex normally measures 17.5 ± 4 mm in the transverse plane immediately proximal to the bladder apex.

Enlargement of the umbilical remnant structures usually indicates infection[1,19] (Fig. 118–8). If excessive hemorrhage was noticed from the umbilicus at parturition, enlargement of the umbilical vein or umbilical arteries may be detected with a large homogeneous echogenic clot in the vessel center. Thickening or edema of the vessel walls may also be imaged. These findings should resolve rapidly if associated only with excessive hemorrhage. Hypoechoic, sonolucent, or echogenic fluid in the lumen of the umbilical remnant

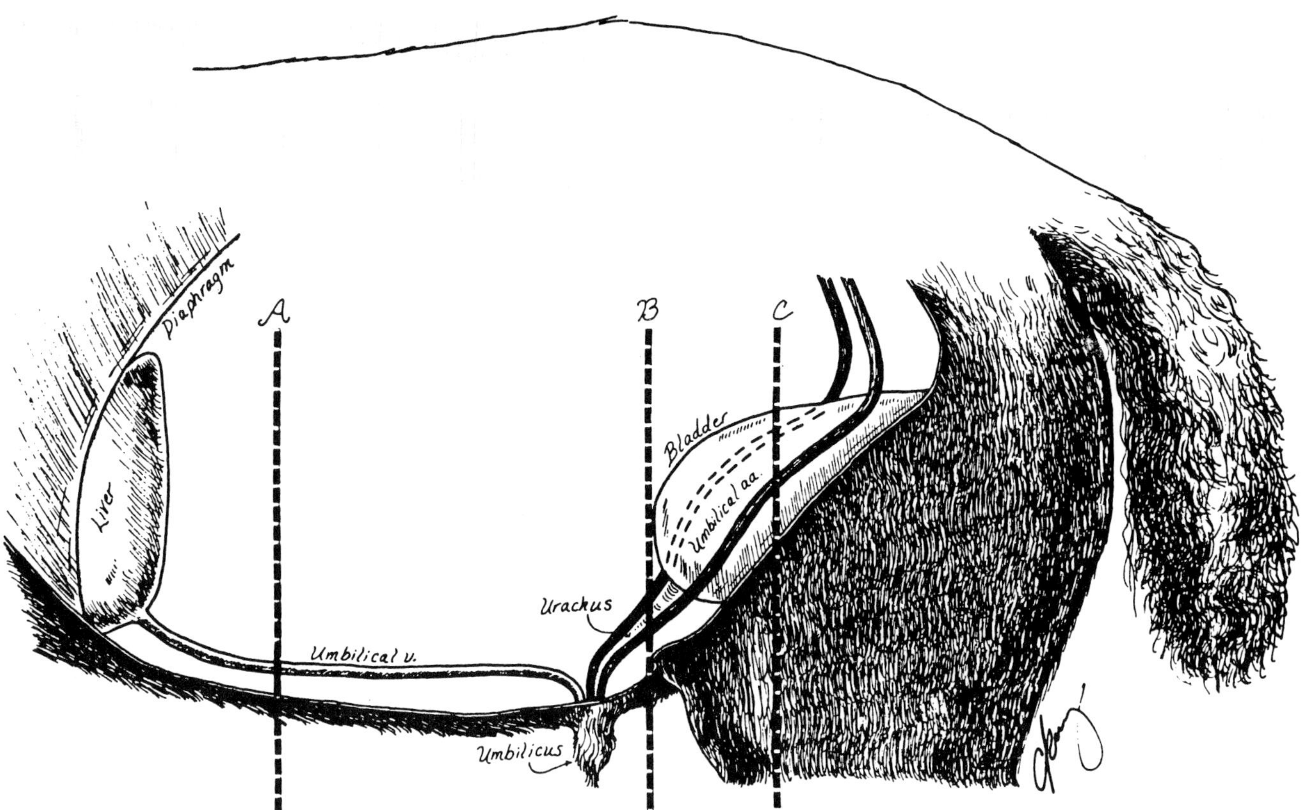

FIG. 118–7. Diagram showing the umbilical vein (v), umbilical arteries (aa), and the urachus and their relationships to the umbilicus, liver, and urinary bladder. The diagram was used to locate umbilical structures ultrasonographically. A, Anatomic region scanned to locate the umbilical vein; B, anatomic region scanned to locate the umbilical arteries and urachus; C, anatomic region scanned to locate the umbilical arteries and the bladder. (From Reef, V.B., and Collatos, C.A.: Ultrasonography of umbilical structures in clinically normal foals. Am. J. Vet. Res., *49:*2143–2146, 1988.)

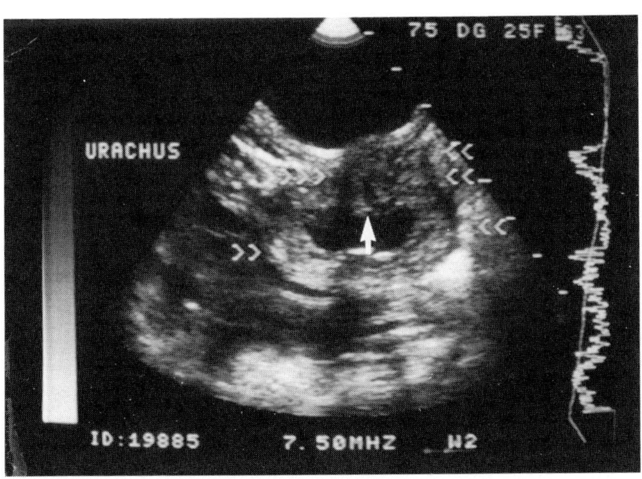

FIG. 118–8. Transverse sonogram from a 2-week-old Thoroughbred colt with a urachal abscess. Arrowheads point to the thick-walled urachus with an anechoic fluid-filled center. The large arrow points to the communication of the abscessed urachus with the external umbilical remnant. This sonogram was obtained with a 7.5-MHz sector scanner transducer containing a built-in fluid bath.

structures is usually associated with the accumulation of purulent debris.[1,19] If anaerobes are involved, free-gas echoes may be seen within the lumen of the internal umbilical structures.[19] Thickening of the wall of the umbilical remnant structure may also be imaged associated with an inflammatory infiltrate. In most affected foals, abnormalities of two or more umbilical remnant structures are detected ultrasonographically.[19]

Infections with multiple organisms are the rule, necessitating broad-spectrum antimicrobial therapy.[19] Medical therapy alone should be considered in foals with fever of unknown origin, an elevated fibrinogen, and/or leukocytosis but who are otherwise healthy.[19] Surgical resection of the infected umbilical remnants should be considered in foals with septicemia, septic arthritis, or other life-threatening infections.[19] Surgery should also be considered in foals whose umbilical remnants are greater than twice normal size or with multiple abnormal internal remnants detected ultrasonographically. The physical examination findings, history, clinical pathologic data, ultrasonographic findings, and previous antimicrobial history should be taken into consideration when deciding between medical or surgi-

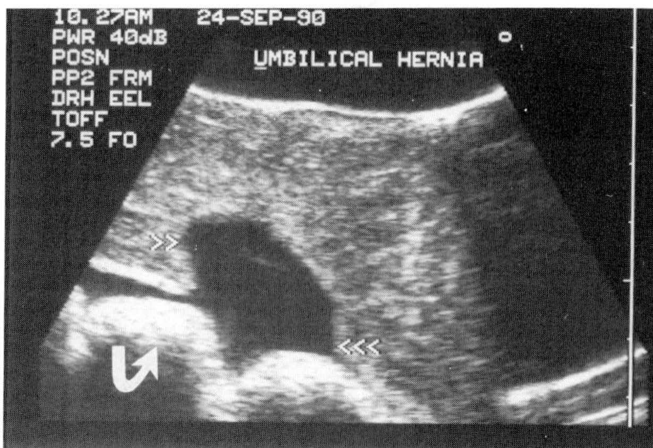

FIG. 118–9. Sagittal sonogram from a 3-month-old Thoroughbred colt with an umbilical hernia and ventral abdominal swelling. The arrowheads point to the cranial (right) and caudal (left) edge of the hernial ring. The anechoic area between the arrowheads is peritoneal fluid within the hernial sac. The hypoechoic to echogenic thickened soft tissue between the ventral abdominal skin surface and the hernial sac is typical of a cellulitis. The semicircular hyperechoic structure (curved arrow) is large colon. This sonogram was obtained with a 7.5-MHz sector scanner transducer containing a built-in fluid bath.

cal therapy. If medical therapy is selected, ultrasonographic re-evaluation should be performed in 3 to 5 days, because changes can occur rapidly. If internal umbilical remnant structures are enlarged from previous examination, a switch in antimicrobial therapy or surgical resection should be considered.

HERNIAS

Ultrasonographic evaluation of a hernia can determine the hernial contents (intestine, omentum, and fluid), size of the hernial ring, and presence of a subcutaneous swelling or abscess[1] (Fig. 118–9). The viability of the intestine within the hernia can be evaluated by assessing wall thickness, echogenicity, distention, and motility.[1] This can be performed successfully for umbilical, inguinal or ventral abdominal wall hernias.

In summary, ultrasonographic evaluation enables the clinician to assess much of the abdominal viscera noninvasively that was previously difficult to assess using other diagnostic techniques. The examination is well tolerated by the neonatal foal and can readily be performed with portable ultrasonographic equipment. The technique can aid in distinguishing between a medical or surgical lesion, obtaining a biopsy or aspirate, and helping to form a diagnostic plan.

REFERENCES

1. Reef, V.B.: The use of diagnostic ultrasound in the horse. Ultrasound Q., *9,* 1–34, 1991.
2. Byars, T.D., and Halley, J.: Uses of ultrasound in equine internal medicine. Vet. Clin. North Am. Equine Pract., *2:*253–258, 1986.
3. Rantanen, N.W.: Diseases of the abdomen. Vet. Clin. North Am. Equine Pract., *2:*67–88, 1986.
4. Bernard, W.V., et al.: Ultrasonographic diagnosis of small-intestinal intussusception in three foals. J. Am. Vet. Med. Assoc., *194:*395–397, 1989.
5. Hanselaer, J.R., and Nyland, T.G.: Chyloabdomen and ultrasonographic detection of an intra-abdominal abscess in a foal. J. Am. Vet. Med. Assoc., *183:*1465–1467, 1983.
6. Reef, V.B., and Collatos, C.A.: Ultrasonography of umbilical structures in clinically normal foals. Am. J. Vet. Res., *49:*2143–2146, 1988.
7. Rantanen, N.W.: Diseases of the kidneys. Vet. Clin. North Am. Equine Pract., *2:*89–103, 1986.
8. James, A.E., et al.: The use of compound B-mode ultrasound in abdominal disease of animals. J. Am. Vet. Radiol. Soc., *17:*106–112, 1976.
9. Yamaga, Y., and Too, K.: Diagnostic ultrasound imaging in domestic animals: Fundamental studies on abdominal organs and fetuses. Jpn. J. Vet. Sci., *46:*203–212, 1984.
10. Pennick, D.G., Eisenberg, H.M., Teuscher, E.E., and Vrins, A.: Equine renal ultrasonography: Normal and abnormal. Vet. Radiol., *27:*81–84, 1986.
11. Modransky, P.D.: Ultrasound-guided renal and hepatic biopsy techniques. Vet. Clin. North Am. Equine Pract., *2:*115–126, 1986.
12. Bayly, W.M., et al.: A reproducible means of studying acute renal failure in horses. Cornell Vet., *76:*287–298, 1986.
13. Kiper, M.L., Traub-Dargatz, J.L., and Wrigley, R.H.: Renal ultrasonography in horses. Compend. Contin. Educ. Practicing Vet., *12:*993–1000, 1990.
14. Ehnen, S.J., Divers, T.J., Gillette, D., and Reef, V.: Obstructive nephrolithiasis and ureterolithiasis associated with chronic renal failure in horses: Eight cases (1981–1987). J. Am. Vet. Med. Assoc., *197:*249–253, 1990.
15. Hope, W.D., et al.: Chronic renal failure associated with bilateral nephroliths and ureteroliths in a two-year-old Thoroughbred colt. Equine Vet. J., *21:*228–231, 1989.
16. Rantanen, N.W.: Ultrasound appearance of normal lung borders and adjacent viscera in the horse. Vet. Radiol., *22:*217–219, 1981.
17. Rantanen, N.W.: Diseases of the liver. Vet. Clin. North Am. Equine Pract., *2:*104–114, 1986.
18. Reef, V.B., Johnston, J.K., Divers, T.J., and Acland, H.: Ultrasonographic findings in horses with cholelithiasis: Eight cases (1985–1987). J. Am. Vet. Med. Assoc., *196:*1836–1840, 1990.
19. Reef, V.B., et al.: Clinical, ultrasonographic and surgical findings in foals with umbilical remnant infections. J. Am. Vet. Med. Assoc., *195:*69–72, 1989.

APPENDICES

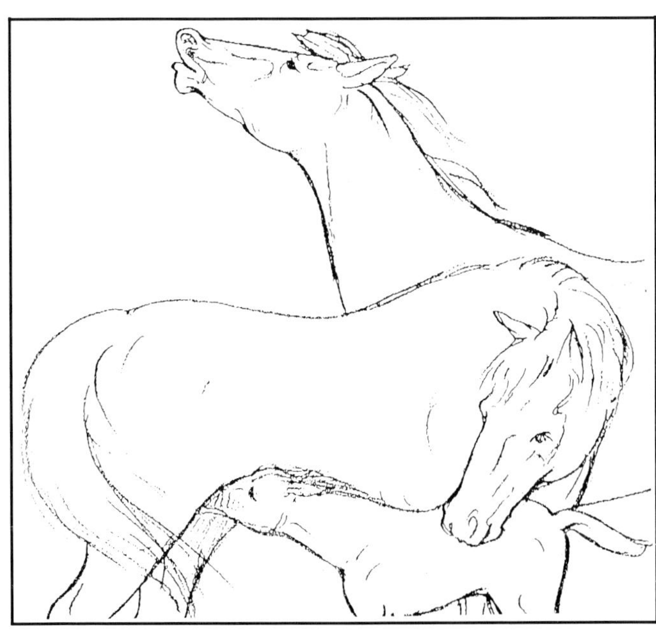

APPENDIX I

BREEDING RECORDS

A. O. McKinnon

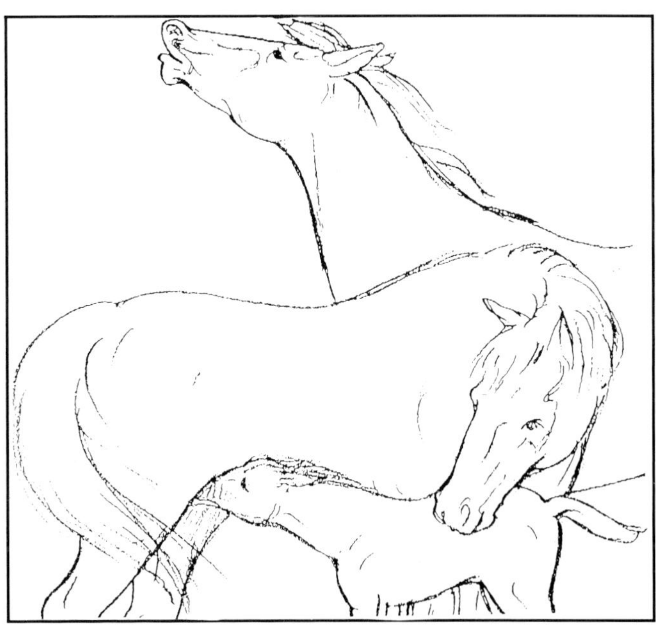

Breeding records are one of the most important records kept by an equine practitioner. They are essential for effective reproductive management, necessary for invoicing, and valuable for historic information and future predictive performance.

Record keeping can be frustrating. Records take time, and most of us struggle throughout our career to find an optimal system. A successful system is one that provides accurate information that is readily available, quick to record, provides permanent information, and can be used expediently for medical, historic, or billing purposes.

Our hospital has managed over 1600 brood mares annually with widely varied levels of both veterinary and breeding farm management. Perhaps one of the most important observations has been that quality of breeding farm management and thus our input varies enormously. Regardless of this, and our perception of economic constraints, our responsibility is to provide accurate information regarding each mare, on each farm, in a manner that facilitates maximizing reproductive efficiency and minimizing costs. To this end, accurate records are essential. This section briefly outlines records used at the Goulburn Valley Equine Hospital (GVEH). It is possible that this system is only appropriate for our use. We understand many other personal preferences exist and that each veterinary practice develops a system with which they are comfortable. We hope that where improvement in these records becomes obvious to readers they take time to communicate their ideas.

REASONS TO KEEP RECORDS

Accurate, complete breeding records are useful and/or necessary for the following reasons:

1. information on the breeding farm for daily management of breeding and treatments
2. monthly or seasonal invoicing
3. litigation
4. permanent records for clients and breeding farms
5. immediate and retrospective analysis of individual breeding problems
6. analysis of current and past breeding performances of stallions, mares (by category—wet, dry, maiden), and breeding farm management
7. retrospective analysis of data for research purposes.

During the height of a busy breeding season, the most important parameters would appear to be accessibility of data for daily decisions and accurate reporting for invoicing. Many possibilities for record keeping exist and range from sophisticated computer management to generic tear off carbon copies that are delivered to the breeding farm and/or practice secretary on a daily basis.

In many cases, the volume of work dictates the level of recording. For example, on a busy breeding farm without a designated record keeper, the recording of data on computer at the time of examination may be detrimental to the speed and efficiency of the operation

(text continues on page 1108)

GOULBURN VALLEY EQUINE HOSPITAL

P.O. BOX 2020, SHEPPARTON, 3630 — TELEPHONE: (058) 299 566 — FAX: (058) 299 307

DR. J. R. VASEY, B.V.Sc., Dip.Vet.Surg., F.A.C.V.Sc.
SPECIALISTS IN EQUINE REPRODUCTION AND SURGERY
AND ASSOCIATES
DR. A. O. McKINNON, B.V.Sc., M.Sc., Dip. Vet. Med., Diplomate A.C.T./A.B.V.P.

Breeding Record

Mare No. ....

Stud: .... **Mare Name:** ....

Address: ....

.... Phone: .... Brand: ....

Arrived at Farm: .... Departed: .... Booked to: ....

Colour: .... Assess. No.: .... Year of Birth: .... Insured: YES / NO

Owner's Name: .... Phone: ....

Address: .... Status of Mare: ....

Due: .... Foaled: .... Foal Sex: M/F Colour: .... Sire: ....

History: Has mare had infection in her reproductive tract, a difficult foaling or any other breeding problems? ....

.... Last Foaled: ....

	1	2	3	4	5	6	7	8	9	10	11	12	13	14	15	16	17	18	19	20	21	22	23	24	25	26	27	28	29	30	31
SEPTEMBER																															
OCTOBER																															
NOVEMBER																															
DECEMBER																															
JANUARY																															
FEBRUARY																															
MARCH																															

Date	Details	Left Ovary	Right Ovary	Cervix	Folds	Fluid

PREGNANCY DATA

Date	Day of Gestation	Vesicle Size	Embryo/Heart Beat	Remarks	Re-examine

The above named mare was confirmed pregnant / non pregnant at or greater than 45 days of gestation on ..../........../..........
On that day she had a normally developing single pregnancy. This was her final pregnancy test.
The mare has / has not been caslicked. It is important to open the caslick prior to foaling.

FIG. A1–1. Breeding records for mares at stud used by the GVEH. Records are produced on cardboard sheets and photostatted monthly or when appropriate for billing purposes.

GOULBURN VALLEY EQUINE HOSPITAL

P.O. BOX 2020, SHEPPARTON, 3630 — TELEPHONE: (058) 299 566 — FAX: (058) 299 307
DR. J. R. VASEY, B.V.Sc., Dip.Vet.Surg., F.A.C.V.Sc.
SPECIALISTS IN EQUINE REPRODUCTION AND SURGERY
AND ASSOCIATES
DR. A. O. McKINNON, B.V.Sc., M.Sc., Dip. Vet. Med., Diplomate A.C.T./A.B.V.P.

Mare Fertility Evaluation

	Name	Address	Phone (work/home)
OWNER	....	....	......../........
		....	
VETERINARIAN	....	....	......../........
		....	

METHOD OF IDENTIFICATION .... **MARE NAME:** ....

DATE .... PLACE OF EXAMINATION ....

AGE .... BREED .... MARKINGS ....

....

Maiden .... Barren .... Foaling* .... EED* .... Abortion* .... *(Date .... Day of gestation ....)

HISTORY OF REPRODUCTIVE PROBLEMS: ....

....

....

....

PREVIOUS REPRODUCTIVE EXAMINATION FINDINGS: ....

....

....

PREVIOUS REPRODUCTIVE SURGERIES, UTERINE TREATMENTS OR HORMONE TREATMENTS: ....

....

....

FERTILITY EVALUATION:

1. Physical Condition: ....
2. External Perineal Conformation: Normal .... Low Pelvis .... Tilted Vulva .... Sunken Anus ....
   Other ....
3. Rectal Examination: ....
   ....
4. Vaginal Examination: ....
   ....
5. Ultrasonographic Examination: ....
   ....
   ....
6. Uterine Culture: ....
   ....
7. Uterine Cytology: ....
   ....
8. Uterine Biopsy (see attached biopsy sheet): ....
   ....

INTERPRETIVE SUMMARY AND RECOMMENDATION: ....

....

....

....

....

....

....

....

....

....

....

....

....

....

....

FIG. A1–2. Mare fertility evaluation form used at the GVEH.

GOULBURN VALLEY EQUINE HOSPITAL

P.O. BOX 2020, SHEPPARTON, 3630 — TELEPHONE: (058) 299 566 — FAX: (058) 299 307

DR. J. R. VASEY, B.V.Sc., Dip.Vet.Surg., F.A.C.V.Sc. — SPECIALISTS IN EQUINE REPRODUCTION AND SURGERY AND ASSOCIATES — DR. A. O. McKINNON, B.V.Sc., M.Sc., Dip. Vet. Med., Diplomate A.C.T./A.B.V.P.

Mare Uterine Biopsy

	Name	Address	Phone (work/home)
OWNER	....	....	......../........
		....	
VETERINARIAN	....	....	......../........
		....	

MARE ....

DATE .... AGE .... BREED .... **MARE NAME:** ....

REPRODUCTIVE HISTORY: ....

REPRODUCTIVE EXAMINATION: ....

ENDOMETRIAL EPITHELIUM

_____ Tall Columnar ....
_____ Columnar ....
_____ Cuboidal ....
_____ Partly Sloughed ....
_____ Vacuolated Cytoplasm with Debris ....
_____ Infiltrated with Neutrophils ....
_____ Elevated Nuclei ....
_____ Laterally Flattened Nuclei ....
_____ Other ....

CONNECTIVE TISSUE

_____ Congested Capillaries ....
_____ Haemmorrhages ....
_____ Relatively Loose, Edematous ....
_____ Relatively Dense ....
_____ Increased Protein Rich Fluid ....
_____ Increased Between Glands ....
_____ Increased Superficially ....
_____ Increased Throughout ....
_____ Focal Necrosis ....
_____ Dilated/Cystic Lymphatics ....
_____ Other ....

UTERINE GLANDS

_____ Numerous ....
_____ Reduced in Number ....
_____ Few ....
_____ Small ....
_____ Epithelium Tall Columnar ....
_____ Epithelium Low Columnar or Cuboidal ....
_____ Frothy Cytoplasm of Epithelium ....
_____ Glands Curcumscribed by Fibrocytes ....
_____ Dilated Lumen ....
_____ Cell Debris in Lumen ....
_____ Luminal Secretion Inspissated ....
_____ Clumped Glands ....
_____ Other ....

INFLAMMATORY CELLS

_____ 1. Neutrophils ....
_____ 2. Lymphocytes ....
_____ 3. Eosinophils ....
_____ 4. Histiocytes ....
_____ 5. Plasma Cells ....
_____ 6. Lightly Pigmented Macrophages ....
_____ 7. Darkly Pigmented Macrophages ....
_____ Occasional ....
_____ Increased Mildly ....
_____ Increased Moderately ....
_____ Increased Severely ....
_____ Scattered ....
_____ Aggregated ....
_____ Immediately Under and/or in Epithelium ....
_____ Around Glands ....
_____ Between Glands ....
_____ Around Blood Vessels ....

SUMMARY OF UTERINE ABNORMALITIES:

Acute	0	1	2	3
Chronic	0	1	2	3
Fibrotic	0	1	2	3

INTERPRETIVE SUMMARY: ....

FIG. A1–3. Mare uterine biopsy form used at the GVEH.

GOULBURN VALLEY EQUINE HOSPITAL

1.

P.O. BOX 2020, SHEPPARTON, 3630 — TELEPHONE: (058) 299 566 — FAX: (058) 299 307

DR. J. R. VASEY, B.V.Sc., Dip.Vet.Surg., F.A.C.V.Sc.

SPECIALISTS IN EQUINE REPRODUCTION AND SURGERY

DR. A. O. McKINNON, B.V.Sc., M.Sc., Dip. Vet. Med., Diplomate A.C.T./A.B.V.P.

AND ASSOCIATES

Stallion Fertility Evaluation

	Name	Address	Phone (work/home)
OWNER	....	....	......../........
		....	
VETERINARIAN	....	....	......../........
		....	

STALLION NAME .... BREED .... BODY CONDITION ....

AGE .... WEIGHT .... METHOD OF IDENTIFICATION ....

....

BREEDING HISTORY ....

....

....

....

....

....

REASON FOR EXAMINATION: 1. Pre-Purchase .... 2. Pre-Breeding Season .... 3. Post-Breeding ....

4. Other ....

PHYSICAL EXAMINATION:

General: ....

....

Specific: ....

....

....

....

GENITAL EXAMINATION:

____ Penis ....

____ Prepuce ....

____ Testicles and Epididymides ....

....

____ Total Scrotal Width ....

____ Internal Reproductive Tract Examination ....

....

____ Special Examinations ....

....

....

FIG. A1–4(a–c). Stallion fertility evaluation form used at the GVEH.

GOULBURN VALLEY EQUINE HOSPITAL

2.

P.O. BOX 2020, SHEPPARTON, 3630 — TELEPHONE: (058) 299 566 — FAX: (058) 299 307

DR. J. R. VASEY, B.V.Sc., Dip.Vet.Surg., F.A.C.V.Sc.

SPECIALISTS IN EQUINE REPRODUCTION AND SURGERY

AND ASSOCIATES

DR. A. O. McKINNON, B.V.Sc., M.Sc., Dip. Vet. Med., Diplomate A.C.T./A.B.V.P.

Stallion Fertility Evaluation

SEMINAL EVALUATION

STALLION NAME .... DATE .... TIME ....

PLACE .... COLLECTOR ....

EJACULATE: .... a) Mount Source .... b) Number of Mounts ....

c) Libido ....

d) Total Seminal Volume .... Gel Volume .... Gel-free Volume ....

e) Concentration of Spermatozoa (10†/ml) ....

f) Total Sperm per Ejaculate (10@) ....

g) Motility: Raw .... Extended .... Cooled ....

h) Morphology: Normal ....• Abnormal ....••

* For specific abnormalities refer to Stallion Spermatozoal Morphologic Examination sheet.

i) Bacterial Examination:

Prepuce .... Urethra .... Semen ....

EJACULATE: .... a) Mount Source .... b) Number of Mounts ....

c) Libido ....

d) Total Seminal Volume .... Gel Volume .... Gel-free Volume ....

e) Concentration of Spermatozoa (10†/ml) ....

f) Total Sperm per Ejaculate (10@) ....

g) Motility: Raw .... Extended .... Cooled ....

h) Morphology: Normal ....• Abnormal ....••

* For specific abnormalities refer to Stallion Spermatozoal Morphologic Examination sheet.

i) Bacterial Examination:

Prepuce .... Urethra .... Semen ....

INTERPRETIVE SUMMARY: ....

....

....

....

....

....

....

....

....

....

....

....

FIG. A1–4(b).

GOULBURN VALLEY EQUINE HOSPITAL

3.

P.). BOX 2020, SHEPPARTON, 3630 — TELEPHONE: (058) 299 566 — FAX: (058) 299 307
DR. J. R. VASEY, B.V.Sc., Dip.Vet.Surg., F.A.C.V.Sc.
SPECIALISTS IN EQUINE REPRODUCTION AND SURGERY
AND ASSOCIATES
DR. A. O. McKINNON, B.V.Sc., M.Sc., Dip. Vet. Med., Diplomate A.C.T./A.B.V.P.

Stallion Fertility Evaluation

STALLION SPERMATOZOAL MORPHOLOGIC EXAMINATION

STALLION NAME .... DATE .... TIME ....

PLACE .... EXAMINER ....

EJACULATE: .... Normal ....• Abnormal ....•

HEAD ABNORMALITY	MIDPIECE ABNORMALITY	TAIL ABNORMALITY
___ microcephalic	___ abaxial*	___ absent
___ macrocephalic	___ separated neck	___ kinked
___ pyriform	___ proximal droplet	___ bent
___ other	___ distal droplet	___ thread-like
	___ swollen	___ two-headed
MISCELLANEOUS	___ thread-like	___ single loop
___ live	___ bent	___ double loop
___ dead	___ looped	___ coiled
	___ other	___ other

EJACULATE: .... Normal ....• Abnormal ....•

HEAD ABNORMALITY	MIDPIECE ABNORMALITY	TAIL ABNORMALITY
___ microcephalic	___ abaxial*	___ absent
___ macrocephalic	___ separated neck	___ kinked
___ pyriform	___ proximal droplet	___ bent
___ other	___ distal droplet	___ thread-like
	___ swollen	___ two-headed
MISCELLANEOUS	___ thread-like	___ single loop
___ live	___ bent	___ double loop
___ dead	___ looped	___ coiled
___	___ other	___ other

COMMENTS/INTERPRETATION: ....

FIG. A1–4(c).

GOULBURN VALLEY EQUINE HOSPITAL

1.

P.O. BOX 2020, SHEPPARTON, 3630 — TELEPHONE: (058) 299 566 — FAX: (058) 299 307

DR. J. R. VASEY, B.V.Sc., Dip.Vet.Surg., F.A.C.V.Sc.

SPECIALISTS IN EQUINE REPRODUCTION AND SURGERY AND ASSOCIATES

DR. A. O. McKINNON, B.V.Sc., M.Sc., Dip. Vet. Med., Diplomate A.C.T./A.B.V.P.

Embryo Donor Information

	Name	Address	Phone (work/home)
OWNER	....	....	......../........
VETERINARIAN	....	....	......../........

MARE NAME .... MARE FERTILITY EVALUATION FORM NUMBER ....

BREED .... AGE .... COLOUR ....

MARKINGS ....

ARRIVAL DATE .... DEPARTURE DATE ....

VACCINATION DATES .... ANTHELMINTHIC TREATMENT DATES ....

REPRODUCTIVE HISTORY: ....

OESTROUS BEHAVIOUR

Month/Day	1	2	3	4	5	6	7	8	9	10	11	12	13	14	15	16	17	18	19	20	21	22	23	24	25	26	27	28	29	30	31

EMBRYO COLLECTION DATA

Date ...., Day After Ovulation ...., Fluid In/Out ..../........,
......../........, .../........, Flush Quality ...., Embryo Recovery ....

Date ...., Day After Ovulation ...., Fluid In/Out ..../........,
......../........, .../........, Flush Quality ...., Embryo Recovery ....

Date ...., Day After Ovulation ...., Fluid In/Out ..../........,
......../........, .../........, Flush Quality ...., Embryo Recovery ....

Date ...., Day After Ovulation ...., Fluid In/Out ..../........,
......../........, .../........, Flush Quality ...., Embryo Recovery ....

Date ...., Day After Ovulation ...., Fluid In/Out ..../........,
......../........, .../........, Flush Quality ...., Embryo Recovery ....

EMBRYO TRANSFER DATA

Embryo Recipient ...., Date ...., Outcome ...., Ipsilateral/Contralateral, Surgical/Non-Surgical,
Surgeon/Technician ..../........, Embryo Age ...., Embryo Size ....,
Embryo Morphology ...., Donor/Recipient Synchrony ....,
Embryo Recipient Synchrony ...., Manipulation Data ....

Embryo Recipient ...., Date ...., Outcome ...., Ipsilateral/Contralateral, Surgical/Non-Surgical,
Surgeon/Technician ..../........, Embryo Age ...., Embryo Size ....,
Embryo Morphology ...., Donor/Recipient Synchrony ....,
Embryo Recipient Synchrony ...., Manipulation Data ....

Embryo Recipient ...., Date ...., Outcome ...., Ipsilateral/Contralateral, Surgical/Non-Surgical,
Surgeon/Technician ..../........, Embryo Age ...., Embryo Size ....,
Embryo Morphology ...., Donor/Recipient Synchrony ....,
Embryo Recipient Synchrony ...., Manipulation Data ....

FIG. A1–5(a–b). Mare embryo transfer form used at the GVEH.

GOULBURN VALLEY EQUINE HOSPITAL 2.

P.O. BOX 2020, SHEPPARTON, 3630 — TELEPHONE: (058) 299 566 — FAX: (058) 299 307

DR. *J. R. VASEY,* B.V.Sc., Dip.Vet.Surg., F.A.C.V.Sc.

SPECIALISTS IN EQUINE REPRODUCTION AND SURGERY

AND *ASSOCIATES*

DR. *A. O. McKINNON,* B.V.Sc., M.Sc., Dip. Vet. Med., Diplomate A.C.T./A.B.V.P.

Embryo Donor Information

REPRODUCTIVE EXAMINATION RECORDS

Date	Left Ovary	Right Ovary	Cervix	Folds	Fluid	Treatment	Bred/Transport/Other

FIG. A1–5(b).

GOULBURN VALLEY EQUINE HOSPITAL

1.

P.O. BOX 2020, SHEPPARTON, 3630 — TELEPHONE: (058) 299 566 — FAX: (058) 299 307

DR. J. R. VASEY,
B.V.Sc., Dip.Vet.Surg., F.A.C.V.Sc.

SPECIALISTS IN EQUINE REPRODUCTION AND SURGERY

DR. A. O. McKINNON,
B.V.Sc., M.Sc., Dip. Vet. Med., Diplomate A.C.T./A.B.V.P.

AND ASSOCIATES

Embryo Recipient Data

MARE DATA

BRAND No. .... COLOUR .... MARKINGS ....

....

BREED .... AGE .... SIZE .... WEIGHT ....

REPRODUCTIVE STATUS .... ACQUISITION DATE ....

VACCINATION DATES .... ANTHELMINTIC TREATMENT (DATES) ....

Transfer Attempt	Date	Donor	Outcome

OESTROUS BEHAVIOUR

Month/Day	1	2	3	4	5	6	7	8	9	10	11	12	13	14	15	16	17	18	19	20	21	22	23	24	25	26	27	28	29	30	31

REPRODUCTIVE EXAMINATION RECORDS

Date	Left Ovary	Right Ovary	Cervix	Folds	Fluid	Transfer Data

FIG. A1–6(a–b). Mare embryo recipient form used at the GVEH.

GOULBURN VALLEY EQUINE HOSPITAL 2.
P.O. BOX 2020, SHEPPARTON, 3630 — TELEPHONE: (058) 299 566 — FAX: (058) 299 307
SPECIALISTS IN EQUINE REPRODUCTION AND SURGERY
DR. J. R. VASEY, B.V.Sc., Dip.Vet.Surg., F.A.C.V.Sc.
DR. A. O. McKINNON, B.V.Sc., M.Sc., Dip. Vet. Med., Diplomate A.C.T./A.B.V.P.
AND ASSOCIATES

Embryo Recipient Data

Date	Left Ovary	Right Ovary	Cervix	Folds	Fluid	Other

TRANSFER DATA

Donor ...., Date ...., Transfer Attempt Number .... (recipient), Ipsilateral/Contralateral,
Surgical/Non-Surgical, Surgeon/Technician ..../.........., Embryo Age ...., Embryo Size ....
Embryo Morphology ....
Donor/Recipient Synchrony ...., Embryo/Recipient Synchrony ...., Manipulation Data ....

Donor ...., Date ...., Transfer Attempt Number .... (recipient), Ipsilateral/Contralateral,
Surgical/Non-Surgical, Surgeon/Technician ..../.........., Embryo Age ...., Embryo Size ....
Embryo Morphology ....
Donor/Recipient Synchrony ...., Embryo/Recipient Synchrony ...., Manipulation Data ....

Donor ...., Date ...., Transfer Attempt Number .... (recipient), Ipsilateral/Contralateral,
Surgical/Non-Surgical, Surgeon/Technician ..../.........., Embryo Age ...., Embryo Size ....
Embryo Morphology ....
Donor/Recipient Synchrony ...., Embryo/Recipient Synchrony ...., Manipulation Data ....

PREGNANCY DATA

Date	Day of Gestation	Vesicle Size	Embryo/Heart Beat	Remarks	Re-examine

FIG. A1–6(b).

and may reduce the actual volume of the work performed by the veterinarian during the course of the day without improving the most important aspect of our management—fertility. In general, computerized records are slow and inappropriate for instant decisions, despite being excellent for billing and retrospective analysis. These programs are not yet either fast enough nor interactive enough, and in addition, many force clients into buying a computer or keeping a second set of records. It is here that our obligations for providing client service and servicing our own needs start to diverge. We hope that in the future the development of faster, less expensive lap-top computers will simplify entering information, and that daily updated disks for each breeding farm can be left with the farm personnel and a copy kept safely with the veterinarian between visits.

Our experiences with carbon-copy records are less than ideal. We found the quality reproduction on the bottom few of the five sheets per record to be poor, and they were not amenable to safe, long-term storage. Multiple (five) sheets were necessary to supply continuous information for billing purposes, and extremely thin sheets were necessary to reduce bulk.

Our current preference is for individual mare records printed on sturdy cardboard (Fig. A1–1), which are left on the farm. This, of course, implies the existence of considerable trust between breeding farm management and the veterinarian; also, there is always a risk of lost or destroyed records. The records are photostatted each month and used for invoicing. This system is typical in that it is not ideal; however, it represents a compromise that works well for us. It is expedient, accurate, and useful. The major drawback relates to record security, but this problem is minimized when breeding farms adopt this record for their own management system.

OTHER RECORDS

Depending on the level of reproductive management and the selection of patients or referral work in each practice, other permanent reproductive records may be necessary. Figures A1–2 through A1–6 are examples of some other records kept at the GVEH.

APPENDIX II

BREEDING EFFICIENCY

J. L. Voss

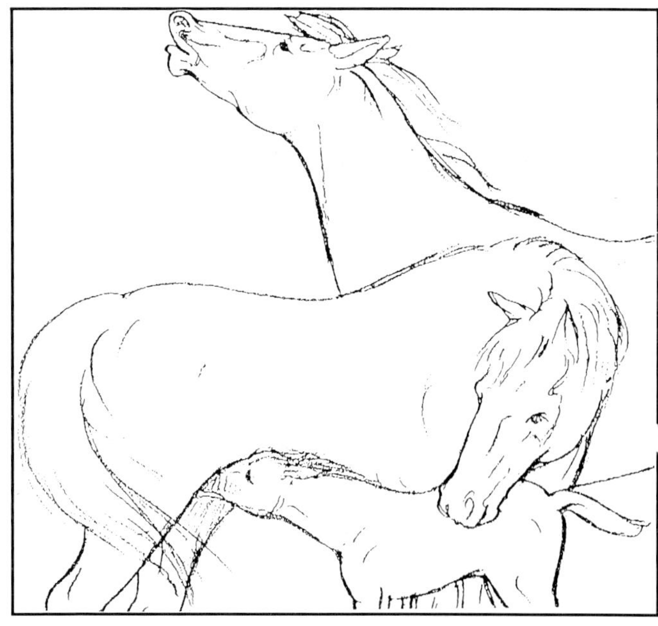

The number of live foals that reach an age for use or sale is the ultimate measure of reproductive efficiency. Without usable, salable offspring, the equine breeder cannot survive economically. Many veterinary clinicians, farm managers, and owners use the overall pregnancy rate (usually determined at or before 50 days of pregnancy) as the primary method of evaluating reproductive efficiency. Unfortunately, although meaningful, such a single criterion has limited management application because many other factors evaluate reproductive efficiency more accurately.

To procure foals born as close to January 1 (Northern Hemisphere) as possible, the artificial breeding season places great stress on a seasonally breeding animal such as the horse. In many instances, breeding begins when the mare has not yet fully entered the normal physiologic breeding season and the stallion is producing only slightly more than half the spermatozoa per ejaculate than it will produce later in the breeding season (June/July). Consequently, careful evaluation of a variety of criteria in both the stallion and the mare is necessary to assess and effectively manage breeding programs.

Fertilization rate is of limited value because present technology in horses does not allow accurate measurement. Pregnancy rate can be accurately measured from about day 7 after ovulation, by means of embryo recovery, or from around day 12 after ovulation, by means of ultrasonography. Fertilization is when a spermatozoon fuses with an ovum. Evidence exists that a high fertilization rate (95+%) occurs in cattle, humans, and horses. A significantly smaller percentage of fertilized ova remains viable and is lost during the first few days and weeks following fertilization. Consequently, other factors such as pregnancy rates per cycle and per month, embryo recovery, early embryonic death, pregnancy loss, and foaling rate should be determined and recorded. In the stallion, these same criteria, in addition to services per pregnancy, services per season, and pregnancy rate per category of mare bred, are helpful evaluators of potential fertility.

Overwhelming evidence in this text indicates a multitude of management procedures and diseases that can reduce reproductive efficiency from fertilization through the neonatal period. Evidence also exists that mares are as fertile as other domestic species and in fact may be improving with time. Perhaps subfertility associated with failure of the corpus luteum, early embryonic death, and other losses of the conceptus has improved with management. If the veterinary profession is to provide necessary leadership, it is essential that clinicians use a variety of criteria to evaluate reproductive efficiency and incorporate results into management practices.

No matter how one evaluates fertility, the stallion contributes 50% to the overall success of any mating. Because a single stallion can mate or inseminate a large number of mares, knowing its fertility will allow management procedures to maximize at least 50% of the potential for breeding success. A subfertile stallion can attain excellent fertility if managed properly. Without proper management, however, subfertile tendencies can be exaggerated and fertility can be highly unsatisfactory, regardless of the fertility of the mares bred. The potential of a disastrous breeding program is much higher without prior warning of a stallion's subfertility, especially if the stallion is mated to a substantial number of subfertile or problem mares. Consequently, the breeding efficiency of a stallion should be established routinely and the information used in managing mares bred to that stallion.

Useful records are necessary to determine reproductive efficiency. In the stallion, records should include baseline seminal characteristics from potential fertility evaluations as well as the reproductive potential of mares. Knowing this information enables one to make comparisons and to determine changes before disastrous breeding results occur. A good example is changes in spermatozoal numbers per ejaculate. Changes in spermatozoal numbers are seldom dramatic and often are reduced over time. Without baseline data for comparison, declining spermatozoal numbers may not be detected until changes are extreme, numerous mares have been bred, and little can be done to improve management to prevent a crisis. The same also applies to other seminal characteristics such as the percentage of progressively motile spermatozoa, spermatozoal morphology, and spermatozoal viability. Without baseline information, intermittent evaluation of a stallion's reproductive potential is of less value. In a properly managed artificial insemination program, changes in seminal characteristics are easily and quickly detected because semen is evaluated at each seminal collection. Consequently, clinicians do not have to wait for mares to return to estrus before a potential problem is recognized and corrective measures taken.

In natural service, baseline seminal characteristics are even more important if the stallion is subfertile. Knowing the number and quality of the spermatozoa a specific stallion normally ejaculates, along with the total scrotal width, is necessary to predict the number of mares a stallion is capable of serving for the entire season and the number of breedings he can perform in a 24-hour period or for an extended number of days. Many stallions with large books are required to cover three or perhaps more mares per day. Only with adequate record keeping, potential fertility evaluation, and measurement of total scrotal width will one be able to predict or determine the number of mares the stallion can breed or inseminate without reducing reproductive efficiency.

Breeding efficiency is best determined on the basis of pregnancy rate per cycle. Assume that 2 separate stallions each attain an overall pregnancy rate of 85% for a given season and that each of these stallions inseminates or covers 100 mares. Assuming that the stallion and management on one farm attain a 30% pregnancy rate per cycle, it would require approximately 6 cycles to attain an overall pregnancy rate of 85%. If the stallion and management on the other farm attain a 75% pregnancy rate per cycle, however, it would require no more than 2 cycles for 85% of the mares to become pregnant. On the first farm, labor would be increased, and it would be much more costly to the mare owner because the mares would stay on the farm longer. Costs associated with routine feeding and care of the mares, as well as increased management activities such as teasing, palpating, treating and in the insemination or breeding processes, would be at least 3 times higher. Further, the average date of foaling would be later, resulting in less marketable foals and creating a group of late breeding mares in that breeding season. Therefore, reproductive efficiency would be much higher on the farm where the pregnancy rate per cycle is 75%. Obviously, breeding efficiency on the 2 farms should not be considered equal although the overall pregnancy rate would be equal.

The fertility of a stallion in addition to the fertility and management of mares allows maximum reproductive efficiency. Mares should be classified by potential fertility (maiden, barren, nursing, foal heat, biopsy grade, etc.) (see Chapter 21). Knowing the potential fertility of mare and stallion will provide management options to enhance fertility. As an example, to maximize the probability of pregnancy, a barren mare with a grade II biopsy perhaps should not be bred to a stallion that only attains a 30% pregnancy rate per cycle. Often, mating decisions are made on the basis of bloodlines and performance with little regard to potential fertility.

The higher the pregnancy rate per cycle, the more efficient the breeding program will be. Moreover, pregnancy rate by month will provide historical data on the type of mares presented to a stallion and/or the potential fertility of an individual stallion early in the season. Normally, on well-managed breeding farms, one would expect to attain at least a 50% pregnancy rate per cycle and per month. Should pregnancy rates per cycle or per month be below 50%, that stallion and/or the quality of mares presented should be immediately evaluated to address potential future problems. Any stallion that is attaining less than a 50% pregnancy rate per cycle or per month should have a potential fertility evaluation. In addition, the management of mares presented to the stallion should be carefully evaluated to determine whether the stallion or mares are most likely at fault.

In natural service, other criteria such as services per pregnancy, cycles per pregnancy, and covers per pregnancy should be determined and records maintained. Where more than one cover per day is necessary, pregnancy rate per specific service of the day should also be determined. If a stallion's pregnancy rate on the third cover of a day is the same as on the first cover, that stallion is not overused, especially if it has satisfactory seminal characteristics and a large total scrotal width. Stallions with a low per cycle pregnancy rate and a low pregnancy per month rate obviously require more covers per pregnancy, and care must be taken not to overuse the stallion and deplete its extragonadal spermatozoal reserves. In such a situation, the number of mares returning to estrus has an adverse impact on the problem as additional mares are presented as the season progresses. Pregnancies early in the season reduce pressure on a breeding program, particularly when large numbers of foaling mares are presented later in the season.

In determining fertility and breeding efficiency, one also should consider the use of newer technology and criteria other than those provided by records. Flushing embryos at day 7 can be used as an indication of the fertility of a particular stallion or mare. The use of ultrasonography to determine pregnancy as early as day 12 may help one more quickly to determine the potential fertility of a stallion for purchase and/or in evaluating the number of mares that it can accommodate in a season. Determining the incidence of early embryonic death for a stallion as well as a mare may provide additional insight on breeding efficiency. These and other newer technologies undoubtedly will find more use in syndication of stallions and in management decisions, particularly in the number of mares that can be efficiently accommodated by a specific stallion or in determining when a stallion is overused.

APPENDIX III

FUTURE RESEARCH

J. L. Voss

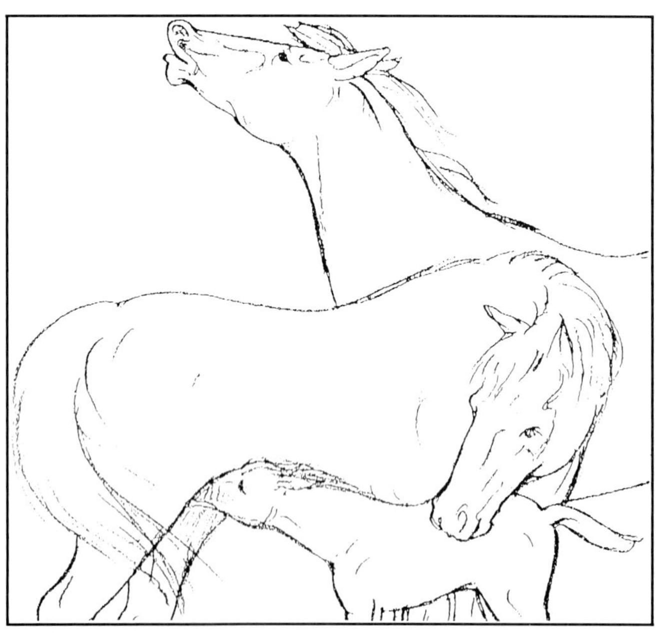

The authors of many of the chapters in this text indicated that additional basic and applied research is needed in virtually all aspects of equine reproduction. Although identifying research needs is relatively easy, the biggest challenge in the future will be to develop a means to finance this research. Governmental agencies in the United States by and large have failed to recognize the value of equine research, and the majority of funds have come from the private sector and industry. In general, research has lagged behind the growth of the equine industry.

MARE

Many aspects of the mare's reproductive physiology remain poorly understood. In the past decade, knowledge of the neuroendocrine system has increased through new and more sophisticated biotechnologic techniques. Additional research is necessary, however, if this information is to be applied to management schemes to improve reproductive efficiency. As examples, little is known about the site(s) of melatonin activity, and newer hormones such as activin and inhibin have not been thoroughly evaluated as to their impact on reproductive management. Many theories of the interaction and complexities of neuroendocrine factors remain unproved. Greater knowledge of cellular and molecular physiology, beyond that described in Chapter 3, is needed to fully understand the factors that regulate and control reproduction.

The normal physiology, hormonal control, and functions of the fallopian tube are not well understood; yet this is the site of fertilization and an area where a high percentage of reproductive failures occur. It is not known why fertilized ova, but not unfertilized ones, pass through the fallopian tube and enter the uterus. If the mechanisms controlling this process, which are undoubtedly chemical in nature, were known, techniques might be developed to prevent embryonic loss in this structure.

In the future, maturation of ova in vitro should become commonplace in horses as it has in humans, cattle, and rodents. When a mare dies, perhaps because of an accident or injury, her ovaries may be removed, and with this technique, oocytes can be recovered and stored for future development. This technology, along with microscopic injection of spermatozoa for fertilization, will allow genetically valuable germ plasma to be preserved into the future.

The mechanisms controlling selection of the primary follicle and methods to promote multiple ovulation need to be determined. If the selection mechanism were clearly known, management techniques to improve reproductive efficiency and methods to improve superovulation might be developed. This information might also be useful in preventing the development of twins, which occur normally from multiple ovulations.

New mare-side diagnostic kits for hormonal profiles to prove competency of follicles and corpora lutea and stage of estrus should be developed and would be of much benefit to the general practitioner. A few such tests currently exist, and others still require adaptation to the horse from other species. The phenomenon of early embryonal death requires additional research and remains one of the greatest deterrents to maximum fertility. Preventing death of a normal embryo would greatly enhance reproductive efficiency.

STALLION

Because the stallion is responsible for 50% of the fertility in any given mating, additional research needs to be directed to the male. Sexual behavior could be the single most important determinant of the number of times a stallion can be used in a breeding program. Unfortunately, the endocrine basis of normal and abnormal sexual behavior in stallions is not understood.

Testicular anomalies also are a problem in the stallion. We must establish the hormonal and physical parameters associated with specific testicular anomalies. Only by doing this will we be able to develop sound treatment methods in clinical cases. Testicular degeneration continues to be a serious problem in stallions. If testicular degeneration can be prevented, the breeding life of many stallions could be extended. In addition, autoimmunity to spermatozoa or testicular tissues is not well understood.

Improved and new methods to evaluate spermatozoa for potential fertility also need to be developed. A clearer relationship between the morphology and motility of spermatozoa from some infertile and fertile stallions needs to be established. In fact, techniques other than determinations of motility and morphology are needed to evaluate seminal quality and to predict potential fertility. Many individual stallions may have excellent spermatozoal motility and morphology but still have lowered fertility or in some instances infertility. The reasons for this need to be elucidated. Computerized motility and morphology estimations may be of some help, but other more specific tests and technologies also need to be developed.

The function of seminal plasma and its importance to stallion spermatozoa has not been fully determined. Some indications are that stallion semen may be more safely stored by extending or freezing if seminal plasma is not present. The role of the secondary sex glands and their contribution to the quality of spermatozoa and fertility should be carefully evaluated.

Because shipping semen is becoming more popular and can significantly affect the economics of the horse industry, better methods are needed to store and transport equine spermatozoa. Factors affecting the survival of stallion spermatozoa during the freezing and thawing process are not understood. Factors such as extenders, antibiotics, freezing and thawing rates, and differences among stallions need to be further evaluated. Why stallion spermatozoa are more fragile to freezing than bull spermatozoa is unknown.

In vitro fertilization and microinjection will become more common, and research in these areas is needed to develop the technology to make these procedures usable at the clinical level. This could be incorporated with ova maturation techniques, so a foal might be produced from a mare and stallion that have been dead for an extended period.

The age-old question concerning the relation of exercise and nutrition to reproduction remains unanswered. More studies are needed to define optimal feeding and exercise regimens to provide maximum reproductive efficiency. Unfortunately, many horses will be required to conduct a meaningful trial, and the expense will be great.

Effective methods to treat stallions that have infections of their reproductive tracts either with viruses or bacteria remain lacking. Many current treatment methods are largely based on personal opinion, bias, and time-honored beliefs that often may be untrue.

The welfare of horses used for research, athletic events, or breeding will also come under more societal scrutiny and potentially increased legislation. The industry needs to conduct well-conceived trials to show whether a horse is being stressed and what the effects are on its well-being and reproductive performance. These studies need to be done with horses and not rats or mice, as is frequently the case with behavioral studies. The social group structure of horses has largely been ignored in most breeding management programs. Undoubtedly, reproductive efficiency could be improved if more were known about behavior and stress.

NEONATE

New technologies have been developed to assess fetal well-being. These technologies are discussed in detail in Chapter 106. Most of these advances have been adopted from human medicine, and much more specific data pertaining to equids are needed. Existing tests must be improved and new technologies need to be developed. Through such technologies, a higher number of foals at risk will be identified, and more efficacious management schemes can be developed. Waiting until a neonate shows signs of disease greatly reduces chances of recovery. New diagnostic kits, especially those that provide mare-side results, are still needed in many areas of neonatology. Tests to determine the degree of maturity or dismaturity more accurately and instantly would be helpful.

FUNDING

To find funding for research in horses is a difficult challenge. In the United States, governmental agencies have largely decided not to fund equine research at a significant level. Prospects for change are not good. Only states with large racing programs that designate a portion of the betting income of their race tracks to research have a sustained funding stream to plan long-range projects. Some other countries have placed more value on horses and have made funding available to help support equine research. In general, however, governmental funding is inadequate to support all the needed research.

In relation to need, only a small number of foundations and industry organizations exist to fund equine research. Most of these solicit requests for proposals, and invariably, many high-quality proposals must be rejected for lack of funds. Many breed organizations simply have insufficient funds to support projects other than small pilot information studies.

Equine researchers, having insufficient sources to which they may turn, often must piece together modest funding from a variety of sources. In many instances, this leads to designing research projects that have too few animals or insufficient design to provide significant results. Much of this type of research, although valuable, may not stand the test of time.

INDEX

Page numbers in *italics* indicate illustrations; numbers followed by "t" indicate tables.